a LANGE medical book

Morgan & Mikhail's Clinical Anesthesiology

FIFTH EDITION

John F. Butterworth IV, MD

...ly
...ersity School of Medicine

...D

...y and Perioperative Medicine
...rson Cancer Center

..., MPH
...for Excellence in Medicine

...Sciences Center

New York
Milan

...rid   Mexico City
...ey   Toronto

Morgan & Mikhail's Clinical Anesthesiology, Fifth Edition

> **Notice**
>
> Medicine is an ever-changing science. As new research and clinical experience broaden our knowledge, changes in treatment and drug therapy are required. The authors and the publisher of this work have checked with sources believed to be reliable in their efforts to provide information that is complete and generally in accord with the standards accepted at the time of publication. However, in view of the possibility of human error or changes in medical sciences, neither the authors nor the publisher nor any other party who has been involved in the preparation or publication of this work warrants that the information contained herein is in every respect accurate or complete, and they disclaim all responsibility for any errors or omissions or for the results obtained from use of the information contained in this work. Readers are encouraged to confirm the information contained herein with other sources. For example and in particular, readers are advised to check the product information sheet included in the package of each drug they plan to administer to be certain that the information contained in this work is accurate and that changes have not been made in the recommended dose or in the contraindications for administration. This recommendation is of particular importance in connection with new or infrequently used drugs.

This book was set in Minion Pro by Thomson Digital.
The editors were Brian Belval and Harriet Lebowitz.
The production supervisor was Sherri Souffrance.
Project management was provided by Charu Bansal, Thomson Digital.
The illustration manager was Armen Ovsepyan; illustrations were provided by Electronic Publishing Services.
The designer was Elise Lansdon; the cover designer was Anthony Landi; cover illustration by Elizabeth Perez.
Quad/Graphics was printer and binder.

McGraw-Hill books are available at special quantity discounts to use as premiums and sales promotions, or for use in corporate training programs. To contact a representative please e-mail us at bulksales@mcgraw-hill.com.

Contents

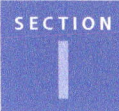
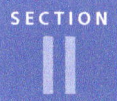
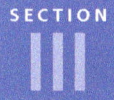

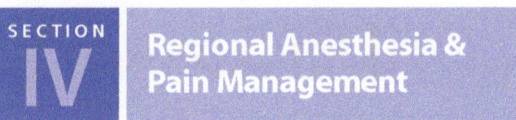

SECTION IV **Regional Anesthesia & Pain Management**

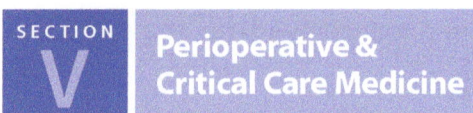

SECTION V **Perioperative & Critical Care Medicine**

Chapter Authors

Gabriele Baldini, MD, MSc
Assistant Professor
Department of Anesthesia
McGill University
Montreal, Quebec

John F. Butterworth IV, MD
Professor and Chairman
Department of Anesthesiology
Virginia Commonwealth University School of Medicine
VCU Health System
Richmond, Virginia

Francesco Carli, MD, MPhil
Professor
Department of Anesthesia
McGill University
Montreal, Quebec

Charles E. Cowles, Jr, MD
Assistant Professor
Department of Anesthesiology
    and Perioperative Medicine
Chief Safety Officer
Perioperative Enterprise
University of Texas MD Anderson Cancer Center
Houston, Texas

Michael A. Frölich, MD, MS
Associate Professor
Department of Anesthesiology
University of Alabama at Birmingham
Birmingham, Alabama

Martin Giesecke, MD
M.T. "Pepper" Jenkins Professor in Anesthesiology
Vice Chair, University Hospitals
Department of Anesthesiology and Pain Management
University of Texas Southwestern Medical Center
Dallas, Texas

Srikanth Hosur, MBBS, MD
Consultant in Intensive Care
QuestCare Intensivists
Dallas, Texas

Brian M. Ilfeld, MD, MS
Professor, In Residence
Department of Anesthesiology
University of California, San Diego
San Diego, California

David C. Mackey, MD
Professor
Department of Anesthesiology and
    Perioperative Medicine
University of Texas M.D. Anderson Cancer Center
Houston, Texas

Sarah J. Madison, MD
Assistant Clinical Professor of Anesthesiology
Department of Anesthesiology
University of California, San Diego
San Diego, California

Edward R. Mariano, MD, MAS (Clinical Research)
Associate Professor of Anesthesia
Stanford University School of Medicine
Chief, Anesthesiology and Perioperative Care Service
VA Palo Alto Health Care System
Palo Alto, California

Brian P. McGlinch, MD
Associate Professor
Department of Anesthesiology
Mayo Clinic
Rochester, Minnesota
Colonel, United States Army Reserve, Medical Corps
452 Combat Support Hospital
Fort Snelling, Minnesota

Michael Ramsay, MD, FRCA
Chairman Department of Anesthesiology
    and Pain Management
Baylor University Medical Center
President Baylor Research Institute
Clinical Professor
University of Texas Southwestern Medical School
Dallas, Texas

Richard W. Rosenquist, MD
Chair, Pain Management Department
Anesthesiology Institute
Cleveland Clinic
Cleveland, Ohio

Bruce M. Vrooman, MD
Department of Pain Management
Anesthesiology Institute
Cleveland Clinic
Cleveland, Ohio

John D. Wasnick, MD, MPH
Steven L. Berk Endowed Chair for
    Excellence in Medicine
Professor and Chair
Department of Anesthesia
Texas Tech University Health Sciences Center
School of Medicine
Lubbock, Texas

Contributors

Kallol Chaudhuri, MD, PhD
Professor
Department of Anesthesia
Texas Tech University Health Sciences Center
Lubbock, Texas

Swapna Chaudhuri, MD, PhD
Professor
Department of Anesthesia
Texas Tech University Health Sciences Center
Lubbock, Texas

John Emhardt, MD
Department of Anesthesia
Indiana University School of Medicine
Indianapolis, Indiana

Suzanne N. Escudier, MD
Associate Professor
Department of Anesthesia
Texas Tech University Health Sciences Center
Lubbock, Texas

Aschraf N. Farag, MD
Assistant Professor
Department of Anesthesia
Texas Tech University Health Sciences Center
Lubbock, Texas

Herbert Gonzalez, MD
Assistant Professor
Department of Anesthesia
Texas Tech University Health Sciences Center
Lubbock, Texas

Kyle Gunnerson, MD
Department of Anesthesiology
VCU School of Medicine
Richmond, Virginia

Robert Johnston, MD
Associate Professor
Department of Anesthesia
Texas Tech University Health Sciences Center
Lubbock, Texas

Sanford Littwin, MD
Assistant Professor
Department of Anesthesiology
St. Luke's Roosevelt Hospital Center and Columbia
    University College of Physicians and Surgeons
New York, New York

Alina Nicoara, MD
Assistant Professor
Department of Anesthesiology
Duke University Medical Center
Durham, North Carolina

Bettina Schmitz, MD, PhD
Associate Professor
Department of Anesthesia
Texas Tech University Health Sciences Center
Lubbock, Texas

Steven L. Shafer, MD
Department of Anesthesia
Stanford University School of Medicine
Palo Alto, California

Christiane Vogt-Harenkamp, MD, PhD
Assistant Professor
Department of Anesthesia
Texas Tech University Health Sciences Center
Lubbock, Texas

Denise J. Wedel, MD
Professor of Anesthesiology
Mayo Clinic
Rochester, Minnesota

Gary Zaloga, MD
Global Medical Affairs
Baxter Healthcare
Deerfield, Illinois

Research and Review

Jacqueline E. Geier, MD
Resident, Department of Anesthesiology
St. Luke's Roosevelt Hospital Center
New York, New York

Brian Hirsch, MD
Resident, Department of Anesthesiology
Texas Tech University Medical Center
Lubbock, Texas

Shane Huffman, MD
Resident, Department of Anesthesiology
Texas Tech University Medical Center
Lubbock, Texas

Rahul K. Mishra, MD
Resident, Department of Anesthesiology
Texas Tech University Medical Center
Lubbock, Texas

Cecilia N. Pena, MD
Resident, Department of Anesthesiology
Texas Tech University Medical Center Hospital
Lubbock, Texas

Charlotte M. Walter, MD
Resident, Department of Anesthesiology
Texas Tech University Medical Center
Lubbock, Texas

Karvier Yates, MD
Resident, Department of Anesthesiology
Texas Tech University Medical Center
Lubbock, Texas

Foreword

A little more than 25 years ago, Alexander Kugushev, then the editor for Lange Medical Publications, approached us to consider writing an introductory textbook in the specialty of anesthesiology that would be part of the popular Lange series of medical books. Mr. Kugushev proved to be a convincing salesman, in part by offering his experience with scores of authors, all of whom opined that their most satisfying career achievement was the fathering of their texts. We could not agree more.

Now in its fifth edition, the overall stylistic goal of *Clinical Anesthesiology* remains unchanged: to be written simply enough so that a third year medical student can understand all essential basic concepts, yet comprehensively enough to provide a strong foundation for a resident in anesthesiology. To quote C. Philip Larson, Jr, MD from the Foreword of the first edition: "The text is complete; nothing of consequence is omitted. The writing style is precise, concise and highly readable."

The fifth edition features three new chapters: Ambulatory, Nonoperating Room, and Office-based Anesthesia; Perioperative Pain Management and Enhanced Outcomes; and Safety, Quality, and Performance Improvement. There are approximately 70 new figures and 20 new tables. The adoption of full color dramatically improves the aesthetic appeal of every page.

However, the biggest and most important change in the fifth edition is the "passing of the baton" to a distinguished and accomplished team of authors and editors. We were thrilled to learn that Drs. Butterworth, Mackey, and Wasnick would be succeeding us. The result of their hard work proves our enthusiasm was justified as they have taken *Clinical Anesthesiology* to a new level. We hope you, the readers, agree!

G. Edward Morgan, Jr, MD
Maged S. Mikhail, MD

Preface

Authors should be proud whenever a book is sufficiently successful to require a new edition. This is especially true when a book's consistent popularity over time leads to the succession of the original authors by a new set of authors. This latter circumstance is the case for the fifth edition of what most of us call "Morgan and Mikhail." We hope that you the reader will find this new edition as readable and useful as you have found the preceding four editions of the work.

This fifth edition, while retaining essential elements of its predecessors, represents a significant revision of the text. Only those who have written a book of this size and complexity will understand just how much effort was involved. Entirely new subjects (eg, Perioperative Pain Management and Enhanced Outcomes) have been added, and many other topics that previously lived in multiple chapters have been moved and consolidated. We have tried to eliminate redundancies and contradictions. The number of illustrations devoted to regional anesthesia and analgesia has been greatly increased to adequately address the rapidly growing importance of this perioperative management topic. The clarity of the illustrations is also enhanced by the widespread use of color throughout the book. We hope the product of this endeavor provides readers with as useful an exercise as was experienced by the authors in composing it.

- **Key Concepts** are listed at the beginning of each chapter and a corresponding numbered icon identifies the section(s) within the chapter in which each concept is discussed. These should help the reader focus on important concepts that underlie the core of anesthesiology.

- **Case Discussions** deal with clinical problems of current interest and are intended to stimulate discussion and critical thinking.

- The suggested reading has been revised and updated to include pertinent Web addresses and references to clinical practice guidelines and practice parameters. We have not tried to provide a comprehensive list of references: we expect that most readers of this text would normally perform their own literature searches on medical topics using Google, PubMed, and other electronic resources. Indeed, we expect that an ever-increasing segment of our readers will access this text in one of its several electronic forms.

- Multiple new illustrations and images have been added to this edition.

Nonetheless, our goal remains the same as that of the first edition: "to provide a concise, consistent presentation of the basic principles essential to the modern practice of anesthesia."

We would like to thank Brian Belval, Harriet Lebowitz, and Marsha Loeb for their invaluable assistance.

Despite our best intentions, various errors may have made their way into the fifth edition. We will be grateful to readers who report these to us at mm5edition@gmail.com so that we can correct them in reprints and future editions.

John F. Butterworth IV, MD
David C. Mackey, MD
John D. Wasnick, MD, MPH

The Practice of Anesthesiology

1. Oliver Wendell Holmes in 1846 was the first to propose use of the term *anesthesia* to denote the state that incorporates amnesia, analgesia, and narcosis to make painless surgery possible.

2. Ether was used for frivolous purposes ("ether frolics") and was not used as an anesthetic agent in humans until 1842, when Crawford W. Long and William E. Clark independently used it on patients. On October 16, 1846, William T.G. Morton conducted the first publicized demonstration of general anesthesia for surgical operation using ether.

3. The original application of modern local anesthesia is credited to Carl Koller, at the time a house officer in ophthalmology, who demonstrated topical anesthesia of the eye with cocaine in 1884.

4. Curare greatly facilitated tracheal intubation and muscle relaxation during surgery. For the first time, operations could be performed on patients without the requirement that relatively deep levels of inhaled general anesthetic be used to produce muscle relaxation.

5. John Snow, often considered the father of the anesthesia specialty, was the first to scientifically investigate ether and the physiology of general anesthesia.

6. The "captain of the ship" doctrine, which held the surgeon responsible for every aspect of the patient's perioperative care (including anesthesia), is no longer a valid notion when an anesthesiologist is present.

The Greek philosopher Dioscorides first used the term *anesthesia* in the first century AD to describe the narcotic-like effects of the plant mandragora. The term subsequently was defined in Bailey's *An Universal Etymological English Dictionary* (1721) as "a defect of sensation" and again in the *Encyclopedia Britannica* (1771) as "privation of the senses."

1 Oliver Wendell Holmes in 1846 was the first to propose use of the term to denote the state that incorporates amnesia, analgesia, and narcosis to make painless surgery possible. In the United States, use of the term *anesthesiology* to denote the practice or study of anesthesia was first proposed in the second decade of the twentieth century to emphasize the growing scientific basis of the specialty.

Although anesthesia now rests on scientific foundations comparable to those of other specialties, the practice of anesthesia remains very much a mixture of science and art. Moreover, the practice has expanded well beyond rendering patients insensible to pain during surgery or obstetric delivery (Table 1–1). The specialty uniquely requires a working familiarity with a long list of other specialties, including surgery and its subspecialties, internal medicine, pediatrics, and obstetrics as well as clinical pharmacology, applied physiology, and biomedical

TABLE 1–1 Definition of the practice of anesthesiology within the practice of medicine.[1]

Assessment and preparation of patients for surgery and anesthesia.
Prevention, diagnosis, and treatment of pain during and following surgical, obstetric, therapeutic, and diagnostic procedures.
Acute care of patients during the perioperative period.
Diagnosis and treatment of critical illness.
Diagnosis and treatment of acute, chronic, and cancer-related pain.
Cardiac, pulmonary, and trauma resuscitation.
Evaluation of respiratory function and application of treatments in respiratory therapy.
Instruction, evaluation of the performance, and supervision of both medical and paramedical personnel involved in perioperative care.
Administration in health care facilities, organizations, and medical schools necessary to implement these responsibilities.
Conduct of clinical, translational, and basic science research.

[1]Data from the American Board of Anesthesiology Booklet of Information, February 2012.

technology. Recent advances in biomedical technology, neuroscience, and pharmacology continue to make anesthesia an intellectually stimulating and rapidly evolving specialty. Many physicians entering residency positions in anesthesiology will already have multiple years of graduate medical education and perhaps even certification in other medical specialties.

This chapter reviews the history of anesthesia, emphasizing its British and American roots, and considers the current scope of the specialty.

The History of Anesthesia

The specialty of anesthesia began in the mid-nineteenth century and became firmly established less than six decades ago. Ancient civilizations had used opium poppy, coca leaves, mandrake root,

alcohol, and even phlebotomy (to the point of unconsciousness) to allow surgeons to operate. Ancient Egyptians used the combination of opium poppy (containing morphine) and hyoscyamus (containing scopolamine); a similar combination, morphine and scopolamine, has been used parenterally for premedication. What passed for regional anesthesia in ancient times consisted of compression of nerve trunks (nerve ischemia) or the application of cold (cryoanalgesia). The Incas may have practiced local anesthesia as their surgeons chewed coca leaves and applied them to operative wounds, particularly prior to trephining for headache.

The evolution of modern surgery was hampered not only by a poor understanding of disease processes, anatomy, and surgical asepsis but also by the lack of reliable and safe anesthetic techniques. These techniques evolved first with inhalation anesthesia, followed by local and regional anesthesia, and finally intravenous anesthesia. The development of surgical anesthesia is considered one of the most important discoveries in human history.

INHALATION ANESTHESIA

Because the hypodermic needle was not invented until 1855, the first general anesthetics were destined to be inhalation agents. Diethyl ether (known at the time as "sulfuric ether" because it was produced by a simple chemical reaction between ethyl alcohol and sulfuric acid) was originally prepared in 1540 by Valerius Cordus. Ether was used for frivolous purposes ("ether frolics"), but not as an anesthetic agent in humans until 1842, when Crawford W. Long and William E. Clark independently used it on patients for surgery and dental extraction, respectively. However, they did not publicize their discovery. Four years later, in Boston, on October 16, 1846, William T.G. Morton conducted the first publicized demonstration of general anesthesia for surgical operation using ether. The dramatic success of that exhibition led the operating surgeon to exclaim to a skeptical audience: "Gentlemen, this is no humbug!"

Chloroform was independently prepared by von Leibig, Guthrie, and Soubeiran in 1831. Although first used by Holmes Coote in 1847, chloroform was introduced into clinical practice by the Scot Sir James Simpson, who administered it to his patients to relieve the pain of labor. Ironically, Simpson had almost abandoned his medical practice after witnessing the terrible despair and agony of patients undergoing operations without anesthesia.

Joseph Priestley produced nitrous oxide in 1772, and Humphry Davy first noted its analgesic properties in 1800. Gardner Colton and Horace Wells are credited with having first used nitrous oxide as an anesthetic for dental extractions in humans in 1844. Nitrous oxide's lack of potency (an 80% nitrous oxide concentration results in analgesia but not surgical anesthesia) led to clinical demonstrations that were less convincing than those with ether.

Nitrous oxide was the least popular of the three early inhalation anesthetics because of its low potency and its tendency to cause asphyxia when used alone (see Chapter 8). Interest in nitrous oxide was revived in 1868 when Edmund Andrews administered it in 20% oxygen; its use was, however, overshadowed by the popularity of ether and chloroform. Ironically, nitrous oxide is the only one of these three agents still in widespread use today. Chloroform superseded ether in popularity in many areas (particularly in the United Kingdom), but reports of chloroform-related cardiac arrhythmias, respiratory depression, and hepatotoxicity eventually caused practitioners to abandon it in favor of ether, particularly in North America.

Even after the introduction of other inhalation anesthetics (ethyl chloride, ethylene, divinyl ether, cyclopropane, trichloroethylene, and fluroxene), ether remained the standard inhaled anesthetic until the early 1960s. The only inhalation agent that rivaled ether's safety and popularity was cyclopropane (introduced in 1934). However, both are highly combustible and both have since been replaced by a succession of nonflammable potent fluorinated hydrocarbons: halothane (developed in 1951; released in 1956), methoxyflurane (developed in 1958; released in 1960), enflurane (developed in 1963; released in 1973), and isoflurane (developed in 1965; released in 1981).

Two newer agents are now the most popular in developed countries. Desflurane (released in 1992), has many of the desirable properties of isoflurane as well as more rapid uptake and elimination (nearly as fast as nitrous oxide). Sevoflurane, has low blood solubility, but concerns about the potential toxicity of its degradation products delayed its release in the United States until 1994 (see Chapter 8). These concerns have proved to be largely theoretical, and sevoflurane, not desflurane, has become the most widely used inhaled anesthetic in the United States, largely replacing halothane in pediatric practice.

LOCAL & REGIONAL ANESTHESIA

The medicinal qualities of coca had been used by the Incas for centuries before its actions were first observed by Europeans. Cocaine was isolated from coca leaves in 1855 by Gaedicke and was purified in 1860 by Albert Niemann. The original application of modern local anesthesia is credited to Carl Koller, at the time a house officer in ophthalmology, who demonstrated topical anesthesia of the eye with cocaine in 1884. Later in 1884 William Halsted used cocaine for intradermal infiltration and nerve blocks (including blocks of the facial nerve, brachial plexus, pudendal nerve, and posterior tibial nerve). August Bier is credited with administering the first spinal anesthetic in 1898. He was also the first to describe intravenous regional anesthesia (Bier block) in 1908. Procaine was synthesized in 1904 by Alfred Einhorn and within a year was used clinically as a local anesthetic by Heinrich Braun. Braun was also the first to add epinephrine to prolong the duration of local anesthetics. Ferdinand Cathelin and Jean Sicard introduced caudal epidural anesthesia in 1901. Lumbar epidural anesthesia was described first in 1921 by Fidel Pages and again (independently) in 1931 by Achille Dogliotti. Additional local anesthetics subsequently introduced include dibucaine (1930), tetracaine (1932), lidocaine (1947), chloroprocaine (1955), mepivacaine (1957), prilocaine (1960), bupivacaine (1963), and etidocaine (1972). The most recent additions, ropivacaine and levobupivacaine, have durations of action similar to bupivacaine but less cardiac toxicity (see Chapter 16).

INTRAVENOUS ANESTHESIA

Induction Agents

Intravenous anesthesia required the invention of the hypodermic syringe and needle by Alexander Wood in 1855. Early attempts at intravenous anesthesia included the use of chloral hydrate (by Oré in 1872), chloroform and ether (Burkhardt in 1909), and the combination of morphine and scopolamine (Bredenfeld in 1916). Barbiturates were first synthesized in 1903 by Fischer and von Mering. The first barbiturate used for induction of anesthesia was diethylbarbituric acid (barbital), but it was not until the introduction of hexobarbital in 1927 that barbiturate induction became popular. Thiopental, synthesized in 1932 by Volwiler and Tabern, was first used clinically by John Lundy and Ralph Waters in 1934 and for many years remained the most common agent for intravenous induction of anesthesia. Methohexital was first used clinically in 1957 by V. K. Stoelting and is the only other barbiturate used for induction of anesthesia in humans. After chlordiazepoxide was discovered in 1955 and released for clinical use in 1960, other benzodiazepines—diazepam, lorazepam, and midazolam—came to be used extensively for premedication, conscious sedation, and induction of general anesthesia. Ketamine was synthesized in 1962 by Stevens and first used clinically in 1965 by Corssen and Domino; it was released in 1970 and continues to be popular today, particular when administered in combination with other agents. Etomidate was synthesized in 1964 and released in 1972. Initial enthusiasm over its relative lack of circulatory and respiratory effects was tempered by evidence of adrenal suppression, reported after even a single dose. The release of propofol in 1986 (1989 in the United States) was a major advance in outpatient anesthesia because of its short duration of action (see Chapter 9). Propofol is currently the most popular agent for intravenous induction worldwide.

Neuromuscular Blocking Agents

The introduction of curare by Harold Griffith and Enid Johnson in 1942 was a milestone in anesthesia. Curare greatly facilitated tracheal intubation and muscle relaxation during surgery. For the first time, operations could be performed on patients without the requirement that relatively deep levels of inhaled general anesthetic be used to produce muscle relaxation. Such large doses of anesthetic often resulted in excessive cardiovascular and respiratory depression as well as prolonged emergence. Moreover, larger doses were often not tolerated by frail patients.

Succinylcholine was synthesized by Bovet in 1949 and released in 1951; it has become a standard agent for facilitating tracheal intubation during rapid sequence induction. Until recently, succinylcholine remained unchallenged in its rapid onset of profound muscle relaxation, but its side effects prompted the search for a comparable substitute. Other neuromuscular blockers (NMBs; discussed in Chapter 11)—gallamine, decamethonium, metocurine, alcuronium, and pancuronium—were subsequently introduced. Unfortunately, these agents were often associated with side effects (see Chapter 11), and the search for the ideal NMB continued. Recently introduced agents that more closely resemble an ideal NMB include vecuronium, atracurium, rocuronium, and *cis*-atracurium.

Opioids

Morphine, isolated from opium in 1805 by Sertürner, was also tried as an intravenous anesthetic. The adverse events associated with large doses of opioids in early reports caused many anesthetists to avoid opioids and favor pure inhalation anesthesia. Interest in opioids in anesthesia returned following the synthesis and introduction of meperidine in 1939. The concept of *balanced anesthesia* was introduced in 1926 by Lundy and others and evolved to include thiopental for induction, nitrous oxide for amnesia, an opioid for analgesia, and curare for muscle relaxation. In 1969, Lowenstein rekindled interest in "pure" opioid anesthesia by reintroducing the concept of large doses of opioids as complete anesthetics. Morphine was the first agent so employed, but fentanyl and sufentanil have been preferred by a large margin as sole agents. As experience grew with this technique, its multiple limitations—unreliably preventing patient awareness, incompletely suppressing autonomic responses during surgery, and prolonged respiratory depression—were realized.

Remifentanil, an opioid subject to rapid degradation by nonspecific plasma and tissue esterases, permits profound levels of opioid analgesia to be employed without concerns regarding the need for postoperative ventilation.

EVOLUTION OF THE SPECIALTY

British Origins

Following its first public demonstration in the United States, ether anesthesia quickly was adopted in England. John Snow, often considered the father of the anesthesia specialty, was the first physician to take a full-time interest in this new anesthetic. He was the first to scientifically investigate ether and the physiology of general anesthesia. Of course, Snow was also a pioneer in epidemiology. He helped stop a cholera epidemic in London by proving that the causative agent was transmitted by ingestion of contaminated well water rather than by inhalation. In 1847, Snow published the first book on general anesthesia, *On the Inhalation of Ether*. When the anesthetic properties of chloroform were made known, he quickly investigated and developed an inhaler for that agent as well. He believed that an inhaler should be used in administering ether or chloroform to control the dose of the anesthetic. His second book, *On Chloroform and Other Anaesthetics*, was published posthumously in 1858.

After Snow's death, Dr. Joseph T. Clover took his place as England's leading anesthetist. Clover emphasized continuously monitoring the patient's pulse during anesthesia, a practice that was not yet standard at the time. He was the first to use the jaw-thrust maneuver for relieving airway obstruction, the first to insist that resuscitation equipment always be available during anesthesia, and the first to use a cricothyroid cannula (to save a patient with an oral tumor who developed complete airway obstruction). After Clover, Sir Frederic Hewitt became England's foremost anesthetist at the turn of the last century. He was responsible for many inventions, including the oral airway. Hewitt also wrote what many consider to be the first true textbook of

anesthesia, which went through five editions. Snow, Clover, and Hewitt established the tradition of physician anesthetists in England. In 1893, the first organization of physician specialists in anesthesia, the London Society of Anaesthetists, was formed in England by J.F. Silk.

The first elective tracheal intubations during anesthesia were performed in the late nineteenth century by surgeons Sir William MacEwen in Scotland, Joseph O'Dwyer in the United States, and Franz Kuhn in Germany. Tracheal intubation during anesthesia was popularized in England by Sir Ivan Magill and Stanley Rowbotham in the 1920s.

American Origins

In the United States, only a few physicians had specialized in anesthesia by 1900. The task of providing general anesthesia was often delegated to junior surgical house officers or medical students, if they were available.

The first organization of physician anesthetists in the United States was the Long Island Society of Anesthetists formed in 1905, which, as it grew, was renamed the New York Society of Anesthetists in 1911. The International Anesthesia Research Society (IARS) was founded in 1922, and in that same year the IARS-sponsored scientific journal *Current Researches in Anesthesia and Analgesia* (now called *Anesthesia and Analgesia*) began publication. In 1936, the New York Society of Anesthetists became the American Society of Anesthetists, and later, in 1945, the American Society of Anesthesiologists (ASA). The scientific journal *Anesthesiology* was first published in 1940.

Four physicians stand out in the early development of anesthesia in the United States after 1900: F.H. McMechan, Arthur E. Guedel, Ralph M. Waters, and John S. Lundy. McMechan was the driving force behind both the IARS and *Current Researches in Anesthesia and Analgesia*, and tirelessly organized physicians specializing in anesthesia into national and international organizations until his death in 1939. Guedel was the first to describe the signs and stages of general anesthesia. He advocated cuffed tracheal tubes and introduced artificial ventilation during ether anesthesia (later termed *controlled respiration* by

Waters). Ralph Waters made a long list of contributions to the specialty, probably the most important of which was his insistence on the proper education of specialists in anesthesia. Waters developed the first academic department of anesthesiology at the University of Wisconsin in Madison. Lundy was instrumental in the formation of the American Board of Anesthesiology and chaired the American Medical Association's Section on Anesthesiology for 17 years.

Because of the scarcity of physicians specializing in anesthesia in the United States and the perceived relative safety of ether anesthesia, surgeons at both the Mayo Clinic and Cleveland Clinic began training and employing nurses as anesthetists in the early 1900s. As the numbers of nurse anesthetists increased, a national organization (now called the American Association of Nurse Anesthetists) was incorporated in 1932. The AANA first offered a certification examination in 1945. In 1969 two Anesthesiology Assistant programs began accepting students, and in 1989 the first certification examinations for AAs were administered. Certified Registered Nurse Anesthetists and Anesthesiologist Assistants represent important members of the anesthesia workforce in the United States and in other countries.

Official Recognition

In 1889 Henry Isaiah Dorr, a dentist, was appointed Professor of the Practice of Dentistry, Anaesthetics and Anaesthesia at the Philadelphia College of Dentistry. Thus he was the first known professor of anesthesia worldwide. Thomas D. Buchanan, of the New York Medical College, was the first physician to be appointed Professor of Anesthesia (in 1905). When the American Board of Anesthesiology was established in 1938, Dr. Buchanan served as its first president. In England, the first examination for the Diploma in Anaesthetics took place in 1935, and the first Chair in Anaesthetics was awarded to Sir Robert Macintosh in 1937 at Oxford University. Anesthesia became an officially recognized specialty in England only in 1947, when the Royal College of Surgeons established its Faculty of Anaesthetists. In 1992 an independent Royal College of Anaesthetists was granted its charter.

The Scope of Anesthesia

The practice of anesthesia has changed dramatically since the days of John Snow. The modern anesthesiologist is now both a perioperative consultant and a primary deliverer of care to patients. In general, anesthesiologists manage nearly all "noncutting" aspects of the patient's medical care in the immediate perioperative period. The "captain of the ship" doctrine, which held the surgeon responsible for every aspect of the patient's perioperative care (including anesthesia), is no longer a valid notion when an anesthesiologist is present. The surgeon and anesthesiologist must function together as an effective team, and both are ultimately answerable to the patient rather than to each other.

The modern practice of anesthesia is not confined to rendering patients insensible to pain (Table 1–1). Anesthesiologists monitor, sedate, and provide general or regional anesthesia outside the operating room for various imaging procedures, endoscopy, electroconvulsive therapy, and cardiac catheterization. Anesthesiologists have traditionally been pioneers in cardiopulmonary resuscitation and continue to be integral members of resuscitation teams.

An increasing number of practitioners pursue a subspecialty in anesthesia for cardiothoracic surgery (see Chapter 22), critical care (see Chapter 57), neuroanesthesia (see Chapter 27), obstetric anesthesia (see Chapter 41), pediatric anesthesia (see Chapter 42), and pain medicine (see Chapter 47). Certification requirements for special competence in critical care and pain medicine already exist in the United States. Fellowship programs in Adult Cardiothoracic Anesthesia and Pediatric Anesthesiology have specific accreditation requirements, and soon those in Obstetric Anesthesiology will as well. A certification examination will soon be available in Pediatric Anesthesiology. Education and certification in anesthesiology can also be used as the basis for certification in Sleep Medicine or in Palliative Medicine.

Anesthesiologists are actively involved in the administration and medical direction of many ambulatory surgery facilities, operating room suites, intensive care units, and respiratory therapy departments. They have also assumed administrative and leadership positions on the medical staffs of many hospitals and ambulatory care facilities. They serve as deans of medical schools and chief executives of health systems.

SUGGESTED READING

The American Board of Anesthesiology Booklet of Information February 2012. Available at: http://www.theaba.org/Home/publications (accessed August 9, 2012).

Bacon DR: The promise of one great anesthesia society. The 1939–1940 proposed merger of the American Society of Anesthetists and the International Anesthesia Research Society. Anesthesiology 1994;80:929.

Bergman N: *The Genesis of Surgical Anesthesia*. Wood Library Museum of Anesthesiology, 1998.

Keys TE: *The History of Surgical Anesthesia*. Schuman's, 1945.

Sykes K, Bunker J: *Anaesthesia and the Practice of Medicine: Historical Perspectives*. Royal Society of Medicine Press, 2007.

CHAPTER

The Operating Room Environment

Charles E. Cowles, MD

2

1 A pressure of 1000 psig indicates an E-cylinder that is approximately half full and represents 330 L of oxygen.

2 The only reliable way to determine residual volume of nitrous oxide is to weigh the cylinder.

3 To discourage incorrect cylinder attachments, cylinder manufacturers have adopted a pin index safety system.

4 A basic principle of radiation safety is to keep exposure "as low as reasonably practical" (ALARP). The principles of ALARP are protection from radiation exposure by the use of time, distance, and shielding.

5 The magnitude of a leakage current is normally imperceptible to touch (<1 mA, and well below the fibrillation threshold of 100 mA). If the current bypasses the high resistance offered by skin, however, and is applied directly to the heart (microshock), current as low as 100 μA may be fatal. The maximum leakage allowed in operating room equipment is 10 μA.

6 To reduce the chance of two coexisting faults, a line isolation monitor measures the potential for current flow from the isolated power supply to the ground. Basically, the line isolation monitor determines the degree of isolation between the two power wires and the ground

and predicts the amount of current that *could* flow if a second short circuit were to develop.

7 Almost all surgical fires can be prevented. Unlike medical complications, fires are a product of simple physical and chemistry properties. Occurrence is guaranteed given the proper combination of factors but can be eliminated almost entirely by understanding the basic principles of fire risk.

8 Likely the most common risk factor for surgical fire relates to the open delivery of oxygen.

9 Administration of oxygen to concentrations of greater than 30% should be guided by clinical presentation of the patient and not solely by protocols or habits.

10 The sequence of stopping gas flow and removal of the endotracheal tube when fire occurs in the airway is not as important as ensuring that both actions are performed quickly.

11 Before beginning laser surgery, the laser device should be in the operating room, warning signs should be posted on the doors, and protective eyewear should be issued. The anesthesia provider should ensure that the warning signs and eyewear match the labeling on the laser device as laser protection is specific to the type of laser.

Anesthesiologists, who spend more time in operating rooms than any other group of physicians, are responsible for protecting patients and operating room personnel from a multitude of dangers during surgery. Some of these threats are unique to the operating room. As a result, the anesthesiologist may be responsible for ensuring proper functioning of the operating room's medical gases, fire prevention and management, environmental factors (eg, temperature, humidity, ventilation, and noise), and electrical safety. The role of the anesthesiologist also may include coordination of or assistance with layout and design of surgical suites, including workflow enhancements. This chapter describes the major operating room features that are of special interest to anesthesiologists and the potential hazards associated with these systems.

Safety Culture

Patients often think of the operating room as a safe place where the care given is centered around protecting the patient. Medical providers such as anesthesia personnel, surgeons, and nurses are responsible for carrying out several critical tasks at a fast pace. Unless members of the operating room team look out for one another, errors can occur. The best way of preventing serious harm to a patient is by creating a culture of safety. When the safety culture is effectively applied in the operating room, unsafe acts are stopped before harm occurs.

One tool that fosters the safety culture is the use of a surgical safety checklist. Such checklists are used prior to incision on every case and can include components agreed upon by the facility as crucial. Many surgical checklists are derived from the surgical safety checklist published by the World Health Organization (WHO). For checklists to be effective, they must first be used; secondly, all members of the surgical team should be engaged when the checklist is being used. Checklists are most effective when performed in an interactive fashion. An example of a suboptimally executed checklist is one that is read in entirety, after which the surgeon asks whether everyone agrees. This format makes it difficult to identify possible problems. A better method is one that elicits a response after each point; eg, "Does everyone agree this is John Doe?",

followed by "Does everyone agree we are performing a removal of the left kidney?", and so forth. Optimal checklists do not attempt to cover every possibility but rather address only key components, allowing them to be completed in less than 90 seconds.

Some practitioners argue that checklists waste too much time; they fail to realize that cutting corners to save time often leads to problems later, resulting in a net loss of time. If safety checklists were followed in every case, significant reductions could be seen in the incidence of surgical complications such as wrong-site surgery, procedures on the wrong patient, retained foreign objects, and other easily prevented mistakes. Anesthesia providers are leaders in patient safety initiatives and should take a proactive role to utilize checklists and other activities that foster the safety culture.

Medical Gas Systems

The medical gases commonly used in operating rooms are oxygen, nitrous oxide, air, and nitrogen. Although technically not a gas, vacuum exhaust for waste anesthetic gas disposal (WAGD or scavenging) and surgical suction must also be provided and is considered an integral part of the medical gas system. Patients are endangered if medical gas systems, particularly oxygen, are misconfigured or malfunction. The main features of such systems are the sources of the gases and the means of their delivery to the operating room. The anesthesiologist must understand both these elements to prevent and detect medical gas depletion or supply line misconnection. Estimates of a particular hospital's peak demand determine the type of medical gas supply system required. Design and standards follow National Fire Protection Association (NFPA) 99 in the United States and HTM 2022 in the United Kingdom.

SOURCES OF MEDICAL GASES

Oxygen

A reliable supply of oxygen is a critical requirement in any surgical area. Medical grade oxygen (99% or 99.5% pure) is manufactured by fractional distillation of liquefied air. Oxygen is stored as a compressed

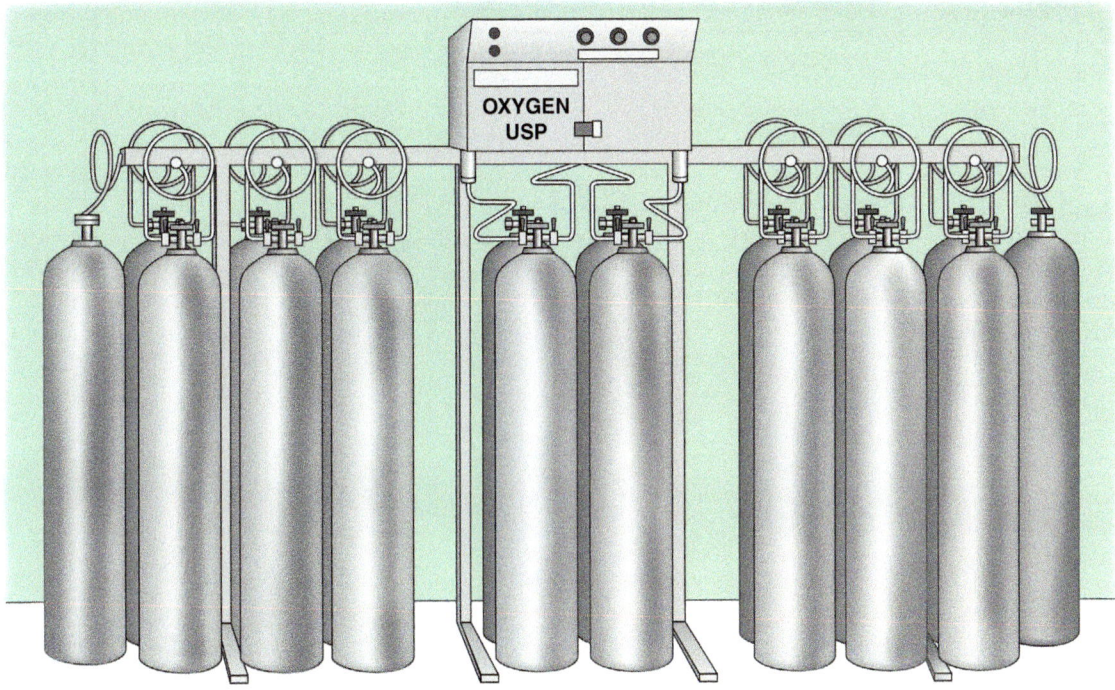

FIGURE 2-1 A bank of oxygen H-cylinders connected by a manifold.

gas at room temperature or refrigerated as a liquid. Most small hospitals store oxygen in two separate banks of high-pressure cylinders (H-cylinders) connected by a manifold (Figure 2–1). Only one bank is utilized at a time. The number of cylinders in each bank depends on anticipated daily demand. The manifold contains valves that reduce the cylinder pressure (approximately 2000 pounds per square inch [psig]) to line pressure (55 ± 5 psig) and automatically switch banks when one group of cylinders is exhausted.

A liquid oxygen storage system (Figure 2–2) is more economical for large hospitals. Liquid oxygen must be stored well below its critical temperature of –119°C because gases can be liquefied by pressure *only* if stored below their critical temperature. A large hospital may have a smaller liquid oxygen supply or a bank of compressed gas cylinders that can provide one day's oxygen requirements as a reserve. To guard against a hospital gas-system failure, the anesthesiologist must always have an emergency (E-cylinder) supply of oxygen available during anesthesia.

Most anesthesia machines accommodate E-cylinders of oxygen (Table 2–1). As oxygen is expended, the cylinder's pressure falls in proportion to its content. A pressure of 1000 psig indicates an E-cylinder that is approximately half full and represents 330 L of oxygen at atmospheric pressure and a temperature of 20°C. If the oxygen is exhausted at a rate of 3 L/min, a cylinder that is half full will be empty in 110 min. Oxygen cylinder pressure should be monitored before use and periodically during use. Anesthesia machines usually also accommodate E-cylinders for medical air and nitrous oxide, and may accept cylinders of helium. Compressed medical gases utilize a pin index safety system for these cylinders to prevent inadvertent crossover and connections for different gas types. As a safety feature of oxygen E-cylinders, the yoke has integral components made from Wood's metal. This metallurgic alloy has a low melting point, which allows dissipation of pressure that might otherwise heat the bottle to the point of ballistic explosion. This pressure-relief "valve" is

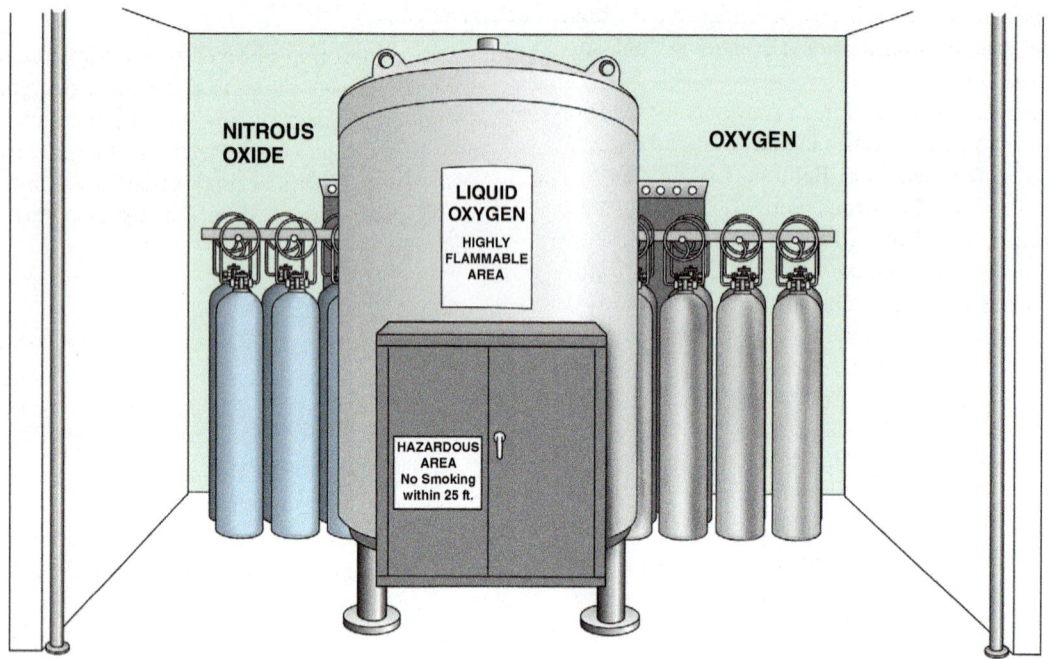

FIGURE 2–2 A liquid storage tank with reserve oxygen tanks in the background.

designed to rupture at 3300 psig, well below the pressure E-cylinder walls should be able to withstand (more than 5000 psig).

Nitrous Oxide

Nitrous oxide is manufactured by heating ammonium nitrate (thermal decomposition). It is almost always stored by hospitals in large H-cylinders connected by a manifold with an automatic crossover feature. Bulk liquid storage of nitrous oxide is economical only in very large institutions.

Because the critical temperature of nitrous oxide (36.5°C) is above room temperature, it can be kept liquefied without an elaborate refrigeration system. If the liquefied nitrous oxide rises above its critical temperature, it will revert to its gaseous phase. Because nitrous oxide is not an ideal gas and is easily compressible, this transformation into a gaseous phase is not accompanied by a great rise in tank pressure. Nonetheless, as with oxygen cylinders, all nitrous oxide E-cylinders are equipped with a Wood's metal yoke to prevent

TABLE 2–1 **Characteristics of medical gas cylinders.**

Gas	E-Cylinder Capacity[1] (L)	H-Cylinder Capacity[1] (L)	Pressure[1] (psig at 20°C)	Color (USA)	Color (International)	Form
O_2	625–700	6000–8000	1800–2200	Green	White	Gas
Air	625–700	6000–8000	1800–2200	Yellow	White and black	Gas
N_2O	1590	15,900	745	Blue	Blue	Liquid
N_2	625–700	6000–8000	1800–2200	Black	Black	Gas

[1]Depending on the manufacturer.

explosion under conditions of unexpectedly high gas pressure (eg, unintentional overfilling), particularly during fires.

Although a disruption in supply is usually not catastrophic, most anesthesia machines have reserve nitrous oxide E-cylinders. Because these smaller cylinders also contain nitrous oxide in its liquid state, the volume remaining in a cylinder is *not* proportional to cylinder pressure. By the time the liquid nitrous oxide is expended and the tank pressure begins to fall, only about 400 L of nitrous oxide remains. **If liquid nitrous oxide is kept at a constant temperature (20°C), it will vaporize at the same rate at which it is consumed and will maintain a constant pressure (745 psig) until the liquid is exhausted**.

2 The only reliable way to determine residual volume of nitrous oxide is to weigh the cylinder. For this reason, the tare weight (TW), or empty weight, of cylinders containing a liquefied compressed gas (eg, nitrous oxide) is often stamped on the shoulder of the cylinder. The pressure gauge of a nitrous oxide cylinder should not exceed 745 psig at 20°C. A higher reading implies gauge malfunction, tank overfill (liquid fill), or a cylinder containing a gas other than nitrous oxide.

Because energy is consumed in the conversion of a liquid to a gas (the latent heat of vaporization), the liquid nitrous oxide cools. The drop in temperature results in a lower vapor pressure and lower cylinder pressure. The cooling is so pronounced at high flow rates that there is often frost on the tank, and pressure regulators may freeze.

Medical Air

The use of air is becoming more frequent in anesthesiology as the popularity of nitrous oxide and unnecessarily high concentrations of oxygen has declined. Cylinder air is medical grade and is obtained by blending oxygen and nitrogen. Dehumidified but unsterile air is provided to the hospital pipeline system by compression pumps. The inlets of these pumps must be distant from vacuum exhaust vents and machinery to minimize contamination. Because the critical temperature of air is −140.6°C, it exists as a gas in cylinders whose pressures fall in proportion to their content.

Nitrogen

Although compressed nitrogen is not administered to patients, it may be used to drive some operating room equipment, such as saws, drills, and surgical handpieces. Nitrogen supply systems either incorporate the use of H-cylinders connected by a manifold or a wall system supplied by a compressor driven central supply.

Vacuum

A central hospital vacuum system usually consists of independent suction pumps, each capable of handling peak requirements. Traps at every user location prevent contamination of the system with foreign matter. The medical-surgical vacuum may be used for waste anesthetic gas disposal (WAGD) providing it does not affect the performance of the system. Medical vacuum receptacles are usually black in color with white lettering. A dedicated WAGD vacuum system is generally required with modern anesthesia machines. The WAGD outlet may incorporate the use of a suction regulator with a float indicator. The float should be maintained between the designated markings. Excess suction may result in inadequate patient ventilation, and insufficient suction levels may result in the failure to evaluate WAGD. WAGD receptacles and tubing are usually lavender in color.

Carbon Dioxide

Many surgical procedures are performed using laparoscopic or robotic-assisted techniques requiring insufflation of body cavities with carbon dioxide, an odorless, colorless, nonflammable and slightly acidic gas. Large cylinders containing carbon dioxide, such as M-cylinders or LK-cylinders, are frequently found in the operating room; these cylinders share a common size orifice and thread with oxygen cylinders and can be inadvertently interchanged.

DELIVERY OF MEDICAL GASES

Medical gases are delivered from their central supply source to the operating room through a piping network. Pipes are sized such that the pressure drop across the whole system never exceeds 5 psig. Gas pipes are usually constructed of seamless copper tubing using a special welding technique. Internal

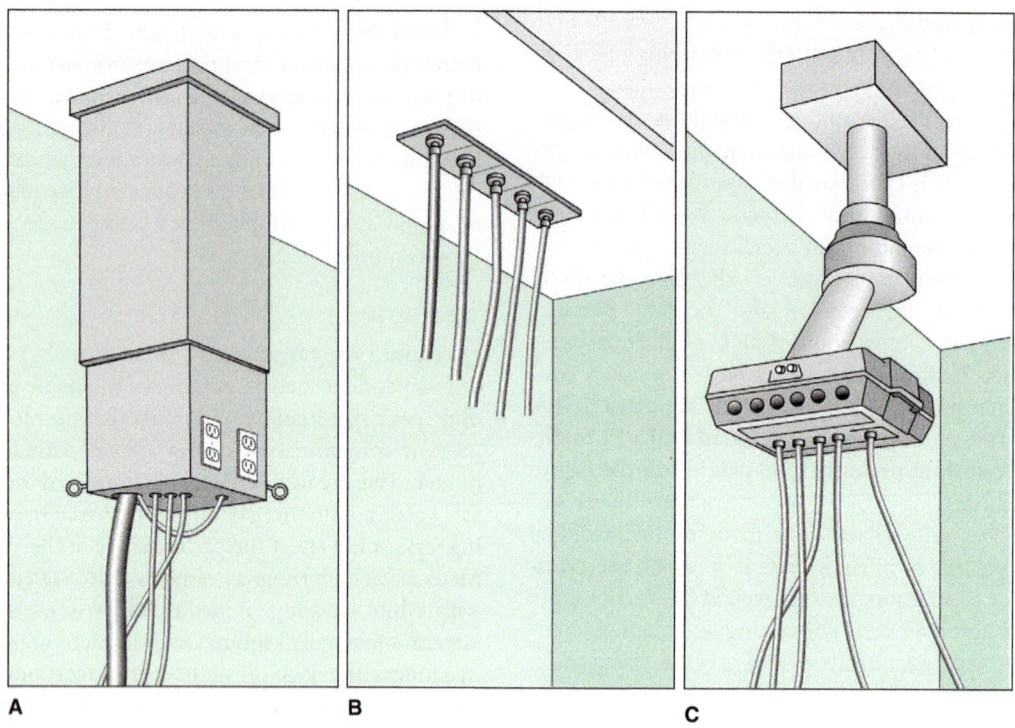

A   **B**   **C**

FIGURE 2–3 Typical examples of (**A**) gas columns, (**B**) ceiling hose drops, and (**C**) articulating arms. One end of a color-coded hose connects to the hospital medical gas supply system by way of a quick-coupler mechanism. The other end connects to the anesthesia machine through the diameter index safety system.

contamination of the pipelines with dust, grease, or water must be avoided. The hospital's gas delivery system appears in the operating room as hose drops, gas columns, or elaborate articulating arms (Figure 2–3). Operating room equipment, including the anesthesia machine, interfaces with these pipeline system outlets by color-coded hoses. Quick-coupler mechanisms, which vary in design with different manufacturers, connect one end of the hose to the appropriate gas outlet. The other end connects to the anesthesia machine through a non-interchangeable diameter index safety system fitting that prevents incorrect hose attachment.

E-cylinders of oxygen, nitrous oxide, and air attach directly to the anesthesia machine. To discourage incorrect cylinder attachments, cylinder manufacturers have adopted a pin index safety system. Each gas cylinder (sizes A–E) has two holes in its cylinder valve that mate with corresponding pins in the yoke of the anesthesia machine (Figure 2–4). The relative positioning of the pins and holes is unique for each gas. Multiple washers placed between the cylinder and yoke, which prevent proper engagement of the pins and holes, have unintentionally defeated this system. The pin index safety system is also ineffective if yoke pins are damaged or the cylinder is filled with the wrong gas.

The functioning of medical gas supply sources and pipeline systems is constantly monitored by central and area alarm systems. Indicator lights and audible signals warn of changeover to secondary gas sources and abnormally high (eg, pressure regulator malfunction) or low (eg, supply depletion) pipeline pressures (Figure 2–5).

Modern anesthesia machines and anesthetic gas analyzers continuously measure the fraction of inspired oxygen (FiO_2). Analyzers have a variable threshold setting for the minimal FiO_2 but should

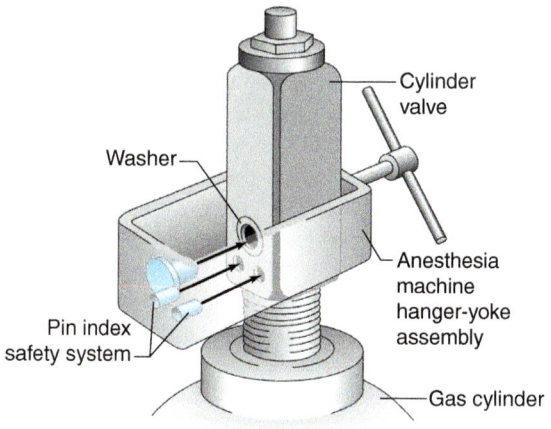

FIGURE 2–4 Pin index safety system interlink between the anesthesia machine and gas cylinder.

be configured to prevent disabling this alarm. The monitoring of FiO_2 does not reflect the oxygen concentration distal to the monitoring port and should not be used to reference the oxygen concentration

within devices such as endotracheal tubes or at the distal tip of the tube. Due to gas exchange, flow rates, and shunting a marked difference can exist between the monitored FiO_2 and oxygen concentration at the tissue level.

Environmental Factors in the Operating Room

TEMPERATURE

The temperature in most operating rooms seems uncomfortably cold to many conscious patients and, at times, to anesthesiologists. However, scrub nurses and surgeons stand in surgical garb for hours under hot operating room lights. As a general principle, the comfort of operating room personnel must be reconciled with patient care. Hypothermia has been associated with an increased incidence of wound infection, greater intraoperative blood loss (impaired coagulation assessed by thromboelastography), and prolonged hospitalization (see Chapter 52).

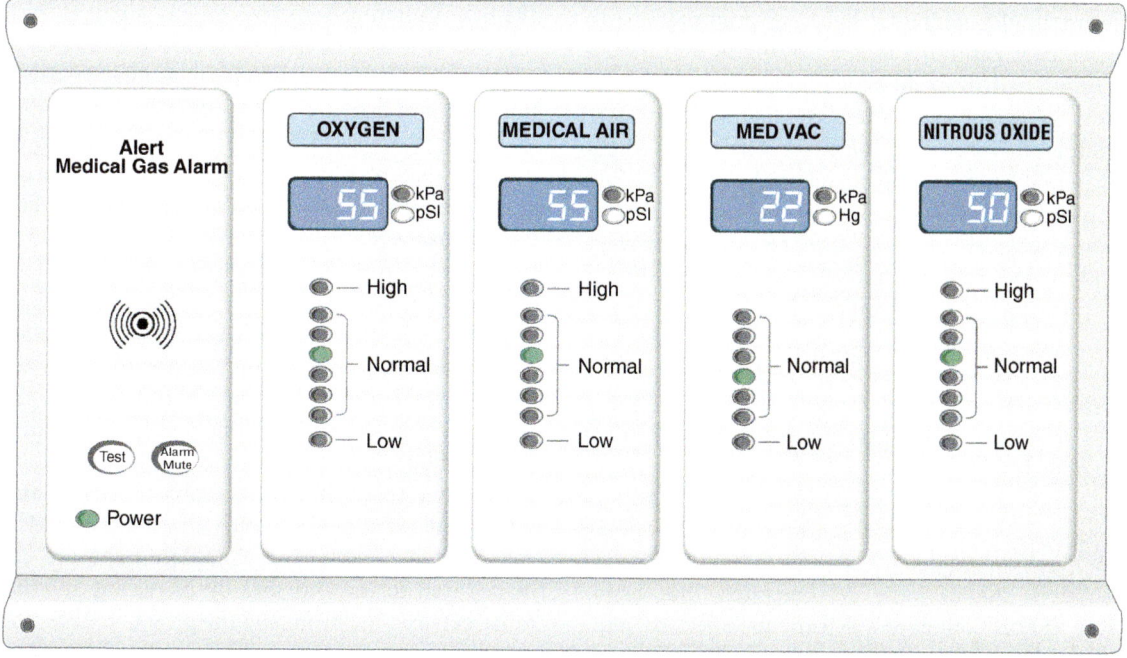

FIGURE 2–5 An example of a master alarm panel that monitors gasline pressure.

HUMIDITY

In past decades, static discharges were a feared source of ignition in an operating room filled with flammable anesthetic vapors. Now humidity control is more relevant to infection control practices. Optimally humidity levels in the operating room should be maintained between 50% and 55%. Below this range the dry air facilitates airborne motility of particulate matter, which can be a vector for infection. At high humidity, dampness can affect the integrity of barrier devices such as sterile cloth drapes and pan liners.

VENTILATION

A high rate of operating room airflow decreases contamination of the surgical site. These flow rates, usually achieved by blending up to 80% recirculated air with fresh air, are engineered in a manner to decrease turbulent flow and be unidirectional. Although recirculation conserves energy costs associated with heating and air conditioning, it is unsuitable for WAGD. Therefore, a separate anesthetic gas scavenging system must always supplement operating room ventilation. The operating room should maintain a slightly positive pressure to drive away gases that escape scavenging and should be designed so fresh air is introduced through or near the ceiling and air return is handled at or near floor level. Ventilation considerations must address air quality and volume changes. The National Fire Protection Agency (NFPA) recommends 25 air volume exchanges per hour to decrease risk of stagnation and bacterial growth. Air quality should be maintained by adequate air filtration using a 90% filter, defined simply as one that filters out 90% of particles presented. High-efficiency particulate filters (HEPA) are frequently used but are not required by engineering or infection control standards.

NOISE

Multiple studies have demonstrated that exposure to noise can have a detrimental effect on multiple human cognitive functions and may result in hearing impairment with prolonged exposure. Operating room noise has been measured at 70–80 decibels (dB) with frequent sound peaks exceeding 80 dB. As a reference, if your speaking voice has to be raised above conversational level, then ambient noise is approximated at 80 dB. Noise levels in the operating room approach the time-weighted average (TWA) for which the Occupational Safety and Health Administration (OSHA) requires hearing protection. Orthopedic air chisels and neurosurgical drills can approach the noise levels of 125 dB, the level at which most human subjects begin to experience pain.

IONIZING RADIATION

Radiation is an energy form that is found in specific beams. For the anesthesia provider radiation is usually a component of either diagnostic imaging or radiation therapy. Examples include fluoroscopy, linear accelerators, computed tomography, directed beam therapy, proton therapy, and diagnostic radiographs. Human effects of radiation are measured by units of absorbed doses such as the gray (Gy) and rads or equivalent dose units such as the Sievert (Sv) and Roentgen equivalent in man (REM). Radiation-sensitive organs such as eyes, thyroid, and gonads must be protected, as well as blood, bone marrow, and fetus. Radiation levels must be monitored if individuals are exposed to greater than 40 REM. The most common method of measurement is by film badge. Lifetime exposure can be tabulated by a required database of film badge wearers.

4 A basic principle of radiation safety is to keep exposure "as low as reasonably practical" (ALARP). The principles of ALARP are protection from radiation exposure by the use of time, distance, and shielding. The length of time of exposure is usually not an issue for simple radiographs such as chest films but can be significant in fluoroscopic procedures such as those commonly performed during interventional radiology, c-arm use, and in the diagnostic gastroenterology lab. Exposure can be reduced to the provider by increasing the distance between the beam and the provider. Radiation exposure over distance follows the inverse square law. To illustrate, intensity is represented as $1/d^2$

(where d = distance) so that 100 mRADs at 1 inch will be 0.01 mRADs at 100 inches. Shielding is the most reliable form of radiation protection; typical personal shielding is in the form of leaded apron and glasses. Physical shields are usually incorporated into radiological suites and can be as simple as a wall to stand behind or a rolling leaded shield to place between the beam and the provider. Although most modern facilities are designed in a very safe manner, providers can still be exposed to scattered radiation as atomic particles are bounced off shielding. For this reason radiation protection should be donned whenever ionizing radiation is used.

As use of reliable shielding has increased, the incidence of radiation-associated diseases of sensitive organs has decreased, with the exception of radiation-induced cataracts. Because protective eyewear has not been consistently used to the same degree as other types of personal protection, radiation-induced cataracts are increasing among employees working in interventional radiology suites. Anesthesia providers who work in these environments should consider the use of leaded goggles or glasses to decrease the risk of such problems.

Electrical Safety

THE RISK OF ELECTROCUTION

The use of electronic medical equipment subjects patients and hospital personnel to the risk of electrocution. Anesthesiologists must have at least a basic understanding of electrical hazards and their prevention.

Body contact with two conductive materials at different voltage potentials may complete a circuit and result in an electrical shock. Usually, one point of exposure is a live 110-V or 240-V conductor, with the circuit completed through a ground contact. For example, a grounded person need contact only one live conductor to complete a circuit and receive a shock. The live conductor could be the frame of a patient monitor that has developed a fault to the hot side of the power line. A circuit is now complete between the power line (which is earth grounded at the utility company's pole-top

transformer) through the victim and back to the ground (Figure 2–6). The physiological effect of electrical current depends on the location, duration, frequency, and magnitude (more accurately, current density) of the shock.

Leakage current is present in all electrical equipment as a result of capacitive coupling, induction between internal electrical components, or defective insulation. Current can flow as a result of capacitive coupling between two conductive bodies (eg, a circuit board and its casing) even though they are not physically connected. Some monitors are doubly insulated to decrease the effect of capacitive coupling. Other monitors are designed to be connected to a low-impedance ground (the safety ground wire) that should divert the current away from a person touching the instrument's case. The magnitude of such leaks is normally imperceptible to touch (<1 mA, and well below the fibrillation threshold of 100 mA). If the current bypasses the high resistance offered by skin, however, and is applied directly to the heart (**microshock**), current as low as 100 μA may be fatal. The maximum leakage allowed in operating room equipment is 10 μA.

Cardiac pacing wires and invasive monitoring catheters provide a conductive pathway to the myocardium. In fact, blood and normal saline can serve as electrical conductors. The exact amount of current required to produce fibrillation depends on the timing of the shock relative to the vulnerable period of heart repolarization (the T wave on the electrocardiogram). Even small differences in potential between the earth connections of two electrical outlets in the same operating room might place a patient at risk for microelectrocution.

PROTECTION FROM ELECTRICAL SHOCK

Most patient electrocutions are caused by current flow from the live conductor of a grounded circuit through the body and back to a ground (Figure 2–6). This would be prevented if everything in the operating room were grounded except the patient. Although direct patient grounds should be avoided, complete patient isolation is not feasible

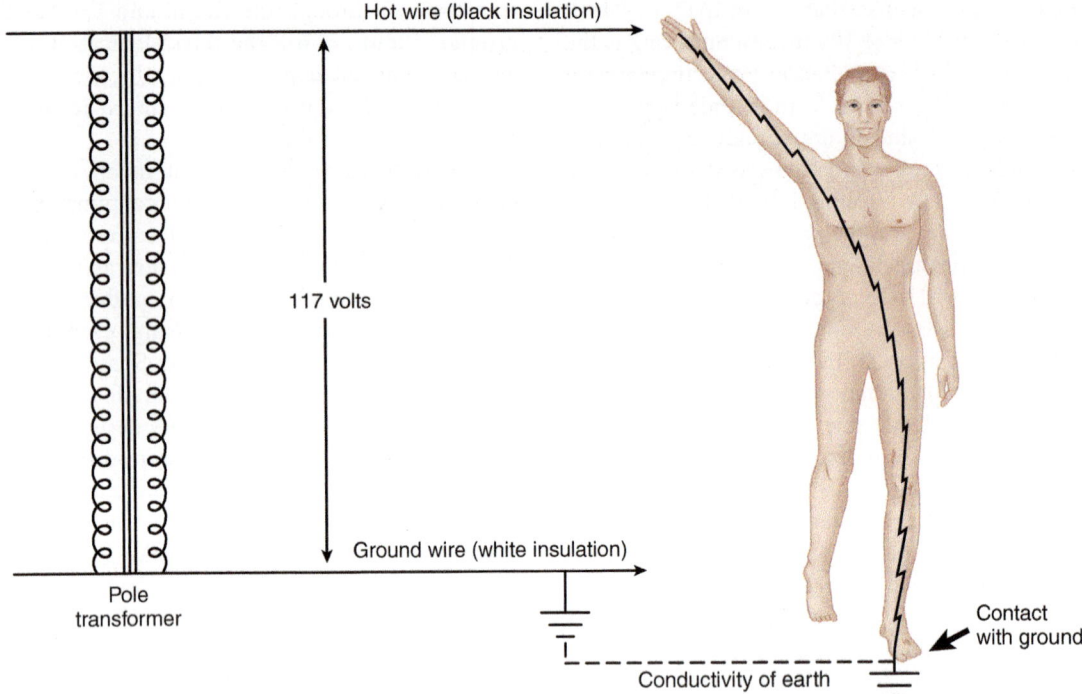

FIGURE 2–6 The setting for the great majority of electric shocks. An accidentally grounded person simultaneously contacts the hot wire of the electric service, usually via defective equipment that provides a pathway linking the hot wire to an exposed conductive surface. The complete electrical loop originates with the secondary of the pole transformer (the voltage source) and extends through the hot wire, the victim and the victim's contact with a ground, the earth itself, the neutral ground rod at the service entrance, and back to the transformer via the neutral (or ground) wire. (Modified and reproduced, with permission, from Bruner J, Leonard PF: *Electricity, Safety, and the Patient*. Mosby Year Book, 1989.)

during surgery. Instead, the operating room power supply can be isolated from grounds by an **isolation transformer** (Figure 2–7).

Unlike the utility company's pole-top transformer, the secondary wiring of an isolation transformer is not grounded and provides two live ungrounded voltage lines for operating room equipment. Equipment casing—but not the electrical circuits—is grounded through the longest blade of a three-pronged plug (the safety ground). If a live wire is then unintentionally contacted by a grounded patient, current will not flow through the patient since no circuit back to the secondary coil has been completed (Figure 2–8).

Of course, if both power lines are contacted, a circuit is completed and a shock is possible. In addition, if either power line comes into contact with a ground through a fault, contact with the other power line will complete a circuit through a grounded patient. To reduce the chance of two coexisting faults, a **line isolation monitor** measures the potential for current flow from the isolated power supply to the ground (Figure 2–9). Basically, the line isolation monitor determines the degree of isolation between the two power wires and the ground and predicts the amount of current that *could* flow if a second short circuit were to develop. An alarm is activated if an unacceptably high current flow to the ground becomes possible (usually 2 mA or 5 mA), but power is not interrupted unless a ground-fault circuit interrupter is also activated. The latter, a feature of household bathrooms, is usually not installed in locations such as operating rooms,

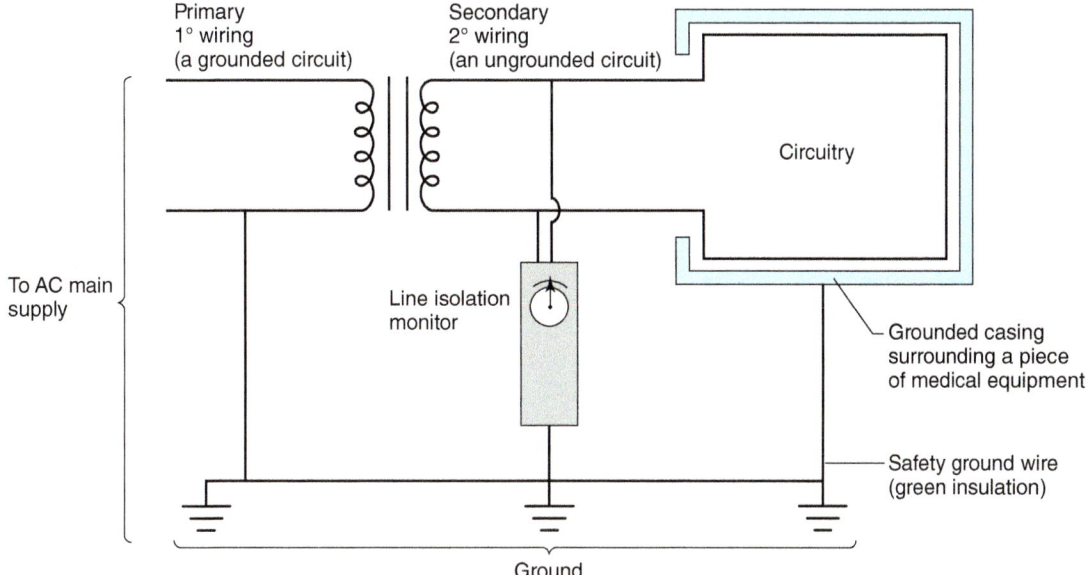

Primary
1° wiring
(a grounded circuit)

Secondary
2° wiring
(an ungrounded circuit)

Circuitry

To AC main
supply

Line isolation
monitor

Grounded casing
surrounding a piece
of medical equipment

Safety ground wire
(green insulation)

Ground

FIGURE 2–7 A circuit diagram of an isolation transformer and monitor.

where discontinuation of life support systems (eg, cardiopulmonary bypass machine) is more hazardous than the risk of electrical shock. The alarm of the line isolation monitor merely indicates that the power supply has partially reverted to a grounded system. In other words, while the line isolation monitor warns of the existence of a single fault (between a power line and a ground), two faults are required for a shock to occur. Since the line isolation monitor alarms when the sum of leakage current exceeds the set threshold, the last piece of equipment is usually the defective one; however, if this item is life-sustaining, other equipment can be removed from the circuit to evaluate whether the life safety item is truly at fault.

Even isolated power circuits do not provide complete protection from the small currents capable of causing microshock fibrillation. Furthermore, the line isolation monitor cannot detect all faults, such as a broken safety ground wire within a piece of equipment. Despite the overall utility of isolated power systems, they add to construction costs. Their requirement in operating rooms was deleted from the National Electrical Code in 1984, and circuits of newer or remodeled operating rooms may offer less

protection from electroshock injury than circuits of a household bathroom.

There are, however, modern equipment designs that decrease the possibility of microelectrocution. These include double insulation of the chassis and casing, ungrounded battery power supplies, and patient isolation from equipment-connected grounds by using optical coupling or transformers.

SURGICAL DIATHERMY

Electrosurgical units (ESUs) generate an ultrahigh-frequency electrical current that passes from a small active electrode (the cautery tip) through the patient and exits by way of a large plate electrode (the dispersal pad, or return electrode). The high current density at the cautery tip is capable of tissue coagulation or cutting, depending on the electrical waveform. Ventricular fibrillation is prevented by the use of ultrahigh electrical frequencies (0.1–3 MHz) compared with line power (50–60 Hz). The large surface area of the low-impedance return electrode avoids burns at the current's point of exit by providing a low current density (the concept of *exit* is technically incorrect, as the current

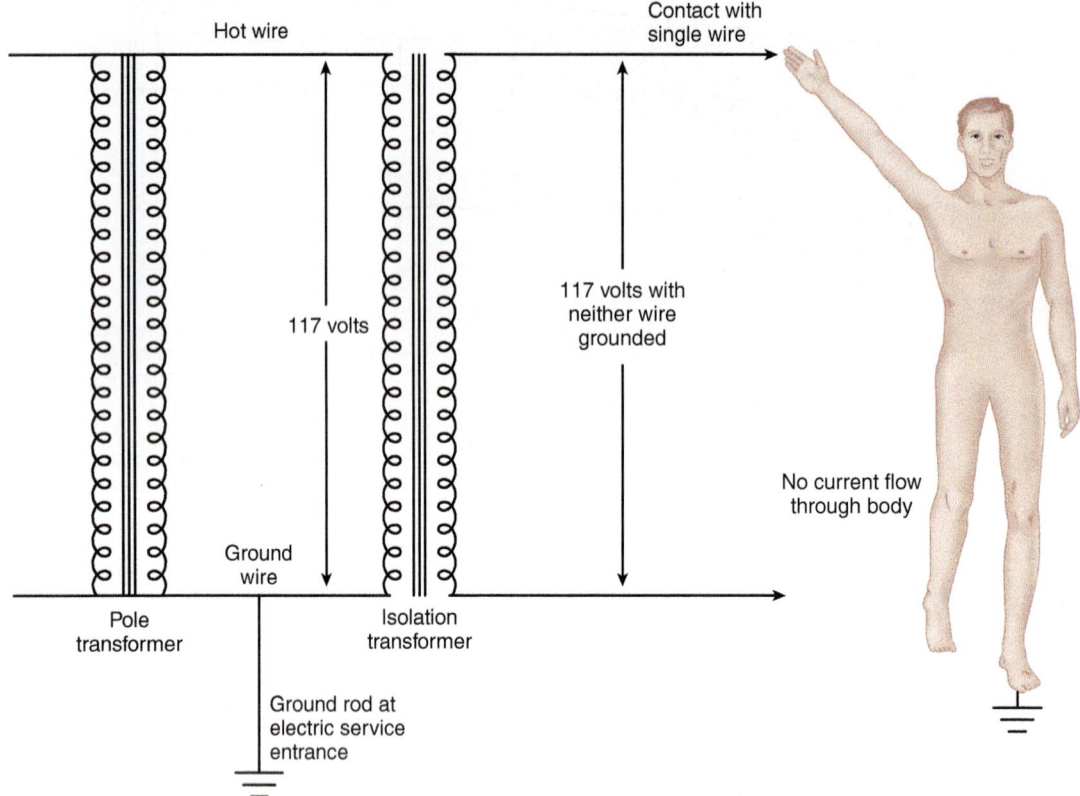

FIGURE 2–8 Even though a person is grounded, no shock results from contact with one wire of an isolated circuit. The individual is in simultaneous contact with two separate voltage sources but does not close a loop including either source. (Modified and reproduced, with permission, from Bruner J, Leonard PF: *Electricity, Safety, and the Patient*. Mosby Year Book, 1989.)

is alternating rather than direct). The high power levels of ESUs (up to 400 W) can cause inductive coupling with monitor cables, leading to electrical interference.

Malfunction of the dispersal pad may result from disconnection from the ESU, inadequate patient contact, or insufficient conductive gel. In these situations, the current will find another place to exit (eg, electrocardiogram pads or metal parts of the operating table), which may result in a burn (Figure 2–10). Precautions to prevent diathermy burns include proper return electrode placement, avoiding prostheses and bony protuberances, and elimination of patient-to-ground contacts. Current flow through the heart may lead to dysfunction of

an implanted cardiac rhythm management device (CRMD). This can be minimized by placing the return electrode as close to the surgical field and as far from the CRMD as practical.

Newer ESUs are isolated from grounds using the same principles as the isolated power supply (isolated output versus ground-referenced units). Because this second layer of protection provides ESUs with their own isolated power supply, the operating room's line isolation monitor may not detect an electrical fault. Although some ESUs are capable of detecting poor contact between the return electrode and the patient by monitoring impedance, many older units trigger the alarm only if the return electrode is unplugged from the machine. Bipolar

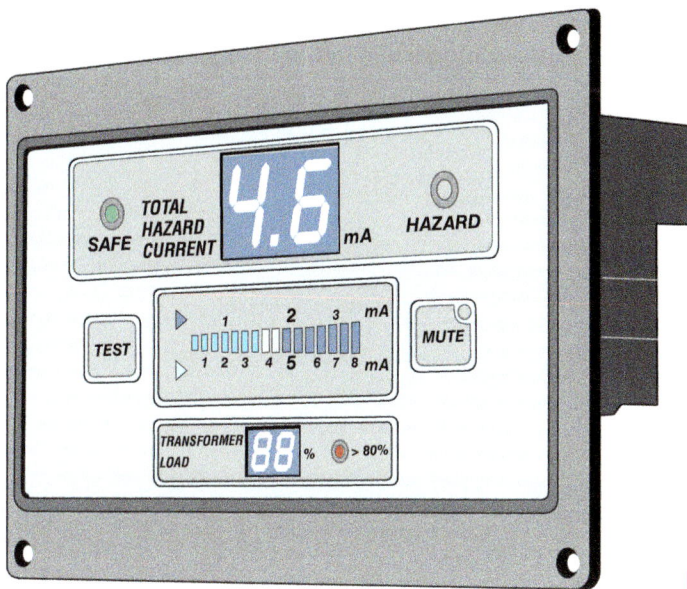

FIGURE 2–9 A line isolation monitor.

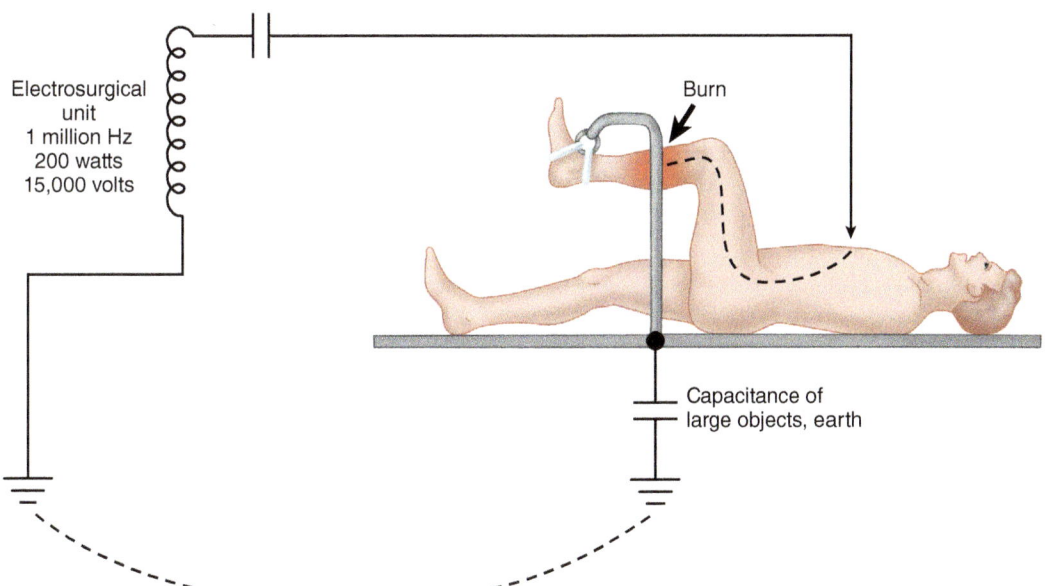

FIGURE 2–10 Electrosurgical burn. If the intended path is compromised, the circuit may be completed through other routes. Because the current is of high frequency, recognized conductors are not essential; capacitances can complete gaps in the circuit. Current passing through the patient to a contact of small area may produce a burn. (A leg drape would not offer protection in the situation depicted.) The isolated output electrosurgical unit (ESU) is much less likely than the ground-referenced ESU to provoke burns at ectopic sites. *Ground-referenced* in this context applies to the ESU output and has nothing to do with isolated versus grounded power systems. (Modified and reproduced, with permission, from Bruner J, Leonard PF: *Electricity, Safety, and the Patient*. Mosby Year Book, 1989.)

electrodes confine current propagation to a few millimeters, eliminating the need for a return electrode. Because pacemaker and electrocardiogram interference is possible, pulse or heart sounds should be closely monitored when any ESU is used. Automatic implanted cardioversion and defibrillator devices may need to be suspended if monopolar ESU is used and any implanted CRMD should be interrogated after use of a monopolar ESU.

Surgical Fires & Thermal Injury

FIRE PREVENTION & PREPARATION

Surgical fires are relatively rare, with an incidence of about 1:87,000 cases, which is close to the incidence rate of other events such as retained foreign objects after surgery and wrong-site surgery. **7** Almost all surgical fires can be prevented. Unlike medical complications, fires are a product of simple physical and chemical properties. Occurrence is guaranteed given the proper combination of factors but can be eliminated almost entirely by understanding the basic principles of fire risk. Likely the most common risk **8** factor for surgical fire relates to the open delivery of oxygen.

Situations classified as carrying a high risk for a surgical fire are those that involve an ignition source used in close proximity to an oxidizer. The simple chemical combination required for any fire is commonly referred to as the fire triad or fire triangle. The triad is composed of fuel, oxidizer, and ignition source (heat). Table 2–2 lists potential contributors to fires and explosions in the operating room. Surgical fires can be managed and possibly avoided completely by incorporating education, fire drills, preparation, prevention, and response into educational programs provided to operating room personnel.

For anesthesia providers, fire prevention education should place a heavy emphasis on the risk relating to the open delivery of oxygen. The Anesthesia Patient Safety Foundation has developed an educational video and online teaching module that

TABLE 2–2 Potential contributors to operating room fires and explosions.

Flammable agents (fuels)
Solutions, aerosols, and ointments
Alcohol
Chlorhexidine
Benzoin
Mastisol
Acetone
Petroleum products
Surgical drapes (paper and cloth)
Surgical gowns
Surgical sponges and packs
Surgical sutures and mesh
Plastic/polyvinyl chloride/latex products
Endotracheal tubes
Masks
Cannulas
Tubing
Intestinal gases
Hair
Gases supporting combustion (oxidizers)
Oxygen
Nitrous oxide
Ignition sources (heat)
Lasers
Electrosurgical units
Fiberoptic light sources (distal tip)
Drills and burrs
External defibrillators

provides fire safety education from the perspective of the anesthesia provider.

Operating room fire drills increase awareness of the fire hazards associated with surgical procedures. In contrast to the typical institutional fire drill, these drills should be specific to the operating room and should place a greater emphasis on the particular risks associated with that setting. For example, consideration should be given to both vertical and horizontal evacuation of surgical patients, movement of patients requiring ventilatory assistance, and unique situations such as prone or lateral positioning and movement of patients who may be fixed in neurosurgical pins.

Preparation for surgical fires can be incorporated into the time-out process of the universal protocol. Team members should be introduced and specific roles agreed upon should a fire erupt. Items needed to properly manage a fire can be assembled or identified beforehand (eg, ensuring the proper endotracheal tube for patients undergoing laser surgery; having water or saline ready on the surgical field; identifying the location of fire extinguishers, gas cutoff valves, and escape routes). A poster or flowsheet to standardize the preparation may be of benefit.

Preventing catastrophic fires in the operating room begins with a strong level of communication among all members of the surgical team. Different aspects of the fire triad are typically under the domain of particular surgical team members. Fuels such as alcohol-based solutions, adhesive removers, and surgical drapes and towels are typically controlled by the circulating nurse. Ignition sources such as electrocautery, lasers, drills, burrs, and light sources for headlamps and laparoscopes are usually controlled by the surgeon. The anesthesia provider maintains control of the oxidizer concentration of oxygen and nitrous oxide. Communication between personnel is evident when a surgeon enters the airway and verifies the concentration of oxygen before using cautery, or when an anesthesiologist asks the circulator to configure drapes to prevent the accumulation of oxygen in a surgical case that involves sedation and use of a nasal cannula.

Administration of oxygen in concentrations of greater than 30% should be guided by clinical presentation of the patient and not solely by protocols or habits. If oxygen is being delivered via nasal cannula or face mask, and if increased oxygen levels are needed, then the airway should be secured by either endotracheal tube or supraglottic device. This is of prime importance when the surgical site is above the level of the xiphoid.

When the surgical site is in or near the airway and a flammable tube is present, the oxygen concentration should be reduced for a sufficient period of time before use of an ignition device (eg, laser or cautery) to allow reduction of oxygen concentration at the site. Laser airway surgery should incorporate either jet ventilation without an endotracheal tube or the appropriate protective tube specific for the wavelength of the laser. Precautions for laser cases are outlined below.

Alcohol-based skin preparations are extremely flammable and require an adequate drying time.

Pooling of solutions must be avoided. Large prefilled swabs of alcohol-based solution should be used with caution on the head or neck to avoid both oversaturation of the product and excess flammable waste. Product inserts are a good source of information about these preparations. Surgical gauze and sponges should be moistened with sterile water or saline if used in close proximity to an ignition source.

Should a fire occur in the operating room it is important to determine whether the fire is located *on the patient, in the airway,* or *elsewhere in the operating room.* For fires occurring in the airway, the delivery of fresh gases to the patient must be stopped. Effective means of stopping fresh gases to the patient can be accomplished by turning off flowmeters, disconnecting the circuit from the machine, or disconnecting the circuit from the endotracheal tube. The endotracheal tube should be removed and either sterile water or saline should be poured into the airway to extinguish any burning embers. The sequence of stopping gas flow and removal of the endotracheal tube when fire occurs in the airway is not as important as ensuring that both actions are performed quickly. Often the two tasks can be accomplished at the same time and even by the same individual. If carried out by different team members, the personnel should act without waiting for a predetermined sequence of events. After these actions are carried out, ventilation may be resumed, preferably using room air and avoiding oxygen or nitrous oxide–enriched gases. The tube should be examined for missing pieces. The airway should be reestablished and, if indicated, examined with a bronchoscope. Treatment for smoke inhalation and possible transfer to a burn center should also be considered.

For fires on the patient, the flow of oxidizing gases should be stopped, the surgical drapes removed, and the fire extinguished by water or smothering. The patient should be assessed for injury. If the fire is not immediately extinguished by first attempts, then a carbon dioxide (CO_2) fire extinguisher may be used. Further actions may include evacuation of the patient and activation of the nearest pull station. As noted previously, prior to an actual emergency, the location of fire extinguishers, emergency exits, and fresh gas cutoff valves should be established by the anesthesia provider.

Fires that result in injuries requiring medical treatment or death must be reported to the fire marshal, who retains jurisdiction over the facility. Providers should gain basic familiarity with local reporting standards, which can vary according to location.

Cases in which supplemental delivery of oxygen is used and the surgical site is above the xiphoid constitute the most commonly reported scenario for surgical fires. Frequently the face or airway is involved, resulting in life-threatening injuries and the potential for severe facial disfigurement. For the most part, these fires can be avoided by the elimination of the open delivery of oxygen, by use of an oxygen blender, or by securing the airway.

FIRE EXTINGUISHERS

For fires not suppressed by initial attempts or those in which evacuation may be hindered by the location or intensity of the fire, the use of a portable fire extinguisher is warranted. A CO_2 extinguisher should be safe during external and internal exposure for fires on the patient in the operating room. CO_2 readily dissipates, is not toxic, and as used in an actual fire is not likely to result in thermal injury. FE-36, manufactured by DuPont, also can be used to extinguish fires but is expensive. Both choices are equally effective and acceptable agents as reflected by manufacturers' product information.

"A"-rated extinguishers contain water, which makes their use in the operating room problematic because of the presence of so much electrical equipment. A water mist "AC"-rated extinguisher is excellent but requires time and an adequate volume of mist over multiple attempts to extinguish the fire. Furthermore, these devices are large and difficult to maneuver. Both can be made cheaply in a nonferromagnetic extinguisher, making them the best choice for fires involving magnetic resonance imagers. Halon extinguishers, although very effective, are being phased out because of concerns about depletion of the ozone layer, as well as the hypoxic atmosphere that results for rescuers. Halotrons are

"greener" halon-type extinguishers that may have fewer effects on the ozone layer.

LASER SAFETY

Lasers are commonly used in operating rooms and procedure areas. When lasers are used for airway surgeries or for procedures involving the neck and face, the case should be considered as high risk for surgical fire and managed as previously discussed. The type of laser (CO_2, neodymium yttrium aluminum garnet [NG:YAG], or potassium titanyl phosphate [KTP]), wavelength, and focal length are all important considerations for the safe operation of medical lasers. Without this vital information, operating room personnel cannot adequately protect themselves or the patient from harm. Before beginning laser surgery, the laser device should be in the operating room, warning signs should be posted on the doors, and protective eyewear should be issued. The anesthesia provider should ensure that the warning signs and eyewear match the labeling on the device as protection is specific to the type of laser. The American National Standards Institute (ANSI) standards specify that eyewear and laser devices must be labeled for the wavelength emitted or protection offered. Some ophthalmologic lasers and vascular mapping lasers have such a short focal length that protective eyewear is not needed. For other devices, protective goggles should be worn by personnel at all times during laser use, and eye protection in the form of either goggles or protective eye patches should be used on the patient.

Laser endotracheal tube selection should be based on laser type and wavelength. The product insert and labeling for each type of tube should be compared to the type of laser used. Certain technical limitations are present when selecting laser tubes. For instance, tubes less than 4.0 mm in diameter are not compatible with the ND:YAG or argon laser nor are ND:YAG-compatible tubes available in half sizes. Attempts to wrap conventional endotracheal tubes with foil should be avoided. This archaic method is not approved by either manufacturers or the U.S. Food and Drug Administration, is prone to breaking or unraveling, and does not confer protection against laser penetration. Alternatively, jet ventilation without an endotracheal tube can offer a reduced risk of airway fire.

CREW RESOURCE MANAGEMENT: CREATING A CULTURE OF SAFETY IN THE OPERATING ROOM

Crew resource management (CRM) was developed in the aviation industry to allow personnel to intervene or call for investigation of any situation thought to be unsafe. Comprising seven principles, its goal is to avoid errors caused by human actions. In the airline model CRM gives any crew member the authority to question situations that fall outside the range of normal practice. Before the implementation of CRM, crew members other that the captain had little or no input on aircraft operations. After CRM was instituted, anyone identifying a safety issue could take steps to ensure adequate resolution of the situation. The benefit of this method in the operating room is clear, given the potential for a deadly mistake to be made.

The seven principles of CRM are (1) adaptability/flexibility, (2) assertiveness, (3) communication, (4) decision making, (5) leadership, (6) analysis, and (7) situational awareness. *Adaptability/flexibility* refers to the ability to alter a course of action when new information becomes available. For example, if a major blood vessel is unintentionally cut in a routine procedure, the anesthesiologist must recognize that the anesthetic plan has changed and volume resuscitation must be made even in presence of medical conditions that typically contraindicate large-volume fluid administration.

Assertiveness is the willingness and readiness to actively participate, state, and maintain a position until convinced by the facts that other options are better; this requires the initiative and the courage to act. For instance, if a senior and well-respected surgeon tells the anesthesiologist that the patient's aortic stenosis is not a problem because it is a chronic condition and the procedure will be relatively quick, the anesthesiologist should respond by voicing concerns about the management of the patient and should not proceed until a safe anesthetic and surgical plan have been agreed upon.

Communication is defined simply as the clear and accurate sending and receiving of information, instructions, or commands, and providing useful feedback. Communication is a two-way process and should continue in a loop fashion.

Decision making is the ability to use logical and sound judgment to make decisions based on available information. Decision-making processes are involved when a less experienced clinician seeks out the advice of a more experienced clinician or when a person defers important clinical decisions because of fatigue. Good decision making is based on realization of personal limitations.

Leadership is the ability to direct and coordinate the activities of other crew members and to encourage the crew to work together as a team. *Analysis* refers to the ability to develop short-term, long-term, and contingency plans, as well as to coordinate, allocate, and monitor crew and operating room resources.

The last and most important principle is *situational awareness*; that is, the accuracy with which a person's perception of the current environment mirrors reality. In the operating room, lack of situational awareness can cost precious minutes, as when readings from a monitor (eg, capnograph or arterial line) suddenly change and the operator focuses on the monitor rather than on the patient, who may have had an embolism. One must decide whether the monitor is correct and the patient is critically ill or the monitor is incorrect and the patient is fine. The problem-solving method utilized should consider both possibilities but quickly eliminate one. In this scenario, tunnel vision can result in catastrophic mistakes. Furthermore, if the sampling line has come loose and the capnograph indicates low end-tidal CO_2, this finding does not exclude the possibility that at the same time or even a bit later, the patient could have a pulmonary embolus resulting in decreased end-tidal CO_2.

If all members of the operating room team apply these seven principles, problems arising from human factors can almost entirely be eliminated. A culture of safety must also exist if the operating room is to be made a safer place. These seven principles serve no purpose when applied in a suppressive surgical environment. Anyone with a concern must be able speak up without fear of repercussion.

Chapter 58 provides further discussion of these and other issues relating to patient safety.

FUTURE DESIGN OF OPERATING ROOMS

Safety Interlock Technology

Despite heightened awareness of safety factors and increased educational efforts among operating room personnel, harm to patients still occurs at a rate that most industries and the public deem unacceptably high. Similarly, despite threats of payment withholding, public scoring of medical personnel and hospital systems, provider rating web sites, and punitive legal consequences, the human factors resulting in medical errors have not been completely eliminated. In future, safety-engineered designs may assist in the reduction of medical errors. One developing area is the use of interlock devices in the operating room. An interlock device is simply a device that cannot be operated until a defined sequence of events occurs. Anesthesia personnel use interlock technology with anesthesia vaporizers that prevent the use of more than one vaporizer at a time. Expansion of this technology might prevent release of a drug from an automated dispensing device until a barcode is scanned from a patient's hospital armband or, at a minimum, the patient's drug allergies have been entered into the machine's database. Other applications might include an electrosurgical device or laser that could not be used when the FiO_2 content was higher than 30%, thus eliminating the risk of fire. Likewise, computers, monitors, and other devices could be designed to be inoperable until patient identification was confirmed.

Workflow Design

Coordinating the activities of surgical personnel, anesthesia providers, and operating room nurses is essential to the day-to-day running of a surgical suite. Clinical directors in facilities ranging from one- or two-room suites to multiroom centers must accommodate surgical procedures of varying durations, requiring varying degrees of surgical skill and efficiency, while allowing for sudden, unplanned, or emergency operations. The need to monitor workflow and analyze data for optimizing scheduling and staffing prompted the development of software systems that anticipate and record the timing of surgical events; these systems are constantly being refined.

Surgical suites are also being designed to augment workflow by incorporating separate induction areas to decrease nonsurgical time spent in operating rooms. Several models exist for induction room design and staffing. Although uncommon in the United States, induction rooms have long been employed in the United Kingdom.

One induction room model uses rotating anesthesia teams. One team is assigned to the first patient of the day; a second team induces anesthesia for the next patient in an adjacent area while the operating room is being turned over. The second team continues caring for that patient after transfer to the operating room, leaving the first team available to induce anesthesia in the third patient as the operating room is being turned over. The advantage of this model is continuity of care; the disadvantage is the need for two anesthesia teams for every operating room.

Another model uses separate induction and anesthesia teams. The induction team induces anesthesia for all patients on a given day and then transfers care to the anesthesia team, which is assigned to an individual operating room. The advantage of this model is the reduction in anesthesia personnel to staff induction rooms; disadvantages include failure to maintain continuity of care and staffing problems that occur when several patients must undergo induction concurrently. This model can utilize either a separate induction room adjacent to each operating room or one common induction room that services several operating rooms.

The final model uses several staffed operating rooms, one of which is kept open. After the first patient of the day is transferred to the initial room, subsequent patients always proceed to the open room, thus eliminating the wait for room turnover and readiness of personnel. All of these models assume that the increased overhead cost of maintaining additional anesthesia personnel can be justified by the increased surgical productivity.

Radio Frequency Identification (RFID)

Radio frequency identification (RFID) technology utilizes a chip with a small transmitter whose signal is read by a reader; each chip yields a unique signal. The technology has many potential applications in the modern operating room. Using RFID in employee identification (ID) badges could enable surgical control rooms to keep track of nursing, surgical faculty, and anesthesia personnel, obviating the need for paging systems and telephony to establish the location of key personnel. Incorporating the technology in patient ID bands and hospital gurneys could allow a patient's flow to be tracked through an entire facility. The ability to project an identifying signal to hospital systems would offer an additional degree of safety for patients unable to communicate with hospital personnel. Finally, RFID could be incorporated into surgical instruments and sponges, allowing surgical counts to be performed by identification of the objects as they are passed on and off the surgical field. In the event that counts are mismatched, a wand could then be placed over the patient to screen for retained objects.

CASE DISCUSSION

Monitored Anesthesia Care with Oxygen Supplementation

You are asked to provide monitored anesthesia care for a patient undergoing simple removal of a lesion on the cheek. The patient is morbidly obese and has a history of sleep apnea. He states, "It bothers me when people are working on my face," and indicates that he does not want to remember anything about the surgery. The surgeon assures you the procedure will not last more than 5 minutes. The patient's wife mentions that they are from out of town and have made flight arrangements to return home soon after the procedure.

What features of this case indicate a high risk for surgical fire?

Patients with a clinical history of obstructive sleep apnea usually have a sensitivity to sedating medications, especially opioid narcotics. Typically administration of even small doses of narcotics obstructs the upper airways, resulting in hypoventilation and hypercapnia. In the obese patient, this response combined with decreased functional reserve capacity results in rapid oxygen desaturation. Most anesthesia providers respond by increasing the amount of oxygen supplementation delivered via face mask or nasal cannula. Open delivery of oxygen in concentrations greater than 30% is one of the elements of the fire triad. Another consideration is the anatomical location of the procedure. A location above the xiphoid process in this patient would place an ignition source (if used) in close proximity to the open delivery of an oxidizer.

What is the safest manner in which to proceed?

There are three strategies that can be implemented to improve safety in this scenario: avoid oxygen supplementation, secure the airway with an endotracheal tube or supraglottic device, or avoid use of an ignition source.

Are there any concerns relating to airway management or selection of the delivery device?

As previously noted, the patient is likely to manifest airway changes associated with obstructive sleep apnea and obesity. Selection of a delivery device should take into consideration the need to prevent the open delivery of oxygen.

How would the length of the procedure affect the management of anesthesia?

Practically speaking, if the patient requires a lengthy procedure, local anesthetics may wear off; the cumulative dose of narcotics provided may exacerbate the patient's obstructive sleep apnea and increase recovery time. Additionally, more complex surgical excision may result in bleeding requiring the use of cautery.

Does the patient's expectation of discharge soon after the procedure affect your anesthesia plans?

The expectation of an accelerated recovery period may not be feasible if the patient requires general anesthesia or significant amounts of opioid narcotics. The American Society of Anesthesiologists (ASA) has published a practice advisory providing direction for the safe postoperative assessment and discharge of patients with obstructive sleep apnea. See www.asahq.org.

> ### *What if the surgeon thinks your plans are "overkill"?*
>
> The first and most effective means for conflict resolution is to communicate your specific concerns to the surgeon. If this fails, the procedure must not be allowed to proceed as long as any team member has a legitimate safety concern. Many ASA safety-related guidelines and advisories are also endorsed by professional societies such as the American College of Surgeons (ACS) and other organizations. The anesthesiologist should also gain familiarity with a facility's methods of dispute resolution before an event occurs.

SUGGESTED READING

Dorsch JA, Dorsch SE: *Understanding Anesthesia Equipment*, 5th ed. Williams & Wilkins, 2008. A detailed discussion of compressed gases and medical gas delivery systems.

Macdonald MR, Wong A, Walker P, Crysdale WS: Electrocautery-induced ignition of tonsillar packing. J Otolaryngol 1994;23:426. An examination of factors that can decrease the risk of airway fire including lower oxygen concentration (using a cuffed tracheal tube), completely soaked tonsil packs, and avoidance of contact between electrocautery and bismuth subgallate.

National Fire Protection Association (NFPA): *Standard for Health Care Facilities*. NFPA, 2002. An updated version of NFPA 99 standards.

WEB SITES

http://www.ansi.org
The American National Standards Institute is the reference source for laser standards and many other protective engineering standards.

http://www.apsf.org
The Anesthesia Patient Safety Foundation provides resources and a newsletter that discusses important safety issues in anesthesia. The web site also contains a link to view or request the video *Prevention and Management of Operating Room Fires*, which is an excellent resource to gain information concerning the risks and prevention of surgical fires.

http://www.asahq.org
The American Society of Anesthesiologists (ASA) web site contains the ASA practice parameters and advisories. Many are oriented around patient safety issues and all can be printed for review.

http://www.cganet.com
The Compressed Gas Association and its web site are dedicated to the development and promotion of safety standards and safe practices in the industrial gas industry.

http://www.ecri.org
The ECRI (formerly the Emergency Care Research Institute) is an independent nonprofit health services research agency that focuses on health care technology, health care risk and quality management, and health care environmental management.

http://www.fda.org
The U.S. Food and Drug Administration (FDA) has an extensive web site covering many broad categories. Two major divisions address patient safety: the Center for Devices and Radiological Health (CDRH), which regulates and evaluates medical devices, and the Center for Drug Evaluation and Research (CDER), which regulates and evaluates drugs.

http://www.nfpa.org
The National Fire Protection Association (NPFA) has a web site with a catalog of publications on fire, electrical, and building safety issues. Some areas require a subscription to access.

http://patientsafetyauthority.org
The Patient Safety Authority maintains data collected from the mandatory reporting of incidents of harm or near harm in the Commonwealth of Pennsylvania. Some data such as surgical fires data can be extrapolated to determine the likely incidence for the entire United States.

http://vam.anest.ufl.edu/
The Virtual Anesthesia Machine web site has extensive interactive modules to facilitate understanding of many processes and equipment. The site, which contains high-quality graphic illustrations and animation, requires free registration.

Breathing Systems

1 Because insufflation avoids any direct patient contact, there is no rebreathing of exhaled gases if the flow is high enough. Ventilation cannot be controlled with this technique, however, and the inspired gas contains unpredictable amounts of entrained atmospheric air.

2 Long breathing tubes with high compliance increase the difference between the volume of gas delivered to a circuit by a reservoir bag or ventilator and the volume actually delivered to the patient.

3 The adjustable pressure-limiting (APL) valve should be fully open during spontaneous ventilation so that circuit pressure remains negligible throughout inspiration and expiration.

4 Because a fresh gas flow equal to minute ventilation is sufficient to prevent rebreathing, the Mapleson A design is the most efficient Mapleson circuit for spontaneous ventilation.

5 The Mapleson D circuit is efficient during controlled ventilation, because fresh gas flow forces alveolar air away from the patient and toward the APL valve.

6 The drier the soda lime, the more likely it will absorb and degrade volatile anesthetics.

7 Malfunction of either unidirectional valve in a circle system may allow rebreathing of carbon dioxide, resulting in hypercapnia.

8 With an absorber, the circle system prevents rebreathing of carbon dioxide at fresh gas flows that are considered low (fresh gas flow ≤ 1 L) or even fresh gas flows equal to the uptake of anesthetic gases and oxygen by the patient and the circuit itself (closed-system anesthesia).

9 Because of the unidirectional valves, apparatus dead space in a circle system is limited to the area distal to the point of inspiratory and expiratory gas mixing at the Y-piece. Unlike Mapleson circuits, the circle system tube length does not directly affect dead space.

10 The fraction of inspired oxygen (F_{IO_2}) delivered by a resuscitator breathing system to the patient is directly proportional to the oxygen concentration and flow rate of the gas mixture supplied to the resuscitator (usually 100% oxygen) and inversely proportional to the minute ventilation delivered to the patient.

Breathing *systems* provide the final conduit for the delivery of anesthetic gases to the patient. Breathing *circuits* link a patient to an anesthesia machine (**Figure 3–1**). Many different circuit designs have been developed, each with varying degrees of efficiency, convenience, and complexity. This chapter reviews the most important breathing systems: insufflation, draw-over, Mapleson circuits, the circle system, and resuscitation systems.

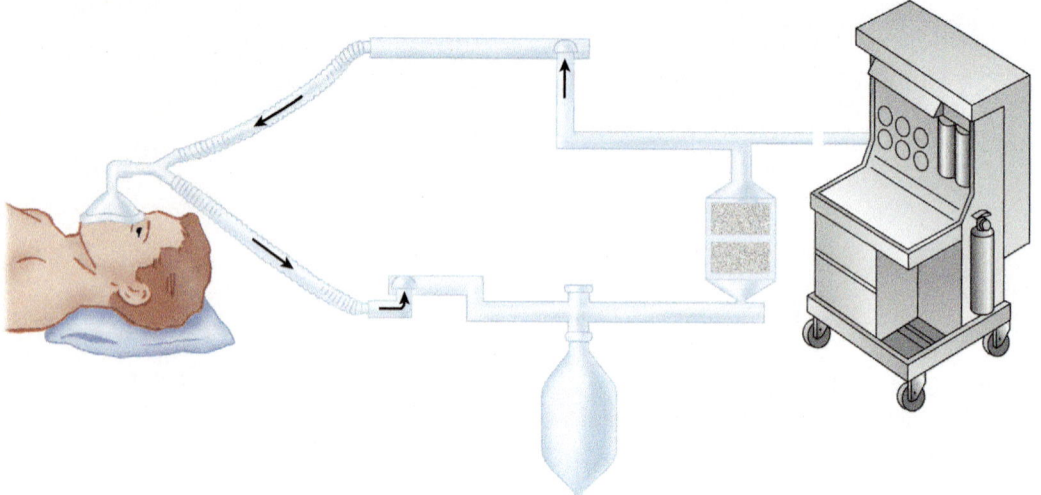

FIGURE 3–1 The relationship between the patient, the breathing system, and the anesthesia machine.

Most classifications of breathing systems artificially consolidate functional characteristics (eg, the extent of rebreathing) with physical characteristics (eg, the presence of unidirectional valves). Because these seemingly contradictory classifications (eg, open, closed, semiopen, semiclosed) often tend to confuse rather than aid understanding, they are avoided in this discussion.

INSUFFLATION

The term insufflation usually denotes the blowing of anesthetic gases across a patient's face. Although insufflation is categorized as a breathing system, it is perhaps better considered a technique that avoids direct connection between a breathing circuit and a patient's airway. Because children often resist the placement of a face mask (or an intravenous line), insufflation is particularly valuable during inductions with inhalation anesthetics in children (Figure 3–2). It is useful in other situations as well. Carbon dioxide accumulation under head and neck draping is a hazard of ophthalmic surgery performed with local anesthesia. Insufflation of air across the patient's face at a high flow rate (>10 L/min) avoids this problem, while not increasing the risk of fire from accumulation of oxygen

1 (Figure 3–3). Because insufflation avoids any direct patient contact, there is no rebreathing of exhaled gases if the flow is high enough. Ventilation cannot be controlled with this technique, however, and the inspired gas contains unpredictable amounts of entrained atmospheric air.

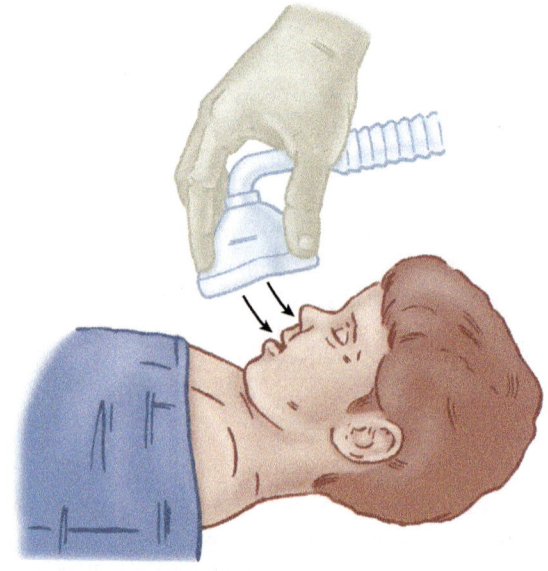

FIGURE 3–2 Insufflation of an anesthetic agent across a child's face during induction.

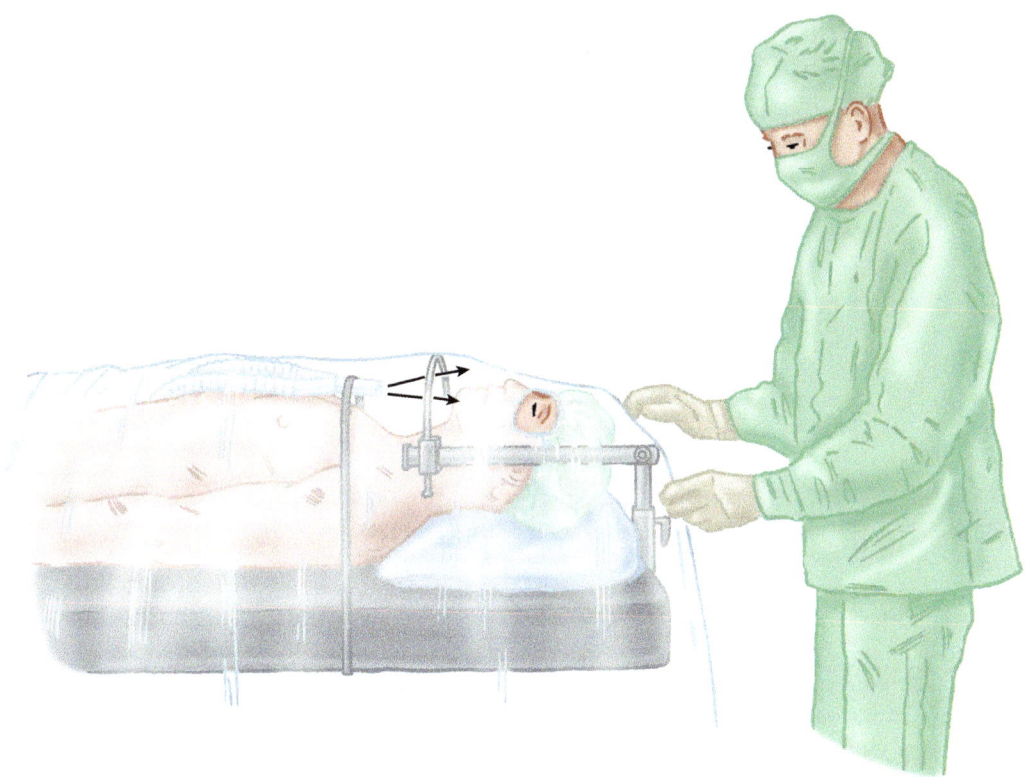

FIGURE 3–3 Insufflation of oxygen and air under a head drape.

Insufflation can also be used to maintain arterial oxygenation during brief periods of apnea (eg, during bronchoscopy). Instead of blowing gases across the face, oxygen is directed into the lungs through a device placed in the trachea.

OPEN-DROP ANESTHESIA

Although open-drop anesthesia is not used in modern medicine, its historic significance warrants a brief description here. A highly volatile anesthetic—historically, ether or chloroform—was dripped onto a gauze-covered mask (Schimmelbusch mask) applied to the patient's face. As the patient inhales, air passes through the gauze, vaporizing the liquid agent, and carrying high concentrations of anesthetic to the patient. The vaporization lowers mask temperature, resulting in moisture condensation and a drop in anesthetic vapor pressure (vapor pressure is proportional to temperature).

A modern derivative of open-drop anesthesia utilizes draw-over vaporizers that depend on the patient's inspiratory efforts to draw ambient air through a vaporization chamber. This technique may be used in locations or situations in which compressed medical gases are unavailable (eg, battlefields).

DRAW-OVER ANESTHESIA

Draw-over devices have nonrebreathing circuits that use ambient air as the carrier gas, although supplemental oxygen can be used, if available. The devices can be fitted with connections and equipment that allow intermittent positive-pressure ventilation (IPPV) and passive scavenging, as well as

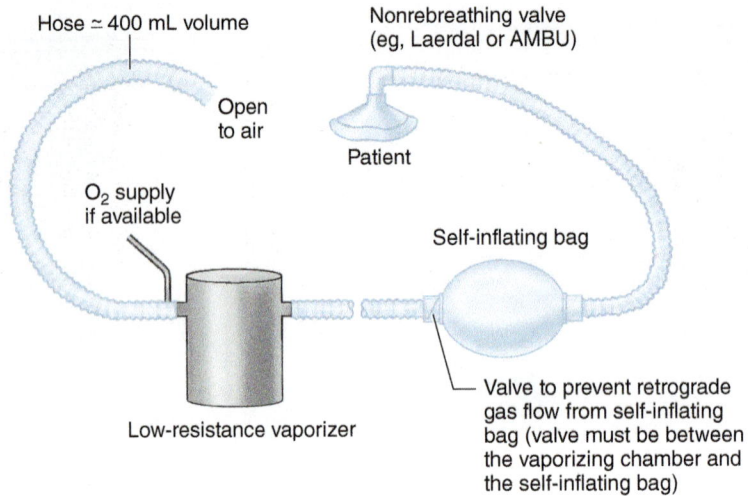

Hose ≈ 400 mL volume

Nonrebreathing valve
(eg, Laerdal or AMBU)

Open
to air

Patient

O₂ supply
if available

Self-inflating bag

Low-resistance vaporizer

Valve to prevent retrograde
gas flow from self-inflating
bag (valve must be between
the vaporizing chamber and
the self-inflating bag)

FIGURE 3–4 Schematic diagram of a draw-over anesthesia device/circuit.

continuous positive airway pressure (CPAP) and positive end-expiratory pressure (PEEP).

In its most basic application (Figure 3–4), air is drawn through a low-resistance vaporizer as the patient inspires. Patients spontaneously breathing room air and a potent halogenated agent often manifest an oxygen saturation (SpO_2) <90%, a situation treated with IPPV, supplemental oxygen, or both. The fraction of inspired oxygen (FIO_2) can be supplemented using an open-ended reservoir tube of about 400 mL, attached to a t-piece at the upstream side of the vaporizer. Across the clinical range of tidal volume and respiratory rate, an oxygen flow rate of 1 L/min gives an FIO_2 of 30% to 40%, or with 4 L/min, an FIO_2 of 60% to 80%. There are several commercial draw-over systems available that share common properties (Table 3–1).

The greatest advantage of draw-over systems is their simplicity and portability, making them useful

TABLE 3–1   Properties of draw-over devices.

Portable
Low resistance to gas flow
Usable with any agent[1]
Controllable vapor output

[1]Halothane cannot be used with the Epstein Mackintosh Oxford device.

in locations where compressed gases or ventilators are not available. The presence of the nonrebreathing valve, PEEP valve, and circuit filter close to the patient's head makes the technique awkward for head and neck surgery and pediatric cases. If the head is draped, the nonrebreathing valve is often covered as well.

The original design of a draw-over system has recently been modified to include a self-inflating bag, a ventilator, and/or a heat and moisture exchanger. The Ohmeda Universal Portable Anesthesia Complete (U-PAC) is one example of a draw-over anesthesia system.

MAPLESON CIRCUITS

The insufflation and draw-over systems have several disadvantages: poor control of inspired gas concentration (and, therefore, poor control of depth of anesthesia), mechanical drawbacks during head and neck surgery, and pollution of the operating room with large volumes of waste gas. The **Mapleson systems** solve some of these problems by incorporating additional components (breathing tubes, fresh gas inlets, adjustable pressure-limiting [APL] valves, and reservoir bags) into the breathing circuit. The relative location of these components determines circuit performance and is the basis of the Mapleson classification (Table 3–2).

TABLE 3–2 Classification and characteristics of Mapleson circuits.

Mapleson Class	Other Names	Configuration[1]	Required Fresh Gas Flows		Comments
			Spontaneous	**Controlled**	
A	Magill attachment		Equal to minute ventilation (≈80 mL/kg/min)	Very high and difficult to predict	Poor choice during cotrolled ventilaton. Enclosed Magill system is a modification that improves efficiency. Coaxial Mapleson A (Lack breathing system) provides waste gas scavenging.
B			2 × minute ventilation	2–2½ × minute ventilation	
C	Waters' to-and-fro		2 × minute ventilation	2–2½ × minute ventilation	
D	Bain circuit		2–3 × minute ventilation	1–2 × minute ventilation	Bain coaxial modifcation: fresh gas tube inside breathing tube (see Figure 3–7).
E	Ayre's T-piece		2–3 × minute ventilation	3 × minute ventilation (I:E-1:2)	Exhalation tubing should provide a larger volume than tidal volume to prevent rebreathing. Scavenging is difficult.
F	Jackson-Rees' modification		2–3 × minute ventilation	2 × minute ventilation	A Mapleson E with a breathing bag connected to the end of the breathing tube to allow controlled ventilation and scavenging.

[1]FGI, fresh gas inlet; APL, adjustable pressure-limiting (value).

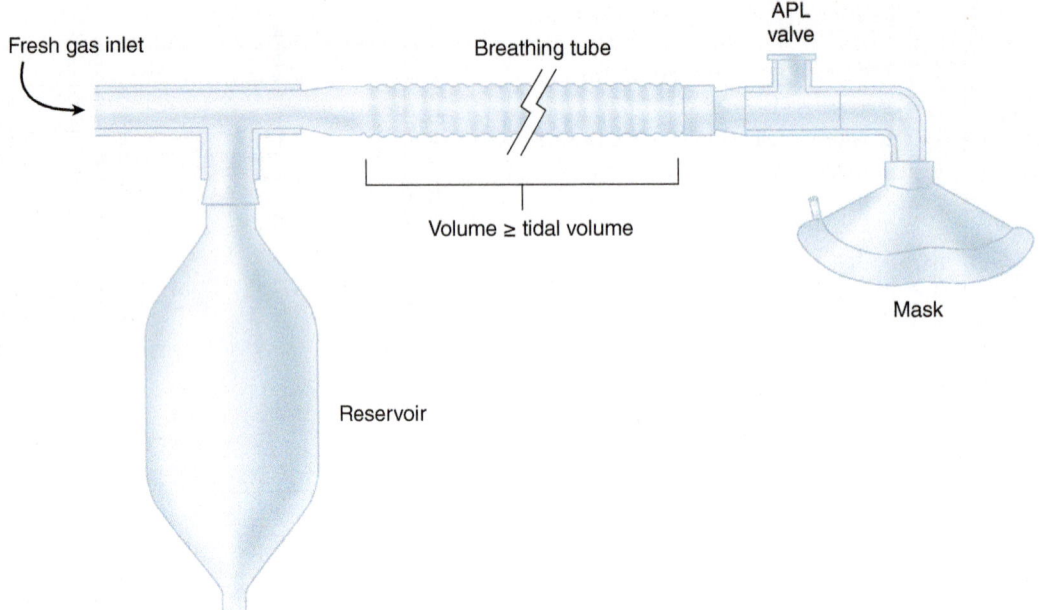

FIGURE 3–5 Components of a Mapleson circuit. APL, adjustable pressure-limiting (valve).

Components of Mapleson Circuits

A. Breathing Tubes

Corrugated tubes—made of rubber (reusable) or plastic (disposable)—connect the components of the Mapleson circuit to the patient (Figure 3–5). The large diameter of the tubes (22 mm) creates a low-resistance pathway and a potential reservoir for anesthetic gases. To minimize fresh gas flow requirements, the volume of gas within the breathing tubes in most Mapleson circuits should be at least as great as the patient's tidal volume.

The compliance of the breathing tubes largely determines the compliance of the circuit. (Compliance is defined as the change of volume produced by a change in pressure.) Long breathing tubes with high compliance increase the difference between the volume of gas delivered to a circuit by a reservoir bag or ventilator and the volume actually delivered to the patient. For example, if a breathing circuit with a compliance of 8 mL gas/cm H_2O is pressurized during delivery of a tidal volume to 20 cm H_2O, 160 mL of the tidal volume will be lost to the circuit. The 160 mL represent a combination of

gas compression and breathing-tube expansion. This is an important consideration in any circuit delivering positive-pressure ventilation through breathing tubes (eg, circle systems).

B. Fresh Gas Inlet

Gases (anesthetics mixed with oxygen or air) from the anesthesia machine continuously enter the circuit through the fresh gas inlet. As discussed below, the relative position of the fresh gas inlet is a key differentiating factor in Mapleson circuit performance.

C. Adjustable Pressure-Limiting Valve (Pressure-Relief Valve, Pop-Off Valve)

As anesthetic gases enter the breathing circuit, pressure will rise if the gas inflow is greater than the combined uptake of the patient and the circuit. Gases may exit the circuit through an APL valve, controlling this pressure buildup. Exiting gases enter the operating room atmosphere or, preferably, a waste-gas scavenging system. All APL valves allow a variable pressure threshold for venting. The APL valve should be fully open during spontaneous ventilation so that circuit pressure remains negligible throughout inspiration and expiration. Assisted and controlled ventilation require positive pressure during inspiration to expand the lungs. Partial closure of the APL valve limits gas exit, permitting positive circuit pressures during reservoir bag compressions.

D. Reservoir Bag (Breathing Bag)

Reservoir bags function as a reservoir of anesthetic gas and a method of generating positive-pressure ventilation. They are designed to increase in compliance as their volume increases. Three distinct phases of reservoir bag filling are recognizable (Figure 3–6). After the nominal 3-L capacity of an adult reservoir bag is achieved (phase I), pressure rises rapidly to a peak (phase II). Further increases in volume result in a plateau or even a slight decrease in pressure (phase III). This ceiling effect provides some minimal protection of the patient's lungs against high airway pressures, if the APL valve is unintentionally left in the closed position while fresh gas continues to flow into the circuit.

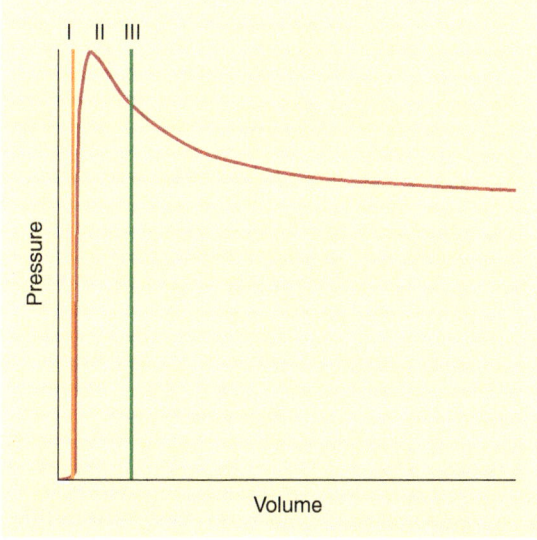

FIGURE 3–6 The increasing compliance and elasticity of breathing bags as demonstrated by three phases of filling (see text). (Reproduced, with permission, from Johnstone RE, Smith TC: Rebreathing bags as pressure limiting devices. Anesthesiology 1973;38:192.)

Performance Characteristics of Mapleson Circuits

Mapleson circuits are lightweight, inexpensive, and simple. Breathing-circuit efficiency is measured by the fresh gas flow required to reduce CO_2 rebreathing to a negligible value. Because there are no unidirectional valves or CO_2 absorption in Mapleson circuits, rebreathing is prevented by adequate fresh gas flow into the circuit and venting exhaled gas through the APL valve before inspiration. There is usually some rebreathing in any Mapleson circuit. The total fresh gas flow into the circuit controls the amount. To attenuate rebreathing, high fresh gas flows are required. The APL valve in Mapleson A, B, and C circuits is located near the face mask, and the reservoir bag is located at the opposite end of the circuit.

Reexamine the drawing of a Mapleson A circuit in Figure 3–5. During spontaneous ventilation, alveolar gas containing CO_2 will be exhaled into the breathing tube or directly vented through an open APL valve. Before inhalation occurs, if the fresh gas flow exceeds alveolar minute ventilation, the inflow of fresh gas will force the alveolar gas remaining in the breathing tube to exit from the APL valve. If the breathing-tube volume is equal to or greater than the patient's tidal volume, the next inspiration will contain only **4** fresh gas. Because a fresh gas flow equal to minute ventilation is sufficient to prevent rebreathing, the Mapleson A design is the most efficient Mapleson circuit for *spontaneous* ventilation.

Positive pressure during *controlled* ventilation, however, requires a partially closed APL valve. Although some alveolar and fresh gas exits through the valve during inspiration, no gas is vented during expiration, since the exhaled gas stagnates during the expiratory phase of positive pressure ventilation. As a result, very high fresh gas flows (greater than three times minute ventilation) are required to prevent rebreathing with a Mapleson A circuit during controlled ventilation. Fresh gas flows are conveniently available because the fresh gas inlet is in close proximity to the APL valve in a Mapleson B circuit.

Interchanging the position of the APL valve and the fresh gas inlet transforms a Mapleson A into a **5** **Mapleson D circuit** (Table 3–2). The Mapleson D circuit is efficient during controlled ventilation, since fresh gas flow forces alveolar air *away*

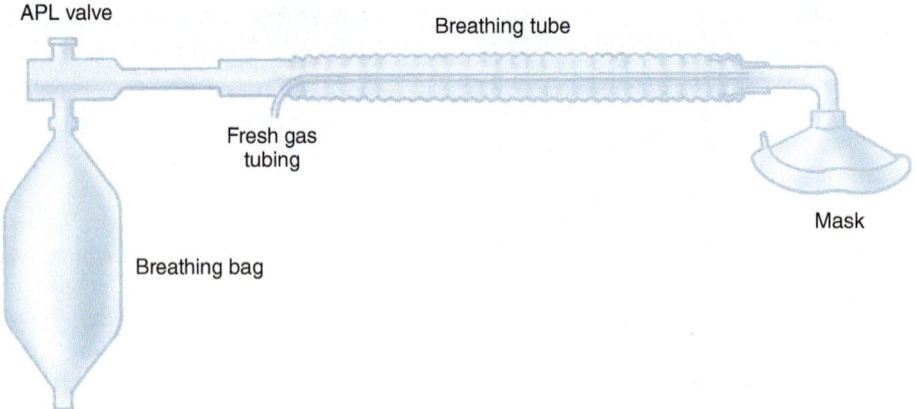

APL valve

Breathing tube

Fresh gas
tubing

Mask

Breathing bag

FIGURE 3–7 A Bain circuit is a Mapleson D circuit design with the fresh gas tubing inside the corrugated breathing tube. APL, adjustable pressure-limiting (valve).

(Redrawn and reproduced, with permission, from Bain JA, Spoerel WE: Flow requirements for a modified Mapleson D system during controlled ventilation. Can Anaesth Soc J 1973;20:629.)

from the patient and *toward* the APL valve. Thus, simply moving components completely alters the fresh gas requirements of the Mapleson circuits.

The **Bain circuit** is a coaxial version of the Mapleson D system that incorporates the fresh gas inlet tubing inside the breathing tube (Figure 3–7). This modification decreases the circuit's bulk and retains heat and humidity better than a conventional Mapleson D circuit as a result of partial warming of the inspiratory gas by countercurrent exchange with the warmer expired gases. A disadvantage of this coaxial circuit is the possibility of kinking or disconnection of the fresh gas inlet tubing. Periodic inspection of the inner tubing is mandatory to prevent this complication; if unrecognized, either of these mishaps could result in significant rebreathing of exhaled gas.

THE CIRCLE SYSTEM

Although Mapleson circuits overcome some of the disadvantages of the insufflation and draw-over systems, the high fresh gas flows required to prevent rebreathing of CO_2 result in waste of anesthetic agent, pollution of the operating room environment, and loss of patient heat and humidity (Table 3–3). In an attempt to avoid these problems, the **circle system** adds more components to the breathing system.

The components of a circle system include: (1) a CO_2 absorber containing CO_2 absorbent; (2) a fresh gas inlet; (3) an inspiratory unidirectional valve and

inspiratory breathing tube; (4) a Y-connector; (5) an expiratory unidirectional valve and expiratory breathing tube; (6) an APL valve; and (7) a reservoir (Figure 3–8).

Components of the Circle System

A. Carbon Dioxide Absorber and the Absorbent

Rebreathing alveolar gas conserves heat and humidity. However, the CO_2 in exhaled gas must be eliminated to prevent hypercapnia. CO_2 chemically

TABLE 3–3 Characteristics of breathing circuits.

	Insufflation and Open Drop	Mapleson	Circle
Complexity	Very simple	Simple	Complex
Control of anesthetic depth	Poor	Variable	Good
Ability to scavenge	Very poor	Variable	Good
Conservation of heat and humidity	No	No	Yes[1]
Rebreathing of exhaled gases	No	No[1]	Yes[1]

[1]These properties depend on the rate of fresh gas flow.

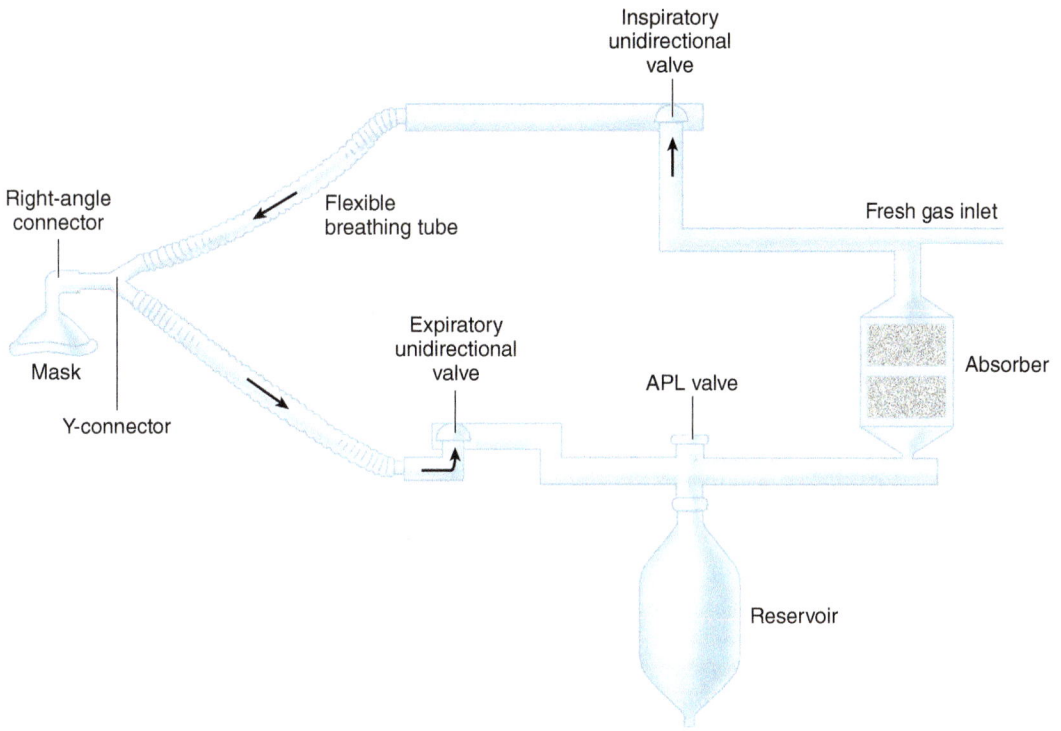

FIGURE 3–8 A circle system. APL, adjustable pressure-limiting (valve).

combines with water to form carbonic acid. CO_2 absorbents (eg, soda lime or calcium hydroxide lime) contain hydroxide salts that are capable of neutralizing carbonic acid (Table 3–4). Reaction end products include heat (the heat of neutralization), water, and calcium carbonate. **Soda lime** is the more common absorbent and is capable of absorbing up to 23 L of CO_2 per 100 g of absorbent. It consists primarily of calcium hydroxide (80%), along with sodium hydroxide, water, and a small amount of potassium hydroxide. Its reactions are as follows:

$$CO_2 + H_2O \rightarrow H_2CO_3$$
$$H_2CO_3 + 2NaOH \rightarrow Na_2CO_3 + 2H_2O + Heat$$
(a fast reaction)
$$Na_2CO_3 + Ca(OH)_2 \rightarrow CaCO_3 + 2NaOH$$
(a slow reaction)

Note that the water and sodium hydroxide initially required are regenerated. Another absorbent, barium hydroxide lime, is no longer used due to the

TABLE 3–4 Comparison of soda lime and barium hydroxide lime.

	Soda Lime	Barium Hydroxide Lime
Mesh size[1]	4–8	4–8
Method of hardness	Silica added	Water of crystallization
Content	Calcium hydroxide Sodium hydroxide Potassium hydroxide	Barium hydroxide Calcium hydroxide
Usual indicator dye	Ethyl violet	Ethyl violet
Absorptive capacity (liters of CO_2/100 g granules)	14–23	9–18

[1]The number of openings per linear inch in a wire screen used to grade particle size.

TABLE 3–5 Indicator dye changes signaling absorbent exhaustion.

Indicator	Color when Fresh	Color when Exhausted
Ethyl violet	White	Purple
Phenolphthalein	White	Pink
Clayton yellow	Red	Yellow
Ethyl orange	Orange	Yellow
Mimosa 2	Red	White

possible increased hazard of fire in the breathing system.

A pH indicator dye (eg, ethyl violet) changes color from white to purple as a consequence of increasing hydrogen ion concentration and absorbent exhaustion (Table 3–5). Absorbent should be replaced when 50% to 70% has changed color. Although exhausted granules may revert to their original color if rested, no significant recovery of absorptive capacity occurs. Granule size is a compromise between the higher absorptive surface area of small granules and the lower resistance to gas flow of larger granules. The granules commonly used as CO_2 absorbent are between 4 and 8 mesh; the number of mesh corresponds to the number of holes per square inch of a screen. The hydroxide salts are irritating to the skin and mucous membranes. Increasing the hardness of soda lime by adding silica minimizes the risk of inhalation of sodium hydroxide dust and also decreases resistance of gas flow. Additional water is added to absorbent during packaging to provide optimal conditions for carbonic acid formation. Commercial soda lime has a water content of 14% to 19%.

Absorbent granules can absorb and later release medically important amounts of volatile anesthetic. This property can be responsible for modest delays of induction or emergence. The drier the soda lime, the more likely it will absorb and degrade volatile anesthetics. Volatile anesthetics can be broken down to carbon monoxide by dry absorbent (eg, sodium or potassium hydroxide) to such a degree that it is capable of causing clinically significant carbon monoxide poisoning. The formation of carbon

monoxide is highest with desflurane; with sevoflurane, it occurs at a higher temperature.

Amsorb is a CO_2 absorbent consisting of calcium hydroxide and calcium chloride (with calcium sulfate and polyvinylpyrrolidone added to increase hardness). It possesses greater inertness than soda lime, resulting in less degradation of volatile anesthetics (eg, sevoflurane into compound A or desflurane into carbon monoxide).

Compound A is one of the by-products of degradation of sevoflurane by absorbent. Higher concentrations of sevoflurane, prolonged exposure, and low-flow anesthetic technique seem to increase the formation of Compound A. Compound A has been shown to produce nephrotoxicity in animals,

The granules of absorbent are contained within one or two canisters that fit snugly between a head and base plate. Together, this unit is called an absorber (Figure 3–9). Although bulky, double

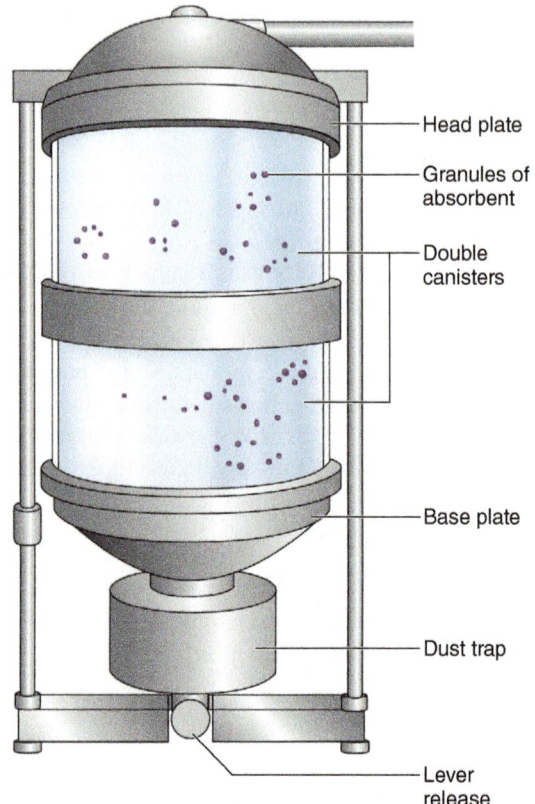

FIGURE 3–9 A carbon dioxide absorber.

canisters permit more complete CO_2 absorption, less frequent absorbent changes, and lower gas flow resistance. To ensure complete absorption, a patient's tidal volume should not exceed the air space between absorbent granules, which is roughly equal to 50% of the absorber's capacity. Indicator dye color is monitored through the absorber's transparent walls. Absorbent exhaustion typically occurs first where exhaled gas enters the absorber and along the canister's smooth inner walls. Channeling through areas of loosely packed granules is minimized by a baffle system, which directs gas flow through the center, thereby allowing greater utilization of the absorbent. A trap at the base of the absorber collects dust and moisture. Newer absorbers are used until CO_2 is found in the inhaled gas on the anesthetic-gas monitor, at which time the canister(s) are replaced.

B. Unidirectional Valves

Unidirectional valves, which function as check valves, contain a ceramic or mica disk resting horizontally on an annular valve seat (**Figure 3–10**). Forward flow displaces the disk upward, permitting the gas to proceed through the circuit. Reverse flow pushes the disk against its seat, preventing reflux. Valve incompetence is usually due to a warped disk or seat irregularities. The expiratory valve is exposed to the humidity of alveolar gas. Condensation and resultant moisture formation may prevent upward displacement of the disks, resulting in incomplete escape of expired gases and rebreathing.

Inhalation opens the inspiratory valve, allowing the patient to breathe a mixture of fresh and exhaled gas that has passed through the CO_2 absorber. Simultaneously, the expiratory valve closes to prevent rebreathing of exhaled gas that still contains CO_2. The subsequent flow of gas away from the patient during exhalation opens the expiratory valve. This gas is vented through the APL valve or rebreathed by the patient after passing through the absorber. Closure of the inspiratory valve during exhalation prevents expiratory gas from mixing with fresh gas in the inspiratory limb. Malfunction of either unidirectional valve may allow rebreathing of CO_2, resulting in hypercapnia.

Optimization of Circle System Design

Although the major components of the circle system (unidirectional valves, fresh gas inlet, APL valve, CO_2 absorber, and a reservoir bag) can be placed in several configurations, the following arrangement is preferred (Figure 3–8):

- Unidirectional valves are relatively close to the patient to prevent backflow into the inspiratory limb if a circuit leak develops. However, unidirectional valves are not placed in the Y-piece, as that makes it difficult to confirm proper orientation and intraoperative function.

- The fresh gas inlet is placed between the absorber and the inspiratory valve. Positioning it downstream from the inspiratory valve would allow fresh gas to bypass the patient during exhalation and be wasted. Fresh gas introduced between the expiratory valve and the absorber would be diluted by recirculating gas. Furthermore, inhalation anesthetics may be absorbed or released by soda lime granules, thus slowing induction and emergence.

- The APL valve is usually placed between the absorber and the expiratory valve and close to the reservoir bag. Positioning of the APL valve in this location (ie, before the absorber) helps to conserve absorption capacity and minimizes the venting of fresh gas.

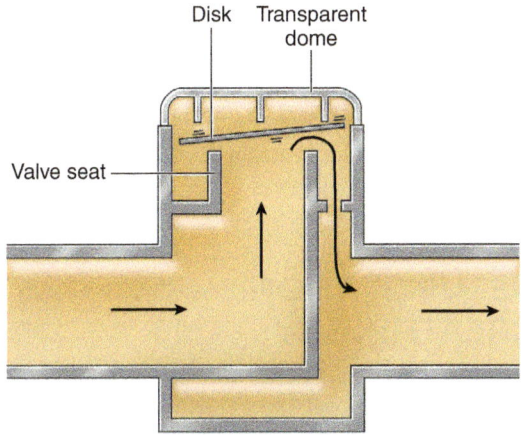

Disk Transparent
dome

Valve seat

FIGURE 3–10 A unidirectional valve.

- Resistance to exhalation is decreased by locating the reservoir bag in the expiratory limb. Bag compression during controlled ventilation will vent expired gas through the APL valve, conserving absorbent.

Performance Characteristics of the Circle System

A. Fresh Gas Requirement

8 With an absorber, the circle system prevents rebreathing of CO_2 at reduced fresh gas flows (≤ 1 L) or even fresh gas flows equal to the uptake of anesthetic gases and oxygen by the patient and the circuit itself (closed-system anesthesia). At fresh gas flows greater than 5 L/min, rebreathing is so minimal that a CO_2 absorber is usually unnecessary.

With low fresh gas flows, concentrations of oxygen and inhalation anesthetics can vary markedly between fresh gas (ie, gas in the fresh gas inlet) and inspired gas (ie, gas in the inspiratory limb of the breathing tubes). The latter is a mixture of fresh gas and exhaled gas that has passed through the absorber. The greater the fresh gas flow rate, the less time it will take for a change in fresh gas anesthetic concentration to be reflected in a change in inspired gas anesthetic concentration. Higher flows speed induction and recovery, compensate for leaks in the circuit, and decrease the risks of unanticipated gas mixtures.

B. Dead Space

That part of a tidal volume that does not undergo alveolar ventilation is referred to as dead space. Thus, any increase in dead space must be accompanied by a corresponding increase in tidal volume, if alveolar ventilation is to remain unchanged.

9 Because of the unidirectional valves, apparatus dead space in a circle system is limited to the area distal to the point of inspiratory and expiratory gas mixing at the Y-piece. Unlike Mapleson circuits, the circle system tube length does not affect dead space. Like Mapleson circuits, length does affect circuit compliance and thus the amount of tidal volume lost to the circuit during positive-pressure ventilation. Pediatric circle systems may have both a septum dividing the inspiratory and expiratory gas in the Y-piece and low-compliance

breathing tubes to further reduce dead space, and are lighter in weight.

C. Resistance

The unidirectional valves and absorber increase circle system resistance, especially at high respiratory rates and large tidal volumes. Nonetheless, even premature neonates can be successfully ventilated using a circle system.

D. Humidity and Heat Conservation

Medical gas delivery systems supply dehumidified gases to the anesthesia circuit at room temperature. Exhaled gas, on the other hand, is saturated with water at body temperature. Therefore, the heat and humidity of inspired gas depend on the relative proportion of rebreathed gas to fresh gas. High flows are accompanied by low relative humidity, whereas low flows allow greater water saturation. Absorbent granules provide a significant source of heat and moisture in the circle system.

E. Bacterial Contamination

The minimal risk of microorganism retention in circle system components could theoretically lead to respiratory infections in subsequent patients. For this reason, bacterial filters are sometimes incorporated into the inspiratory or expiratory breathing tubes or at the Y-piece.

Disadvantages of the Circle System

Although most of the problems of Mapleson circuits are solved by the circle system, the improvements have led to other disadvantages: greater size and less portability; increased complexity, resulting in a higher risk of disconnection or malfunction; complications related to use of absorbent; and the difficulty of predicting inspired gas concentrations during low fresh gas flows.

RESUSCITATION BREATHING SYSTEMS

Resuscitation bags (AMBU bags or bag-mask units) are commonly used for emergency ventilation because of their simplicity, portability, and ability to deliver almost 100% oxygen (**Figure 3–11**). A

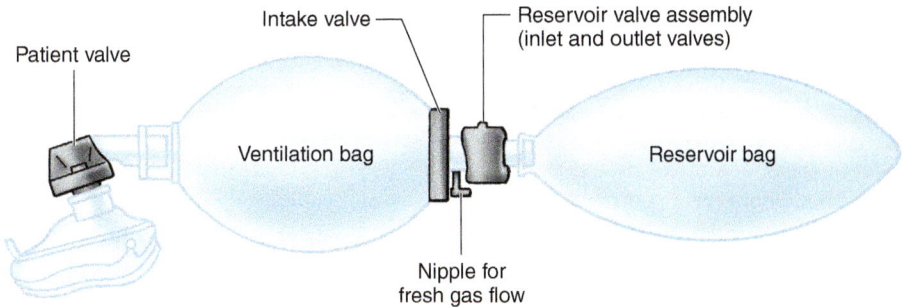

FIGURE 3–11 The Laerdal resuscitator. (Reproduced, with permission, from Laerdal Medical Corp.)

resuscitator is unlike a Mapleson circuit or a circle system because it contains a **nonrebreathing valve**. (Remember that a Mapleson system is considered valveless even though it contains an APL valve, whereas a circle system contains unidirectional valves that direct flow through an absorber but allow rebreathing of exhaled gases.)

High concentrations of oxygen can be delivered to a mask or tracheal tube during spontaneous or controlled ventilation if a source of high fresh gas flow is connected to the inlet nipple. The patient valve opens during controlled or spontaneous inspiration to allow gas flow from the ventilation bag to the patient. Rebreathing is prevented by venting exhaled gas to the atmosphere through exhalation ports in this valve. The compressible, self-refilling ventilation bag also contains an intake valve. This valve closes during bag compression, permitting positive-pressure ventilation. The bag is refilled by flow through the fresh gas inlet and across the intake valve. Connecting a reservoir to the intake valve helps prevent the entrainment of room air. The reservoir valve assembly is really two unidirectional valves: the inlet valve and the outlet valve. The inlet valve allows ambient air to enter the ventilation bag if fresh gas flow is inadequate to maintain reservoir filling. Positive pressure in the reservoir bag opens the outlet valve, which vents oxygen if fresh gas flow is excessive.

There are several disadvantages to resuscitator breathing systems. First, they require high fresh gas flows to achieve a high F_{IO_2}. F_{IO_2} is directly proportional to the oxygen concentration and flow rate of the gas mixture supplied to the resuscitator (usually 100% oxygen) and inversely proportional to the minute ventilation delivered to the patient. For example, a Laerdal resuscitator equipped with a reservoir requires a flow of 10 L/min to achieve an inspired oxygen concentration approaching 100% if a patient with a tidal volume of 750 mL is ventilated at a rate of 12 breaths/min. The maximum achievable tidal volumes are less than those that can be achieved with a system that uses a 3-L breathing bag. In fact, most adult resuscitators have a maximum tidal volume of 1000 mL, which is sufficient for the lower tidal volumes generally employed in patient management. Finally, although a normally functioning patient valve has low resistance to inspiration and expiration, exhaled moisture can cause valve sticking.

CASE DISCUSSION

Unexplained Light Anesthesia

An extremely obese but otherwise healthy 5-year-old girl presents for inguinal hernia repair. After uneventful induction of general anesthesia and tracheal intubation, the patient is placed on a ventilator set to deliver a tidal volume of 7 mL/kg at a rate of 16 breaths/min. Despite delivery of high concentrations of sevoflurane in 50% nitrous oxide, tachycardia (145 beats/min) and mild hypertension (144/94 mm Hg) are noted. To increase anesthetic depth, fentanyl (3 mcg/kg) is administered. Heart rate and blood pressure continue to rise and are accompanied by frequent premature ventricular contractions.

What should be considered in the differential diagnosis of this patient's cardiovascular changes?

The combination of tachycardia and hypertension during general anesthesia should always alert the anesthesiologist to the possibility of hypercapnia or hypoxia, both of which produce signs of increased sympathetic activity. These life-threatening conditions should be quickly and immediately ruled out by end-tidal CO_2 monitoring, pulse oximetry, or arterial blood gas analysis.

A common cause of intraoperative tachycardia and hypertension is an inadequate level of anesthesia. Normally, this is confirmed by movement. If the patient is paralyzed, however, there are few reliable indicators of light anesthesia. The lack of a response to a dose of an opioid should alert the anesthesiologist to the possibility of other, perhaps more serious, causes.

Malignant hyperthermia is rare but must be considered in cases of unexplained tachycardia, especially if accompanied by premature contractions. Certain drugs used in anesthesia (eg, pancuronium, ketamine, ephedrine) stimulate the sympathetic nervous system and can produce or exacerbate tachycardia and hypertension. Diabetic patients who become hypoglycemic from administration of insulin or long-acting oral hypoglycemic agents can have similar cardiovascular changes. Other endocrine abnormalities (eg, pheochromocytoma, thyroid storm, carcinoid) should also be considered.

Could any of these problems be related to an equipment malfunction?

Gas analysis can confirm the delivery of anesthetic gases to the patient.

A misconnection of the ventilator could result in hypoxia or hypercapnia. In addition, a malfunctioning unidirectional valve will increase circuit dead space and allow rebreathing of expired CO_2. Soda lime exhaustion could also lead to rebreathing in the presence of a low fresh gas flow. Rebreathing of CO_2 can be detected during the inspiratory phase on a capnograph. If rebreathing appears to be due to an equipment malfunction, the patient should be disconnected from the anesthesia machine and ventilated with a resuscitation bag until repairs are possible.

What are some other consequences of hypercapnia?

Hypercapnia has a multitude of effects, most of them masked by general anesthesia. Cerebral blood flow increases proportionately with arterial CO_2. This effect is dangerous in patients with increased intracranial pressure (eg, from brain tumor). Extremely high levels of CO_2 (>80 mm Hg) can cause unconsciousness related to a fall in cerebrospinal fluid pH. CO_2 depresses the myocardium, but this direct effect is usually overshadowed by activation of the sympathetic nervous system. During general anesthesia, hypercapnia usually results in an increased cardiac output, an elevation in arterial blood pressure, and a propensity toward arrhythmias.

Elevated serum CO_2 concentrations can overwhelm the blood's buffering capacity, leading to respiratory acidosis. This causes other cations such as Ca^{2+} and K^+ to shift extracellularly. Acidosis also shifts the oxyhemoglobin dissociation curve to the right.

Carbon dioxide is a powerful respiratory stimulant. In fact, for each mm Hg rise of $PaCO_2$ above baseline, normal awake subjects increase their minute ventilation by about 2–3 L/min. General anesthesia markedly decreases this response, and paralysis eliminates it. Finally, severe hypercapnia can produce hypoxia by displacement of oxygen from alveoli.

SUGGESTED READING

Dobson MB: Anaesthesia for difficult locations—developing countries and military conflicts. In: *International Practice of Anaesthesia*. Prys-Roberts C, Brown BR (editors). Butterworth Heinemann, 1996.

Dorsch JA, Dorsch SE: *Understanding Anesthesia Equipment*, 5th ed. Lippincott, Williams & Wilkins, 2008.

The Anesthesia Machine

1. Misuse of anesthesia gas delivery systems is three times more likely than failure of the device to cause equipment-related adverse outcomes. An operator's lack of familiarity with the equipment or a failure to check machine function, or both, are the most frequent causes. These mishaps account for only about 2% of cases in the ASA Closed Claims Project database. The breathing circuit was the most common single source of injury (39%); nearly all damaging events were related to misconnects or disconnects.

2. The anesthesia machine receives medical gases from a gas supply, controls the flow and reduces the pressure of desired gases to a safe level, vaporizes volatile anesthetics into the final gas mixture, and delivers the gases to a breathing circuit that is connected to the patient's airway. A mechanical ventilator attaches to the breathing circuit but can be excluded with a switch during spontaneous or manual (bag) ventilation.

3. Whereas the oxygen supply can pass directly to its flow control valve, nitrous oxide, air, and other gases must first pass through safety devices before reaching their respective flow control valves. These devices permit the flow of other gases only if there is sufficient oxygen pressure in the safety device and help prevent accidental delivery of a hypoxic mixture in the event of oxygen supply failure.

4. Another safety feature of anesthesia machines is a linkage of the nitrous oxide gas flow to the oxygen gas flow; this arrangement helps ensure a minimum oxygen concentration of 25%.

5. All modern vaporizers are agent specific and temperature corrected, capable of delivering a constant concentration of agent regardless of temperature changes or flow through the vaporizer.

6. A rise in airway pressure may signal worsening pulmonary compliance, an increase in tidal volume, or an obstruction in the breathing circuit, tracheal tube, or the patient's airway. A drop in pressure may indicate an improvement in compliance, a decrease in tidal volume, or a leak in the circuit.

7. Traditionally ventilators on anesthesia machines have a double-circuit system design and are pneumatically powered and electronically controlled. Newer machines also incorporate microprocessor control that relies on sophisticated pressure and flow sensors. Some anesthesia machines have ventilators that use a single-circuit piston design.

8. The major advantage of a piston ventilator is its ability to deliver accurate tidal volumes to patients with very poor lung compliance and to very small patients.

—Continued next page

Continued—

9 Whenever a ventilator is used "disconnect alarms" must be passively activated. Anesthesia workstations should have at least three disconnect alarms: low pressure, low exhaled tidal volume, and low exhaled carbon dioxide.

10 Because the ventilator's spill valve is closed during inspiration, fresh gas flow from the machine's common gas outlet normally contributes to the tidal volume delivered to the patient.

11 Use of the oxygen flush valve during the inspiratory cycle of a ventilator must be avoided because the ventilator spill valve will be closed and the adjustable pressure-limiting (APL) valve is excluded; the surge of oxygen (600–1200 mL/s) and circuit pressure will be transferred to the patient's lungs.

12 Large discrepancies between the set and actual tidal volume are often observed in the operating room during volume-controlled ventilation. Causes include breathing circuit compliance, gas compression, ventilator–fresh gas flow coupling, and leaks in the anesthesia machine, the breathing circuit, or the patient's airway.

13 Waste-gas scavengers dispose of gases that have been vented from the breathing circuit by the APL valve and ventilator spill valve. Pollution of the operating room environment with anesthetic gases may pose a health hazard to surgical personnel.

14 A routine inspection of anesthesia equipment before each use increases operator familiarity and confirms proper functioning. The U.S. Food and Drug Administration has made available a generic checkout procedure for anesthesia gas machines and breathing systems.

No piece of equipment is more intimately associated with the practice of anesthesiology than the anesthesia machine (**Figure 4–1**). On the most basic level, the anesthesiologist uses the anesthesia machine to control the patient's ventilation and oxygen delivery and to administer inhalation anesthetics. Proper functioning of the machine is crucial for patient safety. Modern anesthesia machines have become very sophisticated, incorporating many built-in safety features and devices, monitors, and multiple microprocessors that can integrate and monitor all components. Additional monitors can be added externally and often still be fully integrated. Moreover, modular machine designs allow a wide variety of configurations and features within the same product line. The term *anesthesia workstation* is therefore often used for modern anesthesia machines. There are two major manufacturers of anesthesia machines in the United States, Datex-Ohmeda (GE Healthcare) and Dräger Medical. Other manufacturers (eg, Mindray) produce anesthesia delivery systems. Anesthesia providers should carefully review the operations manuals of the machines present in their clinical practice.

Much progress has been made in reducing the number of adverse outcomes arising from anesthetic gas delivery equipment, through redesign of equipment and education. **1** Misuse of anesthesia gas delivery systems is three times more likely than failure of the device to cause equipment-related adverse outcomes. Equipment misuse is characterized as errors in preparation, maintenance, or deployment of a device. Preventable anesthetic mishaps are frequently traced to an operator's lack of familiarity with the equipment or a failure to check machine function, or both. These mishaps account for only about 2% of cases in the American Society of Anesthesiologists' (ASA) Closed Claims Project database. The breathing circuit was the most common single source of injury (39%); nearly all damaging events were related to misconnects or disconnects. A misconnect was defined as a

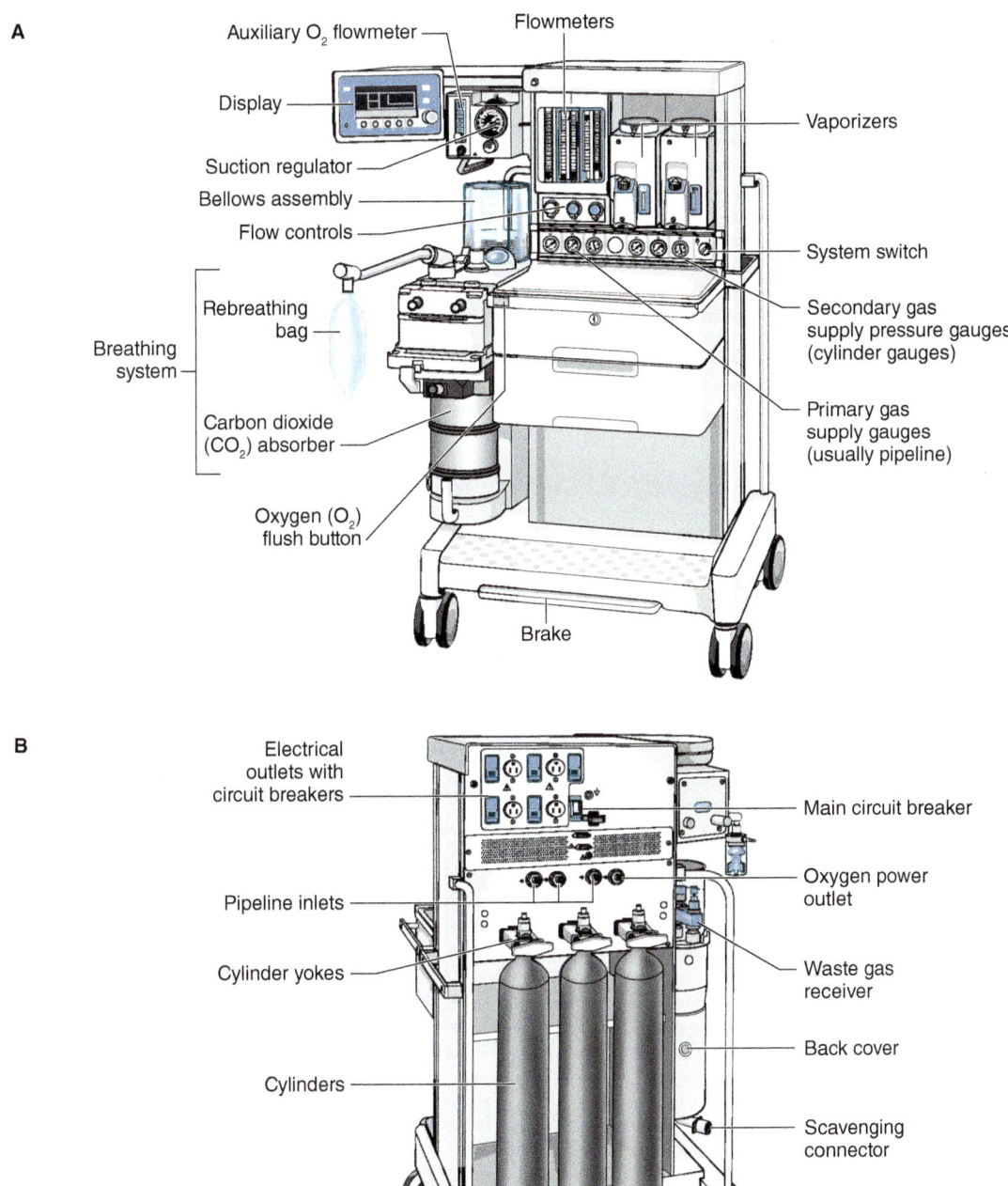

FIGURE 4-1 Modern anesthesia machine (Datex-Ohmeda Aestiva). **A**: Front. **B**: Back.

TABLE 4–1 Essential safety features on a modern anesthesia workstation.

Essential Features	Purpose
Noninterchangeable gas-specific connections to pipeline inlets (DISS)[1] with pressure gauges, filter, and check valve	Prevent incorrect pipeline attachments; detect failure, depletion, or fluctuation
Pin index safety system for cylinders with pressure gauges, and at least one oxygen cylinder	Prevent incorrect cylinder attachments; provide backup gas supply; detect depletion
Low oxygen pressure alarm	Detect oxygen supply failure at the common gas inlet
Minimum oxygen/nitrous oxide ratio controller device (hypoxic guard)	Prevent delivery of less than 21% oxygen
Oxygen failure safety device (shut-off or proportioning device)	Prevent administration of nitrous oxide or other gases when the oxygen supply fails
Oxygen must enter the common manifold downstream to other gases	Prevent hypoxia in event of proximal gas leak
Oxygen concentration monitor and alarm	Prevent administration of hypoxic gas mixtures in event of a low-pressure system leak; precisely regulate oxygen concentration
Automatically enabled essential alarms and monitors (eg, oxygen concentration)	Prevent use of the machine without essential monitors
Vaporizer interlock device	Prevent simultaneous administration of more than one volatile agent
Capnography and anesthetic gas measurement	Guide ventilation; prevent anesthetic overdose; help reduce awareness
Oxygen flush mechanism that does not pass through vaporizers	Rapidly refill or flush the breathing circuit
Breathing circuit pressure monitor and alarm	Prevent pulmonary barotrauma and detect sustained positive, high peak, and negative airway pressures
Exhaled volume monitor	Assess ventilation and prevent hypo- or hyperventilation
Pulse oximetry, blood pressure, and ECG monitoring	Provide minimal standard monitoring
Mechanical ventilator	Control alveolar ventilation more accurately and during muscle paralysis for prolonged periods
Backup battery	Provide temporary electrical power (>30 min) to monitors and alarms in event of power failure
Scavenger system	Prevent contamination of the operating room with waste anesthetic gases

[1]DISS, diameter-index safety system.

nonfunctional and unconventional configuration of breathing circuit components or attachments. In decreasing frequency, other causes involved vaporizers (21%), ventilators (17%), and oxygen supply (11%). Other more basic components of the anesthesia machine (eg, valves) were responsible in only 7% of cases. All malpractice claims in the database that involved the anesthesia machine, oxygen supply tanks or lines, or ventilators occurred before 1990; since then claims involving breathing circuits and vaporizers have continued to occur.

The American National Standards Institute and subsequently the ASTM International (formerly the American Society for Testing and Materials, F1850–00) published standard specifications for anesthesia machines and their components. Table 4–1 lists essential features of a modern anesthesia workstation. Changes in equipment design have been directed at minimizing the probability of breathing circuit misconnects and disconnects and automating machine checks. Because of the durability and functional longevity of anesthesia machines, the ASA has developed guidelines for determining anesthesia machine obsolescence (Table 4–2). This

chapter is an introduction to anesthesia machine design, function, and use.

OVERVIEW

2 In its most basic form, the anesthesia machine receives medical gases from a gas supply, controls the flow and reduces the pressure of desired gases to a safe level, vaporizes volatile anesthetics into the final gas mixture, and delivers the gases to a breathing circuit connected to the patient's airway (Figures 4–2 and 4–3). A mechanical ventilator attaches to the breathing circuit but can be excluded with a switch during spontaneous or manual (bag) ventilation. An auxiliary oxygen supply and suction regulator are also usually built into the workstation. In addition to standard safety features (Table 4–1) top-of-the-line anesthesia machines have additional safety features, enhancements, and built-in computer processors that integrate and monitor all components, perform automated machine checkouts,

TABLE 4–2 Unacceptable/undesirable features of older anesthesia machines.[1]

Unacceptable features
1. Flowmeter-controlled vaporizer (eg, copper kettle, Vernitrol)
2. More than one flow control valve for a single gas
3. Vaporizer with a rotary dial that increases concentration with clockwise rotation
4. Connections in the scavenging system that are the same size as breathing circuit connections

Undesirable features
1. Adjustable pressure-limiting (APL) valve that is not isolated during mechanical ventilation
2. Oxygen flow control knob that is not fluted or larger than other flow control knobs
3. Oxygen flush control that is unprotected from accidental activation
4. Lack of main On/Off switch for electrical power to integral monitors and alarms
5. Lack of antidisconnect device on the fresh gas hose (common gas outlet)
6. Lack of airway pressure alarms

[1]Data from ASA Guidelines for determining Anesthesia Machine Obsolescence.

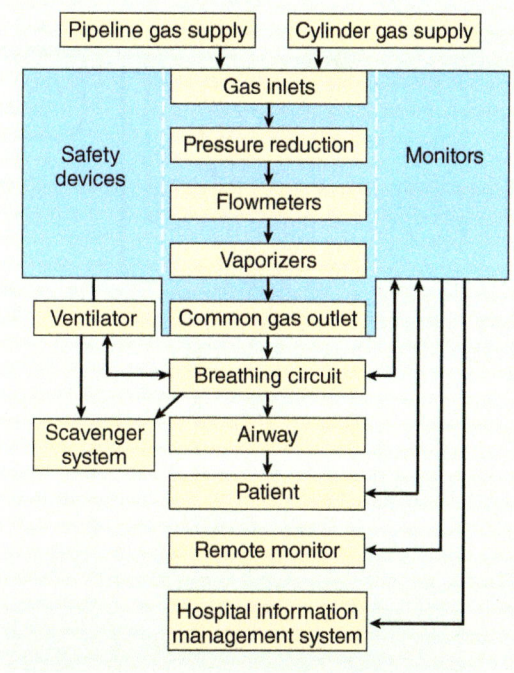

FIGURE 4–2 Functional schematic of an anesthesia machine/workstation.

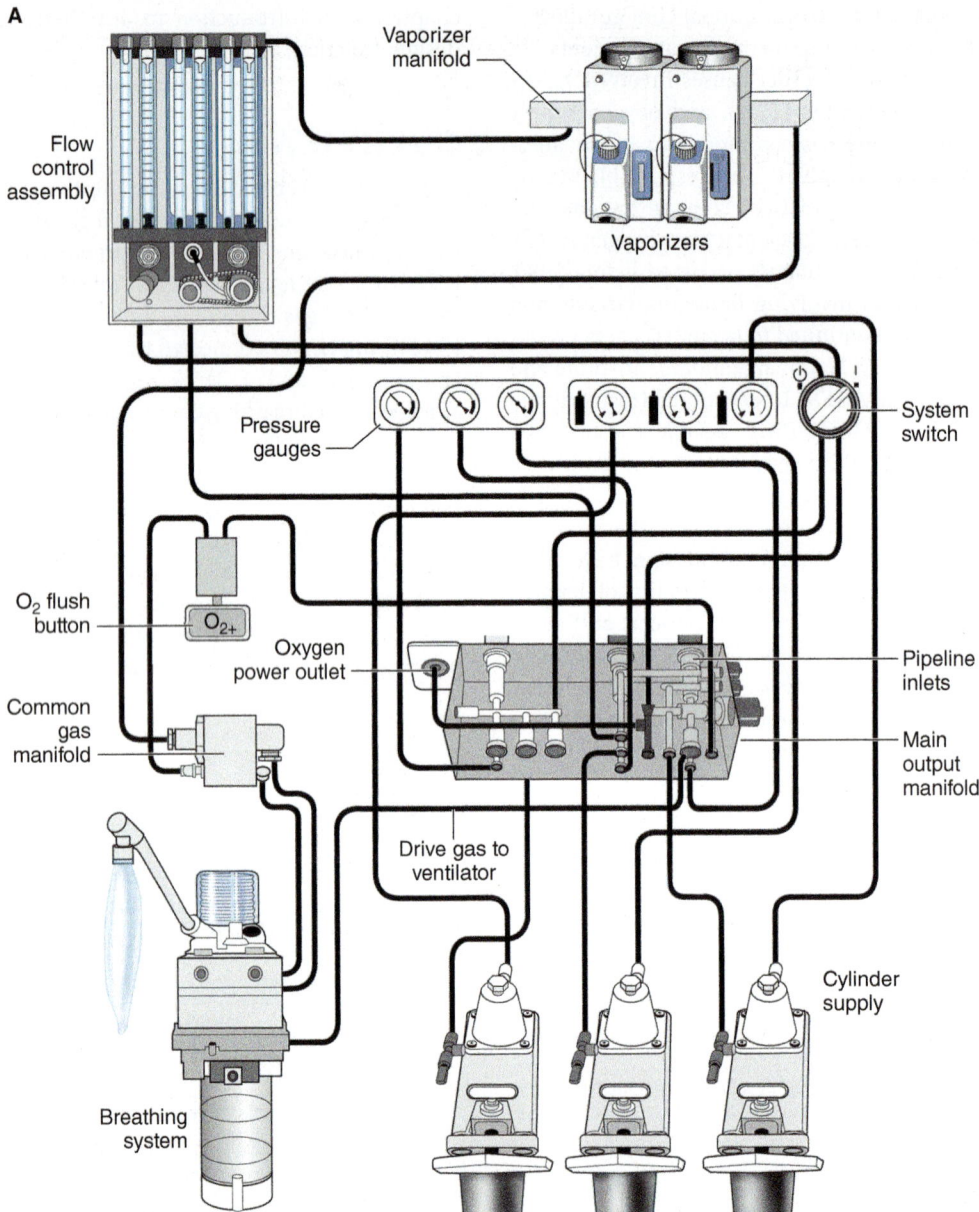

A

Vaporizer manifold

Flow control assembly

Vaporizers

Pressure gauges

System switch

O₂ flush button

Oxygen power outlet

Pipeline inlets

Common gas manifold

Main output manifold

Drive gas to ventilator

Breathing system

Cylinder supply

FIGURE 4–3 Simplified internal schematic of an anesthesia machine. **A**: Datex-Ohmeda Aestiva. (*continued*)

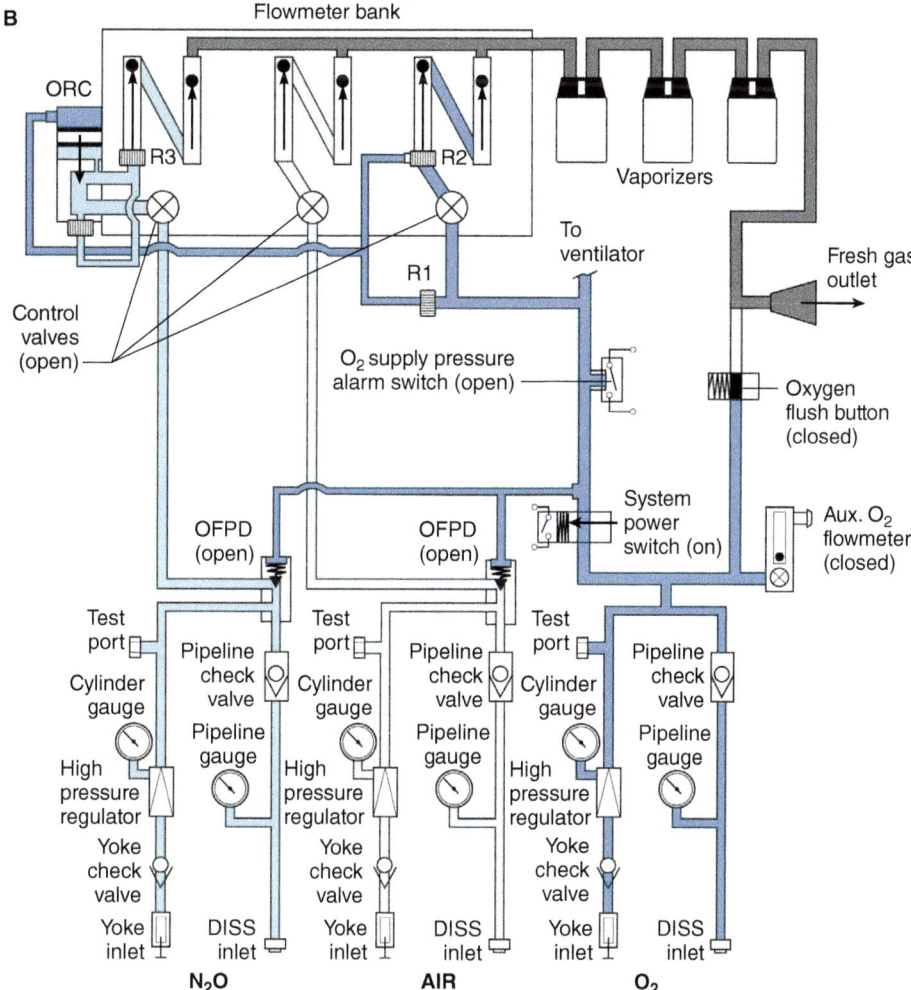

FIGURE 4–3 *(continued)* **B**: Dräger Narkomed. ORC, oxygen ratio controller.

and provide options such as automated record-keeping and networking external monitors and hospital information systems (Figure 4–4). Some machines are designed specifically for mobility, magnetic resonance imaging (MRI) compatibility or compactness.

GAS SUPPLY

Most machines have gas inlets for oxygen, nitrous oxide, and air. Compact models often lack air inlets, whereas other machines may have a fourth inlet for helium, heliox, carbon dioxide, or nitric oxide.

Separate inlets are provided for the primary pipeline gas supply that passes through the walls of health care facilities and the secondary cylinder gas supply. Machines therefore have two gas inlet pressure gauges for each gas: one for pipeline pressure and another for cylinder pressure.

Pipeline Inlets

Oxygen and nitrous oxide (and often air) are delivered from their central supply source to the operating room through a piping network. The tubing is color coded and connects to the anesthesia machine through a noninterchangeable **diameter-index**

A

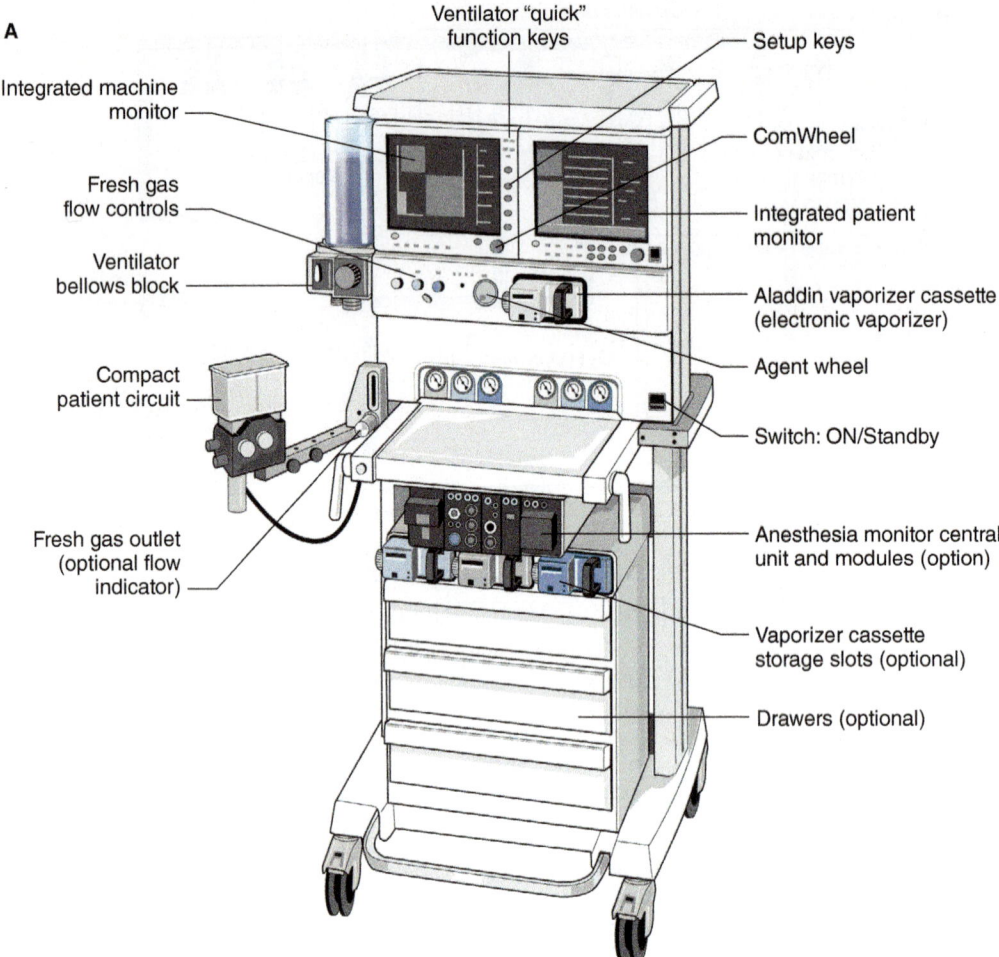

Integrated machine monitor

Fresh gas flow controls

Ventilator bellows block

Compact patient circuit

Fresh gas outlet (optional flow indicator)

Ventilator "quick" function keys

Setup keys

ComWheel

Integrated patient monitor

Aladdin vaporizer cassette (electronic vaporizer)

Agent wheel

Switch: ON/Standby

Anesthesia monitor central unit and modules (option)

Vaporizer cassette storage slots (optional)

Drawers (optional)

FIGURE 4–4 Highly sophisticated anesthesia machines with full integration options. **A:** Datex-Ohmeda S/5 ADU. (*continued*)

B

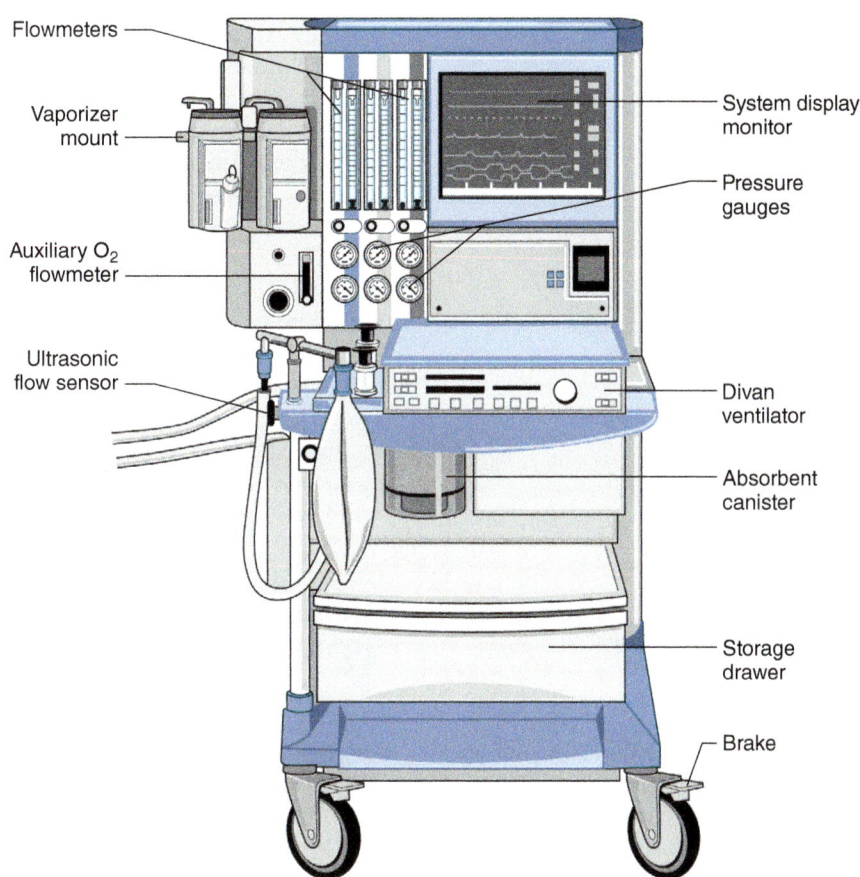

Flowmeters

Vaporizer mount

Auxiliary O₂ flowmeter

Ultrasonic flow sensor

System display monitor

Pressure gauges

Divan ventilator

Absorbent canister

Storage drawer

Brake

FIGURE 4–4 *(continued)* **B**: Dräger 6400.

safety system (DISS) fitting that prevents incorrect hose attachment. The noninterchangeability is achieved by making the bore diameter of the body and that of the connection nipple specific for each supplied gas. A filter helps trap debris from the wall supply and a one-way check valve prevents retrograde flow of gases into the pipeline supplies. It should be noted that most modern machines have an oxygen (pneumatic) power outlet that may be used to drive the ventilator or provide an auxiliary oxygen flowmeter. The DISS fittings for the oxygen inlet and the oxygen power outlet are identical and should not be mistakenly interchanged. The approximate pipeline pressure of gases delivered to the anesthesia machine is 50 psig.

Cylinder Inlets

Cylinders attach to the machine via hanger-yoke assemblies that utilize a **pin index safety system** to prevent accidental connection of a wrong gas cylinder. The yoke assembly includes index pins, a washer, a gas filter, and a check valve that prevents retrograde gas flow. The gas cylinders are also color-coded for specific gases to allow for easy identification. In North America the following color-coding scheme is used: oxygen = green, nitrous oxide = blue, carbon dioxide = gray, air = yellow, helium = brown, nitrogen = black. In the United Kingdom, white is used for oxygen and black and white for air. The E-cylinders attached to the anesthesia machine are

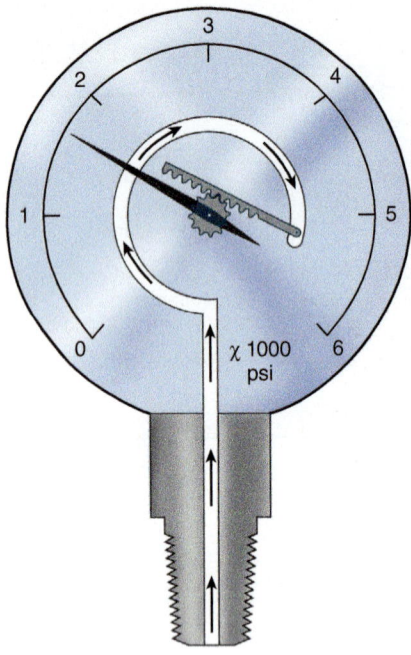

FIGURE 4–5 Bourdon pressure gauge.

a high-pressure source of medical gases and are generally used only as a back-up supply in case of pipeline failure. Pressure of gas supplied from the cylinder to the anesthesia machine is 45 psig. Some machines have two oxygen cylinders so that one cylinder can be used while the other is changed. At 20°C, a full cylinder contains 600 L of oxygen at a pressure of 1900 psig, and 1590 L of nitrous oxide at 745 psig. Cylinder pressure is usually measured by a Bourdon pressure gauge (Figure 4–5). A flexible tube within this gauge straightens when exposed to gas pressure, causing a gear mechanism to move a needle pointer.

FLOW CONTROL CIRCUITS

Pressure Regulators

Unlike the relatively constant pressure of the pipeline gas supply, the high and variable gas pressure in cylinders makes flow control difficult and potentially dangerous. To enhance safety and ensure optimal use of cylinder gases, machines utilize a pressure regulator to reduce the cylinder gas pressure to 45–47 psig[1] before it enters the flow valve (Figure 4–6). This pressure, which is slightly lower than the pipeline supply, allows preferential use of the pipeline supply if a cylinder is left open (unless pipeline pressure drops below 45 psig). After passing through Bourdon pressure gauges and check valves, the pipeline gases share a common pathway with the cylinder gases. A high-pressure relief valve provided for each gas is set to open when the supply pressure exceeds the machine's maximum safety limit (95–110 psig), as might happen with a regulator failure on a cylinder. Some machines also use a second regulator to drop both pipeline and cylinder pressure further (two-stage pressure regulation). A second-stage pressure reduction may also be needed for an auxiliary oxygen flowmeter, the oxygen flush mechanism, or the drive gas to power a pneumatic ventilator.

Oxygen Supply Failure Protection Devices

3 Whereas the oxygen supply can pass directly to its flow control valve, nitrous oxide, air (in some machines), and other gases must first pass through safety devices before reaching their respective flow control valves. In other machines, air passes directly to its flow control valve; this allows administration of air even in the absence of oxygen. These devices permit the flow of other gases only if there is sufficient oxygen pressure in the safety device and help prevent accidental delivery of a hypoxic mixture in the event of oxygen supply failure. Thus in addition to supplying the oxygen flow control valve, oxygen from the common inlet pathway is used to pressurize safety devices, oxygen flush valves, and ventilator power outlets (in some models). Safety devices sense oxygen pressure via a small "piloting pressure" line that may be derived from the gas inlet or secondary regulator. In some anesthesia machine designs (eg, Datex-Ohmeda Excel), if the piloting pressure line falls below a threshold (eg, 20 psig), the shut-off valves close, preventing the administration of any other gases. The terms *fail-safe* and *nitrous cut-off* were previously used for the nitrous oxide shut-off valve.

---

[1]Pressure unit conversions: 1 kiloPascal (kP) = kg/m · s² = 1000 N/m² = 0.01 bar = 0.1013 atmospheres = 0.145 psig = 10.2 cm H₂O = 7.5 mm Hg.

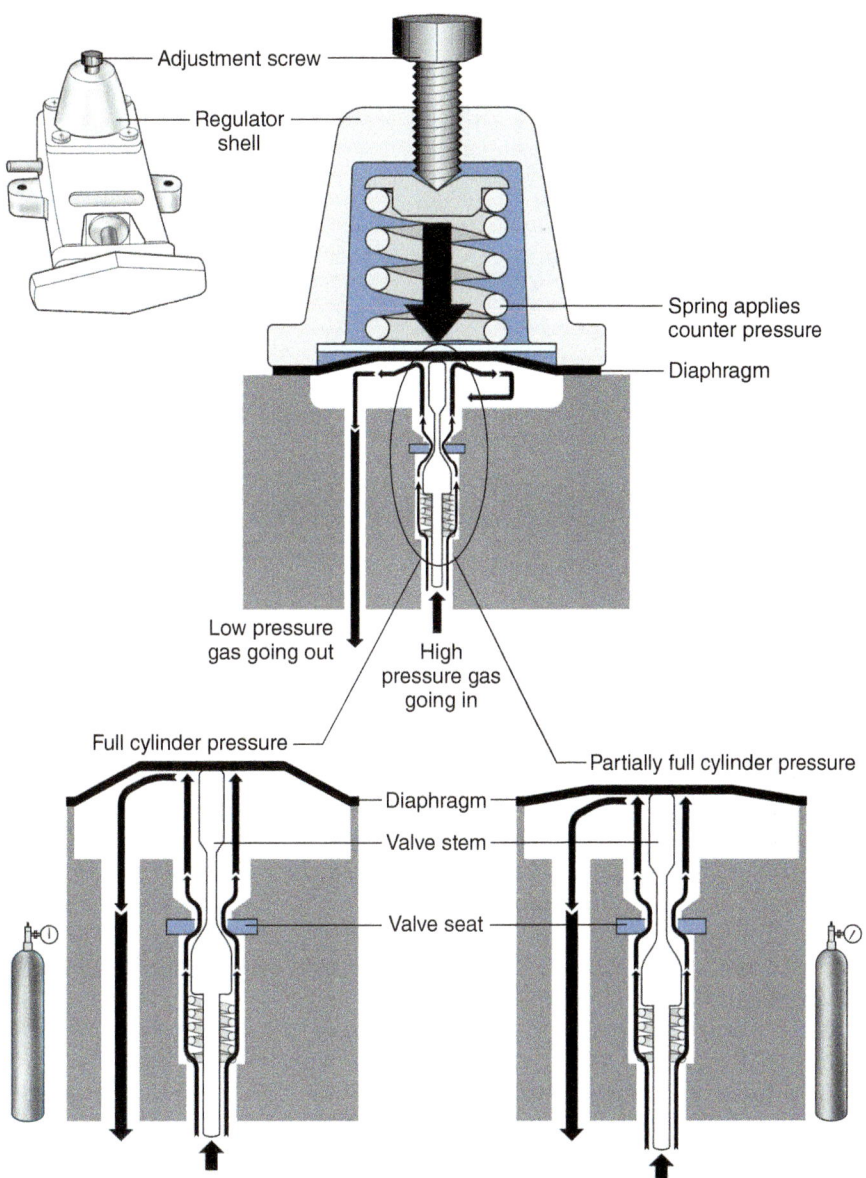

Adjustment screw

Regulator shell

Spring applies counter pressure

Diaphragm

Low pressure gas going out

High pressure gas going in

Full cylinder pressure

Partially full cylinder pressure

Diaphragm

Valve stem

Valve seat

FIGURE 4–6 Cylinder inlet regulator.

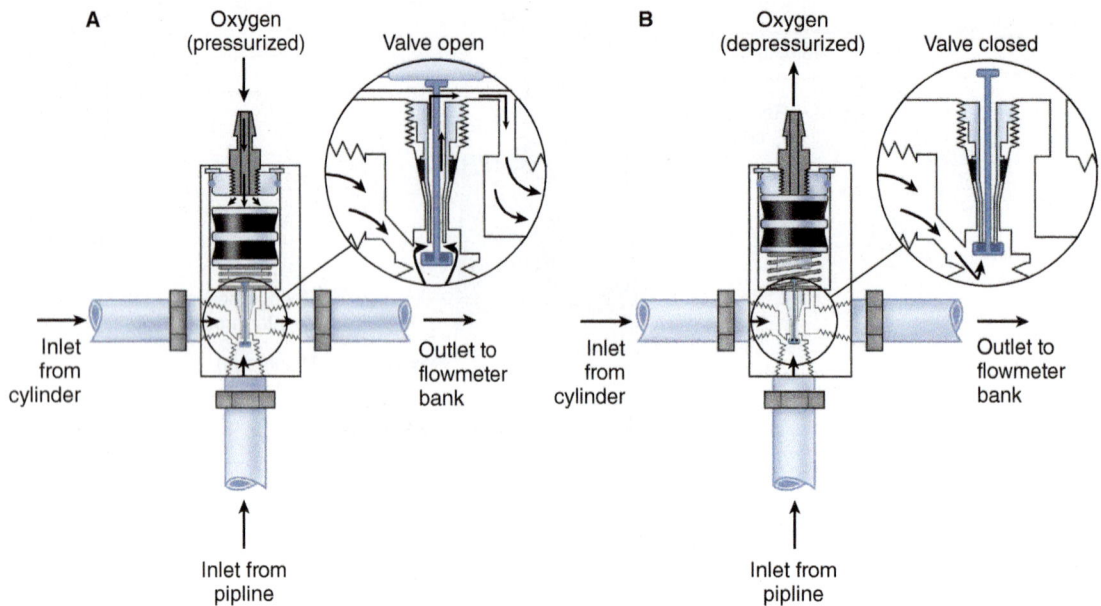

FIGURE 4–7 Dräger oxygen failure protection device (OFPD). **A:** Open. **B:** Closed.

Most modern (particularly Datex-Ohmeda) machines use a proportioning safety device instead of a threshold shut-off valve. These devices, called either an oxygen failure protection device (Dräger) or a balance regulator (Datex-Ohmeda), proportionately reduce the pressure of nitrous oxide and other gases except for air (Figures 4–7 and 4–8). They completely shut off nitrous oxide and other gas flow only below a set minimum oxygen pressure (eg, 0.5 psig for nitrous oxide and 10 psig for other gases).

All machines also have an oxygen supply low-pressure sensor that activates alarm sounds when inlet gas pressure drops below a threshold value (usually 20–30 psig). It must be emphasized that these safety devices do *not* protect against other possible causes of hypoxic accidents (eg, gas line misconnections), in which threshold pressure may be maintained by gases containing inadequate or no oxygen.

Flow Valves & Meters

Once the pressure has been reduced to a safe level, each gas must pass through flow control valves and is measured by flowmeters before mixing with other gases, entering the active vaporizer, and exiting the machine's common gas outlet. **Gas lines proximal to flow valves are considered to be in the high-pressure circuit whereas those between the flow valves and the common gas outlet are considered part of the low-pressure circuit of the machine.** When the knob of the flow control valve is turned counterclockwise, a needle valve is disengaged from its seat, allowing gas to flow through the valve (Figure 4–9). Stops in the full-off and full-on positions prevent valve damage. Touch- and color-coded control knobs make it more difficult to turn the wrong gas off or on. As a safety feature the oxygen knob is usually fluted, larger, and protrudes farther than the other knobs. The oxygen flowmeter is positioned furthest to the right, downstream to the other gases; this arrangement helps to prevent hypoxia if there is leakage from a flowmeter positioned upstream.

Flow control knobs control gas entry into the flowmeters by adjustment via a needle valve. Flowmeters on anesthesia machines are classified as either constant-pressure variable-orifice (rotameter) or electronic. In constant-pressure variable-orifice flowmeters, an indicator ball, bobbin, or float is supported by the flow of gas through a tube (Thorpe

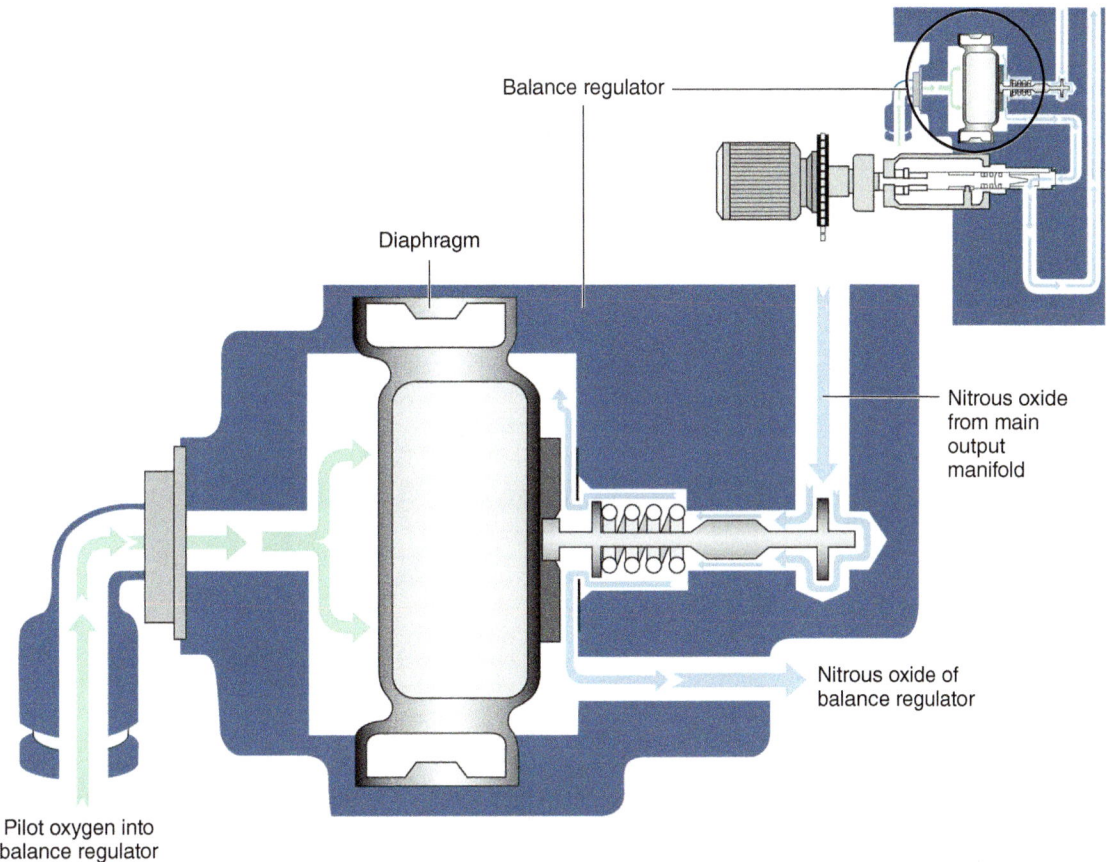

FIGURE 4–8 Datex-Ohmeda balance regulator.

tube) whose bore (orifice) is tapered. Near the bottom of the tube, where the diameter is small, a low flow of gas will create sufficient pressure under the float to raise it in the tube. As the float rises, the (variable) orifice of the tube widens, allowing more gas to pass around the float. The float will stop rising when its weight is just supported by the difference in pressure above and below it. If flow is increased, the pressure under the float increases, raising it higher in the tube until the pressure drop again just supports the float's weight. This pressure drop is constant regardless of the flow rate or the position in the tube and depends on the float weight and tube cross-sectional area.

Flowmeters are calibrated for specific gases, as the flow rate across a constriction depends on the gas's viscosity at low laminar flows (Poiseuille's law) and its density at high turbulent flows. To minimize the effect of friction between them and the tube's wall, floats are designed to rotate constantly, which keeps them centered in the tube. Coating the tube's interior with a conductive substance grounds the system and reduces the effect of static electricity. Some flowmeters have two glass tubes, one for low flows and another for high flows (Figure 4–10A); the two tubes are in series and are still controlled by one valve. A dual taper design can allow a single flowmeter to read both high and low flows (Figure 4–10B). **Causes of flowmeter malfunction include debris in the flow tube, vertical tube misalignment, and sticking or concealment of a float at the top of a tube.**

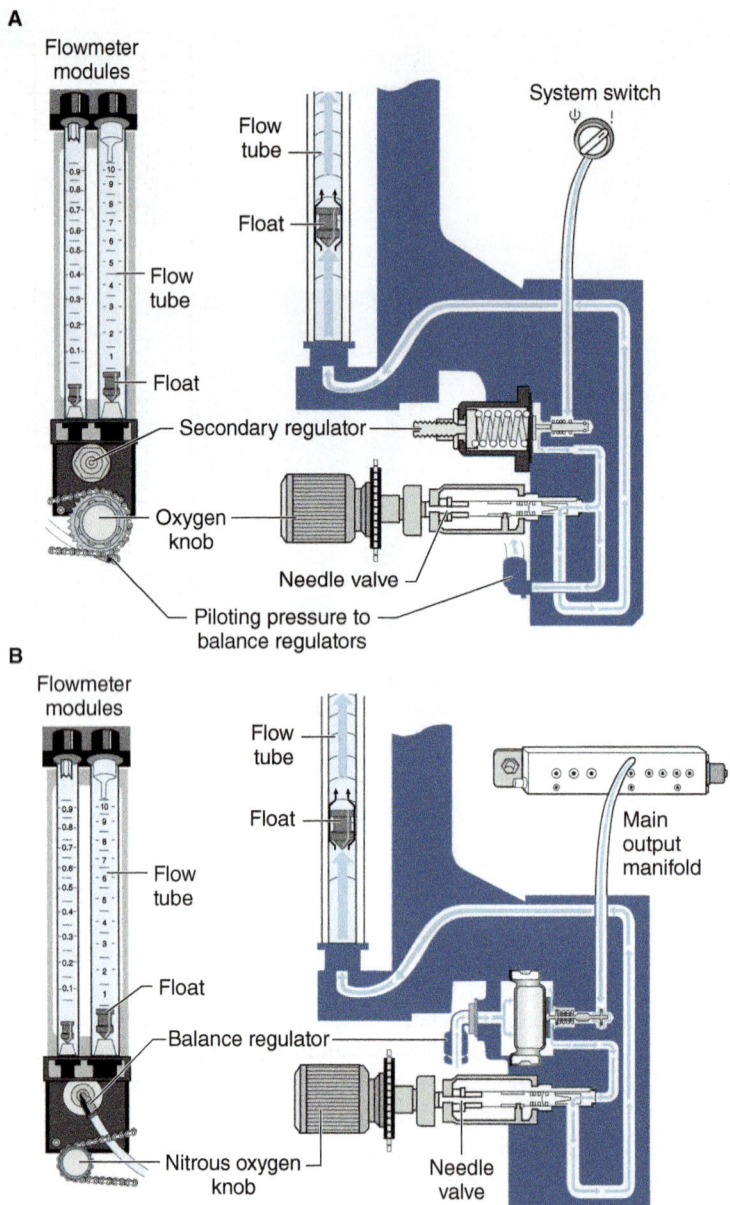

FIGURE 4–9 Gas flow-control needle valve (Datex-Ohmeda). **A**: Oxygen. **B**: Nitrous oxide. Note the secondary pressure regulator in the oxygen circuit and the balance regulator in the nitrous oxide circuit.

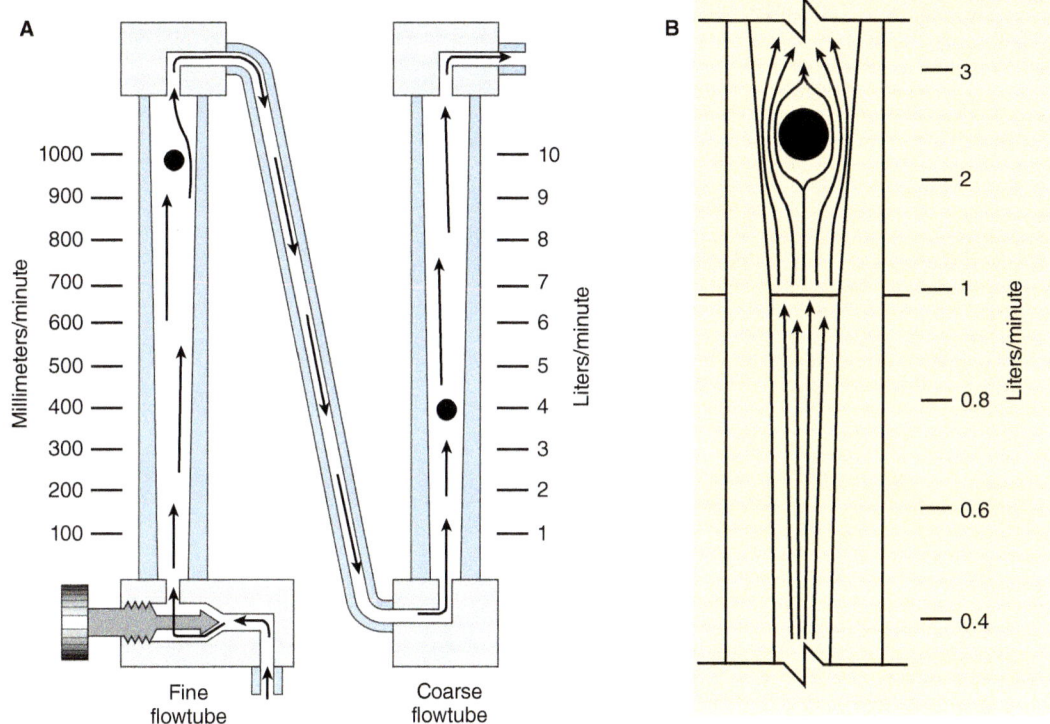

FIGURE 4–10 Constant-pressure variable orifice flowmeters (Thorpe type). **A**: Two tube design. **B**: Dual taper design.

Should a leak develop within or downstream from an oxygen flowmeter, a hypoxic gas mixture can be delivered to the patient (**Figure 4–11**). To reduce this risk, oxygen flowmeters are *always* positioned downstream to all other flowmeters (nearest to the vaporizer).

Some anesthesia machines have electronic flow control and measurement (**Figure 4–12**). In such instances, a back-up conventional (Thorpe) auxiliary oxygen flowmeter is provided. Other models have conventional flowmeters but electronic measurement of gas flow along with Thorpe tubes and

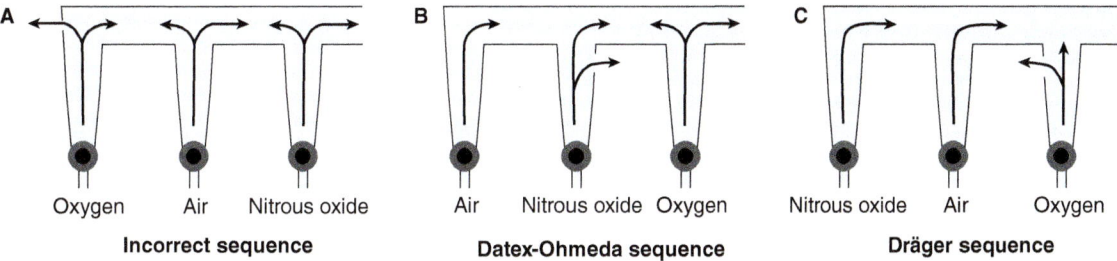

FIGURE 4–11 Sequence of flowmeters in a three-gas machine. **A**: An unsafe sequence. **B**: Typical Datex Ohmeda sequence. **C**: Typical Dräger sequence. Note that regardless of sequence a leak in the oxygen tube or further downstream can result in delivery of a hypoxic mixture.

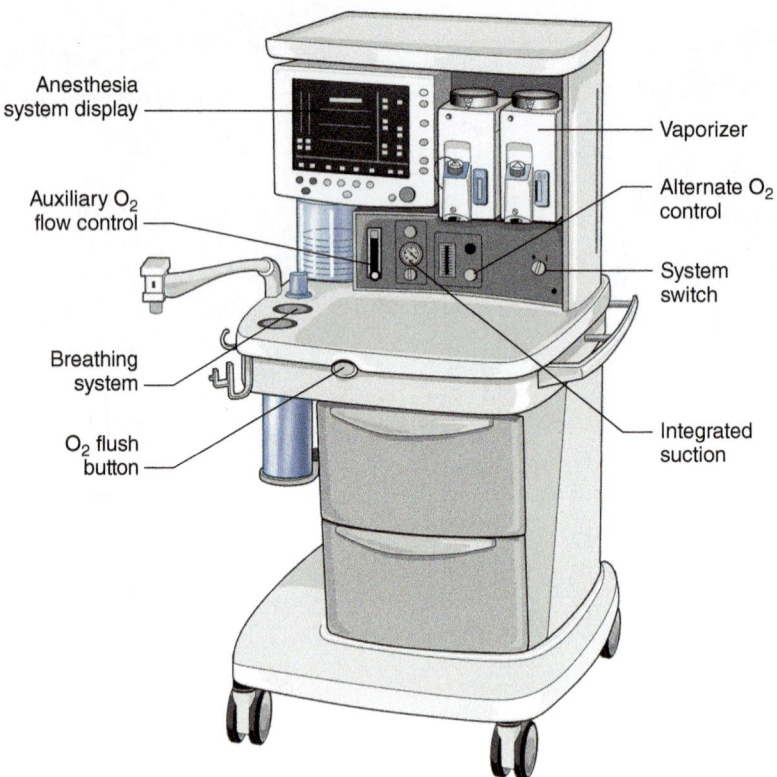

FIGURE 4–12 Datex-Ohmeda S/5 Avance with electronic flow control and measurement. Note the presence of only a single alternate flowmeter for oxygen to be used in a power failure.

digital or digital/graphic displays (Figure 4–13). The amount of pressure drop caused by a flow restrictor is the basis for measurement of gas flow rate in these systems. In these machines oxygen, nitrous oxide, and air each have a separate electronic flow measurement device in the flow control section before they are mixed together. Electronic flowmeters are essential components in workstations if gas flow rate data will be acquired automatically by computerized anesthesia recording systems.

A. Minimum Oxygen Flow

The oxygen flow valves are usually designed to deliver a minimum flow of 150 mL/min when the anesthesia machine is turned on. One method involves the use of a minimum flow resistor (Figure 4–14). This safety feature helps ensure that some oxygen enters the breathing circuit even if the operator forgets

to turn on the oxygen flow. Some machines are designed to deliver minimum flow or low-flow anesthesia (<1 L/min) and have minimum oxygen flows as low as 50 mL/min.

B. Oxygen/Nitrous Oxide Ratio Controller

4 Another safety feature of anesthesia machines is a linkage of the nitrous oxide gas flow to the oxygen gas flow; this arrangement helps ensure a minimum oxygen concentration of 25%. The oxygen/nitrous oxide ratio controller links the two flow valves either pneumatically or mechanically. To maintain the minimum oxygen concentration, the system (Link-25) in Datex-Ohmeda machines increases the flow of oxygen, whereas the oxygen ratio monitor controller (ORMC) in Dräger machines reduces the concentration of nitrous oxide. It should be noted that this safety device does

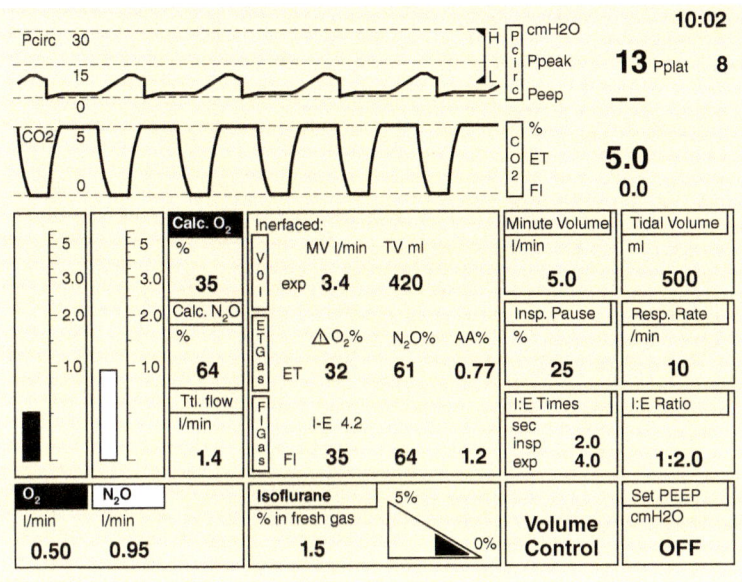

FIGURE 4–13 Graphic and digital flowmeter display of Datex-Ohmeda S/5 ADU.

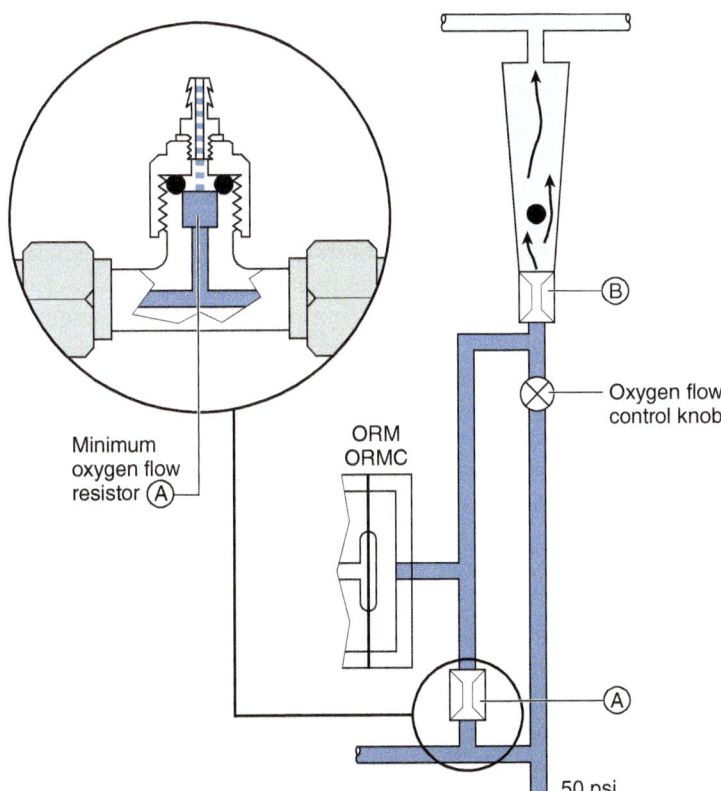

FIGURE 4–14 A bypass tube with minimum flow resistor upstream before the oxygen flow control valve ensures minimum oxygen flow even when the needle valve is turned off. A, B, resistors.

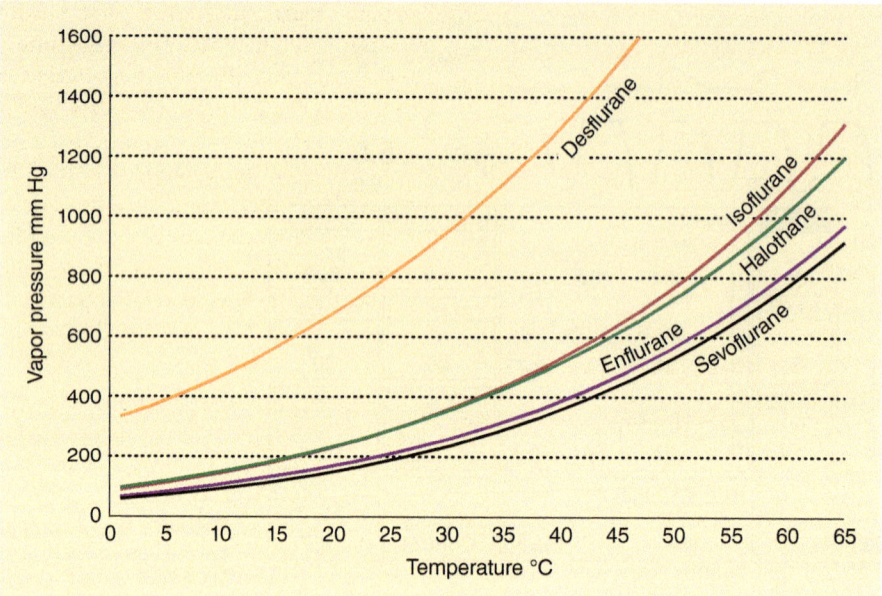

FIGURE 4–15 The vapor pressure of anesthetic gases.

not affect the flow of a third gas (eg, air, helium, or carbon dioxide).

Vaporizers

Volatile anesthetics (eg, halothane, isoflurane, desflurane, sevoflurane) must be vaporized before being delivered to the patient. Vaporizers have concentration-calibrated dials that precisely add volatile anesthetic agents to the combined gas flow from all flowmeters. They must be located between the flowmeters and the common gas outlet. Moreover, unless the machine accepts only one vaporizer at a time, all anesthesia machines should have an interlocking or exclusion device that prevents the concurrent use of more than one vaporizer.

A. Physics of Vaporization

At temperatures encountered in the operating room, the molecules of a volatile anesthetic in a closed container are distributed between the liquid and gaseous phases. The gas molecules bombard the walls of the container, creating the saturated vapor pressure of that agent. Vapor pressure depends on the characteristics of the volatile agent and the temperature. The greater the temperature, the greater the tendency for the liquid molecules to escape into the gaseous phase and the greater the vapor pressure (Figure 4–15). Vaporization requires energy (the latent heat of vaporization), which results in a loss of heat from the liquid. As vaporization proceeds, temperature of the remaining liquid anesthetic drops and vapor pressure decreases unless heat is readily available to enter the system. Vaporizers contain a chamber in which a carrier gas becomes saturated with the volatile agent.

A liquid's boiling point is the temperature at which its vapor pressure is equal to the atmospheric pressure. As the atmospheric pressure decreases (as in higher altitudes), the boiling point also decreases. Anesthetic agents with low boiling points are more susceptible to variations in barometric pressure than agents with higher boiling points. Among the commonly used agents, desflurane has the lowest boiling point (22.8°C at 760 mm Hg).

B. Copper Kettle

The copper kettle vaporizer is no longer used in clinical anesthesia; however, understanding how it works provides invaluable insight into the delivery of volatile anesthetics (Figure 4–16). It is classified as a measured-flow vaporizer (or flowmeter-controlled

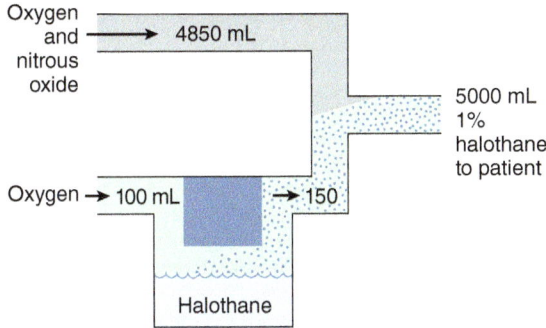

FIGURE 4–16 Schematic of a copper kettle vaporizer. Note that 50 mL/min of halothane vapor is added for each 100 mL/min oxygen flow that passes through the vaporizer.

vaporizer). In a copper kettle, the amount of carrier gas bubbled through the volatile anesthetic is controlled by a dedicated flowmeter. This valve is turned off when the vaporizer circuit is not in use. Copper is used as the construction metal because its relatively high specific heat (the quantity of heat required to raise the temperature of 1 g of substance by 1°C) and high thermal conductivity (the speed of heat conductance through a substance) enhance the vaporizer's ability to maintain a constant temperature. All the gas entering the vaporizer passes through the anesthetic liquid and becomes saturated with vapor. One milliliter of liquid anesthetic is the equivalent of approximately 200 mL of anesthetic vapor. Because the vapor pressure of volatile anesthetics is greater than the partial pressure required for anesthesia, the saturated gas leaving a copper kettle has to be diluted before it reaches the patient.

For example, the vapor pressure of halothane is 243 mm Hg at 20°C, so the concentration of halothane exiting a copper kettle at 1 atmosphere would be 243/760, or 32%. If 100 mL of oxygen enters the kettle, roughly 150 mL of gas exits (the initial 100 mL of oxygen plus 50 mL of saturated halothane vapor), one-third of which would be saturated halothane vapor. To deliver a 1% concentration of halothane (MAC 0.75%), the 50 mL of halothane vapor and 100 mL of carrier gas that left the copper kettle have to be diluted within a total of 5000 mL of fresh gas flow. Thus, every 100 mL of oxygen passing through a halothane vaporizer translates into a 1%

increase in concentration if total gas flow into the breathing circuit is 5 L/min. Therefore when total flow is fixed, flow through the vaporizer determines the ultimate concentration of anesthetic. Isoflurane has an almost identical vapor pressure, so the same relationship between copper kettle flow, total gas flow, and anesthetic concentration exists. However, if total gas flow changes without an adjustment in copper kettle flow (eg, exhaustion of a nitrous oxide cylinder), the delivered volatile anesthetic concentration rises rapidly to potentially dangerous levels.

C. Modern Conventional Vaporizers

5 All modern vaporizers are agent specific and temperature corrected, capable of delivering a constant concentration of agent regardless of temperature changes or flow through the vaporizer. Turning a single calibrated control knob counterclockwise to the desired percentage diverts an appropriate small fraction of the total gas flow into the carrier gas, which flows over the liquid anesthetic in a vaporizing chamber, leaving the balance to exit the vaporizer unchanged (Figure 4–17). Because some of the entering gas is never exposed to anesthetic liquid, this type of agent-specific vaporizer is also known as a variable-bypass vaporizer.

Temperature compensation is achieved by a strip composed of two different metals welded together. The metal strips expand and contract differently in response to temperature changes. When the temperature decreases, differential contraction causes the strip to bend allowing more gas to pass through the vaporizer. Such bimetallic strips are also used in home thermostats. As the temperature rises differential expansion causes the strip to bend the other way restricting gas flow into the vaporizer. Altering total fresh gas flow rates within a wide range does not significantly affect anesthetic concentration because the same proportion of gas is exposed to the liquid. However, the real output of an agent would be lower than the dial setting at extremely high flow (>15 L/min); the converse is true when the flow rate is less than 250 mL/min. Changing the gas composition from 100% oxygen to 70% nitrous oxide may transiently decrease volatile anesthetic concentration due to the greater solubility of nitrous oxide in volatile agents.

A

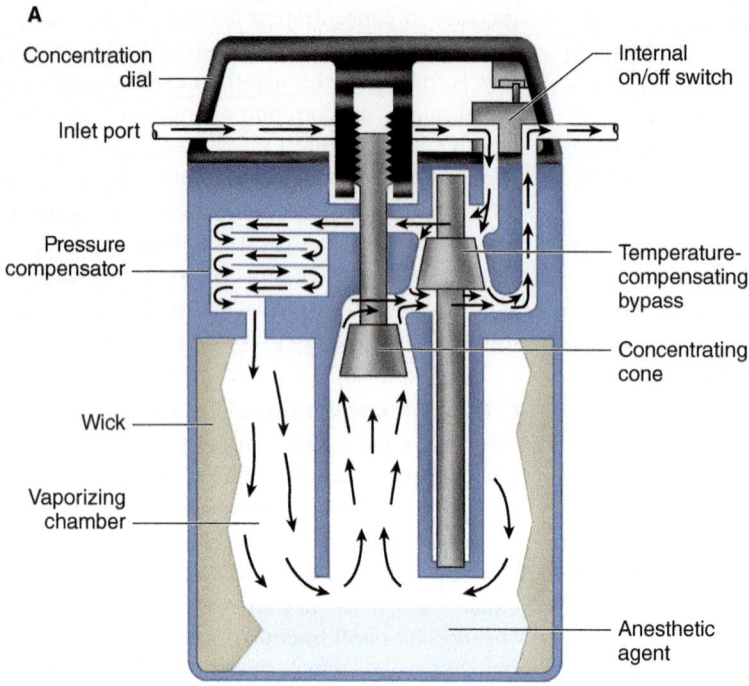

Concentration dial

Inlet port

Internal on/off switch

Pressure compensator

Temperature-compensating bypass

Concentrating cone

Wick

Vaporizing chamber

Anesthetic agent

B

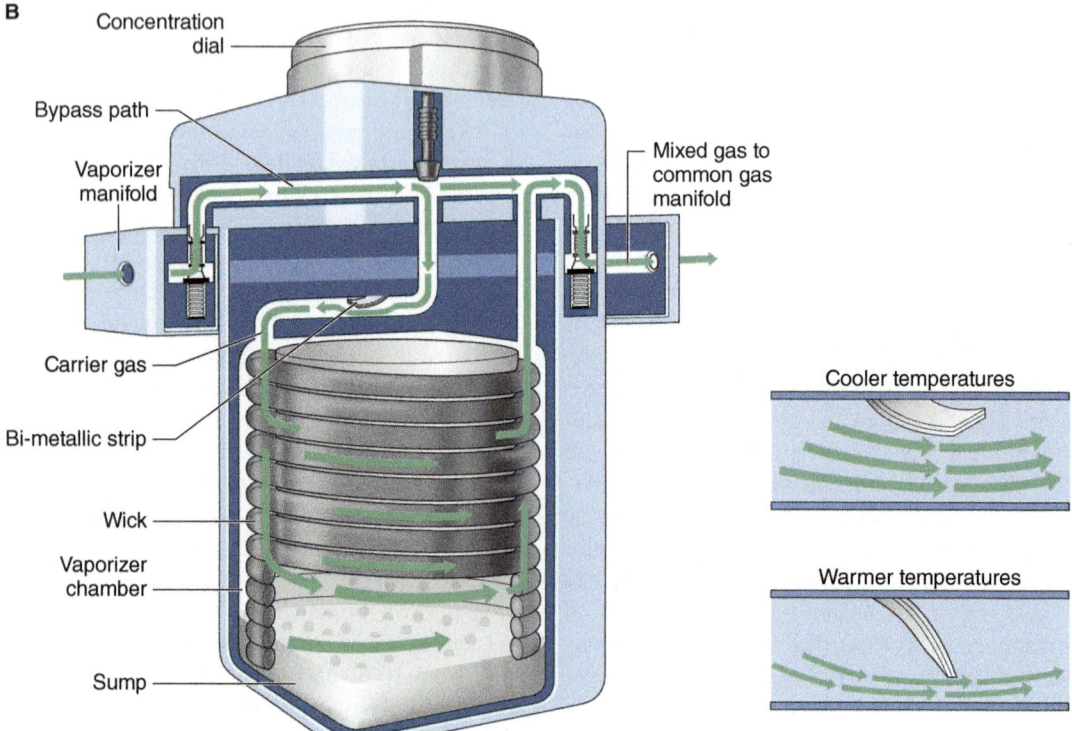

Concentration dial

Bypass path

Vaporizer manifold

Mixed gas to common gas manifold

Carrier gas

Bi-metallic strip

Wick

Vaporizer chamber

Sump

Cooler temperatures

Warmer temperatures

FIGURE 4–17 Schematic of agent-specific variable-bypass vaporizers. **A**: Dräger Vapor 19.n. **B**: Datex-Ohmeda Tec 7.

Given that these vaporizers are agent specific, filling them with the incorrect anesthetic should be avoided. For example, unintentionally filling a sevoflurane-specific vaporizer with halothane could lead to an anesthetic overdose. First, halothane's higher vapor pressure (243 mm Hg versus 157 mm Hg) will cause a 40% greater amount of anesthetic vapor to be released. Second, halothane is more than twice as potent as sevoflurane (MAC 0.75 versus. 2.0). Conversely, filling a halothane vaporizer with sevoflurane will cause an anesthetic underdosage. Modern vaporizers offer agent-specific keyed filling ports to prevent filling with an incorrect agent.

Excessive tilting of older vaporizers (Tec 4, Tec 5, and Vapor 19.n) during transport may flood the bypass area and lead to dangerously high anesthetic concentrations. In the event of tilting and spillage, high flow of oxygen with the vaporizer turned off should be used to vaporize and flush the liquid anesthetic from the bypass area. Fluctuations in pressure from positive-pressure ventilation in older anesthesia machines may cause a transient reversal of flow through the vaporizer, unpredictably changing agent delivery. This "pumping effect" is more pronounced with low gas flows. A one-way check valve between the vaporizers and the oxygen flush valve (Datex-Ohmeda) together with some design modifications in newer units limit the occurrence of some of these problems. Variable bypass vaporizers compensate for changes in ambient pressures (ie, altitude changes maintaining relative anesthetic gas partial pressure).

D. Electronic Vaporizers

Electronically controlled vaporizers must be utilized for desflurane and are used for all volatile anesthetics in some sophisticated anesthesia machines.

1. Desflurane vaporizer—Desflurane's vapor pressure is so high that at sea level it almost boils at room temperature (Figure 4–15). **This high volatility, coupled with a potency only one-fifth that of other volatile agents, presents unique delivery problems.** First, the vaporization required for general anesthesia produces a cooling effect that would overwhelm the ability of conventional vaporizers to maintain a constant temperature. Second, because it vaporizes so extensively, a tremendously high fresh gas flow would be necessary to dilute the carrier gas

to clinically relevant concentrations. These problems have been addressed by the development of special desflurane vaporizers. A reservoir containing desflurane (desflurane sump) is electrically heated to 39°C (significantly higher than its boiling point) creating a vapor pressure of 2 atmospheres. Unlike a variable-bypass vaporizer, no fresh gas flows through the desflurane sump. Rather, pure desflurane vapor joins the fresh gas mixture before exiting the vaporizer. The amount of desflurane vapor released from the sump depends on the concentration selected by turning the control dial and the fresh gas flow rate. Although the Tec 6 Plus maintains a constant desflurane concentration over a wide range of fresh gas flow rates, it cannot automatically compensate for changes in elevation. Decreased ambient pressure (eg, high elevation) does not affect the concentration of agent delivered, but decreases the partial pressure of the agent. Thus, at high elevations, the anesthesiologist must manually increase the concentration control.

2. Aladin cassette vaporizer—This vaporizer is designed for use with the Datex-Ohmeda S/5 ADU and Aisys machines. Gas flow from the flow control is divided into bypass flow and liquid chamber flow (Figure 4–18). The latter is conducted into an agent-specific, color-coded, cassette (Aladin cassette) in which the volatile anesthetic is vaporized. The machine accepts only one cassette at a time and recognizes the cassette through magnetic labeling. The cassette does not contain any bypass flow channels; therefore, unlike traditional vaporizers, liquid anesthetic cannot escape during handling and the cassette can be carried in any position. After leaving the cassette, the now anesthetic-saturated liquid chamber flow reunites with the bypass flow before exiting the fresh gas outlet. A flow restrictor valve near the bypass flow helps to adjust the amount of fresh gas that flows to the cassette. Adjusting the ratio between the bypass flow and liquid chamber flow changes the concentration of volatile anesthetic agent delivered to the patient. In practice, the clinician changes the concentration by turning the agent wheel, which operates a digital potentiometer. Software sets the desired fresh gas agent concentration according to the number of output pulses from the agent wheel. Sensors in the cassette measure pressure and temperature, thus determining agent concentration in the gas leaving the cassette. Correct liquid chamber flow is

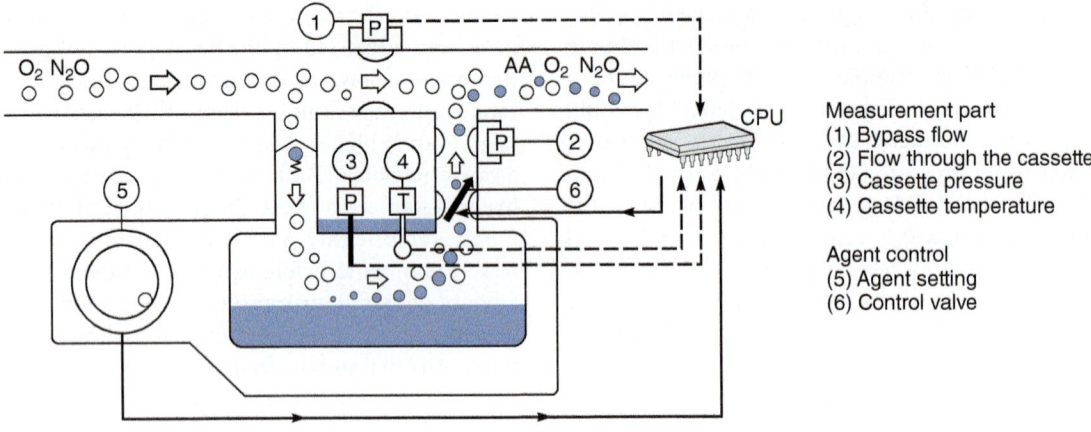

FIGURE 4-18 Schematic of the electronic Datex-Ohmeda Aladin vaporizer.

calculated based on desired fresh gas concentration and determined cassette gas concentration.

Common (Fresh) Gas Outlet

In contrast to the multiple gas inlets, the anesthesia machine has only one common gas outlet that supplies gas to the breathing circuit. The term *fresh gas outlet* is also often used because of its critical role in adding new gas of fixed and known composition to the circle system. Unlike older models, some newer anesthesia machines measure and report common outlet gas flows (Datex-Ohmeda S/5 ADU and Narkomed 6400). An antidisconnect retaining device is used to prevent accidental detachment of the gas outlet hose that connects the machine to the breathing circuit.

The oxygen flush valve provides a high flow (35–75 L/min) of oxygen directly to the common gas outlet, bypassing the flowmeters and vaporizers. It is used to rapidly refill or flush the breathing circuit, but because the oxygen may be supplied at a line pressure of 45–55 psig, there is a real potential of lung barotrauma. For this reason, the flush valve must be used cautiously whenever a patient is connected to the breathing circuit. Moreover, inappropriate use of the flush valve (or a situation of stuck valve) may result in backflow of gases into the low-pressure circuit, causing dilution of inhaled anesthetic concentration. Some machines use a second-stage regulator to drop the oxygen flush pressure to a lower level.

A protective rim around the flush button limits the possibility of unintentional activation. Anesthesia machines (eg, Datex-Ohmeda Aestiva/5) may have an optional auxiliary common gas outlet that is activated with a dedicated switch. It is primarily used for performing the low-pressure circuit leak test (see Anesthesia Machine Checkout List).

THE BREATHING CIRCUIT

The breathing system most commonly used with anesthesia machines is the circle system (Figure 4–19); a Bain circuit is occasionally used. The components and use of the circle system were previously discussed. It is important to note that gas composition at the common gas outlet can be controlled precisely and rapidly by adjustments in flowmeters and vaporizers. In contrast, gas composition, especially volatile anesthetic concentration, in the breathing circuit is significantly affected by other factors, including anesthetic uptake in the patient's lungs, minute ventilation, total fresh gas flow, volume of the breathing circuit, and the presence of gas leaks. Use of high gas flow rates during induction and emergence decreases the effects of such variables and can diminish the magnitude of discrepancies between fresh gas outlet and circle system anesthetic concentrations. Measurement of inspired and expired anesthetic gas concentration also greatly facilitates anesthetic management.

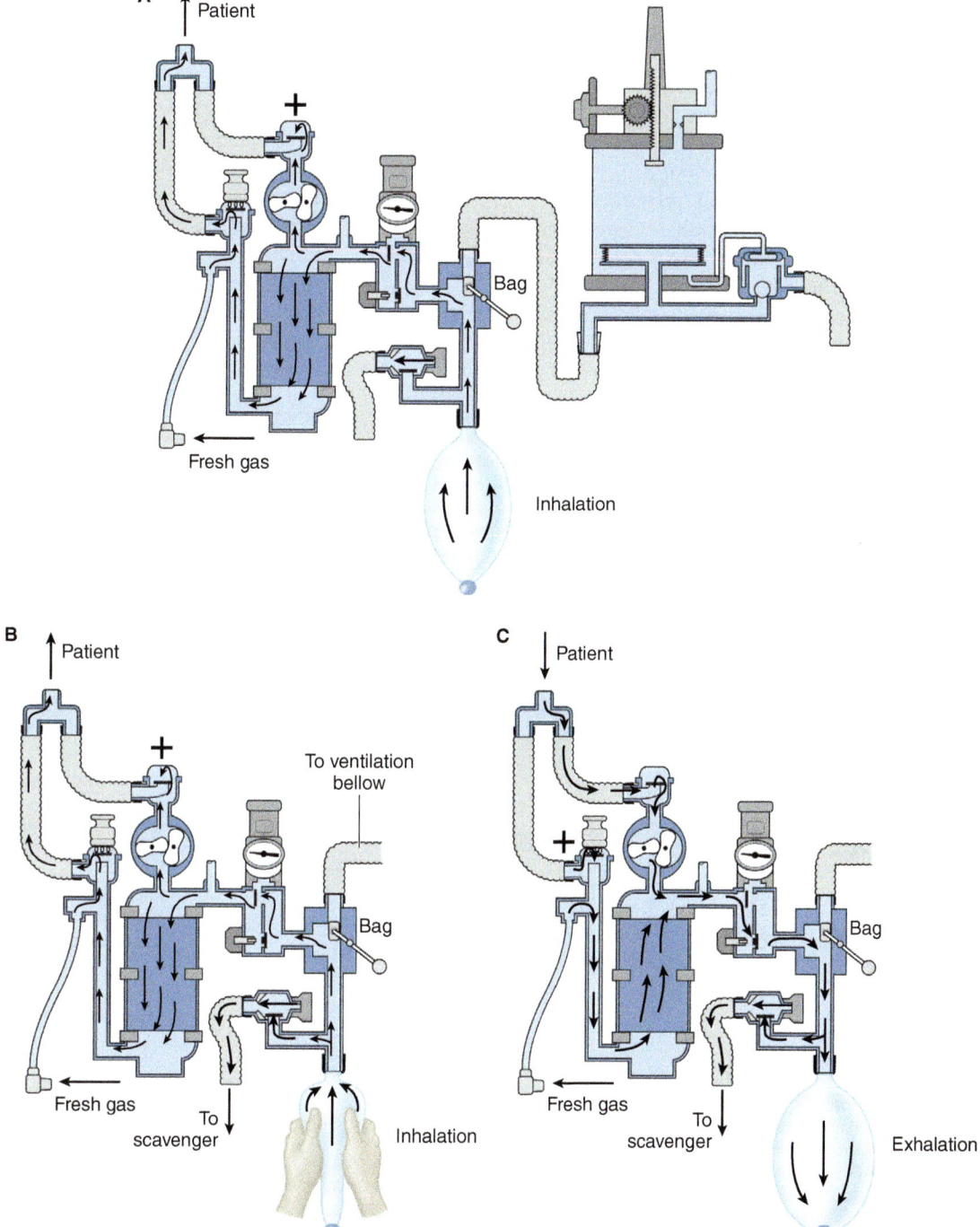

FIGURE 4–19 Diagram of a typical breathing circuit (Dräger Narkomed). Note gas flow during (**A**) spontaneous inspiration, (**B**) manual inspiration ("bagging"), and (**C**) exhalation (spontaneous or bag ventilation).

In most machines the common gas outlet is attached to the breathing circuit just past the exhalation valve to prevent artificially high exhaled tidal volume measurements. When spirometry measurements are made at the Y-connector, fresh gas flow can enter the circuit on the patient side of the inspiratory valve. The latter enhances CO_2 elimination and may help reduce desiccation of the CO_2 absorbent.

Newer anesthesia machines have integrated internalized breathing circuit components (Figure 4–20). The advantages of these designs include reduced probability of breathing circuit misconnects, disconnects, kinks, and leaks. The smaller volume of compact machines can also help conserve gas flow and volatile anesthetics and allow faster

changes in breathing circuit gas concentration. Internal heating of manifolds can reduce precipitation of moisture.

Oxygen Analyzers

General anesthesia should not be administered without an oxygen analyzer in the breathing circuit. **Three types of oxygen analyzers are available: polarographic (Clark electrode), galvanic (fuel cell), and paramagnetic.** The first two techniques utilize electrochemical sensors that contain cathode and anode electrodes embedded in an electrolyte gel separated from the sample gas by an oxygen-permeable membrane (usually Teflon). As oxygen reacts with the electrodes, a current is generated that is proportional

A

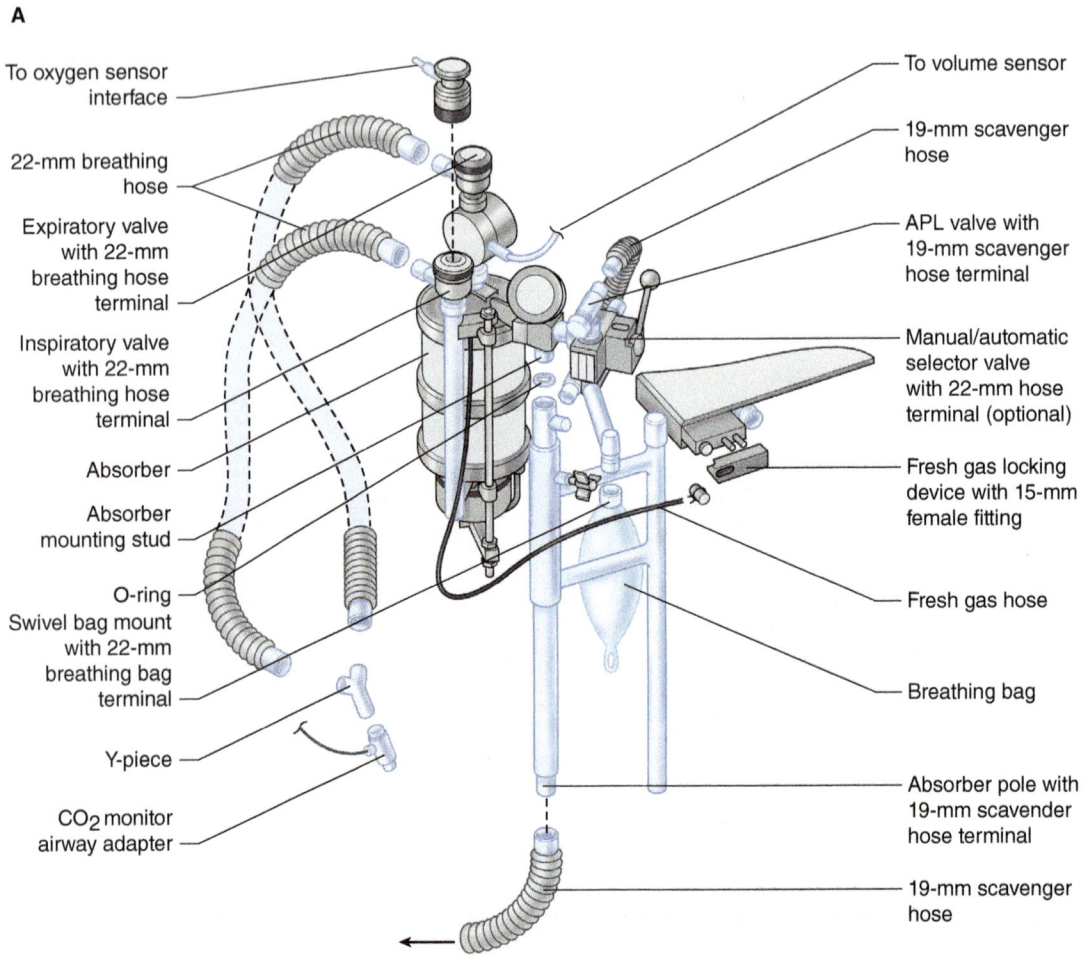

FIGURE 4–20 Breathing circuit design. **A:** Conventional external components. *(continued)*

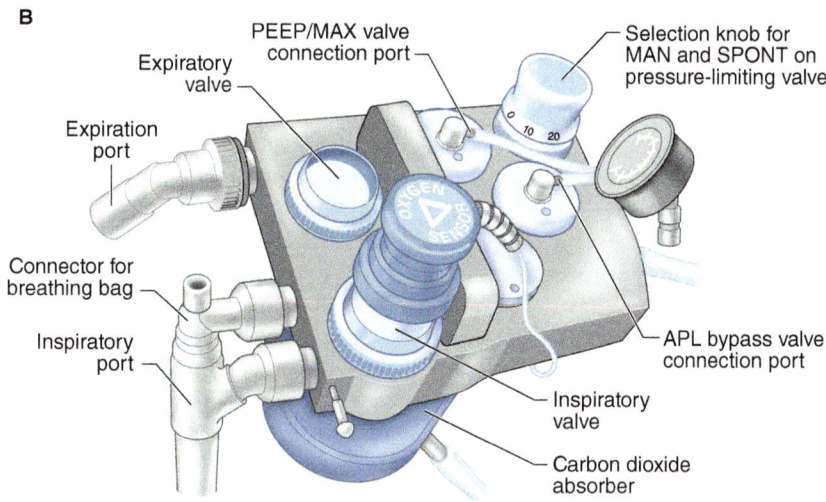

B

PEEP/MAX valve connection port

Expiratory valve

Expiration port

Connector for breathing bag

Inspiratory port

Selection knob for MAN and SPONT on pressure-limiting valve

APL bypass valve connection port

Inspiratory valve

Carbon dioxide absorber

FIGURE 4–20 (*continued*) **B**: Compact design that reduces external connections and circuit volume (Dräger Fabius GS).

to the oxygen partial pressure in the sample gas. The galvanic and polarographic sensors differ in the composition of their electrodes and electrolyte gels. The components of the galvanic cell are capable of providing enough chemical energy so that the reaction does not require an external power source.

Although the initial cost of paramagnetic sensors is greater than that of electrochemical sensors, paramagnetic devices are self-calibrating and have no consumable parts. In addition, their response time is fast enough to differentiate between inspired and expired oxygen concentrations.

All oxygen analyzers should have a low-level alarm that is automatically activated by turning on the anesthesia machine. The sensor should be placed into the inspiratory or expiratory limb of the circle system's breathing circuit—but *not* into the fresh gas line. As a result of the patient's oxygen consumption, the expiratory limb has a slightly lower oxygen partial pressure than the inspiratory limb, particularly at low fresh gas flows. The increased humidity of expired gas does not significantly affect most modern sensors.

Spirometers

Spirometers, also called respirometers, are used to measure exhaled tidal volume in the breathing circuit on all anesthesia machines, typically near the exhalation valve. Some anesthesia machines also measure the inspiratory tidal volume just past the inspiratory valve or the actual delivered and exhaled tidal volumes at the Y-connector that attaches to the patient's airway.

A common method employs a rotating vane of low mass in the expiratory limb in front of the expiratory valve of the circle system (vane anemometer or Wright respirometer, **Figure 4–21A**).

The flow of gas across vanes within the respirometer causes their rotation, which is measured electronically, photoelectrically, or mechanically. In another variation using this turbine principle, the volumeter or displacement meter is designed to measure the movement of discrete quantities of gas over time (**Figure 4–21B**).

Changes in exhaled tidal volumes usually represent changes in ventilator settings, but can also be due to circuit leaks, disconnections, or ventilator malfunction. These spirometers are prone to errors caused by inertia, friction, and water condensation. For example, Wright respirometers underread at low flow rates and over-read at high flow rates. Furthermore, the measurement of exhaled tidal volumes at this location in the expiratory limb includes gas that had been lost to the circuit (and not delivered to the patient; discussed below). The difference between the volume of gas delivered to the circuit and the volume of gas actually reaching the patient becomes very significant with long compliant breathing tubes, rapid respiratory rates, and high airway pressures. These problems are at least partially overcome by measuring the tidal volume at the Y-connector to the patient's airway.

A hot-wire anemometer utilizes a fine platinum wire, electrically heated at a constant temperature, inside the gas flow. The cooling effect of increasing gas flow on the wire electrode causes a change in electrical resistance. In a constant-resistance anemometer, gas flow is determined from the current needed to maintain a constant wire temperature (and resistance). Disadvantages include an inability to detect reverse flow, less accuracy at higher flow rates, and the possibility that the heated wire may be a potential ignition source for fire in the breathing manifold.

Ultrasonic flow sensors rely on discontinuities in gas flow generated by turbulent eddies in the flow stream. Upstream and downstream ultrasonic beams, generated from piezoelectric crystals, are transmitted at an angle to the gas stream. The Doppler frequency shift in the beams is proportional to the flow velocities in the breathing circuit. Major advantages include the absence of moving parts and greater accuracy due to the device's independence from gas density.

Machines with variable-orifice flowmeters usually employ two sensors (Figure 4–21C). One measures flow at the inspiratory port of the breathing system and the other measures flow at the expiratory port. These sensors use a change in internal diameter to generate a pressure drop that is proportional to the flow through the sensor. Clear tubes connect the sensors to differential pressure transducers inside the anesthesia machine (Datex-Ohmeda 7900 SmartVent). The changes in gas flows during the inspiratory and expiratory phases help the ventilator to adjust and provide a constant tidal volume. However, due to excessive condensation sensors can fail when used with heated humidified circuits.

A pneumotachograph is a fixed-orifice flowmeter that can function as a spirometer. A parallel bundle of small-diameter tubes in chamber (Fleisch pneumotachograph) or mesh screen provides a slight resistance to airflow. The pressure drop across this resistance is sensed by a differential pressure transducer and is proportional to the flow rate. Integration

of flow rate over time yields tidal volume. Moreover, analysis of pressure, volume, and time relationships can yield potentially valuable information about airway and lung mechanics. Modifications have been required to overcome inaccuracies due to water condensation and temperature changes. One modification employs two pressure-sensing lines in a Pitot tube at the Y-connection (Figure 4–21D). Gas flowing through the Pitot tube (flow sensor tube) creates a pressure difference between the flow sensor lines. This pressure differential is used to measure flow, flow direction, and airway pressure. Respiratory gases are continuously sampled to correct the flow reading for changes in density and viscosity.

Circuit Pressure

A pressure gauge or electronic sensor is always used to measure breathing-circuit pressure somewhere between the expiratory and inspiratory unidirectional valves; the exact location depends on the model of anesthesia machine. Breathing-circuit pressure usually reflects airway pressure if it is measured as close to the patient's airway as possible. The most accurate measurements of both inspiratory and expiratory pressures can be obtained from the Y-connection (eg, D-lite and Pedi-lite sensors).

6 A rise in airway pressure may signal worsening pulmonary compliance, an increase in tidal volume, or an obstruction in the breathing circuit, tracheal tube, or the patient's airway. A drop in pressure may indicate an improvement in compliance, a decrease in tidal volume, or a leak in the circuit. If circuit pressure is being measured at the CO_2 absorber, however, it will not always mirror the pressure in the patient's airway. For example, clamping the expiratory limb of the breathing tubes during exhalation will prevent the patient's breath from exiting the lungs. Despite this buildup in airway pressure, a pressure gauge at the absorber will read zero because of the intervening one-way valve.

Some machines have incorporated auditory feedback for pressure changes during ventilator use.

Adjustable Pressure-Limiting Valve

The adjustable pressure-limiting (APL) valve, sometimes referred to as the pressure relief or pop-off valve, is usually fully open during spontaneous

A

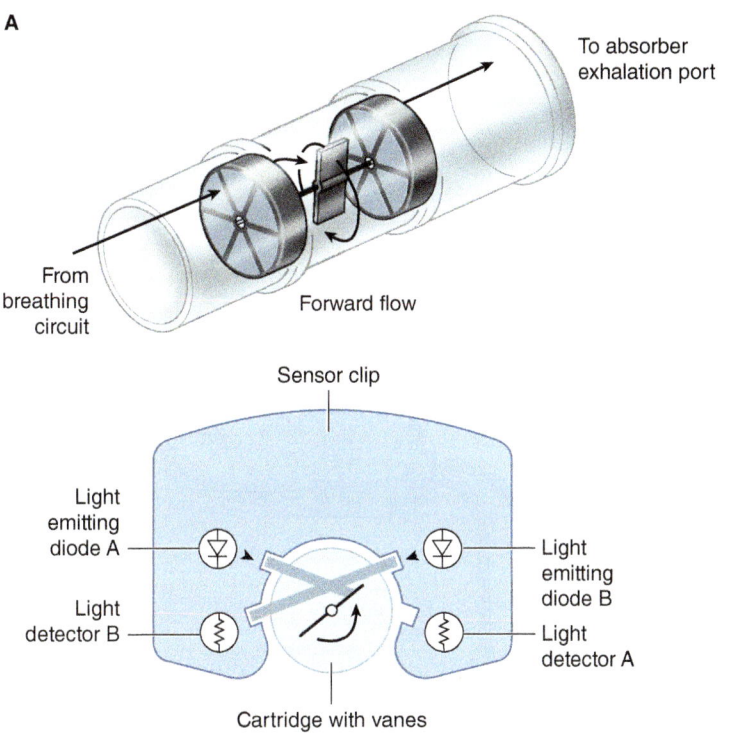

To absorber
exhalation port

From
breathing
circuit

Forward flow

Sensor clip

Light
emitting
diode A

Light
emitting
diode B

Light
detector B

Light
detector A

Cartridge with vanes

B

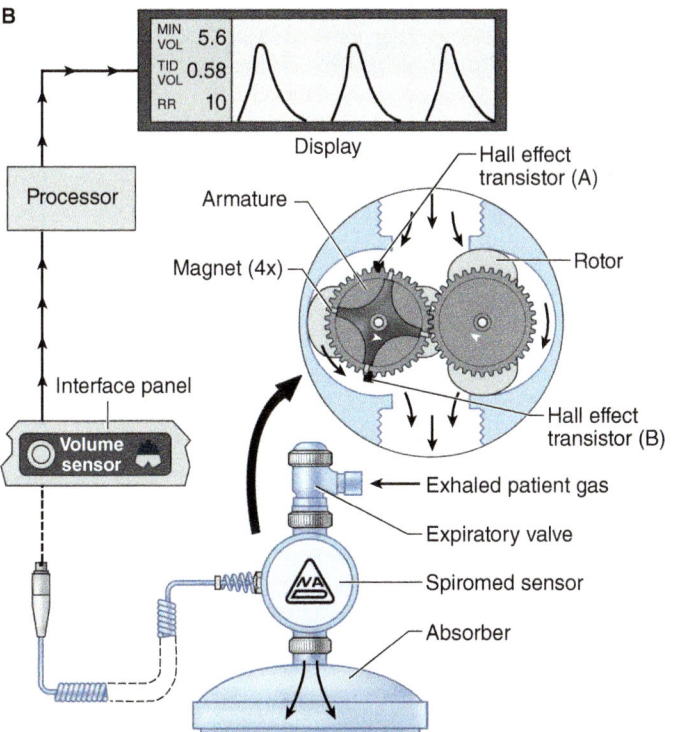

MIN VOL	5.6
TID VOL	0.58
RR	10

Display

Processor

Interface panel

Volume sensor

Hall effect
transistor (A)

Armature

Magnet (4x)

Rotor

Hall effect
transistor (B)

Exhaled patient gas

Expiratory valve

Spiromed sensor

Absorber

FIGURE 4–21 Spirometer designs.
A: Vane anemometer (Datex-Ohmeda).
B: Volumeter (Dräger).

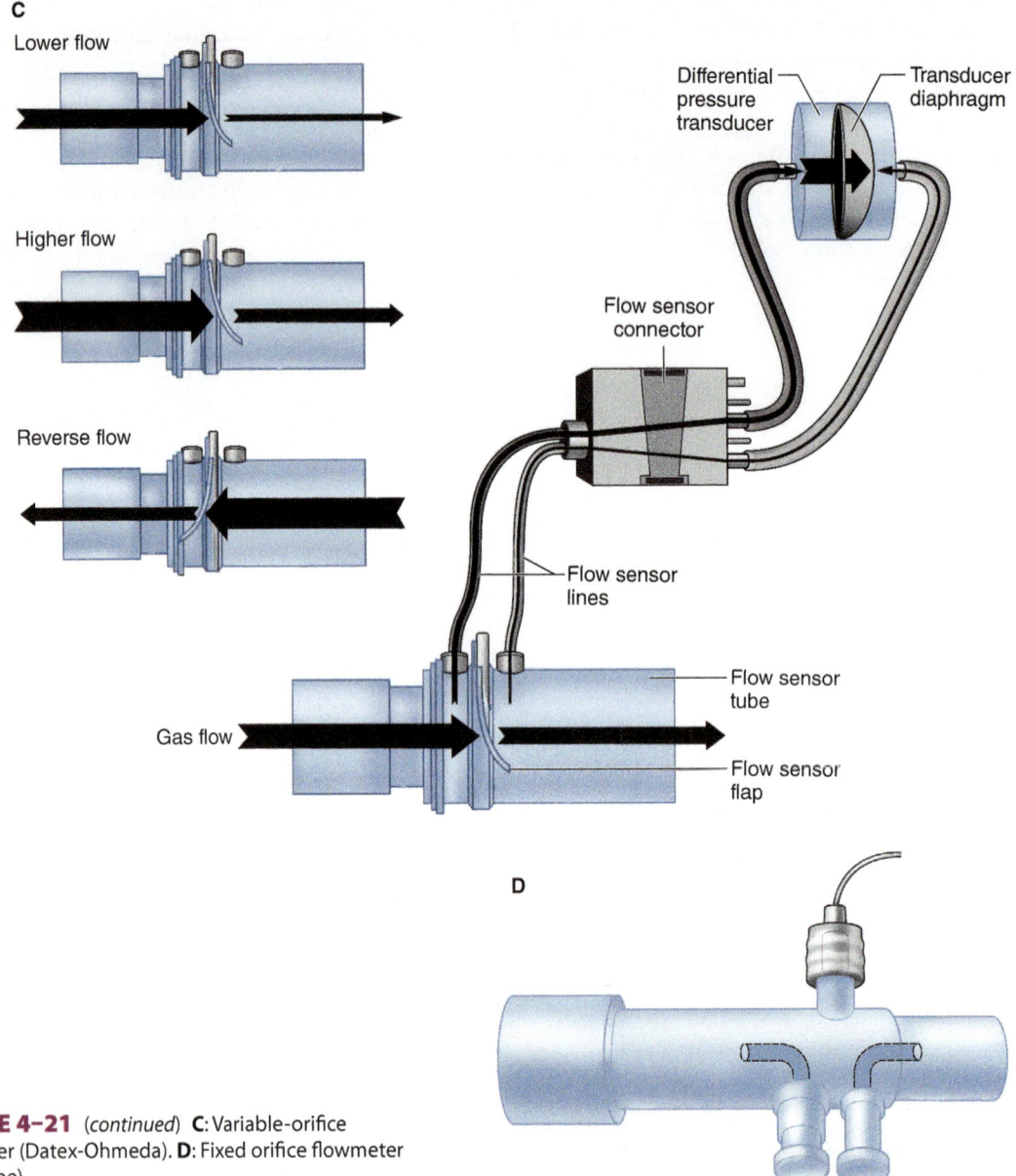

C

Lower flow

Higher flow

Reverse flow

Differential pressure transducer

Transducer diaphragm

Flow sensor connector

Flow sensor lines

Gas flow

Flow sensor tube

Flow sensor flap

D

FIGURE 4–21 (*continued*) **C**: Variable-orifice flowmeter (Datex-Ohmeda). **D**: Fixed orifice flowmeter (Pitot tube).

ventilation but must be partially closed during manual or assisted bag ventilation. The APL valve often requires fine adjustments. If it is not closed sufficiently excessive loss of circuit volume due to leaks prevents manual ventilation. At the same time if it is closed too much or is fully closed a progressive rise in pressure could result in pulmonary barotrauma (eg, pneumothorax) or hemodynamic compromise, or both. As an added safety feature, the APL valves on modern machines act as true pressure-limiting devices that can never be completely closed; the upper limit is usually 70–80 cm H_2O.

Humidifiers

Absolute humidity is defined as the weight of water vapor in 1 L of gas (ie, mg/L). Relative humidity is the ratio of the actual mass of water present in a volume of gas to the maximum amount of water possible at a particular temperature. At 37°C and 100% relative humidity, absolute humidity is 44 mg/L, whereas at room temperature (21°C and 100% humidity) it is 18 mg/L. Inhaled gases in the operating room are normally administered at room temperature with little or no humidification. Gases must therefore be warmed to body temperature and saturated with water by the upper respiratory tract. Tracheal intubation and high fresh gas flows bypass this normal humidification system and expose the lower airways to dry (<10 mg H_2O/L), room temperature gases.

Prolonged humidification of gases by the lower respiratory tract leads to dehydration of mucosa, altered ciliary function, and, if excessively prolonged, could potentially lead to inspissation of secretions, atelectasis, and even ventilation/perfusion mismatching, particularly in patients with underlying lung disease. Body heat is also lost as gases are warmed and even more importantly as water is vaporized to humidify the dry gases. The heat of vaporization for water is 560 cal/g of water vaporized. Fortunately, this heat loss accounts for about only 5–10% of total intraoperative heat loss, is not significant for a short procedure (<1 h), and usually can easily be compensated for with a forced-air warming blanket. Humidification and heating of inspiratory gases may be most important for small pediatric patients and older patients with severe underlying lung pathology, eg, cystic fibrosis.

A. Passive Humidifiers

Humidifiers added to the breathing circuit minimize water and heat loss. The simplest designs are condenser humidifiers or heat and moisture exchanger (HME) units (Figure 4–22). These passive devices do not add heat or vapor but rather contain a hygroscopic material that traps exhaled humidification and heat, which is released upon subsequent inhalation. Depending on the design, they may substantially increase apparatus dead space (more than 60 mL³), which can cause significant rebreathing in pediatric patients. They can also increase breathing-circuit resistance and the work of breathing during spontaneous respirations. Excessive saturation of an HME with water or secretions can obstruct the breathing circuit. Some condenser humidifiers also act as effective filters that may protect the breathing circuit and anesthesia machine from bacterial or viral cross-contamination. This may be particularly important when ventilating patients with respiratory infections or compromised immune systems.

B. Active Humidifiers

Active humidifiers are more effective than passive ones in preserving moisture and heat. Active humidifiers add water to gas by passing the gas over a water chamber (passover humidifier) or through a saturated wick (wick humidifier), bubbling it through water (bubble-through humidifier), or mixing it with vaporized water (vapor-phase humidifier). Because increasing temperature increases the capacity of a gas to hold water vapor, heated humidifiers with thermostatically controlled elements are most effective.

The hazards of heated humidifiers include thermal lung injury (inhaled gas temperature should be monitored and should not exceed 41°C), nosocomial infection, increased airway resistance from excess water condensation in the breathing circuit, interference with flowmeter function, and an increased likelihood of circuit disconnection. These humidifiers are particularly valuable with children as they help prevent both hypothermia and the plugging of small tracheal tubes by dried secretions. Of course, any design that increases airway dead space should be avoided in pediatric patients. Unlike passive humidifiers, active humidifiers do not filter respiratory gases.

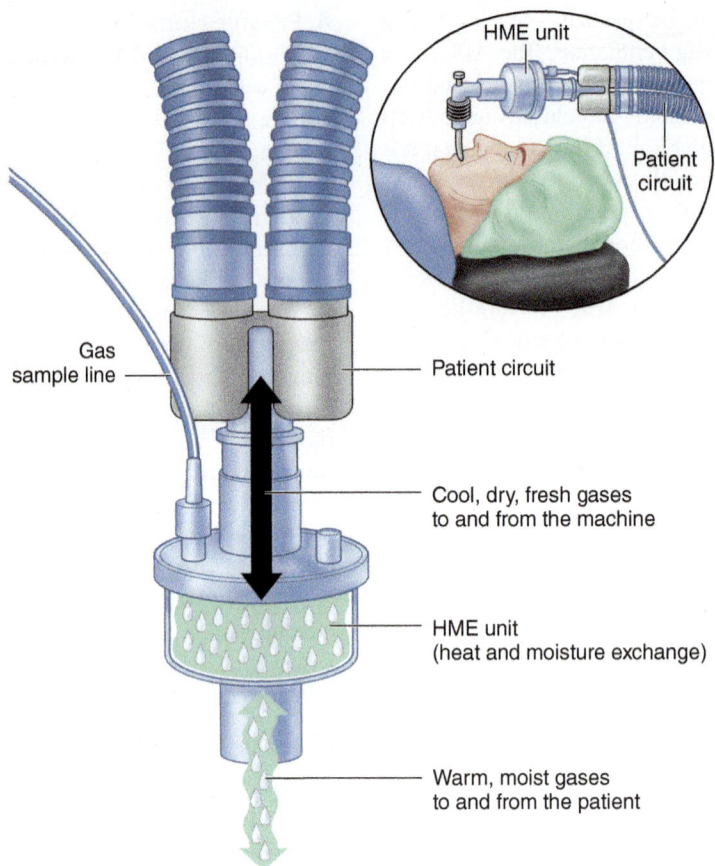

FIGURE 4–22 Heat and moisture exchanger (HME) functions as an "artificial nose" that attaches between the tracheal tube and the right-angle connector of the breathing circuit.

VENTILATORS

Ventilators are used extensively in the operating room (OR) and the intensive care unit (ICU). All modern anesthesia machines are equipped with a ventilator. Historically OR ventilators were simpler and more compact than their ICU counterparts. This distinction has become blurred due to advances in technology together with an increasing need for "ICU-type" ventilators as more critically ill patients come to the OR. The ventilators on some modern machines are just as sophisticated as those in the ICU and have almost the same capabilities. After a general discussion of basic ventilator principles, this section reviews the use of ventilators in conjunction with anesthesia machines.

Overview

Ventilators generate gas flow by creating a pressure gradient between the proximal airway and the alveoli. Older units relied on the generation of negative pressure around (and inside) the chest (eg, iron lungs), whereas modern ventilators generate positive pressure and gas flow in the upper airway.

Ventilator function is best described in relation to the four phases of the ventilatory cycle: inspiration, the transition from inspiration to expiration, expiration, and the transition from expiration to inspiration. Although several classification schemes exist, the most common is based on inspiratory phase characteristics and the method of cycling from inspiration to expiration.

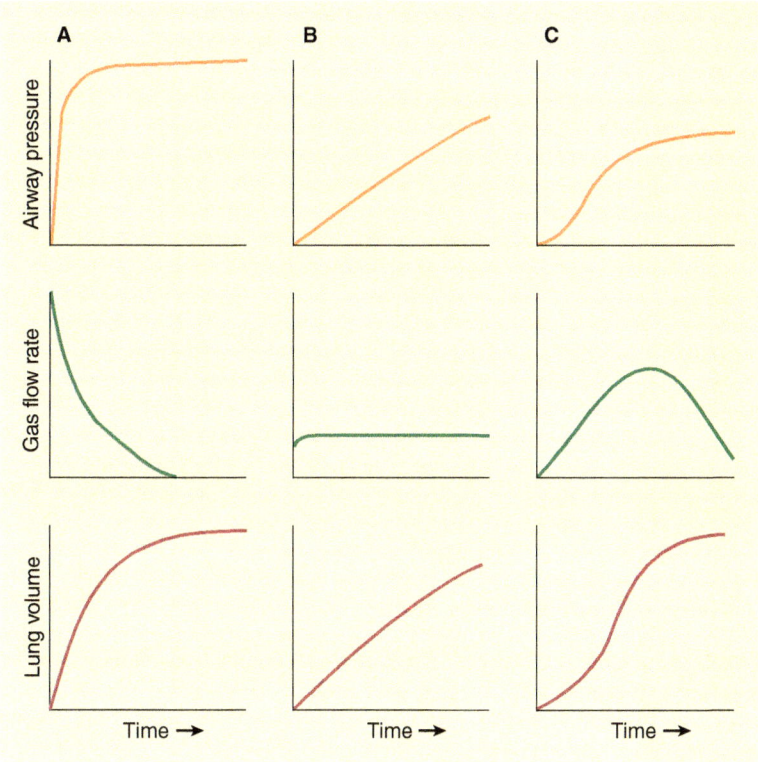

FIGURE 4–23 Pressure, volume, and flow profiles of different types of ventilators. **A**: Constant pressure. **B**: Constant flow. **C**: Nonconstant generator.

Other classification categories may include power source (eg, pneumatic-high pressure, pneumatic-Venturi, or electric), design (single-circuit system, double-circuit system, rotary piston, linear piston), and control mechanisms (eg, electronic timer or microprocessor).

A. Inspiratory Phase

During inspiration, ventilators generate tidal volumes by producing gas flow along a pressure gradient. The machine generates either a constant pressure (constant-pressure generators) or constant gas flow rate (constant-flow generators) during inspiration, regardless of changes in lung mechanics (Figure 4–23). Nonconstant generators produce pressures or gas flow rates that vary during the cycle but remain consistent from breath to breath. For instance, a ventilator that generates a flow pattern resembling a half cycle of a sine wave (eg, rotary piston ventilator) would be classified as a nonconstant-flow generator. An increase in airway resistance or a decrease in lung compliance would increase peak inspiratory pressure but would not alter the flow rate generated by this type of ventilator (Figure 4–24).

B. Transition Phase from Inspiration to Expiration

Termination of the inspiratory phase can be triggered by a preset limit of time (fixed duration), a set inspiratory pressure that must be reached, or a predetermined tidal volume that must be delivered. Time-cycled ventilators allow tidal volume and peak inspiratory pressure to vary depending on lung compliance. Tidal volume is adjusted by setting inspiratory duration and inspiratory flow rate. Pressure-cycled ventilators will not cycle from the inspiratory phase to the expiratory phase until a preset pressure is reached. If a large circuit leak decreases peak pressures significantly,

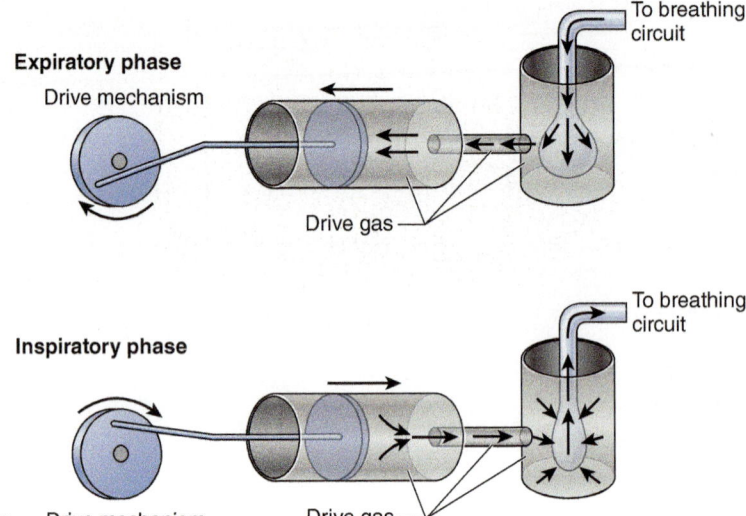

FIGURE 4–24 Rotary piston ventilator.

a pressure-cycled ventilator may remain in the inspiratory phase indefinitely. On the other hand, a small leak may not markedly decrease tidal volume, because cycling will be delayed until the pressure limit is met. Volume-cycled ventilators vary inspiratory duration and pressure to deliver a preset volume. In reality, modern ventilators overcome the many shortcomings of classic ventilator designs by incorporating secondary cycling parameters or other limiting mechanisms. For example, time-cycled and volume-cycled ventilators usually incorporate a pressure-limiting feature that terminates inspiration when a preset, adjustable safety pressure limit is reached. Similarly a volume-preset control that limits the excursion of the bellows allows a time-cycled ventilator to function somewhat like a volume-cycled ventilator, depending on the selected ventilator rate and inspiratory flow rate.

C. Expiratory Phase

The expiratory phase of ventilators normally reduces airway pressure to atmospheric levels or some preset value of positive end-expiratory pressure (PEEP). Exhalation is therefore passive. Flow out of the lungs is determined primarily by airway resistance and lung compliance. Expired gases fill up the bellows; they are then relieved to the scavenging system. PEEP is usually created with an adjustable spring valve mechanism or pneumatic pressurization of the exhalation (spill) valve.

D. Transition Phase from Expiration to Inspiration

Transition into the next inspiratory phase may be based on a preset time interval or a change in pressure. The behavior of the ventilator during this phase together with the type of cycling from inspiration to expiration determines ventilator mode.

During controlled ventilation, the most basic mode of all ventilators, the next breath always occurs after a preset time interval. Thus tidal volume and rate are fixed in volume-controlled ventilation, whereas peak inspiratory pressure is fixed in pressure-controlled ventilation. Controlled ventilation modes are not designed for spontaneous breathing. In the volume-control mode, the ventilator adjusts gas flow rate and inspiratory time based on the set ventilatory rate and I:E ratio (Figure 4–25A). In the pressure-control mode, inspiratory time is also based on the set ventilator rate and inspiratory-to-expiratory (I:E) ratio, but gas flow is adjusted to maintain a constant inspiratory pressure (Figure 4–25B).

A

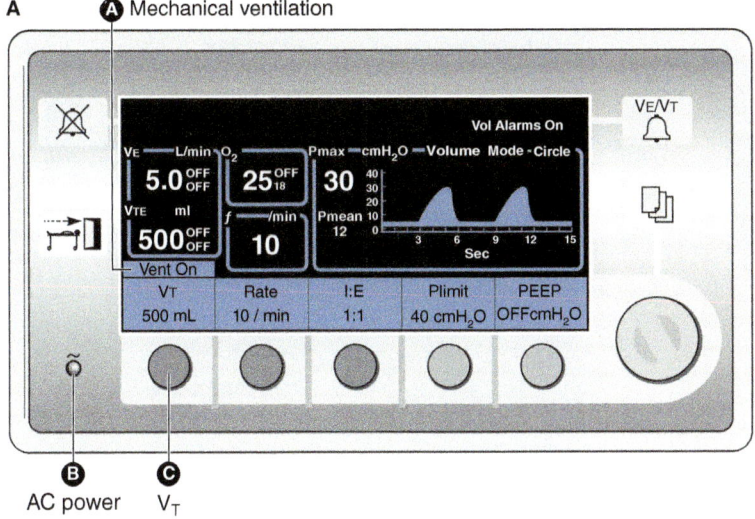

B

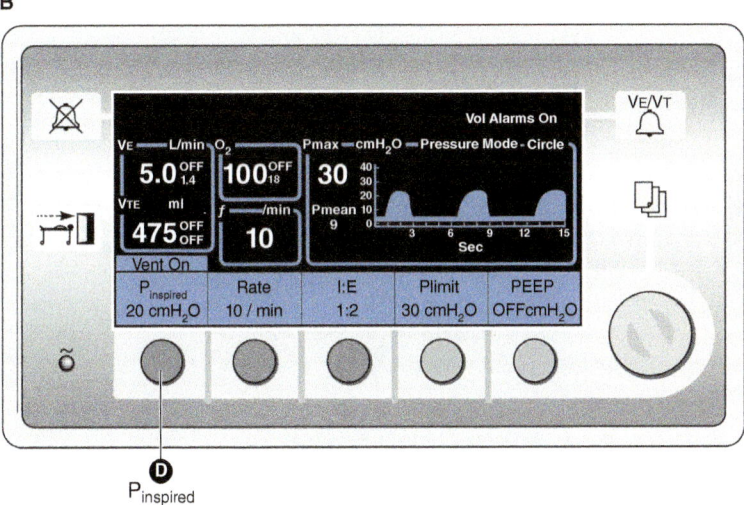

FIGURE 4–25 Ventilator controls (Datex-Ohmeda). **A**: Volume control mode. **B**: Pressure control mode.

In contrast, intermittent mandatory ventilation (IMV) allows patients to breathe spontaneously between controlled breaths. Synchronized intermittent mandatory ventilation (SIMV) is a further refinement that helps prevent "fighting the ventilator" and "breath stacking"; whenever possible, the ventilator tries to time the mandatory mechanical breaths with the drops in airway pressure below the end-expiratory pressure that occur as the patient initiates a spontaneous breath.

Ventilator Circuit Design

7 Traditionally ventilators on anesthesia machines have a double-circuit system design and are pneumatically powered and electronically controlled (Figure 4–26). Newer machines also incorporate microprocessor control that relies on sophisticated pressure and flow sensors. This feature allows multiple ventilatory modes, electronic PEEP, tidal volume modulation, and enhanced safety

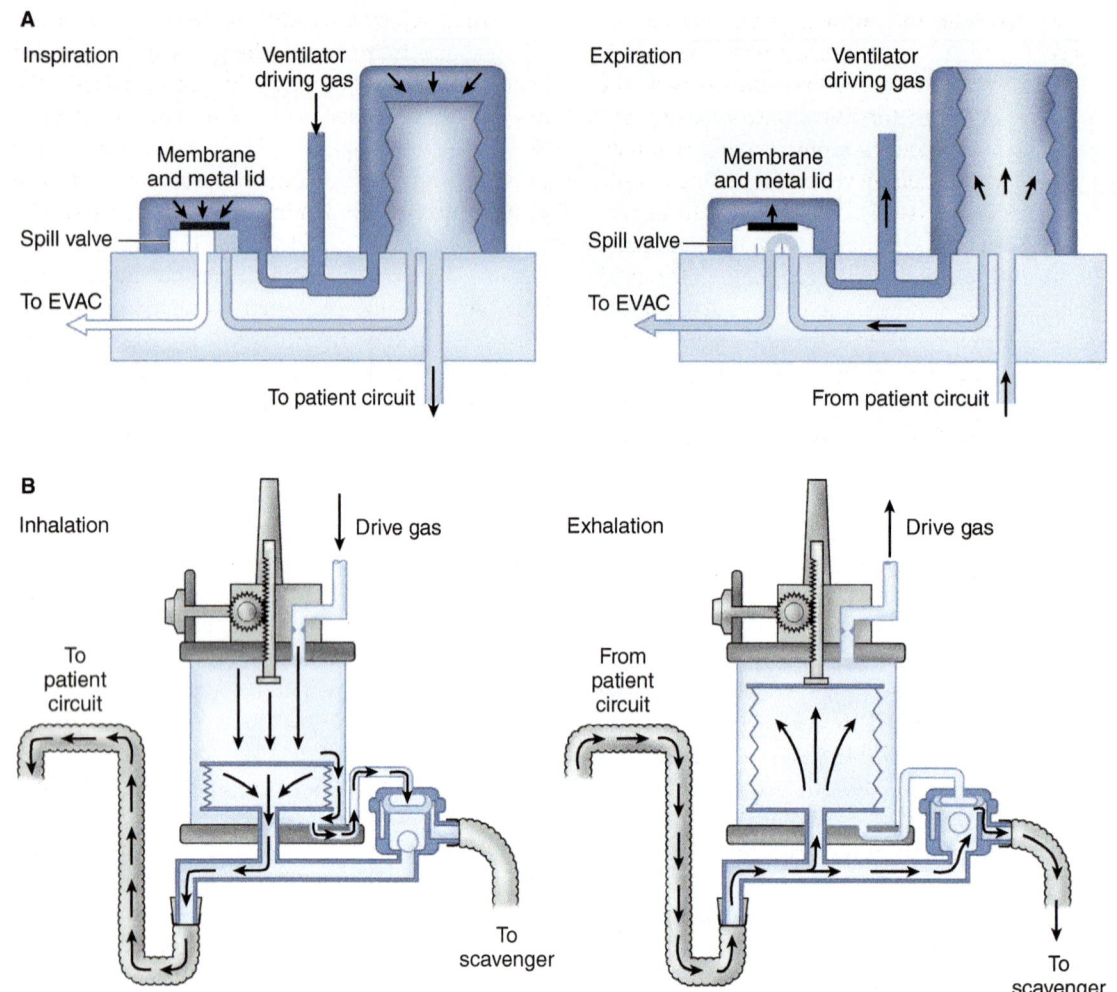

A

Inspiration

Ventilator driving gas

Membrane and metal lid

Spill valve

To EVAC

To patient circuit

Expiration

Ventilator driving gas

Membrane and metal lid

Spill valve

To EVAC

From patient circuit

B

Inhalation

Drive gas

To patient circuit

To scavenger

Exhalation

Drive gas

From patient circuit

To scavenger

FIGURE 4–26 Double-circuit pneumatic ventilator design. **A**: Datex-Ohmeda. **B**: Dräger.

features. Some anesthesia machines have ventilators that use a single-circuit piston design (Figure 4–24).

A. Double-Circuit System Ventilators

In a double-circuit system design, tidal volume is delivered from a bellows assembly that consists of a bellows in a clear rigid plastic enclosure (Figure 4–26). A standing (ascending) bellows is preferred as it readily draws attention to a circuit disconnection by collapsing. Hanging (descending) bellows are rarely used and must not be weighted;

older ventilators with weighted hanging bellows continue to fill by gravity despite a disconnection in the breathing circuit.

The bellows in a double-circuit design ventilator takes the place of the breathing bag in the anesthesia circuit. Pressurized oxygen or air from the ventilator power outlet (45–50 psig) is routed to the space between the inside wall of the plastic enclosure and the outside wall of the bellows. Pressurization of the plastic enclosure compresses the pleated bellows inside, forcing the gas inside into the breathing circuit and patient. In contrast, during exhalation, the bellows ascend as pressure inside the plastic enclosure drops and the bellows fill up with the exhaled gas. A ventilator flow control valve regulates drive gas flow into the pressurizing chamber. This valve is controlled by ventilator settings in the control box (Figure 4–26). Ventilators with microprocessors also utilize feedback from flow and pressure sensors. If oxygen is used for pneumatic power it will be consumed at a rate at least equal to minute ventilation. Thus, if oxygen fresh gas flow is 2 L/min and a ventilator is delivering 6 L/min to the circuit, a total of at least 8 L/min of oxygen is being consumed. This should be kept in mind if the hospital's medical gas system fails and cylinder oxygen is required. Some anesthesia machines reduce oxygen consumption by incorporating a Venturi device that draws in room air to provide air/oxygen pneumatic power. Newer machines may offer the option of using compressed air for pneumatic power. A leak in the ventilator bellows can transmit high gas pressure to the patient's airway, potentially resulting in pulmonary barotrauma. **This may be indicated by a higher than expected rise in inspired oxygen concentration (if oxygen is the sole pressurizing gas).** Some machine ventilators have a built-in drive gas regulator that reduces the drive pressure (eg, to 25 psig) for added safety.

Double-circuit design ventilators also incorporate a free breathing valve that allows outside air to enter the rigid drive chamber and the bellows to collapse if the patient generates negative pressure by taking spontaneous breaths during mechanical ventilation.

B. Piston Ventilators

In a piston design, the ventilator substitutes an electrically driven piston for the bellows (Figure 4–24); the ventilator requires either minimal or no pneumatic (oxygen) power. The major advantage of a piston ventilator is its ability to deliver accurate tidal volumes to patients with very poor lung compliance and to very small patients. During volume-controlled ventilation the piston moves at a constant velocity whereas during pressure-controlled ventilation the piston moves with

decreasing velocity. As with the bellows, the piston fills with gas from the breathing circuit. To prevent generation of significant negative pressure during the downstroke of the piston the circle system configuration has to be modified (Figure 4–27). The ventilator must also incorporate a negative-pressure relief valve or be capable of terminating the piston's downstroke if negative pressure is detected. Introduction of a negative-pressure relief valve to the breathing circuit may introduce the risk of air entrainment and the potential for dilution of oxygen and volatile anesthetic concentrations if the patient breathes during mechanical ventilation and low fresh gas flows.

C. Spill Valve

Whenever a ventilator is used on an anesthesia machine, the circle system's APL valve must be functionally removed or isolated from the circuit. A bag/ventilator switch typically accomplishes this. When the switch is turned to "bag" the ventilator is excluded and spontaneous/manual (bag) ventilation is possible. When it is turned to "ventilator," the breathing bag and the APL are excluded from the breathing circuit. The APL valve may be automatically excluded in some newer anesthesia machines when the ventilator is turned on. The ventilator contains its own pressure-relief (pop-off) valve, called the spill valve, which is pneumatically closed during inspiration so that positive pressure can be generated (Figure 4–26). During exhalation, the pressurizing gas is vented out and the ventilator spill valve is no longer closed. The ventilator bellows or piston refill during expiration; when the bellows is completely filled, the increase in circle system pressure causes the excess gas to be directed to the scavenging system through the spill valve. Sticking of this valve can result in abnormally elevated airway pressure during exhalation.

Pressure & Volume Monitoring

Peak inspiratory pressure is the highest circuit pressure generated during an inspiratory cycle, and provides an indication of dynamic compliance. Plateau pressure is the pressure measured during an inspiratory pause (a time of no gas flow), and mirrors static compliance. During

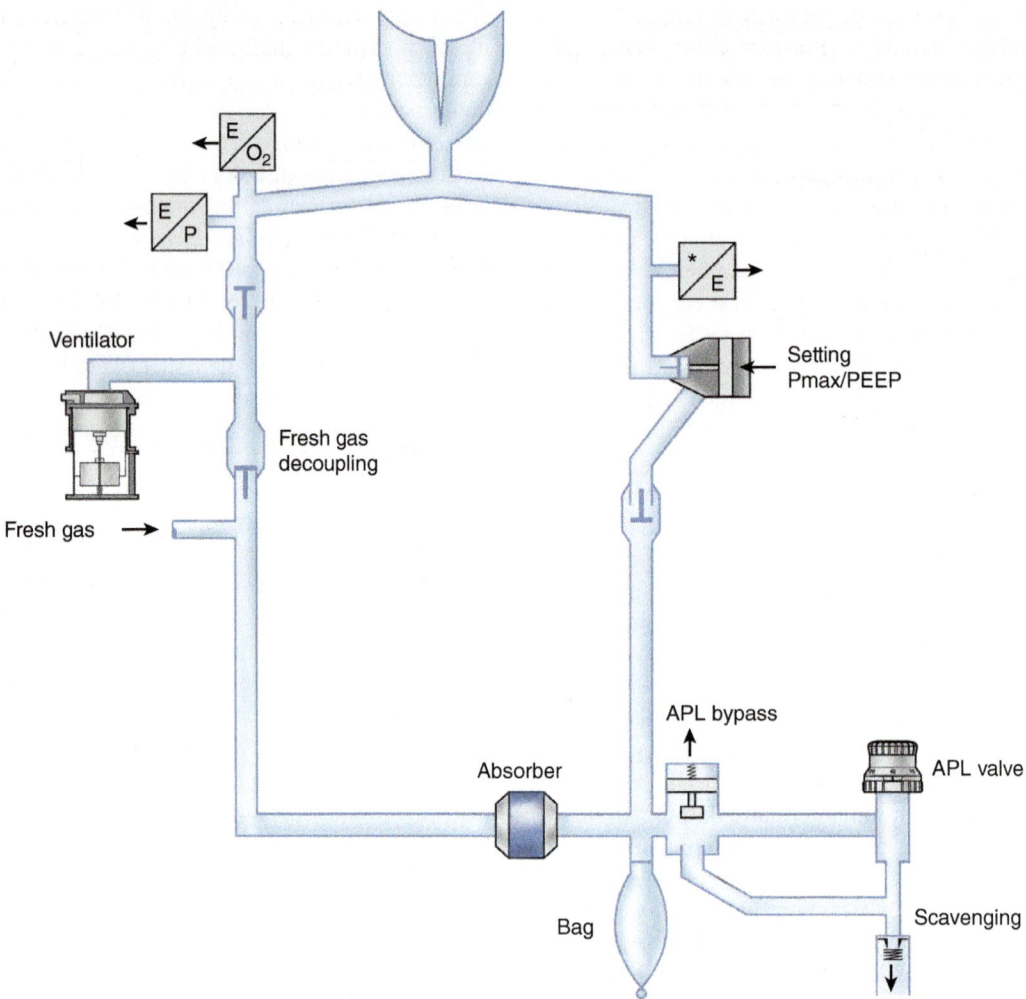

FIGURE 4–27 Modified circle system for a piston ventilator (Dräger Fabius GS).

normal ventilation of a patient without lung disease, peak inspiratory pressure is equal to or only slightly greater than plateau pressure. An increase in both peak inspiratory pressure and plateau pressure implies an increase in tidal volume or a decrease in pulmonary compliance. An increase in peak inspiratory pressure without any change in plateau pressure signals an increase in airway resistance or inspiratory gas flow rate (Table 4–3). Thus, the shape of the breathing-circuit pressure waveform can provide important airway information. Many anesthesia

machines graphically display breathing-circuit pressure (Figure 4–28). Airway secretions or kinking of the tracheal tube can be easily ruled out with the use of a suction catheter. Flexible fiberoptic bronchoscopy will usually provide a definitive diagnosis.

Ventilator Alarms

Alarms are an integral part of all modern anesthesia ventilators. Whenever a ventilator is used "disconnect alarms" must be passively activated. Anesthesia workstations should have at least

TABLE 4–3 **Causes of increased peak inspiratory pressure (PIP), with or without an increased plateau pressure (PP).**

Increased PIP and PP
  Increased tidal volume
  Decreased pulmonary compliance
    Pulmonary edema
    Trendelenburg position
    Pleural effusion
    Ascites
    Abdominal packing
    Peritoneal gas insufflation
    Tension pneumothorax
    Endobronchial intubation

Increased PIP and Unchanged PP
  Increased inspiratory gas flow rate
  Increased airway resistance
    Kinked endotracheal tube
    Bronchospasm
    Secretions
    Foreign body aspiration
    Airway compression
    Endotracheal tube cuff herniation

three disconnect alarms: low peak inspiratory pressure, low exhaled tidal volume, and low exhaled carbon dioxide. The first is always built into the ventilator whereas the latter two may be in separate modules. A small leak or partial breathing-circuit disconnection may be detected by subtle decreases in peak inspiratory pressure, exhaled volume, or end-tidal carbon dioxide before alarm thresholds are reached. Other built-in ventilator alarms include high peak inspiratory pressure, high PEEP, sustained high airway pressure, negative pressure, and low oxygen-supply pressure. Most modern anesthesia ventilators also have integrated spirometers and oxygen analyzers that provide additional alarms.

Problems Associated with Anesthesia Ventilators

A. Ventilator–Fresh Gas Flow Coupling

From the previous discussion, it is important to appreciate that because the ventilator's spill valve is closed during inspiration, fresh gas flow from the machine's common gas outlet normally contributes to the tidal volume delivered to the patient. For example, if the fresh gas flow is 6 L/min, the I:E ratio

is 1:2, and the respiratory rate is 10 breaths/min, each tidal volume will include an extra 200 mL in addition to the ventilator's output:

$$\frac{(6000 \text{ mL/min}) \, (33\%)}{10 \text{ breaths/min}} \approx 200 \text{ mL/breath}$$

Thus, increasing fresh gas flow increases tidal volume, minute ventilation, and peak inspiratory pressure. To avoid problems with ventilator–fresh gas flow coupling, airway pressure and exhaled tidal volume must be monitored closely and excessive fresh gas flows must be avoided.

B. Excessive Positive Pressure

Intermittent or sustained high inspiratory pressures (>30 mm Hg) during positive-pressure ventilation increase the risk of pulmonary barotrauma (eg, pneumothorax) or hemodynamic compromise, or both, during anesthesia. Excessively high pressures may arise from incorrect settings on the ventilator, ventilator malfunction, fresh gas flow coupling (above), or activation of the oxygen flush during the inspiratory phase of the ventilator. Use of the oxygen flush valve during the inspiratory cycle of a ventilator *must be avoided* because the ventilator spill valve will be closed and the APL valve is excluded; the surge of oxygen (600–1200 mL/s) and circuit pressure will be transferred to the patient's lungs.

In addition to a high-pressure alarm, all ventilators have a built-in automatic or APL valve. The mechanism of pressure limiting may be as simple as a threshold valve that opens at a certain pressure or electronic sensing that abruptly terminates the ventilator inspiratory phase.

C. Tidal Volume Discrepancies

Large discrepancies between the set and actual tidal volume that the patient receives are often observed in the operating room during volume control ventilation. Causes include breathing-circuit compliance, gas compression, ventilator–fresh gas flow coupling (above), and leaks in the anesthesia machine, the breathing circuit, or the patient's airway.

The compliance for standard adult breathing circuits is about 5 mL/cm H_2O. Thus, if peak

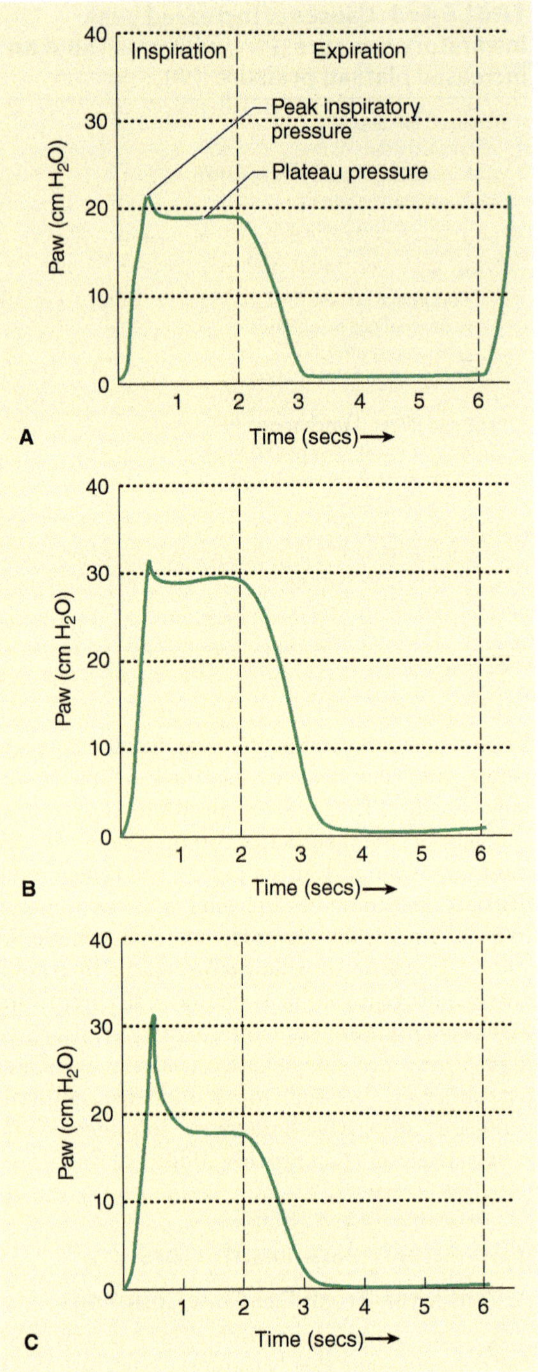

FIGURE 4–28 Airway pressures (Paw) can be diagrammatically presented as a function of time. **A**: In normal persons, the peak inspiratory pressure is equal to or slightly greater than the plateau pressure. **B**: An increase in peak inspiratory pressure and plateau pressure (the difference between the two remains almost constant) can be due to an increase in tidal volume or a decrease in pulmonary compliance. **C**: An increase in peak inspiratory pressure with little change in plateau pressure signals an increase in inspiratory flow rate or an increase in airway resistance.

inspiratory pressure is 20 cm H_2O, about 100 mL of set tidal volume is lost to expanding the circuit. For this reason breathing circuits for pediatric patients are designed to be much stiffer, with compliances as small as 1.5–2.5 mL/cm H_2O.

Compression losses, normally about 3%, are due to gas compression within the ventilator bellows and may be dependent on breathing-circuit volume. Thus if tidal volume is 500 mL another 15 mL of the set tidal gas may be lost. Gas sampling for capnography and anesthetic gas measurements represent additional losses in the form of gas leaks unless the sampled gas is returned to the breathing circuit, as occurs in some machines.

Accurate detection of tidal volume discrepancies is dependent on where the spirometer is placed. Sophisticated ventilators measure both inspiratory and expiratory tidal volumes. It is important to note that unless the spirometer is placed at the Y-connector in the breathing circuit, compliance and compression losses will not be apparent.

Several mechanisms have been built into newer anesthesia machines to reduce tidal volume discrepancies. During the initial electronic self-checkout, some machines measure total system compliance and subsequently use this measurement to adjust the excursion of the ventilator bellows or piston; leaks may also be measured but are usually not compensated. The actual method of tidal volume compensation or modulation varies according to manufacturer and model. In one design a flow sensor measures the tidal volume delivered at the inspiratory valve for the first few breaths and adjusts subsequent metered drive gas flow volumes to compensate for tidal volume losses (feedback adjustment). Another design continually measures fresh gas and vaporizer flow and subtracts this amount from the metered drive gas flow (preemptive adjustment). Alternately, machines that use electronic control of gas flow can decouple fresh gas flow from the tidal volume by delivery of fresh gas flow only during exhalation. Lastly, the inspiratory phase of the ventilator–fresh gas flow may be diverted through a decoupling valve into the breathing bag, which is excluded from the circle system during ventilation. During exhalation the decoupling valve opens, allowing the fresh gas that was temporarily stored in the bag to enter the breathing circuit.

WASTE-GAS SCAVENGERS

Waste-gas scavengers dispose of gases that have been vented from the breathing circuit by the APL valve and ventilator spill valve. Pollution of the operating room environment with anesthetic gases may pose a health hazard to surgical personnel. Although it is difficult to define safe levels of exposure, the National Institute for Occupational Safety and Health (NIOSH) recommends limiting the room concentration of nitrous oxide to 25 ppm and halogenated agents to 2 ppm (0.5 ppm if nitrous oxide is also being used) in time-integrated samples. Reduction to these trace levels is possible only with properly functioning waste-gas scavenging systems.

To avoid the buildup of pressure, excess gas volume is vented through the APL valve in the breathing circuit and the ventilator spill valve. Both valves should be connected to hoses (transfer tubing) leading to the scavenging interface, which may be inside the machine or an external attachment (Figure 4–29). The pressure immediately downstream to the interface should be kept between 0.5 and +3.5 cm H_2O during normal operating conditions. The scavenging interface may be described as either open or closed.

An open interface is open to the outside atmosphere and usually requires no pressure relief valves. In contrast, a closed interface is closed to the outside atmosphere and requires negative- and positive-pressure relief valves that protect the patient from the negative pressure of the vacuum system and positive pressure from an obstruction in the disposal tubing, respectively. The outlet of the scavenging system may be a direct line to the outside via a ventilation duct beyond any point of recirculation (passive scavenging) or a connection to the hospital's vacuum system (active scavenging). A chamber or reservoir bag accepts waste-gas overflow when the capacity of the vacuum is exceeded. The vacuum control valve on an active system should be adjusted to allow the evacuation of 10–15 L of waste gas per minute. This rate is adequate for periods of high fresh gas flow (ie, induction and emergence) yet minimizes the risk of transmitting negative pressure to the breathing circuit during lower flow conditions

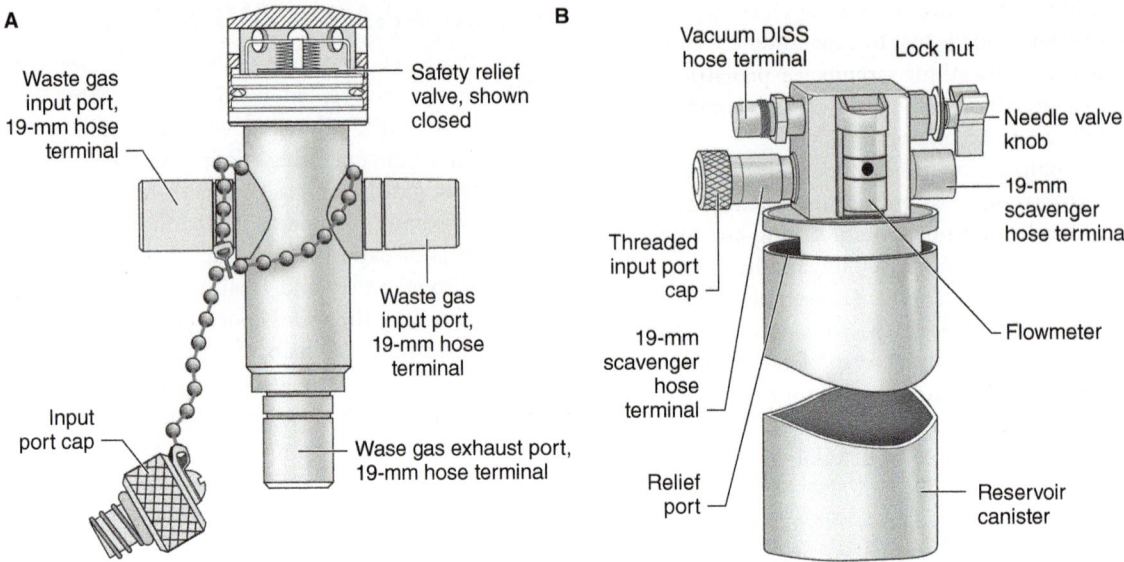

A

Waste gas input port, 19-mm hose terminal

Safety relief valve, shown closed

Waste gas input port, 19-mm hose terminal

Input port cap

Wase gas exhaust port, 19-mm hose terminal

B

Vacuum DISS hose terminal

Lock nut

Needle valve knob

19-mm scavenger hose terminal

Flowmeter

Threaded input port cap

19-mm scavenger hose terminal

Relief port

Reservoir canister

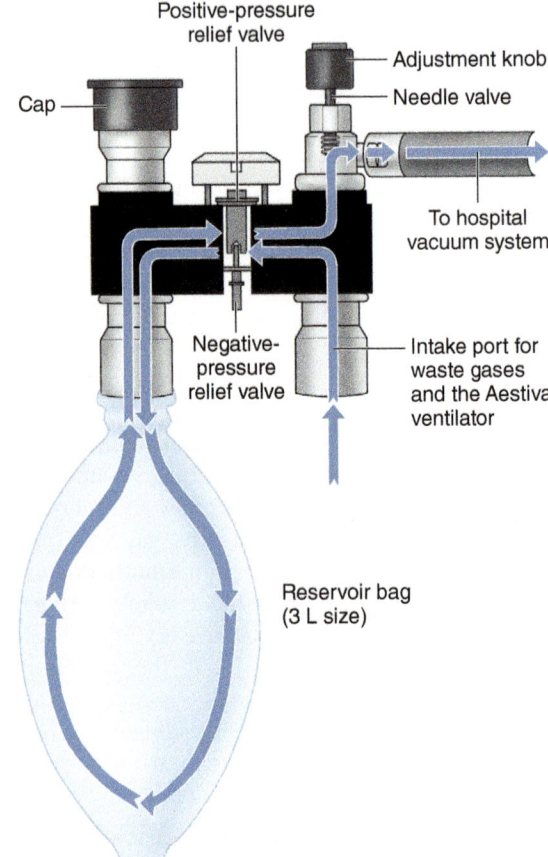

C

Positive-pressure relief valve

Adjustment knob

Needle valve

Cap

To hospital vacuum system

Negative-pressure relief valve

Intake port for waste gases and the Aestiva ventilator

Reservoir bag (3 L size)

FIGURE 4–29 Waste-gas scavenging systems.
A: Closed interface with passive scavenging (Dräger).
B: Open interface with active scavenging (Dräger).
C: Closed interface with active scavenging (Datex-Ohmeda). *(continued)*

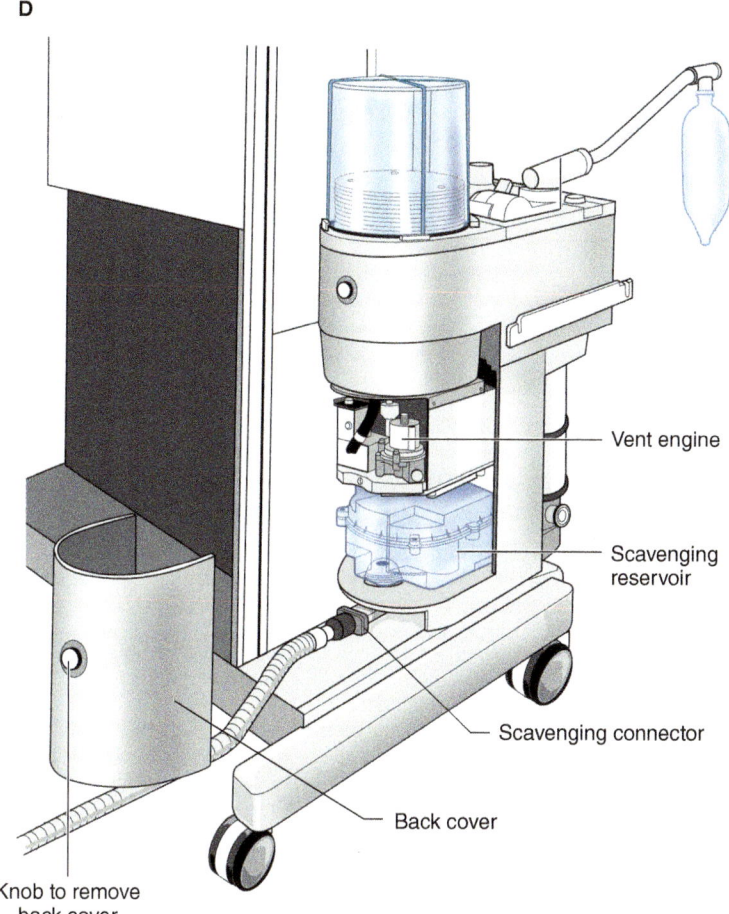

D

Vent engine

Scavenging reservoir

Scavenging connector

Back cover

Knob to remove back cover

FIGURE 4–29 (*continued*) **D:** Built-in scavenging system that can be either active or passive; the active scavenging option has an open interface whereas the passive scavenging option has a closed interface with positive- and negative-pressure relief valves (Datex-Ohmeda).

(maintenance). Unless used correctly the risk of occupational exposure for health care providers is higher with an open interface. Some machines may come with both active and passive scavenger systems.

ANESTHESIA MACHINE CHECKOUT LIST

Misuse or malfunction of anesthesia gas delivery equipment can cause major morbidity or mortality. **14** A routine inspection of anesthesia equipment before each use increases operator familiarity and confirms proper functioning. The U.S. Food and Drug Administration (FDA) has made available a generic checkout procedure for anesthesia gas

machines and breathing systems (Table 4–4). This procedure should be modified as necessary, depending on the specific equipment being used and the manufacturer's recommendations. Note that although the entire checkout does not need to be repeated between cases on the same day, the conscientious use of a checkout list is mandatory before each anesthetic procedure. A mandatory check-off procedure increases the likelihood of detecting anesthesia machine faults. Some anesthesia machines provide an automated system check that requires a variable amount of human intervention. These system checks may include nitrous oxide delivery (hypoxic mixture prevention), agent delivery, mechanical and manual ventilation, pipeline pressures, scavenging, breathing circuit compliance, and gas leakage.

TABLE 4–4 Anesthesia apparatus checkout recommendations.[1,2]

This checkout, or a reasonable equivalent, should be conducted before administration of anesthesia. These recommendations are valid only for an anesthesia system that conforms to current and relevant standards and includes an ascending bellows ventilator and at least the following monitors: capnograph, pulse oximeter, oxygen analyzer, respiratory volume monitor (spirometer), and breathing-system pressure monitor with high- and low-pressure alarms. Users are encouraged to modify this guideline to accommodate differences in equipment design and variations in local clinical practice. Such local modifications should have appropriate peer review. Users should refer to the appropriate operator manuals for specific procedures and precautions.

Emergency Ventilation Equipment
*1. Verify backup ventilation equipment is available and functioning

High-Pressure System
*2. Check O_2 cylinder supply
   a. Open O_2 cylinder and verify at least half full (about 1000 psig).
   b. Close cylinder
*3. Check central pipeline supplies; check that hoses are connected and pipeline gauges read about 50 psig.

Low-Pressure System
*4. Check initial status of low-pressure system
   a. Close flow control valves and turn vaporizers off.
   b. Check fill level and tighten vaporizers' filler caps.
*5. Perform leak check of machine low-pressure system
   a. Verify that the machine master switch and flow control valves are off.
   b. Attach suction bulb to common (fresh) gas outlet.
   c. Squeeze bulb repeatedly until fully collapsed.
   d. Verify bulb stays *fully* collapsed for at least 10 seconds.
   e. Open one vaporizer at a time and repeat steps c and d.
   f. Remove suction bulb, and reconnect fresh gas hose.
*6. Turn on machine master switch and all other necessary electrical equipment.
*7. Test flowmeters
   a. Adjust flow of all gases through their full range, checking for smooth operation of floats and undamaged flowtubes.
   b. Attempt to create a hypoxic O_2/N_2O mixture and verify correct changes in flow and/or alarm.

Scavenging System
*8. Adjust and check scavenging system
   a. Ensure proper connections between the scavenging system and both APL (pop-off) valve and ventilator relief valve.
   b. Adjust waste-gas vacuum (if possible).
   c. Fully open APL valve and occlude Y-piece.
   d. With minimum O_2 flow, allow scavenger reservoir bag to collapse completely and verify that absorber pressure gauge reads about zero.
   e. With the O_2 flush activated, allow scavenger reservoir bag to distend fully, and then verify that absorber pressure gauge reads <10 cm H_2O.

Breathing System
*9. Calibrate O_2 monitor
   a. Ensure monitor reads 21% in room air.
   b. Verify low-O_2 alarm is enabled and functioning.
   c. Reinstall sensor in circuit and flush breathing system with O_2.
   d. Verify that monitor now reads greater than 90%.
10. Check initial status breathing system
   a. Set selector switch to Bag mode.
   b. Check that breathing circuit is complete, undamaged, and unobstructed.
   c. Verify that CO_2 absorbent is adequate.
   d. Install breathing-circuit accessory equipment (eg, humidifier, PEEP valve) to be used during the case.
11. Perform leak check of the breathing system
   a. Set all gas flows to zero (or minimum).
   b. Close APL (pop-off) valve and occlude Y-piece.
   c. Pressurize breathing system to about 30 cm H_2O with O_2 flush.
   d. Ensure that pressure remains fixed for at least 10 seconds.
   e. Open APL (pop-off) valve and ensure that pressure decreases.

Manual and Automatic Ventilation Systems
12. Test ventilation systems and unidirectional valves
   a. Place a second breathing bag on Y-piece.
   b. Set appropriate ventilator parameters for next patient.
   c. Switch to automatic-ventilation (ventilator) mode.
   d. Turn ventilator on and fill bellows and breathing bag with O_2 flush.
   e. Set O_2 flow to minimum, other gas flows to zero.
   f. Verify that during inspiration bellows deliver appropriate tidal volume and that during expiration bellows fill completely.
   g. Set fresh gas flow to about 5 L min⁻¹.
   h. Verify that the ventilator bellows and simulated lungs fill and empty appropriately without sustained pressure at end expiration.
   i. Check for proper action of unidirectional valves.
   j. Exercise breathing circuit accessories to ensure proper function.
   k. Turn ventilator off and switch to manual ventilation (Bag/APL) mode.
   l. Ventilate manually and ensure inflation and deflation of artificial lungs and appropriate feel of system resistance and compliance.
   m. Remove second breathing bag from Y-piece.

(continued)

TABLE 4–4 Anesthesia apparatus checkout recommendations.[1,2] (continued)

Monitors	Final Position
13. Check, calibrate, and/or set alarm limits of all monitors: capnograph, pulse oximeter, O_2 analyzer, respiratory-volume monitor (spirometer), pressure monitor with high and low airway-pressure alarms.	14. Check final status of machine a. Vaporizers off b. APL valve open c. Selector switch to Bag mode d. All flowmeters to zero (or minimum) e. Patient suction level adequate f. Breathing system ready to use

[1]Data from http://www.fda.gov/cdrh/humfac/anesckot.html.
[2]APL, adjust pressure-limiting; PEEP, positive end-expiratory pressure.
*If an anesthesia provider uses the same machine in successive cases, these steps need not be repeated, or they can be abbreviated after the initial checkout.

CASE DISCUSSION

Detection of a Leak

After induction of general anesthesia and intubation of a 70-kg man for elective surgery, a standing bellows ventilator is set to deliver a tidal volume of 500 mL at a rate of 10 breaths/min. Within a few minutes, the anesthesiologist notices that the bellows fails to rise to the top of its clear plastic enclosure during expiration. Shortly thereafter, the disconnect alarm is triggered.

Why has the ventilator bellows fallen and the disconnect alarm sounded?

Fresh gas flow into the breathing circuit is inadequate to maintain the circuit volume required for positive-pressure ventilation. In a situation in which there is no fresh gas flow, the volume in the breathing circuit will slowly fall because of the constant uptake of oxygen by the patient (metabolic oxygen consumption) and absorption of expired CO_2. An absence of fresh gas flow could be due to exhaustion of the hospital's oxygen supply (remember the function of the fail-safe valve) or failure to turn on the anesthesia machine's flow control valves. These possibilities can be ruled out by examining the oxygen Bourdon pressure gauge and the flowmeters. A more likely explanation is a gas leak that exceeds the rate of fresh gas flow. Leaks are particularly important in closed-circuit anesthesia.

How can the size of the leak be estimated?

When the rate of fresh gas inflow equals the rate of gas outflow, the circuit's volume will be maintained. Therefore, the size of the leak can be estimated by increasing fresh gas flows until there is no change in the height of the bellows from one expiration to the next. If the bellows collapse despite a high rate of fresh gas inflow, a complete circuit disconnection should be considered. The site of the disconnection must be determined immediately and repaired to prevent hypoxia and hypercapnia. A resuscitation bag can be used to ventilate the patient if there is a delay in correcting the situation.

Where are the most likely locations of a breathing-circuit disconnection or leak?

Frank disconnections occur most frequently between the right-angle connector and the tracheal tube, whereas leaks are most commonly traced to the base plate of the CO_2 absorber. In the intubated patient, leaks often occur in the trachea around an uncuffed tracheal tube or an inadequately filled cuff. There are numerous potential sites of disconnection or leak within the anesthesia machine and the breathing circuit, however. Every addition to the breathing circuit, such as a humidifier, increases the likelihood of a leak.

How can these leaks be detected?

Leaks usually occur before the fresh gas outlet (ie, within the anesthesia machine) or after the fresh gas inlet (ie, within the breathing circuit). Large leaks within the anesthesia machine are less common and can be ruled out by a simple test. Pinching the tubing that connects the machine's fresh gas outlet to the circuit's fresh gas inlet creates a back pressure that obstructs the forward flow of fresh gas from the anesthesia machine. This is indicated by a drop in the height of the flowmeter floats. When the fresh gas tubing is released, the floats should briskly rebound and settle at their original height. If there is a substantial leak within the machine, obstructing the fresh gas tubing will not result in any back pressure, and the floats will not drop. A more sensitive test for detecting small leaks that occur before the fresh gas outlet involves attaching a suction bulb at the outlet as described in step 5 of Table 4–4. Correcting a leak within the machine usually requires removing it from service.

Leaks within a breathing circuit not connected to a patient are readily detected by closing the APL valve, occluding the Y-piece, and activating the oxygen flush until the circuit reaches a pressure of 20–30 cm H_2O. A gradual decline in circuit pressure indicates a leak within the breathing circuit (Table 4–4, step 11).

How are leaks in the breathing circuit located?

Any connection within the breathing circuit is a potential site of a gas leak. A quick survey of the circuit may reveal a loosely attached breathing tube or a cracked oxygen analyzer adaptor. Less obvious causes include detachment of the tubing used by the disconnect alarm to monitor circuit pressures, an open APL valve, or an improperly adjusted scavenging unit. Leaks can usually be identified audibly or by applying a soap solution to suspect connections and looking for bubble formation.

Leaks within the anesthesia machine and breathing circuit are usually detectable if the machine and circuit have undergone an established checkout procedure. For example, steps 5 and 11 of the FDA recommendations (Table 4–4) will reveal most significant leaks.

SUGGESTED READING

Baum JA, Nunn G: *Low Flow Anaesthesia: The Theory and Practice of Low Flow, Minimal Flow and Closed System Anaesthesia*, 2nd ed. Butterworth-Heinemann, 2001.

Block FE, Schaff C: Auditory alarms during anesthesia monitoring with an integrated monitoring system. Int J Clin Monit Comput 1996;13:81.

Caplan RA, Vistica MF, Posner KL, Cheney FW: Adverse anesthetic outcomes arising from gas delivery equipment: A closed claims analysis. Anesthesiology 1997;87:741.

Dorsch JA, Dorsch SE: *Understanding Anesthesia Equipment,* 5th ed. Lippincott, Williams & Wilkins, 2008.

Eisenkraft JB, Leibowitz AB: Ventilators in the operating room. Int Anesthesiol Clin 1997;35:87.

Klopfenstein CE, Van Gessel E, Forster A: Checking the anaesthetic machine: Self-reported assessment in a university hospital. Eur J Anaesthesiol 1998;15:314. Compliance with recommended safety checklists is low.

Somprakit P, Soontranan P: Low pressure leakage in anaesthetic machines: Evaluation by positive and negative pressure tests. Anaesthesia 1996; 51:461.

WEB SITES

http://www.apsf.org/

The Anesthesia Patient Safety Foundation web site provides resources and a newsletter that discusses important safety issues in anesthesia.

https://www.asahq.org/clinical/fda.aspx

The web site of the American Society of Anesthesiologists includes a link to the 2008 ASA Recommendations for Pre-Anesthesia Checkout.

http://www.simanest.org/

An extremely useful web site of simulations in anesthesia that includes virtual anesthesia machine simulators.

Cardiovascular Monitoring

1. The central venous pressure catheter's tip should not be allowed to migrate into the heart chambers.

2. Although the pulmonary artery catheter can be used to guide goal-directed hemodynamic therapy to ensure organ perfusion in shock states, other less invasive methods to determine hemodynamic performance are available, including transpulmonary thermodilution cardiac output measurements and pulse contour analyses of the arterial pressure waveform.

3. Relative contraindications to pulmonary artery catheterization include left bundle-branch block (because of the concern about complete heart block) and conditions associated with greatly increased risk of arrhythmias, such as Wolff–Parkinson–White syndrome.

4. Pulmonary artery pressure should be continuously monitored to detect an overwedged position indicative of catheter migration.

5. Accurate measurements of cardiac output depend on rapid and smooth injection, precisely known injectant temperature and volume, correct entry of the calibration factors for the specific type of pulmonary artery catheter into the cardiac output computer, and avoidance of measurements during electrocautery.

Vigilant perioperative monitoring of the cardiovascular system is one of the primary duties of anesthesia providers. This chapter focuses on the specific monitoring devices and techniques used by anesthesiologists to monitor cardiac function and circulation in healthy and nonhealthy patients alike.

ARTERIAL BLOOD PRESSURE

The rhythmic contraction of the left ventricle, ejecting blood into the vascular system, results in pulsatile arterial pressures. The peak pressure generated during systolic contraction (in the absence of aortic valve stenosis) approximates the systolic arterial blood pressure (SBP); the lowest arterial pressure during diastolic relaxation is the diastolic blood pressure (DBP). Pulse pressure is the difference between the systolic and diastolic pressures. The time-weighted average of arterial pressures during a pulse cycle is the **mean arterial pressure (MAP)**. MAP can be estimated by application of the following formula:

$$MAP = \frac{(SBP) + 2(DBP)}{3}$$

Arterial blood pressure is greatly affected by where the pressure is measured. **As a pulse moves peripherally through the arterial tree, wave reflection distorts the pressure waveform, leading to**

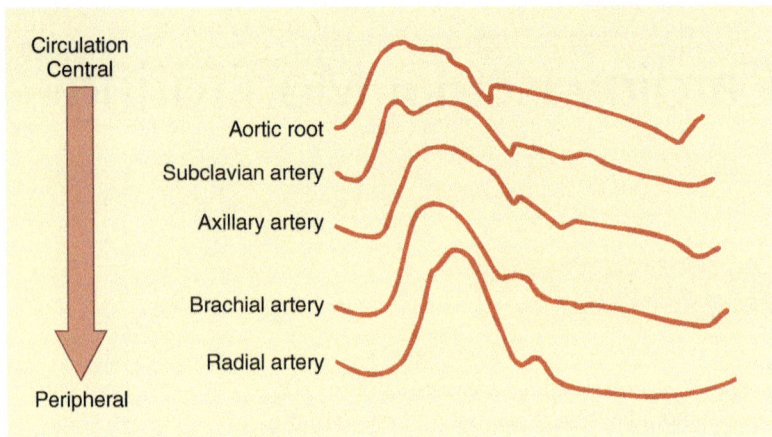

FIGURE 5–1 Changes in configuration as a waveform moves peripherally. (Reproduced, with permission, from Shah N, Bedford RF: Invasive and noninvasive blood pressuring monitoring. In: *Clinical Monitoring: Practical Applications in Anesthesia and Critical Care Medicine.* Lake CL, Hines RL, Blitt CD [editors]. WB Saunders, Philadelphia, 2001.)

an exaggeration of systolic and pulse pressures (Figure 5–1). For example, radial artery systolic pressure is usually greater than aortic systolic pressure because of its more distal location. In contrast, radial artery systolic pressures often underestimate more "central" pressures following hypothermic cardiopulmonary bypass because of changes in hand vascular resistance. Vasodilating drugs may accentuate this discrepancy. The level of the sampling site relative to the heart affects the measurement of blood pressure because of the effect of gravity (Figure 5–2). In patients with severe peripheral vascular disease, there may be a significant difference in blood pressure measurements among the extremities. The higher value should be used in these patients.

Because noninvasive (palpation, Doppler, auscultation, oscillometry, plethysmography) and invasive (arterial cannulation) methods of blood pressure determination differ greatly, they are discussed separately.

1. Noninvasive Arterial Blood Pressure Monitoring

Indications

The use of any anesthetic, no matter how "trivial," is an indication for arterial blood pressure measurement. The techniques and frequency of pressure determination depend on the patient's condition and the type of surgical procedure. An oscillometric

blood pressure measurement every 3–5 min is adequate in most cases.

Contraindications

Although some method of blood pressure measurement is mandatory, techniques that rely on a blood pressure cuff are best avoided in extremities with vascular abnormalities (eg, dialysis shunts) or with intravenous lines. Rarely, it may prove impossible to monitor blood pressure in cases (eg, burns) in which there may be no accessible site from which the blood pressure can be safely recorded.

Techniques & Complications

A. Palpation

SBP can be determined by (1) locating a palpable peripheral pulse, (2) inflating a blood pressure cuff proximal to the pulse until flow is occluded, (3) releasing cuff pressure by 2 or 3 mm Hg per heartbeat, and (4) measuring the cuff pressure at which pulsations are again palpable. This method tends to underestimate systolic pressure, however, because of the insensitivity of touch and the delay between flow under the cuff and distal pulsations. Palpation does not provide a diastolic pressure or MAP. The equipment required is simple and inexpensive.

B. Doppler Probe

When a Doppler probe is substituted for the anesthesiologist's finger, arterial blood pressure

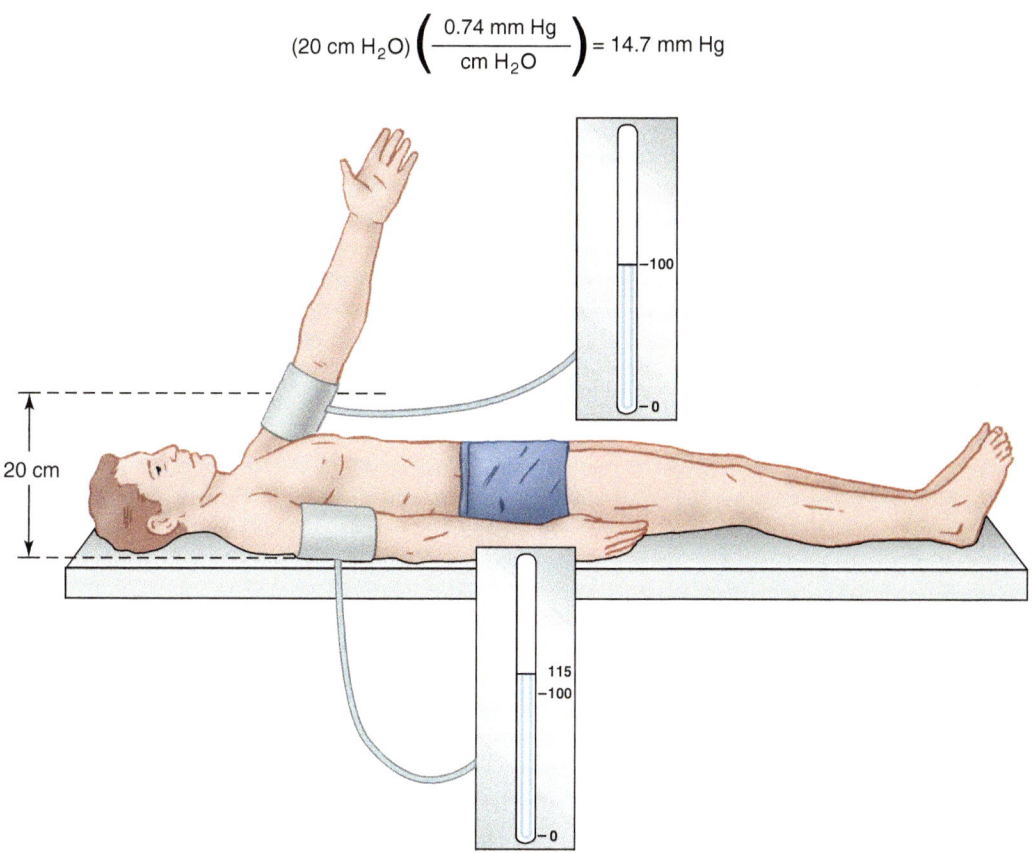

$$(20 \text{ cm H}_2\text{O}) \left(\frac{0.74 \text{ mm Hg}}{\text{cm H}_2\text{O}} \right) = 14.7 \text{ mm Hg}$$

FIGURE 5–2 The difference in blood pressure (mm Hg) at two different sites of measurement equals the height of an interposed column of water (cm H$_2$O) multiplied by a conversion factor (1 cm H$_2$O = 0.74 mm Hg).

measurement becomes sensitive enough to be useful in obese patients, pediatric patients, and patients in shock (**Figure 5–3**). The **Doppler effect** is the shift in the frequency of sound waves when their source moves relative to the observer. For example, the pitch of a train's whistle increases as a train approaches and decreases as it departs. Similarly, the reflection of sound waves off of a moving object causes a frequency shift. A Doppler probe transmits an ultrasonic signal that is reflected by underlying tissue. As red blood cells move through an artery, a Doppler frequency shift will be detected by the probe. The difference between transmitted and received frequency causes the characteristic swishing sound, which indicates blood flow. Because air reflects ultrasound,

a coupling gel (but not corrosive electrode jelly) is applied between the probe and the skin. Positioning the probe directly above an artery is crucial, since the beam must pass through the vessel wall. Interference from probe movement or electrocautery is an annoying distraction. Note that only systolic pressures can be reliably determined with the Doppler technique.

A variation of Doppler technology uses a piezoelectric crystal to detect lateral arterial wall movement to the intermittent opening and closing of vessels between systolic and diastolic pressure. This instrument thus detects both systolic and diastolic pressures. The Doppler effect is routinely employed by perioperative echocardiographers to discern both the directionality and velocity of both blood flow

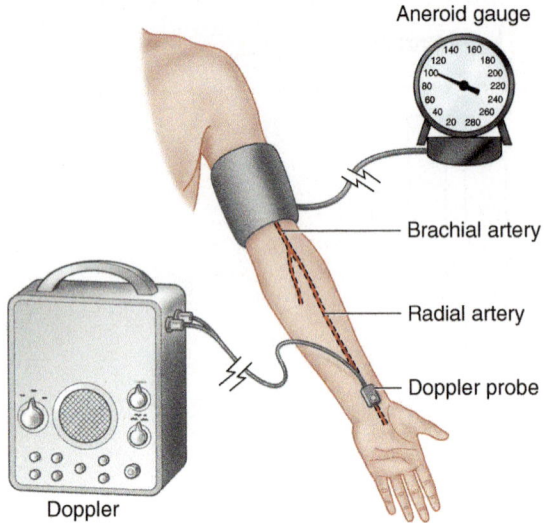

Aneroid gauge

Brachial artery

Radial artery

Doppler probe

Doppler

FIGURE 5–3 A Doppler probe secured over the radial artery will sense red blood cell movement as long as the blood pressure cuff is below systolic pressure. (Reproduced, with permission, from Parks Medical Electronics.)

within the heart and the movement of the heart's muscle tissue (tissue Doppler).

C. Auscultation

Inflation of a blood pressure cuff to a pressure between systolic and diastolic pressures will partially collapse an underlying artery, producing turbulent flow and the characteristic Korotkoff sounds. These sounds are audible through a stethoscope placed under—or just distal to—the distal third of the blood pressure cuff. The clinician measures pressure with an aneroid or mercury manometer.

Occasionally, Korotkoff sounds cannot be heard through part of the range from systolic to diastolic pressure. This auscultatory gap is most common in hypertensive patients and can lead to an inaccurate diastolic pressure measurement. Korotkoff sounds are often difficult to auscultate during episodes of hypotension or marked peripheral vasoconstriction. In these situations, the subsonic frequencies associated with the sounds can be detected by a microphone and amplified to indicate systolic and diastolic pressures. Motion artifact and electrocautery interference limit the usefulness of this method.

D. Oscillometry

Arterial pulsations cause oscillations in cuff pressure. These oscillations are small if the cuff is inflated above systolic pressure. When the cuff pressure decreases to systolic pressure, the pulsations are transmitted to the entire cuff, and the oscillations markedly increase. Maximal oscillation occurs at the MAP, after which oscillations decrease. Because some oscillations are present above and below arterial blood pressure, a mercury or aneroid manometer provides an inaccurate and unreliable measurement. Automated blood pressure monitors electronically measure the pressures at which the oscillation amplitudes change (Figure 5–4). A microprocessor derives systolic, mean, and diastolic pressures using an algorithm. Machines that require identical consecutive pulse waves for measurement confirmation may be unreliable during arrhythmias (eg, atrial fibrillation). Oscillometric monitors should not be used on patients on cardiopulmonary bypass. Nonetheless, the speed, accuracy, and versatility of oscillometric devices have greatly improved, and they have become the preferred noninvasive blood pressure monitors in the United States and worldwide.

E. Arterial Tonometry

Arterial tonometry measures beat-to-beat arterial blood pressure by sensing the pressure required to partially flatten a superficial artery that is supported by a bony structure (eg, radial artery). A tonometer consisting of several independent pressure transducers is applied to the skin overlying the artery (Figure 5–5). The contact stress between the transducer directly over the artery and the skin reflects intraluminal pressure. Continuous pulse recordings produce a tracing very similar to an invasive arterial blood pressure waveform. Limitations to this technology include sensitivity to movement artifact and the need for frequent calibration.

Clinical Considerations

Adequate oxygen delivery to vital organs must be maintained during anesthesia. Unfortunately, instruments to monitor specific organ perfusion and oxygenation are complex, expensive, and often unreliable, and, for that reason, an adequate arterial

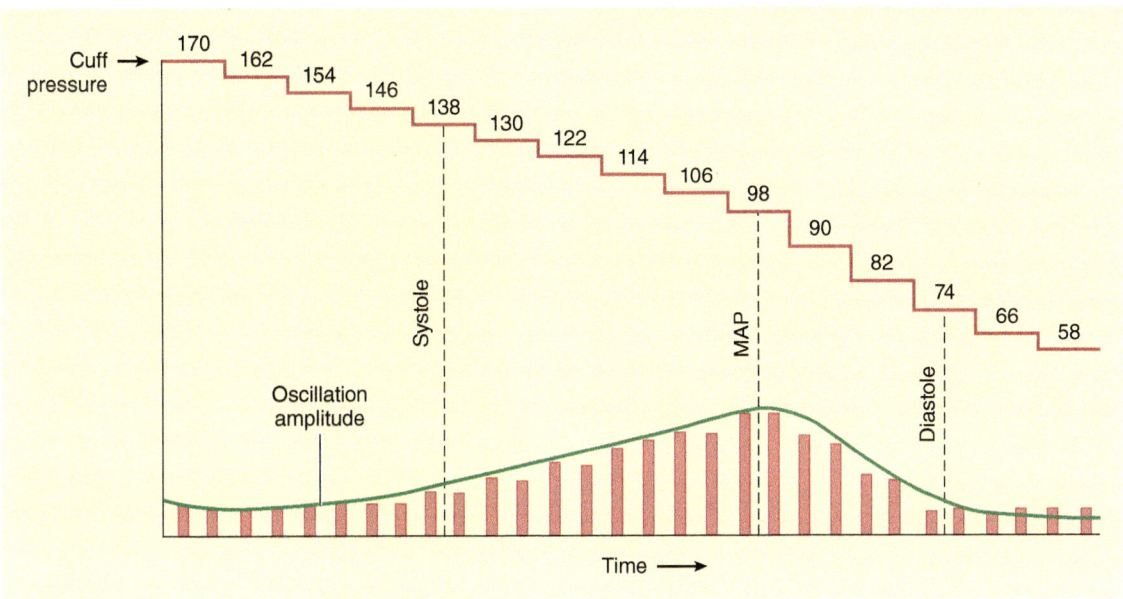

FIGURE 5–4 Oscillometric determination of blood pressure.

blood pressure is assumed to predict adequate organ blood flow. However, flow also depends on vascular resistance:

$$\text{Flow} = \frac{\text{Pressure}}{\text{Resistance}}$$

Even if the pressure is high, when the resistance is also high, flow can be low. Thus, arterial blood pressure should be viewed as an indicator—but not a measure—of organ perfusion.

The accuracy of any method of blood pressure measurement that involves a blood pressure cuff depends on proper cuff size (**Figure 5–6**). The cuff's bladder should extend at least halfway around the extremity, and the width of the cuff should be 20% to 50% greater than the diameter of the extremity.

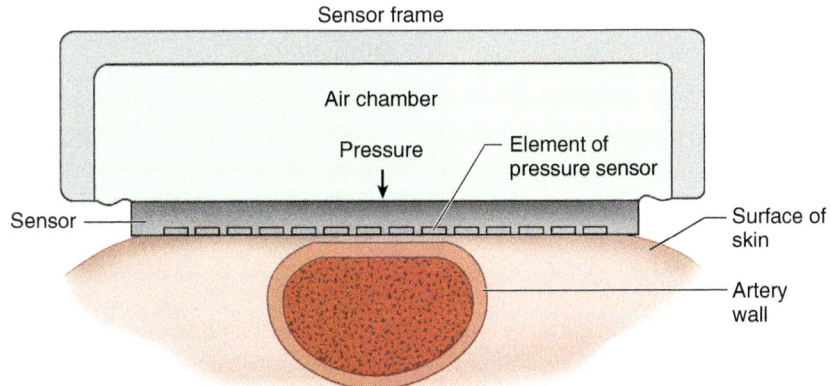

FIGURE 5–5 Tonometry is a method of continuous (beat-to-beat) arterial blood pressure determination. The sensors must be positioned directly over the artery.

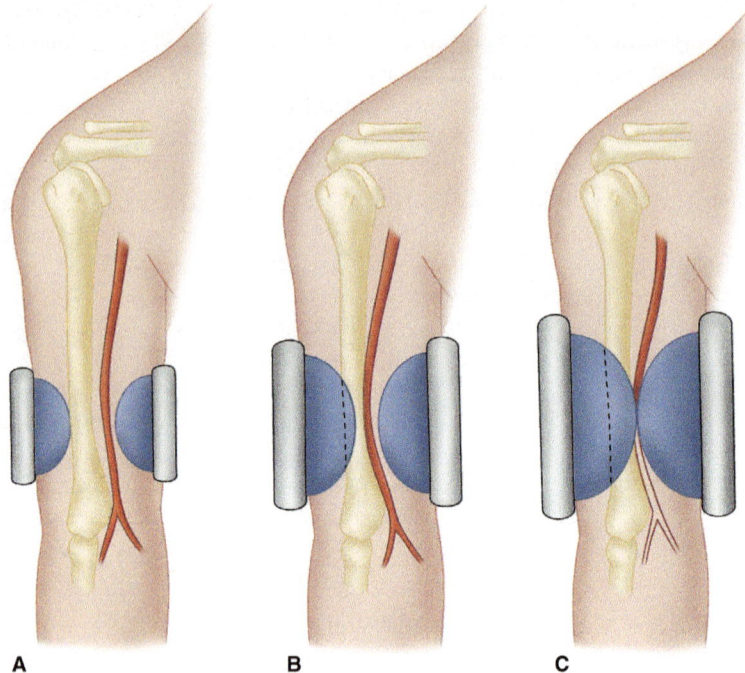

FIGURE 5–6 Blood pressure cuff width influences the pressure readings. Three cuffs, all inflated to the same pressure, are shown. The narrowest cuff (**A**) will require more pressure, and the widest cuff (**C**) less pressure, to occlude the brachial artery for determination of systolic pressure. Too narrow a cuff may produce a large overestimation of systolic pressure. Whereas the wider cuff may underestimate the systolic pressure, the error with a cuff 20% too wide is not as significant as the error with a cuff 20% too narrow. (Reproduced, with permission, from Gravenstein JS, Paulus DA: *Clinical Monitoring Practice*, 2nd ed. Lippincott, Philadelphia, 1987.)

A   **B**   **C**

Automated blood pressure monitors, using one or a combination of the methods described above, are frequently used in anesthesiology. A self-contained air pump inflates the cuff at set intervals. Incorrect or too frequent use of these automated devices has resulted in nerve palsies and extensive extravasation of intravenously administered fluids. In case of equipment failure, an alternative method of blood pressure determination must be immediately available.

2. Invasive Arterial Blood Pressure Monitoring

Indications

Indications for invasive arterial blood pressure monitoring by catheterization of an artery include induced current or anticipated hypotension or wide blood pressure deviations, end-organ disease necessitating precise beat-to-beat blood pressure regulation, and the need for multiple arterial blood gas measurements.

Contraindications

If possible, catheterization should be avoided in smaller end arteries with inadequate collateral blood flow or in extremities where there is a suspicion of preexisting vascular insufficiency.

A. Selection of Artery for Cannulation

Several arteries are available for percutaneous catheterization.

1. The **radial artery** is commonly cannulated because of its superficial location and substantial collateral flow (in most patients the ulnar artery is larger than the radial and there are connections between the two via the palmar arches). Five percent of patients have incomplete palmar arches and lack adequate collateral blood flow. Allen's test is a simple, but not reliable, method for assessing the safety of radial artery cannulation. In this test, the patient exsanguinates his or her hand by making a fist. While the operator occludes

the radial and ulnar arteries with fingertip pressure, the patient relaxes the blanched hand. Collateral flow through the palmar arterial arch is confirmed by flushing of the thumb within 5 sec after pressure on the ulnar artery is released. Delayed return of normal color (5–10 s) indicates an equivocal test or insufficient collateral circulation (>10 s). The Allen's test is of such questionable utility that many practitioners routinely avoid it. Alternatively, blood flow distal to the radial artery occlusion can be detected by palpation, Doppler probe, plethysmography, or pulse oximetry. Unlike Allen's test, these methods of determining the adequacy of collateral circulation do not require patient cooperation.

2. **Ulnar artery** catheterization is usually more difficult than radial catheterization because of the ulnar artery's deeper and more tortuous course. Because of the risk of compromising blood flow to the hand, ulnar catheterization would not normally be considered if the ipsilateral radial artery has been punctured but unsuccessfully cannulated.

3. The **brachial artery** is large and easily identifiable in the antecubital fossa. Its proximity to the aorta provides less waveform distortion. However, being near the elbow predisposes brachial artery catheters to kinking.

4. The **femoral artery** is prone to atheroma formation and pseudoaneurysm, but often provides an excellent access. The femoral site has been associated with an increased incidence of infectious complications and arterial thrombosis. Aseptic necrosis of the head of the femur is a rare, but tragic, complication of femoral artery cannulation in children.

5. The **dorsalis pedis and posterior tibial arteries** are some distance from the aorta and therefore have the most distorted waveforms.

6. The **axillary artery** is surrounded by the axillary plexus, and nerve damage can result from a hematoma or traumatic cannulation. Air or thrombi can quickly gain access to the cerebral circulation during vigorous retrograde flushing of axillary artery catheters.

B. Technique of Radial Artery Cannulation

One technique of radial artery cannulation is illustrated in **Figure 5–7**. Supination and extension of the wrist provide optimal exposure of the radial artery. The pressure–tubing–transducer system should be nearby and already flushed with saline to ensure easy and quick connection after cannulation. The radial pulse is palpated, and the artery's course is determined by lightly pressing the *tips* of the index and middle fingers of the anesthesiologist's nondominant hand over the area of maximal impulse or by use of ultrasound. Using aseptic technique, 1% lidocaine is infiltrated in the skin of awake patients, directly above the artery, with a small gauge needle. A larger gauge needle can then be used as a skin punch, facilitating entry of an 18-, 20-, or 22-gauge catheter over a needle through the skin at a 45° angle, directing it toward the point of palpation. Upon blood flashback, a guidewire may be advanced through the catheter into the artery and the catheter advanced over the guidewire. Alternatively, the needle is lowered to a 30° angle and advanced another 1–2 mm to make certain that the tip of the catheter is well into the vessel lumen. The catheter is advanced off the needle into the arterial lumen, after which the needle is withdrawn. Applying firm pressure over the artery proximal to the catheter tip, with the middle and ring fingertips, prevents blood from spurting from the catheter while the tubing is connected. Waterproof tape or suture can be used to hold the catheter in place.

C. Complications

Complications of intraarterial monitoring include hematoma, bleeding (particularly with catheter tubing disconnections), vasospasm, arterial thrombosis, embolization of air bubbles or thrombi, pseudoaneurysm formation, necrosis of skin overlying the catheter, nerve damage, infection, necrosis of extremities or digits, and unintentional intraarterial drug injection. Factors associated with an increased rate of complications include prolonged cannulation, hyperlipidemia, repeated insertion attempts, female gender, extracorporeal circulation, the use of larger catheters in smaller vessels, and the use of vasopressors. The risks are minimized when the ratio of catheter to artery size is small, saline is

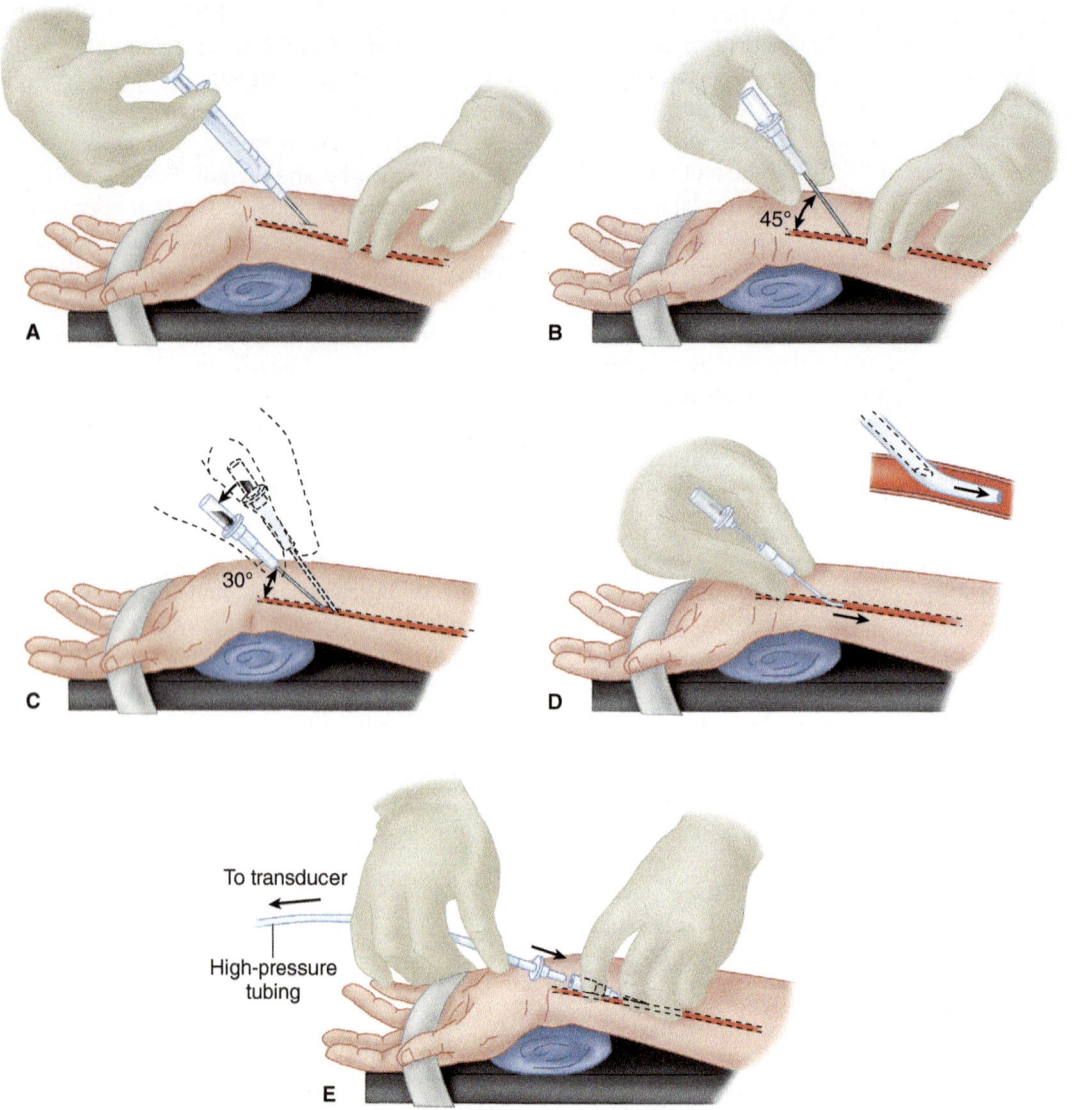

FIGURE 5–7 Cannulation of the radial artery. **A:** Proper positioning and palpation of the artery are crucial. After skin preparation, local anesthetic is infiltrated with a 25-gauge needle. **B:** A 20- or 22-gauge catheter is advanced through the skin at a 45° angle. **C:** Flashback of blood signals entry into the artery, and the catheter– needle assembly is lowered to a 30° angle and advanced 1–2 mm to ensure an intraluminal catheter position. **D:** The catheter is advanced over the needle, which is withdrawn. **E:** Proximal pressure with middle and ring fingers prevents blood loss, while the arterial tubing Luer-lock connector is secured to the intraarterial catheter.

continuously infused through the catheter at a rate of 2–3 mL/hr, flushing of the catheter is limited, and meticulous attention is paid to aseptic technique. Adequacy of perfusion can be continually monitored during radial artery cannulation by placing a pulse oximeter on an ipsilateral finger.

Clinical Considerations

Because intraarterial cannulation allows continuous beat-to-beat blood pressure measurement, it is considered the optimal blood pressure monitoring technique. The quality of the transduced waveform, however, depends on the dynamic characteristics of

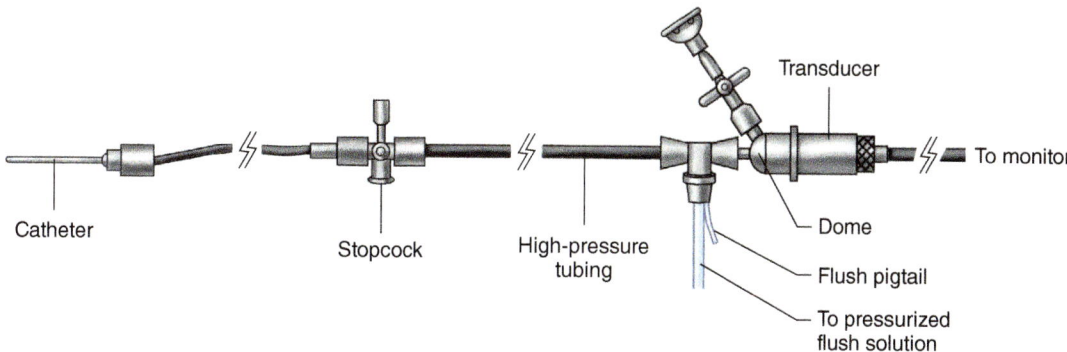

FIGURE 5–8 The catheter–tubing–transducer system.

the catheter–tubing–transducer system (Figure 5–8). False readings can lead to inappropriate therapeutic interventions.

A complex waveform, such as an arterial pulse wave, can be expressed as a summation of simple harmonic waves (according to the Fourier theorem). For accurate measurement of pressure, the catheter–tubing–transducer system must be capable of responding adequately to the highest frequency of the arterial waveform (Figure 5–9). Stated another way, the natural frequency of the measuring system must exceed the natural frequency of the arterial pulse (approximately 16–24 Hz).

Most transducers have frequencies of several hundred Hz (>200 Hz for disposable transducers).

The addition of tubing, stopcocks, and air in the line all decrease the frequency of the system. If the frequency response is too low, the system will be overdamped and will not faithfully reproduce the arterial waveform, underestimating the systolic pressure. Underdamping is also a serious problem, leading to overshoot and a falsely high SBP.

Catheter–tubing–transducer systems must also prevent **hyperresonance,** an artifact caused by reverberation of pressure waves within the system. A **damping coefficient** (β) of 0.6–0.7 is optimal. The natural frequency and damping coefficient can be determined by examining tracing oscillations after a high-pressure flush (Figure 5–10).

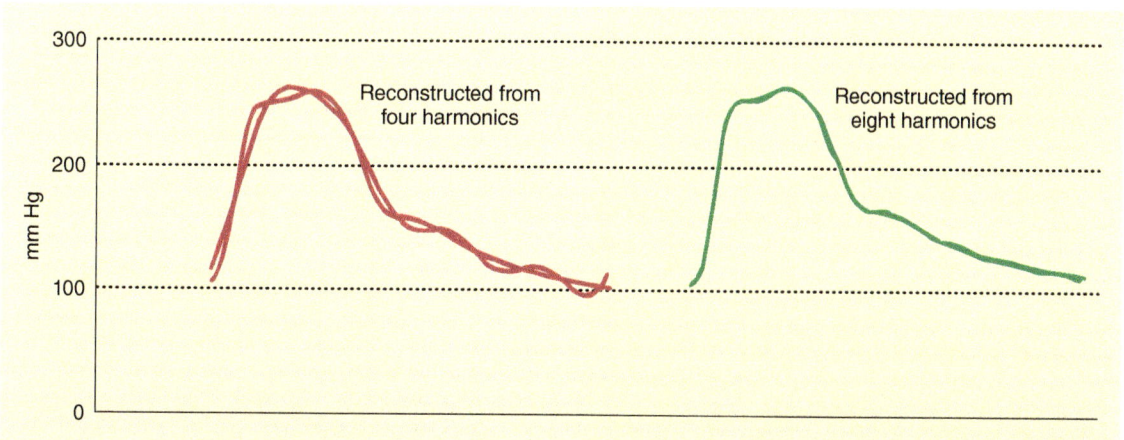

FIGURE 5–9 An original waveform overlays a four-harmonic reconstruction (*left*) and an eight-harmonic reconstruction (*right*). Note that the higher harmonic plot more closely resembles the original waveform. (Reproduced, with permission, from Saidman LS, Smith WT: *Monitoring in Anesthesia.* Butterworth-Heinemann, 1985.)

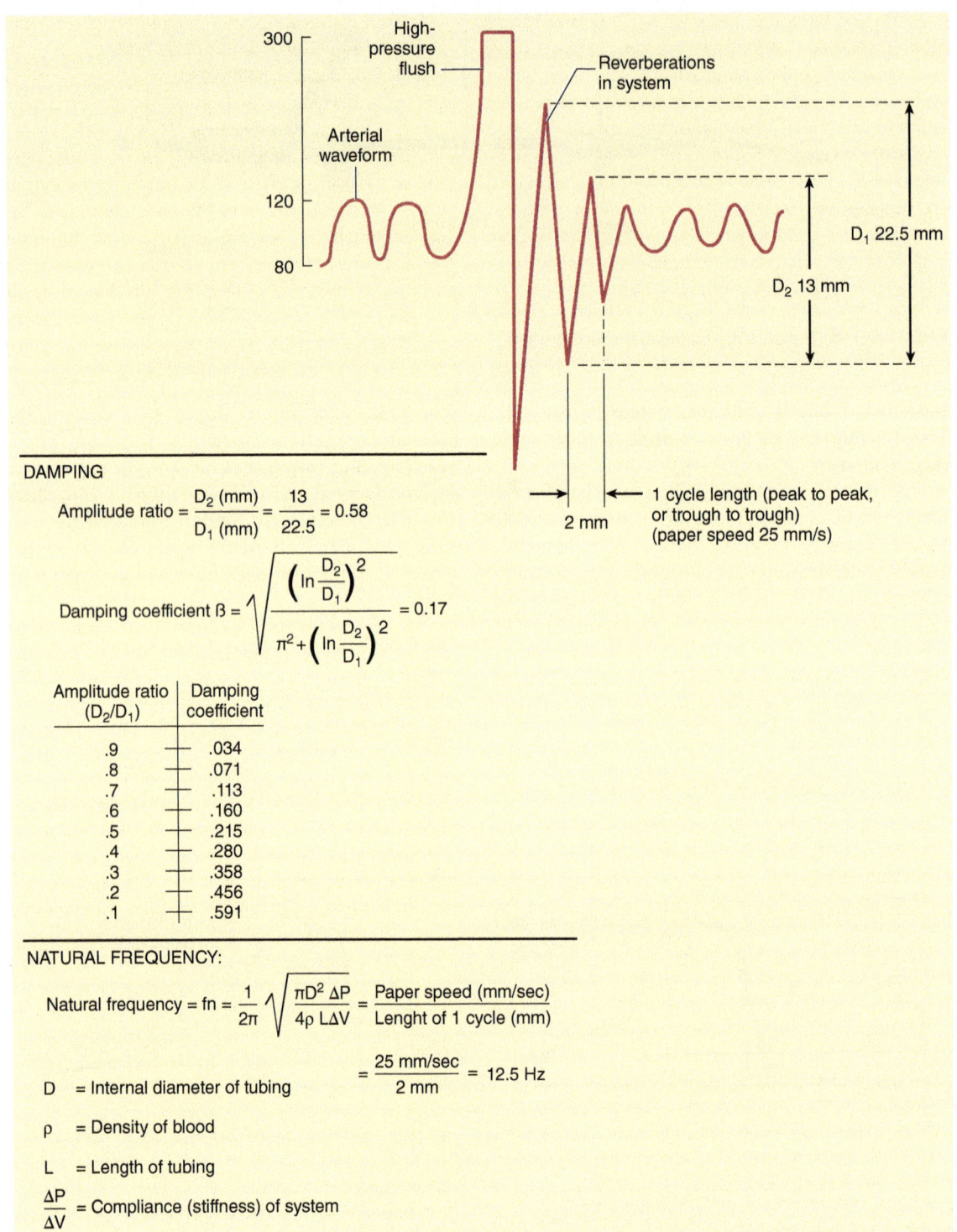

DAMPING

$$\text{Amplitude ratio} = \frac{D_2 \text{ (mm)}}{D_1 \text{ (mm)}} = \frac{13}{22.5} = 0.58$$

$$\text{Damping coefficient } \beta = \sqrt{\frac{\left(\ln\frac{D_2}{D_1}\right)^2}{\pi^2 + \left(\ln\frac{D_2}{D_1}\right)^2}} = 0.17$$

Amplitude ratio (D_2/D_1)	Damping coefficient
.9	.034
.8	.071
.7	.113
.6	.160
.5	.215
.4	.280
.3	.358
.2	.456
.1	.591

NATURAL FREQUENCY:

$$\text{Natural frequency} = fn = \frac{1}{2\pi}\sqrt{\frac{\pi D^2 \, \Delta P}{4\rho \, L\Delta V}} = \frac{\text{Paper speed (mm/sec)}}{\text{Lenght of 1 cycle (mm)}}$$

$$= \frac{25 \text{ mm/sec}}{2 \text{ mm}} = 12.5 \text{ Hz}$$

D = Internal diameter of tubing

ρ = Density of blood

L = Length of tubing

$\dfrac{\Delta P}{\Delta V}$ = Compliance (stiffness) of system

FIGURE 5–10 Damping and natural frequency of a transducer system can be determined by a high-pressure flush test.

System dynamics are improved by minimizing tubing length, eliminating unnecessary stopcocks, removing air bubbles, and using low-compliance tubing. Although smaller diameter catheters lower natural frequency, they improve underdampened systems and are less apt to result in vascular complications. If a large catheter totally occludes an artery, reflected waves can distort pressure measurements.

Pressure transducers have evolved from bulky, reusable instruments to miniaturized, disposable devices. Transducers contain a diaphragm that is distorted by an arterial pressure wave. The mechanical energy of a pressure wave is converted into an electric signal. Most transducers are resistance types that are based on the **strain gauge** principle: stretching a wire or silicone crystal changes its electrical resistance. The sensing elements are arranged as a "Wheatstone bridge" circuit so that the voltage output is proportionate to the pressure applied to the diaphragm (Figure 5–11).

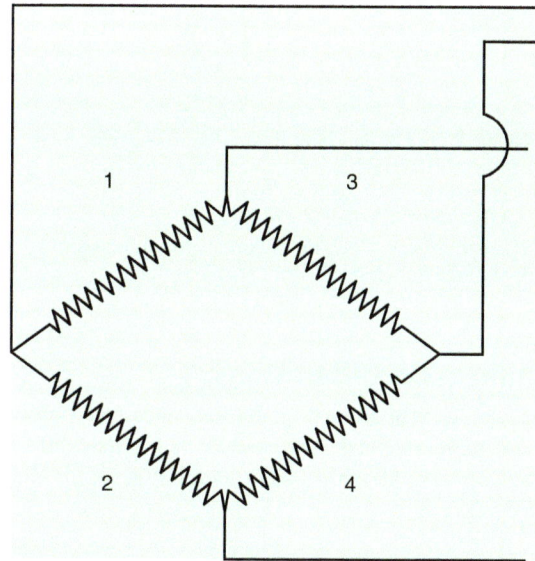

FIGURE 5–11 In the original strain gauge pressure transducers, a deformable diaphragm was connected to a Wheatstone bridge. When pressure was applied to the diaphragm, strain on two of the resistors (No. 2 and No. 3) increased, whereas strain on the other two (No. 1 and No. 4) decreased. The change in total resistance across the bridge was proportional to the change in blood pressure, allowing direct accurate measurement of intravascular blood pressure for the first time.

Transducer accuracy depends on correct calibration and zeroing procedures. A stopcock at the level of the desired point of measurement—usually the midaxillary line—is opened, and the zero trigger on the monitor is activated. If the patient's position is altered by raising or lowering the operating table, the transducer must either be moved in tandem or zeroed to the new level of the midaxillary line. In a seated patient, the arterial pressure in the brain differs significantly from left ventricular pressure. In this circumstance, cerebral pressure is determined by setting the transducer to zero at the level of the ear, which approximates the circle of Willis. The transducer's zero should be checked regularly, as some transducer measurements can "drift" over time.

External calibration of a transducer compares the transducer's reading with a manometer, but modern transducers rarely require external calibration.

Digital readouts of systolic and diastolic pressures are a running average of the highest and lowest measurements within a certain time interval. Because motion or cautery artifacts can result in some very misleading numbers, the arterial waveform should always be monitored. The shape of the arterial wave provides clues to several hemodynamic variables. The rate of upstroke indicates contractility, the rate of downstroke indicates peripheral vascular resistance, and exaggerated variations in size during the respiratory cycle suggest hypovolemia. MAP is calculated by integrating the area under the pressure curve.

Intraarterial catheters also provide access for intermittent arterial blood gas sampling and analysis. The development of fiberoptic sensors that can be inserted through a 20-gauge arterial catheter enables continuous blood gas monitoring. Unfortunately, these sensors are quite expensive and are often inaccurate, so they are rarely used. Analysis of the arterial pressure waveform allows for estimation of cardiac output (CO) and other hemodynamic parameters. These devices are discussed in the section on CO monitoring.

ELECTROCARDIOGRAPHY
Indications & Contraindications

All patients should have intraoperative monitoring of their electrocardiogram (ECG). There are no contraindications.

Techniques & Complications

Lead selection determines the diagnostic sensitivity of the ECG. ECG leads are positioned on the chest and extremities to provide different perspectives of the electrical potentials generated by the heart. At the end of diastole, the atria contract, which provides the atrial contribution to CO, generating the "P" wave. Following atrial contraction, the ventricle is loaded awaiting systole. The QRS complex begins the electrical activity of systole following the 120–200 msec atrioventricular (AV) nodal delay. Depolarization of the ventricle proceeds from the AV node through the interventricular system via the His–Purkinje fibers. The normal QRS lasts approximately 120 msec, which can be prolonged in patients with cardiomyopathies and heart failure. The T wave represents repolarization as the heart prepares to contract again. Prolongation of the QT interval secondary to electrolyte imbalances or drug effects can potentially lead to life-threatening arrhythmias (les torsade de pointes).

The electrical axis of lead II is approximately 60° from the right arm to the left leg, which is parallel to the electrical axis of the atria, resulting in the largest P-wave voltages of any surface lead. This orientation enhances the diagnosis of arrhythmias and the detection of inferior wall ischemia. Lead V_5 lies over the fifth intercostal space at the anterior axillary line; this position is a good compromise for detecting anterior and lateral wall ischemia. A true V_5 lead is possible only on operating room ECGs with at least five lead wires, but a modified V_5 can be monitored by rearranging the standard three-limb lead placement (Figure 5–12). Ideally, because each lead provides unique information, leads II and V_5 should be monitored simultaneously. If only a single-channel machine is available, the preferred lead for monitoring depends on the location of any prior infarction or ischemia. Esophageal leads are even better than lead II for arrhythmia diagnosis, but have not yet gained general acceptance in the operating room.

Electrodes are placed on the patient's body to monitor the ECG (Figure 5–13). Conductive gel lowers the skin's electrical resistance, which can be further decreased by cleansing the site with alcohol. Needle electrodes are used only if the disks are unsuitable (eg, with an extensively burned patient).

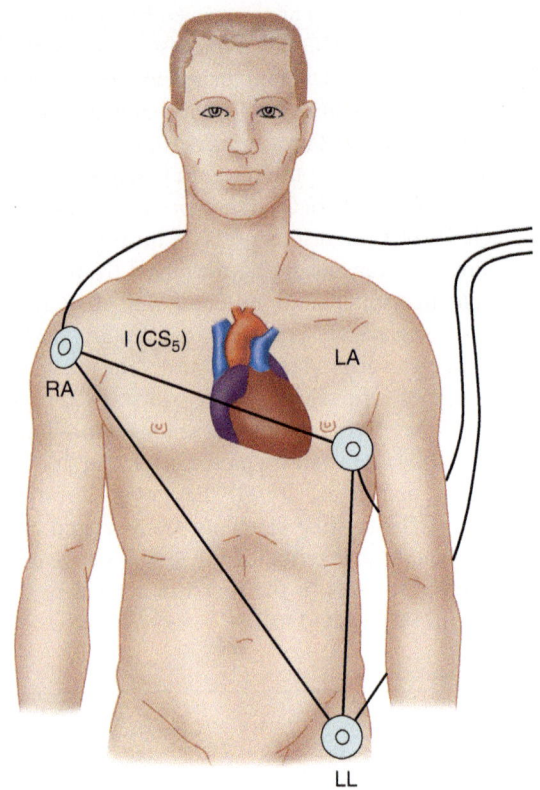

FIGURE 5–12 Rearranged three-limb lead placement. Anterior and lateral ischemia can be detected by placing the left arm lead (LA) at the V_5 position. When lead I is selected on the monitor, a modified V_5 lead (CS_5) is displayed. Lead II allows detection of arrhythmias and inferior wall ischemia. RA, right arm; LL, left leg.

Clinical Considerations

The ECG is a recording of the electrical potentials generated by myocardial cells. Its routine use allows arrhythmias, myocardial ischemia,

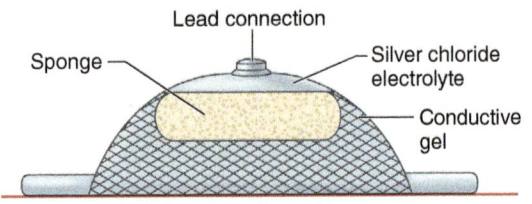

FIGURE 5–13 A cross-sectional view of a silver chloride electrode.

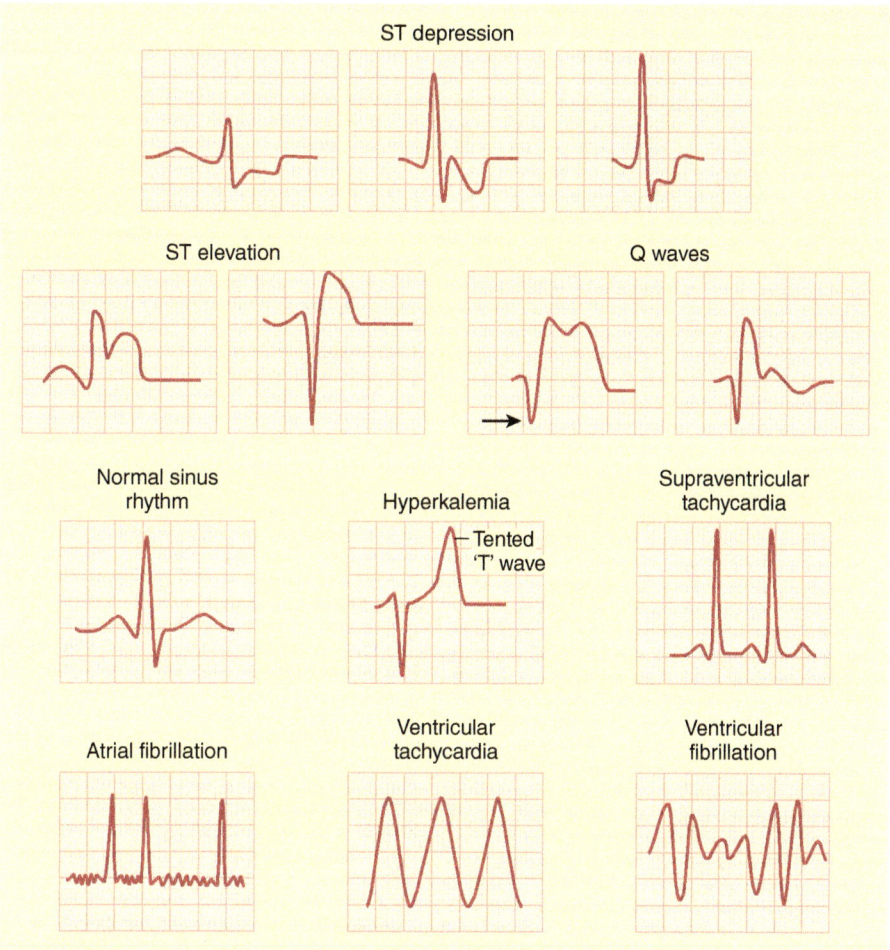

FIGURE 5–14 Common ECG findings during cardiac surgery. (Redrawn and reproduced, with permission, from Wasnick J, Hillel Z, Kramer D, et al: *Cardiac Anesthesia & Transesophageal Echocardiography,* McGraw-Hill, 2011.)

conduction abnormalities, pacemaker malfunction, and electrolyte disturbances to be detected (Figure 5–14). Because of the small voltage potentials being measured, artifacts remain a major problem. Patient or lead-wire movement, use of electrocautery, 60-cycle interference from nearby alternating current devices, and faulty electrodes can simulate arrhythmias. Monitoring filters incorporated into the amplifier to reduce "motion" artifacts will lead to distortion of the ST segment and may impede the diagnosis of ischemia. Digital readouts of the heart rate (HR) may be misleading because of monitor misinterpretation of artifacts or

large T waves—often seen in pediatric patients—as QRS complexes.

Depending on equipment availability, a preinduction rhythm strip can be printed or frozen on the monitor's screen to compare with intraoperative tracings. To interpret ST-segment changes properly, the ECG must be standardized so that a 1-mV signal results in a deflection of 10 mm on a standard strip monitor. Newer units continuously analyze ST segments for early detection of myocardial ischemia. Automated ST-segment analysis increases the sensitivity of ischemia detection, does not require additional physician skill or vigilance, and may help diagnose intraoperative myocardial ischemia.

Commonly accepted criteria for diagnosing myocardial ischemia require that the ECG be recorded in "diagnostic mode" and include a flat or downsloping ST-segment depression exceeding 1 mm, 80 msec after the J point (the end of the QRS complex), particularly in conjunction with T-wave inversion. ST-segment elevation with peaked T waves can also represent ischemia. Wolff–Parkinson–White syndrome, bundle-branch blocks, extrinsic pacemaker capture, and digoxin therapy may preclude the use of ST-segment information. The audible beep associated with each QRS complex should be loud enough to detect rate and rhythm changes when the anesthesiologist's visual attention is directed elsewhere. Some ECGs are capable of storing aberrant QRS complexes for further analysis, and some can even interpret and diagnose arrhythmias. The interference caused by electrocautery units, however, has limited the usefulness of automated arrhythmia analysis in the operating room.

CENTRAL VENOUS CATHETERIZATION

Indications

Central venous catheterization is indicated for monitoring central venous pressure (CVP), administration of fluid to treat hypovolemia and shock, infusion of caustic drugs and total parenteral nutrition, aspiration of air emboli, insertion of transcutaneous pacing leads, and gaining venous access in patients with poor peripheral veins. With specialized catheters, central venous catheterization can be used for continuous monitoring of central venous oxygen saturation.

Contraindications

Relative contraindications include tumors, clots, or tricuspid valve vegetations that could be dislodged or embolized during cannulation. Other contraindications relate to the cannulation site. For example, subclavian vein cannulation is relatively contraindicated in patients who are receiving anticoagulants (due to the inability to provide direct compression in the event of an accidental arterial puncture). Some clinicians avoid central venous cannulation on the side of a previous carotid endarterectomy due to concerns about the possibility of unintentional carotid artery puncture. The presence of other central catheters or pacemaker leads may reduce the number of sites available for central line placement.

Techniques & Complications

Central venous cannulation involves introducing a catheter into a vein so that the catheter's tip lies with the venous system within the thorax. Generally, the optimal location of the catheter tip is just superior to or at the junction of the superior vena cava and the right atrium. When the catheter tip is located within the thorax, inspiration will increase or decrease CVP, depending on whether ventilation is controlled or spontaneous. Measurement of CVP is made with a water column (cm H_2O), or, preferably, an electronic transducer (mm Hg). The pressure should be measured during end expiration.

Various sites can be used for cannulation (Figure 5–15 and Table 5–1). All cannulation sites have an increased risk of line-related infections the longer the catheter remains in place. Compared with other sites, the subclavian vein is associated with a greater risk of pneumothorax during insertion, but a reduced risk of other complications during prolonged cannulations (eg, in critically ill patients). The right internal jugular vein provides a combination of accessibility and safety. Left-sided internal jugular vein catheterization has an increased risk of pleural effusion and chylothorax. The external jugular veins can also be used as entry sites, but due to the acute angle at which they join the great veins of the chest, are associated with a slightly increased likelihood of failure to gain access to the central circulation than the internal jugular veins. Femoral veins can also be cannulated, but are associated with an increased risk of line-related sepsis. There are at least three cannulation techniques: a catheter over a needle (similar to peripheral catheterization), a catheter through a needle (requiring a large-bore needle stick), and a catheter over a guidewire (Seldinger's technique; Figure 5–16). The overwhelming majority of central lines are placed using Seldinger's technique.

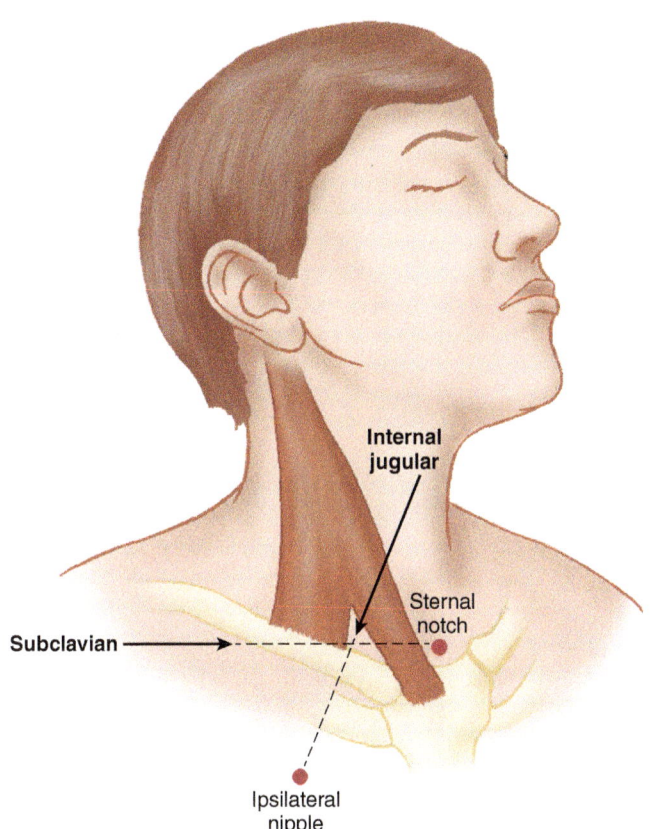

FIGURE 5–15 The subclavian and internal jugular veins are both used for central access perioperatively with the sternal notch and ipsilateral nipple in the direction of needle passage for each, respectively. (Redrawn and reproduced, with permission, from Wasnick J, Hillel Z, Kramer D, et al: *Cardiac Anesthesia & Transesophageal Echocardiography,* McGraw-Hill, 2011.)

The following scenario describes the placement of an internal jugular venous line. The patient is placed in the Trendelenburg position to decrease the risk of air embolism and to distend the internal jugular (or subclavian) vein. Venous catheterization requires full aseptic technique, including scrub, sterile gloves, gown, mask, hat, bactericidal skin preparation (alcohol-based solutions are preferred), and sterile drapes. The two heads of the sternocleidomastoid muscle and the clavicle form the three sides of a triangle (Figure 5–16A). A 25-gauge needle is used to infiltrate the apex of the triangle with local anesthetic. The internal jugular vein can be located using ultrasound, and we strongly

TABLE 5–1   Relative rating of central venous access.[1]

	Basilic	External Jugular	Internal Jugular	Subclavian	Femoral
Ease of cannulation	1	3	2	5	3
Long-term use	4	3	2	1	5
Success rate (pulmonary artery catheter placement)	4	5	1	2	3
Complications (technique-related)	1	2	4	5	3

[1]In each category, 1 = best, 5 = worst.

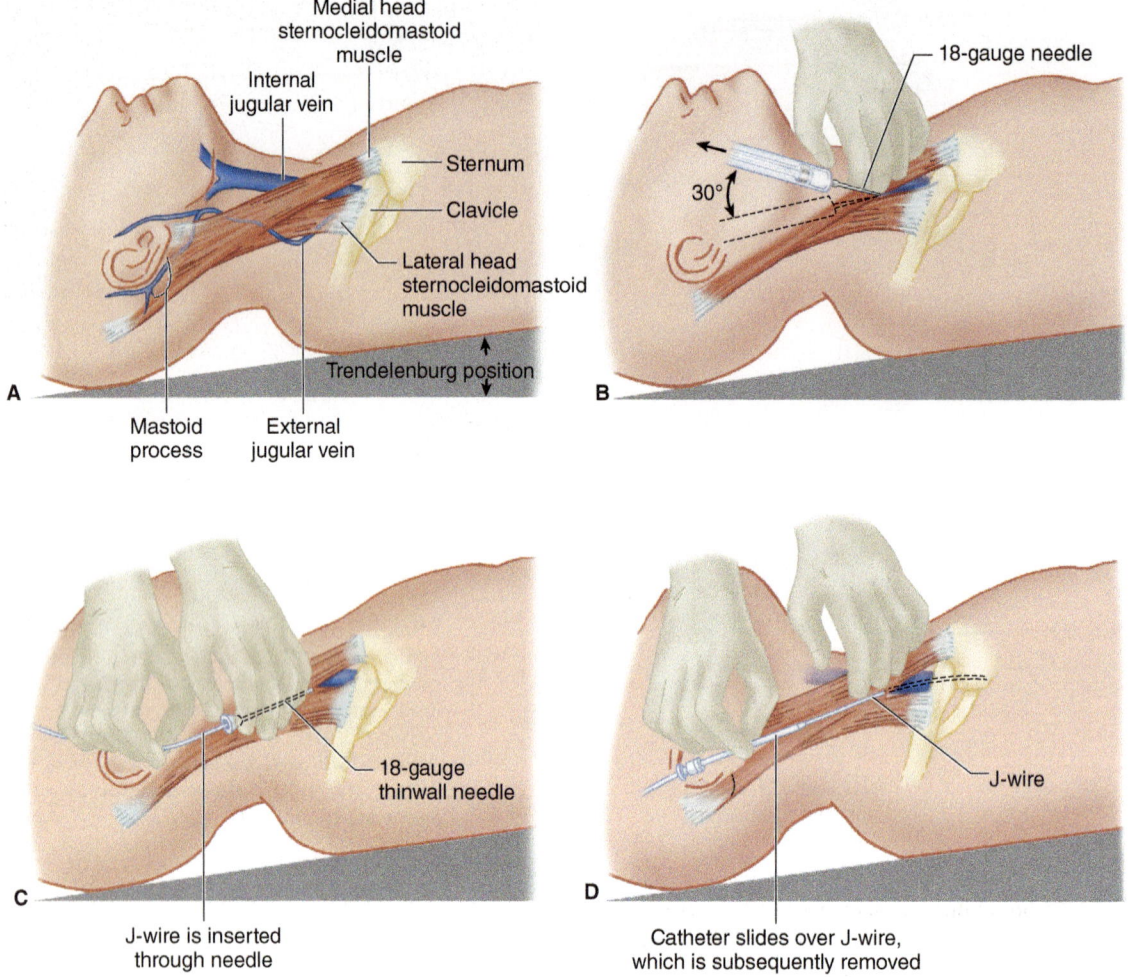

FIGURE 5–16 Right internal jugular cannulation with Seldinger's technique (see text).

recommend that it be used whenever possible (**Figure 5–17**). Alternatively, it may be located by advancing the 25-gauge needle—or a 23-gauge needle in heavier patients—along the medial border of the lateral head of the sternocleidomastoid, toward the ipsilateral nipple, at an angle of 30° to the skin. Aspiration of venous blood confirms the vein's location. It is essential that the vein (and not the artery) be cannulated. Cannulation of the carotid artery can lead to hematoma, stroke, airway compromise, and possibly death. An 18-gauge thin-wall needle or an 18-gauge catheter over needle is advanced along the

same path as the locator needle (Figure 5–16B), and, with the latter apparatus, the needle is removed from the catheter once the catheter has been advanced into the vein. When free blood flow is achieved, a J wire with a 3-mm radius curvature is introduced after confirmation of vein puncture (Figure 5–16C). The needle (or catheter) is removed, and a dilator is advanced over the wire. The catheter is prepared for insertion by flushing all ports with saline, and all distal ports are "capped" or clamped, except the one through which the wire must pass. Next, the dilator is removed, and the final catheter is advanced over

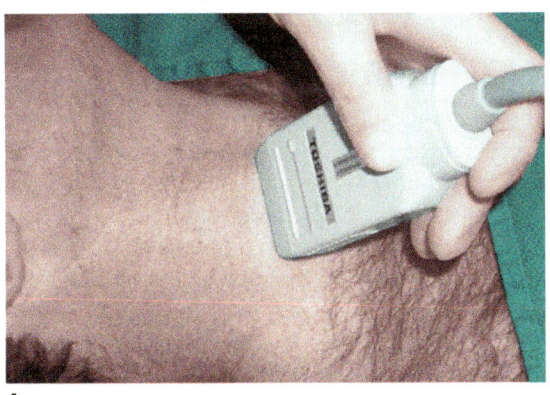

A

FIGURE 5–17 **A**: Probe position for ultrasound of the large internal jugular vein with deeper carotid artery and **B**: corresponding ultrasound image. CA, carotid artery; IJ,

B

internal jugular vein. (Reproduced, with permission, from Tintinalli JE, et al: *Tintinalli's Emergency Medicine: A Comprehensive Study Guide*, 7th edition, McGraw-Hill, 2011.)

the wire (Figure 5–16D). The guidewire is removed, with a thumb placed over the catheter hub to prevent aspiration of air until the intravenous catheter tubing is connected to it. The catheter is then secured, and a sterile dressing is applied. Correct location is confirmed with a chest radiograph. **1** The catheter's tip should not be allowed to migrate into the heart chambers. Fluid-administration sets should be changed frequently, per your medical center protocol.

The possibility of placement of the vein dilator or catheter into the carotid artery can be decreased by transducing the vessel's pressure waveform from the introducer needle (or catheter, if a catheter over needle has been used) before passing the wire (most simply accomplished by using a sterile intravenous extension tubing as a manometer). Alternatively, one may compare the blood's color or Pao_2 with an arterial sample. Blood color and pulsatility can be misleading or inconclusive, and more than one confirmation method should be used. In cases where transesophageal echocardiography (TEE) is used, the guide wire can be seen in the right atrium, confirming venous entry (Figure 5–18).

The risks of central venous cannulation include line infection, blood stream infection, air or thrombus embolism, arrhythmias (indicating that the catheter tip is in the right atrium or ventricle), hematoma, pneumothorax, hemothorax, hydrothorax, chylothorax, cardiac perforation, cardiac tamponade, trauma to nearby nerves and arteries, and thrombosis.

Clinical Considerations

Normal cardiac function requires adequate ventricular filling by venous blood. CVP approximates right atrial pressure. Ventricular volumes are related to pressures through compliance. Highly compliant

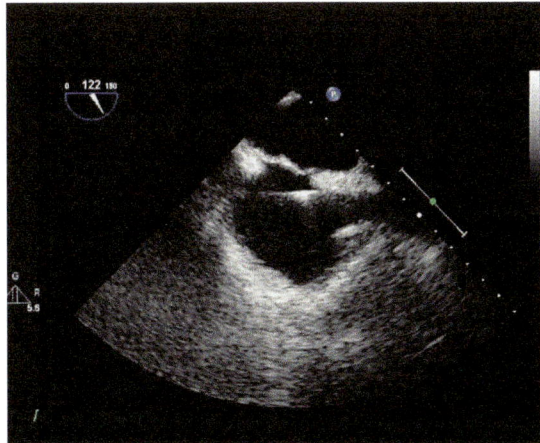

FIGURE 5–18 A wire is seen on this transesophageal echocardiography image of the right atrium.

ventricles accommodate volume with minimal changes in pressure. Noncompliant systems have larger swings in pressure with less volume changes. Consequently, an individual CVP measurement will reveal only limited information about ventricular volumes and filling. Although a very low CVP may indicate a volume-depleted patient, a moderate to high pressure reading may reflect either volume overload or poor ventricular compliance. Changes associated with volume loading coupled with other measures of hemodynamic performance (eg, blood pressure, HR, urine output) may be a better indicator of the patient's volume responsiveness. CVP measurements should always be considered within the context of the patient's overall clinical perspective.

The shape of the central venous waveform corresponds to the events of cardiac contraction (Figure 5–19): *a* waves from *a*trial contraction are absent in atrial fibrillation and are exaggerated in junctional rhythms ("cannon" *a* waves); *c* waves are due to tricuspid valve elevation during early ventricular contraction; *v* waves reflect *v*enous return against a closed tricuspid valve; and the *x* and *y* descents are probably caused by the downward displacement of the tricuspid valve during systole and tricuspid valve opening during diastole.

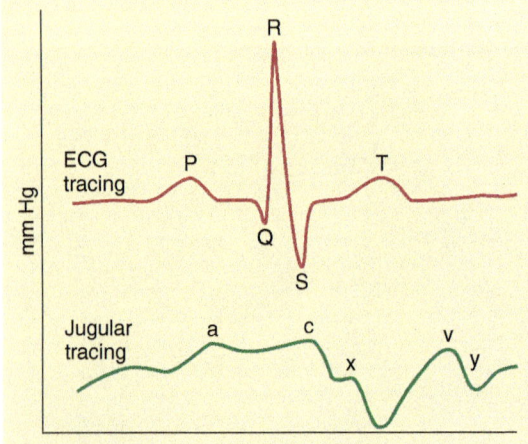

FIGURE 5–19 The upward waves (*a, c, v*) and the downward descents (*x, y*) of a central venous tracing in relation to the electrocardiogram (ECG).

PULMONARY ARTERY CATHETERIZATION

The pulmonary artery (PA) catheter (or Swan-Ganz catheter) was introduced into routine practice in operating rooms and intensive care units in the 1970s. It quickly became common for patients undergoing major surgery to be managed with PA catheterization. The catheter provides measurements of both CO and PA occlusion pressures and was used to guide hemodynamic therapy, especially when patients became unstable. Determination of the PA occlusion or wedge pressure permitted (in the absence of mitral stenosis) an estimation of the left ventricular end-diastolic pressure (LVEDP), and, depending upon ventricular compliance, an estimate of ventricular volume. Through its ability to perform measurements of CO, the patient's stroke volume (SV) was also determined.

$$CO = SV \times HR$$

$$SV = CO/HR$$

Blood pressure = CO × systemic vascular resistance (SVR)

Consequently, hemodynamic monitoring with the PA catheter attempted to discern why a patient was unstable so that therapy could be directed at the underlying problem.

If the SVR is diminished, such as in states of vasodilatory shock (sepsis), the SV may increase. Conversely, a reduction in SV may be secondary to poor cardiac performance or hypovolemia. Determination of the "wedge" or pulmonary capillary occlusion pressure (PCOP) by inflating the catheter balloon estimates the LVEDP. A decreased SV in the setting of a low PCOP/ LVEDP indicates hypovolemia and the need for volume administration. A "full" heart, reflected by a high PCOP/ LVEDP and low SV, indicates the need for a positive inotropic drug. Conversely, a normal or increased SV in the setting of hypotension could be treated with the administration of vasoconstrictor drugs to restore SVR in a vasodilated patient.

Although patients can present concurrently with hypovolemia, sepsis, and heart failure, this basic treatment approach and the use of the

PA catheter to guide therapy became more or less synonymous with perioperative intensive care and cardiac anesthesia. However, numerous large observational studies have shown that patients managed with PA catheters had worse outcomes than similar patients who were managed without PA catheters. Other studies seem to indicate that although PA catheter-guided patient management may do no harm, it offers no specific benefits. Although **2** the PA catheter can be used to guide goal-directed hemodynamic therapy to ensure organ perfusion in shock states, other less invasive methods to determine hemodynamic performance are available, including transpulmonary thermodilution CO measurements and pulse contour analyses of the arterial pressure waveform. Both methods permit calculation of the SV as a guide for hemodynamic management. Moreover, right atrial blood oxygen saturation, as opposed to mixed venous saturation (normal is 75%), can be used as an alternative measure to discern tissue oxygen extraction and the adequacy of tissue oxygen delivery.

Despite numerous reports of its questionable utility and the increasing number of alternative methods to determine hemodynamic parameters, the PA catheter is still employed perioperatively more often in the United States than elsewhere. Although echocardiography can readily inform hemodynamic decision-making through imaging the heart to determine if it is full, compressed, contracting, or empty echocardiography requires a trained individual to obtain and interpret the images. Alternative less invasive hemodynamic monitors have gained acceptance in Europe and may expand in the United States, further decreasing the use of PA catheters.

Until other alternatives are available, PA catheterization should be considered whenever cardiac index, preload, volume status, or the degree of mixed venous blood oxygenation need to be known. These measurements might prove particularly important in surgical patients at high risk for hemodynamic instability (eg, those who recently sustained myocardial infarction) or during surgical procedures associated with an increased incidence of hemodynamic complications (eg, thoracic aortic aneurysm repair).

Contraindications

3 Relative contraindications to pulmonary artery catheterization include left bundle-branch block (because of the concern about complete heart block) and conditions associated with a greatly increased risk of arrhythmias, such as Wolff–Parkinson–White syndrome. A catheter with pacing capability is better suited to these situations. A PA catheter may serve as a nidus of infection in bacteremic patients or thrombus formation in patients prone to hypercoagulation.

Techniques & Complications

Although various PA catheters are available, the most popular design integrates five lumens into a 7.5 FR catheter, 110-cm long, with a polyvinylchloride body (Figure 5–20). The lumens house the

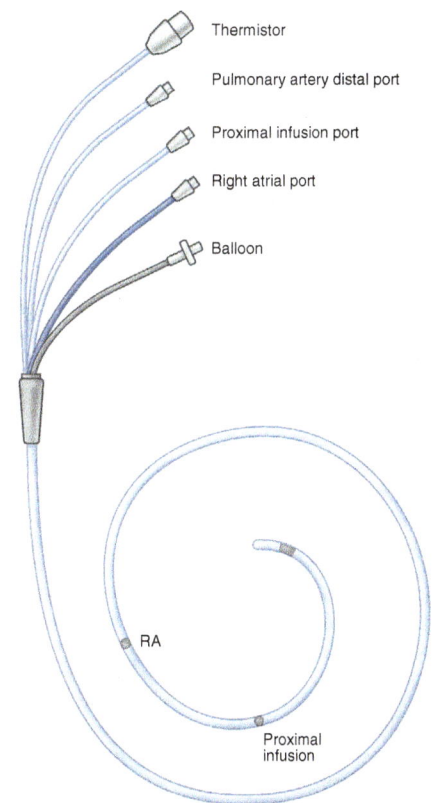

Thermistor

Pulmonary artery distal port

Proximal infusion port

Right atrial port

Balloon

RA

Proximal infusion

FIGURE 5–20 Balloon-tipped pulmonary artery flotation catheter (Swan–Ganz catheter). RA, right atrium.

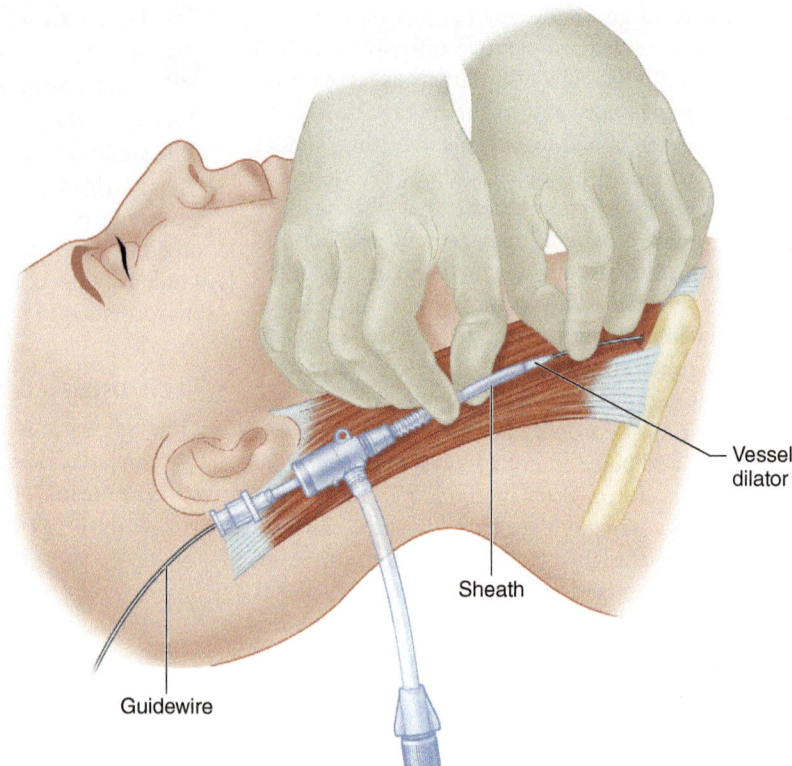

FIGURE 5–21 A percutaneous introducer consisting of a vessel dilator and sheath is passed over the guidewire.

following: wiring to connect the thermistor near the catheter tip to a thermodilution CO computer; an air channel for inflation of the balloon; a proximal port 30 cm from the tip for infusions, CO injections, and measurements of right atrial pressures; a ventricular port at 20 cm for infusion of drugs; and a distal port for aspiration of mixed venous blood samples and measurements of PA pressure.

Insertion of a PA catheter requires central venous access, which can be accomplished using Seldinger's technique, described above. Instead of a central venous catheter, a dilator and sheath are threaded over the guidewire. The sheath's lumen accommodates the PA catheter after removal of the dilator and guidewire (Figure 5–21).

Prior to insertion, the PA catheter is checked by inflating and deflating its balloon and irrigating all three intravascular lumens with saline. The distal port is connected to a transducer that is zeroed to the patient's midaxillary line.

The PA catheter is advanced through the introducer and into the internal jugular vein. At approximately 15 cm, the distal tip should enter the right atrium, and a central venous tracing that varies with respiration confirms an intrathoracic position. The balloon is then inflated with air according to the manufacturer's recommendations (usually 1.5 mL) to protect the endocardium from the catheter tip and to allow the right ventricle's CO to direct the catheter forward. The balloon is always deflated during withdrawal. During the catheter's advancement, the ECG should be monitored for arrhythmias. Transient ectopy from irritation of the right ventricle by the balloon and catheter tip is common and rarely requires treatment. A sudden increase in the *systolic* pressure on the distal tracing indicates a right ventricular location of the catheter tip (Figure 5–22). Entry into the pulmonary artery normally occurs by 35–45 cm and is heralded by a sudden increase in *diastolic* pressure.

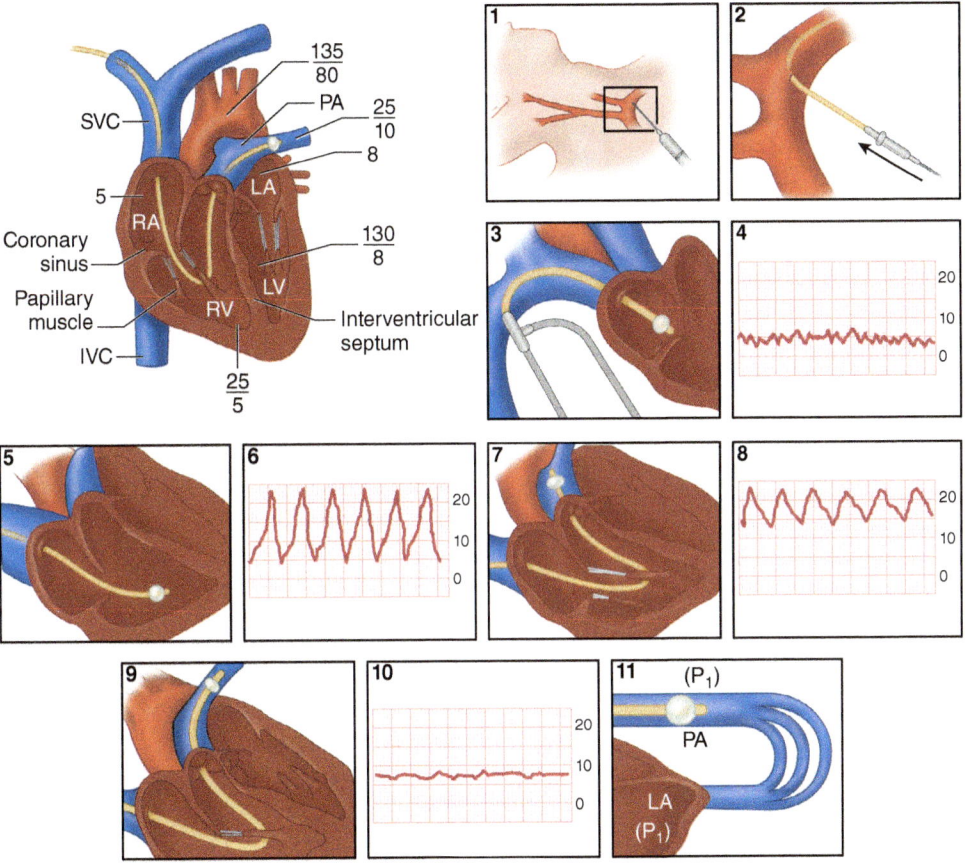

FIGURE 5–22 Although its utility is increasingly questioned, pulmonary artery catheters continue to be a part of perioperative management of the cardiac surgery patient. Following placement of a sheath introducer in the central circulation (panels 1 and 2), the pulmonary artery catheter is floated. Central line placement should always be completed using rigorous sterile technique, full body draping, and only after multiple, redundant confirmations of the correct localization of the venous circulation. Pressure guidance is used to ascertain the localization of the PA catheter in the venous circulation and the heart. Upon entry into the right atrium (panels 3 and 4), the central venous pressure tracing is noted. Passing through the tricuspid valve (panels 5 and 6) right ventricular pressures are detected. At 35 to 50 cm depending upon patient size, the catheter will pass from the right ventricle through the pulmonic valve into the pulmonary artery (panels 7 and 8). This is noted by the measurement of diastolic pressure once the pulmonic valve is passed. Lastly, when indicated the balloon-tipped catheter will wedge or occlude a pulmonary artery branch (panels 9, 10, and 11). When this occurs, the pulmonary artery pressure equilibrates with that of the left atrium which, barring any mitral valve pathology, should be a reflection of left ventricular end-diastolic pressure. (Redrawn and reproduced, with permission, from Soni N. *Practical Procedures in Anaesthesia and Intensive Care.* Butterworth Heinemann, 1994.)

To prevent catheter knotting, the balloon should be deflated and the catheter withdrawn if pressure changes do not occur at the expected distances. In particularly difficult cases (low CO, pulmonary hypertension, or congenital heart anomalies), flotation of the catheter may be enhanced by having the patient inhale deeply; positioning the patient in a head-up, right lateral tilt position; injecting iced saline through the proximal lumen to stiffen the catheter (which also increases the risk of perforation); or administering a small dose of an inotropic agent to increase CO. Occasionally, the insertion may require fluoroscopy or TEE for guidance.

After attaining a PA position, minimal PA catheter advancement results in a pulmonary artery occlusion pressure (PAOP) waveform. The PA tracing should reappear when the balloon is deflated. Wedging before maximal balloon inflation signals an overwedged position, and the catheter should be slightly withdrawn (with the balloon down, of course). Because **PA rupture** may cause mortality and can occur because of balloon overinflation, the frequency of wedge readings should be minimized.

4 PA pressure should be continuously monitored to detect an overwedged position indicative of catheter migration. Furthermore, if the catheter has a right ventricular port 20 cm from the tip, distal migration can often be detected by a change in the pressure tracing that indicates a pulmonary artery location.

Correct catheter position can be confirmed by a chest radiograph.

The numerous complications of PA catheterization include all complications associated with central venous cannulation plus bacteremia, endocarditis, thrombogenesis, pulmonary infarction, PA rupture, and hemorrhage (particularly in patients taking anticoagulants, elderly or female patients, or patients with pulmonary hypertension), catheter knotting, arrhythmias, conduction abnormalities, and pulmonary valvular damage (Table 5–2). Even trace hemoptysis should not be ignored, as it may herald PA rupture. If the latter is suspected, prompt placement of a double-lumen tracheal tube may maintain adequate oxygenation by the unaffected lung. The risk of complications increases with the duration of catheterization, which usually should not exceed 72 hr.

Clinical Considerations

The introduction of PA catheters into the operating room revolutionized the intraoperative management of critically ill patients. PA catheters allow more precise estimation of left ventricular preload than either CVP or physical examination, as well as the sampling of mixed venous blood. Catheters with self-contained thermistors (discussed later in this

TABLE 5–2 Reported incidence of adverse effects of pulmonary artery catheterization.[1]

Complication	Reported Incidence (%)
Central venous access	
Arterial puncture	0.1–13
Bleeding at cut-down site	5.3
Postoperative neuropathy	0.3–1.1
Pneumothorax	0.3–4.5
Air embolism	0.5
Catheterization	
Minor arrhythmias[2]	4.7–68.9
Severe arrhythmias (ventricular tachycardia or fibrillation)[2]	0.3–62.7
Minor increase in tricuspid regurgitation	17
Right bundle-branch block[2]	0.1–4.3
Complete heart block (in patients with prior LBBB)[2]	0–8.5
Catheter residence	
Pulmonary artery rupture[2]	0.03–1.5
Positive catheter tip cultures	1.4–34.8
Catheter-related sepsis	0.7–11.4
Thrombophlebitis	6.5
Venous thrombosis	0.5–66.7
Pulmonary infarction[2]	0.1–5.6
Mural thrombus	28–61
Valvular/endocardial vegetations or endocarditis[2]	2.2–100
Deaths[2]	0.02–1.5

[1]Adapted from Practice guidelines for pulmonary artery catheterization: an updated report by the American Society of Anesthesiologists Task Force on pulmonary artery catheterization. Anesthesiology 2003;99:999.

[2]Complications thought to be more common (or exclusively associated) with pulmonary artery catheterization than with central venous catheterization. LBBB, left bundle-branch block.

chapter) can be used to measure CO, from which a multitude of hemodynamic values can be derived (Table 5–3). Some catheter designs incorporate electrodes that allow intracavitary ECG recording and pacing. Optional fiberoptic bundles allow continuous measurement of the oxygen saturation of mixed venous blood.

Starling demonstrated the relationship between left ventricular function and left ventricular end-diastolic muscle fiber length, which is usually proportionate to end-diastolic volume. If compliance is not abnormally decreased (eg, by myocardial ischemia, overload, ventricular hypertrophy,

TABLE 5–3 Hemodynamic variables derived from pulmonary artery catheterization data.[1]

Variable	Formula	Normal	Units
Cardiac index	$\dfrac{\text{Cardiac output (L/min)}}{\text{Body surface area (m}^2)}$	2.2–4.2	L/min/m²
Total peripheral resistance	$\dfrac{(\text{MAP} - \text{CVP}) \times 80}{\text{Cardiac output (L/min)}}$	1200–1500	dynes · s cm⁻⁵
Pulmonary vascular resistance	$\dfrac{(\overline{\text{PA}} - \text{PAOP}) \times 80}{\text{Cardiac output (L/min)}}$	100–300	dynes · s cm⁻⁵
Stroke volume	$\dfrac{\text{Cardiac output (L/min)} \times 1000}{\text{Heart rate (beats/min)}}$	60–90	mL/beat
Stroke index (SI)	$\dfrac{\text{Stroke volume (mL/beat)}}{\text{Body surface area (m}^2)}$	20–65	mL/beat/m²
Right ventricular stroke-work index	$0.0136\,(\overline{\text{PA}} - \text{CVP}) \times \text{SI}$	30–65	g-m/beat/m²
Left ventricular stroke-work index	$0.0136\,(\text{MAP} - \text{PAOP}) \times \text{SI}$	46–60	g-m/beat/m²

[1]g-m, gram meter; MAP, mean arterial pressure; CVP, central venous pressure; $\overline{\text{PA}}$, mean pulmonary artery pressure; PAOP, pulmonary artery occlusion pressure.

or pericardial tamponade), LVEDP should reflect fiber length. In the presence of a normal mitral valve, left atrial pressure approaches left ventricular pressure during diastolic filling. The left atrium connects with the right side of the heart through the pulmonary vasculature. The distal lumen of a correctly wedged PA catheter is isolated from right-sided pressures by balloon inflation. Its distal opening is exposed only to capillary pressure, which—in the absence of high airway pressures or pulmonary vascular disease—equals left atrial pressure. In fact, aspiration through the distal port during balloon inflation samples arterialized blood. PAOP is an indirect measure of LVEDP which depending upon ventricular compliance approximates left ventricular end diastolic volume.

Whereas central venous pressure may reflect right ventricular function, a PA catheter may be indicated if either ventricle is markedly depressed, causing disassociation of right- and left-sided hemodynamics. CVP is poorly predictive of pulmonary capillary pressures, especially in patients with abnormal left-ventricular function. Even the PAOP does not always predict LVEDP. The relationship between left ventricular end-diastolic volume (actual preload) and PAOP (estimated preload) can become unreliable during conditions associated with changing left atrial or ventricular compliance, mitral valve function, or pulmonary vein resistance. These conditions are common immediately following major cardiac or vascular surgery and in critically ill patients who are on inotropic agents or in septic shock.

Ultimately, the information provided by the PA catheter is like that from any perioperative monitor dependent upon its correct interpretation by the patient's care givers. In this context, the PA catheter is a tool to assist in goal-directed perioperative therapy. Given the increasing number of less invasive methods now available to obtain similar information, we suspect that PA catheterization will become mostly of historic interest.

CARDIAC OUTPUT

Indications

CO measurement to permit calculation of the SV is one of the primary reasons for PA catheterization. Currently, there are a number of alternative, less invasive methods to estimate ventricular function to assist in goal-directed therapy.

Techniques & Complications

A. Thermodilution

The injection of a quantity (2.5, 5, or 10 mL) of fluid that is below body temperature (usually room temperature or iced) into the right atrium changes the temperature of blood in contact with the thermistor at the tip of the PA catheter. The degree of change is inversely proportionate to CO: Temperature change is minimal if there is a high blood flow, whereas temperature change is greater when flow is reduced. After injection, one can plot the temperature as a function of time to produce a **thermodilution curve** (Figure 5–23). CO is determined by a computer program that integrates the area under the curve. Accurate measurements of CO depend on rapid and smooth injection, precisely known injectant temperature and volume, correct entry of the calibration factors for the specific type of PA catheter into the CO computer, and avoidance of measurements during electrocautery. Tricuspid regurgitation and cardiac shunts invalidate results because only right ventricular output into the PA is actually being measured. Rapid infusion of the iced injectant has rarely resulted in cardiac arrhythmias.

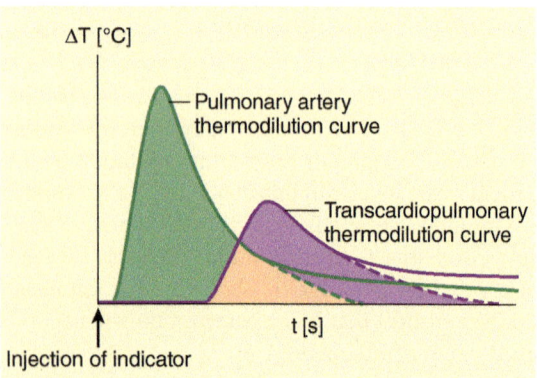

FIGURE 5–23 Comparison of thermodilution curves after injection of cold saline into the superior vena cava. The peak temperature change arrives earlier when measured in the pulmonary artery (a) than if measured in the femoral artery (b). Thereafter, both curves soon reapproximate baseline. (Redrawn and reproduced, with permission from Reuter D, Huang C, Edrich T, et al: Cardiac output monitoring using indicator dilution techniques: basics, limits and perspectives. Anesth Analg 2010;110:799.)

A modification of the thermodilution technique allows continuous CO measurement with a special catheter and monitor system. The catheter contains a thermal filament that introduces small pulses of heat into the blood proximal to the pulmonic valve and a thermistor that measures changes in PA blood temperature. A computer in the monitor determines CO by cross-correlating the amount of heat input with the changes in blood temperature.

Transpulmonary thermodilution (PiCCO® system) relies upon the same principles of thermodilution, but does not require PA catheterization. A central line and a thermistor-equipped arterial catheter (usually placed in the femoral artery) are necessary to perform transpulmonary thermodilution. Thermal measurements from radial artery catheters have been found to be invalid. Transpulmonary thermodilution measurements involve injection of cold indicator into the superior vena cava via a central line (Figure 5–24). A thermistor notes the change in temperature in the arterial system following the cold indicator's transit through the heart and lungs and estimates the CO.

Transpulmonary thermodilution also permits the calculation of both the global-end diastolic volume (GEDV) and the extravascular lung water (EVLW). Through mathematical analysis and extrapolation of the thermodilution curve, it is possible for the transpulmonary thermodilution computer to calculate both the mean transit time of the indicator and its exponential decay time (Figure 5–25). The intrathoracic thermal volume (ITTV) is the product of the CO and the mean transit time (MTT). The ITTV includes the pulmonary blood volume (PBV), EVLW, and the blood contained within the heart. The pulmonary thermal volume (PTV) includes both the EVLW and the PBV and is obtained by multiplying the CO by the exponential decay time (EDT). Subtracting the PTV from the ITTV gives the GEDV (Figure 5–26). The GEDV is a hypothetical volume that assumes that all of the heart's chambers are simultaneously full in diastole. With a normal index between 640 and 800 mL/m², the GEDV can assist in determining volume status. An extra vascular lung water index of less than 10 mL/kg is normative. The EVLW is the ITTV

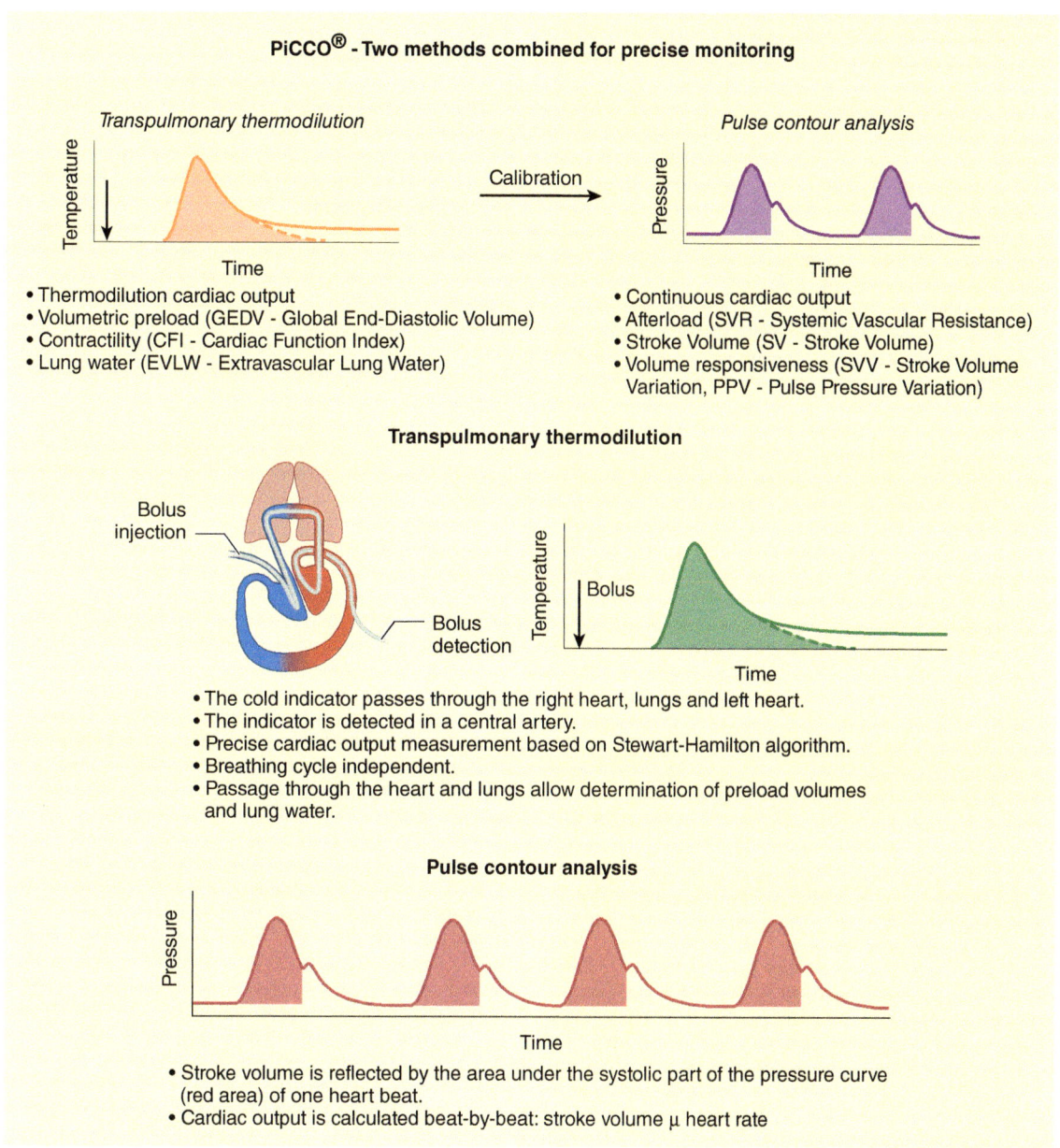

FIGURE 5–24 Two methods combined for precise monitoring. (Reproduced, with permission, from Royal Philips Electronics.)

minus the intrathoracic blood volume (ITBV). The ITBV = GEDV × 1.25.

Thus EVLW = ITTV – ITBV. An increased EVLW can be indicative of fluid overload. Thus, through mathematical analysis of the transpulmonary thermodilution curve, it is possible to obtain volumetric indices to guide fluid replacement therapy. Moreover, the PiCCO® system calculates SV variation and pulse pressure variation through pulse contour analysis, both of which can be used to

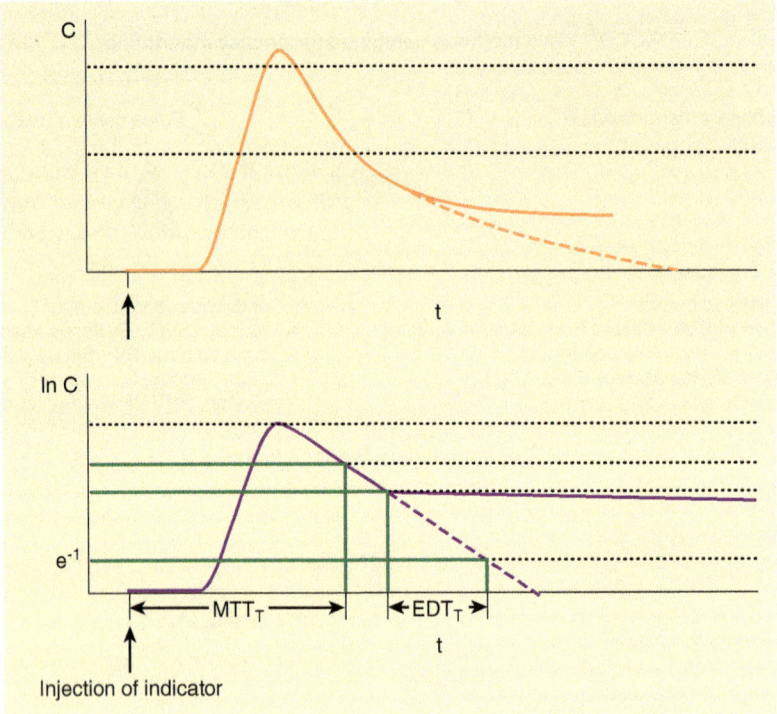

FIGURE 5–25 The upper curve represents the classic thermodilution curve, showing the concentration of an indicator over time at the site of detection. By extrapolation of the curve (dashed line), potential recirculation phenomena are excluded. Logarithmic illustration (lower curve) allows defining the mean transit time (MTT_T) and the exponential decay time (EDT_T) of the indicator. (Redrawn and reproduced, with permission from Reuter D, Huang C, Edrich T, et al: Cardiac output monitoring using indicator dilution techniques: basics, limits and perspectives. Anesth Analg 2010;110:799.)

determine fluid responsiveness. Both SV and pulse pressure are decreased during positive pressure ventilation. The greater the variations over the course of positive pressure inspiration and expiration, the more likely the patient is to improve hemodynamic measures following volume administration.

B. Dye Dilution

If indocyanine green dye (or another indicator such as lithium) is injected through a central venous catheter, its appearance in the systemic arterial circulation can be measured by analyzing arterial samples with an appropriate detector (eg, a densitometer for indocyanine green). The area under the resulting **dye indicator curve** is related to CO. By analyzing arterial blood pressure and integrating it with CO, systems that use lithium (LiDCO™) also calculate

beat-to-beat SV. In the LiDCO™ system, a small bolus of lithium chloride is injected into the circulation. A lithium-sensitive electrode in an arterial catheter measures the decay in lithium concentration over time. Integrating the concentration over time graph permits the machine to calculate the CO. The LiDCO™ device, like the PiCCO® thermodilution device, employs pulse contour analysis of the arterial wave form to provide ongoing beat-to-beat determinations of CO and other calculated parameters. Lithium dilution determinations can be made in patients who have only peripheral venous access. Lithium should not be administered to patients in the first trimester of pregnancy. The dye dilution technique, however, introduces the problems of indicator recirculation, arterial blood sampling, and background tracer buildup, potentially

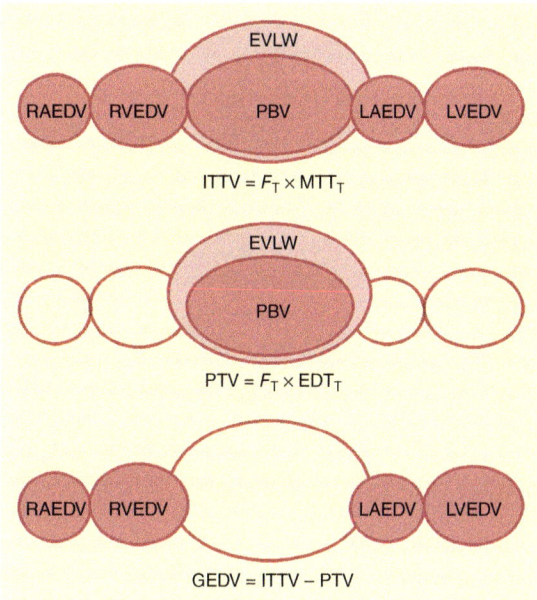

FIGURE 5–26 Assessment of global end-diastolic volume (GEDV) by transcardiopulmonary thermodilution. Upper row: The intrathroacic thermal volume (ITTV) is the complete volume of distribution of the thermal indicator, including the right atrium end-diastolic volume (RAEDV), the right ventricle (RVEDV), the left atrium (LAEDV), the left ventricle (LVEDV), the pulmonary blood volume (PBV), and the extravascular lung water (EVLW). It is calculated by multiplying cardiac output (F_T) with the mean transit time (MTT_T) of the indicator. Middle row: The pulmonary thermal volume (PTV) represents the largest mixing chamber in this system and includes the PBV and the EVLW and is assessed by multiplying F_T with the exponential decay time (EDT_T) of the thermal indicator. Bottom row: The GEDV, including the volumes of the right and the left heart, now is calculated by subtracting PTV from ITTV. (Redrawn and reproduced, with permission from Reuter D, Huang C, Edrich T, et al: Cardiac output monitoring using indicator dilution techniques: basics, limits and perspectives. Anesth Analg 2010;110:799.)

limiting the use of such approaches perioperatively. Nondepolarizing neuromuscular blockers may affect the lithium sensor.

C. Pulse Contour Devices

Pulse contour devices use the arterial pressure tracing to estimate the CO and other dynamic parameters, such as pulse pressure and SV variation with mechanical ventilation. These indices are used to help determine if hypotension is likely to respond to fluid therapy.

Pulse contour devices rely upon algorithms that measure the area of the systolic portion of the arterial pressure trace from end diastole to the end of ventricular ejection. The devices then incorporate a calibration factor for the patient's vascular compliance, which is dynamic and not static. Some pulse contour devices rely first on transpulmonary thermodilution or lithium thermodilution to calibrate the machine for subsequent pulse contour measurements. The FloTrac (Edwards Life Sciences) does not require calibration with another measure and relies upon a statistical analysis of its algorithm to account for changes in vascular compliance occurring as a consequence of changed vascular tone.

D. Esophageal Doppler

Esophageal Doppler relies upon the Doppler principle to measure the velocity of blood flow in the descending thoracic aorta. The Doppler principle is integral in perioperative echocardiography, as discussed below. The Doppler effect has been described previously in this chapter and is the result of the apparent change in sound frequency when the source of the sound wave and the observer of the sound wave are in relative motion. Blood in the aorta is in relative motion compared with the Doppler probe in the esophagus. As red blood cells travel, they reflect a frequency shift, depending upon both the direction and velocity of their movement. When blood flows toward the transducer, its reflected frequency is higher than that which was transmitted by the probe. When blood cells move away from the transducer, the frequency is lower than that which was initially sent by the probe. By using the Doppler equation, it is possible to determine the velocity of blood flow in the aorta. The equation is:

Velocity of blood blow = {frequency change/ cosine of the angle of incidence between the Doppler beam and the blood flow} × {speed of sound in tissue/2 (source frequency)}

For Doppler to provide a reliable estimate of velocity, the angle of incidence should be as close to zero as possible, since the cosine of 0 is 1. As the angle approaches 90°, the Doppler measure is unreliable, as the cosine of 90° is 0.

The esophageal Doppler device calculates the velocity of flow in the aorta. As the velocities of the cells in the aorta travel at different speeds over the cardiac cycle, the machine obtains a measure of all of the velocities of the cells moving over time. Mathematically integrating the velocities represents the distance that the blood travels. Next, using nomograms, the monitor approximates the area of the descending aorta. The monitor thus calculates both the distance the blood travels, as well as the area: area × length = volume.

Consequently, the SV of blood in the descending aorta is calculated. Knowing the HR allows calculation of that portion of the CO flowing through the descending thoracic aorta, which is approximately 70% of total CO. Correcting for this 30% allows the monitor to estimate the patient's total CO. Esophageal Doppler is dependent upon many assumptions and nomograms, which may hinder its ability to accurately reflect CO in a variety of clinical situations.

E. Thoracic Bioimpedance

Changes in thoracic volume cause changes in thoracic resistance (bioimpedance) to low amplitude, high frequency currents. If thoracic changes in bioimpedance are measured following ventricular depolarization, SV can be continuously determined. This noninvasive technique requires six electrodes to inject microcurrents and to sense bioimpedance on both sides of the chest. Increasing fluid in the chest results in less electrical bioimpedance. Mathematical assumptions and correlations are then made to calculate CO from changes in bioimpedance. Disadvantages of thoracic bioimpedance include susceptibility to electrical interference and reliance upon correct electrode positioning. The accuracy of this technique is questionable in several groups of patients, including those with aortic valve disease, previous heart surgery, or acute changes in thoracic sympathetic nervous function (eg, those undergoing spinal anesthesia).

F. Fick Principle

The amount of oxygen consumed by an individual (Vo_2) equals the difference between arterial and venous (a–v) oxygen content (C) (Cao_2 and Cvo_2) multiplied by CO. Therefore

$$CO = \frac{\text{Oxygen consumption}}{\text{a–v } O_2 \text{ content difference}} = \frac{\dot{V}o_2}{Cao_2 - Cvo_2}$$

Mixed venous and arterial oxygen content are easily determined if a PA catheter and an arterial line are in place. Oxygen consumption can also be calculated from the difference between the oxygen content in inspired and expired gas. Variations of the Fick principle are the basis of all indicator–dilution methods of determining CO.

G. Echocardiography

There are no more powerful tools to diagnose and assess cardiac function perioperatively than transthoracic echocardiography (TTE) and transesophageal echocardiography (TEE). Both approaches are increasingly used in the operative setting. In the operating rooms, limited access to the chest makes TEE an ideal option to visualize the heart. Both TTE and TEE can be employed preoperatively and postoperatively. TTE has the advantage of being completely noninvasive; however, acquiring the "windows" to view the heart can be difficult. Disposable TEE probes are now available that can remain in position in critically ill patients for days, during which intermittent TEE examinations can be performed.

Echocardiography can be employed by anesthesia staff in two ways, depending upon degrees of training and certification. Basic (or hemodynamic) TEE permits the anesthesiologist to discern the primary source of a patient's hemodynamic instability. Whereas in past decades the PA flotation catheter would be used to determine why the patient might be hypotensive, the anesthetist performing hemodynamic TEE is attempting to determine if the heart is adequately filled, contracting appropriately, not externally compressed, and devoid of any grossly obvious structural defects. At all times, information obtained from hemodynamic TEE may be correlated with other information as to the patient's general condition.

Anesthesiologists performing advanced TEE make therapeutic and surgical recommendations based upon their TEE interpretations. Various organizations and boards have been established worldwide to certify individuals in all levels of perioperative echocardiography. More importantly, individuals who perform echocardiography should be aware of the credentialing requirements of their respective institutions.

Echocardiography has many uses, including:

- Diagnosis of the source of hemodynamic instability, including myocardial ischemia, systolic and diastolic heart failure, valvular abnormalities, hypovolemia, and pericardial tamponade
- Estimation of hemodynamic parameters, such as SV, CO, and intracavitary pressures
- Diagnosis of structural diseases of the heart, such as valvular heart disease, shunts, aortic diseases
- Guiding surgical interventions, such as mitral valve repair.

Various echocardiographic modalities are employed perioperatively by anesthesiologists, including TTE, TEE, epiaortic and epicardiac ultrasound, and three-dimensional echocardiography. Some advantages and disadvantages of the modalities are as follows:

- TTE has the advantage of being noninvasive and essentially risk free. Limited scope TTE exams are now increasingly common in the intensive care unit (Figure 5–27).
- Unlike TTE, TEE is an invasive procedure with the potential for life-threatening complications (esophageal rupture and mediastinitis) (Figure 5–28). The close proximity of the esophagus to the left atrium eliminates the problem of obtaining "windows" to view the heart and permits great detail. TEE has been used frequently in the cardiac surgical operating room over the past decades. Its use to guide therapy in general cases has been limited by both the cost of the equipment and the learning necessary to correctly interpret the images. Both TTE and TEE generate two-dimensional images of the three-dimensional heart. Consequently, it is necessary to view the heart through many

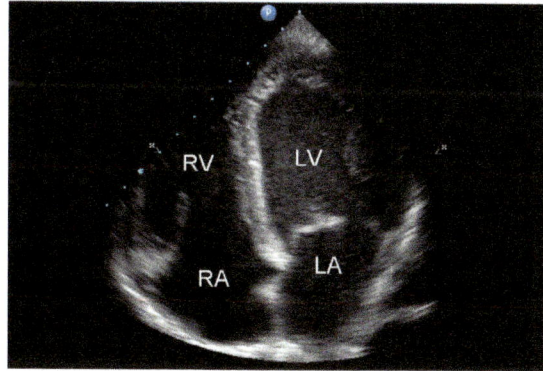

FIGURE 5–27 Normal apical four-chamber view. RV, right ventrical; LV, left ventricle; RA, right atrium; LA, left atrium. (Reproduced, with permission, from Carmody KA, et al: *Handbook of Critical Care and Emergency Ultrasound.* McGraw-Hill, 2011.)

two-dimensional image planes and windows to mentally recreate the three-dimensional anatomy. The ability to interpret these images at the advanced certification level requires much training.

- Epiaortic and epicardiac ultrasound imaging techniques employ an echo probe wrapped in a sterile sheath and manipulated by thoracic surgeons intraoperatively to obtain views of

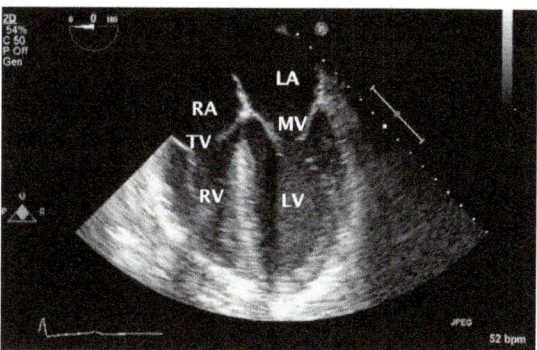

FIGURE 5–28 The structures of the heart as seen on a midesophageal four-chamber view, including the right atrium (RA), tricuspid valve (TV), right ventricle (RV), left atrium (LA), mitral valve (MV), and left ventricle (LV). (Redrawn and reproduced, with permission, from Wasnick J, Hillel Z, Kramer D, et al: *Cardiac Anesthesia & Transesophageal Echocardiography,* McGraw-Hill, 2011.)

the aorta and the heart. The air-filled trachea prevents TEE imaging of the ascending aorta. Because the aorta is manipulated during cardiac surgery, detection of atherosclerotic plaques permits the surgeon to potentially minimize the incidence of embolic stroke. Imaging of the heart with epicardial ultrasound permits intraoperative echocardiography when TEE is contraindicated because of esophageal or gastric pathology.

- Three-dimensional echocardiography (TTE and TEE) has become available in recent years (**Figure 5–29**). These techniques provide a three-dimensional view of the heart's structure. In particular, three-dimensional images can better quantify the heart's volumes and can generate a surgeon's view of the mitral valve to aid in guiding valve repair.

Echocardiography employs ultrasound (sound at frequencies greater than normal hearing) from 2 to 10 MHz. A piezoelectrode in the probe transducer converts electrical energy delivered to the probe into ultrasound waves. These waves then travel

through the tissues, encountering the blood, the heart, and other structures. Sound waves pass readily through tissues of similar acoustic impedance; however, when they encounter different tissues, they are scattered, refracted, or reflected back toward the ultrasound probe. The echo wave then interacts with the ultrasound probe, generating an electrical signal that can be reconstructed as an image. The machine knows the time delay between the transmitted and the reflected sound wave. By knowing the time delay, the location of the source of the reflected wave can be determined and the image generated. The TEE probe contains myriad crystals generating and processing waves, which then create the echo image. The TEE probe can generate images through multiple planes and can be physically manipulated in the stomach and esophagus, permitting visualization of heart structures (**Figure 5–30**). These views can be used to determine if the heart's walls are being delivered adequate blood supply (**Figure 5–31**). In the healthy heart, the heart's walls thicken and move inwardly with each beat. Wall motion abnormalities, in which the heart's walls fail to thicken during systole or move in a dyskinetic fashion, can be associated with myocardial ischemia.

The Doppler effect is routinely used in echocardiographic examinations to determine the heart's function. In the heart, both the blood flowing through the heart and the heart tissue move relative to the echo probe in the esophagus or on the chest wall. By using the Doppler effect, it is possible for echocardiographers to determine both the direction and the velocity of blood flow and tissue movement.

Blood flow in the heart follows the law of the conservation of mass. Therefore, the volume of blood that flows through one point (eg, the left ventricular outflow tract) must be the same volume that passes through the aortic valve. When the pathway through which the blood flows becomes narrowed (eg, aortic stenosis), the blood velocity must increase to permit the volume to pass. The increase in velocity as blood moves toward an esophageal echo probe is detected. The Bernoulli equation (pressure change = $4V^2$) allows echocardiographers to determine the pressure gradient between areas of different velocity, where v represents the area of

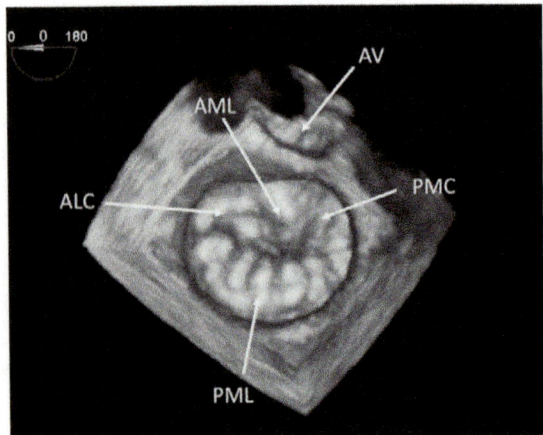

FIGURE 5–29 Three dimensional echocardiography of the mitral valve demonstrates the anterior leaflet (AML), the posterior leaflet (PML), the antero lateral commissure (ALC) and the postero medial commissure (PMC). The aortic valve (AV) is also seem. (Redrawn and reproduced, with permission, from Wasnick J, Hillel Z, Kramer D, et al: *Cardiac Anesthesia & Transesophageal Echocardiography*, McGraw-Hill, 2011.)

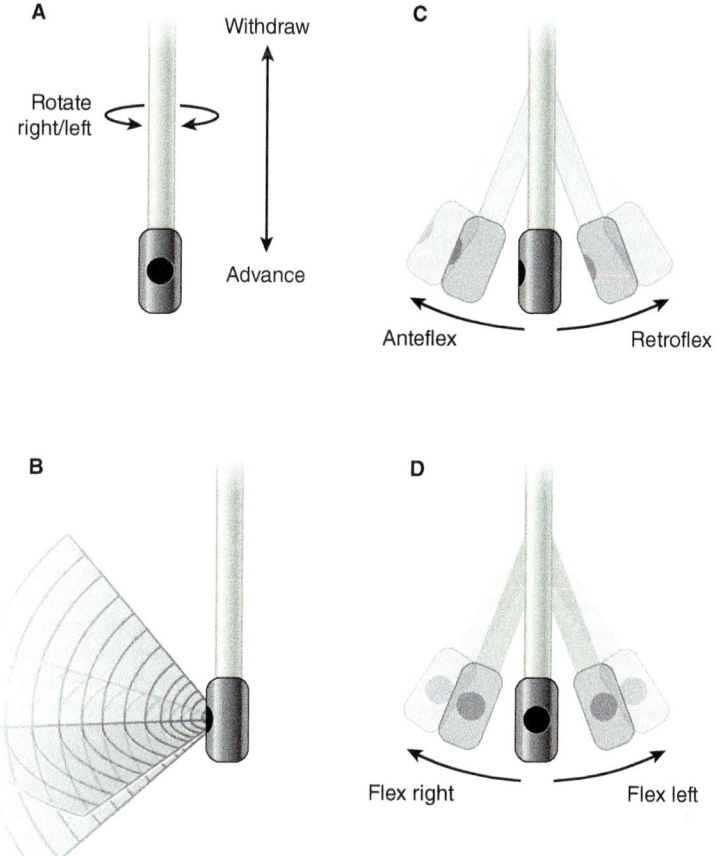

FIGURE 5–30 The echo probe is manipulated by the examiner in multiple ways to create the standard images that constitute the comprehensive perioperative tee examination. At all times never force the probe. If resistance is encountered abandon the examination. Echocardiographic information can be provided by intraoperative epicardial and epiaortic examination. Advancing the probe in the esophagus permits the upper, mid and transgastric examinations (**A**). The probe can be turned in the esophagus from left to right to examine both left and right sided structures (**A**). Using the button located on the probe permits the echocardiographer to rotate the scan beam through 180 degrees thereby creating various two dimensional imaging slices of the three dimensional heart (**B**). Lastly, panels (**C**) and (**D**) demonstrate manipulation of the tip of the probe to permit the beam to be directed to best visualize the image. (Modified and reproduced, with permission, from Shanewise JS, et.al. ASE/SCA guidelines for performing a comprehensive intraoperative multiplane transesophageal echocardiography examination; recommendations of the American Society of Echocardiography Council for Intraoperative Echocardiography and the Society for Cardiovascular Anesthesiologists Task Force for Certification in Perioperative Transesophageal Echocardiography. Anesth Analg 1999;89:870-884.)

maximal velocity (Figure 5–32). Using continuous wave Doppler, it is possible to determine the maximal velocity as blood accelerates through a pathologic heart structure. For example, a blood flow of 4 m/sec reflects a pressure gradient of 84 mm Hg between an area of slow flow (the left ventricular outflow tract) and a region of high flow (a stenotic aortic valve).

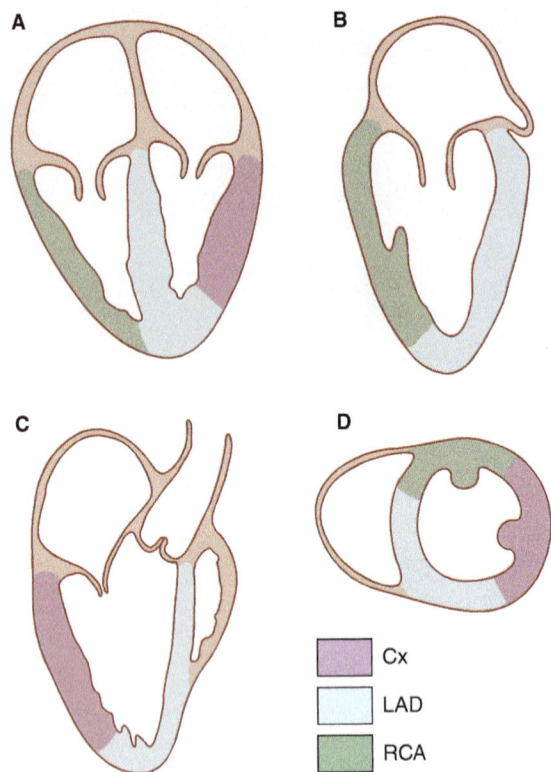

FIGURE 5–31 The midesophageal four-chamber view (**A**), the midesophageal two-chamber view (**B**), the midesophageal long-axis vew (**C**), and the transgastric mid short-axis vew (**D**) are depicted. The different views provide the opportunity to observe the myocardium supplied by each of the three main coronary vessels, the left circumflex (Cx), the left anterior descending (LAD) and the right coronary artery (RCA). Areas of impaired myocardial perfusion are suggested by the inability of the myocardium to both thicken and move inwardly during systole. Image **D** is very useful for monitoring in the operating room because left ventricular myocardium supplied by each of the three vessels can be seen in one image. (Modifed and reproduced, with permission, from Shanewise JS, et.al. ASE/SCA guidelines for performing a comprehensive intraoperative multiplane transesophageal echocardiography examination; recommendations of the American Society of Echocardiography Council for Intraoperative Echocardiography and the Society for Cardiovascular Anesthesiologists Task Force for Certification in Perioperative Transesophageal Echocardiography. Anesth Analg 1999;89:870-884.)

Likewise, the Bernoulli equation permits echocardiographers to estimate PA and other intracavitary pressures, if assumptions are made.

$$\text{Assume } P_1 \gg P_2$$

Blood flow proceeds from an area of high pressure P_1 to an area of low pressure P_2.

The pressure gradient $= 4V^2$, where V is the maximal velocity measured in meters per second. Thus,

$$4V^2 = P_1 - P_2$$

Thus, assuming that there is a jet of regurgitant blood flow from the left ventricle into the left atrium and that left ventricular systolic pressure (P_1) is the same as systemic blood pressure (eg, no aortic stenosis), it is possible to calculate left atrial pressure (P_2). In this manner, echocardiographers can estimate intracavitary pressures when there are pressure gradients, measurable flow velocities between areas

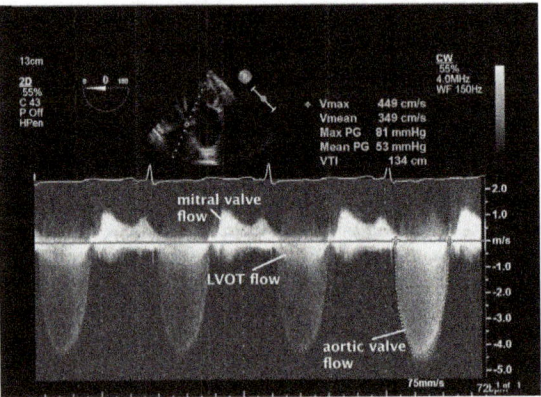

FIGURE 5–32 The time-velocity interval (TVI) of the aortic valve is calculated using continuous wave Doppler, while pulse wave Doppler is useful for measurements at lower blood velocities. This continuous wave Doppler has been aligned parallel to that aortic valve flow as imaged using the deep transgastric view. Of note, the bold velocity across the aortic valve is greater than 4 m/sec. (Redrawn and reproduced, with permission, from Wasnick J, Hillel Z, Kramer D, et al: *Cardiac Anesthesia & Transesophageal Echocardiography*, McGraw-Hill, 2011.)

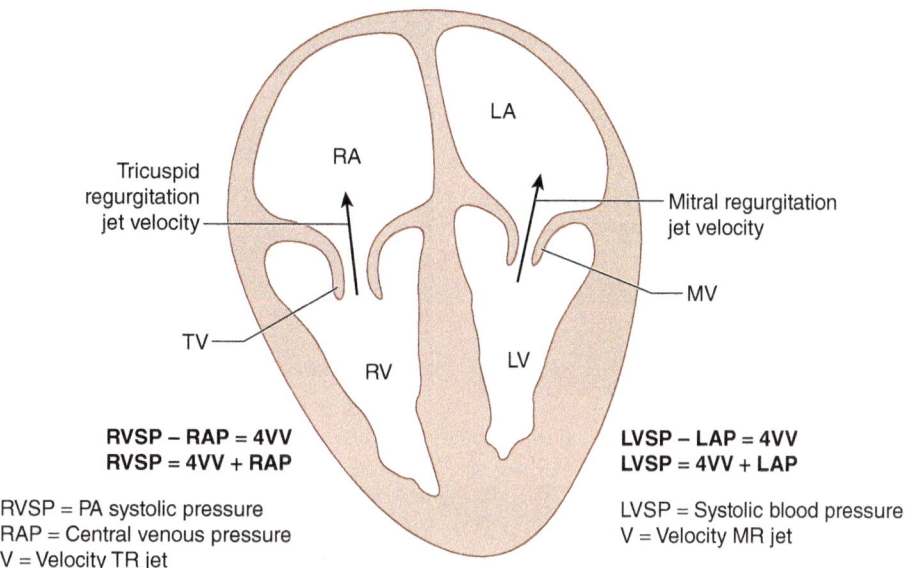

LA

RA

Tricuspid
regurgitation
jet velocity

Mitral regurgitation
jet velocity

MV

TV

LV

RV

RVSP – RAP = 4VV
RVSP = 4VV + RAP

LVSP – LAP = 4VV
LVSP = 4VV + LAP

RVSP = PA systolic pressure
RAP = Central venous pressure
V = Velocity TR jet

LVSP = Systolic blood pressure
V = Velocity MR jet

FIGURE 5–33 Intracavity pressures can be calculated using known pressures and the Bernoulli equation when regurgitant jets are present. The PA systolic pressure is obtained when tricuspid regurgitation is present and the right atrial pressure known. Assuming no pulmonic valve disease, the right ventricular systolic pressure and the pulmonary systolic pressure are the same. The left atrial pressure can be similarly calculated if mitral regurgitation is present. Again, assuming no valvular disease LV systolic pressure should equal systemic systolic blood pressure. Subtracting $4V^2$ from the LVSP estimates the left atrial pressure. (Redrawn and reproduced, with permission, from Wasnick J, Hillel Z, Kramer D, et al: *Cardiac Anesthesia & Transesophageal Echocardiography*, McGraw-Hill, 2011.)

of high and low pressure, and knowledge of either P_1 or P_2 (Figure 5–33).

The Doppler principle is also used by echocardiographers to identify areas of abnormal flow using color flow Doppler. Color flow Doppler creates a visual picture of the heart's blood flow by assigning a color code to the velocities in the heart. Blood flow directed away from the echocardiographic transducer is color-coded blue, whereas that which is moving toward the probe is red. The higher the velocity of flow, the lighter the color hue (Figure 5–34). When the velocity of blood flow becomes greater than that which the machine can measure, flow toward the probe is misinterpreted as flow away from the probe, creating images of turbulent flow and "aliasing" of the image. Such changes in flow pattern are used by echocardiographers to identify areas of pathology.

Doppler can also be used to provide an estimate of SV and CO. Similar to esophageal Doppler probes

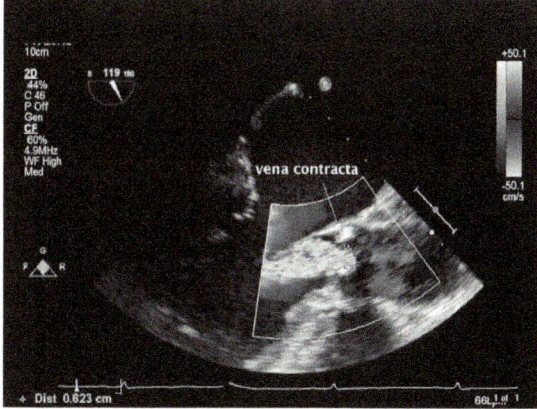

FIGURE 5–34 The color flow Doppler image of the midesophageal aortic valve long-axis view demonstrates measurement of the vena contracta of aortic regurgitation. The vena contracta represents the smallest diameter of the regurgitant jet at the level of the aortic valve. A vena conracta of 6.2 mm grades the aortic regurgitation in this case as severe. (Redrawn and reproduced, with permission, from Wasnick J, Hillel Z, Kramer D, et al: *Cardiac Anesthesia & Transesophageal Echocardiography*, McGraw-Hill, 2011.)

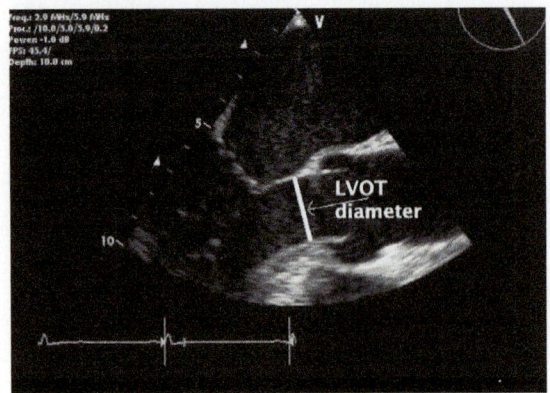

FIGURE 5-35 The midesophageal long-axis view is employed in this image to measure the diameter of the left ventricular outflow track (LVOT). Knowing the diameter of the LVOT permits calculation of the LVOT area ($D^2 \times 0.785$ = LVOT area). (Redrawn and reproduced, with permission, from Wasnick J, Hillel Z, Kramer D, et al: *Cardiac Anesthesia & Transesophageal Echocardiography*, McGraw-Hill, 2011.)

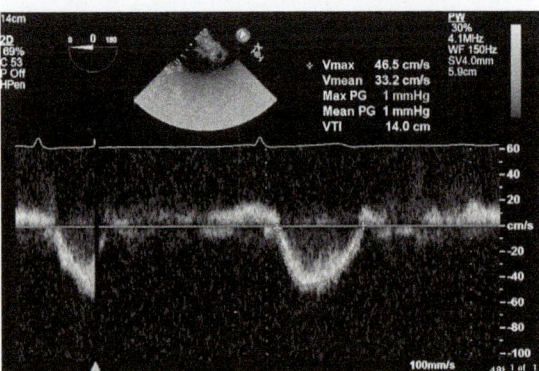

FIGURE 5-36 PW Doppler is employed in this deep transgastric view interrogation of the left ventricular outflow track (LVOT). Blood is flowing in the LVOT away from the esophagus. Therefore, the flow velocities appear below the baseline. Flow velocity through the LVOT is 46.5 cm/s. This is as expected when there is no pathology noted as blood is ejected along the LVOT. Tracing the flow envelope (dotted lines) identifies the time-velocity interval (TVI). In this example the TVI is 14 cm. (Redrawn and reproduced, with permission, from Wasnick J, Hillel Z, Kramer D, et al: *Cardiac Anesthesia & Transesophageal Echocardiography*, McGraw-Hill, 2011.)

previously described, TTE and TEE can be used to estimate CO. Assuming that the left ventricular outflow tract is a cylinder, it is possible to measure its diameter (**Figure 5–35**). Knowing this, it is possible to calculate the area through which blood flows using the following equation:

$$Area = \pi r^2 = 0.785 \times diameter^2$$

Next, the time velocity integral is determined. A Doppler beam is aligned in parallel with the left ventricular outflow tract (**Figure 5–36**). The velocities passing through the left ventricular outflow tract are recorded, and the machine integrates the velocity/time curve to determine the distance the blood traveled.

$$Area \times length = volume$$

In this instance, the SV is calculated:

$$SV \times HR = CO$$

Lastly, Doppler can be used to examine the movement of the myocardial tissue. Tissue velocity is normally 8–15 cm/sec (much less than that of blood, which is 100 cm/s). Using the tissue Doppler function of the echo machine, it is possible to discern both the directionality and velocity of the heart's movement. During diastolic filling, the lateral annulus myocardium will move toward a TEE probe. Reduced myocardial velocities (<8 cm/s) are associated with impaired diastolic function and higher left ventricular end-diastolic pressures.

Ultimately, echocardiography can provide comprehensive cardiovascular monitoring. Its routine use outside of the cardiac operating room has been hindered by both the costs of the equipment and the training required to correctly interpret the images. As equipment becomes more readily available, it is likely that anesthesia staff will perform an increasing number of echocardiographic examinations for hemodynamic monitoring perioperatively. When questions arise beyond those related to hemodynamic guidance, interpretation by an individual credentialed in advanced perioperative echocardiography is warranted.

CASE DISCUSSION

Hemodynamic Monitoring and Management of a Complicated Patient

A 68-year-old male presents with a perforated colon secondary to diverticulitis. Vital signs are: heart rate, 120 beats/min; blood pressure, 80 mm Hg/55 mm Hg; respiratory rate, 28 breaths/min; and body temperature, 38 C°. He is scheduled for emergency exploratory laparotomy. His past history includes placement of a drug-eluting stent in the left anterior descending artery two weeks earlier. His medications include metoprolol and clopidogrel.

What hemodynamic monitors should be employed?

This patient presents with multiple medical issues that could lead to perioperative hemodynamic instability. He has a history of coronary artery disease for which he has been given stents. His previous and current ECGs should be reviewed for signs of new ST- and T-wave changes, heralding ischemia. He is both tachycardic and febrile, and, consequently, may be concurrently ischemic, vasodilated, and hypovolemic. All of these conditions could complicate perioperative management.

Arterial cannulation and monitoring will provide beat-to-beat blood pressure determinations intraoperatively and will also provide for blood gas measurements in a patient likely to be acidotic and hemodynamically unstable. Central venous access is obtained to permit volume resuscitation and to provide a port for delivery of fluid for transpulmonary measurements of CO and SV variation. Alternatively, pulse contour analysis can be employed from an arterial trace to determine volume responsiveness, should the patient become hemodynamically unstable. Echocardiography can be used to determine ventricular function, filling pressures, and CO and to provide surveillance for the development of ischemia-induced wall motion abnormalities.

PA catheters can also be placed to measure CO and pulmonary capillary occlusion pressure.

The choice of hemodynamic monitors remains with the individual physician and the availability of various monitoring techniques. It is important to also consider monitors that will be available in the postoperative setting to insure continuation of goal-directed therapy.

SUGGESTED READING

Alhasemi J, Cecconi M, della Rocca G, et al: Minimally invasive monitoring of cardiac output in the cardiac surgery intensive care unit. Curr Heart Fail Rep 2010;7:116.

Beaulieu Y, Marik P: Bedside ultrasonography in the ICU: part 1. Chest 2005;128:881.

Beaulieu Y, Marik P: Bedside ultrasonography in the ICU: part 2. Chest 2005;128:1766.

Breukers RM, Groeneveld AB, de Wilde RB, Jansen JR: Transpulmonary versus continuous thermodilution cardiac output after valvular and coronary artery surgery. Interact CardioVasc Thorac Surg 2009;9:4.

Chatterjee K: The Swan Ganz catheters: past, present, and future. A viewpoint. Circulation 2009;119:147.

Falyar C: Ultrasound in anesthesia: applying scientific principles to clinical practice. AANA J 2010;78:332.

Funk D, Moretti E, Gan T: Minimally invasive cardiac monitoring in the perioperative setting. Anesth Analg 2009;108:887.

Goepfert M, Reuter D, Akyol D, et al: Goal-directed fluid management reduces vasopressor and catecholamine use in cardiac surgery patients. Intensive Care Med 2007;33:96.

Hadian M, Kim H, Severyn D, Pinsky M: Cross comparison of cardiac output trending accuracy of LiDCO, PiCCO, FloTrac and pulmonary artery catheters. Crit Care 2010;14:R212.

Hett D, Jonas M: Non-invasive cardiac output monitoring. Curr Anaesth Crit Care 2003;14:187.

Hung J, Lang R, Flachskampf F, et al: 3D echocardiography: a review of the current status and future directions. J Am Soc Echocardiogr 2007;20:213.

Leier C: Invasive hemodynamic monitoring the aftermath of the ESCAPE trial. Cardiol Clin 2007; 25:565.

Metzelder S, Coburn M, Fries M, et al: Performance of cardiac output measurement derived from arterial pressure waveform analysis in patients requiring high-dose vasopressor therapy. Br J Anaesth 2011;106:776.

Michard F, Alaya S, Zarka V, et al: Global end diastolic volume as an indicator of cardiac preload in patients with septic shock. Chest 2003;124:1900.

Reuter D, Huang C, Edrich T, et al: Cardiac output monitoring using indicator dilution techniques: basics, limits and perspectives. Anesth Analg 2010;110:799.

Rex S. Brose S, Metzelder S, et al: Prediction of fluid responsiveness in patients during cardiac surgery. Br J Anaesth 2004;93:782.

Shanewise J, Cheung A, Aronson S, et al: ASE/SCA guidelines for performing a comprehensive intraoperative multiplane transesophageal echocardiography examination: recommendations of the American Society of Echocardiography Council for Intraoperative Echocardiography and the Society of Cardiovascular Anesthesiologists Task Force for Certification in Perioperative Transesophageal Echocardiography. Anesth Analg 1999;89:870.

Skubas N: Intraoperative Doppler tissue imaging is a valuable addition to cardiac anesthesiologists' armamentarium: a core review. Anesth Analg 2009;108:48.

Singer M: Oesophageal Doppler monitoring: should it be routine for high-risk surgical patients? Curr Opin Anesthesiol 2011;24:171.

Wouters P: New modalities in echocardiography: tissue Doppler and strain rate imaging. Curr Opin Anaesthesiol 2005;18:47.

Yeates T, Zimmerman J, Cahalan M: Perioperative echocardiography: two-dimensional and three-dimensional applications. Anesthesiol Clin 2008;26:419.

Noncardiovascular Monitoring

KEY CONCEPTS

1. Capnography rapidly and reliably indicates esophageal intubation—a common cause of anesthetic catastrophe—but does not detect bronchial intubation.

2. Close monitoring of neuromuscular blockade using both clinical and quantitative means can reduce the incidence of postoperative curarization.

The previous chapter reviewed routine hemodynamic monitoring used by anesthesiologists. This chapter examines the vast array of techniques and devices used perioperatively to monitor neuromuscular transmission, neurological condition, respiratory gas exchange, and body temperature.

Respiratory Gas Exchange Monitors

PRECORDIAL & ESOPHAGEAL STETHOSCOPES

Indications

Prior to the routine availability of gas exchange monitors, anesthesiologists used a precordial or esophageal stethoscope to ensure that the lungs were being ventilated in the event that the circuit became disconnected. Likewise, the heart tones could be auscultated to confirm a beating heart. Although less essential today because other modalities are available, the finger on the pulse and auscultation remain front-line monitors, especially when technology fails. Chest auscultation remains the primary method to confirm bilateral lung ventilation in the operating room, even if end tidal CO_2 detection

is the primary mechanism to exclude esophageal intubation.

Contraindications

Instrumentation of the esophagus should be avoided in patients with esophageal varices or strictures.

Techniques & Complications

A precordial stethoscope (Wenger chestpiece) is a heavy, bell-shaped piece of metal placed over the chest or suprasternal notch. Although its weight tends to maintain its position, double-sided adhesive disks provide an acoustic seal to the patient's skin. Various chestpieces are available, but the child size works well for most patients. The bell is connected to the anesthesiologist by extension tubing.

The esophageal stethoscope is a soft plastic catheter (8–24F) with balloon-covered distal openings (Figure 6–1). Although the quality of breath and heart sounds is much better than with a precordial stethoscope, its use is limited to intubated patients. Temperature probes, electrocardiogram (ECG) leads, ultrasound probes, and even atrial pacemaker electrodes have been incorporated into esophageal stethoscopes. Placement through the mouth or nose can occasionally cause mucosal irritation and bleeding. Rarely, the stethoscope slides into the trachea

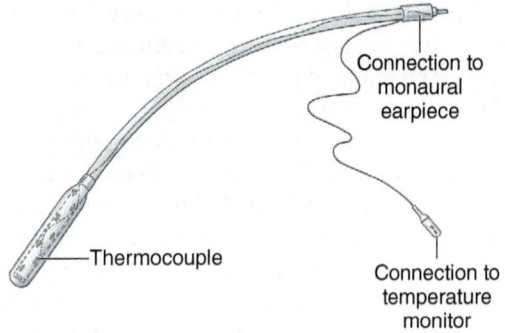

Connection to
monaural
earpiece

Thermocouple

Connection to
temperature
monitor

FIGURE 6-1 Esophageal stethoscope.

instead of the esophagus, resulting in a gas leak around the tracheal tube cuff.

Clinical Considerations

The information provided by a precordial or esophageal stethoscope includes confirmation of ventilation, quality of breath sounds (eg, stridor, wheezing), regularity of heart rate, and quality of heart tones (muffled tones are associated with decreased cardiac output).

The confirmation of bilateral breath sounds after tracheal intubation, however, is made with a binaural stethoscope.

PULSE OXIMETRY

Indications & Contraindications

Pulse oximeters are mandatory monitors for any anesthetic, including cases of moderate sedation. There are no contraindications.

Techniques & Complications

Pulse oximeters combine the principles of oximetry and plethysmography to noninvasively measure oxygen saturation in arterial blood. A sensor containing light sources (two or three light-emitting diodes) and a light detector (a photodiode) is placed across a finger, toe, earlobe, or any other perfused tissue that can be transilluminated. When the light source and detector are opposite one another across the perfused tissue, transmittance oximetry is used. When the light source and detector are placed on

the same side of the patient (eg, the forehead), the backscatter (reflectance) of light is recorded by the detector.

Oximetry depends on the observation that oxygenated and reduced hemoglobin differ in their absorption of red and infrared light (Lambert–Beer law). Specifically, oxyhemoglobin (HbO_2) absorbs more infrared light (940 nm), whereas deoxyhemoglobin absorbs more red light (660 nm) and thus appears blue, or cyanotic, to the naked eye. The change in light absorption during arterial pulsations is the basis of oximetric determinations (Figure 6–2). The ratio of the absorptions at the red and infrared wavelengths is analyzed by a microprocessor to provide the oxygen saturation (Spo_2) of arterial blood based on established norms. The greater the ratio of red/infrared absorption, the lower the arterial saturation. Arterial pulsations are identified by plethysmography, allowing corrections for light absorption by nonpulsating venous blood and tissue. Heat from the light source or sensor pressure may, rarely, result in tissue damage if the monitor is not periodically moved. No user calibration is required.

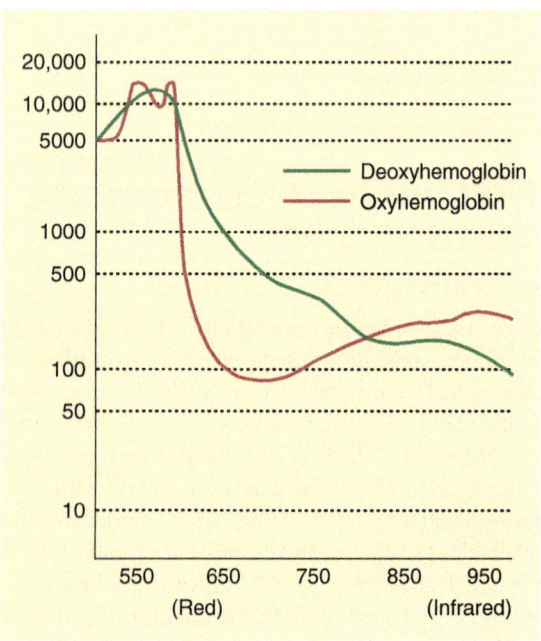

FIGURE 6-2 Oxyhemoglobin and deoxyhemoglobin differ in their absorption of red and infrared light.

Clinical Considerations

In addition to Spo_2, pulse oximeters provide an indication of tissue perfusion (pulse amplitude) and measure heart rate. Because Spo_2 is normally close to 100%, only gross abnormalities are detectable in most anesthetized patients. Depending on a particular patient's oxygen–hemoglobin dissociation curve, a 90% saturation may indicate a Pao_2 of less than 65 mm Hg. This compares with clinically detectable cyanosis, which requires 5 g of desaturated hemoglobin and usually corresponds to an Spo_2 of less than 80%. Bronchial intubation will usually go undetected by pulse oximetry in the absence of lung disease or low fraction of inspired oxygen concentrations (Fio_2).

Because carboxyhemoglobin (COHb) and HbO_2 absorb light at 660 nm identically, pulse oximeters that compare only two wavelengths of light will register a falsely high reading in patients with carbon monoxide poisoning. Methemoglobin has the same absorption coefficient at both red and infrared wavelengths. The resulting 1:1 absorption ratio corresponds to a saturation reading of 85%. **Thus, methemoglobinemia causes a falsely low saturation reading when Sao_2 is actually greater than 85% and a falsely high reading if Sao_2 is actually less than 85%.**

Most pulse oximeters are inaccurate at low Spo_2, and all demonstrate a delay between changes in Sao_2 and Spo_2. **Other causes of pulse oximetry artifact include excessive ambient light, motion, methylene blue dye, venous pulsations in a dependent limb, low perfusion (eg, low cardiac output, profound anemia, hypothermia, increased systemic vascular resistance), malpositioned sensor, and leakage of light from the light-emitting diode to the photodiode, bypassing the arterial bed (optical shunting).** Nevertheless, pulse oximetry can be an invaluable aid to the rapid diagnosis of hypoxia, which may occur in unrecognized esophageal intubation, and it furthers the goal of monitoring oxygen delivery to vital organs. In the recovery room, pulse oximetry helps identify postoperative pulmonary problems, such as severe hypoventilation, bronchospasm, and atelectasis.

Two extensions of pulse oximetry technology are mixed venous blood oxygen saturation (Svo_2) and noninvasive brain oximetry. The former requires the placement of a pulmonary artery catheter containing fiberoptic sensors that continuously determine Svo_2 in a manner analogous to pulse oximetry. Because Svo_2 varies with changes in hemoglobin concentration, cardiac output, arterial oxygen saturation, and whole-body oxygen consumption, its interpretation is somewhat complex. A variation of this technique involves placing the fiberoptic sensor in the internal jugular vein, which provides measurements of jugular bulb oxygen saturation in an attempt to assess the adequacy of cerebral oxygen delivery.

Noninvasive brain oximetry monitors regional oxygen saturation (rSo_2) of hemoglobin in the brain. A sensor placed on the forehead emits light of specific wavelengths and measures the light reflected back to the sensor (near-infrared optical spectroscopy). Unlike pulse oximetry, brain oximetry measures venous and capillary blood oxygen saturation in addition to arterial blood saturation. Thus, its oxygen saturation readings represent the average oxygen saturation of all regional microvascular hemoglobin (approximately 70%). Cardiac arrest, cerebral embolization, deep hypothermia, or severe hypoxia cause a dramatic decrease in rSo_2. (See the section "Neurological System Monitors.")

CAPNOGRAPHY

Indications & Contraindications

Determination of end-tidal CO_2 ($Etco_2$) concentration to confirm adequate ventilation is mandatory during all anesthetic procedures, but particularly so for general anesthesia. A rapid fall of $Etco_2$ is a sensitive indicator of air embolism, a major complication of sitting craniotomies. There are no contraindications.

Techniques & Complications

Capnography is a valuable monitor of the pulmonary, cardiovascular, and anesthetic breathing systems. Capnographs in common use rely on the absorption of infrared light by CO_2 (**Figure 6–3**). As with oximetry, absorption of infrared light by CO_2 is governed by the Beer–Lambert law.

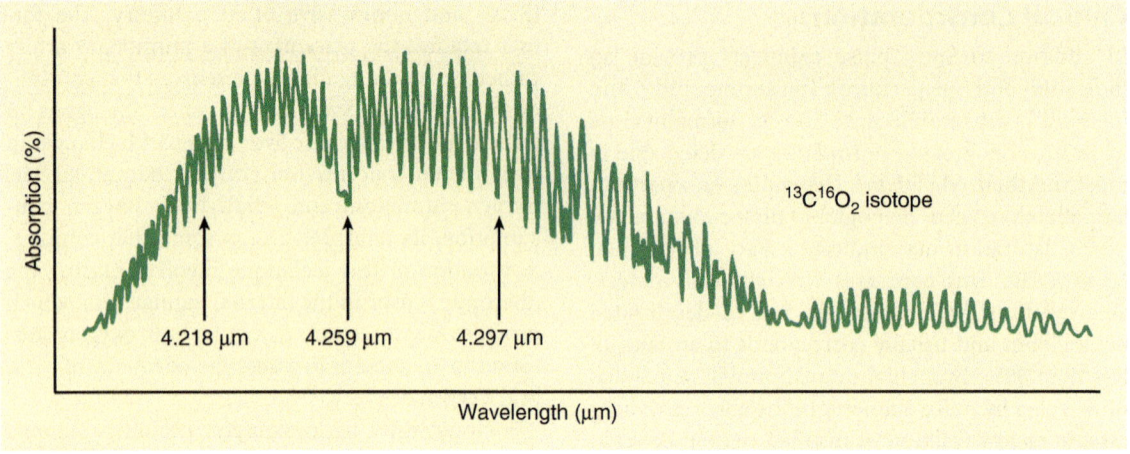

FIGURE 6–3 Absorption spectrum for CO_2. (Reproduced, with permission, from Hill DW: Methods of analysis in the gaseous and vapour phase. In: *Scientific Foundations of Anesthesia*. Scurr C, Feldman S [editors]. Year Book, 1982, p 85.)

A. Nondiverting (Flowthrough)

Nondiverting (mainstream) capnographs measure CO_2 passing through an adaptor placed in the breathing circuit (Figure 6–4). Infrared light transmission through the gas is measured and CO_2 concentration is determined by the monitor. Because of problems with drift, older flowthrough models self-zeroed during inspiration. Thus, they were incapable

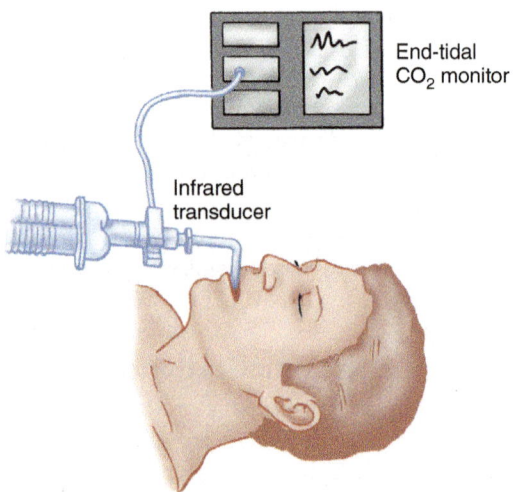

FIGURE 6–4 A nondiverting sensor placed in-line analyzes CO_2 concentration at the sampling site.

of detecting inspired CO_2, such as would occur with a breathing circuit malfunction (eg, absorbent exhaustion, sticking unidirectional valves). The weight of the sensor causes traction on the tracheal tube, and its generation of radiant heat can cause skin burns. Newer designs address these problems.

B. Diverting (Aspiration)

Diverting (sidestream) capnographs continuously suctions gas from the breathing circuit into a sample cell within the monitor. CO_2 concentration is determined by comparing infrared light absorption in the sample cell with a chamber free of CO_2. Continuous aspiration of anesthetic gas essentially represents a leak in the breathing circuit that will contaminate the operating room unless it is scavenged or returned to the breathing system. High aspiration rates (up to 250 mL/min) and low-dead-space sampling tubing usually increase sensitivity and decrease lag time. If tidal volumes (VT) are small (eg, pediatric patients), however, a high rate of aspiration may entrain fresh gas from the circuit and dilute ETCO$_2$ measurement. Low aspiration rates (less than 50 mL/min) can retard ETCO$_2$ measurement and underestimate it during rapid ventilation. New units autocalibrate, but older units must be zeroed to room air and against a known CO_2 concentration (usually 5%). Diverting units are prone to water precipitation in the aspiration tube and sampling cell that can cause obstruction of the sampling line and erroneous readings. Expiratory valve malfunction is detected by the presence of CO_2 in inspired gas. Although inspiratory valve failure also results in rebreathing CO_2, this is not as readily apparent because part of the inspiratory volume will still be free of CO_2, causing the monitor to read zero during part of the inspiratory phase.

Clinical Considerations

Other gases (eg, nitrous oxide) also absorb infrared light, leading to a pressure-broadening effect. To minimize the error introduced by nitrous oxide, various modifications and filters have been incorporated into monitor design. Capnographs rapidly and reliably indicate esophageal intubation—a common cause of anesthetic catastrophe—but do not reliably detect bronchial intubation. Although there may be some CO_2 in the stomach from swallowing expired air, this should be washed out within a few breaths. Sudden cessation of CO_2 during the expiratory phase may indicate a circuit disconnection. The increased metabolic rate caused by malignant hyperthermia causes a marked rise in E_{TCO_2}.

The gradient between Pa_{CO_2} and E_{TCO_2} (normally 2–5 mm Hg) reflects alveolar dead space (alveoli that are ventilated but not perfused). Any significant reduction in lung perfusion (eg, air embolism, decreased cardiac output, or decreased blood pressure) increases alveolar dead space, dilutes expired CO_2, and lessens E_{TCO_2}. True capnographs (as opposed to capnometers) display a waveform of CO_2 concentration that allows recognition of a variety of conditions (Figure 6–5).

ANESTHETIC GAS ANALYSIS

Indications

Analysis of anesthetic gases is essential during any procedure requiring inhalation anesthesia. There are no contraindications to analyzing these gases.

Techniques

Techniques for analyzing multiple anesthetic gases involve mass spectrometry, Raman spectroscopy,

infrared spectrophotometry, or piezoelectric crystal (quartz) oscillation. Mass spectrometry and Raman spectroscopy are primarily of historical interest, as most anesthetic gases are now measured by infrared absorption analysis.

Infrared units use a variety of techniques similar to that described for capnography. These devices are all based on the Beer–Lambert law, which provides a formula for measuring an unknown gas within inspired gas because the absorption of infrared light passing through a solvent (inspired or expired gas) is proportional to the amount of the unknown gas. Oxygen and nitrogen do not absorb infrared light. There are a number of commercially available devices that use a single- or dual-beam infrared light source and positive or negative filtering. Because oxygen molecules do not absorb infrared light, their concentration cannot be measured with monitors that rely on infrared technology and, hence, it must be measured by other means (see below).

Clinical Considerations

A. Piezoelectric Analysis

The piezoelectric method uses oscillating quartz crystals, one of which is covered with lipid. Volatile anesthetics dissolve in the lipid layer and change the frequency of oscillation, which, when compared with the frequency of oscillation of an uncovered crystal, allows the concentration of the volatile anesthetic to be calculated. Neither these devices nor infrared photoacoustic analysis allow different anesthetic agents to be distinguished. New dual-beam infrared optical analyzers do allow gases to be separated and an improperly filled vaporizer to be detected.

B. Oxygen Analysis

To measure the F_{IO_2} of inhaled gas, manufacturers of anesthesia machines have relied on various technologies.

C. Galvanic Cell

Galvanic cell (fuel cell) contains a lead anode and gold cathode bathed in potassium chloride. At the gold terminal, hydroxyl ions are formed that react with the lead electrode (thereby gradually consuming it) to produce lead oxide, causing current, which is proportional to the amount of oxygen being

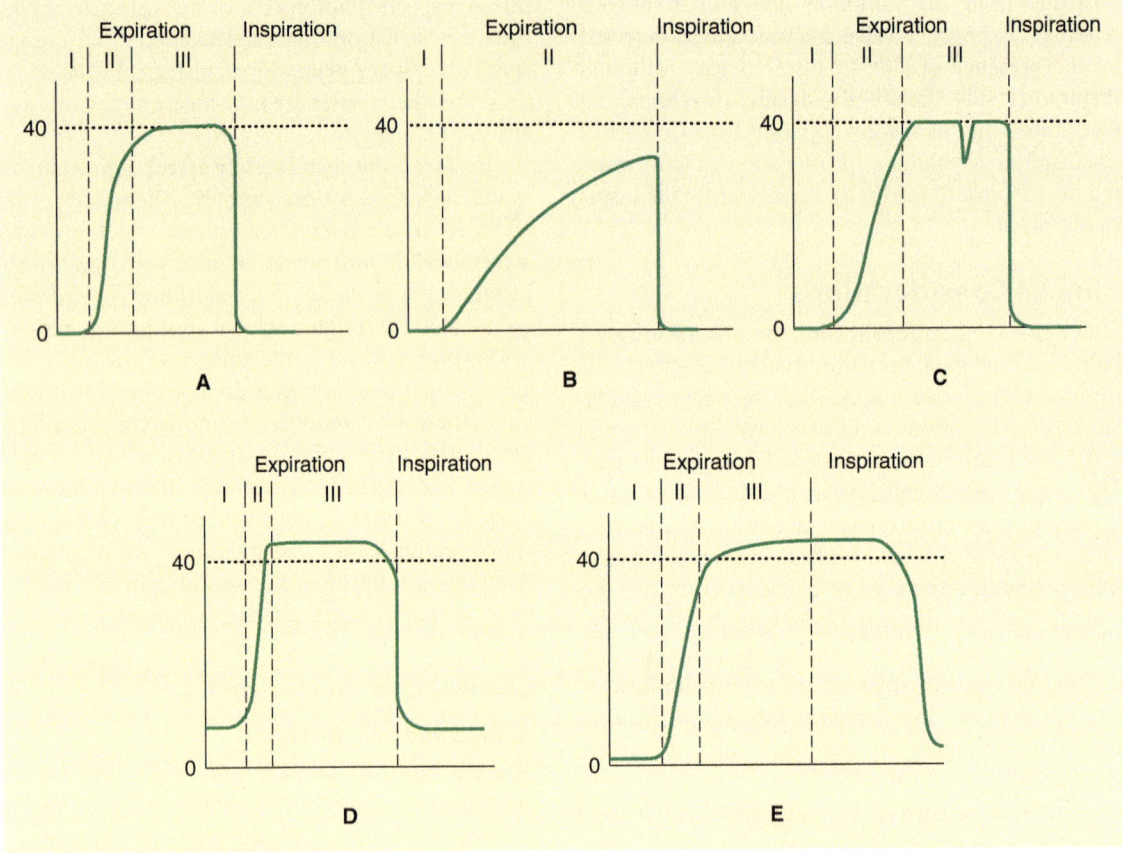

FIGURE 6–5 **A**: A normal capnograph demonstrating the three phases of expiration: phase I—dead space; phase II—mixture of dead space and alveolar gas; phase III—alveolar gas plateau. **B**: Capnograph of a patient with severe chronic obstructive pulmonary disease. No plateau is reached before the next inspiration. The gradient between end-tidal CO_2 and arterial CO_2 is increased. **C**: Depression during phase III indicates spontaneous respiratory effort. **D**: Failure of the inspired CO_2 to return to zero may represent an incompetent expiratory valve or exhausted CO_2 absorbent. **E**: The persistence of exhaled gas during part of the inspiratory cycle signals the presence of an incompetent inspiratory valve.

measured, to flow. Because the lead electrode is consumed, monitor life can be prolonged by exposing it to room air when not in use. These are the oxygen monitors used on many anesthesia machines in the inspiratory limb.

D. Paramagnetic Analysis

Oxygen is a nonpolar gas, but it is paramagnetic, and when placed in a magnetic field, the gas will expand, contracting when the magnet is turned off. By switching the field on and off and comparing the resulting change in volume (or pressure or flow) to a known standard, the amount of oxygen can be measured.

E. Polarographic Electrode

A polarographic electrode has a gold (or platinum) cathode and a silver anode, both bathed in an electrolyte, separated from the gas to be measured by a semipermeable membrane. Unlike the galvanic cell, a polarographic electrode works only if a small voltage is applied to two electrodes. When voltage is applied to the cathode, electrons combine with oxygen to form hydroxide ions. The amount of current that flows between the anode and the cathode is proportional to the amount of oxygen present.

F. Spirometry

Newer anesthesia machines can measure (and therefore manage) airway pressures, volume, and flow to calculate resistance and compliance and to display the relationship of these variables as flow (ie, volume or pressure–volume loops). Measurements of flow and volume are made by mechanical devices that are usually fairly lightweight and are often placed in the inspiratory limb of the anesthesia circuit.

The most fundamental measurements include low peak inspiratory pressure and high peak inspiratory pressure, which indicate either a ventilator or circuit disconnect, or an airway obstruction, respectively. By measuring V_T and breathing frequency (f), exhaled minute ventilation (V_E) can be calculated, providing some sense of security that ventilation requirements are being met.

Spirometric loops and waveforms are characteristically altered by certain disease processes and events. If a normal loop is observed shortly after induction of anesthesia and a subsequent loop is different, the observant anesthesiologist is alerted to the fact that pulmonary and/or airway compliance may have changed. Spirometric loops are usually displayed as flow versus volume and volume versus pressure (Figure 6–6). There are characteristic changes with obstruction, bronchial intubation, reactive airways disease, and so forth.

Neurological System Monitors

ELECTROENCEPHALOGRAPHY

Indications & Contraindications

The electroencephalogram (EEG) is occasionally used during cerebrovascular surgery to confirm the adequacy of cerebral oxygenation. Monitoring the depth of anesthesia with a full 16-lead, 8-channel EEG is not warranted, considering the availability of simpler techniques. There are no contraindications.

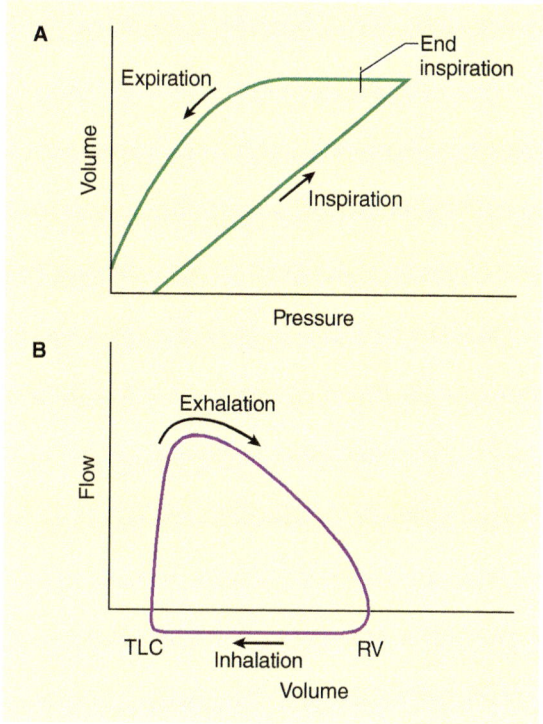

FIGURE 6–6 A: Normal volume–pressure loop. **B:** Normal flow–volume loop.

Techniques & Complications

The EEG is a recording of electrical potentials generated by cells in the cerebral cortex. Although standard ECG electrodes can be used, silver disks containing a conductive gel are preferred. Platinum or stainless steel needle electrodes traumatize the scalp and have high impedance (resistance); however, they can be sterilized and placed in a surgical field. Electrode position (montage) is governed by the international 10–20 system (Figure 6–7). Electric potential differences between combinations of electrodes are filtered, amplified, and displayed by an oscilloscope or pen recorder. EEG activity occurs mostly at frequencies between 1–30 cycles/sec (Hz). Alpha waves have a frequency of 8–13 Hz and are found often in a resting adult with eyes closed. Beta waves at 8–13 Hz are found in concentrating individuals, and at times, in individuals under anesthesia. Delta waves have a frequency of

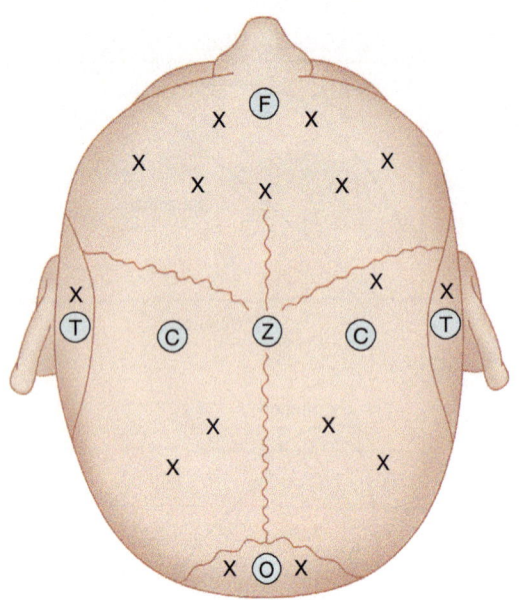

FIGURE 6–7 International 10–20 system. Montage letters refer to cranial location. F, frontal; C, coronal; T, temporal; O, occipital; Z, middle.

0.5–4 Hz and are found in brain injury, deep sleep, and anesthesia. Theta waves (4–7 Hz) are also found in sleeping individuals and during anesthesia. EEG waves are also characterized by their amplitude, which is related to their potential (high amplitude, >50 microV; medium amplitude, 20–50 microV; and low amplitude, <20 microV). Lastly, the EEG is examined as to symmetry between the left and right hemispheres.

Examination of a multichannel EEG is at times performed during surgery to detect areas of cerebral ischemia, such as during carotid endarterectomy as well as during epilepsy surgery. Likewise, it can be used to detect EEG isoelectricity and maximal cerebral protection during hypothermic arrest. The strip chart EEG is cumbersome in the operating room, and often the EEG is processed using power spectral analysis. Frequency analysis divides the EEG into a series of sine waves at different frequencies and then plots the power of the signal at each frequency, allowing for a presentation of EEG activity in a more manageable way than reviewing the raw EEG (Figure 6–8).

During inhalational anesthesia, initial beta activation is followed by slowing, burst suppression, and isoelectricity. Intravenous agents, depending on dose and drug used, can produce a variety of EEG patterns.

To reduce the incidence of anesthesia awareness, devices have been developed in recent years that process two-channel EEG signals and create a dimensionless variable to indicate wakefulness. Bispectral index (BIS) is most commonly used in this regard. BIS monitors examine four components within the EEG that are associated with the anesthetic state: (1) low frequency, as found during deep anesthesia; (2) high-frequency beta activation found during "light" anesthesia; (3) suppressed EEG waves; and (4) burst suppression.

Other devices attempt to include measures of spontaneous muscle activity, as influenced by the activity of subcortical structures not contributing to the EEG to further provide an assessment of anesthetic depth. Various devices, each with its own algorithm to process the EEG and/or incorporate other variables to ascertain patient wakefulness, may become available in the future (Table 6–1).

Controversy still exists as to the exact role of processed EEG devices in assessing anesthetic depth. Some studies have demonstrated a reduced awareness when these devices were used, whereas other studies have failed to reveal any advantage over the use of inhalational gas measurements to ensure a minimal alveolar concentration of anesthetic agent. Because individual EEG responsiveness to anesthetic agents may be variable, EEG monitors to assess anesthesia depth or to titrate anesthetic delivery might not always ensure an absence of wakefulness. Moreover, many monitors have a delay, which might only indicate a risk for the patient being aware after he or she had already become conscious (Table 6–2).

Clinical Considerations

To perform a bispectral analysis, data measured by EEG are taken through a number of steps (Figure 6–9) to calculate a single number that correlates with depth of anesthesia/hypnosis.

BIS values of 65–85 have been advocated as a measure of sedation, whereas values of 40–65

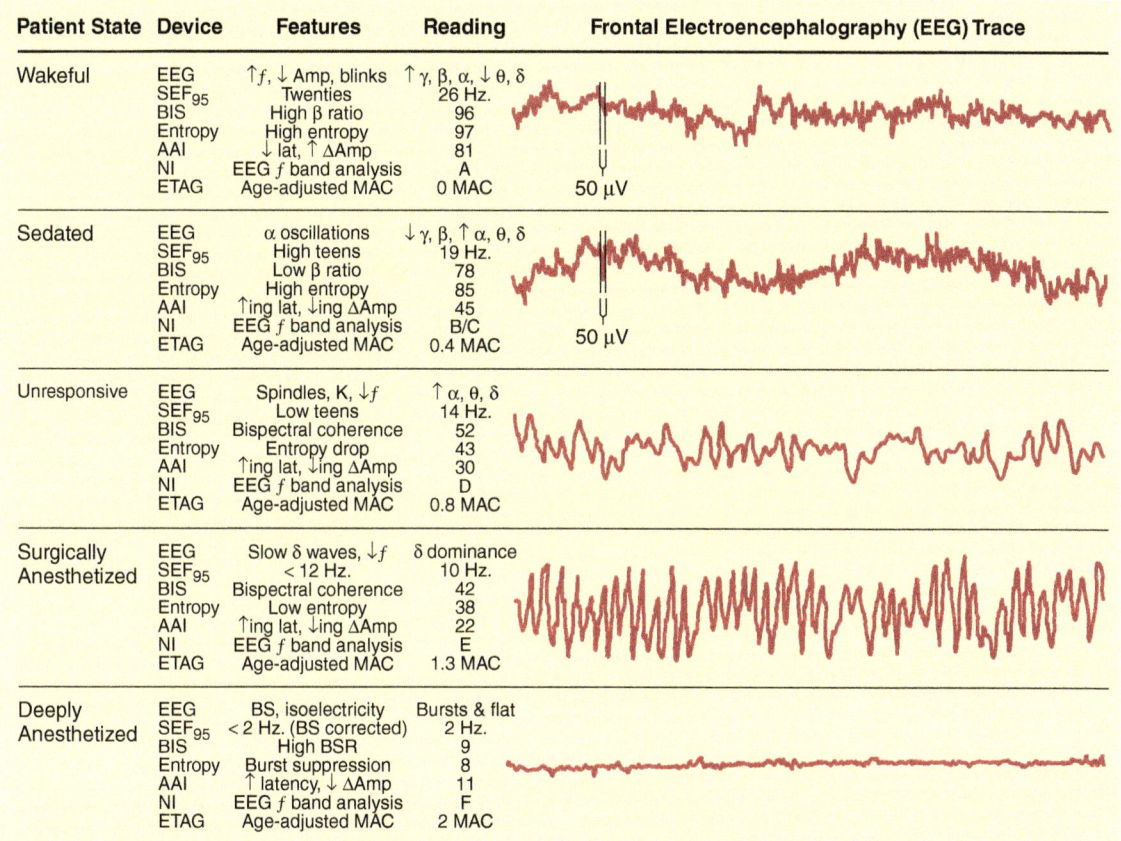

Patient State	Device	Features	Reading	Frontal Electroencephalography (EEG) Trace
Wakeful	EEG	↑f, ↓ Amp, blinks	↑ γ, β, α, ↓ θ, δ	
	SEF$_{95}$	Twenties	26 Hz.	
	BIS	High β ratio	96	
	Entropy	High entropy	97	
	AAI	↓ lat, ↑ ΔAmp	81	
	NI	EEG f band analysis	A	
	ETAG	Age-adjusted MAC	0 MAC	50 µV
Sedated	EEG	α oscillations	↓ γ, β, ↑ α, θ, δ	
	SEF$_{95}$	High teens	19 Hz.	
	BIS	Low β ratio	78	
	Entropy	High entropy	85	
	AAI	↑ing lat, ↓ing ΔAmp	45	
	NI	EEG f band analysis	B/C	
	ETAG	Age-adjusted MAC	0.4 MAC	50 µV
Unresponsive	EEG	Spindles, K, ↓f	↑ α, θ, δ	
	SEF$_{95}$	Low teens	14 Hz.	
	BIS	Bispectral coherence	52	
	Entropy	Entropy drop	43	
	AAI	↑ing lat, ↓ing ΔAmp	30	
	NI	EEG f band analysis	D	
	ETAG	Age-adjusted MAC	0.8 MAC	
Surgically Anesthetized	EEG	Slow δ waves, ↓f	δ dominance	
	SEF$_{95}$	< 12 Hz.	10 Hz.	
	BIS	Bispectral coherence	42	
	Entropy	Low entropy	38	
	AAI	↑ing lat, ↓ing ΔAmp	22	
	NI	EEG f band analysis	E	
	ETAG	Age-adjusted MAC	1.3 MAC	
Deeply Anesthetized	EEG	BS, isoelectricity	Bursts & flat	
	SEF$_{95}$	< 2 Hz. (BS corrected)	2 Hz.	
	BIS	High BSR	9	
	Entropy	Burst suppression	8	
	AAI	↑ latency, ↓ ΔAmp	11	
	NI	EEG f band analysis	F	
	ETAG	Age-adjusted MAC	2 MAC	

FIGURE 6–8 Patient states, candidate depth of anesthesia devices or approaches, key features of different monitoring approaches, and possible readings at different depths of anesthesia. The readings shown represent examples of possible readings that may be seen in conjunction with each frontal electroencephalography trace. The electroencephalography traces show 3-s epochs (x-axis), and the scale (y-axis) is 50 µV. AAI, A-Line Autoregressive Index (a proprietary method of extracting the mid-latency auditory evoked potential from the electroencephalogram); Amp, amplitude of an EEG wave; BIS bispectral index; blinks, eye blink artifacts; BS, burst suppression; BSR, burst suppression ratio; EEG, electroencephalography; ETAG, end-tidal anesthetic gas concentration; f, frequency; γ, β, α, θ, δ, EEG waves in decreasing frequencies (γ more than 30 hertz [Hz]; β, 12–30 Hz; α, 8–12 Hz; θ, 4–8 Hz; δ, 0–4 Hz); K, K complexes; Lat, latency between an auditory stimulus and an evoked EEG waveform response; MAC, minimum alveolar concentration; NI, Narcotrend index; SEF$_{95}$, spectral edge frequency below which 95% of the EEG frequencies reside; Spindles, sleep spindles. (Reproduced, with permission, from Mashour GA, Orser BA, Avidan MS: Intraoperative awareness: from neurobiology to clinical practice. Anesthesiology 2011;114:1218.)

have been recommended for general anesthesia (Figure 6–10). Bispectral analysis may reduce patient awareness during anesthesia, an issue that is important to the public.

Many of the initial studies of its use were not prospective, randomized, controlled trials, but were primarily observational in nature. Artifacts can be a problem. The monitor, in and of itself, costs several thousand dollars and the electrodes are approximately $10 to $15 per anesthetic and cannot be reused.

Some cases with awareness have been identified as having a BIS of less than 65. However, in other cases of awareness, either there were problems with

TABLE 6–1 Characteristics of the commercially available monitors of anesthetic depth.

Parameters	Machine/Manufacturer	Consumable	Physiologic Signals	Recommended Range of Values for Anesthesia	Principles of Measurement
Bispectral index (BIS)	A-2000/Aspect Medical Systems, Newton, MA	BIS sensor	Single channel EEG	40–60	BIS is derived from the weighted sum of three EEG parameters: relative α/β ratio; bio-coherence of the EEG waves; and burst suppression. The relative contribution of these parameters has been tuned to correlate with the degree of sedation produced by various sedative agents. BIS ranges from 0 (asleep)–100 (awake).
Patient state index (PSI)	Patient state analyzer (PSA 400)/ Physiometrix, Inc., N. Billerica, MA	PSArray[2]	4-channel EEG	25–50	PSI is derived from progressive discriminant analysis of several quantitative EEG variables that are sensitive to changes in the level of anesthesia, but insensitive to the specific agents producing such changes. It includes changes in power spectrum in various EEG frequency bands; hemispheric symmetry; and synchronization between brain regions and the inhibition of regions of the frontal cortex. PSI ranges from 0 (asleep)–100 (awake).
Narcotrend stage Narcotrend index	Narcotrend monitor/ Monitor-Technik, Bad Bramstedt, Germany	Ordinary ECG electrode	1–2 channel EEG	Narcotrend stage D_{0-2} to C_1, which corresponds to an index of 40–60	The Narcotrend monitor classifies EEG signals into different stages of anesthesia (A = awake; B_{0-2} = sedated; C_{0-2} = light anesthesia; D_{0-2} = general anesthesia; $E_{0,1}$ = general anesthesia with deep hypnosis; $F_{0,1}$ = burst suppression). The classification algorithm is based on a discriminant analysis of entropy measures and EEG spectral variables. More recently the monitor converts the Narcotrend stages into a dimensionless number from 0 (asleep) to 100 (awake) by nonlinear regression.
Entropy	S/5 Entropy Module, M-ENTROPY/ Datex-Ohmeda, Instrumentarium Corp., Helsinki, Finland	Special entropy sensor	Single-channel EEG	40–60	Entropy described the 'irregularity' of the EEG signal. As the dose of anesthetic is increased, EEG becomes more regular and the entropy value approaches zero. M-ENTROPY calculates the entropy of the EEG spectrum (spectral entropy). In order to shorten the response time, it uses different time windows according to the corresponding EEG frequencies. Two spectral parameters are calculated: state entropy (frequency band 0–32 Hz) and response entropy (0–47 Hz), which also includes muscle activity. Both entropy variables have been re-scaled, so that 0 is asleep and 100 is awake.
Aline autoregressive index (AAI)	AEP/2 monitor/ Danmeter A/S, Odense, Demark	Ordinary ECG electrode	AEP	10–25	AAI is derived from the middle latency AEP (20–80 ms). AAI is extracted from an autoregressive model with exogenous input (ARX model) so that only 18 sweeps are required to reproduce the AEP waveform in 2–6 s. The resultant waveform is then transformed into a numeric index (0–100) that describes the shape of the AEP. AAI > 60 is awake, AAI of 0 indicates deep anesthesia.
Cerebral state index (CSI)	Cerebral state monitor (CSM), Danmeter A/S, Odense, Demark	Ordinary ECG electrode	Single-channel EEG	40–60	CSI is a weighted sum of (1) α ratio, (2) β ratio, (3) difference between the two and (4) burst suppression. It correlates with the degree of sedation by an 'adaptive neuro-fuzzy inference system'. CSI ranges from 0 (asleep) to 100 (awake).

EEG, electroencephalogram; ECG, electrocardiogram; AEP, auditory evoked potential.

Reproduced, with permission, from Chan MTV, Gin T, Goh KYC: Interventional neurophysiologic monitoring. Curr Opin Anaesthesiol 2004;17:389.

TABLE 6–2 Checklist for preventing awareness.

✓ Check all equipment, drugs, and dosages; ensure that drugs are clearly labeled and that infusions are running into veins.
✓ Consider administering an amnesic premedication.
✓ Avoid or minimize the administration of muscle relaxants. Use a peripheral nerve stimulator to guide minimal required dose.
✓ Consider using the isolated forearm technique if intense paralysis is indicated.
✓ Choose potent inhalation agents rather than total intravenous anesthesia, if possible.
✓ Administer at least 0.5 to 0.7 minimum alveolar concentration (MAC) of the inhalation agent.
✓ Set an alarm for a low anesthetic gas concentration.
✓ Monitor anesthetic gas concentration during cardiopulmonary bypass from the bypass machine.
✓ Consider alternative treatments for hypotension other than decreasing anesthetic concentration.
✓ If it is thought that sufficient anesthesia cannot be administered because of concern about hemodynamic compromise, consider the administration of benzodiazepines or scopolamine for amnesia.
✓ Supplement hypnotic agents with analgesic agents such as opioids or local anesthetics, which may help decrease the experience of pain in the event of awareness.
✓ Consider using a brain monitor, such as a raw or processed electroencephalogram but do not try to minimize the anesthetic dose based on the brain monitor because there currently is insufficient evidence to support this practice.
✓ Monitor the brain routinely if using total intravenous anesthesia.
✓ Evaluate known risk factors for awareness, and if specific risk factors are identified consider increasing administered anesthetic concentration.
✓ Redose intravenous anesthesia when delivery of inhalation anesthesia is difficult, such as during a long intubation attempt or during rigid bronchoscopy.

Reproduced, with permission, from Mashour GA, Orser BA, Avidan MS: Intraoperative awareness: from neurobiology to clinical practice. Anesthesiology 2011;114:1218.

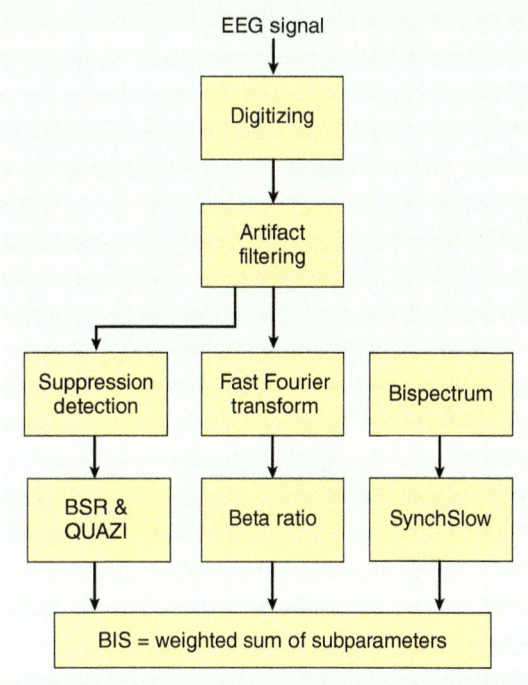

FIGURE 6–9 Calculation of the Bispectral Index. EEG, electroencephalogram; BSR, burst suppression ratio; BIS, Bispectral Index Scale. (Reproduced, with permission, from Rampil IJ: A primer for EEG signal processing in anesthesia. Anesthesiology 1998;89:980.)

the recordings, or awareness could not be related to any specific time or BIS value. Whether this monitoring technique becomes a standard of care in the future remains to be seen, and studies are ongoing.

Detection of awareness often can minimize its consequences. Use of the Brice questions during postoperative visits can alert anesthesia providers of a potential awareness event. Ask patients to recall the following:

• What do you remember before going to sleep?
• What do you remember right when awakening?
• Do you remember anything in between going to sleep and awakening?
• Did you have any dreams while asleep?

Close follow-up and involvement of mental health experts may avoid the traumatic stress that can be associated with awareness events. Increasingly, patients are managed with regional anesthesia and propofol sedation. Patients undergoing such anesthetics should be made aware that they are not having general anesthesia and might recall perioperative events. Clarification of the techniques used may prevent patients so managed from the belief that they "were awake" during anesthesia.

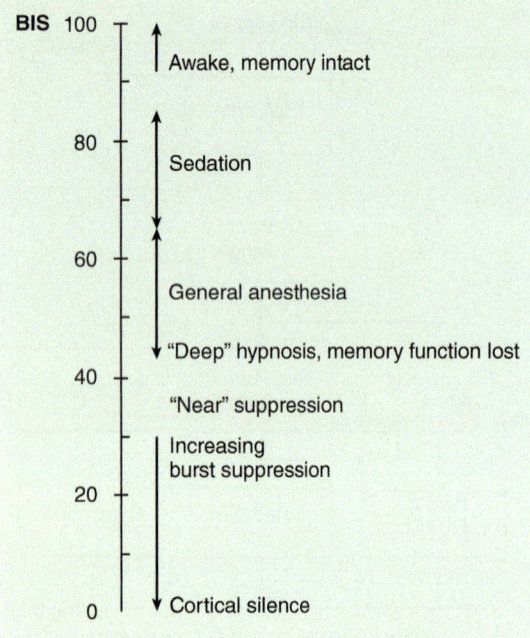

FIGURE 6–10 The Bispectral Index Scale (BIS versions 3.0 and higher) is a dimensionless scale from 0 (complete cortical electroencephalographic suppression) to 100 (awake). BIS values of 65–85 have been recommended for sedation, whereas values of 40–65 have been recommended for general anesthesia. At BIS values lower than 40, cortical suppression becomes discernible in a raw electroencephalogram as a burst suppression pattern. (Reproduced, with permission, from Johansen JW et al: Development and clinical application of electroencephalographic bispectrum monitoring. Anesthesiology 2000;93:1337.)

EVOKED POTENTIALS

Indications

Indications for intraoperative monitoring of **evoked potentials** (EPs) include surgical procedures associated with possible neurological injury: spinal fusion with instrumentation, spine and spinal cord tumor resection, brachial plexus repair, thoracoabdominal aortic aneurysm repair, epilepsy surgery, and cerebral tumor resection. Ischemia in the spinal cord or cerebral cortex can be detected by EPs. EP monitoring facilitates probe localization during stereotactic neurosurgery. Auditory EPs have also been used to assess the effects of general anesthesia on the brain. The middle latency auditory EP may be a more sensitive indicator than BIS in regard to anesthetic depth. The amplitude and latency of this signal following an auditory stimulus is influenced by anesthetics.

Contraindications

Although there are no specific contraindications for somatosensory-evoked potentials (SEPs), this modality is severely limited by the availability of monitoring sites, equipment, and trained personnel. Sensitivity to anesthetic agents can also be a limiting factor, particularly in children. Motor-evoked potentials (MEPs) are contraindicated in patients with retained intracranial metal, a skull defect, and implantable devices, as well as after seizures and any major cerebral insult. Brain injury secondary to repetitive stimulation of the cortex and inducement of seizures is a concern with MEPs.

Techniques & Complications

EP monitoring noninvasively assesses neural function by measuring electrophysiological responses to sensory or motor pathway stimulation. Commonly monitored EPs are brainstem auditory evoked responses (BAERs), SEPs, and increasingly, MEPs (Figure 6–11).

For SEPs, a brief electrical current is delivered to a sensory or mixed peripheral nerve by a pair of electrodes. If the intervening pathway is intact, a nerve action potential will be transmitted to the contralateral sensory cortex to produce an EP. This potential can be measured by cortical surface electrodes, but is usually measured by scalp electrodes. To distinguish the cortical response to a specific stimulus, multiple responses are averaged and background noise is eliminated. EPs are represented by a plot of voltage versus time. The resulting waveforms are analyzed for their poststimulus latency (the time between stimulation and potential detection) and peak amplitude. These are compared with baseline tracings. Technical and physiological causes of a change in an EP must be distinguished from changes due to neural damage. Complications of EP monitoring are rare, but include skin irritation and pressure ischemia at the sites of electrode application.

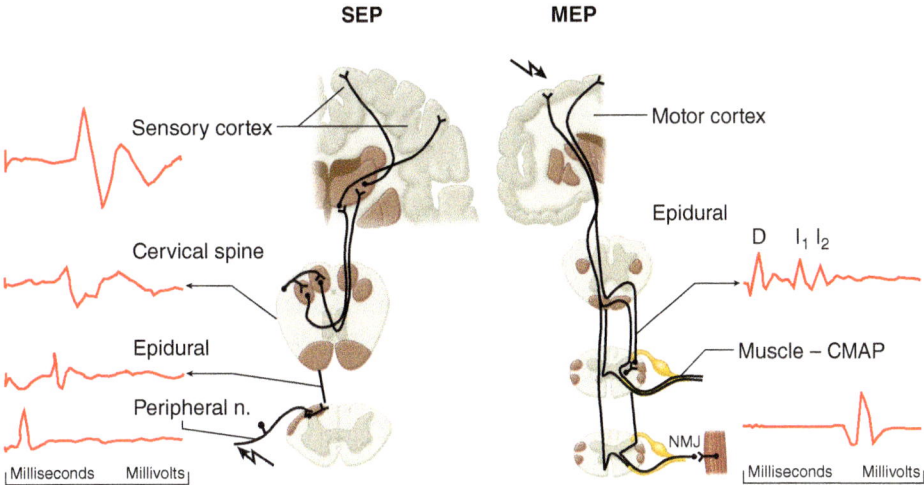

FIGURE 6–11 Neuroanatomic pathways of somatosensory-evoked potential and motor-evoked potential. The somatosensory-evoked potential (SEP) is produced by stimulation of a peripheral nerve wherein a response can be measured. The electrical volley ascends the spinal cord by the posterior columns and can be recorded in the epidural space and over the posterior cervical spine. It crosses the mid-line after synapsing at the cervicomedullary junction and ascends the lemniscal pathways having a second synapse in the thalamus. From there, it travels to the primary sensory cortex where the cortical response is measured. The motor-evoked potential (MEP) is produced by stimulation of the motor cortex leading to an electrical volley that descends to the anterior horn cells of the spinal cord via the corticospinal tract. After synapsing there it travels via a peripheral nerve and crosses the neuromuscular junction (NMJ) to produce a muscle response. The MEP can be measured in the epidural space as D and I waves produced by direct and indirect (via internuncial neurons) stimulation of the motor cortex, respectively. It can also be measured as a compound muscle action potential (CMAP) in the muscle. (Reproduced, with permission, from Sloan TB, Janik D, Jameson L: Multimodality monitoring of the central nervous system using motor-evoked potentials. Curr Opin Anaesthesiol. 2008;21:560.)

Clinical Considerations

EPs are altered by many variables other than neural damage. The effect of anesthetics is complex and not easily summarized. **In general, balanced anesthetic techniques (nitrous oxide, neuromuscular blocking agents, and opioids) cause minimal changes, whereas volatile agents (halothane, sevoflurane, desflurane, and isoflurane) are best avoided or used at a constant low dose**. Early-occurring (specific) EPs are less affected by anesthetics than are late-occurring (nonspecific) responses. Changes in BAERs may provide a measure of the depth of anesthesia. Physiological (eg, blood pressure, temperature, and oxygen saturation) and pharmacological factors should be kept as constant as possible.

Persistent obliteration of EPs is predictive of postoperative neurological deficit. Although SEPs usually identify spinal cord damage, because of their different anatomic pathways, *sensory* (dorsal spinal cord) EP preservation does not guarantee normal *motor* (ventral spinal cord) function (false negative). Furthermore, SEPs elicited from posterior tibial nerve stimulation cannot distinguish between peripheral and central ischemia (false positive). Techniques that elicit MEPs by using transcranial magnetic or electrical stimulation of the cortex allow the detection of action potentials in the muscles if the neural pathway is intact. The advantage of using MEPs as opposed to SEPs for spinal cord monitoring is that MEPs monitor the ventral spinal cord, and if sensitive and specific enough, can be used to indicate which patients might develop a postoperative motor deficit. MEPs are more sensitive to spinal cord ischemia than are SEPs. The same considerations for SEPs are applicable to MEPs in that they are affected by volatile inhalational agents, high-dose benzodiazepines, and moderate hypothermia (temperatures less than 32°C). MEPs require monitoring of the level of neuromuscular blockade. Close communication with a neurophysiologist is essential prior to the start of any case where these monitors are used to review the optimal anesthetic technique to ensure monitoring integrity. MEPs are sensitive to volatile anesthetics. Consequently, intravenous techniques are often preferred.

CEREBRAL OXIMETRY AND OTHER MONITORS OF THE BRAIN

Cerebral oximetry uses near infrared spectroscopy (NIRS). Using reflectance spectroscopy near infrared light is emitted by a probe on the scalp (Figure 6–12). Receptors are likewise positioned to detect the reflected light from both deep and superficial structures. As with pulse oximetry, oxygenated and deoxygenated hemoglobin absorb light at different frequencies. Likewise, cytochrome absorbs infrared light in the mitochondria. The NIRS saturation largely reflects the absorption of venous hemoglobin, as it does not have the ability to identify the pulsatile arterial component. Regional saturations of less than 40% on NIRS measures, or changes of greater than 25% of baseline measures, may herald neurological events secondary to decreased cerebral oxygenation.

Measurements of jugular venous bulb saturation can also provide estimates of cerebral tissue oxygen extraction/decreased cerebral oxygen delivery. Reduced saturations may indicate poor outcomes. Direct tissue oxygen monitoring of the brain is accomplished by placement of a probe to determine the oxygen tension in the brain tissue. In addition to maintaining a cerebral perfusion pressure that is greater than 60 mm Hg and an intracranial pressure that is less than 20 mm Hg, neuroanesthesiologists/intensivists attempt to preserve brain tissue oxygenation by intervening when oxygen tissue tension is less than 20 mm Hg. Such interventions center upon improving oxygen delivery by increasing F_{IO_2}, augmenting hemoglobin, adjusting cardiac output, or decreasing oxygen demand.

Other Monitors

TEMPERATURE

Indications

The temperature of patients undergoing anesthesia must be monitored. Postoperative temperature is increasingly used as a quality anesthesia indicator. Hypothermia is associated with delayed drug metabolism, increased blood glucose, vasoconstriction, impaired coagulation, and impaired resistance to surgical infections. Hyperthermia can likewise

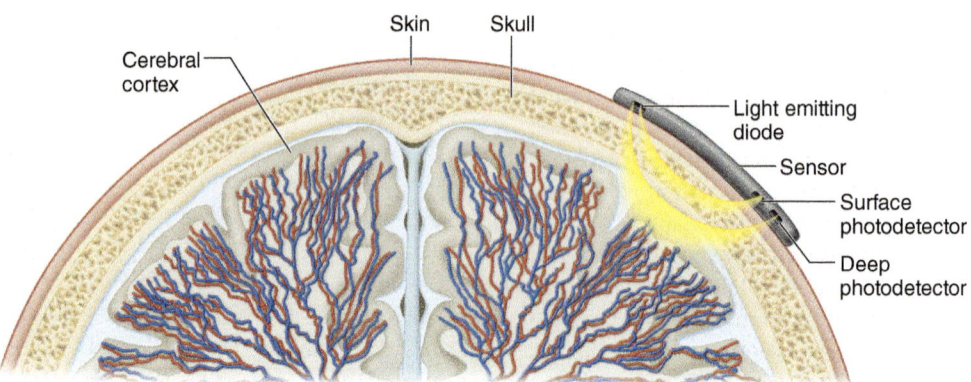

FIGURE 6–12 Principle of the INVOS® near-infrared spectroscopy technique. (Reproduced, with permission, from Rubio A, Hakami L, Münch F, Tandler R, Harig F, Weyand M: Noninvasive control of adequate cerebral oxygenation during low-flow antegrade selective cerebral perfusion on adults and infants in the aortic arch surgery. J Card Surg 2008;23:474.)

have deleterious effects perioperatively, leading to tachycardia, vasodilation, and neurological injury. Consequently, temperature must be measured and recorded perioperatively.

Contraindications

There are no contraindications, although a particular monitoring site may be unsuitable in certain patients.

Techniques & Complications

Intraoperatively, temperature is usually measured using a thermistor or thermocouple. Thermistors are semiconductors whose resistance decreases predictably with warming. A thermocouple is a circuit of two dissimilar metals joined so that a potential difference is generated when the metals are at different temperatures. Disposable thermocouple and thermistor probes are available for monitoring the temperature of the tympanic membrane, nasopharynx, esophagus, bladder, rectum, and skin. Infrared sensors estimate temperature from the infrared energy that is produced. Tympanic membrane temperatures reflect core body temperature; however, the devices used may not reliably measure the temperature at the tympanic membrane. Complications of temperature monitoring are usually related to trauma caused by the probe (eg, rectal or tympanic membrane perforation).

Each monitoring site has advantages and disadvantages. The tympanic membrane theoretically reflects brain temperature because the auditory canal's blood supply is the external carotid artery. Trauma during insertion and cerumen insulation detract from the routine use of tympanic probes. Rectal temperatures have a slow response to changes in core temperature. Nasopharyngeal probes are prone to cause epistaxis, but accurately measure core temperature if placed adjacent to the nasopharyngeal mucosa. The thermistor on a pulmonary artery catheter also measures core temperature. There is a variable correlation between axillary temperature and core temperature, depending on skin perfusion. Liquid crystal adhesive strips placed on the skin are inadequate indicators of core body temperature during surgery. Esophageal temperature sensors, often incorporated into esophageal stethoscopes, provide

the best combination of economy, performance, and safety. To avoid measuring the temperature of tracheal gases, the temperature sensor should be positioned behind the heart in the lower third of the esophagus. Conveniently, heart sounds are most prominent at this location. For more on the clinical considerations of temperature control, see Chapter 52.

URINARY OUTPUT

Indications

Urinary bladder catheterization is the only reliable method of monitoring urinary output. Insertion of a urinary catheter is indicated in patients with congestive heart failure, renal failure, advanced hepatic disease, or shock. Catheterization is routine in some surgical procedures such as cardiac surgery, aortic or renal vascular surgery, craniotomy, major abdominal surgery, or procedures in which large fluid shifts are expected. Lengthy surgeries and intraoperative diuretic administration are other possible indications. Occasionally, postoperative bladder catheterization is indicated in patients having difficulty voiding in the recovery room after general or regional anesthesia.

Contraindications

Bladder catheterization should be done with utmost care in patients at high risk for infection.

Techniques & Complications

Bladder catheterization is usually performed by surgical or nursing personnel. To avoid unnecessary trauma, a urologist should catheterize patients suspected of having abnormal urethral anatomy. A soft rubber Foley catheter is inserted into the bladder transurethrally and connected to a disposable calibrated collection chamber. To avoid urine reflux and minimize the risk of infection, the chamber should remain at a level below the bladder. Complications of catheterization include urethral trauma and urinary tract infections. Rapid decompression of a distended bladder can cause hypotension. Suprapubic catheterization of the bladder with tubing inserted through a large-bore needle is an uncommon alternative.

Clinical Considerations

An additional advantage of placing a Foley catheter is the ability to include a thermistor in the catheter tip so that bladder temperature can be monitored. As long as urinary output is high, bladder temperature accurately reflects core temperature. An added value with more widespread use of urometers is the ability to electronically monitor and record urinary output and temperature.

Urinary output is a reflection of kidney perfusion and function and an indicator of renal, cardiovascular, and fluid volume status. Inadequate urinary output (oliguria) is often arbitrarily defined as urinary output of less than 0.5 mL/kg/hr, but actually is a function of the patient's concentrating ability and osmotic load. Urine electrolyte composition, osmolality, and specific gravity aid in the differential diagnosis of oliguria.

PERIPHERAL NERVE STIMULATION

Indications

Because of the variation in patient sensitivity to neuromuscular blocking agents, the neuromuscular function of all patients receiving intermediate- or long-acting neuromuscular blocking agents should be monitored. In addition, peripheral nerve stimulation is helpful in assessing paralysis during rapid-sequence inductions or during continuous infusions of short-acting agents. Furthermore, peripheral nerve stimulators can help locate nerves to be blocked by regional anesthesia.

Contraindications

There are no contraindications to neuromuscular monitoring, although certain sites may be precluded by the surgical procedure. Additionally, atrophied muscles in areas of hemiplegia or nerve damage may appear refractory to neuromuscular blockade secondary to the proliferation of receptors. Determining the degree of neuromuscular blockade using such an extremity could lead to potential overdosing of competitive neuromuscular blocking agents.

Techniques & Complications

A peripheral nerve stimulator delivers current (60-80 mA) to a pair of either ECG silver chloride pads or subcutaneous needles placed over a peripheral motor nerve. The evoked mechanical or electrical response of the innervated muscle is observed. Although electromyography provides a fast, accurate, and quantitative measure of neuromuscular transmission, visual or tactile observation of muscle contraction is usually relied upon in clinical practice. Ulnar nerve stimulation of the adductor pollicis muscle and facial nerve stimulation of the orbicularis oculi are most commonly monitored (**Figure 6–13**). Because it is the inhibition of the

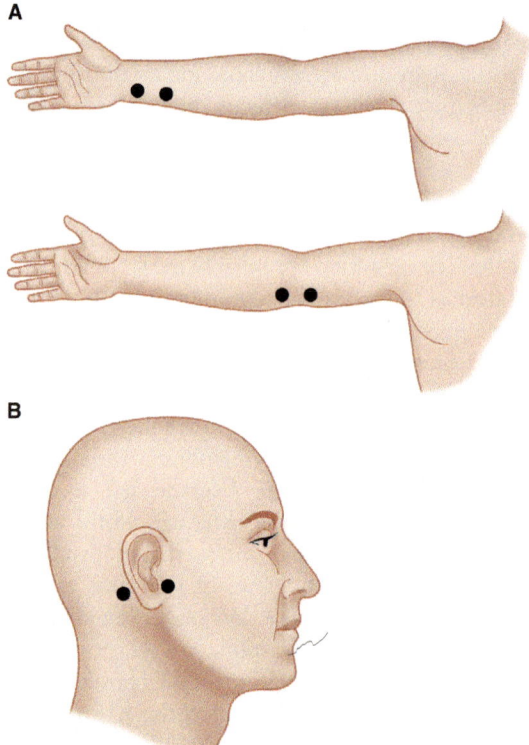

FIGURE 6–13 **A:** Stimulation of the ulnar nerve causes contraction of the adductor pollicis muscle. **B:** Stimulation of the facial nerve leads to orbicularis oculi contraction. The orbicularis oculi recovers from neuromuscular blockade before the adductor pollicis. (Reproduced, with permission, from Dorsch JA, Dorsch SE: *Understanding Anesthesia Equipment*, 4th ed. Williams & Wilkins, 1999.)

neuromuscular receptor that needs to be monitored, direct stimulation of muscle should be avoided by placing electrodes over the course of the nerve and not over the muscle itself. To deliver a supramaximal stimulation to the underlying nerve, peripheral nerve stimulators must be capable of generating at least a 50-mA current across a 1000-Ω load. This current is uncomfortable for a conscious patient. Complications of nerve stimulation are limited to skin irritation and abrasion at the site of electrode attachment.

Because of concerns of residual neuromuscular blockade, increased attention has been focused on providing quantitative measures of the degree of neuromuscular blockade perioperatively. Acceleromyography uses a piezoelectric transducer on the muscle to be stimulated. Movement of the muscle generates an electrical current that can be quantified and displayed. Indeed, acceleromyography can better predict residual paralysis, compared with routine tactile train-of-four monitoring used in most operating rooms, if calibrated from the beginning of the operative period to establish baselines prior to administration of neuromuscular blocking agents.

Clinical Considerations

The degree of neuromuscular blockade is monitored by applying various patterns of electrical stimulation (Figure 6–14). All stimuli are 200 μs in duration and of square-wave pattern and equal current intensity. A twitch is a single pulse that is delivered from every 1 to every 10 sec (1–0.1 Hz). Increasing block results in decreased evoked response to stimulation.

Train-of-four stimulation denotes four successive 200-μs stimuli in 2 sec (2 Hz). The twitches in a train-of-four pattern progressively fade as nondepolarizing muscle relaxant block increases. The ratio of the responses to the first and fourth twitches is a sensitive indicator of nondepolarizing muscle paralysis. Because it is difficult to estimate the train-of-four ratio, it is more convenient to visually observe the sequential disappearance of the twitches, as this also correlates with the extent of blockade. Disappearance of the fourth twitch represents a 75% block, the third twitch an 80% block,

and the second twitch a 90% block. Clinical relaxation usually requires 75% to 95% neuromuscular blockade.

Tetany at 50 or 100 Hz is a sensitive test of neuromuscular function. Sustained contraction for 5 sec indicates adequate—but not necessarily complete—reversal from neuromuscular blockade. Double-burst stimulation (DBS) represents two variations of tetany that are less painful to the patient. The DBS$_{3,3}$ pattern of nerve stimulation consists of three short (200-μs) high-frequency bursts separated by 20 ms intervals (50 Hz) followed 750 ms later by another three bursts. DBS$_{3,2}$ consists of three 200-μs impulses at 50 Hz followed 750 ms later by two such impulses. DBS is more sensitive than train-of-four stimulation for the clinical (ie, visual) evaluation of fade.

Because muscle groups differ in their sensitivity to neuromuscular blocking agents, use of the peripheral nerve stimulator cannot replace direct observation of the muscles (eg, the diaphragm) that need to be relaxed for a specific surgical procedure. Furthermore, recovery of adductor pollicis function does not exactly parallel recovery of muscles required to maintain an airway. **The diaphragm, rectus abdominis, laryngeal adductors, and orbicularis oculi muscles recover from neuromuscular blockade sooner than do the adductor pollicis.** Other indicators of adequate recovery include sustained (≥ 5 s) head lift, the ability to generate an inspiratory pressure of at least –25 cm H_2O, and a forceful hand grip. Twitch tension is reduced by hypothermia of the monitored muscle group (6%/°C). Decisions regarding adequacy of reversal of neuromuscular blockade, as well as timing of extubation, should be made only by considering both the patient's clinical presentation and assessments determined by peripheral nerve stimulation. Postoperative residual curarization (PORC) remains a problem in postanesthesia care, producing potentially injurious airway and respiratory function compromise. Reversal of neuromuscular blocking agents is warranted, as is the use of intermediate acting neuromuscular blocking agents instead of longer acting drugs.

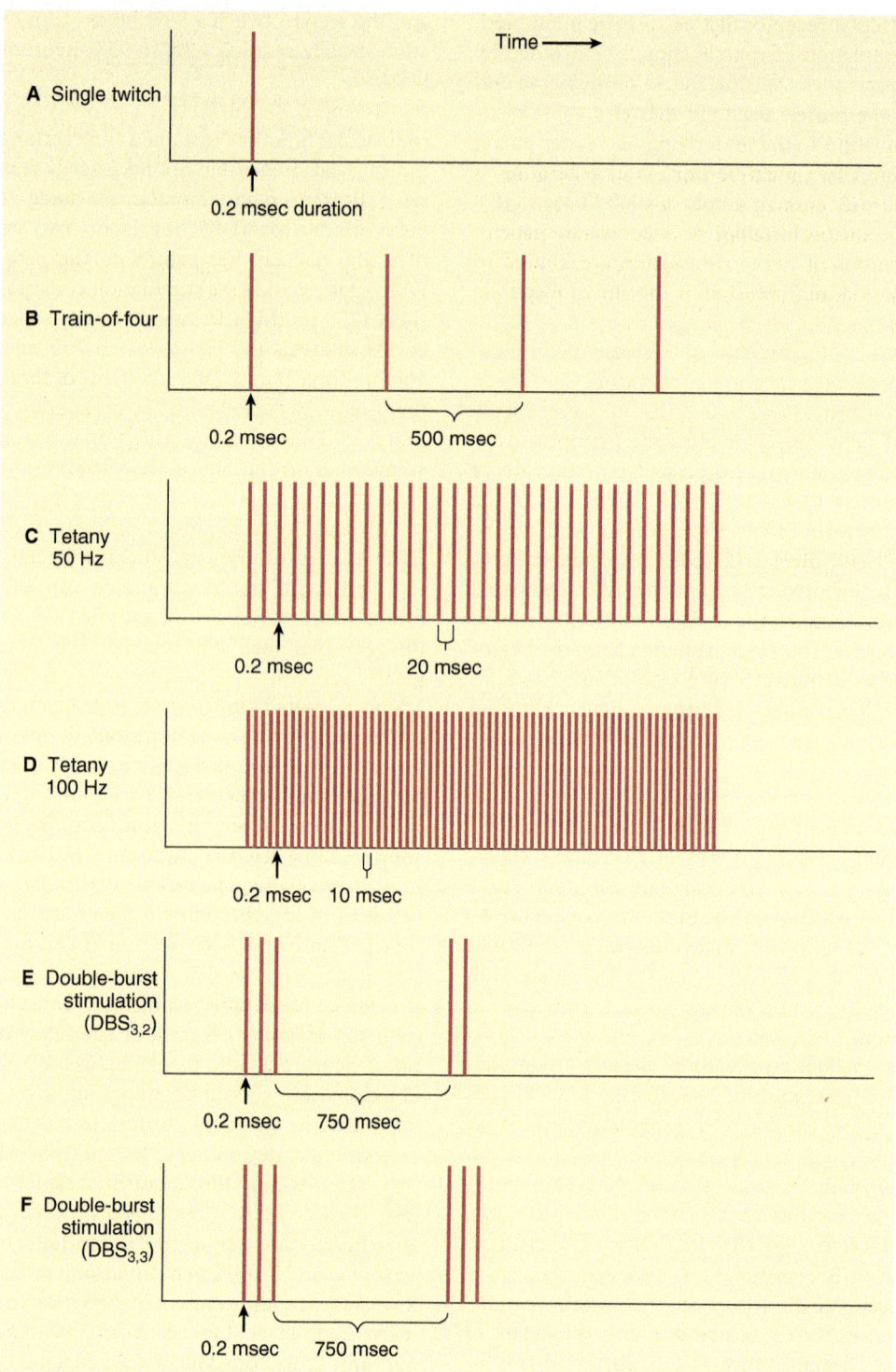

FIGURE 6–14 Peripheral nerve stimulators can generate various patterns of electrical impulses.

CASE DISCUSSION

Monitoring During Magnetic Resonance Imaging

A 50-year-old man with recent onset of seizures is scheduled for magnetic resonance imaging (MRI). A prior MRI attempt was unsuccessful because of the patient's severe claustrophobic reaction. The radiologist requests your help in providing either sedation or general anesthesia.

Why does the MRI suite pose special problems for the patient and the anesthesiologist?

MRI studies tend to be long (often more than 1 h) and many scanners totally surround the body, causing a high incidence of claustrophobia in patients already anxious about their health. Good imaging requires immobility, something that is difficult to achieve in many patients without sedation or general anesthesia.

Because the MRI uses a powerful magnet, no ferromagnetic objects can be placed near the scanner. This includes implanted prosthetic joints, artificial pacemakers, surgical clips, batteries, ordinary anesthesia machines, watches, pens, or credit cards. Ordinary metal lead wires for pulse oximeters or electrocardiography act as antennas and may attract enough radiofrequency energy to distort the MRI image or even cause patient burns. In addition, the scanner's magnetic field causes severe monitor artifact. The more powerful the scanner's magnet, as measured in Tesla units (1 T = 10,000 gauss), the greater the potential problem. Other obstacles include poor access to the patient during the imaging (particularly the patient's airway), hypothermia in pediatric patients, dim lighting within the patient tunnel, and very loud noise (up to 100 dB).

How have these monitoring and anesthesia machine problems been addressed?

Equipment manufacturers have modified monitors so that they are compatible with the MRI environment. These modifications include non-ferromagnetic electrocardiographic electrodes, graphite and copper cables, extensive filtering and gating of signals, extra-long blood pressure cuff tubing, and use of fiberoptic technologies. Anesthesia machines with no ferromagnetic components (eg, aluminum gas cylinders) have been fitted with MRI-compatible ventilators and long circle systems or Mapleson D breathing circuits.

What factors influence the choice between general anesthesia and intravenous sedation?

Although most patients will tolerate an MRI study with sedation, head injured and pediatric patients present special challenges and will often require general anesthesia. Because of machine and monitoring limitations, an argument could be made that sedation, when possible, would be a safer choice. On the other hand, loss of airway control from deep sedation could prove catastrophic because of poor patient access and delayed detection. Other important considerations include the monitoring modalities available at a particular facility and the general medical condition of the patient.

Which monitors should be considered mandatory in this case?

The patient should receive at least the same level of monitoring and care in the MRI suite as in the operating room for a similarly noninvasive procedure. Thus, the American Society of Anesthesiologists Standards for Basic Anesthetic Monitoring (see Guidelines on next page) apply as they would to a patient undergoing general anesthesia.

Continuous auscultation of breath sounds with a plastic (not metal) precordial stethoscope can help to identify airway obstruction caused by excessive sedation. Palpation of a peripheral pulse or listening for Korotkoff sounds is impractical in this setting. Ensuring adequacy of circulation depends on electrocardiographic and oscillometric blood pressure monitoring. End-tidal CO_2 analyzers can be adapted to sedation cases by connecting the sampling line to a site near the patient's mouth or nose if nasal cannula with a CO_2 sampling channel are not available. Because room air entrainment precludes exact measurements, this technique provides a qualitative indicator of ventilation. Whenever sedation is planned, equipment for emergency conversion to general anesthesia (eg, tracheal tubes, resuscitation bag) must be immediately available.

Is the continuous presence of anesthesia personnel required during these cases?

Absolutely, yes. Sedated patients need to have continuous monitored anesthesia care to prevent a multitude of unforeseen complications, such as apnea or emesis.

GUIDELINES

American Society of Anesthesiologists Standards for basic anesthetic monitoring, July 2011. http://www.asahq.org/For-Members/Standards-Guidelines-and-Statements.aspx. Accessed January 9, 2013.

SUGGESTED READING

Avidan M, Zhang L, Burnside B, et al: Anesthesia awareness and bispectral index. New Eng J Med 2008;358:1097.

Ben Julian A, Mashour G, Avidan M: Processed electroencephalogram in depth of anesthesia monitoring. Curr Opin Anaesthesiol 2009;22:553.

Fenelly M: Spinal cord monitoring. Anaesthesia 1998;53:41.

Frye E, Levy J: Cerebral monitoring in the operating and the intensive care unit—an introductory for the clinician and a guide for the novice wanting to open a window to the brain. Part I: The electroencephalogram. J Clin Monit Comput 2005;19:1.

Fuchs-Binder T, Schreiber J, Meistelman C: Monitoring neuromuscular block: an update. Anaesthesia 2009;64:82.

Grocott J, Davie S, Fedorow C: Monitoring of brain function in anesthesia and intensive care. Curr Opin Anesthesiol 2010; 23:759.

Jubran A: Advances in respiratory monitoring during mechanical ventilation. Chest 1999;116:1416.

Kasman N, Brady K: Cerebral oximetry for pediatric anesthesia: why do intelligent clinicians disagree? Pediatr Anaesth 2011;21:473.

Mashour G, Orser B, Avidan M: Intraoperative awareness. Anesthiology 2011;114:1218.

Moritz S, Kasprzak P, Arit M, et al: Accuracy of cerebral monitoring in detecting cerebral ischemia during carotid endarterectomy. Anesthiology 2007;107:563.

Myles P, Leslie K, McNeil J: Bispectral function monitoring to prevent awareness during anaesthesia. The B-Aware randomized controlled trial. Lancet 2004;363:1757.

Naguib M, Koman A, Ensor J: Neuromuscular monitoring and postoperative residual curarization: a meta analysis. Br J Anaesth 2007;98:302.

Nishiyama T: Recent advance in patient monitoring. Korean J Anesthesiol 2010;59:144.

Pellicer A, Bravo Mdel C: Near infrared spectroscopy: a methodology focused review. Semin Fetal Neonatal Med 2011;16:42.

Rubio A, Hakami L, Munch F, et al: Noninvasive control of adequate cerebral oxygenation during low flow antegrade selective cerebral perfusion on adults and infants in the aortic arch surgery. J Card Surg 2008;23:474.

Saidi N, Murkin J: Applied neuromonitoring in cardiac surgery; patient specific management. Semin Cardiothorac Vasc Anesth 2005;9:17.

Schell RM, Cole DJ: Cerebral monitoring: jugular venous oximetry. Anesth Analg 2000;90:559.

Sessler D: Temperature monitoring and perioperative thermoregulation. Anesthesiology 2008;109:318.

Sloan T, Janik D, Jameson L: Multimodality monitoring of the central nervous system using motor evoked potentials. Curr Opin Anaesthesiol 2008;21:560.

Tortoriello T, Stayer S, Mott A, et al: A noninvasive estimation of mixed venous oxygen saturation using near infrared spectroscopy by cerebral oximetry in pediatric cardiac surgery patients. Pediatr Anesth 2005;15:495.

Pharmacological Principles

1 Drug molecules obey the law of mass action. When the plasma concentration exceeds the tissue concentration, the drug moves from the plasma into tissue. When the plasma concentration is less than the tissue concentration, the drug moves from the tissue back to plasma.

2 Most drugs that readily cross the blood–brain barrier (eg, lipophilic drugs like hypnotics and opioids) are avidly taken up in body fat.

3 Biotransformation is the chemical process by which the drug molecule is altered in the body. The liver is the primary organ of metabolism for drugs.

4 Small unbound molecules freely pass from plasma into the glomerular filtrate. The nonionized (uncharged) fraction of drug is reabsorbed in the renal tubules, whereas the ionized (charged) portion is excreted in urine.

5 Elimination half-life is the time required for the drug concentration to fall by 50%. For drugs described by multicompartment pharmacokinetics (eg, all drugs used in anesthesia), there are multiple elimination half-lives.

6 The offset of a drug's effect cannot be predicted from half-lives. The context-sensitive half-time is a clinically useful concept to describe the rate of decrease in drug concentration and should be used instead of half-lives to compare the pharmacokinetic properties of intravenous drugs used in anesthesia.

The clinical practice of anesthesiology is connected more directly than any other specialty to the science of clinical pharmacology. One would think, therefore, that the study of pharmacokinetics and pharmacodynamics would receive attention comparable to that given to airway assessment, choice of inhalation anesthetic for ambulatory surgery, or neuromuscular blockade in anesthesiology curricula and examinations. The frequent misidentification or misuse of pharmacokinetic principles and measurements suggests that this is not the case.

PHARMACOKINETICS

Pharmacokinetics defines the relationships among drug dosing, drug concentration in body fluids and tissues, and time. It consists of four linked processes: absorption, distribution, biotransformation, and excretion.

Absorption

Absorption defines the processes by which a drug moves from the site of administration to the bloodstream. There are many possible routes of drug administration: oral, sublingual, rectal, inhalational, transdermal, transmucosal, subcutaneous, intramuscular, and intravenous. Absorption is influenced by the physical characteristics of the drug (solubility, pK_a, diluents, binders, and formulation), dose, and the site of absorption (eg, gut, lung, skin, muscle). Bioavailability is the fraction of the administered dose reaching the systemic circulation. For example, nitroglycerin is well absorbed by the gastrointestinal tract but has low bioavailability when administered orally. The reason is that nitroglycerin undergoes extensive first-pass hepatic metabolism as it transits the liver before reaching the systemic circulation.

Oral drug administration is convenient, inexpensive, and relatively tolerant of dosing errors. However, it requires cooperation of the patient, exposes the drug to first-pass hepatic metabolism, and permits gastric pH, enzymes, motility, food, and other drugs to potentially reduce the predictability of systemic drug delivery.

Nonionized (uncharged) drugs are more readily absorbed than ionized (charged) forms. Therefore, an acidic environment (stomach) favors the absorption of acidic drugs ($A^- + H^+ \rightarrow AH$), whereas a more alkaline environment (intestine) favors basic drugs ($BH^+ \rightarrow H^+ + B$). Most drugs are largely absorbed from the intestine rather than the stomach because of the greater surface area of the small intestine and longer transit duration.

All venous drainage from the stomach and small intestine flows to the liver. As a result, the bioavailability of highly metabolized drugs may be significantly reduced by first-pass hepatic metabolism. Because the venous drainage from the mouth and esophagus flows into the superior vena cava rather than into the portal system, sublingual or buccal drug absorption bypasses the liver and first-pass metabolism. Rectal administration partly bypasses the portal system, and represents an alternative route in small children or patients who are unable to tolerate oral ingestion.

However, rectal absorption can be erratic, and many drugs irritate the rectal mucosa.

Transdermal drug administration can provide prolonged continuous administration for some drugs. However, the stratum corneum is an effective barrier to all but small, lipid-soluble drugs (eg, clonidine, nitroglycerin, scopolamine, fentanyl, and free-base local anesthetics [EMLA]).

Parenteral routes of drug administration include subcutaneous, intramuscular, and intravenous injection. Subcutaneous and intramuscular absorption depend on drug diffusion from the site of injection to the bloodstream. The rate at which a drug enters the bloodstream depends on both blood flow to the injected tissue and the injectate formulation. Drugs dissolved in solution are absorbed faster than those present in suspensions. Irritating preparations can cause pain and tissue necrosis (eg, intramuscular diazepam). Intravenous injections completely bypass the process of absorption.

Distribution

Once absorbed, a drug is distributed by the bloodstream throughout the body. Highly perfused organs (the so-called vessel-rich group) receive a disproportionate fraction of the cardiac output (Table 7–1). Therefore, these tissues receive a disproportionate amount of drug in the first minutes following drug administration. These tissues approach equilibration with the plasma concentration more quickly than less well perfused tissues due to the differences in

TABLE 7–1 Tissue group composition, relative body mass, and percentage of cardiac output.

Tissue Group	Composition	Body Mass (%)	Cardiac Output (%)
Vessel-rich	Brain, heart, liver, kidney, endocrine glands	10	75
Muscle	Muscle, skin	50	19
Fat	Fat	20	6
Vessel-poor	Bone, ligament, cartilage	20	0

blood flow. However, less well perfused tissues such as fat and skin may have enormous capacity to absorb lipophilic drugs, resulting in a large reservoir of drug following long infusions.

① Drug molecules obey the law of mass action. When the plasma concentration exceeds the concentration in tissue, the drug moves from the plasma into tissue. When the plasma concentration is less than the concentration in tissue, the drug moves from the tissue back to plasma.

Distribution is a major determinant of end-organ drug concentration. The rate of rise in drug concentration in an organ is determined by that organ's perfusion and the relative drug solubility in the organ compared with blood. The equilibrium concentration in an organ relative to blood depends only on the relative solubility of the drug in the organ relative to blood, unless the organ is capable of metabolizing the drug.

Molecules in blood are either free or bound to plasma proteins and lipids. The free concentration equilibrates between organs and tissues. However, the equilibration between bound and unbound molecules is instantaneous. As unbound molecules of drug diffuse into tissue, they are instantly replaced by previously bound molecules. Plasma protein binding does not affect the rate of transfer directly, but it does affect relative solubility of the drug in blood and tissue. If the drug is highly bound in tissues, and unbound in plasma, then the relative solubility favors drug transfer into tissue. Put another way, a drug that is highly bound in tissue, but not in blood, will have a very large free drug concentration gradient driving drug into the tissue. Conversely, if the drug is highly bound in plasma and has few binding sites in the tissue, then transfer of a small amount of drug may be enough to bring the free drug concentration into equilibrium between blood and tissue. Thus, high levels of binding in blood relative to tissues increase the rate of onset of drug effect, because fewer molecules need to transfer into the tissue to produce an effective free drug concentration.

Albumin binds many acidic drugs (eg, barbiturates), whereas α_1-acid glycoprotein (AAG) binds basic drugs (local anesthetics). If the concentrations of these proteins are diminished or (typically less important) if the protein-binding sites are occupied by other drugs, then the relative solubility of the drugs in blood is decreased, increasing tissue uptake. Kidney disease, liver disease, chronic congestive heart failure, and malignancies decrease albumin production. Trauma (including surgery), infection, myocardial infarction, and chronic pain increase AAG levels. Pregnancy is associated with reduced AAG concentrations. Note that these changes will have very little effect on propofol, which is administered with its own binding molecules (the lipid in the emulsion).

Lipophilic molecules can readily transfer between the blood and organs. Charged molecules are able to pass in small quantities into most organs. However, the blood–brain barrier is a special case. Permeation of the central nervous system by ionized drugs is limited by pericapillary glial cells and endo-**②** thelial cell tight junctions. Most drugs that readily cross the blood–brain barrier (eg, lipophilic drugs like hypnotics and opioids) are avidly taken up in body fat.

The time course of distribution of drugs into peripheral tissues is complex and can only be assessed with computer models. Following intravenous bolus administration, rapid distribution of drug from the plasma into peripheral tissues accounts for the profound decrease in plasma concentration observed in the first few minutes. For each tissue, there is a point in time at which the apparent concentration in the tissue is the same as the concentration in the plasma. The redistribution phase (for each tissue) follows this moment of equilibration. During redistribution, drug returns from peripheral tissues back into the plasma. This return of drug back to the plasma slows the rate of decline in plasma drug concentration.

Distribution generally contributes to rapid emergence by removing drug from the plasma for many minutes following administration of a bolus infusion. Following prolonged infusions, *redistri*bution generally delays emergence as drug returns from tissue reservoirs to the plasma for many hours.

The complex process of drug distribution into and out of tissues is one reason that half-lives are clinically useless. The offset of a drug's clinical actions are best predicted by computer models using the context-sensitive half-time or decrement times. The *context-sensitive half-time* is the time required for a 50% decrease in plasma drug concentration to occur following a pseudo steady-state infusion (in other words, an infusion that has continued long enough to yield nearly steady-state concentrations). Here the "context" is the duration of the infusion. The *context-sensitive decrement time* is a more generalized concept referring to any clinically relevant decreased concentration in any tissue, particularly the brain or effect site.

The volume of distribution, V_d, is the *apparent* volume into which a drug has "distributed" (ie, mixed). This volume is calculated by dividing a bolus dose of drug by the plasma concentration at time 0. In practice, the concentration used to define the V_d is often obtained by extrapolating subsequent concentrations back to "0 time" when the drug was injected, as follows:

$$V_d = \frac{\text{Bolus dose}}{\text{Concentration}_{time0}}$$

The concept of a single V_d does not apply to any intravenous drugs used in anesthesia. All intravenous anesthetic drugs are better modeled with at least two compartments: a central compartment and a peripheral compartment. The behavior of many of these drugs is best described using three compartments: a central compartment, a rapidly equilibrating peripheral compartment, and a slowly equilibrating peripheral compartment. The central compartment may be thought of as including the blood and any ultra-rapidly equilibrating tissues such as the lungs. The peripheral compartment is composed of the other body tissues. For drugs with two peripheral compartments, the rapidly equilibrating compartment comprises the organs and muscles, while the slowly equilibrating compartment roughly represents distribution of the drug into fat and skin. These compartments are designated V_1 (central), V_2 (rapid distribution), and V_3 (slow distribution). The volume of distribution at steady state, V_{dss} is the algebraic sum of these compartment volumes. V_1 is calculated by the above equation showing the relationship between volume, dose, and concentration. The other volumes are calculated through pharmacokinetic modeling.

A small V_{dss} implies that the drug has high aqueous solubility and will remain largely within the intravascular space. For example, the V_{dss} of pancuronium is about 15 L in a 70-kg person, indicating that pancuronium is mostly present in body water, with little distribution into fat. However, the typical anesthetic drug is lipophilic, resulting in a V_{dss} that exceeds total body water (approximately 40 L). For example, the V_{dss} for fentanyl is about 350 L in adults, and the V_{dss} for propofol may exceed 5000 L. V_{dss} does not represent a real volume but rather reflects the volume into which the drug would need to distribute to account for the observed plasma concentration given the dose that was administered.

Biotransformation

3 Biotransformation is the chemical process by which the drug molecule is altered in the body. The liver is the primary organ of metabolism for drugs. The exception is esters, which undergo hydrolysis in the plasma or tissues. The end products of biotransformation are often (but not necessarily) inactive and water soluble. Water solubility allows excretion by the kidneys.

Metabolic biotransformation is frequently divided into phase I and phase II reactions. Phase I reactions convert a parent compound into more polar metabolites through oxidation, reduction, or hydrolysis. Phase II reactions couple (conjugate) a parent drug or a phase I metabolite with an endogenous substrate (eg, glucuronic acid) to form water-soluble metabolites that can be eliminated in the urine or stool. Although this is usually a sequential process, phase I metabolites may be excreted without undergoing phase II biotransformation, and a phase II reaction can precede or occur without a phase I reaction.

Hepatic clearance is the volume of blood or plasma (whichever was measured in the assay) cleared of drug per unit of time. The units of clearance are units of flow: volume per unit time. Clearance may be expressed in milliliters per minute, liters per hour, or any other convenient unit of flow.

If every molecule of drug that enters the liver is metabolized, then hepatic clearance will equal liver blood flow. This is true for very few drugs, although it is very nearly the case for propofol. For most drugs, only a fraction of the drug that enters the liver is removed. The fraction removed is called the *extraction ratio*. The hepatic clearance can therefore be expressed as the liver blood flow times the extraction ratio. If the extraction ratio is 50%, then hepatic clearance is 50% of liver blood flow. The clearance of drugs efficiently removed by the liver (ie, having a high hepatic extraction ratio) is proportional to hepatic blood flow. For example, because the liver removes almost all of the propofol that goes through it, if the hepatic blood flow doubles, then the clearance of propofol doubles. Induction of liver enzymes has no effect on propofol clearance, because the liver so efficiently removes all of the propofol that goes through it. Even severe loss of liver tissue, as occurs in cirrhosis, has little effect on propofol clearance. Drugs such as propofol have flow-dependent clearance.

Many drugs have low hepatic extraction ratios and are slowly cleared by the liver. For these drugs, the rate-limiting step is not the flow of blood to the liver, but rather the metabolic capacity of the liver itself. Changes in liver blood flow have little effect on the clearance of such drugs. However, if liver enzymes are induced, then clearance will increase because the liver has more capacity to metabolize the drug. Conversely, if the liver is damaged, then less capacity is available for metabolism and clearance is reduced. Drugs with low hepatic extraction ratios thus have capacity-dependent clearance. The extraction ratios of methadone and alfentanil are 10% and 15% respectively, making these capacity-dependent drugs.

Excretion

Some drugs and many drug metabolites are excreted by the kidneys. Renal clearance is the rate of elimination of a drug from the body by kidney excretion. This concept is analogous to hepatic clearance, and similarly, renal clearance can be expressed as the renal blood flow times the renal extraction ratio. **4** Small unbound drugs freely pass from plasma into the glomerular filtrate. The nonionized (uncharged) fraction of drug is reabsorbed in the renal tubules, whereas the ionized (charged) portion is excreted in urine. The fraction of drug ionized depends on the pH; thus renal elimination of drugs that exist in ionized and nonionized forms depends in part on urinary pH. The kidney actively secretes some drugs into the renal tubules.

Many drugs and drug metabolites pass from the liver into the intestine via the biliary system. Some drugs excreted into the bile are then reabsorbed in the intestine, a process called *enterohepatic recirculation*. Occasionally metabolites excreted in bile are subsequently converted back to the parent drug. For example, lorazepam is converted by the liver to lorazepam glucuronide. In the intestine, β-glucuronidase breaks the ester linkage, converting lorazepam glucuronide back to lorazepam.

Compartment Models

Multicompartment models provide a mathematical framework that can be used to relate drug dose to changes in drug concentrations over time. Conceptually, the compartments in these models are tissues with a similar distribution time course. For example, the plasma and lungs are components of the central compartment. The organs and muscles, sometimes called the vessel-rich group, could be the second, or rapidly equilibrating, compartment. Fat and skin have the capacity to bind large quantities of lipophilic drug but are poorly perfused. These could represent the third, or slowly equilibrating, compartment. This is an intuitive definition of compartments, and it is important to recognize that the compartments of a pharmacokinetic model are mathematical abstractions that relate dose to observed concentration. A one-to-one relationship does not exist between any compartment and any organ or tissue in the body.

Many drugs used in anesthesia are well described by a two-compartment model. This is generally the case if the studies used to characterize the pharmacokinetics do not include rapid arterial sampling over the first few minutes (Figure 7–1). Without rapid arterial sampling the ultra-rapid initial drop in plasma concentration immediately after a bolus injection is missed, and the central compartment volume is blended into the rapidly equilibrating compartment. When rapid arterial sampling is used in pharmacokinetic experiments, the results are generally a three-compartment model. In these cases the number of identifiable compartments is a function of the experimental design and not a characteristic of the drug.

In compartmental models the instantaneous concentration at the time of a bolus injection is assumed to be the amount of the bolus divided by the central compartment volume. This is not

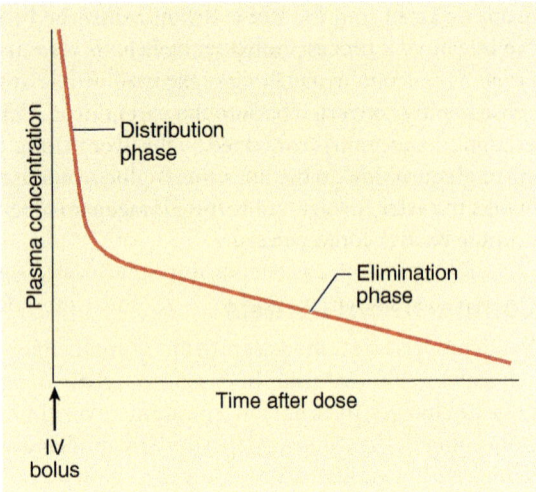

FIGURE 7–1 Two-compartment model demonstrates the distribution phase (α phase) and the elimination phase (β phase). During the distribution phase, the drug moves from the central compartment to the peripheral compartment. The elimination phase consists of metabolism and excretion.

correct. If the bolus is given over a few seconds, the instantaneous concentration is 0, because the drug is all in the vein, still flowing to the heart. It takes only a minute or two for the drug to mix in the central compartment volume. This misspecification is common to conventional pharmacokinetic models. More physiologically based models, sometimes called *front-end kinetic models*, can characterize the initial delay in concentration. These models are useful only if the concentrations over the first few minutes are clinically important. After the first few minutes, front-end models resemble conventional compartmental models.

In the first few minutes following initial bolus administration of a drug, the concentration drops very rapidly as the drug quickly diffuses into peripheral compartments. The decline is typically an order of magnitude over 10 minutes. For drugs with very rapid hepatic clearance (eg, propofol) or those that are metabolized in the blood (eg, remifentanil), metabolism contributes significantly to the rapid initial drop in concentration. Following this very rapid drop there is a period of slower decrease in plasma concentration. During this period, the rapidly

equilibrating compartment is no longer removing drug from the plasma. Instead, drug returns to the plasma from the rapidly equilibrating compartment. The reversed role of the rapidly equilibrating tissues from extracting drug to returning drug accounts for the slower rate of decline in plasma concentration in this intermediate phase. Eventually there is an even slower rate of decrease in plasma concentration, which is log-linear until the drug is completely eliminated from the body. This terminal log-linear phase occurs after the slowly equilibrating compartment shifts from net removal of drug from the plasma to net return of drug to the plasma. During this terminal phase the organ of elimination (typically the liver) is exposed to the body's entire body drug load, which accounts for the very slow rate of decrease in plasma drug concentration during this final phase.

The mathematical models used to describe a drug with two or three compartments are, respectively:

$$Cp(t) = Ae^{-\alpha t} + Be^{-\beta t}$$

and

$$Cp(t) = Ae^{-\alpha t} + Be^{-\beta t} + Ce^{-\gamma t}$$

where $Cp(t)$ equals plasma concentration at time t, and α, β, and γ are the exponents that characterize the very rapid (ie, very steep), intermediate, and slow (ie, log-linear) portions of the plasma concentration over time, respectively. Drugs described by two-compartment and three-compartment models will have two or three half-lives. Each half-life is calculated as the natural log of 2 (0.693), divided by the exponent. The coefficients A, B, and C represent the contribution of each of the exponents to the overall decrease in concentration over time.

The two-compartment model is described by a curve with two exponents and two coefficients, whereas the three-compartment model is described by a curve with three exponents and three coefficients. The mathematical relationships among compartments, clearances, coefficients, and exponents are complex. Every coefficient and every exponent is a function of every volume and every clearance.

⑤   Elimination half-life is the time required for the drug concentration to fall by 50%. For drugs described by multicompartment pharmacokinetics (eg, all drugs used in anesthesia), there are multiple elimination half-lives, in other words the elimination half-time is context dependent. The offset of a drug's effect cannot be predicted from half-lives. Moreover, one cannot easily determine how rapidly a drug effect will disappear simply by looking at coefficients, exponents, and half-lives. For example, the terminal half-life of sufentanil is about 10 h, whereas that of alfentanil is 2 h. This does not mean that recovery from alfentanil will be faster, because clinical recovery from clinical dosing will be influenced by all half-lives, not just the terminal one. Computer models readily demonstrate that recovery from an infusion lasting several hours will be faster when the drug administered is sufentanil than it will be when the infused drug is alfentanil. The time required for a 50% decrease in concentration depends on the duration or "context" of the infusion. The context-sensitive half-time, discussed earlier, captures this concept and should be used instead of half-lives to compare the pharmacokinetic properties of intravenous drugs used in anesthesia.

PHARMACODYNAMICS

Pharmacodynamics, the study of how drugs affect the body, involves the concepts of potency, efficacy, and therapeutic window. Pharmacokinetic models can range from entirely empirical dose versus response relationships to mechanistic models of ligand–receptor binding. The fundamental pharmacodynamic concepts are captured in the relationship between exposure to a drug and physiological response to the drug, often called the *dose–response* or *concentration–response relationship*.

Exposure–Response Relationships

As the body is exposed to an increasing amount of a drug, the response to the drug similarly increases, typically up to a maximal value. This fundamental concept in the exposure versus response relationship is captured graphically by plotting exposure (usually dose or concentration) on the *x* axis as the independent variable, and the body's response on the *y* axis as the dependent variable. Depending on the circumstances, the dose or concentration may be plotted on a linear scale (Figure 7–2A) or a logarithmic

scale (Figure 7–2B), while the response is typically plotted either as the actual measured response (Figure 7–2A) or as a fraction of the baseline or maximum physiological measurement (Figure 7–2B). For our purposes here, basic pharmacodynamic properties are described in terms of concentration, but any metric of drug exposure (dose, area under the curve, etc) could be used.

The shape of the relationship is typically sigmoidal, as shown in Figure 7–2. The sigmoidal

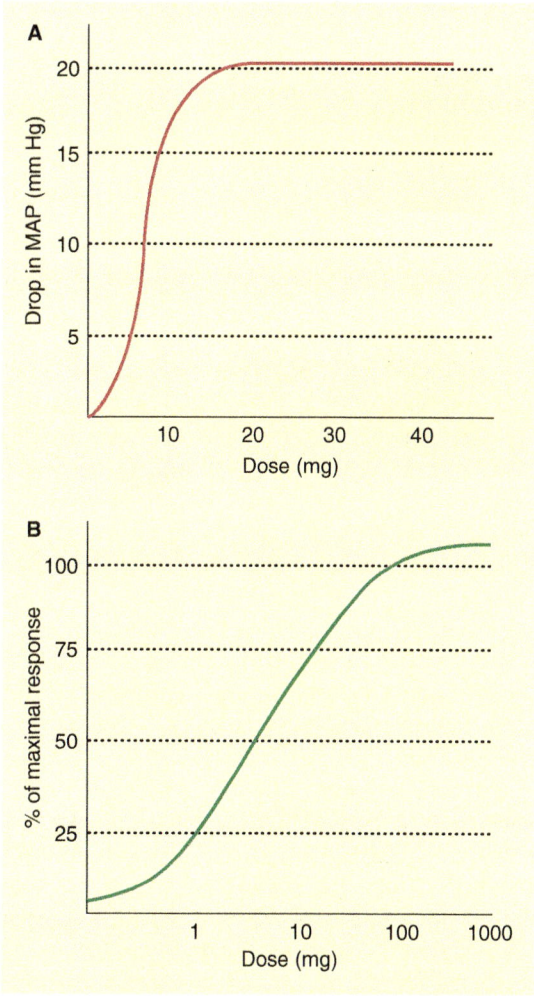

FIGURE 7–2 The shape of the dose–response curve depends on whether the dose or steady-state plasma concentration (C_{cpss}) is plotted on a linear **A**: or logarithmic **B**: scale. MAP, mean arterial pressure.

shape reflects the observation that often a certain amount of drug must be present before there is any measurable physiological response. Thus, the left side of the curve is flat until the drug concentration reaches a minimum threshold. The right side is also flat, reflecting the maximum physiological response of the body, beyond which the body simply cannot respond to additional drug (with the possible exception of eating and weight). Thus, the curve is flat on both the left and right sides. A sigmoidal curve is required to connect the baseline to the asymptote, which is why sigmoidal curves are ubiquitous when modeling pharmacodynamics

The sigmoidal relationship between exposure and response is defined by one of two interchangeable relationships:

$$\text{Effect} = E_0 + E_{max} \frac{C^{\gamma}}{C_{50}^{\gamma} + C^{\gamma}}$$

or

$$\text{Effect} = E_0 + (E_{max} - E_0) \frac{C^{\gamma}}{C_{50}^{\gamma} + C^{\gamma}}$$

In both cases, E_0 is the baseline effect in the absence of drug, C is drug concentration, C_{50} is the concentration associated with half-maximal effect, and γ describes the steepness of the concentration versus response relationship. For the first equation, E_{max} is the maximum change from baseline. In the second equation, E_{max} is the maximum physiological measurement, not the maximum change from baseline.

Once defined in this fashion, each parameter of the pharmacodynamic model speaks to the specific concepts mentioned earlier. E_{max} is related to the intrinsic efficacy of a drug. Highly efficacious drugs have a large maximum physiological effect, characterized by a large E_{max}. For drugs that lack efficacy, E_{max} will equal E_0. C_{50} is a measure of drug potency. Highly potent drugs have a low C_{50}; thus small amounts produce the drug effect. Drugs lacking potency have a high C_{50}, indicating that a large amount of drug is required to achieve the drug effect. The parameter γ indicates steepness of the relationship between concentration and effect. A γ value less than 1 indicates a very gradual increase in drug effect with increasing concentration. A

γ value greater than 4 suggests that once drug effect is observed, small increases in drug concentration produce large increases in drug effect until the maximum effect is reached.

The curve described above represents the relationship of drug concentration to a continuous physiological response. The same relationship can be used to characterize the probability of a binary (yes/no) response to a drug dose:

$$\text{Probability} = P_0 + (P_{max} - P_0) \frac{C^{\gamma}}{C_{50}^{\gamma} + C^{\gamma}}$$

In this case, the probability (P) ranges from 0 (no chance) to 1 (certainty). P_0 is the probability of a "yes" response in the absence of drug. P_{max} is the maximum probability, necessarily less than or equal to 1. As before, C is the concentration, C_{50} is the concentration associated with half-maximal effect, and γ describes the steepness of the concentration versus response relationship. Half-maximal effect is the same as 50% probability of a response when P_0 is 0 and P_{max} is 1.

The *therapeutic window* for a drug is the range between the concentration associated with a desired therapeutic effect and the concentration associated with a toxic drug response. This range can be measured either between two different points on the same concentration versus response curve, or the distance between two distinct curves. For a drug such as sodium nitroprusside, a single concentration versus response curve defines the relationship between concentration and decrease in blood pressure. The therapeutic window might be the difference in the concentration producing a desired 20% decrease in blood pressure and a toxic concentration that produces a 60% decrease in blood pressure. However, for a drug such as lidocaine, the therapeutic window might be the difference between the C_{50} for local anesthesia and the C_{50} for lidocaine-induced seizures, the latter being a separate concentration versus response relationship. The therapeutic index is the C_{50} for toxicity divided by the C_{50} for the desired therapeutic effect. Because of the risk of ventilatory and cardiovascular depression (even at concentrations only slightly greater than those producing anesthesia), most inhaled and intravenous hypnotics are considered to have very low therapeutic indices relative to other drugs.

Drug Receptors

Drug receptors are macromolecules, typically proteins, that bind a drug (agonist) and mediate the drug response. Pharmacological antagonists reverse the effects of the agonist but do not otherwise exert an effect of their own. Competitive antagonism occurs when the antagonist competes with the agonist for the binding site, each potentially displacing the other. Noncompetitive antagonism occurs when the antagonist, through covalent binding or another process, permanently impairs the drug's access to the receptor.

The drug effect is governed by the fraction of receptors that are occupied by an agonist. That fraction is based on the concentration of the drug, the concentration of the receptor, and the strength of binding between the drug and the receptor. This binding is described by the law of mass action, which states that the reaction rate is proportional to the concentrations of the reactants:

$$[D][RU] \underset{k_{off}}{\overset{k_{on}}{\rightleftharpoons}} [DR]$$

where $[D]$ is the concentration of the drug, $[RU]$ is the concentration of unbound receptor, and $[DR]$ is the concentration of bound receptor. The rate constant k_{on} defines the rate of ligand binding to the receptor. The rate constant k_{off} defines the rate of ligand unbinding from the receptor. According to the law of mass action, the rate of receptor binding, $d[DR]/dt$ is:

$$\frac{d[DR]}{dt} = [D][RU]\,k_{on} - [DR]k_{off}$$

Steady state occurs almost instantly. Because the rate of formation at steady state is 0, it follows that:

$$[D][RU]\,k_{on} = [DR]k_{off}$$

In this equation, k_d is the dissociation rate constant, defined as k_{on}/k_{off}. If we define f, fractional receptor occupancy, as:

$$\frac{[DR]}{[DR] + [RU]}$$

then we can solve for receptor occupancy as:

$$f = \frac{[D]}{k_d + [D]}$$

The receptors are half occupied when $[D] = k_d$. Thus, k_d is the concentration of drug associated with 50% receptor occupancy.

Receptor occupancy is only the first step in mediating drug effect. Binding of the drug to the receptor can trigger a myriad of subsequent steps, including opening or closing of an ion channel, activation of a G protein, activation of an intracellular kinase, direct interaction with a cellular structure, or direct binding to DNA.

Like the concentration versus response curve, the shape of the curve relating fractional receptor occupancy to drug concentration is intrinsically sigmoidal. However, the concentration associated with 50% receptor occupancy and the concentration associated with 50% of maximal drug effect are not necessarily the same. Maximal drug effect could occur at very low receptor occupancy, or (for partial agonists) at greater than 100% receptor occupancy.

Prolonged binding and activation of a receptor by an agonist may lead to hyporeactivity ("desensitization") and tolerance. If the binding of an endogenous ligand is chronically blocked, then receptors may proliferate resulting in hyperreactivity and increased sensitivity.

SUGGESTED READING

Bauer LA (Ed): *Applied Clinical Pharmacokinetics*, 2nd ed. McGraw-Hill, 2008: Chaps 1, 2.

Brunton LL, Chabner BA, Knollman BC (Eds): *Goodman & Gilman's The Pharmacological Basis of Therapeutics*, 12th ed. McGraw-Hill, 2010: Chap 2.

Keifer J, Glass P: Context-sensitive half-time and anesthesia: How does theory match reality? Curr Opin Anaesthesiol 1999;12:443.

Shargel L, Yu AB, Wu-Pong S (Eds): *Applied Biopharmaceutics & Pharmacokinetics*, 6th ed. McGraw-Hill, 2012.

Inhalation Anesthetics

1 The greater the uptake of anesthetic agent, the greater the difference between inspired and alveolar concentrations, and the slower the rate of induction.

2 Three factors affect anesthetic uptake: solubility in the blood, alveolar blood flow, and the difference in partial pressure between alveolar gas and venous blood.

3 Low-output states predispose patients to overdosage with soluble agents, as the rate of rise in alveolar concentrations will be markedly increased.

4 Many of the factors that speed induction also speed recovery: elimination of rebreathing, high fresh gas flows, low anesthetic-circuit volume, low absorption by the anesthetic circuit, decreased solubility, high cerebral blood flow, and increased ventilation.

5 The unitary hypothesis proposes that all inhalation agents share a common mechanism of action at the molecular level. This is supported by the observation that the anesthetic potency of inhalation agents correlates directly with their lipid solubility (Meyer–Overton rule). There is an ongoing debate as to the mechanism of anesthetic action. Anesthetic interactions at specific protein ion channels, as well as more nonspecific membrane effects, may combine to produce the anesthetized state.

6 The minimum alveolar concentration (MAC) is the alveolar concentration of an inhaled anesthetic that prevents movement in 50% of patients in response to a standardized stimulus (eg, surgical incision).

7 Prolonged exposure to anesthetic concentrations of nitrous oxide can result in bone marrow depression (megaloblastic anemia) and even neurological deficiencies (peripheral neuropathies).

8 Halothane hepatitis is extremely rare (1 per 35,000 cases). Patients exposed to multiple halothane anesthetics at short intervals, middle-aged obese women, and persons with a familial predisposition to halothane toxicity or a personal history of toxicity are considered to be at increased risk. Desflurane and isoflurane undergo much less metabolism than halothane, resulting in fewer of the metabolite protein adducts that lead to immunologically mediated hepatic injury.

9 Isoflurane dilates coronary arteries, but is not nearly as potent a dilator as nitroglycerin or adenosine. Dilation of normal coronary arteries could theoretically divert blood away from fixed stenotic lesions.

10 The low solubility of desflurane in blood and body tissues causes a very rapid induction of and emergence from anesthesia.

—Continued next page

Continued—

 11 Rapid increases in desflurane concentration lead to transient but sometimes worrisome elevations in heart rate, blood pressure, and catecholamine levels that are more pronounced than occur with isoflurane, particularly in patients with cardiovascular disease.

12 Nonpungency and rapid increases in alveolar anesthetic concentration make sevoflurane an excellent choice for smooth and rapid inhalation inductions in pediatric and adult patients.

Nitrous oxide, chloroform, and ether were the first universally accepted general anesthetics. Methoxyflurane and enflurane, two potent halogenated agents, were used for many years in North American anesthesia practice. Methoxyflurane was the most potent inhalation agent, but its high solubility and low vapor pressure yielded longer inductions and emergences. Up to 50% of it was metabolized by cytochrome P-450 (CYP) enzymes to free fluoride (F^-), oxalic acid, and other nephrotoxic compounds. Prolonged anesthesia with methoxyflurane was associated with a vasopressin-resistant, high-output, renal failure that was most commonly seen when F^- levels increased to greater than 50 μmol/L. Enflurane has a nonpungent odor and is nonflammable at clinical concentrations. It depresses myocardial contractility. It also increases the secretion of cerebrospinal fluid (CSF) and the resistance to CSF outflow. During deep anesthesia with hypocarbia electroencephalographic changes can progress to a spike-and-wave pattern producing tonic–clonic seizures. Because of these concerns, methoxyflurane and enflurane are no longer used.

Five inhalation agents continue to be used in clinical anesthesiology: nitrous oxide, halothane, isoflurane, desflurane, and sevoflurane.

The course of a general anesthetic can be divided into three phases: (1) induction, (2) maintenance, and (3) emergence. Inhalation anesthetics, such as halothane and sevoflurane, are particularly useful in the induction of pediatric patients in whom it may be difficult to start an intravenous line. Although adults are usually induced with intravenous agents, the nonpungency and rapid onset of sevoflurane make inhalation induction practical for them as well. Regardless of the patient's age, anesthesia is often maintained with inhalation agents. Emergence depends primarily upon redistribution from the brain and pulmonary elimination of these agents.

Because of their unique route of administration, inhalation anesthetics have useful pharmacological properties not shared by other anesthetic agents. For instance, administration via the pulmonary circulation allows a more rapid appearance of the drug in arterial blood than intravenous administration.

Pharmacokinetics of Inhalation Anesthetics

Although the mechanism of action of inhalation anesthetics is complex, likely involving numerous membrane proteins and ion channels, it is clear that producing their ultimate effect depends on attainment of a therapeutic tissue concentration in the central nervous system (CNS). There are many steps in between the anesthetic vaporizer and the anesthetic's deposition in the brain (**Figure 8–1**).

FACTORS AFFECTING INSPIRATORY CONCENTRATION (F_I)

The fresh gas leaving the anesthesia machine mixes with gases in the breathing circuit before being inspired by the patient. Therefore, the patient is not necessarily receiving the concentration set on the

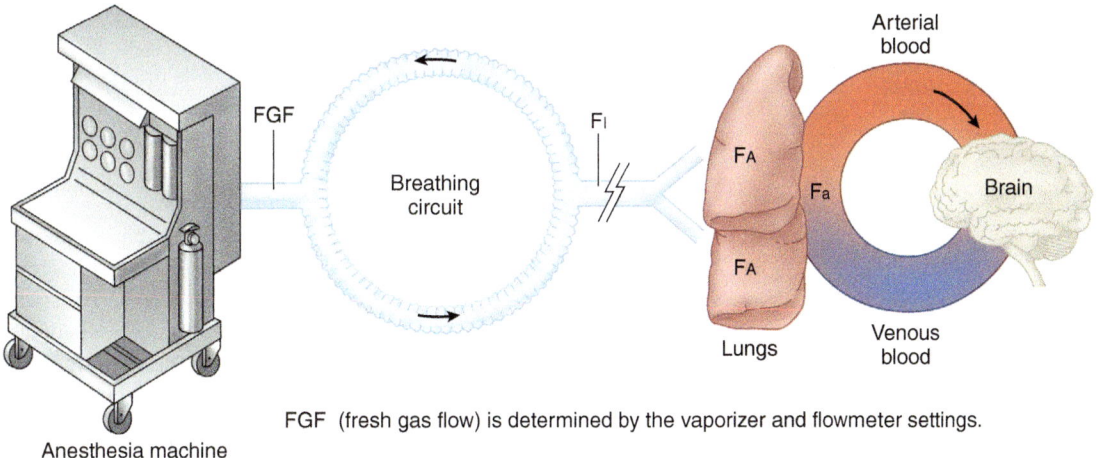

FGF (fresh gas flow) is determined by the vaporizer and flowmeter settings.

FI (inspired gas concentration) is determined by (1) FGF rate; (2) breathing-circuit volume; and (3) circuit absorption.

FA (aveolar gas concentration) is determined by (1) uptake (uptake = $\lambda b/g \times C(A-V) \times Q$); (2) ventilation; and (3) the concentration effect and second gas effect:
    a) concentrating effect
    b) augmented inflow effect

Fa (arterial gas concentration) is affected by ventilation/perfusion mismatching.

FIGURE 8–1 Inhalation anesthetic agents must pass through many barriers between the anesthesia machine and the brain.

vaporizer. The actual composition of the inspired gas mixture depends mainly on the fresh gas flow rate, the volume of the breathing system, and any absorption by the machine or breathing circuit. The higher the fresh gas flow rate, the smaller the breathing system volume, and the lower the circuit absorption, the closer the inspired gas concentration will be to the fresh gas concentration. Clinically, these attributes translate into faster induction and recovery times.

FACTORS AFFECTING ALVEOLAR CONCENTRATION (FA)

Uptake

If there were no uptake of anesthetic agent by the body, the alveolar gas concentration (FA) would rapidly approach the inspired gas concentration (FI). Because anesthetic agents are taken up by the pulmonary circulation during induction, alveolar concentrations lag behind inspired concentrations (FA/FI <1.0). The greater the uptake, the slower the rate of rise of the alveolar concentration and the lower the FA:FI ratio.

Because the concentration of a gas is directly proportional to its partial pressure, the alveolar partial pressure will also be slow to rise. The alveolar partial pressure is important because it determines the partial pressure of anesthetic in the blood and, ultimately, in the brain. Similarly, the partial pressure of the anesthetic in the brain is directly proportional to its brain tissue concentration, which determines clinical effect.

1 Therefore, the greater the uptake of anesthetic agent, the greater the difference between inspired and alveolar concentrations, and the slower the rate of induction.

TABLE 8–1 Partition coefficients of volatile anesthetics at 37°C.[1]

Agent	Blood/ Gas	Brain/ Blood	Muscle/ Blood	Fat/ Blood
Nitrous oxide	0.47	1.1	1.2	2.3
Halothane	2.4	2.9	3.5	60
Isoflurane	1.4	2.6	4.0	45
Desflurane	0.42	1.3	2.0	27
Sevoflurane	0.65	1.7	3.1	48

[1]These values are averages derived from multiple studies and should be used for comparison purposes, not as exact numbers.

2 Three factors affect anesthetic uptake: solubility in the blood, alveolar blood flow, and the difference in partial pressure between alveolar gas and venous blood.

Relatively soluble agents, such as nitrous oxide, are taken up by the blood less avidly than more soluble agents, such as halothane. As a consequence, the alveolar concentration of nitrous oxide rises faster than that of halothane, and induction is faster. The relative solubilities of an anesthetic in air, blood, and tissues are expressed as partition coefficients (Table 8–1). Each coefficient is the ratio of the concentrations of the anesthetic gas in each of two phases at steady state. Steady state is defined as equal partial pressures in the two phases. For instance, the blood/gas partition coefficient ($\lambda_{b/g}$) of nitrous oxide at 37°C is 0.47. In other words, at steady state, 1 mL of blood contains 0.47 as much nitrous oxide as does 1 mL of alveolar gas, even though the partial pressures are the same. Stated another way, blood has 47% of the capacity for nitrous oxide as alveolar gas. Nitrous oxide is much less soluble in blood than is halothane, which has a blood/gas partition coefficient at 37°C of 2.4. Thus, almost five times more halothane than nitrous oxide must be dissolved to raise the partial pressure of blood. The higher the blood/gas coefficient, the greater the anesthetic's solubility and the greater its uptake by the pulmonary circulation. As a consequence of this increased solubility, alveolar partial pressure rises more slowly, and induction is prolonged. Because fat/blood partition coefficients are greater than 1, blood/gas solubility is

increased by postprandial lipidemia and is decreased by anemia.

The second factor that affects uptake is alveolar blood flow, which—in the absence of pulmonary shunting—is essentially equal to cardiac output. If the cardiac output drops to zero, so will anesthetic uptake. As cardiac output increases, anesthetic uptake increases, the rise in alveolar partial pressure slows, and induction is delayed. The effect of changing cardiac output is less pronounced for insoluble anesthetics, as so little is taken up regardless of alveolar blood flow. Low-output states predispose **3** patients to overdosage with soluble agents, as the rate of rise in alveolar concentrations will be markedly increased.

The final factor affecting uptake of anesthetic by the pulmonary circulation is the partial pressure difference between alveolar gas and venous blood. This gradient depends on tissue uptake. If anesthetics did not pass into organs such as the brain, venous and alveolar partial pressures would become identical, and there would be no pulmonary uptake. The transfer of anesthetic from blood to tissues is determined by three factors analogous to systemic uptake: tissue solubility of the agent (tissue/blood partition coefficient), tissue blood flow, and the difference in partial pressure between arterial blood and the tissue.

To better understand inhaled anesthetic uptake and distribution, tissues have been classified into four groups based on their solubility and blood flow (Table 8–2). The highly perfused vessel-rich group (brain, heart, liver, kidney, and endocrine organs) is

TABLE 8–2 Tissue groups based on perfusion and solubilities.

Characteristic	Vessel Rich	Muscle	Fat	Vessel Poor
Percentage of body weight	10	50	20	20
Percentage of cardiac output	75	19	6	0
Perfusion (mL/ min/100 g)	75	3	3	0
Relative solubility	1	1	20	0

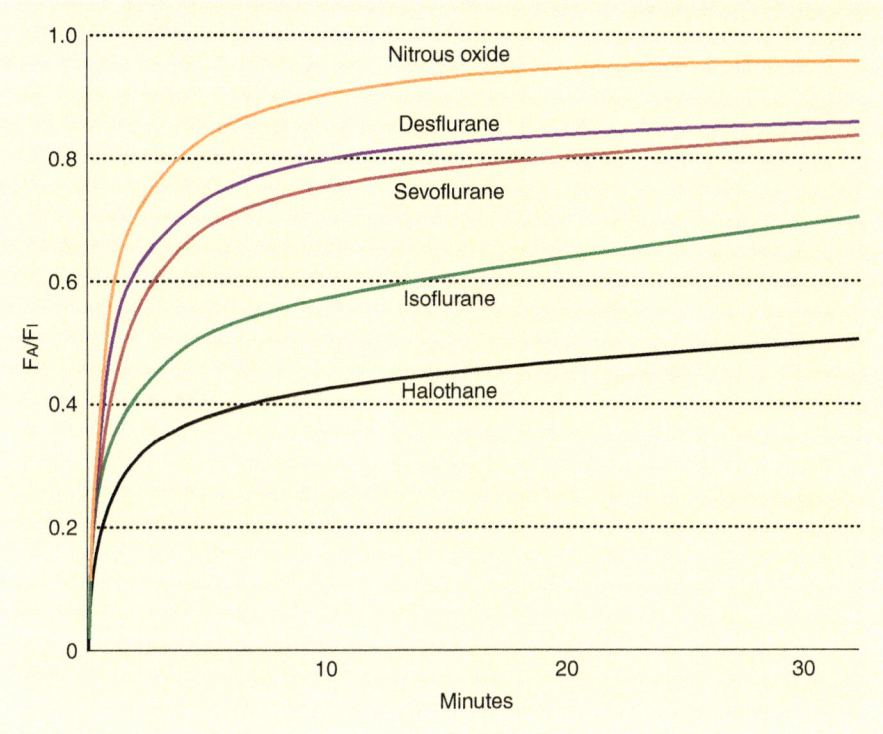

FIGURE 8–2 FA rises toward FI faster with nitrous oxide (an insoluble agent) than with halothane (a soluble agent). See Figure 8–1 for an explanation of FA and FI.

the first to encounter appreciable amounts of anesthetic. Moderate solubility and small volume limit the capacity of this group, so it is also the first to reach steady state (ie, arterial and tissue partial pressures are equal). The muscle group (skin and muscle) is not as well perfused, so uptake is slower. In addition, it has a greater capacity due to a larger volume, and uptake will be sustained for hours. Perfusion of the fat group nearly equals that of the muscle group, but the tremendous solubility of anesthetic in fat leads to a total capacity (tissue/blood solubility × tissue volume) that would take days to approach steady state. The minimal perfusion of the vessel-poor group (bones, ligaments, teeth, hair, and cartilage) results in insignificant uptake.

Anesthetic uptake produces a characteristic curve that relates the rise in alveolar concentration to time (Figure 8–2). The shape of this graph is determined by the uptakes of individual tissue groups (Figure 8–3). The initial steep rate of uptake is due to unopposed filling of the alveoli by ventilation. The rate of rise slows as the vessel-rich group—and eventually the muscle group—approach steady state levels of saturation.

Ventilation

The lowering of alveolar partial pressure by uptake can be countered by increasing alveolar ventilation. In other words, constantly replacing anesthetic taken up by the pulmonary bloodstream results in better maintenance of alveolar concentration. The effect of increasing ventilation will be most obvious in raising the FA/FI for soluble anesthetics, as they are more subject to uptake. Because the FA/FI very rapidly approaches 1.0 for insoluble agents, increasing ventilation has minimal effect. In contrast to the effect of anesthetics on cardiac output, anesthetics that depress spontaneous ventilation (eg, ether or

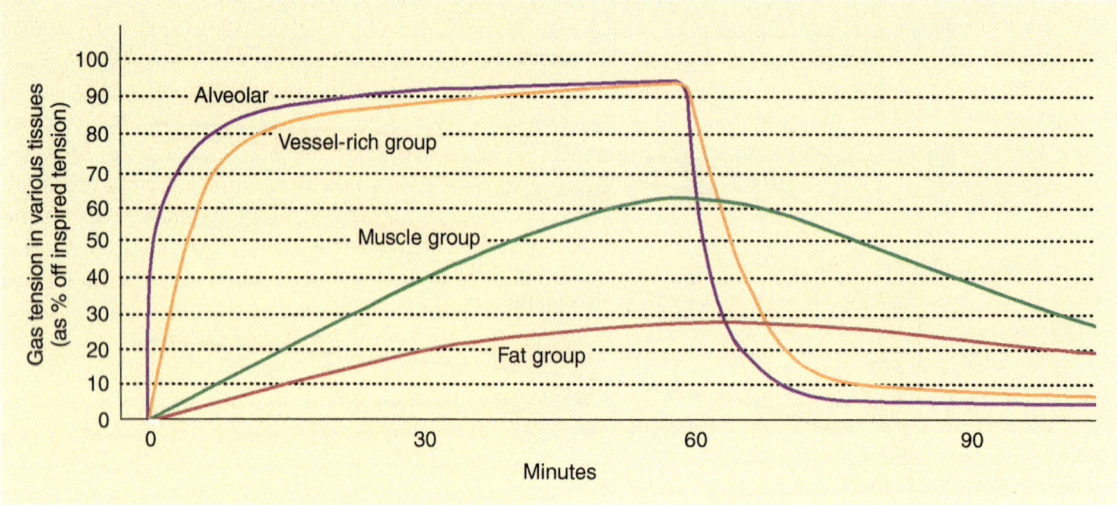

FIGURE 8–3 The rise and fall in alveolar partial pressure precedes that of other tissues. (Modified and reproduced, with permission, from Cowles AL et al: Uptake and distribution of inhalation anesthetic agents in clinical practice. Anesth Analg 1968;4:404.)

halothane) will decrease the rate of rise in alveolar concentration and create a negative feedback loop.

Concentration

The slowing of induction due to uptake from alveolar gas can be reduced by increasing the inspired concentration. Interestingly, increasing the inspired concentration not only increases the alveolar concentration, but also increases its rate of rise (ie, increases F_A/F_I), because of two phenomena (see Figure 8–1) that produce a so-called "concentrating effect." First, if 50% of an anesthetic is taken up by the pulmonary circulation, an inspired concentration of 20% (20 parts of anesthetic per 100 parts of gas) will result in an alveolar concentration of 11% (10 parts of anesthetic remaining in a total volume of 90 parts of gas). On the other hand, if the inspired concentration is raised to 80% (80 parts of anesthetic per 100 parts of gas), the alveolar concentration will be 67% (40 parts of anesthetic remaining in a total volume of 60 parts of gas). Thus, even though 50% of the anesthetic is taken up in both examples, a higher inspired concentration results in a disproportionately higher alveolar concentration. In this example, increasing the inspired concentration 4-fold results in a 6-fold increase in alveolar concentration. The extreme case is an inspired concentration of 100%

(100 parts of 100), which, despite a 50% uptake, will result in an alveolar concentration of 100% (50 parts of anesthetic remaining in a total volume of 50 parts of gas).

The second phenomenon responsible for the concentration effect is the augmented inflow effect. Using the example above, the 10 parts of absorbed gas must be replaced by an equal volume of the 20% mixture to prevent alveolar collapse. Thus, the alveolar concentration becomes 12% (10 plus 2 parts of anesthetic in a total of 100 parts of gas). In contrast, after absorption of 50% of the anesthetic in the 80% gas mixture, 40 parts of 80% gas must be inspired. This further increases the alveolar concentration from 67% to 72% (40 plus 32 parts of anesthetic in a volume of 100 parts of gas).

The concentration effect is more significant with nitrous oxide, than with the volatile anesthetics, as the former can be used in much higher concentrations. Nonetheless, a high concentration of nitrous oxide will augment (by the same mechanism) not only its own uptake, but theoretically that of a concurrently administered volatile anesthetic. The concentration effect of one gas upon another is called the second gas effect, which is probably insignificant in the clinical practice of anesthesiology.

FACTORS AFFECTING ARTERIAL CONCENTRATION (Fa)

Ventilation/Perfusion Mismatch

Normally, alveolar and arterial anesthetic partial pressures are assumed to be equal, but in fact, the arterial partial pressure is consistently less than end-expiratory gas would predict. Reasons for this may include venous admixture, alveolar dead space, and nonuniform alveolar gas distribution. Furthermore, the existence of ventilation/perfusion mismatching will increase the alveolar–arterial difference. Mismatch acts as a restriction to flow: It raises the pressure in front of the restriction, lowers the pressure beyond the restriction, and reduces the flow through the restriction. The overall effect is an increase in the alveolar partial pressure (particularly for highly soluble agents) and a decrease in the arterial partial pressure (particularly for poorly soluble agents). Thus, a bronchial intubation or a right-to-left intracardiac shunt will slow the rate of induction with nitrous oxide more than with halothane.

FACTORS AFFECTING ELIMINATION

Recovery from anesthesia depends on lowering the concentration of anesthetic in brain tissue. Anesthetics can be eliminated by biotransformation, transcutaneous loss, or exhalation. Biotransformation usually accounts for a minimal increase in the rate of decline of alveolar partial pressure. Its greatest impact is on the elimination of soluble anesthetics that undergo extensive metabolism (eg, methoxyflurane). The greater biotransformation of halothane compared with isoflurane accounts for halothane's faster elimination, even though it is more soluble. The CYP group of isozymes (specifically CYP 2EI) seems to be important in the metabolism of some volatile anesthetics. Diffusion of anesthetic through the skin is insignificant.

4   The most important route for elimination of inhalation anesthetics is the alveolus. Many of the factors that speed induction also speed recovery: elimination of rebreathing, high fresh gas

flows, low anesthetic-circuit volume, low absorption by the anesthetic circuit, decreased solubility, high cerebral blood flow (CBF), and increased ventilation. Elimination of nitrous oxide is so rapid that alveolar oxygen and CO_2 are diluted. The resulting **diffusion hypoxia** is prevented by administering 100% oxygen for 5–10 min after discontinuing nitrous oxide. The rate of recovery is usually faster than induction because tissues that have not reached equilibrium will continue to take up anesthetic until the alveolar partial pressure falls below the tissue partial pressure. For instance, fat will continue to take up anesthetic and hasten recovery until the partial pressure exceeds the alveolar partial pressure. This redistribution is not as useful after prolonged anesthesia (fat partial pressures of anesthetic will have come "closer" to arterial partial pressures at the time the anesthetic was removed from fresh gas)—thus, the speed of recovery also depends on the length of time the anesthetic has been administered.

Pharmacodynamics of Inhalation Anesthetics

THEORIES OF ANESTHETIC ACTION

General anesthesia is an altered physiological state characterized by reversible loss of consciousness, analgesia, amnesia, and some degree of muscle relaxation. The multitude of substances capable of producing general anesthesia is remarkable: inert elements (xenon), simple inorganic compounds (nitrous oxide), halogenated hydrocarbons (halothane), ethers (isoflurane, sevoflurane, desflurane), and complex organic structures (propofol). A unifying theory explaining anesthetic action would have to accommodate this diversity of structure. In fact, the various agents probably produce anesthesia by differing sets of molecular mechanisms. Inhalational agents interact with numerous ion channels present in the CNS and peripheral nervous system. Nitrous oxide and xenon are believed to inhibit *N*-methyl-D-aspartate (NMDA) receptors. NMDA receptors are excitatory receptors in the brain. Other inhalational agents may interact at other receptors (eg, gamma-aminobutyric acid [GABA]-activated chloride channel conductance) leading to anesthetic effects. Additionally, some studies suggest that inhalational agents continue to act in a nonspecific manner, thereby affecting the membrane bilayer. It is possible that inhalational anesthetics act on multiple protein receptors that block excitatory channels and promote the activity of inhibitory channels affecting neuronal activity, as well as by some nonspecific membrane effects.

There does not seem to be a single macroscopic site of action that is shared by all inhalation agents. Specific brain areas affected by various anesthetics include the reticular activating system, the cerebral cortex, the cuneate nucleus, the olfactory cortex, and the hippocampus; however, to be clear, general anesthetics bind throughout the CNS. Anesthetics have also been shown to depress excitatory transmission in the spinal cord, particularly at the level of the dorsal horn interneurons that are involved in pain transmission. Differing aspects of anesthesia may be related to different sites of anesthetic action. For example, unconsciousness and amnesia are probably mediated by cortical anesthetic action, whereas the suppression of purposeful withdrawal from pain may be related to subcortical structures, such as the spinal cord or brain stem. One study in rats revealed that removal of the cerebral cortex did not alter the potency of the anesthetic! Indeed, measures of minimal alveolar concentration (MAC), the anesthetic concentration that prevents movement in 50% of subjects or animals, are dependent upon anesthetic effects at the spinal cord and not at the cortex.

5 Past understanding of anesthetic action attempted to identify a unitary hypothesis of anesthetic effects. This hypothesis proposes that all inhalation agents share a common mechanism of action at the molecular level. This was previously supported by the observation that the anesthetic potency of inhalation agents correlates directly with their lipid solubility (Meyer–Overton rule). The implication is that anesthesia results from molecules dissolving at specific lipophilic sites. Of course, not all lipid-soluble molecules are anesthetics (some are actually convulsants), and the correlation between anesthetic potency and lipid solubility is only approximate (**Figure 8–4**).

Neuronal membranes contain a multitude of hydrophobic sites in their phospholipid bilayer. Anesthetic binding to these sites could expand the bilayer beyond a critical amount, altering membrane function (critical volume hypothesis). Although this theory is almost certainly an oversimplification, it explains an interesting phenomenon: the reversal of anesthesia by increased pressure. Laboratory animals exposed to elevated hydrostatic pressure develop a resistance to anesthetic effects. Perhaps the pressure is displacing a number of molecules from the membrane or distorting the anesthetic binding sites in the membrane, increasing anesthetic requirements. However, studies in the 1980s demonstrated the ability of anesthetics to inhibit protein actions, shifting attention to the numerous ion channels that might affect neuronal transmission and away from the critical volume hypothesis.

General anesthetic action could be due to alterations in any one (or a combination) of several cellular systems, including voltage-gated ion channels, ligand-gated ion channels, second messenger functions, or neurotransmitter receptors. For example, many anesthetics enhance GABA inhibition of the CNS. Furthermore, GABA receptor agonists seem to enhance anesthesia, whereas GABA antagonists reverse some anesthetic effects. There seems to be a strong correlation between anesthetic potency and potentiation of GABA receptor activity. Thus, anesthetic action may relate to binding in relatively hydrophobic domains in channel proteins (GABA receptors). Modulation of GABA function may prove to be a principal mechanism of action for many anesthetic drugs.

The glycine receptor α_1-subunit, whose function is enhanced by inhalation anesthetics, is another potential anesthetic site of action.

The tertiary and quaternary structure of amino acids within an anesthetic-binding pocket could be modified by inhalation agents, perturbing the receptor itself, or indirectly producing an effect at a distant site.

Other ligand-gated ion channels whose modulation may play a role in anesthetic action include nicotinic acetylcholine receptors and NMDA receptors.

Investigations into mechanisms of anesthetic action are likely to remain ongoing for many years,

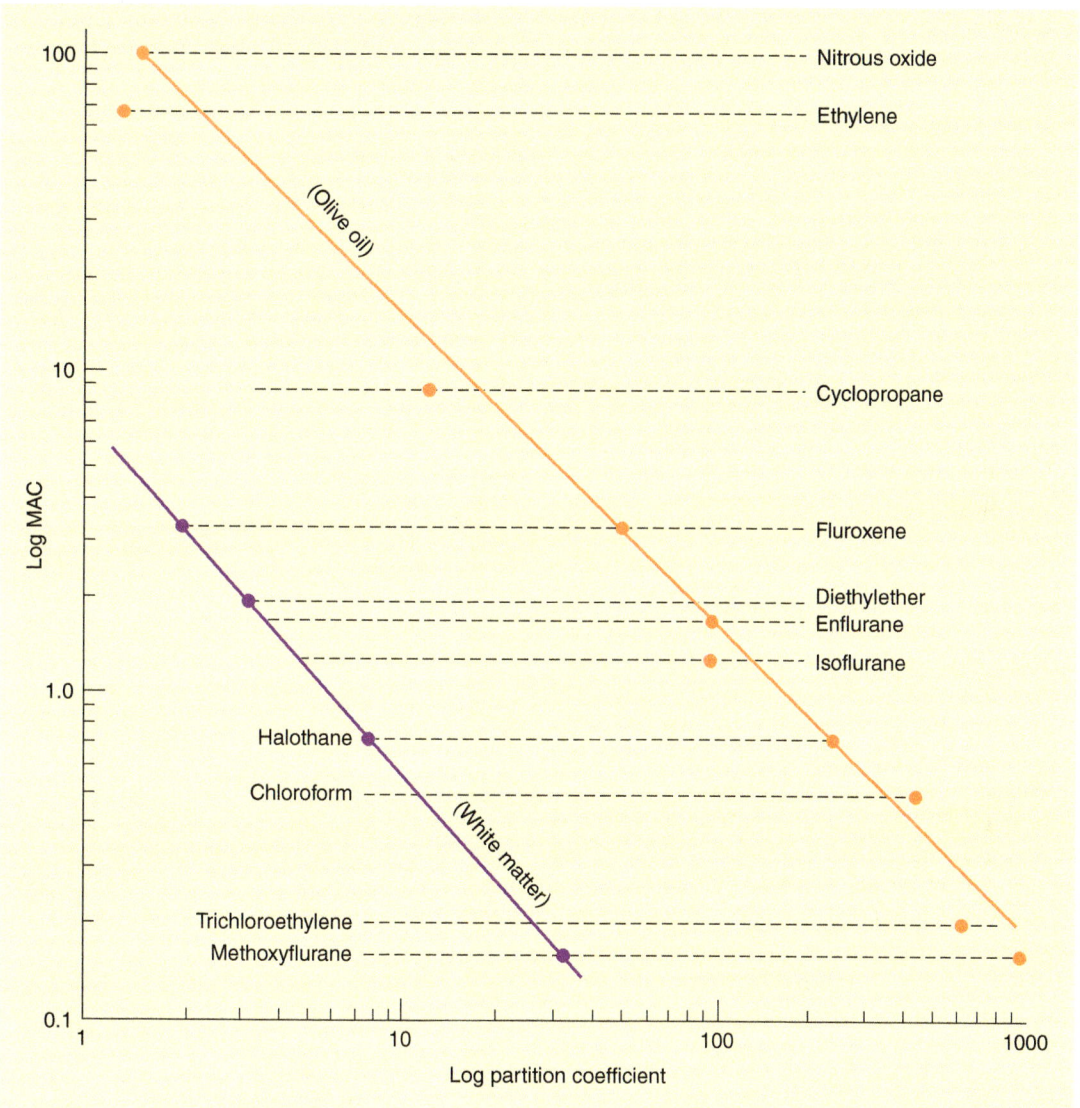

FIGURE 8–4 There is a good but not perfect correlation between anesthetic potency and lipid solubility. MAC, minimum alveolar concentration. (Modified and reproduced, with permission, from Lowe HJ, Hagler K: *Gas Chromatography in Biology and Medicine.* Churchill, 1969.)

as many protein channels may be affected by individual anesthetic agents, and no obligatory site has yet been identified. Selecting among so many molecular targets for the one(s) that provide optimum effects with minimal adverse actions will be the challenge in designing better inhalational agents.

ANESTHETIC NEUROTOXICITY

In recent years, there has been ongoing concern that general anesthetics damage the developing brain. It has been suggested that early exposure to anesthetics can promote cognitive impairment in later life. Concern has been raised that anesthetic exposure affects the development and the elimination of synapses in the infant brain. For example, animal studies have demonstrated that isoflurane exposure promotes neuronal apoptosis and subsequent learning disability. Volatile anesthetics have been shown to promote apoptosis by altering cellular calcium homeostatic mechanisms.

Human studies exploring whether anesthesia is harmful in children are difficult, as conducting a randomized controlled trial for that purpose only would be unethical. Studies that compare populations of children who have had anesthetics with those who have not are also complicated by the reality that the former population is likewise having surgery and receiving the attention of the medical community. Consequently, children receiving anesthetics may be more likely to be diagnosed with learning difficulties in the first place. Data from one large study demonstrated that children who underwent surgery and anesthesia had a greater likelihood of carrying the diagnosis of a developmental disorder; however, the finding was not supported in twins (ie, the incidence of developmental disability was not greater in a twin who was exposed to anesthesia and surgery than in one who was not).

Human, animal, and laboratory trials demonstrating or refuting that anesthetic neurotoxicity leads to developmental disability in children are underway. As of this writing, there is insufficient and conflicting evidence to warrant changes in anesthetic practice (see: www.smarttots.org).

ANESTHETIC NEUROPROTECTION AND CARDIAC PRECONDITIONING

Although inhalational agents have been suggested as contributing to neurotoxicity, they have also been shown to provide both neurologic and cardiac protective effects against ischemia-reperfusion injury. Ischemic preconditioning implies that a brief ischemic episode protects a cell from future, more pronounced ischemic events. Various molecular mechanisms have been suggested to protect cells preconditioned either through ischemic events or secondary to pharmacologic mechanisms, such as

through the use of inhalational anesthetics. In the heart, preconditioning in part arises from actions at ATP-sensitive potassium (K_{ATP}) channels.

The exact mechanism of anesthetic preconditioning is likely to be multifocal and includes the opening of K_{ATP} channels, resulting in less mitochondrial calcium ion concentration and reduction of reactive oxygen species (ROS) production. ROS are associated with cellular injury. For example, excitatory NMDA receptors are linked to the development of neuronal injury. NMDA antagonists, such as the noble anesthetic gas Xenon, have been shown to be neuroprotective. Xenon has an anti-apoptotic effect that may be secondary to its inhibition of calcium ion influx following cell injury. Other inhalational agents, such as sevoflurane, have been shown to reduce markers of myocardial cell injury (eg, troponin T), compared with intravenous anesthetic techniques.

As with neurotoxicity, the role of inhalational anesthetics in tissue protection is the subject of ongoing investigation.

MINIMUM ALVEOLAR CONCENTRATION

The minimum alveolar concentration (MAC) of an inhaled anesthetic is the alveolar concentration that prevents movement in 50% of patients in response to a standardized stimulus (eg, surgical incision). MAC is a useful measure because it mirrors brain partial pressure, allows comparisons of potency between agents, and provides a standard for experimental evaluations (Table 8–3). Nonetheless, it should be remembered that this is a median value with limited usefulness in managing individual patients, particularly during times of rapidly changing alveolar concentrations (eg, induction).

The MAC values for different anesthetics are roughly additive. For example, a mixture of 0.5 MAC of nitrous oxide (53%) and 0.5 MAC of halothane (0.37%) produces the same likelihood that movement in response to surgical incision will be suppressed as 1.0 MAC of isoflurane (1.7%) or 1.0 MAC of any other single agent. In contrast to CNS depression, the degree of myocardial depression may not be equivalent at the same MAC: 0.5 MAC of halothane causes more myocardial depression than 0.5 MAC

TABLE 8–3 Properties of modern inhalation anesthetics.

Agent	Structure	MAC%[1]	Vapor Pressure (mm Hg at 20°C)
Nitrous oxide	$N=N$ $\diagdown O \diagup$	105[2]	—
Halothane (Fluothane)	F–C–C–H with F, Cl, F, Br substituents	0.75	243
Isoflurane (Forane)	H–C–O–C–C–F with F, H, F, Cl, F substituents	1.2	240
Desflurane (Suprane)	H–C–O–C–C–F with F, H, F, F, F substituents	6.0	681
Sevoflurane (Ultane)	H–C–O–C with F–C–F groups	2.0	160

[1]These minimum alveolar concentration (MAC) values are for 30- to 55-year old human subjects and are expressed as a percentage of 1 atmosphere. High altitude requires a higher inspired concentration of anesthetic to achieve the same partial pressure.

[2]A concentration greater than 100% means that hyperbaric conditions are required to achieve 1.0 MAC.

of nitrous oxide. MAC represents only one point on the dose–response curve—it is the equivalent of a median effective dose (ED_{50}). MAC multiples are clinically useful if the concentration–response curves of the anesthetics being compared are parallel, nearly linear, and continuous for the effect being predicted. Roughly 1.3 MAC of any of the volatile anesthetics (eg, for halothane: $1.3 \times 0.74\% = 0.96\%$) has been found to prevent movement in about 95% of patients (an approximation of the ED_{95}); 0.3–0.4 MAC is associated with awakening from anesthesia (MAC awake) when the inhaled drug is the only agent maintaining anesthetic (a rare circumstance).

MAC can be altered by several physiological and pharmacological variables (Table 8–4). **One of the most striking is the 6% decrease in MAC per decade of age, regardless of volatile anesthetic.**

MAC is relatively unaffected by species, sex, or duration of anesthesia. Surprisingly, MAC is not altered after spinal cord transection in rats, leading to the hypothesis that the site of anesthetic inhibition of motor responses lies in the spinal cord.

Clinical Pharmacology of Inhalation Anesthetics

NITROUS OXIDE

Physical Properties

Nitrous oxide (N_2O; laughing gas) is colorless and essentially odorless. Although nonexplosive and nonflammable, nitrous oxide is as capable as oxygen of supporting combustion. Unlike the potent volatile

TABLE 8–4 Factors affecting MAC.[1]

Variable	Effect on MAC	Comments	Variable	Effect on MAC	Comments
Temperature			Electrolytes		
Hypothermia	↓		Hypercalcemia	↓	
Hyperthermia	↓	↑ if > 42°C	Hypernatremia	↑	Caused by altered CSF[2]
			Hyponatremia	↓	Caused by altered CSF
Age			Pregnancy	↓	MAC decreased by one-third at 8 weeks' gestation; normal by 72 h postpartum
Young	↑				
Elderly	↓				
Alcohol			Drugs		
Acute intoxication	↓		Local anesthetics	↓	Except cocaine
Chronic abuse	↑		Opioids	↓	
			Ketamine	↓	
			Barbiturates	↓	
Anemia			Benzodiazepines	↓	
Hematocrit < 10%	↓		Verapamil	↓	
			Lithium	↓	
PaO_2	↓		Sympatholytics		
<40 mm Hg			Methyldopa	↓	
			Clonidine	↓	
$Paco_2$			Dexmedetomidine	↓	
>95 mm Hg	↓	Caused by < pH in CSF	Sympathomimetics		
			Amphetamine		
			Chronic	↓	
Thyroid			Acute	↑	
Hyperthyroid	No change		Cocaine	↑	
Hypothyroid	No change		Ephedrine	↑	
Blood pressure					
Mean arterial pressure <40 mm Hg	↓				

[1]These conclusions are based on human and animal studies.
[2]CSF, cerebrospinal fluid.

agents, nitrous oxide is a gas at room temperature and ambient pressure. It can be kept as a liquid under pressure because its critical temperature lies above room temperature. Nitrous oxide is a relatively inexpensive anesthetic; however, concerns regarding its safety have led to continued interest in alternatives such as **xenon** (Table 8–5). As noted earlier, nitrous oxide, like xenon, is an NMDA receptor antagonist.

Effects on Organ Systems

A. Cardiovascular

Nitrous oxide has a tendency to stimulate the sympathetic nervous system. Thus, even though nitrous oxide directly depresses myocardial contractility in

TABLE 8–5 Advantages and disadvantages of xenon (Xe) anesthesia.

Advantages
  Inert (probably nontoxic with no metabolism)
  Minimal cardiovascular effects
  Low blood solubility
  Rapid induction and recovery
  Does not trigger malignant hyperthermia
  Environmentally friendly
  Nonexplosive

Disadvantages
  High cost
  Low potency (MAC = 70%)[1]

[1]MAC, minimum alveolar concentration.

TABLE 8–6 Clinical pharmacology of inhalational anesthetics.

	Nitrous Oxide	Halothane	Isoflurane	Desflurane	Sevoflurane
Cardiovascular					
Blood pressure	N/C[1]	↓↓	↓↓	↓↓	↓
Heart rate	N/C	↓	↑	N/C or ↑	N/C
Systemic vascular resistance	N/C	N/C	↓↓	↓↓	↓
Cardiac output[2]	N/C	↓	N/C	N/C or ↓	↓
Respiratory					
Tidal volume	↓	↓↓	↓↓	↓	↓
Respiratory rate	↑	↑↑	↑	↑	↑
Paco$_2$					
Resting	N/C	↑	↑	↑↑	↑
Challenge	↑	↑	↑	↑↑	↑
Cerebral					
Blood flow	↑	↑↑	↑	↑	↑
Intracranial pressure	↑	↑↑	↑	↑	↑
Cerebral metabolic rate	↑	↓	↓↓	↓↓	↓↓
Seizures	↓	↓	↓	↓	↓
Neuromuscular					
Nondepolarizing blockade[3]	↑	↑↑	↑↑↑	↑↑↑	↑↑
Renal					
Renal blood flow	↓↓	↓↓	↓↓	↓	↓
Glomerular filtration rate	↓↓	↓↓	↓↓	↓	↓
Urinary output	↓↓	↓↓	↓↓	↓	↓
Hepatic					
Blood flow	↓	↓↓	↓	↓	↓
Metabolism[4]	0.004%	15% to 20%	0.2%	<0.1%	5%

[1]N/C, no change.

[2]Controlled ventilation.

[3]Depolarizing blockage is probably also prolonged by these agents, but this is usually not clinically significant.

[4]Percentage of absorbed anesthetic undergoing metabolism.

vitro, arterial blood pressure, cardiac output, and heart rate are essentially unchanged or slightly elevated in vivo because of its stimulation of catecholamines (Table 8–6). Myocardial depression may be unmasked in patients with coronary artery disease or severe hypovolemia. Constriction of pulmonary vascular smooth muscle increases pulmonary vascular resistance, which results in a generally modest elevation of right ventricular end-diastolic pressure. Despite vasoconstriction of cutaneous vessels, peripheral vascular resistance is not significantly altered.

B. Respiratory

Nitrous oxide increases respiratory rate (tachypnea) and decreases tidal volume as a result of CNS stimulation and, perhaps, activation of pulmonary stretch receptors. The net effect is a minimal change in minute ventilation and resting arterial CO_2 levels. Hypoxic drive, the ventilatory response to arterial hypoxia that is mediated by peripheral chemoreceptors in the carotid bodies, is markedly depressed by even small amounts of nitrous oxide. This is a concern in the recovery room.

C. Cerebral

By increasing CBF and cerebral blood volume, nitrous oxide produces a mild elevation of intracranial pressure. Nitrous oxide also increases cerebral oxygen consumption (CMRO$_2$). These two effects make nitrous oxide theoretically less attractive than other agents for neuroanesthesia. Concentrations of nitrous oxide below MAC may provide analgesia in dental surgery, labor, traumatic injury, and minor surgical procedures.

D. Neuromuscular

In contrast to other inhalation agents, nitrous oxide does not provide significant muscle relaxation. In fact, at high concentrations in hyperbaric chambers, nitrous oxide causes skeletal muscle rigidity. Nitrous oxide is not a triggering agent of malignant hyperthermia.

E. Renal

Nitrous oxide seems to decrease renal blood flow by increasing renal vascular resistance. This leads to a drop in glomerular filtration rate and urinary output.

F. Hepatic

Hepatic blood flow probably falls during nitrous oxide anesthesia, but to a lesser extent than with the volatile agents.

G. Gastrointestinal

Use of nitrous oxide in adults increases the risk of postoperative nausea and vomiting, presumably as a result of activation of the chemoreceptor trigger zone and the vomiting center in the medulla.

Biotransformation & Toxicity

During emergence, almost all nitrous oxide is eliminated by exhalation. A small amount diffuses out through the skin. Biotransformation is limited to the less than 0.01% that undergoes reductive metabolism in the gastrointestinal tract by anaerobic bacteria.

By irreversibly oxidizing the cobalt atom in vitamin B_{12}, nitrous oxide inhibits enzymes that are vitamin B_{12} dependent. These enzymes include methionine synthetase, which is necessary for myelin formation, and thymidylate synthetase, which is necessary for DNA synthesis. Prolonged exposure to anesthetic concentrations of nitrous oxide can result in bone marrow depression (megaloblastic anemia) and even neurological deficiencies (peripheral neuropathies). However, administration of nitrous oxide for bone marrow harvest does not seem to affect the viability of bone marrow mononuclear cells. Because of possible teratogenic effects, nitrous oxide is often avoided in pregnant patients who are not yet in the third trimester. Nitrous oxide may also alter the immunological response to infection by affecting chemotaxis and motility of polymorphonuclear leukocytes.

Contraindications

Although nitrous oxide is insoluble in comparison with other inhalation agents, it is 35 times more soluble than nitrogen in blood. Thus, it tends to diffuse into air-containing cavities more rapidly than nitrogen is absorbed by the bloodstream. For instance, if a patient with a 100-mL pneumothorax inhales 50% nitrous oxide, the gas content of the pneumothorax will tend to approach that of the bloodstream. Because nitrous oxide will diffuse into the cavity more rapidly than the air (principally nitrogen) diffuses out, the pneumothorax expands until it contains 100 mL of air and 100 mL of nitrous oxide. If the walls surrounding the cavity are rigid, pressure rises instead of volume. **Examples of conditions in which nitrous oxide might be hazardous include venous or arterial air embolism, pneumothorax, acute intestinal obstruction with bowel distention, intracranial air (pneumocephalus following dural closure or pneumoencephalography), pulmonary air cysts, intraocular air bubbles, and tympanic membrane grafting.** Nitrous oxide will even diffuse into tracheal tube cuffs, increasing the pressure against the tracheal mucosa. Obviously, nitrous oxide is of limited value in patients requiring high inspired oxygen concentrations.

Drug Interactions

Because the high MAC of nitrous oxide prevents its use as a complete general anesthetic, it is frequently used in combination with the more potent volatile agents. The addition of nitrous oxide decreases the requirements of these other agents (65% nitrous oxide decreases the MAC of the volatile anesthetics by approximately 50%). Although nitrous oxide should not be considered a benign carrier gas, it does attenuate the circulatory and respiratory effects of volatile anesthetics in adults. Nitrous oxide potentiates neuromuscular blockade, but less so than the volatile agents. The concentration of nitrous oxide flowing through a vaporizer can influence the concentration of volatile anesthetic delivered. For example, decreasing nitrous oxide concentration (ie, increasing oxygen concentration) increases the concentration of volatile agent despite a constant vaporizer setting. This disparity is due to the relative solubilities of nitrous oxide and oxygen in liquid volatile anesthetics. The second gas effect was discussed earlier. Nitrous oxide is an ozone-depleting gas with greenhouse effects.

HALOTHANE

Physical Properties

Halothane is a halogenated alkane (see Table 8–3). The carbon–fluoride bonds are responsible for its nonflammable and nonexplosive nature. Thymol preservative and amber-colored bottles retard spontaneous oxidative decomposition. It is rarely used in the United States.

Effects on Organ Systems

A. Cardiovascular

A dose-dependent reduction of arterial blood pressure is due to direct myocardial depression; 2.0 MAC of halothane in patients not undergoing surgery results in a 50% decrease in blood pressure and cardiac output. Cardiac depression—from interference with sodium–calcium exchange and intracellular calcium utilization—causes an increase in right atrial pressure. Although halothane is a coronary artery vasodilator, coronary blood flow decreases, due to the drop in systemic arterial pressure. Adequate myocardial perfusion is usually maintained, as oxygen demand also drops. Normally, hypotension inhibits baroreceptors in the aortic arch and carotid bifurcation, causing a decrease in vagal stimulation and a compensatory rise in heart rate. Halothane blunts this reflex. Slowing of sinoatrial node conduction may result in a junctional rhythm or bradycardia. In infants, halothane decreases cardiac output by a combination of decreased heart rate and depressed myocardial contractility. Halothane sensitizes the heart to the arrhythmogenic effects of epinephrine, so that doses of epinephrine above 1.5 mcg/kg should be avoided. Although organ blood flow is redistributed, systemic vascular resistance is unchanged.

B. Respiratory

Halothane typically causes rapid, shallow breathing. The increased respiratory rate is not enough to counter the decreased tidal volume, so alveolar ventilation drops, and resting $Paco_2$ is elevated. **Apneic threshold**, the highest $Paco_2$ at which a patient remains apneic, also rises because the difference between it and resting $Paco_2$ is not altered by general anesthesia. Similarly, halothane limits the increase in minute ventilation that normally accompanies a rise in $Paco_2$. Halothane's ventilatory effects are probably due to central (medullary depression) and peripheral (intercostal muscle dysfunction) mechanisms. These changes are exaggerated by preexisting lung disease and attenuated by surgical stimulation. The increase in $Paco_2$ and the decrease in intrathoracic pressure that accompany spontaneous ventilation with halothane partially reverse the depression in cardiac output, arterial blood pressure, and heart rate described above. Hypoxic drive is severely depressed by even low concentrations of halothane (0.1 MAC).

Halothane is considered a potent bronchodilator, as it often reverses asthma-induced bronchospasm. This action is not inhibited by β-adrenergic blocking agents. Halothane attenuates airway reflexes and relaxes bronchial smooth muscle by inhibiting intracellular calcium mobilization. Halothane also depresses clearance of mucus from the respiratory tract (mucociliary function), promoting postoperative hypoxia and atelectasis.

C. Cerebral

By dilating cerebral vessels, halothane lowers cerebral vascular resistance and increases CBF. **Autoregulation**, the maintenance of constant CBF during changes in arterial blood pressure, is blunted. Concomitant rises in intracranial pressure can be prevented by establishing hyperventilation *prior to* administration of halothane. Cerebral activity is decreased, leading to electroencephalographic slowing and modest reductions in metabolic oxygen requirements.

D. Neuromuscular

Halothane relaxes skeletal muscle and potentiates nondepolarizing neuromuscular-blocking agents (NMBA). Like the other potent volatile anesthetics, it is a triggering agent of malignant hyperthermia.

E. Renal

Halothane reduces renal blood flow, glomerular filtration rate, and urinary output. Part of this decrease can be explained by a fall in arterial blood pressure and cardiac output. Because the reduction in renal blood flow is greater than the reduction in glomerular filtration rate, the filtration fraction is increased. Preoperative hydration limits these changes.

F. Hepatic

Halothane causes hepatic blood flow to decrease in proportion to the depression of cardiac output. Hepatic artery vasospasm has been reported during halothane anesthesia. The metabolism and clearance of some drugs (eg, fentanyl, phenytoin, verapamil) seem to be impaired by halothane. Other evidence of hepatic cellular dysfunction includes sulfobromophthalein (BSP) dye retention and minor liver transaminase elevations.

Biotransformation & Toxicity

Halothane is oxidized in the liver by a particular isozyme of CYP (2EI) to its principal metabolite, trifluoroacetic acid. This metabolism can be inhibited by pretreatment with disulfiram. Bromide, another oxidative metabolite, has been incriminated in (but is an improbable cause of) postanesthetic changes in mental status. In the absence of oxygen, reductive metabolism may result in a small amount of hepatotoxic end products that covalently bind to tissue macromolecules. This is more apt to occur following enzyme induction by phenobarbital. Elevated fluoride levels signal significant anaerobic metabolism.

Postoperative hepatic dysfunction has several causes: viral hepatitis, impaired hepatic perfusion, preexisting liver disease, hepatocyte hypoxia, sepsis, hemolysis, benign postoperative intrahepatic cholestasis, and drug-induced hepatitis. "**Halothane hepatitis**" is extremely rare (1 per 35,000 cases). Patients exposed to multiple halothane anesthetics at short intervals, middle-aged obese women, and persons with a familial predisposition to halothane toxicity or a personal history of toxicity are considered to be at increased risk. Signs are mostly related to hepatic injury, such as increased serum alanine and aspartate transferase, elevated bilirubin (leading to jaundice), and encephalopathy.

The hepatic lesion seen in humans—centrilobular necrosis—also occurs in rats pretreated with an enzyme inducer (phenobarbital) and exposed to halothane under hypoxic conditions ($FIO_2 < 14\%$). This *halothane hypoxic model* implies hepatic damage from reductive metabolites or hypoxia.

More likely evidence points to an immune mechanism. For instance, some signs of the disease indicate an allergic reaction (eg, eosinophilia, rash, fever) and do not appear until a few days after exposure. Furthermore, an antibody that binds to hepatocytes previously exposed to halothane has been isolated from patients with halothane-induced hepatic dysfunction. This antibody response may involve liver microsomal proteins that have been modified by trifluoroacetic acid as the triggering antigens (trifluoroacetylated liver proteins such as microsomal carboxylesterase). As with halothane, other inhalational agents that undergo oxidative metabolism can likewise lead to hepatitis. However, newer agents undergo little to no metabolism, and therefore do not form trifluroacetic acid protein adducts or produce the immune response leading to hepatitis.

Contraindications

It is prudent to withhold halothane from patients with unexplained liver dysfunction following previous anesthetic exposure.

Halothane, like all inhalational anesthetics, should be used with care in patients with intracranial mass lesions because of the possibility of intracranial hypertension secondary to increased cerebral blood volume and blood flow.

Hypovolemic patients and some patients with severe reductions in left ventricular function may not tolerate halothane's negative inotropic effects. Sensitization of the heart to catecholamines limits the usefulness of halothane when exogenous epinephrine is administered or in patients with pheochromocytoma.

Drug Interactions

The myocardial depression seen with halothane is exacerbated by β-adrenergic-blocking agents and calcium channel-blocking agents. Tricyclic antidepressants and monoamine oxidase inhibitors have been associated with fluctuations in blood pressure and arrhythmias, although neither represents an absolute contraindication. The combination of halothane and aminophylline has resulted in serious ventricular arrhythmias.

ISOFLURANE

Physical Properties

Isoflurane is a nonflammable volatile anesthetic with a pungent ethereal odor. Although it is a chemical isomer with the same molecular weight as enflurane, it has different physicochemical properties (see Table 8–3).

Effects on Organ Systems

A. Cardiovascular

Isoflurane causes minimal left ventricular depression in vivo. Cardiac output is maintained by a rise in heart rate due to partial preservation of carotid baroreflexes. Mild β-adrenergic stimulation increases skeletal muscle blood flow, decreases systemic vascular resistance, and lowers arterial blood pressure. Rapid increases in isoflurane concentration lead to transient increases in heart rate, arterial blood pressure, and plasma levels of norepinephrine. Isoflurane dilates coronary arteries, but not nearly as potently as nitroglycerin or adenosine. Dilation of normal coronary arteries could theoretically divert blood away from fixed stenotic lesions, which was the basis for concern about coronary "steal" with this agent, a concern that has largely been forgotten.

B. Respiratory

Respiratory depression during isoflurane anesthesia resembles that of other volatile anesthetics, except that tachypnea is less pronounced. The net effect is a more pronounced fall in minute ventilation. Even low levels of isoflurane (0.1 MAC) blunt the normal ventilatory response to hypoxia and hypercapnia.

Despite a tendency to irritate upper airway reflexes, isoflurane is considered a good bronchodilator, but may not be as potent a bronchodilator as halothane.

C. Cerebral

At concentrations greater than 1 MAC, isoflurane increases CBF and intracranial pressure. These effects are thought to be less pronounced than with halothane and are reversed by hyperventilation. In contrast to halothane, the hyperventilation does not have to be instituted prior to the use of isoflurane to prevent intracranial hypertension. Isoflurane reduces cerebral metabolic oxygen requirements, and at 2 MAC, it produces an electrically silent electroencephalogram (EEG).

D. Neuromuscular

Isoflurane relaxes skeletal muscle.

E. Renal

Isoflurane decreases renal blood flow, glomerular filtration rate, and urinary output.

F. Hepatic

Total hepatic blood flow (hepatic artery and portal vein flow) may be reduced during isoflurane anesthesia. Hepatic oxygen supply is better maintained with isoflurane than with halothane, however, because hepatic artery perfusion is preserved. Liver function tests are usually not affected.

Biotransformation & Toxicity

Isoflurane is metabolized to trifluoroacetic acid. Although serum fluoride fluid levels may rise, nephrotoxicity is extremely unlikely, even in the presence of enzyme inducers. Prolonged sedation (>24 h at 0.1–0.6% isoflurane) of critically ill patients has resulted in elevated plasma fluoride levels (15–50 μmol/L) without evidence of renal impairment. Similarly, up to 20 MAC-hours of isoflurane may lead to fluoride levels exceeding 50 μmol/L without detectable postoperative renal dysfunction. Its limited oxidative metabolism also minimizes any possible risk of significant hepatic dysfunction.

Contraindications

Isoflurane presents no unique contraindications. Patients with severe hypovolemia may not tolerate its vasodilating effects. It can trigger malignant hyperthermia.

Drug Interactions

Epinephrine can be safely administered in doses up to 4.5 mcg/kg. Nondepolarizing NMBAs are potentiated by isoflurane.

DESFLURANE

Physical Properties

The structure of desflurane is very similar to that of isoflurane. In fact, the only difference is the substitution of a fluorine atom for isoflurane's chlorine atom. That "minor" change has profound effects on the physical properties of the drug, however. For instance, because the vapor pressure of desflurane at 20°C is 681 mm Hg, at high altitudes (eg, Denver, Colorado) it boils at room temperature. This problem necessitated the development of a special desflurane vaporizer. Furthermore, the low solubility of desflurane in blood and body tissues causes a very rapid induction and emergence of anesthesia. Therefore, the alveolar concentration of desflurane approaches the inspired concentration much more rapidly than the other volatile agents, giving the anesthesiologist tighter control over anesthetic levels. **Wakeup times are approximately 50% less than those observed following isoflurane.** This is principally attributable to a blood/gas partition coefficient (0.42) that is even lower than that of nitrous oxide (0.47). Although desflurane is roughly one-fourth as potent as the other volatile agents, it is 17 times more potent than nitrous oxide. A high vapor pressure, an ultrashort duration of action, and moderate potency are the most characteristic features of desflurane.

Effects on Organ Systems

A. Cardiovascular

The cardiovascular effects of desflurane seem to be similar to those of isoflurane. Increasing the dose is associated with a decline in systemic vascular resistance that leads to a fall in arterial blood pressure. Cardiac output remains relatively unchanged or slightly depressed at 1–2 MAC. There is a moderate rise in heart rate, central venous pressure, and pulmonary artery pressure that often does not become apparent at low doses. Rapid increases in desflurane concentration lead to transient but sometimes worrisome elevations in heart rate, blood pressure, and catecholamine levels that are more pronounced than occur with isoflurane, particularly in patients with cardiovascular disease. These cardiovascular responses to rapidly increasing desflurane concentration can be attenuated by fentanyl, esmolol, or clonidine.

B. Respiratory

Desflurane causes a decrease in tidal volume and an increase in respiratory rate. There is an overall decrease in alveolar ventilation that causes a rise in resting $Paco_2$. Like other modern volatile anesthetic agents, desflurane depresses the ventilatory response to increasing $Paco_2$. Pungency and airway irritation during desflurane induction can be manifested by salivation, breath-holding, coughing, and laryngospasm. Airway resistance may increase in children with reactive airway susceptibility. These problems make desflurane a poor choice for inhalation induction.

C. Cerebral

Like the other volatile anesthetics, desflurane directly vasodilates the cerebral vasculature, increasing CBF, cerebral blood volume, and intracranial pressure at normotension and normocapnia. Countering the decrease in cerebral vascular resistance is a marked decline in the cerebral metabolic rate of oxygen ($CMRO_2$) that tends to cause cerebral vasoconstriction and moderate any increase in CBF. The cerebral vasculature remains responsive to changes in $Paco_2$, however, so that intracranial pressure can be lowered by hyperventilation. Cerebral oxygen consumption is decreased during desflurane anesthesia. Thus, during periods of desflurane-induced hypotension (mean arterial pressure = 60 mm Hg), CBF is adequate to maintain aerobic metabolism despite a low cerebral perfusion pressure. The effect on the EEG is similar to that of isoflurane. Initially, EEG frequency is increased, but as anesthetic depth is increased, EEG slowing becomes manifest, leading to burst suppression at higher inhaled concentrations.

D. Neuromuscular

Desflurane is associated with a dose-dependent decrease in the response to train-of-four and tetanic peripheral nerve stimulation.

E. Renal

There is no evidence of any significant nephrotoxic effects caused by exposure to desflurane. However, as cardiac output declines, decreases in urine output and glomerular filtration should be expected with desflurane and all other anesthetics.

F. Hepatic

Hepatic function tests are generally unaffected by desflurane, assuming that organ perfusion is maintained perioperatively. Desflurane undergoes minimal metabolism, therefore the risk of anesthetic-induced hepatitis is likewise minimal. As with isoflurane and sevoflurane, hepatic oxygen delivery is generally maintained.

Biotransformation & Toxicity

Desflurane undergoes minimal metabolism in humans. Serum and urine inorganic fluoride levels following desflurane anesthesia are essentially unchanged from preanesthetic levels. There is insignificant percutaneous loss. Desflurane, more than other volatile anesthetics, is degraded by desiccated CO_2 absorbent (particularly barium hydroxide lime, but also sodium and potassium hydroxide) into potentially clinically significant levels of carbon monoxide. Carbon monoxide poisoning is difficult to diagnose under general anesthesia, but the presence of carboxyhemoglobin may be detectable by arterial blood gas analysis or lower than expected pulse oximetry readings (although still falsely high). Disposing of dried out absorbent or use of calcium hydroxide can minimize the risk of carbon monoxide poisoning.

Contraindications

Desflurane shares many of the contraindications of other modern volatile anesthetics: severe hypovolemia, malignant hyperthermia, and intracranial hypertension.

Drug Interactions

Desflurane potentiates nondepolarizing neuromuscular blocking agents to the same extent as isoflurane. Epinephrine can be safely administered in doses up to 4.5 mcg/kg as desflurane does not sensitize the myocardium to the arrhythmogenic effects of epinephrine. Although emergence is more rapid following desflurane anesthesia than after isoflurane anesthesia, switching from isoflurane to desflurane toward the end of anesthesia does not significantly accelerate recovery, nor does faster emergence translate into faster discharge times from the post-anesthesia care unit. Desflurane emergence has been associated with delirium in some pediatric patients.

SEVOFLURANE

Physical Properties

Like desflurane, sevoflurane is halogenated with fluorine. Sevoflurane's solubility in blood is slightly greater than desflurane ($\lambda_{b/g}$ 0.65 versus 0.42)

12 (see Table 8–3). Nonpungency and rapid increases in alveolar anesthetic concentration make sevoflurane an excellent choice for smooth and rapid inhalation inductions in pediatric and adult patients. In fact, inhalation induction with 4% to 8% sevoflurane in a 50% mixture of nitrous oxide and oxygen can be achieved within 1 min. Likewise, its low blood solubility results in a rapid fall in alveolar anesthetic concentration upon discontinuation and a more rapid emergence compared with isoflurane (although not an earlier discharge from the post-anesthesia care unit). Sevoflurane's modest vapor pressure permits the use of a conventional variable bypass vaporizer.

Effects on Organ Systems

A. Cardiovascular

Sevoflurane mildly depresses myocardial contractility. Systemic vascular resistance and arterial blood pressure decline slightly less than with isoflurane or desflurane. Because sevoflurane causes little, if any, rise in heart rate, cardiac output is not maintained as well as with isoflurane or desflurane. Sevoflurane may prolong the QT interval, the clinical significance of which is unknown. QT prolongation may be manifest 60 min following anesthetic emergence in infants.

B. Respiratory

Sevoflurane depresses respiration and reverses bronchospasm to an extent similar to that of isoflurane.

C. Cerebral

Similar to isoflurane and desflurane, sevoflurane causes slight increases in CBF and intracranial pressure at normocarbia, although some studies show a decrease in cerebral blood flow. High concentrations of sevoflurane (>1.5 MAC) may impair autoregulation of CBF, thus allowing a drop in CBF during hemorrhagic hypotension. This effect on CBF autoregulation seems to be less pronounced than with isoflurane. Cerebral metabolic oxygen requirements decrease, and seizure activity has not been reported.

D. Neuromuscular

Sevoflurane produces adequate muscle relaxation for intubation of children following an inhalation induction.

E. Renal

Sevoflurane slightly decreases renal blood flow. Its metabolism to substances associated with impaired renal tubule function (eg, decreased concentrating ability) is discussed below.

F. Hepatic

Sevoflurane decreases portal vein blood flow, but increases hepatic artery blood flow, thereby maintaining total hepatic blood flow and oxygen delivery. It is generally not associated with immune-mediated anesthetic hepatotoxicity

Biotransformation & Toxicity

The liver microsomal enzyme P-450 (specifically the 2E1 isoform) metabolizes sevoflurane at a rate one-fourth that of halothane (5% versus 20%), but 10 to 25 times that of isoflurane or desflurane and may be induced with ethanol or phenobarbital pretreatment. The potential nephrotoxicity of the resulting

rise in inorganic fluoride (F^-) was discussed earlier. Serum fluoride concentrations exceed 50 μmol/L in approximately 7% of patients who receive sevoflurane, yet clinically significant renal dysfunction has not been associated with sevoflurane anesthesia. The overall rate of sevoflurane metabolism is 5%, or 10 times that of isoflurane. Nonetheless, there has been no association with peak fluoride levels following sevoflurane and any renal concentrating abnormality.

Alkali such as barium hydroxide lime or soda lime (but not calcium hydroxide) can degrade sevoflurane, producing another proven (at least in rats) nephrotoxic end product (*compound A*, fluoromethyl-2,2-difluoro-1-[trifluoromethyl]vinyl ether). Accumulation of compound A increases with increased respiratory gas temperature, low-flow anesthesia, dry barium hydroxide absorbent (Baralyme), high sevoflurane concentrations, and anesthetics of long duration.

Most studies have not associated sevoflurane with any detectable postoperative impairment of renal function that would indicate toxicity or injury. Nonetheless, some clinicians recommend that fresh gas flows be at least 2 L/min for anesthetics lasting more than a few hours and that sevoflurane not be used in patients with preexisting renal dysfunction.

Sevoflurane can also be degraded into hydrogen fluoride by metal and environmental impurities present in manufacturing equipment, glass bottle packaging, and anesthesia equipment. Hydrogen fluoride can produce an acid burn on contact with respiratory mucosa. The risk of patient injury has been substantially reduced by inhibition of the degradation process by adding water to sevoflurane during the manufacturing process and packaging it in a special plastic container. The manufacturer has also distributed a "Dear Provider" letter warning of isolated incidents of fire in the respiratory circuits of anesthesia machines with desiccated CO_2 absorbent when sevoflurane was used.

Contraindications

Contraindications include severe hypovolemia, susceptibility to malignant hyperthermia, and intracranial hypertension.

Drug Interactions

Like other volatile anesthetics, sevoflurane potentiates NMBAs. It does not sensitize the heart to catecholamine-induced arrhythmias.

XENON

Xenon is a "noble" gas that has long been known to have anesthetic properties. It is an inert element that does not form chemical bonds. Xenon is scavenged from the atmosphere through a costly distillation process. It is an odorless, nonexplosive, naturally occurring gas with a MAC of .71 and a blood/gas coefficient of 0.115, giving it very fast onset and emergence parameters. As previously mentioned, xenon's anesthetic effects seem to be mediated by NMDA inhibition by competing with glycine at the glycine binding site. Xenon seems to have little effect on cardiovascular, hepatic, or renal systems and has been found to be protective against neuronal ischemia. As a natural element, it has no effect upon the ozone layer compared with another NMDA antagonist, nitrous oxide. Cost and limited availability have prevented its widespread use.

SUGGESTED READING

Banks P, Franks N, Dickinson R: Competitive inhibition at the glycine site of the *N*-methyl-D-aspartate receptor mediates xenon neuroprotection against hypoxia ischemia. Anesthesiology 2010;112:614.

Bantel C, Maze M, Trapp S: Neuronal preconditioning by inhalational anesthetics. Anesthesiology 2009;11:986.

Cittanova M-L, Lelongt B, Verpont M-C: Fluoride ion toxicity in human kidney collecting duct cells. Anesthesiology 1996;84:428.

Coburn M, Maze M, Franks N: The neuroprotective effects of xenon and helium in an in vitro model of traumatic brain injury. Crit Care Med 2008;36:588.

De Hert S, Preckel B, Schlack W: Update on inhalational anaesthetics. Curr Opin Anaesthesiol 2009;22:491.

DiMaggio C, Sun L, Li G: Early childhood exposure to anesthesia and risk of developmental and behavioral disorders in a sibling birth cohort. Anesth Analg 2011; 113:1143.

Ebert TJ: Myocardial ischemia and adverse cardiac outcomes in cardiac patients undergoing noncardiac surgery with sevoflurane and isoflurane. Anesth Analg 1997;85:993.

Eger EI 2nd, Bowland T, Ionescu P, et al: Recovery and kinetic characteristics of desflurane and sevoflurane in volunteers after 8-h exposure, including kinetics of degradation products. Anesthesiology 1997;87:517.

Eger EI 2nd, Raines DE, Shafer SL, Hemmings HC Jr, Sonner JM: Is a new paradigm needed to explain how inhaled anesthetics produce immobility? Anesth Analg 2008;107: 832.

Ghatge S, Lee J, Smith I: Sevoflurane: an ideal agent for adult day-case anesthesia? Acta Anaesthesiol Scand 2003;47:917.

Ishizawa Y: General anesthetic gases and the global environment. Anesth Analg 2011; 112:213.

Jevtovic-Todorovic V: Pediatric anesthesia neurotoxicity: an overview of the 2011 Smart Tots panel. Anesth Analg 2011;113:965.

Jordan BD, Wright EL: Xenon as an anesthetic agent. AANA J 2010;78:387.

Loeckinger A, Kleinsasser A, Maier S, et.al: Sustained prolongation of the QTc interval after anesthesia with sevoflurane in infants during the first 6 months of life. Anesthesiology 2003;98:639.

Njoku D, Laster MJ, Gong DH: Biotransformation of halothane, enflurane, isoflurane, and desflurane to trifluoroacetylated liver proteins: association between protein acylation and hepatic injury. Anesth Analg 1997;84:173.

Preckel B, Weber N, Sanders R, et al: Molecular mechanisms transducing the anesthetic analgesic and organ protective actions of Xenon. Anesthesiology 2006;105:187.

Stratmann G: Neurotoxicity of anesthetic drugs in the developing brain. Anesth Analg 2011;113:1170.

Summors AC, Gupta AK, Matta BF: Dynamic cerebral autoregulation during sevoflurane anesthesia: a comparison with isoflurane. Anesth Analg 1999;88:341.

Sun X, Su F, Shi Y, Lee C: The "second gas effect" is not a valid concept. Anesth Analg 1999;88:188.

Thomas J, Crosby G, Drummond J, et.al: Anesthetic neurotoxicity: a difficult dragon to slay. Anesth Analg 2011;113;969.

Torri G: Inhalational anesthetics: a review. Minerva Anestesiol 2010;76:215.

Wang L, Traystman R, Murphy S: Inhalational agents in ischemic brain. Curr Opin Pharmacol 2008;8:104.

Wei H: The role of calcium dysregulation in anesthetic mediated neurotoxicity. Anesth Analg 2011;113:972.

Intravenous Anesthetics

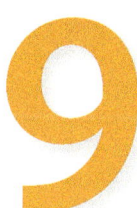

9

1 Repetitive administration of barbiturates (eg, infusion of thiopental for "barbiturate coma" and brain protection) saturates the peripheral compartments, minimizing any effect of redistribution, and rendering the duration of action more dependent on elimination. This is an example of context sensitivity.

2 Barbiturates constrict the cerebral vasculature, causing a decrease in cerebral blood flow, cerebral blood volume, and intracranial pressure.

3 Although apnea may be relatively uncommon after benzodiazepine induction, even small intravenous doses of diazepam and midazolam have resulted in respiratory arrest.

4 In contrast to other anesthetic agents, ketamine increases arterial blood pressure, heart rate, and cardiac output, particularly after rapid bolus injections.

5 Induction doses of etomidate transiently inhibit enzymes involved in cortisol and aldosterone synthesis. Etomidate was often used in the past for ICU sedation before reports of its consistent ability to produce adrenocortical suppression in that circumstance appeared.

6 Propofol formulations can support the growth of bacteria, so sterile technique must be observed in preparation and handling. Propofol should be administered within 6 h of opening the ampule.

General anesthesia began with inhaled agents but now can be induced and maintained with drugs that enter the patient through a wide range of routes. Drug administration can be oral, rectal, transdermal, transmucosal, intramuscular, or intravenous for the purpose of producing or enhancing an anesthetic state. Preoperative sedation of adults is usually accomplished by way of oral or intravenous routes. Induction of general anesthesia in adults usually includes intravenous drug administration. Effective topical anesthesia with EMLA (eutectic mixture of local anesthetic) cream, LMX (plain lidocaine cream 4% and 5%), or 2% lidocaine jelly has increased the ease of intravenous inductions in children. Maintenance of general anesthesia is

feasible with a total intravenous anesthesia (TIVA) technique. This chapter focuses on the intravenous agents used to produce hypnosis, including barbiturates, benzodiazepines, ketamine, etomidate, and propofol.

BARBITURATES

Mechanisms of Action

Barbiturates depress the reticular activating system in the brainstem, which controls multiple vital functions, including consciousness. In clinical concentrations, barbiturates more potently affect the function of nerve synapses than axons. Their primary

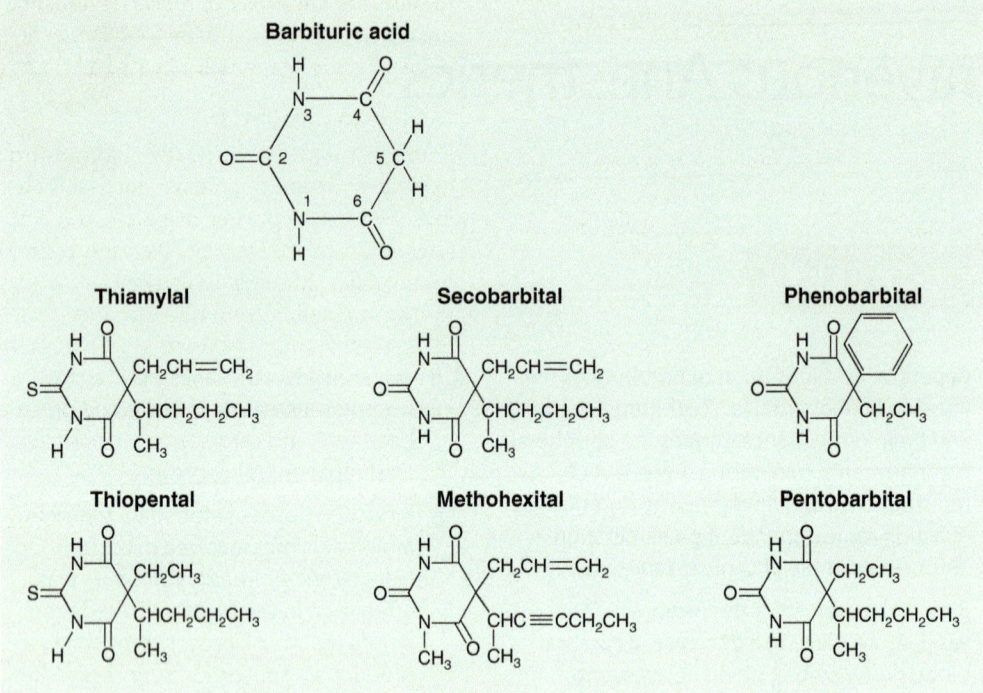

FIGURE 9–1 Barbiturates share the structure of barbituric acid and differ in the C_2, C_3, and N_1 substitutions.

mechanism of action is believed to be through binding to the γ-aminobutyric acid type A ($GABA_A$) receptor. Barbiturates potentiate the action of GABA in increasing the duration of openings of a chloride-specific ion channel.

Structure–Activity Relationships

Barbiturates are derived from barbituric acid (Figure 9–1). Substitution at carbon C_5 determines hypnotic potency and anticonvulsant activity. A long-branched chain conveys more potency than does a short straight chain. Likewise, the phenyl group in *phenobarbital* is anticonvulsive, whereas the methyl group in *methohexital* is not. Replacing the oxygen at C_2 (*oxy*barbiturates) with a sulfur atom (*thiobarbiturates*) increases lipid solubility. As a result, thiopental and thiamylal have a greater potency, more rapid onset of action, and shorter durations of action (after a single "sleep dose") than pentobarbital. The sodium salts of the barbiturates are water soluble but markedly alkaline (pH of 2.5% thiopental >10) and relatively unstable (2-week shelf-life for

2.5% thiopental solution). Concentrations greater than recommended cause an unacceptable incidence of pain on injection and venous thrombosis.

Pharmacokinetics

A. Absorption
In clinical anesthesiology, thiopental, thiamylal, and methohexital were frequently administered intravenously for induction of general anesthesia in adults and children (prior to the introduction of propofol). Rectal thiopental or, more often, methohexital has been used for induction in children, and intramuscular (or oral) pentobarbital was often used in the past for premedication of all age groups.

B. Distribution
The duration of sleep doses of the highly lipid-soluble barbiturates (thiopental, thiamylal, and methohexital) is determined by redistribution, not by metabolism or elimination. For example, although thiopental is highly protein bound (80%), its great lipid solubility and high nonionized fraction (60%)

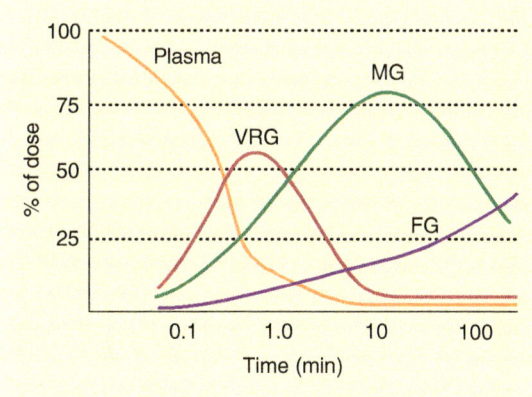

FIGURE 9–2 Distribution of thiopental from plasma to the vessel-rich group (VRG; brain, heart, liver, kidney, endocrine glands), to the muscle group (MG), and finally to the fat group (FG). (Modified and reproduced, with permission, from Price HL et al: The uptake of thiopental by body tissues and its relation to the duration of narcosis. Clin Pharmacol Ther 1960;1:16.)

account for rapid brain uptake (within 30 s). If the central compartment is contracted (eg, hypovolemic shock), if the serum albumin is low (eg, severe liver disease or malnutrition), or if the nonionized fraction is increased (eg, acidosis), larger brain and heart concentrations will be achieved for a given dose. Redistribution to the peripheral compartment—specifically, the muscle group—lowers plasma and brain concentration to 10% of peak levels within 20–30 min (Figure 9–2). This pharmacokinetic profile correlates with clinical experience—patients typically lose consciousness within 30 s and awaken within 20 min.

The minimal induction dose of thiopental will depend on body weight and age. Reduced induction doses are required for elderly patients primarily due to slower redistribution. In contrast to the rapid initial distribution half-life of a few minutes, elimination of thiopental is prolonged (elimination half-life ranges of 10–12 h). Thiamylal and methohexital have similar distribution patterns, whereas less lipid-soluble barbiturates have much longer distribution half-lives and durations of action after a sleep dose. Repetitive administration of barbiturates (eg, infusion of thiopental for "barbiturate coma" and brain protection) saturates the peripheral compartments,

minimizing any effect of redistribution, and rendering the duration of action more dependent on elimination. This is an example of context sensitivity.

C. Biotransformation
Barbiturates are principally biotransformed via hepatic oxidation to inactive water-soluble metabolites. Because of greater hepatic extraction, methohexital is cleared by the liver more rapidly than thiopental. Although redistribution is responsible for the awakening from a single sleep dose of any of these lipid-soluble barbiturates, full recovery of psychomotor function is more rapid following methohexital due to its enhanced metabolism.

D. Excretion
Increased protein binding decreases barbiturate glomerular filtration, whereas increased lipid solubility tends to increase renal tubular reabsorption. Except for the less protein-bound and less lipid-soluble agents such as phenobarbital, renal excretion is limited to water-soluble end products of hepatic biotransformation. Methohexital is excreted in the feces.

Effects on Organ Systems

A. Cardiovascular
Intravenous bolus induction doses of barbiturates cause a decrease in blood pressure and an increase in heart rate. Hemodynamic responses to barbiturates are reduced by slower rates of induction. Depression of the medullary vasomotor center produces vasodilation of peripheral capacitance vessels, which increases peripheral pooling of blood, mimicking a reduced blood volume. Tachycardia following administration is probably due to a central vagolytic effect and reflex responses to decreases in blood pressure. Cardiac output is often maintained by an increased heart rate and increased myocardial contractility from compensatory baroreceptor reflexes. Sympathetically induced vasoconstriction of resistance vessels (particularly with intubation under light planes of general anesthesia) may actually increase peripheral vascular resistance. However, in situations where the baroreceptor response will be blunted or absent (eg, hypovolemia, congestive heart failure, β-adrenergic blockade), **cardiac output and arterial blood pressure may fall dramatically due**

to uncompensated peripheral pooling of blood and direct myocardial depression. Patients with poorly controlled hypertension are particularly prone to wide swings in blood pressure during anesthesia induction. The cardiovascular effects of barbiturates therefore vary markedly, depending on rate of administration, dose, volume status, baseline autonomic tone, and preexisting cardiovascular disease. A slow rate of injection and adequate preoperative hydration attenuates or eliminates these changes in most patients.

B. Respiratory

Barbiturates depress the medullary ventilatory center, decreasing the ventilatory response to hypercapnia and hypoxia. Deep barbiturate sedation often leads to upper airway obstruction; apnea often follows an induction dose. During awakening, tidal volume and respiratory rate are decreased following barbiturate induction. Barbiturates incompletely depress airway reflex responses to laryngoscopy and intubation, and airway instrumentation may lead to bronchospasm (in asthmatic patients) or laryngospasm in lightly anesthetized patients.

C. Cerebral

2 Barbiturates constrict the cerebral vasculature, causing a decrease in cerebral blood flow, cerebral blood volume, and intracranial pressure. Intracranial pressure decreases to a greater extent than arterial blood pressure, so cerebral perfusion pressure (CPP) usually increases. (CPP

equals cerebral artery pressure minus the greater of jugular venous pressure or intracranial pressure.) Barbiturates induce a greater decline in cerebral oxygen consumption (up to 50% of normal) than in cerebral blood flow; therefore the decline in cerebral blood flow is not detrimental. Barbiturate-induced reductions in oxygen requirements and cerebral metabolic activity are mirrored by changes in the electroencephalogram (EEG), which progress from low-voltage fast activity with small doses to high-voltage slow activity, burst suppression, and electrical silence with larger doses. Barbiturates may protect the brain from transient episodes of focal ischemia (eg, cerebral embolism) but probably do not protect from global ischemia (eg, cardiac arrest). Abundant animal data document these effects but the clinical data are sparse and inconsistent. Furthermore, thiopental doses required to maintain EEG suppression (most often burst suppression or flat line) are associated with prolonged awakening, delayed extubation, and the need for inotropic support.

The degree of central nervous system depression induced by barbiturates ranges from mild sedation to unconsciousness, depending on the dose administered (Table 9–1). Some patients relate a taste sensation of garlic, onions, or pizza during induction with thiopental. Barbiturates do not impair the perception of pain. In fact, they sometimes appear to lower the pain threshold. Small doses occasionally cause a state of excitement and disorientation that can be disconcerting when sedation is the objective. Barbiturates do not produce

TABLE 9–1 Uses and dosages of common barbiturates.

Agent	Use	Route[1]	Concentration (%)	Dose (mg/kg)
Thiopental, thiamylal	Induction	IV	2.5	3–6
Methohexital	Induction	IV	1	1–2
	Sedation	IV	1	0.2–0.4
	Induction	Rectal (children)	10	25
Secobarbital, pentobarbital	Premedication	Oral	5	2–4[2]
		IM		2–4[2]
		Rectal suppository		3

[1]IV, intravenous; IM, intramuscular.
[2]Maximum dose is 150 mg.

muscle relaxation, and some induce involuntary skeletal muscle contractions (eg, methohexital). Relatively small doses of thiopental (50–100 mg intravenously) rapidly (but temporarily) control most grand mal seizures. Unfortunately, acute tolerance and physiological dependence on the sedative effect of barbiturates develop quickly.

D. Renal
Barbiturates reduce renal blood flow and glomerular filtration rate in proportion to the fall in blood pressure.

E. Hepatic
Hepatic blood flow is decreased. Chronic exposure to barbiturates has opposing effects on drug biotransformation. Induction of hepatic enzymes increases the rate of metabolism of some drugs, whereas binding of barbiturates to the cytochrome P-450 enzyme system interferes with the biotransformation of other drugs (eg, tricyclic antidepressants). Barbiturates promote aminolevulinic acid synthetase, which stimulates the formation of **porphyrin** (an intermediary in heme synthesis). This may precipitate acute intermittent porphyria or variegate porphyria in susceptible individuals.

F. Immunological
Anaphylactic or anaphylactoid allergic reactions are rare. Sulfur-containing thiobarbiturates evoke mast cell histamine release in vitro, whereas oxybarbiturates do not. For this reason, some anesthesiologists prefer induction agents other than thiopental or thiamylal in asthmatic or atopic patients, but the evidence for this choice is sparse. There is no question that airway instrumentation with light anesthesia is troublesome in patients with reactive airways.

Drug Interactions
Contrast media, sulfonamides, and other drugs that occupy the same protein-binding sites as thiopental may displace the barbiturate, increasing the amount of free drug available and potentiating the organ system effects of a given dose.

Ethanol, opioids, antihistamines, and other central nervous system depressants potentiate the sedative effects of barbiturates. The common clinical impression that chronic alcohol abuse is associated with increased thiopental requirements during induction lacks scientific proof.

BENZODIAZEPINES
Mechanisms of Action
Benzodiazepines bind the same set of receptors in the central nervous system as barbiturates but bind to a different site on the receptors. Benzodiazepine binding to the $GABA_A$ receptor increases the frequency of openings of the associated chloride ion channel. For example, benzodiazepine-receptor binding facilitates binding of GABA to its receptor. **Flumazenil** (an imidazobenzodiazepine) is a specific benzodiazepine–receptor antagonist that effectively reverses most of the central nervous system effects of benzodiazepines (see Chapter 17).

Structure–Activity Relationships
The chemical structure of benzodiazepines includes a benzene ring and a seven-member diazepine ring (Figure 9–3). Substitutions at various positions on these rings affect potency and biotransformation. The imidazole ring of midazolam contributes to its water solubility at low pH. Diazepam and lorazepam are insoluble in water so parenteral preparations contain propylene glycol, which can produce venous irritation.

Pharmacokinetics
A. Absorption
Benzodiazepines are commonly administered orally, intramuscularly, and intravenously to provide sedation or, less commonly, to induce general anesthesia (Table 9–2). Diazepam and lorazepam are well absorbed from the gastrointestinal tract, with peak plasma levels usually achieved in 1 and 2 h, respectively. Oral midazolam has not been approved by the U.S. Food and Drug Administration, nevertheless this route of administration has been popular for pediatric premedication. Likewise, intranasal (0.2–0.3 mg/kg), buccal (0.07 mg/kg), and sublingual (0.1 mg/kg) midazolam provide effective preoperative sedation.

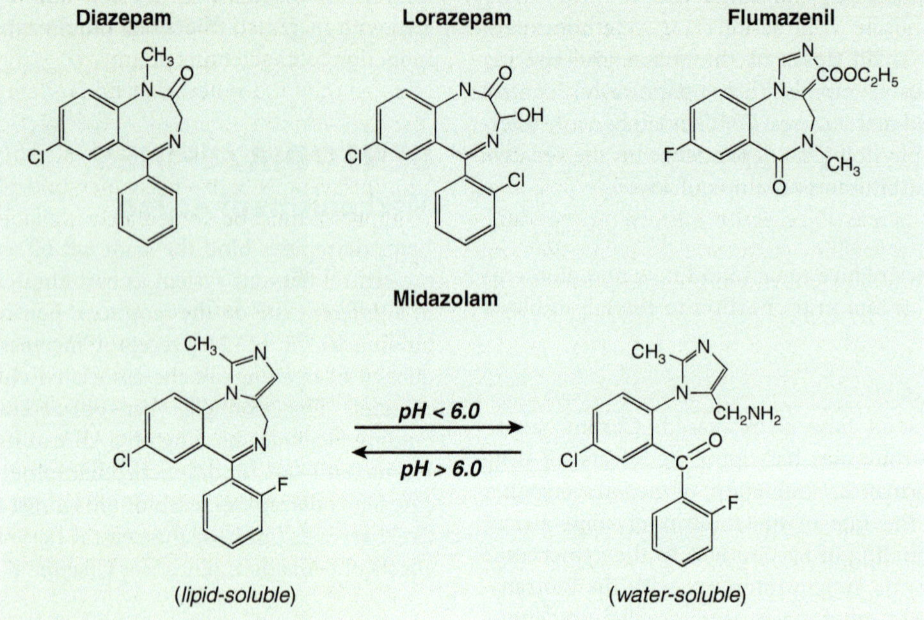

Diazepam

Lorazepam

Flumazenil

Midazolam

pH < 6.0
pH > 6.0

(*lipid-soluble*)

(*water-soluble*)

FIGURE 9–3 The structures of commonly used benzodiazepines and their antagonist, flumazenil, share a seven-member diazepine ring. (Modified and reproduced, with permission, from White PF: Pharmacologic and clinical aspects of preoperative medication. Anesth Analg 1986;65:963. With permission from the International Anesthesia Research Society.)

Intramuscular injections of diazepam are painful and unreliably absorbed. In contrast, midazolam and lorazepam are well absorbed after intramuscular injection, with peak levels achieved in 30 and 90 min, respectively. Induction of general anesthesia with midazolam is convenient only with intravenous administration.

TABLE 9–2 Uses and doses of commonly used benzodiazepines.

Agent	Use	Route[1]	Dose (mg/kg)
Diazepam	Premedication	Oral	0.2–0.5[2]
	Sedation	IV	0.04–0.2
Midazolam	Premedication	IM	0.07–0.15
	Sedation	IV	0.01–0.1
	Induction	IV	0.1–0.4
Lorazepam	Premedication	Oral	0.05

[1]IV, intravenous; IM, intramuscular.
[2]Maximum dose is 15 mg.

B. Distribution

Diazepam is relatively lipid soluble and readily penetrates the blood–brain barrier. Although midazolam is water soluble at reduced pH, its imidazole ring closes at physiological pH, increasing its lipid solubility (see Figure 9–3). The moderate lipid solubility of lorazepam accounts for its slower brain uptake and onset of action. Redistribution is fairly rapid for the benzodiazepines (the initial distribution half-life is 3–10 min) and, like the barbiturates, is responsible for awakening. Although midazolam has been used as an induction agent, neither midazolam nor any other of the benzodiazepines can match the rapid onset and short duration of action of propofol or even thiopental. All three benzodiazepines are highly protein bound (90–98%).

C. Biotransformation

The benzodiazepines rely on the liver for biotransformation into water-soluble glucuronidated end products. The phase I metabolites of diazepam are pharmacologically active.

Slow hepatic extraction and a large volume of distribution (V_d) result in a long elimination half-life for diazepam (30 h). Although lorazepam also has a low hepatic extraction ratio, its lower lipid solubility limits its V_d, resulting in a shorter elimination half-life (15 h). Nonetheless, the clinical duration of lorazepam is often quite prolonged due to increased receptor affinity. These differences between lorazepam and diazepam illustrate the low utility of individual pharmacokinetic half-lives in guiding clinical practice. Midazolam shares diazepam's V_d, but its elimination half-life (2 h) is the shortest of the group because of its increased hepatic extraction ratio.

D. Excretion

The metabolites of benzodiazepine biotransformation are excreted chiefly in the urine. Enterohepatic circulation produces a secondary peak in diazepam plasma concentration 6–12 h following administration. Kidney failure may lead to prolonged sedation in patients receiving larger doses of midazolam due to the accumulation of a conjugated metabolite (α-hydroxymidazolam).

Effects on Organ Systems

A. Cardiovascular

The benzodiazepines display minimal cardiovascular depressant effects even at general anesthetic doses, except when they are coadministered with opioids (these agents interact to produce myocardial depression and arterial hypotension). Benzodiazepines given alone decrease arterial blood pressure, cardiac output, and peripheral vascular resistance slightly, and sometimes increase heart rate. Intravenous midazolam tends to reduce blood pressure and peripheral vascular resistance more than diazepam. Changes in heart rate variability during midazolam sedation suggest decreased vagal tone (ie, drug-induced vagolysis).

B. Respiratory

Benzodiazepines depress the ventilatory response to CO_2. This depression is usually insignificant unless the drugs are administered intravenously or in association with other respiratory depressants. Although apnea may be relatively uncommon after benzodiazepine induction, even small intravenous doses of diazepam and midazolam have resulted in respiratory arrest. The steep dose–response curve, slightly prolonged onset (compared with propofol or thiopental), and potency of midazolam necessitate careful titration to avoid overdosage and apnea. Ventilation must be monitored in all patients receiving intravenous benzodiazepines, and resuscitation equipment must be immediately available.

C. Cerebral

Benzodiazepines reduce cerebral oxygen consumption, cerebral blood flow, and intracranial pressure but not to the extent the barbiturates do. They are effective in preventing and controlling grand mal seizures. Oral sedative doses often produce antegrade amnesia, a useful premedication property. The mild muscle-relaxing property of these drugs is mediated at the spinal cord level, not at the neuromuscular junction. The antianxiety, amnestic, and sedative effects seen at lower doses progress to stupor and unconsciousness at induction doses. Compared with propofol or thiopental, induction with benzodiazepines is associated with a slower rate of loss of consciousness and a longer recovery. Benzodiazepines have no direct analgesic properties.

Drug Interactions

Cimetidine binds to cytochrome P-450 and reduces the metabolism of diazepam. Erythromycin inhibits metabolism of midazolam and causes a two- to threefold prolongation and intensification of its effects. Heparin displaces diazepam from protein-binding sites and increases the free drug concentration.

As previously mentioned, the combination of opioids and benzodiazepines markedly reduces arterial blood pressure and peripheral vascular resistance. This synergistic interaction has often been observed in patients with ischemic or valvular heart disease who often receive benzodiazepines for premedication and during induction of anesthesia with opioids.

Benzodiazepines reduce the minimum alveolar concentration of volatile anesthetics as much as 30%.

Ethanol, barbiturates, and other central nervous system depressants potentiate the sedative effects of the benzodiazepines.

KETAMINE

Mechanisms of Action

Ketamine has multiple effects throughout the central nervous system, inhibiting polysynaptic reflexes in the spinal cord as well as excitatory neurotransmitter effects in selected areas of the brain. In contrast to the depression of the reticular activating system induced by the barbiturates, ketamine functionally "dissociates" the thalamus (which relays sensory impulses from the reticular activating system to the cerebral cortex) from the limbic cortex (which is involved with the awareness of sensation). Clinically, this state of dissociative anesthesia may cause the patient to appear conscious (eg, eye opening, swallowing, muscle contracture) but unable to process or respond to sensory input. Ketamine has been demonstrated to be an N-methyl-D-aspartate (NMDA) receptor (a subtype of the glutamate receptor) antagonist.

Structure–Activity Relationships

Ketamine (**Figure 9–4**) is a structural analogue of phencyclidine (an anesthetic that has been used in veterinary medicine, and a drug of abuse). It is one-tenth as potent, yet retains many of phencyclidine's psychotomimetic effects. Ketamine is used for intravenous induction of anesthesia, particularly in settings where its tendency to produce sympathetic stimulation are useful (hypovolemia, trauma). When intravenous access is lacking, ketamine is useful for intramuscular induction of general anesthesia in children and uncooperative adults. Ketamine can be combined with other agents (eg, propofol or midazolam) in small bolus doses or infusions for deep conscious sedation during nerve blocks, endoscopy, etc. Even subanesthetic doses of ketamine may cause hallucinogenic effects but usually do not do so in clinical practice, where many patients will have received at least a small dose of midazolam (or a related agent) for amnesia and sedation. The increased anesthetic potency and decreased psychotomimetic side effects of one isomer (S[+] versus R[−]) are the result of stereospecific receptors. The single S(+) stereoisomer preparation is not available in the United States (but widely available throughout the world), and it has considerably greater affinity than the racemic mixture for the NMDA receptor as well as several-fold greater potency as a general anesthetic.

Pharmacokinetics

A. Absorption

Ketamine has been administered orally, nasally, rectally, subcutaneously, and epidurally, but in usual clinical practice it is given intravenously or intramuscularly (**Table 9–3**). Peak plasma levels are usually achieved within 10–15 min after intramuscular injection.

B. Distribution

Ketamine is more lipid soluble and less protein bound than thiopental. These characteristics, along with ketamine-induced increase in cerebral blood flow and cardiac output, lead to rapid brain uptake and subsequent redistribution (the distribution half-life is 10–15 min). Awakening is due to redistribution from brain to peripheral compartments.

C. Biotransformation

Ketamine is biotransformed in the liver to several metabolites, one of which (norketamine) retains

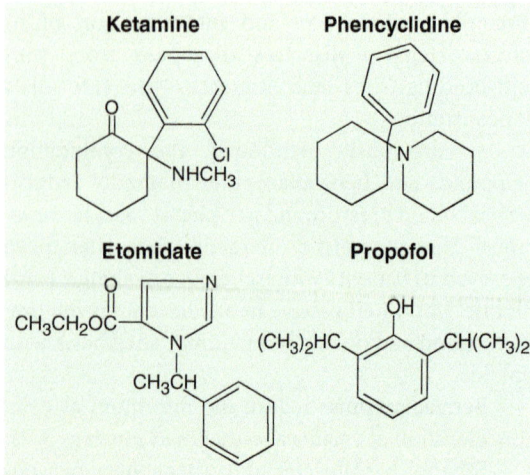

FIGURE 9–4 The structures of ketamine, etomidate, and propofol. Note the similarities between ketamine and phencyclidine.

TABLE 9–3 Uses and doses of ketamine, etomidate, and propofol.

Agent	Use	Route[1]	Dose
Ketamine	Induction	IV	1–2 mg/kg
		IM	3–5 mg/kg
	Sedation[2]	IV	2.5–15 mcg/kg/min
Etomidate	Induction	IV	0.2–0.5 mg/kg
Propofol	Induction	IV	1–2.5 mg/kg
	Maintenance infusion	IV	50–200 mcg/kg/min
	Sedation infusion	IV	25–100 mcg/kg/min

[1]IV, intravenous; IM, intramuscular.

[2]Almost always in combination with propofol.

anesthetic activity. Induction of hepatic enzymes only partially explains the tolerance that patients who receive multiple doses of ketamine will develop. Extensive hepatic uptake (hepatic extraction ratio of 0.9) explains ketamine's relatively short elimination half-life (2 h).

D. Excretion

End products of ketamine biotransformation are excreted renally.

Effects on Organ Systems

A. Cardiovascular

In contrast to other anesthetic agents, ketamine increases arterial blood pressure, heart rate, and cardiac output (Table 9–4), particularly after rapid bolus injections. These indirect cardiovascular effects are due to central stimulation of the sympathetic nervous system and inhibition of the reuptake of norepinephrine after release at nerve terminals. Accompanying these changes are increases in pulmonary artery pressure and myocardial work. For these reasons, large bolus injections of ketamine should be administered cautiously in patients with coronary artery disease, uncontrolled hypertension, congestive heart failure, or arterial aneurysms. The **direct myocardial depressant** effects of large doses of ketamine, probably due to inhibition of calcium transients, are unmasked by sympathetic blockade (eg, spinal cord transection) or exhaustion of catecholamine stores (eg, severe end-stage shock). On the other hand, ketamine's **indirect stimulatory effects** may be beneficial to patients with acute shock.

B. Respiratory

Ventilatory drive is minimally affected by induction doses of ketamine, although rapid intravenous bolus

TABLE 9–4 Summary of nonvolatile anesthetic effects on organ systems.[1]

Agent	Cardiovascular		Respiratory		Cerebral		
	HR	MAP	Vent	B'dil	CBF	CMRO$_2$	ICP
Barbiturates							
Thiopental	↑↑	↓↓	↓↓↓	↓	↓↓↓	↓↓↓	↓↓↓
Thiamylal	↑↑	↓↓	↓↓↓	↓	↓↓↓	↓↓↓	↓↓↓
Methohexital	↑↑	↓↓	↓↓↓	0	↓↓↓	↓↓↓	↓↓↓
Benzodiazepines							
Diazepam	0/↑	↓	↓↓	0	↓↓	↓↓	↓↓
Lorazepam	0/↑	↓	↓↓	0	↓↓	↓↓	↓↓
Midazolam	↑	↓↓	↓↓	0	↓↓	↓↓	↓↓
Ketamine	↑↑	↑↑	↓	↑↑↑	↑↑[2]	↑	↑↑[2]
Etomidate	0	↓	↓	0	↓↓↓	↓↓↓	↓↓↓
Propofol	0	↓↓	↓↓↓	0	↓↓↓	↓↓↓	↓↓↓

[1]HR, heart rate; MAP, mean arterial pressure; Vent, ventilatory drive; B'dil, bronchodilation; CBF, cerebral blood flow; CMRO$_2$, cerebral oxygen consumption; ICP, intracranial pressure; 0, no effect; 0/↑, no change or mild increase; ↓, decrease (mild, moderate, marked); ↑, increase (mild, moderate, marked).

[2]Minimal change in CBF and ICP when coadministered with other agents (see text).

administration or combinations of ketamine with opioids occasionally produce apnea. Racemic ketamine is a potent bronchodilator, making it a good induction agent for asthmatic patients; however, S(+) ketamine produces minimal bronchodilation. Upper airway reflexes remain largely intact, but partial airway obstruction may occur, and patients at increased risk for aspiration pneumonia ("full stomachs") should be intubated during ketamine general anesthesia (see Case Discussion, Chapter 17). The increased salivation associated with ketamine can be attenuated by premedication with an anticholinergic agent such as glycopyrrolate

C. Cerebral

The received dogma about ketamine is that it increases cerebral oxygen consumption, cerebral blood flow, and intracranial pressure. These effects would seem to preclude its use in patients with space-occupying intracranial lesions such as occur with head trauma; however, recent publications offer convincing evidence that when combined with a benzodiazepine (or another agent acting on the same GABA receptor system) and controlled ventilation, but not with nitrous oxide, ketamine is *not* associated with increased intracranial pressure. Myoclonic activity is associated with increased subcortical electrical activity, which is not apparent on surface EEG. Undesirable psychotomimetic side effects (eg, disturbing dreams and delirium) during emergence and recovery are less common in children and in patients premedicated with benzodiazepines or those in whom ketamine is combined with propofol in a TIVA technique. Of the nonvolatile agents, ketamine comes closest to being a "complete" anesthetic as it induces analgesia, amnesia, and unconsciousness.

Drug Interactions

Ketamine interacts synergistically (more than additive) with volatile anesthetics but in an additive way with propofol, benzodiazepines, and other GABA-receptor–mediated agents. In animal experiments nondepolarizing neuromuscular blocking agents are minimally potentiated by ketamine (see Chapter 11). Diazepam and midazolam attenuate ketamine's cardiostimulatory effects and diazepam prolongs ketamine's elimination half-life.

α-Adrenergic and β-adrenergic antagonists (and other agents and techniques that diminish sympathetic stimulation) unmask the direct myocardial depressant effects of ketamine, which are normally overwhelmed by sympathetic stimulation. Concurrent infusion of ketamine and propofol, often in a fixed infusion rate ratio of 1:10, has achieved great popularity for sedation with local and regional anesthesia, particularly in office-based settings.

ETOMIDATE

Mechanisms of Action

Etomidate depresses the reticular activating system and mimics the inhibitory effects of GABA. Specifically, etomidate—particularly the R(+) isomer—appears to bind to a subunit of the $GABA_A$ receptor, increasing the receptor's affinity for GABA. Unlike barbiturates, etomidate may have disinhibitory effects on the parts of the nervous system that control extrapyramidal motor activity. This disinhibition offers a potential explanation for the 30–60% incidence of myoclonus with etomidate induction of anesthesia.

Structure–Activity Relationships

Etomidate contains a carboxylated imidazole and is structurally unrelated to other anesthetic agents (see Figure 9–4). The imidazole ring provides water solubility in acidic solutions and lipid solubility at physiological pH. Therefore etomidate is dissolved in propylene glycol for injection. This solution often causes pain on injection that can be lessened by a prior intravenous injection of lidocaine.

Pharmacokinetics

A. Absorption

Etomidate is available only for intravenous administration and is used primarily for induction of general anesthesia (see Table 9–3). It is sometimes used for brief production of deep (unconscious) sedation such as prior to placement of retrobulbar blocks.

B. Distribution

Although it is highly protein bound, etomidate is characterized by a very rapid onset of action due to its great lipid solubility and large nonionized fraction at physiological pH. Redistribution is responsible for decreasing the plasma concentration to awakening levels. Etomidate plasma kinetics are well explained by a two-compartment model.

C. Biotransformation

Hepatic microsomal enzymes and plasma esterases rapidly hydrolyze etomidate to an inactive metabolite.

D. Excretion

The end products of etomidate hydrolysis are primarily excreted in the urine.

Effects on Organ Systems

A. Cardiovascular

Etomidate has minimal effects on the cardiovascular system. A mild reduction in peripheral vascular resistance is responsible for a slight decline in arterial blood pressure. Myocardial contractility and cardiac output are usually unchanged. Etomidate does not release histamine. However, etomidate by itself, even in large doses, produces relatively light anesthesia for laryngoscopy, and marked increases in heart rate and blood pressure may be recorded when etomidate provides the only anesthetic depth for intubation.

B. Respiratory

Ventilation is affected less with etomidate than with barbiturates or benzodiazepines. Even induction doses usually do not result in apnea unless opioids have also been administered.

C. Cerebral

Etomidate decreases cerebral metabolic rate, cerebral blood flow, and intracranial pressure. Because of minimal cardiovascular effects, CPP is well maintained. Although changes on EEG resemble those associated with barbiturates, etomidate increases the amplitude of somatosensory evoked potentials. Postoperative nausea and vomiting are more common following etomidate than following propofol or barbiturate induction. Etomidate lacks analgesic properties.

D. Endocrine

5 Induction doses of etomidate transiently inhibit enzymes involved in cortisol and aldosterone synthesis. It was used in the past for sedation in the intensive care unit (ICU) before reports of its consistent ability to produce adrenocortical suppression in that circumstance appeared. Long-term infusion and **adrenocortical suppression** were associated with an increased mortality rate in critically ill (particularly septic) patients.

Drug Interactions

Fentanyl increases the plasma level and prolongs the elimination half-life of etomidate. Opioids decrease the myoclonus characteristic of an etomidate induction.

PROPOFOL
Mechanisms of Action

Propofol induction of general anesthesia may involve facilitation of inhibitory neurotransmission mediated by $GABA_A$ receptor binding. Propofol allosterically increases binding affinity of GABA for the $GABA_A$ receptor. This receptor, as previously noted, is coupled to a chloride channel, and activation of the receptor leads to hyperpolarization of the nerve membrane. Propofol (like most general anesthetics) binds multiple ion channels and receptors. Propofol actions are not reversed by the specific benzodiazepine antagonist flumazenil.

Structure–Activity Relationships

Propofol consists of a phenol ring substituted with two isopropyl groups (see Figure 9–4). Propofol is not water soluble, but a 1% aqueous solution (10 mg/mL) is available for intravenous administration as an oil-in-water emulsion containing soybean oil, glycerol, and egg lecithin. A history of egg allergy does not necessarily contraindicate the use of propofol because most egg allergies involve a reaction to egg white (egg albumin), whereas egg lecithin is extracted from egg yolk. This formulation will often cause pain during injection that can be decreased by prior injection of lidocaine or less effectively by mixing lidocaine with propofol prior to injection (2 mL of 1% lidocaine in 18 mL propofol). Propofol formulations can support the growth of bacteria, so sterile technique must be observed in preparation and handling. Propofol should be administered within 6 h of opening the ampule. Sepsis and death have been linked to contaminated propofol preparations. Current formulations of propofol contain 0.005% disodium edetate or 0.025% sodium metabisulfite to help retard the rate of growth of microorganisms; however, these additives do not render the product "antimicrobially preserved" under United States Pharmacopeia standards.

Pharmacokinetics

A. Absorption

Propofol is available only for intravenous administration for the induction of general anesthesia and for moderate to deep sedation (see Table 9–3).

B. Distribution

Propofol has a rapid onset of action. Awakening from a single bolus dose is also rapid due to a very short initial distribution half-life (2–8 min). Most investigators believe that recovery from propofol is more rapid and is accompanied by less "hangover" than recovery from methohexital, thiopental, ketamine, or etomidate. This makes it a good agent for outpatient anesthesia. A smaller induction dose is recommended in elderly patients because of their smaller V_d. Age is also a key factor determining required propofol infusion rates for TIVA. In countries other than the United States, a device called the Diprifusor is often used to provide target (concentration) controlled infusion of propofol. The user must enter the patient's age and weight and the desired target concentration. The device uses these data, a microcomputer, and standard pharmacokinetic parameters to continuously adjust the infusion rate.

C. Biotransformation

The clearance of propofol exceeds hepatic blood flow, implying the existence of extrahepatic metabolism. This exceptionally high clearance rate probably contributes to relatively rapid recovery after continuous infusions. Conjugation in the liver results in inactive metabolites that are eliminated by renal clearance. The pharmacokinetics of propofol do not appear to be affected by obesity, cirrhosis, or kidney failure. Use of propofol infusion for long-term sedation of children who are critically ill or young adult

neurosurgical patients has been associated with sporadic cases of lipemia, metabolic acidosis, and death, the so-termed *propofol infusion syndrome*.

D. Excretion

Although metabolites of propofol are primarily excreted in the urine, chronic kidney failure does not affect clearance of the parent drug.

Effects on Organ Systems

A. Cardiovascular

The major cardiovascular effect of propofol is a decrease in arterial blood pressure due to a drop in systemic vascular resistance (inhibition of sympathetic vasoconstrictor activity), preload, and cardiac contractility. Hypotension following induction is usually reversed by the stimulation accompanying laryngoscopy and intubation. Factors associated with propofol-induced hypotension include large doses, rapid injection, and old age. Propofol markedly impairs the normal arterial baroreflex response to hypotension. Rarely, a marked drop in preload may lead to a vagally mediated reflex bradycardia. Changes in heart rate and cardiac output are usually transient and insignificant in healthy patients but may be severe in patients at the extremes of age, those receiving β-adrenergic blockers, or those with impaired ventricular function. Although myocardial oxygen consumption and coronary blood flow usually decrease comparably, coronary sinus lactate production increases in some patients, indicating some mismatch between myocardial oxygen supply and demand.

B. Respiratory

Propofol is a profound respiratory depressant that usually causes apnea following an induction dose. Even when used for conscious sedation in subanesthetic doses, propofol inhibits hypoxic ventilatory drive and depresses the normal response to hypercarbia. As a result, only properly educated and qualified personnel should administer propofol for sedation. Propofol-induced depression of upper airway reflexes exceeds that of thiopental, allowing intubation, endoscopy, or laryngeal mask placement in the absence of neuromuscular blockade. Although propofol can cause histamine release, induction with propofol is accompanied by a lower incidence of wheezing in asthmatic and nonasthmatic patients compared with barbiturates or etomidate.

C. Cerebral

Propofol decreases cerebral blood flow and intracranial pressure. In patients with elevated intracranial pressure, propofol can cause a critical reduction in CPP (<50 mm Hg) unless steps are taken to support mean arterial blood pressure. Propofol and thiopental probably provide a similar degree of cerebral protection during experimental focal ischemia. Unique to propofol are its antipruritic properties. Its antiemetic effects (requiring a blood propofol concentration of 200 ng/mL) provide yet another reason for it to be a preferred drug for outpatient anesthesia. Induction is occasionally accompanied by excitatory phenomena such as muscle twitching, spontaneous movement, opisthotonus, or hiccupping. Although these reactions may occasionally mimic tonic–clonic seizures, propofol has anticonvulsant properties and has been used successfully to terminate status epilepticus. Propofol may be safely administered to epileptic patients. Propofol decreases intraocular pressure. Tolerance does not develop after long-term propofol infusions. Propofol is an uncommon agent of physical dependence or addiction; however, both anesthesia personnel and medically untrained individuals have died while using propofol inappropriately to induce sleep in nonsurgical settings.

Drug Interactions

Fentanyl and alfentanil concentrations may be increased with concomitant administration of propofol. Many clinicians administer a small amount of midazolam (eg, 30 mcg/kg) prior to induction with propofol; midazolam can reduce the required propofol dose by more than 10%.

FOSPROPOFOL

Fospropofol is a water-soluble prodrug that is metabolized in vivo to propofol, phosphate, and formaldehyde. It has been released in the United States and other countries based on studies showing that it produces more complete amnesia and better conscious sedation for endoscopy than midazolam plus fentanyl. It has a slower onset and azolam plus fentanyl. It has a slower onset and slower recovery than propofol, offering little reason for anesthesiologists to use fospropofol in place of propofol. The place (if any) of fospropofol relative to other competing agents has not yet been established in clinical practice.

CASE DISCUSSION

Premedication of the Surgical Patient

An extremely anxious 17-year-old woman presents for dilation and curettage. She demands to be asleep before going to the operating room and does not want to remember anything.

What are the goals of administering preoperative medication?

Anxiety is a normal response to impending surgery. Diminishing anxiety is usually the major goal of preoperative medication. For many patients, the preoperative interview with the anesthesiologist allays fears more effectively than sedative drugs. Preoperative medication may also provide relief of preoperative pain or perioperative amnesia.

There may also be specific medical indications for preoperative medication: prophylaxis against postoperative nausea and vomiting (5-HT$_3$s) and against aspiration pneumonia (eg, antacids), prevention of allergic reactions (eg, antihistamines), or decreasing upper airway secretions (eg, anticholinergics). The goals of preoperative medication depend on many factors, including the health and emotional status of the patient, the proposed surgical procedure, and the anesthetic plan. For this reason, the choice of anesthetic premedication must be individualized and must follow a thorough preoperative evaluation.

Do all patients require preoperative medication?

No—customary levels of preoperative anxiety do not harm most patients. Some patients dread intramuscular injections, and others find altered states of consciousness more unpleasant than nervousness. If the surgical procedure is brief, the effects of some sedatives may extend into the postoperative period and prolong recovery time. This is particularly troublesome for patients undergoing ambulatory surgery. Specific contraindications for sedative premedication include severe lung disease, hypovolemia, impending airway obstruction, increased intracranial pressure, and depressed baseline mental status. Premedication with sedative drugs should never be given before informed consent has been obtained.

Which patients are most likely to benefit from preoperative medication?

Some patients are quite anxious despite the preoperative interview. Separation of young children from their parents is often a traumatic ordeal, particularly if they have endured multiple prior surgeries. Medical conditions such as coronary artery disease or hypertension may be aggravated by psychological stress.

How does preoperative medication influence the induction of general anesthesia?

Some medications often given preoperatively (eg, opioids) decrease anesthetic requirements and can smooth induction. However, intravenous administration of these medications just prior to induction is a more reliable method of achieving the same benefits.

What governs the choice among the preoperative medications commonly administered?

After the goals of premedication have been determined, the clinical effects of the agents dictate choice. For instance, in a patient experiencing preoperative pain from a femoral fracture, the analgesic effects of an opioid (eg, fentanyl, morphine, hydromorphone) will decrease the discomfort associated with transportation to the operating room and positioning on the operating room table. On the other hand, respiratory depression, orthostatic hypotension, and nausea and vomiting may result from opioid premedication.

Benzodiazepines relieve anxiety, often provide amnesia, and are relatively free of side effects; however, they are not analgesics. Diazepam and

lorazepam are available orally. Intramuscular midazolam has a rapid onset (30 min) and short duration (90 min), but intravenous midazolam has an even better pharmacokinetic profile.

Which factors must be considered in selecting the anesthetic premedication for this patient?

First, it must be made clear to the patient that in most centers, lack of necessary equipment and concern for patient safety preclude anesthesia being induced in the preoperative holding room. Long-acting agents such as morphine or lorazepam are poor choices for an outpatient procedure. Diazepam can also affect mental function for several hours. One alternative is to establish an intravenous line in the preoperative holding area and titrate small doses of midazolam using slurred speech as an end point. At that time, the patient can be taken to the operating room. Vital signs—particularly respiratory rate—must be continuously monitored.

SUGGESTED READING

Domino EF: Taming the ketamine tiger. Anesthesiology 2010;113:678.

Garnock-Jones KP, Scott LJ: Fospropofol. Drugs 2010;70:469.

Jensen LS, Merry AF, Webster CS, et al: Evidence-based strategies for preventing drug administration errors during anaesthesia. Anaesthesia 2004;59:493.

Leslie K, Clavisi O, Hargrove J: Target-controlled infusion versus manually-controlled infusion of propofol for general anaesthesia or sedation in adults. Cochrane Database Syst Rev 2008;(3):CD006059.

Raeder J: Ketamine, revival of a versatile intravenous anaesthetic. Adv Exp Med Biol 2003;523:269.

Short TG, Young R: Toxicity of intravenous anaesthetics. Best Pract Res Clin Anaesthesiol 2003;17:77.

Vanlersberghe C, Camu F: Etomidate and other non-barbiturates. Handb Exp Pharmacol 2008;(182):267.

Vanlersberghe C, Camu F: Propofol. Handb Exp Pharmacol 2008;(182):227.

Analgesic Agents

1. The accumulation of morphine metabolites (morphine 3-glucuronide and morphine 6-glucuronide) in patients with kidney failure has been associated with narcosis and ventilatory depression lasting several days.

2. Rapid administration of larger doses of opioids (particularly fentanyl, sufentanil, remifentanil, and alfentanil) can induce chest wall rigidity severe enough to prevent adequate bag-and-mask ventilation.

3. Prolonged dosing of opioids can produce "opioid-induced hyperalgesia," in which patients become more sensitive to painful stimuli. Infusion of large doses of (in particular) remifentanil during general anesthesia can produce acute tolerance, in which much larger than usual doses

of opioids are required for postoperative analgesia.

4. The neuroendocrine stress response to surgical stimulation is measured in terms of the secretion of specific hormones, including catecholamines, antidiuretic hormone, and cortisol. Large doses of opioids block the release of these hormones in response to surgery more completely than volatile anesthetics.

5. Aspirin is unique in that it irreversibly inhibits COX-1 by acetylating a serine residue in the enzyme. The irreversible nature of its inhibition underlies the nearly 1-week duration of its clinical effects (eg, return of platelet aggregation to normal) after drug discontinuation.

Regardless of how expertly surgical and anesthetic procedures are performed, appropriate prescription of analgesic drugs, especially opioids and cyclooxygenase (COX) inhibitors, can make the difference between a satisfied and an unsatisfied postoperative patient. Studies have shown that outcomes can be improved when analgesia is provided in a "multimodal" format (typically emphasizing COX inhibitors and local anesthetic techniques while minimizing opioid use) as one part of a well-defined and well-organized plan for postoperative care (see Chapter 48).

OPIOIDS

Mechanisms of Action

Opioids bind to specific receptors located throughout the central nervous system and other tissues. Four major opioid receptor types have been identified (Table 10–1): mu (μ, with subtypes μ_1 and μ_2), kappa (κ), delta (δ), and sigma (σ). All opioid receptors couple to G proteins; binding of an agonist to an opioid receptor causes membrane hyperpolarization. Acute opioid effects are mediated by inhibition of adenylyl cyclase (reductions in intracellular cyclic

TABLE 10–1   Classification of opioid receptors.[1]

Receptor	Clinical Effect	Agonists
μ	Supraspinal analgesia (μ_1) Respiratory depression (μ_2) Physical dependence Muscle rigidity	Morphine Met-enkephalin[2] β-Endorphin[2] Fentanyl
κ	Sedation Spinal analgesia	Morphine Nalbuphine Butorphanol Dynorphin[2] Oxycodone
δ	Analgesia Behavioral Epileptogenic	Leu-enkephalin[2] β-Endorphin[2]
σ	Dysphoria Hallucinations Respiratory stimulation	Pentazocine Nalorphine Ketamine

[1]Note: The relationships among receptor, clinical effect, and agonist are more complex than indicated in this table. For example, pentazocine is an antagonist at μ receptors, a partial agonist at κ receptors, and an agonist at σ receptors.

[2]Endogenous opioid.

adenosine monophosphate concentrations) and activation of phospholipase C. Opioids inhibit voltage-gated calcium channels and activate inwardly rectifying potassium channels. Opioid effects vary based on the duration of exposure, and opioid tolerance leads to changes in opioid responses.

Although opioids provide some degree of sedation and (in many species) can produce general anesthesia when given in large doses, they are principally used to provide analgesia. The properties of specific opioids depend on which receptor is bound (and in the case of spinal and epidural administration of opioids, the location in the neuraxis where the receptor is located) and the binding affinity of the drug. Agonist–antagonists (eg, nalbuphine, nalorphine, butorphanol, and pentazocine) have less efficacy than so-called full agonists (eg, fentanyl) and under some circumstances will antagonize the actions of full agonists. The pure opioid antagonists are discussed in Chapter 17.

The opioid drugs mimic endogenous compounds. Endorphins, enkephalins, and dynorphins are endogenous peptides that bind to opioid receptors. These three families of opioid peptides differ in their amino acid sequences, anatomic distributions, and receptor affinities.

Opioid receptor activation inhibits the presynaptic release and postsynaptic response to excitatory neurotransmitters (eg, acetylcholine, substance P) from nociceptive neurons. The cellular mechanism for this action was described at the beginning of this chapter. Transmission of pain impulses can be *selectively* modified at the level of the dorsal horn of the spinal cord with intrathecal or epidural administration of opioids. Opioid receptors also respond to systemically administered opioids. Modulation through a descending inhibitory pathway from the periaqueductal gray matter to the dorsal horn of the spinal cord may also play a role in opioid analgesia. Although opioids exert their greatest effect within the central nervous system, opiate receptors have also been identified on somatic and sympathetic peripheral nerves. Certain opioid side effects (eg, depression of gastrointestinal motility) are the result of opioid binding to receptors in peripheral tissues (eg, the wall of the gastrointestinal tract), and there are now selective antagonists for opioid actions outside the central nervous system (alvimopan and oral naltrexone). The distribution of opioid receptors on axons of primary sensory nerves and the clinical importance of these receptors (if present) remains speculative, despite the persisting practice of compounding of opioids in local anesthetic solutions applied to peripheral nerves.

Structure–Activity Relationships

Opioid receptor binding is a property shared by a chemically diverse group of compounds. Nonetheless, there are common structural characteristics, which are shown in Figure 10–1. As is true for most classes of drugs, small molecular changes can convert an agonist into an antagonist. The levorotatory isomers are generally more potent than the dextrorotatory opioid isomers.

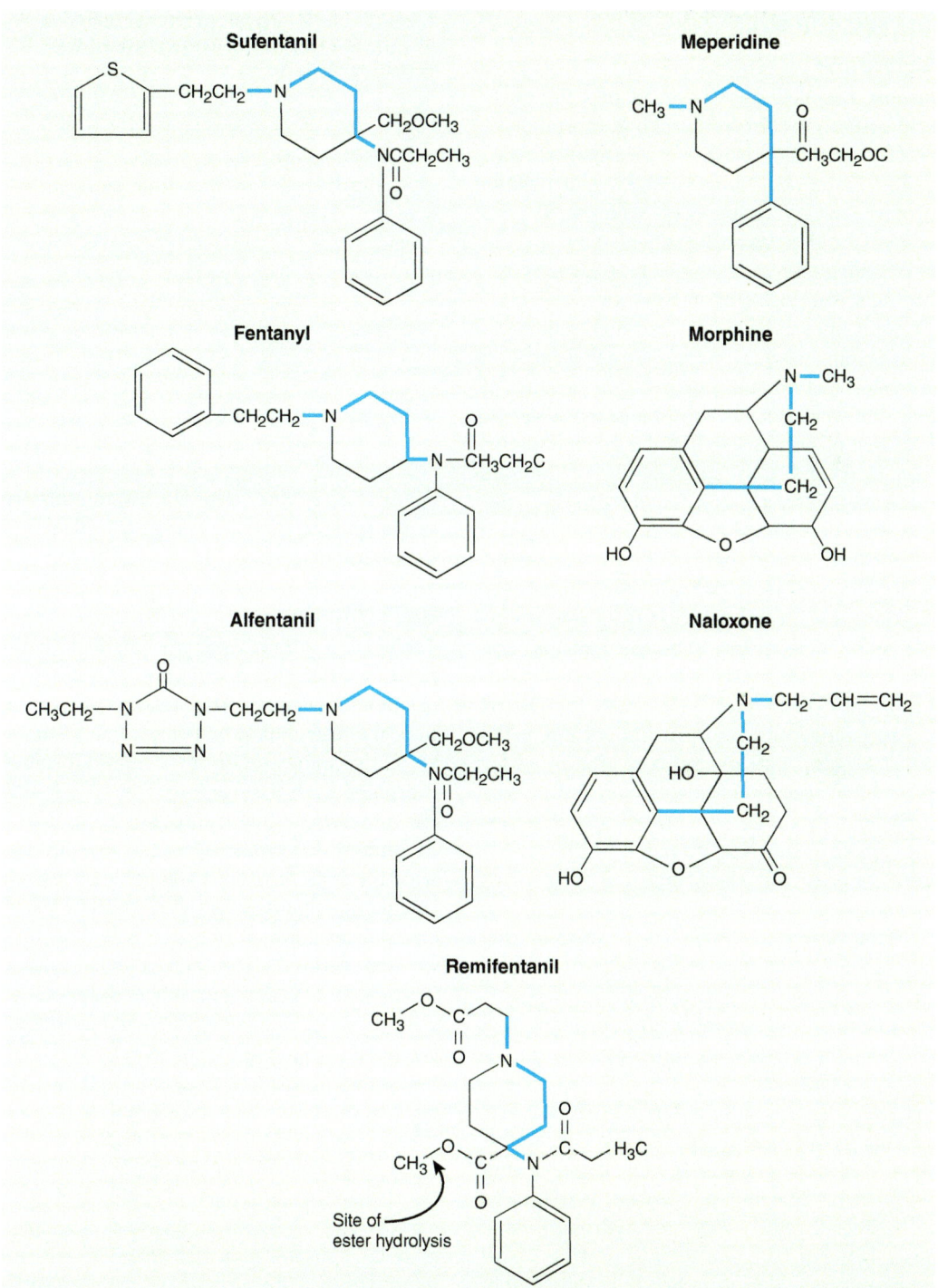

FIGURE 10–1 Opioid agonists and antagonists share part of their chemical structure, which is outlined in cyan.

Pharmacokinetics

A. Absorption

Rapid and complete absorption follows the intramuscular injection of hydromorphone, morphine, or meperidine, with peak plasma levels usually reached after 20–60 min. Oral transmucosal fentanyl citrate absorption (fentanyl "lollipop") provides rapid onset of analgesia and sedation in patients who are not good candidates for conventional oral, intravenous, or intramuscular dosing of opioids.

The low molecular weight and high lipid solubility of fentanyl also favor transdermal absorption (the transdermal fentanyl "patch"). The amount of fentanyl absorbed per unit of time depends on the surface area of skin covered by the patch and also on local skin conditions (eg, blood flow). The time required to establish a reservoir of drug in the upper dermis delays by several hours the achievement of effective blood concentrations. Serum concentrations of fentanyl reach a plateau within 14–24 h of application (with peak levels occurring after a longer delay in elderly than in younger patients) and remain constant for up to 72 h. Continued absorption from the dermal reservoir accounts for persisting measurable serum levels many hours after patch removal. Fentanyl patches are most often used for outpatient management of chronic pain and are particularly appropriate for patients who require continuous opioid dosing but cannot take the much less expensive, but equally efficacious, oral agents such as methadone.

A wide variety of opioids are effective by oral administration, including oxycodone, hydrocodone (most often in combination with acetaminophen), codeine, tramadol, morphine, hydromorphone, and methadone. These agents are much used for outpatient pain management.

Fentanyl is often administered in small doses (10–25 mcg) with local anesthetics for spinal anesthesia, and adds to the analgesia when included with local anesthetics in epidural infusions. Morphine in doses between 0.1 and 0.5 mg and hydromorphone in doses between 0.05 and 0.2 mg provide 12–18 hours of analgesia after intrathecal administration. Morphine and hydromorphone are commonly included in local anesthetic solutions infused for postoperative epidural analgesia. Extended-release

TABLE 10–2 **Physical characteristics of opioids that determine distribution.[1]**

Agent	Nonionized Fraction	Protein Binding	Lipid Solubility
Morphine	++	++	+
Meperidine	+	+++	++
Fentanyl	+	+++	++++
Sufentanil	++	++++	++++
Alfentanil	++++	++++	+++
Remifentanil	+++	+++	++

[1]+, very low; ++, low; +++, high; ++++, very high.

epidural morphine (DepoDur) is administered as a single epidural dose (5–15 mg), the effects of which persist for 48 h.

B. Distribution

Table 10–2 summarizes the physical characteristics that determine distribution and tissue binding of opioid analgesics. After intravenous administration, the distribution half-lives of all of the opioids are fairly rapid (5–20 min). The low fat solubility of morphine slows passage across the blood–brain barrier, however, so that its onset of action is slow and its duration of action is prolonged. This contrasts with the increased lipid solubility of fentanyl and sufentanil, which are associated with a faster onset and shorter duration of action **when administered in small doses**. Interestingly, alfentanil has a more rapid onset of action and shorter duration of action than fentanyl following a bolus injection, even though it is less lipid soluble than fentanyl. The high nonionized fraction of alfentanil at physiological pH and its small volume of distribution (V_d) increase the amount of drug (as a percentage of the administered dose) available for binding in the brain.

Significant amounts of lipid-soluble opioids can be retained by the lungs (first-pass uptake); as systemic concentrations fall they will return to the bloodstream. The amount of pulmonary uptake is reduced by prior accumulation of other drugs, increased by a history of tobacco use, and decreased by concurrent inhalation anesthetic administration.

Unbinding of opioid receptors and redistribution (of drug from effect sites) terminate the clinical effects of all opioids. After smaller doses of the lipid-soluble drugs (eg, fentanyl or sufentanil), redistribution alone is the driver for reducing blood concentrations, whereas after larger doses biotransformation becomes an important driver in reducing plasma levels below those that have clinical effects. Thus, the time required for fentanyl or sufentanil concentrations to decrease by half is *context sensitive;* in other words, the half-time depends on the total dose of drug and duration of exposure (see Chapter 7).

C. Biotransformation

With the exception of remifentanil, all opioids depend primarily on the liver for biotransformation and are metabolized by the cytochrome P (CYP) system, conjugated in the liver, or both. Because of the high hepatic extraction ratio of opioids, their clearance depends on liver blood flow. The small V_d of alfentanil contributes to a short elimination half-life (1.5 h). Morphine and hydromorphone undergo conjugation with glucuronic acid to form, in the former case, morphine 3-glucuronide and morphine 6-glucuronide, and in the latter case, hydromorphone 3-glucuronide. Meperidine is N-demethylated to normeperidine, an active metabolite associated with seizure activity, particularly after very large meperidine doses. The end products of fentanyl, sufentanil, and alfentanil are inactive. Norfentanyl, the metabolite of fentanyl, can be measured in urine long after the native compound is no longer detectable in blood to determine chronic fentanyl ingestion. This has its greatest importance in diagnosing fentanyl abuse.

Codeine is a prodrug that becomes active after it is metabolized by CYP to morphine. Tramadol similarly must be metabolized by CYP to O-desmethyltramadol to be active. Oxycodone is metabolized by CYP to series of active compounds that are less potent than the parent one.

The ester structure of remifentanil makes it susceptible to hydrolysis (in a manner similar to esmolol) by nonspecific esterases in red blood cells and tissue (see Figure 10–1), yielding a terminal elimination half-life of less than 10 min. Remifentanil biotransformation is rapid and the duration of a

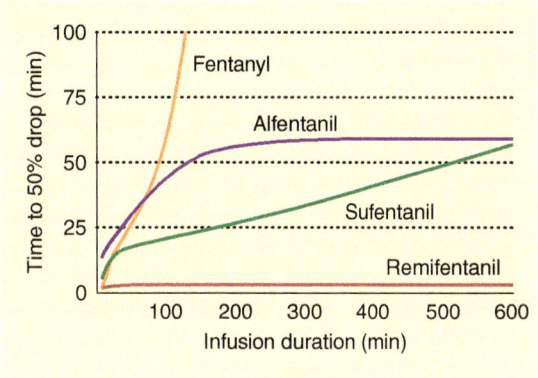

FIGURE 10–2 In contrast to other opioids, the time necessary to achieve a 50% decrease in the plasma concentration of remifentanil (its **context-sensitive half-time**) is very short and is not influenced by the duration of the infusion. (Reproduced, with permission, from Egan TD: The pharmacokinetics of the new short-acting opioid remifentanil [GI87084B] in healthy adult male volunteers. Anesthesiology 1993;79:881.)

remifentanil infusion has little effect on wake-up time (**Figure 10–2**). The context-sensitive half-time of remifentanil remains approximately 3 min regardless of the dose or duration of infusion. In its lack of accumulation remifentanil differs from other currently available opioids. Hepatic dysfunction requires no adjustment in remifentanil dosing. Finally, patients with pseudocholinesterase deficiency have a normal response to remifentanil (as also appears true for esmolol).

D. Excretion

The end products of morphine and meperidine biotransformation are eliminated by the kidneys, with less than 10% undergoing biliary excretion. Because 5–10% of morphine is excreted unchanged in the urine, kidney failure prolongs morphine duration of action. The accumulation of morphine metabolites (morphine 3-glucuronide and morphine 6-glucuronide) in patients with kidney failure has been associated with prolonged narcosis and ventilatory depression. In fact, morphine 6-glucuronide is a more potent and longer-lasting opioid agonist than morphine. As previously noted, normeperidine at increased concentrations may produce seizures; these are not reversed by naloxone. Renal dysfunction increases the likelihood of toxic effects from normeperidine accumulation. However, both morphine and meperidine have been used safely and successfully in patients with kidney failure. Metabolites of sufentanil are excreted in urine and bile. The main metabolite of remifentanil is eliminated in urine, is several thousand times less potent than its parent compound, and thus is unlikely to produce any clinical opioid effects.

Effects on Organ Systems

A. Cardiovascular

In general, opioids have few direct effects on the heart. Meperidine tends to increase heart rate (it is structurally similar to atropine and was originally synthesized as an atropine replacement), whereas larger doses of morphine, fentanyl, sufentanil, remifentanil, and alfentanil are associated with a vagus nerve-mediated bradycardia. With the exception of meperidine (and only then at very large doses), the opioids do not depress cardiac contractility provided they are administered alone (which is almost never the circumstance in surgical anesthetic settings). Nonetheless, arterial blood pressure often falls as a result of bradycardia, venodilation, and decreased sympathetic reflexes, sometimes requiring vasopressor support. These effects are more pronounced when opioids are administered in combination with benzodiazepines, in which case drugs such as sufentanil and fentanyl can be associated with reduced cardiac output. Bolus doses of meperidine, hydromorphone, and morphine evoke histamine release in some individuals that can lead to profound drops in systemic vascular resistance and arterial blood pressure. The potential hazards of histamine release can be minimized in susceptible patients by infusing opioids slowly or by pretreatment with H_1 and H_2 antagonists, or both. The end effects of histamine release can be reversed by infusion of intravenous fluid and vasopressors.

Intraoperative hypertension during large-dose opioid anesthesia or nitrous oxide–opioid anesthesia is common. Such hypertension is often attributed to inadequate anesthetic depth, thus it is conventionally treated by the addition of other anesthetic agents (benzodiazepines, propofol, or potent inhaled agents). If depth of anesthesia is adequate and hypertension persists, vasodilators or other antihypertensives may be used. The inherent cardiac

stability provided by opioids is greatly diminished in actual practice when other anesthetic drugs, including nitrous oxide, benzodiazepines, propofol, or volatile agents, are typically added. The end result of polypharmacy can include myocardial depression.

B. Respiratory

Opioids depress ventilation, particularly respiratory rate. Thus, monitoring of respiratory rate provides a convenient, simple way of detecting early respiratory depression in patients receiving opioid analgesia. Opioids increase the partial pressure of carbon dioxide ($Paco_2$) and blunt the response to a CO_2 challenge, resulting in a shift of the CO_2 response curve downward and to the right (Figure 10–3). These effects result from opioid binding to neurons in the respiratory centers of the brainstem. **The apneic threshold—the greatest $Paco_2$ at which a patient remains apneic—rises, and hypoxic drive is decreased**. Morphine and meperidine can cause histamine-induced bronchospasm in susceptible **❷ patients. Rapid administration of larger doses of opioids (particularly fentanyl, sufentanil, remifentanil, and alfentanil) can induce chest wall rigidity severe enough to prevent adequate bag-and-mask ventilation**. This centrally

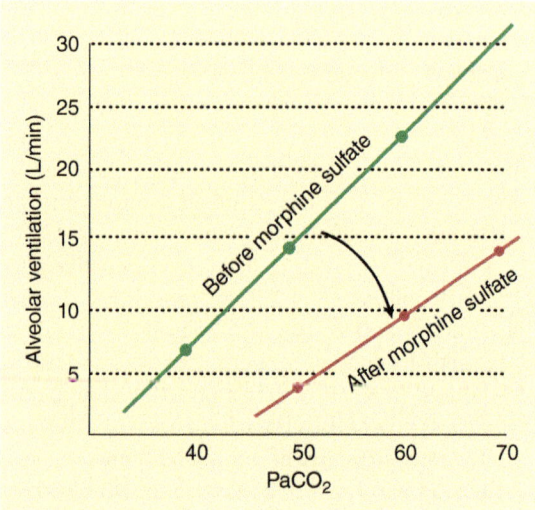

FIGURE 10–3 Opioids depress ventilation. This is graphically displayed by a shift of the CO_2 curve downward and to the right.

mediated muscle contraction is effectively treated with neuromuscular blocking agents. This problem is rarely seen now that large-dose opioid anesthesia is less often used in cardiovascular anesthesia practice. Opioids can effectively blunt the bronchoconstrictive response to airway stimulation such as occurs during tracheal intubation.

C. Cerebral

The effects of opioids on cerebral perfusion and intracranial pressure must be separated from any effects of opioids on $Paco_2$. In general, opioids reduce cerebral oxygen consumption, cerebral blood flow, cerebral blood volume, and intracranial pressure, but to a much lesser extent than barbiturates, propofol, or benzodiazepines. These effects will occur during maintenance of normocarbia by artificial ventilation; however, there are some reports of mild—but transient and almost certainly unimportant—increases in cerebral artery blood flow velocity and intracranial pressure following opioid boluses in patients with brain tumors or head trauma. If combined with hypotension, the resulting fall in cerebral perfusion pressure *could* be deleterious to patients with abnormal intracranial pressure–volume relationships. Nevertheless, the important clinical message is that any trivial opioid-induced increase in intracranial pressure would likely be much less important than the much more likely large increases in intracranial pressure associated with intubation that might be observed in an inadequately anesthetized patient (from whom opioids were withheld). Opioids usually have almost no effects on the electroencephalogram (EEG), although large doses are associated with slow δ-wave activity. There are curious sporadic case reports that large doses of fentanyl may rarely cause seizure activity; however, some of these apparent seizures have been retrospectively diagnosed as severe opioid-induced muscle rigidity. EEG activation and seizures have been associated with the meperidine metabolite normeperidine, as previously noted.

Stimulation of the medullary chemoreceptor trigger zone is responsible for opioid-induced nausea and vomiting. Curiously, nausea and vomiting are more common following smaller (analgesic) than very large (anesthetic) doses of opioids. Prolonged oral dosing of opioids or infusion of large doses of remifentanil during general anesthesia can produce the phenomenon of opioid-induced tolerance. Repeated dosing of opioids will reliably produce tolerance, a phenomenon in which larger doses are required to produce the same response. This is not the same as physical dependence or addiction, which may also be associated with repeated opioid administration.

3 Prolonged dosing of opioids can also produce "opioid-induced hyperalgesia," in which patients become more sensitive to painful stimuli. Infusion of large doses of (in particular) remifentanil during general anesthesia can produce acute tolerance, in which much larger than usual doses of opioids will be required for postoperative analgesia. Relatively large doses of opioids are required to render patients unconscious (Table 10–3). Regardless of the dose, however, opioids will not reliably produce amnesia. Parenteral opioids have been the mainstay of pain control for more than a century. The relatively recent use of opioids in epidural and intrathecal spaces has revolutionized acute and chronic pain management (see Chapters 47 and 48).

Unique among the commonly used opioids, meperidine has minor local anesthetic qualities, particularly when administered into the subarachnoid space. Meperidine's clinical use as a local anesthetic has been limited by its relatively low potency and propensity to cause typical opioid side effects (nausea, sedation, and pruritus) at the doses required to induce local anesthesia. **Intravenous meperidine (10–25 mg) is more effective than morphine or fentanyl for decreasing shivering in the postanesthetic care unit and meperidine appears to be the best agent for this indication.**

D. Gastrointestinal

Opioids slow gastrointestinal motility by binding to opioid receptors in the gut and reducing peristalsis. Biliary colic may result from opioid-induced contraction of the sphincter of Oddi. Biliary spasm, which can mimic a common bile duct stone on cholangiography, is reversed with the opioid antagonist naloxone or glucagon. Patients receiving long-term opioid therapy (eg, for cancer pain) usually become tolerant to many of the side effects but rarely to constipation. This is the basis for

TABLE 10–3 **Uses and doses of common opioids.**

Agent	Use	Route[1]	Dose[2]
Morphine	Postoperative analgesia	IM IV	0.05–0.2 mg/kg 0.03–0.15 mg/kg
Hydromorphone	Postoperative analgesia	IM IV	0.02–0.04 mg/kg 0.01–0.02 mg/kg
Fentanyl	Intraoperative anesthesia Postoperative analgesia	IV IV	2–50 mcg/kg 0.5–1.5 mcg/kg
Sufentanil	Intraoperative anesthesia	IV	0.25–20 mcg/kg
Alfentanil	Intraoperative anesthesia Loading dose Maintenance infusion	IV IV	8–100 mcg/kg 0.5–3 mcg/kg/min
Remifentanil	Intraoperative anesthesia Loading dose Maintenance infusion Postoperative analgesia/sedation	IV IV IV	1.0 mcg/kg 0.5–20 mcg/kg/min 0.05–0.3 mcg/kg/min

[1]IM, intramuscular; IV, intravenous.

[2]Note: The wide range of opioid doses reflects a large therapeutic index and depends upon which other anesthetics are simultaneously administered. For obese patients, dose should be based on ideal body weight or lean body mass, not total body weight. Tolerance can develop rapidly (ie, within 2 h) during IV infusion of opioids, necessitating higher infusion rates. Dose correlates with other variables besides body weight that need to be considered (eg, age). The relative potencies of fentanyl, sufentanil, and alfentanil are estimated to be 1:9:1/7.

the recent development of the peripheral opioid antagonists methylnaltrexone and alvimopan, and for their salutary effects in promoting motility in patients with opioid bowel syndrome, those receiving chronic opioid treatment of cancer pain, and those receiving intravenous opioids after abdominal surgery.

E. Endocrine

4 The neuroendocrine stress response to surgical stimulation is measured in terms of the secretion of specific hormones, including catecholamines, antidiuretic hormone, and cortisol. Large doses of opioids (typically fentanyl or sufentanil) block the release of these hormones in response to surgery more completely than volatile anesthetics. Although much discussed, the actual clinical outcome benefit produced by attenuating the stress response, even in high-risk cardiac patients, remains speculative (and possibly nonexistent).

Drug Interactions

The combination of meperidine and monoamine oxidase inhibitors should be avoided as it may result in hypertension, hypotension, hyperpyrexia, coma, or respiratory arrest. The cause of this catastrophic interaction is incompletely understood. (The results of failure to appreciate this drug interaction in the celebrated Libby Zion case led to changes in work rules for house officers in the United States.)

Propofol, barbiturates, benzodiazepines, and other central nervous system depressants can have synergistic cardiovascular, respiratory, and sedative effects with opioids.

The biotransformation of alfentanil may be impaired following treatment with erythromycin, leading to prolonged sedation and respiratory depression.

CYCLOOXYGENASE INHIBITORS

Mechanisms of Action

Many over-the-counter nonsteroidal antiinflammatory agents (NSAIDs) work through inhibition of cyclooxygenase (COX), the key step in prostaglandin synthesis. COX catalyzes the production of prostaglandin H_1 from arachidonic acid. The two forms of the enzyme, COX-1 and COX-2, have differing distribution in tissue. COX-1 receptors are widely distributed throughout the body, including the gut and platelets. COX-2 is produced in response to inflammation.

COX-1 and COX-2 enzymes differ further in the size of their binding sites: the COX-2 site can accommodate larger molecules that are restricted from binding at the COX-1 site. This distinction is in part responsible for selective COX-2 inhibition. Agents that inhibit COX nonselectively (eg, aspirin) will control fever, inflammation, pain, and thrombosis. COX-2 selective agents (eg, acetaminophen [paracetamol], celecoxib, etoricoxib) can be used perioperatively without concerns about platelet inhibition or gastrointestinal upset. Curiously, while COX-1 inhibition decreases thrombosis, selective COX-2 inhibition increases the risk of heart attack, thrombosis, and stroke.

Aspirin, the first of the so-called NSAIDs, formerly was used as an antipyretic and analgesic. Now it is used almost exclusively for prevention of thrombosis in susceptible individuals or for treatment of acute myocardial infarction. Aspirin is unique in that it irreversibly inhibits COX-1 by acetylating a serine residue in the enzyme. The irreversible nature of its inhibition underlies the nearly 1-week duration of its clinical effects (eg, return of platelet aggregation to normal) after drug discontinuation.

The first relatively selective COX-2 agent to be developed was acetaminophen (paracetamol). Curiously, this agent, while effective for analgesia, produces almost no effects on inflammation relative to other COX-2 selective agents. With few exceptions, the COX inhibitors are oral agents. Acetaminophen and ketorolac are available in an intravenous form for perioperative use.

Multimodal analgesia typically includes the use of COX inhibitors, regional or local anesthesia techniques, and other approaches aimed at reducing the requirement for opioids in postoperative patients. The hope is that reduced exposure to opioids will hasten and improve recovery from surgical procedures.

Structure–Activity Relationships

The COX enzyme is inhibited by an unusually diverse group of compounds that can be grouped into salicylic acids (eg, aspirin), acetic acid derivatives (eg, ketorolac), propionic acid derivatives (eg, ibuprofen), heterocyclics (eg, celecoxib), and others. Thus a conventional discussion of structure to potency (and other factors) is not useful for these chemicals, other than to note that the heterocyclics tend to be the compounds with the greatest selectivity for the COX-2 rather than COX-1 form of the enzyme.

Pharmacokinetics

A. Absorption

All COX inhibitors (save for ketorolac) are well absorbed after oral administration and all will typically achieve their peak blood concentrations in less than 3 hours. Some COX inhibitors are formulated for topical application (eg, as a gel to be applied over joints or as liquid drops to be instilled on the eye).

B. Distribution

After absorption, COX inhibitors are highly bound by plasma proteins, chiefly albumin. Their lipid solubility allows them to readily permeate the blood–brain barrier to produce a central analgesia and antipyresis, and to penetrate joint spaces to produce (with the exception of acetaminophen) an antiinflammatory effect.

C. Biotransformation

Most COX inhibitors undergo hepatic biotransformation. The agent with the most notable metabolite is acetaminophen which at toxic, increased doses yields sufficiently large concentrations of N-acetyl-p-benzoquinone imine to produce hepatic failure.

D. Excretion

Nearly all COX inhibitors are excreted in urine after biotransformation.

Effects on Organ Systems

A. Cardiovascular

COX inhibitors do not act directly on the cardiovascular system. Any cardiovascular effects result from the actions of these agents on coagulation. Prostaglandins maintain the patency of the ductus arteriosus, thus prostaglandin inhibitors have been administered to neonates to promote closure of a persistently patent ductus arteriosus.

B. Respiratory

At appropriate clinical doses, none of the COX inhibitors have effects on respiration or lung function. Aspirin overdosage has complex effects on acid–base balance and respiration.

C. Gastrointestinal

The classical complication of COX-1 inhibition is gastrointestinal upset. In its most extreme form this can cause upper gastrointestinal bleeding. Both complications result from direct actions of the drug, in the former case, on protective effects of prostaglandins in the mucosa, and in the latter case, on the combination of mucosal effects and inhibition of platelet aggregation.

Acetaminophen abuse or overdosage is a common cause of fulminant hepatic failure resulting in need for hepatic transplantation in western societies.

SUGGESTED READING

Brunton LL, Chabner BA, Knollmann BC (Eds): *Goodman & Gilman's The Pharmacological Basis of Therapeutics*, 12th ed. McGraw-Hill, 2010: Chaps 18, 34.

Chu LF, Angst MS, Clark D: Opioid-induced hyperalgesia in humans: Molecular mechanisms and clinical considerations. Clin J Pain 2008;24:479.

Jahr JS, Lee VK: Intravenous acetaminophen. Anesthesiol Clin 2010;28:619.

Myles PS, Power I: Clinical update: Postoperative analgesia. Lancet 2007;369:810.

Parvizi J, Miller AG, Gandhi K: Multimodal pain management after total joint arthroplasty. J Bone Joint Surg Am 2011;93:1075.

Neuromuscular Blocking Agents

1. It is important to realize that muscle relaxation does not ensure unconsciousness, amnesia, or analgesia.

2. Depolarizing muscle relaxants act as acetylcholine (ACh) receptor agonists, whereas nondepolarizing muscle relaxants function as competitive antagonists.

3. Because depolarizing muscle relaxants are not metabolized by acetylcholinesterase, they diffuse away from the neuromuscular junction and are hydrolyzed in the plasma and liver by another enzyme, pseudocholinesterase (nonspecific cholinesterase, plasma cholinesterase, or butyrylcholinesterase).

4. With the exception of mivacurium, nondepolarizing agents are not significantly metabolized by either acetylcholinesterase or pseudocholinesterase. Reversal of their blockade depends on redistribution, gradual metabolism, and excretion of the relaxant by the body, or administration of specific reversal agents (eg, cholinesterase inhibitors) that inhibit acetylcholinesterase enzyme activity.

5. Muscle relaxants owe their paralytic properties to mimicry of ACh. For example, succinylcholine consists of two joined ACh molecules.

6. Compared with patients with low enzyme levels or heterozygous atypical enzyme in whom blockade duration is doubled or tripled, patients with homozygous atypical enzyme will have a very long blockade (eg, 4–8 h) following succinylcholine administration.

7. Succinylcholine is considered contraindicated in the routine management of children and adolescents because of the risk of hyperkalemia, rhabdomyolysis, and cardiac arrest in children with undiagnosed myopathies.

8. Normal muscle releases enough potassium during succinylcholine-induced depolarization to raise serum potassium by 0.5 mEq/L. Although this is usually insignificant in patients with normal baseline potassium levels, a life-threatening potassium elevation is possible in patients with burn injury, massive trauma, neurological disorders, and several other conditions.

9. Doxacurium, pancuronium, vecuronium, and pipecuronium are partially excreted by the kidneys, and their action is prolonged in patients with renal failure.

10. Cirrhotic liver disease and chronic renal failure often result in an increased volume of distribution and a lower plasma concentration for a given dose of water-soluble drugs, such as muscle relaxants. On the other hand, drugs dependent on hepatic or renal excretion may demonstrate prolonged clearance. Thus, depending on

—Continued next page

Continued—

the drug, a greater initial dose—but smaller maintenance doses—might be required in these diseases.

11 Atracurium and cisatracurium undergo degradation in plasma at physiological pH and temperature by organ-independent Hofmann elimination. The resulting metabolites (a monoquaternary acrylate and laudanosine) have no intrinsic neuromuscular blocking effects.

12 Hypertension and tachycardia may occur in patients given pancuronium. These cardiovascular effects are caused by the combination of vagal blockade and catecholamine release from adrenergic nerve endings.

13 Long-term administration of vecuronium to patients in intensive care units has resulted in prolonged neuromuscular blockade (up to several days), possibly from accumulation of its active 3-hydroxy metabolite, changing drug clearance, or the development of a polyneuropathy.

14 Rocuronium (0.9–1.2 mg/kg) has an onset of action that approaches succinylcholine (60–90 s), making it a suitable alternative for rapid-sequence inductions, but at the cost of a much longer duration of action.

Skeletal muscle relaxation can be produced by deep inhalational anesthesia, regional nerve block, or neuromuscular blocking agents (commonly called *muscle relaxants*). In 1942, Harold Griffith published the results of a study using an extract of curare (a South American arrow poison) during anesthesia. Following the introduction of succinylcholine as a "new approach to muscular relaxation," these agents rapidly became a routine part of the anesthesiologist's drug arsenal. However, as noted by Beecher and Todd in 1954: "[m]uscle relaxants given inappropriately may provide the surgeon with optimal [operating] conditions in . . . a patient [who] is paralyzed but not anesthetized—a state [that] is **1** wholly unacceptable for the patient." In other words, muscle relaxation does not ensure unconsciousness, amnesia, or analgesia. This chapter reviews the principles of neuromuscular transmission and presents the mechanisms of action, physical structures, routes of elimination, recommended dosages, and side effects of several muscle relaxants.

Neuromuscular Transmission

Association between a motor neuron and a muscle cell occurs at the neuromuscular junction (**Figure 11–1**). The cell membranes of the neuron and muscle fiber are separated by a narrow (20-nm) gap, the synaptic cleft. As a nerve's action potential depolarizes its terminal, an influx of calcium ions through voltage-gated calcium channels into the nerve cytoplasm allows storage vesicles to fuse with the terminal plasma membrane and release their contents

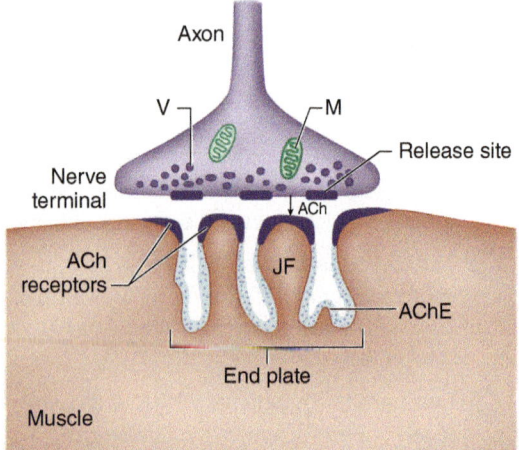

FIGURE 11–1 The neuromuscular junction. V, transmitter vesicle; M, mitochondrion; ACh, acetylcholine; AChE, acetylcholinesterase; JF, junctional folds. (Reproduced, with permission, from Drachman DB: Myasthenia gravis. N Engl J Med 1978;298:135.)

(acetylcholine [ACh]). The ACh molecules diffuse across the synaptic cleft to bind with nicotinic cholinergic receptors on a specialized portion of the muscle membrane, the motor end-plate. Each neuromuscular junction contains approximately 5 million of these receptors, but activation of only about 500,000 receptors is required for normal muscle contraction.

The structure of ACh receptors varies in different tissues and at different times in development. Each ACh receptor in the neuromuscular junction normally consists of five protein subunits; two α subunits; and single β, δ, and ε subunits. Only the two identical α subunits are capable of binding ACh molecules. If both binding sites are occupied by ACh, a conformational change in the subunits briefly (1 ms) opens an ion channel in the core of the receptor (**Figure 11–2**). The channel will not open if ACh binds on only one site. In contrast to the normal (or

mature) junctional ACh receptor, another isoform contains a γ subunit instead of the ε subunit. This isoform is referred to as the fetal or immature receptor because it is in the form initially expressed in fetal muscle. It is also often referred to as extrajunctional because, unlike the mature isoform, it may be located anywhere in the muscle membrane, inside or outside the neuromuscular junction when expressed in adults.

Cations flow through the open ACh receptor channel (sodium and calcium in; potassium out), generating an **end-plate potential**. The contents of a single vesicle, a quantum of ACh (10^4 molecules per quantum), produce a miniature end-plate potential. The number of quanta released by each nerve impulse, normally at least 200, is very sensitive to extracellular ionized calcium concentration; increasing calcium concentration increases the

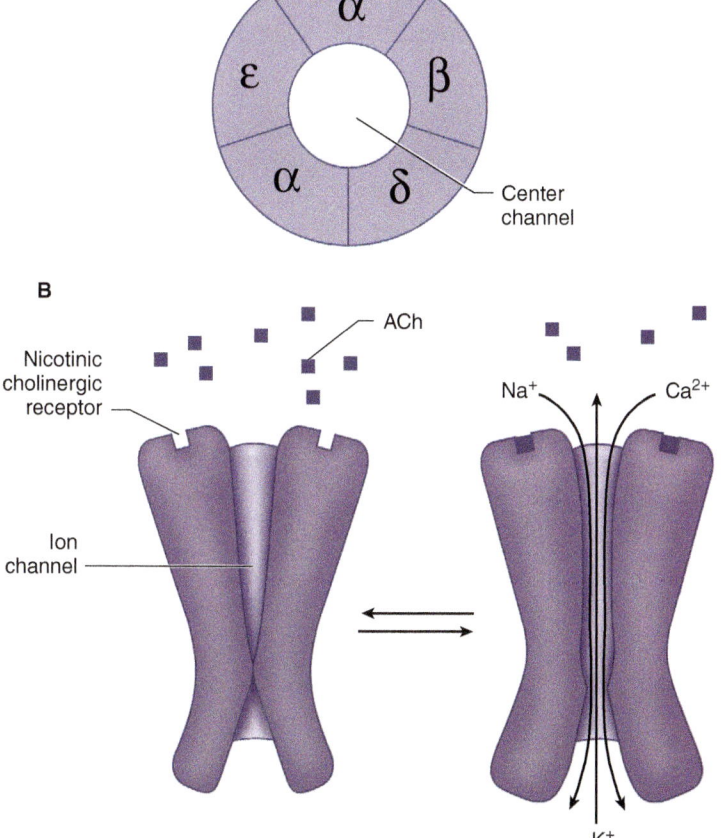

FIGURE 11–2 **A**: Structure of the ACh receptor. Note the two α subunits that actually bind ACh and the center channel. **B**: Binding of ACh to receptors on muscle end-plate causes channel opening and ion flux.

number of quanta released. When enough receptors are occupied by ACh, the end-plate potential will be sufficiently strong to depolarize the perijunctional membrane. Voltage-gated sodium channels within this portion of the muscle membrane open when a threshold voltage is developed across them, as opposed to end-plate receptors that open when ACh is applied (Figure 11–3). Perijunctional areas of muscle membrane have a higher density of these sodium channels than other parts of the membrane. The resulting action potential propagates along the muscle membrane and T-tubule system, opening sodium channels and releasing calcium from the sarcoplasmic reticulum. This intracellular calcium allows the contractile proteins actin and myosin to interact, bringing about muscle contraction. The

amount of ACh released and the number of receptors subsequently activated will normally far exceed the minimum required for the initiation of an action potential. The nearly 10-fold margin of safety is lost in Eaton–Lambert myasthenic syndrome (decreased release of ACh) and myasthenia gravis (decreased number of receptors).

ACh is rapidly hydrolyzed into acetate and choline by the substrate-specific enzyme **acetylcholinesterase**. This enzyme (also called specific cholinesterase or true cholinesterase) is embedded into the motor end-plate membrane immediately adjacent to the ACh receptors. After unbinding ACh, the receptors' ion channels close, permitting the end-plate to repolarize. Calcium is resequestered in the sarcoplasmic reticulum, and the muscle cell relaxes.

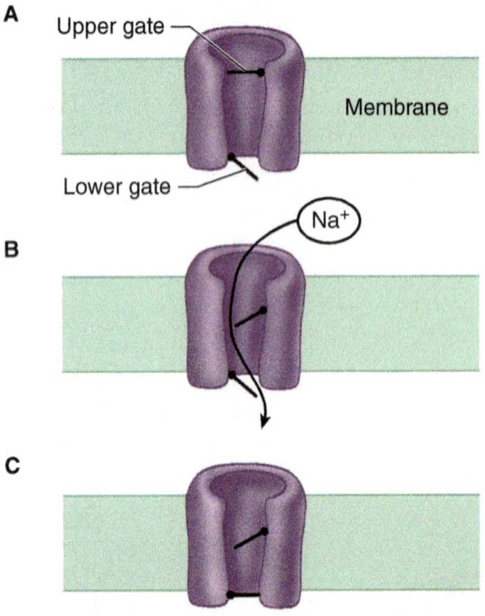

FIGURE 11–3 Schematic of the sodium channel. The sodium channel is a transmembrane protein that can be conceptualized as having two gates. Sodium ions pass only when both gates are open. Opening of the gates is time dependent and voltage dependent. The channel therefore possesses three functional states. At rest, the lower gate is open but the upper gate is closed (**A**). When the muscle membrane reaches threshold voltage depolarization, the upper gate opens and sodium can pass (**B**). Shortly after the upper gate opens the time-dependent lower gate closes (**C**). When the membrane repolarizes to its resting voltage, the upper gate closes and the lower gate opens (A).

Distinctions Between Depolarizing & Nondepolarizing Blockade

Neuromuscular blocking agents are divided into two classes: depolarizing and nondepolarizing (Table 11–1). This division reflects distinct differences in the mechanism of action, response to peripheral nerve stimulation, and reversal of block.

MECHANISM OF ACTION

Similar to ACh, all neuromuscular blocking agents are quaternary ammonium compounds whose positively charged nitrogen imparts an affinity to

TABLE 11–1 Depolarizing and nondepolarizing muscle relaxants.

Depolarizing	Nondepolarizing
Short acting	Short-acting
Succinylcholine	Gantacurium[1]
	Intermediate-acting
	Atracurium
	Cisatracurium
	Vecuronium
	Rocuronium
	Long-acting
	Pancuronium

[1]Not yet commercially available in the United States.

nicotinic ACh receptors. Whereas most agents have two quaternary ammonium atoms, a few have one quaternary ammonium cation and one tertiary amine that is protonated at physiological pH.

Depolarizing muscle relaxants very closely resemble ACh and readily bind to ACh receptors, generating a muscle action potential. Unlike ACh, however, these drugs are *not* metabolized by acetylcholinesterase, and their concentration in the synaptic cleft does not fall as rapidly, resulting in a prolonged depolarization of the muscle end-plate.

Continuous end-plate depolarization causes muscle relaxation because opening of perijunctional sodium channels is time limited (sodium channels rapidly "inactivate" with continuing depolarization) (Figure 11–3). After the initial excitation and opening (Figure 11–3B), these sodium channels inactivate (Figure 11–3C) and cannot reopen until the end-plate repolarizes. The end-plate cannot repolarize as long as the depolarizing muscle relaxant continues to bind to ACh receptors; this is called a phase I block. After a period of time, prolonged end-plate depolarization can cause poorly understood changes in the ACh receptor that result in a phase II block, which clinically resembles that of nondepolarizing muscle relaxants.

Nondepolarizing muscle relaxants bind ACh receptors but are incapable of inducing the conformational change necessary for ion channel opening. Because ACh is prevented from binding to its receptors, no end-plate potential develops. Neuromuscular blockade occurs even if only one α subunit is blocked.

2 Thus, depolarizing muscle relaxants act as ACh receptor agonists, whereas nondepolarizing muscle relaxants function as competitive antagonists. This basic difference in mechanism of action explains their varying effects in certain disease states. For example, conditions associated with a chronic decrease in ACh release (eg, muscle denervation injuries) stimulate a compensatory increase in the number of ACh receptors within muscle membranes. These states also promote the expression of the immature (extrajunctional) isoform of the ACh receptor, which displays low channel conductance properties and prolonged open-channel time. This up-regulation causes an exaggerated response to depolarizing muscle relaxants (with more receptors being depolarized), but a resistance to nondepolarizing relaxants (more receptors that must be blocked). In contrast, conditions associated with fewer ACh receptors (eg, downregulation in myasthenia gravis) demonstrate a resistance to depolarizing relaxants and an increased sensitivity to nondepolarizing relaxants.

OTHER MECHANISMS OF NEUROMUSCULAR BLOCKADE

Some drugs may interfere with the function of the ACh receptor without acting as an agonist or antagonist. They interfere with normal functioning of the ACh receptor binding site or with the opening and closing of the receptor channel. These may include inhaled anesthetic agents, local anesthetics, and ketamine. The ACh receptor–lipid membrane interface may be an important site of action.

Drugs may also cause either closed or open channel blockade. During closed channel blockade, the drug physically plugs up the channel, preventing passage of cations whether or not ACh has activated the receptor. Open channel blockade is use dependent, because the drug enters and obstructs the ACh receptor channel only after it is opened by ACh binding. The clinical relevance of open channel blockade is unknown. Based on laboratory experiments, one would expect that increasing the concentration of ACh with a cholinesterase inhibitor would not overcome this form of neuromuscular blockade. Drugs that may cause channel block in the laboratory include neostigmine, some antibiotics, cocaine, and quinidine. Other drugs may impair the presynaptic release of ACh. Prejunctional receptors play a role in mobilizing ACh to maintain muscle contraction. Blocking these receptors can lead to a fading of the train-of-four response.

REVERSAL OF NEUROMUSCULAR BLOCKADE

3 Because succinylcholine is not metabolized by acetylcholinesterase, it unbinds the receptor and diffuses away from the neuromuscular junction to be hydrolyzed in the plasma and liver by another enzyme, pseudocholinesterase (nonspecific cholinesterase, plasma cholinesterase, or butyrylcholinesterase). Fortunately, this is a fairly rapid process, because no specific agent to reverse a depolarizing blockade is available.

④ With the exception of the discontinued drug mivacurium, nondepolarizing agents are not metabolized by either acetylcholinesterase or pseudocholinesterase. Reversal of their blockade depends on unbinding the receptor, redistribution, metabolism, and excretion of the relaxant by the body, or administration of specific reversal agents (eg, cholinesterase inhibitors) that inhibit acetylcholinesterase enzyme activity. Because this inhibition increases the amount of ACh that is available at the neuromuscular junction and can compete with the nondepolarizing agent, clearly, the reversal agents are of no benefit in reversing a depolarizing block. In fact, by increasing neuromuscular junction ACh concentration and inhibiting pseudocholinesterase-induced metabolism of succinylcholine, *cholinesterase inhibitors can prolong neuromuscular blockade produced by succinylcholine.* The ONLY time neostigmine reverses neuromuscular block after succinylcholine is when there is a phase II block (fade of the train-of-four) AND sufficient time has passed for the circulating concentration of succinylcholine to be negligible.

Sugammadex, a cyclodextrin, is the first selective relaxant-binding agent; it exerts its reversal effect by forming tight complexes in a 1:1 ratio with steroidal nondepolarizing agents (vecuronium, rocuronium,). This drug has been in use in the European Union for the past few years, but is not yet commercially available in the United States.

The newer neuromuscular blocking agents, such as gantacurium, which are still under investigation, show promise as ultrashort-acting nondepolarizing agents; they undergo chemical degradation by rapid adduction with L-cysteine.

RESPONSE TO PERIPHERAL NERVE STIMULATION

The use of peripheral nerve stimulators to monitor neuromuscular function is discussed in Chapter 6. Four patterns of electrical stimulation with supramaximal square-wave pulses are considered:

Tetany: A sustained stimulus of 50–100 Hz, usually lasting 5 sec.

Single twitch: A single pulse 0.2 ms in duration.

Train-of-four: A series of four twitches in 2 s (2-Hz frequency), each 0.2 ms long.

Double-burst stimulation (DBS): Three short (0.2 ms) high-frequency stimulations separated by a 20-ms interval (50 Hz) and followed 750 ms later by two ($DBS_{3,2}$) or three ($DBS_{3,3}$) additional impulses.

The occurrence of fade, a gradual diminution of evoked response during prolonged or repeated nerve stimulation, is indicative of a nondepolarizing block (Table 11–2), or of a phase II block if only succinylcholine has been administered. Fade may be due to a prejunctional effect of nondepolarizing relaxants that reduces the amount of ACh in the nerve terminal available for release during stimulation (blockade of ACh mobilization). Adequate clinical recovery correlates well with the absence of fade. Because fade is more obvious during sustained tetanic stimulation or double-burst stimulation than following a train-of-four pattern or repeated twitches, the first two patterns are the preferred methods for determining adequacy of recovery from a nondepolarizing block.

The ability of tetanic stimulation during a partial nondepolarizing block to increase the evoked response to a subsequent twitch is termed posttetanic potentiation. This phenomenon may relate to a transient increase in ACh mobilization following tetanic stimulation.

In contrast, a phase I depolarization block from succinylcholine does not exhibit fade during tetanus or train-of-four; neither does it demonstrate posttetanic potentiation. With longer infusions of succinylcholine, however, the quality of the block will sometimes change to resemble a nondepolarizing block (phase II block).

Newer quantitative methods of assessment of neuromuscular blockade, such as acceleromyography, permit determination of exact train-of-four ratios, as opposed to subjective interpretations. Acceleromyography may reduce the incidence of

TABLE 11–2 Evoked responses during depolarizing (phase I and phase II) and nondepolarizing block.

	Depolarizing Block		
Normal Evoked Stimulus	**Phase I**	**Phase II**	**Nondepolarizing Block**
Train-of-four	Constant but diminished	Fade	Fade
Tetany	Constant but diminished	Fade	Fade
Double-burst stimulation (DBS$_{3,2}$)	Constant but diminished	Fade	Fade
Posttetanic potentiation	Absent	Present	Present

unexpected postoperative residual neuromuscular blockade.

Depolarizing Muscle Relaxants

SUCCINYLCHOLINE

The only depolarizing muscle relaxant in clinical use today is succinylcholine.

Physical Structure

5 Succinylcholine—also called diacetylcholine or suxamethonium—consists of two joined ACh molecules (Figure 11–4). This structure underlies succinylcholine's mechanism of action, side effects, and metabolism.

Metabolism & Excretion

The popularity of succinylcholine is due to its rapid onset of action (30–60 s) and short duration

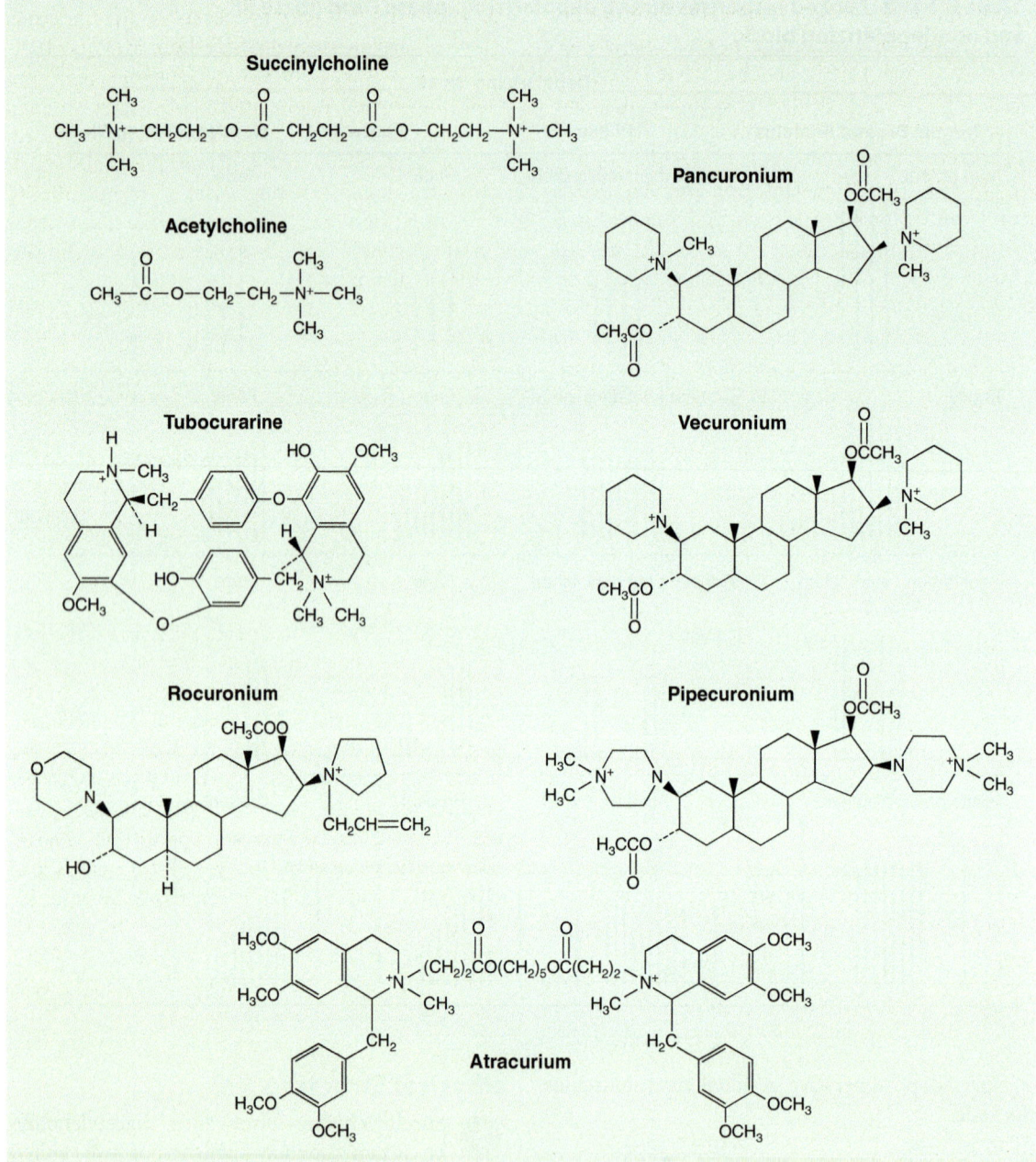

FIGURE 11–4 Chemical structures of neuromuscular blocking agents.

of action (typically less than 10 min). Its rapid onset of action relative to other neuromuscular blockers is largely due to the relative overdose that is usually administered. Succinylcholine, like all neuromuscular blockers, has a small volume of distribution due to its very low lipid solubility, and this also underlies a rapid onset of action. As succinylcholine enters the circulation, most of it is rapidly metabolized by pseudocholinesterase into succinylmonocholine. This process is so efficient that only a small fraction of the injected dose ever reaches the neuromuscular junction. As drug levels fall in blood, succinylcholine molecules diffuse away from the neuromuscular junction, limiting the duration of action. However, this duration of action can be prolonged by high doses, infusion of succinylcholine, or abnormal metabolism. The latter may result from hypothermia, reduced pseudocholinesterase levels, or a genetically aberrant enzyme. Hypothermia decreases the rate of hydrolysis. Reduced levels of pseudocholinesterase (measured as units per liter) accompany pregnancy, liver disease, renal failure, and certain drug therapies (Table 11–3). Reduced pseudocholinesterase levels generally produce only modest prolongation of succinylcholine's actions (2–20 min).

One in 25-30 patients of European extraction is a heterozygote with one normal and one abnormal (atypical) pseudocholinesterase gene, resulting in a slightly prolonged block (20–30 min). Even fewer (1 in 3000) patients have two copies of the most prevalent abnormal gene (homozygous atypical) that produce an enzyme with little or no affinity for succinylcholine. In contrast to the doubling or tripling of blockade duration seen in

6

patients with low enzyme levels or heterozygous atypical enzyme, patients with homozygous atypical enzyme will have a *very* long blockade (eg, 4–8 h) following administration of succinylcholine. Of the recognized abnormal pseudocholinesterase genes, the dibucaine-resistant (variant) allele, which produces an enzyme with 1/100 of normal affinity for succinylcholine, is the most common. Other variants include fluoride-resistant and silent (no activity) alleles.

Dibucaine, a local anesthetic, inhibits normal pseudocholinesterase activity by 80%, but inhibits atypical enzyme activity by only 20%. Serum from an individual who is heterozygous for the atypical enzyme is characterized by an intermediate 40% to 60% inhibition. The percentage of inhibition of pseudocholinesterase activity is termed the **dibucaine number**. A patient with normal pseudocholinesterase has a dibucaine number of 80; a homozygote for the most common abnormal allele will have a dibucaine number of 20. The dibucaine number measures pseudocholinesterase function, not the amount of enzyme. Therefore, adequacy of pseudocholinesterase can be determined in the laboratory quantitatively in units per liter (a minor factor) and qualitatively by dibucaine number (the major factor). **Prolonged paralysis from succinylcholine caused by abnormal pseudocholinesterase (atypical cholinesterase) should be treated with continued mechanical ventilation and sedation until muscle function returns to normal by clinical signs. Such unsedated patients do NOT appreciate unnecessary, repetitive use of nerve stimulation when all members of a department come by to confirm the diagnosis.**

TABLE 11–3 Drugs known to decrease pseudocholinesterase activity.

Drug	Description
Echothiophate	Organophosphate use for glaucoma
Neostigmine Pyridostigmine	Cholinesterase inhibitors
Phenelzine	Monoamine oxidase inhibitor
Cyclophosphamide	Antineoplastic agent
Metoclopramide	Antiemetic/prokinetic agent
Esmolol	β-Blocker
Pancuronium	Nondepolarizing muscle relaxant
Oral contraceptives	Various agents

Drug Interactions

The effects of muscle relaxants can be modified by concurrent drug therapy (Table 11–4). Succinylcholine is involved in two interactions deserving special comment.

A. Cholinesterase Inhibitors

Although cholinesterase inhibitors reverse nondepolarizing paralysis, they markedly prolong a depolarizing phase I block by two mechanisms. By inhibiting acetylcholinesterase, they lead to a

TABLE 11–4 Potentiation (+) and resistance (–) of neuromuscular blocking agents by other drugs.

Drug	Effect on Depolarizing Blockade	Effect on Nondepolarizing Blockade	Comments
Antibiotics	+	+	Streptomycin, aminoglycosides, kanamycin, neomycin, colistin, polymyxin, tetracycline, lincomycin, clindamycin
Anticonvulsants	?	–	Phenytoin, carbamazepine, primidone, sodium valproate
Antiarrhythmics	+	+	Quinidine, calcium channel blockers
Cholinesterase inhibitors	+	–	Neostigmine, pyridostigmine
Dantrolene	?	+	Used in treatment of malignant hyperthermia (has quaternary ammonium group)
Inhalational anesthetics	+	+	Volatile anesthetics
Ketamine	?	+	
Local anesthetics	+	+	High doses only
Lithium carbonate	+	?	Prolongs onset and duration of succinylcholine
Magnesium sulfate	+	+	Doses used to treat preeclampsia and eclampsia of pregnancy

higher ACh concentration at the nerve terminal, which intensifies depolarization. They also reduce the hydrolysis of succinylcholine by inhibiting pseudocholinesterase. Organophosphate pesticides, for example, cause an irreversible inhibition of acetylcholinesterase and can prolong the action of succinylcholine by 20–30 min. Echothiophate eye drops, used in the past for glaucoma, can markedly prolong succinylcholine by this mechanism.

B. Nondepolarizing Relaxants

In general, small doses of nondepolarizing relaxants antagonize a depolarizing phase I block. Because the drugs occupy some ACh receptors, depolarization by succinylcholine is partially prevented.

If enough depolarizing agent is administered to develop a phase II block, a nondepolarizer will potentiate paralysis.

Dosage

Because of the rapid onset, short duration, and low cost of succinylcholine, many clinicians believe that it is still a good choice for routine intubation in adults. The usual adult dose of succinylcholine for intubation is 1–1.5 mg/kg intravenously. Doses as small as 0.5 mg/kg will often provide acceptable intubating conditions if a defasciculating dose of a nondepolarizing agent is not used. Repeated small boluses (10 mg) or a succinylcholine drip (1 g in 500 or 1000 mL, titrated to effect) can be used during surgical procedures that require brief but intense paralysis (eg, otolaryngological endoscopies). Neuromuscular function should be frequently monitored with a nerve stimulator to prevent overdosing and to watch for phase II block. The availability of intermediate-acting nondepolarizing muscle relaxants has reduced the popularity of succinylcholine infusions. In the past, these infusions were a mainstay of ambulatory practice in the United States.

Because succinylcholine is not lipid soluble, it has a small volume of distribution. Per kilogram, infants and neonates have a larger extracellular space than adults. Therefore, dosage requirements for pediatric patients are often greater than for adults. If succinylcholine is administered *intramuscularly* to children, a dose as high as 4–5 mg/kg does not always produce complete paralysis.

Succinylcholine should be stored under refrigeration (2–8°C), and should generally be used within 14 days after removal from refrigeration and exposure to room temperature.

Side Effects & Clinical Considerations

Succinylcholine is a relatively safe drug—assuming that its many potential complications are understood and avoided. Because of the risk of hyperkalemia, rhabdomyolysis, and cardiac arrest in children with undiagnosed myopathies, succinylcholine is considered relatively contraindicated in the routine management of children and adolescent patients. Most clinicians have also abandoned the *routine* use of succinylcholine for adults. Succinylcholine is still useful for rapid sequence induction and for short periods of intense paralysis because none of the presently available nondepolarizing muscle relaxants can match its very rapid onset and short duration.

A. Cardiovascular

Because of the resemblance of muscle relaxants to ACh, it is not surprising that they affect cholinergic receptors in addition to those at the neuromuscular junction. The entire parasympathetic nervous system and parts of the sympathetic nervous system (sympathetic ganglions, adrenal medulla, and sweat glands) depend on ACh as a neurotransmitter.

Succinylcholine not only stimulates nicotinic cholinergic receptors at the neuromuscular junction, it stimulates all ACh receptors. The cardiovascular actions of succinylcholine are therefore very complex. Stimulation of nicotinic receptors in parasympathetic and sympathetic ganglia, and muscarinic receptors in the sinoatrial node of the heart, can increase or decrease blood pressure and heart rate. Low doses of succinylcholine can produce negative chronotropic and inotropic effects, but higher doses usually increase heart rate and contractility and elevate circulating catecholamine levels. In most patients, the hemodynamic consequences are

inconsequential in comparison to the effects of the induction agent and laryngoscopy.

Children are particularly susceptible to profound bradycardia following administration of succinylcholine. Bradycardia will sometimes occur in adults when a second bolus of succinylcholine is administered approximately 3–8 min after the first dose. The dogma (based on no real evidence) is that the succinylcholine metabolite, succinylmonocholine, sensitizes muscarinic cholinergic receptors in the sinoatrial node to the second dose of succinylcholine, resulting in bradycardia. Intravenous atropine (0.02 mg/kg in children, 0.4 mg in adults) is normally given prophylactically to children prior to the first and subsequent doses, and *usually* before a second dose of succinylcholine is given to adults. Other arrhythmias, such as nodal bradycardia and ventricular ectopy, have been reported.

B. Fasciculations

The onset of paralysis by succinylcholine is usually signaled by visible motor unit contractions called fasciculations. These can be prevented by pretreatment with a small dose of nondepolarizing relaxant. Because this pretreatment usually antagonizes a depolarizing block, a larger dose of succinylcholine is required (1.5 mg/kg). Fasciculations are typically not observed in young children and elderly patients.

C. Hyperkalemia

Normal muscle releases enough potassium during succinylcholine-induced depolarization to increase serum potassium by 0.5 mEq/L. Although this is usually insignificant in patients with normal baseline potassium levels, it can be life-threatening in patients with preexisting hyperkalemia. The increase in potassium in patients with burn injury, massive trauma, neurological disorders, and several other conditions (Table 11–5) can be large and catastrophic. Hyperkalemic cardiac arrest can prove to be quite refractory to routine cardiopulmonary resuscitation, requiring calcium, insulin, glucose, bicarbonate, and even cardiopulmonary bypass to support the circulation while reducing serum potassium levels.

TABLE 11–5   Conditions causing susceptibility to succinylcholine-induced hyperkalemia.

Burn injury
Massive trauma
Severe intraabdominal infection
Spinal cord injury
Encephalitis
Stroke
Guillain-Barré syndrome
Severe Parkinson's disease
Tetanus
Prolonged total body immobilization
Ruptured cerebral aneurysm
Polyneuropathy
Closed head injury
Hemorrhagic shock with metabolic acidosis
Myopathies (eg, Duchenne's dystrophy)

Following denervation injuries (spinal cord injuries, larger burns), the immature isoform of the ACh receptor may be expressed inside and outside the neuromuscular junction (up-regulation). These extrajunctional receptors allow succinylcholine to effect widespread depolarization and extensive potassium release. Life-threatening potassium release is *not* reliably prevented by pretreatment with a nondepolarizer. The risk of hyperkalemia usually seems to peak in 7–10 days following the injury, but the exact time of onset and the duration of the risk period vary. The risk of hyperkalemia from succinylcholine is minimal in the first 2 days after spinal cord or burn injury.

D. Muscle Pains

Patients who have received succinylcholine have an increased incidence of postoperative myalgia. The efficacy of nondepolarizing pretreatment is controversial. Administration of rocuronium (0.06–0.1 mg/kg) prior to succinylcholine has been reported to be effective in preventing fasciculations and reducing postoperative myalgias. The relationship between fasciculations and postoperative myalgias is also inconsistent. The myalgias are theorized to be due to the initial unsynchronized contraction of muscle groups; myoglobinemia and increases in serum creatine kinase can be detected following administration of succinylcholine. Perioperative use of nonsteroidal antiinflammatory drugs may reduce the incidence and severity of myalgias.

E. Intragastric Pressure Elevation

Abdominal wall muscle fasciculations increase intragastric pressure, which is offset by an increase in lower esophageal sphincter tone. Therefore, despite being much discussed, there is no evidence that the risk of gastric reflux or pulmonary aspiration is increased by succinylcholine.

F. Intraocular Pressure Elevation

Extraocular muscle differs from other striated muscle in that it has multiple motor end-plates on each cell. Prolonged membrane depolarization and contraction of extraocular muscles following administration of succinylcholine transiently raise intraocular pressure and theoretically could compromise an injured eye. However, there is no evidence that succinylcholine leads to worsened outcome in patients with "open" eye injuries. The elevation in intraocular pressure is not always prevented by pretreatment with a nondepolarizing agent.

G. Masseter Muscle Rigidity

Succinylcholine transiently increases muscle tone in the masseter muscles. Some difficulty may initially be encountered in opening the mouth because of incomplete relaxation of the jaw. A marked increase in tone preventing laryngoscopy is abnormal and can be a premonitory sign of malignant hyperthermia.

H. Malignant Hyperthermia

Succinylcholine is a potent triggering agent in patients susceptible to malignant hyperthermia, a hypermetabolic disorder of skeletal muscle (see Chapter 52). Although some of the signs and symptoms of neuroleptic malignant syndrome (NMS) resemble those of malignant hyperthermia, the pathogenesis is completely different and there is no need to avoid use of succinylcholine in patients with NMS.

I. Generalized Contractions

Patients afflicted with myotonia may develop myoclonus after administration of succinylcholine.

J. Prolonged Paralysis

As discussed above, patients with reduced levels of normal pseudocholinesterase may have a longer than normal duration of action, whereas patients with atypical pseudocholinesterase will experience markedly prolonged paralysis.

K. Intracranial Pressure

Succinylcholine may lead to an activation of the electroencephalogram and slight increases in cerebral blood flow and intracranial pressure in some patients. Muscle fasciculations stimulate muscle stretch receptors, which subsequently increase cerebral activity. The increase in intracranial pressure can be attenuated by maintaining good airway control and instituting hyperventilation. It can also be prevented by pretreating with a nondepolarizing muscle relaxant and administering intravenous lidocaine (1.5–2.0 mg/kg) 2–3 min prior to intubation. The effects of intubation on intracranial pressure far outweigh any increase caused by succinylcholine, and succinylcholine is NOT contraindicated for rapid sequence induction of patients with intracranial mass lesions or other causes of increased intracranial pressure.

L. Histamine Release

Slight histamine release may be observed following succinylcholine in some patients.

Nondepolarizing Muscle Relaxants

Unique Pharmacological Characteristics

In contrast to depolarizing muscle relaxants, there is a wide selection of nondepolarizing muscle relaxants (Tables 11–6 and 11–7). Based on their chemical structure, they can be classified as benzylisoquinolinium, steroidal, or other compounds. It is often said that choice of a particular drug depends on its unique characteristics, which are often related to its structure; however, for most patients, the differences among the intermediate-acting neuromuscular blockers are inconsequential. In general, steroidal compounds can be vagolytic, but this property is most notable with pancuronium and clinically unimportant with vecuronium or rocuronium. Benzylisoquinolines tend to release histamine. Because of structural similarities, an allergic history to one muscle relaxant strongly suggests the possibility of allergic reactions to other muscle relaxants, particularly those in the same chemical class.

A. Suitability for Intubation

None of the currently available nondepolarizing muscle relaxants equals succinylcholine's rapid onset of action or short duration. However, the

TABLE 11–6 A summary of the pharmacology of nondepolarizing muscle relaxants.

Relaxant	Chemical Structure[1]	Metabolism	Primary Excretion	Onset[2]	Duration[3]	Histamine Release[4]	Vagal Blockade[5]
Atracurium	B	+++	Insignificant	++	++	+	0
Cisatracurium	B	+++	Insignificant	++	++	0	0
Pancuronium	S	+	Renal	++	+++	0	++
Vecuronium	S	+	Biliary	++	++	0	0
Rocuronium	S	Insignificant	Biliary	+++	++	0	+
Gantacurium	C	+++	Insignificant	+++	+	+	0

[1]B, benzylisoquinolone; S, steroidal; C, chlorofumarate.
[2]Onset: +, slow; ++, moderately rapid; +++, rapid.
[3]Duration: +, short; ++, intermediate; +++, long.
[4]Histamine release: 0, no effect; +, slight effect; ++, moderate effect; +++, marked effect.
[5]Vagal blockade: 0, no effect; +, slight effect; ++, moderate effect.

TABLE 11–7 Clinical characteristics of nondepolarizing muscle relaxants.

Drug	ED_{95} for Adductor Pollicis During Nitrous Oxide/Oxygen/Intravenous Anesthesia (mg/kg)	Intubation Dose (mg/kg)	Onset of Action for Intubating Dose (min)	Duration of Intubating Dose (min)	Maintenance Dosing by Boluses (mg/kg)	Maintenance Dosing by Infusion (µg/kg/min)
Succinylcholine	0.5	1.0	0.5	5–10	0.15	2–15 mg/min
Gantacurium[1]	0.19	0.2	1–2	4–10	N/A	—
Rocuronium	0.3	0.8	1.5	35–75	0.15	9–12
Mivacurium[2]	0.08	0.2	2.5–3.0	15–20	0.05	4–15
Atracurium	0.2	0.5	2.5–3.0	30–45	0.1	5–12
Cisatracurium	0.05	0.2	2.0–3.0	40–75	0.02	1–2
Vecuronium	0.05	0.12	2.0–3.0	45–90	0.01	1–2
Pancuronium	0.07	0.12	2.0–3.0	60–120	0.01	—
Pipecuronium[2]	0.05	0.1	2.0–3.0	80–120	0.01	—
Doxacurium[2]	0.025	0.07	4.0–5.0	90–150	0.05	—

[1]Not commercially available in the United States.
[2]No longer available in the United States.

onset of nondepolarizing relaxants can be quickened by using either a larger dose or a priming dose. The ED_{95} of any drug is the effective dose of a drug in 95% of individuals. For neuromuscular blockers, one often specifies the dose that produces 95% twitch depression in 50% of individuals. One to two times the ED_{95} or twice the dose that produces 95% twitch depression is usually used for intubation. Although a larger intubating dose speeds onset, it exacerbates side effects and prolongs the duration of blockade. For example, a dose of 0.15 mg/kg of pancuronium may produce intubating conditions in 90 sec, but at the cost of more pronounced tachycardia—and a block that may be irreversible (by neostigmine) for more than 60 min. The consequence of a long duration of action is the ensuing difficulty in completely reversing the blockade and a subsequent increased incidence of postoperative pulmonary complications. As a general rule, the more potent the nondepolarizing muscle relaxant, the slower its speed of onset; the "explanatory dogma" is that greater potency necessitates a smaller dose, with fewer total drug molecules, which in turn, decreases the rate of drug binding opportunities at the neuromuscular junction.

The introduction of short- and intermediate-acting agents has resulted in the greater use of priming doses. Theoretically, giving 10% to 15% of the usual intubating dose 5 min before induction will occupy enough receptors so that paralysis will quickly follow when the balance of relaxant is administered. Use of a priming dose can produce conditions suitable for intubation as soon as 60 sec following administration of rocuronium or 90 sec following administration of other intermediate-acting nondepolarizers. A priming dose does not *usually* lead to clinically significant paralysis, which requires that 75% to 80% of the receptors be blocked (a neuromuscular margin of safety). In some patients, however, the priming dose produces distressing dyspnea, diplopia, or dysphagia; in such instances, the patient should be reassured, and induction of anesthesia should proceed without delay. Priming can additionally cause measureable deterioration in respiratory function (eg, decreased forced vital capacity) and may lead to oxygen desaturation in patients with marginal pulmonary reserve. These negative side effects are more common in older, sicker patients.

Muscle groups vary in their sensitivity to muscle relaxants. For example, the laryngeal muscles—whose relaxation is important during intubation—recover from blockade more quickly than the adductor pollicis, which is commonly monitored by the peripheral nerve stimulator.

B. Suitability for Preventing Fasciculations

To prevent fasciculations and myalgias, 10% to 15% of a nondepolarizer intubating dose can be administered 5 min before succinylcholine. When administered only shortly before succinylcholine, myalgias, but not fasciculations, will be inhibited. Although most nondepolarizers have been successfully used for this purpose, tubocurarine and rocuronium have been most popular (precurarization); tubocurarine is no longer available in the United States.

C. Maintenance Relaxation

Following intubation, muscle paralysis may need to be maintained to facilitate surgery, (eg, abdominal operations), to permit a reduced depth of anesthesia, or to control ventilation. There is great variability among patients in response to muscle relaxants. Monitoring neuromuscular function with a nerve stimulator helps to prevent over- and underdosing and to reduce the likelihood of serious residual muscle paralysis in the recovery room. Maintenance doses, whether by intermittent boluses or continuous infusion (Table 11–7), should be guided by the nerve stimulator *and* clinical signs (eg, spontaneous respiratory efforts or movement). In some instances, clinical signs may precede twitch recovery because of differing sensitivities to muscle relaxants between muscle groups or technical problems with the nerve stimulator. Some return of neuromuscular transmission should be evident prior to administering each maintenance dose, if the patient needs to resume spontaneous ventilation at the end of the anesthetic. When an infusion is used for maintenance, the rate should be adjusted at or just above the rate that allows some return of neuromuscular transmission so that drug effects can be monitored.

D. Potentiation by Inhalational Anesthetics

Volatile agents decrease nondepolarizer dosage requirements by at least 15%. The actual degree of this postsynaptic augmentation depends on both the inhalational anesthetic (desflurane > sevoflurane > isoflurane and enflurane > halothane > N_2O/O_2/narcotic) and the muscle relaxant employed (pancuronium > vecuronium and atracurium).

E. Potentiation by Other Nondepolarizers

Some combinations of nondepolarizers produce a greater than additive (synergistic) neuromuscular blockade. The lack of synergism (ie, the drugs are only additive) by closely related compounds (eg, vecuronium and pancuronium) lends credence to the theory that synergism results from slightly differing mechanisms of action.

F. Autonomic Side Effects

In clinical doses, the nondepolarizers differ in their relative effects on nicotinic and muscarinic cholinergic receptors. Some older agents (tubocurarine and, to a lesser extent, metocurine) blocked autonomic ganglia, reducing the ability of the sympathetic nervous system to increase heart contractility and rate in response to hypotension and other intraoperative stresses. In contrast, pancuronium (and gallamine) block vagal muscarinic receptors in the sinoatrial node, resulting in tachycardia. All newer nondepolarizing relaxants, including atracurium, cisatracurium, vecuronium, and rocuronium, are devoid of significant autonomic effects in their recommended dosage ranges.

G. Histamine Release

Histamine release from mast cells can result in bronchospasm, skin flushing, and hypotension from peripheral vasodilation. Both atracurium and mivacurium are capable of triggering histamine release, particularly at higher doses. Slow injection rates and H_1 and H_2 antihistamine pretreatment ameliorate these side effects.

H. Hepatic Clearance

Only pancuronium and vecuronium are metabolized to any significant degree by the liver. Active metabolites likely contribute to their clinical effect. Vecuronium and rocuronium depend heavily on biliary excretion. Clinically, liver failure prolongs pancuronium and rocuronium blockade, with less effect on vecuronium, and no effect on pipecuronium. Atracurium, cisatracurium, and mivacurium, although extensively metabolized, depend on extrahepatic mechanisms. Severe liver disease does not significantly affect clearance of atracurium or cisatracurium, but the associated decrease in pseudocholinesterase levels may slow the metabolism of mivacurium.

I. Renal Excretion

9 Doxacurium, pancuronium, vecuronium, and pipecuronium are partially excreted by the kidneys, and their action is prolonged in patients with renal failure. The elimination of atracurium, cisatracurium, mivacurium, and rocuronium is independent of kidney function.

General Pharmacological Characteristics

Some variables affect all nondepolarizing muscle relaxants.

A. Temperature

Hypothermia prolongs blockade by decreasing metabolism (eg, mivacurium, atracurium, and cisatracurium) and delaying excretion (eg, pancuronium and vecuronium).

B. Acid–Base Balance

Respiratory acidosis potentiates the blockade of most nondepolarizing relaxants and antagonizes its reversal. This could prevent complete neuromuscular recovery in a hypoventilating postoperative patient. Conflicting findings regarding the neuromuscular effects of other acid–base changes may be due to coexisting alterations in extracellular pH, intracellular pH, electrolyte concentrations, or structural differences between drugs (eg, monoquaternary versus bisquaternary; steroidal versus isoquinolinium).

C. Electrolyte Abnormalities

Hypokalemia and hypocalcemia augment a nondepolarizing block. The responses of patients with hypercalcemia are unpredictable. Hypermagnesemia, as may be seen in preeclamptic patients being managed with magnesium sulfate (or after intravenous magnesium administered in the operating room), potentiates a nondepolarizing blockade by competing with calcium at the motor end-plate.

TABLE 11–8 Additional considerations in special populations.

Pediatric	Succinylcholine – should not be used routinely Nondepolarizing agents – faster onset Vecuronium – long-acting in neonates
Elderly	Decreased clearance – prolonged duration, except with cisatracurium
Obese	Dosage 20% more than lean body weight; onset unchanged Prolonged duration, except with cisatracurium
Hepatic disease	Increased volume of distribution Pancuronium and vecuronium – prolonged elimination due to hepatic metabolism and biliary excretion Cisatracurium – unchanged Pseudocholinesterase decreased; prolonged action may be seen with succinylcholine in severe disease
Renal failure	Vecuronium – prolonged Rocuronium – relatively unchanged Cisatracurium – safest alternative
Critically ill	Myopathy, polyneuropathy, nicotinic acetylcholine receptor up-regulation

D. Age

Neonates have an increased sensitivity to nondepolarizing relaxants because of their immature neuromuscular junctions (Table 11-8). This sensitivity does not necessarily decrease dosage requirements, as the neonate's greater extracellular space provides a larger volume of distribution.

E. Drug Interactions

As noted earlier, many drugs augment nondepolarizing blockade (see Table 11–4). They have multiple sites of interaction: prejunctional structures, postjunctional cholinergic receptors, and muscle membranes.

F. Concurrent Disease

The presence of neurological or muscular disease can have profound effects on an individual's response **10** to muscle relaxants (Table 11–9). Cirrhotic liver disease and chronic renal failure often result in an increased volume of distribution and a lower plasma concentration for a given dose of

TABLE 11–9 Diseases with altered responses to muscle relaxants.

Disease	Response to Depolarizers	Response to Nondepolarizers
Amyotrophic lateral sclerosis	Contracture	Hypersensitivity

Autoimmune disorders
    Systemic lupus erythematosus
    Polymyositis
    Dermatomyositis
	Hypersensitivity	Hypersensitivity

Burn injury	Hyperkalemia	Resistance
Cerebral palsy	Slight hypersensitivity	Resistance
Familial periodic paralysis (hyperkalemic)	Myotonia and hyperkalemia	Hypersensitivity?
Guillain–Barré syndrome	Hyperkalemia	Hypersensitivity
Hemiplegia	Hyperkalemia	Resistance on affected side
Muscular denervation (peripheral nerve injury)	Hyperkalemia and contracture	Normal response or resistance
Muscular dystrophy (Duchenne type)	Hyperkalemia and malignant hyperthermia	Hypersensitivity
Myasthenia gravis	Resistance	Hypersensitivity
Myasthenic syndrome	Hypersensitivity	Hypersensitivity

Myotonia
    Dystrophica
    Congenital
    Paramyotonia
	Generalized muscular contractions	Normal or hypersensitivity

Severe chronic infection
    Tetanus
    Botulism
	Hyperkalemia	Resistance

water-soluble drugs, such as muscle relaxants. On the other hand, drugs dependent on hepatic or renal excretion may demonstrate prolonged clearance (Table 11-8). Thus, depending on the drug chosen, a greater initial (loading) dose—but smaller maintenance doses—might be required in these diseases.

G. Muscle Groups

The onset and intensity of blockade vary among muscle groups. This may be due to differences in blood flow, distance from the central circulation, or different fiber types. Furthermore, the relative sensitivity of a muscle group may depend on the choice of muscle relaxant. In general, the diaphragm, jaw, larynx, and facial muscles (orbicularis oculi) respond to and recover from muscle relaxation sooner than the thumb. Although they are a fortuitous safety feature,

persistent diaphragmatic contractions can be disconcerting in the face of complete adductor pollicis paralysis. Glottic musculature is also quite resistant to blockade, as is often confirmed during laryngoscopy. The ED_{95} for laryngeal muscles is nearly two times that for the adductor pollicis muscle. Good intubating conditions are usually associated with visual loss of the orbicularis oculi twitch response.

Considering the multitude of factors influencing the duration and magnitude of muscle relaxation, it becomes clear that an individual's response to neuromuscular blocking agents should be monitored. Dosage recommendations, including those in this chapter, should be considered guidelines that require modification for individual patients. Wide variability in sensitivity to nondepolarizing muscle relaxants is often encountered in clinical practice.

ATRACURIUM

Physical Structure

Like all muscle relaxants, atracurium has a quaternary group; however, a benzylisoquinoline structure is responsible for its unique method of degradation. The drug is a mixture of 10 stereoisomers.

Metabolism & Excretion

Atracurium is so extensively metabolized that its pharmacokinetics are independent of renal and hepatic function, and less than 10% is excreted unchanged by renal and biliary routes. Two separate processes are responsible for metabolism.

A. Ester Hydrolysis

This action is catalyzed by nonspecific esterases, not by acetylcholinesterase or pseudocholinesterase.

B. Hofmann Elimination

A spontaneous nonenzymatic chemical breakdown occurs at physiological pH and temperature.

Dosage

A dose of 0.5 mg/kg is administered intravenously for intubation. After succinylcholine, intraoperative relaxation is achieved with 0.25 mg/kg initially, then in incremental doses of 0.1 mg/kg every 10–20 min. An infusion of 5–10 mcg/kg/min can effectively replace intermittent boluses.

Although dosage requirements do not significantly vary with age, atracurium may be shorter acting in children and infants than in adults.

Atracurium is available as a solution of 10 mg/mL. It must be stored at 2–8°C, as it loses 5% to 10% of its potency for each month it is exposed to room temperature. At room temperature, it should be used within 14 days to preserve potency.

Side Effects & Clinical Considerations

Atracurium triggers dose-dependent histamine release that becomes significant at doses above 0.5 mg/kg.

A. Hypotension and Tachycardia

Cardiovascular side effects are unusual unless doses in excess of 0.5 mg/kg are administered. Atracurium may also cause a transient drop in systemic vascular resistance and an increase in cardiac index independent of any histamine release. A slow rate of injection minimizes these effects.

B. Bronchospasm

Atracurium should be avoided in asthmatic patients. Severe bronchospasm is occasionally seen in patients without a history of asthma.

C. Laudanosine Toxicity

Laudanosine, a tertiary amine, is a breakdown product of atracurium's Hofmann elimination and has been associated with central nervous system excitation, resulting in elevation of the minimum alveolar concentration and even precipitation of seizures. Concerns about laudanosine are probably irrelevant unless a patient has received an extremely large total dose or has hepatic failure. Laudanosine is metabolized by the liver and excreted in urine and bile.

D. Temperature and pH Sensitivity

Because of its unique metabolism, atracurium's duration of action can be markedly prolonged by hypothermia and to a lesser extent by acidosis.

E. Chemical Incompatibility

Atracurium will precipitate as a free acid if it is introduced into an intravenous line containing an alkaline solution such as thiopental.

F. Allergic Reactions

Rare anaphylactoid reactions to atracurium have been described. Proposed mechanisms include direct immunogenicity and acrylate-mediated immune activation. IgE-mediated antibody reactions directed against substituted ammonium compounds, including muscle relaxants, have been described. Reactions to acrylate, a metabolite of atracurium and a structural component of some dialysis membranes, have also been reported in patients undergoing hemodialysis.

CISATRACURIUM

Physical Structure

Cisatracurium is a stereoisomer of atracurium that is four times more potent. Atracurium contains approximately 15% cisatracurium.

Metabolism & Excretion

11 Like atracurium, cisatracurium undergoes degradation in plasma at physiological pH and temperature by organ-independent Hofmann elimination. The resulting metabolites (a monoquaternary acrylate and laudanosine) have no neuromuscular blocking effects. Because of cisatracurium's greater potency, the amount of laudanosine produced for the same extent and duration of neuromuscular blockade is much less than with atracurium. Nonspecific esterases are not involved in the metabolism of cisatracurium. Metabolism and elimination are independent of renal or liver failure. Minor variations in pharmacokinetic patterns due to age result in no clinically important changes in duration of action.

Dosage

Cisatracurium produces good intubating conditions following a dose of 0.1–0.15 mg/kg within 2 min and results in muscle blockade of intermediate duration. The typical maintenance infusion rate ranges from 1.0–2.0 mcg/kg/min. Thus, it is more potent than atracurium.

Cisatracurium should be stored under refrigeration (2–8°C) and should be used within 21 days after removal from refrigeration and exposure to room temperature.

Side Effects & Clinical Considerations

Unlike atracurium, cisatracurium does not produce a consistent, dose-dependent increase in plasma histamine levels following administration. Cisatracurium does not alter heart rate or blood pressure, nor does it produce autonomic effects, even at doses as high as eight times ED_{95}.

Cisatracurium shares with atracurium the production of laudanosine, pH and temperature sensitivity, and chemical incompatibility.

PANCURONIUM

Physical Structure

Pancuronium consists of a steroid ring on which two modified ACh molecules are positioned (a bisquaternary relaxant). The steroid ring serves as a "spacer" between the two quaternary amines. Pancuronium resembles ACh enough to bind (but not activate) the nicotinic ACh receptor.

Metabolism & Excretion

Pancuronium is metabolized (deacetylated) by the liver to a limited degree. Its metabolic products have some neuromuscular blocking activity. Excretion is primarily renal (40%), although some of the drug is cleared by the bile (10%). Not surprisingly, elimination of pancuronium is slowed and neuromuscular blockade is prolonged by renal failure. Patients with cirrhosis may require a larger initial dose due to an increased volume of distribution but have reduced maintenance requirements because of a decreased rate of plasma clearance.

Dosage

A dose of 0.08–0.12 mg/kg of pancuronium provides adequate relaxation for intubation in 2–3 min. Intraoperative relaxation is achieved by administering 0.04 mg/kg initially followed every 20–40 min by 0.01 mg/kg.

Children may require moderately larger doses of pancuronium. Pancuronium is available as a solution of 1 or 2 mg/mL and is stored at 2–8°C but may be stable for up to 6 months at normal room temperature.

Side Effects & Clinical Considerations

A. Hypertension and Tachycardia

12 These cardiovascular effects are caused by the combination of vagal blockade and sympathetic stimulation. The latter is due to a combination of ganglionic stimulation, catecholamine release from adrenergic nerve endings, and decreased catecholamine reuptake. Large bolus doses of pancuronium should be given with caution to patients in whom an increased heart rate would be particularly detrimental (eg, coronary artery disease, hypertrophic cardiomyopathy, aortic stenosis).

B. Arrhythmias

Increased atrioventricular conduction and catecholamine release increase the likelihood of ventricular arrhythmias in predisposed individuals. The combination of pancuronium, tricyclic antidepressants, and halothane has been reported to be particularly arrhythmogenic.

C. Allergic Reactions

Patients who are hypersensitive to bromides may exhibit allergic reactions to pancuronium (pancuronium bromide).

VECURONIUM

Physical Structure

Vecuronium is pancuronium minus a quaternary methyl group (a monoquaternary relaxant). This minor structural change beneficially alters side effects without affecting potency.

Metabolism & Excretion

Vecuronium is metabolized to a small extent by the liver. It depends primarily on biliary excretion and secondarily (25%) on renal excretion. Although it is a satisfactory drug for patients with renal failure, its duration of action is somewhat prolonged. Vecuronium's brief duration of action is explained by its shorter elimination half-life and more rapid clearance compared with pancuronium. Long-term administration of vecuronium to patients in intensive care units has resulted in prolonged neuromuscular blockade (up to several days), possibly from accumulation of its active 3-hydroxy metabolite, changing drug clearance, and in some patients, leading to the development of a polyneuropathy. Risk factors seem to include female gender, renal failure, long-term or high-dose corticosteroid therapy, and sepsis. Thus, these patients must be closely monitored, and the dose of vecuronium carefully titrated. Long-term relaxant administration and the subsequent prolonged lack of ACh binding at the postsynaptic nicotinic ACh receptors may mimic a chronic denervation state and cause lasting receptor dysfunction and paralysis. Tolerance to nondepolarizing muscle relaxants can also develop after long-term use. Fortunately, the use of unnecessary paralysis has greatly declined in critical care units.

Dosage

Vecuronium is equipotent with pancuronium, and the intubating dose is 0.08–0.12 mg/kg. A dose of 0.04 mg/kg initially followed by increments of 0.01 mg/kg every 15–20 min provides intraoperative relaxation. Alternatively, an infusion of 1–2 mcg/kg/min produces good maintenance of relaxation.

Age does not affect initial dose requirements, although subsequent doses are required less frequently in neonates and infants. Women seem to be approximately 30% more sensitive than men to vecuronium, as evidenced by a greater degree of blockade and longer duration of action (this has also been seen with pancuronium and rocuronium). The cause for this sensitivity may be related to gender-related differences in fat and muscle mass, protein binding, volume of distribution, or metabolic activity. The duration of action of vecuronium may be further prolonged in postpartum patients due to alterations in hepatic blood flow or liver uptake.

Side Effects & Clinical Considerations

A. Cardiovascular

Even at doses of 0.28 mg/kg, vecuronium is devoid of significant cardiovascular effects. Potentiation of opioid-induced bradycardia may be observed in some patients.

B. Liver Failure

Although it is dependent on biliary excretion, the duration of action of vecuronium is usually not significantly prolonged in patients with cirrhosis unless doses greater than 0.15 mg/kg are given. Vecuronium requirements are reduced during the anhepatic phase of liver transplantation.

ROCURONIUM

Physical Structure

This monoquaternary steroid analogue of vecuronium was designed to provide a rapid onset of action.

Metabolism & Excretion

Rocuronium undergoes no metabolism and is eliminated primarily by the liver and slightly by the kidneys. Its duration of action is not significantly affected by renal disease, but it is modestly prolonged by severe hepatic failure and pregnancy. Because rocuronium does not have active metabolites, it may be a better choice than vecuronium in the rare patient requiring prolonged infusions in the intensive care unit setting. Elderly patients may experience a prolonged duration of action due to decreased liver mass.

Dosage

Rocuronium is less potent than most other steroidal muscle relaxants (potency seems to be inversely related to speed of onset). It requires 0.45–0.9 mg/kg intravenously for intubation and 0.15 mg/kg boluses for maintenance. A lower dose of 0.4 mg/kg may allow reversal as soon as 25 min after intubation. Intramuscular rocuronium (1 mg/kg for infants; 2 mg/kg for children) provides adequate vocal cord and diaphragmatic paralysis for intubation, but not until after 3–6 min (deltoid injection has a faster onset than quadriceps), and can be reversed after about 1 hr. The infusion requirements for rocuronium range from 5–12 mcg/kg/min. Rocuronium can produce a prolonged duration of action in elderly patients. Initial dosage requirements are modestly increased in patients with advanced liver disease, presumably due to a larger volume of distribution.

Side Effects & Clinical Considerations

14 Rocuronium (at a dose of 0.9–1.2 mg/kg) has an onset of action that *approaches* succinylcholine (60–90 s), making it a suitable alternative for rapid-sequence inductions, but at the cost of a much longer duration of action. This intermediate duration of action is comparable to vecuronium or atracurium.

Rocuronium (0.1 mg/kg) has been shown to be a rapid (90 s) and effective agent (decreased fasciculations and postoperative myalgias) for precurarization prior to administration of succinylcholine. It has slight vagolytic tendencies.

OTHER RELAXANTS

Muscle relaxants, primarily of historical interest, are either no longer manufactured or not clinically used. They include tubocurarine, metocurine,

gallamine, alcuronium, rapacuronium, and decamethonium. Tubocurarine, the first muscle relaxant used clinically, often produced hypotension and tachycardia through histamine release; its ability to block autonomic ganglia was of secondary importance. Histamine release could also produce or exacerbate bronchospasm. Tubocurarine is not metabolized significantly, and its elimination is primarily renal and secondarily biliary. Metocurine, a closely related agent, shares many of the side effects of tubocurarine. It is primarily dependent on renal function for elimination. Patients allergic to iodine (eg, shellfish allergies) could exhibit hypersensitivity to metocurine preparations, as they contain iodide. Gallamine has the most potent vagolytic properties of any relaxant, and it is entirely dependent on renal function for elimination. Alcuronium, a long-acting nondepolarizer with mild vagolytic properties, is also primarily dependent on renal function for elimination. Rapacuronium has a rapid onset of action, minimal cardiovascular side effects, and a short duration of action. It was withdrawn by the manufacturer following multiple reports of serious bronchospasm, including a few unexplained fatalities. Histamine release may have been a factor. Decamethonium was an older depolarizing agent.

More recently, doxacurium, pipecuronium, and mivacurium are no longer commercially available in the United States. Mivacurium is a benzylisoquinolinium derivative, which is metabolized by pseudocholinesterase; therefore, its duration of action may be prolonged in pathophysiological states that result in low pseudocholinesterase levels. The usual intubating dose is 0.2 mg/kg, with the steady state infusion rate being 4-10 mcg/kg/min. Mivacurium releases histamine to about the same degree as atracurium; the resulting cardiovascular effects can be minimized by slow injection. Doxacurium is a potent long-acting benzylisoquinolinium compound that is primarily eliminated by renal excretion. Adequate intubating conditions are achieved in 5 min with 0.05 mg/kg. It is essentially devoid of cardiovascular and histamine-releasing side effects. Pipecuronium, on the other hand, is a bisquaternary steroidal compound similar to pancuronium, without the vagolytic effects. Onset and duration of action are also similar to pancuronium; elimination is primarily through renal (70%) and biliary (20%) excretion. The usual intubating dose ranges from 0.06-0.1 mg/kg; its pharmacologic profile is relatively unchanged in elderly patients.

NEWER MUSCLE RELAXANTS

Gantacurium belongs to a new class of nondepolarizing neuromuscular blockers called chlorofumarates. It is provided as a lyophilized powder, because it is not stable as an aqueous solution; therefore, it requires reconstitution prior to administration. In preclinical trials, gantacurium demonstrated an ultrashort duration of action, similar to that of succinylcholine. Its pharmacokinetic profile is explained by the fact that it undergoes nonenzymatic degradation by two chemical mechanisms: rapid formation of inactive cysteine adduction product and ester hydrolysis. At a dose of 0.2 mg/kg (ED_{95}), the onset of action has been estimated to be 1-2 min, with a duration of blockade similar to that of succinylcholine. Its clinical duration of action ranged from 5-10 min; recovery can be accelerated by edrophonium, as well as by the administration of exogenous cysteine. Cardiovascular effects suggestive of histamine release were observed following the use of three times the ED_{95} dosage.

AV002 (CW002) is another investigational nondepolarizing agent. It is a benzylisoquinolinium fumarate ester-based compound with an intermediate duration of action that undergoes metabolism and elimination similar to that of gantacurium.

CASE DISCUSSION

Delayed Recovery from General Anesthesia

A 72-year-old man has undergone general anesthesia for transurethral resection of the prostate. Twenty minutes after conclusion of the procedure, he is still intubated and shows no evidence of spontaneous respiration or consciousness.

What is your general approach to this diagnostic dilemma?

Clues to the solution of complex clinical problems are usually found in a pertinent review of the medical and surgical history, the history of drug ingestions, the physical examination, and laboratory results. In this case, the perioperative anesthetic management should also be considered.

What medical illnesses predispose a patient to delayed awakening or prolonged paralysis?

Chronic hypertension alters cerebral blood flow autoregulation and decreases the brain's tolerance to episodes of hypotension. Liver disease reduces hepatic drug metabolism and biliary excretion, resulting in prolonged drug action. Reduced serum albumin concentrations increase free drug (active drug) availability. Hepatic encephalopathy can alter consciousness. Kidney disease decreases the renal excretion of many drugs. Uremia can also affect consciousness. Diabetic patients are prone to hypoglycemia and hyperosmotic, hyperglycemic, and nonketotic coma. A prior stroke or symptomatic carotid bruit increases the risk of intraoperative cerebral vascular accident. Right-to-left heart shunts, particularly in children with congenital heart disease, allow air emboli to pass directly from the venous circulation to the systemic (possibly cerebral) arterial circulation. A paradoxic air embolism can result in permanent brain damage. Severe hypothyroidism is associated with impaired drug metabolism and, rarely, myxedema coma.

Does an uneventful history of general anesthesia narrow the differential?

Hereditary atypical pseudocholinesterase is ruled out by uneventful prior general anesthesia, assuming succinylcholine was administered. Decreased levels of normal enzyme would not result in postoperative apnea unless the surgery was of very short duration. Malignant hyperthermia does not typically present as delayed awakening, although prolonged somnolence is not unusual. Uneventful prior anesthetics do not, however, rule out malignant hyperthermia. Persons unusually sensitive to anesthetic agents (eg, geriatric patients) may have a history of delayed emergence.

How do drugs that a patient takes at home affect awakening from general anesthesia?

Drugs that decrease minimum alveolar concentration, such as methyldopa, predispose patients to anesthetic overdose. Acute ethanol intoxication decreases barbiturate metabolism and acts independently as a sedative. Drugs that decrease liver blood flow, such as cimetidine, will limit hepatic drug metabolism. Antiparkinsonian drugs and tricyclic antidepressants have anticholinergic side effects that augment the sedation produced by scopolamine. Long-acting sedatives, such as the benzodiazepines, can delay awakening.

Does anesthetic technique alter awakening?

Preoperative medications can affect awakening. In particular, anticholinergics (with the exception of glycopyrrolate, which does not cross the blood–brain barrier), opioids, and sedatives can interfere with postoperative recovery. Patients with low cardiac output may have delayed absorption of intramuscular injections.

Intraoperative hyperventilation is a common cause of postoperative apnea. Because volatile agents raise the apneic threshold, the Pa_{CO_2} level at which spontaneous ventilation ceases, moderate postoperative hypoventilation may be required to stimulate the respiratory centers. Severe intraoperative hypotension or hypertension may lead to cerebral hypoxia and edema.

Hypothermia decreases minimum alveolar concentration, antagonizes muscle relaxation reversal, and limits drug metabolism. Arterial hypoxia or severe hypercapnia ($Pa_{CO_2} > 70$ mm Hg) can alter consciousness.

Certain surgical procedures, such as carotid endarterectomy, cardiopulmonary bypass, and intracranial procedures, are associated with an increased incidence of postoperative neurological deficits. Subdural hematomas can occur in severely coagulopathic patients. Transurethral resection of the prostate is associated with hyponatremia from the dilutional effects of absorbed irrigating solution.

What clues does a physical examination provide?

Pupil size is not always a reliable indicator of central nervous system integrity. Fixed and dilated pupils in the absence of anticholinergic medication or ganglionic blockade (eg, the formerly used hypotensive agent, trimethaphan), however, may be an ominous sign. Response to physical stimulation, such as a forceful jaw thrust, may differentiate somnolence from paralysis. Peripheral nerve stimulation also differentiates paralysis from coma.

What specific laboratory findings would you order?

Arterial blood gases and serum electrolytes, particularly sodium, may be helpful. Computed tomographic scanning may be necessary if unresponsiveness is prolonged. Increased concentrations of inhalational agent provided by respiratory gas analysis, as well as processed electroencephalogram (EEG) measurements, may assist in determining if the patient is still under the effects of anesthesia. Slow EEG signals can be indicative of both anesthesia and cerebral pathology. Processed EEG awareness monitors can also be employed with the realization that low numbers on the bispectral index can be caused both by anesthetic suppression of the EEG and ischemic brain injury.

What therapeutic interventions should be considered?

Supportive mechanical ventilation should be continued in the unresponsive patient. Naloxone, flumazenil, and physostigmine may be indicated, depending on the probable cause of the delayed emergence, if drug effects are suspected and reversal is considered both safe and desirable.

SUGGESTED READING

Donati F, Bevan D: Neuromuscular Blocking Agents. In: *Clinical Anesthesia*, 6th ed. Barash PG, Cullen BF, Stoelting RK, Cahalan MK, Stock MC (editors). Lippincott, Williams & Wilkins, 2009.

Foldes FF, McNall PG, Borrego-Hinojosa JM: Succinylcholine: a new approach to muscular relaxation in anesthesiology. N Engl J Med 1952;247:596.

Fuchs-Buder, Schreiber JU, Meistelman C: Monitoring neuromuscular block: an update. Anaesthesia 2009;64:82.

Hunter JM: New neuromuscular blocking drugs. N Engl J Med 1995;22:1691.

Lee C: Structure, conformation, and action of neuromuscular blocking drugs. Br J Anaesth 2001;87:755.

Naguib M, Brull SJ: Update on neuromuscular pharmacology. Curr Opin Anaesthesiol 2009;22:483.

Murphy G, Szokol J, Avram M, et al: Intraoperative acceleromyography monitoring reduces symptoms of muscle weakness and improves quality recovery in the early postoperative period. Anesthesiology 2011;115:946.

Naguib M, Lien CA: Pharmacology of muscle relaxants and their antagonists. In: *Miller's Anesthesia*, 7th ed. Miller RD, Eriksson LI, Wiener-Kronish JP, Young WL (editors). Churchill Livingstone, 2010.

Cholinesterase Inhibitors & Other Pharmacologic Antagonists to Neuromuscular Blocking Agents

KEY CONCEPTS

1. The primary clinical use of cholinesterase inhibitors, also called anticholinesterases, is to reverse nondepolarizing muscle blockade.

2. Acetylcholine is the neurotransmitter for the entire parasympathetic nervous system (parasympathetic ganglions and effector cells), parts of the sympathetic nervous system (sympathetic ganglions, adrenal medulla, and sweat glands), some neurons in the central nervous system, and somatic nerves innervating skeletal muscle.

3. Neuromuscular transmission is blocked when nondepolarizing muscle relaxants compete with acetylcholine to bind to nicotinic cholinergic receptors. The cholinesterase inhibitors indirectly increase the amount of acetylcholine available to compete with the nondepolarizing agent, thereby reestablishing neuromuscular transmission.

4. In excessive doses, acetylcholinesterase inhibitors can paradoxically potentiate a nondepolarizing neuromuscular blockade. In addition, these drugs prolong the depolarization blockade of succinylcholine.

5. Any prolongation of action of a nondepolarizing muscle relaxant from renal or hepatic insufficiency will probably be accompanied by a corresponding increase

in the duration of action of a cholinesterase inhibitor.

6. The time required to fully reverse a nondepolarizing block depends on several factors, including the choice and dose of cholinesterase inhibitor administered, the muscle relaxant being antagonized, and the extent of the blockade before reversal.

7. A reversal agent should be routinely given to patients who have received nondepolarizing muscle relaxants unless full reversal can be demonstrated or the postoperative plan includes continued intubation and ventilation.

8. In monitoring a patient's recovery from neuromuscular blockade, the suggested end points are sustained tetanus for 5 sec in response to a 100-Hz stimulus in anesthetized patients or sustained head lift in awake patients. If neither of these end points is achieved, the patient should remain intubated and ventilation should be continued.

9. Sugammadex exerts its effects by forming tight complexes in a 1:1 ratio with steroidal neuromuscular blocking agents.

10. Cysteine causes inactivation of gantacurium via metabolic degradation and adduct formation.

Incomplete reversal of neuromuscular blocking agents and residual post-procedure paralysis are associated with morbidity; therefore, careful evaluation of neuromuscular blockade and appropriate pharmacologic antagonism are strongly recommended whenever muscle relaxants are administered. The primary clinical use of cholinesterase inhibitors, also called anticholinesterases, is to reverse nondepolarizing muscle blockade. Some of these agents are also used to diagnose and treat myasthenia gravis. More recently, newer agents, such as cyclodextrins and cysteine, with superior ability to reverse neuromuscular blockade from specific agents, are being investigated with promising results. This chapter reviews cholinergic pharmacology and mechanisms of acetylcholinesterase inhibition and presents the clinical pharmacology of commonly used cholinesterase inhibitors (neostigmine, edrophonium, pyridostigmine, and physostigmine). It concludes with a brief description and mechanisms of action of some unique reversal agents.

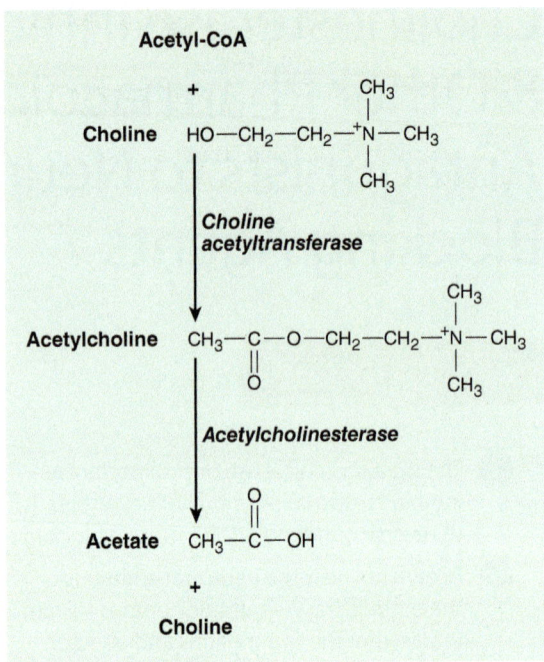

FIGURE 12–1 The synthesis and hydrolysis of acetylcholine.

Cholinergic Pharmacology

The term cholinergic refers to the effects of the neurotransmitter acetyl*choline*, as opposed to the adrenergic effects of nor*adrenaline* (norepinephrine). Acetylcholine is synthesized in the nerve terminal by the enzyme cholineacetyltransferase, which catalyzes the reaction between acetylcoenzyme A and choline (Figure 12–1). After its release, acetylcholine is rapidly hydrolyzed by acetylcholinesterase (true cholinesterase) into acetate and choline.

Acetylcholine is the neurotransmitter for the entire parasympathetic nervous system (parasympathetic ganglions and effector cells), parts of the sympathetic nervous system (sympathetic ganglions, adrenal medulla, and sweat glands), some neurons in the central nervous system, and somatic nerves innervating skeletal muscle (Figure 12–2).

Cholinergic receptors have been subdivided into two major groups based on their reaction to the alkaloids muscarine and nicotine (Figure 12–3). Nicotine stimulates the autonomic ganglia and skeletal muscle receptors (nicotinic receptors), whereas muscarine activates end-organ effector cells in

bronchial smooth muscle, salivary glands, and the sinoatrial node (muscarinic receptors). The central nervous system has both nicotinic and muscarinic receptors. Nicotinic receptors are blocked by muscle relaxants (also called neuromuscular blockers), and muscarinic receptors are blocked by anticholinergic drugs, such as atropine. Although nicotinic and muscarinic receptors differ in their response to some agonists (eg, nicotine, muscarine) and some antagonists (eg, vecuronium vs atropine), they both respond to acetylcholine (Table 12–1). Clinically available cholinergic agonists resist hydrolysis by cholinesterase. Methacholine and bethanechol are primarily muscarinic agonists, whereas carbachol has both muscarinic and nicotinic agonist activities. Methacholine by inhalation has been used as a provocative test in asthma, bethanechol is used for bladder atony, and carbachol may be used topically for wide-angle glaucoma.

When reversing neuromuscular blockade, the primary goal is to maximize nicotinic transmission with a minimum of muscarinic side effects.

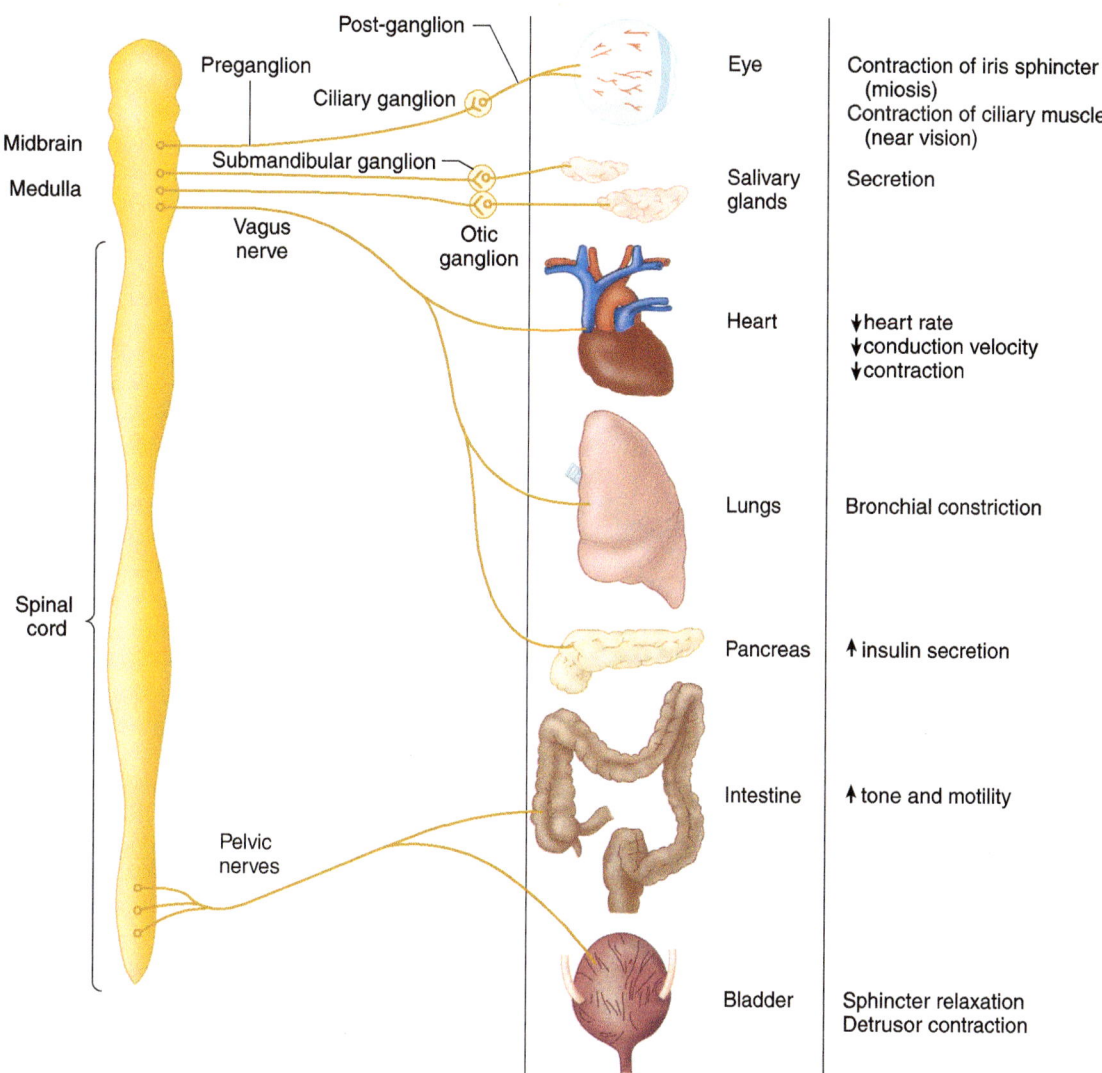

FIGURE 12–2 The parasympathetic nervous system uses acetylcholine as a preganglionic and postganglionic neurotransmitter.

MECHANISM OF ACTION

3 Normal neuromuscular transmission critically depends on acetylcholine binding to nicotinic cholinergic receptors on the motor endplate. Nondepolarizing muscle relaxants act by competing with acetylcholine for these binding sites, thereby blocking neuromuscular transmission. Reversal of blockade depends on gradual diffusion, redistribution, metabolism, and excretion from the body of the nondepolarizing relaxant (*spontaneous reversal*), often assisted by the administration of specific reversal agents (*pharmacological reversal*). Cholinesterase inhibitors *indirectly* increase the amount of acetylcholine available to compete with the nondepolarizing agent, thereby reestablishing normal neuromuscular transmission.

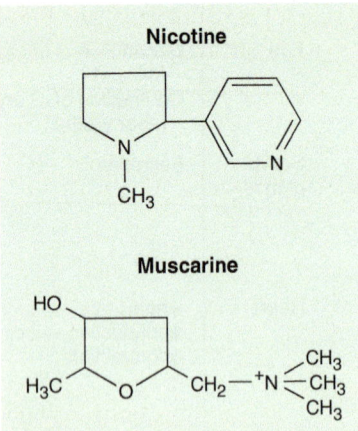

FIGURE 12–3 The molecular structures of nicotine and muscarine. Compare these alkaloids with acetylcholine (Figure 12–1).

Cholinesterase inhibitors inactivate acetylcholinesterase by reversibly binding to the enzyme. The stability of the bond influences the duration of action. The electrostatic attraction and hydrogen bonding of edrophonium are short-lived; the

TABLE 12–1 Characteristics of cholinergic receptors.

	Nicotinic	Muscarinic

Location	Autonomic ganglia
	  Sympathetic
	    ganglia
	  Parasympathetic
	    ganglia
	Skeletal muscle
		Glands
		  Lacrimal
		  Salivary
		  Gastric
		Smooth muscle
		  Bronchial
		  Gastrointestinal
		  Bladder
		  Blood vessels
		Heart
		  Sinoatrial node
		  Atrioventricular
		    node

Agonists	Acetylcholine Nicotine	Acetylcholine Muscarine
Antagonists	Nondepolarizing relaxants	Antimuscarinics Atropine Scopolamine Glycopyrrolate

covalent bonds of neostigmine and pyridostigmine are longer lasting.

Organophosphates, a special class of cholinesterase inhibitors, form very stable, irreversible bonds to the enzyme. They are used in ophthalmology and more commonly as pesticides. The clinical duration of the cholinesterase inhibitors used in anesthesia, however, is probably most influenced by the rate of drug disappearance from the plasma. Differences in duration of action can be overcome by dosage adjustments. Thus, the normally short duration of action of edrophonium can be partially overcome by increasing the dosage. Cholinesterase inhibitors are also used in the diagnosis and treatment of myasthenia gravis.

Mechanisms of action other than acetylcholinesterase inactivation may contribute to the restoration of neuromuscular function. Edrophonium seems to have prejunctional effects that enhance the release of acetylcholine. Neostigmine has a direct (but weak) agonist effect on nicotinic receptors. Acetylcholine mobilization and release by the nerve may also be enhanced (a presynaptic mechanism).

4 In excessive doses, acetylcholinesterase inhibitors paradoxically potentiate a nondepolarizing neuromuscular blockade. Standard dogma states that neostigmine in high doses may cause receptor channel blockade; however, clinical evidence of this is lacking. In addition, these drugs prolong the depolarization blockade of succinylcholine. Two mechanisms may explain this latter effect: an increase in acetylcholine (which increases motor end-plate depolarization) and inhibition of pseudocholinesterase activity. Neostigmine and to some extent pyridostigmine display some limited pseudocholinesterase-inhibiting activity, but their effect on acetylcholinesterase is much greater. Edrophonium has little or no effect on pseudocholinesterase. In large doses, neostigmine can cause a weak depolarizing neuromuscular blockade.

CLINICAL PHARMACOLOGY

General Pharmacological Characteristics

The increase in acetylcholine caused by cholinesterase inhibitors affects more than the nicotinic receptors of skeletal muscle (Table 12–2). Cholinesterase

TABLE 12–2 Muscarinic side effects of cholinesterase inhibitors.

Organ System	Muscarinic Side Effects
Cardiovascular	Decreased heart rate, bradyarrhythmias
Pulmonary	Bronchospasm, bronchial secretions
Cerebral	Diffuse excitation[1]
Gastrointestinal	Intestinal spasm, increased salivation
Genitourinary	Increased bladder tone
Ophthalmological	Pupillary constriction

[1]Applies only to physostigmine.

inhibitors can act at cholinergic receptors of several other organ systems, including the cardiovascular and gastrointestinal systems.

Cardiovascular receptors—The predominant muscarinic effect on the heart is bradycardia that can progress to sinus arrest.

Pulmonary receptors—Muscarinic stimulation can result in bronchospasm (smooth muscle contraction) and increased respiratory tract secretions.

Cerebral receptors—Physostigmine is a cholinesterase inhibitor that crosses the blood–brain barrier and can cause diffuse activation of the electroencephalogram by stimulating muscarinic and nicotinic receptors within the central nervous system. Inactivation of nicotinic acetylcholine receptors in the central nervous system may play a role in the action of general anesthetics. Unlike physostigmine, cholinesterase inhibitors used to reverse neuromuscular blockers do not cross the blood–brain barrier.

Gastrointestinal receptors—Muscarinic stimulation increases peristaltic activity (esophageal, gastric, and intestinal) and glandular secretions (eg, salivary). Postoperative nausea, vomiting, and fecal

incontinence have been attributed to the use of cholinesterase inhibitors.

Unwanted muscarinic side effects are minimized by prior or concomitant administration of anticholinergic medications, such as atropine sulfate or glycopyrrolate. The duration of action is similar among the cholinesterase inhibitors. Clearance is due to both hepatic metabolism (25% to 50%) and renal excretion (50% to 75%). Thus, any prolongation of action of a nondepolarizing muscle relaxant from renal or hepatic insufficiency will probably be accompanied by a corresponding increase in the duration of action of a cholinesterase inhibitor.

As a rule, no amount of cholinesterase inhibitor can immediately reverse a block that is so intense that there is no response to tetanic peripheral nerve stimulation. Moreover, the absence of any palpable single twitches following 5 sec of tetanic stimulation at 50 Hz implies a very intensive blockade that cannot be reversed. Excessive doses of cholinesterase inhibitors may actually prolong recovery. Some evidence of spontaneous recovery (ie, the first twitch of the train-of-four [TOF]) should be present before reversal is attempted. The posttetanic count (the number of palpable twitches after tetanus) generally correlates with the time of return of the first twitch of the TOF and therefore the ability to reverse intense paralysis. For intermediate-acting agents, such as atracurium and vecuronium, a palpable posttetanic twitch appears about 10 min before spontaneous recovery of the first twitch of the TOF. In contrast, for longer-acting agents, such as pancuronium, the first twitch of the TOF appears about 40 min after a palpable posttetanic twitch.

The time required to fully reverse a nondepolarizing block depends on several factors, including the choice and dose of cholinesterase inhibitor administered, the muscle relaxant being antagonized, and the extent of the blockade before reversal. For example, reversal with edrophonium is usually faster than with neostigmine; large doses of neostigmine lead to faster reversal than small doses; intermediate-acting relaxants reverse sooner than long-acting relaxants; and a shallow block is easier to reverse than a deep block (ie, twitch height >10%). Intermediate-acting muscle relaxants therefore require a lower dose of reversal agent (for the same degree of blockade) than long-acting agents, and concurrent excretion or metabolism provides a proportionally faster reversal of the short- and intermediate-acting agents. These advantages can be lost in conditions associated with severe end-organ disease (eg, the use of vecuronium in a patient with liver failure) or enzyme deficiencies (eg, mivacurium in a patient with homozygous atypical pseudocholinesterase). Depending on the dose of muscle relaxant that has been given, spontaneous recovery to a level adequate for pharmacological reversal may take more than 1 hr with long-acting muscle relaxants because of their insignificant metabolism and slow excretion. Factors associated with faster reversal are also associated with a lower incidence of residual paralysis in the recovery room and a lower risk of postoperative respiratory complications.

7 A reversal agent should be routinely given to patients who have received nondepolarizing muscle relaxants unless full reversal can be demonstrated or the postoperative plan includes continued intubation and ventilation. In the latter situation, adequate sedation must also be provided.

A peripheral nerve stimulator should also be used to monitor the progress and confirm the adequacy of reversal. In general, the higher the frequency of stimulation, the greater the sensitivity of the test (100-Hz tetany > 50-Hz tetany or TOF > single-twitch height). Clinical signs of adequate reversal also vary in sensitivity (sustained head lift > inspiratory force > vital capacity > tidal volume).

8 Therefore, the suggested end points of recovery are sustained tetanus for 5 sec in response to a 100-Hz stimulus in anesthetized patients or sustained head or leg lift in awake patients. Newer quantitative methods for assessing recovery from neuromuscular blockade, such as acceleromyography, may further reduce the incidence of residual postoperative neuromuscular paralysis.

Specific Cholinesterase Inhibitors

NEOSTIGMINE

Physical Structure

Neostigmine consists of a carbamate moiety and a quaternary ammonium group (Figure 12–4). The former provides covalent bonding to acetylcholinesterase. The latter renders the molecule lipid insoluble, so that it cannot pass through the blood–brain barrier.

Dosage & Packaging

The maximum recommended dose of neostigmine is 0.08 mg/kg (up to 5 mg in adults), but smaller

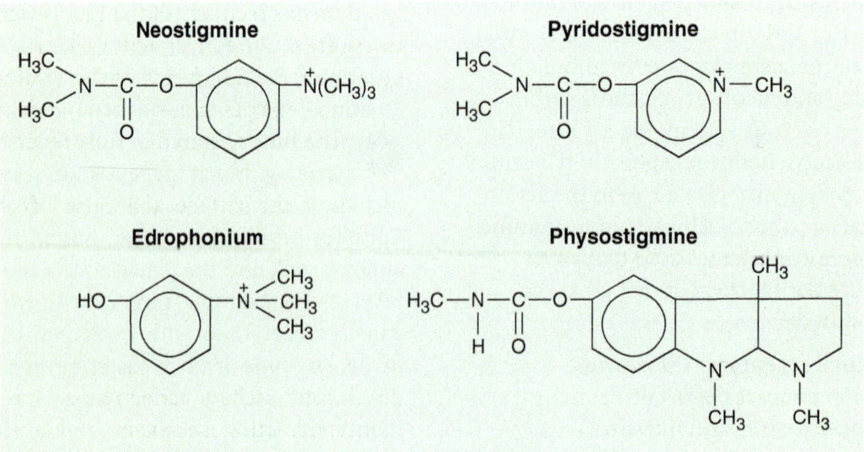

FIGURE 12–4 The molecular structures of neostigmine, pyridostigmine, edrophonium, and physostigmine.

TABLE 12–3 The choice and dose of cholinesterase inhibitor determine the choice and dose of anticholinergic.

Cholinesterase Inhibitor	Usual Dose of Cholinesterase Inhibitor	Recommended Anticholinergic	Usual Dose of Anticholinergic per mg of Cholinesterase Inhibitor
Neostigmine	0.04–0.08 mg/kg	Glycopyrrolate	0.2 mg
Pyridostigmine	0.1–0..25 mg/kg	Glycopyrrolate	0.05 mg
Edrophonium	0.5–1 mg/kg	Atropine	0.014 mg
Physostigmine[1]	0.01–0.03 mg/kg	Usually not necessary	NA

[1]Not used to reverse muscle relaxants.

amounts often suffice and larger doses have also been given safely (Table 12–3). Neostigmine is most commonly packaged as 10 mL of a 1 mg/mL solution, although 0.5 mg/mL and 0.25 mg/mL concentrations are also available.

Clinical Considerations

The effects of neostigmine (0.04 mg/kg) are usually apparent in 5min, peak at 10 min, and last more than 1 hr. If reversal is not complete in 10 min after 0.08 mg/kg, the time for full recovery of neuromuscular function will depend on the nondepolarizing agent used and the intensity of blockade. In practice, many clinicians use a dose of 0.04 mg/kg (or 2.5 mg) if the preexisting blockade is mild to moderate and a dose of 0.08 mg/kg (or 5 mg) if intense paralysis is being reversed. The duration of action is prolonged in geriatric patients. Muscarinic side effects are minimized by prior or concomitant administration of an anticholinergic agent. The onset of action of glycopyrrolate (0.2 mg glycopyrrolate per 1 mg of neostigmine) is similar to that of neostigmine and is associated with less tachycardia than is experienced with atropine (0.4 mg of atropine per 1 mg of neostigmine). It has been reported that neostigmine crosses the placenta, resulting in fetal bradycardia. Thus, *theoretically*, atropine may be a better choice of an anticholinergic agent than glycopyrrolate in pregnant patients receiving neostigmine, but there is no evidence that this makes any difference in patient outcomes. Neostigmine is also used to treat myasthenia gravis, urinary bladder atony, and paralytic ileus.

PYRIDOSTIGMINE
Physical Structure

Pyridostigmine is structurally similar to neostigmine except that the quaternary ammonium is incorporated into the phenol ring. Pyridostigmine shares neostigmine's covalent binding to acetylcholinesterase and its lipid insolubility.

Dosage & Packaging

Pyridostigmine is 20% as potent as neostigmine and may be administered in doses up to 0.25 mg/kg (a total of 20 mg in adults). It is available as a solution of 5 mg/mL.

Clinical Considerations

The onset of action of pyridostigmine is slower (10–15 min) than that of neostigmine, and its duration is slightly longer (>2 h). Glycopyrrolate (0.05 mg per 1 mg of pyridostigmine) or atropine (0.1 mg per 1 mg of pyridostigmine) must also be administered to prevent bradycardia. Glycopyrrolate is preferred because its slower onset of action better matches that of pyridostigmine, again resulting in less tachycardia.

EDROPHONIUM
Physical Structure

Because it lacks a carbamate group, edrophonium must rely on noncovalent bonding to the acetylcholinesterase enzyme. The quaternary ammonium group limits lipid solubility.

Dosage & Packaging

Edrophonium is less than 10% as potent as neostigmine. The recommended dosage is 0.5–1 mg/kg. Edrophonium is available as a solution containing 10 mg/mL; it is available with atropine as a combination drug (Enlon-Plus; 10 mg edrophonium and 0.14 mg atropine per mL).

Clinical Considerations

Edrophonium has the most rapid onset of action (1–2 min) and the shortest duration of effect of any of the cholinesterase inhibitors. Reduced doses should not be used, because longer-acting muscle relaxants may outlast the effects of edrophonium. Higher doses prolong the duration of action to more than 1 hr. Edrophonium may not be as effective as neostigmine at reversing intense neuromuscular blockade. In equipotent doses, muscarinic effects of edrophonium are less pronounced than those of neostigmine or pyridostigmine, requiring only half the amount of anticholinergic agent. Edrophonium's rapid onset is well matched to that of atropine (0.014 mg of atropine per 1 mg of edrophonium). Although glycopyrrolate (0.007 mg per 1 mg of edrophonium) can also be used, it should be given several minutes prior to edrophonium to avoid the possibility of bradycardia.

PHYSOSTIGMINE

Physical Structure

Physostigmine, a tertiary amine, has a carbamate group but no quaternary ammonium. Therefore, it is lipid soluble and is the only clinically available cholinesterase inhibitor that freely passes the blood–brain barrier.

Dosage & Packaging

The dose of physostigmine is 0.01–0.03 mg/kg. It is packaged as a solution containing 1 mg/mL.

Clinical Considerations

The lipid solubility and central nervous system penetration of physostigmine limit its usefulness as a reversal agent for nondepolarizing blockade, but make it effective in the treatment of central anticholinergic toxicity caused by overdoses of atropine or scopolamine. In addition, it reverses some of the central nervous system depression and delirium associated with use of benzodiazepines and volatile anesthetics. Physostigmine (0.04 mg/kg) has been shown to be effective in preventing postoperative shivering. It reportedly partially antagonizes morphine-induced respiratory depression, presumably because morphine reduces acetylcholine release in the brain. These effects are transient, and repeated doses may be required. Bradycardia is infrequent in the recommended dosage range, but atropine should be immediately available. Because glycopyrrolate does not cross the blood–brain barrier, it will not reverse the central nervous system effects of physostigmine. Other possible muscarinic side effects include excessive salivation, vomiting, and convulsions. In contrast to other cholinesterase inhibitors, physostigmine is almost completely metabolized by plasma esterases, so renal excretion is not important.

OTHER CONSIDERATIONS

Recovery from neuromuscular blockade is influenced by the depth of block at the time of antagonism, clearance and half-life of the relaxant used, and other factors that affect neuromuscular blockade (Table 12–4), such as drugs and electrolyte

TABLE 12–4 Factors potentiating neuromuscular blockade.

Drugs
Volatile anesthetics
Antibiotics: Aminoglycosides, polymyxin B, neomycin, tetracycline, clindamycin
Dantrolene
Verapamil
Furosemide
Lidocaine

Electrolytes and acid–base disorders
Hypermagnesemia
Hypocalcemia
Hypokalemia
Respiratory acidosis

Temperature
Hypothermia

disturbances. In addition, some specific agents with the potential of reversing the neuromuscular blocking effects of nondepolarizing muscle relaxants merit brief discussion.

NON-CLASSIC REVERSAL AGENTS

Besides cholinesterase inhibitors, two unique drugs (sugammadex and L-cysteine) are currently under investigation in the United States; these agents act as selective antagonists of nondepolarizing neuromuscular blockade. Sugammadex is able to reverse aminosteroid-induced neuromuscular blockade, whereas cysteine has been shown to reverse the neuromuscular blocking effects of gantacurium and other fumarates.

SUGAMMADEX

Sugammadex is a novel selective relaxant-binding agent that is currently available for clinical use in Europe. It is a modified gamma-cyclodextrin (*su* refers to sugar, and *gammadex* refers to the structural molecule gamma-cyclodextrin).

Physical Structure

Its three-dimensional structure resembles a hollow truncated cone or doughnut with a hydrophobic cavity and a hydrophilic exterior. Hydrophobic interactions trap the drug (eg, rocuronium) in the cyclodextrin cavity (doughnut hole), resulting in tight formation of a water-soluble guest–host complex in a 1:1 ratio. This terminates the neuromuscular blocking action and restrains the drug in extracellular fluid where it cannot interact with nicotinic acetylcholine receptors. Sugammadex is essentially eliminated unchanged via the kidneys.

Clinical Considerations

Sugammadex has been administered in doses of 4–8 mg/kg. With an injection of 8 mg/kg, given 3 min after administration of 0.6 mg/kg of rocuronium, recovery of TOF ratio to 0.9 was observed within 2 min. It produces rapid and effective reversal of both shallow and profound

rocuronium-induced neuromuscular blockade in a consistent manner. Because of some concerns about hypersensitivity and allergic reactions, sugammadex has not yet been approved by the US Food and Drug Administration.

L-CYSTEINE

L-cysteine is an endogenous amino acid that is often added to total parenteral nutrition regimens to enhance calcium and phosphate solubility. The ultrashort-acting neuromuscular blocker, gantacurium, and other fumarates rapidly combine with L-cysteine *in vitro* to form less active degradation products (adducts). Exogenous administration of L-cysteine (10–50 mg/kg intravenously) given to anesthetized monkeys 1 min after these neuromuscular blocking agents abolished the block within 2–3 min; this antagonism was found to be superior to that produced by anticholinesterases. This unique method of antagonism by adduct formation and inactivation is still in the investigative stage, especially in terms of its safety and efficacy in humans.

CASE DISCUSSION

Respiratory Failure in the Recovery Room

A 66-year-old woman weighing 85 kg is brought to the recovery room following cholecystectomy. The anesthetic technique included the use of iso-flurane and vecuronium for muscle relaxation. At the conclusion of the procedure, the anesthesiologist administered 6 mg of morphine sulfate for postoperative pain control and 3 mg of neostigmine with 0.6 mg of glycopyrrolate to reverse any residual neuromuscular blockade. The dose of cholinesterase inhibitor was empirically based on clinical judgment. Although the patient was apparently breathing normally on arrival in the recovery room, her tidal volume progressively diminished. Arterial blood gas measurements revealed a Pa_{CO_2} of 62 mm Hg, a Pa_{O_2} of 110 mm Hg, and a pH of 7.26 on a fraction of inspired oxygen (F_{IO_2}) of 40%.

Which drugs administered to this patient could explain her hypoventilation?

Isoflurane, morphine sulfate, and vecuronium all interfere with a patient's ability to maintain a normal ventilatory response to an elevated Pa_{CO_2}.

Why would the patient's breathing worsen in the recovery room?

Possibilities include the delayed onset of action of morphine sulfate, a lack of sensory stimulation in the recovery area, fatigue of respiratory muscles, and splinting as a result of upper abdominal pain.

Could the patient still have residual neuromuscular blockade?

If the dose of neostigmine was not determined by the response to a peripheral nerve stimulator, or if the recovery of muscle function was inadequately tested after the reversal drugs were given, persistent neuromuscular blockade is possible. Assume, for example, that the patient had minimal or no response to initial tetanic stimulation at 100 Hz. Even the maximal dose of neostigmine (5 mg) might not yet have adequately reversed the paralysis. Because of enormous patient variability, the response to peripheral nerve stimulation must always be monitored when intermediate- or long-acting muscle relaxants are administered. Even if partial reversal is achieved, paralysis may worsen if the patient hypoventilates. **Other factors (in addition to respiratory acidosis) that impair the reversal of nondepolarizing muscle relaxants include intense neuromuscular paralysis, electrolyte disturbances (hypermagnesemia, hypokalemia, and hypocalcemia), hypothermia (temperature <32°C), drug interactions (see Table 11–4), metabolic alkalosis (from accompanying hypokalemia and hypocalcemia), and coexisting diseases (see Table 11–8).**

How could the extent of reversal be tested?

Tetanic stimulation is a sensitive but uncomfortable test of neuromuscular transmission in an awake patient. Because of its shorter duration, double-burst stimulation is tolerated better than tetany by conscious patients. Many other tests of neuromuscular transmission, such as vital capacity and tidal volume, are insensitive as they may still seem normal when 70% to 80% of receptors are blocked. In fact, 70% of receptors may remain blocked despite an apparently normal response to TOF stimulation. The ability to sustain a head lift for 5 sec, however, indicates that fewer than 33% of receptors are occupied by muscle relaxant.

What treatment would you suggest?

Ventilation should be assisted to reduce the respiratory acidosis. Even if diaphragmatic function seems to be adequate, residual blockade can lead to airway obstruction and poor airway protection. More neostigmine (with an anticholinergic) could be administered up to a maximum recommended dose of 5 mg. If this does not adequately reverse paralysis, mechanical ventilation and airway protection should be instituted and continued until neuromuscular function is fully restored.

SUGGESTED READING

Naguib M: Sugammadex: another milestone in clinical neuromuscular pharmacology. Anesth Analg 2007;104:575.

Naguib M, Lien CA: Pharmacology of muscle relaxants and their antagonists. In: *Miller's Anesthesia*, 7th ed. Miller RD, Eriksson LI, Wiener-Kronish JP, Young WL (editors). Churchill Livingstone, 2010.

Savarese JJ, McGilvra JD, Sunaga H, et al: Rapid chemical antagonism of neuromuscular blockade by L-cysteine adduction to and inactivation of the olefinic (double-bonded) isoquinoliniumdiester compounds gantacurium (AV430A), CW 002, and CW 011. Anesthesiology 2010;113:58.

Stoelting RK: *Pharmacology and Physiology in Anesthetic Practice*, 4th ed. Lippincott, William & Wilkins, 2005.

Taylor P: Anticholinesterase agents. In: *Goodman and Gilman'sPharmacological Basis of Therapeutics*, 12th ed. Hardman JG (editor). McGraw-Hill, 2011.

Anticholinergic Drugs

1 The ester linkage is essential for effective binding of the anticholinergics to the acetylcholine receptors. This competitively blocks binding by acetylcholine and prevents receptor activation. The cellular effects of acetylcholine, which are mediated through second messengers, are inhibited.

2 Anticholinergics relax the bronchial smooth musculature, which reduces airway resistance and increases anatomic dead space.

3 Atropine has particularly potent effects on the heart and bronchial smooth muscle and is the most efficacious anticholinergic for treating bradyarrhythmias.

4 Ipratropium solution (0.5 mg in 2.5 mL) seems to be particularly effective in the treatment of acute chronic obstructive pulmonary disease when combined with a β-agonist drug (eg, albuterol).

5 Scopolamine is a more potent antisialagogue than atropine and causes greater central nervous system effects.

6 Because of its quaternary structure, glycopyrrolate cannot cross the blood–brain barrier and is almost devoid of central nervous system and ophthalmic activity.

One group of cholinergic antagonists has already been discussed: the nondepolarizing neuromuscular-blocking agents. These drugs act primarily at the nicotinic receptors in skeletal muscle. This chapter presents the pharmacology of drugs that block muscarinic receptors. Although the classification *anticholinergic* usually refers to this latter group, a more precise term would be *antimuscarinic*.

In this chapter, the mechanism of action and clinical pharmacology are introduced for three common anticholinergics: atropine, scopolamine, and glycopyrrolate. The clinical uses of these drugs in anesthesia relate to their effect on the cardiovascular, respiratory, cerebral, gastrointestinal, and other organ systems (Table 13–1).

MECHANISMS OF ACTION

Anticholinergics are esters of an aromatic acid combined with an organic base (Figure 13–1). The ester linkage is essential for effective binding of the anticholinergics to the acetylcholine receptors. **This competitively blocks binding by acetylcholine and prevents receptor activation.** The cellular effects of acetylcholine, which are mediated through second messengers, are inhibited. The tissue receptors vary in their sensitivity to blockade. In fact, muscarinic receptors are not homogeneous, and receptor subgroups have been identified including: neuronal (M_1), cardiac (M_2), and glandular (M_3) receptors.

TABLE 13–1 Pharmacological characteristics of anticholinergic drugs.[1]

	Atropine	Scopolamine	Glycopyrrolate
Tachycardia	+++	+	++
Bronchodilatation	++	+	++
Sedation	+	+++	0
Antisialagogue effect	++	+++	+++

[1]0, no effect; +, minimal effect; ++, moderate effect; +++, marked effect.

CLINICAL PHARMACOLOGY

General Pharmacological Characteristics

In normal clinical doses, only muscarinic receptors are blocked by the anticholinergic drugs discussed in this chapter. The extent of the anticholinergic effect depends on the degree of baseline vagal tone. Several organ systems are affected.

A. Cardiovascular

Blockade of muscarinic receptors in the sinoatrial node produces tachycardia. This effect is especially useful in reversing bradycardia due to vagal reflexes (eg, baroreceptor reflex, peritoneal traction, or oculocardiac reflex). A transient slowing of heart rate in response to smaller intravenous doses of atropine (<0.4 mg) has been reported. The mechanism of this paradoxical response is unclear. Facilitation of

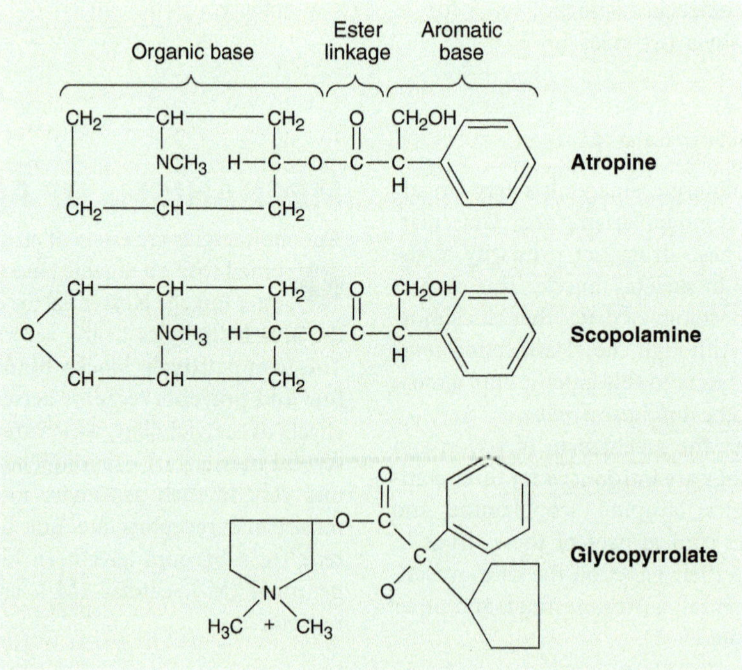

FIGURE 13–1 Physical structures of anticholinergic drugs.

conduction through the atrioventricular node shortens the P–R interval on the electrocardiogram and often decreases heart block caused by vagal activity. Atrial arrhythmias and nodal (junctional) rhythms occasionally occur. Anticholinergics generally have little effect on ventricular function or peripheral vasculature because of the paucity of direct cholinergic innervation of these areas despite the presence of cholinergic receptors. Presynaptic muscarinic receptors on adrenergic nerve terminals are known to inhibit norepinephrine release, so muscarinic antagonists may modestly enhance sympathetic activity. Large doses of anticholinergic agents can result in dilation of cutaneous blood vessels (atropine flush).

B. Respiratory

The anticholinergics inhibit the secretions of the respiratory tract mucosa, from the nose to the bronchi, a valuable property during airway endoscopic or surgical procedures. Relaxation of the bronchial smooth musculature reduces airway resistance and increases anatomic dead space. These effects are particularly pronounced in patients with chronic obstructive pulmonary disease or asthma.

C. Cerebral

Anticholinergic medications can cause a spectrum of central nervous system effects ranging from stimulation to depression, depending on drug choice and dosage. Cerebral stimulation may present as excitation, restlessness, or hallucinations. Cerebral depression, including sedation and amnesia, are prominent after scopolamine. Physostigmine, a cholinesterase inhibitor that crosses the blood–brain barrier, promptly reverses anticholinergic actions on the brain.

D. Gastrointestinal

Salivary secretions are markedly reduced by anticholinergic drugs. Gastric secretions are also decreased, but larger doses are necessary. Decreased intestinal motility and peristalsis prolong gastric emptying time. Lower esophageal sphincter pressure is reduced. Overall, the anticholinergic drugs do not prevent aspiration pneumonia.

E. Ophthalmic

Anticholinergics cause mydriasis (pupillary dilation) and cycloplegia (an inability to accommodate to near vision); acute angle-closure glaucoma is unlikely following systemic administration of most anticholinergic drugs.

F. Genitourinary

Anticholinergics may decrease ureter and bladder tone as a result of smooth muscle relaxation and lead to urinary retention, particularly in elderly men with prostatic hypertrophy.

G. Thermoregulation

Inhibition of sweat glands may lead to a rise in body temperature (atropine fever).

Specific Anticholinergic Drugs

ATROPINE

Physical Structure

Atropine is a tertiary amine. The naturally occurring levorotatory form is active, but the commercial mixture is racemic (Figure 13–1).

Dosage & Packaging

As a premedication, atropine is administered intravenously or intramuscularly in a range of 0.01–0.02 mg/kg, up to the usual adult dose of 0.4–0.6 mg. Larger intravenous doses up to 2 mg may be required to completely block the cardiac vagal nerves in treating severe bradycardia. Atropine sulfate is available in a multitude of concentrations.

Clinical Considerations

Atropine has particularly potent effects on the heart and bronchial smooth muscle and is the most efficacious anticholinergic for treating bradyarrhythmias. Patients with coronary artery disease may not tolerate the increased myocardial oxygen demand and decreased oxygen supply associated with the tachycardia caused by atropine. A derivative of atropine, ipratropium bromide, is available in a metered-dose inhaler for the treatment of bronchospasm. Its quaternary ammonium structure significantly limits systemic absorption. Ipratropium solution (0.5 mg in 2.5 mL) seems to be particularly effective in the treatment of acute chronic obstructive pulmonary disease when combined with a β-agonist drug (eg, albuterol). The central nervous system effects of atropine are minimal after the usual doses, even though this tertiary amine can rapidly cross the blood–brain barrier. Atropine has been associated with mild postoperative memory deficits, and toxic doses are usually associated with excitatory reactions. An intramuscular dose of 0.01–0.02 mg/kg reliably provides an antisialagogue effect. Atropine should be used cautiously in patients with narrow-angle glaucoma, prostatic hypertrophy, or bladder-neck obstruction.

SCOPOLAMINE

Physical Structure

Scopolamine, a tertiary amine, differs from atropine by the addition of an epoxide to the heterocyclic ring.

Dosage & Packaging

The premedication dose of scopolamine is the same as that of atropine, and it is usually given intramuscularly. Scopolamine hydrobromide is available as solutions containing 0.3, 0.4, and 1 mg/mL.

Clinical Considerations

5 Scopolamine is a more potent antisialagogue than atropine and causes greater central nervous system effects. Clinical dosages usually result in drowsiness and amnesia, although restlessness, dizziness, and delirium are possible. The sedative effects may be desirable for premedication but can interfere with awakening following short procedures. Scopolamine has the added virtue of preventing motion sickness. The lipid solubility allows transdermal absorption, and transdermal scopolamine has been used to prevent postoperative nausea and vomiting. Because of its pronounced ocular effects, scopolamine is best avoided in patients with closed-angle glaucoma.

GLYCOPYRROLATE

Physical Structure

Glycopyrrolate is a synthetic product that differs from atropine in being a quaternary amine and having both cyclopentane and a pyridine moieties in the compound.

Dosage & Packaging

The usual dose of glycopyrrolate is one-half that of atropine. For instance, the premedication dose is 0.005–0.01 mg/kg up to 0.2–0.3 mg in adults. Glycopyrrolate for injection is packaged as a solution of 0.2 mg/mL.

Clinical Considerations

6 Because of its quaternary structure, glycopyrrolate cannot cross the blood–brain barrier and is almost devoid of central nervous system and ophthalmic activity. Potent inhibition of salivary gland and respiratory tract secretions is the primary rationale for using glycopyrrolate as a premedication. Heart rate usually increases after intravenous—but not intramuscular—administration. Glycopyrrolate has a longer duration of action than atropine (2–4 h vs 30 min after intravenous administration).

CASE DISCUSSION

Central Anticholinergic Syndrome

An elderly patient is scheduled for enucleation of a blind, painful eye. Scopolamine, 0.4 mg intramuscularly, is administered as premedication. In the preoperative holding area, the patient becomes agitated and disoriented. The only other medication the patient has received is 1% atropine eye drops.

How many milligrams of atropine are in one drop of a 1% solution?

A 1% solution contains 1 g dissolved in 100 mL, or 10 mg/mL. Eyedroppers vary in the number of drops formed per milliliter of solution, but average 20 drops/mL. Therefore, one drop usually contains 0.5 mg of atropine.

How are ophthalmic drops systemically absorbed?

Absorption by vessels in the conjunctival sac is similar to subcutaneous injection. More rapid absorption is possible by the nasolacrimal duct mucosa.

What are the signs and symptoms of anticholinergic poisoning?

Reactions from an overdose of anticholinergic medication involve several organ systems. The central anticholinergic syndrome refers to central nervous system changes that range from unconsciousness to hallucinations. Agitation and delirium are not unusual in elderly patients. Other systemic manifestations include dry mouth, tachycardia, atropine flush, atropine fever, and impaired vision.

What other drugs possess anticholinergic activity that could predispose patients to the central anticholinergic syndrome?

Tricyclic antidepressants, antihistamines, and antipsychotics have antimuscarinic properties that could potentiate the side effects of anticholinergic drugs.

What drug is an effective antidote to anticholinergic overdosage?

Cholinesterase inhibitors indirectly increase the amount of acetylcholine available to compete with anticholinergic drugs at the muscarinic receptor. Neostigmine, pyridostigmine, and edrophonium possess a quaternary ammonium group that prevents penetration of the blood–brain barrier. Physostigmine, a tertiary amine, is lipid soluble and effectively reverses central anticholinergic toxicity. An initial dose of 0.01–0.03 mg/kg may have to be repeated after 15–30 min.

Should this case be canceled or allowed to proceed?

Enucleation to relieve a painful eye is clearly an elective procedure. The most important question that must be addressed for elective cases is whether the patient is optimally medically managed. In other words, would canceling surgery allow further fine-tuning of any medical problems? For example, if this anticholinergic overdose were accompanied by tachycardia, it would probably be prudent to postpone surgery in this elderly patient. On the other hand, if the patient's mental status responds to physostigmine and there seems to be no other significant anticholinergic side effects, surgery could proceed.

SUGGESTED READING

Brown JH: Muscarinic receptor agonists and antagonists. In: *Goodman and Gilman's The Pharmacological Basis of Therapeutics*, 12th ed. Brunton LL (editor). McGraw-Hill, 2011.

Katzung BG (editor): Cholinoceptor-blocking drugs. In: *Basic and Clinical Pharmacology*, 11th ed. McGraw-Hill, 2009.

Adrenergic Agonists & Antagonists

1. Adrenergic agonists can be categorized as direct or indirect. Direct agonists bind to the receptor, whereas indirect agonists increase endogenous neurotransmitter activity.

2. The primary effect of phenylephrine is peripheral vasoconstriction with a concomitant rise in systemic vascular resistance and arterial blood pressure.

3. Clonidine seems to decrease anesthetic and analgesic requirements and to provide sedation and anxiolysis.

4. Dexmedetomidine is a lipophylic α-methylol derivative with a higher affinity for α_2-receptors than clonidine. It has sedative, analgesic, and sympatholytic effects that blunt many of the cardiovascular responses seen during the perioperative period.

5. Long-term use of these agents, particularly clonidine and dexmedetomidine, leads to supersensitization and up-regulation of receptors; with abrupt discontinuation of either drug, an acute withdrawal syndrome manifested by a hypertensive crisis can occur.

6. Ephedrine is commonly used as a vasopressor during anesthesia. As such, its administration should be viewed as a temporizing measure while the cause of hypotension is determined and remedied.

7. Small doses (approximately 2 mcg/kg/min) of dopamine (DA) have minimal adrenergic effects but activate dopaminergic receptors. Stimulation of these nonadrenergic receptors (specifically, DA_1 receptors) vasodilates the renal vasculature and promotes diuresis.

8. Favorable effects on myocardial oxygen balance are believed to make dobutamine a good choice for patients with the combination of congestive heart failure and coronary artery disease, particularly if peripheral vascular resistance is elevated. (There are some recent debates regarding this beneficial effect.)

9. Labetalol lowers blood pressure without reflex tachycardia because of its combination of α- and β-effects.

10. Esmolol is an ultrashort-acting selective β_1-antagonist that reduces heart rate and, to a lesser extent, blood pressure.

11. Discontinuation of β-blocker therapy for 24–48 hr may trigger a withdrawal syndrome characterized by hypertension, tachycardia, and angina pectoris.

Adrenergic agonists and antagonists produce their clinical effects by interacting with the adrenergic receptors (ie, adrenoceptors). The clinical effects of these drugs can be deduced from an understanding of the adrenoceptor physiology and a knowledge of which receptors each drug activates or blocks.

ADRENOCEPTOR PHYSIOLOGY

The term "adrenergic" originally referred to the effects of epinephrine (*adren*aline), although norepinephrine (noradrenaline) is the primary neurotransmitter responsible for most of the adrenergic activity of the sympathetic nervous system. With the exception of eccrine sweat glands and some blood vessels, norepinephrine is released by postganglionic sympathetic fibers at end-organ tissues (Figure 14–1). In contrast, acetylcholine is released by preganglionic sympathetic fibers and all parasympathetic fibers.

Norepinephrine is synthesized in the cytoplasm of sympathetic postganglionic nerve endings and stored in the vesicles (Figure 14–2). After release by a process of exocytosis, the action of norepinephrine is primarily terminated by reuptake into the postganglionic nerve ending (inhibited by tricyclic antidepressants), but also by diffusion from receptor sites, or via metabolism by monoamine oxidase (inhibited by monoamine oxidase inhibitors) and catechol-O-methyltransferase (Figure 14–3). Prolonged adrenergic activation leads to desensitization and hyporesponsiveness to further stimulation.

Adrenergic receptors are divided into two general categories: α and β. Each of these has been further subdivided into at least two subtypes: α_1 and α_2, and β_1, β_2, and β_3. The α-receptors have been further divided using molecular cloning techniques into α_{1A}, α_{1B}, α_{1D}, α_{2A}, α_{2B}, and α_{2C}. These receptors are linked to G proteins (Figure 14–4; Drs. Rodbell and Gilman received the Nobel Prize in physiology or medicine in 1994 for their discovery)—heterotrimeric receptors with α, β, and γ subunits. The different adrenoceptors are linked to specific G proteins, each with a unique effector, but each using guanosine triphosphate (GTP) as a cofactor. α_1 is linked to G_q, which activates phospholipases; α_2 is linked to

G_i, which inhibits adenylate cyclase, and β is linked to G_s, which activates adenylate cyclase.

α_1-Receptors

α_1-Receptors are postsynaptic adrenoceptors located in smooth muscle throughout the body (in the eye, lung, blood vessels, uterus, gut, and genitourinary system). Activation of these receptors increases intracellular calcium ion concentration, which leads to contraction of smooth muscles. Thus, α_1-agonists are associated with mydriasis (pupillary dilation due to contraction of the radial eye muscles), bronchoconstriction, vasoconstriction, uterine contraction, and constriction of sphincters in the gastrointestinal and genitourinary tracts. α_1-stimulation also inhibits insulin secretion and lipolysis. The myocardium possesses α_1-receptors that have a positive inotropic effect, which might play a role in catecholamine-induced arrhythmia. During myocardial ischemia, enhanced α_1-receptor coupling with agonists is observed. Nonetheless, the most important cardiovascular effect of α_1-stimulation is vasoconstriction, which increases peripheral vascular resistance, left ventricular afterload, and arterial blood pressure.

α_2-Receptors

In contrast to α_1-receptors, α_2-receptors are located primarily on the presynaptic nerve terminals. Activation of these adrenoceptors inhibits adenylate cyclase activity. This decreases the entry of calcium ions into the neuronal terminal, which limits subsequent exocytosis of storage vesicles containing norepinephrine. Thus, α_2-receptors create a negative feedback loop that inhibits further norepinephrine release from the neuron. In addition, vascular smooth muscle contains postsynaptic α_2-receptors that produce vasoconstriction. More importantly, stimulation of postsynaptic α_2-receptors in the central nervous system causes sedation and reduces sympathetic outflow, which leads to peripheral vasodilation and lower blood pressure.

β_1-Receptors

β-Adrenergic receptors are classified into β_1, β_2, and β_3 receptors. The catecholamines, norepinephrine,

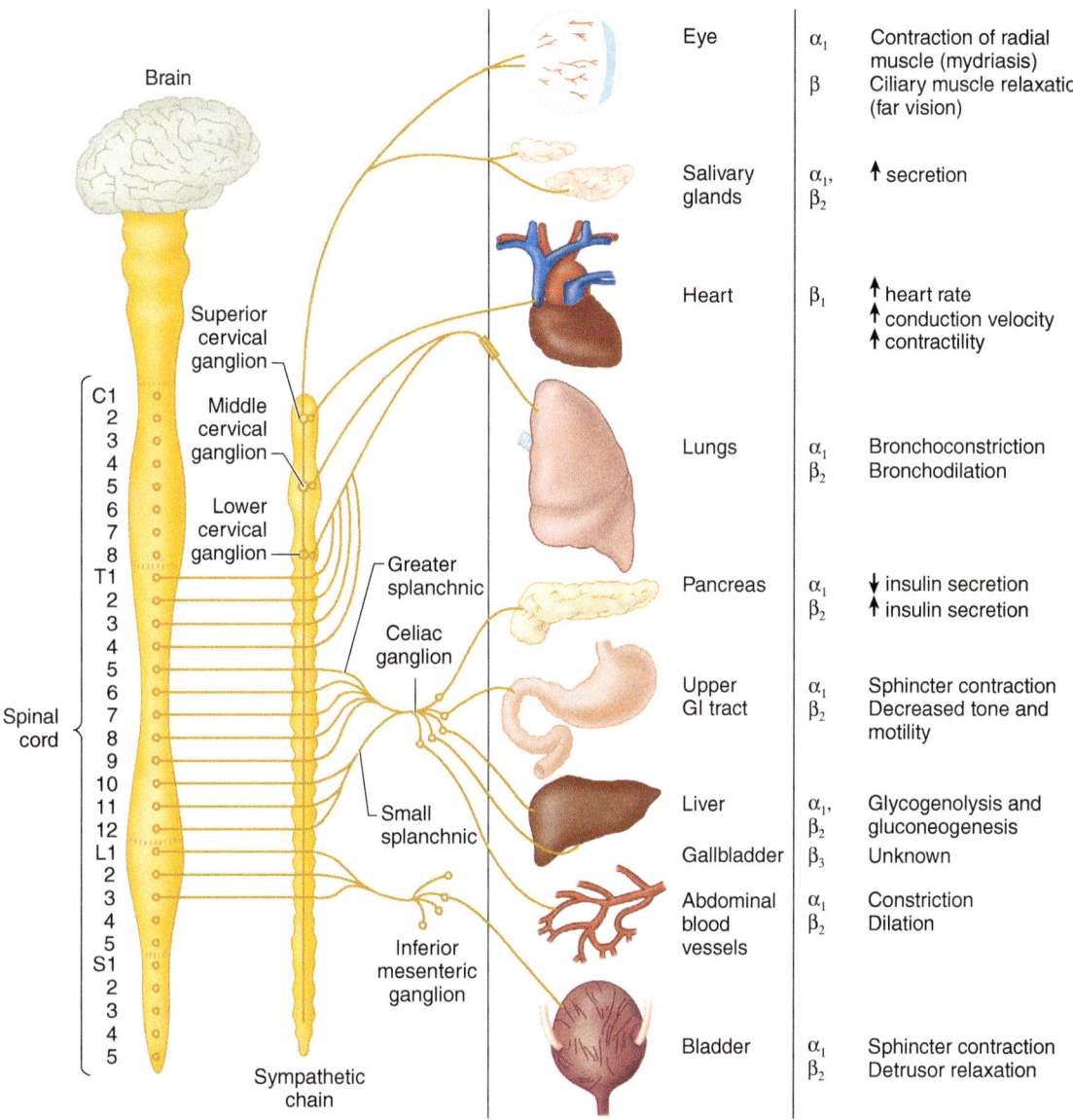

Eye	α_1	Contraction of radial muscle (mydriasis)	
	β	Ciliary muscle relaxation (far vision)	
Salivary glands	α_1, β_2	↑ secretion	
Heart	β_1	↑ heart rate ↑ conduction velocity ↑ contractility	
Lungs	α_1 β_2	Bronchoconstriction Bronchodilation	
Pancreas	α_1 β_2	↓ insulin secretion ↑ insulin secretion	
Upper GI tract	α_1 β_2	Sphincter contraction Decreased tone and motility	
Liver	α_1, β_2	Glycogenolysis and gluconeogenesis	
Gallbladder	β_3	Unknown	
Abdominal blood vessels	α_1 β_2	Constriction Dilation	
Bladder	α_1 β_2	Sphincter contraction Detrusor relaxation	

FIGURE 14–1 The sympathetic nervous system. Organ innervation, receptor type, and response to stimulation. The origin of the sympathetic chain is the thoracoabdominal (T1–L3) spinal cord, in contrast to the craniosacral distribution of the parasympathetic nervous system. Another anatomic difference is the greater distance from the sympathetic ganglion to the visceral structures.

and epinephrine are equipotent on β_1 receptors, but epinephrine is significantly more potent than norepinephrine on β_2 receptors.

The most important β_1-receptors are located on the postsynaptic membranes in the heart. Stimulation of these receptors activates adenylate cyclase, which converts adenosine triphosphate to cyclic adenosine monophosphate and initiates a kinase phosphorylation cascade. Initiation of the cascade has positive chronotropic (increased heart

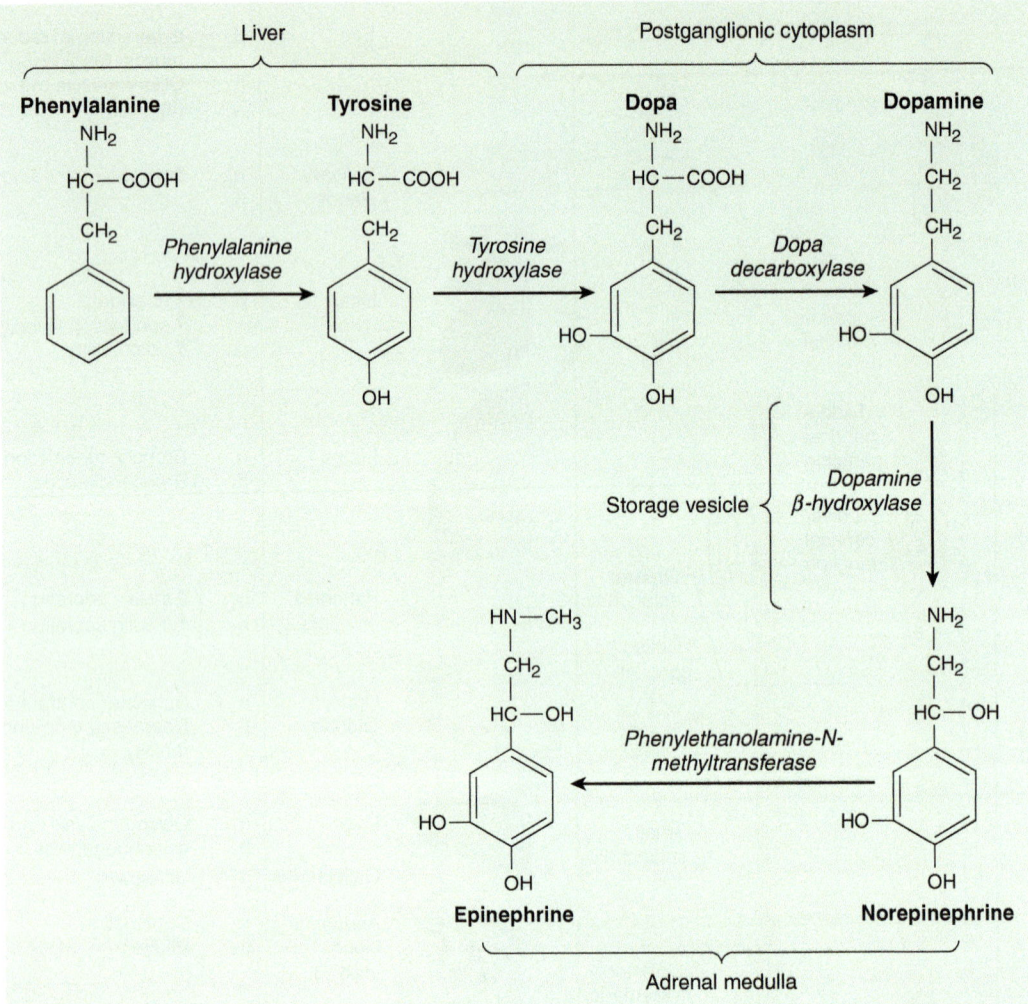

FIGURE 14–2 The synthesis of norepinephrine. Hydroxylation of tyrosine to dopa is the rate-limiting step. Dopamine is actively transported into storage vesicles. Norepinephrine can be converted to epinephrine in the adrenal medulla.

rate), dromotropic (increased conduction), and inotropic (increased contractility) effects.

β₂-Receptors

β_2-Receptors are primarily postsynaptic adrenoceptors located in smooth muscle and gland cells. They share a common mechanism of action with β_1-receptors: adenylate cyclase activation. Despite this commonality, β_2 stimulation relaxes smooth muscle, resulting in bronchodilation, vasodilation, and relaxation of the uterus (tocolysis), bladder, and

gut. Glycogenolysis, lipolysis, gluconeogenesis, and insulin release are stimulated by β_2-receptor activation. β_2-agonists also activate the sodium–potassium pump, which drives potassium intracellularly and can induce hypokalemia and dysrhythmias.

β₃-Receptors

β_3-Receptors are found in the gallbladder and brain adipose tissue. Their role in gallbladder physiology is unknown, but they are thought to play a role in lipolysis and thermogenesis in brown fat.

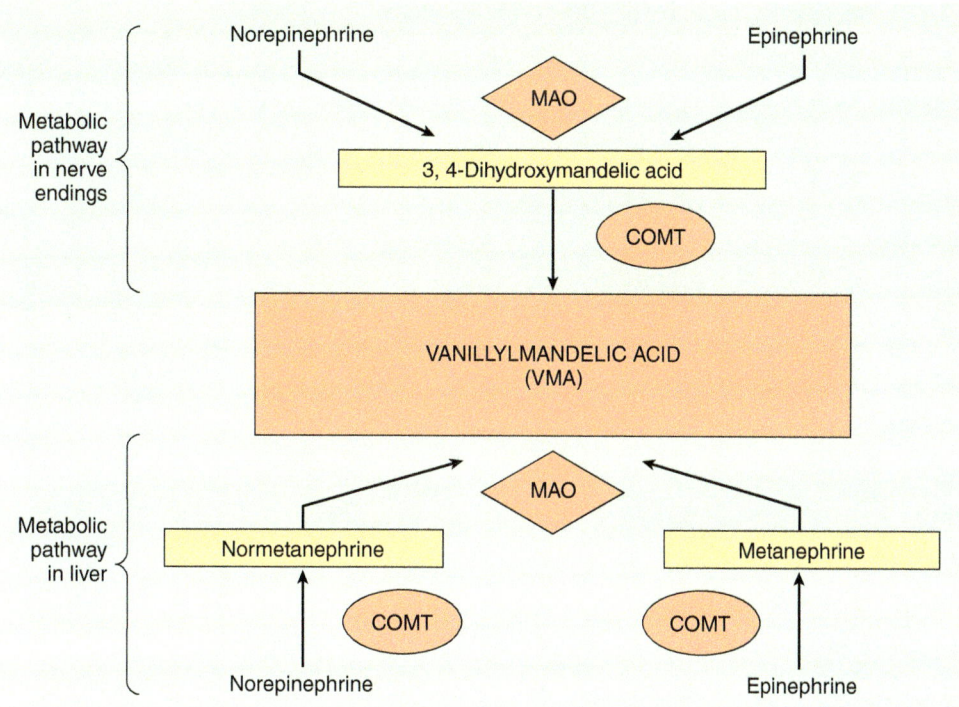

FIGURE 14–3 Sequential metabolism of norepinephrine and epinephrine. Monoamine oxidase (MAO) and catechol-*O*-methyltransferase (COMT) produce a common end product, vanillylmandelic acid (VMA).

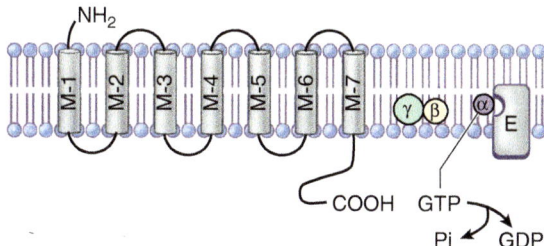

FIGURE 14–4 The adrenoceptor is a transmembrane-spanning receptor made up of seven subunits, which is linked to a G protein. G proteins are trimeric endoplasmic membrane proteins made of α, β, and γ units. With activation, GTP on the α-subunit is replaced by GDP, stimulating a conformational change, disassociating the α, β, and γ units. Either the Gα or Gβγ subunits can activate (or inhibit) the enzyme effector for that adrenoceptor. M1–M7, membrane-spanning units; α, β, γ, subunits of G protein; GTP, guanosine triphosphate; P_i, inorganic phosphate—quickly assimilated; GDP, guanosine diphosphate; E, effector; cyclophosphatase for G_q, adenylate cyclase for G_i and G_s.

Dopaminergic Receptors

Dopamine (DA) receptors are a group of adrenergic receptors that are activated by dopamine; these receptors are classified as D_1 and D_2 receptors. Activation of D_1 receptors mediates vasodilation in the kidney, intestine, and heart. D_2 receptors are believed to play a role in the antiemetic action of droperidol.

Adrenergic Agonists

Adrenergic agonists interact with varying specificity (selectivity) at α- and β-adrenoceptors (Tables 14–1 and 14–2).

Overlapping of activity complicates the prediction of clinical effects. For example, epinephrine stimulates α_1-, α_2-, β_1-, and β_2-adrenoceptors. Its net effect on arterial blood pressure depends on the balance between α_1-vasoconstriction, α_2- and

TABLE 14–1 Receptor selectivity of adrenergic agonists.[1]

Drug	α_1	α_2	β_1	β_2	DA_1	DA_2
Phenylephrine	+++	+	0	0	0	0
Methyldopa	+	+	0	0	0	0
Clonidine	+	++	0	0	0	0
Dexmedetomidine	+	+++	0	0	0	0
Epinephrine[2]	++	++	+++	++	0	0
Ephedrine[3]	++	?	++	+	0	0
Fenoldopam	0	0	0	0	+++	0
Norepinephrine[2]	++	++	++	0	0	0
Dopamine[2]	++	++	++	+	+++	+++
Dopexamine	0	0	+	+++	++	+++
Dobutamine	0/+	0	+++	+	0	0
Terbutaline	0	0	+	+++	0	0

[1]0, no effect; +, agonist effect (mild, moderate, marked); ?, unknown effect; DA_1 and DA_2, dopaminergic receptors.
[2]The α_1-effects of epinephrine, norepinephrine, and dopamine become more prominent at high doses.
[3]The primary mode of action of ephedrine is indirect stimulation.

β_2-vasodilation, and β_1-inotropic influences. Moreover, this balance changes at different doses.

① Adrenergic agonists can be categorized as direct or indirect. Direct agonists bind to the receptor, whereas indirect agonists increase endogenous neurotransmitter activity. Mechanisms of indirect action include increased release or decreased reuptake of norepinephrine. The differentiation between direct and indirect mechanisms of action is particularly important in patients who

TABLE 14–2 Effects of adrenergic agonists on organ systems.[1]

Drug	Heart Rate	Mean Arterial Pressure	Cardiac Output	Peripheral Vascular Resistance	Bronchodilation	Renal Blood Flow
Phenylephrine	↓	↑↑↑	↓	↑↑↑	0	↓↓↓
Epinephrine	↑↑	↑	↑↑	↑/↓	↑↑	↓↓
Ephedrine	↑↑	↑↑	↑↑	↑	↑↑	↓↓
Fenoldopam	↑↑	↓↓↓	↓/↑	↓↓	0	↑↑↑
Norepinephrine	↓	↑↑↑	↓/↑	↑↑↑	0	↓↓↓
Dopamine	↑/↑↑	↑	↑↑↑	↑	0	↑↑↑
Dopexamine	↑/↑↑	↓/↑	↑↑	↑	0	↑
Isoproterenol	↑↑↑	↓	↑↑↑	↓↓	↑↑↑	↓/↑
Dobutamine	↑	↑	↑↑↑	↓	0	↑

[1]0, no effect; ↑, increase (mild, moderate, marked); ↓, decrease (mild, moderate, marked); ↓/↑, variable effect; ↑/↑↑, mild-to-moderate increase.

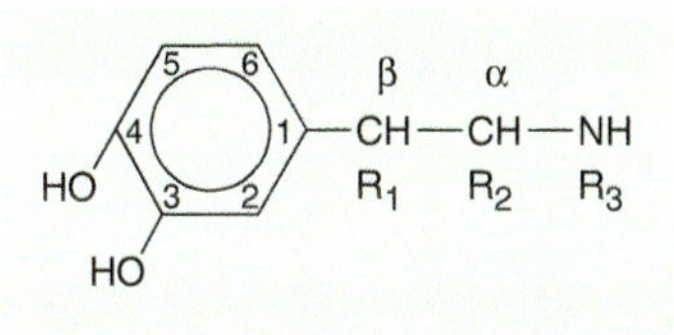

FIGURE 14–5 Adrenergic agonists that have a 3,4-dihydroxybenzene structure are known as catecholamines. Substitutions at the R_1, R_2, and R_3 sites affect activity and selectivity.

have abnormal endogenous norepinephrine stores, as may occur with use of some antihypertensive medications or monoamine oxidase inhibitors. Intraoperative hypotension in these patients should be treated with direct agonists, as their response to indirect agonists will be altered.

Another feature distinguishing adrenergic agonists from each other is their chemical structure. Adrenergic agonists that have a 3,4-dihydroxybenzene structure (Figure 14–5) are known as catecholamines. These drugs are typically short-acting because of their metabolism by monoamine oxidase and catechol-O-methyltransferase. Patients taking monoamine oxidase inhibitors or tricyclic antidepressants may therefore demonstrate an exaggerated response to catecholamines. The naturally occurring catecholamines are epinephrine, norepinephrine, and DA. Changing the side-chain structure (R_1, R_2, R_3) of naturally occurring catecholamines has led to the development of synthetic catecholamines (eg, isoproterenol and dobutamine), which tend to be more receptor specific.

Adrenergic agonists commonly used in anesthesiology are discussed individually below. Note that the recommended doses for continuous infusion are expressed as mcg/kg/min for some agents and mcg/min for others. In either case, these recommendations should be regarded only as guidelines, as individual responses are quite variable.

PHENYLEPHRINE
Clinical Considerations

Phenylephrine is a noncatecholamine with predominantly selective α_1-agonist activity. The primary effect of phenylephrine is peripheral

vasoconstriction with a concomitant rise in systemic vascular resistance and arterial blood pressure. Reflex bradycardia mediated by the vagus nerve can reduce cardiac output. Phenylephrine is also used topically as a decongestant and a mydriatic agent.

Dosing & Packaging

Small intravenous boluses of 50–100 μg (0.5–1 mcg/kg) of phenylephrine rapidly reverse reductions in blood pressure caused by peripheral vasodilation (eg, spinal anesthesia). The duration of action is short, lasting approximately 15 min after administration of a single dose. A continuous infusion (100 mcg/mL at a rate of 0.25–1 mcg/kg/min) will maintain arterial blood pressure, but at the expense of renal blood flow. Tachyphylaxis occurs with phenylephrine infusions requiring upward titration of the infusion. Phenylephrine must be diluted from a 1% solution (10 mg/1-mL ampule), usually to a 100 mcg/mL solution.

α_2-AGONISTS
Clinical Considerations

Clonidine is an α_2-agonist that is commonly used for its antihypertensive and negative chronotropic effects. More recently, it and other α_2-agonists are increasingly being used for their sedative properties. Various studies have examined the anesthetic effects of oral (3–5 mcg/kg), intramuscular (2 mcg/kg), intravenous (1–3 mcg/kg), transdermal (0.1–0.3 mg released per day), intrathecal (75–150 mcg), and epidural (1–2 mcg/kg) clonidine administration. In general, clonidine seems to decrease anesthetic and analgesic requirements (decreases minimum alveolar concentration) and provides sedation and anxiolysis. During general anesthesia, clonidine reportedly enhances intraoperative circulatory stability by reducing catecholamine levels. During regional anesthesia, including peripheral nerve block, clonidine prolongs the duration of the block. Direct effects on the spinal cord may be mediated by α_2-postsynaptic receptors within the dorsal horn. Other possible benefits include decreased postoperative shivering, inhibition of opioid-induced muscle rigidity, attenuation of opioid withdrawal symptoms, and the treatment of some chronic pain syndromes. Side effects include bradycardia, hypotension, sedation, respiratory depression, and dry mouth.

4 Dexmedetomidine is a lipophylic α-methylol derivative with a higher affinity for α_2-receptors than clonidine. Compared with clonidine, dexmedetomidine is more selective to α_2-receptors ($\alpha_2:\alpha_1$ specificity ratio is 200:1 for clonidine and 1600:1 for dexmedetomidine). Dexmedetomidine has a shorter half-life (2–3 h) than clonidine (12–24 h). It has sedative, analgesic, and sympatholytic effects that blunt many of the cardiovascular responses seen during the perioperative period. The sedative and analgesic effects are mediated by α_2-adrenergic receptors in the brain (locus ceruleus) and spinal cord. When used intraoperatively, dexmedetomidine reduces intravenous and volatile anesthetic requirements; when used postoperatively, it reduces concurrent analgesic and sedative requirements. Dexmedetomidine is useful in sedating patients in preparation for awake fiberoptic intubation. It is also a useful agent for sedating patients postoperatively in postanesthesia and intensive care units, because it does so without significant ventilatory depression. Rapid administration may elevate blood pressure, but hypotension and bradycardia can occur during ongoing therapy. The recommended dosing of dexmedetomidine consists of a loading dose at 1 mcg/kg over 10 min followed by an infusion at 0.2–0.7 mcg/kg/hr.

Although these agents are adrenergic agonists, they are also considered to be sympatholytic because **5** sympathetic outflow is reduced. Long-term use of these agents, particularly clonidine and dexmedetomidine, leads to supersensitization and up-regulation of receptors; with abrupt discontinuation of either drug, an acute withdrawal syndrome manifested by a hypertensive crisis can occur. Because of the increased affinity of dexmedetomidine for the α_2-receptor, compared with that of clonidine, this syndrome may manifest after only 48 hr of dexmedetomidine use when the drug is discontinued.

Dosing & Packaging

Clonidine is available as an oral, transdermal, or parenteral preparation. Dexmedetomidine is available as an injectable solution (100 mcg/mL), which should be diluted to 5–10 mcg/mL for bolus administration and titrated to effect.

EPINEPHRINE

Clinical Considerations

Epinephrine is an endogenous catecholamine synthesized in the adrenal medulla. Direct stimulation of β_1-receptors of the myocardium by epinephrine raises blood pressure, cardiac output, and myocardial oxygen demand by increasing contractility and heart rate (increased rate of spontaneous phase IV depolarization). α_1-stimulation decreases splanchnic and renal blood flow but increases coronary perfusion pressure by increasing aortic diastolic pressure. Systolic blood pressure rises, although β_2-mediated vasodilation in skeletal muscle may lower diastolic pressure. β_2-stimulation also relaxes bronchial smooth muscle.

Administration of epinephrine is the principal pharmacological treatment for anaphylaxis and can be used to treat ventricular fibrillation. Complications include cerebral hemorrhage, coronary ischemia, and ventricular dysrhythmias. Volatile anesthetics, particularly halothane, potentiate the dysrhythmic effects of epinephrine.

Dosing & Packaging

In emergency situations (eg, cardiac arrest and shock), epinephrine is administered as an intravenous bolus of 0.05–1 mg, depending on the severity of cardiovascular compromise. In major anaphylactic reactions, epinephrine should be used at a dose of 100–500 mcg (repeated, if necessary) followed by infusion. To improve myocardial contractility or heart rate, a continuous infusion is prepared (1 mg in 250 mL [4 mcg/mL]) and run at a rate of 2–20 mcg/min. Epinephrine is also used to reduce bleeding from the operative sites. Some local anesthetic solutions containing epinephrine at a concentration of 1:200,000 (5 mcg/mL) or 1:400,000 (2.5 mcg/mL) are characterized by less systemic absorption and a longer duration of action. Epinephrine is available in vials at a concentration of 1:1000 (1 mg/mL) and prefilled syringes at a concentration of 1:10,000 (0.1 mg/mL [100 mcg/mL]). A 1:100,000 (10 mcg/mL) concentration is available for pediatric use.

EPHEDRINE
Clinical Considerations

The cardiovascular effects of ephedrine, a noncatecholamine sympathomimetic, are similar to those of epinephrine: increase in blood pressure, heart rate, contractility, and cardiac output. Likewise, ephedrine is also a bronchodilator. There are important differences, however: ephedrine has a longer duration of action, is much less potent, has indirect and direct actions, and stimulates the central nervous system (it raises minimum alveolar concentration). The indirect agonist properties of ephedrine may be due to peripheral postsynaptic norepinephrine release, or by inhibition of norepinephrine reuptake.

6 Ephedrine is commonly used as a vasopressor during anesthesia. As such, its administration should be viewed as a temporizing measure while the cause of hypotension is determined and remedied. Unlike direct-acting α_1-agonists, ephedrine is believed not to decrease uterine blood flow, and thus was regarded as the preferred vasopressor for most obstetric uses. Recently, however, phenylephrine has been argued to be a better vasopressor in obstetric patients undergoing neuroaxial anesthesia due its faster onset, shorter duration of action, and better titratability and maintenance of fetal pH. Ephedrine has also been reported to possess antiemetic properties, particularly in association with hypotension following spinal anesthesia. Clonidine premedication augments the effects of ephedrine.

Dosing & Packaging

In adults, ephedrine is administered as a bolus of 2.5–10 mg; in children, it is given as a bolus of 0.1 mg/kg. Subsequent doses are increased to offset the development of tachyphylaxis, which is probably due to depletion of norepinephrine stores. Ephedrine is available in 1-mL ampules containing 25 or 50 mg of the agent.

NOREPINEPHRINE
Clinical Considerations

Direct α_1-stimulation with little β_2-activity induces intense vasoconstriction of arterial and venous vessels. Increased myocardial contractility from β_1-effects, along with peripheral vasoconstriction, contributes to a rise in arterial blood pressure. Both systolic and diastolic pressures usually rise, but increased afterload and reflex bradycardia prevent any elevation in cardiac output. Decreased renal and splanchnic blood flow and increased myocardial oxygen requirements limit the outcome benefits of norepinephrine in the management of refractory shock. Norepinephrine has been used with an α-blocker (eg, phentolamine) in an attempt to take advantage of its β-activity without the profound vasoconstriction caused by its α-stimulation. Extravasation of norepinephrine at the site of intravenous administration can cause tissue necrosis.

Dosing & Packaging

Norepinephrine is administered as a bolus (0.1 mcg/kg) or usually as a continuous infusion due to its short half-life at a rate of 2–20 mcg/min. Ampules contain 4 mg of norepinephrine in 4 mL of solution.

DOPAMINE
Clinical Considerations

The clinical effects of DA, an endogenous nonselective direct and indirect adrenergic and dopaminergic agonist, vary markedly with the dose. At

7 low doses (0.5–3 mcg/kg/min), DA primarily activates dopaminergic receptors (specifically, DA_1 receptors); stimulation of these receptors vasodilates the renal vasculature and promotes diuresis and natriuresis. Although this action increases renal blood flow, use of this "renal dose" does not impart any beneficial effect on renal function. When used in moderate doses (3–10 mcg/kg/min), β_1-stimulation increases myocardial contractility, heart rate, systolic blood pressure, and cardiac output. Myocardial oxygen demand typically increases more than supply. The α_1-effects become prominent at higher doses (10–20 mcg/kg/min), causing an increase in peripheral vascular resistance and a fall in renal blood flow. The indirect effects of DA are due to release of norepinephrine from presynaptic sympathetic nerve ganglion.

DA is commonly used in the treatment of shock to improve cardiac output, support blood pressure, and maintain renal function. It is often used in combination with a vasodilator (eg, nitroglycerin or nitroprusside), which reduces afterload and further improves cardiac output. The chronotropic and proarrhythmic effects of DA limit its usefulness in some patients.

Dosing & Packaging

DA is administered as a continuous infusion at a rate of 1–20 mcg/kg/min. It is most commonly supplied in 5–10 mL vials containing 200 or 400 mg of DA.

ISOPROTERENOL

Isoproterenol is of interest because it is a pure β-agonist. $β_1$-Effects increase heart rate, contractility, and cardiac output. Systolic blood pressure may increase or remain unchanged, but $β_2$-stimulation decreases peripheral vascular resistance and diastolic blood pressure. Myocardial oxygen demand increases while oxygen supply falls, making isoproterenol or any pure β-agonist a poor inotropic choice in most situations.

DOBUTAMINE

Clinical Considerations

Dobutamine is a racemic mixture of two isomers with affinity for both $β_1$ and $β_2$ receptors, with relatively higher selectivity for $β_1$ receptors. Its primary cardiovascular effect is a rise in cardiac output as a result of increased myocardial contractility. A decline in peripheral vascular resistance caused by $β_2$-activation usually prevents much of a rise in arterial blood pressure. Left ventricular filling pressure decreases, whereas coronary blood flow increases. Favorable effects on myocardial oxygen balance are believed to make dobutamine a choice for patients with the combination of congestive heart failure and coronary artery disease, particularly if peripheral vascular resistance is elevated. However, because it has been shown to increase myocardial oxygen consumption, such as during stress testing (rationale for its use in perfusion imaging), some concern remains regarding its use in patients with myocardial ischemia. Moreover, dobutamine should not be routinely used without specific indications to facilitate separation from cardiopulmonary bypass.

Dosing & Packaging

Dobutamine is administered as an infusion at a rate of 2–20 mcg/kg/min. It is supplied in 20-mL vials containing 250 mg.

DOPEXAMINE

Clinical Considerations

Dopexamine, a structural analogue of DA, has potential advantages over DA because it has less $β_1$-adrenergic (arrhythmogenic) and α-adrenergic effects. Because of the decreased β-adrenergic effects and its specific effect on renal perfusion, it may have advantages over dobutamine. The drug has been clinically available in many countries since 1990, but has not gained widespread acceptance in practice.

Dosing & Packaging

Dopexamine infusion should be started at a rate of 0.5 mcg/kg/min, increasing to 1 mcg/kg/min at intervals of 10–15 min to a maximum infusion rate of 6 mcg/kg/min.

FENOLDOPAM

Clinical Considerations

Fenoldopam is a selective D_1-receptor agonist that has many of the benefits of DA but with little or no α- or β-adrenoceptor or D_2-receptor agonist activity. Fenoldopam has been shown to exert hypotensive effects characterized by a decrease in peripheral vascular resistance, along with an increase in renal blood flow, diuresis, and natriuresis. It is indicated for patients undergoing cardiac surgery and aortic aneurysm repair with potential risk of perioperative renal impairment. Fenoldopam exerts an antihypertensive effect, but helps to maintain renal blood flow. It is also indicated for patients who have severe hypertension, particularly those with renal impairment. Along with its recommended use in hypertensive emergencies, fenoldopam is also indicated in the prevention of contrast media-induced nephropathy. Fenoldopam has a fairly rapid onset of action and is easily titratable because of its short elimination half-life. The ability of fenoldopam to "protect" the kidney perioperatively remains the subject of ongoing studies.

Dosing & Packaging

Fenoldopam is supplied in 1-, 2-, and 5-mL ampules, 10 mg/mL. It is started as a continuous infusion of 0.1 mcg/kg/min, increased by increments of 0.1 mcg/kg/min at 15- to 20-min intervals until target blood pressure is achieved. Lower doses have been associated with less reflex tachycardia.

Adrenergic Antagonists

Adrenergic antagonists bind but do not activate adrenoceptors. They act by preventing adrenergic agonist activity. Like the agonists, the antagonists differ in their spectrum of receptor interaction.

α-BLOCKERS—PHENTOLAMINE

Clinical Considerations

Phentolamine produces a competitive (reversible) blockade of both α_1- and α_2- receptors. α_1-Antagonism and direct smooth muscle relaxation are responsible for peripheral vasodilation and a decline in arterial blood pressure. The drop in blood pressure provokes reflex tachycardia. This tachycardia is augmented by antagonism of presynaptic α_2-receptors in the heart because α_2-blockade promotes norepinephrine release by eliminating negative feedback. These cardiovascular effects are usually apparent within 2 min and last up to 15 min. As with all of the adrenergic antagonists, the extent of the response to receptor blockade depends on the degree of existing sympathetic tone. Reflex tachycardia and postural hypotension limit the usefulness of phentolamine to the treatment of hypertension caused by excessive α-stimulation (eg, pheochromocytoma, clonidine withdrawal). Prazosin and phenoxybenzamine are examples of other alpha antagonists.

Dosing & Packaging

Phentolamine is administered intravenously as intermittent boluses (1–5 mg in adults) or as a continuous infusion. To prevent tissue necrosis following extravasation of intravenous fluids containing an α-agonist (eg, norepinephrine), 5–10 mg of phentolamine in 10 mL of normal saline can be locally infiltrated. Phentolamine is packaged as a lyophilized powder (5 mg).

MIXED ANTAGONISTS—LABETALOL

Clinical Considerations

Labetalol blocks α_1-, β_1-, and β_2-receptors. The ratio of α-blockade to β-blockade has been estimated to be approximately 1:7 following intravenous administration. This mixed blockade reduces peripheral vascular resistance and arterial blood pressure. Heart rate and cardiac output are usually slightly depressed or unchanged. Thus, labetalol lowers blood pressure without reflex tachycardia because of its combination of α- and β-effects, which is beneficial to patients with coronary artery disease. Peak effect usually occurs within 5 min after an intravenous dose. Left ventricular failure, paradoxical hypertension, and bronchospasm have been reported.

Dosing & Packaging

The initial recommended dose of labetalol is 2.5–10 mg administered intravenously over 2 min. Twice this amount may be given at 10-min intervals until the desired blood pressure response is obtained. Labetalol can also be administered as a slow continuous infusion at a rate of 0.5–2 mg/min. However, due to its long elimination half-life (>5 h), prolonged infusions are not recommended.

β-BLOCKERS

β-Receptor blockers have variable degrees of selectivity for the β_1-receptors. Those that are more β_1 selective have less influence on bronchopulmonary and vascular β_2-receptors (Table 14–3). Theoretically, a selective β_1-blocker would have less of an inhibitory effect on β_2-receptors and, therefore, might be preferred in patients with chronic obstructive lung disease or peripheral vascular disease. Patients with peripheral vascular disease could potentially have a decrease in blood flow if β_2-receptors, which dilate the arterioles, are blocked. β-Receptor blocking agents also reduce intraocular pressure in patients with glaucoma.

TABLE 14–3 Pharmacology of β-blockers.[1]

	Selectivity for β_1-Receptors	ISA	α-Blockade	Hepatic Metabolism	$t_{1/2}$
Atenolol	+	0	0	0	6–7
Esmolol	+	0	0	0	–¼
Labetalol	0	0	+	+	4
Metoprolol	+	0	0	+	3–4
Propranolol	0	0	0	+	4–6

[1]ISA, intrinsic sympathomimetic activity; +, mild effect; 0, no effect.

β-Blockers are also classified by the amount of intrinsic sympathomimetic activity (ISA) they have. Many of the β-blockers have some agonist activity; although they would not produce effects similar to full agonists (such as epinephrine), β-blockers with ISA may not be as beneficial as β-blockers without ISA in treating patients with cardiovascular disease.

β-Blockers can be further classified as those that are eliminated by hepatic metabolism (such as metoprolol), those that are excreted by the kidneys unchanged (such as atenolol), or those that are hydrolyzed in the blood (such as esmolol).

ESMOLOL

Clinical Considerations

10 Esmolol is an ultrashort-acting selective β_1-antagonist that reduces heart rate and, to a lesser extent, blood pressure. It has been successfully used to prevent tachycardia and hypertension in response to perioperative stimuli, such as intubation, surgical stimulation, and emergence. For example, esmolol (0.5–1 mg/kg) attenuates the rise in blood pressure and heart rate that usually accompanies electroconvulsive therapy, without significantly affecting seizure duration. Esmolol is as effective as propranolol in controlling the ventricular rate of patients with atrial fibrillation or flutter. Although esmolol is considered to be cardioselective, at higher doses it inhibits β_2-receptors in bronchial and vascular smooth muscle.

The short duration of action of esmolol is due to rapid redistribution (distribution half-life is 2 min) and hydrolysis by red blood cell esterase (elimination half-life is 9 min). Side effects can be reversed within minutes by discontinuing its infusion. As with all β_1-antagonists, esmolol should be avoided in patients with sinus bradycardia, heart block greater than first degree, cardiogenic shock, or overt heart failure.

Dosing & Packaging

Esmolol is administered as a bolus (0.2–0.5 mg/kg) for short-term therapy, such as attenuating the cardiovascular response to laryngoscopy and intubation. Long-term treatment is typically initiated with a loading dose of 0.5 mg/kg administered over 1 min, followed by a continuous infusion of 50 mcg/kg/min to maintain therapeutic effect. If this fails to produce a sufficient response within 5 min, the loading dose may be repeated and the infusion increased by increments of 50 mcg/kg/min every 5 min to a maximum of 200 mcg/kg/min.

Esmolol is supplied as multidose vials for bolus administration containing 10 mL of drug (10 mg/mL). Ampules for continuous infusion (2.5 g in 10 mL) are also available but must be diluted prior to administration to a concentration of 10 mg/mL.

METOPROLOL

Clinical Considerations

Metoprolol is a selective β_1-antagonist with no intrinsic sympathomimetic activity. It is available for both oral and intravenous use. It can be administered intravenously in 2–5 mg increments every 2 to 5 min, titrated to blood pressure and heart rate.

PROPRANOLOL

Clinical Considerations

Propranolol nonselectively blocks β_1- and β_2-receptors. Arterial blood pressure is lowered by several mechanisms, including decreased myocardial contractility, lowered heart rate, and diminished renin release. Cardiac output and myocardial oxygen demand are reduced. Propranolol is particularly useful during myocardial ischemia related to increased blood pressure and heart rate. Impedance of ventricular ejection is beneficial in patients with obstructive cardiomyopathy and aortic aneurysm. Propranolol slows atrioventricular conduction and stabilizes myocardial membranes, although the latter effect may not be significant at clinical doses. Propranolol is particularly effective in slowing the ventricular response to supraventricular tachycardia, and it occasionally controls recurrent ventricular tachycardia or fibrillation caused by myocardial ischemia. Propranolol blocks the β-adrenergic effects of thyrotoxicosis and pheochromocytoma.

Side effects of propranolol include bronchospasm (β_2-antagonism), congestive heart failure, bradycardia, and atrioventricular heart block (β_1-antagonism). Propranolol may worsen the myocardial depression of volatile anesthetics (eg, halothane) or unmask the negative inotropic characteristics of indirect cardiac stimulants (eg, isoflurane). Concomitant administration of propranolol and verapamil (a calcium channel blocker) can synergistically depress heart rate, contractility, and atrioventricular node conduction.

Propranolol is extensively protein bound and is cleared by hepatic metabolism. Its elimination half-life of 100 min is quite long compared with that of esmolol.

Dosing & Packaging

Individual dosage requirements of propranolol depend on baseline sympathetic tone. Generally, propranolol is titrated to the desired effect, beginning with 0.5 mg and progressing by 0.5-mg increments every 3–5 min. Total doses rarely exceed 0.15 mg/kg. Propranolol is supplied in 1-mL ampules containing 1 mg.

NEBIVOLOL

Clinical Considerations

Nebivolol is a newer generation β-blocker with high affinity for β_1-receptors. The drug is unique in its ability to cause direct vasodilation via its stimulatory effect on endothelial nitric oxide synthase. It is presently available only in oral formulation; the recommended dose is 5–40 mg daily.

CARVEDILOL

Carvedilol is a mixed β- and α-blocker used in the management of chronic heart failure secondary to cardiomyopathy, left ventricular dysfunction following acute myocardial infarction, and hypertension. Carvedilol dosage is individualized and gradually increased up to 25 mg twice daily, as required and tolerated.

PERIOPERATIVE β-BLOCKER THERAPY

Management of β-blockers perioperatively is a key anesthesia performance indicator and is closely monitored by various "quality management" agencies. Although studies regarding the perioperative administration of β-blockers have yielded conflicting results as to benefit, maintenance of β-blockers in patients already being treated with them is essential, unless contraindicated by other clinical concerns.

β-Blocker therapy in the perioperative period has the potential to reduce the perioperative cardiovascular complications (myocardial ischemia, stroke, cardiac failure) due to counteraction of catecholamine-induced tachycardia and hypertension. However, these beneficial effects have not been widely demonstrated in recent clinical trials. Perioperative β-blocker therapy was associated with a reduced risk of in-hospital death in a small group of high-risk patients (ie, those with a Revised Cardiac Score Index of 3 or higher), but showed no improvement or even an increase in stroke and overall mortality in low-risk patients undergoing noncardiac surgery.

Current American Heart Association/American College of Cardiology guidelines recommend continuation of β-blocker therapy during the perioperative period in patients who are receiving β-blockers for the treatment of angina, symptomatic arrhythmia, heart failure, and hypertension. In addition, β-blocker therapy should be initiated in patients undergoing vascular surgery who are at high risk of cardiac events because of findings of myocardial ischemia during perioperative testing. The guidelines also note that β-blockers titrated to heart rate and blood pressure are "reasonable" in patients undergoing vascular surgery who have more than one cardiac risk factor. Additionally, the guidelines suggest that perioperative β-blockers are likewise "reasonable" in patients undergoing intermediate-risk procedures who have more than one cardiac disease risk factor. The routine administration of high-dose β-blockers in the absence of dose titration may be harmful in patients not currently taking β-blockers who are undergoing noncardiac surgery.

(11) Discontinuation of β-blocker therapy for 24–48 hr may trigger a withdrawal syndrome characterized by hypertension (rebound hypertension), tachycardia, and angina pectoris. This effect seems to be caused by an increase in the number of β-adrenergic receptors (up-regulation).

CASE DISCUSSION

Pheochromocytoma

A 45-year-old man with a history of paroxysmal attacks of headache, hypertension, sweating, and palpitations is scheduled for resection of an abdominal pheochromocytoma.

What is a pheochromocytoma?

A pheochromocytoma is a vascular tumor of chromaffin tissue (most commonly the adrenal medulla) that produces and secretes norepinephrine and epinephrine. The diagnosis and management of pheochromocytoma are based on the effects of abnormally high circulating levels of these endogenous adrenergic agonists.

How is the diagnosis of pheochromocytoma made in the laboratory?

Urinary excretion of vanillylmandelic acid (an end product of catecholamine metabolism), norepinephrine, and epinephrine is often markedly increased. Elevated levels of urinary catecholamines and metanephrines (Figure 14–3) provide a highly accurate diagnosis. Fractionated plasma-free metanephrine levels may be superior to urinary studies in making the diagnosis. The location of the tumor can be determined by magnetic resonance imaging or computed tomographic scan with or without contrast.

What pathophysiology is associated with chronic elevations of norepinephrine and epinephrine?

α_1-Stimulation increases peripheral vascular resistance and arterial blood pressure. Hypertension can lead to intravascular volume depletion (increasing hematocrit), renal failure, and cerebral hemorrhage. Elevated peripheral vascular resistance also increases myocardial work, which predisposes patients to myocardial ischemia, ventricular hypertrophy, and congestive heart failure. Prolonged exposure to epinephrine and norepinephrine may lead to a catecholamine-induced cardiomyopathy. Hyperglycemia results from decreased insulin secretion in the face of increased glycogenolysis and gluconeogenesis. β_1-Stimulation increases automaticity and ventricular ectopy.

Which adrenergic antagonists might be helpful in controlling the effects of norepinephrine and epinephrine hypersecretion?

Phenoxybenzamine, an α_1-antagonist, effectively reverses the vasoconstriction, resulting in a drop in arterial blood pressure and an increase in intravascular volume (hematocrit drops). Glucose intolerance is often corrected. Phenoxybenzamine can be administered orally and is longer acting than phentolamine, another α_1-antagonist. For these reasons, phenoxybenzamine is often administered preoperatively to control symptoms.

Intravenous phentolamine is often used intraoperatively to control hypertensive episodes. Compared with some other hypotensive agents, however, phentolamine has a slow onset and long duration of action; furthermore, tachyphylaxis often develops.

β_1-Blockade with an agent such as labetalol is recommended for patients with tachycardia or ventricular arrhythmias.

Why should α_1-receptors be blocked with phenoxybenzamine before administration of a β-antagonist?

If β-receptors are blocked first, norepinephrine and epinephrine will produce unopposed α-stimulation. β_2-Mediated vasodilation will not be able to offset α_1-vasoconstriction, and peripheral vascular resistance would increase. This may explain the paradoxical hypertension that has been reported in a few patients with pheochromocytoma treated only with labetalol. Finally, the myocardium might not be able to handle its already elevated workload without the inotropic effects of β_1-stimulation.

Which anesthetic agents should be specifically avoided?

Succinylcholine-induced fasciculations of the abdominal musculature will increase intraabdominal pressure, which theoretically might cause release of catecholamines from the tumor. Ketamine is a sympathomimetic and would exacerbate the effects of adrenergic agonists. Halothane sensitizes the myocardium to the arrhythmogenic effects of epinephrine. Vagolytic drugs (eg, anticholinergics and pancuronium) will worsen the imbalance of autonomic tone. Because histamine provokes catecholamine secretion by the tumor, drugs associated with histamine release (eg, atracurium) are best avoided. Vecuronium and rocuronium are probably the neuromuscular blocking agents of choice.

Would an epidural or spinal technique effectively block sympathetic hyperactivity?

A major regional block—such as an epidural or spinal anesthetic—could block sensory (afferent) nerves and sympathetic (efferent) discharge in the area of the surgical field. The catecholamines released from a pheochromocytoma during surgical manipulation would still be able to bind and activate adrenergic receptors throughout the body, however.

GUIDELINES

Fleisher LA, Beckman JA, Brown KA, et al: 2009 ACCF/AHA focused update on perioperative beta blockade incorporated into the ACC/AHA 2007 guidelines on perioperative cardiovascular evaluation and care for noncardiac surgery: a report of the American College of Cardiology Foundation/American Heart Association task force on practice guidelines. Circulation 2009;120:2123.

SUGGESTED READING

Bonet S, Agusti A, Arnau JM, et al: β-Adrenergic blocking agents in heart failure: Benefits of vasodilating and nonvasodilating agents according to patients' characteristics: A meta-analysis of clinical trials. Arch Intern Med 2000;160:621.

Ebert TJ: Is gaining control of the autonomic nervous system important to our specialty? Anesthesiology 1999;90:651.

Glick DB: The autonomic nervous system. In: *Miller's Anesthesia*, 7th ed. Miller RD, Eriksson LI, Fleisher LI, et al (editors). Churchill Livingstone, 2010.

Insel PA: Adrenergic receptors—evolving concepts and clinical implications. N Engl J Med 1996; 334:580.

Johnson JO, Grecu L, Lawson NW: Autonomic nervous system. In: *Clinical Anesthesia*, 6th ed. Barash PG, Cullen BF, Stoelting RK, et al. (editors). Lippincott Williams & Wilkins, 2009.

Stoelting RK: *Pharmacology and Physiology in Anesthetic Practice*, 4th ed. Lippincott-Raven, 2005.

Hypotensive Agents

1. Clinical trials have shown that inhaled nitric oxide is a selective pulmonary vasodilator that is beneficial in the treatment of reversible pulmonary hypertension. By improving perfusion only in ventilated areas of the lung, inhaled nitric oxide may improve oxygenation in patients with acute respiratory distress syndrome or during one-lung ventilation.

2. Acute cyanide toxicity is characterized by metabolic acidosis, cardiac arrhythmias, and increased venous oxygen content (as a result of the inability to utilize oxygen). Another early sign of cyanide toxicity is the acute resistance to the hypotensive effects of increasing doses of sodium nitroprusside (tachyphylaxis).

3. By dilating pulmonary vessels, sodium nitroprusside may prevent the normal vasoconstrictive response of the pulmonary vasculature to hypoxia (hypoxic pulmonary vasoconstriction).

4. Preload reduction makes nitroglycerin an excellent drug for the relief of cardiogenic pulmonary edema.

5. Hydralazine relaxes arteriolar smooth muscle, causing dilatation of precapillary resistance vessels via increased cyclic guanosine 3′,5′-monophosphate.

6. The body reacts to a hydralazine-induced fall in blood pressure by increasing heart rate, myocardial contractility, and cardiac output. These compensatory responses can be detrimental to patients with coronary artery disease and are minimized by the concurrent administration of a β-adrenergic antagonist.

7. Fenoldopam mesylate (infusion rates studied in clinical trials range from 0.01–1.6 mcg/kg/min) reduces systolic and diastolic blood pressure in patients with malignant hypertension to an extent comparable to nitroprusside.

8. Dihydropyridine calcium channel blockers preferentially dilate arterial vessels, often preserving or increasing cardiac output.

A multitude of drugs are capable of lowering blood pressure, including volatile anesthetics, sympathetic antagonists and agonists, calcium channel blockers, β-blockers, and angiotensin-converting enzyme inhibitors. This chapter examines agents that may be useful to the anesthesiologist for intraoperative control of arterial blood pressure.

Patients with an increasing "vascular age" routinely present for anesthesia and surgery. As patients chronologically age, so too does their vasculature. When a pulse wave is generated by ventricular contraction, it is propagated through the arterial system. At branch points of the aorta, the wave is reflected back toward the heart. In patients of young vascular age, the reflected wave tends to augment diastole, improving diastolic pressure. In patients with "older" vasculature, the wave arrives sooner, being conducted back by the noncompliant vasculature during late systole, which causes an increase in cardiac workload and a decrease in diastolic pressure (Figure 15–1). Thus, older patients develop increased systolic pressure and decreased diastolic pressure.

Widened pulse pressures (the difference between systolic and diastolic pressures) have been associated with both increased incidence of postoperative renal dysfunction and increased risk of cerebral events in patients undergoing coronary bypass

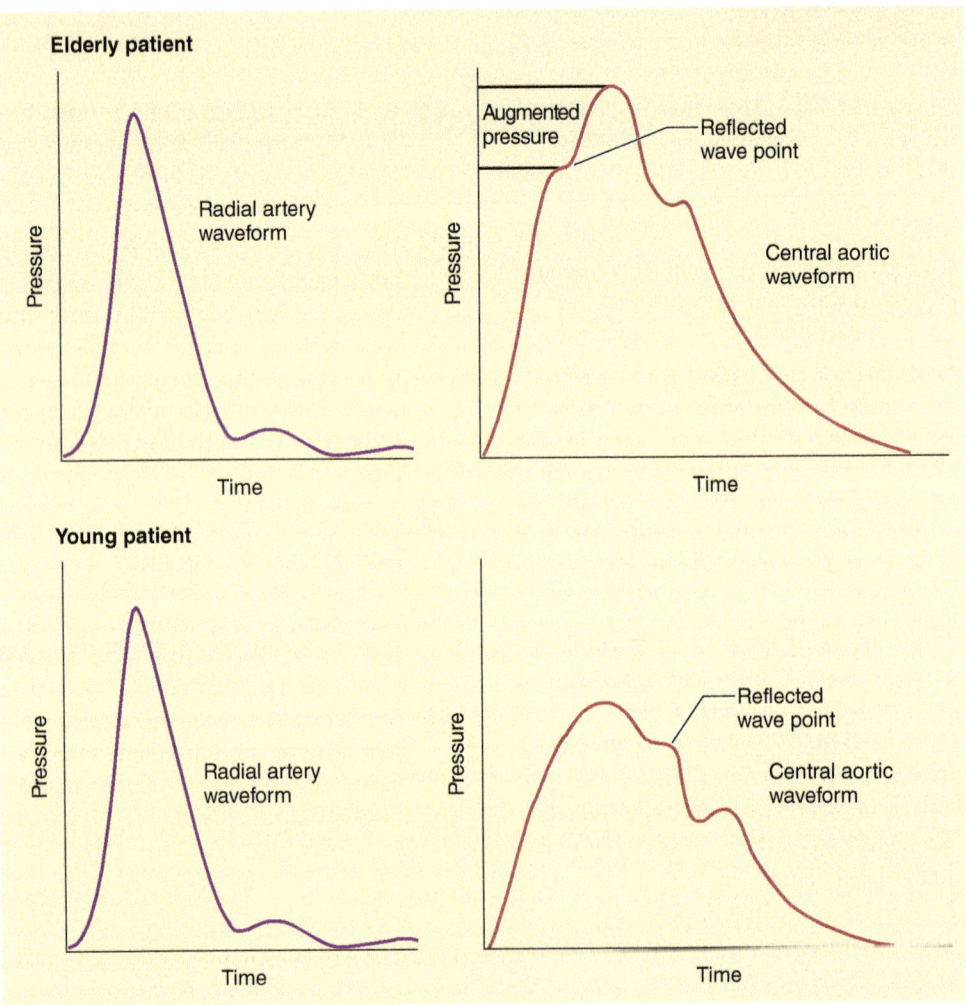

FIGURE 15–1 Illustration of the influence of increased vascular stiffness on peripheral (radial) and central (aortic) pressures. Note the similarity of peripheral radial pressures in individuals with normal (lower left panel) and increased (upper left panel) vascular stiffness. In young individuals with normal vascular stiffness, central aortic pressures are lower than radial pressures (lower panels). In contrast, in older individuals with increased vascular stiffness, central aortic pressures are increased and can approach or equal peripheral pressures as a result of wave reflection and central wave augmentation during systole (top panels). (Reproduced, with permission, from Barodka V, Joshi B, Berkowitz D, Hogue CW Jr, Nyhan D: Implications of vascular aging. Anesth Analg 2011;112:1048.)

surgery. Consequently, control of blood pressure is essential to mitigate postoperative morbidity, especially as patients of advanced vascular age present for surgery.

β-Blocker therapy should be maintained perioperatively in patients who are being treated with β-blockers as a part of their routine medical regimen. Furthermore, according to the American College of Cardiology, β-blockers are also of potential benefit to patients with more than one cardiac risk factor, especially those who are undergoing vascular surgery. However, the routine administration of high-dose β-blocker therapy may, in the absence of dose titration, be harmful in patients not taking β-blockers. The American College of Cardiology/American Heart Association guidelines for β-blocker use perioperatively should be closely followed. Adherence to such guidelines is used by third parties as a "quality" performance indicator for anesthesia delivery. Thus, anesthesia providers should periodically review recommendations regarding β-blocker therapy, as guidelines evolve as new evidence becomes available and older evidence is refuted. β-Blockers (esmolol, metoprolol, and others) were previously discussed for the treatment of transient perioperative hypertension and are routinely used by anesthesia providers. This chapter discusses antihypertensive agents other than β-blockers that are used perioperatively.

Along with increased vascular age, diastolic dysfunction is often underestimated in patients, as it can present in individuals with preserved systolic function. Acute diastolic heart failure can develop in the perioperative period secondary to hypertensive crisis. Diastolic dysfunction occurs due to the inability of the heart to relax effectively. Failure to actively sequester calcium ion into the sarcoplasmic reticulum (an energy-dependent process) impedes relaxation. Acute hypertension can produce diastolic dysfunction perioperatively, leading to elevated left ventricular end-diastolic pressures, myocardial ischemia, and pulmonary edema. Consequently, as increasing numbers of patients have diastolic dysfunction, tight control of blood pressure perioperatively is essential for safe anesthetic practice.

Blood pressure is essentially the product of cardiac output and systemic vascular resistance. Agents that lower blood pressure either reduce the force of myocardial contraction and/or produce vasodilation of the arterial and venous capacitance vessels. Agents used to lower blood pressure include nitrovasodilators, calcium antagonists, dopamine agonists, anesthetic agents, and angiotensin-converting enzyme inhibitors. β-Blockers have been previously discussed.

Nitrovasodilators

SODIUM NITROPRUSSIDE
Mechanism of Action

Sodium nitroprusside and other nitrovasodilators relax both arteriolar and venous smooth muscle. Its primary mechanism of action is shared with other nitrates (eg, hydralazine and nitroglycerin). As these drugs are metabolized, they release **nitric oxide**, which activates guanylyl cyclase. This enzyme is responsible for the synthesis of cyclic guanosine 3′,5′-monophosphate (cGMP), which controls the phosphorylation of several proteins, including some involved in the control of free intracellular calcium and smooth muscle contraction.

Nitric oxide, a naturally occurring potent vasodilator released by endothelial cells (endothelium-derived relaxing factor), plays an important role in regulating vascular tone throughout the body. Its ultrashort half-life (<5 s) provides sensitive endogenous control of regional blood flow.

1 Inhaled nitric oxide is a selective pulmonary vasodilator that is beneficial and routinely used in the treatment of reversible pulmonary hypertension.

Clinical Uses

Sodium nitroprusside is a potent and reliable antihypertensive. It is usually diluted to a concentration of 100 mcg/mL and administered as a continuous intravenous infusion (0.5–10 mcg/kg/min). Its extremely rapid onset of action (1–2 min) and fleeting duration of action allow precise titration of arterial blood pressure. A bolus of 1–2 mcg/kg minimizes blood pressure elevation during laryngoscopy but can cause transient hypotension in some patients. The potency of this drug requires frequent blood pressure measurements—or, preferably, intraarterial monitoring—and the use of mechanical infusion pumps. Solutions of sodium nitroprusside must be protected from light because of photodegradation.

Metabolism

After parenteral injection, sodium nitroprusside enters red blood cells, where it receives an electron from the iron (Fe^{2+}) of oxyhemoglobin. This nonenzymatic electron transfer results in an unstable nitroprusside radical and methemoglobin (Hgb Fe^{3+}). The former moiety spontaneously decomposes into five cyanide ions and the active nitroso ($N = O$) group.

The cyanide ions can be involved in one of three possible reactions: binding to methemoglobin to form **cyanmethemoglobin**; undergoing a reaction in the liver and kidney catalyzed by the enzyme rhodanase (thiosulfate + cyanide → thiocyanate); or binding to tissue cytochrome oxidase, which interferes with normal oxygen utilization (Figure 15–2).

2 The last of these reactions is responsible for the development of **acute cyanide toxicity**, characterized by metabolic acidosis, cardiac arrhythmias, and increased venous oxygen content (as a result of the inability to utilize oxygen). Another early sign of cyanide toxicity is the acute resistance to the hypotensive effects of increasing doses of sodium nitroprusside (tachyphylaxis). It should be noted that tachyphylaxis implies acute tolerance to the drug following multiple rapid injections, as opposed to tolerance, which is caused by more chronic exposure. Cyanide toxicity is more likely

if the cumulative dose of sodium nitroprusside is greater than 500 mcg/kg administered at an infusion rate faster than 2 mcg/kg/min. Patients with cyanide toxicity should be mechanically ventilated with 100% oxygen to maximize oxygen availability. The pharmacological treatment of cyanide toxicity depends on increasing the kinetics of the two reactions by administering sodium thiosulfate (150 mg/kg over 15 min) or 3% sodium nitrate (5 mg/kg over 5 min), which oxidizes hemoglobin to methemoglobin. Hydroxocobalamin combines with cyanide to form cyanocobalamin (vitamin B_{12}).

Thiocyanate is slowly cleared by the kidney. Accumulation of large amounts of thiocyanate (eg, in patients with renal failure) may result in a milder toxic reaction that includes thyroid dysfunction, muscle weakness, nausea, hypoxia, and an acute toxic psychosis. The risk of cyanide toxicity is not increased by renal failure, however. Methemoglobinemia from excessive doses of sodium nitroprusside or sodium nitrate can be treated with methylene blue (1–2 mg/kg of a 1% solution over 5 min), which reduces methemoglobin to hemoglobin.

Effects on Organ Systems

The combined dilation of venous and arteriolar vascular beds by sodium nitroprusside results in reductions of preload and afterload. Arterial blood pressure falls due to the decrease in peripheral vascular resistance. Although cardiac output is usually unchanged in normal patients, the reduction in afterload may increase cardiac output in patients with congestive heart failure, mitral regurgitation, or aortic regurgitation. In opposition to any favorable changes in myocardial oxygen requirements are reflex-mediated responses to the fall in arterial blood pressure. These include tachycardia and increased myocardial contractility. In addition, dilation of coronary arterioles by sodium nitroprusside may result in an **intracoronary** steal of blood flow away from ischemic areas that are already maximally dilated.

Sodium nitroprusside dilates cerebral vessels and abolishes cerebral autoregulation. Cerebral blood flow is maintained or increases unless arterial blood pressure is markedly reduced. The resulting increase in cerebral blood volume tends to increase intracranial pressure, particularly in patients with

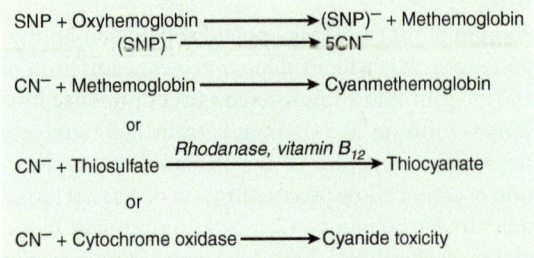

FIGURE 15–2 The metabolism of sodium nitroprusside.

reduced intracranial compliance (eg, brain tumors). This intracranial hypertension can be minimized by slow administration of sodium nitroprusside and institution of hypocapnia.

The pulmonary vasculature also dilates in response to sodium nitroprusside infusion. Reductions in pulmonary artery pressure may decrease the perfusion of some normally ventilated alveoli, increasing physiological dead space. By dilating pulmonary vessels, sodium nitroprusside may prevent the normal vasoconstrictive response of the pulmonary vasculature to hypoxia (hypoxic pulmonary vasoconstriction). Both of these effects tend to mismatch pulmonary ventilation to perfusion and decrease arterial oxygenation.

In response to decreased arterial blood pressure, renin and catecholamines are released during administration of nitroprusside. Renal function is fairly well maintained during sodium nitroprusside infusion, despite moderate drops in arterial blood pressure and renal perfusion.

Sodium nitroprusside does not directly interact with neuromuscular blocking agents. Nonetheless, a decrease in muscle blood flow caused by arterial hypotension could indirectly delay the onset and prolong the duration of neuromuscular blockade.

NITROGLYCERIN

Mechanism of Action

Nitroglycerin relaxes vascular smooth muscle, with venous dilation predominating over arterial dilation. Its mechanism of action is presumably similar to that of sodium nitroprusside: metabolism to nitric oxide, which activates guanylyl cyclase, leading to increased cGMP, decreased intracellular calcium, and vascular smooth muscle relaxation.

Clinical Uses

Nitroglycerin relieves myocardial ischemia, hypertension, and ventricular failure. Like sodium nitroprusside, nitroglycerin is commonly diluted to a concentration of 100 mcg/mL and administered as a continuous intravenous infusion (0.5–10 mcg/kg/min). Glass containers and special intravenous tubing are recommended because of the adsorption of nitroglycerin to polyvinylchloride. Nitroglycerin can also be administered by a sublingual (peak effect in 4 min) or transdermal (sustained release for 24 h) route. Some patients seem to require higher than expected doses of nitroglycerin to achieve a given drop in blood pressure, particularly after chronic administration (tolerance). Tolerance may be due to depletion of reactants necessary for nitric oxide formation, compensatory secretion of vasoconstrictive substances, or volume expansion. Dosing regimens that provide for intermittent periods of low or no drug exposure may minimize the development of tolerance.

Metabolism

Nitroglycerin undergoes rapid reductive hydrolysis in the liver and blood by glutathione-organic nitrate reductase. One metabolic product is nitrite, which can convert hemoglobin to methemoglobin. Significant methemoglobinemia is rare and can be treated with intravenous methylene blue (1–2 mg/kg over 5 min).

Nitroglycerin reduces myocardial oxygen demand and increases myocardial oxygen supply by several mechanisms:

- The pooling of blood in the large-capacitance vessels reduces venous return and preload. The accompanying decrease in ventricular end-diastolic pressure reduces myocardial oxygen demand and increases endocardial perfusion.

- Any afterload reduction from arteriolar dilation will decrease both end-systolic pressure and oxygen demand. Of course, a fall in diastolic pressure may lower coronary perfusion pressure and actually decrease myocardial oxygen supply.

- Nitroglycerin redistributes coronary blood flow to ischemic areas of the subendocardium.

- Coronary artery spasm may be relieved.

The beneficial effect of nitroglycerin in patients with coronary artery disease contrasts with the coronary steal phenomenon seen with sodium nitroprusside. Preload reduction makes nitroglycerin an excellent drug for the relief of cardiogenic pulmonary edema. Heart rate is unchanged or minimally increased. Rebound hypertension is less likely after discontinuation of nitroglycerin than following discontinuation of sodium nitroprusside. The prophylactic administration of low-dose nitroglycerin (0.5–2.0 mcg/kg/min) during anesthesia of patients at high risk for perioperative myocardial ischemia remains controversial.

The effects of nitroglycerin on cerebral blood flow and intracranial pressure are similar to those of sodium nitroprusside. Headache from dilation of cerebral vessels is a common side effect of nitroglycerin.

In addition to the dilating effects on the pulmonary vasculature (previously described for sodium nitroprusside), nitroglycerin relaxes bronchial smooth muscle.

Nitroglycerin (50–100 mcg boluses) has been demonstrated to be an effective (but transient) uterine relaxant that can be beneficial during certain obstetrical procedures if the placenta is still present in the uterus (eg, retained placenta, uterine inversion, uterine tetany, breech extraction, and external version of the second twin). Nitroglycerin therapy has been shown to diminish platelet aggregation, an effect enhanced by administration of *N*-acetylcysteine.

HYDRALAZINE

5 Hydralazine relaxes arteriolar smooth muscle, causing dilation of precapillary resistance vessels via increased cGMP.

Intraoperative hypertension is usually controlled with an intravenous dose of 5–20 mg of hydralazine. The onset of action is within 15 min, and the antihypertensive effect usually lasts 2–4 hr. Hydralazine can be used to control pregnancy-induced hypertension.

Hydralazine undergoes acetylation and hydroxylation in the liver.

Effects on Organ Systems

The lowering of peripheral vascular resistance causes **6** a drop in arterial blood pressure. The body reacts to a hydralazine-induced fall in blood pressure by increasing heart rate, myocardial contractility, and cardiac output. These compensatory responses can be detrimental to patients with coronary artery disease and are minimized by the concurrent administration of a β-adrenergic antagonist. Conversely, the decline in afterload often proves beneficial to patients in congestive heart failure.

Hydralazine is a potent cerebral vasodilator and inhibitor of cerebral blood flow autoregulation. Unless blood pressure is markedly reduced, cerebral blood flow and intracranial pressure will rise.

Renal blood flow is usually maintained or increased by hydralazine.

Non-Nitrovasodilator Hypotensive Agents

FENOLDOPAM
Mechanism of Action

Fenoldopam mesylate causes rapid vasodilation by selectively activating D_1-dopamine receptors. It has also demonstrated moderate affinity for α_2-adrenoceptors. The R-isomer is responsible for the racemic mixture's biological activity due to its much greater receptor affinity, compared with the S-isomer.

Clinical Uses

7 Fenoldopam mesylate (infusion rates studied in clinical trials range from 0.01–1.6 mcg/kg/min) reduces systolic and diastolic blood pressure in patients with malignant hypertension to an extent comparable to nitroprusside. Side effects include headache, flushing, nausea, tachycardia, hypokalemia, and hypotension. The onset of the hypotensive effect occurs within 15 min, and discontinuation of an infusion quickly reverses this effect without rebound hypertension. Some degree of tolerance may develop 48 hr after the infusion. Studies are conflicted as to fenolodopam's ability to "protect" and "maintain" renal function in perioperative patients with hypertension at risk of perioperative kidney injury.

Metabolism

Fenoldopam undergoes conjugation without participation of the cytochrome P-450 enzymes, and its metabolites are inactive. Clearance of fenoldopam remains unaltered despite the presence of renal or hepatic failure, and no dosage adjustments are necessary for these patients.

Effects on Organ Systems

Fenoldopam decreases systolic and diastolic blood pressure. Heart rate typically increases. Low initial doses (0.03–0.1 mcg/kg/min) titrated slowly have been associated with less reflex tachycardia than higher doses (>0.3 mcg/kg/min). Tachycardia decreases over time but remains substantial at higher doses.

Fenoldopam can lead to rises in intraocular pressure and should be administered with caution or avoided in patients with a history of glaucoma or intraocular hypertension.

As would be expected from a D_1-dopamine receptor agonist, fenoldopam markedly increases renal blood flow. Despite a drop in arterial blood pressure, the glomerular filtration rate is well maintained. Fenoldopam increases urinary flow rate, urinary sodium extraction, and creatinine clearance compared with sodium nitroprusside.

CALCIUM ANTAGONISTS

8 Dihydropyridine calcium channel blockers (nicardipine, clevidipine) are arterial selective vasodilators routinely used for perioperative blood pressure control in patients undergoing cardiothoracic surgery. Clevidipine is a relatively new drug with a short half-life, which facilitates its rapid titration. Unlike verapamil and diltiazem, the dihydropyridine calcium channel blockers have minimal effects on cardiac conduction and ventricular contractility. Calcium channel blockers bind to L-type calcium channel and impair calcium entry into the vascular smooth muscle. These L-type receptors are more prevalent on arterial vessels than venous capacitance vessels. Consequently, cardiac filling and preload is less affected by these agents than nitrates, which might dilate both arterial and venous systems. With preload maintained, cardiac output often increases when vascular tone is reduced by use of dihydropyridine calcium

blockers. Nicardipine infusion is titrated to effect (5–15 mg/h).

Other intravenous agents that can produce hypotension perioperatively include the intravenous angiotensin-converting enzyme inhibitor enalaprilat (0.625–1.25 mg). The role of enalaprilat as a nondirect-acting agent in the acute treatment of a hypertensive crisis is limited.

CASE DISCUSSION

Controlled Hypotension

A 59-year-old man is scheduled for total hip arthroplasty under general anesthesia. The surgeon requests a controlled hypotensive technique.

What is controlled hypotension, and what are its advantages?

Controlled hypotension is the elective lowering of arterial blood pressure. The primary advantages of this technique are minimization of surgical blood loss and better surgical visualization.

How is controlled hypotension achieved?

The primary methods of electively lowering blood pressure are proper positioning, positive-pressure ventilation, and the administration of hypotensive drugs. Positioning involves elevation of the surgical site so that the blood pressure at the wound is selectively reduced. The increase in intrathoracic pressure that accompanies positive-pressure ventilation lowers venous return, cardiac output, and mean arterial pressure. Numerous pharmacological agents effectively lower blood pressure: volatile anesthetics, spinal and epidural anesthesia, sympathetic antagonists, calcium channel blockers, and the peripheral vasodilators discussed in this chapter.

What surgical procedures might benefit most from a controlled hypotensive technique?

Controlled hypotension has been successfully used during cerebral aneurysm repair, brain tumor resection, total hip arthroplasty, radical neck dissection, radical cystectomy, and other operations associated with significant blood loss. Controlled hypotension may allow safer surgery of patients whose religious beliefs prohibit blood transfusions (eg, Jehovah's Witnesses). Decreasing extravasation of blood may improve the result of some plastic surgery procedures.

What are some relative contraindications to controlled hypotension?

Some patients have predisposing illnesses that decrease the margin of safety for adequate organ perfusion: severe anemia, hypovolemia, atherosclerotic cardiovascular disease, renal or hepatic insufficiency, cerebrovascular disease, or uncontrolled glaucoma.

What are the possible complications of controlled hypotension?

As the above list of contraindications suggests, the risks of low arterial blood pressure include cerebral thrombosis, hemiplegia (due to decreased spinal cord perfusion), acute tubular necrosis, massive hepatic necrosis, myocardial infarction, cardiac arrest, and blindness (from retinal artery thrombosis or ischemic optic neuropathy). These complications are more likely in patients with coexisting anemia. Consequently, the use of induced or controlled hypotension continues to decline.

What is a safe level of hypotension?

This depends on the patient. Healthy young individuals tolerate mean arterial pressures as low as 50–60 mm Hg without complications. On the other hand, chronically hypertensive patients have altered autoregulation of cerebral blood flow and may tolerate a mean arterial pressure of no more than 20% to 30% lower than baseline. Patients with a history of transient ischemic attacks may not tolerate any decline in cerebral perfusion.

What special monitoring is indicated during controlled hypotension?

Intraarterial blood pressure monitoring and electrocardiography with ST-segment analysis are strongly recommended. Central venous monitoring and measurement of urinary output by an indwelling catheter are indicated if extensive surgery is anticipated.

GUIDELINES

Fleisher LA, Beckman JA, Brown KA, et al: 2009 ACCF/AHA focused update on perioperative beta blockade incorporated into the ACC/AHA 2007 guidelines on perioperative cardiovascular evaluation and care for noncardiac surgery: a report of the American College of Cardiology Foundation/American Heart Association task force on practice guidelines. Circulation 2009;120:2123.

SUGGESTED READING

Barodka V, Joshi B, Berkowitz D, Hogue CW Jr, Nyhan D: Implications of vascular aging. Anesth Analg 2011; 112:1048.

Lauretti GR, de Oliveira R, Reis MP: Transdermal nitroglycerine enhances spinal sufentanil postoperative analgesia following orthopedic surgery. Anesthesiology 1999;90:734.

Marshman LAG, Morice AH, Thompson JS: Increased efficacy of sodium nitroprusside in middle cerebral arteries following acute subarachnoid hemorrhage: Indications for its use after rupture. J Neurosurg Anesthesiol 1998;10:171.

Parker JD, Parker JO: Nitrate therapy for stable angina pectoris. N Engl J Med 1998;338:520.

Pirracchio R, Cholley B, De Hert S, Solal AC, Mebazaa A: Diastolic heart failure in anaesthesia and critical care. Br J Anaesth 2007;98:707.

Tobias JD: Fenoldopam: Applications in anesthesiology, perioperative medicine, and critical care medicine. Am J Anesthesiol 2000;27:395.

Williams-Russo P, Sharrock NE, Mattis S: Randomized trial of hypotensive epidural anesthesia in older adults. Anesthesiology 1999;91:926.

Local Anesthetics

1. Sodium (Na) channels are membrane-bound proteins that are composed of one large α subunit, through which Na ions pass, and one or two smaller β subunits. Voltage-gated Na channels exist in (at least) three states—resting (nonconducting), open (conducting), and inactivated (nonconducting). Local anesthetics bind a specific region of the α subunit and inhibit voltage-gated Na channels, preventing channel activation and the Na influx associated with membrane depolarization.

2. Sensitivity of nerve fibers to inhibition by local anesthetics is determined by axonal diameter, myelination, and other anatomic and physiological factors.

3. Potency correlates with octanol solubility, which in turn reflects the ability of the local anesthetic molecule to permeate lipid membranes. Potency is increased by adding large alkyl groups to a parent molecule. There is no measurement of local anesthetic potency that is analogous to the minimum alveolar concentration of inhalation anesthetics.

4. Onset of action depends on many factors, including lipid solubility and the relative concentration of the nonionized lipid-soluble form (B) and the ionized water-soluble form (BH$^+$), expressed by the pK_a. The pK_a is the pH at which the fraction of ionized and nonionized drug is equal. Less potent, less lipid-soluble agents generally have a faster onset than more potent, more lipid-soluble agents.

5. Duration of action correlates with potency and lipid solubility. Highly lipid-soluble local anesthetics have a longer duration of action, presumably because they more slowly diffuse from a lipid-rich environment to the aqueous bloodstream.

6. In regional anesthesia local anesthetics are typically injected or applied very close to their intended site of action; thus their pharmacokinetic profiles are much more important determinants of elimination and toxicity than of their desired clinical effect.

7. The rate of systemic absorption is related to the vascularity of the site of injection: intravenous (or intraarterial) > tracheal > intercostal > paracervical > epidural > brachial plexus > sciatic > subcutaneous.

8. Ester local anesthetics are predominantly metabolized by pseudocholinesterase. Amide local anesthetics are metabolized (N-dealkylation and hydroxylation) by microsomal P-450 enzymes in the liver.

9. The central nervous system is vulnerable to local anesthetic toxicity and is the site of premonitory signs of rising blood concentrations in awake patients.

—Continued next page

Continued—

10 Major cardiovascular toxicity usually requires about three times the local anesthetic concentration in blood as that required to produce seizures.

11 Unintentional intravascular injection of bupivacaine during regional anesthesia may produce severe cardiovascular toxicity, including left ventricular depression, atrioventricular heart block, and life-threatening arrhythmias such as ventricular tachycardia and fibrillation.

12 True hypersensitivity reactions to local anesthetic agents—as distinct from systemic toxicity caused by excessive plasma concentration—are uncommon. Esters appear more likely to induce a true allergic reaction (due to IgG or IgE antibodies) especially if they are derivatives (eg, procaine or benzocaine) of *p*-aminobenzoic acid, a known allergen.

Local and regional anesthesia and analgesia techniques depend on a group of drugs—local anesthetics—that transiently inhibit sensory, motor, or autonomic nerve function, or a combination of these functions, when the drugs are injected or applied near neural tissue. This chapter presents the mechanism of action, structure–activity relationships, and clinical pharmacology of local anesthetic drugs. The more commonly used regional anesthetic techniques are presented in Section IV (see Chapters 45 and 46).

MECHANISMS OF LOCAL ANESTHETIC ACTION

Neurons (and all other living cells) maintain a resting membrane potential of −60 to −70 mV by active transport and passive diffusion of ions. The electrogenic, energy-consuming sodium–potassium pump (Na^+-K^+-ATPase) couples the transport of three sodium (Na) ions out of the cell for every two potassium (K) ions it moves into the cell. This creates an ionic disequilibrium (concentration gradient) that favors the movement of K ions from an intracellular to an extracellular location, and the movement of Na ions in the opposite direction. The cell membrane is normally much more "leaky" to K ions than to Na ions, so a relative excess of negatively charged ions (anions) accumulates intracellularly. This accounts for the negative resting potential difference (−70 mV polarization).

Unlike most other types of tissue, excitable cells (eg, neurons or cardiac myocytes) have the capability of generating **action potentials**. Membrane-bound, voltage-gated Na channels in peripheral nerve axons can produce and transmit membrane depolarizations following chemical, mechanical, or electrical stimuli. When a stimulus is sufficient to depolarize a patch of membrane, the signal can be transmitted as a wave of depolarization along the nerve membrane (an impulse). Activation of voltage-gated Na channels causes a very brief (roughly 1 msec) change in the conformation of the channel, allowing an influx of Na ions and generating an action potential (Figure 16–1). The increase in Na permeability causes temporary depolarization of the membrane potential to +35 mV. The Na current is brief and is terminated by inactivation of voltage-gated Na channels, which do not conduct Na ions. Subsequently the membrane returns to its resting potential. Baseline concentration gradients are maintained by the sodium–potassium pump, and only a minuscule number of Na ions pass into the cell during an action potential.

1 Na channels are membrane-bound proteins that are composed of one large α subunit, through which Na ions pass, and one or two smaller β subunits. Voltage-gated Na channels exist in (at least) three states—resting (nonconducting), open

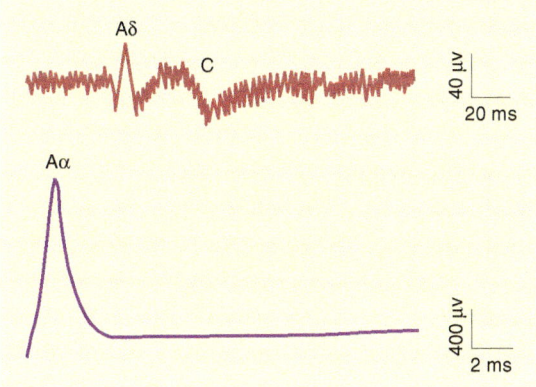

FIGURE 16–1 Compound Aα, Aδ, and C fiber action potentials recorded after supramaximal stimulation of a rat sciatic nerve. Note the differing time scale of the recordings. In peripheral nerves, Aδ and C fibers have much slower conduction velocities, and their compound action potentials are longer and of less amplitude when compared with those from Aα fibers. (Reproduced, with permission, from Butterworth JF 4th, Strichartz GR: The alpha 2-adrenergic agonists clonidine and guanfacine produce tonic and phasic block of conduction in rat sciatic nerve fibers. Anesth Analg 1993;76:295.)

(conducting), and inactivated (nonconducting) (Figure 16–2). Local anesthetics bind a specific region of the α subunit and inhibit voltage-gated Na channels, preventing channel activation and

inhibiting the Na influx associated with membrane depolarization. Local anesthetic binding to Na channels does not alter the resting membrane potential. With increasing local anesthetic concentrations, an increasing fraction of the Na channels in the membrane bind a local anesthetic molecule and cannot conduct Na ions. As a consequence, impulse conduction slows, the rate of rise and the magnitude of the action potential decrease, and the threshold for excitation and impulse conduction increases progressively. At high enough local anesthetic concentrations and with a sufficient fraction of local anesthetic-bound Na channels, an action potential can no longer be generated and impulse propagation is abolished. Local anesthetics have a greater affinity for the channel in the open or inactivated state than in the resting state. Local anesthetic binding to open or inactivated channels, or both, is facilitated by depolarization. The fraction of Na channels that have bound a local anesthetic increases with frequent depolarization (eg, during trains of impulses). This phenomenon is termed *use-dependent block*. Put another way, local anesthetic inhibition is both voltage and frequency dependent, and is greater when nerve fibers are firing rapidly than with infrequent depolarizations.

Local anesthetics may also bind and inhibit calcium (Ca), K, transient receptor potential

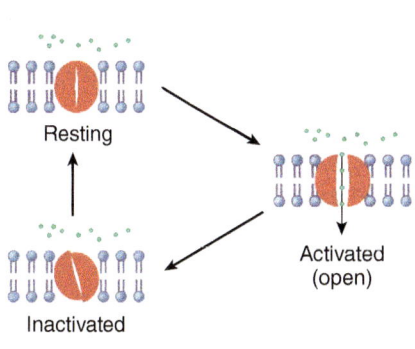

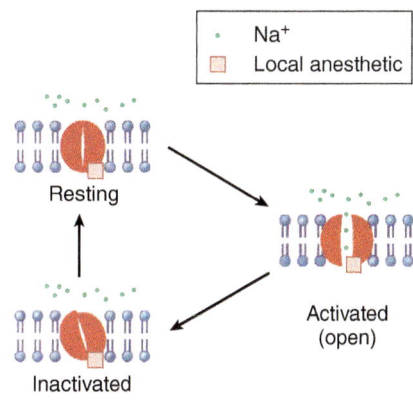

FIGURE 16–2 Voltage-gated sodium (Na) channels exist in (at least) three states—resting, activated (open), and inactivated. Note that local anesthetics bind and inhibit the voltage-gated Na channel from a site that is not directly accessible from outside the cell, interfering with the large transient Na influx associated with membrane depolarization.

TABLE 16–1 Nerve fiber classification.[1]

Fiber Type	Modality Served	Diameter (mm)	Conduction (m/s)	Myelinated?
Aα	Motor efferent	12–20	70–120	Yes
Aα	Proprioception	12–20	70–120	Yes
Aβ	Touch, pressure	5–12	30–70	Yes
Aγ	Motor efferent (muscle spindle)	3–6	15–30	Yes
Aδ	Pain Temperature Touch	2–5	12–30	Yes
B	Preganglionic autonomic fibers	<3	3–14	Some
C Dorsal root	Pain Temperature	0.4–1.2	0.5–2	No
C Sympathetic	Postganglionic sympathetic fibers	0.3–1.3	0.7–2.3	No

[1]An alternative numerical system is sometimes used to classify sensory fibers.

vanilloid 1 (TRPV1), and many other channels and receptors. Conversely, other classes of drugs, most notably tricyclic antidepressants (amitriptyline), meperidine, volatile anesthetics, Ca channel blockers, and ketamine, also may inhibit Na channels. Tetrodotoxin is a poison that specifically binds Na channels but at a site on the exterior of the plasma membrane. Human studies are under way with similar toxins to determine whether they might provide effective, prolonged analgesia after local infiltration.

2 Sensitivity of nerve fibers to inhibition by local anesthetics is determined by axonal diameter, myelination, and other anatomic and physiological factors. Table 16–1 lists the most commonly used classification for nerve fibers. In comparing nerve fibers of the same type, small diameter increases sensitivity to local anesthetics. Thus, larger, faster Aα fibers are less sensitive to local anesthetics than smaller, slower-conducting Aδ fibers, and larger unmyelinated fibers are less sensitive than smaller unmyelinated fibers. On the other hand, small unmyelinated C fibers are relatively resistant to inhibition by local anesthetics as compared with larger myelinated fibers. In spinal nerves local anesthetic inhibition (and conduction failure) generally follows the sequence autonomic > sensory > motor, but at steady state if sensory anesthesia is present all fibers are inhibited.

STRUCTURE–ACTIVITY RELATIONSHIPS

Local anesthetics consist of a lipophilic group (usually an aromatic benzene ring) separated from a hydrophilic group (usually a tertiary amine) by an intermediate chain that includes an ester or amide linkage. Articaine, the most popular local anesthetic for dentistry in several European countries, is an amide but it contains a thiophene ring rather than a benzene ring. Local anesthetics are weak bases that usually carry a positive charge at the tertiary amine group at physiological pH. The nature of the intermediate chain is the basis of the classification of local anesthetics as either esters or amides (Table 16–2). Physicochemical properties of local anesthetics depend on the substitutions in the aromatic ring, the type of linkage in the intermediate

TABLE 16–2 Physicochemical properties of local anesthetics.

Generic (Proprietary)	Structure	Relative Lipid Solubility of Unchanged Local Anesthetic	pK_a	Protein Binding (%)
Amides				
Bupivacaine (Marcaine, Sensorcaine)		8	8.2	96
Etidocaine (Duranest)		16	8.1	94
Lidocaine (Xylocaine)		1	8.2	64
Mepivacaine (Carbocaine)		0.3	7.9	78
Prilocaine (Citanest)		0.4	8.0	53
Ropivacaine (Naropin)		2.5	8.2	94

(continued)

TABLE 16–2 **Physicochemical properties of local anesthetics. (continued)**

Generic (Proprietary)	Structure	Relative Lipid Solubility of Unchanged Local Anesthetic	pK$_a$	Protein Binding (%)
Esters				
Chloroprocaine (Nesacaine)		2.3	9.1	NA[1]
Cocaine		NA	8.7	91
Procaine (Novocaine)		0.3	9.1	NA
Tetracaine (Pontocaine)		12	8.6	76

*Carbon atom responsible for optical isomerism.
[1]NA, not available.

chain, and the alkyl groups attached to the amine nitrogen.

3 Potency correlates with octanol solubility, which in turn reflects the ability of the local anesthetic molecule to permeate lipid membranes. Potency is increased by adding large alkyl groups to a parent molecule (compare tetracaine to procaine or bupivacaine to mepivacaine). There is no measurement of local anesthetic potency that is analogous to the minimum alveolar concentration (MAC) of inhalation anesthetics. The minimum concentration of local anesthetic that will block nerve impulse conduction is affected by several factors, including fiber size, type, and myelination; pH (acidic pH antagonizes block); frequency of nerve stimulation; and electrolyte concentrations (hypokalemia and hypercalcemia antagonize blockade).

4 Onset of local anesthetic action depends on many factors, including lipid solubility and the relative concentration of the nonionized lipid-soluble form (B) and the ionized water-soluble form (BH$^+$), expressed by the pK$_a$. The pK$_a$ is the pH at which the fraction of ionized and nonionized drug is equal. Less potent, less lipid-soluble agents generally have a faster onset than more potent, more lipid-soluble agents.

Local anesthetics with a pK_a closest to physiological pH will have (at physiological pH) a greater fraction of nonionized base that more readily permeates the nerve cell membrane, generally facilitating a more rapid onset of action. It is the lipid-soluble form that more readily diffuses across the neural sheath (epineurium) and passes through the nerve membrane. Curiously, once the local anesthetic molecule gains access to the cytoplasmic side of the Na channel, it is the charged cation (rather than the nonionized base) that more avidly binds the Na channel. For instance, the pK_a of lidocaine exceeds physiological pH. Thus, at physiological pH (7.40) more than half the lidocaine will exist as the charged cation form (BH^+).

It is often stated that the onset of action of local anesthetics directly correlates with pK_a. This assertion is not supported by actual data; in fact, the agent of fastest onset (2-chloroprocaine) has the greatest pK_a of all clinically used agents. Other factors, such as ease of diffusion through connective tissue, can affect the onset of action in vivo. Moreover, not all local anesthetics exist in a charged form (eg, benzocaine).

The importance of the ionized and nonionized forms has many clinical implications, at least for those agents that exist in both forms. Local anesthetic solutions are prepared commercially as water-soluble hydrochloride salts (pH 6–7). Because epinephrine is unstable in alkaline environments, commercially formulated, epinephrine-containing, local anesthetic solutions are generally more acidic (pH 4–5) than the comparable "plain" solutions lacking epinephrine. As a direct consequence, these commercially formulated, epinephrine-containing preparations may have a lower concentration of free base and a slower onset than when the epinephrine is added by the clinician at the time of use. Similarly, the extracellular base-to-cation ratio is decreased and onset is delayed when local anesthetics are injected into acidic (eg, infected) tissues. Tachyphylaxis—the decreased efficacy of repeated doses—could be partly explained by the eventual consumption of the local extracellular buffering capacity by repeat injections

of the acidic local anesthetic solution, but data are lacking. Some researchers have found that alkalinization of local anesthetic solutions (particularly commercially prepared, epinephrine-containing ones) by the addition of sodium bicarbonate (eg, 1 mL 8.4% sodium bicarbonate per 10 mL local anesthetic) speeds the onset and improves the quality of the block by increasing the amount of free base available. Interestingly, alkalinization also decreases pain during subcutaneous infiltration.

5 Duration of action correlates with potency and lipid solubility. Highly lipid-soluble local anesthetics have a longer duration of action, presumably because they more slowly diffuse from a lipid-rich environment to the aqueous bloodstream. Lipid solubility of local anesthetics is correlated with plasma protein binding. Local anesthetics are mostly bound by α_1-acid glycoprotein and to a lesser extent to albumin. Sustained-release systems using liposomal encapsulation or microspheres for delivery of local anesthetics can significantly prolong their duration of action, but these approaches are not yet being used for prolonged anesthesia in the way that extended-duration epidural morphine is being used for single-shot, prolonged epidural analgesia.

Differential block of sensory rather than motor function would be desirable. Unfortunately, only bupivacaine and ropivacaine display *some* selectively (mostly during onset and offset of block) for sensory nerves; however, the concentrations required for surgical anesthesia almost always result in some motor blockade.

CLINICAL PHARMACOLOGY

Pharmacokinetics

6 In regional anesthesia local anesthetics are typically injected or applied very close to their intended site of action; thus their pharmacokinetic profiles are much more important determinants of elimination and toxicity than of their desired clinical effect.

A. Absorption

Most mucous membranes (eg, ocular conjunctiva, tracheal mucosa) provide a minimal barrier to local anesthetic penetration, leading to a rapid onset of action. Intact skin, on the other hand, requires a high concentration of lipid-soluble local anesthetic base to ensure permeation and analgesia. EMLA cream consists of a 1:1 mixture of 5% lidocaine and 5% prilocaine bases in an oil-in-water emulsion. Dermal analgesia sufficient for beginning an intravenous line requires a contact time of at least 1 h under an occlusive dressing. Depth of penetration (usually 3–5 mm), duration of action (usually 1–2 h), and amount of drug absorbed depend on application time, dermal blood flow, keratin thickness, and total dose administered. Typically, 1–2 g of cream is applied per 10-cm^2 area of skin, with a maximum application area of 2000 cm^2 in an adult (100 cm^2 in children weighing less than 10 kg). Split-thickness skin-graft harvesting, laser removal of portwine stains, lithotripsy, and circumcision have been successfully performed with EMLA cream. Side effects include skin blanching, erythema, and edema. EMLA cream should not be used on mucous membranes, broken skin, infants younger than 1 month of age, or patients with a predisposition to methemoglobinemia (see Biotransformation and Excretion, below).

Systemic absorption of injected local anesthetics depends on blood flow, which is determined by the following factors.

1. Site of injection—The rate of systemic absorption is related to the vascularity of the site of injection: intravenous (or intraarterial) > tracheal > intercostal > paracervical > epidural > brachial plexus > sciatic > subcutaneous.

2. Presence of vasoconstrictors—Addition of epinephrine—or less commonly phenylephrine—causes vasoconstriction at the site of administration. The consequent decreased absorption reduces the peak local anesthetic concentration in blood, facilitates neuronal uptake, enhances the quality of analgesia, prolongs the duration of action, and limits toxic side effects. Vasoconstrictors have more pronounced effects on shorter-acting than longer-acting agents. For example, addition of epinephrine to lidocaine usually extends the duration of anesthesia by at least 50%, but epinephrine has little or no effect on the duration of bupivacaine peripheral nerve blocks. Epinephrine and clonidine

can also augment analgesia through activation of α_2-adrenergic receptors.

3. Local anesthetic agent—More lipid-soluble local anesthetics that are highly tissue bound are also more slowly absorbed. The agents also vary in their intrinsic vasodilator properties.

B. Distribution

Distribution depends on organ uptake, which is determined by the following factors.

1. Tissue perfusion—The highly perfused organs (brain, lung, liver, kidney, and heart) are responsible for the initial rapid uptake (α phase), which is followed by a slower redistribution (β phase) to moderately perfused tissues (muscle and gut). In particular, the lung extracts significant amounts of local anesthetic; consequently, the threshold for systemic toxicity involves much lower doses following arterial injections than venous injections (and children with right-to-left shunts are more susceptible to toxic side effects of lidocaine injected as an antiarrhythmic agent).

2. Tissue/blood partition coefficient—Increasing lipid solubility is associated with greater plasma protein binding and also greater tissue uptake from an aqueous compartment.

3. Tissue mass—Muscle provides the greatest reservoir for distribution of local anesthetic agents in the bloodstream because of its large mass.

C. Biotransformation and Excretion

The biotransformation and excretion of local anesthetics is defined by their chemical structure.

1. Esters—Ester local anesthetics are predominantly metabolized by pseudocholinesterase (plasma cholinesterase or butyrylcholinesterase). Ester hydrolysis is very rapid, and the water-soluble metabolites are excreted in the urine. Procaine and benzocaine are metabolized to *p*-aminobenzoic acid (PABA), which has been associated with rare anaphylactic reactions. Patients with genetically abnormal pseudocholinesterase would theoretically be at increased risk for toxic side effects, as metabolism is slower, but clinical evidence for this is lacking. Cerebrospinal fluid lacks esterase enzymes, so the termination of action of intrathecally injected ester local anesthetics, eg, tetracaine, depends on their redistribution into the bloodstream, as it does for all other nerve blocks. In contrast to other ester anesthetics, cocaine is partially metabolized (N-methylation and ester hydrolysis) in the liver and partially excreted unchanged in the urine.

2. Amides—Amide local anesthetics are metabolized (N-dealkylation and hydroxylation) by microsomal P-450 enzymes in the liver. The rate of amide metabolism depends on the specific agent (prilocaine > lidocaine > mepivacaine > ropivacaine > bupivacaine) but overall is consistently slower than ester hydrolysis of ester local anesthetics. Decreases in hepatic function (eg, cirrhosis of the liver) or liver blood flow (eg, congestive heart failure, β blockers, or H_2-receptor blockers) will reduce the metabolic rate and potentially predispose patients to having greater blood concentrations and a greater risk of systemic toxicity. Very little unmetabolized local anesthetic is excreted by the kidneys, although water-soluble metabolites are dependent on renal clearance.

Prilocaine is the only local anesthetic that is metabolized to *o*-toluidine, which produces methemoglobinemia in a dose-dependent fashion. Classical teaching was that a defined minimal dose of prilocaine was needed to produce clinically important methemoglobinemia (in the range of 10 mg/kg); however, recent studies have shown that younger, healthier patients develop medically important methemoglobinemia after lower doses of prilocaine (and at lower doses than needed in older, sicker patients). Prilocaine is generally not used for epidural anesthesia during labor or in larger doses in patients with limited cardiopulmonary reserve. **Benzocaine, a common ingredient in topical local anesthetic sprays, can also cause dangerous levels of methemoglobinemia**. For this reason, many hospitals no longer permit benzocaine spray during endoscopic procedures. Treatment of medically important methemoglobinemia includes intravenous methylene blue (1–2 mg/kg of a 1% solution over 5 min). Methylene blue reduces methemoglobin (Fe^{3+}) to hemoglobin (Fe^{2+}).

Effects on Organ Systems

Because inhibition of voltage-gated Na channels from circulating local anesthetics might affect action potentials in neurons throughout the body as well as impulse generation and conduction in the heart, it is not surprising that local anesthetics in high circulating concentrations could have the propensity for systemic toxicity. Although organ system effects are discussed for these drugs as a group, individual drugs differ.

Potency at most toxic side effects correlates with potency at nerve blocks. Maximum safe doses are listed in Table 16–3, but it must be recognized that the maximum safe dose depends on the patient, the specific nerve block, the rate of injection, and a long list of other factors. In other words, tables of purported maximal safe doses are nearly nonsensical. Mixtures of local anesthetics should be considered to have additive toxic effects; therefore, a solution containing 50% of the toxic dose of lidocaine and 50% of the toxic dose of bupivacaine if injected by accident intravenously will produce toxic effects.

A. Neurological

The central nervous system is vulnerable to local anesthetic toxicity and is the site of premonitory signs of rising blood concentrations in awake patients. Early symptoms include circumoral numbness, tongue paresthesia, dizziness, tinnitus, and blurred vision. Excitatory signs include restlessness, agitation, nervousness, garrulousness, and a feeling of "impending doom." Muscle twitching heralds the onset of tonic–clonic seizures. Still higher blood concentrations may produce central nervous system depression (eg, coma and respiratory arrest). The excitatory reactions are thought to be the result of selective blockade of inhibitory pathways. Potent, highly lipid-soluble local anesthetics produce seizures at lower blood concentrations than less potent agents. Benzodiazepines and hyperventilation raise the threshold of local anesthetic-induced seizures. Both respiratory and metabolic acidosis reduce the seizure threshold. Propofol (0.5–2 mg/kg) quickly and reliably terminates seizure activity (as do comparable doses of benzodiazepines or barbiturates). Maintaining a clear airway with adequate ventilation and oxygenation is of key importance.

Infused local anesthetics have a variety of actions. Systemically administered local anesthetics such as lidocaine (1.5 mg/kg) can decrease cerebral

TABLE 16–3 Clinical use of local anesthetic agents.

Agent	Techniques	Concentrations Available	Maximum Dose (mg/kg)	Typical Duration of Nerve Blocks[1]
Esters				
Benzocaine	Topical[2]	20%	NA[3]	NA
Chloroprocaine	Epidural, infiltration, peripheral nerve block, spinal[4]	1%, 2%, 3%	12	Short
Cocaine	Topical	4%, 10%	3	NA
Procaine	Spinal, local infiltration	1%, 2%, 10%	12	Short
Tetracaine (amethocaine)	Spinal, topical (eye)	0.2%, 0.3%, 0.5%, 1%, 2%	3	Long
Amides				
Bupivacaine	Epidural, spinal, infiltration, peripheral nerve block	0.25%, 0.5%, 0.75%	3	Long
Lidocaine (lignocaine)	Epidural, spinal, infiltration, peripheral nerve block, intravenous regional, topical	0.5%, 1%, 1.5%, 2%, 4%, 5%	4.5 7 (with epinephrine)	Medium
Mepivacaine	Epidural, infiltration, peripheral nerve block, spinal	1%, 1.5%, 2%, 3%	4.5 7 (with epinephrine)	Medium
Prilocaine	EMLA (topical), epidural, intravenous regional (outside North America)	0.5%, 2%, 3%, 4%	8	Medium
Ropivacaine	Epidural, spinal, infiltration, peripheral nerve block	0.2%, 0.5%, 0.75%, 1%	3	Long

[1]Wide variation depending on concentration, location, technique, and whether combined with a vasoconstrictor (epinephrine). Generally the shortest duration is with spinal anesthesia and the longest with peripheral nerve blocks.
[2]No longer recommended for topical anesthesia.
[3]NA, not applicable.
[4]Recent literature describes this agent for short-duration spinal anesthesias.

blood flow and attenuate the rise in intracranial pressure that may accompany intubation in patients with decreased intracranial compliance. Infusions of lidocaine and procaine have been used to supplement general anesthetic techniques, as they are capable of reducing the MAC of volatile anesthetics by up to 40%. Infusions of lidocaine inhibit inflammation and reduce postoperative pain. Infused lidocaine reduces postoperative opioid requirements sufficiently to reduce length of stay after colorectal or open prostate surgery.

Cocaine stimulates the central nervous system and at moderate doses usually causes a sense of euphoria. An overdose is heralded by restlessness, emesis, tremors, convulsions, arrhythmias, respiratory failure, and cardiac arrest.

Local anesthetics temporarily inhibit neuronal function. **In the past, unintentional injection of large volumes of chloroprocaine into the subarachnoid space (during attempts at epidural anesthesia), produced total spinal anesthesia and marked hypotension, and caused prolonged**

neurological deficits. The cause of this neural toxicity may be direct neurotoxicity or a combination of the low pH of chloroprocaine and a preservative, sodium bisulfite. The latter has been replaced in some formulations by an antioxidant, a derivative of disodium ethylenediaminetetraacetic acid (EDTA). Chloroprocaine has also been occasionally associated with severe back pain following epidural administration. The etiology is unclear. Chloroprocaine is available in a preservative-free formulation, which has been used in recent studies safely and successfully for short duration, outpatient spinal anesthetics.

Administration of 5% lidocaine has been associated with neurotoxicity (cauda equina syndrome) following infusion through small-bore catheters used in continuous spinal anesthesia. This may be due to pooling of drug around the cauda equina, resulting in high concentrations and permanent neuronal damage. Animal data suggest that the extent of histological evidence of neurotoxicity following repeat intrathecal injection is lidocaine = tetracaine > bupivacaine > ropivacaine.

Transient neurological symptoms, which consist of dysesthesia, burning pain, and aching in the lower extremities and buttocks, have been reported following spinal anesthesia with a variety of local anesthetic agents, most commonly after use of lidocaine for outpatient spinal anesthesia in men undergoing surgery in the lithotomy position. These symptoms have been attributed to radicular irritation and typically resolve within 1–4 weeks. Many clinicians have substituted 2-chloroprocaine, mepivacaine, or small doses of bupivacaine for lidocaine in spinal anesthesia in the hope of avoiding these transient symptoms.

B. Respiratory

Lidocaine depresses hypoxic drive (the ventilatory response to low PaO_2). Apnea can result from phrenic and intercostal nerve paralysis or depression of the medullary respiratory center following direct exposure to local anesthetic agents (as may occur after retrobulbar blocks; see Chapter 36). Apnea after administration of a "high" spinal or epidural anesthetic is nearly always the result of hypotension, rather than phrenic block. Local anesthetics relax bronchial smooth muscle. Intravenous lidocaine (1.5 mg/kg) may be effective in blocking the reflex bronchoconstriction sometimes associated with intubation. Lidocaine (or any other inhaled agent) administered as an aerosol can lead to bronchospasm in some patients with reactive airway disease.

C. Cardiovascular

All local anesthetics depress myocardial automaticity (spontaneous phase IV depolarization). Myocardial contractility and conduction velocity are also depressed at higher concentrations. These effects result from direct cardiac muscle membrane changes (ie, cardiac Na channel blockade) and in intact organisms from inhibition of the autonomic nervous system. All local anesthetics except cocaine produce smooth muscle relaxation at higher concentrations, which may cause some degree of arteriolar vasodilation. At low concentrations all local anesthetics inhibit nitric oxide, causing vasoconstriction. At increased blood concentrations the combination of arrhythmias, heart block, depression of ventricular contractility, and hypotension may culminate in cardiac arrest. Major cardiovascular toxicity usually requires about three times the local anesthetic concentration in blood as that required to produce seizures. Cardiac arrhythmias or circulatory collapse are the usual presenting signs of local anesthetic overdose during general anesthesia. Particularly in awake subjects, signs of transient cardiovascular stimulation (tachycardia and hypertension) may occur with central nervous system excitation at local anesthetic concentrations producing central nervous system toxic side effects.

Intravenous amiodarone provides effective treatment for some forms of ventricular arrhythmias. Myocardial contractility and arterial blood pressure are generally unaffected by the usual intravenous doses. The hypertension associated with laryngoscopy and intubation is attenuated in some patients by intravenous administration of lidocaine (1.5 mg/kg) 1–3 min prior to instrumentation. On the other hand, overdoses of lidocaine can lead to marked left ventricular contractile dysfunction.

11 Unintentional intravascular injection of bupivacaine during regional anesthesia may produce severe cardiovascular toxicity, including left ventricular depression, atrioventricular heart block, and life-threatening arrhythmias such as ventricular tachycardia and fibrillation. Pregnancy, hypoxemia, and respiratory acidosis are predisposing risk factors. Young children may also be at increased risk of toxicity. Multiple studies have demonstrated that bupivacaine is associated with more pronounced changes in conduction and a greater risk of terminal arrhythmias than comparable doses of lidocaine. Mepivacaine, ropivacaine, and bupivacaine have chiral carbons and therefore can exist in either of two optical isomers (enantiomers). The R(+) optical isomer of bupivacaine blocks more avidly and dissociates more slowly from cardiac Na channels than does the S(−) optical isomer. Resuscitation from bupivacaine-induced cardiac toxicity is often difficult and resistant to standard resuscitation drugs. Recent reports suggest that bolus administration of nutritional lipid solutions at 1.5 mL/kg can resuscitate bupivacaine-intoxicated patients who do not respond to standard therapy. Ropivacaine shares many physicochemical properties with bupivacaine. Onset time and duration of action are similar, but ropivacaine produces less motor block when injected at the same volume and concentration as bupivacaine (which may reflect an overall lower potency as compared with bupivacaine). Ropivacaine appears to have a greater therapeutic index than bupivacaine. This improved safety profile likely reflects its formulation as a pure S(−) isomer—that is, having no R(+) isomer—as opposed to racemic bupivacaine. Levobupivacaine, the S(−) isomer of bupivacaine, which is no longer available in the United States, was reported to have fewer cardiovascular and cerebral side effects than the racemic mixture; studies suggest its cardiovascular effects may approximate those of ropivacaine.

Cocaine's cardiovascular reactions are unlike those of any other local anesthetic. Adrenergic nerve terminals normally reabsorb norepinephrine after its release. Cocaine inhibits this reuptake, thereby potentiating the effects of adrenergic stimulation. Cardiovascular responses to cocaine include hypertension and ventricular ectopy. The latter contraindicated its use in patients anesthetized with halothane. **Cocaine-induced arrhythmias** have been successfully treated with adrenergic and Ca channel antagonists. Cocaine produces vasoconstriction when applied topically and is a useful agent to reduce pain and epistaxis related to nasal intubation in awake patients.

D. Immunological

12 True hypersensitivity reactions to local anesthetic agents—as distinct from systemic toxicity caused by excessive plasma concentration—are uncommon. Esters appear more likely to induce a true allergic reaction (due to IgG or IgE antibodies) especially if they are derivatives (eg, procaine or benzocaine) of p-aminobenzoic acid, a known allergen. Commercial multidose preparations of amides often contain **methylparaben**, which has a chemical structure vaguely similar to that of PABA. As a consequence, generations of anesthesiologists have speculated whether this preservative may be responsible for most of the apparent allergic responses to amide agents. The signs and treatment of allergic drug reactions are discussed in Chapter 55.

E. Musculoskeletal

When directly injected into skeletal muscle (eg, trigger-point injection treatment of myofascial pain), local anesthetics are mildly myotoxic. Regeneration usually occurs 3–4 weeks after local anesthetic injection into muscle. Concomitant steroid or epinephrine injection worsens the myonecrosis.

F. Hematological

Lidocaine mildly depresses normal blood coagulation (reduced thrombosis and decreased platelet aggregation) and enhances fibrinolysis of whole blood as measured by thromboelastography. These effects may underlie the reduced efficacy of an epidural autologous blood patch shortly after local anesthetic administration and the lower incidence of embolic events in patients receiving epidural anesthetics (in older studies of patients not receiving prophylaxis against deep vein thrombosis).

Drug Interactions

Local anesthetics potentiate nondepolarizing muscle relaxant blockade in laboratory experiments, but the clinical importance of this observation is unknown (and probably nil).

Succinylcholine and ester local anesthetics depend on pseudocholinesterase for metabolism. Concurrent administration might conceivably increase the time that both drugs remain unmetabolized in the bloodstream. There is likely no actual clinical importance of this potential interaction.

Dibucaine, an amide local anesthetic, inhibits pseudocholinesterase, and the extent of inhibition by dibucaine defines one family of genetically abnormal pseudocholinesterases (see Chapter 11). Pseudocholinesterase inhibitors (eg, organophosphate poisons) can prolong the metabolism of ester local anesthetics (see Table 11–3).

Histamine (H_2) receptor blockers and β blockers (eg, propranolol) decrease hepatic blood flow and lidocaine clearance. Opioids potentiate epidural and spinal analgesia produced by local anesthetics. Similarly α_2-adrenergic agonists (eg, clonidine) potentiate local anesthetic analgesia produced after epidural or peripheral nerve block injections. Epidural chloroprocaine may interfere with the analgesic actions of neuraxial morphine, notably after cesarean delivery.

CASE DISCUSSION

Local Anesthetic Overdose

An 18-year-old woman in the active stage of labor requests an epidural anesthetic. Immediately following the epidural injection of 2 mL and 5 mL test doses of 2% lidocaine, the patient complains of lip numbness and becomes very apprehensive.

What is your presumptive diagnosis?

Circumoral numbness and apprehension immediately following administration of lidocaine suggest an intravascular injection. These signs will not always be followed by a seizure.

What prophylactic measures should be immediately taken?

The patient should already be receiving supplemental oxygen. She should be closely observed for a possible (but unlikely) seizure.

If symptoms progress to a generalized convulsion, what treatment should be initiated?

The laboring patient is always considered to be at risk for aspiration (see Chapter 41). Therefore, protecting the airway is an important concern. Immediate administration of succinylcholine should be followed by a rapid-sequence intubation (see Case Discussion, Chapter 17). Although the succinylcholine will eliminate tonic–clonic activity, it will not address the underlying cerebral excitability. An anticonvulsant such as midazolam (1–2 mg) or propofol (20–50 mg) should be administered with or before succinylcholine. It is clear from this sequence of events that wherever conduction anesthetics are administered, comparable resuscitation drugs and equipment must be available as for a general anesthetic.

What could have been expected if a large dose of bupivacaine (eg, 15 mL 0.5% bupivacaine)—instead of lidocaine—had been given intravascularly?

When administered at "comparably anesthetizing" doses bupivacaine is more cardiotoxic than lidocaine. Acute acidosis (nearly universal after a seizure) tends to potentiate local anesthetic toxicity. Ventricular arrhythmias and conduction disturbances may lead to cardiac arrest and death. Bupivacaine is considered a more potent cardiac Na channel inhibitor because Na channels unbind bupivacaine more slowly than lidocaine. Amiodarone should be considered the preferred alternative to lidocaine in the treatment of local anesthetic-induced ventricular tachyarrhythmias. Vasopressors may include epinephrine and vasopressin. The reason for the apparent greater susceptibility to local anesthetic cardiotoxicity during pregnancy is unclear. Although total dose (not concentration) of local anesthetic determines toxicity, the Food and

Drug Administration recommends against use of 0.75% bupivacaine in pregnant and elderly patients.

What could have prevented the toxic reaction described?

The risk from an accidental intravascular injection of local anesthetic during attempted epidural anesthesia is reduced by using test doses and administering the anesthetic dose in smaller, safer aliquots. Finally, one should administer only the minimum appropriate total dose of local anesthetic for a given regional anesthetic procedure.

SUGGESTED READING

Cousins MJ, Carr DB, Horlocker TT, Bridenbaugh PO (editors): *Cousins & Bridenbugh's Neural Blockade in Clinical Anesthesia and Pain Medicine*, 4th ed. Lippincott, Williams & Wilkins, 2009.

Hadzic A (editor): *Textbook of Regional Anesthesia and Acute Pain Management*. McGraw-Hill, 2007. Includes discussions of the selection of local anesthetic agents.

Hardman J, Limbird L, Gilman A: *Goodman and Gilman's The Pharmacological Basis of Therapeutics*, 12th ed. McGraw-Hill, 2011.

Rosenblatt MA, Abel M, Fischer GW, et al: Successful use of a 20% lipid emulsion to resuscitate a patient after a presumed bupivacaine–related cardiac arrest. Anesthesiology 2006;105:217-218.

Strichartz GR, Sanchez V, Arthur GR, et al: Fundamental properties of local anesthetics. II. Measured octanol: buffer partition coefficients and pK_a values of clinically used drugs. Anesth Analg 1990;71:158.

WEB SITE

http://www.lipidrescue.org

This web site provides up-to-date information about the use of lipid for rescue from local anesthetic toxicity.

Adjuncts to Anesthesia

1 Diphenhydramine is one of a diverse group of drugs that competitively blocks H_1 receptors. Many drugs with H_1-receptor antagonist properties have considerable antimuscarinic, or atropine-like, activity (eg, dry mouth), or antiserotonergic activity (antiemetic).

2 H_2 blockers reduce the perioperative risk of aspiration pneumonia by decreasing gastric fluid volume and raising the pH of gastric contents.

3 Metoclopramide increases lower esophageal sphincter tone, speeds gastric emptying, and lowers gastric fluid volume by enhancing the stimulatory effects of acetylcholine on intestinal smooth muscle.

4 Ondansetron, granisetron, and dolasetron selectively block serotonin 5-HT_3 receptors, with little or no effect on dopamine receptors. 5-HT_3 receptors, which are located peripherally and centrally, appear to play an important role in the initiation of the vomiting reflex.

5 Ketorolac is a parenterally administered nonsteroidal antiinflammatory drug that provides analgesia by inhibiting prostaglandin synthesis.

6 Clonidine is a commonly used antihypertensive agent but in anesthesia it is used as an adjunct for epidural and peripheral nerve block anesthesia and analgesia. It is often used in the management of patients with chronic neuropathic pain to increase the efficacy of epidural opioid infusions.

7 Dexmedetomidine is a parenteral selective α_2 agonist with sedative properties. It appears to be more selective for the α_2 receptor than clonidine.

8 Selective activation of carotid chemoreceptors by low doses of doxapram stimulates hypoxic drive, producing an increase in tidal volume and a slight increase in respiratory rate. However, doxapram is not a specific reversal agent and should not replace standard supportive therapy (ie, mechanical ventilation).

9 Naloxone reverses the agonist activity associated with endogenous or exogenous opioid compounds.

10 Flumazenil is useful in the reversal of benzodiazepine sedation and the treatment of benzodiazepine overdose.

11 Aspiration does not necessarily result in aspiration pneumonia. The seriousness of the lung damage depends on the volume and composition of the aspirate. Patients are at risk if their gastric volume is greater than 25 mL (0.4 mL/kg) and their gastric pH is less than 2.5.

Many drugs are routinely administered by anesthetists perioperatively to protect against aspiration pneumonitis, to prevent or reduce the incidence of perianesthetic nausea and vomiting, and to reverse respiratory depression secondary to narcotics or benzodiazepines. This chapter discusses these agents along with other unique classes of drugs that are often administered as adjuvants during anesthesia or analgesia.

Aspiration

Aspiration of gastric contents is a rare, potentially fatal, and often litigious event that can complicate anesthesia. Based on an animal study, it is often stated that aspiration of 25 mL of volume at a pH of less than 2.5 will be sufficient to produce aspiration pneumonia. Many factors place patients at risk for aspiration, including "full" stomach, intestinal obstruction, hiatal hernia, obesity, pregnancy, reflux disease, emergency surgery, and inadequate depth of anesthesia.

Many approaches are employed to reduce the potential for aspiration perioperatively. Many of these interventions, such as the holding of cricoid pressure (Sellick's maneuver) and rapid sequence induction, may only offer limited protection. Cricoid pressure can be applied incorrectly and fail to occlude the esophagus. Whether it has *any* beneficial effect on outcomes even when it is applied correctly remains unproven. Anesthetic agents can decrease lower esophageal sphincter tone and decrease or obliterate the gag reflex, theoretically increasing the risk for passive aspiration. Additionally, inadequately anesthetized patients can vomit with an unprotected airway, likewise leading to aspiration. Different combinations of premedications have been advocated to reduce gastric volume, increase gastric pH, or augment lower esophageal sphincter tone. These agents include antihistamines, antacids, and metoclopramide.

HISTAMINE-RECEPTOR ANTAGONISTS

Histamine Physiology

Histamine is found in the central nervous system, in the gastric mucosa, and in other peripheral tissues. It is synthesized by decarboxylation of the amino

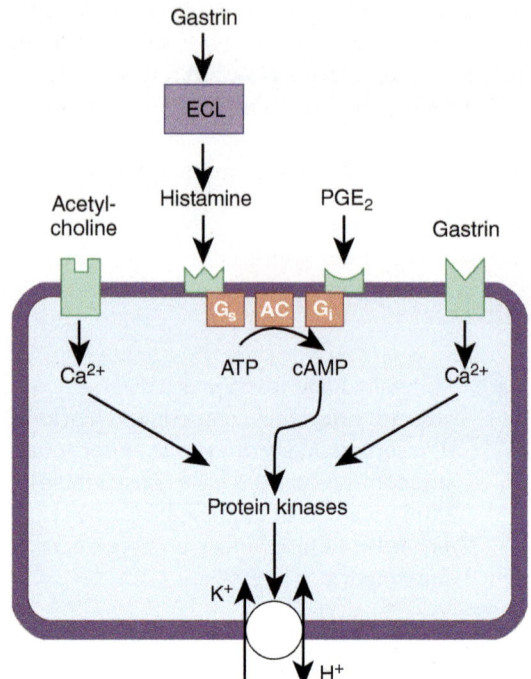

FIGURE 17–1 Secretion of hydrochloric acid is normally mediated by gastrin-induced histamine release from enterochromaffin-like cells (ECL) in the stomach. Note that acid secretion by gastric parietal cells can also be increased indirectly by acetylcholine (AC) via stimulation of M_3 receptors and directly by gastrin through an increase in intracellular Ca^{2+} concentration. Prostaglandin E_2 (PGE_2) can inhibit acid secretion by decreasing cyclic adenosine monophosphate (cAMP) activity. ATP, adenosine triphosphate; G_i, G inhibitory protein; G_s, G stimulatory protein.

acid histidine. Histaminergic neurons are primarily located in the posterior hypothalamus but have wide projections in the brain. Histamine also normally plays a major role in the secretion of hydrochloric acid by parietal cells in the stomach (Figure 17–1). The highest concentrations of histamine are found in the storage granules of circulating basophils and mast cells throughout the body. Mast cells tend to be concentrated in connective tissue just beneath epithelial (mucosal) surfaces. Histamine release (degranulation) from these cells can be triggered by chemical, mechanical, or immunological stimulation

Multiple receptors mediate the effects of histamine. The H_1 receptor activates phospholipase C, whereas the H_2 receptor increases intracellular cyclic adenosine monophosphate (cAMP). An H_3 receptor is primarily located on histamine-secreting cells and mediates negative feedback, inhibiting the synthesis and release of additional histamine. Histamine-*N*-methyltransferase metabolizes histamine to inactive metabolites that are excreted in the urine.

A. Cardiovascular

Histamine reduces arterial blood pressure but increases heart rate and myocardial contractility. H_1-Receptor stimulation increases capillary permeability and enhances ventricular irritability, whereas H_2-receptor stimulation increases heart rate and increases contractility. Both types of receptors mediate peripheral arteriolar dilation and some coronary vasodilation.

B. Respiratory

Histamine constricts bronchiolar smooth muscle via the H_1 receptor. H_2-Receptor stimulation may produce mild bronchodilation. Histamine has variable effects on the pulmonary vasculature; the H_1 receptor appears to mediate some pulmonary vasodilation, whereas the H_2 receptor may be responsible for histamine-mediated pulmonary vasoconstriction.

C. Gastrointestinal

Activation of H_2 receptors in parietal cells increases gastric acid secretion. Stimulation of H_1 receptors leads to contraction of intestinal smooth muscle.

D. Dermal

The classic wheal-and-flare response of the skin to histamine results from increased capillary permeability and vasodilation, primarily via H_1-receptor activation.

E. Immunological

Histamine is a major mediator of type 1 hypersensitivity reactions. H_1-Receptor stimulation attracts leukocytes and induces synthesis of prostaglandin. In contrast, the H_2 receptor appears to activate suppressor T lymphocytes.

1. H_1-Receptor Antagonists

Mechanism of Action

Diphenhydramine (an ethanolamine) is one of a diverse group of drugs that competitively blocks H_1 receptors (Table 17–1). Many drugs with

TABLE 17–1 Properties of commonly used H_1-receptor antagonists.[1]

Drug	Route	Dose (mg)	Duration (h)	Sedation	Antiemesis
Diphenhydramine (Benadryl)	PO, IM, IV	25–50	3–6	+++	++
Dimenhydrinate (Dramamine)	PO, IM, IV	50–100	3–6	+++	++
Chlorpheniramine (Chlor-Trimeton)	PO IM, IV	2–12 5–20	4–8	++	0
Hydroxyzine (Atarax, Vistaril)	PO, IM	25–100	4–12	+++	++
Promethazine (Phenergan)	PO, IM, IV	12.5–50	4–12	+++	+++
Cetirizine (Zyrtec)	PO	5–10	24	+	
Cyproheptadine (Periactin)	PO	4	6–8	++	
Dimenhydrinate (Dramamine)	PO	50	6–12	++	
Fexofenadine (Allegra)	PO	30–60	12	0	
Meclizine (Antivert)	PO	12.5–50	8–24	+	
Loratadine (Claritin)	PO	10	24	0	

[1]0, no effect; ++, moderate activity; +++, marked activity.

H_1-receptor antagonist properties have considerable antimuscarinic, or atropine-like, activity (eg, dry mouth), or antiserotonergic activity (antiemetic). Promethazine is a phenothiazine derivative with H_1-receptor antagonist activity as well as antidopaminergic and α-adrenergic–blocking properties.

Clinical Uses

Like other H_1-receptor antagonists, diphenhydramine has a multitude of therapeutic uses: suppression of allergic reactions and symptoms of upper respiratory tract infections (eg, urticaria, rhinitis, conjunctivitis); vertigo, nausea, and vomiting (eg, motion sickness, Ménière's disease); sedation; suppression of cough; and dyskinesia (eg, parkinsonism, drug-induced extrapyramidal side effects). Some of these actions are predictable from an understanding of histamine physiology, whereas others are the result of the drugs' antimuscarinic and antiserotonergic effects (Table 17–1). Although H_1 blockers prevent the bronchoconstrictive response to histamine, they are ineffective in treating bronchial asthma, which is primarily due to other mediators. Likewise, H_1 blockers will not completely prevent the hypotensive effect of histamine unless an H_2 blocker is administered concomitantly.

The antiemetic and mild hypnotic effects of antihistaminic drugs (particularly diphenhydramine, promethazine, and hydroxyzine) have led to their use for premedication. Although many H_1 blockers cause significant sedation, ventilatory drive is usually unaffected in the absence of other sedative medications. Promethazine and hydroxyzine were often combined with opioids to potentiate analgesia. Newer (second-generation) antihistamines tend to produce little or no sedation because of limited penetration across the blood–brain barrier. This group of drugs is used primarily for allergic rhinitis and urticaria. They include loratadine, fexofenadine, and cetirizine. Many preparations for allergic rhinitis often also contain vasoconstrictors such as pseudoephedrine. Meclizine and dimenhydrinate are used primarily as an antiemetic, particularly for motion sickness, and in the management of vertigo. Cyproheptadine, which also has significant serotonin antagonist activity, has been used in the management of Cushing's Disease, carcinoid syndrome, and vascular (cluster) headaches.

Dosage

The usual adult dose of diphenhydramine is 25–50 mg (0.5–1.5 mg/kg) orally, intramuscularly, or intravenously every 4–6 h. The doses of other H_1-receptor antagonists are listed in Table 17–1.

Drug Interactions

The sedative effects of H_1-receptor antagonists can potentiate other central nervous system depressants such as barbiturates, benzodiazepines, and opioids.

2. H_2-Receptor Antagonists

Mechanism of Action

H_2-Receptor antagonists include cimetidine, famotidine, nizatidine, and ranitidine (Table 17–2). These agents competitively inhibit histamine binding to H_2 receptors, thereby reducing gastric acid output and raising gastric pH.

Clinical Uses

All H_2-receptor antagonists are equally effective in the treatment of peptic duodenal and gastric ulcers, hypersecretory states (Zollinger–Ellison syndrome), and gastroesophageal reflux disease (GERD). Intravenous preparations are also used to prevent stress ulceration in critically ill patients. Duodenal and gastric ulcers are usually associated with *Helicobacter pylori* infection, which is treated with combinations of bismuth, tetracycline, and metronidazole. By decreasing gastric fluid volume and hydrogen ion content, H_2 blockers reduce the perioperative risk of aspiration pneumonia. These drugs affect the pH of only those gastric secretions that occur after their administration.

The combination of H_1- and H_2-receptor antagonists provides some protection against drug-induced allergic reactions (eg, intravenous radiocontrast, chymopapain injection for lumbar disk disease, protamine, vital blue dyes used for sentinel node biopsy). Although pretreatment with these agents does not reduce histamine release, it may decrease subsequent hypotension.

TABLE 17–2 **Pharmacology of aspiration pneumonia prophylaxis.**[1]

Drug	Route	Dose	Onset	Duration	Acidity	Volume	LES Tone
Cimetidine (Tagamet)	PO IV	300–800 mg 300 mg	1–2 h	4–8 h	↓↓↓	↓↓	0
Ranitidine (Zantac)	PO IV	150–300 mg 50 mg	1–2 h	10–12 h	↓↓↓	↓↓	0
Famotidine (Pepcid)	PO IV	20–40 mg 20 mg	1–2 h	10–12 h	↓↓↓	↓↓	0
Nizatidine (Axid)	PO	150–300 mg	0.5–1 h	10–12 h	↓↓↓	↓↓	0
Nonparticulate antacids (Bicitra, Polycitra)	PO	15–30 mL	5–10 min	30–60 min	↓↓↓	↑	0
Metoclopramide (Reglan)	IV PO	10 mg 10–15 mg	1–3 min	1–2 h 30–60 min[2]	0	↓↓	↑↑

[1]0, no effect; ↓↓, moderate decrease; ↓↓↓, marked decrease; ↑, slight increase; ↑↑, moderate increase; LES, lower esophageal sphincter.
[2]Oral metoclopramide has a quite variable onset of action and duration of action.

Side Effects

Rapid intravenous injection of cimetidine or ranitidine has been rarely associated with hypotension,
bradycardia, arrhythmias, and cardiac arrest. These
adverse cardiovascular effects have been reported
following the administration of cimetidine to critically ill patients. In contrast, famotidine can be
safely injected intravenously over a 2-min period.
H_2-Receptor antagonists change the gastric flora by
virtue of their pH effects. Complications of long-
term cimetidine therapy include hepatotoxicity (elevated serum transaminases), interstitial nephritis
(elevated serum creatinine), granulocytopenia, and
thrombocytopenia. Cimetidine also binds to androgen receptors, occasionally causing gynecomastia
and impotence. Finally, cimetidine has been associated with changes in mental status ranging from
lethargy and hallucinations to seizures, particularly
in elderly patients. In contrast, ranitidine, nizatidine,
and famotidine do not affect androgen receptors and
penetrate the blood–brain barrier poorly.

Dosage

As a premedication to reduce the risk of aspiration pneumonia, H_2-receptor antagonists should
be administered at bedtime and again at least 2 h
before surgery (Table 17–2). Because all four drugs

are eliminated primarily by the kidneys, the dose
should be reduced in patients with significant renal
dysfunction.

Drug Interactions

Cimetidine may reduce hepatic blood flow and binds
to the cytochrome P-450 mixed-function oxidases.
These effects slow the metabolism of a multitude of
drugs, including lidocaine, propranolol, diazepam,
theophylline, phenobarbital, warfarin, and phenytoin. Ranitidine is a weak inhibitor of the cytochrome
P-450 system, and no significant drug interactions
have been demonstrated. Famotidine and nizatidine
do not appear to affect the cytochrome P-450 system.

ANTACIDS
Mechanism of Action

Antacids neutralize the acidity of gastric fluid by
providing a base (usually hydroxide, carbonate,
bicarbonate, citrate, or trisilicate) that reacts with
hydrogen ions to form water.

Clinical Uses

Common uses of antacids include the treatment of
gastric and duodenal ulcers, GERD, and Zollinger–
Ellison syndrome. In anesthesiology, antacids

provide protection against the harmful effects of aspiration pneumonia by raising the pH of gastric contents. Unlike H_2-receptor antagonists, antacids have an immediate effect. Unfortunately, they increase intragastric volume. Aspiration of particulate antacids (aluminum or magnesium hydroxide) produces abnormalities in lung function comparable to those that occur following acid aspiration. Nonparticulate antacids (sodium citrate or sodium bicarbonate) are much less damaging to lung alveoli if aspirated. Furthermore, nonparticulate antacids mix with gastric contents better than particulate solutions. Timing is critical, as nonparticulate antacids lose their effectiveness 30–60 min after ingestion.

Dosage

The usual adult dose of a 0.3 M solution of sodium citrate—Bicitra (sodium citrate and citric acid) or Polycitra (sodium citrate, potassium citrate, and citric acid)—is 15–30 mL orally, 15–30 min prior to induction.

Drug Interactions

Because antacids alter gastric and urinary pH, they change the absorption and elimination of many drugs. The rate of absorption of digoxin, cimetidine, and ranitidine is slowed, whereas the rate of phenobarbital elimination is quickened.

METOCLOPRAMIDE

Mechanism of Action

Metoclopramide acts peripherally as a cholinomimetic (ie, facilitates acetylcholine transmission at selective muscarinic receptors) and centrally as a dopamine receptor antagonist. Its action as a prokinetic agent in the upper gastrointestinal (GI) tract is not dependent on vagal innervation but is abolished by anticholinergic agents. It does not stimulate secretions.

Clinical Uses

3 By enhancing the stimulatory effects of acetylcholine on intestinal smooth muscle, metoclopramide increases lower esophageal sphincter tone, speeds gastric emptying, and lowers gastric fluid volume. These properties account for its efficacy in the treatment of patients with diabetic gastroparesis and GERD, as well as prophylaxis for those at risk for aspiration pneumonia. Metoclopramide does not affect the secretion of gastric acid or the pH of gastric fluid.

Metoclopramide produces an antiemetic effect by blocking dopamine receptors in the chemoreceptor trigger zone of the central nervous system. However, at doses used clinically during the perioperative period, the drug's ability to reduce postoperative nausea and vomiting is negligible.

Side Effects

Rapid intravenous injection may cause abdominal cramping, and metoclopramide is contraindicated in patients with complete intestinal obstruction. It can induce a hypertensive crisis in patients with pheochromocytoma by releasing catecholamines from the tumor. Sedation, nervousness, and extrapyramidal signs from dopamine antagonism (eg, akathisia) are uncommon and reversible. Nonetheless, metoclopramide is best avoided in patients with Parkinson's disease. Metoclopramide-induced increases in aldosterone and prolactin secretion are probably inconsequential during short-term therapy. Metoclopramide may rarely result in hypotension and arrhythmias.

Dosage

An adult dose of 10–20 mg of metoclopramide (0.25 mg/kg) is effective orally, intramuscularly, or intravenously (injected over 5 min). Larger doses (1–2 mg/kg) have been used to prevent emesis during chemotherapy. The onset of action is much more rapid following parenteral (3–5 min) than oral (30–60 min) administration. Because metoclopramide is excreted in the urine, its dose should be decreased in patients with renal dysfunction.

Drug Interactions

Antimuscarinic drugs (eg, atropine, glycopyrrolate) block the GI effects of metoclopramide. Metoclopramide decreases the absorption of orally administered cimetidine. Concurrent use of phenothiazines or butyrophenones (droperidol) increases the likelihood of extrapyramidal side effects.

PROTON PUMP INHIBITORS

Mechanism of Action

These agents, including omeprazole (Prilosec), lansoprazole (Prevacid), rabeprazole (Aciphex), esomeprazole (Nexium), and pantoprazole (Protonix), bind to the proton pump of parietal cells in the gastric mucosa and inhibit secretion of hydrogen ions.

Clinical Uses

Proton pump inhibitors (PPIs) are indicated for the treatment of duodenal ulcer, GERD, and Zollinger–Ellison syndrome. They may promote healing of peptic ulcers and erosive GERD more quickly than H_2-receptor blockers. There are ongoing questions regarding the safety of PPIs in patients taking clopidogrel (Plavix) because of concerns of inadequate antiplatelet therapy when these drugs are combined.

Side Effects

PPIs are generally well tolerated, causing few side effects. Adverse side effects primarily involve the GI system (nausea, abdominal pain, constipation, diarrhea). On rare occasions, these drugs have been associated with myalgias, anaphylaxis, angioedema, and severe dermatological reactions. Long-term use of PPIs has also been associated with gastric enterochromaffin-like cell hyperplasia and an increased risk of pneumonia secondary to bacterial colonization in the higher-pH environment.

Dosage

Recommended oral doses for adults are omeprazole, 20 mg; lansoprazole, 15 mg; rabeprazole, 20 mg; and pantoprazole, 40 mg. Because these drugs are primarily eliminated by the liver, repeat doses should be decreased in patients with severe liver impairment.

Drug Interactions

PPIs can interfere with hepatic P-450 enzymes, potentially decreasing the clearance of diazepam, warfarin, and phenytoin. Concurrent administration can decrease clopidogrel (Plavix) effectiveness, as the latter medication is dependent on hepatic enzymes for activation.

Postoperative Nausea & Vomiting (PONV)

Without any prophylaxis, PONV occurs in approximately 20–30% of the general surgical population and up to 70–80% in patients with predisposing risk factors (Table 17–3). As anesthetic duration increases, so, too, does PONV risk. When the risk is sufficiently great, prophylactic antiemetic medications are administered and strategies to reduce its incidence are initiated. The Society of Ambulatory Anesthesia (SAMBA) provides simplified risk scoring systems, which assign points for specific risk factors, as well as guidelines that assist in the management of at-risk patients (Table 17–4). Obesity, anxiety, and reversal of neuromuscular blockade are not independent risk factors for PONV.

Drugs used in the prophylaxis and treatment of PONV include 5-HT$_3$ antagonists, butyrophenones, dexamethasone, neurokinin-1 receptor antagonists (aprepitant, Emend); antihistamines and transdermal scopolamine may also be used. At-risk patients often benefit from one or more prophylactic measures.

TABLE 17–3 **Risk factors for postoperative nausea and vomiting (PONV).**[1,2]

Patient-specific risk factors:
Female gender
Nonsmoking status
History of PONV/motion sickness
Anesthetic risk factors:
Use of volatile anesthetics
Use of nitrous oxide
Use of intraoperative and postoperative opioids
Surgical risk factors:
Duration of surgery (each 30-min increase in duration increases PONV risk by 60%, so that a baseline risk of 10% is increased by 16% after 30 min)
Type of surgery

[1]Reproduced, with permission, from Gan TJ, Meyer TA, Apfel CC, et al: Society for ambulatory anesthesia guidelines for management of postoperative nausea and vomiting. Anesth Analg 2007;105:1615.

[2]Risk factors are assigned points and an increasing number of points increases the likelihood of PONV. Refer to the Society of Ambulatory Anesthesia (SAMBA) guidelines.

TABLE 17–4 **SAMBA guidelines to reduce the risk of postoperative nausea and vomiting (PONV).[1]**

1. Identify patients at risk for PONV.
2. Employ management strategies to reduce PONV risk.
3. Employ one to two prophylactic measures in adults at moderate PONV risk.
4. Use multiple interventions in patients at high PONV risk.
5. Administer prophylactic antiemetic therapy to children at high risk using combination therapy.
6. Provide antiemetic therapy to patients with PONV who did not receive prophylactic therapy or in whom prophylaxis failed. Therapy should be with a drug from a different class than that which failed to provide prophylaxis.

[1]Data based on guidelines from the Society of Ambulatory Anesthesia (SAMBA). Refer to Gan TJ, Meyer TA, Apfel CC, et al: Society for ambulatory anesthesia guidelines for management of postoperative nausea and vomiting. Anesth Analg 2007;105:1615.

5-HT$_3$ RECEPTOR ANTAGONISTS

Serotonin Physiology

Serotonin, 5-hydroxytryptamine (5-HT), is present in large quantities in platelets and the GI tract (enterochromaffin cells and the myenteric plexus). It is also an important neurotransmitter in multiple areas of the central nervous system. Serotonin is formed by hydroxylation and decarboxylation of tryptophan. Monoamine oxidase inactivates serotonin into 5-hydroxyindoleacetic acid (5-HIAA). The physiology of serotonin is very complex because there are at least seven receptor types, most with multiple subtypes. The 5-HT$_3$ receptor mediates vomiting and is found in the GI tract and the brain (area postrema). The 5-HT$_{2A}$ receptors are responsible for smooth muscle contraction and platelet aggregation, the 5-HT$_4$ receptors in the GI tract mediate secretion and peristalsis, and the 5-HT$_6$ and 5-HT$_7$ receptors are located primarily in the limbic system where they appear to play a role in depression. All except the 5-HT$_3$ receptor are coupled to G proteins and affect either adenylyl cyclase or phospholipase C; effects of the 5-HT$_3$ receptor are mediated via an ion channel.

A. Cardiovascular

Except in the heart and skeletal muscle, serotonin is a powerful vasoconstrictor of arterioles and veins. Its vasodilator effect in the heart is endothelium dependent. When the myocardial endothelium is damaged following injury, serotonin produces vasoconstriction. The pulmonary and renal vasculatures are very sensitive to the arterial vasoconstrictive effects of serotonin. Modest and transient increases in cardiac contractility and heart rate may occur immediately following serotonin release; reflex bradycardia often follows. Vasodilation in skeletal muscle can subsequently cause hypotension.

B. Respiratory

Contraction of smooth muscle increases airway resistance. Bronchoconstriction from released serotonin is often a prominent feature of carcinoid syndrome

C. Gastrointestinal

Direct smooth muscle contraction (via 5-HT$_2$ receptors) and serotonin-induced release of acetylcholine in the myenteric plexus (via 5-HT$_3$ receptors) greatly augment peristalsis. Secretions are unaffected.

D. Hematological

Activation of 5-HT$_2$ receptors causes platelet aggregation.

Mechanism of Action

4 Ondansetron (Zofran), granisetron (Kytril), and dolasetron (Anzemet) selectively block serotonin 5-HT$_3$ receptors, with little or no effect on dopamine receptors (**Figure 17–2**). 5-HT$_3$

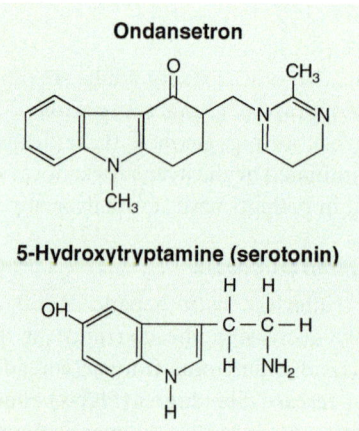

Ondansetron

5-Hydroxytryptamine (serotonin)

FIGURE 17–2 Ondansetron is structurally related to serotonin.

receptors, which are located peripherally (abdominal vagal afferents) and centrally (chemoreceptor trigger zone of the area postrema and the nucleus tractus solitarius), appear to play an important role in the initiation of the vomiting reflex. The 5-HT$_3$ receptors of the chemoreceptor trigger zone in the area postrema reside outside the blood–brain barrier. The trigger zone is activated by substances such as anesthetics and opioids and signals the nucleus tractus solitarius, resulting in PONV. Emetogenic stimuli from the GI tract similarly stimulate the development of PONV.

Clinical Uses

5-HT$_3$-receptor antagonists are generally administered at the end of surgery. All these agents are effective antiemetics in the postoperative period. In comparison with other antiemetic agents such as droperidol (1.25 mg) and dexamethasone (4 mg), ondansetron appears equally effective. A new agent, palonosetron (Aloxi), has an extended duration of action and may reduce the incidence of postdischarge nausea and vomiting (PDNV).

Side Effects

5-HT$_3$ receptor antagonists are essentially devoid of serious side effects, even in amounts several times the recommended dose. They do not appear to cause sedation, extrapyramidal signs, or respiratory depression. The most commonly reported side effect is headache. All three drugs can slightly prolong the QT interval on the electrocardiogram. This effect may be more frequent with dolasetron, although it has not been associated with any adverse arrhythmias. Nonetheless, these drugs, particularly dolasetron, should be used cautiously in patients who are taking antiarrhythmic drugs or who have a prolonged QT interval.

Ondansetron undergoes extensive metabolism in the liver via hydroxylation and conjugation by cytochrome P-450 enzymes. Liver failure impairs clearance several-fold, and the dose should be reduced accordingly. The recommended intravenous dose is 12.5 mg for dolasetron and 1 mg for granisetron. All three drugs are available in oral formulations for PONV prophylaxis.

BUTYROPHENONES

Droperidol (0.625–1.25 mg) was previously used routinely for PONV prophylaxis. Given at the end of the procedure it blocks dopamine receptors that contribute to the development of PONV. Despite its effectiveness, many practitioners no longer routinely administer this medication because of a U.S. Food and Drug Administration (FDA) black box warning related to concerns that doses described in the product labeling ("package insert") may lead to QT prolongation and development of torsades des pointes dysrhythmia. However, the doses relevant to the FDA warning, as acknowledged by the FDA, were those used for neurolept anesthesia (5–15 mg), not the much smaller doses employed for PONV. Cardiac monitoring is warranted when large doses of the drug are used. There is no evidence that use of droperidol at the doses routinely employed for PONV management increases the risk of sudden cardiac death in the perioperative population.

As with other drugs that antagonize dopamine, droperidol use in patients with Parkinson's disease and in patients manifesting extrapyramidal signs should be carefully considered.

The phenothiazine, prochlorperazine (Compazine), which affects multiple receptors (histaminergic, dopaminergic, muscarinic), may be used for PONV management. It may cause extrapyramidal and anticholinergic side effects. Promethazine (Phenergan) works primarily as an anticholinergic agent and antihistamine and likewise can be used to treat PONV. As with other agents of this class, anticholinergic effects (sedation, delirium, confusion, vision changes) can complicate the postoperative period.

DEXAMETHASONE

Dexamethasone (Decadron) in doses as small as 4 mg has been shown to be as effective as ondansetron in reducing the incidence of PONV. Dexamethasone should be given at induction as opposed to the end of surgery, and its mechanism of action is unclear. There appear to be no significant or long-lasting systemic effects from this dose of glucocorticoid.

NEUROKININ-1 RECEPTOR ANTAGONIST

Substance P is a neuropeptide that interacts at neurokinin-1 (NK_1) receptors. NK_1 antagonists inhibit substance P at central and peripheral receptors. Aprepitant (Emend), an NK_1 antagonist, has been found to reduce PONV perioperatively and is additive with ondansetron for this indication.

OTHER PONV STRATEGIES

Several other agents and techniques have been employed to reduce the incidence of PONV. Transdermal scopolamine has been used effectively, although it may produce central anticholinergic effects (confusion, blurred vision, and dry mouth). Acupuncture, acupressure, and transcutaneous electrical stimulation of the P6 acupuncture point can reduce PONV incidence and medication requirements.

As no single agent will both treat and prevent PONV, perioperative management centers on identifying patients at greatest risk so that prophylaxis, often with multiple agents, may be initiated.

Other Drugs Used as Adjuvants to Anesthesia

KETOROLAC

Mechanism of Action

5 Ketorolac is a parenteral nonsteroidal antiinflammatory drug (NSAID) that provides analgesia by inhibiting prostaglandin synthesis.

Clinical Uses

Ketorolac is indicated for the short-term (<5 days) management of pain, and appears to be particularly useful in the immediate postoperative period. A standard dose of ketorolac provides analgesia equivalent to 6–12 mg of morphine administered by the same route. Its time to onset is also similar to morphine, but ketorolac has a longer duration of action (6–8 h).

Ketorolac, a peripherally acting drug, has become a popular alternative to opioids for postoperative analgesia because of its minimal central nervous system side effects. Specifically, ketorolac does not cause respiratory depression, sedation, or nausea and vomiting. In fact, ketorolac does not cross the blood–brain barrier to any significant degree. Numerous studies have shown that oral and parenteral NSAIDs have an opioid-sparing effect. They may be most beneficial in patients at increased risk for postoperative respiratory depression or emesis.

Side Effects

As with other NSAIDs, ketorolac inhibits platelet aggregation and prolongs bleeding time. It and other NSAIDs should therefore be used with caution in patients at risk for postoperative hemorrhage. Long-term administration may lead to renal toxicity (eg, papillary necrosis) or GI tract ulceration with bleeding and perforation. Because ketorolac depends on elimination, it should not be given to patients with kidney failure. Ketorolac is contraindicated in patients allergic to aspirin or NSAIDs. Patients with asthma have an increased incidence of aspirin sensitivity (approximately 10%), particularly if they also have a history of nasal polyps (approximately 20%).

Dosage

Ketorolac has been approved for administration as either a 60 mg intramuscular or 30 mg intravenous loading dose; a maintenance dose of 15–30 mg every 6 h is recommended. Elderly patients clear ketorolac more slowly and should receive reduced doses.

Drug Interactions

Aspirin decreases the protein binding of ketorolac, increasing the amount of active unbound drug. Ketorolac does not affect minimum alveolar concentration of inhalation anesthetic agents, and its administration does not alter the hemodynamics of anesthetized patients. It decreases the postoperative requirement for opioid analgesics.

Other NSAID Adjuvant Drugs

Other NSAID agents are used perioperatively. Ketorolac and other NSAIDs inhibit cyclooxygenase

(COX) isoenzymes. COX-1 maintains gastric mucosa and stimulates platelet aggregation. COX-2 is expressed during inflammation. Whereas ketorolac is a nonselective COX inhibitor, other agents such as parecoxib (Dynastat), celecoxib (Celebrex), and rofecoxib (Vioxx) are specific for COX-2. COX-2 inhibitors spare both the gastric mucosa and platelet function. However, their use is associated with an increased risk of cardiovascular thromboembolic events. Because nonspecific NSAIDs such as ketorolac also inhibit COX-2, their use following cardiac bypass surgery is contraindicated.

Intravenous acetaminophen (Ofirmev) has recently become available for perioperative use in the United States. Acetaminophen is a centrally acting analgesic with likely central COX inhibition and with weak peripheral COX effects resulting in a lack of gastric irritation and clotting abnormalities. A maximal adult (>50 kg weight) dose of 1 g is infused to a maximum total dose of 4 g/d. Patients weighing 50 kg or less should receive a maximal dose of 15 mg/kg and a maximal total dose of 75 mg/kg/d. Hepatoxicity is a known risk of overdosage, and the drug should be used with caution in patients with hepatic disease or undergoing hepatic surgery.

CLONIDINE
Mechanism of Action

Clonidine (Catapres, Duraclon) is an imidazoline derivative with predominantly α_2-adrenergic agonist activity. It is highly lipid soluble and readily penetrates the blood–brain barrier and the placenta. Studies indicate that binding of clonidine to receptors is highest in the rostral ventrolateral medulla in the brainstem (the final common pathway for sympathetic outflow) where it activates inhibitory neurons. The overall effect is to decrease sympathetic activity, enhance parasympathetic tone, and reduce circulating catecholamines. There is also evidence that much of clonidine's antihypertensive action occurs via binding to a nonadrenergic (imidazoline) receptor. In contrast, its analgesic effects, particularly in the spinal cord, are mediated entirely via pre- and possibly postsynaptic α_2-adrenergic receptors that block nociceptive transmission. Clonidine also has local anesthetic effects when applied to

peripheral nerves and is frequently added to local anesthetic solutions.

Clinical Uses

6 Clonidine is a commonly used antihypertensive agent that reduces sympathetic tone, decreasing systemic vascular resistance, heart rate, and blood pressure. In anesthesia, clonidine is used as an adjunct for epidural, caudal, and peripheral nerve block anesthesia and analgesia. It is often used in the management of patients with chronic neuropathic pain to increase the efficacy of epidural opioid infusions. When given epidurally, the analgesic effect of clonidine is segmental, being localized to the level at which it is injected or infused. When added to local anesthetics of intermediate duration (eg, mepivacaine or lidocaine) administered for epidural or peripheral nerve block, clonidine will markedly prolong both the anesthetic and analgesic effects.

Unlabeled/investigational uses of clonidine include serving as an adjunct in premedication, control of withdrawal syndromes (nicotine, opioids, alcohol, and vasomotor symptoms of menopause), and treatment of glaucoma as well as various psychiatric disorders.

Side Effects

Sedation, dizziness, bradycardia, and dry mouth are common side effects. Less commonly, bradycardia, orthostatic hypotension, nausea, and diarrhea may be observed. Abrupt discontinuation of clonidine following long-term administration (>1 mo) can produce a withdrawal phenomenon characterized by rebound hypertension, agitation, and sympathetic overactivity.

Dosage

Epidural clonidine is usually started at 30 mcg/h in a mixture with an opioid or a local anesthetic. Oral clonidine is readily absorbed, has a 30–60 min onset, and lasts 6–12 h. In the treatment of acute hypertension, 0.1 mg can be given orally every hour until the blood pressure is controlled, or up to a maximum of 0.6 mg; the maintenance dose is 0.1–0.3 mg twice daily. Transdermal preparations of clonidine can also be used for maintenance therapy. They are available as 0.1, 0.2, and 0.3 mg/d patches that are replaced every 7 days. Clonidine is metabolized by the liver and excreted renally. Dosages should be reduced for patients with renal insufficiency.

Drug Interactions

Clonidine enhances and prolongs sensory and motor blockade from local anesthetics. Additive effects with hypnotic agents, general anesthetics, and sedatives can potentiate sedation, hypotension, and bradycardia. The drug should be used cautiously, if at all, in patients who take β-adrenergic blockers and in those with significant cardiac conduction system abnormalities. Lastly, clonidine can mask the symptoms of hypoglycemia in diabetic patients.

DEXMEDETOMIDINE

Mechanism of Action

7 Dexmedetomidine (Precedex) is a parenteral selective α_2 agonist with sedative properties. It appears to be more selective for the α_2 receptor than clonidine. At higher doses it loses its selectivity and also stimulates α_1-adrenergic receptors.

Clinical Uses

Dexmedetomidine causes dose-dependent sedation anxiolysis and some analgesia and blunts the sympathetic response to surgery and other stress. Most importantly, it has an opioid-sparing effect and does not significantly depress respiratory drive; excessive sedation, however, may cause airway obstruction. The drug is used for short-term (<24 h), intravenous sedation of mechanically ventilated patients. Discontinuation after more prolonged use can potentially cause a withdrawal phenomenon similar to that of clonidine. It has also been used for intraoperative sedation and as an adjunct to general anesthetics.

Side Effects

The principal side effects are bradycardia, heart block, and hypotension. It may also cause nausea.

Dosage

The recommended initial loading dose is 1 mcg/kg intravenously over 10 min with a maintenance infusion rate of 0.2–0.7 mcg/kg/h. Dexmedetomidine has a rapid onset and terminal half-life of 2 h. The drug is metabolized in the liver and its metabolites are eliminated in the urine. Dosage should be reduced in patients with renal insufficiency or hepatic impairment.

Drug Interactions

Caution should be used when dexmedetomidine is administered with vasodilators, cardiac depressants, and drugs that decrease heart rate. Reduced requirements of hypnotics/anesthetic agents should prevent excessive hypotension.

DOXAPRAM

Mechanism of Action

8 Doxapram (Dopram) is a peripheral and central nervous system stimulant. Selective activation of carotid chemoreceptors by low doses of doxapram stimulates hypoxic drive, producing an increase in tidal volume and a slight increase in respiratory rate. At larger doses, the central respiratory centers in the medulla are stimulated.

Clinical Uses

Because doxapram mimics a low Pa_{O_2}, it may be useful in patients with chronic obstructive pulmonary disease who are dependent on hypoxic drive yet require supplemental oxygen. Drug-induced respiratory and central nervous system depression, including that seen immediately postoperatively, can be *temporarily* overcome. Doxapram is not a specific reversal agent, however, and should not replace standard supportive therapy (mechanical ventilation). For example, doxapram will not reverse paralysis caused by muscle relaxants, although it may transiently mask respiratory failure. The most common cause of postoperative hypoventilation—airway obstruction—will not be alleviated by doxapram. For these reasons, many anesthesiologists believe that the usefulness of doxapram is very limited.

Side Effects

Stimulation of the central nervous system leads to a variety of possible side effects: changes in mental status (confusion, dizziness, seizures), cardiac abnormalities (tachycardia, dysrhythmias, hypertension), and pulmonary dysfunction (wheezing, tachypnea). Vomiting and laryngospasm are of particular concern to the anesthesiologist in the postoperative period. Doxapram should not be used in patients with a history of epilepsy, cerebrovascular disease, acute head injury, coronary artery disease, hypertension, or bronchial asthma.

Dosage

Bolus intravenous administration (0.5–1 mg/kg) results in transient increases in minute ventilation (the onset of action is 1 min; the duration of action is 5–12 min). Continuous intravenous infusions (1–3 mg/min) provide longer-lasting effects (the maximum dose is 4 mg/kg).

Drug Interactions

The sympathetic stimulation produced by doxapram may exaggerate the cardiovascular effects of monoamine oxidase inhibitors or adrenergic agents. Doxapram should probably not be used in patients awakening from halothane anesthesia, as halothane sensitizes the myocardium to catecholamines.

NALOXONE

Mechanism of Action

Naloxone (Narcan) is a competitive opioid receptor antagonist. Its affinity for opioid μ receptors appears to be much greater than for opioid κ or δ receptors Naloxone has no significant agonist activity.

Clinical Uses

9 Naloxone reverses the agonist activity associated with endogenous (enkephalins, endorphins) or exogenous opioid compounds. A dramatic example is the reversal of unconsciousness that occurs in a patient with opioid overdose who has received naloxone. Perioperative respiratory depression caused by excessive opioid administration is rapidly antagonized (1–2 min). Some degree of opioid analgesia can often be spared if the dose of naloxone is limited to the minimum required to maintain adequate ventilation. Low doses of intravenous naloxone reverse the side effects of epidural opioids without necessarily reversing the analgesia.

Side Effects

Abrupt reversal of opioid analgesia can result in sympathetic stimulation (tachycardia, ventricular irritability, hypertension, pulmonary edema) caused by severe, acute pain, and an acute withdrawal syndrome in patients who are opioid-dependent. The extent of these side effects is proportional to the amount of opioid being reversed and the speed of the reversal.

Dosage

In postoperative patients experiencing respiratory depression from excessive opioid administration, intravenous naloxone (0.4 mg/mL vial diluted in 9 mL saline to 0.04 mg/mL) can be titrated in increments of 0.5–1 mcg/kg every 3–5 min until adequate ventilation and alertness are achieved. Doses in excess of 0.2 mg are rarely indicated. The brief duration of action of intravenous naloxone (30–45 min) is due to rapid redistribution from the central nervous system. A more prolonged effect is almost always necessary to prevent the recurrence of respiratory depression from longer-acting opioids. Therefore, intramuscular naloxone (twice the required intravenous dose) or a continuous infusion (4–5 mcg/kg/h) is recommended. Neonatal respiratory depression resulting from maternal opioid administration is treated with 10 mcg/kg, repeated in 2 min if necessary. Neonates of opioid-dependent mothers will exhibit withdrawal symptoms if given naloxone. The primary treatment of respiratory depression is always establishment of an adequate airway to permit spontaneous, assisted, or controlled ventilation.

Drug Interactions

The effect of naloxone on nonopioid anesthetic agents such as nitrous oxide is insignificant. Naloxone may antagonize the antihypertensive effect of clonidine.

NALTREXONE

Naltrexone is also a pure opioid antagonist with a high affinity for the μ receptor, but with a significantly longer half-life than naloxone. Naltrexone is used orally for maintenance treatment of opioid addicts and for ethanol abuse. In the latter instance, it appears to block some of the pleasant effects of alcohol in some individuals.

FLUMAZENIL

Mechanism of Action

Flumazenil (Romazicon), an imidazobenzodiazepine, is a specific and competitive antagonist of benzodiazepines at benzodiazepine receptors.

Clinical Uses

10 Flumazenil is useful in the reversal of benzodiazepine sedation and the treatment of benzodiazepine overdose. Although it promptly (onset <1 min) reverses the hypnotic effects of benzodiazepines, amnesia has proved to be less reliably prevented. Some evidence of respiratory depression may linger despite an alert and awake appearance. Specifically, tidal volume and minute ventilation return to normal, but the slope of the carbon dioxide response curve remains depressed. Effects in elderly patients appear to be particularly difficult to reverse fully, and these patients are more prone to resedation.

Side Effects & Drug Interactions

Rapid administration of flumazenil may cause anxiety reactions in previously sedated patients and symptoms of withdrawal in those on long-term benzodiazepine therapy. Flumazenil reversal has been associated with increases in intracranial pressure in patients with head injuries and abnormal intracranial compliance. Flumazenil may induce seizure activity if benzodiazepines have been given as anticonvulsants or in conjunction with an overdose of tricyclic antidepressants. Flumazenil reversal following a midazolam–ketamine anesthetic technique may increase the incidence of emergence dysphoria and hallucinations. Nausea and vomiting are not uncommon following administration of flumazenil. The reversal effect of flumazenil is based on its strong antagonist affinity for benzodiazepine receptors. Flumazenil does not affect the minimum alveolar concentration of inhalation anesthetics.

Dosage

Gradual titration of flumazenil is usually accomplished by intravenous administration of 0.2 mg/min until reaching the desired degree of reversal. The usual total dose is 0.6–1.0 mg. Because of flumazenil's rapid hepatic clearance, repeat doses may be required after 1–2 h to avoid resedation and premature recovery room or outpatient discharge. A continuous infusion (0.5 mg/h) may be helpful in the case of an overdose of a longer-acting benzodiazepine. Liver failure prolongs the clearance of flumazenil and benzodiazepines.

CASE DISCUSSION

Management of Patients at Risk for Aspiration Pneumonia

A 58-year-old man is scheduled for elective inguinal hernia repair. His past history reveals a persistent problem with heartburn and passive regurgitation of gastric contents into the pharynx. He has been told by his internist that these symptoms are due to a hiatal hernia.

Why would a history of hiatal hernia concern the anesthesiologist?

Perioperative aspiration of gastric contents (Mendelson's syndrome) is a potentially fatal complication of anesthesia. Hiatal hernia is commonly associated with symptomatic GERD, which is considered a predisposing factor for aspiration. Mild or occasional heartburn may not significantly increase the risk of aspiration. In contrast, symptoms related to passive reflux of gastric fluid, such as acid taste or sensation of refluxing liquid into the mouth, should alert the clinician to a high risk of pulmonary aspiration. Paroxysms of coughing or wheezing, particularly at night or when the patient is flat, may be indicative of chronic aspiration. Aspiration can occur on induction, during maintenance, or upon emergence from anesthesia.

Which patients are predisposed to aspiration?

Patients with altered airway reflexes (eg, drug intoxication, general anesthesia, encephalopathy, neuromuscular disease) or abnormal pharyngeal or esophageal anatomy (eg, large hiatal hernia, Zenker's diverticulum, scleroderma, pregnancy, obesity) are prone to pulmonary aspiration.

 ### Does aspiration consistently result in aspiration pneumonia?

Not necessarily. The seriousness of the lung damage depends on the volume and composition of the aspirate. Traditionally, patients are considered to be at risk if their gastric volume is greater than 25 mL (0.4 mL/kg) and their gastric pH is less than 2.5. Some investigators believe that controlling acidity is more important than volume and that the criteria should be revised to a pH less than 3.5 with a volume greater than 50 mL.

Patients who have eaten immediately prior to emergency surgery are obviously at risk. Traditionally, "NPO after midnight" implied a preoperative fast of at least 6 h. Current opinion allows clear liquids until 2–4 h before induction of anesthesia, although solids are still taboo for 6 h in adult patients. Some patients who have fasted for 8 h or more before elective surgery also meet the at-risk criteria, however. Certain patient populations are particularly likely to have large volumes of acidic gastric fluid: patients with an acute abdomen or peptic ulcer disease, children, the elderly, diabetic patients, pregnant women, and obese patients. Furthermore, pain, anxiety, or opioid-agonists may delay gastric emptying. Note that pregnancy and obesity place patients in double jeopardy by increasing the chance of aspiration (increased intraabdominal pressure and distortion of the lower esophageal sphincter) and the risk of aspiration pneumonia (increased acidity and volume of gastric contents). Aspiration is more common in patients undergoing esophageal, upper abdominal, or emergency laparoscopic surgery.

Which drugs lower the risk of aspiration pneumonia?

H_2-Receptor antagonists decrease gastric acid secretion. Although they will not affect gastric contents already in the stomach, they will inhibit further acid production. Both gastric pH and volume are affected. In addition, the long duration of action of ranitidine and famotidine may provide protection in the recovery room.

Metoclopramide shortens gastric emptying time and increases lower esophageal sphincter tone. It does not affect gastric pH, and it cannot clear large volumes of food in a few hours. Nonetheless, metoclopramide with ranitidine is a good combination for most at-risk patients. Antacids usually raise gastric fluid pH, but, at the same time, they increase gastric volume. Although antacid administration technically removes a patient from the at-risk category, aspiration of a substantial volume of particulate matter will lead to serious physiological damage. For this reason, clear antacids (eg, sodium citrate) are strongly preferred. In contrast to H_2 antagonists, antacids are immediately effective and alter the acidity of existing gastric contents. Thus, they are useful in emergency situations and in patients who have recently eaten.

Anticholinergic drugs, particularly glycopyrrolate, decrease gastric secretions if large doses are administered; however, lower esophageal sphincter tone is reduced. Overall, anticholinergic drugs do not reliably reduce the risk of aspiration pneumonia and can reverse the protective effects of metoclopramide. Proton pump inhibitors are generally as effective as H_2 antagonists.

What anesthetic techniques are used in full-stomach patients?

If the full stomach is due to recent food intake and the surgical procedure is elective, the operation should be postponed. If the risk factor is not reversible (eg, large hiatal hernia) or the case is emergent, proper anesthetic technique can minimize the risk of aspiration pneumonia. Regional anesthesia with minimal sedation should be considered in patients at increased risk for aspiration pneumonia. If local anesthetic techniques are impractical, the patient's airway must be protected. Delivering anesthesia by mask or laryngeal mask airway is contraindicated. As in every anesthetic case, the availability of suction must be confirmed before induction. If there are signs suggesting a difficult airway, intubation should precede induction. Otherwise, a rapid-sequence induction is indicated.

How does a rapid-sequence induction differ from a routine induction?

- The patient is always preoxygenated prior to induction. Patients with lung disease require 3–5 min of preoxygenation.
- Prior curarization with a nondepolarizing muscle relaxant may prevent the increase in intraabdominal pressure that accompanies the fasciculations caused by succinylcholine. This step is often omitted, however, as it can decrease lower esophageal sphincter tone. If rocuronium has been selected for relaxation, a small priming dose (0.1 mg/kg) given 2–3 min prior to induction may speed its onset of action.
- A wide assortment of blades, video laryngoscopes, and endotracheal tubes are prepared in advance.
- An assistant may apply firm pressure over the cricoid cartilage prior to induction (Sellick's maneuver). Because the cricoid cartilage forms an uninterrupted and incompressible ring, pressure over it is transmitted to underlying tissue. The esophagus is collapsed, and passively regurgitated gastric fluid cannot reach the hypopharynx. Excessive cricoid pressure (beyond what can be tolerated by a conscious person) applied during active regurgitation has been associated with rupture of the posterior wall of the esophagus. The effectiveness of Sellick's maneuver has been questioned.
- A propofol induction dose is given as a bolus. Obviously, this dose must be modified if there is any indication that the patient's cardiovascular system is unstable. Other rapid-acting induction agents can be substituted (eg, etomidate, ketamine).
- Succinylcholine (1.5 mg/kg) or rocuronium (0.9–1.2 mg/kg) is administered immediately following the induction dose, even if the patient has not yet lost consciousness.

- The patient is not artificially ventilated, to avoid filling the stomach with gas and thereby increasing the risk of emesis. Once spontaneous efforts have ceased or muscle response to nerve stimulation has disappeared, the patient is rapidly intubated. Cricoid pressure is maintained until the endotracheal tube cuff is inflated and tube position is confirmed. A modification of the classic rapid-sequence induction allows gentle ventilation as long as cricoid pressure is maintained.
- If the intubation proves difficult, cricoid pressure is maintained and the patient is gently ventilated with oxygen until another intubation attempt can be performed. If intubation is still unsuccessful, spontaneous ventilation should be allowed to return and an awake intubation performed.
- After surgery, the patient should remain intubated until airway reflexes have returned and consciousness has been regained.

What are the relative contraindications to rapid-sequence inductions?

Rapid-sequence inductions are usually associated with increases in intracranial pressure, arterial blood pressure, and heart rate. Contraindications to succinylcholine also apply (eg, thermal burns).

Describe the pathophysiology and clinical findings associated with aspiration pneumonia.

The pathophysiological changes depend on the composition of the aspirate. Acid solutions cause atelectasis, alveolar edema, and loss of surfactant. Particulate aspirate will also result in small-airway obstruction and alveolar necrosis. Granulomas may form around food or antacid particles. The earliest physiological change following aspiration is intrapulmonary shunting, resulting in hypoxia. Other changes may include pulmonary edema, pulmonary hypertension, and hypercapnia.

Wheezing, rhonchi, tachycardia, and tachypnea are common physical findings. Decreased lung compliance can make ventilation difficult. Hypotension signals significant fluid shifts into the alveoli and is associated with massive lung injury.

Chest roentgenography may not demonstrate diffuse bilateral infiltrates for several hours after the event. Arterial blood gases reveal hypoxemia, hypercapnia, and respiratory acidosis.

What is the treatment for aspiration pneumonia?

As soon as regurgitation is suspected, the patient should be placed in a head-down position so that gastric contents drain out of the mouth instead of into the trachea. The pharynx and, if possible, the trachea should be thoroughly suctioned. The mainstay of therapy in patients who subsequently become hypoxic is positive-pressure ventilation. Intubation and the institution of positive end-expiratory pressure or continuous positive airway pressure are often required. Bronchoscopy and pulmonary lavage are usually indicated when particulate aspiration has occurred. Use of corticosteroids is generally not recommended and antibiotics are administered depending upon culture results.

GUIDELINES

Gan TJ, Meyer TA, Apfel CC, et al: Society for ambulatory anesthesia guidelines for management of postoperative nausea and vomiting. Anesth Analg 2007;105:1615.

Practice guidelines for preoperative fasting and the use of pharmacologic agents to reduce the risk of pulmonary aspiration: Application to healthy patients undergoing elective procedures. A report by the American Society of Anesthesiologists Task Force on Preoperative Fasting. Anesthesiology 1999;90:896.

SUGGESTED READING

De Souza D, Doar L, Mehta S, et al: Aspiration prophylaxis and rapid sequence induction for elective cesarean delivery; time to reassess old dogma. Anesth Analg 2010;110:1503.

Ferrari LR, Rooney FM, Rockoff MA: Preoperative fasting practices in pediatrics. Anesthesiology 1999;90:978.

Gan T, Apfel C, Kovac A, et al: A randomized double blind comparison of the NK$_1$ antagonist, aprepitant, versus ondansetron for the prevention of post operative nausea and vomiting. Anesth Analg 2007;104:1082.

Gan T, Coop A, Philip B, et al: A randomized double blind study of granisetron plus dexamethasone versus ondansetron plus dexamethasone to prevent postoperative nausea and vomiting in patients undergoing abdominal hysterectomy. Anesth Analg 2005;101:1323.

Glass P: Postoperative nausea and vomiting: We don't know everything yet. Anesth Analg 2010;110:299.

Glass P, White P: Practice guidelines for the management of postoperative nausea and vomiting: Past, present and future. Anesth Analg 2007;105:1528.

George E, Hornuss C, Apfel C: Neurokinin 1 and novel serotonin antagonists for postoperative and postdischarge nausea and vomiting. Curr Opin Anesth 2010;23:714.

Joshi GP, Gertler R, Fricer R: Cardiovascular thromboembolic adverse effects associated with cyclooxygenase 2 selective inhibitors and nonselective anti inflammatory drugs. Anesth Analg 2007;105:1793.

Lipp A, Kaliappan A: Focus on quality: managing pain and PONV in day surgery. Curr Anaesth Crit Care 2007;18:200.

Schug S, Joshi G, Camu F, et al: Cardiovascular safety of the cyclooxygenase 2 selective inhibitors parecoxib and valdecoxib in the postoperative setting; an analysis of integrated data. Anesth Analg 2009;108:299.

Smith H: Perioperative intravenous acetaminophen and NSAIDS. Pain Medicine 2011;12:961.

Steeds C, Orme R: Premedication. Anaesth Intensive Care Med 2006;7:393–396.

Warner MA, Warner ME, Warner DO, et al: Clinical significance of pulmonary aspiration during the perioperative period. Anesthesiology 1993;78:56.

Young A, Buvanendran A: Multimodal systemic and intra articular analgesics. Int Anesth Clin 2011;49:117.

Preoperative Assessment, Premedication, & Perioperative Documentation

KEY CONCEPTS

1. The cornerstones of an effective preoperative evaluation are the history and physical examination, which should include a complete account of all medications taken by the patient in the recent past, all pertinent drug and contact allergies, and responses and reactions to previous anesthetics.

2. The anesthesiologist should not be expected to provide the risk-versus-benefit discussion for the proposed procedure; this is the responsibility and purview of the responsible surgeon or "proceduralist."

3. By convention physicians in many countries use the American Society of Anesthesiologists' classification to identify relative risk prior to conscious sedation and surgical anesthesia.

4. In general, the indications for cardiovascular investigations are the same in surgical patients as in any other patient.

5. Adequacy of long-term blood glucose control can be easily and rapidly assessed by measurement of hemoglobin A_{1c}.

6. In patients deemed at high risk for thrombosis (eg, those with certain mechanical heart valve implants or with atrial fibrillation and a prior thromboembolic stroke), warfarin should be replaced by intravenous heparin or, more commonly, by intramuscular heparinoids to minimize the risk.

7. Current guidelines recommend postponing all but mandatory emergency surgery until at least 1 month after any coronary intervention and suggest that treatment options *other* than a drug-eluting stent (which requires prolonged dual antiplatelet therapy) be used in patients expected to undergo a surgical procedure within 12 months after the intervention.

8. There are no good outcomes data to support restricting fluid intake (of any kind or any amount) more than 2 h before induction of general anesthesia in healthy patients undergoing elective procedures; indeed, there is evidence that nondiabetic patients should be encouraged to drink glucose-containing fluids up to 2 h before induction of anesthesia.

9. To be valuable, preoperative testing must discriminate: an increased perioperative risk exists when the results are abnormal (and unknown); a reduced risk exists when the abnormality is absent or detected (and perhaps corrected).

—*Continued next page*

Continued—

10 The utility of a test depends on its sensitivity and specificity. Sensitive tests have a low rate of false-negative results and rarely fail to identify an abnormality when one is present, whereas specific tests have a low rate of false-positive results and rarely identify an abnormality when one is not present.

11 Premedication should be given purposefully, not as a mindless routine.

12 Incomplete, inaccurate, or illegible records unnecessarily complicate defending a physician against otherwise unjustified allegations of malpractice.

PREOPERATIVE EVALUATION

1 The cornerstones of an effective preoperative evaluation are the medical history and physical examination, which should include a complete account of all medications taken by the patient in the recent past, all pertinent drug and contact allergies, and responses and reactions to previous anesthetics. Additionally, this evaluation should include any indicated diagnostic tests, imaging procedures, or consultations from other physicians. The preoperative evaluation guides the anesthetic plan: inadequate preoperative planning and incomplete patient preparation are commonly associated with anesthetic complications.

The preoperative evaluation serves multiple purposes. One purpose is to identify those few patients whose outcomes likely will be improved by implementation of a specific medical treatment (which in rare circumstances may require that the planned surgery be rescheduled). For example, a 60-year-old patient scheduled for elective total hip arthroplasty who also has unstable angina from left main coronary artery disease would more likely survive if coronary artery bypass grafting is performed before the elective procedure. Another purpose is to identify patients whose condition is so poor that the proposed surgery might only hasten death without improving the quality of life. For example, a patient with severe chronic lung disease, end-stage kidney failure, liver failure, and heart failure likely would not survive to derive benefit from an 8-hour, complex, multilevel spinal fusion with instrumentation.

The preoperative evaluation can identify patients with specific characteristics that likely will influence the proposed anesthetic plan (Table 18–1). For example, the anesthetic plan may need to be reassessed for a patient whose trachea appears difficult to intubate, one with a family history of malignant hyperthermia, or one with an infection near where a proposed regional anesthetic would be

TABLE 18–1 The anesthetic plan.

Will sedative-hypnotic premedication be useful?

What type(s) of anesthesia will be employed?
  General[1]
    Airway management
    Induction drugs
    Maintenance drugs
  Regional
    Technique(s)
    Agent(s)
  Sedation and monitored anesthesia care
    Supplemental oxygen
    Specific sedative drugs

Are there special intraoperative management issues?
  Nonstandard monitors
  Positions other than supine
  Relative or absolute contraindications to specific
    anesthetic drugs
  Fluid management
  Special techniques
  Site (anesthetizing location) concerns

How will the patient be managed postoperatively?
  Management of acute pain
  Intensive care
    Postoperative ventilation
    Hemodynamic monitoring

[1]Including need for (or need for avoidance of) muscle relaxation.

administered. Another purpose of the evaluation is to provide the patient with an estimate of anesthetic

2 risk. However, the anesthesiologist should not be expected to provide the risk-versus-benefit discussion for the proposed procedure; this is the responsibility and purview of the responsible surgeon or "proceduralist." For example, a discussion of the risks and benefits of robotic prostatectomy versus radiation therapy versus "watchful waiting" requires knowledge of both the medical literature and the morbidity–mortality statistics of an individual surgeon, and it would be most unusual for an anesthesiologist to have access to the necessary data for this discussion. Finally, the preoperative evaluation is an opportunity for the anesthesiologist to describe the proposed anesthetic plan in the context of the overall surgical and postoperative plan, provide the patient with psychological support, and obtain informed consent for the proposed anesthetic plan from the surgical patient.

3 By convention, physicians in many countries use the American Society of Anesthesiologists' (ASA) classification to define relative risk prior to conscious sedation and surgical anesthesia (Table 18–2). The ASA physical status classification has many advantages over all other risk classification tools: it is time honored, simple, reproducible, and, most importantly, it has been shown to be strongly associated with perioperative risk. But, many other risk assessment tools are available.

Elements of the Preoperative History

Patients presenting for elective surgery and anesthesia typically require a focused preoperative medical history emphasizing cardiac and pulmonary function, kidney disease, endocrine and metabolic diseases, musculoskeletal and anatomic issues relevant to airway management and regional anesthesia, and responses and reactions to previous anesthetics. The ASA publishes and periodically updates general guidelines for preoperative assessment (see Guidelines at end of Chapter).

A. Cardiovascular Issues

Guidelines for preoperative cardiac assessment are available from the American College of Cardiology/

TABLE 18–2 American Society of Anesthesiologists' physical status classification of patients.[1]

Class	Definition
1	Normal healthy patient
2	Patient with mild systemic disease (no functional limitations)
3	Patient with severe systemic disease (some functional limitations)
4	Patient with severe systemic disease that is a constant threat to life (functionality incapacitated)
5	Moribund patient who is not expected to survive without the operation
6	Brain-dead patient whose organs are being removed for donor purposes
E	If the procedure is an emergency, the physical status is followed by "E" (for example, "2E")

[1]Data from Committee on Standards and practice Parameters, Apfelbaum JL, Connis RT, et al: Practice advisory for preanesthesia evaluation: An updated report by the American Society of Anesthesiologists Task Force on Preanesthesia Evaluation. Anesthesiology 2012;116:522.

American Heart Association and from the European Society of Cardiology (see Guidelines). A more complete discussion of cardiovascular assessment is provided in Chapter 21. The focus of preoperative cardiac assessment should be on determining whether the patient's condition can and must be improved prior to the scheduled procedure, and whether the patient meets criteria for further cardiac evaluation prior to the scheduled surgery. Clearly the criteria for what must be done before elective arthroplasty will differ from what must be done before an operation for resectable pancreatic cancer, given the benign results of a delay in the former procedure and the potential life-shortening effects of a

4 delay in the latter procedure. In general, the indications for cardiovascular investigations are the same in surgical patients as in any other patient. Put another way, the fact that a patient is scheduled to undergo surgery does not change the indications for such measures as noninvasive stress testing to diagnose coronary artery disease.

B. Pulmonary Issues

Perioperative pulmonary complications, most notably postoperative respiratory depression and respiratory failure, are vexing problems that have become seemingly more common as severe obesity and obstructive sleep apnea have increased in incidence. A recent guideline developed by the American College of Physicians takes an aggressive stance; it identifies patients 60 years of age or older, those with chronic obstructive lung disease, those with markedly reduced exercise tolerance and functional dependence, and those with heart failure as potentially requiring preoperative and postoperative interventions to avoid complications. The risk of postoperative pulmonary complications is closely associated with these factors, and with the following: ASA class (class 3 and 4 patients have a markedly increased risk of pulmonary complications relative to class 1 patients), cigarette smoking, longer surgeries (>4 h), certain types of surgery (abdominal, thoracic, aortic aneurysm, head and neck, and emergency surgery), and general anesthesia (compared with cases in which general anesthesia was not used).

Efforts at prevention of pulmonary complications should focus on cessation of cigarette smoking prior to surgery and on lung expansion techniques (eg, incentive spirometry) after surgery in patients at risk. Patients with asthma, particularly those receiving suboptimal medical management, have a greater risk for bronchospasm during airway manipulation. Appropriate use of analgesia and monitoring are key strategies for avoiding postoperative respiratory depression in patients with obstructive sleep apnea. Further discussion of this topic appears in Chapter 44.

C. Endocrine and Metabolic Issues

Appropriate targets for control of diabetes mellitus and of blood glucose in critically ill patients have been subjects of great debate over the past decade. "Tight" control of blood glucose, with a target level in the normal range, was shown in the Diabetes Control and Complications Trial to improve outcomes in ambulatory patients with type 1 diabetes mellitus. It has become the usual practice to obtain a blood glucose measurement on the morning of elective surgery. Unfortunately, many diabetic patients presenting for elective surgery do not maintain blood glucose within the desired range. Other patients, who may be unaware that they have type 2 diabetes, present with blood glucose measurements above the normal range. Adequacy of long-term blood glucose control can be easily and rapidly assessed by measurement of hemoglobin A_{1c}. In patients with abnormally elevated hemoglobin A_{1c}, referral to a diabetology service for education about the disease and adjustment of diet and medications to improve metabolic control may be beneficial. Elective surgery should be delayed in patients presenting with marked hyperglycemia; this delay might consist only of rearranging the order of scheduled cases to allow insulin infusion to bring the blood glucose concentration closer to the normal range before surgery begins. A more complete discussion of diabetes mellitus and other perioperative endocrine concerns is provided in Chapter 34.

D. Coagulation Issues

Three important coagulation issues that must be addressed during the preoperative evaluation are (1) how to manage patients who are taking warfarin on a long-term basis; (2) how to manage patients who are taking clopidogrel and related agents; and (3) how to safely provide regional anesthesia to patients who either are receiving long-term anticoagulation therapy or who will receive anticoagulation perioperatively. In the first circumstance, most patients who undergoing anything more involved than minor surgery will require discontinuation of warfarin 5 days in advance of surgery to avoid excessive blood loss. The key question to be answered is whether the patient will require "bridging" therapy with another agent while warfarin is discontinued. In patients deemed at high risk for thrombosis (eg, those with certain mechanical heart valve implants or with atrial fibrillation and a prior thromboembolic stroke), warfarin should be replaced by intravenous heparin or, more commonly, by intramuscular heparinoids to minimize the risk. In patients receiving bridging therapy for a high risk of thrombosis, the risk of death from excessive bleeding is an order of magnitude lower than the risk of death or disability from stroke if the bridging therapy is omitted. Patients at lower risk for thrombosis may have warfarin discontinued and then reinitiated after successful surgery. Decisions regarding bridging therapy often require consultation with the physician who initiated the warfarin therapy.

Clopidogrel and related agents are most often administered with aspirin (so-called dual antiplatelet therapy) to patients with coronary artery disease who have received intracoronary stenting. Immediately after stenting, such patients are at increased risk of acute myocardial infarction if clopidogrel (or related agents) and aspirin are abruptly discontinued for a surgical procedure.

7 Therefore, current guidelines recommend postponing all but mandatory emergency surgery until at least 1 month after any coronary intervention and suggest that treatment options *other* than a drug-eluting stent (which will require prolonged dual antiplatelet therapy) be used in patients expected to undergo a surgical procedure within 12 months after the intervention (eg, in a patient with colon cancer who requires treatment for coronary disease). As the available drugs, treatment options, and consensus guidelines are updated relatively frequently, we recommend consultation with a cardiologist regarding safe management of patients receiving these agents who require a surgical procedure.

The third circumstance—when it may be safe to perform regional (particularly neuraxial) anesthesia in patients who are or will be receiving anticoagulation therapy—has also been the subject of debate among hematologists and regional anesthetists. The American Society of Regional Anesthesia publishes a periodically updated consensus guideline on this topic, and other prominent societies (eg, the European Society of Anaesthesiologists) also provide guidance on this topic. This topic is considered in greater detail in Chapter 45.

E. Gastrointestinal Issues

Since Mendelson's 1946 report, aspiration of gastric contents has been recognized as a potentially disastrous pulmonary complication of surgical anesthesia. It has also been long recognized that the risk of aspiration is increased in certain groups of patients: pregnant women in the second and third trimesters, those whose stomachs have not emptied after a recent meal, and those with serious gastroesophageal reflux disease (GERD).

Although there is a consensus that pregnant women and those who have recently (within 6 h) consumed a full meal should be treated as if they have "full" stomachs, there is less consensus as to the necessary period of time in which patients must fast before elective surgery. Proof of the lack of consensus is the fact that the ASA's guideline on this topic was voted down by the ASA House of Delegates several years in a row before it was presented in a form that received majority approval. The guideline as approved is more permissive of fluid intake than many anesthesiologists would prefer, and many medical centers have policies that are more restric-

8 tive than the ASA guideline on this topic. The truth is that there are no good outcomes data to support restricting fluid intake (of any kind or any amount) more than 2 h before induction of general anesthesia in healthy patients undergoing elective procedures; indeed, there is evidence that nondiabetic patients should be encouraged to drink glucose-containing fluids up to 2 h before induction of anesthesia.

Patients with a history of GERD present vexing problems. Some of these patients will clearly be at increased risk for aspiration; others may carry this "self-diagnosis" based on television advertisements or conversations with friends and family, or may have been given this diagnosis by a physician who did not follow the standard diagnostic criteria. Our approach is to treat patients who have only occasional symptoms like any other patient without GERD, and to treat patients with consistent symptoms (multiple times per week) with medications (eg, nonparticulate antacids such as sodium citrate) and techniques (eg, tracheal intubation rather than laryngeal mask airway) as if they were at increased risk for aspiration.

Elements of the Preoperative Physical Examination

The preoperative history and physical examination complement one another: The physical examination may detect abnormalities not apparent from the history, and the history helps focus the physical examination. Examination of healthy asymptomatic patients should include measurement of vital signs (blood pressure, heart rate, respiratory rate, and temperature) and examination of the airway, heart, lungs, and musculoskeletal system using standard techniques of inspection, auscultation, palpation, and percussion. Before procedures such as a nerve block, regional anesthesia, or invasive monitoring the relevant anatomy should be examined; evidence of infection near the site or of anatomic abnormalities may contraindicate the planned procedure (see Chapters 5, 45, and 46). An abbreviated neurological examination is important when regional anesthesia will likely be used. The preoperative neurological examination serves to document whether any neurological deficits may be present *before* the block is performed.

The anesthesiologist must examine the patient's airway before every anesthetic procedure. The patient's dentition should be inspected for loose or chipped teeth, caps, bridges, or dentures. Poor fit of the anesthesia mask should be expected in edentulous patients and those with significant facial abnormalities. Micrognathia (a short distance between the chin and the hyoid bone), prominent upper incisors, a large tongue, limited range of motion of the temporomandibular joint or cervical spine, or a short or thick neck suggest that difficulty may be encountered in direct laryngoscopy for tracheal intubation (see Chapter 19).

Preoperative Laboratory Testing

Routine laboratory testing when patients are fit and asymptomatic is not recommended. Testing should be guided by the history and physical examination. "Routine" testing is expensive and rarely alters perioperative management; moreover, abnormal values often are overlooked or if recognized may result in unnecessary delays. Nonetheless, despite the lack of evidence of benefit, many physicians order a hematocrit or hemoglobin concentration, urinalysis, serum electrolyte measurements, coagulation studies, an electrocardiogram, and a chest radiograph for all patients, perhaps in the misplaced hope of reducing their exposure to litigation.

⑨ To be valuable, preoperative testing must discriminate: there must be an increased perioperative risk when the results are abnormal (and unknown when the test is not performed), and there must be a reduced risk when the abnormality is not

detected (or it has been corrected). This requires that the test have a very low rate of false-positive and **⑩** false-negative results. **The utility of a test depends on its sensitivity and specificity. Sensitive tests have a low rate of false-negative results and rarely fail to identify an abnormality when one is present, whereas specific tests have a low rate of false-positive results and rarely identify an abnormality when one is not present.** The prevalence of a disease or of an abnormal test result varies with the population tested. Testing is therefore most effective when sensitive and specific tests are used in patients in whom the abnormality will be detected frequently enough to justify the expense and inconvenience of the test procedure. Accordingly, laboratory testing should be based on the presence or absence of underlying diseases and drug therapy as detected by the history and physical examination. The nature of the proposed surgery or procedure should also be taken into consideration. Thus, a baseline hemoglobin or hematocrit measurement is desirable in any patient about to undergo a procedure that may result in extensive blood loss and require transfusion, particularly when there is sufficient time to correct anemia preoperatively (eg, with iron supplements).

Testing fertile women for an undiagnosed early pregnancy is controversial and should not be done without the permission of the patient; pregnancy testing involves detection of chorionic gonadotropin in urine or serum. Routine testing for HIV antibody is not indicated. Routine coagulation studies and urinalysis are not cost-effective in asymptomatic healthy patients; nevertheless, a preoperative urinalysis is required by state law in at least one U.S. jurisdiction.

PREMEDICATION

A classic study showed that a preoperative visit from an anesthesiologist resulted in a greater reduction in patient anxiety than preoperative sedative drugs. Yet, there was a time when virtually every patient received premedication before arriving in the preoperative area in anticipation of surgery. Despite the evidence, the belief was that all patients benefitted from sedation and anticholinergics, and most patients would benefit from a preoperative opioid. After such premedication, some patients arrived in a nearly anesthetized state. With the move to outpatient surgery and "same-day" hospital admission, the practice has shifted. Today, preoperative sedative-hypnotics or opioids are almost never administered before patients arrive in the preoperative holding area (other than for intubated patients who have been previously sedated in the intensive care unit). Children, especially those aged 2–10 years who will experience separation anxiety on being removed from their parent, may benefit from premedication administered in the preoperative holding area. This topic is discussed in Chapter 42. Midazolam, administered either intravenously or orally, is a common method. Adults often receive intravenous midazolam (2–5 mg) once an intravenous line has been established, and if a painful procedure (eg, regional block or a central venous line) will be performed while the patient remains awake, small doses of opioid (typically fentanyl) will often be given. Patients who will undergo airway surgery or extensive airway manipulations benefit from preoperative administration of an anticholinergic agent (glycopyrrolate or atropine) to reduce airway secretions before and during surgery. The fundamental **(11)** message here is that premedication should be given purposefully, not as a mindless routine.

DOCUMENTATION

Physicians should first and foremost provide high-quality and efficient medical care. Secondly, they must document the care that has been provided. Adequate documentation provides guidance to those who may encounter the patient in the future. It permits others to assess the quality of the care that was given and to provide risk adjustment of outcomes. Adequate documentation is required for a physician to submit a bill for his or her services. Finally, adequate and well-organized documentation (as opposed to inadequate and sloppy documentation) supports a potential defense case should a claim for medical malpractice be filed.

Preoperative Assessment Note

The preoperative assessment note should appear in the patient's permanent medical record and should describe pertinent findings, including the medical history, anesthetic history, current medications (and whether they were taken on the day of surgery), physical examination, ASA physical status class, laboratory results, interpretation of imaging, electrocardiograms, and recommendations of any consultants. A comment is particularly important when the consultant's recommendation will not be followed. As most North American hospitals are transitioning to electronic medical records, the preanesthetic note will often appear as a standardized form.

The preoperative note should briefly describe the anesthetic plan and include a statement regarding informed consent from the patient (or guardian). The plan should indicate whether regional or general anesthesia (or sedation) will be used, and whether invasive monitoring or other advanced techniques will be employed. Documentation of the informed consent discussion sometimes takes the form of a narrative indicating that the plan, alternative plans, and their advantages and disadvantages (including their relative risks) were presented, understood, and accepted by the patient. Alternatively, the patient may be asked to sign a special anesthesia consent form that contains the same information. A sample preanesthetic report form is illustrated in Figure 18–1.

In the United States, The Joint Commission (TJC) requires an immediate preanesthetic reevaluation to determine whether the patient's status has changed in the time since the preoperative evaluation was performed. Even when the elapsed time is less than a minute, the bureaucracy will not be denied: the "box" must be checked to indicate that there has been no interval change.

Intraoperative Anesthesia Record

The intraoperative anesthesia record (Figure 18–2) serves many purposes. It functions as documentation of intraoperative monitoring, a reference for future anesthetics for that patient, and a source of data for quality assurance. This record should be terse, pertinent, and accurate. Increasingly, parts of the anesthesia record are generated automatically and recorded electronically. Such anesthesia information management systems (commonly abbreviated AIMS) have many theoretical and practical advantages over the traditional paper record but also introduce all the common pitfalls of

ANESTHESIOLOGY PREOPERATIVE NOTE

DATE:	TIME:	HT.	PREOP DIAGNOSIS:
AGE:	SEX: M F	WT.	PROPOSED OPERATION:

MEDICAL HISTORY   **MEDICATIONS:**
ALLERGIES:
INTOLERANCES:
DRUG USE: TOBACCO: ETOH:

PRESENT PROBLEM:

CARDIOVASCULAR

RESPIRATORY

DIABETES

NEUROLOGIC   RENAL

ARTHRITIS/MUSCULO-SKELETAL   HEPATIC

                                                  OTHER

PREVIOUS ANESTHETICS:

FAMILY HISTORY

LAST ORAL INTAKE

PHYSICAL EXAMINATION   BP   P   R   T

   HEART   EXTREMITIES

   LUNGS   NEUROLOGIC

   AIRWAY   OTHER

   TEETH

LABORATORY

   Hct/Hgb   ECG   CHEST X-RAY
   URINE
   LYTES: Na   Cl
           K   GLUCOSE   OTHER
           CO_2 BUN: CREATININE

PLAN   ☐ GENERAL   INVASIVE MONITORS
            ☐ REGIONAL
            ☐ MONITORED ANESTHESIA CARE   SPECIAL TECHNIQUES

ASA CLASS   SIGNATURE _____ M.D.
                                              (RESIDENT)   (STAFF)

PATIENT CONSENT
ANESTHETIC ALTERNATIVES AND RISKS RANGING FROM TOOTH DAMAGE
TO LIFE-THREATENING EVENTS HAVE BEEN EXPLAINED AND ACCEPTED.

                                              PATIENT
                                              NAME

PATIENT'S SIGNATURE   #

FIGURE 18–1 A sample preoperative note.

ANESTHESIA RECORD

AGE:_____ SEX: M F   PRE MED: S U _____ ASA _____

DENTITION _____ NPO _____ PROPOSED SURGERY _____

☐ PT. IDED ☐ CONSENT ✓ED ☐ CHART REVIEWED SURGEON _____

OPERATION PERFORMED _____

PRE OP: BP_____ P_____ R _____ T _____ Hct _____ ALLERGIES _____

TIME		TOTALS
OXYGEN		
NITROUS OXIDE		
HALO/ENFL/ISOFL/DES/SEVO		
TEMP		
URINE		
FLUIDS/BLOOD		

IV # _____

BP ⋀ SYS ∨ DIA

PULSE •

RESP. ⊘ ASSISTED ○ SPONT. ● CONTROLLED

ECG
FiO₂ — FiO_2
EtCO₂ — $EtCO_2$
SaO₂ — SaO_2
Et_A — Et_A
Temp

MONITORS:

☐ MACHINE ✓ED   ☐ RAPID TRANSFER
☐ OXIMETER   ☐ FORCED AIR WARMER
☐ BP. SITE   ☐ FiO₂
☐ EKG   ☐ EtCO₂
☐ FLUID WARMER   ☐ ESOPH
☐ PRECORDIAL   ☐ NERVE STIM
☐ TEMP   ☐ CVP
☐ HUMIDIFIER   ☐ A-LINE
☐ BLANKET WARM/COOL   ☐ PA CATHETER

Scale: 240 220 200 180 160 140 120 100 80 60 40 20 0

VENT.	VT/RR	
	AIRWAY	P
BLOOD LOSS		
POSITION		

☐ MONITORED ANESTHESIA CARE
☐ REGIONAL
☐ GENERAL
BLADE _____
ETT# _____
BBS _____
CUFF _____ cc.
☐ ATRAUMATIC
☐ CO₂

COMMENTS:

EYE PROTECTION:

ANESTH. START _____
ANESTH. INDUC _____
SURG. START _____
SURG. END _____
ANESTH. END _____
ANESTH. NET _____

REMARKS: _____

_____

RECOVERY ROOM B.P. _____ P. _____ R.R. _____ TIME _____ O₂ SAT. _____

CONDITION _____

_____ M.D.

SIGNED (RESIDENT)

_____ M.D.

SIGNED (STAFF)

_____

DATE

PAGE _____ OF _____

PATIENT NAME

#

FIGURE 18–2 A representative intraoperative anesthesia record. These paper "charts" are rapidly being replaced by computerized anesthesia information management systems.

computerization, including the potential for unrecognized recording of artifactual data, the possibility that practitioners will find attending to the computer more interesting than attending to the patient, and the inevitable occurrence of device and software shutdowns. Regardless of whether the record is on paper or electronic it should document the anesthetic care in the operating room by including the following elements:

- Whether there has been a preoperative check of the anesthesia machine and other relevant equipment.

- Whether there has been a reevaluation of the patient immediately prior to induction of anesthesia (a TJC requirement); this generally includes a review of the medical record to search for any new laboratory results or consultation reports.

- Time of administration, dosage, and route of drugs given intraoperatively.

- Intraoperative estimates of blood loss and urinary output.

- Results of laboratory tests obtained during the operation.

- Intravenous fluids and any blood products administered.

- Pertinent procedure notes (such as for tracheal intubation or insertion of invasive monitors).

- A notation regarding specialized intraoperative techniques such as the mode of ventilation, or special techniques such as the use of hypotensive anesthesia, one-lung ventilation, high-frequency jet ventilation, or cardiopulmonary bypass.

- Timing and conduct of intraoperative events such as induction, positioning, surgical incision, and extubation.

- Unusual events or complications (eg, arrhythmias).

- Condition of the patient at the time of release to the postanesthesia or intensive care unit nurse.

By tradition and convention (and, in the United States, according to practice guidelines) arterial blood pressure and heart rate are recorded graphically no less frequently than at 5-min intervals. Data from other monitors are also usually entered graphically, whereas descriptions of techniques or complications are described in text. In some anesthetizing locations of most hospitals the computerized AIMS will be unavailable. Unfortunately, the conventional, handwritten intraoperative anesthetic record often proves inadequate for documenting critical incidents, such as a cardiac arrest. In such cases, a separate text note inserted in the patient's medical record may be necessary. Careful recording of the timing of events is needed to avoid discrepancies between multiple simultaneous records (anesthesia record, nurses' notes, cardiopulmonary resuscitation record, and other physicians' entries in the medical record). Such discrepancies are frequently targeted by malpractice attorneys as evidence of incompetence, inaccuracy, or deceit. Incomplete, inaccurate, or illegible records unnecessarily complicate defending a physician against otherwise unjustified allegations of malpractice.

Postoperative Notes

The anesthesiologist's immediate responsibility to the patient does not end until the patient has recovered from the effects of the anesthetic. After accompanying the patient to the postanesthesia care unit (PACU), the anesthesiologist should remain with the patient until normal vital signs have been measured and the patient's condition is deemed stable. Before discharge from the PACU, a note should be written by the anesthesiologist to document the patient's recovery from anesthesia, any apparent anesthesia-related complications, the immediate postoperative condition of the patient, and the patient's disposition (discharge to an outpatient area, an inpatient ward, an intensive care unit, or home). In the United States, as of 2009, the Centers for Medicare and Medicaid Services require that certain elements be included in all postoperative notes (Table 18–3). Recovery from anesthesia should be assessed at least once within 48 h after discharge from the PACU in all inpatients. Postoperative notes should document the general condition of the patient, the presence or absence of any anesthesia-related complications, and any measures undertaken to treat such complications.

TABLE 18–3 **Elements required by the Center for Medicare and Medicaid Services in all postoperative notes.**[1]

Respiratory function, including respiratory rate, airway patency, and oxygen saturation
Cardiovascular function, including pulse rate and blood pressure
Mental status
Temperature
Pain
Nausea and vomiting
Postoperative hydration

[1]Data from the Centers for Medicare and Medicaid Services (CMS): *Revised Anesthesia Services Interpretive Guidelines,* issued December 2009. Available at: http://www.kdheks.gov/bhfr/download/Appendix_L.pdf (accessed September 1, 2012).

CASE DISCUSSION

Medical Malpractice (also see Chapter 54)

A healthy 45-year-old man has a cardiac arrest during an elective laparoscopic inguinal hernia repair. Although cardiopulmonary resuscitation is successful, the patient is left with permanent changes in mental status that preclude his return to work. One year later, the patient files a complaint against the anesthesiologist, surgeon, and hospital.

What four elements must be proved by the plaintiff (patient) to establish negligence on the part of the defendant (physician or hospital)?

1. *Duty:* Once a physician establishes a professional relationship with a patient, the physician owes that patient certain obligations, such as adhering to the "standard of care."
2. *Breach of Duty:* If these obligations are not fulfilled, the physician has breached his duties to the patient.
3. *Injury:* An injury must result. The injury may result in general damages (eg, pain and suffering) or special damages (eg, loss of income).
4. *Causation:* The plaintiff must demonstrate that the breach of duty was causally related to the injury. But for the breach of duty, the injury

should not have occurred. This proximate cause does not have to be the most important or immediate cause of the injury.

How is the standard of care defined and established?

Individual physicians are expected to perform as any prudent and reasonable physician would in similar circumstances. This does *not* require "best" care or optimal care, only that the care meet the minimum standard of a prudent and reasonable physician. As a specialist, the anesthesiologist is held to a higher standard of knowledge and skill with respect to the subject matter of that specialty than would a general practitioner or a physician in another specialty. Expert witnesses usually provide testimony to define the standard of care in legal proceedings. Although most jurisdictions have extended the "locality rule" to encompass a national standard of care, medical malpractice cases are governed by the laws of the jurisdiction in which the event took place and these may differ from state to state. The specific circumstances pertaining to each individual case are taken into account. The law recognizes that there are differences of opinion and varying schools of thought within the medical profession.

How is causation determined?

It is usually the plaintiff who bears the burden of proving that the injury would not have occurred "but for" the negligence of the physician, or that the physician's action was a "substantial factor" in causing the injury. An exception is the doctrine of *res ipsa loquitur* ("the thing speaks for itself"), which permits a finding of negligence based solely on the evidence. For example, if a set of car keys were visualized inside a patient on a chest radiograph after a thoracotomy, the doctrine of res ipsa loquitur would apply. Res ipsa loquitur could not be used in the case under discussion because the plaintiff would have to establish that cardiac arrest could not occur in the absence of negligence and that cardiac arrest could not have been due to something outside the control of the anesthesiologist. An important concept is that causation in civil cases need only be established by a preponderance of the evidence ("more likely than not")—as opposed to criminal cases, in which all elements of a charged offense must be proved "beyond a reasonable doubt."

What factors influence the likelihood of a malpractice suit?

1. *The Physician–Patient Relationship:* This is particularly important for the anesthesiologist, who usually does not meet the patient until immediately before the operation. Another problem is that the patient is unconscious while under the anesthesiologist's care. Thus, the preoperative and postoperative visits with the patient are often the only opportunities to establish a good relationship with the patient. Family members should also be included during these meetings with patients (provided the patient does not object), particularly during the postoperative visit if there has been an intraoperative complication.

2. *Adequacy of Informed Consent:* Rendering care to a competent patient who does not consent constitutes assault and battery. Consent is not enough, however. The patient should be informed of the contemplated procedure, including its reasonably anticipated risks, its possible benefits, and the therapeutic alternatives. The physician may be liable for a complication—even if it is not due to the negligent performance of a procedure—if a jury is convinced that a reasonable person would have refused treatment if properly informed of the possibility of the complication. This does not mean, of course, that a documented consent relieves from liability physicians who violate the standard of care.

3. *Quality of Documentation:* Careful documentation of the perioperative visits, informed consent, consultations with other specialists, intraoperative events, and postoperative care is essential. The viewpoint of many courts and juries, reinforced by plaintiff's attorneys, is that "if it isn't written, it wasn't done." It goes without saying that medical records should never be intentionally destroyed or altered.

GUIDELINES

American College of Cardiology Foundation/American Heart Association Task Force on Practice Guidelines; American Society of Echocardiography; American Society of Nuclear Cardiology; et al: 2009 ACCF/AHA focused update on perioperative beta blockade incorporated into the ACC/AHA 2007 guidelines on perioperative cardiovascular evaluation and care for noncardiac surgery. J Am Coll Cardiol 2009;54:e13.

American Society of Anesthesiologists Committee: Practice guidelines for preoperative fasting and the use of pharmacologic agents to reduce the risk of pulmonary aspiration: Application to healthy patients undergoing elective procedures: An updated report by the American Society of Anesthesiologists Committee on Standards and Practice Parameters. Anesthesiology 2011;114:495.

Committee on Standards and practice Parameters, Apfelbaum JL, Connis RT, et al: Practice advisory for preanesthesia evaluation: An updated report by the American Society of Anesthesiologists Task Force on Preanesthesia Evaluation. Anesthesiology 2012;116:522.

Gogarten W, Vandermeulen E, Van Aken H, et al: Regional anaesthesia and antithrombotic agents: Recommendations of the European Society of Anaesthesiology. Eur J Anaesthesiol 2010;27:999.

Horlocker TT, Wedel DJ, Rowlingson JC, et al: Regional anesthesia in the patient receiving antithrombotic or thrombolytic therapy: American Society of Regional Anesthesia and Pain Medicine evidence-based guidelines (third edition). Reg Anesth Pain Med 2010;35:64.

Keeling D, Baglin T, Tait C, et al: British Committee for Standards in Haematology: Guidelines on oral anticoagulation with warfarin—fourth edition. Br J Haematol 2011;154:311.

Korte W, Cattaneo M, Chassot PG, et al: Peri-operative management of antiplatelet therapy in patients with coronary artery disease: Joint position paper by members of the working group on Perioperative Haemostasis of the Society on Thrombosis and Haemostasis Research (GTH), the working group on Perioperative Coagulation of the Austrian Society for Anesthesiology, Resuscitation and Intensive Care (ÖGARI) and the Working Group Thrombosis of the European Society for Cardiology (ESC). Thromb Haemost 2011;105:743.

Qaseem A, Snow V, Fitterman N, et al: Risk assessment for and strategies to reduce perioperative pulmonary complications for patients undergoing noncardiothoracic surgery: A guideline from the American College of Physicians. Ann Intern Med 2006;144:575.

Smith I, Kranke P, Murat I, et al: Perioperative fasting in adults and children: Guidelines from the European Society of Anaesthesiology. Eur J Anaesthesiol. 2011;28:556.

SUGGESTED READING

Centers for Medicare & Medicaid Services (CMS): CMS Manual System. Pub 100-07 State Operations Provider Certification. DHHS. Available at: http://www.kdheks.gov/bhfr/download/Appendix_L.pdf (accessed September 1, 2012).

Douketis JD: Perioperative management of patients who are receiving warfarin therapy: An evidence-based and practical approach. Blood 2011;117:5044.

Egbert LD, Battit G, Turndorf H, Beecher HK: The value of the preoperative visit by an anesthetist. A study of doctor-patient rapport. JAMA 1963;185:553.

Mendelson CL: The aspiration of stomach contents into the lungs during obstetric anesthesia. Am J Obstet Gynecol 1946;52:191.

Airway Management

1. Improper face mask technique can result in continued deflation of the anesthesia reservoir bag when the adjustable pressure-limiting valve is closed, usually indicating a substantial leak around the mask. In contrast, the generation of high breathing circuit pressures with minimal chest movement and breath sounds implies an obstructed airway or obstructed tubing.

2. The laryngeal mask airway partially protects the larynx from pharyngeal secretions, but not gastric regurgitation.

3. After insertion of a tracheal tube (TT), the cuff is inflated with the least amount of air necessary to create a seal during positive-pressure ventilation to minimize the pressure transmitted to the tracheal mucosa.

4. Although the persistent detection of CO_2 by a capnograph is the best confirmation of tracheal placement of a TT, it cannot exclude bronchial intubation. The earliest evidence of bronchial intubation often is an increase in peak inspiratory pressure.

5. After intubation, the cuff of a TT should not be felt above the level of the cricoid cartilage, because a prolonged intralaryngeal location may result in

postoperative hoarseness and increases the risk of accidental extubation.

6. Unrecognized esophageal intubation can produce catastrophic results. Prevention of this complication depends on direct visualization of the tip of the TT passing through the vocal cords, careful auscultation for the presence of bilateral breath sounds and the absence of gastric gurgling while ventilating through the TT, analysis of exhaled gas for the presence of CO_2 (the most reliable automated method), chest radiography, or use of fiberoptic bronchoscopy.

7. Clues to the diagnosis of bronchial intubation include unilateral breath sounds, unexpected hypoxia with pulse oximetry (unreliable with high inspired oxygen concentrations), inability to palpate the TT cuff in the sternal notch during cuff inflation, and decreased breathing bag compliance (high peak inspiratory pressures).

8. The large negative intrathoracic pressures generated by a struggling patient in laryngospasm can result in the development of negative-pressure pulmonary edema even in healthy patients.

Expert airway management is an essential skill in anesthetic practice. This chapter reviews the anatomy of the upper respiratory tract: describes the necessary equipment for successful management, presents various management techniques: and discusses complications of laryngoscopy, intubation, and extubation. Patient safety depends on a thorough understanding of each of these topics.

ANATOMY

The upper airway consists of the pharynx, nose, mouth, larynx, trachea, and main-stem bronchi. The mouth and pharynx are also a part of the upper gastrointestinal tract. The laryngeal structures in part serve to prevent aspiration into the trachea.

There are two openings to the human airway: the nose, which leads to the nasopharynx, and the mouth, which leads to the oropharynx. These passages are separated anteriorly by the palate, but they join posteriorly in the pharynx (**Figure 19–1**). The pharynx is a U-shaped fibromuscular structure that extends from the base of the skull to the cricoid cartilage at the entrance to the esophagus. It opens anteriorly into the nasal cavity, the mouth, the larynx, and the nasopharynx, oropharynx, and laryngopharynx, respectively. The nasopharynx is separated from the oropharynx by an imaginary plane that extends posteriorly. At the base of the tongue, the epiglottis functionally separates the oropharynx from the laryngopharynx (or hypopharynx).

The epiglottis prevents aspiration by covering the glottis—the opening of the larynx—during swallowing. The larynx is a cartilaginous skeleton held together by ligaments and muscle. The larynx is composed of nine cartilages (**Figure 19–2**): thyroid, cricoid, epiglottic, and (in pairs) arytenoid, corniculate, and cuneiform. The thyroid cartilage shields the conus elasticus, which forms the vocal cords.

The sensory supply to the upper airway is derived from the cranial nerves (**Figure 19–3**). The mucous membranes of the nose are innervated by the ophthalmic division (V_1) of the trigeminal nerve anteriorly (anterior ethmoidal nerve) and by the maxillary division (V_2) posteriorly (sphenopalatine nerves). The palatine nerves provide sensory fibers from the trigeminal nerve (V) to the superior and inferior surfaces of the hard and soft palate. The **olfactory nerve** (cranial nerve I) innervates the nasal mucosa to provide the sense of smell. The lingual nerve (a branch of the mandibular division [V_3] of the trigeminal nerve) and the glossopharyngeal nerve (the ninth cranial nerve) provide general sensation to the anterior two-thirds and posterior one-third of the tongue, respectively. Branches of the facial nerve (VII) and glossopharyngeal nerve provide the sensation of taste to those areas, respectively. The **glossopharyngeal nerve** also innervates the roof of the pharynx, the tonsils, and the undersurface of the soft palate. The **vagus nerve** (the tenth cranial nerve) provides sensation to the airway below the epiglottis. The superior laryngeal branch of the vagus divides into an external (motor) nerve and an internal (sensory) laryngeal nerve that provide sensory supply to the larynx between the epiglottis and the vocal cords. Another branch of the vagus, the **recurrent laryngeal nerve**, innervates the larynx below the vocal cords and the trachea.

The muscles of the larynx are innervated by the recurrent laryngeal nerve, with the exception of the cricothyroid muscle, which is innervated by the external (motor) laryngeal nerve, a branch of the superior laryngeal nerve. The posterior cricoarytenoid muscles abduct the vocal cords, whereas the lateral cricoarytenoid muscles are the principal adductors.

Phonation involves complex simultaneous actions by several laryngeal muscles. Damage to the motor nerves innervating the larynx leads

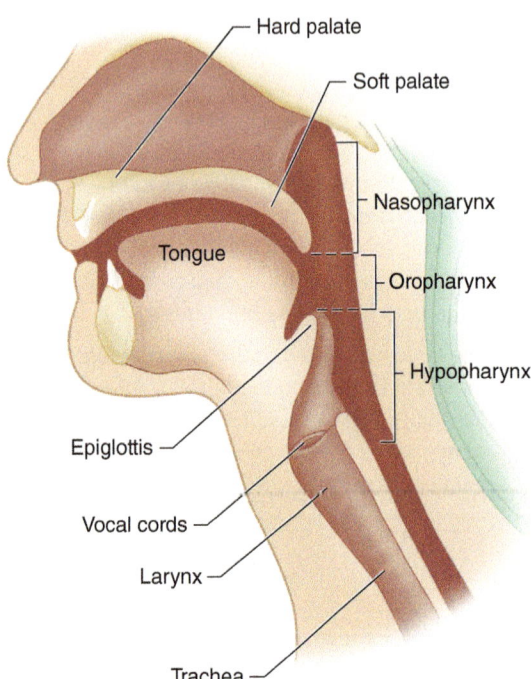

- Hard palate
- Soft palate
- Nasopharynx
- Tongue
- Oropharynx
- Hypopharynx
- Epiglottis
- Vocal cords
- Larynx
- Trachea

FIGURE 19–1 Anatomy of the airway.

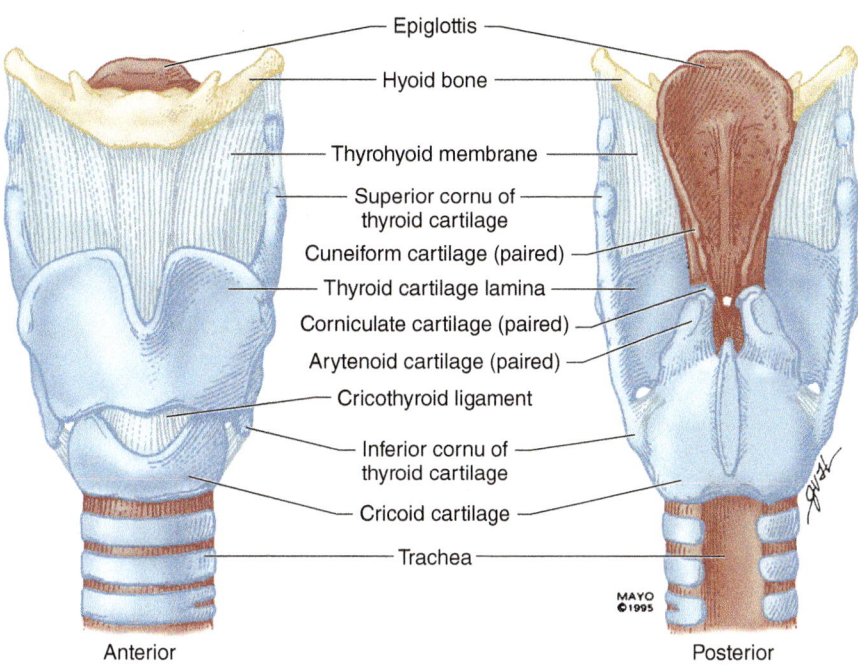

FIGURE 19–2 Cartilaginous structures comprising the larynx. (With permission, from The Mayo Foundation.)

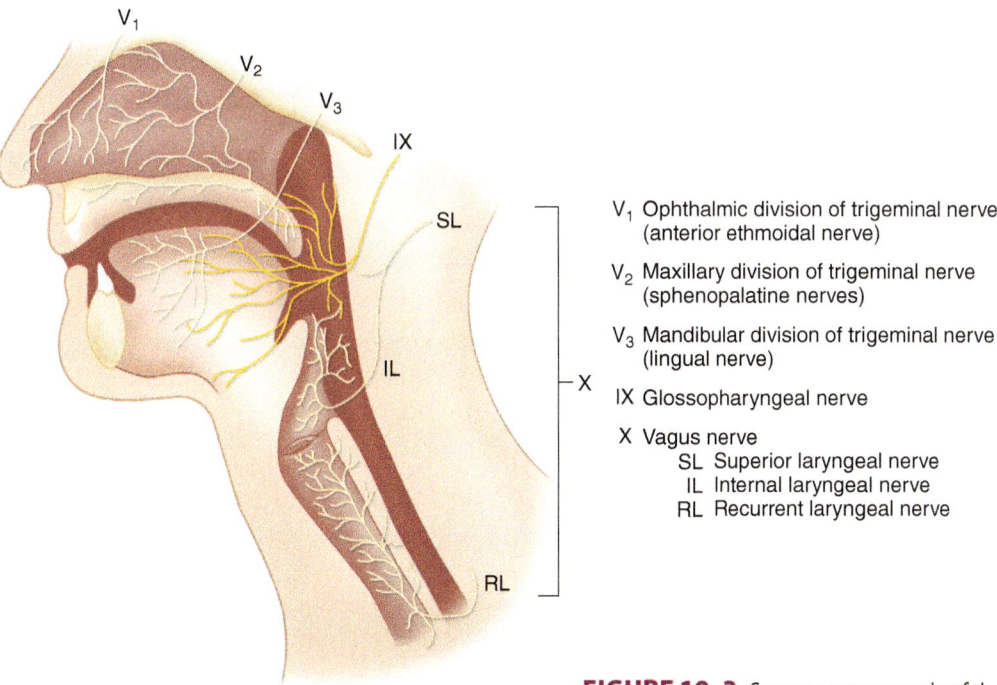

V_1 Ophthalmic division of trigeminal nerve
(anterior ethmoidal nerve)

V_2 Maxillary division of trigeminal nerve
(sphenopalatine nerves)

V_3 Mandibular division of trigeminal nerve
(lingual nerve)

IX Glossopharyngeal nerve

X Vagus nerve
  SL Superior laryngeal nerve
  IL Internal laryngeal nerve
  RL Recurrent laryngeal nerve

FIGURE 19–3 Sensory nerve supply of the airway.

TABLE 19–1 The effects of laryngeal nerve injury on the voice.

Nerve	Effect of Nerve Injury
Superior laryngeal nerve	
Unilateral	Minimal effects
Bilateral	Hoarseness, tiring of voice
Recurrent laryngeal nerve	
Unilateral	Hoarseness
Bilateral	
Acute	Stridor, respiratory distress
Chronic	Aphonia
Vagus nerve	
Unilateral	Hoarseness
Bilateral	Aphonia

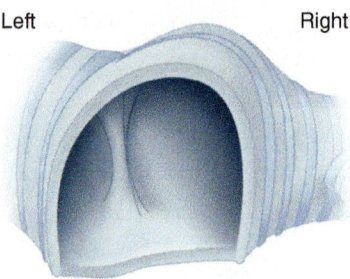

Left   Right

FIGURE 19–4 Carina.

to a spectrum of speech disorders (Table 19–1). Unilateral denervation of a cricothyroid muscle causes very subtle clinical findings. Bilateral palsy of the superior laryngeal nerve may result in hoarseness or easy tiring of the voice, but airway control is not jeopardized.

Unilateral paralysis of a recurrent laryngeal nerve results in paralysis of the ipsilateral vocal cord, causing deterioration in voice quality. Assuming intact superior laryngeal nerves, *acute* bilateral recurrent laryngeal nerve palsy can result in stridor and respiratory distress because of the remaining unopposed tension of the cricothyroid muscles. Airway problems are less frequent in *chronic* bilateral recurrent laryngeal nerve loss because of the development of various compensatory mechanisms (eg, atrophy of the laryngeal musculature).

Bilateral injury to the vagus nerve affects both the superior and the recurrent laryngeal nerves. Thus, bilateral vagal denervation produces flaccid, midpositioned vocal cords similar to those seen after administration of succinylcholine. Although phonation is severely impaired in these patients, airway control is rarely a problem.

The blood supply of the larynx is derived from branches of the thyroid arteries. The cricothyroid artery arises from the superior thyroid artery itself, the first branch given off from the external carotid artery, and crosses the upper cricothyroid membrane (CTM), which extends from the cricoid cartilage to the thyroid cartilage. The superior thyroid artery is found along the lateral edge of the CTM.

The trachea begins beneath the cricoid cartilage and extends to the carina, the point at which the right and left main-stem bronchi divide (Figure 19–4). Anteriorly, the trachea consists of cartilaginous rings; posteriorly, the trachea is membranous.

ROUTINE AIRWAY MANAGEMENT

Routine airway management associated with general anesthesia consists of:

- Airway assessment
- Preparation and equipment check
- Patient positioning
- Preoxygenation
- Bag and mask ventilation (BMV)
- Intubation (if indicated)
- Confirmation of endotracheal tube placement
- Intraoperative management and troubleshooting
- Extubation

AIRWAY ASSESSMENT

Airway assessment is the first step in successful airway management. Several anatomical and functional maneuvers can be performed to estimate the difficulty of endotracheal intubation; however, it is important to note that successful ventilation (with or without intubation) must be achieved by

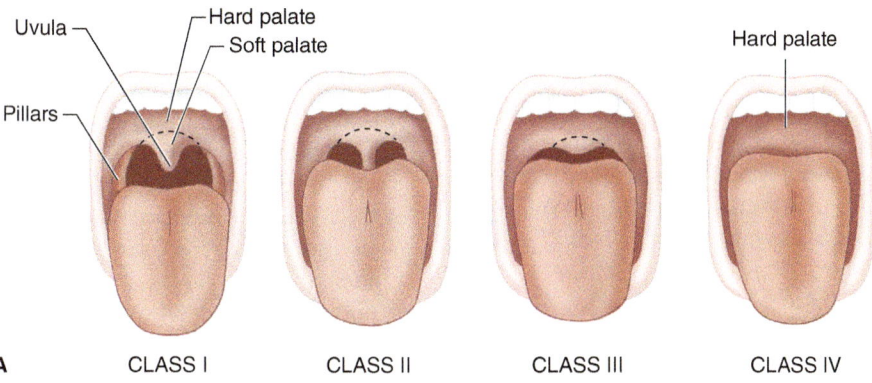

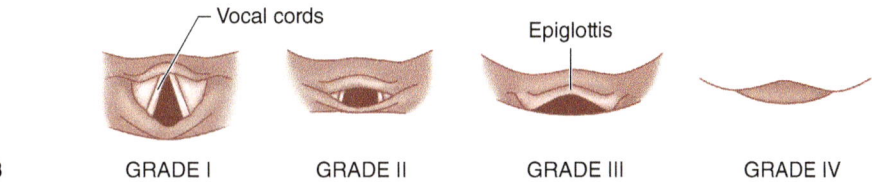

FIGURE 19–5 A: Mallampati classification of oral opening. **B**: Grading of the laryngeal view. A difficult orotracheal intubation (grade III or IV) may be predicted by the inability to visualize certain pharyngeal structures (class III or IV) during the preoperative examination of a seated patient. (Reproduced, with permission, from Mallampati SR: Clinical signs to predict difficult tracheal intubation [hypothesis]. Can Anaesth Soc J 1983;30:316.)

the anesthetist if mortality and morbidity are to be avoided. Assessments include:

- Mouth opening: an incisor distance of 3 cm or greater is desirable in an adult.

- Upper lip bite test: the lower teeth are brought in front of the upper teeth. The degree to which this can be done estimates the range of motion of the temperomandibular joints.

- Mallampati classification: a frequently performed test that examines the size of the tongue in relation to the oral cavity. The greater the tongue obstructs the view of the pharyngeal structures, the more difficult intubation may be (Figure 19–5).

  - Class I: the entire palatal arch, including the bilateral faucial pillars, are visible down to their bases.

  - Class II: the upper part of the faucial pillars and most of the uvula are visible.
  - Class III: only the soft and hard palates are visible.
  - Class IV: only the hard palate is visible.

- Thyromental distance: the distance between the mentum and the superior thyroid notch. A distance greater than 3 fingerbreadths is desirable.

- Neck circumference: a neck circumference of greater than 27 in is suggestive of difficulties in visualization of the glottic opening.

Although the presence of these findings may not be particularly sensitive for detecting a difficult intubation, the absence of these findings is predictive for relative ease of intubation.

Increasingly, patients present with morbid obesity and body mass indices of 30 kg/m² or greater. Although some morbidly obese patients have relatively normal head and neck anatomy, others have much redundant pharyngeal tissue and increased neck circumference. Not only may these patients prove to be difficult to intubate, but routine ventilation with bag and mask also may be problematic.

EQUIPMENT

Preparation is mandatory for all airway management scenarios. The following equipment is routinely needed in airway management situations:

- An oxygen source
- BMV capability
- Laryngoscopes (direct and video)
- Several endotracheal tubes of different sizes
- Other (not endotracheal tube) airway devices (eg, oral, nasal airways)
- Suction
- Oximetry and CO_2 detection
- Stethoscope
- Tape
- Blood pressure and electrocardiography (ECG) monitors
- Intravenous access

Oral & Nasal Airways

Loss of upper airway muscle tone (eg, weakness of the genioglossus muscle) in anesthetized patients allows the tongue and epiglottis to fall back against the posterior wall of the pharynx. Repositioning the head or a jaw thrust is the preferred technique for opening the airway. To maintain the opening, an artificial airway can be inserted through the mouth or nose to maintain an air passage between the tongue and the posterior pharyngeal wall (**Figure 19–6**). Awake or lightly anesthetized patients with intact laryngeal reflexes may cough or even develop laryngospasm during airway insertion. Placement of an oral airway is sometimes facilitated by suppressing airway reflexes, and, in addition, sometimes by depressing the tongue with a tongue blade. Adult oral airways typically come in small (80 mm [Guedel No. 3]), medium (90 mm [Guedel No. 4]), and large (100 mm [Guedel No. 5]) sizes.

The length of a nasal airway can be estimated as the distance from the nares to the meatus of the ear and should be approximately 2–4 cm longer than oral airways. Because of the risk of epistaxis, nasal airways are less desirable in anticoagulated or thrombocytopenic patients. Also, nasal airways (and nasogastric tubes) should be used with caution in patients with basilar skull fractures, where there has been a case report of a nasogastric tube entering the cranial vault. All tubes inserted through the nose (eg, nasal airways, nasogastric

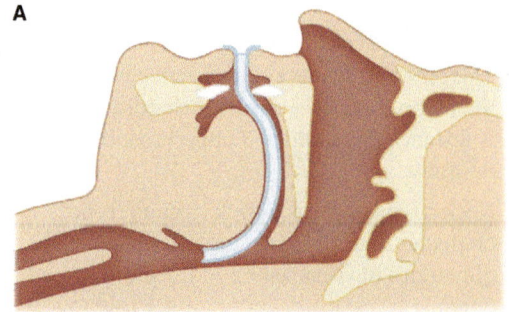

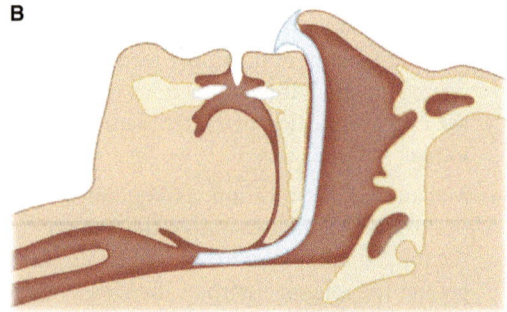

FIGURE 19–6 **A**: The oropharyngeal airway in place. The airway follows the curvature of the tongue, pulling it and the epiglottis away from the posterior pharyngeal wall and providing a channel for air passage. **B**: The nasopharyngeal airway in place. The airway passes

through the nose and extends to just above the epiglottis.
(Modified and reproduced, with permission, from Face masks and airways. In: *Understanding Anesthesia Equipment*, 4th ed. Dorsch JA, Dorsch SE, eds. Williams & Wilkins, 1999.)

catheters, nasotracheal tubes) should be lubricated before being advanced along the floor of the nasal passage.

Face Mask Design & Technique

The use of a face mask can facilitate the delivery of oxygen or an anesthetic gas from a breathing system to a patient by creating an airtight seal with the patient's face (Figure 19–7). The rim of the mask is contoured and conforms to a variety of facial features. The mask's 22-mm orifice attaches to the breathing circuit of the anesthesia machine through a right-angle connector. Several mask designs are available. Transparent masks allow observation of exhaled humidified gas and immediate recognition of vomitus. Retaining hooks surrounding the orifice can be attached to a head strap so that the mask does not have to be continually held in place. Some pediatric masks are specially designed to minimize apparatus dead space (Figure 19–8).

Effective mask ventilation requires both a gastight mask fit and a patent airway. Improper face mask technique can result in continued deflation of the anesthesia reservoir bag when the adjustable pressure-limiting valve is closed, usually indicating a substantial leak around the mask. In contrast, the generation of high breathing circuit pressures with minimal chest movement and breath sounds implies an obstructed airway or obstructed tubing.

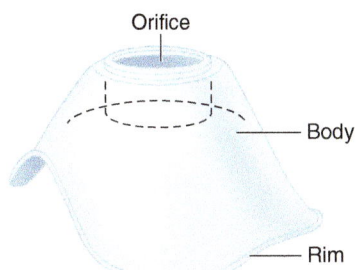

FIGURE 19–8 The Rendell–Baker–Soucek pediatric face mask has a shallow body and minimal dead space.

If the mask is held with the left hand, the right hand can be used to generate positive-pressure ventilation by squeezing the breathing bag. The mask is held against the face by downward pressure on the mask body exerted by the left thumb and index finger (Figure 19–9). The middle and ring finger grasp the mandible to facilitate extension of the atlanto-occipital joint. This is a maneuver that is easier to teach than to describe. Finger pressure should be placed on the bony mandible and not on the soft tissues supporting the base of the tongue, which may obstruct the airway. The little finger is placed under the angle of the jaw and used to thrust the jaw anteriorly, the most important maneuver to allow ventilation to the patient.

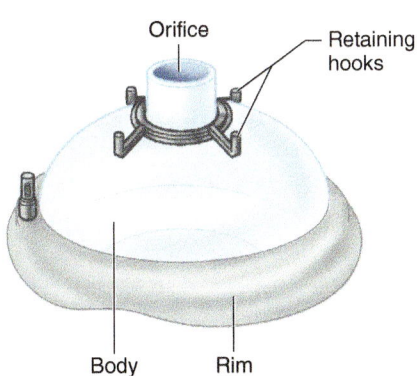

FIGURE 19–7 Clear adult face mask.

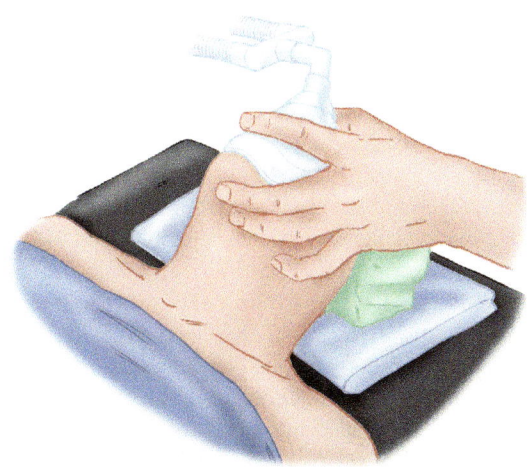

FIGURE 19–9 One-handed face mask technique.

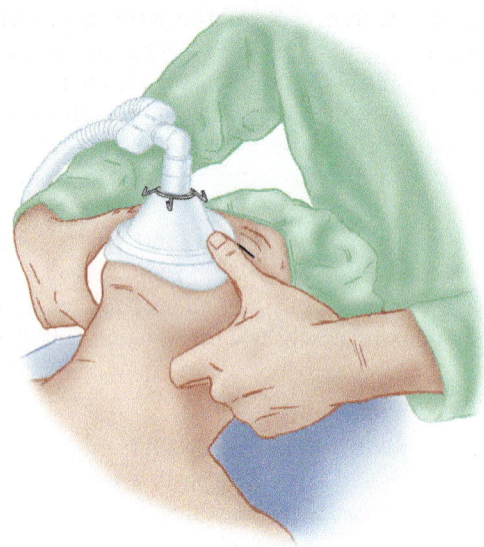

FIGURE 19–10 A difficult airway can often be managed with a two-handed technique.

In difficult situations, two hands may be needed to provide adequate jaw thrust and to create a mask seal. Therefore, an assistant may be needed to squeeze the bag, or the machine's ventilator can be used. In such cases, the thumbs hold the mask down, and the fingertips or knuckles displace the jaw forward (Figure 19–10). Obstruction during expiration may be due to excessive downward pressure from the mask or from a ball-valve effect of the jaw thrust. The former can be relieved by decreasing the pressure on the mask, and the latter by releasing the jaw thrust during this phase of the respiratory cycle. It is often difficult to form an adequate mask fit with the cheeks of edentulous patients. Positive-pressure ventilation using a mask should normally be limited to 20 cm of H_2O to avoid stomach inflation.

Most patients' airways can be maintained with a face mask and an oral or nasal airway. Mask ventilation for long periods may result in pressure injury to branches of the trigeminal or facial nerves. Because of the absence of positive airway pressures during spontaneous ventilation, only minimal downward force on the face mask is required to create an adequate seal. If the face mask and mask straps are used for extended periods, the position should be

regularly changed to prevent injury. Care should be used to avoid mask or finger contact with the eye, and the eyes should be taped shut to minimize the risk of corneal abrasions.

POSITIONING

When manipulating the airway, correct patient positioning is required. Relative alignment of the oral and pharyngeal axes is achieved by having the patient in the "sniffing" position. When cervical spine pathology is suspected, the head must be kept in a neutral position during all airway manipulations. In-line stabilization of the neck must be maintained during airway management in these patients, unless appropriate films have been reviewed and cleared by a radiologist or neurological or spine surgeon. Patients with morbid obesity should be positioned on a 30° upward ramp, as the functional residual capacity (FRC) of obese patients deteriorates in the supine position, leading to more rapid deoxygenation should ventilation be impaired.

PREOXYGENATION

When possible, preoxygenation with face mask oxygen should precede all airway management interventions. Oxygen is delivered by mask for several minutes prior to anesthetic induction. In this way, the functional residual capacity, the patient's oxygen reserve, is purged of nitrogen. Up to 90% of the normal FRC of 2 L following preoxygenation is filled with O_2. Considering the normal oxygen demand of 200–250 mL/min, the preoxygenated patient may have a 5–8 min oxygen reserve. Increasing the duration of apnea without desaturation improves safety, if ventilation following anesthetic induction is delayed. Conditions that increase oxygen demand (eg, sepsis, pregnancy) and decrease FRC (eg, morbid obesity, pregnancy) reduce the apneic period before desaturation ensues.

BAG AND MASK VENTILATION

Bag and mask ventilation (BMV) is the first step in airway management in most situations, with the exception of patients undergoing rapid sequence intubation. Rapid sequence inductions avoid BMV to avoid stomach inflation and to reduce the potential for the aspiration of gastric contents in nonfasted patients and those with delayed gastric emptying. In emergency situations, BMV precedes attempts at intubation in an effort to oxygenate the patient, with the understanding that there is an implicit risk of aspiration.

As noted above, the anesthetist's left hand supports the mask on the patient's face. The face is lifted into the mask with the third, fourth, and fifth fingers of the anesthesia provider's left hand. The fingers are placed on the mandible, and the jaw is thrust forward, lifting the base of the tongue away from the posterior pharynx opening the airway. The thumb and index finger sit on top of the mask. If the airway is patent, squeezing the bag will result in the rise of the chest. If ventilation is ineffective (no sign of chest rising, no end-tidal CO_2 detected, no mist in the clear mask), oral or nasal airways can be placed to relieve airway obstruction secondary to redundant pharyngeal tissues. Difficult mask ventilation is often found in patients with morbid obesity, beards, and craniofacial deformities.

In years past, anesthetics were routinely delivered solely by mask administration. In recent decades, a variety of supraglottic devices has permitted both airway rescue (when BMV is not possible) and routine anesthetic airway management (when intubation is not thought to be necessary).

SUPRAGLOTTIC AIRWAY DEVICES

Supraglottic airway devices (SADs) are used with both spontaneously and ventilated patients during anesthesia. They have also been employed as conduits to aid endotracheal intubation when both BMV and endotracheal intubation have failed. All SADs consist of a tube that is connected to a respiratory circuit or breathing bag, which is attached to a hypopharyngeal device that seals and directs airflow to the glottis, trachea, and lungs. Additionally, these airway devices occlude the esophagus with varying degrees of effectiveness, reducing gas distension of the stomach. Different sealing devices to prevent airflow from exiting through the mouth are also available. Some are equipped with a port to suction gastric contents. None offer the protection from aspiration pneumonitis offered by a properly sited, cuffed endotracheal tube.

Laryngeal Mask Airway

A laryngeal mask airway (LMA) consists of a wide-bore tube whose proximal end connects to a breathing circuit with a standard 15-mm connector, and whose distal end is attached to an elliptical cuff that can be inflated through a pilot tube. The deflated cuff is lubricated and inserted blindly into the hypopharynx so that, once inflated, the cuff forms a low-pressure seal around the entrance to the larynx. This requires anesthetic depth and muscle relaxation slightly greater than that required for the insertion of an oral airway. Although insertion is relatively simple (Figure 19–11), attention to detail will improve the success rate (Table 19–2). An ideally positioned cuff is bordered by the base of the tongue superiorly, the pyriform sinuses laterally, and the upper esophageal sphincter inferiorly. If the esophagus lies within the rim of the cuff, gastric distention and regurgitation become possible. Anatomic variations prevent adequate functioning in some patients. However, if an LMA is not functioning properly after attempts to improve the "fit" of the LMA have failed, most practitioners will try another LMA one size larger or smaller. The shaft can be secured with tape to the skin of the face.

2 The LMA partially protects the larynx from pharyngeal secretions (but *not* gastric regurgitation), and it should remain in place until the patient has regained airway reflexes. This is usually signaled by coughing and mouth opening on command. The LMA is available in many sizes (Table 19–3).

The LMA provides an alternative to ventilation through a face mask or TT (Table 19–4). Relative contraindications for the LMA include patients with pharyngeal pathology (eg, abscess), pharyngeal obstruction, full stomachs (eg, pregnancy, hiatal hernia), or low pulmonary compliance (eg, restrictive airways disease) requiring peak inspiratory pressures greater than 30 cm H_2O. Traditionally, the LMA has been avoided in patients

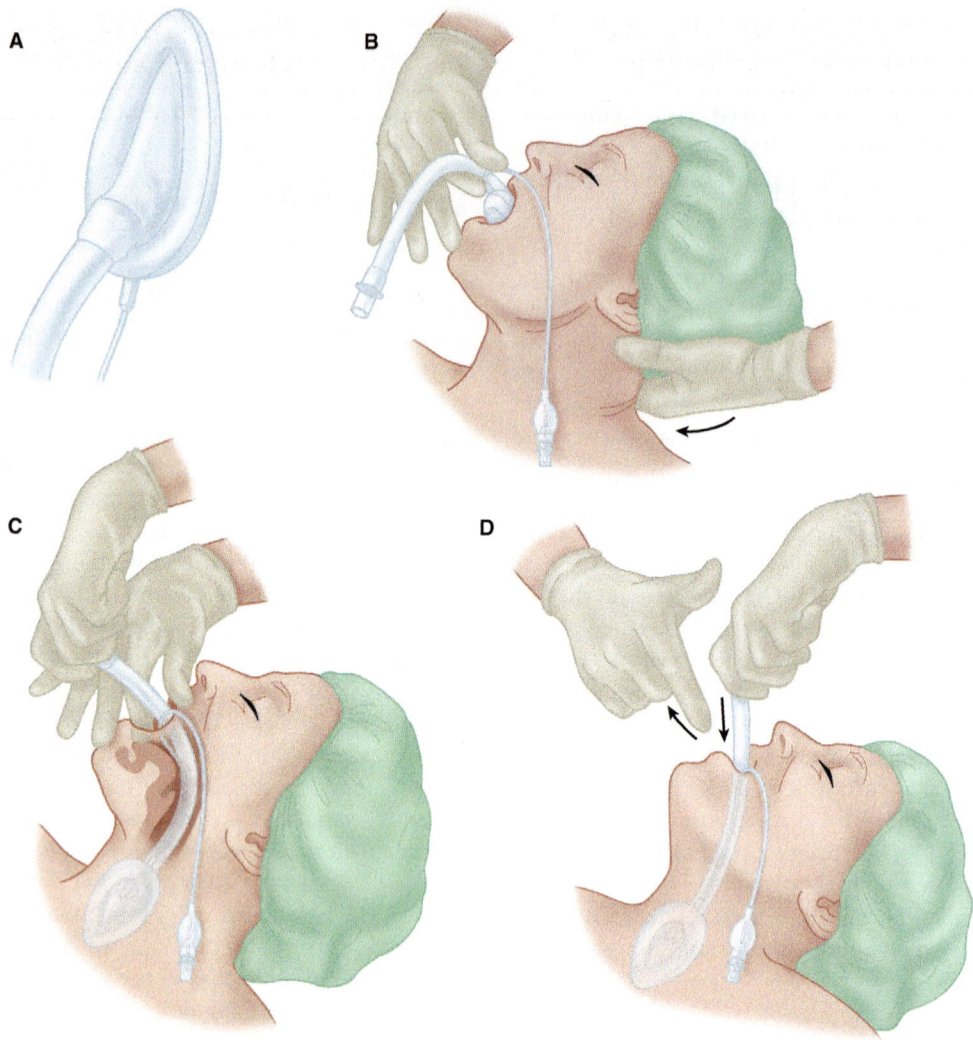

FIGURE 19–11 **A:** The laryngeal mask ready for insertion. The cuff should be deflated tightly with the rim facing away from the mask aperture. There should be no folds near the tip. **B:** Initial insertion of the laryngeal mask. Under direct vision, the mask tip is pressed upward against the hard palate. The middle finger may be used to push the lower jaw downward. The mask is pressed forward as it is advanced into the pharynx to ensure that the tip remains flattened and avoids the tongue. The jaw should not be held open once the mask is inside the mouth. The nonintubating hand can be used to stabilize the occiput. **C:** By withdrawing the other fingers and with a slight pronation of the forearm, it is usually possible to push the mask fully into position in one fluid movement. Note that the neck is kept flexed and the head extended. **D:** The laryngeal mask is grasped with the other hand and the index finger withdrawn. The hand holding the tube presses gently downward until resistance is encountered. (Reproduced, with permission, from LMA North America.)

with bronchospasm or high airway resistance, but new evidence suggests that because it is not placed in the trachea, use of an LMA is associated with less bronchospasm than a TT. Although it is clearly not a substitute for tracheal intubation, the LMA has proven particularly helpful as a life-saving temporizing measure in patients with difficult airways (those who cannot be ventilated or intubated) because of

TABLE 19–2 Successful insertion of a laryngeal mask airway depends upon attention to several details.

1. Choose the appropriate size (Table 19–3) and check for leaks before insertion.
2. The leading edge of the deflated cuff should be wrinkle free and facing away from the aperture (Figure 19–11A).
3. Lubricate only the back side of the cuff.
4. Ensure adequate anesthesia before attempting insertion.
5. Place patient's head in sniffing position (Figure 19–11B and Figure 19–23).
6. Use your index finger to guide the cuff along the hard palate and down into the hypopharynx until an increased resistance is felt (Figure 19–11C). The longitudinal black line should *always* be pointing directly cephalad (ie, facing the patient's upper lip).
7. Inflate with the correct amount of air (Table 19–3).
8. Ensure adequate anesthetic depth during patient positioning.
9. Obstruction after insertion is usually due to a down-folded epiglottis or transient laryngospasm.
10. Avoid pharyngeal suction, cuff deflation, or laryngeal mask removal until the patient is awake (eg, opening mouth on command).

TABLE 19–3 A variety of laryngeal masks with different cuff volumes are available for different sized patients.

Mask Size	Patient Size	Weight (kg)	Cuff Volume (mL)
1	Infant	<6.5	2–4
2	Child	6.5–20	Up to 10
2½	Child	20–30	Up to 15
3	Small adult	>30	Up to 20
4	Normal adult	<70	Up to 30
5	Larger adult	>70	Up to 30

performed under topical anesthesia and bilateral superior laryngeal nerve blocks, if the airway must be secured while the patient is awake.

Variations in LMA design include:

- The ProSeal LMA, which permits passage of a gastric tube to decompress the stomach
- The I-Gel, which uses a gel occluder rather than inflatable cuff
- The Fastrach intubation LMA, which is designed to facilitate endotracheal intubation through the LMA device
- The LMA CTrach, which incorporates a camera to facilitate passage of an endotracheal tube

its ease of insertion and relatively high success rate (95% to 99%). It has been used as a conduit for an intubating stylet (eg, gum-elastic bougie), ventilating jet stylet, flexible FOB, or small-diameter (6.0-mm) TT. Several LMAs are available that have been modified to facilitate placement of a larger TT, with or without the use of a FOB. Insertion can be

TABLE 19–4 Advantages and disadvantages of the laryngeal mask airway compared with face mask ventilation or tracheal intubation.[1]

	Advantages	Disadvantages
Compared with face mask	Hands-free operation Better seal in bearded patients Less cumbersome in ENT surgery Often easier to maintain airway Protects against airway secretions Less facial nerve and eye trauma Less operating room pollution	More invasive More risk of airway trauma Requires new skill Deeper anesthesia required Requires some TMJ mobility N₂O diffusion into cuff Multiple contraindications
Compared with tracheal intubation	Less invasive Very useful in difficult intubations Less tooth and laryngeal trauma Less laryngospasm and bronchospasm Does not require muscle relaxation Does not require neck mobility No risk of esophageal or endobronchial intubation	Increased risk of gastrointestinal aspiration Less safe in prone or jackknife positions Limits maximum PPV Less secure airway Greater risk of gas leak and pollution Can cause gastric distention

[1]ENT, ear, nose, and throat; TMJ, temporomandibular joint; PPV, positive-pressure ventilation.

Sore throat is a common side effect following SAD use. Injuries to the lingual, hypoglossal, and recurrent laryngeal nerve have been reported. Correct device sizing, avoidance of cuff hyperinflation, and gentle movement of the jaw during placement may reduce the likelihood of such injuries.

Esophageal–Tracheal Combitube

The esophageal–tracheal Combitube consists of two fused tubes, each with a 15-mm connector on its proximal end (Figure 19–12). The longer blue tube has an occluded distal tip that forces gas to exit through a series of side perforations. The shorter clear tube has an open tip and no side perforations. The Combitube is usually inserted blindly through the mouth and advanced until the two black rings on the shaft lie between the upper and lower teeth. The Combitube has two inflatable cuffs, a 100-mL proximal cuff and a 15-mL distal cuff, both of which should be fully inflated after placement. The distal lumen of the Combitube usually comes to lie in the esophagus approximately 95% of the time so that ventilation through the longer blue tube will force gas out of the side perforations and into the larynx. The shorter, clear tube can be used for gastric

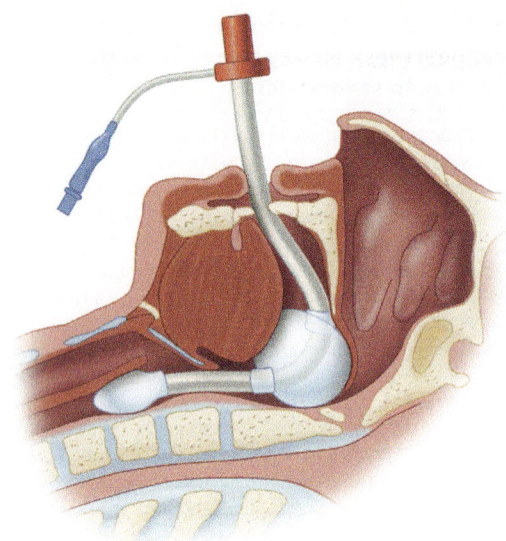

FIGURE 19–13 King laryngeal tube.

decompression. Alternatively, if the Combitube enters the trachea, ventilation through the clear tube will direct gas into the trachea.

King Laryngeal Tube

King laryngeal tubes (LTs) consist of tube with a small esophageal balloon and a larger balloon for placement in the hypopharynx (Figure 19–13). Both tubes inflate through one inflation line. The lungs are inflated from air that exits between the two balloons. A suction port distal to the esophageal balloon is present, permitting decompression of the stomach. The LT is inserted and the cuffs inflated. Should ventilation prove difficult, the LT is likely inserted too deep. Slightly withdrawing the device until compliance improves ameliorates the situation.

ENDOTRACHEAL INTUBATION

Endotracheal intubation is employed both for the conduct of general anesthesia and to facilitate the ventilator management of the critically ill.

Tracheal Tubes

Standards govern TT manufacturing (American National Standard for Anesthetic Equipment; ANSI Z–79). TTs are most commonly made from polyvinyl chloride. In the past, TTs were marked "I.T." or

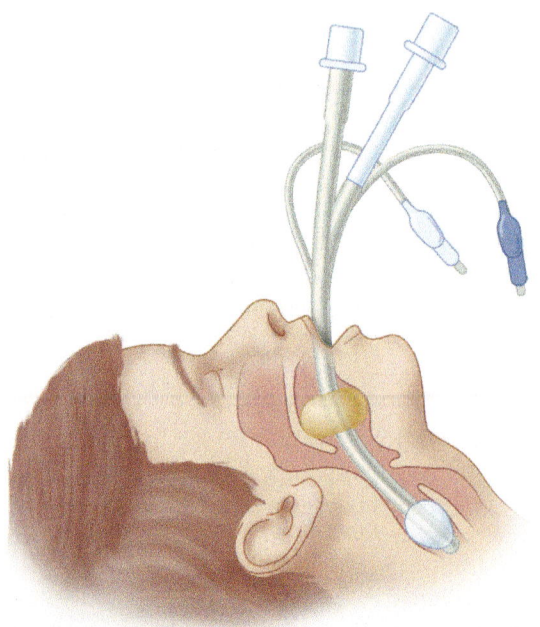

FIGURE 19–12 Combitube.

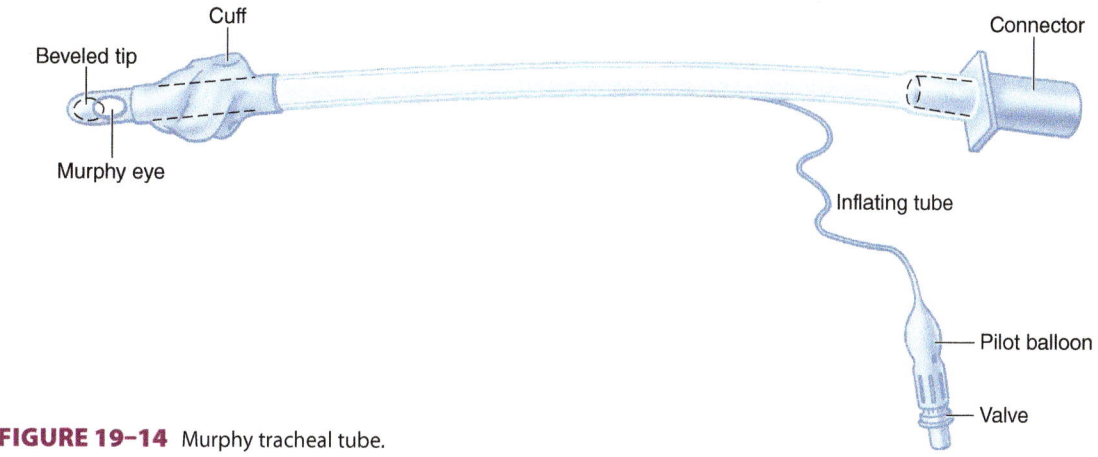

FIGURE 19–14 Murphy tracheal tube.

"Z–79" to indicate that they had been implant tested to ensure nontoxicity. The shape and rigidity of TTs can be altered by inserting a stylet. The patient end of the tube is beveled to aid visualization and insertion through the vocal cords. Murphy tubes have a hole (the Murphy eye) to decrease the risk of occlusion, should the distal tube opening abut the carina or trachea (Figure 19–14).

Resistance to airflow depends primarily on tube diameter, but is also affected by tube length and curvature. TT size is usually designated in millimeters of internal diameter, or, less commonly, in the French scale (external diameter in millimeters multiplied by 3). The choice of tube diameter is always a compromise between maximizing flow with a larger size and minimizing airway trauma with a smaller size (Table 19–5).

Most adult TTs have a cuff inflation system consisting of a valve, pilot balloon, inflating tube, and cuff (Figure 19–14). The valve prevents air loss after cuff inflation. The pilot balloon provides a gross indication of cuff inflation. The inflating tube connects the valve to the cuff and is incorporated into the tube's wall. By creating a tracheal seal, TT cuffs permit positive-pressure ventilation and reduce the likelihood of aspiration. Uncuffed tubes are often used in infants and young children to minimize the risk of pressure injury and postintubation croup; however, in recent years, cuffed pediatric tubes have been increasingly favored.

There are two major types of cuffs: high pressure (low volume) and low pressure (high volume). High-pressure cuffs are associated with more ischemic damage to the tracheal mucosa and are less suitable for intubations of long duration. Low-pressure cuffs may increase the likelihood of sore throat (larger mucosal contact area), aspiration, spontaneous extubation, and difficult insertion (because of the floppy cuff). Nonetheless, because of their lower incidence of mucosal damage, low-pressure cuffs are generally employed.

Cuff pressure depends on several factors: inflation volume, the diameter of the cuff in relation to the trachea, tracheal and cuff compliance, and intrathoracic pressure (cuff pressures increase with coughing). Cuff pressure may increase during general anesthesia from diffusion of nitrous oxide from the tracheal mucosa into the TT cuff.

TTs have been modified for a variety of specialized applications. Flexible, spiral-wound, wire-reinforced TTs (armored tubes) resist kinking and

TABLE 19–5 Oral tracheal tube size guidelines.

Age	Internal Diameter (mm)	Cut Length (cm)
Full-term infant	3.5	12
Child	$4 + \dfrac{Age}{4}$	$14 + \dfrac{Age}{2}$
Adult		
Female	7.0–7.5	24
Male	7.5–9.0	24

may prove valuable in some head and neck surgical procedures or in the prone patient. If an armored tube becomes kinked from extreme pressure (eg, an awake patient biting it), however, the lumen will often remain permanently occluded, and the tube will need replacement. Other specialized tubes include microlaryngeal tubes, double-lumen endotracheal tubes (to facilitate lung isolation and one-lung ventilation), endotracheal tubes equipped with bronchial blockers (to facilitate lung isolation and one-lung ventilation), metal tubes designed for laser airway surgery to reduce fire hazards, and preformed curved tubes for nasal and oral intubation in head and neck surgery.

LARYGOSCOPES

A laryngoscope is an instrument used to examine the larynx and to facilitate intubation of the trachea. The handle usually contains batteries to light a bulb on the blade tip (Figure 19–15), or, alternately, to power a fiberoptic bundle that terminates at the tip of the blade. Light from a fiberoptic bundle tends to be more precisely directed and less diffuse. Also, laryngoscopes with fiberoptic light bundles in their blades can be made magnetic resonance imaging compatible. The Macintosh and Miller blades are the most popular curved and straight designs, respectively, in

the United States. The choice of blade depends on personal preference and patient anatomy. Because no blade is perfect for all situations, the clinician should become familiar and proficient with a variety of blade designs (Figure 19–16).

VIDEO LARYNGOSCOPES

In recent years, a myriad of laryngoscopy devices that utilize video technology have revolutionized management of the airway. Direct laryngoscopy with a Macintosh or Miller blade mandates appropriate alignment of the oral, pharyngeal, and laryngeal structures to facilitate a direct view of the glottis. Various maneuvers, such as the "sniffing" position and external movement of the larynx with cricoid pressure during direct laryngoscopy, are used to improve the view. Video- or optically-based laryngoscopes have either a video chip (DCI system, GlideScope, McGrath, Airway) or a lens/mirror (Airtraq) at the tip of the intubation blade to transmit a view of the glottis to the operator. These devices differ in the angulation of the blade, the presence of a channel to guide the tube to the glottis, and the single use or multiuse nature of the device.

Video or indirect laryngoscopy most likely offers minimal advantage in patients with uncomplicated airways. However, use in these patients is valuable as a training guide for learners, especially when the trainee is performing a direct laryngoscopy with the device while the instructor views the glottis on the video screen. Additionally, use in uncomplicated airway management patients improves familiarity with the device for times when direct laryngoscopy is not possible.

Indirect laryngoscopes generally improve visualization of laryngeal structures in difficult airways; however, visualization does not always lead to successful intubation. An endotracheal tube stylet is recommended when video laryngoscopy is to be performed. Some devices come with stylets designed to facilitate intubation with that particular device. Bending the stylet and endotracheal tube in a manner similar to the bend in the curve of the blade often facilitates passage of the endotracheal tube into the trachea. Even when the glottic opening is seen clearly, directing the endotracheal tube into

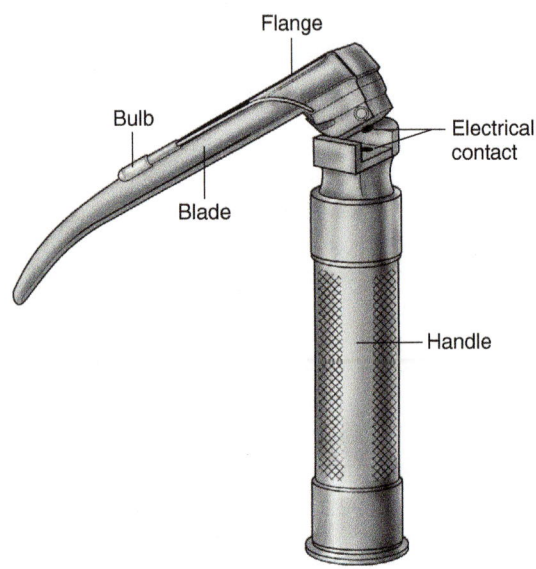

FIGURE 19–15 A rigid laryngoscope.

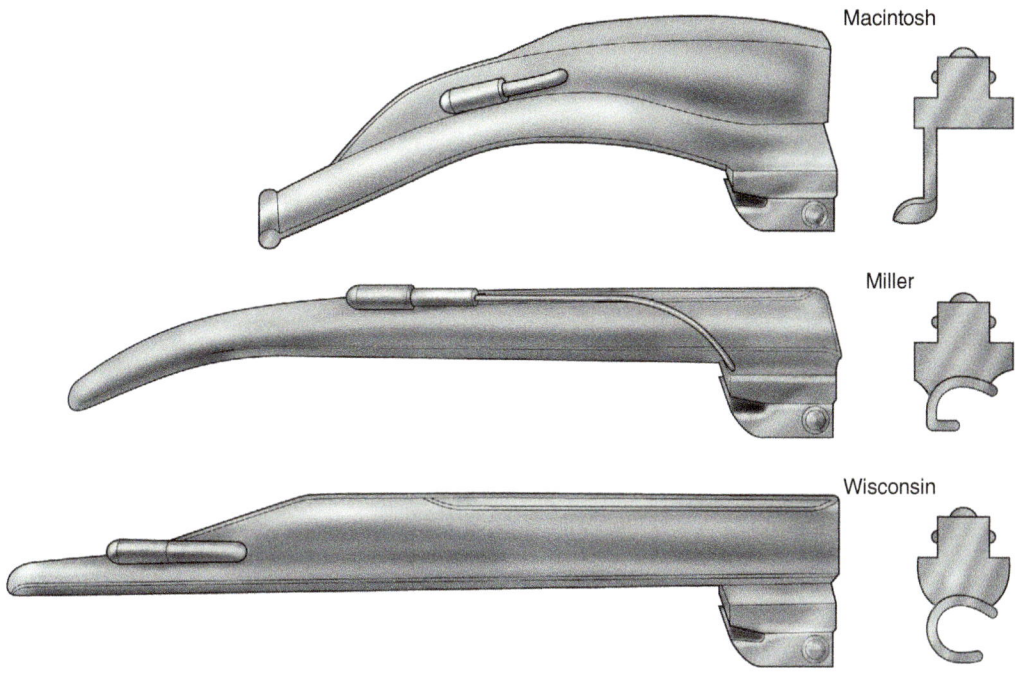

Macintosh

Miller

Wisconsin

FIGURE 19–16 An assortment of laryngoscope blades.

the trachea can be difficult. Should the tube become caught on the arytenoids, slightly pulling the blade farther out may better permit tube passage.

Indirect laryngoscopy may result in less displacement of the cervical spine; however, all precautions associated with airway manipulation in a patient with a possible cervical spine fracture should be maintained.

Varieties of indirect laryngoscopes include:

- Various Macintosh and Miller blades in pediatric and adult sizes have video capability in the Storz DCI system. The system can also incorporate an optical intubating stylet (Figure 19–17). The blades are similar to conventional intubation blades, permitting direct laryngoscopy and indirect video laryngoscopy. Assistants and instructors are able to see the view obtained by the operator and adjust their maneuvers accordingly to facilitate intubation or to provide instruction, respectively.

- The McGrath laryngoscope is a portable video laryngoscope with a blade length that can be adjusted to facilitate a child of age 5 years up to an adult (Figure 19–18). The blade can be disconnected from the handle to facilitate its insertion in morbidly obese patients in whom the space between the upper chest and head is reduced. The blade is inserted midline, with the laryngeal structures viewed at a distance to enhance intubation success.

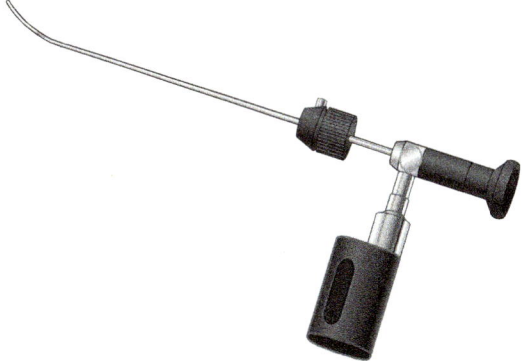

FIGURE 19–17 Optical intubating stylet.

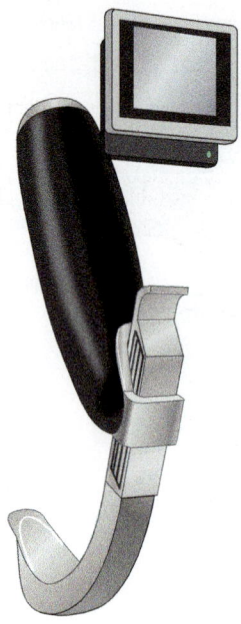

FIGURE 19–18 McGrath laryngoscope.

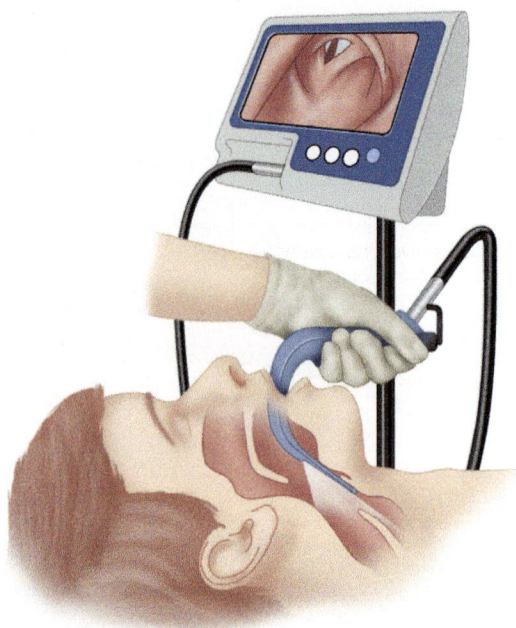

FIGURE 19–19 Glidescope.

- The GlideScope comes with disposable adult- and pediatric-sized blades (Figure 19–19). The blade is inserted midline and advanced until glottic structures are identified. The GlideScope has a 60° angle, preventing direct laryngoscopy and necessitating the use of stylet that is similar in shape to the blade.

- Airtraq is a single-use optical laryngoscope available in pediatric and adult sizes (Figure 19–20). The device has a channel to guide the endotracheal tube to the glottis. This device is inserted midline. Success is more likely when the device is not positioned too close to the glottis.

- Video intubating stylets have a video capability and light source. The stylet is introduced, and the glottis identified. Intubation with a video stylet may result in less cervical spine movement than with other techniques.

Flexible Fiberoptic Bronchoscopes

In some situations—for example, patients with unstable cervical spines, poor range of motion of the temporomandibular joint, or certain congenital or acquired upper airway anomalies—laryngoscopy with direct or indirect laryngoscopes may be undesirable or impossible. A flexible FOB allows indirect visualization of the larynx in such cases or in any situation in which awake intubation is planned (Figure 19–21). Bronchoscopes are constructed of coated glass fibers that transmit light and images by internal reflection (ie, a light beam becomes trapped

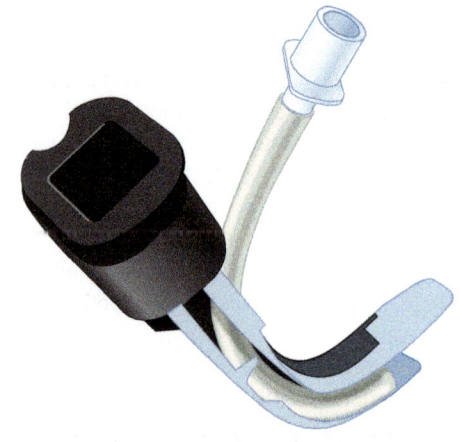

FIGURE 19–20 Airtraq optical laryngoscope.

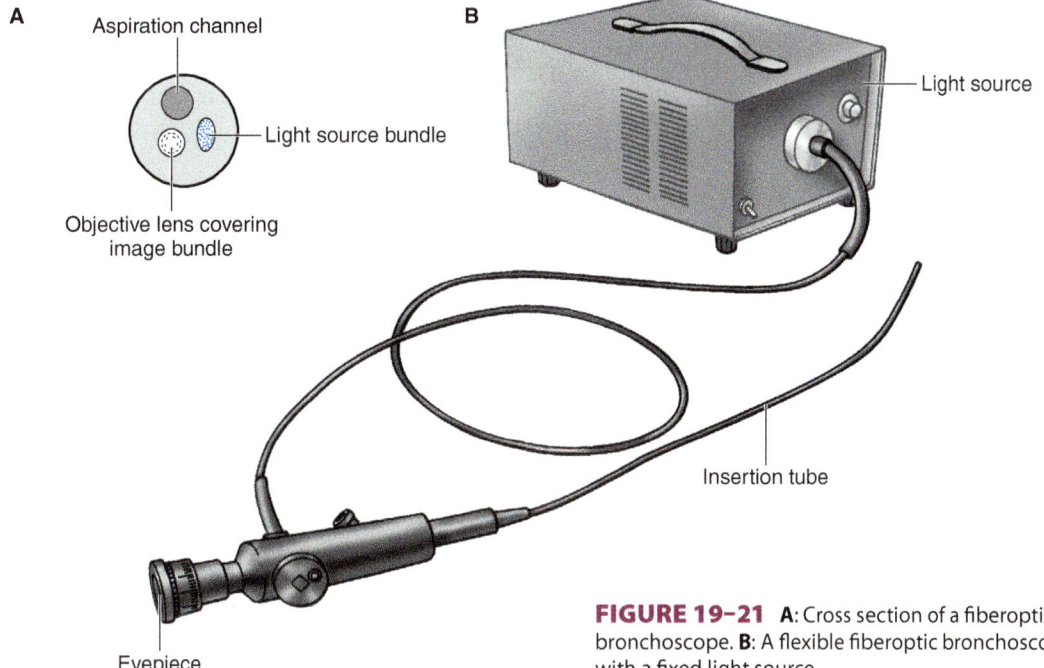

A   Aspiration channel

Light source bundle

Objective lens covering image bundle

B

Light source

Insertion tube

Eyepiece

FIGURE 19–21 **A**: Cross section of a fiberoptic bronchoscope. **B**: A flexible fiberoptic bronchoscope with a fixed light source.

within a fiber and exits unchanged at the opposite end). The insertion tube contains two bundles of fibers, each consisting of 10,000 to 15,000 fibers. One bundle transmits light from the light source (light source or incoherent bundle), which is either external to the device or contained within the handle (Figure 19–21B), whereas the other provides a high-resolution image (image or coherent bundle). Directional manipulation of the insertion tube is accomplished with angulation wires. Aspiration channels allow suctioning of secretions, insufflation of oxygen, or instillation of local anesthetic. Aspiration channels can be difficult to clean, and, if not properly cleaned and sterilized after each use, may provide a nidus for infection.

TECHNIQUES OF DIRECT AND INDIRECT LARYNGOSCOPY & INTUBATION

Indications for Intubation

Inserting a tube into the trachea has become a routine part of delivering a general anesthetic. Intubation is

not a risk-free procedure, and not all patients receiving general anesthesia require it. A TT is generally placed to protect the airway and for airway access. Intubation is indicated in patients who are at risk of aspiration and in those undergoing surgical procedures involving body cavities or the head and neck. Mask ventilation or ventilation with an LMA is usually satisfactory for short minor procedures such as cystoscopy, examination under anesthesia, inguinal hernia repairs, extremity surgery, and so forth.

Preparation for Direct Laryngoscopy

Preparation for intubation includes checking equipment and properly positioning the patient. The TT should be examined. The tube's cuff inflation system can be tested by inflating the cuff using a 10-mL syringe. Maintenance of cuff pressure *after detaching the syringe* ensures proper cuff and valve function. Some anesthesiologists cut the TT to a preset length to decrease the dead space, the risk of bronchial intubation, and the risk of occlusion from tube kinking (Table 19–5). The connector should be pushed firmly into the tube to decrease the likelihood of disconnection. If a stylet is used, it should be inserted

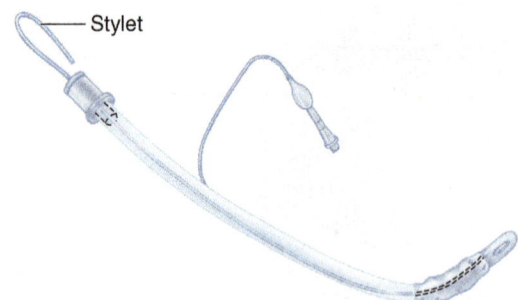

FIGURE 19–22 A tracheal tube with a stylet bent to resemble a hockey stick.

into the TT, which is then bent to resemble a hockey stick (**Figure 19–22**). This shape facilitates intubation of an anteriorly positioned larynx. The desired blade is locked onto the laryngoscope handle, and bulb function is tested. The light intensity should remain constant even if the bulb is jiggled. A blinking light signals a poor electrical contact, whereas

fading indicates depleted batteries. An extra handle, blade, TT (one size smaller than the anticipated optimal size), and stylet should be immediately available. A functioning suction unit is needed to clear the airway in case of unexpected secretions, blood, or emesis.

Successful intubation often depends on correct patient positioning. The patient's head should be level with the anesthesiologist's waist or higher to prevent unnecessary back strain during laryngoscopy.

Direct laryngoscopy displaces pharyngeal soft tissues to create a direct line of vision from the mouth to the glottic opening. Moderate head elevation (5–10 cm above the surgical table) and extension of the atlantooccipital joint place the patient in the desired sniffing position (**Figure 19–23**). The lower portion of the cervical spine is flexed by resting the head on a pillow or other soft support.

Preparation for induction and intubation also involves routine preoxygenation. Administration of 100% oxygen provides an extra margin of safety in

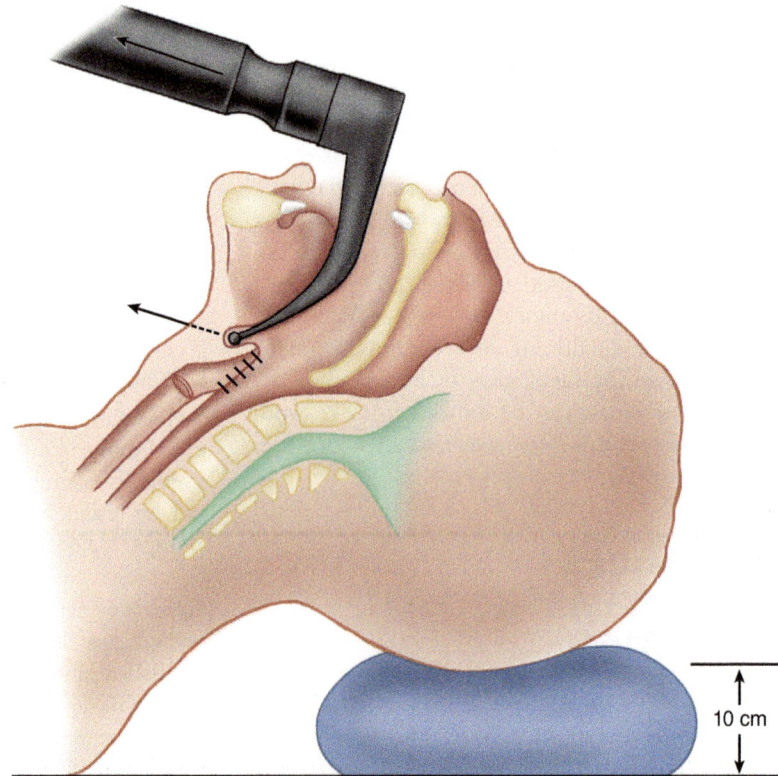

FIGURE 19–23 The sniffing position and intubation with a Macintosh blade. (Modified and reproduced, with permission, from Dorsch JA, Dorsch SE: *Understanding Anesthesia Equipment: Construction, Care, and Complications.* Williams & Wilkins, 1991.)

10 cm

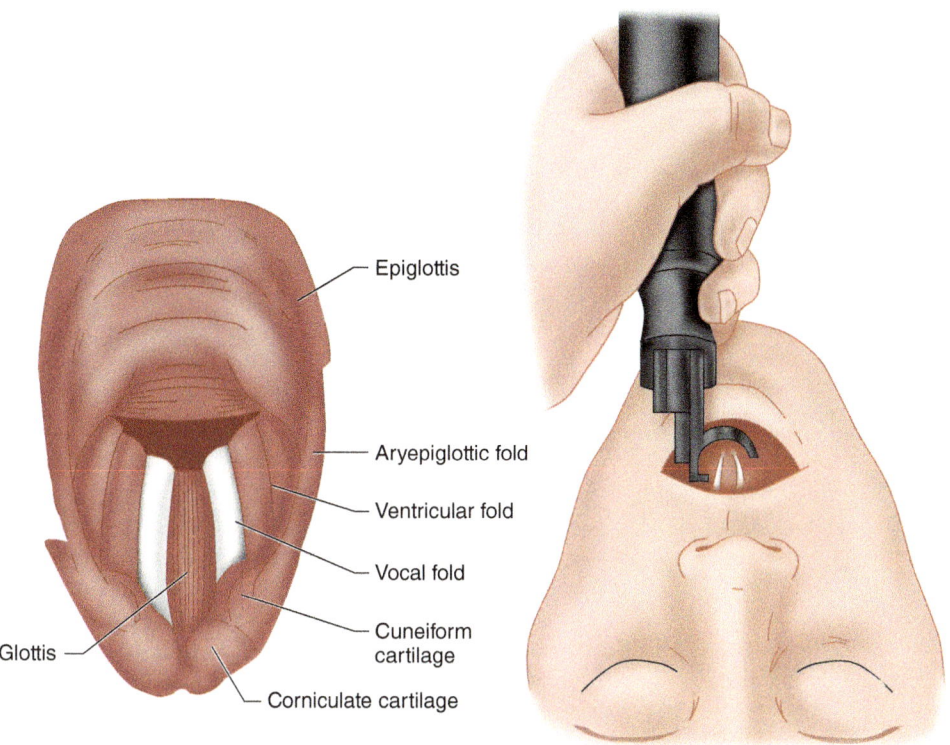

Epiglottis

Aryepiglottic fold

Ventricular fold

Vocal fold

Cuneiform cartilage

Corniculate cartilage

Glottis

FIGURE 19–24 Typical view of the glottis during laryngoscopy with a curved blade. (Modified and reproduced, with permission, from Barash PG: *Clinical Anesthesia*, 4th ed. Lippincott, 2001.)

case the patient is not easily ventilated after induction. Preoxygenation can be omitted in patients who object to the face mask; however, failing to preoxygenate increases the risk of rapid desaturation following apnea.

Because general anesthesia abolishes the protective corneal reflex, care must be taken during this period not to injure the patient's eyes by unintentionally abrading the cornea. Thus, the eyes are routinely taped shut, often after applying an ophthalmic ointment before manipulation of the airway.

Orotracheal Intubation

The laryngoscope is held in the left hand. With the patient's mouth opened the blade is introduced into the right side of the oropharynx—with care to avoid the teeth. The tongue is swept to the left and up into the floor of the pharynx by the blade's flange. Successful sweeping of the tongue leftward

clears the view for TT placement. The tip of a curved blade is usually inserted into the vallecula, and the straight blade tip covers the epiglottis. With either blade, the handle is raised up and away from the patient in a plane perpendicular to the patient's mandible to expose the vocal cords (Figure 19–24). Trapping a lip between the teeth and the blade and leverage on the teeth are avoided. The TT is taken with the right hand, and its tip is passed through the abducted vocal cords. The "backward, upward, rightward, pressure" (BURP) maneuver applied externally moves an anteriorly positioned glottis posterior to facilitate visualization of the glottis. The TT cuff should lie in the upper trachea, but beyond the larynx. The laryngoscope is withdrawn, again with care to avoid tooth damage. The cuff is inflated with the least amount of air necessary to create a seal during positive-pressure ventilation to minimize the

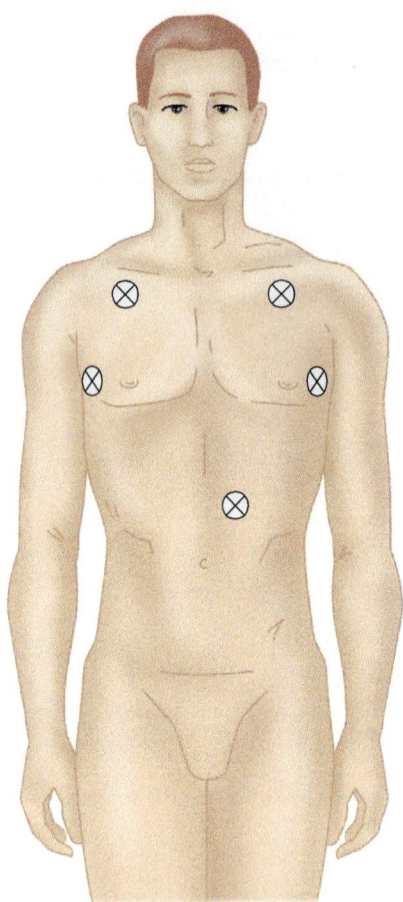

FIGURE 19–25 Sites for auscultation of breath sounds at the apices and over the stomach.

visualization of the tracheal rings and carina will likewise confirm correct placement. Otherwise, the tube is taped or tied to secure its position. **4** Although the persistent detection of CO_2 by a capnograph is the best confirmation of tracheal placement of a TT, it cannot exclude bronchial intubation. The earliest evidence of bronchial intubation often is an increase in peak inspiratory pressure. Proper tube location can be reconfirmed by palpating the cuff in the sternal notch while compressing the pilot balloon with the other hand. **5** The cuff should not be felt above the level of the cricoid cartilage, because a prolonged intralaryngeal location may result in postoperative hoarseness and increases the risk of accidental extubation. Tube position can also be documented by chest radiography.

The description presented here assumes an unconscious patient. Oral intubation is usually poorly tolerated by awake, fit patients. Intravenous sedation, application of a local anesthetic spray in the oropharynx, regional nerve block, and constant reassurance will improve patient acceptance.

A failed intubation should not be followed by identical repeated attempts. Changes must be made to increase the likelihood of success, such as repositioning the patient, decreasing the tube size, adding a stylet, selecting a different blade, using an indirect laryngoscope, attempting a nasal route, or requesting the assistance of another anesthesiologist. If the patient is also difficult to ventilate with a mask, alternative forms of airway management (eg, LMA, Combitube, cricothyrotomy with jet ventilation, tracheostomy) must be immediately pursued. The guidelines developed by the American Society of Anesthesiologists for the management of a difficult airway include a treatment plan algorithm (**Figure 19–26**).

Use of video or indirect laryngoscopes is dependent upon the design of the device. Some devices are placed midline without the requirement to sweep the tongue from view. Other devices contain channels to direct the endotracheal tube to the glottic opening. Practitioners should be familiar with the features of available devices well in advance of using one in a difficult airway situation. The combined use of a video laryngoscope and an intubation

pressure transmitted to the tracheal mucosa. Overinflation beyond 30 mm Hg may inhibit capillary blood flow, injuring the trachea. Compressing the pilot balloon with the fingers is *not* a reliable method of determining whether cuff pressure is either sufficient or excessive.

After intubation, the chest and epigastrium are immediately auscultated, and a capnographic tracing (the definitive test) is monitored to ensure intratracheal location (**Figure 19–25**). If there is doubt as to whether the tube is in the esophagus or trachea, repeat the laryngoscopy to confirm placement. End-tidal CO_2 will not be produced if there is no cardiac output. FOB through the tube and

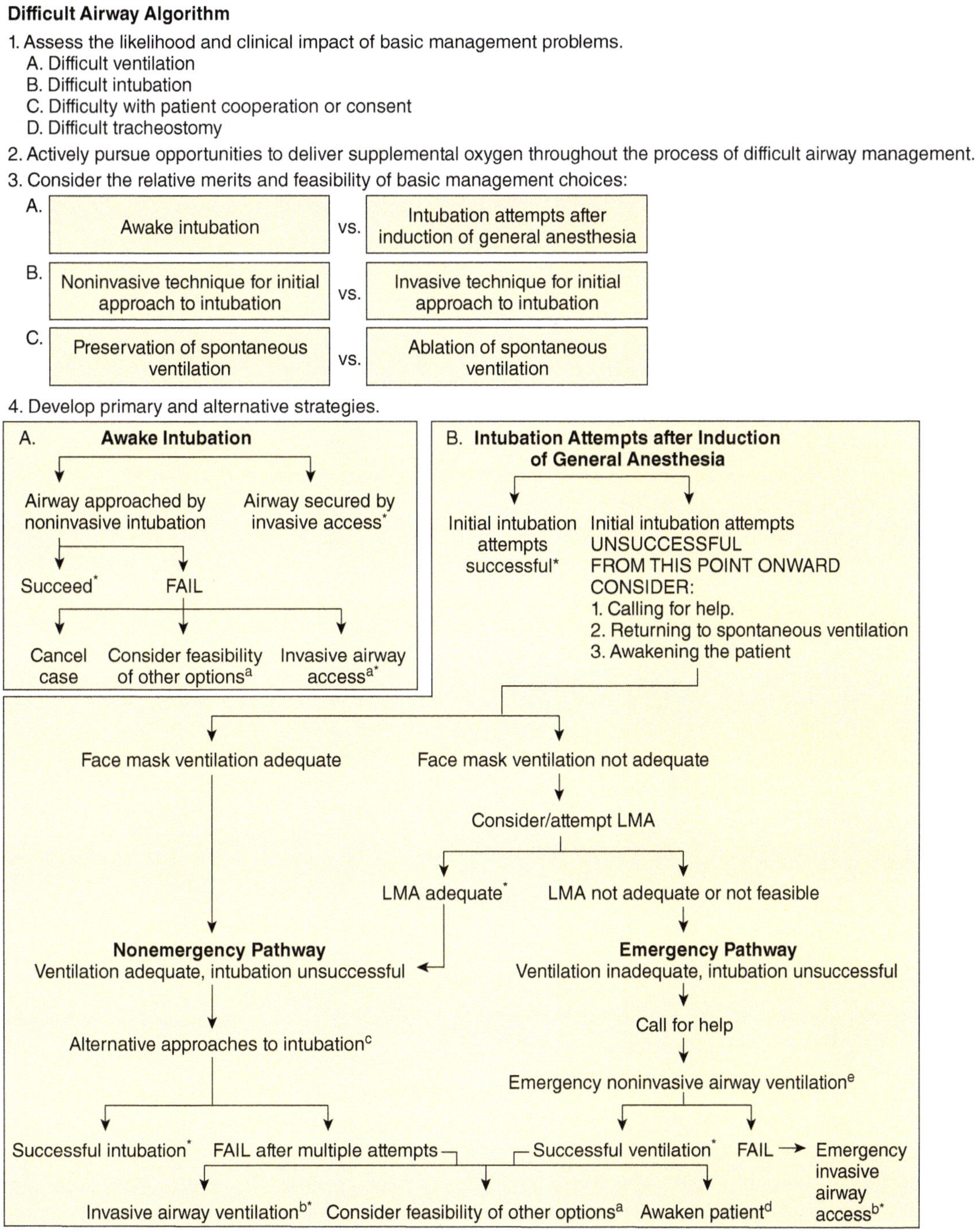

Difficult Airway Algorithm
1. Assess the likelihood and clinical impact of basic management problems.
A. Difficult ventilation
B. Difficult intubation
C. Difficulty with patient cooperation or consent
D. Difficult tracheostomy
2. Actively pursue opportunities to deliver supplemental oxygen throughout the process of difficult airway management.
3. Consider the relative merits and feasibility of basic management choices:
A.
Awake intubation
vs.
Intubation attempts after induction of general anesthesia
B.
Noninvasive technique for initial approach to intubation
vs.
Invasive technique for initial approach to intubation
C.
Preservation of spontaneous ventilation
vs.
Ablation of spontaneous ventilation
4. Develop primary and alternative strategies.
A. Awake Intubation
Airway approached by noninvasive intubation
Airway secured by invasive access*
Succeed*
FAIL
Cancel case
Consider feasibility of other options[a]
Invasive airway access[a]*
B. Intubation Attempts after Induction of General Anesthesia
Initial intubation attempts successful*
Initial intubation attempts UNSUCCESSFUL
FROM THIS POINT ONWARD CONSIDER:
1. Calling for help.
2. Returning to spontaneous ventilation
3. Awakening the patient
Face mask ventilation adequate
Face mask ventilation not adequate
Consider/attempt LMA
LMA adequate*
LMA not adequate or not feasible
Nonemergency Pathway
Ventilation adequate, intubation unsuccessful
Emergency Pathway
Ventilation inadequate, intubation unsuccessful
Call for help
Alternative approaches to intubation[c]
Emergency noninvasive airway ventilation[e]
Successful intubation*
FAIL after multiple attempts
Successful ventilation*
FAIL
Emergency invasive airway access[b]*
Invasive airway ventilation[b]*
Consider feasibility of other options[a]
Awaken patient[d]

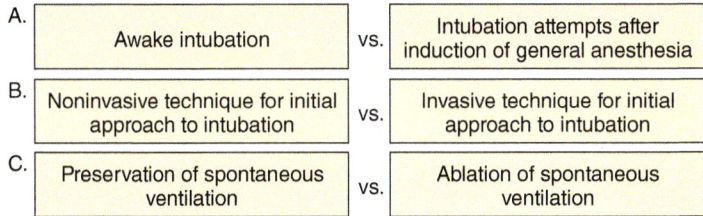

FIGURE 19–26 Difficult Airway Algorithm developed by the American Society of Anesthesiologists. *Confirm tracheal intubation or LMA placement with exhaled CO_2. (Reproduced, with permission, from the American Society of Anesthesiologists Task Force on Management of the Difficult Airway. Practice guidelines for management of the difficult airway: an updated report by the American Society of Anesthesiologists Task Force on Management of the Difficult Airway. Anesthesiology 2003;98:1269.)

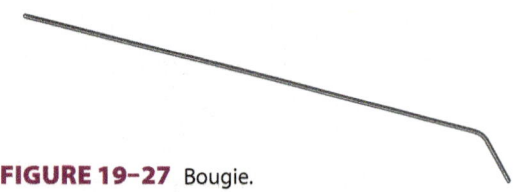

FIGURE 19–27 Bougie.

bougie often can facilitate intubation, when the endotracheal tube cannot be directed into the glottis despite good visualization of the laryngeal opening (Figure 19–27).

Nasotracheal Intubation

Nasal intubation is similar to oral intubation except that the TT is advanced through the nose and nasopharynx into the oropharynx before laryngoscopy. The nostril through which the patient breathes most easily is selected in advance and prepared. Phenylephrine nose drops (0.5% or 0.25%) vasoconstrict vessels and shrink mucous membranes. If the patient is awake, local anesthetic ointment (for the nostril), spray (for the oropharynx), and nerve blocks can also be utilized.

A TT lubricated with water-soluble jelly is introduced along the floor of the nose, below the inferior turbinate, *at an angle perpendicular to the face*. The tube's bevel should be directed laterally away from the turbinates. To ensure that the tube passes along the floor of the nasal cavity, the proximal end of the TT should be pulled cephalad. The tube is gradually advanced, until its tip can be visualized in the oropharynx. Laryngoscopy, as discussed, reveals the abducted vocal cords. Often the distal end of the TT can be pushed into the trachea without difficulty. If difficulty is encountered, the tip of the tube may be directed through the vocal cords with Magill forceps, being careful not to damage the cuff. Nasal passage of TTs, airways, or nasogastric catheters carries greater risk in patients with severe mid-facial trauma because of the risk of intracranial placement (Figure 19–28).

Although less used today, blind nasal intubation of spontaneously breathing patients can be employed. In this technique, after applying topical anesthetic to the nostril and pharynx, a breathing tube is passed through the nasopharynx. Using

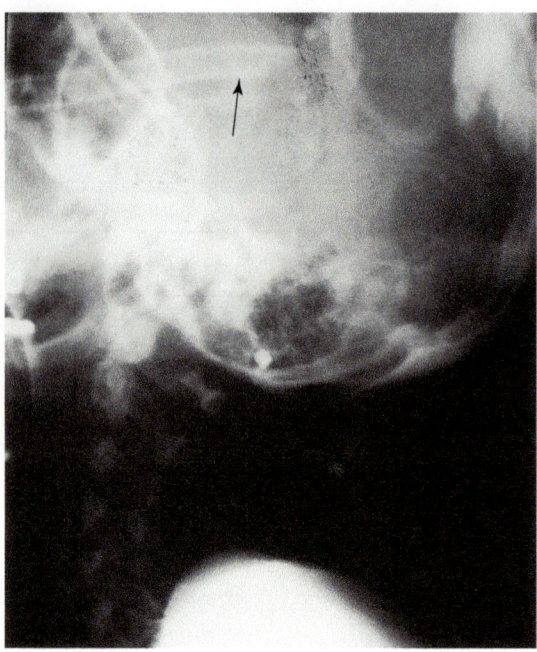

FIGURE 19–28 Radiograph demonstrating a 7.0-mm tracheal tube placed through the cribriform plate into the cranial vault in a patient with a basilar skull fracture.

breath sounds as a guide, it is directed toward the glottis. When breath sounds are maximal, the anesthetist advances the tube during inspiration in an effort to blindly pass the tube into the trachea.

Flexible Fiberoptic Intubation

Fiberoptic intubation (FOI) is routinely performed in awake or sedated patients with problematic airways. FOI is ideal for:

- A small mouth opening

- Minimizing cervical spine movement in trauma or rheumatoid arthritis

- Upper airway obstruction, such as angioedema or tumor mass

- Facial deformities, facial trauma

FOI can be performed awake or asleep via oral or nasal routes.

- Awake FOI: predicted inability to ventilate by mask, upper airway obstruction

- Asleep FOI: Failed intubation, desire for minimal C spine movement in patients who refuse awake intubation
- Oral FOI: Facial, skull injuries
- Nasal FOI: A poor mouth opening

When FOI is considered, careful planning is necessary, as it will likely add to the anesthesia time prior to surgery. Patients should be informed of the need for awake intubation as a part of the informed consent process.

The airway is anesthetized with a local anesthetic spray, and patient sedation is provided, as tolerated. Dexmedetomidine has the advantage of preserving respiration while providing sedation. Airway anesthesia is discussed in the Case Discussion below.

If nasal FOI is planned, both nostrils are prepared with vasoconstrictive drops. The nostril through which the patient breathes more easily is identified. Oxygen can be insufflated through the suction port and down the aspiration channel of the FOB to improve oxygenation and blow secretions away from the tip.

Alternatively, a large nasal airway (eg, 36F) can be inserted in the contralateral nostril. The breathing circuit can be directly connected to the end of this nasal airway to administer 100% oxygen during laryngoscopy. If the patient is unconscious and not breathing spontaneously, the mouth can be closed and ventilation attempted through the single nasal airway. When this technique is used, adequacy of ventilation and oxygenation should be confirmed by capnography and pulse oximetry. The lubricated shaft of the FOB is introduced into the TT lumen. It is important to keep the shaft of the broncho-scope relatively straight (Figure 19–29) so that if the head of the bronchoscope is rotated in one direction, the distal end will move to a similar degree and in the same direction. As the tip of the FOB passes through the distal end of the TT, the epiglottis or glottis should be visible. The tip of the bronchoscope is manipulated, as needed, to pass the abducted cords.

Having an assistant thrust the jaw forward or apply cricoid pressure may improve visualization in difficult cases. If the patient is breathing

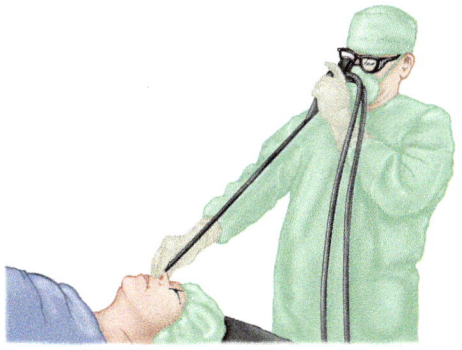

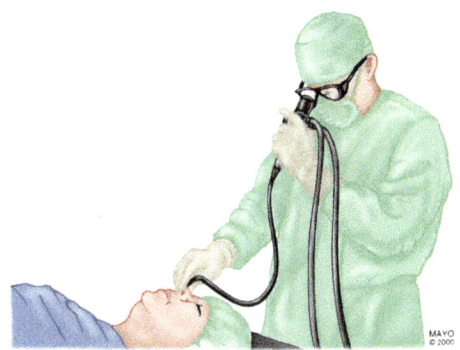

FIGURE 19–29 Correct technique for manipulating a fiberoptic bronchoscope through a tracheal tube is shown in the top panel; avoid curvature in the bronchoscope, which makes manipulation difficult.

spontaneously, grasping the tongue with gauze and pulling it forward may also facilitate intubation.

Once in the trachea, the FOB is advanced to within sight of the carina. The presence of tracheal rings and the carina is proof of proper positioning. The TT is pushed off the FOB. The acute angle around the arytenoid cartilage and epiglottis may prevent easy advancement of the tube. Use of an armored tube usually decreases this problem due to its greater lateral flexibility and more obtusely angled distal end. Proper TT position is confirmed by viewing the tip of the tube an appropriate distance (3 cm in adults) above the carina before the FOB is withdrawn.

Oral FOI proceeds similarly, with the aid of various oral airway devices to direct the FOB toward the glottis and to reduce obstruction of the view by the tongue.

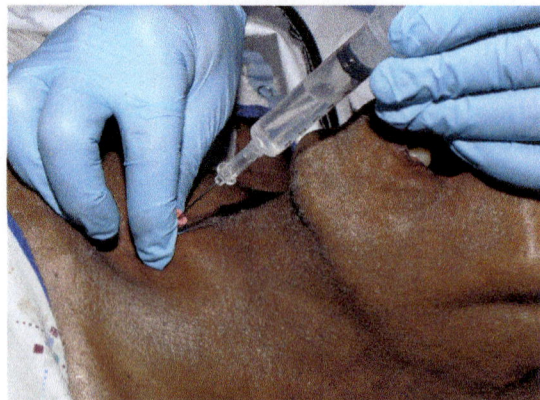

FIGURE 19–30 Cricothyrotomy. Slide catheter into trachea. (Photo contributor: Lawrence B. Stack, MD.)

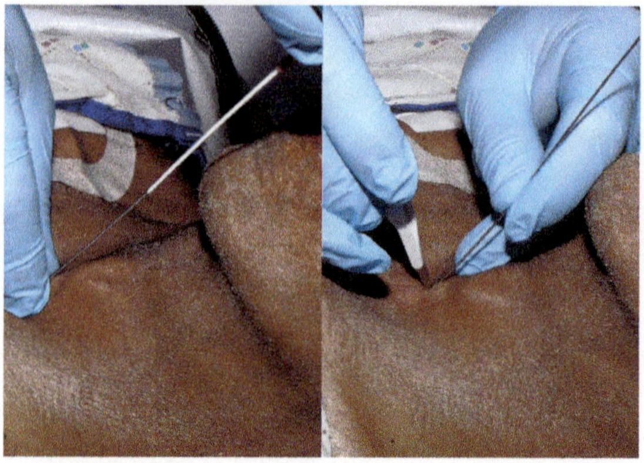

FIGURE 19–31 Cricothyrotomy. Incision at wire entry site. Remove catheter and make incision at the wire entry site. (Photo contributor: Lawrence B. Stack, MD.)

SURGICAL AIRWAY TECHNIQUES

"Invasive" airways are required when the "can't intubate, can't ventilate" scenario presents and may be performed in anticipation of such circumstances in selected patients. The options include: surgical cricothyrotomy, catheter or needle cricothyrotomy, transtracheal catheter with jet ventilation, and retrograde intubation.

Surgical cricothyrotomy refers to surgical incision of the CTM and placement of a breathing tube. More recently, several needle/dilator cricothyrotomy kits have become available. Unlike surgical cricothyrotomy, where a horizontal incision is made across the CTM, these kits utilize the Seldinger catheter/wire/dilator technique. A catheter attached to a syringe is inserted across the CTM (**Figure 19–30**). When air is aspirated, a guidewire is passed through the catheter into the trachea (**Figure 19–31**). A dilator is then passed over the guidewire, and a breathing tube placed (**Figure 19–32**).

Catheter-based salvage procedures can also be performed. A 16- or 14-gauge intravenous cannula is attached to a syringe and passed through the CTM toward the carina. Air is aspirated. If a jet ventilation system is available, it can be attached. The catheter MUST be secured, otherwise the jet pressure will push the catheter out of the airway, leading to potentially disastrous subcutaneous emphysema. Short (1 s) bursts of oxygen ventilate the patient. Sufficient outflow of expired air must be assured to avoid barotrauma. Patients ventilated in this manner may develop subcutaneous or mediastinal emphysema and may become hypercapneic despite adequate oxygenation. Transtracheal jet ventilation will usually require conversion to a surgical airway or tracheal intubation.

Should a jet ventilation system not be available, a 3-mL syringe can be attached to the catheter and the syringe plunger removed. A 7.0-mm internal

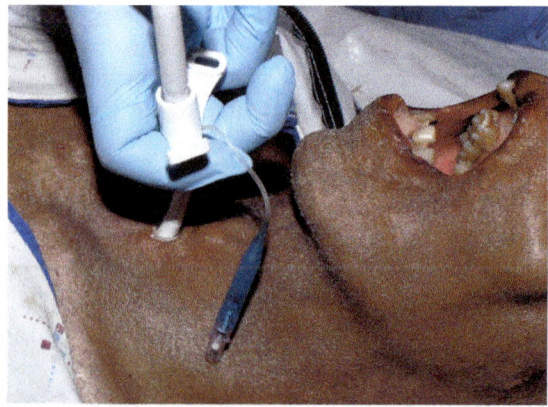

FIGURE 19–32 Cricothyrotomy. Insert tracheostomy tube/introducer. Insert both devices over the wire and into the trachea. (Photo contributor: Lawrence B. Stack, MD.)

diameter TT connector can be inserted into the syringe and attached to a breathing circuit or an ambu bag. As with the jet ventilation system, adequate exhalation must occur to avoid barotraumas.

Retrograde intubation is another approach to secure an airway. A wire is passed via a catheter placed in the CTM. The wire is angulated cephalad and emerges either through the mouth or nose. The distal end of the wire is secured with a clamp to prevent it from passing through the CTM. The wire can then be threaded into an FOB with a loaded endotracheal tube to facilitate and confirm placement. Conversely, a small endotracheal tube can be guided by the wire into the trachea. Once placed, the wire is removed. Alternatively, an epidural catheter can be placed via an epidural needle in the CTM. After the distal end is retrieved from the mouth, an endotracheal tube may be passed over the catheter into the trachea.

PROBLEMS FOLLOWING INTUBATION

Following apparently successful intubation, several scenarios may develop that require immediate attention. Anesthesia staff MUST confirm that the tube is correctly placed with bilateral ventilation immediately following placement. Detection of end-tidal CO_2 remains the gold standard in this regard, with the caveat that cardiac output must be present for end-tidal CO_2 production.

Decreases in oxygen saturation can occur following tube placement. This is often secondary to endobronchial intubation, especially in small children and babies. Decreased oxygen saturation perioperatively may be due to inadequate oxygen delivery (oxygen not turned on, patient not ventilated) or to ventilation/perfusion mismatch (almost any form of lung disease). When saturation declines, the patient's chest is auscultated to confirm bilateral tube placement and to listen for wheezes, rhonchi, and rales consistent with lung pathology. The breathing circuit is checked. An intraoperative chest radiograph may be needed to identify the cause of desaturation. Intraoperative fiberoptic bronchoscopy can also be performed and used to confirm proper tube placement and to clear mucous plugs. Bronchodilators and deeper planes of inhalation anesthetics are

administered to treat bronchospasm. Obese patients may desaturate secondary to a reduced FRC and atelectasis. Application of positive end-expiratory pressure may improve oxygenation.

Should the end-tidal CO_2 decline suddenly, pulmonary (thrombus) or venous air embolism should be considered. Likewise, other causes of a sudden decline in cardiac output or a leak in the circuit should be considered.

A rising end-tidal CO_2 may be secondary to hypoventilation or increased CO_2 production, as occurs with malignant hyperthermia, sepsis, a depleted CO_2 absorber, or breathing circuit malfunction.

Increases in airway pressure may indicate an obstructed or kinked endotracheal tube or reduced pulmonary compliance. The endotracheal tube should be suctioned to confirm that it is patent and the lungs auscultated to detect signs of bronchospasm, pulmonary edema, endobronchial intubation, or pneumothorax.

Decreases in airway pressure can occur secondary to leaks in the breathing circuit or inadvertent extubation.

TECHNIQUES OF EXTUBATION

Most often, extubation should be performed when a patient is either deeply anesthetized or awake. In either case, adequate recovery from neuromuscular blocking agents should be established prior to extubation. If neuromuscular blocking agents are used, the patient has at least a period of controlled mechanical ventilation and likely must be weaned from the ventilator before extubation can occur.

Extubation during a light plane of anesthesia (ie, a state between deep and awake) is avoided because of an increased risk of laryngospasm. The distinction between deep and light anesthesia is usually apparent during pharyngeal suctioning: any reaction to suctioning (eg, breath holding, coughing) signals a light plane of anesthesia, whereas no reaction is characteristic of a deep plane. Similarly, eye opening or purposeful movements imply that the patient is sufficiently awake for extubation.

Extubating an awake patient is usually associated with coughing (bucking) on the TT. This reaction increases the heart rate, central venous pressure, arterial blood pressure, intracranial pressure, intraabdominal pressure, and intraocular pressure. It may also cause wound dehiscence and increased bleeding. The presence of a TT in an awake asthmatic patient may trigger bronchospasm. Some practitioners attempt to decrease the likelihood of these effects by administering 1.5 mg/kg of intravenous lidocaine 1–2 min before suctioning and extubation; however, extubation during deep anesthesia may be preferable in patients who cannot tolerate these effects (provided such patients are not at risk of aspiration and/or do not have airways that may be difficult to control after removal of the TT).

Regardless of whether the tube is removed when the patient is deeply anesthetized or awake, the patient's pharynx should be thoroughly suctioned before extubation to decrease the potential for aspiration of blood and secretions. In addition, patients should be ventilated with 100% oxygen in case it becomes difficult to establish an airway after the TT is removed. Just prior to extubation, the TT is untaped or untied and its cuff is deflated. The tube is withdrawn in a single smooth motion, and a face mask is applied to deliver oxygen. Oxygen delivery by face mask is maintained during the period of transportation to the postanesthesia care area.

COMPLICATIONS OF LARYNGOSCOPY & INTUBATION

The complications of laryngoscopy and intubation include hypoxia, hypercarbia, dental and airway trauma, tube malpositioning, physiological responses to airway instrumentation, or tube malfunction. These complications can occur during laryngoscopy and intubation, while the tube is in place, or following extubation (Table 19–6).

Airway Trauma

Instrumentation with a metal laryngoscope blade and insertion of a stiff TT often traumatizes delicate airway tissues. Tooth damage is a common cause of (relatively small) malpractice claims against anesthesiologists. Laryngoscopy and intubation can lead

TABLE 19–6 Complications of intubation.

During laryngoscopy and intubation
  Malpositioning
    Esophageal intubation
    Bronchial intubation
    Laryngeal cuff position
  Airway trauma
    Dental damage
    Lip, tongue, or mucosal laceration
    Sore throat
    Dislocated mandible
    Retropharyngeal dissection
  Physiological reflexes
    Hypoxia, hypercarbia
    Hypertension, tachycardia
    Intracranial hypertension
    Intraocular hypertension
    Laryngospasm
  Tube malfunction
    Cuff perforation
While the tube is in place
  Malpositioning
    Unintentional extubation
    Bronchial intubation
    Laryngeal cuff position
  Airway trauma
    Mucosal inflammation and ulceration
    Excoriation of nose
  Tube malfunction
    Fire/explosion
    Obstruction
Following extubation
  Airway trauma
    Edema and stenosis (glottic, subglottic, or tracheal)
    Hoarseness (vocal cord granuloma or paralysis)
    Laryngeal malfunction and aspiration
  Laryngospasm
  Negative-pressure pulmonary edema

to a range of complications from sore throat to tracheal stenosis. Most of these are due to prolonged external pressure on sensitive airway structures. When these pressures exceed the capillary–arteriolar blood pressure (approximately 30 mm Hg), tissue ischemia can lead to a sequence of inflammation, ulceration, granulation, and stenosis. Inflation of a TT cuff to the minimum pressure that creates a seal during routine positive-pressure ventilation (usually at least 20 mm Hg) reduces tracheal blood flow by 75% at the cuff site. Further cuff inflation or induced hypotension can totally eliminate mucosal blood flow.

Postintubation croup caused by glottic, laryngeal, or tracheal edema is particularly serious in children. The efficacy of corticosteroids (eg, dexamethasone—0.2 mg/kg, up to a maximum of 12 mg) in preventing postextubation airway edema remains controversial; however, corticosteroids have been demonstrated to be efficacious in children with croup from other causes. Vocal cord paralysis from cuff compression or other trauma to the recurrent laryngeal nerve results in hoarseness and increases the risk of aspiration. The incidence of postoperative hoarseness seems to increase with obesity, difficult intubations, and anesthetics of long duration. Curiously, applying a water-soluble lubricant or a local anesthetic-containing gel to the tip or cuff of the TT does not decrease the incidence of postoperative sore throat or hoarseness, and, in some studies, actually increased the incidence of these complications. Smaller tubes (size 6.5 in women and size 7.0 in men) are associated with fewer complaints of postoperative sore throat. Repeated attempts at laryngoscopy during a difficult intubation may lead to periglottic edema and the inability to ventilate with a face mask, thus turning a bad situation into a life-threatening one.

Errors of Tracheal Tube Positioning

6 Unrecognized esophageal intubation can produce catastrophic results. Prevention of this complication depends on direct visualization of the tip of the TT passing through the vocal cords, careful auscultation for the presence of bilateral breath sounds and the absence of gastric gurgling while ventilating through the TT, analysis of exhaled gas for the presence of CO_2 (the most reliable automated method), chest radiography, or the use of an FOB.

Even though it is confirmed that the tube is in the trachea, it may not be correctly positioned. Overly "deep" insertion usually results in intubation of the right (rather than left) main-stem bronchus because of the right bronchus' less acute angle with
7 the trachea. Clues to the diagnosis of bronchial intubation include unilateral breath sounds, unexpected hypoxia with pulse oximetry (unreliable with high inspired oxygen concentrations), inability to palpate the TT cuff in the sternal notch during cuff inflation, and decreased breathing-bag compliance (high peak inspiratory pressures).

In contrast, inadequate insertion depth will position the cuff in the larynx, predisposing the patient to laryngeal trauma. Inadequate depth of insertion can be detected by palpating the cuff over the thyroid cartilage.

Because no one technique protects against all possibilities for misplacing a TT, minimal testing should include chest auscultation, routine capnography, and occasionally cuff palpation.

If the patient is repositioned, tube placement must be reconfirmed. Neck extension or lateral rotation most often moves a TT away from the carina, whereas neck flexion most often moves the tube toward the carina.

At no time should excessive force be employed during intubation. Esophageal intubations can result in esophageal rupture and mediastinitis. Mediastinitis presents as severe sore throat, fever, sepsis, and subcutaneous air often manifesting as crepitus. Early intervention is necessary to avoid mortality. If esophageal perforation is suspected, consultation with an otolaryngologist or thoracic surgeon is recommended.

Physiological Responses to Airway Instrumentation

Laryngoscopy and tracheal intubation violate the patient's protective airway reflexes and predictably lead to hypertension and tachycardia when performed under "light" planes of general anesthesia. The insertion of an LMA is typically associated with less hemodynamic change. Hemodynamic changes can be attenuated by intravenous administration of lidocaine, opioids, or β-blockers or deeper planes of inhalation anesthesia in the minutes before laryngoscopy. Hypotensive agents, including sodium nitroprusside, nitroglycerin, esmolol and nicardipine, have also been shown to effectively attenuate the transient hypertensive response associated with laryngoscopy and intubation. Cardiac arrhythmias—particularly ventricular bigeminy—sometimes occur during intubation and may indicate light anesthesia.

Laryngospasm is a forceful involuntary spasm of the laryngeal musculature caused by sensory stimulation of the superior laryngeal nerve. Triggering stimuli include pharyngeal secretions or passing a TT through the larynx during extubation. Laryngospasm is usually prevented by extubating patients either deeply asleep or fully awake, but it can occur—albeit rarely—in an awake patient. Treatment of laryngospasm includes providing gentle positive-pressure ventilation with an anesthesia bag and mask using 100% oxygen or administering intravenous lidocaine (1–1.5 mg/kg). If laryngospasm persists and hypoxia develops, small doses of succinylcholine (0.25–0.5 mg/kg) may be required (perhaps in combination with small doses of propofol or another anesthetic) to relax the laryngeal muscles and to allow controlled **8** ventilation. The large negative intrathoracic pressures generated by a struggling patient during laryngospasm can result in the development of negative-pressure pulmonary edema, even in healthy patients.

Whereas laryngospasm may result from an abnormally sensitive reflex, aspiration can result from depression of laryngeal reflexes following prolonged intubation and general anesthesia.

Bronchospasm is another reflex response to intubation and is most common in asthmatic patients. Bronchospasm can sometimes be a clue to bronchial intubation. Other pathophysiological effects of intubation include increased intracranial and intraocular pressures.

Tracheal Tube Malfunction

TTs do not always function as intended. Polyvinyl chloride tubes may be ignited by cautery or laser in an oxygen/nitrous oxide-enriched environment. Valve or cuff damage is not unusual and should be excluded prior to insertion. TT obstruction can result from kinking, from foreign body aspiration, or from thick or inspissated secretions in the lumen.

CASE DISCUSSION

Evaluation & Management of a Difficult Airway

A 17-year-old girl presents for emergency drainage of a submandibular abscess.

TABLE 19–7 Conditions associated with difficult intubations.

Tumors
Cystic hygroma
Hemangioma
Hematoma[1]
Infections
Submandibular abscess
Peritonsillar abscess
Epiglottitis
Congenital anomalies
Pierre Robin syndrome
Treacher Collins syndrome
Laryngeal atresia
Goldenhar syndrome
Craniofacial dysostosis
Foreign body
Trauma
Laryngeal fracture
Mandibular or maxillary fracture
Inhalation burn
Cervical spine injury
Obesity
Inadequate neck extension
Rheumatoid arthritis[2]
Ankylosing spondylitis
Halo traction
Anatomic variations
Micrognathia
Prognathism
Large tongue
Arched palate
Short neck
Prominent upper incisors

[1]Can occur postoperatively in patients who have had any neck surgery.
[2]Also affects arytenoids making them immobile.

What are some important anesthetic considerations during the preoperative evaluation of a patient with an abnormal airway?

Induction of general anesthesia followed by direct laryngoscopy and oral intubation is dangerous, if not impossible, in several situations. (Table 19–7). To determine the optimal intubation technique, the anesthesiologist must elicit an airway history and carefully examine the patient's head and neck. Any available prior anesthesia records should be reviewed for previous problems in airway management. If a facial deformity is severe enough to preclude a good mask seal, positive-pressure ventilation may be impossible.

Furthermore, patients with hypopharyngeal disease are more dependent on awake muscle tone to maintain airway patency. These two groups of patients should generally not be allowed to become apneic—including induction of anesthesia, sedation, or muscle paralysis—until their airway is secured.

If there is an abnormal limitation of the temporomandibular joint that may not improve with muscle paralysis, a nasal approach with an FOB should be considered. Infection confined to the floor of the mouth usually does not preclude nasal intubation. If the hypopharynx is involved to the level of the hyoid bone, however, any translaryngeal attempt will be difficult. Other clues to a potentially difficult laryngoscopy include limited neck extension (<35°), a distance between the tip of the patient's mandible and hyoid bone of less than 7 cm, a sternomental distance of less than 12.5 cm with the head fully extended and the mouth closed, and a poorly visualized uvula during voluntary tongue protrusion. It must be stressed that because no examination technique is foolproof and the signs of a difficult airway may be subtle, the anesthesiologist must always be prepared for unanticipated difficulties.

The anesthesiologist should also evaluate the patient for signs of airway obstruction (eg, chest retraction, stridor) and hypoxia (agitation, restlessness, anxiety, lethargy). Aspiration pneumonia is more likely if the patient has recently eaten or if pus is draining from an abscess into the mouth. In either case, techniques that ablate laryngeal reflexes (eg, topical anesthesia) should be avoided.

Cervical trauma or disease is a factor that should be evaluated prior to direct laryngoscopy. Cervical arthritis or previous cervical fusion may make it difficult for the head to be put in the sniffing position; these patients are candidates for bronchoscopy to secure the airway, as discussed previously. Trauma patients with unstable necks or whose neck has not yet been "cleared" are also candidates for bronchoscopy for tracheal intubation. Alternatively, laryngoscopy with in-line stabilization can be performed (**Figure 19–33**).

In the case under discussion, physical examination reveals extensive facial edema that limits the mandible's range of motion. Mask fit does not seem to be impaired, however. Lateral radiographs of the head and neck suggest that the infection has spread over the larynx. Frank pus is observed in the mouth.

Which intubation technique is indicated?

Routine oral and nasal intubations have been described for anesthetized patients. Both of these can also be performed in awake patients. Whether the patient is awake or asleep or whether intubation is to be oral or nasal, it can be performed with

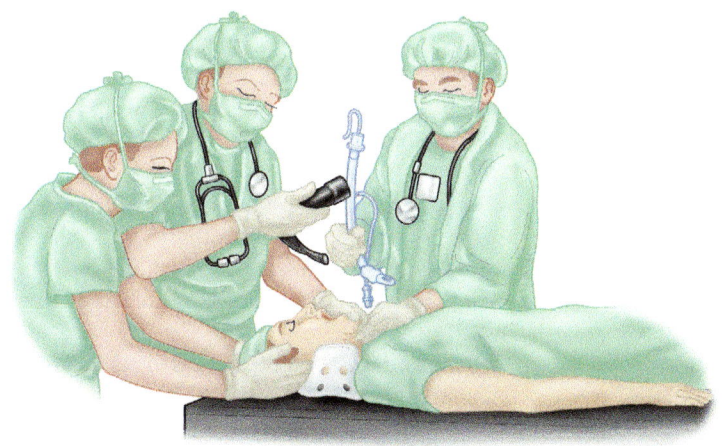

FIGURE 19–33 Technique for airway management of a patient with suspected spinal cord injury. One individual holds the head firmly with the patient on a backboard, the cervical collar left alone if in place, ensuring that neither the head nor neck moves with direct laryngoscopy. A second person applies cricoid pressure and the third performs laryngoscopy and intubation.

direct laryngoscopy, fiberoptic visualization, or video laryngoscopy techniques.

Intubation may be difficult in this patient; however, there is pus draining into the mouth, and positive-pressure ventilation may be impossible. Induction of anesthesia should, therefore, be delayed until after the airway has been secured. Therefore, the alternatives are awake fiberoptic intubation, awake video laryngoscopy, or awake use of optical stylets. The final decision depends on the availability of equipment and the experiences and preferences of the anesthesia caregivers.

Regardless of which alternative is chosen, an emergency surgical airway may be necessary. Therefore, an experienced team, including a surgeon, should be in the operating room, all necessary equipment should be available and unwrapped, and the neck should be prepped and draped.

What premedication would be appropriate for this patient?

Any loss of consciousness or interference with airway reflexes could result in airway obstruction or aspiration. Glycopyrrolate would be a good choice of premedication because it minimizes upper airway secretions without crossing the blood–brain barrier. Parenteral sedatives should be very carefully titrated. Dexmedetomidine and ketamine preserve respiratory effort and are frequently used as sedatives. Psychological preparation of the patient, including explaining each step planned in securing the airway, may improve patient cooperation.

What nerve blocks could be helpful during an awake intubation?

The lingual and some pharyngeal branches of the glossopharyngeal nerve that provide sensation to the posterior third of the tongue and oropharynx are easily blocked by bilateral injection of 2 mL of local anesthetic into the base of the palatoglossal arch (also known as the anterior tonsillar pillar) with a 25-gauge spinal needle (**Figure 19–34**).

Bilateral **superior laryngeal nerve blocks** and a transtracheal block would anesthetize the airway

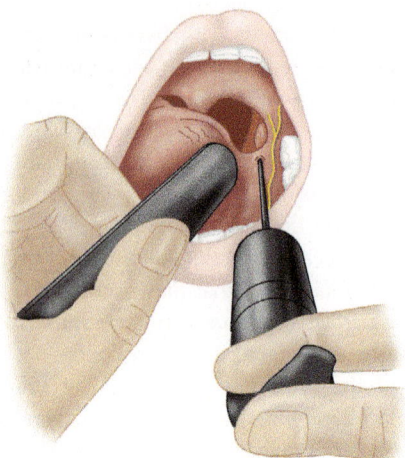

FIGURE 19–34 Nerve block. While the tongue is laterally retracted with a tongue blade, the base of the palatoglossal arch is infiltrated with local anesthetic to block the lingual and pharyngeal branches of the glossopharyngeal nerve. Note that the lingual branches of the glossopharyngeal nerve are not the same as the lingual nerve, which is a branch of the trigeminal nerve.

below the epiglottis (**Figure 19–35**). The hyoid bone is located, and 3 mL of 2% lidocaine is infiltrated 1 cm below each greater cornu, where the internal branch of the superior laryngeal nerves penetrates the thyrohyoid membrane.

A transtracheal block is performed by identifying and penetrating the CTM while the neck is extended. After confirmation of an intratracheal position by aspiration of air, 4 mL of 4% lidocaine is injected into the trachea at end expiration. A deep inhalation and cough immediately following injection distribute the anesthetic throughout the trachea. Although these blocks may allow the awake patient to tolerate intubation better, they also obtund protective cough reflexes, depress the swallowing reflex, and may lead to aspiration. Topical anesthesia of the pharynx may induce a transient obstruction from the loss of reflex regulation of airway caliber at the level of the glottis.

Because of this patient's increased risk for aspiration, local anesthesia might best be limited to

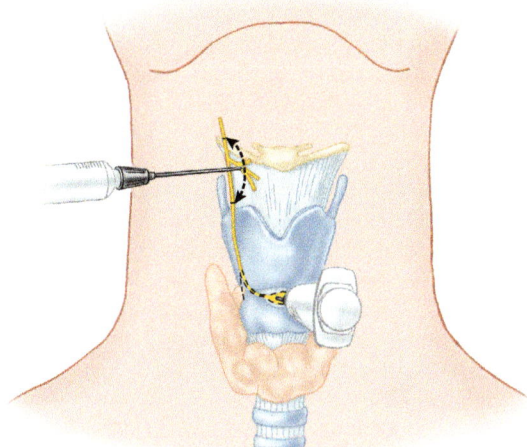

FIGURE 19–35 Superior laryngeal nerve block and transtracheal block.

the nasal passages. Four percent cocaine has no advantages compared with a mixture of 4% lidocaine and 0.25% phenylephrine and can cause cardiovascular side effects. The maximum safe dose of local anesthetic should be calculated—and not exceeded. Local anesthetic is applied to the nasal mucosa with cotton-tipped applicators until a nasal airway that has been lubricated with lidocaine jelly can be placed into the naris with minimal discomfort. Benzocaine spray is frequently used to topicalize the airway, but can produce methemoglobinemia.

Why is it necessary to be prepared for a surgical airway?

Laryngospasm is always a possible complication of intubation in the nonparalyzed patient, even if the patient remains awake. Laryngospasm may make positive-pressure ventilation with a mask impossible. If succinylcholine is administered to break the spasm, the consequent relaxation of pharyngeal muscles may lead to upper airway obstruction and continued inability to ventilate. In this situation, an emergency cricothyrotomy may be lifesaving.

What are some alternative techniques that might be successful?

Other possible strategies include the retrograde passage of a long guidewire or epidural catheter through a needle inserted across the CTM. The catheter is guided cephalad into the pharynx and out through the nose or mouth. A TT is passed over the catheter, which is withdrawn after the tube has entered the larynx. Variations of this technique include passing the retrograde wire through the suction port of a flexible FOB or the lumen of a reintubation stylet that has been preloaded with a TT. These thicker shafts help the TT negotiate the bend into the larynx more easily. Obviously, a vast array of specialized airway equipment exists and must be readily available for management of difficult airways (**Table 19–8**). Either of these techniques would have been difficult in the patient described in this case

TABLE 19–8 Suggested contents of the portable storage unit for difficult airway management.[1,2]

- Rigid laryngoscope blades of alternate design and size from those routinely used.
- Tracheal tubes of assorted size.
- Tracheal tube guides. Examples include (but are not limited to) semirigid stylets with or without a hollow core for jet ventilation, light wands, and forceps designed to manipulate the distal portion of the tracheal tube.
- Laryngeal mask airways of assorted sizes.
- Fiberoptic intubation equipment and assorted video and indirect laryngoscopes.
- Retrograde intubation equipment.
- At least one device suitable for emergency nonsurgical airway ventilation. Examples include (but are not limited to) transtracheal jet ventilator, hollow jet ventilation stylet, and Combitube.
- Equipment suitable for emergency surgical airway access (eg, cricothyrotomy).
- An exhaled CO_2 detector.

[1]Modified and used, with permission, from the American Society of Anesthesiologists: Practice guidelines for management of the difficult airway: A report by the American Society of Anesthesiologists Task Force on Management of the Difficult Airway. Anesthesiology 2003; 98:1272.
[2]The items listed in this table are suggestions. The contents of the portable storage unit should be customized to meet the specific needs, preferences, and skills of the practitioner and healthcare facility.

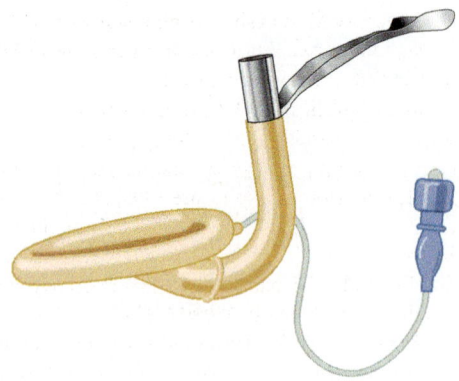

FIGURE 19–36 Intubating laryngeal mask airway.

because of the swelling and anatomic distortion of the neck that can accompany a submandibular abscess.

What are some approaches when the airway is unexpectedly difficult?

The unexpected difficult airway can present both in elective surgical patients and also in emergency intubations in intensive care units, the emergency department, or general hospital wards. Should video laryngoscopy fail even after attempts with an intubating bougie, an intubating LMA should be attempted (Figure 19–36). If ventilation is adequate, an FOB can be loaded with a TT and passed through the LMA into the trachea. Correct tube position is confirmed by visualization of the carina.

SUGGESTED READING

Armstrong J, John J Karsli C: A comparison between the GlideScope Video Laryngoscope and direct laryngoscope in paediatric patients with difficult airways—a pilot study. Anaesthesia 2010;65:353.

Aziz M, Healy D, Kheterpal S, et al: Routine clinical practice effectiveness of the GlideScope in difficult airway management. Anesthesiology 2011;114:34.

Bercker S, Schmidbauer W, Volk T, et al: A comparison of seal in seven supraglottic airway devices using a cadaver model of elevated esophageal pressure. Anesth Analg 2008;106:445.

Brain A: Pressure in laryngeal mask airway cuffs. Anaesthesia 1996;51:603.

Cheney FW, Posner KL, Lee LA, Caplan RA, Domino KB: Trends in anesthesia-related death and brain damage. A closed claims analysis. Anesthesiology 2006;105:1081.

Cook TM: A new practical classification of laryngeal view. Anaesthesia 2000;55:274.

Cooper R: Complications associated with the use of the GlideScope video laryngoscope. Can J Anesth 2007;54:54.

El-Orbany M, Woehlck H, Ramez Salem M: Head and neck position for direct laryngoscopy. Anesth Analg 2011;113:103.

Galvin E, van Doorn M, Blazques J, et al: A randomized prospective study comparing cobra perilaryngeal airway and laryngeal mask airway classic during controlled ventilation for gynecological laparoscopy. Anesth Analg 2007;104:102.

Hagberg C, Johnson S, Pillai D: Effective use of the esophageal tracheal Combitube TN following severe burn injury. J Clin Anesth 2003;15:463.

Hohlrieder M, Brimacombe J, Von Goedecke A, et al: Postoperative nausea, vomiting, airway morbidity, and analgesic requirements are lower for the ProSeal laryngeal mask airway than the tracheal tube in females undergoing breast and gynaecological surgery. Br J Anaesth 2007;99:576.

Holst B, Hodzovic I, Francis V: Airway trauma caused by the Airtraq laryngoscope. Anaesthesia 2008;63:889.

Houston G, Bourke P, Wilson G, et al: Bonfils intubating fiberscope in normal paediatric airways. Br J Anaesth 2010;105:546.

Hurford WE: Orotracheal intubation outside the operating room: anatomic considerations and techniques. Respir Care 1999;44:615.

Jaeger JM, Durbin CG Jr: Special purpose endotracheal tubes. Respir Care 1999;44:661.

Jefferson M, Riffat F, McGuinness J, et al: The laryngeal mask airway and otorhinolaryngology head and neck surgery. Laryngoscope 2011;121:1620.

Kaplan M, Ward D, Hagberg C, et al: Seeing is believing: the importance of video laryngoscopy in teaching and in managing the difficult airway. Surg Endosc 2006;20:S479.

Kim ES, Bishop MJ: Endotracheal intubation, but not laryngeal mask airway insertion, produces reversible bronchoconstriction. Anesthesiology 1999;90:391.

Langeron O, Masso E, Huraux C, et al: Prediction of difficult mask ventilation. Anesthesiology 2000;92:1217.

Maharaj C, Costello J, McDonnell J, et al: The Airtraq as a rescue airway device following failed direct laryngoscopy: a case series. Anaesthesia 2007;67:598.

Malik M, Maharaj C, Harte B, et al: Comparison of Macintosh, Trueview EVO2, GlideScope, and Airwayscope laryngoscope use in patients with cervical spine immobilization. Br J Anaesth 2008;101:723.

Malik M, Subramanian R, Maharaj C, et al: Randomized controlled trial of the Pentax AWS, GlideScope, and Macintosh laryngoscopes in predicted difficult intubations. Br J Anaesth 2009;103:761.

Noppens R, Möbus S, Heid F, Schmidtmann I, Werner C, Piepho T: Use of the McGrath Series 5 videolaryngoscope after failed direct laryngoscopy. Anaesthesia 2010;65:716.

Robitaille A, Williams S, Trembaly M, et al: Cervical spine motion during tracheal intubation with manual in-line stabilization direct laryngoscopy versus GlideScope video laryngoscopy. Anesth Analg 2008;106:935.

Russi C, Hartley M, Buresh C: A pilot study of the King LT supralaryngeal airway use in a rural Iowa EMS system. Int J Emerg Med 2008;1:135.

Shelly MP, Nightingale P: ABC of intensive care. Respiratory support. BMJ 1999;318:1674.

Stauffer JL: Complications of endotracheal intubation and tracheostomy. Respir Care 1999;44:828.

Stix MS, O'Connor CJ Jr: Depth of insertion of the ProSeal laryngeal mask airway. Br J Anaesth 2003;90:235.

Tanoubi I, Drolet P, Donati F: Optimizing preoxygenation in adults. Can J Anesth 2009;56:449.

Ting J: Temporomandibular joint dislocation after use of a laryngeal mask airway. Anaesthesia 2006;61:190.

Thompson AE: Issues in airway management in infants and children. Respir Care 1999;44:650.

Verghese C, Ramaswamy B: LMA-Supreme—a new single-use LMA with gastric access: a report on its clinical efficacy. Br J Anaesth 2008;101:405.

Watson CB: Prediction of a difficult intubation: methods for successful intubation. Respir Care 1999;44:777.

Cardiovascular Physiology & Anesthesia

KEY CONCEPTS

1 In contrast to action potentials in axons, the spike in cardiac action potentials is followed by a plateau phase that lasts 0.2–0.3 sec. Whereas the action potential for skeletal muscle and nerves is due to the abrupt opening of voltage-gated sodium channels in the cell membrane, in cardiac muscle it is initiated by voltage-gated sodium channels (the spike) and maintained by voltage-gated calcium channels (the plateau).

2 Potent inhalational agents depress sinoatrial (SA) node automaticity. These agents seem to have only modest direct effects on the atrioventricular (AV) node, prolonging conduction time and increasing refractoriness. This combination of effects likely explains the frequent occurrence of junctional tachycardia when an anticholinergic agent is administered for sinus bradycardia during inhalation anesthesia; junctional pacemakers are accelerated more than those in the SA node.

3 Studies suggest that volatile anesthetics depress cardiac contractility by decreasing the entry of Ca^{2+} into cells during depolarization (affecting T- and L-type calcium channels), altering the kinetics of its release and uptake into the sarcoplasmic reticulum,

and decreasing the sensitivity of contractile proteins to calcium.

4 Because the normal cardiac index (CI) has a wide range, it is a relatively insensitive measurement of ventricular performance. Abnormalities in CI therefore usually reflect gross ventricular impairment.

5 In the absence of hypoxia or severe anemia, measurement of mixed venous oxygen tension (or saturation) is an excellent estimate of the adequacy of cardiac output.

6 Patients with reduced ventricular compliance are most affected by loss of a normally timed atrial systole.

7 Cardiac output in patients with marked right or left ventricular impairment is very sensitive to acute increases in afterload.

8 The ventricular ejection fraction, the fraction of the end-diastolic ventricular volume ejected, is the most commonly used clinical measurement of systolic function.

9 Left ventricular diastolic function can be assessed clinically by Doppler echocardiography in a transthoracic or transesophageal examination.

—Continued next page

Continued—

 10 Because the endocardium is subjected to the greatest intramural pressures during systole, it tends to be most vulnerable to ischemia during decreases in coronary perfusion pressure.

11 The failing heart becomes increasingly dependent on circulating catecholamines. Abrupt withdrawal in sympathetic outflow or decreases in circulating catecholamine levels, such as can occur following induction of anesthesia, may lead to acute cardiac decompensation.

Anesthesiologists must have a thorough understanding of cardiovascular physiology both for its scientific significance in anesthesia and for its practical applications to patient management. Anesthetic successes and failures are often directly related to the skill of the practitioner in manipulating cardiovascular physiology. This chapter reviews the physiology of the heart and the systemic circulation and the pathophysiology of heart failure.

The circulatory system consists of the heart, blood vessels, and blood. Its function is to provide oxygen and nutrients to the tissues and to carry away the products of metabolism. The heart propels blood through two vascular systems arranged in series. In the normally low-pressure pulmonary circulation, venous blood flows past the alveolar–capillary membrane, takes up oxygen, and eliminates CO_2. In the high pressure systemic circulation, oxygenated arterial blood is pumped to metabolizing tissues, and the by-products of metabolism are taken up for elimination by the lungs, kidneys, or liver.

The Heart

Although anatomically one organ, the heart can be functionally divided into right and left pumps, each consisting of an atrium and a ventricle. The atria serve as both conduits and priming pumps, whereas the ventricles act as the major pumping chambers. The right ventricle receives systemic venous (deoxygenated) blood and pumps it into the pulmonary circulation, whereas the left ventricle receives pulmonary venous (oxygenated) blood and

pumps it into the systemic circulation. Four valves normally ensure unidirectional flow through each chamber. The normal pumping action of the heart is the result of a complex series of electrically driven and mechanical events. Electrical events precede mechanical ones.

The heart consists of specialized striated muscle in a connective tissue skeleton. Cardiac muscle can be divided into atrial, ventricular, and specialized pacemaker and conducting cells. The self-excitatory nature of cardiac muscle cells and their unique organization allow the heart to function as a highly efficient pump. Serial low-resistance connections (intercalated disks) between individual myocardial cells allow the rapid and orderly spread of depolarization in each pumping chamber. Electrical activity readily spreads from one atrium to another and from one ventricle to another via specialized conduction pathways. The normal absence of direct connections between the atria and ventricles except through the atrioventricular (AV) node delays conduction and enables atrial contraction to prime the ventricle.

CARDIAC ACTION POTENTIALS

At rest, the myocardial cell membrane is nominally permeable to K^+, but is relatively impermeable to Na^+. A membrane-bound Na^+–K^+-adenosine triphosphatase (ATPase) concentrates K^+ intracellularly in exchange for extrusion of Na^+ out of the cell. Intracellular Na^+ concentration is kept low, whereas intracellular K^+ concentration is kept high relative to the extracellular space. The relative impermeability of the membrane to calcium also maintains a high extracellular to cytoplasmic calcium gradient. Movement of K+ out of the cell and down its concentration gradient results in a net loss of positive charges from inside the cell. An electrical potential is established across the cell membrane, with the inside of the cell negative with respect to the extracellular environment, because anions do not accompany K+. Thus, the resting membrane potential represents the balance between two opposing forces: the movement of K+ down its concentration gradient and the electrical attraction of the negatively charged intracellular space for the positively charged potassium ions.

The normal ventricular cell resting membrane potential is –80 to –90 mV. As with other excitable tissues (nerve and skeletal muscle), when the cell membrane potential becomes less negative and reaches a threshold value, a characteristic action potential (depolarization) develops (**Figure 20–1** and **Table 20–1**). The action potential transiently raises the membrane potential of the myocardial cell to +20 mV. In contrast to action potentials in axons, the spike in cardiac action potentials is followed by a plateau phase that lasts 0.2–0.3 sec. Whereas the action potential for skeletal muscle and nerves is due to the abrupt opening of voltage-gated sodium channels in the cell membrane, in cardiac muscle, it is initiated by voltage-gated sodium channels (the spike) and maintained by voltage-gated calcium channels (the plateau). Depolarization is also accompanied by a transient decrease in potassium permeability. Subsequent restoration of normal potassium permeability and termination of sodium and calcium channel permeability eventually restores the membrane potential to its resting value.

Following depolarization, the cells are typically refractory to subsequent normal depolarizing stimuli until "phase 4." The effective refractory period is the minimum interval between two depolarizing impulses that will propagate. In fast-conducting myocardial cells, this period is generally closely correlated with the duration of the action potential. In contrast, the effective refractory period in more slowly conducting myocardial cells can outlast the duration of the action potential.

Table 20–2 lists some of the multiple types of ion channels in cardiac muscle membrane. Some are activated by a change in cell membrane voltage, whereas others open only when bound by ligands. T-type (transient) voltage-gated calcium channels play a role in phase 0 of depolarization. During the plateau phase (phase 2), Ca^{2+} inflow occurs through slow L-type (long-lasting), voltage-gated calcium channels. Three major types of potassium channels are responsible for repolarization. The first results in a transient outward K+ current (I_{To}), the second is responsible for a short rectifying current (I_{Kr}), and the third produces a slowly acting rectifying current (I_{Ks}) that helps to restore the cell membrane potential to its resting value.

INITIATION & CONDUCTION OF THE CARDIAC IMPULSE

The cardiac impulse normally originates in the sinoatrial (SA) node, a group of specialized pacemaker cells in the sulcus terminalis, located posteriorly at the junction of the right atrium and the superior vena cava. These cells seem to have an outer membrane that leaks Na+ (and possibly Ca^{2+}). The slow influx of Na+, which results in a less negative resting membrane potential (–50 to –60 mV), has three important consequences: near constant inactivation of voltage-gated sodium channels, an action potential with a threshold of –40 mV that is primarily due to ion movement across the slow calcium channels, and regular spontaneous depolarizations. During each cycle, intracellular leakage of Na+ causes the cell membrane to become progressively less negative; when the threshold potential is reached, calcium channels open, K+ permeability decreases, and an action potential develops. Restoration of normal K+ permeability returns the cells in the SA node to their normal resting membrane potential.

The impulse generated at the SA node is normally rapidly conducted across the atria and to the AV node. Specialized atrial fibers may speed up conduction to both the left atrium and the AV node. The AV node, which is located in the septal wall of the right atrium, just anterior to the opening of the coronary sinus and above the insertion of the septal leaflet of the tricuspid valve, is actually made up of three distinct areas: an upper junctional (AN) region, a middle nodal (N) region, and a lower junctional (NH) region. Although the N region does not

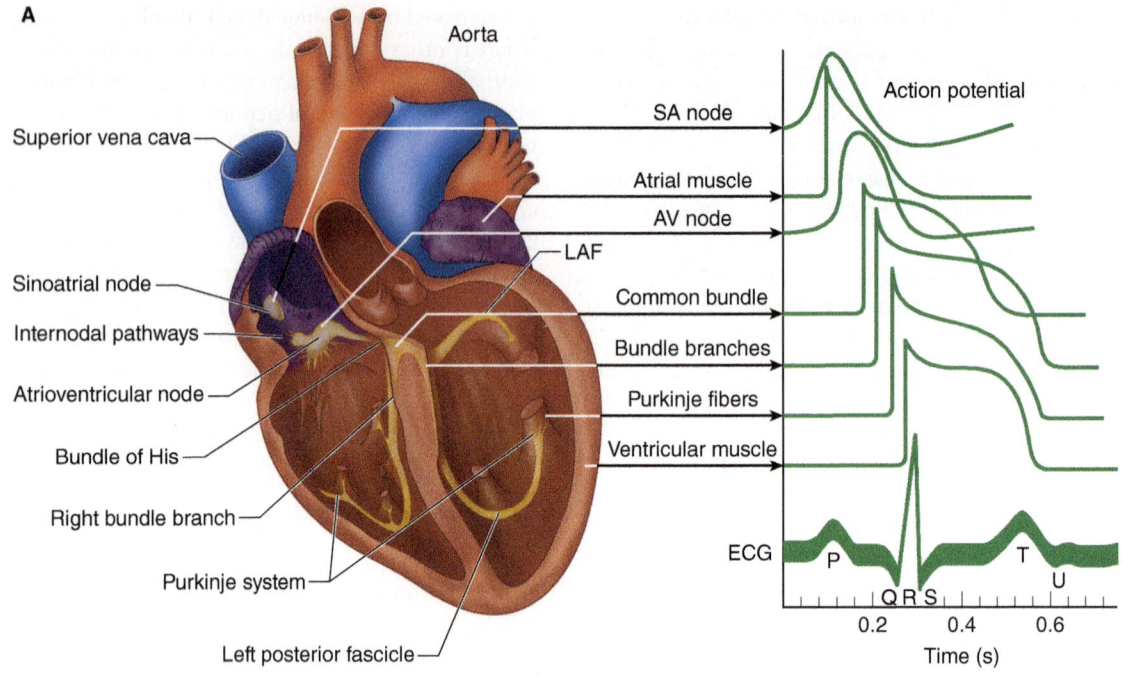

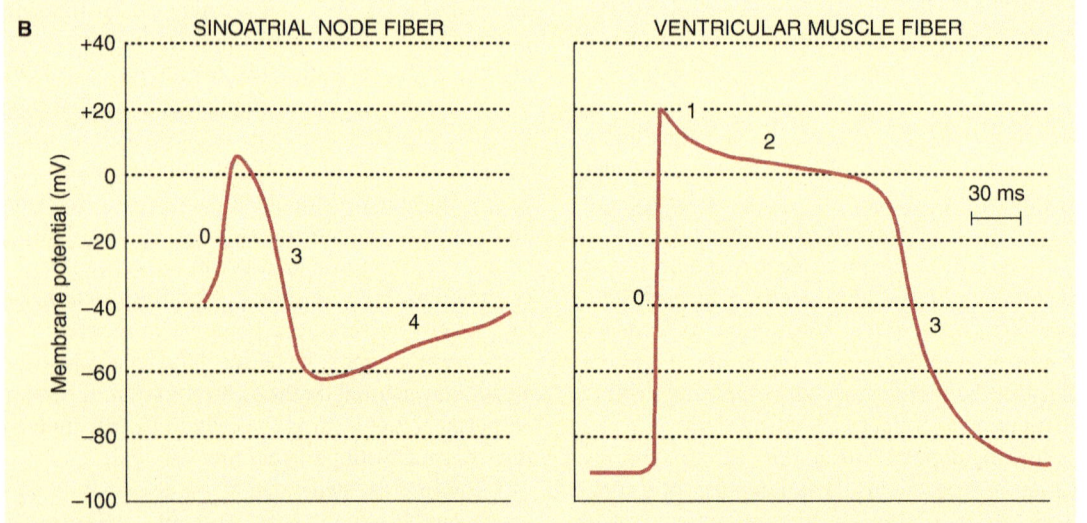

FIGURE 20–1 Cardiac action potentials. **A:** Note the characteristic contours of action potentials recorded from different parts of the heart. **B:** Pacemaker cells in the sinoatrial (SA) node lack the same distinct phases as atrial and ventricular muscle cells and display prominent spontaneous diastolic depolarization. See Table 20–1 for an explanation of the different phases of the action potential. (Modified and reproduced, with permission, from Barrett KE: Ganong's *Review of Medical Physiology*, 24th ed., McGraw-Hill, 2012.)

TABLE 20-1 Cardiac action potential.

Phase	Name	Event	Cellular Ion Movement
0	Upstroke	Activation (opening) of voltage-gated Na+ channels	Na+ entry and decreased permeability to K+
1	Early rapid repolarization	Inactivation of Na+ channel and transient increase in K+ permeability	K+ out (I_{To})
2	Plateau	Activation of slow calcium channels	Ca2+ entry
3	Final repolarization	Inactivation of calcium channels and increased permeability to K+	K+ out
4	Resting potential	Normal permeability restored (atrial and ventricular cells)	Na+–K+-ATPase pumps K+ in and Na+ out
	Diastolic repolarization	Intrinsic slow leakage of Ca2+ into cells that spontaneously depolarize	Ca2+ in

TABLE 20-2 Cardiac ion channels.[1]

Voltage-gated channels
  Na+
  T Ca2+
  L Ca2+
  K+
    Transient outward
    Inward rectifying
    Slow (delayed) rectifying

Ligand-gated K+ channels
  Ca2+ activated
  Na+ activated
  ATP sensitive[2]
  Acetylcholine activated
  Arachadonic acid activated

[1]From Ganong WF: *Review of Medical Physiology*, 21st ed. McGraw-Hill, 2003.

[2]ATP, adenosine triphosphate.

possess intrinsic spontaneous activity (automaticity), both junctional areas do. The normally slower rate of spontaneous depolarization in AV junctional areas (40–60 times/min) allows the faster SA node to control heart rate. Any factor that decreases the rate of SA node depolarization or increases the automaticity of AV junctional areas allows the junctional areas to function as the pacemaker for the heart.

Impulses from the SA node normally reach the AV node after about 0.04 sec, but leave after another 0.11 sec. This delay is the result of the slowly conducting small myocardial fibers within the AV node, which depend on slow calcium channels for propagation of the action potential. In contrast, conduction of the impulse between adjoining cells in the atria and in the ventricles is due primarily to activation of sodium channels. The lower fibers of the AV node combine to form the common bundle of His. This specialized group of fibers passes into the

interventricular septum before dividing into left and right branches to form the complex network of Purkinje fibers that depolarizes both ventricles. In sharp contrast to AV nodal tissue, His–Purkinje fibers have the fastest conduction velocities in the heart, resulting in nearly simultaneous depolarization of the entire endocardium of both ventricles (normally within 0.03 s). Synchronized depolarization of the lateral and septal walls of the left ventricle promotes effective ventricular contraction. The spread of the impulse from the endocardium to the epicardium through ventricular muscle requires an additional 0.03 sec. Thus, an impulse arising from the SA node normally requires less than 0.2 sec to depolarize the entire heart.

Potent inhaled anesthetics depress SA node automaticity. These agents seem to have only modest direct effects on the AV node, prolonging conduction time and increasing refractoriness. This combination of effects likely explains the occurrence of junctional tachycardia when an anticholinergic is administered for sinus bradycardia during inhalation anesthesia; junctional pacemakers are accelerated more than those in the SA node. The electrophysiological effects of volatile agents on Purkinje fibers and ventricular muscle are complex due to autonomic interactions. Both antiarrhythmic and arrhythmogenic properties are described. The former may be due to direct depression of Ca2+ influxes, whereas the latter generally involves potentiation of catecholamines, especially with halothane. The arrhythmogenic effect requires activation of both α_1- and β-adrenergic receptors. Intravenous induction agents have limited electrophysiological effects in usual clinical doses. Opioids, particularly fentanyl and sufentanil, can depress cardiac conduction, increasing AV node conduction and the refractory period and prolonging the duration of the Purkinje fiber action potential.

Local anesthetics have important electrophysiological effects on the heart at blood concentrations that are generally associated with systemic toxicity. In the case of lidocaine, electrophysiological effects at low blood concentrations can be therapeutic. At high blood concentrations, local anesthetics depress conduction by binding to sodium channels; at extremely high concentrations, they also depress the SA node. The most potent local anesthetics—bupivacaine, etidocaine, and to a lesser degree, ropivacaine—seem to have the most potent effects on the heart, particularly on Purkinje fibers and ventricular muscle. Bupivacaine binds open or inactivated sodium channels and dissociates from them slowly. It can cause profound sinus bradycardia and sinus node arrest and malignant ventricular arrhythmias; furthermore, it can depress left ventricular contractility. Twenty percent lipid emulsions have been used to treat local anesthetic cardiac toxicity. The mechanisms of action of this therapy are unclear, although possibilities include serving as a lipid reservoir and decreasing lipophilic toxic local anesthetics in the myocardium.

Calcium channel blockers are organic compounds that block Ca^{2+} influx through L-type but not T-type channels. Dihydropyridine blockers, such as nifedipine, simply plug the channel, whereas other agents, such as verapamil, and to a lesser extent, diltiazem, preferentially bind the channel in its depolarized inactivated state (use-dependent blockade).

MECHANISM OF CONTRACTION

Myocardial cells contract as a result of the interaction of two overlapping, rigid contractile proteins, actin and myosin. These proteins are fixed in position within each cell during both contraction and relaxation. Dystrophin, a large intracellular protein, connects actin to the cell membrane (sarcolemma). Cell shortening occurs when the actin and myosin are allowed to fully interact and slide over one another. This interaction is normally prevented by two regulatory proteins, troponin and tropomyosin; troponin is composed of three subunits (troponin I, troponin C, and troponin T). Troponin is attached to actin at regular intervals, whereas tropomyosin lies within the center of the actin structure. An increase in intracellular Ca^{2+} concentration (from about 10^{-7} to 10^{-5} mol/L) promotes contraction as Ca^{2+} ions bind troponin C. The resulting conformational change in these regulatory proteins exposes the active sites on actin that allow interaction with myosin bridges (points of overlapping). The active site on myosin functions as a magnesium-dependent ATPase whose activity is enhanced by the increase in intracellular Ca^{2+} concentration. A series of attachments and disengagements occur as each myosin bridge advances over successive active sites on actin. Adenosine triphosphate (ATP) is consumed during each attachment. Relaxation occurs as Ca^{2+} is actively pumped back into the sarcoplasmic reticulum by a Ca^{2+}–Mg^{2+}-ATPase; the resulting drop in intracellular Ca^{2+} concentration allows the troponin–tropomyosin complex to again prevent the interaction between actin and myosin.

Excitation–Contraction Coupling

The quantity of Ca^{2+} ions required to initiate contraction exceeds that entering the cell through slow calcium channels during phase 2. The small amount that does enter through slow calcium channels triggers the release of much larger amounts of Ca^{2+} stored intracellularly (calcium-dependent calcium release) within cisterns in the sarcoplasmic reticulum.

The action potential of muscle cells depolarizes their T systems, tubular extensions of the cell membrane that transverse the cell in close approximation to the muscle fibrils, via dihydropyridine receptors (voltage-gated calcium channels). This initial increase in intracellular Ca^{2+} triggers an even greater Ca^{2+} inflow across ryanodine receptors, a nonvoltage-dependent calcium channel in the sarcoplasmic reticulum. The force of contraction is directly dependent on the magnitude of the initial Ca^{2+} influx. During relaxation, when the slow channels close, a membrane-bound ATPase actively transports Ca^{2+} back into the sarcoplasmic reticulum. Ca^{2+} is also extruded extracellularly by an exchange of intracellular Ca^{2+} for extracellular sodium by an ATPase in the cell membrane. Thus, relaxation of the heart also requires ATP.

The quantity of intracellular Ca^{2+} available, its rate of delivery, and its rate of removal determine, respectively, the maximum tension developed, the rate of contraction, and the rate of relaxation. Sympathetic stimulation increases the force of contraction by raising intracellular Ca^{2+} concentration via a β_1-adrenergic receptor-mediated increase in intracellular cyclic adenosine monophosphate (cAMP) through the action of a stimulatory G protein. The increase in cAMP recruits additional open calcium channels. Moreover, adrenergic agonists enhance the rate of relaxation by enhancing Ca^{2+} reuptake by the sarcoplasmic reticulum. Phosphodiesterase inhibitors, such as inamrinone, enoximone, and milrinone, produce similar effects by preventing the breakdown of intracellular cAMP. Digitalis glycosides increase intracellular Ca^{2+} concentration through inhibition of the membrane-bound Na^+–K^+-ATPase; the resulting small increase in intracellular Na^+ allows for a greater influx of Ca^{2+} via the Na^+–Ca^{2+} exchange mechanism. Glucagon enhances contractility by increasing intracellular cAMP levels via activation of a specific nonadrenergic receptor. The new agent levosimendan is a calcium sensitizer that enhances contractility by binding to troponin C. In contrast, release of acetylcholine following vagal stimulation depresses contractility through increased cyclic guanosine monophosphate (cGMP) levels and inhibition of adenylyl cyclase; these effects are mediated by an inhibitory G protein. Acidosis blocks slow calcium channels and therefore also depresses cardiac contractility by unfavorably altering intracellular Ca^{2+} kinetics.

3 Studies suggest that volatile anesthetics depress cardiac contractility by decreasing the entry of Ca^{2+} into cells during depolarization (affecting T- and L-type calcium channels), altering the kinetics of its release and uptake into the sarcoplasmic reticulum, and decreasing the sensitivity of contractile proteins to Ca^{2+}. Halothane and enflurane seem to depress contractility more than isoflurane, sevoflurane, and desflurane. Anesthetic-induced cardiac depression is potentiated by hypocalcemia, β-adrenergic blockade, and calcium channel blockers. Nitrous oxide also produces concentration-dependent decreases in contractility by reducing the availability of intracellular Ca^{2+} during contraction. The mechanisms of direct cardiac depression from intravenous anesthetics are not well established, but presumably involve similar actions. Of all the major intravenous induction agents, ketamine seems to have the least direct depressant effect on contractility. Local anesthetic agents also depress cardiac contractility by reducing Ca^{2+} influx and release in a dose-dependent fashion. The more potent (at nerve block) agents, such as bupivacaine, tetracaine, and ropivacaine, more significantly depress left ventricular contractility than less potent (at nerve block) agents, such as lidocaine or chloroprocaine.

INNERVATION OF THE HEART

Parasympathetic fibers primarily innervate the atria and conducting tissues. Acetylcholine acts on specific cardiac muscarinic receptors (M_2) to produce negative chronotropic, dromotropic, and inotropic effects. In contrast, sympathetic fibers are more widely distributed throughout the heart. Cardiac sympathetic fibers originate in the thoracic spinal cord (T1–T4) and travel to the heart initially through the cervical (stellate) ganglia and from the ganglia as the cardiac nerves. Norepinephrine release causes positive chronotropic, dromotropic, and inotropic effects primarily through activation of β_1-adrenergic receptors. β_2-Adrenergic receptors are normally fewer in number and are found primarily in the atria; activation increases heart rate and, to a lesser extent, contractility.

Cardiac autonomic innervation has an apparent *sidedness*, because the right sympathetic and right vagus nerves primarily affect the SA node, whereas the left sympathetic and vagus nerves principally affect the AV node. Vagal effects frequently have a very rapid onset and resolution, whereas sympathetic influences generally have a more gradual onset and dissipation. Sinus arrhythmia is a cyclic variation in heart rate that corresponds to respiration (increasing with inspiration and decreasing during expiration); it is due to cyclic changes in vagal tone.

THE CARDIAC CYCLE

The cardiac cycle can be defined by both electrical and mechanical events (**Figure 20–2**). *Systole* refers to contraction and *diastole* refers to relaxation. Most diastolic ventricular filling occurs passively before atrial contraction. Contraction of the atria normally contributes 20% to 30% of ventricular filling. **Three waves can generally be identified on atrial pressure tracings** (Figure 20–2). The *a* wave is due to

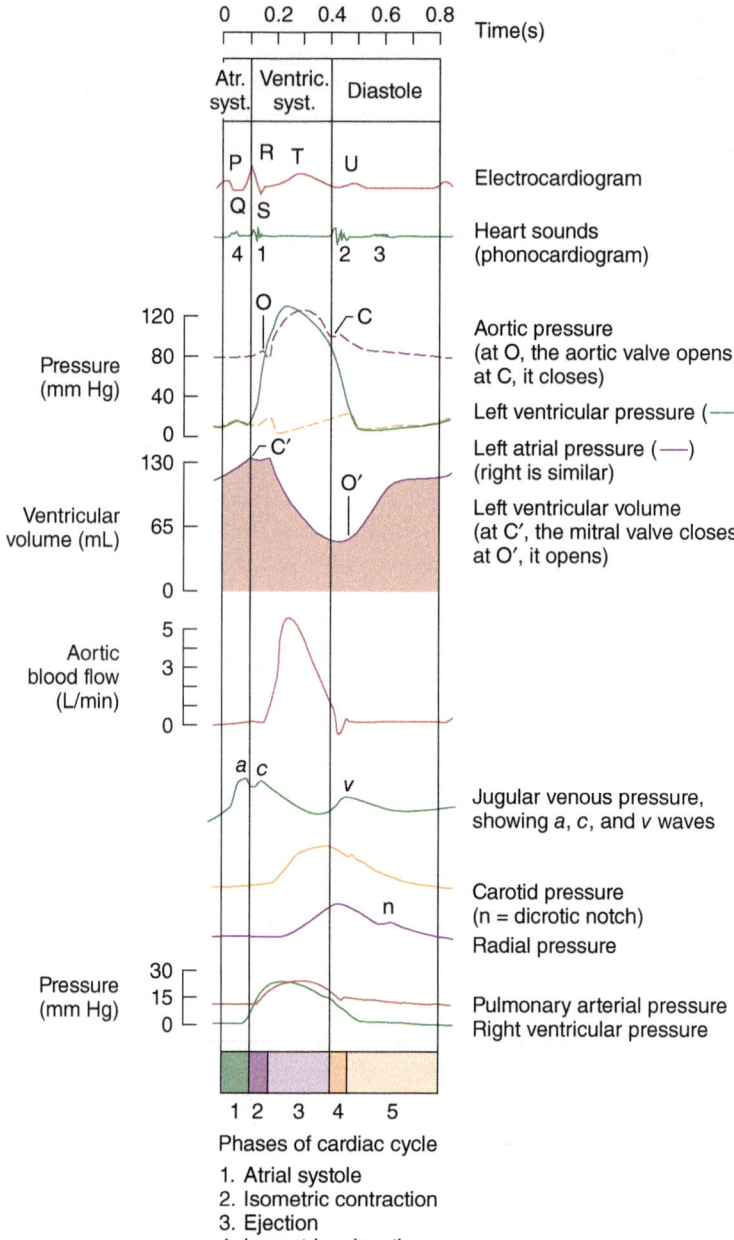

FIGURE 20–2 The normal cardiac cycle. Note the correspondence between electrical and mechanical events. (Modified and reproduced, with permission, from Barrett KE: *Ganong's Review of Medical Physiology*, 24th ed. McGraw-Hill, 2012.)

Phases of cardiac cycle
1. Atrial systole
2. Isometric contraction
3. Ejection
4. Isometric relaxation
5. Filling

atrial systole. The *c* wave coincides with ventricular contraction and is said to be caused by bulging of the AV valve into the atrium. The *v* wave is the result of pressure buildup from venous return before the AV valve opens again. The *x* descent is the decline in pressure between the *c* and *v* waves and is thought to be due to a pulling down of the atrium by ventricular contraction. Incompetence of the AV valve on either side of the heart abolishes the *x* descent on that side, resulting in a prominent *cv* wave. The *y* descent follows the *v* wave and represents the decline in atrial pressure as the AV valve opens. The notch in the aortic pressure tracing is referred to as the *incisura* and is said to represent the brief pressure change from transient backflow of blood into the left ventricle just before aortic valve closure.

DETERMINANTS OF VENTRICULAR PERFORMANCE

Discussions of ventricular function usually refer to the left ventricle, but the same concepts apply to the right ventricle. Although the ventricles are often thought of as functioning separately, their interdependence has clearly been demonstrated. Moreover, factors affecting systolic and diastolic functions can be differentiated: Systolic function involves ventricular ejection, whereas diastolic function is related to ventricular filling.

Ventricular systolic function is often (erroneously) equated with cardiac output, which can be defined as the volume of blood pumped by the heart per minute. Because the two ventricles function in series, their outputs are normally equal. Cardiac output (CO) is expressed by the following equation:

$$CO = SV \times HR$$

where SV is the stroke volume (the volume pumped per contraction) and HR is heart rate. To compensate for variations in body size, CO is often expressed in terms of total body surface area:

$$CI = \frac{CO}{BSA}$$

where CI is the cardiac index and BSA is body surface area. BSA is usually obtained from nomograms

based on height and weight (**Figure 20–3**). Normal **4** CI is 2.5–4.2 L/min/m². Because the normal CI has a wide range, it is a relatively insensitive measurement of ventricular performance. Abnormalities in CI therefore usually reflect gross ventricular impairment. A more accurate assessment can be obtained if the response of the cardiac output to exercise is evaluated. Under these conditions, failure of the cardiac output to increase and keep up with oxygen consumption is reflected by a decreasing mixed venous oxygen saturation. A decrease in mixed venous oxygen saturation in response to increased demand usually reflects inad-**5** equate tissue perfusion. Thus, in the absence of hypoxia or severe anemia, measurement of mixed venous oxygen tension (or saturation) is an excellent estimate of the adequacy of cardiac output.

1. Heart Rate

When stroke volume remains constant, cardiac output is directly proportional to heart rate. Heart rate is an intrinsic function of the SA node (spontaneous depolarization), but is modified by autonomic, humoral, and local factors. The normal intrinsic rate of the SA node in young adults is about 90–100 beats/min, but it decreases with age based on the following formula:

$$\text{Normal intrinsic heart rate} = 118 \text{ beats/min} - (0.57 \times \text{age})$$

Enhanced vagal activity slows the heart rate via stimulation of M_2 cholinergic receptors, whereas enhanced sympathetic activity increases the heart rate mainly through activation of β_1-adrenergic receptors and, to lesser extent, β_2-adrenergic receptors (see above).

2. Stroke Volume

Stroke volume is normally determined by three major factors: preload, afterload, and contractility. This analysis is analogous to laboratory observations on skeletal muscle preparations. Preload is muscle length prior to contraction, whereas afterload is the tension against which the muscle must

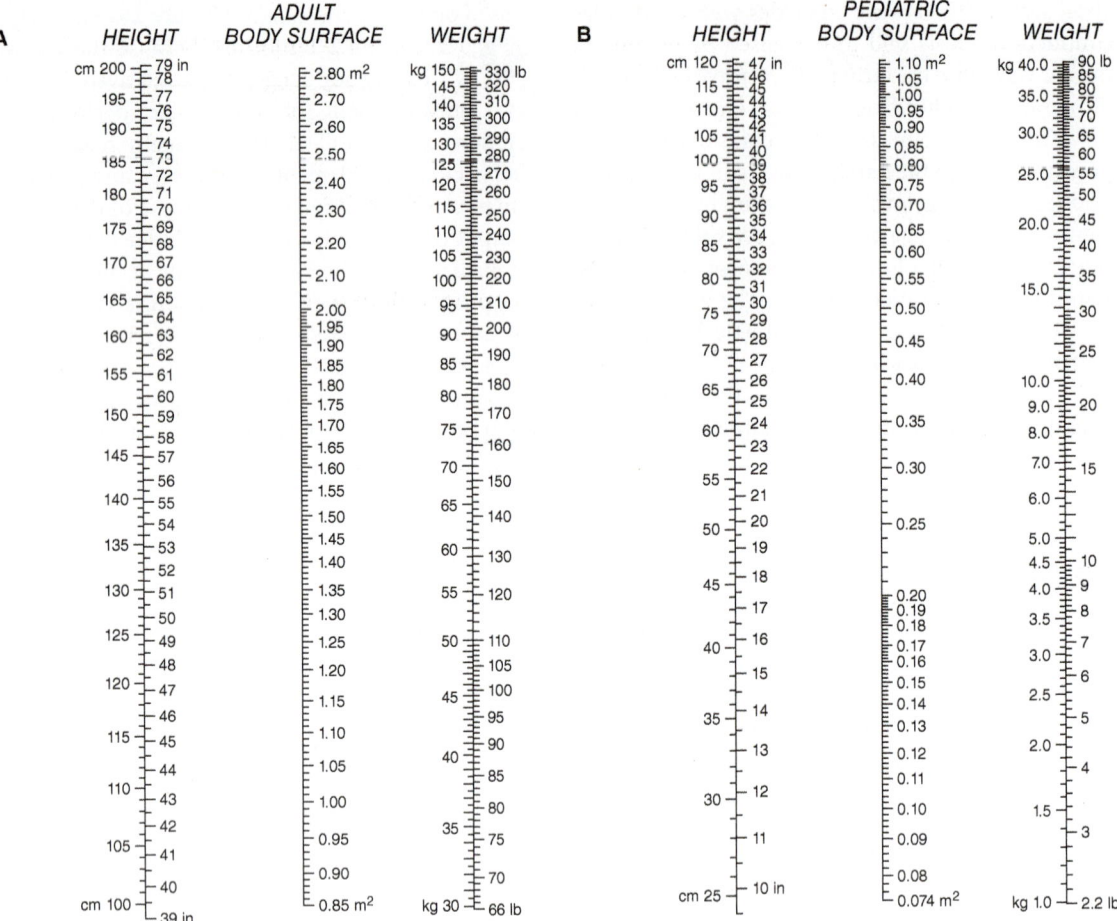

FIGURE 20–3 Nomograms for calculating body surface area (BSA) in adult (**A**) and pediatric (**B**) patients. (Data from the formula of Du Bois and Du Bois: Arch Intern Med 1916;17:863. Copyright 1916, American Medical Association.)

contract. Contractility is an intrinsic property of the muscle that is related to the force of contraction but is independent of both preload and afterload. Because the heart is a three-dimensional multichambered pump, both ventricular geometric form and valvular dysfunction can also affect stroke volume (Table 20–3).

Preload

Ventricular preload is end-diastolic volume, which is generally dependent on ventricular filling. The relationship between cardiac output and left ventricular end-diastolic volume is known as Starling's

law of the heart (Figure 20–4). Note that when the heart rate and contractility remain constant, cardiac output is directly proportional to preload until excessive end-diastolic volumes are reached. At that

TABLE 20–3 Major factors affecting cardiac stroke volume.

Preload
Afterload
Contractility
Wall motion abnormalities
Valvular dysfunction

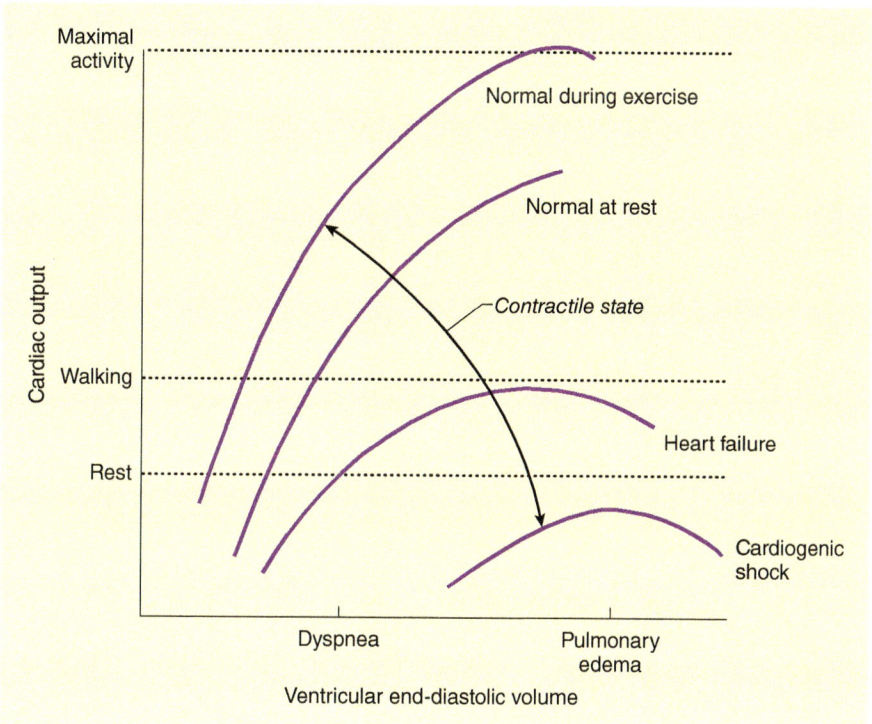

FIGURE 20–4 Starling's law of the heart.

point, cardiac output does not appreciably change— or may even decrease. Excessive distention of either ventricle can lead to excessive dilatation and incompetence of the AV valves.

A. Determinants of Ventricular Filling

Ventricular filling can be influenced by a variety of factors (Table 20–4), of which the most important is venous return. Because most of the other

TABLE 20–4 Factors affecting ventricular preload.

Blood volume
Distribution of blood volume
   Posture
   Intrathoracic pressure
   Pericardial pressure
   Venous tone
Rhythm (atrial contraction)
Heart rate

factors affecting venous return are usually fixed, vascular capacity is normally its major determinant. Increases in metabolic activity reduce vascular capacity, so that venous return to the heart increases as the volume of venous capacitance vessels decreases. Changes in blood volume and venous tone are important causes of intraoperative and postoperative changes in ventricular filling and cardiac output. Any factor that alters the normally small venous pressure gradient favoring blood return to the heart also affects cardiac filling. Such factors include changes in intrathoracic pressure (positive-pressure ventilation or thoracotomy), posture (positioning during surgery), and pericardial pressure (pericardial disease).

The most important determinant of right ventricular preload is venous return. **In the absence of significant pulmonary or right ventricular dysfunction, venous return is also the major determinant of left ventricular preload.** Normally, the end-diastolic volumes of both ventricles are similar, and, normally, the venous return is numerically equivalent to the cardiac output.

Both heart rate and rhythm can also affect ventricular preload. Increases in heart rate are associated with proportionately greater reductions in diastole than systole. Ventricular filling therefore progressively becomes impaired at increased heart rates (>120 beats/min in adults). Absent (atrial fibrillation), ineffective (atrial flutter), or altered timing of atrial contraction (low atrial or junctional rhythms) can also reduce ventricular filling by 20% to 30%. Patients with reduced ventricular compliance are more affected by the loss of a normally timed atrial systole than are those with normal ventricular compliance.

B. Diastolic Function and Ventricular Compliance

Left ventricular end-diastolic pressure (LVEDP) can be used as a measure of preload only if the relationship between ventricular volume and pressure (ventricular compliance) is constant. However, ventricular compliance is normally nonlinear (**Figure 20–5**). Impaired diastolic function reduces ventricular compliance. Therefore, the same LVEDP that corresponds to a normal preload in a normal patient may correspond to a decreased preload in a patient with impaired diastolic function.

Many factors are known to influence ventricular diastolic function and compliance. Nonetheless, measurement of LVEDP or other pressures approximating LVEDP (such as pulmonary artery occlusion pressure) are potential means of estimating left ventricular preload. Changes in central venous pressure can be used as a rough index for changes in right and left ventricular preload in most normal individuals.

Factors affecting ventricular compliance can be separated into those related to the rate of relaxation (early diastolic compliance) and passive stiffness of the ventricles (late diastolic compliance). Hypertrophy (from hypertension or aortic valve stenosis), ischemia, and asynchrony reduce early compliance; hypertrophy and fibrosis reduce late compliance. Extrinsic factors (such as pericardial disease, excessive distention of the contralateral ventricle, increased airway or pleural pressure, tumors, and surgical compression) can also reduce ventricular compliance. Because of its normally thinner wall, the right ventricle is more compliant than the left.

Afterload

Afterload for the intact heart is commonly equated with either ventricular wall tension during systole or arterial impedance to ejection. Wall tension may be thought of as the pressure the ventricle must overcome to reduce its cavity volume. If the ventricle is assumed to be spherical, ventricular wall tension can be expressed by Laplace's law:

$$\text{Circumferential stress} = \frac{P \times R}{2 \times H}$$

where P is intraventricular pressure, R is the ventricular radius, and H is wall thickness. Although the normal ventricle is usually ellipsoidal, this relationship is still useful. The larger the ventricular radius, the greater the wall tension required to develop the same ventricular pressure. Conversely, an increase in wall thickness reduces ventricular wall tension.

Systolic intraventricular pressure is dependent on the force of ventricular contraction; the viscoelastic properties of the aorta, its proximal branches,

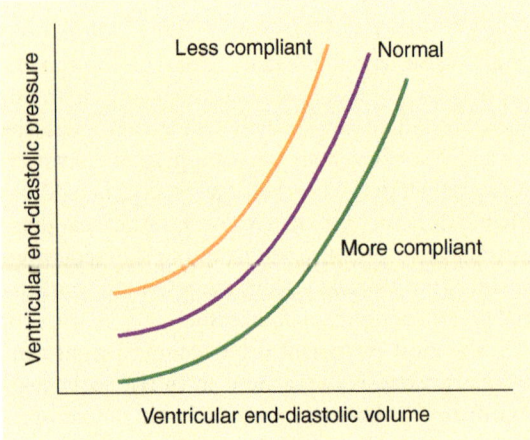

FIGURE 20–5 Normal and abnormal ventricular compliance.

and blood (viscosity and density); and **systemic vascular resistance (SVR)**. Arteriolar tone is the primary determinant of SVR. Because viscoelastic properties are generally fixed in any given patient, left ventricular afterload is usually equated clinically with SVR, which is calculated by the following equation:

$$SVR = 80 \times \frac{MAP - CVP}{CO}$$

where MAP is mean arterial pressure in millimeters of mercury, CVP is central venous pressure in millimeters of mercury, and CO is cardiac output in liters per minute. Normal SVR is 900–1500 dyn · s cm^{-5}. Systolic blood pressure may also be used as an approximation of left ventricular afterload in the absence of chronic changes in the size, shape, or thickness of the ventricular wall or acute changes in systemic vascular resistance. Some clinicians prefer to use CI instead of CO in calculating a systemic vascular resistance index (SVRI), so that SVRI = SVR × BSA.

Right ventricular afterload is mainly dependent on pulmonary vascular resistance (PVR) and is expressed by the following equation:

$$PVR = 80 \times \frac{PAP - LAP}{CO}$$

where PAP is mean pulmonary artery pressure and LAP is left atrial pressure. In practice, pulmonary capillary wedge pressure (PCWP) is usually substituted as an approximation for LAP. Normal PVR is 50–150 dyn · s cm^{-5}.

Cardiac output is inversely related to large changes in afterload on the left ventricle; however, small increases or decreases in afterload may have no effect at all on cardiac output. Because of its thinner wall, the right ventricle is more sensitive to changes in afterload than is the left ventricle. **7** Cardiac output in patients with marked right or left ventricular impairment is very sensitive to acute increases in afterload. The latter is particularly true in the presence of drug- or ischemia-induced myocardial depression or chronic heart failure.

Contractility

Cardiac contractility (inotropy) is the intrinsic ability of the myocardium to pump in the absence of changes in preload or afterload. Contractility is related to the rate of myocardial muscle shortening, which is, in turn, dependent on the intracellular Ca^{2+} concentration during systole. Increases in heart rate can also enhance contractility under some conditions, perhaps because of the increased availability of intracellular Ca^{2+}.

Contractility can be altered by neural, humoral, or pharmacological influences. Sympathetic nervous system activity normally has the most important effect on contractility. Sympathetic fibers innervate atrial and ventricular muscle, as well as nodal tissues. In addition to its positive chronotropic effect, norepinephrine release also enhances contractility primarily via β$_1$-receptor activation. α-Adrenergic receptors are also present in the myocardium, but seem to have only minor positive inotropic and chronotropic effects. Sympathomimetic drugs and secretion of epinephrine from the adrenal glands similarly increase contractility via β$_1$-receptor activation.

Myocardial contractility is depressed by hypoxia, acidosis, depletion of catecholamine stores within the heart, and loss of functioning muscle mass as a result of ischemia or infarction. At large enough doses, most anesthetics and antiarrhythmic agents are negative inotropes (ie, they decrease contractility).

Wall Motion Abnormalities

Regional wall motion abnormalities cause a breakdown of the analogy between the intact heart and skeletal muscle preparations. Such abnormalities may be due to ischemia, scarring, hypertrophy, or altered conduction. When the ventricular cavity does not collapse symmetrically or fully, emptying becomes impaired. Hypokinesis (decreased contraction), akinesis (failure to contract), and dyskinesis (paradoxic bulging) during systole reflect increasing degrees of contraction abnormalities. Although contractility may be normal or even enhanced in some areas, abnormalities in other areas of the ventricle can impair emptying and reduce stroke volume. The severity of the impairment depends on the size and number of abnormally contracting areas.

Valvular Dysfunction

Valvular dysfunction can involve any one of the four valves in the heart and can include stenosis, regurgitation (incompetence), or both. Stenosis of an AV valve (tricuspid or mitral) reduces stroke volume primarily by decreasing ventricular preload, whereas stenosis of a semilunar valve (pulmonary or aortic) reduces stroke volume primarily by increasing ventricular afterload. In contrast, valvular regurgitation can reduce stroke volume without changes in preload, afterload, or contractility and without wall motion abnormalities. The effective stroke volume is reduced by the regurgitant volume with every contraction. When an AV valve is incompetent, a significant part of the ventricular end-diastolic volume can flow backward into the atrium during systole; the stroke volume is reduced by the regurgitant volume. Similarly, when a semilunar valve is incompetent, a fraction of end-diastolic volume arises from backward flow into the ventricle during diastole.

ASSESSMENT OF VENTRICULAR FUNCTION

1. Ventricular Function Curves

Plotting cardiac output or stroke volume against preload is useful in evaluating pathological states and understanding drug therapy. Normal right and left ventricular function curves are shown in Figure 20–6.

Ventricular pressure–volume diagrams are useful because they dissociate contractility from both preload and afterload. Two points are identified on such diagrams: the end-systolic point (ESP) and the end-diastolic point (EDP) (Figure 20–7). ESP is reflective of systolic function, whereas EDP is more reflective of diastolic function. For any given contractile state, all ESPs are on the same line (ie, the relationship between end-systolic volume and end-systolic pressure is fixed).

2. Assessment of Systolic Function

The change in ventricular pressure over time during systole (*dP/dt*) is defined by the first derivative of the ventricular pressure curve and is often used

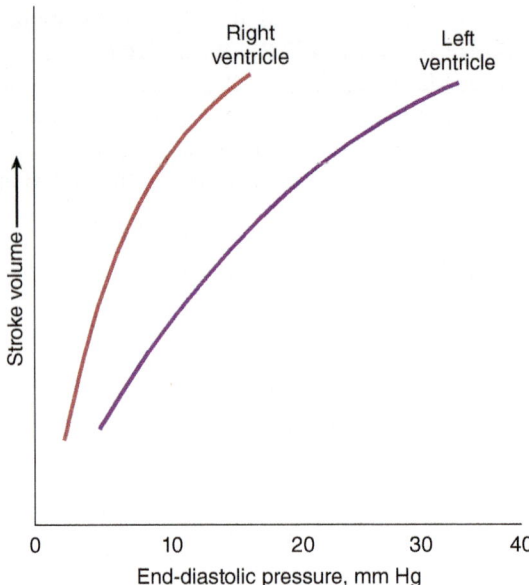

FIGURE 20–6 Function curves for the left and right ventricles.

as a measure of contractility. Contractility is directly proportional to *dP/dt*, but accurate measurement of this value requires a high-fidelity ("Millar") ventricular catheter; however, it can be estimated with echocardiography. Although arterial pressure tracings are distorted due to properties of the vascular tree, the initial rate of rise in pressure (the slope) can serve as a rough approximation; the more proximally the arterial line catheter is located in the arterial tree, the more accurate the extrapolation will be. The usefulness of *dP/dt* is also limited in that it may be affected by preload, afterload, and heart rate.

Ejection Fraction

8 The ventricular ejection fraction (EF), the fraction of the end-diastolic ventricular volume ejected, is the most commonly used clinical measurement of systolic function. EF can be calculated by the following equation:

$$EF = \frac{EDV - ESV}{EDV}$$

where EDV is left ventricular diastolic volume and ESV is end-systolic volume. Normal EF is

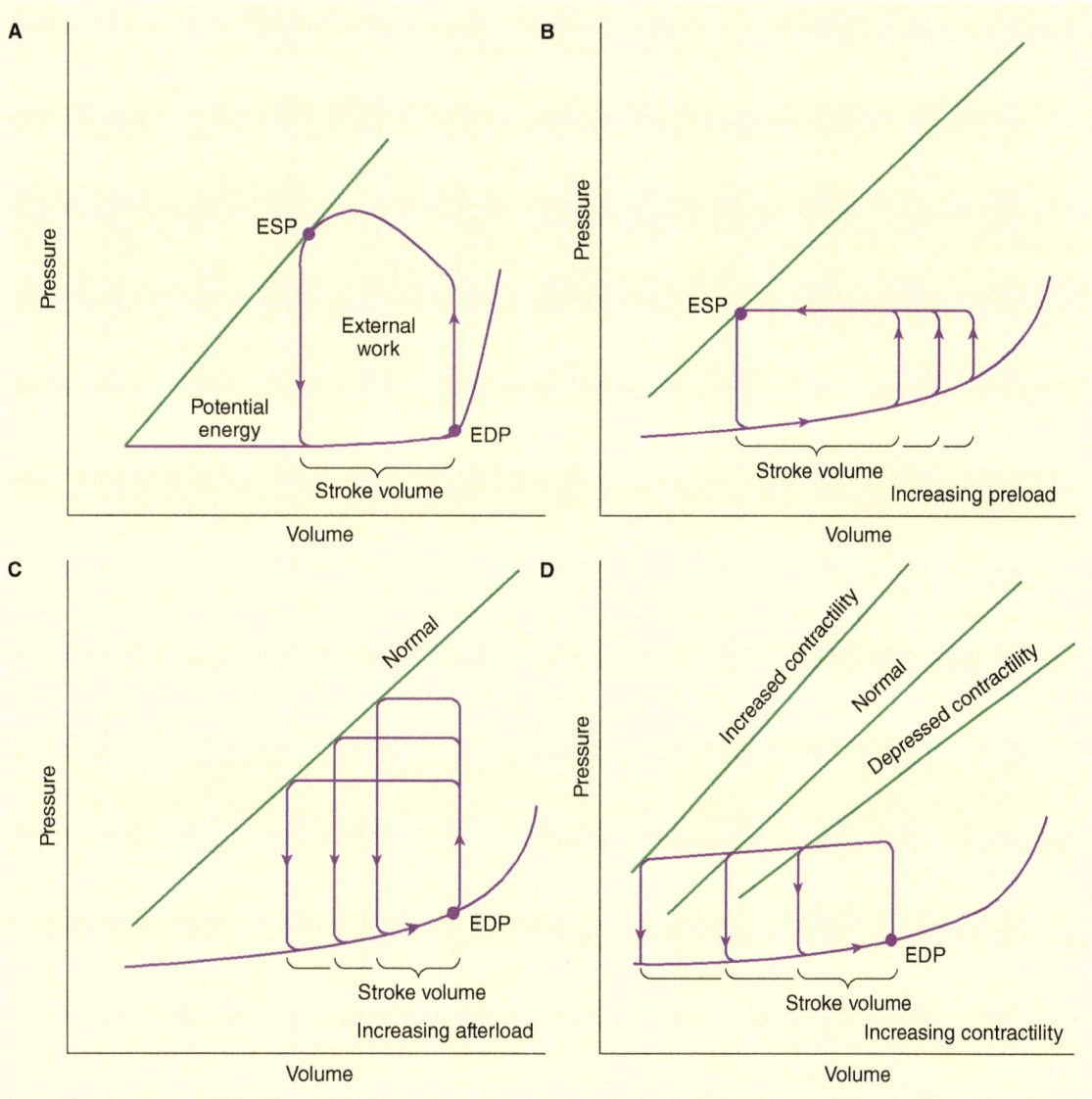

FIGURE 20–7 Ventricular pressure-volume diagrams. **A:** A single ventricular contraction. Note that stroke volume represents change in volume on the x-axis (difference between end-systolic volume and end-diastolic volume). Note also that the circumscribed area represents external work performed by the ventricle.
B: Increasing preload with constant contractility and afterload. **C:** Increasing afterload with constant preload and contractility. **D:** Increasing contractility with constant preload and afterload. ESP, end-systolic point; EDP, end-diastolic point.

approximately 0.67 ± 0.08. Measurements can be made preoperatively from cardiac catheterization, radionucleotide studies, or transthoracic (TTE) or transesophageal echocardiography (TEE).

Pulmonary artery catheters with fast-response thermistors allow measurement of the right ventricular EF. Unfortunately, when pulmonary vascular resistance increases, decreases in right ventricular

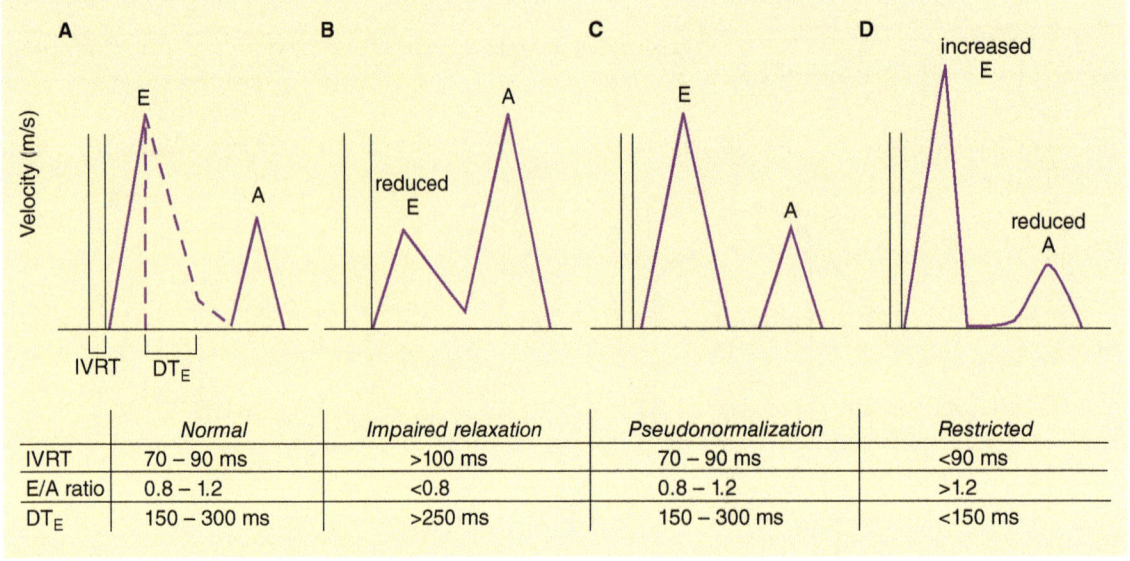

	Normal	Impaired relaxation	Pseudonormalization	Restricted
IVRT	70 – 90 ms	>100 ms	70 – 90 ms	<90 ms
E/A ratio	0.8 – 1.2	<0.8	0.8 – 1.2	>1.2
DT$_E$	150 – 300 ms	>250 ms	150 – 300 ms	<150 ms

FIGURE 20–8 Doppler echocardiography of diastolic flow across the mitral valve. **A–D** (from left to right) represents increasing severity of diastolic dysfunction. E, early diastolic flow; A, peak atrial systolic flow; IVRT, isovolumic relaxation time; DT$_E$, deceleration time of E.

EF may reflect afterload rather than contractility. Left ventricular EF is not an accurate measure of ventricular contractility in the presence of mitral insufficiency.

3. Assessment of Diastolic Function

9 Left ventricular diastolic function can be assessed clinically by Doppler echocardiography on a transthoracic or transesophageal examination. Flow velocities are measured across the mitral valve during diastole. Three patterns of diastolic dysfunction are generally recognized based on isovolumetric relaxation time, the ratio of peak early diastolic flow (E) to peak atrial systolic flow (A), and the deceleration time (DT) of E (DT$_E$) (Figure 20–8). Tissue Doppler is frequently used to distinguish "pseudonormal" from normal diastolic function. Tissue Doppler is also an excellent way to detect "conventional" diastolic dysfunction. An e' wave peak velocity of less than 8 cm/sec is associated with impaired diastolic function. An E/e' wave ratio that is greater than 15 is consistent with elevated left ventricular end-diastolic pressure (Figure 20–9).

Systemic Circulation

The systemic vasculature can be divided functionally into arteries, arterioles, capillaries, and veins. Arteries are the high-pressure conduits that supply the various organs. Arterioles are the small vessels that directly feed and control blood flow through each capillary bed. Capillaries are thin-walled vessels that allow the exchange of nutrients between blood and tissues. Veins return blood from capillary beds to the heart.

The distribution of blood between the various components of the circulatory system is shown in Table 20–5. Note that most of the blood volume is in the systemic circulation—specifically, within systemic veins. Changes in systemic venous tone allow these vessels to function as a reservoir for blood. Following significant blood or fluid losses, a sympathetically mediated increase in venous tone reduces the caliber of these vessels and shifts blood into other parts of the vascular system. Conversely, venodilation allows these vessels to accommodate increases in blood volume. Sympathetic control of venous tone is an important determinant of venous

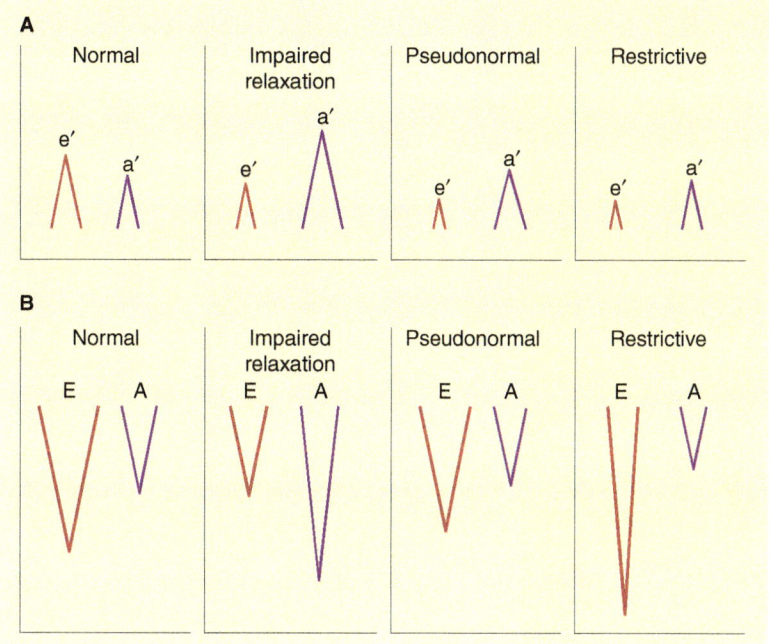

FIGURE 20–9 Tissue Doppler. **A**: Tissue Doppler at the lateral mitral annulus. During diastole the annulus moves toward the transesophageal examination transducer in the esophagus. Thus the e′ and a′ waves of diastolic filling are positive deflections above the baseline. **B**: When transesophageal examination is used to measure transmitral diastolic inflow, the E and A waves of early and late filling are below the baseline because flow is moving away from the Doppler probe in the esophagus. Tissue Doppler can be used to distinguish normal from pseudonormal diastolic inflow pattern because the e′ wave remains depressed as diastolic dysfunction progresses. (Reproduced with permission from Wasnick JD, et al: *Cardiac Anesthesia and Transesophageal Echocardiography*, McGraw-Hill, 2011.)

return to the heart. Reduced venous tone following induction of anesthesia frequently results in venous pooling of blood and contributes to hypotension.

A multiplicity of factors influences blood flow in the vascular tree. These include mechanisms of local and metabolic control, endothelium-derived factors, the autonomic nervous system, and circulating hormones.

TABLE 20–5 Distribution of blood volume.

Heart	7%
Pulmonary circulation	9%
Systemic circulation	
Arterial	15%
Capillary	5%
Venous	64%

AUTOREGULATION

Most tissue beds regulate their own blood flow (autoregulation). Arterioles generally dilate in response to reduced perfusion pressure or increased tissue demand. Conversely, arterioles constrict in response to increased pressure or reduced tissue demand. These phenomena are likely due to both an intrinsic response of vascular smooth muscle to stretch and the accumulation of vasodilatory metabolic by-products. The latter may include K^+, H^+, CO_2, adenosine, and lactate.

ENDOTHELIUM-DERIVED FACTORS

The vascular endothelium is metabolically active in elaborating or modifying substances that directly or indirectly play a major role in controlling blood pressure and flow. These include vasodilators (eg, nitric oxide, prostacyclin [PGI_2]), vasoconstrictors (eg, endothelins, thromboxane A_2), anticoagulants (eg, thrombomodulin, protein C), fibrinolytics (eg, tissue plasminogen activator), and factors that inhibit platelet aggregation (eg, nitric oxide and PGI_2). Nitric oxide is synthesized from arginine by nitric oxide synthetase. This substance has a number of functions In the circulation, it is a potent vasodilator. It binds guanylate cyclase, increasing cGMP levels and producing vasodilation. Endothelially derived vasoconstrictors (endothelins) are released in response to thrombin and epinephrine.

AUTONOMIC CONTROL OF THE SYSTEMIC VASCULATURE

Although the parasympathetic system can exert important influences on the circulation, autonomic control of the vasculature is primarily sympathetic. Sympathetic outflow to the circulation passes out of the spinal cord at all thoracic segments and the first two lumbar segments. These fibers reach blood vessels via specific autonomic nerves or by traveling along spinal nerves. Sympathetic fibers innervate all parts of the vasculature except for capillaries. Their principal function is to regulate vascular tone. Variations of arterial vascular tone serve to regulate blood pressure and the distribution of blood flow to the various organs, whereas variations in venous tone alter vascular capacity, venous pooling, and venous return to the heart.

The vasculature has sympathetic vasoconstrictor and vasodilator fibers, but the former are more important physiologically in most tissue beds. Sympathetic-induced vasoconstriction (via α_1-adrenergic receptors) can be potent in skeletal muscle, kidneys, gut, and skin; it is least active in the brain and heart. The most important vasodilatory fibers are those feeding skeletal muscle, mediating increased blood flow (via β_2-adrenergic receptors) in response to exercise. Vasodepressor (vasovagal) syncope, which can occur following intense emotional strain associated with high sympathetic tone, results from reflex activation of both vagal and sympathetic vasodilator fibers.

Vascular tone and autonomic influences on the heart are controlled by vasomotor centers in the reticular formation of the medulla and lower pons. Distinct vasoconstrictor and vasodilator areas have been identified. Vasoconstriction is mediated by the anterolateral areas of the lower pons and upper medulla. They are also responsible for adrenal secretion of catecholamines, as well as the enhancement of cardiac automaticity and contractility. Vasodilatory areas, which are located in the lower medulla, are also adrenergic, but function by projecting inhibitory fibers upward to the vasoconstrictor areas. Vasomotor output is modified by inputs from throughout the central nervous system, including the hypothalamus, cerebral cortex, and the other areas in the brainstem. Areas in the posterolateral medulla receive input from both the vagal and the glossopharyngeal nerves and play an important role in mediating a variety of circulatory reflexes. The sympathetic system normally maintains some tonic vasoconstriction on the vascular tree. Loss of this tone following induction of anesthesia or sympathectomy frequently contributes to perioperative hypotension.

ARTERIAL BLOOD PRESSURE

Systemic blood flow is pulsatile in large arteries because of the heart's cyclic activity; by the time blood reaches the systemic capillaries, flow is continuous (laminar). The mean pressure falls to less than 20 mm Hg in the large systemic veins that return blood to the heart. The largest pressure drop, nearly 50%, is across the arterioles, and the arterioles account for the majority of SVR.

MAP is proportionate to the product of SVR × CO. This relationship is based on an analogy to Ohm's law, as applied to the circulation:

$$MAP - CVP \approx SVR \times CO$$

Because CVP is normally very small compared with MAP, the former can usually be ignored. From this relationship, it is readily apparent that hypotension is the result of a decrease in SVR, CO, or both: To maintain arterial blood pressure, a decrease in either SVR or CO must be compensated by an increase in the other. MAP can be measured as the integrated mean of the arterial pressure waveform.

Alternatively, MAP may be estimated by the following formula:

$$MAP = Diastolic\ pressure + \frac{Pulse\ pressure}{3}$$

where pulse pressure is the difference between systolic and diastolic blood pressure. Arterial pulse pressure is directly related to stroke volume, but is inversely proportional to the compliance of the arterial tree. Thus, decreases in pulse pressure may be due to a decrease in stroke volume, an increase in SVR, or both. Increased pulse pressure increases shear stress on vessel walls, potentially leading to atherosclerotic plaque rupture and thrombosis or rupture of aneurysms. Increased pulse pressure in patients undergoing cardiac surgery has been associated with adverse renal and neurological outcomes.

Transmission of the arterial pressure wave from large arteries to smaller vessels in the periphery is faster than the actual movement of blood; the pressure wave velocity is 15 times the velocity of blood in the aorta. Moreover, reflections of the propagating waves off arterial walls widen pulse pressure before the pulse wave is completely dampened in very small arteries.

Control of Arterial Blood Pressure

Arterial blood pressure is regulated by a series of immediate, intermediate, and long-term adjustments that involve complex neural, humoral, and renal mechanisms.

A. Immediate Control

Minute-to-minute control of blood pressure is primarily the function of autonomic nervous system reflexes. Changes in blood pressure are sensed both centrally (in hypothalamic and brainstem areas) and peripherally by specialized sensors (baroreceptors). Decreases in arterial blood pressure result in increased sympathetic tone, increased adrenal secretion of epinephrine, and reduced vagal activity. **The resulting systemic vasoconstriction, increased heart rate, and enhanced cardiac contractility serve to increase blood pressure**.

Peripheral baroreceptors are located at the bifurcation of the common carotid arteries and the aortic arch. Elevations in blood pressure increase baroreceptor discharge, inhibiting systemic vasoconstriction and enhancing vagal tone (**baroreceptor reflex**). Reductions in blood pressure decrease baroreceptor discharge, allowing vasoconstriction and reduction of vagal tone. Carotid baroreceptors send afferent signals to circulatory brainstem centers via Hering's nerve (a branch of the glossopharyngeal nerve), whereas aortic baroreceptor afferent signals travel along the vagus nerve. Of the two peripheral sensors, the carotid baroreceptor is physiologically more important and is primarily responsible for minimizing changes in blood pressure that are caused by acute events, such as a change in posture. Carotid baroreceptors sense MAP most effectively between pressures of 80 and 160 mm Hg. Adaptation to acute changes in blood pressure occurs over the course of 1–2 days, rendering this reflex ineffective for longer term blood pressure control. All volatile anesthetics depress the normal baroreceptor response, but isoflurane and desflurane seem to have less effect. Cardiopulmonary stretch receptors located in the atria, left ventricle, and pulmonary circulation can cause a similar effect.

B. Intermediate Control

In the course of a few minutes, sustained decreases in arterial pressure, together with enhanced sympathetic outflow, activate the renin–angiotensin–aldosterone system, increase secretion of arginine vasopressin (AVP), and alter normal capillary fluid exchange. Both angiotensin II and AVP are potent arteriolar vasoconstrictors. Their immediate action is to increase SVR. In contrast to formation of angiotensin II, which responds to relatively smaller changes, sufficient AVP secretion to produce vasoconstriction will only occur in response to more marked degrees of hypotension. Angiotensin constricts arterioles via AT_1 receptors. AVP mediates vasoconstriction via V_1 receptors and exerts its antidiuretic effect via V_2 receptors.

Sustained changes in arterial blood pressure can also alter fluid exchange in tissues by their secondary effects on capillary pressures. Hypertension increases interstitial movement of intravascular fluid, whereas hypotension increases reabsorption of interstitial fluid. Such compensatory changes in intravascular volume can reduce fluctuations in blood pressure, particularly in the absence of adequate renal function (see below).

C. Long-Term Control

The effects of slower renal mechanisms become apparent within hours of sustained changes in arterial pressure. As a result, the kidneys alter total body sodium and water balance to restore blood pressure to normal. Hypotension results in sodium (and water) retention, whereas hypertension generally increases sodium excretion in normal individuals.

ANATOMY & PHYSIOLOGY OF THE CORONARY CIRCULATION

1. Anatomy

Myocardial blood supply is derived entirely from the right and left coronary arteries (**Figure 20–10**). Blood flows from epicardial to endocardial vessels. After perfusing the myocardium, blood returns to the right atrium via the coronary sinus and the anterior cardiac veins. A small amount of blood returns directly into the chambers of the heart by way of the thebesian veins.

The right coronary artery (RCA) normally supplies the right atrium, most of the right ventricle, and a variable portion of the left ventricle (inferior wall). In 85% of persons, the RCA gives rise to the posterior descending artery (PDA), which supplies the superior–posterior interventricular septum and inferior wall—a right dominant circulation; in the remaining 15% of persons, the PDA is a branch of the left coronary artery—a left dominant circulation.

The left coronary artery normally supplies the left atrium and most of the interventricular septum and left ventricle (septal, anterior, and lateral walls). After a short course, the left main coronary artery bifurcates into the left anterior descending artery (LAD) and the circumflex artery (CX); the LAD supplies the septum and anterior wall and the CX supplies the lateral wall. In a left dominant circulation, the CX wraps around the AV groove and continues down as the PDA to also supply most of the posterior septum and inferior wall.

The arterial supply to the SA node may be derived from either the RCA (60% of individuals)

or the LAD (the remaining 40%). The AV node is usually supplied by the RCA (85% to 90%) or, less frequently, by the CX (10% to 15%); the bundle of His has a dual blood supply derived from the PDA and LAD. The anterior papillary muscle of the mitral valve also has a dual blood supply that is fed by diagonal branches of the LAD and marginal branches of the CX. In contrast, the posterior papillary of the mitral valve is usually supplied only by the PDA and is therefore much more vulnerable to ischemic dysfunction.

2. Determinants of Coronary Perfusion

Coronary perfusion is unique in that it is intermittent rather than continuous, as it is in other organs. During contraction, intramyocardial pressures in the left ventricle approach systemic arterial pressure. The force of left ventricular contraction almost completely occludes the intramyocardial part of the coronary arteries; in fact, blood flow may transiently reverse in epicardial vessels. Even during the latter part of diastole, left ventricular pressure eventually exceeds venous (right atrial) pressure. **Thus, coronary perfusion pressure is usually determined by the difference between aortic pressure and ventricular pressure**, and the left ventricle is perfused almost entirely during diastole. In contrast, the right ventricle is perfused during both systole and diastole (**Figure 20–11**). Moreover, as a determinant of myocardial blood flow, arterial diastolic pressure is more important than MAP:

$$\text{Coronary perfusion pressure} = \text{Arterial diastolic pressure} - \text{LVEDP}$$

Decreases in aortic pressure or increases in ventricular end-diastolic pressure can reduce coronary perfusion pressure. Increases in heart rate also decrease coronary perfusion because of the disproportionately greater reduction in diastolic time as heart rate increases (**Figure 20–12**). Because it is subjected to the greatest intramural pressures during systole, the endocardium tends to be most vulnerable to ischemia during decreases in coronary perfusion pressure.

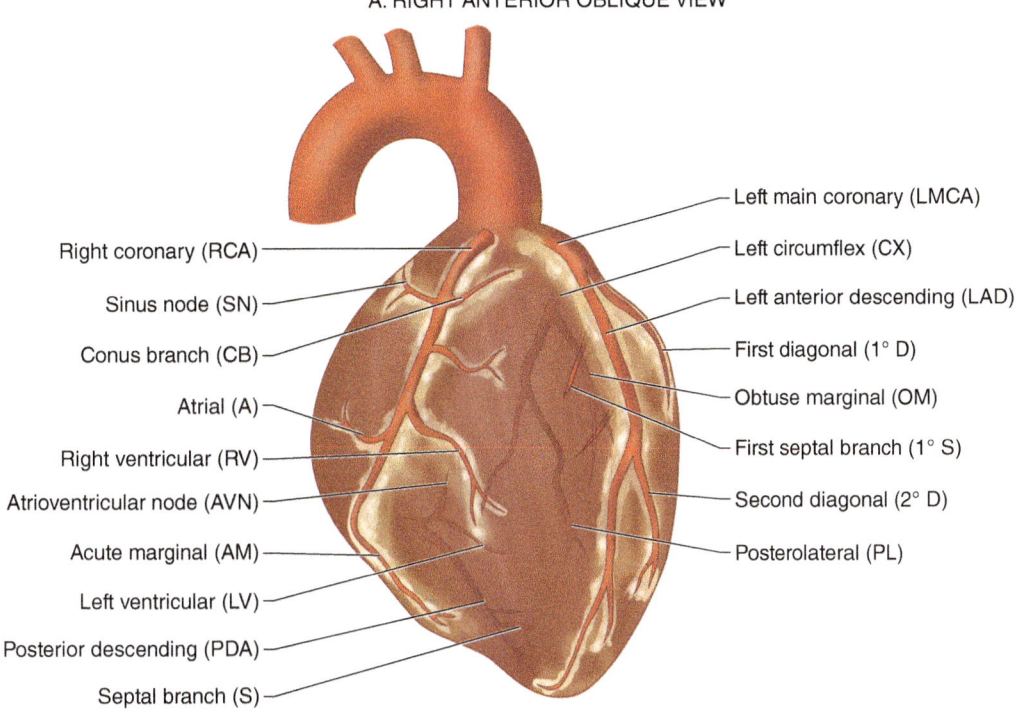

A. RIGHT ANTERIOR OBLIQUE VIEW

Right coronary (RCA)
Sinus node (SN)
Conus branch (CB)
Atrial (A)
Right ventricular (RV)
Atrioventricular node (AVN)
Acute marginal (AM)
Left ventricular (LV)
Posterior descending (PDA)
Septal branch (S)

Left main coronary (LMCA)
Left circumflex (CX)
Left anterior descending (LAD)
First diagonal (1° D)
Obtuse marginal (OM)
First septal branch (1° S)
Second diagonal (2° D)
Posterolateral (PL)

B. LEFT ANTERIOR OBLIQUE VIEW

CB
SN
RCA
RV
AVN
AM
PD

LMCA
CX
LAD
1° D
OM
2° D
PL
LV

FIGURE 20–10 Anatomy of the coronary arteries in a patient with a right dominant circulation. **A:** Right anterior oblique view. **B:** Left anterior oblique view.

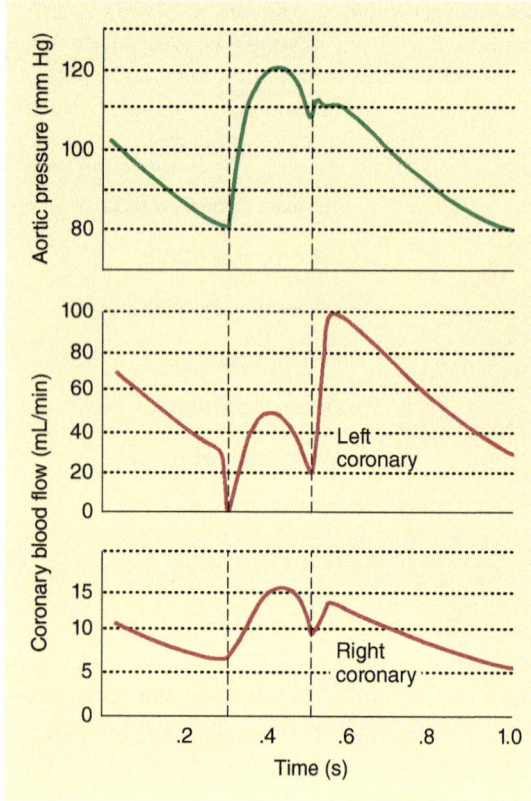

FIGURE 20–11 Coronary blood flow during the cardiac cycle. (Modified and reproduced, with permission, from Pappano A, Wier W: *Cardiovascular Physiology*, 10th ed. Mosby, 2013.)

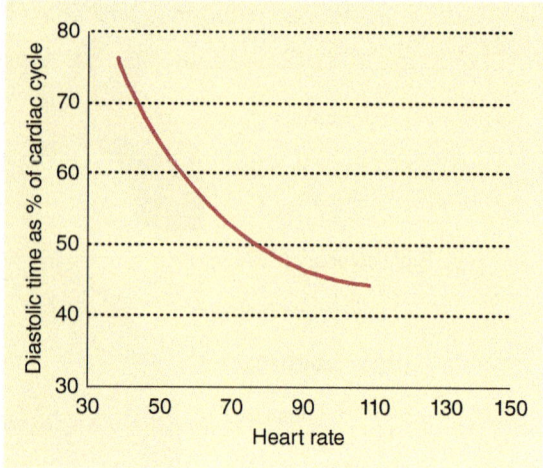

FIGURE 20–12 The relationship between diastolic time and heart rate.

Control of Coronary Blood Flow

Coronary blood flow normally parallels myocardial metabolic demand. In the average adult man, coronary blood flow is approximately 250 mL/min at rest. The myocardium regulates its own blood flow closely between perfusion pressures of 50 and 120 mm Hg. Beyond this range, blood flow becomes increasingly pressure dependent.

Under normal conditions, changes in blood flow are entirely due to variations in coronary arterial tone (resistance) in response to metabolic demand. Hypoxia—either directly, or indirectly through the release of adenosine—causes coronary vasodilation. Autonomic influences are generally weak. Both α_1- and β_2-adrenergic receptors are present in the coronary arteries. The α_1-receptors are primarily located on larger epicardial vessels, whereas the β_2-receptors are mainly found on the smaller intramuscular and subendocardial vessels. Sympathetic stimulation generally increases myocardial blood flow because of an increase in metabolic demand and a predominance of β_2-receptor activation. Parasympathetic effects on the coronary vasculature are generally minor and weakly vasodilatory.

3. Myocardial Oxygen Balance

Myocardial oxygen demand is usually the most important determinant of myocardial blood flow. Relative contributions to oxygen requirements include basal requirements (20%), electrical activity (1%), volume work (15%), and pressure work (64%). The myocardium usually extracts 65% of the oxygen in arterial blood, compared with 25% in most other tissues. Coronary sinus oxygen saturation is usually 30%. Therefore, the myocardium (unlike other tissues) cannot compensate for reductions in blood flow by extracting more oxygen from hemoglobin. Any increases in myocardial metabolic demand must be met by an increase in coronary blood flow. Table 20–6 lists the most important factors in myocardial oxygen demand and supply. Note that the heart rate and, to a lesser extent, ventricular

TABLE 20–6 Factors affecting myocardial oxygen supply–demand balance.

Supply
   Heart rate (diastolic filling time)
   Coronary perfusion pressure
      Aortic diastolic blood pressure
      Ventricular end-diastolic pressure
   Arterial oxygen content
      Arterial oxygen tension
      Hemoglobin concentration
   Coronary vessel diameter

Demand
   Basal metabolic requirements
   Heart rate
   Wall tension
      Preload (ventricular radius)
      Afterload
   Contractility

end-diastolic pressure are important determinants of both supply and demand.

EFFECTS OF ANESTHETIC AGENTS

Most volatile anesthetic agents are coronary vasodilators. Their effect on coronary blood flow is variable because of their direct vasodilating properties, reduction of myocardial metabolic requirements (and secondary decrease due to autoregulation), and effects on arterial blood pressure. The mechanism is not clear, and these effects are unlikely to have any clinical importance. Halothane and isoflurane seem to have the greatest effect; the former primarily affects large coronary vessels, whereas the latter affects mostly smaller vessels. Vasodilation due to desflurane seems to be primarily autonomically mediated, whereas sevoflurane seems to lack coronary vasodilating properties. Dose-dependent abolition of autoregulation may be greatest with isoflurane.

Volatile agents exert beneficial effects in experimental myocardial ischemia and infarction. They reduce myocardial oxygen requirements and protect against reperfusion injury; these effects are mediated by activation of ATP-sensitive K^+ (K_{ATP}) channels. Some evidence also suggests that volatile anesthetics enhance recovery of the "stunned" myocardium (hypocontractile, but recoverable, myocardium after ischemia). Moreover, although volatile anesthetics decrease myocardial contractility, they can be potentially beneficial in patients with heart failure because most of them decrease preload and afterload.

The Pathophysiology of Heart Failure

Systolic heart failure occurs when the heart is unable to pump a sufficient amount of blood to meet the body's metabolic requirements. Clinical manifestations usually reflect the effects of the low cardiac output on tissues (eg, fatigue, dyspnea, oxygen debt, acidosis), the damming-up of blood behind the failing ventricle (dependent edema or pulmonary venous congestion), or both. The left ventricle is most commonly the primary cause, often with secondary involvement of the right ventricle. Isolated right ventricular failure can occur in the setting of advanced disease of the lung parenchyma or pulmonary vasculature. Left ventricular failure is most commonly the result of myocardial dysfunction, usually from coronary artery disease, but may also be the result of viral disease, toxins, untreated hypertension, valvular dysfunction, arrhythmias, or pericardial disease.

Diastolic dysfunction can be present in the absence of signs or symptoms of heart failure. Symptoms arising from diastolic dysfunction are the result of atrial hypertension (Figure 20–13). Failure of the heart to relax during diastole leads to elevated left ventricular end-diastolic pressure, which is transmitted to the left atrium and pulmonary vasculature. Common causes of diastolic dysfunction include hypertension, coronary artery disease, hypertrophic cardiomyopathy, valvular heart disease, and pericardial disease. Although diastolic dysfunction can occasionally cause symptoms of heart failure, even in the presence of normal systolic function (normal left ventricular ejection fraction), it nearly always occurs in association with systolic dysfunction in patients with heart failure.

Diastolic dysfunction is diagnosed echocardiographically. Placing the pulse wave Doppler sample gate at the tips of the mitral valve during

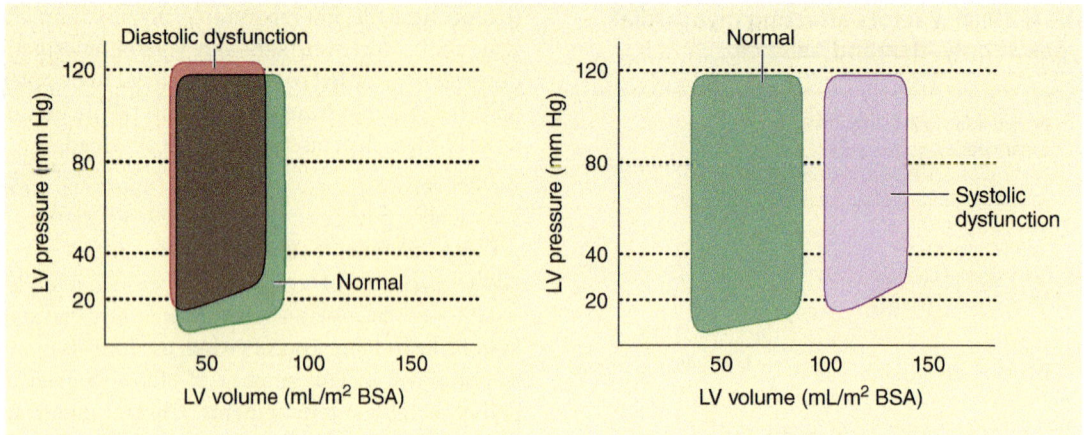

FIGURE 20–13 Ventricular pressure–volume relationships in isolated systolic and diastolic dysfunction.

left ventricular filling will produce the characteristic diastolic flow pattern (Figure 20–9). In patients with normal diastolic function, the ratio between the peak velocities of the early (E) and the atrial (A) waves is from 0.8 to 2. In the early stages of diastolic dysfunction, the primary abnormality is impaired relaxation. When left ventricular relaxation is delayed, the initial pressure gradient between the left atrium and the left ventricle is reduced, resulting in a decline in early filling, and, consequently, a reduced peak E wave velocity. The A wave velocity is increased relative to the E wave, and the E/A ratio is reduced. As diastolic dysfunction advances, the left atrial pressure increases, restoring the gradient between the left atrium and left ventricle with an apparent restoration of the normal E/A ratio. This pattern is characterized as "pseudonormalized." Using the E/A ratio alone cannot distinguish between a normal and pseudonormalized pattern of diastolic inflow. As diastolic dysfunction worsens further, a restrictive pattern is obtained. In this scenario, the left ventricle is so stiff that pressure builds in the left atrium, resulting in a dramatic peak of early filling and a prominent, tall, narrow E wave. Because the ventricle is so poorly compliant, the atrial contraction contributes little to filling, resulting in a diminished A wave and an E/A ratio greater than 2:1.

Doppler patterns of pulmonary venous flow have been used to distinguish between a pseudonormalized and normal E/A ratio. Currently, most echocardiographers use tissue Doppler to examine the movement of the lateral annulus of the mitral valve during ventricular filling (Figure 20–9). Tissue Doppler allows the echocardiographer to determine both the velocity and the direction of the movement of the heart. During systole, the heart contracts toward the apex, away from a TEE transducer in the esophagus. This motion produces the s' wave of systole. During early and late diastolic filling, the heart moves toward the transducer producing the e' and a' waves. Like the inflow patterns achieved with pulse wave Doppler, characteristic patterns of diastolic dysfunction are reflected in the tissue Doppler trace. An e' wave less than 8 cm/sec is consistent with diastolic dysfunction. Of note, the tissue Doppler trace does not produce a pseudonormalized pattern permitting the echocardiographer to readily distinguish between normal and abnormal diastolic function.

Cardiac output *may* be reduced at rest with heart failure, but the key point is that the heart is incapable of appropriately *increasing* cardiac output and oxygen delivery in response to demand. Inadequate oxygen delivery to tissues is reflected by a low mixed venous oxygen tension and an increase in the arteriovenous oxygen content difference. In compensated heart failure, the arteriovenous difference may be normal at rest, but it rapidly widens during stress or exercise.

Heart failure is less commonly associated with an elevated cardiac output. This form of heart failure is most often seen with sepsis, thyrotoxicosis, and other hypermetabolic states, which are typically associated with a low SVR.

COMPENSATORY MECHANISMS

Compensatory mechanisms generally present in patients with heart failure include increased preload, activation of the sympathetic nervous system and the renin–angiotensin–aldosterone system, and increased release of AVP. Although these mechanisms can initially compensate for mild to moderate cardiac dysfunction, with increasing severity of dysfunction, they may actually contribute to the cardiac impairment. Many of the drug treatments of chronic heart failure serve to counteract these mechanisms.

Increased Preload

An increase in ventricular size not only reflects an inability to keep up with an increased circulating blood volume, but also serves to increase stroke volume by moving the heart up the Starling curve (see Figure 20–4). Even when EF is reduced, an increase in ventricular end-diastolic volume can maintain a normal stroke volume. Worsening venous congestion caused by the pooling of blood behind the failing ventricle and excessive ventricular dilatation can rapidly lead to clinical deterioration. Left ventricular failure results in pulmonary vascular congestion and progressive transudation of fluid, first into the pulmonary interstitium and then into alveoli (pulmonary edema). Right ventricular failure leads to systemic venous hypertension, which results in peripheral edema, hepatic congestion and dysfunction, and ascites. Dilatation of the annulus of either AV valve leads to valvular regurgitation, further impairing ventricular output.

Increased Sympathetic Tone

Sympathetic activation increases release of norepinephrine from nerve endings in the heart and the adrenal secretion of epinephrine into the circulation. Plasma catecholamine levels are generally directly proportional to the degree of left ventricular dysfunction. Although enhanced sympathetic outflow can initially maintain cardiac output by increasing heart rate and contractility, worsening ventricular function elicits increasing degrees of vasoconstriction in an effort to maintain arterial blood pressure. The associated increase in afterload, however, reduces cardiac output and exacerbates the ventricular failure.

Chronic sympathetic activation in patients with heart failure eventually decreases the response of adrenergic receptors to catecholamines (receptor uncoupling), the number of receptors (downregulation), and cardiac catecholamine stores. **11** Nonetheless, the failing heart becomes increasingly dependent on circulating catecholamines. Abrupt withdrawal in sympathetic outflow or decreases in circulating catecholamine levels, such as can occur following induction of anesthesia, may lead to acute cardiac decompensation. A reduced density of M_2 receptors also decreases parasympathetic influences on the heart.

Sympathetic activation tends to redistribute systemic blood flow output away from the skin, gut, kidneys, and skeletal muscle to the heart and brain. Decreased renal perfusion, together with β_1-adrenergic activity at the juxtaglomerular apparatus, activates the renin–angiotensin–aldosterone axis, which leads to sodium retention and interstitial edema. Moreover, vasoconstriction secondary to elevated angiotensin II levels increases left ventricular afterload and causes further deterioration of systolic function. The latter partially accounts for the efficacy of angiotensin-converting enzyme (ACE) inhibitors and angiotensin receptor blockers in heart failure. Symptoms may also improve in some patients with careful, low-dose β-adrenergic blockade. Outcomes in heart failure are improved by administration of ACE inhibitors (and/or angiotensin receptor blockers), certain long-acting β-blockers (carvedilol or extended release metoprolol), and aldosterone inhibitors (spironolactone or eplerenone).

Circulating AVP levels, often markedly increased in patients with severe heart failure, will increase ventricular afterload and are responsible for a defect in free water clearance that is commonly associated with hyponatremia.

Brain natriuretic peptide (BNP) is produced in the heart in response to myocyte distention. Elevated BNP concentration (>500 pg/mL) usually indicates heart failure, and measurement of BNP concentration can be used to distinguish between heart failure and lung disease as a cause of dyspnea. Recombinant BNP was developed as a vasodilator and inhibitor of the renin–angiotensin–aldosterone system for use in patients with severe decompensated heart failure, but outcomes were not improved with its use.

Ventricular Hypertrophy

Ventricular hypertrophy can occur with or without dilatation, depending on the type of stress imposed on the ventricle. When the heart is subjected to either pressure or volume overload, the initial response is to increase sarcomere length and optimally overlap actin and myosin. With time, ventricular muscle mass begins to increase in response to the abnormal stress.

In the volume-overloaded ventricle, the problem is an increase in diastolic wall stress. The increase in ventricular muscle mass is sufficient only to compensate for the increase in diameter: The ratio of the ventricular radius to wall thickness is unchanged. Sarcomeres replicate mainly in series, resulting in eccentric hypertrophy. Although ventricular EF remains depressed, the increase in end-diastolic volume can maintain normal at-rest stroke volume (and cardiac output).

The problem in a pressure-overloaded ventricle is an increase in systolic wall stress. In this case, sarcomeres mainly replicate in parallel, resulting in concentric hypertrophy: The hypertrophy is such that the ratio of myocardial wall thickness to ventricular radius increases. As can be seen from Laplace's law, systolic wall stress can then be normalized. Ventricular hypertrophy, particularly that caused by pressure overload, usually results in progressive diastolic dysfunction. The most common reasons for isolated left ventricular hypertrophy are hypertension and aortic stenosis.

CASE DISCUSSION

A Patient With a Short P–R Interval

A 38-year-old man is scheduled for endoscopic sinus surgery following a recent onset of headaches. He gives a history of having passed out at least once during one of these headaches. A preoperative electrocardiogram (ECG) is normal, except for a P–R interval of 0.116 sec with normal P-wave morphology.

What is the significance of the short P–R interval?

The P–R interval, which is measured from the beginning of atrial depolarization (P wave) to the beginning of ventricular depolarization (QRS complex), usually represents the time required for depolarization of both atria, the AV node, and the His–Purkinje system. Although the P–R interval can vary with heart rate, it is normally 0.12–0.2 sec in duration. Abnormally short P–R intervals can be seen with either low atrial (or upper AV junctional) rhythms or preexcitation phenomena. The two can usually be differentiated by P-wave morphology: With a low atrial rhythm, atrial depolarization is retrograde, resulting in an inverted P wave in leads II, III, and aVF; with preexcitation, the P wave is normal during sinus rhythm. If the pacemaker rhythm originates from a lower AV junctional focus, the P wave may be lost in the QRS complex or may follow the QRS.

What is preexcitation?

Preexcitation usually refers to early depolarization of the ventricles by an abnormal conduction pathway from the atria. Rarely, more than one such pathway is present. The most common form of preexcitation is due to the presence of an accessory pathway (bundle of Kent) that connects one of the atria with one of the ventricles. This abnormal connection between the atria and ventricles allows electrical impulses to bypass the AV node (hence the term bypass tract). The ability to conduct impulses along the bypass tract can be quite variable and may be only intermittent or rate dependent. Bypass tracts can conduct in both directions, retrograde only (ventricle to atrium), or, rarely, anterograde only (atrium to ventricle). The name Wolff–Parkinson–White (WPW) syndrome is often applied to ventricular preexcitation associated with tachyarrhythmias.

How does preexcitation shorten the P–R interval?

In patients with preexcitation, the normal cardiac impulse originating from the SA node is conducted simultaneously through the normal (AV nodal) and anomalous (bypass tract) pathways. Because conduction is more rapid in the anomalous pathway than in the AV nodal pathway, the cardiac impulse rapidly reaches and depolarizes the area of the ventricles where the bypass tract ends. This early depolarization of the ventricle is reflected by a short P–R interval and a slurred initial deflection (δ wave) in the QRS complex. The spread of the anomalous impulse to the rest of the ventricle is delayed because it must be conducted by ordinary ventricular muscle, not by the much faster Purkinje system. The remainder of the ventricle is then depolarized by the normal impulse from the AV node as it catches up with the preexcitation front. Although the P–R interval is shortened, the resulting QRS is slightly prolonged and represents a fusion complex of normal and abnormal ventricular depolarizations.

The P–R interval in patients with preexcitation depends on relative conduction times between the AV nodal pathway and the bypass pathway. If conduction through the former is fast, preexcitation (and the δ wave) is less prominent, and QRS will be relatively normal. If conduction is delayed in the AV nodal pathway, preexcitation is more prominent, and more of the ventricle will be depolarized by the abnormally conducted impulse. When the AV nodal pathway is completely blocked, the entire ventricle is depolarized by the bypass pathway, resulting in a very short P–R interval, a very prominent δ wave, and a wide, bizarre QRS complex. Other factors that can affect the degree of preexcitation include interatrial conduction time, the distance of the atrial end of the bypass tract from the SA node, and autonomic tone. The P–R interval is often normal or only slightly shortened with a left lateral bypass tract (the most common location). Preexcitation may be more apparent at fast heart rates because conduction slows through the AV node with increasing heart rates. Secondary ST-segment and T-wave changes are also common because of abnormal ventricular repolarization.

What is the clinical significance of preexcitation?

Preexcitation occurs in approximately 0.3% of the general population. An estimated 20% to 50% of affected persons develop paroxysmal tachyarrhythmias, typically paroxysmal supraventricular tachycardia (PSVT). Although most patients are otherwise normal, preexcitation can be associated with other cardiac anomalies, including Ebstein's anomaly, mitral valve prolapse, and cardiomyopathies. Depending on its conductive properties, the bypass tract in some patients may predispose them to tachyarrhythmias and even sudden death. Tachyarrhythmias include PSVT, atrial fibrillation, and, less commonly, atrial flutter. Ventricular fibrillation can be precipitated by a critically timed premature atrial beat that travels down the bypass tract and catches the ventricle at a vulnerable period. Alternatively, very rapid conduction of impulses into the ventricles by the bypass tract during atrial fibrillation can rapidly lead to myocardial ischemia, hypoperfusion, and hypoxia and culminate in ventricular fibrillation.

Recognition of the preexcitation phenomenon is also important because its QRS morphology on the surface ECG can mimic bundle branch block, right ventricular hypertrophy, ischemia, myocardial infarction, and ventricular tachycardia (during atrial fibrillation).

What is the significance of the history of syncope in this patient?

This patient should be evaluated preoperatively by a cardiologist for possible electrophysiological studies, curative radiofrequency ablation of the bypass tract, and the need for perioperative drug therapy. Such studies can identify the location of the bypass tracts, reasonably predict the potential for malignant arrhythmias by programmed pacing, and assess the efficacy of antiarrhythmic therapy if curative ablation is not possible. Ablation is reported to be curative in over 90% of patients. A history of syncope may be ominous because it may indicate the ability to conduct impulses very rapidly through the bypass tract, leading to systemic hypoperfusion and perhaps predisposing the patient to sudden death.

Patients with only occasional asymptomatic tachyarrhythmias generally do not require investigation or prophylactic drug therapy. Those with frequent episodes of tachyarrhythmias or arrhythmias associated with significant symptoms require drug therapy and close evaluation.

How do tachyarrhythmias generally develop?

Tachyarrhythmias develop as a result of either abnormal impulse formation or abnormal impulse propagation (reentry). Abnormal impulses result from enhanced automaticity, abnormal automaticity, or triggered activity. Usually, only cells of the SA node, specialized atrial conduction pathways, AV nodal junctional areas, and the His–Purkinje system depolarize spontaneously. Because diastolic repolarization (phase 4) is fastest in the SA node, other areas of automaticity are suppressed. Enhanced or abnormal automaticity in other areas, however, can usurp pacemaker function from the SA node and lead to tachyarrhythmias. Triggered activity is the result of either early after-depolarizations (phase 2 or 3) or delayed after-depolarizations (after phase 3). It consists of small-amplitude depolarizations that can follow action potentials under some conditions in atrial, ventricular, and His–Purkinje tissue. If these after-depolarizations reach threshold potential, they can result in an extrasystole or repetitive sustained tachyarrhythmias. Factors that can promote the formation of abnormal impulses include increased catecholamine levels, electrolyte disorders (hyperkalemia, hypokalemia, and hypercalcemia), ischemia, hypoxia, mechanical stretch, and drug toxicity (particularly digoxin).

The most common mechanism for tachyarrhythmias is reentry. Four conditions are necessary to initiate and sustain reentry (**Figure 20–14**): (1) two areas in the myocardium that differ in

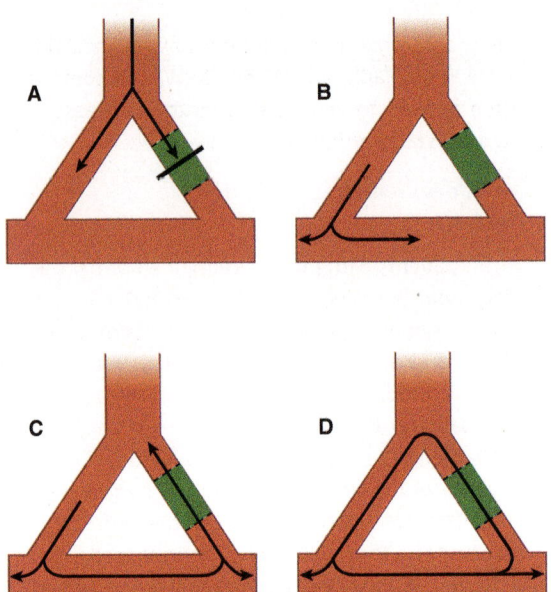

FIGURE 20–14 A–D: The mechanism of reentry. See text for description.

conductivity or refractoriness and that can form a closed electrical loop; (2) unidirectional block in one pathway (Figure 20–14A and B); (3) slow conduction or sufficient length in the circuit to allow recovery of the conduction block in the first pathway (Figure 20–14C); and (4) excitation of the initially blocked pathway to complete the loop (Figure 20–14D). Reentry is usually precipitated by a premature cardiac impulse.

What is the mechanism of PSVT in patients with WPW syndrome?

If the bypass tract is refractory during antegrade conduction of a cardiac impulse, as during a critically timed atrial premature contraction (APC), and the impulse is conducted by the AV node, the same impulse can be conducted retrograde from the ventricle back into the atria via the bypass tract. The retrograde impulse can then depolarize the atrium and travel down the AV nodal pathway again, establishing a continuous repetitive circuit (circus movement). The impulse reciprocates between the atria and ventricles and conduction alternates between the AV nodal pathway and the bypass tract. The term "concealed conduction" is often applied because the absence of preexcitation during this arrhythmia results in a normal QRS that lacks a δ wave.

The circus movement less commonly involves anterograde conduction through the bypass tract and retrograde conduction through the AV nodal pathway. In such instances, the QRS has a δ wave and is completely abnormal; the arrhythmia can be mistaken for ventricular tachycardia.

What other mechanisms may be responsible for PSVT?

In addition to the WPW syndrome, PSVT can be caused by AV reentrant tachycardia, AV nodal reentrant tachycardia, and SA node and atrial reentrant tachycardias. Patients with AV reentrant tachycardia have an extranodal bypass tract similar to patients with WPW syndrome, but the bypass tract conducts only retrograde; preexcitation and a δ wave are absent. The PSVT may be initiated either by an APC or a ventricular premature contraction (VPC). A retrograde P wave is usually visible because atrial depolarization always follows ventricular depolarization.

Functional differences in conduction and refractoriness may occur within the AV node, SA node, or atria; a large bypass tract is not necessary. Thus, the circus movement may occur on a smaller scale within the AV node, SA node, or atria, respectively. PSVT is always induced during AV nodal reentry by an APC with a prolonged P–R interval; a retrograde P wave is either absent or buried in the QRS complex. Another APC may terminate the arrhythmia.

PSVT associated with SA node or atrial reentry is always triggered by an APC. The P wave is usually visible and has a prolonged P–R interval. Its morphology is normal with SA nodal reentry and abnormal with atrial reentry.

How does atrial fibrillation in patients with WPW syndrome differ from the arrhythmia in other patients?

Atrial fibrillation can occur when a cardiac impulse is conducted rapidly retrograde up into the atria and arrives to find different parts of the atria out of phase in recovery from the impulse. Once atrial fibrillation is established, conduction into the ventricles most commonly occurs through the bypass tract only; because of the accessory pathway's ability to conduct very rapidly (unlike the AV nodal pathway), the ventricular rate is typically very rapid (180–300 beats/min). The majority of QRS complexes are bizarre, but periodic conduction of an impulse through the AV nodal pathway results in occasional normal-looking QRS complexes. Less commonly, impulses during atrial fibrillation are conducted mainly through the AV nodal pathway (resulting in mostly normal QRS complexes) or through both the bypass tract and the AV nodal pathway (resulting in a mixture of normal, fusion, and bizarre QRS complexes). As stated previously, atrial fibrillation in patients with WPW syndrome is a very dangerous arrhythmia.

What anesthetic agents can safely be used in patients with preexcitation?

Few data are available comparing the use of different anesthetic agents or techniques in patients with preexcitation. Almost all the volatile and intravenous agents have been used with equal success. Volatile anesthetics increase antegrade refractoriness in both normal and accessory pathways and increase the coupling interval (a measure of the ability of an extrasystole to induce tachycardia). Propofol, opioids, and benzodiazepines seem to have little direct electrophysiological effects, but can alter autonomic tone, generally reducing sympathetic outflow. Factors that tend to cause sympathetic stimulation and increased cardiac automaticity are undesirable. Premedication with a benzodiazepine helps reduce high sympathetic tone preoperatively. Agents that can increase sympathetic tone, such as ketamine and perhaps pancuronium in large bolus doses, should generally be avoided. Anticholinergics should be used cautiously; glycopyrrolate may be preferable to atropine. Endotracheal intubation should be carried out only after the patient is deeply anesthetized; pretreatment with a β-adrenergic blocker, such as esmolol, may be useful. Light anesthesia, hypercapnia, acidosis, and even transient hypoxia will activate the sympathetic system and are to be avoided. A deep extubation and good postoperative analgesia (without respiratory acidosis) may also help prevent the onset of arrhythmias. When patients with preexcitation are anesthetized for electrophysiological study and surgical ablation, opioids, propofol, and benzodiazepines may be the agents least likely to alter conduction characteristics.

How are antiarrhythmic agents selected for tachyarrhythmias?

Most antiarrhythmic agents act by altering myocardial cell conduction (phase 0), repolarization (phase 3), or automaticity (phase 4). Prolongation of repolarization increases the refractoriness of cells. Many antiarrhythmic drugs also exert direct or indirect autonomic effects. Although antiarrhythmic agents are generally classified according to broad mechanisms of action or electrophysiological effects (Table 20–7), the most commonly

TABLE 20–7 Classification of antiarrhythmic agents.[1]

Class	Mechanism of Action	Agents	Intravenous Loading Dose
I	Blocks voltage-gated sodium channels; decreases slope of phase 0 (V_{max})		
Ia	Moderate depression of V_{max}, prolongs APD	Quinidine[2–4]	NR
		Procainamide (Pronestyl)[1,4]	5–10 mg/kg
		Disopyramide (Norpace)[1,4]	NA
Ib	Minimal effect on V_{max}, shorten APD	Lidocaine	1–2 mg/kg
		Phenytoin	5–15 mg/kg
		Tocainide (Tonocard)	NA
		Mexiletine (Mexitil)	NA
		Moricizine (Ethmozine)	NA
Ic	Marked depression of V_{max}, minimal effect of APD	Flecainide (Tambacor)	NA
		Propafenone (Rythmol)	NA
II	Blocks β-adrenergic receptors	Esmolol (Brevibloc)	0.5 mg/kg
		Metoprolol (Lopressor)	5–10 mg
III	Prolongs repolarization	Amiodarone (Cordarone)[5–7]	150 mg
		Sotalol (Betapace)[8]	NA
		Ibutilide (Corvert)	1 mg
		Dofetilide (Tikosyn)	NA
IV	Blocks slow calcium channels	Verapamil (Calan)	2.5–10 mg
		Diltiazem (Cardizem)	0.25–0.35 mg/kg
V	Various (miscellaneous agents)	Digoxin	0.5–0.75 mg
		Adenosine (Adenocard)	6–12 mg

[1]V_{max}, maximum velocity; APD, action potential duration; NR, not recommended; NA, not available for intravenous use.
[2]Also has antimuscarinic (vagolytic activity).
[3]Also blocks α-adrenergic receptors.
[4]Also prolongs repolarization.
[5]Also binds inactivated sodium channels.
[6]Also causes noncompetitive α- and β-adrenergic blockade.
[7]Also blocks slow calcium channels.
[8]Also has nonselective β-adrenergic blocking activity.

used classification system is not perfect because some agents have more than one mechanism of action.

Selection of an antiarrhythmic agent generally depends on whether the arrhythmia is ventricular or supraventricular and whether acute control or chronic therapy is required. Intravenous agents are usually employed in the acute management of arrhythmias, whereas oral agents are reserved for chronic therapy (Table 20–8).

TABLE 20–8 Clinical pharmacological properties of antiarrhythmic drugs.[1]

Drug	Effect on SA Nodal Rate	Effect on AV Nodal Refractory Period	PR Interval	QRS Duration	QT Interval	Usefulness in Arrhythmias Supraventricular	Ventricular	Half-Life
Adenosine	Little	↑↑↑	↑↑↑	0	0	++++	?	<10 s
Amiodarone	↓↓[2]	↑↑	↑↑	↑	↑↑↑↑	+++	+++	(Weeks)
Bretylium	↑↓[3]	↑↓[3]	0	0	0	0	+	4 h
Diltiazem	↑↓	↑↑	↑	0	0	+++	–	4–8 h
Disopyramide	↑↓[2,4]	↑↓[4]	↑↓[4]	↑↑	↑↑	+	+++	6–8 h
Dofetilide	↓?	0	0	0	↑↑	++	None	7 h
Esmolol	↓↓	↑↑	↑↑	0	0	+	+	10 min
Flecainide	None	↑	↑	↑↑↑	0	+[5]	++++	20 h
Ibutilide	↓(?)	0	0	0	↑↑	++	?	6 h
Lidocaine	None[2]	None	0	0	0	None[6]	+++	1–2 h
Metopolol	↓↓	↑↑	↑↑	0	0	+	+	8 h
Mexiletine	None[2]	None	0	0	0	None[7]	+++	12 h
Moricizine	None	None	↑	↑↑	0	None	+++	2–6 h[7]
Procainamide	↓[2]	↑↓[4]	↑↓[4]	↑↑	↑↑	+	+++	3–4 h
Propafenone	0	↑	↑	↑↑↑	0	+	+++	5–7 h
Quinidine	↑↓[2,4]	↑↓[4]	↑↓[4]	↑↑	↑↑	+	+++	6 h
Sotalol	↓↓	↑↑	↑↑	0	↑↑↑	+++	+++	7 h
Tocainide	None[2]	None	0	0	0	None[6]	+++	12 h
Verapamil	↓↓	↑↑	↑↑	0	0	+++	–	7 h

[1]Data from Katzung BG: *Basic and Clinical Pharmacology*, 12th ed. McGraw-Hill, 2012.
[2]May suppress diseased sinus nodes.
[3]Initial stimulation by release of endogenous norepinephrine followed by depression.
[4]Anticholinergic effect and direct depressant action.
[5]Particularly in Wolff–Parkinson–White syndrome.
[6]May be effective in atrial arrhythmias caused by digitalis.
[7]Half-life of active metabolites is much longer.

Which agents are most useful for tachyarrhythmias in patients with WPW syndrome?

Cardioversion is the treatment of choice in hemodynamically compromised patients. Adenosine is the drug of choice for PSVT because of its short duration of action. Small doses of phenylephrine (100 mcg), together with vagal maneuvers (carotid massage if not contraindicated by carotid occulsive disease), help support arterial blood pressure and may terminate the arrhythmia. The most useful pharmacological agents are class Ia drugs (eg, procainamide). These agents increase the refractory period and decrease conduction in the accessory pathway. Moreover, class Ia drugs frequently terminate and can suppress the recurrence of PSVT and atrial fibrillation. Class Ic drugs and amiodarone are also useful because they slow conduction and prolong refractoriness in both the AV node and the accessory pathway. β-Adrenergic blocking agents may also be useful, particularly in controlling ventricular rate once these rhythms are established. Verapamil and digoxin are contraindicated during atrial fibrillation or flutter in these patients because they can dangerously accelerate the ventricular response. Both types of agents decrease conduction through the AV node, favoring conduction of impulses down the accessory pathway. The bypass tract is capable of conducting impulses into the ventricles much faster than the AV nodal pathway. Digoxin may also increase the ventricular response by shortening the refractory period and increasing conduction in accessory pathways. Although verapamil can terminate PSVT, its use in this setting may be hazardous because patients can subsequently develop atrial fibrillation or flutter. Moreover, atrial fibrillation may not be readily distinguishable from ventricular tachycardia in these patients if wide-QRS tachycardia develops.

SUGGESTED READING

Balser JR: The rational use of intravenous amiodarone in the perioperative period. Anesthesiology 1997;86:974.

Colson P, Ryckwaert F, Coriat P: Renin angiotensin system antagonists and anesthesia. Anesth Analg 1999;89:1143.

Eriksson H, Jalonen J, Heikkinen L: Levosimendan facilitates weaning from cardiopulmonary bypass in high risk coronary patients. Eur J Cardiothorac Surg 1997;11:1097.

Fontes M, Aronson S, Mathew J, et al: Pulse pressure and risk of adverse outcome in coronary bypass surgery. Anesth Analg 2008;107:1122.

Ganong WF: *Review of Medical Physiology*, 23rd ed. McGraw-Hill, 2009.

Gomez MN: Magnesium and cardiovascular disease. Anesthesiology 1998;89:222.

Groban L, Butterworth J: Perioperative management of chronic heart failure. Anesth Analg 2006;103:557.

Jacobsohn E, Chorn R, O'Connor M: The role of the vasculature in regulating venous return and cardiac output: Historical and graphical approach. Can J Anaesth 1997;44:849.

Ross S, Foex P: Protective effects of anaesthetics in reversible and irreversible ischemia-reperfusion injury. Br J Anaesth 1999;82:622.

Van Gelder IC, Tuinenburg AE, Schoonderwoerd BS, et al: Pharmacologic versus direct-current electrical cardioversion of atrial flutter and fibrillation. Am J Cardiol 1999;84:147R.

Woods J, Monteiro P, Rhodes A: Right ventricular dysfunction. Curr Opin Crit Care 2007;13:535.

Yost CS: Potassium channels. Basic aspects, functional roles and medical significance. Anesthesiology 1999;90:1186.

Anesthesia for Patients with Cardiovascular Disease

1. Cardiovascular complications account for 25% to 50% of deaths following noncardiac surgery. Perioperative myocardial infarction (MI), pulmonary edema, congestive heart failure, arrhythmias, and thromboembolism are most commonly seen in patients with preexisting cardiovascular disease.

2. Regardless of the level of preoperative blood pressure control, many patients with hypertension display an accentuated hypotensive response to induction of anesthesia, followed by an exaggerated hypertensive response to intubation. Hypertensive patients may display an exaggerated response to both endogenous catecholamines (from intubation or surgical stimulation) and exogenously administered sympathetic agonists.

3. Patients with extensive (three-vessel or left main) coronary artery disease, a history of MI, or ventricular dysfunction are at greatest risk of cardiac complications.

4. Holter monitoring, exercise electrocardiography, myocardial perfusion scans, and echocardiography are important in determining perioperative risk and the need for coronary angiography; however, these tests are indicated only if their outcome would alter patient care.

5. Sudden withdrawal of antianginal medication perioperatively—particularly β-blockers—can precipitate a sudden, rebound increase in ischemic episodes.

6. The overwhelming priority in managing patients with ischemic heart disease is maintaining a favorable myocardial supply–demand relationship. Autonomic-mediated increases in heart rate and blood pressure should be controlled by deep anesthesia or adrenergic blockade, and excessive reductions in coronary perfusion pressure or arterial oxygen content are to be avoided.

7. Intraoperative detection of ischemia depends on recognition of electrocardiographic changes, hemodynamic manifestations, or regional wall motion abnormalities on transesophageal echocardiography. New ST-segment elevations are rare during noncardiac surgery and are indicative of severe ischemia, vasospasm, or infarction.

8. The principal hemodynamic goals in managing mitral stenosis are to maintain a sinus rhythm (if present preoperatively) and to avoid tachycardia, large increases in cardiac output, and both hypovolemia and fluid overload by judicious administration of intravenous fluids.

9. Anesthetic management of mitral regurgitation should be tailored to the severity of regurgitation and to the underlying left ventricular function. Factors that exacerbate the regurgitation, such as slow heart rates and acute increases in afterload, should be avoided. Excessive volume expansion can also worsen the regurgitation by dilating the left ventricle.

—Continued next page

Continued—

10 Maintenance of normal sinus rhythm, heart rate, vascular resistance and intravascular volume is critical in patients with aortic stenosis. Loss of a normally timed atrial systole often leads to rapid deterioration, particularly when associated with tachycardia. Spinal and epidural anesthesia are relatively contraindicated in patients with severe aortic stenosis.

11 Bradycardia and increase in systemic vascular resistance (SVR) increase the regurgitant volume in patients with aortic regurgitation, whereas tachycardia can contribute to myocardial ischemia. Excessive myocardial depression should also be avoided. The compensatory increase in cardiac preload should be maintained, but excessive fluid replacement can readily result in pulmonary edema.

12 In patients with congenital heart disease, an increase in SVR relative to pulmonary vascular resistance (PVR) favors left-to-right shunting, whereas an increase in PVR relative to SVR favors right-to-left shunting.

13 The presence of shunt flow between the right and left hearts, regardless of the direction of blood flow, mandates the meticulous exclusion of air bubbles or particulate material from intravenous fluids to prevent paradoxical embolism into the cerebral or coronary circulations.

14 The goals of anesthetic management in patients with tetralogy of Fallot should be to maintain intravascular volume and SVR. Increases in PVR, such as might occur from acidosis or excessive airway pressures, should be avoided. The right-to-left shunting tends to slow the uptake of inhalation anesthetics; in contrast, it may accelerate the onset of intravenous agents.

15 The transplanted heart is totally denervated, so direct autonomic influences are absent. Moreover, the absence of reflex increases in heart rate can make patients particularly sensitive to rapid vasodilatation. Indirect vasopressors, such as ephedrine, are less effective than direct-acting agents because of the absence of catecholamine stores in myocardial neurons.

Cardiovascular diseases—particularly hypertensive, ischemic, congenital, and valvular heart disease—are among the medical illnesses most frequently encountered in anesthetic practice and are a major cause of perioperative morbidity and mortality. Management of patients with these diseases continues to challenge the ingenuity and resources of the anesthesiologist. The adrenergic response to surgical stimulation and the circulatory effects of anesthetic agents, endotracheal intubation, positive-pressure ventilation, blood loss, fluid shifts, and alterations in body temperature impose additional burdens on an often already compromised cardiovascular system. Most anesthetic agents cause cardiac depression, vasodilatation, or both. Even anesthetics that have no direct circulatory effects may cause apparent circulatory depression in severely compromised patients who are dependent on the enhanced sympathetic activity characteristic of heart failure or acute blood loss. Decreased sympathetic activity as a consequence of the anesthetized state can lead to acute circulatory collapse.

Good anesthetic management of patients with cardiovascular disease requires a thorough knowledge of normal cardiac physiology, the circulatory effects of the various anesthetic agents, and the pathophysiology and treatment of these diseases. The same principles used in treating cardiovascular diseases in patients not undergoing surgery should be used perioperatively. In most instances, the choice of anesthetic agent is not terribly important; on the other hand, knowing how the agent is used, understanding the underlying pathophysiology, and understanding how the two interact are critical.

Patients with severe cardiovascular illnesses commonly undergo both cardiac and noncardiac surgery. The American College of Cardiology (ACC), in collaboration with the American Heart Association (AHA), have issued numerous guidelines related to the management of patients with heart disease, and many of their recommendations are relevant to patients undergoing anesthesia and invasive procedures. Because guidelines change as new evidence becomes available, anesthesiologists are advised to review the AHA website for current evidence-based indications for the management of heart disease.

Perioperative Cardiovascular Evaluation and Preparation for Noncardiac Surgery

The prevalence of cardiovascular disease increases progressively with advancing age. Moreover, the number of patients over 65 years of age is expected to increase by 25% to 35% over the next two decades. Cardiovascular complications account for 25% to 50% of deaths following noncardiac surgery. Perioperative myocardial infarction (MI), pulmonary edema, systolic and diastolic heart failure, arrhythmias, and thromboembolism are the most common diagnoses in patients with preexisting cardiovascular disease. The incidence of postoperative cardiogenic pulmonary edema is approximately 2% in all patients over 40 years of age, but it is 6% in patients with a history of heart failure and 16% in patients with poorly compensated heart failure. The relatively high prevalence of cardiovascular disorders in surgical patients has given rise to attempts to define *cardiac risk* or the likelihood of intraoperative or postoperative fatal or life-threatening cardiac complications.

In 2007, the ACC/AHA Task Force Report produced revised guidelines for perioperative evaluation. The revised guidelines stated that the patient's medical history is critical in determining the requirements for preoperative cardiac evaluation and that certain conditions (eg, unstable coronary syndromes and decompensated heart failure) warrant cardiology intervention prior to all but emergency procedures (Table 21–1). The history should also review any past procedures, such as cardioverter defibrillator implants, coronary stents, and other interventions.

TABLE 21–1 Active cardiac conditions for which the patient should undergo evaluation and treatment before noncardiac surgery (class I, level of evidence: B).

Condition	Examples
Unstable coronary syndromes	Unstable or severe angina[1] (CCS class III or IV)[2] Recent MI[3]
Decompensated HF (NYHA functional class IV; worsening or new-onset HF)	
Significant arrhythmias	High-grade atrioventricular block Mobitz II atrioventricular block Third-degree atrioventricular heart block Symptomatic ventricular arrhythmias Supraventricular arrhythmias (including atrial fibrillation) with uncontrolled ventricular rate (HR greater than 100 bpm at rest) Symptomatic bradycardia Newly recognized ventricular tachycardia
Severe valvular disease	Severe aortic stenosis (mean pressure gradient greater than 40 mm Hg, aortic valve area less than 1.0 cm², or symptomatic) Symptomatic mitral stenosis (progressive dyspnea on exertion, exertional presyncope, or HF)

CCS indicates Canadian Cardiovascular Society; HF, heart failure; HR, heart rate; MI, myocardial infarction; NYHA, New York Heart Association.

[1]According to Campeau L. Letter: Grading of angina pectoris. Circulation. 1976;54:522-523.

[2]May include "stable" angina in patients who are unusually sedentary.

[3]The American College of Cardiology National Database Library defines recent MI as more than 7 days but less than or equal to 1 month (within 30 days).

Reproduced, with permission from Fleisher L, Beckman J, Brown K, et al: ACC/AHA 2007 guidelines on perioperative cardiovascular evaluation and care for noncardiac surgery. Circulation 2007;116: 1971-1996.

TABLE 21–2 Estimated energy requirements for various activities.

	Can you ...		Can you ...
1 MET	Take care of yourself?	4 METs	Climb a flight of stairs or walk up a hill?
	Eat, dress, or use the toilet?		Walk on level ground at 4 mph (6.4 kph)?
	Walk indoors around the house?		Run a short distance?
	Walk a block or 2 on level ground at 2 to 3 mph (3.2 to 4.8 kph)?		Do heavy work around the house like scrubbing floors or lifting or moving heavy furniture?
4 METs	Do light work around the house like dusting or washing dishes?		Participate in moderate recreational activities like golf, bowling, dancing, doubles tennis, or throwing a baseball or football?
		Greater than 10 METs	Participate in strenuous sports like swimming, singles tennis, football, basketball, or skiing?

kph indicates kilometers per hour; MET, metabolic equivalent; and mph, miles per hour.

Modified and reproduced, with permission, from Hlatky MA, Boineau RE, Higginbotham MB, et al. A brief self-administered questionnaire to determine functional capacity (the Duke Activity Status Index). Am J Cardiol. 1989;64:651-654.

Additionally, the patient's ability to perform the tasks of daily living should be assessed as a guide to determine functional capacity. A patient with a history of cardiac disease and advanced age, but good exercise tolerance, will likely have a lower perioperative risk than a similar individual with dyspnea after minimal physical activity (Table 21–2).

The patient's history should also seek signs of other disease processes that frequently accompany heart disease. Cardiac patients often present with obstructive pulmonary disease, reduced renal function, and diabetes mellitus.

A physical examination should be performed on all patients, and the heart and lungs should be auscultated. The physical examination is especially useful in patients with certain conditions. For example, if a murmur suggestive of aortic stenosis is detected, additional ultrasound evaluation will likely be warranted, as aortic stenosis substantially increases the risks in patients undergoing noncardiac surgery.

The following conditions are associated with increased risk:

- Ischemic heart disease (history of MI, evidence on electrocardiogram [ECG], chest pain)
- Congestive heart failure (dyspnea, pulmonary edema)
- Cerebral vascular disease (stroke)
- High-risk surgery (vascular, thoracic, abdominal, orthopedic)
- Diabetes mellitus
- Preoperative creatinine >2 mg/dL

Recent ACC/AHA guidelines identify conditions that are a major cardiac risk and warrant intensive management prior to all but emergent surgery. These conditions include: unstable coronary syndromes (recent MI, unstable angina), decompensated heart failure, significant arrhythmias, and severe valvular heart disease. The ACC/AHA guidelines identify an MI within 7 days, or one within 1 month with myocardium at risk for ischemia, as "active" cardiac conditions. On the other hand, evidence of past MI with no myocardium thought at ischemic risk is considered a low risk for perioperative infarction after noncardiac surgery.

The ACC/AHA guidelines suggest a stepwise approach to preoperative cardiac evaluation. Their recommendations are classified as follows:

- Class I: Benefits >> risk
- Class IIa: Benefits >> risk, but scientific evidence incomplete

- Class IIb: Benefits ≥ risk, and scientific evidence incomplete
- Class III: Risks >>benefits

Class I recommendations are as follows:

- Patients who have a need for emergency noncardiac surgery should proceed to the operating room with perioperative surveillance and postoperative risk factor management
- Patients with active cardiac conditions should be evaluated by a cardiologist and treated according to ACC/AHA guidelines
- Patients undergoing low-risk procedures should proceed to surgery
- Patients with poor exercise tolerance (<4 metabolic equivalents [METs]) and no known risk factors should proceed to surgery

Class IIa recommendations are as follows:

- Patients with a functional capacity >4 METs and without symptoms should proceed to surgery
- Patients with a functional capacity <4 METs or those with an unknown functional capacity with three or more clinical risk factors scheduled for vascular surgery should be tested, if management is likely to change based on the results
- Patients with a functional capacity <4 METs or those with an unknown functional capacity with three or more clinical risk factors scheduled for intermediate-risk surgery should proceed to surgery with heart rate control
- Patients with a functional capacity <4 METs or those with an unknown functional capacity with one or two clinical risk factors who are scheduled for vascular or intermediate-risk surgery should proceed to surgery with heart rate control

The ACC/AHA guidelines also note, as class IIb recommendations, that noninvasive testing might be considered *if* patient management changes in patients with poor or unknown functional capacity or in patients undergoing intermediate-risk surgery

TABLE 21–3 Cardiac risk[1] stratification for noncardiac surgical procedures.

Risk Stratification	Procedure Examples
Vascular (reported cardiac risk often more than 5%)	Aortic and other major vascular surgery Peripheral vascular surgery
Intermediate (reported cardiac risk generally 1% to 5%)	Intraperitoneal and intrathoracic surgery Carotid endarterectomy Head and neck surgery Orthopedic surgery Prostate surgery
Low[2] (reported cardiac risk generally less than 1%)	Endoscopic procedures Superficial procedure Cataract surgery Breast surgery Ambulatory surgery

[1]Combined incidence of cardiac death and nonfatal myocardial infarction.

[2]These procedures do not generally require further preoperative cardiac testing.

Fleisher L, Beckman J, Brown K, et al: ACC/AHA 2007 guidelines on perioperative cardiovascular evaluation and care for noncardiac surgery. Circulation 2007;116:1971-1996.

with three clinical risk factors. Likewise, such testing might be indicated in patients with one or two clinical risk factors scheduled for vascular or intermediate-risk surgery. Table 21–3 classifies surgical procedures according to risk.

The ACC/AHA guidelines also provide specific recommendations regarding various conditions likely to be encountered perioperatively.

CORONARY ARTERY DISEASE

The ACC/AHA guidelines note that only the subset of patients with coronary artery disease (CAD) who would benefit from revascularization, irrespective of their need for a nonemergent surgical procedure, would likely benefit from preoperative coronary interventions. Consequently, the indications for the testing of such patients as candidates for a coronary intervention are unrelated to their presenting for surgery and depend only on whether such evaluation would be indicated as part of general medical management.

HYPERTENSION

Patients with hypertension frequently present for elective surgical procedures. Some will have been effectively managed, but unfortunately, many others will not have been. Hypertension is a leading cause of death and disability in most Western societies and the most prevalent preoperative medical abnormality in surgical patients, with an overall prevalence of 20% to 25%. Long-standing uncontrolled hypertension accelerates atherosclerosis and hypertensive organ damage. Hypertension is a major risk factor for cardiac, cerebral, renal, and vascular disease. **Complications of hypertension include MI, congestive heart failure, stroke, renal failure, peripheral occlusive disease, and aortic dissection.** The presence of left ventricular hypertrophy (LVH) in hypertensive patients may be an important predictor of cardiac mortality. However, systolic blood pressures below 180 mm Hg, and diastolic pressures below 110 mm Hg, have not been associated with increased perioperative risks. When patients present with systolic blood pressures greater than 180 mm Hg and diastolic pressures greater than 110 mm Hg, anesthesiologists face the dilemma of delaying surgery to allow optimization of oral antihypertensive therapy, but adding the risk of a surgical delay versus proceeding with surgery and achieving blood pressure control with rapidly acting intravenous agents. Intravenous β-blockers can be useful to treat preoperative hypertension. Of note, patients with preoperative hypertension are more likely than others to develop intraoperative hypotension. This is particularly frequent in patients treated with angiotensin receptor blockers and/or angiotensin-converting enzyme (ACE) inhibitors.

Blood pressure measurements are affected by many variables, including posture, time of day or night, emotional state, recent activity, and drug intake, as well as the equipment and technique used. A diagnosis of hypertension cannot be made by one preoperative reading, but requires confirmation by a history of consistently elevated measurements. Although preoperative anxiety or pain may produce some degree of hypertension in normal patients, patients with a history of hypertension generally exhibit greater preoperative elevations in blood pressure.

TABLE 21–4 Classification of blood pressure (adults).

Category of Blood Pressure	Systolic Pressure (mm Hg)	Diastolic Pressure (mm Hg)
Normal	<130	<85
High normal	130–139	85–89
Hypertension		
Stage 1/mild	140–159	90–99
Stage 2/moderate	160–179	100–109
Stage 3/severe	180–209	110–119
Stage 4/very severe	>210	>120

Epidemiological studies demonstrate a direct and continuous correlation between both diastolic and systolic blood pressures and mortality rates. The definition of systemic hypertension is arbitrary: a consistently elevated diastolic blood pressure greater than 90 mm Hg or a systolic pressure greater than 140 mm Hg. A common classification scheme is listed in Table 21–4. Borderline hypertension is said to exist when the diastolic pressure is 85–89 mm Hg or the systolic pressure is 130–139 mm Hg. Whether patients with borderline hypertension are at some increased risk for cardiovascular complications remains unclear. Accelerated, or severe hypertension (stage 3), is defined as a recent, sustained, and progressive increase in blood pressure, usually with diastolic blood pressures in excess of 110–119 mm Hg. Renal dysfunction is often present in such patients. Malignant hypertension is a true medical emergency characterized by severe hypertension (>210/120 mm Hg) often associated with papilledema and encephalopathy.

Pathophysiology

Hypertension can be either idiopathic (essential), or, less commonly, secondary to other medical conditions such as renal disease, renal artery stenosis, primary hyperaldosteronism, Cushing's disease, acromegaly, pheochromocytoma, pregnancy, or estrogen therapy. Essential hypertension accounts for 80% to 95% of cases and may be associated with an abnormal baseline elevation of cardiac output, systemic vascular resistance (SVR), or both. An evolving pattern is commonly seen over the course of the disease, where cardiac output returns to (or remains) normal, but SVR becomes abnormally high. The chronic increase in cardiac afterload results in concentric LVH and altered diastolic function. Hypertension also alters cerebral autoregulation, such that normal cerebral blood flow is maintained in the face of high blood pressures; autoregulation limits may be in the range of mean blood pressures of 110–180 mm Hg.

The mechanisms responsible for the changes observed in hypertensive patients seem to involve vascular hypertrophy, hyperinsulinemia, abnormal increases in intracellular calcium, and increased intracellular sodium concentrations in vascular smooth muscle and renal tubular cells. The increased intracellular calcium presumably results in increased arteriolar tone, whereas the increased sodium concentration impairs renal excretion of sodium. Sympathetic nervous system overactivity and enhanced responses to sympathetic agonists are present in some patients. Hypertensive patients sometimes display an exaggerated response to vasopressors and vasodilators. Overactivity of the renin–angiotensin–aldosterone system seems to play an important role in patients with accelerated hypertension.

Long-Term Treatment

Effective drug therapy reduces the progression of hypertension and the incidence of stroke, congestive heart failure, CAD, and renal damage. Effective treatment can also delay and sometimes reverse concomitant pathophysiological changes, such as LVH and altered cerebral autoregulation.

Some patients with mild hypertension require only single-drug therapy, which may consist of a thiazide diuretic, ACE inhibitor, angiotensin-receptor blocker (ARB), β-adrenergic blocker, or calcium channel blocker, although guidelines and outcome studies favor the first three options. Concomitant illnesses should guide drug selection. All patients with a prior MI should receive a β-adrenergic blocker and an ACE inhibitor (or ARB) to improve

outcomes, irrespective of the presence of hypertension. In many patients, the "guideline specified" agents will also be more than sufficient to control hypertension.

Patients with moderate to severe hypertension often require two or three drugs for control. The combination of a diuretic with a β-adrenergic blocker and an ACE inhibitor is often effective when single-drug therapy is not. As previously noted, ACE inhibitors (or ARBs) prolong survival in patients with congestive heart failure, left ventricular dysfunction, or a prior MI. Familiarity with the names, mechanisms of action, and side effects of commonly used antihypertensive agents is important for anesthesiologists (Table 21–5).

PREOPERATIVE MANAGEMENT

A recurring question in anesthetic practice is the degree of preoperative hypertension that is acceptable for patients scheduled for elective surgery. Except for optimally controlled patients, most hypertensive patients present to the operating room with some degree of hypertension. Although data suggest that even moderate preoperative hypertension (diastolic pressure <90–110 mm Hg) is not clearly statistically associated with *postoperative* complications, other data indicate that the untreated or poorly controlled hypertensive patient is more apt to experience *intraoperative* episodes of myocardial ischemia, arrhythmias, or both hypertension and hypotension. Intraoperative adjustments in anesthetic depth and use of vasoactive drugs should reduce the incidence of postoperative complications referable to poor preoperative control of hypertension.

Although patients should ideally undergo elective surgery only when rendered normotensive, this is not always feasible or necessarily desirable because of altered cerebral autoregulation. Excessive reductions in blood pressure can compromise cerebral perfusion. Moreover, the decision to delay or to proceed with surgery should be individualized, based on the severity of the preoperative blood pressure elevation; the likelihood of coexisting myocardial ischemia, ventricular dysfunction, or cerebrovascular or renal complications; and the surgical procedure (whether major

TABLE 21–5 Oral antihypertensive agents.

Category	Class	Subclass	Agent
Diuretics	Thiazide		Chlorothiazide (Diuril) Chlorthalidone (Thalitone) Hydrochlorothiazide (Microzide) Indapamide (Lozol) Metolazone (Zaroxolyn)
	Potassium sparing		Spironolactone (Aldactone) Triamterene (Dyrenium) Amiloride (Midamor)
	Loop		Bumetanide (Bumex) Ethacrynic acid (Edecrin) Furosemide (Lasix) Torasemide (Demadex)
Sympatholytics	Adrenergic-receptor blockers	B	Acebutolol (Sectral) Atenolol (Tenormin) Betaxolol (Kerlone) Bisoprolol (Zebeta) Carteolol (Cartrol) Metoprolol (Lopressor) Nadolol (Corgard) Penbutolol (Levatol) Pindolol (Visken) Propranolol (Inderal) Timolol (Blocadren)
		A	α_1 Doxazosin (Cardura) Prazosin (Minipress) Terazosin (Hytrin) $\alpha_1 + \alpha_2$ Phenoxybenzamine (Dibenzyline)
		α and β	Labetalol (Trandate) Carvedilol (Coreg)
	Central α_2-agonists		Clonidine (Catapres) Guanabenz (Wytensin) Guanfacine (Tenex) Methyldopa (Aldomet)

(continued)

surgically induced changes in cardiac preload or afterload are anticipated). With rare exceptions, antihypertensive drug therapy should be continued up to the time of surgery. Some clinicians withhold ACE inhibitors and ARBs on the morning of surgery because of their association with an increased incidence of intraoperative hypotension; however, withholding these agents increases the risk of marked perioperative hypertension and the need for parenteral antihypertensive agents. It also requires the surgical team to remember to restart the medication after surgery. The decision to delay elective surgical procedures in patients with sustained preoperative diastolic blood pressures higher than 110 mm Hg should be made when the perceived benefits of delayed surgery exceed the risks. Unfortunately, there are few appropriate studies to guide the decision-making.

History

The preoperative history should inquire into the severity and duration of the hypertension, the

TABLE 21–5 Oral antihypertensive agents. (continued)

Category	Class	Subclass	Agent
Vasodilators	Calcium channel blockers	Benzothiazepine	
			Diltiazem[1] (Tiazac)
		Phenylalkylamines	
			Verapamil[1] (Calan SR)
		Dihydropyridines	
			Amlodipine (Norvasc)
			Felodipine (Plendil)
			Isradipine[1] (Dynacirc)
			Nicardipine[1] (Cardene)
			Nifedipine[1] (Procardia XL)
			Nisoldipine (Sular)
		ACE inhibitors[2]	Benazepril (Lotensin)
			Captopril (Capoten)
			Enalapril (Vasotec)
			Fosinopril (Monopril)
			Lisinopril (Zestril)
			Moexipril (Univasc)
			Perindopril (Aceon)
			Quinapril (Accupril)
			Ramipril (Altace)
			Trandopril (Mavik)
		Angiotensin-receptor antagonists	Candesartan (Atacand)
			Eprosartan (Tevetan)
			Irbesartan (Avapro)
			Losartan (Cozaar)
			Olmesartan (Benicar)
			Telmisartan (Micardis)
			Valsartan (Diovan)
	Direct vasodilators		Hydralazine (Apresoline)
			Minoxidil

[1]Extended release.
[2]ACE, angiotensin-converting enzyme.

drug therapy currently prescribed, and the presence or absence of hypertensive complications. Symptoms of myocardial ischemia, ventricular failure, impaired cerebral perfusion, or peripheral vascular disease should be elicited, as well as the patient's record of compliance with the drug regimen. The patient should be questioned regarding chest pain, exercise tolerance, shortness of breath (particularly at night), dependent edema, postural lightheadedness, syncope, episodic visual disturbances or episodic neurologic symptoms, and claudication. Adverse effects of current antihypertensive drug therapy (Table 21–6) should also be identified.

Physical Examination & Laboratory Evaluation

Ophthalmoscopy is useful in hypertensive patients. Visible changes in the retinal vasculature usually parallel the severity and progression of arteriosclerosis and hypertensive damage in other organs. An S_4 cardiac gallop is common in patients with LVH. Other physical findings, such as pulmonary rales and an S_3 cardiac gallop, are late findings and indicate congestive heart failure. Blood pressure can be measured in both the supine and standing positions. Orthostatic changes can be due to volume depletion, excessive vasodilatation, or sympatholytic drug

TABLE 21–6 Adverse effects of long-term antihypertensive therapy.

Class	Adverse Effects
Diuretics	
Thiazide	Hypokalemia, hyponatremia, hyperglycemia, hyperuricemia, hypomagnesemia, hyperlipidemia, hypercalcemia
Loop	Hypokalemia, hyperglycemia, hypocalcemia, hypomagnesemia, metabolic alkalosis
Potassium sparing	Hyperkalemia
Sympatholytics	
β-Adrenergic blockers	Bradycardia, conduction blockade, myocardial depression, enhanced bronchial tone, sedation, fatigue, depression
α-Adrenergic blockers	Postural hypertension, tachycardia, fluid retention
Central α_2-agonists	Postural hypotension, sedation, dry mouth, depression, decreased anesthetic requirements, bradycardia, rebound hypertension, positive Coombs test and hemolytic anemia (methyldopa), hepatitis (methyldopa)
Ganglionic blockers	Postural hypotension, diarrhea, fluid retention, depression (reserpine)
Vasodilators	
Calcium channels blockers	Cardiac depression, bradycardia, conduction blockade (verapamil, diltiazem), peripheral edema (nifedipine), tachycardia (nifedipine), enhanced neuromuscular nondepolarizing blockade
ACE inhibitors[1]	Cardiac depression, bradycardia, conduction blockade (verapamil, diltiazem), peripheral edema (nifedipine), tachycardia (nifedipine), enhanced neuromuscular nondepolarizing blockade
Angiotensin-receptor antagonists	Hypotension, renal failure in bilateral renal artery stenosis, hyperkalemia
Direct vasodilators	Reflex tachycardia, fluid retention, headache, systemic lupus erythematosus-like syndrome (hydralazine), pleural or pericardial effusion (minoxidil)

[1]ACE, angiotensin-converting enzyme.

therapy; preoperative fluid administration can prevent severe hypotension after induction of anesthesia in these patients. Although asymptomatic carotid bruits are usually hemodynamically insignificant, they may be reflective of atherosclerotic vascular disease that may affect the coronary circulation. When a bruit is detected, further workup should be guided by the urgency of the scheduled surgery and the likelihood that further investigations, if diagnostic, would result in a change in therapy. Doppler studies of the carotid arteries can be used to define the extent of carotid disease.

The ECG is often normal, but in patients with a long history of hypertension, it may show evidence of ischemia, conduction abnormalities, an old infarction, or LVH or strain. A normal ECG does not exclude CAD or LVH. Similarly, a normal heart size on a chest radiograph does not exclude ventricular hypertrophy. Echocardiography is a sensitive test of LVH and can be used to evaluate ventricular systolic and diastolic functions in patients with symptoms of heart failure. Chest radiographs are rarely useful in an asymptomatic patient, but may show a boot-shaped heart (suggestive of LVH), frank cardiomegaly, or pulmonary vascular congestion.

Renal function is best evaluated by measurement of serum creatinine and blood urea nitrogen levels. Serum electrolyte levels (K) should be determined in patients taking diuretics or digoxin or those with renal impairment. Mild to moderate hypokalemia (3–3.5 mEq/L) is often seen in patients taking diuretics, but does not have adverse outcome effects. Potassium replacement should be undertaken only in patients who are symptomatic or who are also taking digoxin. Hypomagnesemia is often present and may be a cause of perioperative arrhythmias. Hyperkalemia may be encountered in patients who are taking potassium-sparing diuretics or ACE inhibitors, particularly those with impaired renal function.

Premedication

Premedication reduces preoperative anxiety and is desirable in hypertensive patients. Mild to moderate preoperative hypertension often resolves following administration of an agent such as midazolam.

INTRAOPERATIVE MANAGEMENT
Objectives

The overall anesthetic plan for a hypertensive patient is to maintain an appropriate stable blood pressure range. Patients with borderline hypertension may be treated as normotensive patients. Those with long-standing or poorly controlled hypertension, however, have altered autoregulation of cerebral blood flow; higher than normal mean blood pressures may be required to maintain adequate cerebral blood flow. Because most patients with long-standing hypertension are assumed to have some element of CAD and cardiac hypertrophy, excessive blood pressure elevations are undesirable. Hypertension, particularly in association with tachycardia, can precipitate or exacerbate myocardial ischemia, ventricular dysfunction, or both. Arterial blood pressure should generally be kept within 20% of preoperative levels. If marked hypertension (>180/ 120 mm Hg) is present preoperatively, arterial blood pressure should be maintained in the high-normal range (150–140/90–80 mm Hg).

Monitoring

Most hypertensive patients do not require special intraoperative monitors. Direct intraarterial pressure monitoring should be reserved for patients with wide swings in blood pressure and those undergoing major surgical procedures associated with rapid or marked changes in cardiac preload or afterload.

Electrocardiographic monitoring should focus on detecting signs of ischemia. Urinary output should generally be monitored with an indwelling urinary catheter in patients with a preexisting renal impairment who are undergoing procedures expected to last more than 2 hr. When invasive hemodynamic monitoring is used, reduced ventricular compliance (see Chapter 20) is often apparent in patients with ventricular hypertrophy; these patients may require more intravenous fluid to produce a higher filling pressure to maintain adequate left ventricular end-diastolic volume and cardiac output. Volume administration in patients with decreased ventricular compliance can also result in elevated pulmonary arterial pressures and pulmonary congestion.

Induction

Induction of anesthesia and endotracheal intubation are often associated with hemodynamic instability in hypertensive patients. Regardless of the level of preoperative blood pressure control, many patients with hypertension display an accentuated hypotensive response to induction of anesthesia, followed by an exaggerated hypertensive response to intubation. Many, if not most, antihypertensive agents and general anesthetics are vasodilators, cardiac depressants, or both. In addition, many hypertensive patients present for surgery in a volume-depleted state. Sympatholytic agents attenuate the normal protective circulatory reflexes, reducing sympathetic tone and enhancing vagal activity.

Up to 25% of hypertensive patients may exhibit severe hypertension following endotracheal intubation. Prolonged laryngoscopy should be avoided. Moreover, intubation should generally be performed under deep anesthesia (provided hypotension can be avoided). One of several techniques may be used before intubation to attenuate the hypertensive response:

- Deepening anesthesia with a potent volatile agent
- Administering a bolus of an opioid (fentanyl, 2.5–5 mcg/kg; alfentanil, 15–25 mcg/kg; sufentanil, 0.5–1.0 mcg/kg; or remifentanil, 0.5–1 mcg/kg).

- Administering lidocaine, 1.5 mg/kg intravenously, intratracheally, or topically in the airway
- Achieving β-adrenergic blockade with esmolol, 0.3–1.5 mg/kg; metoprolol 1–5 mg; or labetalol, 5–20 mg.

Choice of Anesthetic Agents

A. Induction Agents

The superiority of any one agent or technique over another has not been established. Propofol, barbiturates, benzodiazepines, and etomidate are equally safe for inducing general anesthesia in most hypertensive patients. Ketamine by itself can precipitate marked hypertension; however, it is almost never used as a single agent. When administered with a small dose of another agent, such as a benzodiazepine or propofol, ketamine's sympathetic stimulating properties can be blunted or eliminated.

B. Maintenance Agents

Anesthesia may be safely continued with volatile agents (alone or with nitrous oxide), a balanced technique (opioid + nitrous oxide + muscle relaxant), or a total intravenous technique. Regardless of the primary maintenance technique, addition of a volatile agent or intravenous vasodilator generally allows convenient intraoperative blood pressure control.

C. Muscle Relaxants

With the possible exception of large bolus doses of pancuronium, any muscle relaxant can be used. Pancuronium-induced vagal blockade and neural release of catecholamines could exacerbate hypertension in poorly controlled patients, but, if given slowly, in small increments, pancuronium is unlikely to cause medically important increases in heart rate or blood pressure. Moreover, pancuronium can be useful in offsetting excessive vagal tone induced by opioids or surgical manipulations. Hypotension following large (intubating) doses of atracurium may be accentuated in hypertensive patients.

D. Vasopressors

Hypertensive patients may display an exaggerated response to both endogenous catecholamines (from intubation or surgical stimulation) and exogenously administered sympathetic agonists. If a vasopressor is necessary to treat excessive hypotension, a small dose of a direct-acting agent, such as phenylephrine (25–50 mcg), may be useful. Patients taking sympatholytics preoperatively may exhibit a decreased response to ephedrine. Vasopressin as a bolus or infusion can also be employed to restore vascular tone in the hypotensive patient.

Intraoperative Hypertension

Intraoperative hypertension not responding to an increase in anesthetic depth (particularly with a volatile agent) can be treated with a variety of parenteral agents (Table 21–7). Readily reversible causes— such as inadequate anesthetic depth, hypoxemia, or hypercapnia—should always be excluded before initiating antihypertensive therapy. Selection of a hypotensive agent depends on the severity, acuteness, and cause of hypertension; the baseline ventricular function; the heart rate; the presence of bronchospastic pulmonary disease; and the anesthetist's familiarity with each of the drug options. β-Adrenergic blockade alone or as a supplement is a good choice for a patient with good ventricular function and an elevated heart rate, but is relatively contraindicated in a patient with bronchospastic disease. Metoprolol, esmolol, or labetolol are readily used intraoperatively. Nicardipine or clevidipine may be preferable to β-blockers for patients with bronchospastic disease. Nitroprusside remains the most rapid and effective agent for the intraoperative treatment of moderate to severe hypertension. Nitroglycerin may be less effective, but is also useful in treating or preventing myocardial ischemia. Fenoldopam, a dopamine agonist, is also a useful hypotensive agent; furthermore, it increases renal blood flow. Hydralazine provides sustained blood pressure control, but also has a delayed onset and can cause reflex tachycardia. The latter is not seen with labetalol because of a combined α- and β-adrenergic blockade.

TABLE 21–7 Parenteral agents for the acute treatment of hypertension.

Agent	Dosage Range	Onset	Duration
Nitroprusside	0.5–10 mcg/kg/min	30–60	1–5 min
Nitroglycerin	0.5–10 mcg/kg/min	1 min	3–5 min
Esmolol	0.5 mg/kg over 1 min; 50–300 mcg/kg/min	1 min	12–20 min
Labetalol	5–20 mg	1–2 min	4–8 hr
Metoprolol	2.5–5 mg	1–5 min	5–8 hr
Hydralazine	5–20 mg	5–20 min	4–8 hr
Clevidipine	1–32 mg/hr	1–3 min	5–15 min
Nicardipine	0.25–0.5 mg 5–15 mg/hr	1–5 min	3–4 hr
Enalaprilat	0.625–1.25 mg	6–15 min	4–6 hr
Fenoldopam	0.1–1.6 mg/kg/min	5 min	5 min

POSTOPERATIVE MANAGEMENT

Postoperative hypertension is common and should be anticipated in patients who have poorly controlled hypertension. Close blood pressure monitoring should be continued in both the recovery room and the early postoperative period. In addition to myocardial ischemia and congestive heart failure, marked sustained elevations in blood pressure can contribute to the formation of wound hematomas and the disruption of vascular suture lines.

Hypertension in the recovery period is often multifactorial and enhanced by respiratory abnormalities, anxiety and pain, volume overload, or bladder distention. Contributing causes should be corrected and parenteral antihypertensive agents given if necessary. Intravenous labetalol is particularly useful in controlling hypertension and tachycardia, whereas vasodilators are useful in controlling blood pressure in the setting of a slow heart rate. When the patient resumes oral intake, preoperative medications should be restarted.

ISCHEMIC HEART DISEASE
Preoperative Considerations

Myocardial ischemia is characterized by a metabolic oxygen demand that exceeds the oxygen supply. Ischemia can therefore result from a marked increase in myocardial metabolic demand, a reduction in myocardial oxygen delivery, or a combination of both. Common causes include coronary arterial vasospasm or thrombosis; severe hypertension or tachycardia (particularly in the presence of ventricular hypertrophy); severe hypotension, hypoxemia, or anemia; and severe aortic stenosis or regurgitation.

By far, the most common cause of myocardial ischemia is atherosclerosis of the coronary arteries. CAD is responsible for about 25% of all deaths in Western societies and is a major cause of perioperative morbidity and mortality. The overall incidence of CAD in surgical patients is estimated to be between 5% and 10%. Major risk factors for CAD include hyperlipidemia, hypertension, diabetes, cigarette smoking, increasing age, male sex, and a positive family history. Other risk factors include obesity, a history of cerebrovascular or peripheral vascular disease, menopause, use of high-estrogen oral contraceptives (in women who smoke), and a sedentary lifestyle.

CAD may be clinically manifested by symptoms of myocardial necrosis (infarction), ischemia (usually angina), arrhythmias (including sudden death), or ventricular dysfunction (congestive heart failure). When symptoms of congestive heart failure predominate, the term "ischemic cardiomyopathy" is often used.

Unstable Angina

Unstable angina is defined as (1) an abrupt increase in severity, frequency (more than three episodes per day), or duration of anginal attacks (crescendo angina): (2) angina at rest; or (3) new onset of angina (within the past 2 months) with severe or frequent episodes (more than three per day). Unstable angina may occur following MI or be precipitated by noncardiac medical conditions (including severe anemia, fever, infections, thyrotoxicosis, hypoxemia, and emotional distress) in previously stable patients.

Unstable angina, particularly when it is associated with significant ST-segment changes at rest, usually reflects severe underlying coronary disease and frequently precedes MI. Plaque disruption with platelet aggregates or thrombi and vasospasm are frequent pathological correlates. Critical stenosis in one or more major coronary arteries is present in more than 80% of patients with these symptoms. Patients with unstable angina require evaluation and treatment, which may include admission to a coronary care unit and some form of coronary intervention.

Chronic Stable Angina

Anginal chest pains are most often substernal, exertional, radiating to the neck or arm, and relieved by rest or nitroglycerin. Variations are common, including epigastric, back, or neck pain, or transient shortness of breath from ventricular dysfunction (anginal equivalent). Nonexertional ischemia and silent (asymptomatic) ischemia are recognized as fairly common occurrences. Patients with diabetes have an increased incidence of silent ischemia.

Symptoms are generally absent until the atherosclerotic lesions cause 50% to 75% occlusion of the coronary circulation. When a stenotic segment reaches 70% occlusion, maximum compensatory dilatation is usually present distally: blood flow is generally adequate at rest, but becomes inadequate with increased metabolic demand. An extensive collateral blood supply allows some patients to remain relatively asymptomatic in spite of severe disease. Coronary vasospasm is also a cause of transient transmural ischemia in some patients; 90% of vasospastic episodes occur at preexisting stenotic lesions in epicardial vessels and are often precipitated by a variety of factors, including emotional upset and hyperventilation (Prinzmetal's angina). Coronary spasm is most often observed in patients who have angina with varying levels of activity or emotional stress (variable-threshold); it is least common with classic exertional (fixed-threshold) angina.

The overall prognosis of patients with CAD is related to both the number and severity of coronary obstructions, as well as to the extent of ventricular dysfunction.

Treatment of Ischemic Heart Disease

The general approach in treating patients with ischemic heart disease is five-fold:

- Correction of risk factors, with the hope of slowing disease progression.
- Modification of the patient's lifestyle to reduce stress and improve exercise tolerance.
- Correction of complicating medical conditions that can exacerbate ischemia (ie, hypertension, anemia, hypoxemia, hyperthyroidism, fever, infection, or adverse drug effects).
- Pharmacological manipulation of the myocardial oxygen supply–demand relationship.
- Correction of coronary lesions by percutaneous coronary intervention (angioplasty [with or without stenting] or atherectomy) or coronary artery bypass surgery.

The last three approaches are of direct relevance to anesthesiologists. The same principles should be applied in the care of these patients in both the operating room and the intensive care unit.

TABLE 21–8 Comparison of antianginal agents.[1]

| | | Calcium Channel Blockers | | | |
Cardiac Parameter	Nitrates	Verapamil	Nifedipine Nicardipine Nimodipine	Diltiazem	β-Blockers
Preload	↓↓	—	—	—	—/↑
Afterload	↓	↓	↓↓	↓	—/↓
Contractility	—	↓↓	—	↓	↓↓↓
SA node automaticity	↑/—	↓↓	↑/—	↓↓	↓↓↓
AV conduction	—	↓↓↓	—	↓↓	↓↓↓

Vasodilatation
  Coronary
  Systemic
	↑
	↑↑
		↑↑
		↑
			↑↑↑
			↑↑
				↑↑
				↑
					—/↓
					—/↓

[1]SA, sinoatrial; AV, atrioventricular; ↑, increases; —, no change; ↓, decreases.

The most commonly used pharmacological agents are nitrates, β-blockers, and calcium channel blockers. These drugs also have potent circulatory effects, which are compared in Table 21–8. Any of these agents can be used for mild angina. Calcium channel blockers are the drugs of choice for patients with predominantly vasospastic angina. β-Blockers improve the long-term outcome of patients with CAD. Nitrates are good agents for both types of angina.

A. Nitrates

Nitrates relax all vascular smooth muscle, but have a much greater effect on venous than on arterial vessels. Decreasing venous and arteriolar tone and reducing the effective circulating blood volume (cardiac preload) reduce wall tension afterload. These effects tend to reduce myocardial oxygen demand. The prominent venodilatation makes nitrates excellent agents when congestive heart failure is also present.

Perhaps equally important, nitrates dilate the coronary arteries. Even minor degrees of dilatation at stenotic sites may be sufficient to increase blood flow, because flow is directly related to the fourth power of the radius. Nitrate-induced coronary vasodilatation preferentially increases subendocardial blood flow in ischemic areas. This favorable redistribution of coronary blood flow to ischemic areas may

be dependent on the presence of collaterals in the coronary circulation.

Nitrates can be used for both the treatment of acute ischemia and prophylaxis against frequent anginal episodes. Unlike β-blockers and calcium channel blockers, nitrates do not have a negative inotropic effect—a desirable feature in the presence of ventricular dysfunction. Intravenous nitroglycerin can also be used for controlled hypotensive anesthesia.

B. Calcium Channel Blockers

The effects and uses of the most commonly used calcium channel blockers are shown in Table 21–9. Calcium channel blockers reduce myocardial oxygen demand by decreasing cardiac afterload and augment oxygen supply by increasing blood flow (coronary vasodilatation). Verapamil and diltiazem also reduce demand by slowing the heart rate.

Nifedipine's potent effects on the systemic blood pressure may precipitate hypotension, reflex tachycardia, or both; its fast-onset preparations (eg, sublingual) have been associated with MI in some patients. Its tendency to decrease afterload generally offsets any negative inotropic effect. The slow-release form of nifedipine is associated with much less reflex tachycardia and is more suitable than other agents for patients with ventricular

TABLE 21-9 Comparison of calcium channel blockers.

Agent	Route	Dosage[1]	Half-life	Clinical Use			
				Angina	Hypertension	Cerebral Vasospasm	Supraventricular Tachycardia
Verapamil	PO	40–240 mg	5 hr	+	+		+
	IV	5–15 mg	5 hr	+			+
Nifedipine	PO	30–180 mg	2 hr	+	+		
	SL	10 mg	2 hr	+	+		
Diltiazem	PO	30–60 mg	4 hr	+	+		+
	IV	0.25–0.35 mg/kg	4 hr	+			+
Nicardipine	PO	60–120 mg	2–4 hr	+	+		
	IV	0.25–0.5 mg/kg	2–4 hr	+	+		
Nimodipine	PO	240 mg	2 hr			+	
Bepridil[2]	PO	200–400 mg	24 hr	+	+		
Isradipine	PO	2.5–5.0 mg	8 hr		+		
Felodipine	PO	5–20 mg	9 hr		+		
Amlodipine	PO	2.5–10 mg	30–50 hr	+	+		

[1]Total oral dose per day divided into three doses unless otherwise stated.
[2]Also possesses antiarrhythmic properties.

dysfunction. In contrast, verapamil and diltiazem have greater effects on cardiac contractility and atrioventricular (AV) conduction and therefore should be used cautiously, if at all, in patients with ventricular dysfunction, conduction abnormalities, or bradyarrhythmias. Diltiazem seems to be better tolerated than verapamil in patients with impaired ventricular function. Nicardipine, nimodipine, and clevidipine generally have the same effects as nifedipine; nimodipine is primarily used in preventing cerebral vasospasm following subarachnoid hemorrhage, whereas nicardipine is used as an intravenous arterial vasodilator. Clevidipine is an ultrashort–acting arterial vasodilator.

Calcium channel blockers can have significant interactions with anesthetic agents. All calcium channel blockers potentiate both depolarizing and nondepolarizing neuromuscular blocking agents and the circulatory effects of volatile agents. Both verapamil and diltiazem can potentiate depression of cardiac contractility and conduction in the AV node by volatile anesthetics. Nifedipine and similar agents can potentiate systemic vasodilatation by volatile and intravenous agents.

C. β-Adrenergic Blocking Agents

These drugs decrease myocardial oxygen demand by reducing heart rate and contractility, and, in some cases, afterload (via their antihypertensive effect). Optimal blockade results in a resting heart rate between 50 and 60 beats/min and prevents appreciable increases with exercise (<20 beats/min increase during exercise). Available agents differ in receptor selectivity, intrinsic sympathomimetic (partial agonist) activity, and membrane-stabilizing properties (Table 21–10). Membrane stabilization, often described as a quinidine-like effect, results in antiarrhythmic activity. Agents with

TABLE 21–10 Comparison of β-adrenergic blocking agents.

Agent	β₁-Receptor Selectivity	Half-life	Sympathomimetic	α-Receptor Blockade	Membrane Stabilizing
Acebutolol	+	2–4 hr	+		+
Atenolol	++	5–9 hr			
Betaxlol	++	14–22 hr			
Esmolol	++	9 min			
Metoprolol	++	3–4 hr			±
Bisoprolol	+	9–12 hr			
Oxprenolol		1–2 hr	+		+
Alprenolol		2–3 hr	+		+
Pindolol		3–4 hr	++		±
Penbutolol		5 hr	+		+
Carteolol		6 hr	+		
Labetalol		4–8 hr		+	±
Propranolol		3–6 hr			++
Timolol		3–5 hr			
Sotalol¹		5–13 hr			
Nadolol		10–24 hr			
Carvedilol		6–8 hr		+	±

¹Also possesses unique antiarrhythmic properties.

intrinsic sympathomimetic properties are better tolerated by patients with mild to moderate ventricular dysfunction. Certain β-blockers (carvedilol and extended-duration metoprolol) improve survival in patients with chronic heart failure. This has not been shown to be a drug class effect. Blockade of β₂-adrenergic receptors also can mask hypoglycemic symptoms in patients with diabetes, delay metabolic recovery from hypoglycemia, and impair the handling of large potassium loads. Cardioselective (β₁-receptor-specific) agents, although generally better tolerated than nonselective agents in patients with reactive airways, must still be used cautiously in such patients. The selectivity of cardioselective agents tends to be dose dependent. Patients on

long-standing β-blocker therapy should have these agents continued perioperatively. Acute β-blocker withdrawal in the perioperative period places patients at a markedly increased risk of cardiac morbidity and mortality.

Documentation of avoidance of β-blocker withdrawal is a frequent tool by which "quality" of anesthesia services can be assessed by regulatory agencies.

D. Other Agents

ACE inhibitors prolong survival in patients with congestive heart failure or left ventricular dysfunction. Chronic aspirin therapy reduces coronary events in patients with CAD and prevents coronary and ischemic cerebral events in at-risk patients. Antiarrhythmic therapy in patients with complex ventricular ectopy who have significant CAD and left ventricular dysfunction should be guided by an electrophysiological study. Patients with inducible sustained ventricular tachycardia (VT) or ventricular fibrillation are candidates for an automatic internal cardioverter-defibrillator (ICD). Treatment of ventricular ectopy (with the exception of sustained VT) in patients with good ventricular function does not improve survival and may increase mortality. In contrast, ICDs have been shown to improve survival in patients with advanced cardiomyopathy (ejection fraction <30%), even in the absence of demonstrable arrhythmias.

E. Combination Therapy

Moderate to severe angina frequently requires combination therapy with two or all three classes of agents. Patients with ventricular dysfunction may not tolerate the combined negative inotropic effect of a β-blocker and a calcium channel blocker together; an ACE inhibitor is better tolerated and seems to improve survival. Similarly, the additive effect of a β-blocker and a calcium channel blocker on the AV node may precipitate heart block in susceptible patients.

PREOPERATIVE MANAGEMENT

The importance of ischemic heart disease—particularly a history of MI—as a risk factor for perioperative morbidity and mortality was discussed earlier in the chapter. Most studies confirm that perioperative outcome is related to disease severity, ventricular function, and the type of surgery to be undertaken. Patients with extensive (three-vessel or left main) CAD, a recent history of MI, or ventricular dysfunction are at greatest risk of cardiac complications. As mentioned above, current guidelines recommend revascularization when such treatment would be indicated irrespective of the patient's need for surgery.

Chronic stable (mild to moderate) angina does not seem to increase perioperative risk substantially. Similarly, a history of prior coronary artery bypass

surgery or coronary angioplasty alone does not seem to substantially increase perioperative risk. In some studies, maintenance of chronic β-receptor blockers in the perioperative period has been shown to reduce perioperative mortality and the incidence of postoperative cardiovascular complications; however, other studies have shown an increase in stroke and death following preoperative introduction of β-blockers to "at risk" patients. Consequently, as with all drugs, the risks and benefits of initiating therapy with β-blockers in at risk patients must be considered. Like β-blockers, statins should be continued perioperatively in patients so routinely treated, as acute perioperative withdrawal of statins is associated with adverse outcomes. ACC/AHA guidelines suggest that β-blockers are useful in patients undergoing vascular surgery with evidence of ischemia on their evaluative workup (class I).

History

The history is of prime importance in patients with ischemic heart disease. Questions should encompass symptoms, current and past treatment, complications, and the results of previous evaluations. This information alone is usually enough to provide some estimate of disease severity and ventricular function.

The most important symptoms to elicit include chest pains, dyspnea, poor exercise tolerance, syncope, or near syncope. The relationship between symptoms and activity level should be established. Activity should be described in terms of everyday tasks, such as walking or climbing stairs. Patients may be relatively asymptomatic despite severe CAD if they have a sedentary lifestyle. Patients with diabetes are particularly prone to silent ischemia. The patient's description of chest pains may suggest a major role for vasospasm (variable-threshold angina). Easy fatigability or shortness of breath suggests impaired ventricular function.

A history of unstable angina or MI should include the time of its occurrence and whether it was complicated by arrhythmias, conduction disturbances, or heart failure. Localization of the areas of ischemia is invaluable in deciding which electrocardiographic leads to monitor intraoperatively. Arrhythmias and conduction abnormalities are more common in patients with previous infarction and in those with poor ventricular function. This latter group of patients will often have ICDs.

Physical Examination & Routine Laboratory Evaluation

Evaluation of patients with CAD is similar to that of patients with hypertension. Laboratory evaluation in patients who have a history compatible with recent unstable angina and are undergoing emergency procedures should include cardiac enzymes. Serum levels of cardiac-specific troponins, creatine kinase (MB isoenzyme), and lactate dehydrogenase (type 1 isoenzyme) are useful in excluding MI.

The baseline ECG is normal in 25% to 50% of patients with CAD but no prior MI. Electrocardiographic evidence of ischemia often becomes apparent only during chest pain. The most common baseline abnormalities are nonspecific ST-segment and T-wave changes. Prior infarction is often manifested by Q waves or loss of R waves in the leads closest to the infarct. First-degree AV block, bundle-branch block, or hemiblock may be present. Persistent ST-segment elevation following MI may be indicative of a left ventricular aneurysm. A long rate-corrected QT interval ($QT_c > 0.44$ s) may reflect the underlying ischemia, drug toxicity (usually class Ia antiarrhythmic agents, antidepressants, or phenothiazines), electrolyte abnormalities (hypokalemia or hypomagnesemia), autonomic dysfunction, mitral valve prolapse, or, less commonly, a congenital abnormality. Patients with a long QT interval are at risk of developing ventricular arrhythmias—particularly polymorphic VT (torsade de pointes), which can lead to ventricular fibrillation. The long QT interval reflects nonuniform prolongation of ventricular repolarization and predisposes patients to reentry phenomena. In contrast to polymorphic ventricular arrhythmias with a normal QT interval, which respond to conventional antiarrhythmics, polymorphic tachyarrhythmias with a long QT interval generally respond best to pacing or magnesium salts. Patients with congenital prolongation generally respond to β-adrenergic blocking agents. Left stellate ganglion blockade is also effective and suggests that autonomic imbalance plays an important role in this group of patients.

The chest film can be used to exclude cardiomegaly or pulmonary vascular congestion secondary to ventricular dysfunction. Rarely, calcification of the coronaries, aorta, or the aortic valve may be seen on the chest radiograph; such is a more common finding on CT.

Specialized Studies

When used as screening tests for the general population, noninvasive stress tests have a low predictability in asymptomatic patients, but are sufficiently reliable in symptomatic patients with suspect lesions.

4 Holter monitoring, exercise electrocardiography, myocardial perfusion scans, and echocardiography are important in determining perioperative risk and the need for coronary angiography; however, these tests are indicated only if their outcome would alter patient care.

Current ACC/AHA guidelines recommend noninvasive stress testing in patients scheduled for noncardiac surgery with active cardiac conditions (class I). The current guidelines also suggest that there may be benefit of such testing in patients with three or more clinical risk factors and poor functional capacity (class IIa). Likewise, they suggest that noninvasive testing can be of some possible benefit in patients with one or two clinical risk factors undergoing intermediate risk or vascular surgery (class IIb). What they do not recommend is the indiscriminate use of noninvasive cardiac testing in patients with no risk factors undergoing intermediate-risk surgery. Consequently, indications for preoperative cardiac screening tests continue to narrow.

A. Holter Monitoring

Continuous ambulatory electrocardiographic (Holter) monitoring is useful in evaluating arrhythmias, antiarrhythmic drug therapy, and severity and frequency of ischemic episodes. Silent (asymptomatic) ischemic episodes are frequently found in patients with CAD. Frequent ischemic episodes on preoperative Holter monitoring correlate well with intraoperative and postoperative ischemia. Holter monitoring has an excellent negative predictive value for postoperative cardiac complications.

B. Exercise Electrocardiography

The usefulness of this test is limited in patients with baseline ST-segment abnormalities and those who are unable to increase their heart rate (>85% of maximal predicted) because of fatigue, dyspnea, or drug therapy. Overall sensitivity is 65%, and specificity is 90%. The test is most sensitive (85%) in patients with three-vessel or left main CAD. Disease that is limited to the left circumflex artery may also be missed because ischemia in its distribution may not be evident on the standard surface ECG. A normal test does not necessarily exclude CAD, but suggests that severe disease is not likely. The degree of ST-segment depression, its severity and configuration, the time of onset in the test, and the time required for resolution are important findings. A myocardial ischemic response at low levels of exercise is associated with a significantly increased risk of perioperative complications and long-term cardiac events. Other significant findings include changes in blood pressure and the occurrence of arrhythmias. Exercise-induced ventricular ectopy frequently indicates severe CAD associated with ventricular dysfunction. The ischemia presumably leads to electrical instability in myocardial cells. Given that risk seems to be associated with the degree of myocardium potentially ischemic, testing often includes perfusion scans or echocardiographic assessments; however, in ambulatory patients, exercise ECG testing is useful because it estimates functional capacity and detects myocardial ischemia.

C. Myocardial Perfusions Scans and Other Imaging Techniques

Myocardial perfusion imaging using thallium-201 or technetium-99m is used in evaluating patients who cannot exercise (eg, peripheral vascular disease) or who have underlying ECG abnormalities that preclude interpretation during exercise (eg, left bundle-branch block). If the patient cannot exercise, images are obtained before and after injection of an intravenous coronary dilator (eg, dipyridamole or adenosine) to produce a hyperemic response similar to exercise. Myocardial perfusion studies following exercise or injection of dipyridamole or adenosine have a high sensitivity, but only fairly good specificity for CAD. They are best for

detecting two- or three-vessel disease. These scans can locate and quantitate areas of ischemia or scarring and differentiate between the two. Perfusion defects that fill in on the redistribution phase represent ischemia, not previous infarction. The negative predictive value of a normal perfusion scan is approximately 99%.

MRI, PET, and CT scans are increasingly being used to define coronary artery anatomy and determine myocardial viability.

D. Echocardiography

This technique provides information about both regional and global ventricular function and may be carried out at rest, following exercise, or with administration of dobutamine. Detectable regional wall motion abnormalities and the derived left ventricular ejection fraction correlate well with angiographic findings. Moreover, dobutamine stress echocardiography seems to be a reliable predictor of adverse cardiac complications in patients who cannot exercise. New or worsening wall motion abnormalities following dobutamine infusion are indicative of significant ischemia. Patients with an ejection fraction of less than 50% tend to have more severe disease and increased perioperative morbidity. Dobutamine stress echocardiography, however, may not be reliable in patients with left bundle-branch block because septal motion may be abnormal, even in the absence of left anterior descending CAD in some patients.

E. Coronary Angiography

Coronary angiography remains the definitive way to evaluate CAD and is associated with a low complication rate (<1%). Nonetheless, coronary angiography should be performed only to determine if the patient may benefit from percutaneous coronary angioplasty or coronary artery bypass grafting prior to noncardiac surgery. The location and severity of occlusions can be defined, and coronary vasospasm may also be observed on angiography. In evaluating fixed stenotic lesions, occlusions greater than 50% to 75% are generally considered significant. The severity of disease is often expressed according to the number of major coronary vessels affected (one-, two-, or three-vessel disease). Significant stenosis of the left main coronary artery is of great concern because disruption of flow in this vessel will have adverse effects on almost the entire left ventricle.

Ventriculography, measurement of the ejection fraction, and measurement of intracardiac pressures, also provide important information. Indicators of significant ventricular dysfunction include an ejection fraction <50%, a left ventricular end-diastolic pressure >18 mm Hg, a cardiac index <2.2 L/min/m², and marked or multiple wall motion abnormalities.

Guidelines suggest that patients with stable angina and significant left main disease, stable angina and three-vessel disease, stable angina and two-vessel disease with an ejection fraction <50%, unstable angina, non-ST segment elevation MI, and acute ST segment elevation MI benefit from revascularization. This recommendation also applies to patients who are scheduled for noncardiac surgery (class I). Conversely, revascularization is not indicated in patients with stable angina (class III). Moreover, elective noncardiac surgery is not recommended within 4–6 weeks following bare metal stent placement or within 12 months of placement of a drug-eluting stent, if the surgery requires that antiplatelet therapy be discontinued.

Premedication

Allaying fear, anxiety, and pain preoperatively are desirable goals in patients with CAD. Satisfactory premedication prevents sympathetic activation, which adversely affects the myocardial oxygen supply–demand balance. Overmedication is equally detrimental and should be avoided because it may result in hypoxemia, respiratory acidosis, and hypotension. A benzodiazepine, alone or in combination with an opioid, is commonly used. (The concomitant administration of oxygen via nasal cannula helps avoid hypoxemia following premedication.) Patients with poor ventricular function and coexistent lung disease should receive reduced doses. Preoperative medications should generally be continued until the time of surgery. They may be given orally (with a small sip of water), intramuscularly, intravenously, sublingually, or transdermally.

5 The sudden withdrawal of antianginal medication perioperatively—particularly β-blockers—can precipitate a sudden, rebound increase in ischemic episodes. In the past, some clinicians prophylactically administered nitrates intravenously or transdermally to patients with CAD in the perioperative period. Although this practice may be theoretically advantageous, there is no evidence of its efficacy in patients not previously on long-term nitrate therapy and without evidence of ongoing ischemia. Transdermal absorption of nitroglycerin may be erratic in the perioperative period.

INTRAOPERATIVE MANAGEMENT

The intraoperative period is regularly associated with factors and events that can adversely affect the myocardial oxygen demand–supply relationship. Activation of the sympathetic system plays a major role. Hypertension and enhanced contractility increase myocardial oxygen demand, whereas tachycardia increases demand and reduces supply. Although myocardial ischemia is commonly associated with tachycardia, it can occur in the absence of any apparent hemodynamic derangement.

Objectives

6 The overwhelming priority in managing patients with ischemic heart disease is maintaining a favorable myocardial supply–demand relationship. Autonomic-mediated increases in heart rate and blood pressure should be controlled by deep anesthesia or adrenergic blockade. Excessive reductions in coronary perfusion pressure or arterial oxygen content are to be avoided. Although exact limits are not defined or predictable, diastolic arterial pressure should generally be maintained at 50 mm Hg or above. Higher diastolic pressures may be preferable in patients with high-grade coronary occlusions. Excessive increases—such as those caused by fluid overload—in left ventricular end-diastolic pressure should be avoided because they increase ventricular wall tension (afterload) and can reduce subendocardial perfusion (see Chapter 20). Transfusion carries its own risks and consequently there is no set transfusion trigger in patients with

CAD; however, anemia can lead to tachycardia, worsening the balance between myocardial oxygen supply and demand.

MONITORING

Intraarterial pressure monitoring is reasonable for all patients with severe CAD and major or multiple cardiac risk factors who are undergoing any but the most minor procedures. Central venous (or rarely pulmonary artery) pressure can be monitored during prolonged or complicated procedures involving large fluid shifts or blood loss. Less invasive methods of cardiac output determination and volume assessment have been previously discussed in this text. Transesophageal echocardiography (TEE) and transthoracic echocardiography (TTE) can provide valuable information, both qualitative and quantitative, on contractility and ventricular chamber size (preload) perioperatively. Intensive care unit staff increasingly use ultrasound to assist in hemodynamic management. Numerous "basic" courses in TEE and TTE are available to assist practitioners in performing "hemodynamic," as opposed to cardiac diagnostic TEE.

7 Intraoperative detection of ischemia depends on recognition of electrocardiographic changes, hemodynamic manifestations, or regional wall motion abnormalities on TEE. Doppler TEE also allows detection of the onset of mitral regurgitation caused by ischemic papillary muscle dysfunction.

A. Electrocardiography

Early ischemic changes are subtle and can often be overlooked. They involve changes in T-wave morphology, including inversion, tenting, or both (Figure 21–1). More obvious ischemia may be seen in the form of progressive ST-segment depression. Down-sloping and horizontal ST depressions are of greater specificity for ischemia than is up-sloping depression. New ST-segment elevations are rare during noncardiac surgery and are indicative of severe ischemia, vasospasm, or infarction. However, the increasing number of individuals treated with drug-eluting stents can be problematic perioperatively, especially if surgical concerns necessitate discontinuation of antiplatelet therapy (eg, emergency spine

surgery). Such patients are at very increased risk of thrombosis and perioperative MI. Anesthesia staff should never for nonsurgical reasons (eg, desire to perform a spinal anesthetic) discontinue antiplatelet or anti thrombotic agents perioperatively without first discussing the risks and benefits of the proposed anesthetic requiring suspension of antiplatelet therapy with the patient and his or her cardiologist. ACC/AHA offers recommendations on the approach of bringing patients to surgery following percutaneous coronary interventions and the type of interventions suggested when subsequent surgery is expected (Figures 21–2 and 21–3). It should be noted that an isolated minor ST elevation in the mid-precordial leads (V_3 and V_4) can be a normal variant in young patients. Ischemia may also present as an unexplained intraoperative atrial or ventricular arrhythmia or the onset of a new conduction abnormality. The sensitivity of the ECG in detecting ischemia is related to the number of leads monitored. Studies suggest that the V_5, V_4, II, V_2, and V_3 leads (in decreasing sensitivity) are most useful. Ideally, at least two leads should be monitored simultaneously. Usually, lead II is monitored for inferior wall ischemia and arrhythmias, and V_5 is monitored for anterior wall ischemia. When only one channel can be monitored, a modified V_5 lead provides the highest sensitivity.

B. Hemodynamic Monitoring

The most common hemodynamic abnormalities observed during ischemic episodes are hypertension and tachycardia. They are almost always a cause (rather than the result) of ischemia. Hypotension is a late and ominous manifestation of progressive ventricular dysfunction. TEE readily will demonstrate a dysfunctional ventricle and ventricular wall motion changes associated with myocardial ischemia. Ischemia is frequently, but not always, associated with an abrupt increase in pulmonary capillary wedge pressure. The sudden appearance of a prominent *v* wave on the wedge waveform is usually indicative of acute mitral regurgitation from ischemic papillary muscle dysfunction or acute left ventricular dilatation.

C. Transesophageal Echocardiography

TEE can be helpful in detecting global and regional cardiac dysfunction, as well as valvular function in selected patients. Moreover, detection of new

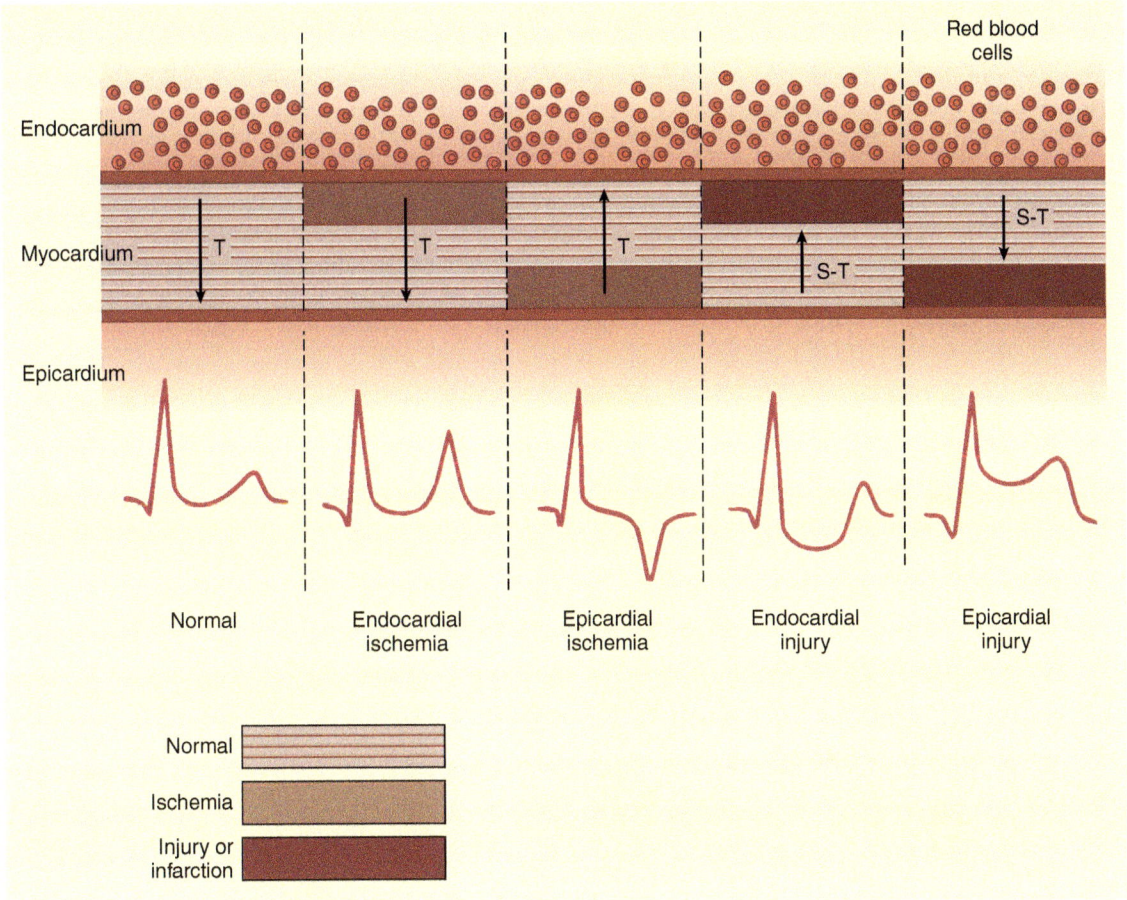

FIGURE 21–1 Electrocardiographic signs of ischemia. Patterns of ischemia and injury. (Information compiled from Schamroth L: *The 12 Lead Electrocardiogram.* Blackwell, 1989.)

regional wall motion abnormalities is a rapid and more sensitive indicator of myocardial ischemia than the ECG. In animal studies in which coronary blood flow is gradually reduced, regional wall motion abnormalities develop before the ECG changes. Although the occurrence of new intraoperative abnormalities correlates with postoperative MIs in some studies, not all such abnormalities are necessarily ischemic. Both regional and global abnormalities can be caused by changes in heart rate, altered conduction, preload, afterload, or drug-induced changes in contractility. Decreased systolic wall thickening may be a more reliable index for ischemia than endocardial wall motion alone.

Arrhythmias, Pacemakers, and Internal Cardioverter-Defibrillator Management

Electrolyte disorders, heart structure defects, inflammation, myocardial ischemia, cardiomyopathies, and conduction abnormalities can all contribute to the development of perioperative arrhythmias and heart block. Consequently, the anesthesia staff must be prepared to manage both chronic and new-onset cardiac rhythm problems.

Supraventricular tachycardias (SVTs) can have hemodynamic consequences secondary to loss of AV synchrony and decreased diastolic filling time.

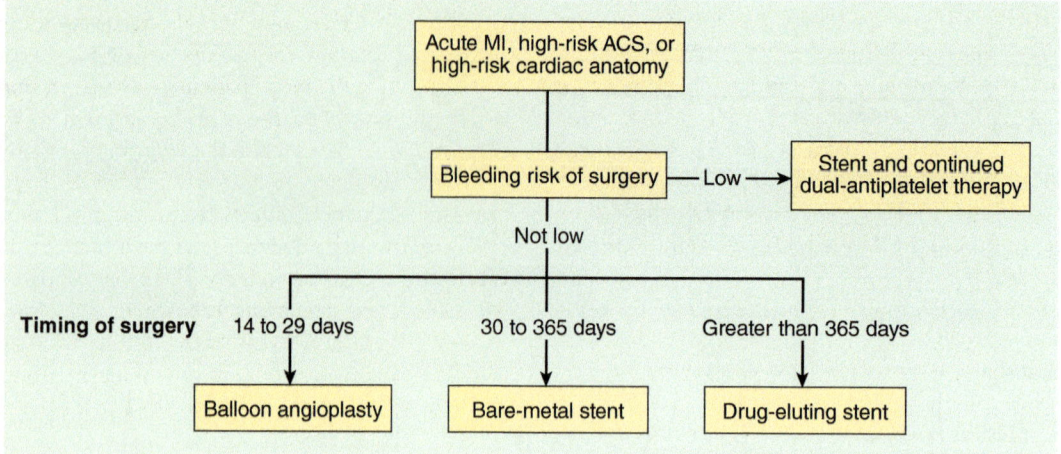

FIGURE 21–2 Proposed treatment for patients requiring percutaneous coronary intervention (PCI) who need subsequent surgery. ACS, acute coronary syndrome; COR, class of recommendation; LOE, level of evidence; MI, myocardial infarction. (Reproduced, with permission, from Fleisher L, Beckman J, Brown K, et al: ACC/AHA 2007 guidelines on perioperative cardiovascular evaluation and care for noncardiac surgery. Circulation 2007;116: e418.)

Loss of the "P" wave on the ECG with a fast ventricular response is consistent with SVTs. Most SVTs occur secondary to a reentrant mechanism. Reentrant arrhythmias occur when conduction tissues in the heart depolarize or repolarize at varying rates. In this manner, a self-perpetuating loop of repolarization and depolarization can occur in the conduction pathways and/or AV node. SVTs producing hemodynamic collapse are treated perioperatively with synchronized cardioversion. Adenosine can likewise be given to slow AV node conduction and potentially disrupt the reentrant loop. SVTs

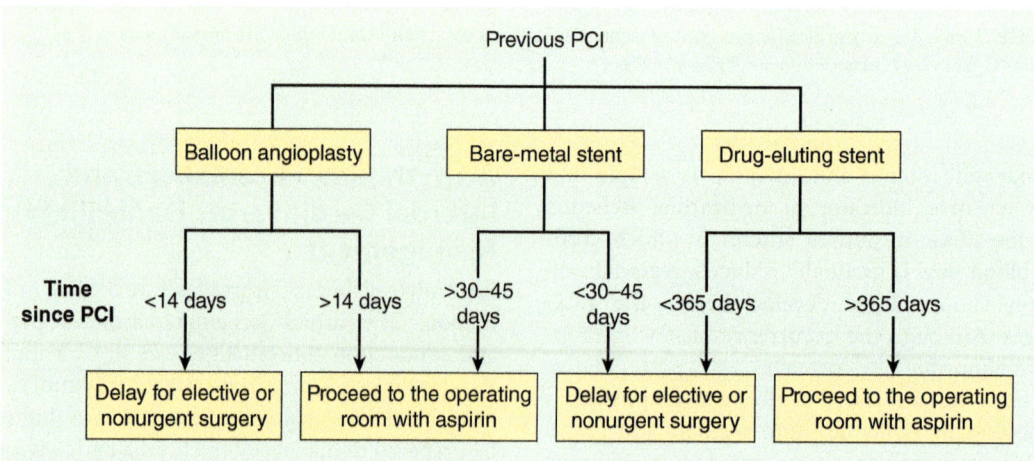

FIGURE 21–3 Proposed approach to the management of patients with previous percutaneous coronary intervention (PCI) who require non-cardiac surgery, based on expert opinion. (Reproduced, with permission, from Fleisher L, Beckman J, Brown K, et al: ACC/AHA 2007 guidelines on perioperative cardiovascular evaluation and care for noncardiac surgery. Circulation 2007;116: e418.)

in patients without accessory conduction bundles (Wolff–Parkinson–White [WPW] syndrome) are treated with β-blockers and calcium channel blockers. In patients with known WPW, procainamide or amiodarone can be used to treat SVTs. At times, SVTs manifest with a broad QRS complex and seem to be similar to VTs. Such rhythms, when they present, should be treated like VT, until proven otherwise.

Atrial fibrillation (AF) can complicate the perioperative period (Figure 21–4) Up to 35% of cardiac surgery patients develop postoperative AF. Moreover, many patients present with AF for anesthesia and noncardiac surgery. The ACC/AHA has issued voluminous guidelines for the outpatient management of AF. The guidelines recommend use of β-blockers or nondihydropyridine calcium antagonists for ventricular rate control in patients without accessory conduction pathways. Amiodarone, procainamide, disopyramide, and ibutilide are suggested for ventricular rate control in patients with accessory pathways. The use of digitalis and nondihyropryidine calcium channel blockers is contraindicated in patients with accessory pathways.

The ACC/AHA guidelines also recommend antithrombotic therapy in patients with long-standing AF. Consequently, many patients with AF will present to the operating room on some form of antithrombotic therapy—often the vitamin K antagonist warfarin. However, ACC/AHA guidelines suggest that aspirin can be an alternative to vitamin K antagonists in low-risk patients or those with contraindications to oral anticoagulation. Likewise, in patients with AF without mechanical prosthetic heart valves, the guidelines suggest that it is acceptable to discontinue anticoagulation for up to 1 week in advance of surgical procedures, without instituting heparin anticoagulation.

When AF develops perioperatively, rate control with β-blockers can often be instituted. Chemical cardioversion can be attempted with amiodarone or procainamide. Of note, if the duration of AF is greater than 48 hours, or unknown, ACC/AHA guidelines recommend anticoagulation for 3 weeks prior to and 4 weeks following either electrical or chemical cardioversion. Alternatively, TEE can be performed to rule out the presence of left atrial or left atrial appendage thrombus.

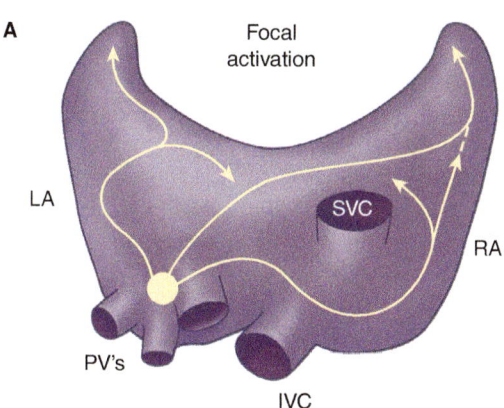 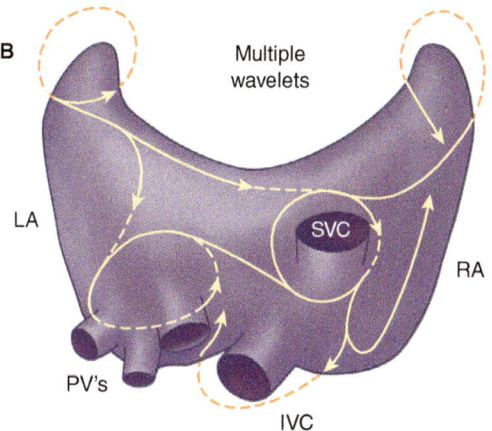

FIGURE 21–4 Posterior view of principal electrophysiological mechanisms of atrial fibrillation. **A**: Focal activation. The initiating focus (indicated by the dot) often lies within the region of the pulmonary veins. The resulting wavelets represent fibrillatory conduction, as in multiple-wavelet reentry. **B**: Multiple-wavelet reentry. Wavelets (indicated by arrows) randomly reenter tissue previously activated by the same or another wavelet. The routes the wavelets travel vary. LA, left atrium; PV, pulmonary vein; ICV, inferior vena cava; SCV, superior vena cava; RA, right atrium. (Reproduced with permission, from Konings KT, Kirchhof CJ, Smeets JR, et al: High-density mapping of electrically induced atrial fibrillation in humans. Circulation 1994 Apr;89(4):1665-1680.)

Should AF develop postoperatively, ventricular rate response can be controlled with AV nodal blocking agents, unless contraindicated. Should AF result in hemodynamic instability, synchronized cardioversion can be attempted. Patients at high risk of AF following cardiac surgery can be treated with prophylactic amiodarone.

AF is most frequently associated with loss of atrial muscle and the development of fibrosis. Fibrosis may contribute to reentrant mechanisms of AF as depolarization/repolarization becomes nonhomogeneous. AF may also develop from a focal source often located in the pulmonary veins. In patients with an accessory bundle, AF can produce rapid ventricular responses and hemodynamic collapse. Drugs that slow conduction across the AV node (eg, digitalis, verapamil, diltiazem) do not slow conduction across the accessory pathway, potentially leading to hemodynamic collapse. The ACC/AHA guidelines likewise recommend caution in the use of β-blockers for AF in patients with preexcitation syndromes.

Ventricular arrhythmias have been the subject of much review by the AHA (Table 21–11). Ventricular premature contractions (VPCs) can appear perioperatively secondary to electrolyte abnormalities (hypokalemia, hypomagnesium, hypocalcemia), acidosis, ischemia, embolic phenomenon, mechanical irritation of the heart from central lines, cardiac manipulation, and drug effects. Correction of the underlying source of any arrhythmia should be addressed. Patients can likewise present with VPCs secondary to various cardiomyopathies (dilated, hypertrophic, and arrhythmogenic right ventricular).

The incidence of sudden cardiac death (SCD) is estimated at 1-2/1000 per year. Consequently, some patients will experience an unexpected death in the perioperative period. All anesthesia providers must be prepared to resuscitate and manage patients with ventricular arrhythmias, including VT (nonsustained and sustained) and ventricular fibrillation.

Nonsustained ventricular tachycardia is a short run of ventricular ectopy that lasts <30 sec and spontaneously terminates, whereas sustained VT persists longer than 30 seconds. VT is either monomorphic or polymorphic, depending on the QRS complex. If the QRS complex morphology changes, it is designated as polymorphic VT. Torsades de pointes is a form of VT associated with a prolonged QT interval, producing a sine wave-like VT pattern on the ECG. Ventricular fibrillation requires immediate resuscitative efforts and defibrillation.

Patients presenting with ventricular ectopy and nonsustained runs of VT should undergo investigation prior to surgery. Supraventricular and ventricular arrhythmias constitute active cardiac conditions that warrant evaluation and treatment prior to elective, noncardiac surgery. Exercise testing, echocardiography, and nuclear perfusion studies are all recommended by the ACC/AHA in patients with ventricular arrhythmias as part of their workup and management. Electrophysiologic studies are undertaken to determine the possibility for catheter-mediated ablation of ventricular tachycardias.

Should VT present perioperatively, cardioversion is recommended at any point where hemodynamic compromise occurs. Otherwise, treatment with amiodarone or procainamide can be attempted. At all times, therapy should also be directed at identifying any causative sources of the arrhythmia. β-Blockers are useful in the treatment of VT, especially if ischemia is a suspected causative factor in the development of rhythm. The use of β-blockers following myocardial infarction has reduced the incidence of post-MI ventricular fibrillation.

Torsades de pointes is associated with conditions that lengthen the QT interval. If the arrhythmia develops in association with pauses, pacing can be effective. Likewise, some patients may benefit from isoproterenol infusions, if they develop pause-dependent torsades de pointes. Magnesium sulfate may be useful in patients with long QT syndrome and episodes of torsades.

The development of perioperative ventricular fibrillation (VF) requires defibrillation and the use of resuscitation algorithms. Amiodarone can be used to stabilize the rhythm following successful defibrillation.

Following VF, patients can present to surgery for both ICD placement and other surgical procedures. ICDs are recommended in patients with a history of survived sudden cardiac death (SCD), decreased ventricular function following

TABLE 21–11 Classification of ventricular arrhythmias.

Classification by Clinical Presentation		
Hemodynamically stable	Asymptomatic	The absence of symptoms that could result from an arrhythmia.
	Minimal symptoms, e.g., palpitations	Patient reports palpitations felt in either the chest, throat, or neck as described by the following: • Heartbeat sensations that feel like pounding or racing • An unpleasant awareness of heartbeat • Feeling skipped beats or a pause
Hemodynamically unstable	Presyncope	Patient reports presyncope as described by the following: • Dizziness • Lightheadedness • Feeling faint • "Graying out"
	Syncope	Sudden loss of consciousness with loss of postural tone, not related to anesthesia, with spontaneous recovery as reported by the patient or observer. Patient may experience syncope when supine.
	Sudden cardiac death	Death from an unexpected circulatory arrest, usually due to a cardiac arrhythmia occurring within an hour of the onset of symptoms.
	Sudden cardiac arrest	Death from an unexpected circulatory arrest, usually due to a cardiac arrhythmia occurring within an hour of the onset of symptoms, in whom medical intervention (e.g., defibrillation) reverses the event.
Classification by Electrocardiography		
Nonsustained VT		Three or more beats in duration, terminating spontaneously in less than 30 s.
		VT is a cardiac arrhythmia of three or more consecutive complexes in duration emanating from the ventricles at a rate of greater than 100 bpm (cycle length less than 600 ms)
	Monomorphic	Nonsustained VT with a single QRS morphology.
	Polymorphic	Nonsustained VT with a changing QRS morphology at cycle length between 600 and 180 ms.
Sustained VT		VT greater than 30 s in duration and/or requiring termination due to hemodynamic compromise in less than 30 s.
	Monomorphic	Sustained VT with a stable single QRS morphology.
	Polymorphic	Sustained VT with a changing or multiform QRS morphology at cycle length between 600 and 180 ms.
Bundle-branch reentrant tachycardia		VT due to reentry involving the His-Purkinje system, usually with LBBB morphology; this usually occurs in the setting of cardiomyopathy.
Bidirectional VT		VT with a beat-to-beat alternans in the QRS frontal plane axis, often associated with digitalis toxicity.
Torsades de pointes		Characterized by VT associated with a long QT or QTc, and electrocardiographically characterized by twisting of the peaks of the QRS complexes around the isoelectric line during the arrhythmia: • "Typical," initiated following "short-long-short" coupling intervals. • Short coupled variant initiated by normal-short coupling.

(continued)

TABLE 21–11 **Classification of ventricular arrhythmias. (continued)**

Classification by Electrocardiography	
Ventricular flutter	A regular (cycle length variability 30 ms or less) ventricular arrhythmia approximately 300 bpm (cycle length—200 ms) with a monomorphic appearance; no isoelectric interval between successive QRS complexes.
Ventricular fibrillation	Rapid, usually more than 300 bpm/200 ms (cycle length 180 ms or less), grossly irregular ventricular rhythm with marked variability in QRS cycle length, morphology, and amplitude.
Classification by Disease Entity	

Chronic coronary heart disease
Heart failure
Congenital heart disease
Neurological disorders
Structurally normal hearts
Sudden infant death syndrome
Cardiomyopathies:
  Dilated cardiomyopathy
  Hypertrophic cardiomyopathy
  Arrhythmogenic right ventricular
    cardiomyopathy	

LBBB, left bundle-branch block; VT, ventricular tachycardia.

Reproduced, with permission, from Zipes DP, Camm AJ, Borggrefe M, et al: ACC/AHA/ESC 2006 guidelines for management of patients with ventricular arrhythmias and the prevention of sudden cardiac death—executive summary. Circulation 2006;114:1088.

MI, and left ventricular ejection fractions <35%. Additionally, ICDs are used to treat potential sudden cardiac death in patients with dilated, hypertrophic, arrhythmogenic right ventricular, and genetic cardiomyopathies.

ICDs usually have a biventricular pacing function that improves the effectiveness of left ventricular contraction. Patients with heart failure frequently have a widened QRS complex >120 msec. In such patients, ventricular systole is less efficient, as the lateral and septal left ventricular walls do not effectively contract because of the conduction delay. Cardiac resynchronizaton therapy (CRT) has been shown to improve functional status in patients with heart failure (Table 21–12).

Anesthetic management for the placement of ICDs and other electrophysiologic procedures (eg, catheter ablation) depends on the patient's underlying conditions. Many patients present with systolic and diastolic heart failure, and, as such, are dependent on sympathetic tone to maintain blood pressure. Many patients tolerate ICD placement using deep sedation rather than general anesthesia. However, catheter-based electrophysiologic studies can be quite time consuming, and patients can develop atelectasis and airway obstruction. Should the patient's blood pressure suddenly decline during electrophysiololgic studies, development of pericardial tamponade should be ruled out. Emergent drainage of tamponade may be necessary.

TABLE 21–12 **Functional benefits of CRT.**

↑ 6-Minute walking distance
↑ Health-related quality-of-life score
↑ Peak oxygen consumption
↓ Hospitalizations for decompensated heart failure
↓ NYHA functional classification

↑ indicates increased; ↓, decreased.

Reproduced, with permission, from Strickberger SA, Conti J, Daoud EG, et al: Patient selection for cardiac resynchronization therapy: from the Council on Clinical Cardiology Subcommittee on Electrocardiogrpahy and Arrhythmias and the Quality of Care and Outcomes Research Interdisciplinary Working Group, in Collaboration with the Heart Rhythm Society. Circulation 2005;111:2146.

Many patients present to surgery with ICDs in place. Published guidelines of the American Society of Anesthesiologists can provide assistance in the management of such patients.

Management is a three-step process, as follows:

- *Preoperative.* Identify the type of device and determine if it is used for antibradycardia functions. Consult with the patient's cardiologist preoperatively as to the device's function and use history.

- *Intraoperative.* Determine what electromagnetic interference is likely to present intraoperatively and advise the use of bipolar electrocautery where possible. Assure the availability of temporary pacing and defibrillation equipment and apply pads as necessary. Patients who are pacer dependent can be programmed to an asynchronous mode to mitigate electrical interference. Magnet application to ICDs may disable the antitachycardia function, but not convert to an asynchronous pacemaker. Consultation with the patient's cardiologist and interrogation of the device is advised.

- *Postoperative.* The device must be interrogated to ensure that therapeutic functions have been restored. Patients should be continuously monitored until the antitachycardia functions of the device are restored and its function has been confirmed.

ICDs are particularly problematic intraoperatively when electrocautery is used because the device may (1) interpret cautery as ventricular fibrillation; (2) inhibit pacemaker function due to cautery artifact; (3) increase the pacing rate due to activation of a rate-responsive sensor; or (4) temporarily or permanently reset to a backup or reset mode. Use of bipolar cautery, placement of the grounding pad far from the ICD device, and limiting use of the cautery to only short bursts help to reduce the likelihood of problems, but will not eliminate them.

ICD devices should have the defibrillator function programmed off immediately before surgery and reprogrammed back on immediately afterward. External defibrillation pads should be applied and attached to a defibrillator machine intraoperatively.

Careful monitoring of the arterial pulse with pulse oximetry or an arterial waveform is necessary to ensure that the pacemaker is not inhibited and that there is arterial perfusion during episodes of ECG artifact from surgical cautery. The manufacturer should be contacted to determine the best method for managing the device (eg, reprogramming or applying a magnet) prior to surgery. A large number of ICD models are in use; however, most suspend their antitachycardia function in response to a magnet.

HEART FAILURE

An increasing number of patients present for surgery with either systolic and/or diastolic heart failure. Congestive heart failure affects more than 5 million Americans. Heart failure may be secondary to ischemia, valvular heart disease, infectious agents, and many types of cardiomyopathy. Most patients seek medical attention secondary to heart failure because of complaints of dyspnea and fatigue. Heart failure develops over time, as symptoms worsen (Figure 21–5). Patients generally undergo echocardiography to diagnose structural heart defects, to detect signs of cardiac "remodeling", to determine the left ventricular ejection fraction, and to assess the heart's diastolic function. Laboratory evaluations of concentration of brain natriuretic peptide (BNP) are likewise obtained to distinguish heart failure from other causes of dyspnea. BNP is released from the heart, and its elevation is associated with impaired ventricular function.

In response to ventricular failure, the body attempts to compensate for LV systolic function through the sympathetic and renin–angiotensin–aldosterone system. Consequently, patients experience salt retention, volume expansion, sympathetic stimulation, and vasoconstriction. The heart dilates to maintain the stroke volume in spite of decreased contractility. Over time, compensatory mechanisms fail and contribute to the symptoms associated with heart failure (eg, edema, tachycardia, decreased tissue perfusion). Patients with systolic heart failure are likely to present to surgery having been previously treated with diuretics, ACE inhibitors, angiotensin receptor blockers, and

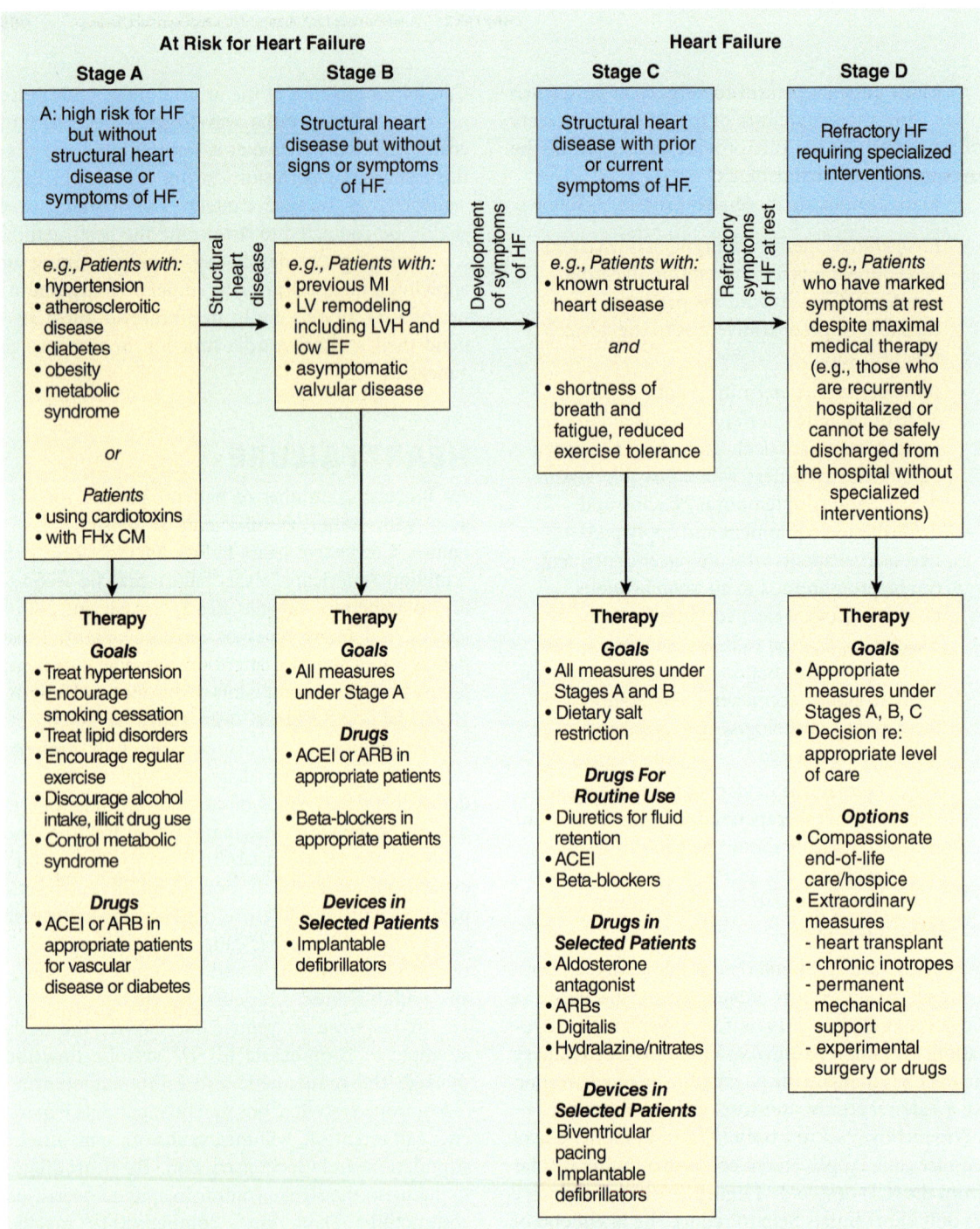

FIGURE 21-5 Stages in the development of heart failure/recommended therapy by stage. ACEI, angiotensin-converting enzyme inhibitor; ARB, angiotensin II receptor blocker; EF, ejection fraction; FHx CM, family history of cardiomyopathy; HF, heart failure; LVH, left ventricular hypertrophy; MI, myocardial infarction. (Reproduced, with permission, from Jessup M, Abraham W, Casey D, et al: 2009 Focused update: ACCF/AHA guidelines for the diagnosis and management of heart failure in adults: a report of the American College of Cardiology Foundation/American Heart Association Task Force on Practice Guidelines. Circulation 2009;119:1977.)

possibly aldosterone antagonists. Electrolytes must be measured, as heart failure therapies frequently lead to changes in serum potassium concentration. Angiotensin receptor blocker or ACE inhibitor use may contribute to periinduction hypotension in the patient with heart failure. ACE inhibitors are rarely associated with angioedema requiring emergent airway management.

Diastolic ventricular dysfunction produces symptoms of congestion and heart failure. Myocardial relaxation is a dynamic, not passive, process. The heart with preserved diastolic function accommodates volume during diastole, with minimal increases in left ventricular end-diastolic pressure. Conversely, the heart with diastolic dysfunction relaxes poorly and produces increased left ventricular end-diastolic pressure. The left ventricular end-diastolic pressure is transmitted to the left atrium and pulmonary vasculature resulting in symptoms of congestion.

Anesthetic management of the patient with heart failure requires careful assessment and optimization of intravascular fluid volume—especially if positive inotropic agents, vasoconstrictors, or vasodilators are used. In particular, patients with diastolic dysfunction may tolerate increases in volume poorly, leading to pulmonary congestion.

HYPERTROPHIC CARDIOMYOPATHY

Hypertrophic cardiomyopathy (HCM) is an autosomal dominant trait that affects 1 in 500 adults. Many patients are unaware of the condition, and some will present with SCD as an initial manifestation. Symptoms include dyspnea, exercise intolerance, palpitations, and chest pain. Clinically, HCM is detected by the murmur of dynamic left ventricular outflow tract (LVOT) obstruction in late systole. Symptomatic patients frequently have a thickened intraventricular septum of 20 to 30 mm. Mutations in the genes that code for the cardiac sarcomeres and their supporting proteins are implicated. The myocardium of the intraventricular septum is abnormal, and many patients can develop diastolic dysfunction and SCD without pronounced dynamic obstructive gradients. During systole, the anterior leaflet of

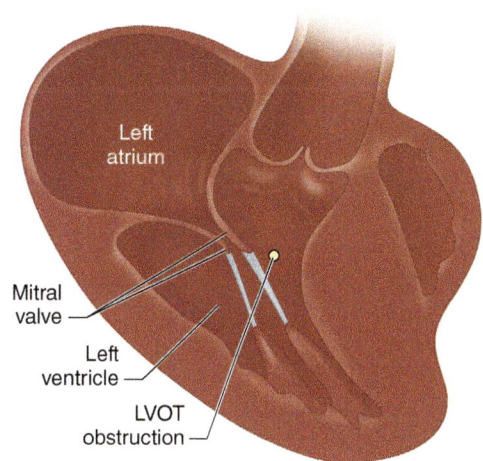

FIGURE 21–6 The midesophageal long axis view is shown. As a consequence of the hypertrophied interventricular septum, flow patterns within the heart are altered so that the anterior leaflet of the mitral valve is drawn during ventricular systole into the left ventricular outflow tract (LOVT), producing obstruction. This is known as systolic anterior motion of the mitral valve (SAM). (Reproduced, with permission, from Wasnick J, Hillel Z, Kramer D, et al: *Cardiac Anesthesia & Transesophageal Echocardiography,* McGraw-Hill, 2011.)

the mitral valve abuts the intraventricular septum (Figure 21–6), producing obstruction and a late systolic murmur.

Perioperative management is aimed at minimizing the degree of LVOT obstruction. This is accomplished by maintaining adequate intravascular volume, avoiding vasodilatation, and reducing myocardial contractility through the use of β-blockers.

Valvular Heart Disease

1. General Evaluation of Patients

Regardless of the lesion or its cause, preoperative evaluation should be primarily concerned with determining the identity and severity of the lesion and its hemodynamic significance, residual ventricular function, and the presence of any secondary effects on pulmonary, renal, and hepatic function.

Concomitant CAD should not be overlooked, particularly in older patients and those with known risk factors (see above). Myocardial ischemia may also occur in the absence of significant coronary occlusion in patients with severe aortic stenosis or regurgitation.

History

The preanesthesia history should focus on symptoms related to decreased ventricular function. Symptoms and signs should be correlated with laboratory data. Questions should evaluate exercise tolerance, fatigability, and pedal edema and shortness of breath in general (dyspnea), when lying flat (orthopnea), or at night (paroxysmal nocturnal dyspnea). The New York Heart Association functional classification of heart disease (Table 21–13) is useful for grading the severity of heart failure symptoms and estimating prognosis. Patients should also be questioned about chest pains and neurological symptoms. Some valvular lesions are associated with thromboembolic phenomena. Prior procedures, such as valvotomy or valve replacement and their effects, should also be well documented.

A review of medications should evaluate efficacy and exclude serious side effects. Commonly used agents include diuretics, vasodilators, ACE inhibitors, β-blockers, antiarrhythmics, and anticoagulants. Preoperative vasodilator therapy may be used to decrease preload, afterload, or both. Excessive vasodilatation worsens exercise tolerance and is often first manifested as postural (orthostatic) hypotension.

TABLE 21–13 Modified New York Association functional classification of heart disease.

Class	Description
I	Asymptomatic except during severe exertion
II	Symptomatic with moderate activity
III	Symptomatic with minimal activity
IV	Symptomatic at rest

Physical Examination

The most important signs to identify on physical examination are those of congestive heart failure. Left-sided (S_3 gallop or pulmonary rales) and right-sided (jugular venous distention, hepatojugular reflux, hepatosplenomegaly, or pedal edema) signs may be present. Auscultatory findings may confirm the valvular dysfunction (Figure 21–7), but echocardiographic studies are more reliable. Neurological deficits, usually secondary to embolic phenomena, should be documented.

Laboratory Evaluation

In addition to the laboratory studies discussed for patients with hypertension and CAD, liver function tests may be useful in assessing hepatic dysfunction caused by passive hepatic congestion in patients with severe or chronic right-sided failure. Arterial blood gases can be measured in patients with significant pulmonary symptoms. Reversal of warfarin or heparin should be documented with a prothrombin time and international normalized ratio (INR) or partial thromboplastin time, respectively, prior to surgery.

Electrocardiographic findings are generally nonspecific. The chest radiograph is useful to assess cardiac size and pulmonary vascular congestion.

Special Studies

Echocardiography, imaging studies, and cardiac catheterization provide important diagnostic and prognostic information about valvular lesions, but should only be obtained if the results will change therapy or outcomes. More than one valvular lesion is often found. In many instances, noninvasive studies obviate the need for cardiac catheterization, unless there are concerns about CAD. Information from these studies is best reviewed with a cardiologist. The following questions must be answered:

- Which valvular abnormality is most important hemodynamically?
- What is the severity of an identified lesion?
- What degree of ventricular impairment is present?
- What is the hemodynamic significance of other identified abnormalities?
- Is there any evidence of CAD?

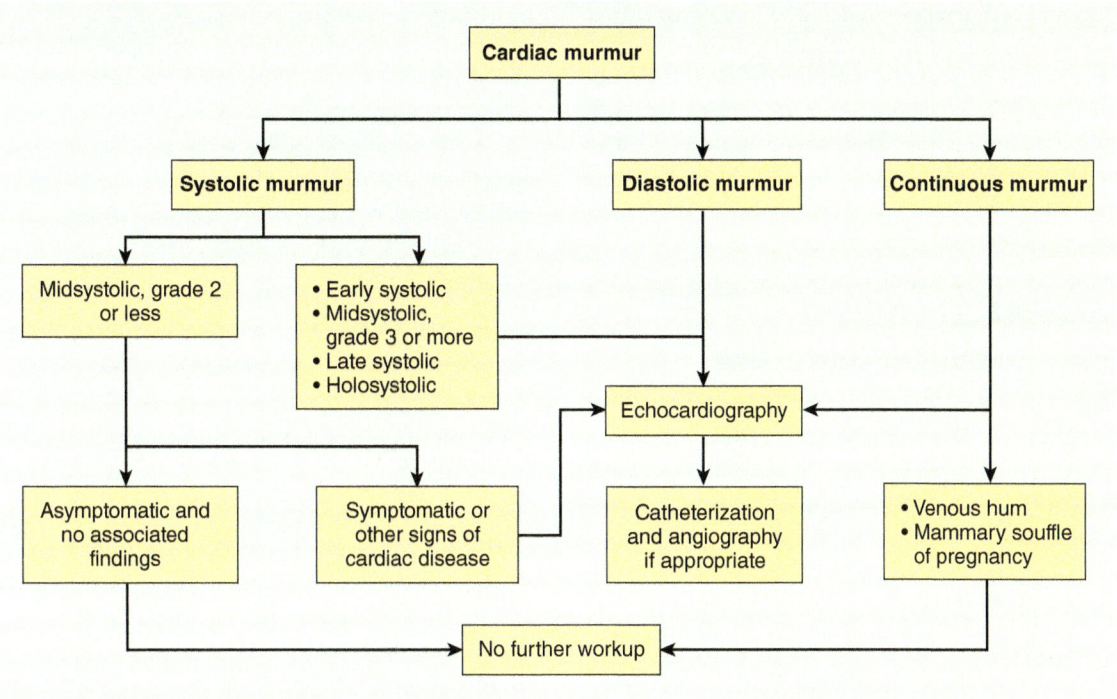

FIGURE 21–7 Strategy for evaluating heart murmurs. (Reproduced, with permission, from Bonow RO, Carabello BA, Chatterjee K, et al: 2008 focused update incorporated in the ACC/AHA 2006 guidelines for the management of patients with valvular heart disease: a report of the American College of Cardiology/American Heart Association Task Force on Practice Guidelines (writing committee to revise the 1998 guidelines for the management of patients with valvular heart disease): endorsed by the Society of Cardiovascular Anesthesiologists, Society for Cardiovascular Angiography and Interventions, and Society of Thoracic Surgeons. Circulation 2008;118:e523.)

The ACC/AHA have prepared detailed guidelines to assist in the management of the patient with valvular heart disease. Although the evaluation of the patient with a heart murmur generally rests with the cardiologist, anesthesia providers will on occasion discover the presence of a previously undetected murmur on preanesthetic examination. In particular, anesthetists are concerned that undiagnosed, critical aortic stenosis might be present, which could potentially lead to hemodynamic collapse with either regional or general anesthesia. In the past, most valvular heart diseases were a consequence of rheumatic heart disease; however, with an aging surgical population, increasing numbers of patients have degenerative valve problems. More than one in eight patients older than age 75 years may manifest at least one form of moderate to severe valvular heart disease.

A study conducted in the Netherlands reported that the prevalence of aortic stenosis was 2.4% in patients older than age 60 years who were scheduled for elective surgery. Underdiagnosed valvular disease is particularly prevalent in elderly females.

According to the ACC/AHA guidelines, auscultation of the heart is the most widely used method to detect valvular heart disease. Murmurs occur as a consequence of the accelerated blood flow through narrowed openings in stenotic and regurgitant lesions. Although systolic murmurs may be related to increased blood flow velocity, the ACC/AHA guidelines note that all diastolic and continuous murmurs reflect pathology. Other than murmurs that are thought to be innocent, such as mid-systolic flow murmurs (grade 2 or softer), the ACC/AHA guidelines recommend echocardiographic evaluation.

When new murmurs are detected in a preoperative evaluation, consultation with the patient's personal physician is helpful to determine the need for echo-cardiographic evaluation. In many centers, immediate echocardiographic evaluation can be performed in the preoperative area.

2. Specific Valvular Disorders

MITRAL STENOSIS

Preoperative Considerations

Mitral stenosis almost always occurs as a delayed complication of rheumatic fever. However, mitral stenosis can also occur in dialysis-dependent patients. Two-thirds of patients with mitral stenosis are female. The stenotic process is estimated to begin after a minimum of 2 years following rheumatic heart disease and results from progressive fusion and calcification of the valve leaflets. Symptoms generally develop after 20–30 years, when the mitral valve orifice is reduced from its normal 4–6 cm^2 opening to less than 1.5 cm^2. Less than 50% of patients have isolated mitral stenosis; the remaining patients also have mitral regurgitation, and up to 25% of patients also have rheumatic involvement of the aortic valve (stenosis or regurgitation).

Pathophysiology

The rheumatic process causes the valve leaflets to thicken, calcify, and become funnel shaped; annular calcification may also be present. The mitral commissures fuse, the chordae tendinae fuse and shorten, and the valve cusps become rigid; as a result, the valve leaflets typically display bowing or doming during diastole on echocardiography.

Significant restriction of blood flow through the mitral valve results in a transvalvular pressure gradient that depends on cardiac output, heart rate (diastolic time), and cardiac rhythm. Increases in either cardiac output or heart rate (decreased diastolic time) necessitate higher flows across the valve and result in higher transvalvular pressure gradients. The left atrium is often markedly dilated, promoting SVTs, particularly AF. Blood flow stasis in the atrium promotes the formation of thrombi, usually in the left atrial appendage. Loss of normal atrial systole with

AF (which is usually responsible for 20% to 30% of ventricular filling) necessitates even higher diastolic flow across the valve to maintain the same cardiac output and increases the transvalvular gradient.

Acute elevations in left atrial pressure are rapidly transmitted back to the pulmonary capillaries. If mean pulmonary capillary pressure acutely and significantly rises transudation of capillary fluid may result in pulmonary edema. Chronic elevations in pulmonary capillary pressure are partially compensated by increases in pulmonary lymph flow, but eventually result in pulmonary vascular changes, leading to irreversible increases in pulmonary vascular resistance (PVR) and pulmonary hypertension. Reduced lung compliance and a secondary increase in the work of breathing contribute to chronic dyspnea. Right ventricular failure is frequently precipitated by acute or chronic elevations in right ventricular afterload. Marked dilatation of the right ventricle can result in tricuspid or pulmonary valve regurgitation.

Embolic events are common in patients with mitral stenosis and AF. Dislodgment of clots from the left atrium results in systemic emboli, most commonly to the cerebral circulation. Patients also have an increased incidence of pulmonary emboli, pulmonary infarction, hemoptysis, and recurrent bronchitis. Hemoptysis most commonly results from rupture of pulmonary–bronchial venous communications. Chest pain occurs in 10% to 15% of patients with mitral stenosis, even in the absence of CAD; its etiology often remains unexplained, but may be emboli in the coronary circulation or acute right ventricular pressure overload. Patients may develop hoarseness as a result of compression of the left recurrent laryngeal nerve by the enlarged left atrium.

Left ventricular function is normal in the majority of patients with pure mitral stenosis (**Figure 21–8**), but impaired left ventricular function may be encountered in up to 25% of patients and presumably represents residual damage from rheumatic myocarditis or coexistent hypertensive or ischemic heart disease.

The left ventricle is chronically underloaded in the patient with mitral stenosis. At the same time, the left atrium, right ventricle, and right atrium are frequently dilated and dysfunctional. Vasodilatation that occurs following both neuraxial and general

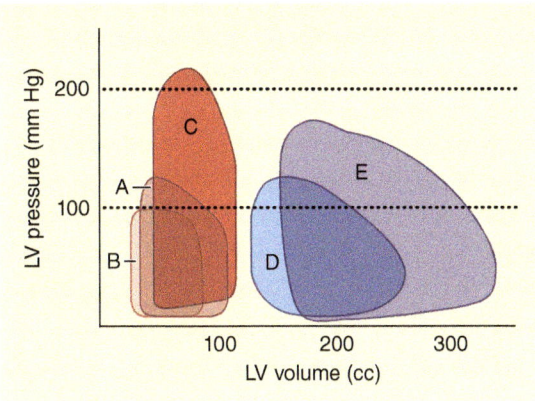

FIGURE 21–8 Pressure–volume loops in patients with valvular heart disease. A, normal; B, mitral stenosis; C, aortic stenosis; D, mitral regurgitation (chronic); E, aortic regurgitation (chronic). LV, left ventricular. (Reproduced, with permission, from Jackson JM, Thomas SJ, Lowenstein E: Anesthetic management of patients with valvular heart disease. Semin Anesth 1982;1:239.)

anesthesia can lead to peripheral venous blood pooling and inadequate volume delivery to the left ventricle. This can precipitate hemodynamic collapse.

Calculating Mitral Valve Area & Transvalvular Gradient

Two-dimensional and Doppler echocardiography can be used to estimate both the pressure drop across a stenotic valve and the valve area. Based on the assumption that the velocity of blood flow is much greater distal than proximal to an obstruction, the Bernoulli equation can be simplified:

$$\Delta P = 4V^2$$

where ΔP is the pressure gradient (mm Hg) and V is blood flow velocity (m/s) distal to the obstruction. Valve orifice can be estimated from the time it takes for the initial peak pressure gradient to fall to one-half of its original value, the pressure half-time ($T_{1/2}$). This relationship is approximated by

$$A = \frac{220}{T_{1/2}}$$

where A is valve orifice (cm^2) and $T_{1/2}$ is the time from peak flow velocity (V_{max}) to $V_{max}/1.4$. This relationship

is based on the observation that $T_{1/2}$ remains relatively constant for a given orifice over a wide range of flows. A pressure half-time of 220 msec corresponds to a mitral valve area of 1 cm^2.

Mitral valve areas less than 1 cm^2 are typically associated with transvalvular gradients of 20 mm Hg at rest and dyspnea with minimal exertion; a mitral valve area less than 1 cm^2 is often referred to as critical mitral stenosis. Patients with valve areas between 1.5 and 2.0 cm^2 are generally asymptomatic or have only mild symptoms with exertion. When the mitral valve area is between 1 and 1.5 cm^2, most patients are symptomatic with mild to moderate exertion. Although cardiac output may be normal at rest, it fails to increase appropriately during exertion because of decreased left ventricular preload.

Treatment

The time from onset of symptoms to incapacitation averages 5–10 years. At that stage, most patients die within 2–5 years. Surgical correction is therefore usually undertaken once significant symptoms develop. Percutaneous transseptal balloon valvuloplasty may be used in selected young or pregnant patients, as well as older patients who are poor surgical candidates. Medical management is primarily supportive and includes limitation of physical activity, sodium restriction, and diuretics. Small doses of a β-adrenergic blocking drug may also be useful in controlling heart rate in patients with mild to moderate symptoms. Patients with a history of emboli and those at high risk (age older than 40 years; a large atrium with chronic atrial fibrillation) are usually anticoagulated.

Anesthetic Management

A. Objectives

8 The principal hemodynamic goals are to maintain a sinus rhythm (if present preoperatively) and to avoid tachycardia, large increases in cardiac output, and both hypovolemia and fluid overload by judicious administration of intravenous fluids.

B. Monitoring

Invasive hemodynamic monitoring is often used for major surgical procedures, particularly those associated with large fluid shifts. TEE can also be used to help guide perioperative management. Overzealous fluid replacement readily precipitates pulmonary edema in patients with severe disease. Pulmonary capillary wedge pressure measurements in the presence of mitral stenosis reflect the transvalvular gradient and not necessarily left ventricular end-diastolic pressure. Prominent *a* waves and a decreased *y* descent are typically present on the pulmonary capillary wedge pressure waveform in patients who are in sinus rhythm. A prominent *cv* wave on the central venous pressure waveform is usually indicative of secondary tricuspid regurgitation. The ECG typically shows a notched P wave in patients who are in sinus rhythm.

C. Choice of Agents

Patients may be very sensitive to the vasodilating effects of spinal and epidural anesthesia. Epidural anesthesia may be easier to manage than spinal anesthesia because of the more gradual onset of sympathetic blockade. There is no "ideal" general anesthetic, and agents should be employed to achieve the desired effects of permitting sufficient diastolic time to adequately load the left ventricle. Vasopressors are often needed to maintain vascular tone following anesthetic induction.

Intraoperative tachycardia may be controlled by deepening anesthesia with an opioid (excluding meperidine) or β-blocker (esmolol or metoprolol). In the presence of atrial fibrillation, ventricular rate should be controlled. **Marked hemodynamic deterioration from sudden SVT necessitates cardioversion.** Phenylephrine is preferred over ephedrine as a vasopressor because the former lacks β-adrenergic agonist activity. Vasopressin can also be employed to restore vascular tone should hypotension develop secondary to anesthetic induction.

MITRAL REGURGITATION

Preoperative Considerations

Mitral regurgitation can develop acutely or insidiously as a result of a large number of disorders. Chronic mitral regurgitation is usually the result of rheumatic fever (often with concomitant mitral stenosis); congenital or developmental abnormalities of the valve apparatus; or dilatation, destruction, or calcification of the mitral annulus. Acute mitral regurgitation is usually due to myocardial ischemia or infarction (papillary muscle dysfunction or rupture of a chorda tendinea), infective endocarditis, or chest trauma.

Pathophysiology

The principal derangement is a reduction in forward stroke volume due to backward flow of blood into the left atrium during systole. The left ventricle compensates by dilating and increasing end-diastolic volume (Figure 21–8). Regurgitation thorugh the mitral valve initially maintains a normal end systolic volume in spite of an increased end diastolic volume. However, as the disease progresses the end systolic volume increases. By increasing end-diastolic volume, the volume-overloaded left ventricle can maintain a normal cardiac output despite blood being ejected retrograde into the atrium. With time, patients with chronic mitral regurgitation eventually develop eccentric left ventricular hypertrophy and progressive impairment in contractility. In patients with severe mitral regurgitation, the regurgitant volume may exceed the forward stroke volume. In time, wall stress increases, resulting in an increased demand for myocardial oxygen supply.

The regurgitant volume passing through the mitral valve is dependent on the size of the mitral valve orifice (which can vary with ventricular cavity size), the heart rate (systolic time), and the left ventricular–left atrial pressure gradient during systole. The last factor is affected by the relative resistances of the two outflow paths from the left ventricle, namely, SVR and left atrial compliance. Thus, a decrease in SVR or an increase in mean left atrial pressure will reduce the regurgitant volume. Atrial compliance also determines the predominant clinical manifestations. Patients with normal or reduced atrial compliance (acute mitral regurgitation) have primarily pulmonary vascular congestion and edema. Patients with increased atrial compliance (long-standing mitral regurgitation resulting in a large dilated left atrium) primarily show signs of a reduced cardiac output. Most patients are between the two extremes and exhibit symptoms of both pulmonary congestion and low cardiac output. Patients with a regurgitant fraction of less than 30% of the total stroke volume generally have mild symptoms. Regurgitant fractions of 30% to 60% generally cause

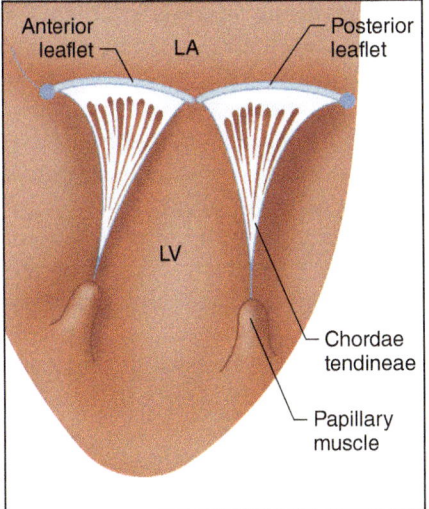

Anterior leaflet — LA — Posterior leaflet

LV

Chordae tendineae

Papillary muscle

Normal motion

Regurgitant jet

Prolapse (excessive motion)

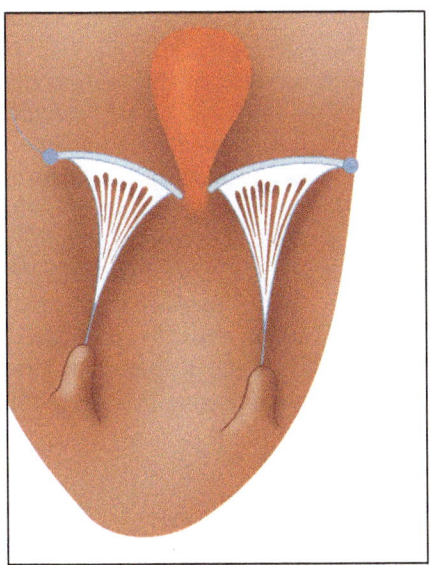

Restricted motion

Bileaflet prolapse

FIGURE 21–9 Classification of mitral valve leaflet motion (as seen from transesophageal echocardiography). Note that with prolapse, the free edge of the leaflet(s) extends beyond the plane of the mitral annulus producing an eccentric jet. With restricted motion, the leaflets fail to coapt, resulting in a central jet.

moderate symptoms, whereas fractions greater than 60% are associated with severe disease.

Echocardiography, particularly TEE, is useful in delineating the underlying pathophysiology of mitral regurgitation and guiding treatment. Mitral valve leaflet motion is often described as normal, prolapsing, or restrictive (Figure 21–9). Excessive motion or prolapse is defined by systolic movement of a leaflet beyond the plane of the mitral valve and into the left atrium (see the section below on mitral valve prolapse).

Calculating Regurgitant Fraction

To calculate regurgitant fraction (RF), forward stroke volume (SV) and the regurgitant stroke volume (RSV) must be measured. Although they can both be estimated by catheterization data, pulsed Doppler echocardiography provides reasonably acute calculations. Stroke volume is measured at the left ventricular outflow tract (LVOT) and at the mitral valve (MV), where

Stroke volume = cross-sectional area $(A) \times$ (TVI)

and cross-sectional area (A) can be approximated as,

$$A = 0.785 \times (\text{diameter})^2$$

The time–velocity integral (TVI) is the integral of the velocity versus the time signal obtained with pulsed Doppler. The TVI reflects the distance the blood has traveled during a heart beat. By knowing the area through which the blood travels and the distance traveled, it is possible to estimate the stroke volume. This is the case because the area is expressed in centimeters squared, and the distance is expressed in centimeters. The product of these measures is cubic centimeters or milliliters—hence, the stroke volume for each heartbeat.

Thus, the volume of blood that enters through the mitral valve must be the same as that passing through the left ventricular outflow track. Any difference between the two represents the amount of the volume that initially entered the left ventricle, but that did not pass the LVOT. This is the volume that regurgitated into the left atrium.

$$\text{RSV}_{\text{mitral regurgitation}} = (A_{\text{MV}} \times \text{VTI}_{\text{MV}}) - (A_{\text{LVOT}} \times \text{TVI}_{\text{LVOT}}),$$

and

$$\text{RF} = \text{RSV/SV}$$

An RSV greater than 65 mL usually correlates with severe mitral regurgitation.

Treatment

Afterload reduction is beneficial in most patients and may even be lifesaving in patients with acute mitral regurgitation. Reduction of SVR increases forward SV and decreases the regurgitant volume. Surgical treatment is usually reserved for patients with moderate to severe symptoms. Valvuloplasty or valve repair are performed whenever possible to avoid the problems associated with valve replacement (eg, thromboembolism, hemorrhage, and prosthetic failure). Catheter-mediated valve repairs are continually being refined, potentially reducing the need for "open" surgery. Anesthesiologists skilled in advanced perioperative echocardiography assist in correctly identifying the leaflet(s) to be repaired and determining the repair's success. Three-dimensional echocardiography is increasingly employed to assist in the assessment of the mitral valve (see Figure 5-29).

Anesthetic Management

A. Objectives

9 Anesthetic management should be tailored to the severity of mitral regurgitation as well as the underlying left ventricular function. Factors that exacerbate the regurgitation, such as slow heart rates and acute increases in afterload, should be avoided. Bradycardia can increase the regurgitant volume by increasing left ventricular end-diastolic volume and acutely dilating the mitral annulus. The heart rate should ideally be kept between 80 and 100 beats/min. Acute increases in left ventricular afterload, such as with endotracheal intubation and surgical stimulation under "light" anesthesia, should be treated rapidly but without excessive myocardial depression. Excessive volume expansion can also worsen the regurgitation by dilating the left ventricle.

B. Monitoring

Monitors are based on the severity of ventricular dysfunction, as well as the procedure. Mitral regurgitation may be recognized on the pulmonary artery wedge waveform as a large v wave and a rapid y descent (Figure 21–10). The height of the v wave is inversely related to atrial and pulmonary vascular compliance, but is directly proportional to pulmonary blood flow and the regurgitant volume; thus, the v wave may not be prominent in patients with chronic mitral regurgitation, except during acute deterioration. Very large v waves are often apparent on the pulmonary artery pressure waveform, even without wedging the catheter. Color-flow Doppler TEE can be invaluable in quantitating the severity of

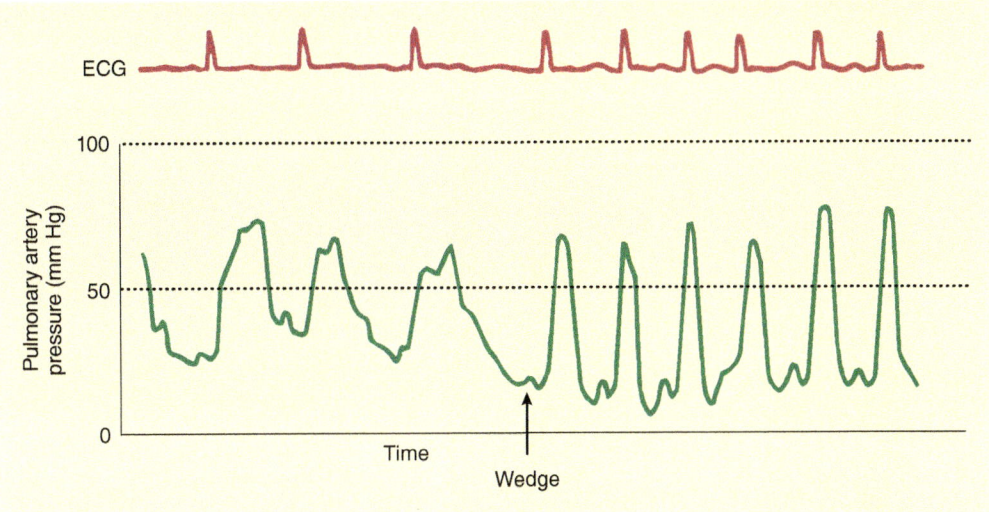

FIGURE 21–10 The pulmonary capillary wedge waveform in mitral regurgitation, demonstrating a large *v* wave.

the regurgitation and guiding therapeutic interventions in patients with severe mitral regurgitation. By definition, blood flow reverses in the pulmonary veins during systole with severe mitral regurgitation.

C. Choice of Agents

Patients with relatively well-preserved ventricular function tend to do well with most anesthetic techniques. Spinal and epidural anesthesia are well tolerated, provided bradycardia is avoided. Patients with moderate to severe ventricular impairment may be sensitive to depression from high concentrations of volatile agents. An opioid-based anesthetic may be more suitable for those patients—again, provided bradycardia is avoided.

MITRAL VALVE PROLAPSE

Preoperative Considerations

Mitral valve prolapse is classically characterized by a mid-systolic click, with or without a late apical systolic murmur on auscultation. It is a relatively common abnormality that is present in up to 1% to 2.5% of the general population. The diagnosis is based on auscultatory findings and is confirmed by echocardiography, which shows systolic prolapse of mitral valve leaflets into the left atrium. Patients with the murmur often have some element of mitral regurgitation. The posterior mitral leaflet is more commonly affected than the anterior leaflet. The mitral annulus may also be dilated. Pathologically, most patients have redundancy or some myxomatous degeneration of the valve leaflets. Most cases of mitral valve prolapse are sporadic or familial, affecting otherwise normal persons. A high incidence of mitral valve prolapse is found in patients with connective tissue disorders (particularly Marfan syndrome).

The overwhelming majority of patients with mitral valve prolapse are asymptomatic, but in a small percentage of patients, the myxomatous degeneration is progressive. Manifestations, when they occur, can include chest pains, arrhythmias, embolic events, florid mitral regurgitation, infective endocarditis, and, rarely, sudden death. The diagnosis can be made preoperatively by auscultation of the characteristic click, but must be confirmed by echocardiography. The prolapse is accentuated by maneuvers that decrease ventricular volume (preload). Both atrial and ventricular arrhythmias are common. Although bradyarrhythmias have been reported, paroxysmal supraventricular tachycardia is the most commonly encountered sustained arrhythmia. An increased incidence of abnormal AV bypass tracts is reported in patients with mitral valve prolapse.

Most patients have a normal life span. About 15% develop progressive mitral regurgitation. A smaller percentage develops embolic phenomena or infective endocarditis. Patients with both a click and a systolic murmur seem to be at greater risk of developing complications. Anticoagulation or anti-platelet agents may be used for patients with a history of emboli, whereas β-adrenergic blocking drugs are commonly used for arrhythmias.

Anesthetic Management

The management of these patients is based on their clinical course. Most patients are asymptomatic and do not require special care. Ventricular arrhythmias may occur intraoperatively, particularly following sympathetic stimulation, and will generally respond to lidocaine or β-adrenergic blocking agents. Mitral regurgitation caused by prolapse is generally exacerbated by decreases in ventricular size. Hypovolemia and factors that increase ventricular emptying or decrease afterload should be avoided. Vasopressors with pure α-adrenergic agonist activity (such as phenylephrine) may be preferable to those that are primarily β-adrenergic agonists (ephedrine).

AORTIC STENOSIS

Preoperative Considerations

Valvular aortic stenosis is the most common cause of obstruction to left ventricular outflow. Left ventricular outflow obstruction is less commonly due to hypertrophic cardiomyopathy, discrete congenital subvalvular stenosis, or, rarely, supravalvular stenosis. Valvular aortic stenosis is nearly always congenital, rheumatic, or degenerative. Abnormalities in the number of cusps (most commonly a bicuspid valve) or their architecture produce turbulence that traumatizes the valve and eventually leads to stenosis. Rheumatic aortic stenosis is rarely isolated; it is more commonly associated with aortic regurgitation or mitral valve disease. In the most common degenerative form, calcific aortic stenosis, wear and tear results in the buildup of calcium deposits on normal cusps, preventing them from opening completely (Figure 21–11).

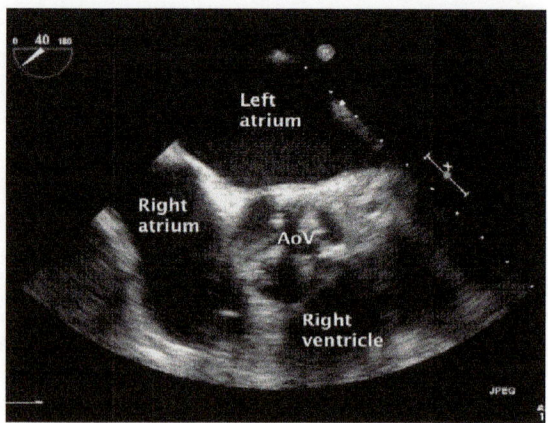

FIGURE 21–11 A stenotic aortic valve is clearly seen in this midesophageal short axis aortic valve view. Calcification of the aortic valve is usually associated with senile degeneration. However, congenitally abnormal (bicuspid) and rheumatic presentations also occur. (Reproduced, with permission, from Wasnick J, Hillel Z, Kramer D, et al: *Cardiac Anesthesia & Transesophageal Echocardiography,* McGraw-Hill, 2011.)

Pathophysiology

Left ventricular outflow obstruction caused by valvular aortic stenosis is almost always gradual, allowing the ventricle, at least initially, to compensate and maintain SV. Concentric left ventricular hypertrophy enables the ventricle to maintain SV by generating the needed transvalvular pressure gradient and to reduce ventricular wall stress.

Critical aortic stenosis is said to exist when the aortic valve orifice is reduced to 0.5–0.7 cm² (normal is 2.5–3.5 cm²). With this degree of stenosis, patients generally have a transvalvular gradient of approximately 50 mm Hg at rest (with a normal cardiac output) and are unable to increase cardiac output in response to exertion. Moreover, further increases in the transvalvular gradient do not significantly increase SV. With long-standing aortic stenosis, myocardial contractility progressively deteriorates and compromises left ventricular function.

Classically, patients with advanced aortic stenosis have the triad of dyspnea on exertion, angina, and orthostatic or exertional syncope. A prominent feature of aortic stenosis is a decrease in left ventricular compliance as a result of hypertrophy.

Diastolic dysfunction is the result of an increase in ventricular muscle mass, fibrosis, or myocardial ischemia. In contrast to left ventricular end-diastolic volume, which remains normal until very late in the disease, left ventricular end-diastolic pressure is elevated early in the disease. The decreased diastolic pressure gradient between the left atrium and left ventricle impairs ventricular filling, which becomes quite dependent on a normal atrial contraction. Loss of atrial systole can precipitate congestive heart failure or hypotension in patients with aortic stenosis. Cardiac output may be normal in symptomatic patients at rest, but characteristically, it does not appropriately increase with exertion. Patients may experience angina even in the absence of CAD. Myocardial oxygen demand increases because of ventricular hypertrophy, whereas myocardial oxygen supply decreases as a result of the marked compression of intramyocardial coronary vessels caused by high intracavitary systolic pressures (up to 300 mm Hg). Exertional syncope or near-syncope is thought to be due to an inability to tolerate the vasodilatation in muscle tissue during exertion. Arrhythmias leading to severe hypoperfusion may also account for syncope and sudden death in some patients.

CALCULATING AORTIC VALVE AREA & TRANSVALVULAR GRADIENT

As with mitral stenosis, the pressure gradient across the aortic valve can be determined noninvasively using continuous wave Doppler echocardiography:

$$\Delta P = 4V^2$$

where ΔP is the peak pressure gradient (mm Hg) and V is peak blood flow velocity (m/s) distal to the obstruction. Peak velocities greater than 4.5 m/sec are usually indicative of severe stenosis. Moreover, if the area proximal to the stenosis (LVOT) can be measured, the continuity equation can then be applied to estimate valve area. Either TVIs or maximum velocities can be used:

$$A_2 = \frac{A_1 V_1}{V_2}$$

where A_2 is valve area, A_1 is the cross-sectional area of the LVOT, V_1 is maximum blood flow velocity in LVOT, and V_2 is maximum flow velocity through the aortic valve.

Treatment

Once symptoms develop, most patients, without surgical treatment, will die within 2–5 years. Percutaneous balloon valvuloplasty is generally used in younger patients with congenital aortic stenosis; it can also be used in elderly patients with calcific aortic stenosis who are poor candidates for aortic valve replacement. Its efficacy for the latter group is short-lived, however, and restenosis usually occurs within 6–12 months. Catheter-delivered aortic valves are increasingly being perfected and deployed in the treatment of aortic valve disease. Surgical replacement of the stenotic aortic valve remains the mainstay of therapy.

Anesthetic Management

A. Objectives

10 Maintenance of normal sinus rhythm, heart rate, vascular resistance, and intravascular volume is critical in patients with aortic stenosis. Loss of a normally timed atrial systole often leads to rapid deterioration, particularly when associated with tachycardia. The combination of the two (AF with rapid ventricular response) seriously impairs ventricular filling and necessitates immediate cardioversion. The reduced ventricular compliance also makes the patient very sensitive to abrupt changes in intravascular volume. Many patients behave as though they have a fixed SV in spite of adequate hydration; under these conditions, cardiac output becomes very rate dependent. Extreme bradycardia (<50 beats/min) is therefore poorly tolerated. Heart rates between 60 and 90 beats/min are optimal in most patients.

B. Monitoring

Close monitoring of the ECG and blood pressure is crucial. Monitoring for ischemia is complicated by baseline ST-segment and T-wave abnormalities. Intraarterial pressure monitoring is desirable in patients with severe aortic stenosis, as many of these patients do not tolerate even brief episodes of hypotension. Pulmonary artery catheterization data should be interpreted carefully; a higher than normal pulmonary capillary wedge pressure is often required to maintain adequate left ventricular end-diastolic volume and cardiac output. Prominent *a* waves are often visible on the pulmonary artery wedge pressure waveform. Vasodilators should generally be used cautiously because patients are often very sensitive to these agents. TEE can be useful in these patients for monitoring ischemia, ventricular preload, contractility, valvular function, and the effects of therapeutic interventions.

C. Choice of Agents

Patients with mild to moderate aortic stenosis (generally asymptomatic) may tolerate spinal or epidural anesthesia. These techniques should be employed very cautiously, however, because hypotension readily occurs as a result of reductions in preload, afterload, or both. Epidural anesthesia may be preferable to single-shot spinal anesthesia in many situations because of its slower onset of hypotension, which allows more timely correction. Continuous spinal catheters can similarly be used to gradually increase the level of regional anesthesia and limit the possibility of blood pressure collapse. Spinal and epidural anesthesia are relatively contraindicated in patients with severe aortic stenosis.

In the patient with severe aortic stenosis the choice of general anesthetic agents is less important than managing their hemodynamic effects. Most general anesthetics can produce both vasodilation and hypotension, which require treatment post induction. If a volatile agent is used, the concentration should be controlled to avoid excessive vasodilatation, myocardial depression, or loss of normal atrial systole. Significant tachycardia and severe hypertension, which can precipitate ischemia, should be treated immediately by increasing anesthetic depth or administration of a β-adrenergic blocking agent. Most patients with aortic stenosis tolerate moderate hypertension and are sensitive to vasodilators. Moreover, because of an already precarious myocardial oxygen demand–supply balance, they tolerate even mild degrees of hypotension

poorly. Hypotension should generally be promptly treated with escalating doses (25–100 mcg) of phenylephrine. Intraoperative supraventricular tachycardias with hemodynamic compromise should be treated with immediate synchronized cardioversion. Frequent ventricular ectopy (which often reflects ischemia) is usually poorly tolerated hemodynamically and should be treated. Amiodarone is generally effective for both supraventricular and ventricular arrhythmias.

AORTIC REGURGITATION

Preoperative Considerations

Aortic regurgitation usually develops slowly and is progressive (chronic), but it can also develop quickly (acute). Chronic aortic regurgitation may be caused by abnormalities of the aortic valve, the aortic root, or both. Abnormalities in the valve are usually congenital (bicuspid valve) or due to rheumatic fever. Diseases affecting the ascending aorta cause regurgitation by dilating the aortic annulus; they include syphilis, annuloaortic ectasia, cystic medial necrosis (with or without Marfan syndrome), ankylosing spondylitis, rheumatoid and psoriatic arthritis, and a variety of other connective tissue disorders. Acute aortic insufficiency most commonly follows infective endocarditis, trauma, or aortic dissection.

Pathophysiology

Regardless of the cause, aortic regurgitation produces volume overload of the left ventricle. The effective forward SV is reduced because of backward (regurgitant) flow of blood into the left ventricle during diastole. Systemic arterial diastolic pressure and SVR are typically low. The decrease in cardiac afterload helps facilitate ventricular ejection. Total SV is the sum of the effective stroke volume and the regurgitant volume. The regurgitant volume depends on the heart rate (diastolic time) and the diastolic pressure gradient across the aortic valve (diastolic aortic pressure minus left ventricular end-diastolic pressure). Slow heart rates increase regurgitation because of the associated disproportionate increase in diastolic time, whereas increases in diastolic arterial pressure favor regurgitant volume by increasing the pressure gradient for backward flow.

With chronic aortic regurgitation, the left ventricle progressively dilates and undergoes eccentric hypertrophy. Patients with severe aortic regurgitation have the largest end-diastolic volumes of any heart disease. The resulting increase in end-diastolic volume maintains an effective SV. Any increase in the regurgitant volume is compensated by an increase in end-diastolic volume. Left ventricular end-diastolic pressure is usually normal or only slightly elevated, because ventricular compliance initially increases. Eventually, as ventricular function deteriorates, the ejection fraction declines, and impaired ventricular emptying is manifested as gradual increases in left ventricular end-diastolic pressure and end-systolic volume.

Sudden incompetence of the aortic valve does not allow compensatory dilatation or hypertrophy of the left ventricle. Effective SV rapidly declines because the normal-sized ventricle is unable to accommodate a sudden large regurgitant volume. The sudden rise in left ventricular end-diastolic pressure is transmitted back to the pulmonary circulation and causes acute pulmonary venous congestion.

Acute aortic regurgitation typically presents as the sudden onset of pulmonary edema and hypotension, whereas chronic regurgitation usually presents insidiously as congestive heart failure. Symptoms are generally minimal (in the chronic form) when the regurgitant volume remains under 40% of SV, but become severe when it exceeds 60%. Angina can occur even in the absence of coronary disease. The myocardial oxygen demand is increased from muscle hypertrophy and dilatation, whereas the myocardial blood supply is reduced by low diastolic pressures in the aorta as a result of the regurgitation.

Calculating Regurgitant Fraction & Other Measurements of Severity

As with mitral regurgitation, RSV and RF for aortic regurgitation can be estimated by pulsed Doppler echocardiography. Stroke volume is measured at the left ventricular outflow tract (LVOT) and at the mitral valve (MV). The stroke volume ejected at the LVOT includes both the stroke volume that entered the left ventricle through the mitral valve and the volume of blood that entered the left ventricle through the leaky aortic valve.

Thus,

$$RSV_{aortic\ regurgitation} = (A_{LOVT} \times TVI_{LVOT}) - (A_{MV} \times TVI_{MV})$$

and

$$RF = RSV/SV$$

Pressure half-time ($T_{1/2}$, see the section on mitral stenosis above) of the regurgitant jet is another useful echocardiographic parameter for clinically assessing the severity of aortic regurgitation. The shorter the half-time, the more severe the regurgitation; severe regurgitation rapidly raises left ventricular diastolic pressure and results in more rapid pressure equilibration. Unfortunately, $T_{1/2}$ is affected not only by the regurgitant orifice area, but also by aortic and ventricular pressure. An aortic regurgitation jet with a $T_{1/2}$ less than 240 msec is associated with severe regurgitation.

Treatment

Most patients with chronic aortic regurgitation remain asymptomatic for 10–20 years. Once significant symptoms develop, the expected survival time is about 5 years without valve replacement. Diuretics and afterload reduction, particularly with ACE inhibitors, generally benefit patients with advanced chronic aortic regurgitation. The decrease in arterial blood pressure reduces the diastolic gradient for regurgitation. Patients with chronic aortic regurgitation should receive valve replacement before irreversible ventricular dysfunction occurs.

Patients with acute aortic regurgitation typically require intravenous inotropic and vasodilator therapy. Early intervention is indicated in patients with acute aortic regurgitation: medical management alone is associated with a high mortality rate.

Anesthetic Management

A. Objectives

The heart rate should be maintained toward the upper limits of normal (80–100 beats/min). **11** Bradycardia and increases in SVR increase the regurgitant volume in patients with aortic regurgitation, whereas tachycardia can contribute to myocardial ischemia. Excessive myocardial depression should also be avoided. The compensatory increase in cardiac preload should be maintained, but overzealous fluid replacement can readily result in pulmonary edema.

B. Monitoring

Invasive hemodynamic monitoring should be employed in patients with acute aortic regurgitation and in those with severe chronic regurgitation. Premature closure of the mitral valve often occurs during acute aortic regurgitation and may cause pulmonary capillary wedge pressure to give a falsely high estimate of left ventricular end-diastolic pressure. The appearance of a large *v* wave suggests mitral regurgitation secondary to dilatation of the left ventricle. The arterial pressure wave in patients with aortic regurgitation characteristically has a very wide pulse pressure. *Pulsus bisferiens* may also be present in patients with moderate to severe aortic insufficiency and is thought to result from the rapid ejection of a large SV. Color-flow Doppler TEE can be invaluable in quantitating the severity of the regurgitation and guiding therapeutic interventions. By definition, some reversal of blood flow is present in the aorta during all of diastole (holodiastolic) with severe aortic regurgitation; moreover, the more distal the detection of holodiastolic flow reversal is in the aorta, the more severe the regurgitation.

C. Choice of Agents

Most aortic insufficiency patients tolerate spinal and epidural anesthesia well, provided intravascular volume is maintained. When general anesthesia is required, inhalational agents may be ideal because of the associated vasodilatation. Phenylephrine (25–50 mcg) can be used to treat hypotension secondary to anesthetic-induced vasodilatation. Large doses of phenylephrine increase SVR (and arterial diastolic pressure) and may exacerbate the regurgitation.

TRICUSPID REGURGITATION

Preoperative Considerations

Up to 70% to 90% of patients have trace to mild tricuspid regurgitation on echocardiography; the regurgitant volume in these cases is almost always insignificant. Clinically significant tricuspid regurgitation, however, is most commonly due to dilatation of the right ventricle from pulmonary hypertension that is associated with chronic left ventricular failure. Tricuspid regurgitation can also follow infective endocarditis (usually in injecting drug abusers), rheumatic fever, carcinoid syndrome, or chest trauma or may be due to Ebstein's anomaly (downward displacement of the valve because of abnormal attachment of the valve leaflets).

Pathophysiology

Chronic left ventricular failure often leads to sustained increases in pulmonary vascular pressures. The chronic increase in afterload causes progressive dilatation of the thin-walled right ventricle, and excessive dilatation of the tricuspid annulus eventually results in regurgitation. An increase in end-diastolic volume allows the right ventricle to compensate for the regurgitant volume and maintain an effective forward flow. Because the right atrium and the vena cava are compliant and can usually accommodate the volume overload, mean right atrial and central venous pressures are generally only slightly elevated. Acute or marked elevations in pulmonary artery pressures increase the regurgitant volume and are reflected by an increase in central venous pressure. Moreover, sudden marked increases in right ventricular afterload sharply reduce the effective right ventricular output, reduce left ventricular preload, and can precipitate systemic hypotension.

Chronic venous hypertension leads to passive congestion of the liver and progressive hepatic dysfunction. Severe right ventricular failure with underloading of the left heart may also produce right-to-left shunting through a patent foramen ovale, which can result in marked hypoxemia.

The normal right ventricle does not extend to the apex of the heart when visualized using echocardiography. As the right heart dilates, it acquires a more spherical shape, the right ventricle extends to the apex of the heart, and the interventricular septum is flattened. These changes can impair left heart function.

Calculating Pulmonary Artery Pressure

With severe tricuspid regurgitation, the normal systolic inflow into the right atrium is reversed, and the reversal of flow is also observed in the hepatic veins.

Systolic pulmonary artery pressure (PAS) can be estimated from the peak velocity of the regurgitant jet:

$$\Delta P = 4 \times V^2$$

where ΔP is the systolic pressure gradient (mm Hg) between the right ventricle and right atrium, and V is peak blood flow velocity (m/s) of the regurgitant jet. If the central venous pressure (CVP) is known or assumed, then

$$PAS = CVP + \Delta P$$

Treatment

Tricuspid regurgitation is generally well tolerated by most patients. Because the underlying disorder is generally more important than the tricuspid regurgitation itself, treatment is aimed at the underlying disease process. With moderate to severe regurgitation, tricuspid annuloplasty may be performed in conjunction with replacement of another valve. Recent studies suggest that correction of significant tricuspid regurgitation is beneficial when patients are brought to surgery for replacement of another valve.

Anesthetic Management

A. Objectives

Hemodynamic goals should be directed primarily toward the underlying disorder. Hypovolemia and factors that increase right ventricular afterload, such as hypoxia and acidosis, should be avoided to maintain effective right ventricular SV and left ventricular preload. Positive end-expiratory pressure and high mean airway pressures may also be undesirable during mechanical ventilation because they reduce venous return and increase right ventricular afterload.

B. Monitoring

In these patients, invasive monitoring may be useful. Pulmonary artery catheterization is not always possible; rarely a large regurgitant flow may make passage of a pulmonary artery catheter across the tricuspid valve difficult. Increasing CVP implies worsening right ventricular dysfunction. The x descent is absent, and a prominent cv wave is usually present on the CVP waveform. Thermodilution cardiac output measurements are falsely elevated because of the tricuspid regurgitation. Color-flow Doppler TEE is useful in evaluating the severity of the regurgitation and other associated abnormalities.

C. Choice of Agents

The selection of anesthetic agents should be based on the underlying disorder. Most patients tolerate spinal

and epidural anesthesia well. Coagulopathy secondary to hepatic dysfunction should be excluded prior to any regional technique. During general anesthesia, nitrous oxide may exacerbate pulmonary hypertension and should be administered cautiously, if at all.

ENDOCARDITIS PROPHYLAXIS

The ACC/AHA guidelines regarding prophylactic antibiotic regimens in patients with prosthetic heart valves and other structural heart abnormalities have dramatically changed in recent years, decreasing the number of indications for antibiotic administration. The risk of antibiotic administration is often considered greater than the potential for developing perioperative endocarditis. At present, the ACC/AHA guidelines suggest the use of endocarditis prophylaxis in the highest risk patients undergoing dental procedures involving gingival manipulation or perforation of the oral mucosa (class IIa); see Tables 21–14 and 21–15. Such conditions include:

- Patients with prosthetic cardiac valves or prosthetic heart materials
- Patients with a past history of endocarditis

TABLE 21–14 Endocarditis prophylaxis for dental procedures (UPDATED)[1].

Reasonable	Not Recommended
Endocarditis prophylaxis is reasonable for patients with the highest risk of adverse outcomes who undergo dental procedures that involve manipulation of either gingival tissue or the periapical region of teeth or perforation of the oral mucosa.	Endocarditis prophylaxis is not recommended for: • Routine anesthetic injections through noninfected tissue • Dental radiographs • Placement or removal of prosthodontic or orthodontic appliances • Adjustment of orthodontic appliances • Placement of orthodontic brackets • Shedding of deciduous teeth • Bleeding from trauma to the lips or oral mucosa

[1]Corresponds to the 2008 focused update incorporated into the ACC/AHA 2006 guidelines for the management of patients with valvular heart disease.

Reproduced, with permission, from Dajani AS, Taubert KA, Wilson W, et al: Prevention of bacterial endocarditis: recommendations by the American Heart Association. Circulation. 1997;96:358.

TABLE 21–15 Regimens for a dental procedure (UPDATED).

| Situation | Agent | Regimen: Single Dose 30 to 60 min Before Procedure | |
		Adults	Children
Oral	Amoxicillin	2 g	50 mg/kg
Unable to take oral medication	Ampicillin	2 g IM or IV	50 mg/kg IM or IV
	OR		
	Cefazolin or ceftriaxone	1 g IM or IV	50 mg/kg IM or IV
Allergic to penicillins or ampicillin—oral	Cephalexin[1,2]	2 g	50 mg/kg
	OR		
	Clindamycin	600 mg	20 mg/kg
	OR		
	Azithromycin or clarithromycin	500 mg	15 mg/kg
Allergic to penicillins or ampicillin and unable to take oral medication	Cefazolin or ceftriaxone[‡]	1 g IM or IV	50 mg/kg IM or IV
	OR		
	Clindamycin	600 mg IM or IV	20 mg/kg IM or IV

[1]Or use other first- or second-generation oral cephalosporin in equivalent adult or pediatric dosage.

[2]Cephalosporins should not be used in an individual with a history of anaphylaxis, angioedema, or urticaria with penicillins or ampicillin.

IM indicates intramuscular; and IV, intravenous.

Reproduced, with permission, from Nishimura RA, Carabello BA, Faxon DP, et al: ACC/AHA 2008 guideline update on valvular heart disease: focused update on infective endocarditis prophylaxis. J Am Coll Cardiol 2008;52:676.

- Patients with congenital heart disease that is either partially repaired or unrepaired
- Patients with congenital heart disease with residual defects following repair
- Patients with congenital heart disease within 6 months of a complete repair, whether catheter-based or surgical
- Cardiac transplant patients with structurally abnormal valves

Class III recommendations indicate that prophylaxis is not necessary for nondental procedures, including TEE and esophagogastroduodenoscopy, except in the presence of an active infection.

Endocarditis is believed to occur in areas of cardiac endothelial damage, where in cases of bacteremia, bacteria can be deposited and multiply. Areas of increased myocardial blood flow velocity lead to damaged endothelium, providing a template for bacterial adherence and growth. Indeed, the latest ACC/AHA guidelines do not suggest prophylaxis for genitourinary or gastrointestinal procedures; however, the AHA does note that it is reasonable to administer antibiotics to prevent wound infection. Moreover, they note that although prophylaxis is not suggested for respiratory tract procedures, it is a reasonable strategy in high-risk patients in whom an incision has been made in the respiratory tract (eg, in tonsillectomy).

In spite of these much reduced indications, the ACC/AHA notes that many patients and physicians expect the administration of endocarditis prophylaxis in patients with valvular heart disease, aortic coarctation, and hypertrophic cardiomyopathy. As always, the risk of antibiotic administration must be considered in offering prophylaxis to patients outside of the ACC/AHA high-risk category. Guidelines are ever changing, and although not considered to be "standard of care," they are increasingly present in medical practice; furthermore, deviation from guidelines often requires explanation as being outside of "evidenced-based" practice. Review of ACC/AHA guidelines, which are now available online, are recommended when high-risk patients are encountered.

ANTICOAGULATION

Patients with mechanical prosthetic heart valves require anticoagulation, which is currently accomplished with warfarin. Aspirin is also indicated in this population, as well as in patients with bioprosthetic valves, to prevent thrombus formation. Warfarin is sometimes also used initially for mitral bioprosthetic valves (Table 21–16).

Patients with prosthetic valves often present for noncardiac surgery that will require temporary discontinuation of anticoagulation. The ACC/AHA guidelines indicate that patients at low risk of thrombosis, such as those with bileaflet mechanical valves

TABLE 21–16 Recommendations for antithrombotic therapy in patients with prosthetic heart valves.

	Aspirin (75–100 mg)	Warfarin (INR 2.0–3.0)	Warfarin (INR 2.5–3.5)	No Warfarin
Mechanical prosthetic valves				
AVR–low risk				
Less than 3 months	Class I	Class I	Class IIa	
Greater than 3 months	Class I	Class I		
AVR–high risk	Class I		Class I	
MVR	Class I		Class I	
Biological prosthetic valves				
AVR–low risk				
Less than 3 months	Class I	Class IIa		Class IIb
Greater than 3 months	Class I			Class IIa
AVR–high risk	Class I	Class I		
MVR–low risk				
Less than 3 months	Class I	Class IIa		
Greater than 3 months	Class I			Class IIa
MVR–high risk	Class I	Class I		

Depending on patients' clinical status, antithrombotic therapy must be individualized (see special situations in text). In patients receiving warfarin, aspirin is recommended in virtually all situations. Risk factors: atrial fibrillation, left ventricular dysfunction, previous thromboembolism, and hypercoagulable condition. International normalized ratio (INR) should be maintained between 2.5 and 3.5 for aortic disc valves and Starr-Edwards valves.

AVR indicates aortic valve replacement; and MVR, mitral valve replacement.

Data from McAnuty JH, Rahimtoola SH. Antithrombotic therapy in valvular heart disease. In: Schlant R, Alexander RW. editors. *Hurst's The Heart.* New York, McGraw-Hill, 1998:1867-1874.

in the aortic position with no additional problems (eg, no AF or no hypercoaguable state) can discontinue warfarin 48–72 hours preoperatively so that the INR falls below 1.5. In patients at greater risk of thrombosis, warfarin should be discontinued and heparin, either unfractionated or low molecular weight, started when the INR falls below 2.0. Heparin can be discontinued 4–6 hours prior to surgery and then restarted as soon as surgical bleeding permits, until the patient can be restarted on warfarin therapy. Fresh frozen plasma may be given, if needed, in an emergency situation to interrupt warfarin therapy. Vitamin K should not be administered, as it could potentially lead to a hypercoaguable state. Anesthesia staff should always consult with the patient's surgeon and the physician responsible for prescribing the anticoagulation before adjusting anticoagulation or antiplatelet regimens perioperatively.

Congenital Heart Disease

Preoperative Considerations

Congenital heart disease encompasses a seemingly endless list of abnormalities that may be detected in infancy, early childhood, or, less commonly, adulthood. The incidence of congenital heart disease in all live births approaches 1%. The natural history of some defects is such that patients often survive to adulthood (Table 21–17). Moreover, the number of surviving adults with congenital heart disease is steadily increasing, possibly as a result of advances in surgical and medical treatment. An increasing number of patients with congenital heart disease may therefore be encountered during noncardiac surgery and obstetric deliveries. Knowledge of the

TABLE 21–17 Common congenital heart defects in which patients typically survive to adulthood without treatment.

Bicuspid aortic valve
Coarctation of the aorta
Pulmonic valve stenosis
Ostium secundum atrial septal defect
Ventricular septal defect
Patent ductus arteriosus

TABLE 21–18 Classification of congenital heart disease.

Lesions causing outflow obstruction
Left ventricle
Coarctation of the aorta
Aortic stenosis
Right ventricle
Pulmonic valve stenosis
Lesions causing left-to-right shunting
Ventricular septal defect
Patent ductus arteriosus
Atrial septal defect
Endocardial cushion defect
Partial anomalous pulmonary venous return
Lesions causing right-to-left shunting
With decreased pulmonary blood flow
Tetralogy of Fallot
Pulmonary atresia
Tricuspid atresia
With increased pulmonary blood flow
Transposition of the great vessels
Truncus arteriosus
Single ventricle
Double-outlet right ventricle
Total anomalous pulmonary venous return
Hypoplastic left heart

anatomy of the original heart structure defect and of any corrective repairs is essential prior to anesthetizing the patient with congental heart disease (CHD).

The complex nature and varying pathophysiology of congenital heart defects make classification difficult. A commonly used scheme is presented in Table 21–18. Most patients present with cyanosis, congestive heart failure, or an asymptomatic abnormality. Cyanosis is typically the result of an abnormal intracardiac communication that allows unoxygenated blood to reach the systemic arterial circulation (right-to-left shunting). Congestive heart failure is most prominent with defects that either obstruct left ventricular outflow or markedly increase pulmonary blood flow. The latter is usually due to an abnormal intracardiac communication that returns oxygenated blood to the right heart (left-to-right shunting). Whereas right-to-left shunts generally decrease pulmonary blood flow, some complex lesions increase pulmonary blood flow—even in the presence of right-to-left shunting. In many cases, more than one lesion is present.

In fact, survival (prior to surgical correction) with some anomalies (eg, transposition, total anomalous venous return, pulmonary atresia) depends on the simultaneous presence of another shunting lesion (eg, patent ductus arteriosus, patent foramen ovale, ventricular septal defect). Chronic hypoxemia in patients with cyanotic heart disease typically results in erythrocytosis. This increase in red cell mass, which is due to enhanced erythropoietin secretion from the kidneys, serves to restore tissue oxygen concentration to normal. Unfortunately, blood viscosity can also rise to the point at which it may interfere with oxygen delivery. When tissue oxygenation is restored to normal, the hematocrit is stable (usually <65%), and symptoms of the hyperviscosity syndrome are absent, the patient is said to have compensated erythrocytosis. Patients with uncompensated erythrocytosis do not establish this equilibrium; they have symptoms of hyperviscosity and may be at risk of thrombotic complications, particularly stroke. The last is aggravated by dehydration. Children younger than age 4 years seem to be at greatest risk of stroke. Phlebotomy is generally not recommended if symptoms of hyperviscosity are absent and the hematocrit is <65%.

Coagulation abnormalities are common in patients with cyanotic heart disease. Platelet counts tend to be low-normal, and many patients have subtle or overt defects in the coagulation cascade. Phlebotomy may improve hemostasis in some patients. Hyperuricemia often occurs because of increased urate reabsorption secondary to renal hypoperfusion. Gouty arthritis is uncommon, but the hyperuricemia can result in progressive renal impairment.

Preoperative Doppler echocardiography is invaluable in helping to define the anatomy of the defect(s) and to confirm or exclude the existence of other lesions or complications, their physiological significance, and the effects of any therapeutic interventions.

Anesthetic Management

This population of patients includes four groups: those who have undergone corrective cardiac surgery and require no further operations, those who have had only palliative surgery, those who have not yet undergone any cardiac surgery, and those whose conditions are inoperable and may be awaiting cardiac transplantation. Although the management of the first group of patients may be the same as that of normal patients (except for consideration of prophylactic antibiotic therapy), the care of others requires familiarity with the complex pathophysiology of these defects. Even patients who have had corrective surgery may be prone to the development of perioperative problems (Tables 21–19 and 21–20). Some surgical procedures eliminate the risk of endocarditis, whereas others increase the risk through the use of prosthetic valves or conduits or the creation of new shunts.

For the purpose of anesthetic management, congenital heart defects may be divided into obstructive lesions, predominantly left-to-right shunts, or predominantly right-to-left shunts. In reality, shunts can also be bidirectional and may reverse under certain conditions.

TABLE 21–19 Common problems in survivors of surgery for congenital heart defects.

Arrhythmias
Hypoxemia
Pulmonary hypertension
Existing shunts
Paradoxical embolism
Bacterial endocarditis

TABLE 21–20 Congenital cardiac lesions and perioperative risk for noncardiac surgery.

High risk
    Pulmonary hypertension, primary or secondary
    Cyanotic congenital heart disease
    New York Heart Association class III or IV
    Severe systemic ventricular dysfunction (ejection
        fraction less than 35%)
    Severe left-sided heart obstructive lesions
Moderate risk
    Prosthetic valve or conduit
    Intracardiac shunt
    Moderate left-sided heart obstruction
    Moderate systemic ventricular dysfunction

Warnes C, Williams R, Bashore T, et al: ACC/AHA 2008 guidelines for the management of adults with congenital heart disease. Circulation 2008;118:2395.

1. Obstructive Lesions

Pulmonic Stenosis

Pulmonary valve stenosis obstructs right ventricular outflow and causes concentric right ventricular hypertrophy. Severe obstruction presents in the neonatal period, whereas lesser degrees of obstruction may go undetected until adulthood. The valve is usually deformed and is either bicuspid or tricuspid. Valve leaflets are often partially fused and display systolic doming on echocardiography. The right ventricle undergoes hypertrophy, and poststenotic dilatation of the pulmonary artery is often present. Symptoms are those of right ventricular heart failure. Symptomatic patients readily develop fatigue, dyspnea, and peripheral cyanosis with exertion as a result of the limited pulmonary blood flow and increased oxygen extraction by tissues. With severe stenosis, the pulmonic valve gradient exceeds 60–80 mm Hg, depending on the age of the patient. Right-to-left shunting may also occur in the presence of a patent foramen ovale or atrial septal defect. Cardiac output is very dependent on an elevated heart rate, but excessive increases in the latter can compromise ventricular filling. Percutaneous balloon valvuloplasty is generally considered the initial treatment of choice in most patients with symptomatic pulmonic stenosis. Anesthetic management for patients undergoing surgery should maintain a normal or slightly high heart rate, augment preload, and avoid factors that increase PVR.

2. Predominantly Left-to-Right (Simple) Shunts

Simple shunts are isolated abnormal communications between the right and left sides of the heart. Because pressures are normally higher on the left side of the heart, blood usually flows across from left to right, and blood flow through the right heart and the lungs increases. Depending on the size and location of the communication, the right ventricle may also be subjected to the higher left-sided pressures, resulting in both pressure and volume overload. Right ventricular afterload is normally 5% that of the left ventricle, so even small left-to-right pressure gradients can produce large increases in

pulmonary blood flow. The ratio of pulmonary (Qp) to systemic (Qs) blood flow is useful to determine the directionality of the shunt.

A ratio greater than 1 usually indicates a left-to-right shunt, whereas a ratio less than 1 indicates a right-to-left shunt. A ratio of 1 indicates either no shunting or a bidirectional shunt of opposing magnitudes.

Large increases in pulmonary blood flow produce pulmonary vascular congestion and increase extravascular lung water. The latter interferes with gas exchange, decreases lung compliance, and increases the work of breathing. Left atrial distention also compresses the left bronchus, whereas distention of pulmonary vessels compresses smaller bronchi.

Over the course of several years, chronic increases in pulmonary blood flow produce vascular changes that irreversibly increase PVR. Elevation of right ventricular afterload produces hypertrophy and progressively raises right-sided cardiac pressures. With advanced disease, the pressures within the right heart can exceed those within the left heart. Under these conditions, the intracardiac shunt reverses and becomes a right-to-left shunt (Eisenmenger syndrome).

When a communication is small, shunt flow depends primarily on the size of the communication (restrictive shunt). When the communication is large (nonrestrictive shunt), shunt flow depends on the relative balance between PVR and SVR. **12** An increase in SVR relative to PVR favors left-to-right shunting, whereas an increase in PVR relative to SVR favors right-to-left shunting. Common chamber lesions (eg, single atrium, single ventricle, truncus arteriosus) represent the extreme form of nonrestrictive shunts; shunt flow with these lesions is bidirectional and totally dependent on relative changes in the ventricular afterload.

13 The presence of shunt flow between the right and left hearts, regardless of the direction of blood flow, mandates the meticulous exclusion of air bubbles and particulate material from intravenous fluids to prevent paradoxical embolism into the cerebral or coronary circulations.

Atrial Septal Defects

Ostium secundum atrial septal defects (ASDs) are the most common type and usually occur as isolated lesions in the area of the fossa ovalis. The defect is sometimes associated with partial anomalous pulmonary venous return, most commonly of the right upper pulmonary vein. A secundum ASD may result in single or multiple (fenestrated) openings between the atria. The less common sinus venosus and ostium primum ASDs are typically associated with other cardiac abnormalities. Sinus venosus defects are located in the upper interatrial septum close to the superior vena cava; one or more of the right pulmonary veins often abnormally drains into the superior vena cava. In contrast, ostium primum ASDs are located in the lower interatrial septum and overlie the mitral and tricuspid valves; most patients also have a cleft in the anterior leaflet of the mitral, valve and some have an abnormal septal leaflet in the tricuspid valve.

Most children with ASDs are minimally symptomatic; some have recurrent pulmonary infections. Congestive heart failure and pulmonary hypertension are more commonly encountered in adults with ASDs. Patients with ostium primum defects often have large shunts and may also develop significant mitral regurgitation. In the absence of heart failure, anesthetic responses to inhalation and intravenous agents are generally not significantly altered in patients with ASDs. **Large increases in SVR should be avoided because they may worsen the left-to-right shunting**.

Ventricular Septal Defects

Ventricular septal defect (VSD) is a common congenital heart defect, accounting for up to 25% to 35% of congenital heart disease. The defect is most frequently found in the membranous part of the interventricular septum (membranous or infracristal VSD) in a posterior position and anterior to the septal leaflet of the tricuspid valve. Muscular VSDs are the next most frequent type and are located in the mid or apical portion of the interventricular septum, where there may be a single defect or multiple openings (resembling Swiss cheese). Defects in the subpulmonary (supracristal) septum are often associated with aortic regurgitation because the right coronary cusp can prolapse into the VSD. Septal defects at the ventricular inlet are usually similar in development and location to AV septal defects (see the following section).

The resulting functional abnormality of a VSD is dependent on the size of the defect, PVR, and the presence or absence of other abnormalities. Small VSDs, particularly of the muscular type, often close during childhood. Restrictive defects are associated with only small left-to-right shunts (pulmonary–systemic blood flow ratios less than 1.75:1). Large defects produce large left-to-right shunts (shunts larger than 2:1) that vary directly with SVR and indirectly with PVR. Recurrent pulmonary infections and congestive heart failure are common with pulmonary–systemic flow ratios of 3–5:1. Patients with small VSDs are treated medically and followed by electrocardiography (for signs of right ventricular hypertrophy) and echocardiography. Surgical closure is usually undertaken in patients with large VSDs before pulmonary vascular disease and Eisenmenger physiology develop. As with atrial defects, in the absence of heart failure, anesthetic responses to inhalation and intravenous agents are generally not significantly altered. Similarly, increases in SVR worsen the left-to-right shunting. **When right-to-left shunting is present, abrupt increases in PVR or decreases in SVR are poorly tolerated.**

Atrioventricular Septal Defects

Endocardial cushion (AV canal) defects produce contiguous atrial and ventricular septal defects, often with very abnormal AV valves. This is a common lesion in patients with Down syndrome. The defect can produce large shunts both at the atrial and ventricular levels. Mitral and tricuspid regurgitation exacerbate the volume overload on the ventricles. Initially, shunting is predominately left to right; however, with increasing pulmonary hypertension, Eisenmenger syndrome with obvious cyanosis develops.

Patent Ductus Arteriosus

Persistence of the communication between the main pulmonary artery and the aorta can produce restrictive or nonrestrictive left-to-right shunts. This abnormality is commonly responsible for the cardiopulmonary deterioration of premature infants and occasionally presents later in life when it can be corrected thoracoscopically. Anesthetic goals should be similar to atrial and ventricular septal defects.

Partial Anomalous Venous Return

This defect is present when one or more pulmonary veins drains into the right side of the heart; the anomalous veins are usually from the right lung. Possible anomalous entry sites include the right atrium, the superior or inferior vena cava, and the coronary sinus. The resulting abnormality produces a variable amount of left-to-right shunting. The clinical course and prognosis are usually excellent and similar to that of a secundum ASD. A very large coronary sinus on TEE suggests anomalous drainage into the coronary sinus, which may complicate the management of cardioplegia during cardiac surgery. Total anomalous venous return is corrected immediately after birth.

3. Predominantly Right-to-Left (Complex) Shunts

Lesions within this group (some also called **mixing lesions**) often produce both ventricular outflow obstruction and shunting. The obstruction favors shunt flow toward the unobstructed side. When the obstruction is relatively mild, the amount of shunting is affected by the ratio of SVR to PVR, but increasing degrees of obstruction fix the direction and magnitude of the shunt. Atresia of any one of the cardiac valves represents the extreme form of obstruction. Shunting occurs proximal to the atretic valve and is completely fixed; survival depends on another distal shunt (usually a patent ductus arteriosus [PDA], patent foramen ovale, ASD, or VSD), where blood flows in the opposite direction. This group of defects may also be divided according to whether they increase or decrease pulmonary blood flow.

Tetralogy of Fallot

This anomaly classically includes right ventricular outflow obstruction, right ventricular hypertrophy, and a VSD with an overriding aorta. Right ventricular obstruction in most patients is due to infundibular stenosis, which is due to hypertrophy of the subpulmonic muscle (crista ventricularis).

At least 20% to 25% of patients also have pulmonic stenosis, and a small percentage of patients has some element of supravalvular obstruction. The pulmonic valve is often bicuspid, or, less commonly, atretic. Infundibular obstruction may be increased by sympathetic tone and is therefore dynamic; this obstruction is likely responsible for the hypercyanotic spells observed in very young patients. **The combination of right ventricular outflow obstruction and a VSD results in ejection of unoxygenated right ventricular blood, as well as oxygenated left ventricular blood into the aorta.** The right-to-left shunting across the VSD has both fixed and variable components. The fixed component is determined by the severity of the right ventricular obstruction, whereas the variable component depends on SVR and PVR.

Neonates with severe right ventricular obstruction may deteriorate quickly, as pulmonary blood flow decreases when a PDA starts to close. Intravenous prostaglandin E$_1$ (0.05–0.2 mcg/kg/min) is used to prevent ductal closure in such instances. Surgical palliation with a left-to-right systemic shunt or complete correction is then usually undertaken. For the former, a modified Blalock–Taussig (systemic–pulmonary artery) shunt is most often used to increase pulmonary blood flow. In this procedure, a synthetic graft is anastomosed between a subclavian artery and an ipsilateral pulmonary artery. Complete correction involves closure of the VSD, removal of obstructing infundibular muscle, and pulmonic valvulotomy or valvuloplasty, when necessary.

The goals of anesthetic management in patients with tetralogy of Fallot should be to maintain intravascular volume and SVR. Increases in PVR, such as might occur from acidosis or excessive airway pressures, should be avoided. **Ketamine (intramuscular or intravenous) is a commonly used induction agent because it maintains or increases SVR and therefore does not aggravate the right-to-left shunting.** Patients with milder degrees of shunting generally tolerate inhalation induction. The right-to-left shunting tends to slow the uptake of inhalation anesthetics; in contrast, it may accelerate the onset of intravenous agents. Oxygenation often improves following induction of anesthesia. Muscle relaxants that release histamine should be avoided. Hypercyanotic spells may be treated with intravenous fluid and phenylephrine (5 mcg/kg). Beta blockers (eg, propranolol) may also be effective in relieving infundibular spasm. Sodium bicarbonate to correct the resulting metabolic acidosis, may also be helpful when the hypoxemia is severe and prolonged.

Tricuspid Atresia

With tricuspid atresia, blood can flow out of the right atrium only via a patent foramen ovale (or an ASD). Moreover, a PDA (or VSD) is necessary for blood to flow from the left ventricle into the pulmonary circulation. Cyanosis is usually evident at birth, and its severity depends on the amount of pulmonary blood flow that is achieved. Early survival is dependent on prostaglandin E_1 infusion, with or without a percutaneous Rashkind balloon atrial septostomy. Severe cyanosis requires a modified Blalock–Taussig shunt early in life. The preferred surgical management is a modified Fontan procedure, in which the venous drainage is directed to the pulmonary circulation. In some centers, a superior vena cava to the main pulmonary artery (bidirectional Glenn) shunt may be employed before or instead of a Fontan procedure. With both procedures, blood from the systemic veins flows to the left atrium without the assistance of the right ventricle. Success of the procedure depends on a high systemic venous pressure and maintaining both low PVR and a low left atrial pressure. Heart transplantation may be necessary for a failed Fontan procedure.

Transposition of the Great Arteries

In patients with transposition of the great arteries, pulmonary and systemic venous return flows normally back to the right and left atrium, respectively, but the aorta arises from the right ventricle, and the pulmonary artery arises from the left ventricle. Thus, deoxygenated blood returns back into the systemic circulation, and oxygenated blood returns back to the lungs. Survival is possible only through mixing of oxygenated and deoxygenated blood across the foramen ovale and a PDA. The presence of a VSD increases mixing and reduces the level of hypoxemia. Prostaglandin E_1 infusion is usually necessary. Rashkind septostomy may be necessary

if surgical correction is delayed. Corrective surgical treatment involves an arterial switch procedure in which the aorta is divided and reanastomosed to the left ventricle, and the pulmonary artery is divided and reanastomosed to the right ventricle. The coronary arteries must also be reimplanted into the old pulmonary artery root. A VSD, if present, is closed. Less commonly, an atrial switch (Senning) procedure may be carried out if an arterial switch is not possible. In this latter procedure, an intraatrial baffle is created from the atrial wall, and blood from the pulmonary veins flows across an ASD to the right ventricle, from which it is ejected into the systemic circulation.

Transposition of the great vessels may occur with a VSD and pulmonic stenosis. This combination of defects mimics tetralogy of Fallot; however, the obstruction affects the left ventricle, not the right ventricle. Corrective surgery involves patch closure of the VSD, directing left ventricular outflow into the aorta, ligation of the proximal pulmonary artery, and connecting the right ventricular outflow to the pulmonary artery with a valved conduit (Rastelli procedure).

Truncus Arteriosus

With a truncus arteriosus defect, a single arterial trunk supplies the pulmonary and systemic circulation. The truncus always overrides a VSD, allowing both ventricles to eject into it. As PVR gradually decreases after birth, pulmonary blood flow increases greatly, resulting in heart failure. If left untreated, PVR increases, and cyanosis develops again, along with Eisenmenger physiology. Surgical correction closes the VSD, separates the pulmonary artery from the truncus, and connects the right ventricle to the pulmonary artery with a conduit (Rastelli repair).

Hypoplastic Left Heart Syndrome

This syndrome describes a group of defects characterized by aortic valve atresia and marked underdevelopment of the left ventricle. The right ventricle is the main pumping chamber for both systemic and pulmonary circulations. It ejects normally into the pulmonary artery, and all (or nearly all) blood flow entering the aorta is usually derived from a PDA. Surgical treatment includes both the Norwood repair and a hybrid approach to palliation. In the Norwood repair, a new aorta is created from the hypoplastic aorta and the main pulmonary artery. Pulmonary blood flow is delivered via a Blalock–Taussig shunt. The right ventricle becomes the heart's systemic pumping ventricle. A hybrid approach has also been advocated for the treatment of hypoplastic left heart syndrome. In this approach, the pulmonary arteries are banded to reduce pulmonary blood flow, and the PDA is stented to provide for systemic blood flow.

The Patient with a Transplanted Heart

Preoperative Considerations

The number of patients with cardiac transplants is increasing because of both the increasing frequency of transplantation and improved post-transplant survival rates. These patients may present to the operating room early in the postoperative period for mediastinal exploration or retransplantation, or they may appear later for incision and drainage of infections, orthopedic surgery, or unrelated procedures.

15 The transplanted heart is totally denervated, so direct autonomic influences are absent. Cardiac impulse formation and conduction are normal, but the absence of vagal influences causes a relatively high resting heart rate (100–120 beats/min). Although sympathetic fibers are similarly interrupted, the response to circulating catecholamines is normal or even enhanced because of denervation sensitivity (increased receptor density). Cardiac output tends to be low-normal and increases relatively slowly in response to exercise because the response is dependent on an increase in circulating catecholamines. Because the Starling relationship between end-diastolic volume and cardiac output is normal, the transplanted heart is also often said to be preload dependent. Coronary autoregulation is preserved.

Preoperative evaluation should focus on evaluating the functional status of the transplanted organ and detecting complications of immunosuppression.

Rejection may be heralded by arrhythmias (in the first 6 months) or decreased exercise tolerance from a progressive deterioration of myocardial performance. Periodic echocardiographic evaluations are commonly used to monitor for rejection, but the most reliable technique is endomyocardial biopsy. Accelerated atherosclerosis in the graft is a very common and serious problem that limits the life of the transplant. Moreover, myocardial ischemia and infarction are almost always silent because of the denervation. Because of this, patients must undergo periodic evaluations, including angiography, for assessment of coronary atherosclerosis.

Immunosuppressive therapy usually includes cyclosporine, azathioprine, and prednisone. Important side effects include nephrotoxicity, bone marrow suppression, hepatotoxicity, opportunistic infections, and osteoporosis. Hypertension and fluid retention are common and typically require treatment with a diuretic and an ACE inhibitor. Stress doses of corticosteroids are needed when patients undergo major procedures.

Anesthetic Management

Almost all anesthetic techniques, including regional anesthesia, have been used successfully for transplanted patients. The preload-dependent function of the graft makes maintenance of a normal or high cardiac preload desirable. Moreover, the absence of reflex increases in heart rate can make patients particularly sensitive to rapid vasodilatation. Indirect vasopressors, such as ephedrine, are less effective than direct-acting agents because of the absence of catecholamine stores in myocardial neurons. Isoproterenol or epinephrine infusions should be readily available to increase the heart rate if necessary.

Careful electrocardiographic monitoring for ischemia is necessary. The ECG usually demonstrates two sets of P waves, one representing the recipient's own sinoatrial node (SA) (which is left intact), and the other representing the donor's SA node. The recipient's SA node may still be affected by autonomic influences, but it does not affect cardiac function. Direct arterial pressure monitoring should be used for major operations; strict asepsis should be observed during placement.

In a recently transplanted patient, the right ventricle of the transplanted heart may not be able to overcome the resistance of the pulmonary vasculature. Right ventricular failure can occur perioperatively, requiring the use of inhaled nitric oxide, inotropes, and, at times, right ventricular assist devices.

CASE DISCUSSION

Hip Fracture in an Elderly Woman who Fell

A 71-year-old woman presents for open reduction and internal fixation of a left hip fracture. She gives a history of two episodes of lightheadedness several days prior to her fall today. When questioned about her fall, she can only recall standing in her bathroom while brushing her teeth and then awakening on the floor with hip pain. The preoperative ECG shows a sinus rhythm with a P–R interval of 220 msec and a right bundle-branch block (RBBB) pattern.

Why should the anesthesiologist be concerned about a history of syncope?

A history of syncope in elderly patients should always raise the possibility of arrhythmias and underlying organic heart disease. Although arrhythmias can occur in the absence of organic heart disease, the two are commonly related. Cardiac syncope usually results from an abrupt arrhythmia that suddenly compromises cardiac output and impairs cerebral perfusion. Lightheadedness and presyncope, may reflect lesser degrees of cerebral impairment. Both bradyarrhythmias and tachyarrhythmias (see Chapter 20) can produce syncope. Table 21–21 lists other cardiac and noncardiac causes of syncope.

How do bradyarrhythmias commonly arise?

Bradyarrhythmias may arise from either SA node dysfunction or abnormal AV conduction of the cardiac impulse. A delay or block of the impulse can occur anywhere between the SA node and the distal His-Purkinje system). Reversible abnormalities may be due to abnormal vagal tone, electrolyte

TABLE 21–21 Causes of syncope.

Cardiac
  Arrhythmias
    Tachyarrhythmias (usually >180 beats/min)
    Bradyarrhythmias (usually <40 beats/min)
  Impairment of left ventricular ejection
    Aortic stenosis
    Hypertrophic cardiomyopathy
    Massive myocardial infarction
    Atrial myxoma
  Impairment of right ventricular output
    Tetralogy of Fallot
    Primary pulmonary hypertension
    Pulmonary embolism
    Pulmonic valve stenosis
  Biventricular impairment
    Cardiac tamponade
    Massive myocardial infarction

Noncardiac
  Accentuated reflexes
    Vasodepressor reflex (ie, vasovagal syncope)
    Carotid sinus hypersensitivity
    Neuralgias
  Postural hypotension
    Hypovolemia
    Sympathectomy
    Autonomic dysfunction
  Sustained Valsalva maneuver
  Cerebrovascular disease
  Seizures
  Metabolic
    Hypoxia
    Marked hypocapnia
    Hypoglycemia

abnormalities, drug toxicity, hypothermia, or myocardial ischemia. Irreversible abnormalities, which initially may be only intermittent before they become permanent, reflect either isolated conduction system abnormalities or underlying heart disease (most commonly hypertensive, coronary artery, or valvular heart disease).

What is the pathophysiology of sinus node dysfunction?

Patients with sinus node dysfunction may have a normal baseline 12-lead ECG but abrupt pauses in SA node activity (sinus arrest) or intermittent block of conduction of the SA impulse to the surrounding tissue (exit block). Symptoms are usually present when pauses are prolonged

(>3 s) or the effective ventricular rate is less than 40 beats/min. Patients may experience intermittent dizziness, syncope, confusion, fatigue, or shortness of breath. Symptomatic SA node dysfunction, or sick sinus syndrome, is often unmasked by β-adrenergic blocking agents, calcium channel blockers, digoxin, or quinidine. The term tachycardia–bradycardia syndrome is often used when patients experience paroxysmal tachyarrhythmias (usually atrial flutter or fibrillation) followed by sinus pauses or bradycardia. The latter, bradycardia, probably represents failure of the SA node to recover normal automaticity following suppression by the tachyarrhythmia. The diagnosis must be based on electrocardiographic recordings made during symptoms (Holter monitoring) or after provocative tests (carotid baroreceptor stimulation or rapid atrial pacing).

How are AV conduction abnormalities manifested on the surface 12-lead ECG?

AV conduction abnormalities are usually manifested by abnormal ventricular depolarization (bundle-branch block), prolongation of the P–R interval (first-degree AV block), failure of some atrial impulses to depolarize the ventricles (second-degree AV block), or AV dissociation (third-degree AV block; also called complete heart block).

What determines the significance of these conduction abnormalities?

The significance of a conduction system abnormality depends on its location, its likelihood for progression to complete heart block, and the likelihood that a more distal pacemaker site will be able to maintain a stable and adequate escape rhythm (>40 beats/min). The His bundle is normally the lowest area in the conduction system that can maintain a stable rhythm (usually 40–60 beats/min). When conduction fails anywhere above it, a normal His bundle can take over the pacemaker function of the heart and maintain a normal QRS complex, unless a distal intraventricular conduction defect is present. When the escape rhythm arises farther down the His-Purkinje system, the rhythm is usually slower

(<40 beats/min) and is often unstable; it results in a wide QRS complex.

What is the significance of isolated bundle-branch block with a normal P–R interval?

A conduction delay or block in the right bundle-branch results in a typical RBBB QRS pattern on the surface ECG (M-shape or rSR' in V_1) and may represent a congenital abnormality or underlying organic heart disease. In contrast, a delay or block in the main left bundle-branch results in a left bundle-branch block (LBBB) QRS pattern (wide R with a delayed upstroke in V_5) and nearly always represents underlying heart disease. The term hemiblock is often used if only one of the two fascicles of the left bundle-branch is blocked (left anterior or left posterior hemiblock). When the P–R interval is normal—and in the absence of an acute MI—a conduction block in either the left or right bundle rarely leads to complete heart block.

Can the site of an AV block always be determined from a 12-lead ECG?

No. A first-degree AV block (P–R interval >200 ms) can reflect abnormal conduction anywhere between the atria and the distal His-Purkinje system. Mobitz type I second-degree AV block, which is characterized by progressive lengthening of the P–R interval before a P wave is not conducted (a QRS does not follow the P wave), is usually due to a block in the AV node itself, and can be caused by digitalis toxicity or myocardial ischemia; progression to a third-degree AV block is uncommon.

In patients with Mobitz type II second-degree AV block, atrial impulses are periodically not conducted into the ventricle without progressive prolongation of the P–R interval. The conduction block is nearly always in or below the His bundle and frequently progresses to complete (third-degree) AV block, particularly following an acute anteroseptal MI. The QRS is typically wide.

In patients with a third-degree AV block, the atrial rate and ventricular depolarization rates are independent (AV dissociation) because atrial impulses completely fail to reach the ventricles. If the site of the block is in the AV node, a stable His bundle rhythm will result in a normal QRS complex, and the ventricular rate will often increase following administration of atropine. If the block involves the His bundle, the origin of the ventricular rhythm is more distal, resulting in wide QRS complexes. A wide QRS complex does not necessarily exclude a normal His bundle, as it may represent a more distal block in one of the bundle branches.

Can AV dissociation occur in the absence of AV block?

Yes. AV dissociation may occur during anesthesia with volatile agents in the absence of AV block and results from sinus bradycardia or an accelerated AV junctional rhythm. During isorhythmic dissociation, the atria and ventricles beat independently at nearly the same rate. The P wave often just precedes or follows the QRS complex, and their relationship is generally maintained. In contrast, interference AV dissociation results from a junctional rhythm that is faster than the sinus rate—such that sinus impulses always find the AV node refractory.

How do bifascicular and trifascicular blocks present?

A bifascicular block exists when two of the three major His bundle-branches (right, left anterior, or left posterior) are partially or completely blocked. If one fascicle is completely blocked and the others are only partially blocked, a bundle-branch block pattern will be associated with either first-degree or second-degree AV block. If all three are affected, a trifascicular block is said to exist. A delay or partial block in all three fascicles results in either a prolonged P–R interval (first-degree AV block) or alternating LBBB and RBBB. Complete block in all three fascicles results in third-degree AV block.

What is the significance of the electrocardiographic findings in this patient?

The electrocardiographic findings (first-degree AV block plus RBBB) suggest a bifascicular block. Extensive disease of the conduction system is likely. Moreover, the patient's syncopal and near-syncopal episodes suggest that she may be at risk of life-threatening bradyarrhythmias (third-degree AV block). Intracardiac electrocardiographic recordings would be necessary to confirm the site of the conduction delay.

What is appropriate management for this patient?

Cardiological evaluation is required because of the symptomatic bifascicular block. One of two approaches can be recommended, depending on the urgency of the surgery. If the surgery is truly emergent, a temporary transvenous pacing catheter or a transcutaneous pacemaker is indicated prior to induction of general or regional anesthesia. If the surgery can be postponed 24–48 hr (as in this case), continuous electrocardiographic monitoring, serial 12-lead ECGs, and measurements of cardiac isoenzymes are required to exclude myocardial ischemia or infarction and to try to record findings during symptoms.

What are general perioperative indications for temporary pacing?

Suggested indications include the following: any documented symptomatic bradyarrhythmia; second-degree (type II) AV block, or third-degree AV block and refractory supraventricular tachyarrhythmias.

The first three indications generally require ventricular pacing, whereas the fourth requires atrial pacing electrodes and a programmable rapid atrial pulse generator.

How can temporary cardiac pacing be established?

Pacing can be established by transvenous, transcutaneous, epicardial, or transesophageal electrodes. The most reliable method is generally via a transvenous pacing electrode in the form of a pacing wire or a balloon-tipped pacing catheter. A pacing wire should always be positioned fluoroscopically, but a flow-directed pacing catheter can also be placed in the right ventricle under pressure monitoring. A pacing wire must be used when blood flow has ceased. If the patient has a rhythm, intracardiac electrocardiographic recording showing ST-segment elevation when the electrode comes in contact with the right ventricular endocardium confirms placement of either type of electrode. Specially designed pulmonary artery catheters have an extra port for passage of a right ventricular pacing wire. These catheters are particularly useful in patients with LBBB, who can theoretically develop complete heart block during catheter placement. Transcutaneous ventricular pacing is also possible via large stimulating adhesive pads placed on the chest and should be used whenever transvenous pacing Is not readily available. Epicardial electrodes are usually used during cardiac surgery. Pacing the left atrium via an esophageal electrode is a simple, relatively noninvasive technique, but it is useful only for symptomatic sinus bradycardias and for terminating some supraventricular tachyarrhythmias.

Once positioned, the pacing electrodes are attached to an electrical pulse generator that periodically delivers an impulse at a set rate and magnitude. Most pacemaker generators can also sense the heart's spontaneous (usually ventricular) electrical activity: when activity is detected, the generator suppresses its next impulse. By altering the generator's sensing threshold, the pacemaker generator can function in a fixed (asynchronous) mode or in a demand mode (by increasing sensitivity). The lowest current through the electrode that can depolarize the myocardium is called the threshold current (usually <2 mA for transvenous electrodes).

What is AV sequential pacing?

Ventricular pacing often reduces cardiac output because the atrial contribution to ventricular filling is lost. When the AV conducting system is diseased, atrial contraction can still be maintained by sequential stimulation by separate atrial and ventricular electrodes. The P–R interval can be varied by adjusting the delay between the atrial and ventricular impulses (usually set at 150–200 ms).

How are pacemakers classified?

Pacemakers are categorized by a five-letter code, according to the chambers paced, chambers sensed, response to sensing, programmability, and arrhythmia function (Table 21–22). The two most commonly used pacing modes are VVI and DDD (the last two letters are frequently omitted).

If a pacemaker is placed in this patient, how can its function be evaluated?

If the patient's underlying rhythm is slower than the rate of a demand pacemaker, pacing spikes should be seen on the ECG. The spike rate should be identical to the programmed (permanent pacemaker—usually 72/min) or set (temporary) pacemaker rate; a slower rate may indicate a low battery. Every pacing spike should be followed by a QRS complex (100% capture). Moreover, every impulse should be followed by a palpable arterial pulse. If the patient has a temporary pacemaker, the escape rhythm can be established by temporarily slowing the pacing rate or decreasing the current output.

When the patient's heart rate is faster than the set pacemaker rate, pacing spikes should not be observed if the generator is sensing properly. In this instance, ventricular capture cannot be evaluated

TABLE 21–22   Classification of pacemakers.

Chamber-Paced	Chamber-Sensed	Response to Sensing	Programmability	Antitacharrhythmia Function
O = none	O = none	O = none	O = none	O = none
A = atrium	A = atrium	T = triggered	P = simple	P = pacing
V = ventricle	V = ventricle	I = inhibited	M = multi-programmable	S = shock
D = dual (atrium and ventricle)	D = dual (atrium and ventricle)	D = dual (triggered and inhibited)	C = communicating R = rate modulation	D = dual (pacing and shock)

unless the pacemaker rate increases or the spontaneous heart rate decreases. Fortunately, when the battery is low, sensing is generally affected before pacing output decreases. A chest radiograph is useful in excluding fracture or displacement of pacing leads. If pacemaker malfunction is suspected, cardiological consultation is essential.

What intraoperative conditions may cause the pacemaker to malfunction?

Electrical interference from surgical electrocautery units can be interpreted as myocardial electrical activity and can suppress the pacemaker generator. Problems with electrocautery may be minimized by limiting its use to short bursts, limiting its power output, placing its grounding plate as far from the pacemaker generator as possible, and using bipolar cautery. Moreover, continuous monitoring of an arterial pulse wave (pressure, plethysmogram, or oximetry signal) is mandatory to ensure continuous perfusion during electrocautery.

Both hypokalemia and hyperkalemia can alter the pacing electrodes' threshold for depolarizing the myocardium and can result in failure of the pacing impulse to depolarize the ventricle. Myocardial ischemia, infarction, or scarring can also increase the electrodes' threshold and cause failure of ventricular capture.

What are appropriate measures if a pacemaker fails intraoperatively?

If a temporary pacemaker fails intraoperatively, the inspired oxygen concentration should be increased to 100%. All connections and the generator battery should be checked. Most units have a battery-level indicator and a light that flashes with every impulse. The generator should be set into the asynchronous mode, and the ventricular output should be set on maximum. Failure of a temporary transvenous electrode to capture the ventricle is usually due to displacement of the electrode away from the ventricular endocardium; careful slow advancement of the catheter or wire while pacing often results in capture. Pharmacological management (atropine, isoproterenol, or epinephrine)

may be useful until the problem is resolved. If an adequate arterial blood pressure cannot be maintained with adrenergic agonists, cardiopulmonary resuscitation should be instituted until another pacing electrode is placed or a new generator box is obtained. Transcutaneous pacing can be employed.

If a permanent pacemaker malfunctions (as with electrocautery), it should generally be converted to an asynchronous mode. Some units will automatically reprogram themselves to the asynchronous mode if malfunction is detected. Other pacemaker units must be reprogrammed by placing either an external magnet, or, preferably, a programming device over the generator. The effect of an external magnet on some pacemakers—particularly during electrocautery—may be unpredictable and should generally be determined prior to surgery.

Which anesthetic agents are appropriate for patients with pacemakers?

All anesthetic agents have been safely used in patients who already have pacemakers. Even volatile agents seem to have no effect on pacing electrode thresholds. Local anesthesia with moderate to deep intravenous sedation is usually used for placement of permanent pacemakers.

GUIDELINES

Bonow RO, Carabello BA, Chatterjee K, et al: 2008 focused update incorporated in the ACC/AHA 2006 guidelines for the management of patients with valvular heart disease: a report of the American College of Cardiology/American Heart Association Task Force on Practice Guidelines (writing committee to revise the 1998 guidelines for the management of patients with valvular heart disease): endorsed by the Society of Cardiovascular Anesthesiologists, Society for Cardiovascular Angiography and Interventions, and Society of Thoracic Surgeons. Circulation 2008;118:e523.

Eagle KA, Berger PB, Calkins H, et al: ACC/AHA guideline update for perioperative cardiovascular evaluation for noncardiac surgery—Executive summary. Anesth Analg 2002;94:1052.

Fleisher L, Beckman J, Brown K, et al: ACC/AHA 2007 guidelines on perioperative cardiovascular evaluation and care for noncardiac surgery. Circulation 2007;116: e418.

Fuster V, Rydén L, Cannom D, et al: ACC/AHA/ESC 2006 guidelines for the management of patients with atrial fibrillation-executive summary: a report of the American College of Cardiology/ American Heart Association Task Force on Practice Guidelines and European Society of Cardiology Committee for Practice Guidelines. Circulation. 2006;114:700.

Jessup M, Abraham W, Casey D, et al: 2009 Focused update: ACCF/AHA guidelines for the diagnosis and management of heart failure in adults: a report of the American College of Cardiology Foundation/ American Heart Association Task Force on Practice Guidelines. Circulation 2009;119:1977.

Strickberger S, Conti J, Daoud E, et al: Patient selection for cardiac resynchronization therapy: from the Council of Clinical Cardiology Subcommittee on Electrocardiography and Arrhythmias and the Quality of Care and Outcomes Research Interdisciplinary Working Group in Collaboration with the Heart Rhythm Society. Circulation 2005;111:2146.

Warnes C, Williams R, Bashore T, et al: ACC/AHA 2008 guidelines for the management of adults with congenital heart disease: a report of the American College of Cardiology/American Heart Association Task Force on Practice Guidelines (writing committee to develop guidelines on the management of adults with congenital heart disease). Circulation 2008;118:e714.

Zipes D, Camm A, Borggrefe M, et al: ACC/AHA/ESC 2006 guidelines for management of patients with ventricular arrhythmias and the prevention of sudden cardiac death—executive summary. Circulation 2006;114:1088.

SUGGESTED READING

Amar D: Perioperative atrial tachyarrhythmias. Anesthesiology 2002;97:1618.

Atlee JL, Bernstein AD: Cardiac rhythm management devices (part I). Indications, device selection, and function. Anesthesiology 2001;95:1265.

Atlee JL, Bernstein AD: Cardiac rhythm management devices (part II). Perioperative management. Anesthesiology 2001;95:1492.

Braunwald E, Zipes DP, Libby P: *Heart Disease*, 9th ed. W.B. Saunders, 2011.

Chassot PG, Delabays A, Spahn DR: Preoperative evaluation of patients with, or at risk of, CAD undergoing non-cardiac surgery. Br J Anaesth 2002;89:747.

Howell SJ, Sear JW, Foex P: Hypertension, hypertensive heart disease and perioperative cardiac risk. Br J Anaesth 2004;92:570.

Lake CL: *Pediatric Cardiac Anesthesia*, 4th ed. LWW, 2004.

Otto CM: *Valvular Heart Disease*, 3rd ed. W.B. Saunders, 2009.

Otto CM: *Textbook of Clinical Echocardiography*, 4th ed. W.B. Saunders, 2009.

Park KW: Preoperative cardiac evaluation. Anesth Clin North Am 2004;22:199.

Wasnick J, Hillel Z, Kramer D, et al: *Cardiac Anesthesia & Transesophageal Echocardiography*, McGraw-Hill, 2011.

Anesthesia for Cardiovascular Surgery

KEY CONCEPTS

1 Cardiopulmonary bypass (CPB) is a technique that diverts venous blood away from the heart (most often from one or more cannulas in the right atrium), adds oxygen, removes CO_2, and returns the blood through a cannula in a large artery (usually the ascending aorta or a femoral artery). As a result, nearly all blood bypasses the heart and lungs.

2 The fluid level in the reservoir is critical. If a "roller" pump is used and the reservoir is allowed to empty, air can enter the main pump and be embolized into the patient where it may cause organ damage or fatality.

3 Initiation of CPB is associated with a variable increase in stress hormones and systemic inflammatory response.

4 Establishing the adequacy of the patient's preoperative cardiac function should be based on exercise (activity) tolerance, measurements of myocardial contractility such as ejection fraction, the severity and location of coronary stenoses, ventricular wall motion abnormalities, cardiac end-diastolic pressures, cardiac output, and valvular areas and gradients.

5 Blood should be immediately available for transfusion if the patient has already had a midline sternotomy (a "redo"); in these cases, the right ventricle or coronary grafts may be adherent to the sternum and may be accidentally entered during the repeat sternotomy.

6 In general, pulmonary artery catheterization has been most often used in patients with compromised ventricular function (ejection fraction <40–50%) or pulmonary hypertension and in those undergoing complicated procedures.

7 Transesophageal echocardiography (TEE) provides valuable information about cardiac anatomy and function during surgery. Two-dimensional, multiplane TEE can detect regional and global ventricular abnormalities, chamber dimensions, valvular anatomy, and the presence of intracardiac air. Three-dimensional TEE provides a more complete description of valvular anatomy and pathology.

8 Anesthetic dose requirements are variable and patient tolerance of inhaled anesthetics generally declines with declining ventricular function. Severely compromised patients should be given anesthetic agents in incremental, small doses.

9 Anticoagulation must be established before CPB to prevent acute disseminated intravascular coagulation and formation of clots in the CPB pump.

—Continued next page

Continued—

10 Antifibrinolytic therapy may be particularly useful for patients who are undergoing a repeat operation; who refuse blood products, such as Jehovah's Witnesses; who are at high risk for postoperative bleeding because of recent administration of glycoprotein IIb/IIIa inhibitors (abciximab, eptifibatide, or tirofiban); who have preexisting coagulopathy; and who are undergoing long and complicated procedures involving the heart or aorta.

11 Hypotension from impaired ventricular filling may occur during manipulation of the venae cavae and the heart.

12 Hypothermia (<34°C) potentiates general anesthetic potency, but failure to give anesthetic agents, particularly during rewarming on CPB, may result in awareness and recall.

13 Protamine administration can result in a number of adverse hemodynamic effects, some of which are immunological in origin. Protamine given slowly (5–10 min) usually has few effects; when given more rapidly it produces a fairly consistent vasodilation that is easily treated with blood from the pump oxygenator and small doses of phenylephrine. Catastrophic protamine reactions often include myocardial depression and marked pulmonary hypertension. Diabetic patients previously maintained on protamine-containing insulin (such as NPH) may be at increased risk for adverse reactions to protamine.

14 Persistent bleeding often follows prolonged durations of bypass (>2 h) and in most instances has multiple causes. Inadequate surgical control of bleeding sites, incomplete reversal of heparin, thrombocytopenia, platelet dysfunction, hypothermia-induced coagulation defects, undiagnosed preoperative hemostatic defects, or newly acquired factor deficiency or hypofibrinogenemia may be responsible.

15 Chest tube drainage in the first 2 h of more than 250–300 mL/h (10 mL/kg/h)—in the absence of a hemostatic defect—is excessive and may require surgical reexploration. Intrathoracic bleeding at a site not adequately drained may cause cardiac tamponade, requiring immediate reopening of the chest.

16 Factors known to increase pulmonary vascular resistance (PVR) such as acidosis, hypercapnia, hypoxia, enhanced sympathetic tone, and high mean airway pressures are to be avoided for patients with right-to-left shunting; hyperventilation (hypocapnia) with 100% oxygen is usually effective in lowering PVR. Conversely, patients with left-to-right shunting benefit from systemic vasodilation and increases in PVR, although specific hemodynamic manipulation is generally not attempted.

17 Induction of general anesthesia in patients with cardiac tamponade can precipitate severe hypotension and cardiac arrest.

18 The sudden increase in left ventricular afterload after application of the aortic cross-clamp during aortic surgery may precipitate acute left ventricular failure and myocardial ischemia, particularly in patients with underlying ventricular dysfunction or coronary disease. The period of greatest hemodynamic instability follows the release of the aortic cross-clamp; the abrupt decrease in afterload together with bleeding and the release of vasodilating acid metabolites from the ischemic lower body can precipitate severe systemic hypotension.

19 The emphasis of anesthetic management during carotid surgery is on maintaining adequate perfusion to the brain and heart.

Anesthesia for cardiovascular surgery requires an understanding of circulatory physiology, pharmacology, and pathophysiology as well as a familiarity with cardiopulmonary bypass (CPB) pumps, filters, and circuitry; transesophageal echocardiography (TEE); and techniques of myocardial preservation. Because surgical manipulations often have a profound impact on circulatory function, the anesthesiologist must understand the rationale behind the surgical techniques, follow the progress of the surgery, and anticipate the potential problems associated with each step.

This chapter presents an overview of anesthesia for cardiovascular surgery and of the principles, techniques, and physiology of CPB. Surgery on the aorta, the carotid arteries, and the pericardium presents problems that require special anesthetic considerations, which are also discussed herein.

Cardiopulmonary Bypass

1 CPB is a technique that diverts venous blood away from the heart (most often from one or more cannulas in the right atrium), adds oxygen, removes CO_2, and returns the blood through a cannula in a large artery (usually the ascending aorta or a femoral artery). As a result, nearly all blood bypasses the heart and lungs. When CPB is fully established, the extracorporeal circuit is in series with the systemic circulation and provides both artificial ventilation and perfusion. This technique provides distinctly nonphysiological conditions, because arterial pressure is usually less than normal and blood flow is usually nonpulsatile. To minimize organ damage during this stressful period, various degrees of systemic hypothermia may be employed. Topical hypothermia (an ice-slush solution) and cardioplegia (a chemical solution for arresting myocardial electrical activity) may also be used to protect the heart.

The operation of the CPB machine is a complex task requiring the attention of a perfusionist—a specialized (and certified) technician. Optimal results with CPB require close cooperation and communication between the surgeon, anesthesiologist, and perfusionist.

BASIC CIRCUIT

The typical CPB machine has six basic components: a venous reservoir, an oxygenator, a heat exchanger, a main pump, an arterial filter, tubing that conducts venous blood to the venous reservoir, and tubing that conducts oxygenated blood back to the patient (Figure 22–1). Modern machines use a single disposable unit that includes the reservoir, oxygenator, and heat exchanger. Most machines also have

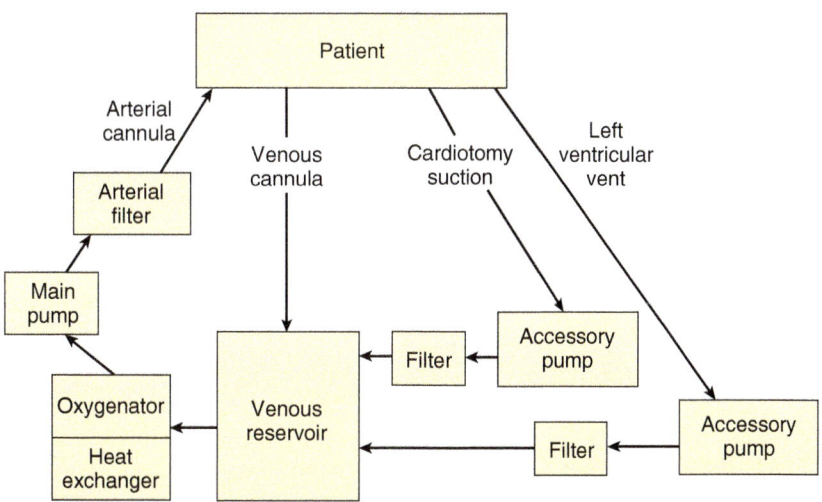

FIGURE 22–1 The basic design of cardiopulmonary bypass machines.

separate accessory pumps that can be used for blood salvage (cardiotomy suction), venting (draining) the left ventricle, and administration of cardioplegia solutions. A number of other filters, alarms, and in-line pressure, oxygen-saturation, and temperature monitors are also typically used.

Prior to use, the CPB circuit must be primed with fluid (typically 1200–1800 mL for adults) that is devoid of bubbles. A balanced salt solution, such as lactated Ringer's solution, is generally used, but other components are frequently added, including colloid (albumin or starch), mannitol (to promote diuresis), heparin (500–5000 units), and bicarbonate. At the onset of bypass, hemodilution decreases the hematocrit to about 22–27% in most patients. Blood is included in priming solutions for smaller children and severely anemic adults to prevent severe hemodilution.

Reservoir

The reservoir of the CPB machine receives blood from the patient via one or two venous cannulas placed in the right atrium, the superior and inferior vena cava, or a femoral vein. With most circuits blood returns to the reservoir by gravity drainage. During extracorporeal circulation the patient's venous pressure is normally low. Thus, the driving force for flow into the pump is directly related to the difference in height between the patient and the reservoir and inversely proportional to the resistance of the cannulas and tubing. An appropriately primed CPB machine draws in blood like a siphon. Entrainment of air in the venous line can produce an air lock that may prevent blood flow. With some circuits (eg, use of an unusually small venous cannula) assisted venous drainage may be required; a regulated vacuum together with a hard shell venous reservoir or centrifugal pump (see below) is used in such instances. The fluid level in the reservoir is critical. If a "roller" pump is used and the reservoir is allowed to empty, air can enter the main pump and be embolized into the patient where it may cause organ damage or fatality. A low reservoir level alarm is typically present. Centrifugal pumps will not pump air but have the disadvantage of not impelling a well-defined volume with each turn of the head (unlike roller pumps).

Oxygenator

Blood is drained by gravity from the bottom of the venous reservoir into the oxygenator, which contains a blood–gas interface that allows blood to equilibrate with the gas mixture (primarily oxygen). A volatile anesthetic is frequently added to the oxygenator gas mixture. The blood–gas interface in a modern, membrane-type oxygenator is a very thin, gas-permeable silicone membrane. Arterial CO_2 tension during CPB is dependent on total gas flow past the oxygenator. By varying the inspired oxygen concentration, a membrane oxygenator allows independent control of Pa_{O_2} and Pa_{CO_2}.

Heat Exchanger

Blood from the oxygenator enters the heat exchanger and can either be cooled or warmed, depending on the temperature of the water flowing through the exchanger; heat transfer occurs by conduction. Because gas solubility decreases as blood temperature rises, a filter is built into the unit to catch any bubbles that may form during rewarming.

Main Pump

Modern CPB machines use either an electrically driven double-arm roller (positive displacement) or a centrifugal pump to propel blood through the CPB circuit.

A. Roller Pumps

Roller pumps produce flow by compressing large-bore tubing in the main pumping chamber as the roller heads turn. Subtotal occlusion of the tubing prevents excessive red cell trauma. The rollers pump blood regardless of the resistance encountered, and produce a nearly continuous nonpulsatile flow. Flow is directly proportional to the number of revolutions per minute. In some pumps, an emergency back-up battery provides power in case of an electrical power failure. All roller pumps have a hand crank to allow manual pumping, but those who have hand cranked a roller pump head will confirm that this is not a good long-term solution.

B. Centrifugal Pumps

Centrifugal pumps consist of a series of cones in a plastic housing. As the cones spin, the centrifugal forces created propel the blood from the centrally located inlet to the periphery. In contrast to roller pumps, blood flow with centrifugal pumps is pressure sensitive and must be monitored by an electromagnetic flowmeter. Increases in distal pressure will decrease flow and must be compensated for by increasing the pump speed. Because these pumps are nonocclusive, they are less traumatic to blood than roller pumps. Unlike roller pumps, which are placed after the oxygenator (Figure 22–1), centrifugal pumps are normally located between the venous reservoir and the oxygenator. Centrifugal (unlike roller) pumps have the advantage of not being able to pump air.

C. Pulsatile Flow

Pulsatile blood flow is possible with some roller pumps. Pulsations can be produced by instantaneous variations in the rate of rotation of the roller heads; they can also be added after flow is generated. Pulsatile flow is not available with centrifugal pumps. Although there is no consensus and the data are contradictory, some clinicians believe that pulsatile flow improves tissue perfusion, enhances oxygen extraction, attenuates the release of stress hormones, and results in lower systemic vascular resistances (SVRs) during CPB.

Arterial Filter

Particulate matter (eg, thrombi, fat globules, tissue debris) may enter the CPB circuit via the cardiotomy suction line. Although filters are often used at other locations, a final, in-line, arterial filter (27–40 μm) helps to reduce systemic embolism. Once filtered, the propelled blood returns to the patient, usually via a cannula in the ascending aorta, or less commonly in the femoral artery. A normally functioning aortic valve prevents blood from regurgitating into the left ventricle.

The filter is always in parallel with a (normally clamped) bypass limb in case the filter becomes clogged or develops increased resistance. For the same reason, arterial inflow pressure is measured before the filter. The filter is also designed to trap air, which can be bled out through a built-in stopcock.

Accessory Pumps & Devices

A. Cardiotomy Suction

The cardiotomy suction pump aspirates blood from the surgical field during CPB and returns it directly to the main pump reservoir. This is a potential port of entry for fat and other debris to the pump that could embolize to organs. A so-called cell-saver suction device may also be used to aspirate blood from the surgical field, in which case blood is returned to a separate reservoir on a separate device. When sufficient blood has accumulated (or at the end of the procedure), the cell-saver blood is centrifuged, washed, and returned to the patient. Excessive suction pressure can theoretically contribute to red cell trauma. Use of cell-saver suction (instead of cardiotomy suction) during bypass will deplete CPB circuit volume if blood loss is brisk. The high negative pressure of ordinary wall suction devices produces excessive red cell trauma precluding blood salvage from that source.

B. Left Ventricular Vent

With time, even with "total" CPB, blood reaccumulates in the left ventricle as a result of residual pulmonary flow from the bronchial arteries (which arise directly from the aorta or the intercostal arteries) or thebesian vessels (see Chapter 20), or sometimes as a result of aortic valvular regurgitation. Aortic regurgitation can occur as a result of either (structural) valvular abnormalities or surgical manipulation of the heart (functional). Distention by blood of the left ventricle compromises myocardial preservation (see below) and requires decompression (venting). Most surgeons accomplish this by inserting a catheter via the right superior pulmonary vein and left atrium into the left ventricle. Venting may also be accomplished using a catheter placed in the left ventricular apex or across the aortic valve. The blood aspirated by the vent pump normally passes through a filter before being returned to the venous reservoir.

C. Cardioplegia Pump

Cardioplegic solutions are most often administered via an accessory pump on the CPB machine. This technique allows optimal control over the infusion pressure, rate, and temperature. A separate heat exchanger ensures control of the temperature of the cardioplegia solution. Less commonly, cardioplegic solutions may be infused from a cold intravenous fluid bag given under pressure or by gravity.

D. Ultrafiltration

Ultrafiltration can be used during CPB to increase the patient's hematocrit without transfusion. Ultrafilters consist of hollow capillary fibers that can function as membranes, allowing separation of the aqueous phase of blood from its cellular and proteinaceous elements. Blood can be diverted to pass through the fibers either from the arterial side of the main pump or from the venous reservoir using an accessory pump. Hydrostatic pressure forces water and electrolytes across the fiber membrane. Effluents of up to 40 mL/min may be removed.

SYSTEMIC HYPOTHERMIA

Intentional hypothermia is often used following the initiation of CPB. Core body temperature may be reduced to 20–32°C. In recent years, so-called tepid bypass has been used; this may be accomplished by allowing the patient's temperature to "drift" downward to 30–35°C. Metabolic oxygen requirements are generally halved with each reduction of 10°C in body temperature. At the end of the surgical procedure, rewarming via the heat exchanger restores normal body temperature.

For complex repairs, profound hypothermia to temperatures of 15–18°C allows total circulatory arrest for durations of as long as 60 min. During that time, both the heart and the CPB machine are stopped.

The adverse effects of hypothermia include platelet dysfunction; reversible coagulopathy; and depression of myocardial contractility.

MYOCARDIAL PRESERVATION

Optimal results in cardiac surgery require an expeditious and complete surgical repair with minimal physical trauma to the heart. Meanwhile, several techniques are used to prevent myocardial damage and maintain normal cellular integrity and function during CPB. Nearly all patients sustain at least minimal myocardial injury during cardiac surgery. With good preservation techniques, however, most of the injury is reversible. Although myocardial injury can be related to the hemodynamic instability or surgical technique, it most commonly appears to be related to incomplete myocardial preservation during CPB. Injury related to hemodynamic instability results from an imbalance between oxygen demand and supply, producing cell ischemia. After ischemia, reperfusion injury may also play a role. Reperfusion following a period of ischemia may produce excess oxygen-derived free radicals, intracellular calcium overload, abnormal endothelial–leukocyte interactions, and myocardial cellular edema. Patients at greatest risk are those with poor ventricular function (as measured preoperatively) (see Table 21–13) those with ventricular hypertrophy, and those with diffuse severe coronary artery disease. Inadequate myocardial preservation is usually manifested at the end of bypass as a persistently reduced cardiac output, worsened ventricular function by TEE, or cardiac arrhythmias. Electrocardiographic signs of myocardial ischemia are often difficult to detect due to frequent use of electrical pacing. Myocardial "stunning," resulting from ischemia and reperfusion, produces systolic and diastolic dysfunction that is reversible with time. The stunned myocardium usually responds to positive inotropic drugs. Myocardial necrosis, on the other hand, produces irreversible injury.

Aortic cross-clamping during CPB completely excludes the coronary arteries from the generalized bypass machine flow to the body, reducing coronary blood flow to 0. Although it is difficult to estimate a safe period for cross-clamping because of differing vulnerabilities among patients and differing techniques for myocardial preservation, CPB times longer than 120 min (while often unavoidable) increase risk relative to shorter bypass times. Myocardial ischemia during bypass may occur not only during aortic clamping, but also after release of the cross-clamp. Low arterial pressures, coronary embolism (from thrombi, platelets, air, fat, or atheromatous debris), reperfusion injury, coronary artery or bypass graft vasospasm, and contortion of the heart—causing compression or distortion of the coronary vessels—are all possible causes. Areas of the myocardium distal to a high-grade coronary obstruction are at greatest risk.

Ischemia causes depletion of high-energy phosphate compounds and an accumulation of intracellular calcium. When coronary blood flow ceases, creatine phosphate and anaerobic metabolism become the principal sources of cellular energy; fatty acid oxidation is impaired. Unfortunately, these energy stores rapidly become depleted, and the progressive acidosis that develops limits glycolysis.

Cardioplegic solutions maintain normal cellular integrity and function during CPB by reducing energy expenditure and preserving the availability of high-energy phosphate compounds. Although measures directed at increasing or replenishing energy substrates in the form of glucose or glutamate/aspartate infusions are used, the emphasis of myocardial preservation has been on reducing cellular energy requirements to minimal levels. This is accomplished initially by the use of potassium cardioplegia (below). The initial dose of cardioplegic solution may be hypothermic or may start warm ("hot shot") and progress to cold. Maintenance of myocardial protection may be facilitated by systemic and topical cardiac hypothermia (ice slush). Myocardial hypothermia reduces basal metabolic oxygen consumption, and potassium cardioplegia minimizes energy expenditure by arresting both electrical and mechanical activity. Myocardial temperature is often monitored directly; 10–15°C is usually considered desirable. Cardioplegic solutions can be administered either antegrade through a catheter placed in the proximal aorta between the aortic clamp and the aortic valve, or retrograde through a catheter placed through the right atrium into the coronary sinus.

Ventricular fibrillation and distention (previously discussed) are important causes of myocardial damage. Ventricular fibrillation can dangerously increase myocardial oxygen demand, whereas distention not only increases oxygen demand but also reduces oxygen supply by interfering with subendocardial blood flow. The combination of the two is particularly bad. Other factors that might contribute to perioperative myocardial damage include the use of excessive doses of positive inotropes or calcium salts. In open heart procedures, de-airing of cardiac chambers and venting before and during initial cardiac ejection are critically important in preventing cerebral or coronary air embolism (and strokes—see below). Removing air from coronary grafts during bypass procedures is similarly important.

Depending on the amount and the location of coronary emboli, even small air bubbles can cause varying degrees of ventricular dysfunction at the end of CPB. To some extent, air emboli may preferentially find their way into the right (versus left) coronary ostium because of its superior location on the aortic root in the supine patient.

Potassium Cardioplegia

The most widely used method of arresting myocardial electrical activity is the administration of potassium-rich crystalloid or blood–crystalloid solutions. Following initiation of CPB and aortic cross-clamping, the coronary circulation is perfused intermittently with (usually cold) cardioplegic solutions. The resulting increase in extracellular potassium concentration reduces the transmembrane potential. Eventually, the heart is arrested in diastole. Usually, cold cardioplegia must be repeated at intervals (about every 30 min) because of gradual washout and rewarming of the myocardium. The heart is subject to warming by contact with blood in the adjacent descending aorta and by contact with warmer ambient air in the surgical theater. Moreover, multiple doses of cardioplegia solutions may improve myocardial preservation by preventing an excessive accumulation of metabolites that inhibit anaerobic metabolism.

Although the exact recipe varies from center to center, the essential ingredient of the induction dose of cardioplegic solution is the same: an elevated potassium (10–40 mEq/L) concentration. Potassium concentration is kept below 40 mEq/L, because higher levels can be associated with an excessive potassium load and excessive potassium concentrations at the end of termination of bypass perfusion. Sodium concentration in cardioplegic solutions is usually less than in plasma (<140 mEq/L) because ischemia tends to increase intracellular sodium content. A small amount of calcium (0.7–1.2 mmol/L) is needed to maintain cellular integrity, whereas magnesium (1.5–15 mmol/L) is usually added to control excessive intracellular influxes of calcium. A buffer—most commonly bicarbonate—is necessary to prevent excessive buildup of acid metabolites; in fact, alkalotic perfusates are reported to produce better myocardial preservation. Alternative buffers include histidine and tromethamine (also known as THAM). Other components may include hypertonic agents to control cellular edema (mannitol) and agents thought to have membrane-stabilizing effects (lidocaine or glucocorticoids). Energy substrates are provided as glucose, glutamate, or aspartate. The question of whether to use crystalloid or blood as a vehicle for achieving cardioplegia remains controversial, although blood cardioplegia has become very common in North America. Evidence suggests that at least some groups of high-risk patients may do better with blood cardioplegia. Certainly, oxygenated blood cardioplegia may contain more oxygen than crystalloid cardioplegia.

Because cardioplegia may not reach areas distal to high-grade coronary obstructions (the areas that need it most), many surgeons administer retrograde cardioplegia through a coronary sinus catheter. Some centers have reported that the combination of antegrade plus retrograde cardioplegia is superior to either technique alone. Others have suggested that continuous warm blood cardioplegia is superior to intermittent hypothermic cardioplegia for myocardial preservation, but many surgeons avoid continuous cardioplegia so that they can operate in a "bloodless" surgical field. Moreover, warm cardiac surgery raises additional concerns about loss of the potentially protective effects of systemic hypothermia against cerebral injury, when true normothermia (rather than tepid bypass) is maintained.

As discussed previously, with prolonged myocardial ischemic times (cross-clamp time), reperfusion of the myocardium can lead to extensive cell injury, rapid accumulation of intracellular calcium, and potentially irreversible cellular necrosis. This process has long been attributed to depletion of endogenous free radical scavengers during CPB and accumulation of deleterious oxygen-derived free radicals. Free radical scavengers, such as mannitol, may help decrease reperfusion injury and are typical constituents of cardioplegic solutions and bypass "priming" solutions. Several steps may help limit reperfusion injury before unclamping of the aorta. Just prior to reperfusion, the heart may be perfused by a reduced potassium cardioplegic solution that serves to wash out accumulated metabolic byproducts. Alternatively, a "hot shot" or warm blood cardioplegic solution may

be administered to wash out byproducts and replenish metabolic substrates. Hypercalcemia should be avoided in the immediate reperfusion period. Reperfusion pressures should be controlled closely because of altered coronary autoregulation. Systemic perfusion pressure is reduced just prior to clamp release; it is then brought up initially to about 40 mm Hg before gradually being increased and maintained at about 70 mm Hg. To further minimize metabolic requirement, the heart should have the opportunity to recover and resume contracting in an empty state for some additional time (5–10 min), and acidosis and hypoxia should be corrected before attempting to wean the patient from bypass perfusion.

Inadequate myocardial protection or inadequate washout and recovery from cardioplegia can result in asystole, atrioventricular conduction block, or a poorly contracting heart at the end of bypass. Excessive volumes of hyperkalemic cardioplegic solutions may produce persisting systemic hyperkalemia. Although calcium salt administration partially offsets hyperkalemia, excessive calcium can promote and enhance myocardial damage. In the usual patient myocardial performance improves with time as the contents of the cardioplegia are cleared from the heart.

PHYSIOLOGICAL EFFECTS OF CARDIOPULMONARY BYPASS
Hormonal, Humoral, & Immunological Responses

3 Initiation of CPB is associated with a variable increase in stress hormones and systemic inflammatory response. Elevated levels of catecholamines, cortisol, arginine vasopressin, and angiotensin are observed. These neurohormonal responses are variously influenced by depth of anesthesia, blood pressure, type of surgical repair, or presence of pulsatile CPB.

Multiple humoral systems are also activated, including complement, coagulation, fibrinolysis, and the kallikrein system. Contact of blood with the internal surfaces of the CPB system activates complement via the alternate pathway (C3) as well as the classic pathway; the latter also activates the coagulation cascade, platelets, plasminogen, and kallikrein. Mechanical trauma from blood contact with the bypass apparatus also activates platelets and leukocytes. Increased amounts of oxygen-derived free radicals are generated. A systemic inflammatory response syndrome similar to that seen with sepsis and trauma can develop. When this response is intense or prolonged, patients can develop the same complications, including generalized edema, the acute respiratory distress syndrome, coagulopathy, and acute kidney failure.

CPB alters and depletes glycoprotein receptors on the surface of platelets. The resulting platelet dysfunction likely increases perioperative bleeding and potentiates other coagulation abnormalities (activation of plasminogen and the inflammatory response described above).

Animal and clinical research has demonstrated that the inflammatory response to CPB can be modulated by various therapies. Leukocyte depletion reduces inflammation and may similarly reduce complications. Leukocyte-depleted blood cardioplegia has been shown to improve myocardial preservation in some studies. Hemofiltration (ultrafiltration) during CPB, which presumably removes inflammatory cytokines, appears beneficial in pediatric patients. Administration of free radical scavengers such as high-dose vitamins C and E and mannitol has improved outcome in some studies. Systemic corticosteroids before and during CPB can modulate the inflammatory response during CPB but improved outcome is not well established. Two large randomized clinical trials are underway to test whether there is an outcome benefit to the routine use of systemic corticosteroids with CPB.

One once-promising agent, aprotinin, reduced inflammation and surgical bleeding following CPB. Unfortunately, it increased mortality and is no longer available in North America.

CPB Effects on Pharmacokinetics

Plasma and serum concentrations of most water-soluble drugs (eg, nondepolarizing muscle relaxants) acutely decrease at the onset of CPB, but the change can be minimal and inconsequential for most lipid-soluble drugs (eg, fentanyl and sufentanil). The effects of CPB are complex because of the sudden increase in volume of distribution with hemodilution, decreased protein binding, and changes in perfusion and redistribution between peripheral and central compartments. Some drugs, such as opioids, also bind CPB components (but this is also minimal and inconsequential). Heparin potentially alters protein binding of drugs and ions by releasing and activating lipoprotein lipase, which hydrolyzes plasma triglycerides into free fatty acids; the latter can competitively inhibit drug binding to plasma proteins and bind free calcium ions. With the possible exception of propofol, constant infusion of a drug during CPB (even when adjusted to maintain a constant "effect site" concentration using data from patients *not* undergoing CPB) generally causes progressively increasing blood levels as a result of reduced hepatic and renal perfusion (reduced elimination) and hypothermia (reduced metabolism).

Anesthetic Management of Cardiac Surgery

ADULTS

The preoperative evaluation and anesthetic management of common cardiovascular diseases are discussed in Chapter 21. The same principles apply whether these patients are undergoing cardiac or noncardiac surgery. An important distinction is that patients undergoing cardiac procedures will by definition have advanced disease. Establishing the adequacy of the patient's preoperative cardiac function should be based on exercise (activity) tolerance, measurements of myocardial contractility such as ejection fraction, the severity and location of coronary stenoses, ventricular wall motion abnormalities, cardiac end-diastolic pressures, cardiac output, and valvular areas and gradients. Fortunately, unlike noncardiac surgery, cardiac surgery improves cardiac function in the majority of patients, and these patients have usually been extensively evaluated before being offered surgical repair. The anesthetic preoperative evaluation should also include a focus on pulmonary, neurological, and renal function, as preoperative impairment of these organ systems predisposes patients to myriad postoperative complications.

1. Preinduction Period

Premedication

The prospect of heart surgery is frightening, and relatively "heavy" oral or intramuscular premedication was often given in the past, particularly when patients had coronary artery disease with good left ventricular function (see Chapter 21). However, in current practice, most patients receive no sedative-hypnotic premedication until their arrival on the surgical unit, at which time most will receive small doses of intravenous midazolam.

Benzodiazepine sedative-hypnotics (diazepam, 5–10 mg orally), alone or in combination with an opioid (morphine, 5–10 mg intramuscularly or hydromorphone, 1–2 mg intramuscularly), were often used in the past. Longer acting premedicant agents (eg, lorazepam) are avoided by most practitioners to permit "fast tracking" of patients through their recovery.

Preparation

The best practitioners of cardiac anesthesia formulate a simple anesthetic plan that includes adequate preparations for contingencies. Many patients are critically ill, and there is little time intraoperatively to have an assistant search for drugs and equipment. At the same time, the anesthetic plan should not be excessively rigid; when problems are encountered with one technique, one should be ready to change to another without delay. Preparation, organization, and attention to detail permit one to more efficiently deal with unexpected intraoperative problems. The anesthesia machine, monitors, infusion pumps, and blood warmer should all be checked before the patient arrives. Drugs—including anesthetic and vasoactive agents—should be immediately available. Many clinicians prepare one vasoconstrictor and one vasodilator infusion before the start of the procedure.

Venous Access

Cardiac surgery is sometimes associated with large and rapid blood loss, and with the need for multiple drug infusions. Ideally, two large-bore (16-gauge or larger) intravenous catheters should be placed. One of these should be in a large central vein, usually an internal or external jugular or subclavian vein. Central venous cannulations may be accomplished while the patient is awake but sedated or after induction of anesthesia. Studies show no benefit from placing either central venous or pulmonary arterial catheters in awake (versus anesthetized) patients undergoing cardiovascular surgery.

Drug infusions should ideally be given into a central catheter, preferably directly into the catheter or into the injection port closest to the catheter (to minimize dead space). Multilumen central venous catheters and multilumen pulmonary artery catheter introducer sheaths allow for multiple drug infusions with simultaneous measurement of vascular pressures. One intravenous port should be dedicated for drug infusions and nothing else; drug and fluid boluses should be administered through another site. The side port of the introducer sheath used for a pulmonary catheter can be used for drug infusions but serves better as a fluid bolus line when a large-bore introducer (9F) is used.

5 Blood should be immediately available for transfusion if the patient has already had a midline sternotomy (a "redo"); in these cases, the right ventricle or coronary grafts may be adherent to the sternum and may be accidentally entered during the repeat sternotomy.

Monitoring

A. Electrocardiography

The electrocardiogram (ECG) is continuously monitored with two leads, usually leads II and V_5. Baseline tracings of all leads may be recorded on paper for further reference. The advent of monitors with computerized ST-segment analysis and the use of additional monitoring leads (V_4, aVF, and V_{4R}) have greatly improved detection of ischemic episodes, as has the frequent intraoperative use of TEE.

B. Arterial Blood Pressure

In addition to all basic monitoring, arterial cannulation is always performed either prior to or immediately after induction of anesthesia, as the induction period represents a time when major hemodynamic alterations may occur. Radial arterial catheters may occasionally give falsely low readings following sternal retraction as a result of compression of the subclavian artery between the clavicle and the first rib. They may also provide falsely low values early after CPB due to the opening of atrioventricular shunts in the hand during rewarming. The radial artery on the side of a previous brachial artery cutdown should be avoided, because its use is associated with a greater incidence of arterial thrombosis and wave distortion. Obviously, if a radial artery will be harvested for a coronary bypass conduit, it cannot be used as a site for arterial pressure monitoring. Other useful catheterization sites include the ulnar, axillary, and especially brachial and femoral arteries. A backup manual or automatic blood pressure cuff should also be placed on the opposite side for comparison with direct measurements.

C. Central Venous and Pulmonary Artery Pressure

Central venous pressure is not terribly useful for diagnosis of hypovolemia but has been customarily monitored in nearly all patients undergoing cardiac surgery. The decision about whether to use a pulmonary artery catheter is based on the patient, the procedure, and the preferences of the surgical team. Routine use of a pulmonary artery catheter, once nearly universal in adult cardiovascular practice, is controversial. Pulmonary artery catheterization has declined precipitously in nearly all circumstances except adult cardiac surgery due to lack of evidence of a positive effect on patient outcomes. Left ventricular filling pressures can be measured with a left atrial pressure line inserted by the surgeon during bypass. In general, pulmonary artery catheterization has been most often used in patients with compromised ventricular function (ejection fraction <40–50%) or pulmonary hypertension and in those undergoing complicated procedures. The most useful data are pulmonary artery pressures, the pulmonary artery occlusion ("wedge") pressure, and thermodilution cardiac outputs. Specialized catheters provide extra infusion ports, continuous measurements of mixed venous oxygen saturation and cardiac output, and the capability for right ventricular or atrioventricular sequential pacing. Given the risk associated with placing any pulmonary artery catheter, some clinicians opine that it makes sense to restrict pulmonary artery catheterization only to devices that offer these advanced capabilities.

The right internal jugular vein is the preferred approach for intraoperative central venous cannulation. Catheters placed through the other sites, particularly on the left side, are more likely to kink following sternal retraction (above) and are not nearly as likely to pass into the superior vena cava as those placed through the right internal jugular vein.

Pulmonary artery catheters migrate distally during CPB and may spontaneously wedge without balloon inflation. Inflation of the balloon under these conditions can rupture a pulmonary artery causing lethal hemorrhage. Pulmonary artery catheters should be routinely retracted 2–3 cm during CPB and the balloon subsequently inflated slowly. If the catheter wedges with less than 1.5 mL of air in the balloon, it should be withdrawn farther.

D. Urinary Output

Once the patient is anesthetized, an indwelling urinary catheter is placed to monitor the hourly output. Bladder temperature is often monitored as a measure of core temperature but may not track core temperature well with reduced urinary flow. The sudden appearance of reddish urine may indicate excessive red cell hemolysis caused by CPB or a transfusion reaction.

E. Temperature

Multiple temperature monitors are usually placed once the patient is anesthetized. Bladder (or rectal), esophageal, and pulmonary artery (blood) temperatures are often simultaneously monitored. Because of the heterogeneity of readings during cooling and rewarming, bladder and rectal readings are generally taken to represent an average body temperature, whereas esophageal represents core temperature. Pulmonary artery temperature provides an accurate estimate of blood temperature, which should be the same as core temperature in the absence of active cooling or warming. Nasopharyngeal and tympanic probes may most closely approximate brain temperature. Myocardial temperature is often measured directly during CPB.

F. Laboratory Parameters

Intraoperative laboratory monitoring is mandatory during cardiac surgery. Blood gases, hematocrit, serum potassium, ionized calcium, and glucose measurements should be immediately available. The **activated clotting time (ACT)** approximates the Lee–White clotting time and is used to monitor heparin anticoagulation. Some centers routinely use thromboelastography (TEG) to identify causes of bleeding after CPB.

G. Surgical Field

One of the most important actions in intraoperative monitoring is inspection of the surgical field. Once the sternum is opened, lung expansion can be observed through the pleura. When the pericardium is opened, the heart (primarily the right ventricle) is visible; thus cardiac rhythm, volume, and contractility can often be judged visually. Blood loss and surgical maneuvers must be closely watched and related to changes in hemodynamics and rhythm.

H. Transesophageal Echocardiography

 TEE provides valuable information about cardiac anatomy and function during surgery.

Two-dimensional, multiplane TEE can detect regional and global ventricular abnormalities, chamber dimensions, valvular anatomy, and the presence of intracardiac air. Three-dimensional TEE provides a more complete description of valvular anatomy and pathology. TEE can also be helpful in confirming cannulation of the coronary sinus for cardioplegia. Multiple views should be obtained from the upper esophagus, mid-esophagus, and transgastric positions in the transverse, sagittal, and in-between planes (**Figure 22–2**). The two views most commonly used for monitoring during cardiac surgery are the four-chamber view (**Figure 22–3**) and the transgastric (short-axis) view (**Figure 22–4**). Three-dimensional echocardiography offers great promise for better visualization of complex anatomic features, particularly of cardiac valves. The following represent the most important applications of intraoperative TEE.

1. Assessment of valvular function—Valvular morphology can be assessed by multiplane and three-dimensional TEE. Pressure gradients, area and severity of stenosis, and severity of valvular regurgitation can be assessed by Doppler echocardiography and

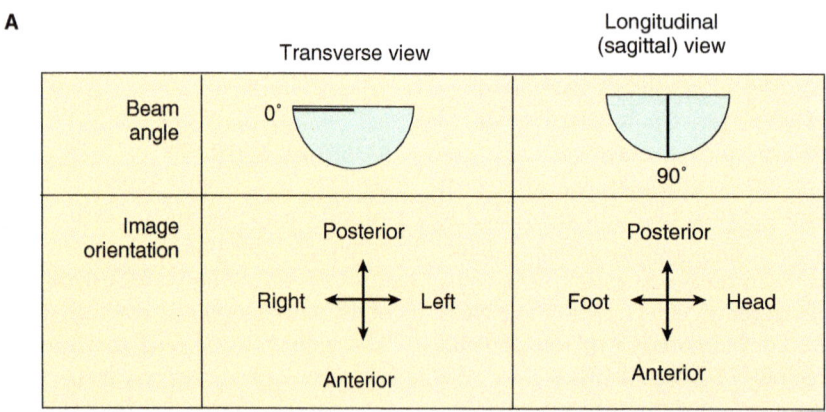

FIGURE 22–2 Useful views during transesophageal echocardiography. **A:** The relationship between the angle of the ultrasound beam and image orientation relative to the patient. **B–D:** Echocardiographic views from the upper mid-esophagus, lower mid-esophagus, and transgastric position (C). Note that different views can be obtained in each position as the tip of the probe is tilted either upward (anteflexion) or backward (retroflexion) and the angle of the beam is changed from 0° to 180°. The angle of the beam is shown in the upper left-hand corner of each image. The probe is also rotated clockwise or counterclockwise to optimize viewing of the various structures. AO, aorta; AV, aortic valve; CS, coronary sinus; IVC, inferior vena cava; LA, left atrium; LAA, left atrial appendage; LUPV, left upper pulmonary vein; LV, left ventricle; MPA, main pulmonary artery; MV, mitral valve; PA, pulmonary artery; RA, right atrium; RPA, right pulmonary artery; RV, right ventricle; SVC, superior vena cava. (*continued*)

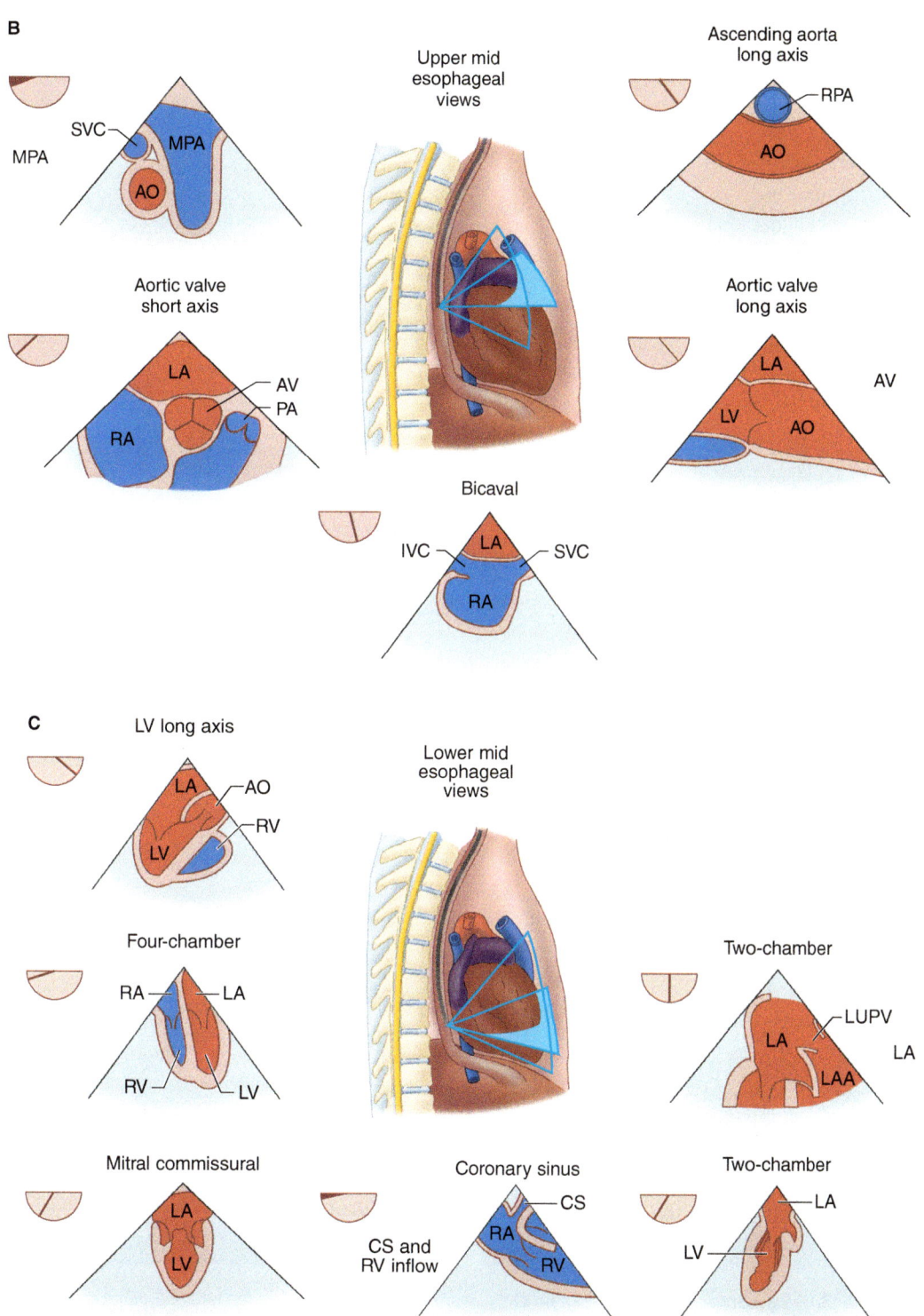

FIGURE 22–2 (*continued*)

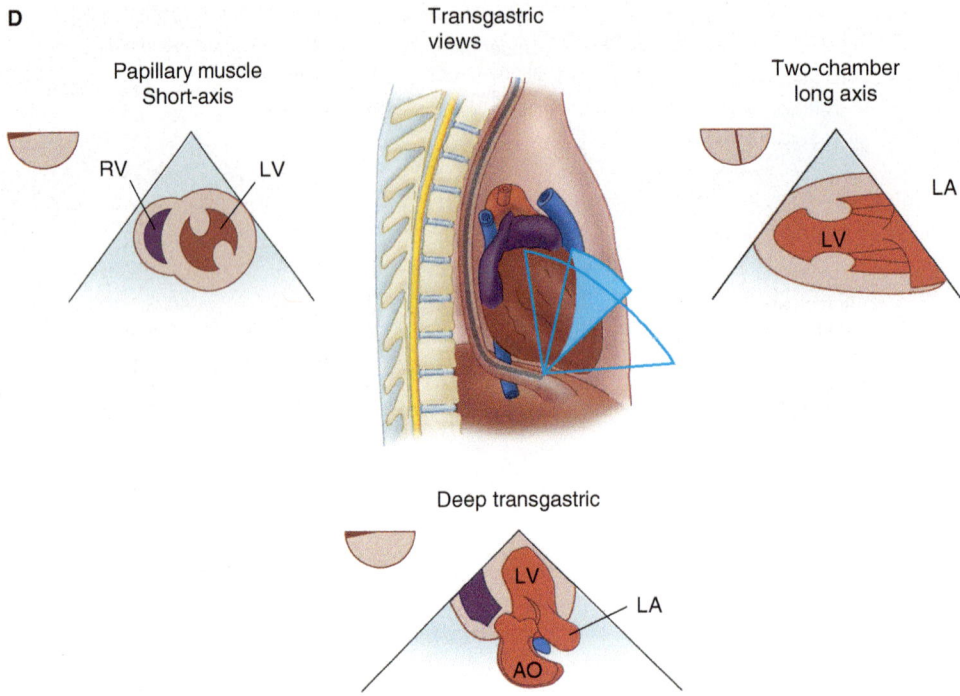

FIGURE 22–2 (continued)

color-flow imaging (Figure 22–5). Colors are usually adjusted so that flow toward the probe is red and flow in the opposite direction is blue. TEE also can detect prosthetic valve dysfunction, such as obstruction or

regurgitation, and can detect vegetations from endocarditis. The TEE images in the upper mid-esophagus at 40–60° and 110–130° are useful for examining the aortic valve and ascending aorta (Figure 22–6). The

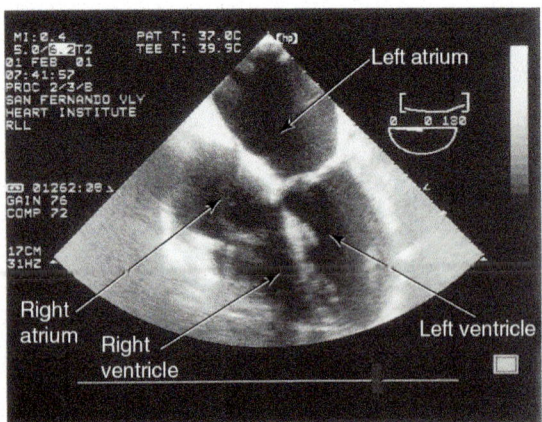

FIGURE 22–3 Transesophageal echocardiogram of the mid-esophageal four-chamber view, showing the right and left atria and ventricles.

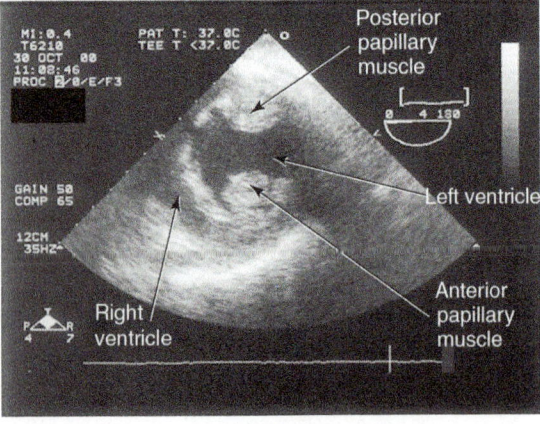

FIGURE 22–4 Transesophageal echocardiogram at the lower esophageal/transgastric level looking up at the left ventricle at the level of the papillary muscles.

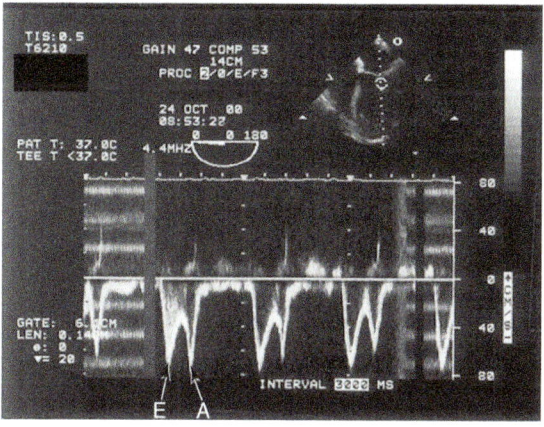

A

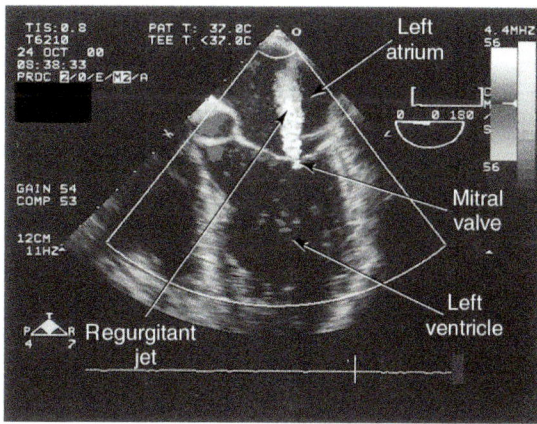

B

FIGURE 22–5 Transesophageal echocardiography Doppler and color-flow imaging. Pulse-wave Doppler recording of mitral valve inflow showing two phases, E (early filling) and A (atrial filling) (**A**). Color-flow imaging demonstrates backward flow (regurgitant jet) across the mitral valve during systole (mitral regurgitation) (**B**).

valve annular diameter can also be estimated with reasonable accuracy. Doppler flow across the aortic valve must be measured looking up from the deep transgastric view (Figure 22–7). The anatomic features of the mitral valve relevant to TEE are shown in Figure 22–8. The mitral valve is examined from the mid-esophageal position, looking at the mitral valve apparatus with and without color in the 0° through 150° views (Figure 22–9). TEE is an invaluable aid to guide and assess the quality of mitral valve repair surgery. The commissural view (at about 60°) is particularly helpful because it cuts across many scallops of the mitral valve.

2. Assessment of ventricular function—Ventricular function can be assessed by global systolic function, estimated by means of ejection fraction (often calculated using Simpson's method of disks) and left ventricular end-diastolic volume; diastolic function

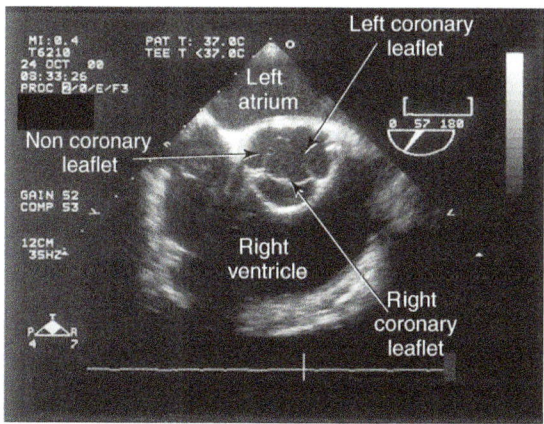

A

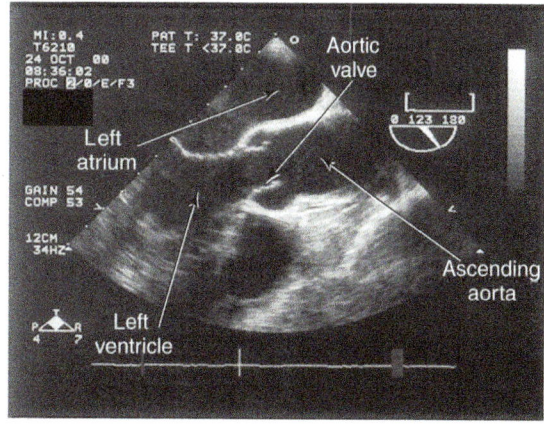

B

FIGURE 22–6 Two views of the aortic valve. Between 40° and 60°, all three leaflets are usually visualized (**A**). Between 110° and 130°, the left ventricular outflow, aortic valve, and ascending aorta are clearly visualized (**B**).

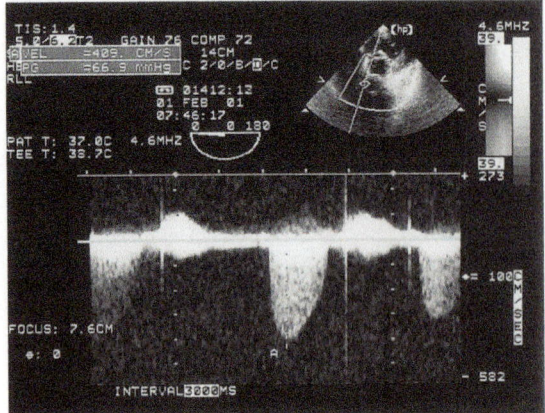

FIGURE 22–7 Transesophageal echocardiographic recording of continuous-wave Doppler from the transgastric view looking up at the aortic valve, demonstrating severe aortic stenosis. Peak velocity of 409 cm/s indicates a gradient of 66.9 mm Hg.

(ie, looking for abnormal relaxation and restrictive diastolic patterns by checking mitral flow velocity or by measuring movements of the mitral valve annulus using tissue Doppler techniques); and regional systolic function (by assessing wall motion and thickening abnormalities). Regional wall abnormalities from myocardial ischemia often appear before ECG changes. Regional wall motion abnormalities can be classified into three categories based on severity (**Figure 22–10**): hypokinesis (reduced wall motion), akinesis (no wall motion), and dyskinesis (paradoxical wall motion). The location of a regional wall motion abnormality can indicate which coronary artery is experiencing reduced flow. The left ventricular myocardium is supplied by three major arteries: the left anterior descending artery, the left circumflex artery, and the right coronary artery (**Figure 22–11**). The areas of distribution of these arteries on echocardiographic views

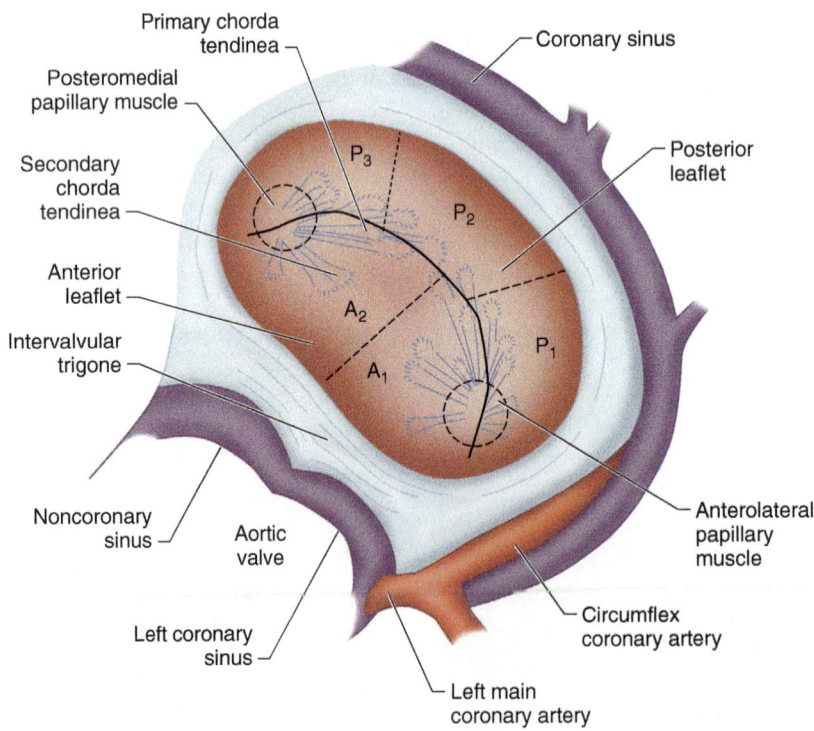

FIGURE 22–8 The anatomy of the mitral valve and its anatomic relationships to the aortic valve and left circumflex coronary artery. The posterior leaflet has three scallops, P_1, P_2, and P_3. The anterior leaflet is usually divided into A₁ and A₂ regions; in some classifications the anterior leaflet is divided into three areas (A_1, A_2, A_3), corresponding to the opposing corresponding areas of the posterior leaflet.

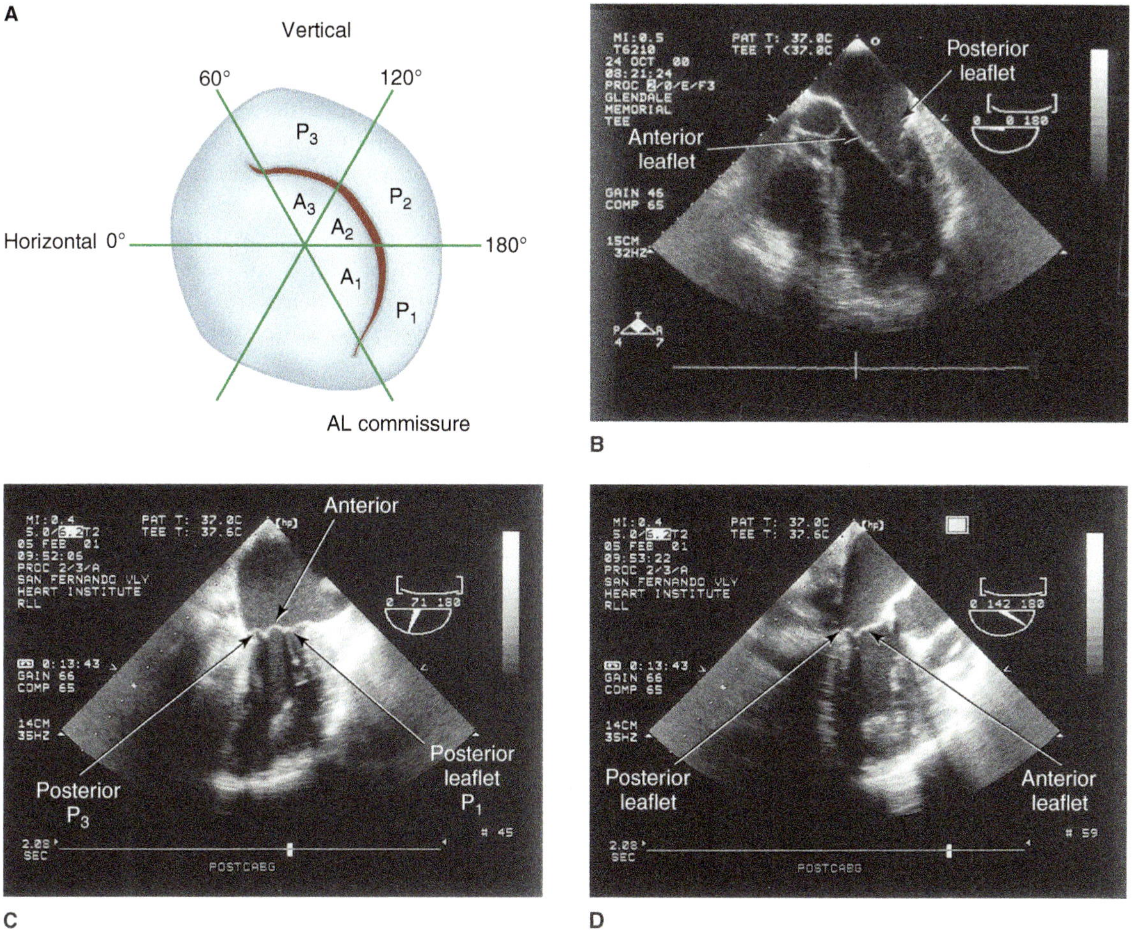

A

Vertical

60°   120°

P₃

P₂

A₃

A₂

Horizontal 0° ——————————— 180°

A₁

P₁

AL commissure

B

C

Anterior

Posterior
leaflet
P₃

Posterior
leaflet
P₁

D

Posterior
leaflet

Anterior
leaflet

FIGURE 22–9 Multiplane imaging cuts across different segments of the mitral valve apparatus between 0° and 180° (**A**). Images of the mitral valve at 0°, 71°, and 142° (**B**, **C**, and **D**, respectively).

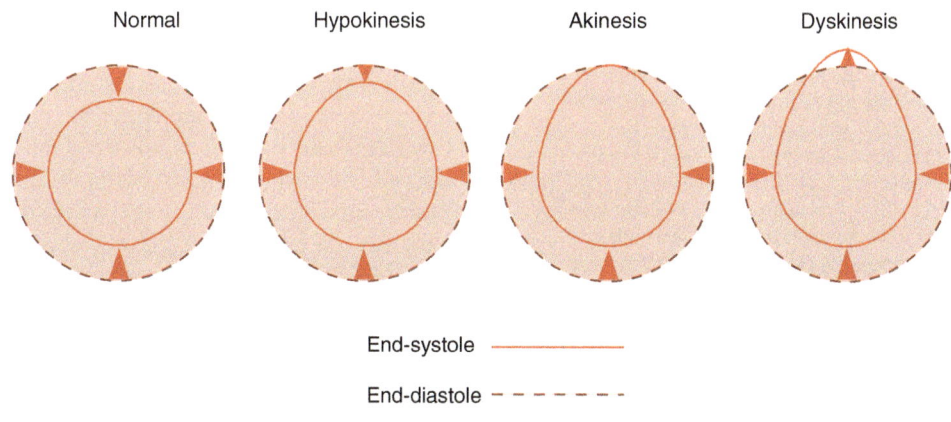

| Normal | Hypokinesis | Akinesis | Dyskinesis |

End-systole ——————

End-diastole – – – – – –

FIGURE 22–10 Classification of regional wall motion abnormalities.

A

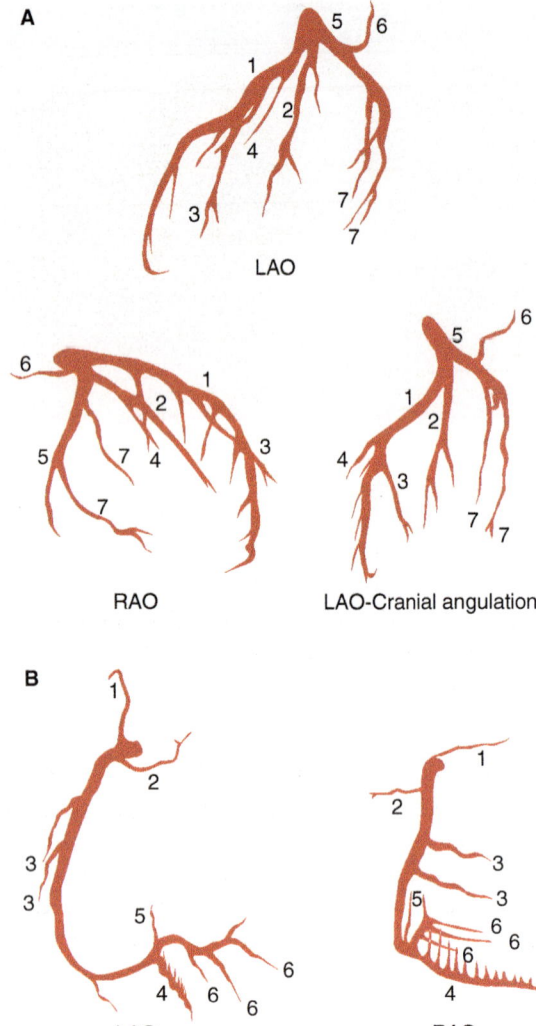

LAO

RAO

LAO-Cranial angulation

B

LAO

RAO

FIGURE 22–11 Standard angiographic views of the left (**A**) and right (**B**) coronary arteries. Note the left main coronary artery quickly divides into the left anterior descending and the left circumflex arteries. A: (1) Left anterior descending artery with septal branches; (2) ramus medianus; (3) diagonal artery; (4) first septal branch; (5) left circumflex artery; (6) left atrial circumflex artery; (7) obtuse marginal artery. B: (1) Conus artery; (2) SA node artery; (3) acute marginal artery; (4) posterior descending artery with septal branches; (5) AV node artery; (6) posterior left ventricular artery.

are shown in Figure 22–12. The ventricular short-axis mid view at the mid-papillary muscle level contains all three blood supplies from the major coronary arteries.

3. Assessment of other cardiac structures and abnormalities—In an adult undergoing elective cardiac surgery TEE can help diagnose previously undetected congenital defects such as an atrial or ventricular septal defect; pericardial diseases such as pericardial effusions and constrictive pericarditis; and cardiac tumors. Doppler color-flow imaging helps delineate abnormal intracardiac blood flows and shunts. TEE can assess the extent of myomectomy in patients with hypertrophic cardiomyopathy (idiopathic hypertrophic subaortic stenosis). Upper-, mid-, and lower-esophageal views are valuable in diagnosing aortic disease processes such as dissection, aneurysm, and atheroma (Figure 22–13). The extent of dissections in the ascending and descending aorta can be accurately defined; however, airway structures prevent complete visualization of the aortic arch. The presence of protruding atheroma in the ascending aorta increases the risk of postoperative stroke and should prompt the use of epiaortic scanning to identify an atheroma-free cannulation site or a change in surgical plans.

4. Examination for residual air—Air is introduced into the cardiac chambers during all "open" heart procedures, such as valve surgery. Residual amounts of air often remain in the left ventricular apex even after the best deairing maneuvers. TEE is helpful in defining the volume of residual air, to determine whether additional surgical maneuvers need to be undertaken to help avoid cerebral or coronary embolism.

I. Electroencephalography

Computer-processed electroencephalographic (EEG) recordings can be used to assess anesthetic depth during cardiac surgery, and either the processed or "raw" EEG can be used to ensure complete drug-induced electrical silence (for brain protection) prior to circulatory arrest. These recordings are generally not useful in detecting neurological insults during CPB. Progressive hypothermia (or progressively deepened anesthesia) is typically associated with EEG slowing, burst suppression, and, finally, an isoelectric recording. Most strokes during CPB are due to small emboli that are not likely to produce changes in the EEG. Artifacts from the CPB roller pump may be seen on the raw EEG (due to

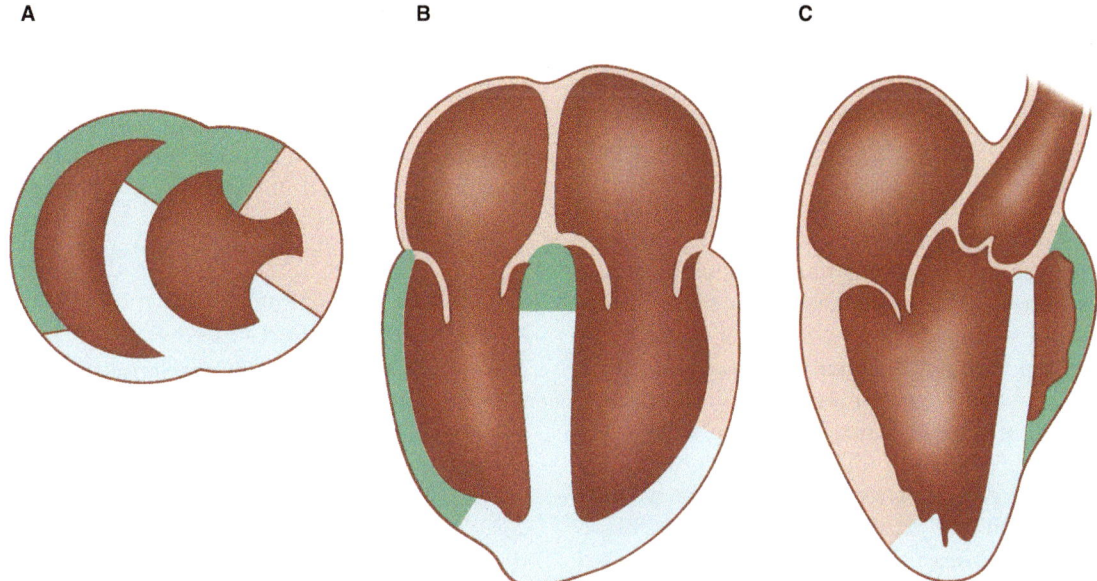

FIGURE 22–12 Coronary artery supply of the left and right ventricles in three views: the short-axis view (**A**), the four-chamber view (**B**), and the three-chamber view (**C**). Green, right coronary artery; blue, left anterior descending artery; pink, left circumflex artery.

piezoelectric effects from compression of the pump tubing) but can usually be identified as such by computer processing.

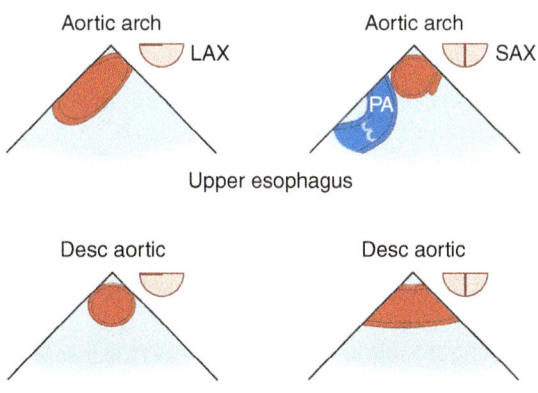

FIGURE 22–13 Upper esophageal TEE views of the aortic arch and descending aorta. The ascending aorta can be visualized in the upper mid-esophagus at 110–130° with anteflexion at the aortic valve level (see Figures 22–2B and 22–6B).

J. Transcranial Doppler (TCD)

This modality provides noninvasive measurements of blood flow velocity in the middle cerebral artery, which is insonated through the temporal bone. TCD is useful for detecting cerebral emboli. Increased numbers of emboli detected by TCD or Doppler interrogation of the carotid artery have been associated with an increased risk of postoperative neurobehavioral dysfunction.

Induction of Anesthesia

Cardiac operations usually require general anesthesia, endotracheal intubation, and controlled ventilation. Some centers have used thoracic epidural anesthesia alone for minimally invasive surgery without CPB or combined thoracic epidural with light general endotracheal anesthesia for other forms of cardiac surgery. These techniques have never been popular in North America due to concerns about the risk of spinal hematomas following heparinization, the associated medical–legal consequences, and the limited evidence of an outcome benefit. Other centers use a single intrathecal morphine injection to provide postoperative analgesia.

For elective procedures, induction of general anesthesia should be performed in a smooth, controlled (but not necessarily "slow") fashion often referred to as a cardiac induction. The principles are discussed in Chapter 21. Selection of anesthetic agents is generally less important than the way they are used. Indeed, studies have failed to show differences in long-term outcome with various anesthetic techniques. Anesthetic dose requirements are variable and patient tolerance of inhaled anesthetics generally declines with declining ventricular function. Severely compromised patients should be given anesthetic agents in incremental, small doses. A series of challenges may be used to judge when anesthetic depth will allow intubation without a marked hypertensive response, while also avoiding hypotension from excessive anesthetic dosing. Blood pressure and heart rate are continuously evaluated following unconsciousness, insertion of an oral airway, urinary catheterization, and tracheal intubation. A sudden increase in heart rate or blood pressure may indicate light anesthesia and the need for more anesthetic prior to the next challenge, whereas a decrease or no change suggests that the patient is ready for the subsequent stimulus. Muscle relaxant is given after consciousness is lost. Reductions in blood pressure greater than 20% generally call for administration of a vasopressor (see below).

The period following intubation is often characterized by a gradual decrease in blood pressure resulting from the anesthetized state (often associated with vasodilation and decreased sympathetic tone) and a lack of surgical stimulation. Patients will usually respond to fluid boluses or a vasoconstrictor. Nevertheless, the administration of large amounts of intravenous fluids prior to the bypass may serve to accentuate the hemodilution associated with CPB (below). Small doses of phenylephrine (25–100 mcg), vasopressin (1–3 units), or ephedrine (5–10 mg) may be useful to avoid excessive hypotension. Following intubation and institution of controlled ventilation; arterial blood gases, hematocrit, serum potassium, and glucose concentrations are measured. The baseline ACT (normal <130 s) is best measured after skin incision.

Choice of Anesthetic Agents

Anesthetic techniques for cardiac surgery have evolved over the years. Successful techniques range from primarily volatile inhalation anesthesia to high-dose opioid totally intravenous techniques. In recent years, total intravenous anesthesia with short-acting agents and combinations of intravenous and volatile agents have become most popular.

A. "High-Dose" Opioid Anesthesia

This technique was originally developed to circumvent the myocardial depression associated with older volatile anesthetics, particularly halothane. But pure high-dose opioid anesthesia (eg, fentanyl, 50–100 mcg/kg, or sufentanil, 15–25 mcg/kg) produces prolonged postoperative respiratory depression (12–24 h), is associated with an unacceptably high incidence of patient awareness (recall) during surgery, and often fails to control the hypertensive response to stimulation in many patients with preserved left ventricular function. Other undesirable effects include skeletal muscle rigidity during induction and prolonged postoperative ileus. Moreover, simultaneous administration of benzodiazepines with large doses of opioids can produce hypotension and myocardial depression. Patients anesthetized with sufentanil (and other shorter acting agents) generally regain consciousness and can be extubated sooner than those anesthetized with fentanyl.

B. Total Intravenous Anesthesia (TIVA)

The drive for cost containment in cardiac surgery was a major impetus for development of anesthesia techniques with short-acting agents. Although the drugs may be costlier, large economic benefits resulted from earlier extubation, decreased intensive care unit (ICU) stays, earlier ambulation, and earlier hospital discharge ("fast-track" management). One technique employs induction with propofol (0.5–1.5 mg/kg followed by 25–100 mcg/kg/min), and modest doses of fentanyl (total doses of 5–7 mcg/kg) or remifentanil (0–1 mcg/kg bolus followed by 0.25–1 mcg/kg/min). Target controlled infusion (TCI) employs software and hardware (computerized infusion pump) to deliver a drug and achieve a set concentration at the effect site based on pharmacokinetic modeling. For propofol the clinician sets only the patient's age and weight, and the desired blood concentration on the Diprifusor, a TCI device widely available in countries outside North America. During cardiac surgery, this technique can be used for propofol with a target concentration of 1.5–2 mcg/mL. Whenever the very short-acting remifentanil is used for painful surgery, provision must be made for postoperative analgesia after its discontinuation.

C. Mixed Intravenous/Inhalation Anesthesia

Renewed interest in volatile agents came about following studies demonstrating the protective effects of volatile agents on ischemic myocardium and an increased emphasis on fast-track recovery of cardiac patients. Selection of anesthetic agents is oriented to hemodynamic stability as well as early extubation (1–6 h). Propofol (0.5–1.5 mg/kg) or etomidate (0.1–0.3 mg/kg) is often used for induction. Induction usually follows sedation with small doses of midazolam (0.05 mg/kg). Opioids are given in small doses together with a volatile agent (0.5–1.5 minimum alveolar concentration [MAC]) for maintenance anesthesia and to blunt the sympathetic response to stimulation. The opioid may be given in small intermittent boluses, by continuous infusion, or both (Table 22–1). To facilitate fast-track management, typical total doses of fentanyl and sufentanil generally do not exceed 15 and 5 mcg/kg, respectively, and some clinicians combine much smaller doses of fentanyl or sufentanil with an analgesic dose of hydromorphone or morphine administered toward the end of CPB. Some clinicians also administer a low-dose infusion of propofol (25–50 mcg/kg/min) for maintenance.

TABLE 22–1 Opioid dosing compatible with early extubation after cardiac surgery.

Opioid	Loading Dose (mcg/kg)	Maintenance Infusion	Boluses (mcg/kg)
Fentanyl	1–5	1–3 mcg/kg/h	0.5–1
Sufentanil	0.25–1.25	0.25–0.75 mcg/kg/h	0.125–0.25
Remifentanil	0.5–1	0.1–1 mcg/kg/min	0.25–1

The major advantage of volatile agents or infusions of remifentanil or propofol, or both, is the ability to change the anesthetic concentration and depth rapidly. Isoflurane, sevoflurane, and desflurane are the most commonly used volatile anesthetics. Early laboratory reports of isoflurane inducing intracoronary steal have been overshadowed by later reports of myocardial protection. Isoflurane remains a commonly used volatile agent. Nitrous oxide is generally not used, particularly during the time interval between cannulation and decannulation, because of its tendency to expand any intravascular air bubbles that may form.

D. Other Techniques

The combination of ketamine with midazolam (or diazepam or propofol) for induction and maintenance of anesthesia is a useful technique, particularly in frail patients with hemodynamic compromise. It is associated with stable hemodynamics, reliable amnesia and analgesia, minimal postoperative respiratory depression, and rare (if any) psychotomimetic side effects. Ketamine and midazolam are compatible in solution, and may be mixed together in the same syringe or infusion bag in a 20:1 ratio. For induction, ketamine, 1–2 mg/kg, with midazolam, 0.05–0.1 mg/kg, is given as a slow intravenous bolus. Anesthesia can then be maintained by infusion of ketamine, 1.3–1.5 mg/kg/h, and midazolam, 0.065–0.075 mg/kg/h, or more easily with an inhaled agent. Hypertension following intubation or surgical stimulation can be treated with propofol or a volatile agent.

E. Muscle Relaxants

Muscle relaxation is helpful for intubation, to facilitate sternal retraction, and to prevent patient movement and shivering. Unless airway difficulties are expected, intubation may be accomplished after administration of a nondepolarizing muscle relaxant. The choice of muscle relaxant in the past was often based on the desired hemodynamic response. Modern, shorter acting agents such as rocuronium, vecuronium, and cisatracurium are commonly used and have almost no hemodynamic side effects of their own. Vecuronium, however, has been reported to markedly enhance bradycardia associated with large doses of opioids, particularly sufentanil. Because of its vagolytic effects, pancuronium was often used in patients with marked bradycardia who were taking β-blocking agents, Succinylcholine remains appropriate for endotracheal intubation, particularly for rapid sequence induction. Judicious dosing and appropriate use of a peripheral nerve stimulator allow fast-tracking with any of these agents.

2. Prebypass Period

Following induction and intubation, the anesthetic course is typically characterized by an initial period of minimal stimulation (skin preparation and draping) that is frequently associated with hypotension, followed by discrete periods of intense stimulation that can produce tachycardia and hypertension. These periods of stimulation include the skin incision, sternotomy and sternal retraction, opening the pericardium, and, sometimes, aortic dissection. The anesthetic agent should be adjusted appropriately in anticipation of these events.

Accentuated vagal responses resulting in marked bradycardia and hypotension may occasionally be seen during sternal retraction or opening of the pericardium, perhaps more commonly in patients who have been taking β-adrenergic blocking agents or diltiazem.

Myocardial ischemia in the prebypass period is not always associated with hemodynamic perturbations such as tachycardia, hypertension, or hypotension. Prophylactic infusion of nitroglycerin (1–2 mcg/kg/min) has been studied many times and continues to be used but does not appear to reduce the incidence of ischemic episodes or to alter outcomes.

Anticoagulation

9 Anticoagulation must be established before CPB to prevent acute disseminated intravascular coagulation and formation of clots in the CPB pump. In most centers the adequacy of anticoagulation will be confirmed by measuring the ACT. An ACT longer than 400–480 s is considered adequate at most centers. Heparin, 300–400 units/kg, is usually given while the aortic pursestring sutures are placed before cannulation. Some surgeons prefer

to administer the heparin themselves directly into the right atrium. If heparin is administered by the anesthesiologist, it should be given through a reliable (usually central) intravenous line, and the ACT should be measured 3–5 min later. If the ACT is less than 400 s, additional heparin (100 units/kg) is given. Some drugs (eg, aprotinin) prolong the celite-activated ACT but not the kaolin-activated ACT; the kaolin-ACT should be used to assess adequacy of anticoagulation in these circumstances. Heparin concentration assays (see Reversal of Anticoagulation, below) measure heparin levels and not necessarily effect; these assays are therefore not reliable for measuring the degree of anticoagulation but can be used as an adjunct. A whole blood heparin concentration of 3–4 units/mL is usually sufficient for CPB. The high-dose thrombin time (HiTT) is not influenced by aprotinin but is more complicated to perform than a kaolin-ACT. HiTT cannot provide a preheparin control and does not provide an index for the adequacy of reversal with protamine (see below).

Resistance to heparin is occasionally encountered; many such patients have antithrombin III deficiency (acquired or congenital). Antithrombin III is a circulating serine protease that irreversibly binds and inactivates thrombin (as well as the activated forms of factors X, XI, XII, and XIII). When heparin complexes with antithrombin III, the anticoagulant activity of antithrombin III is enhanced 1000-fold. Patients with antithrombin III deficiency will achieve adequate anticoagulation following infusion of 2 units of fresh frozen plasma or antithrombin III concentrate. Alternatively, recombinant human antithrombin III may be administered. Milder forms of heparin resistance can be managed by administration of a modestly larger than normal dose of heparin.

Patients with a history of heparin-induced thrombocytopenia (HIT) require special consideration. These patients produce heparin-dependent (platelet factor 4) antibodies that agglutinate platelets and produce thrombocytopenia, sometimes associated with thromboembolism. If the history of HIT is remote and antibodies can no longer be demonstrated, heparin may safely used for CPB. Other anticoagulants should be preferred in other circumstances. When significant antibody titers are detected, alternative anticoagulants including hirudin, bivalirudin, ancrod, and argatroban may be considered, but experience with them is limited. Consultation with a hematologist may be helpful.

Bleeding Prophylaxis

Bleeding prophylaxis with antifibrinolytic agents may be initiated before or after anticoagulation. Some clinicians prefer to administer antifibrinolytic agents after heparinization to reduce the possible incidence of thrombotic complications; others fear that delayed administration may reduce antifibrino-lytic efficacy. Antifibrinolytic therapy may be particularly useful for patients who are under-going a repeat operation; who refuse blood products (such as Jehovah's Witnesses); who are at high risk for postoperative bleeding because of recent admin-istration of glycoprotein IIb/IIIa inhibitors (abcix-imab [RheoPro], eptifibatide [Integrilin], or tirofiban [Aggrastat]); who have preexisting coagulopathy; and who are undergoing long and complicated pro-cedures involving the heart or aorta. The antiplatelet effect of abciximab typically lasts 24–48 h; those of eptifibatide and tirofiban are 2–4 and 4–8 h, respec-tively. The combination of aspirin and the adenosine diphosphate receptor antagonist clopidogrel (Plavix) is also associated with excessive bleeding.

The antifibrinolytic agents currently avail-able, ε-aminocaproic acid and tranexamic acid, do not affect the ACT and only rarely induce allergic reactions. ε-Aminocaproic acid is usually adminis-tered as a 50–75 mg/kg loading dose followed by a 20–25 mg/kg/h maintenance infusion (some clini-cians use a standard 5–10 g loading dose followed by 1 g/h). Tranexamic acid is often dosed at 10 mg/kg followed by 1 mg/kg/h, although pharmacokinetic studies suggest that larger doses may more reliably maintain effective blood concentrations. Intra-operative collection of platelet-rich plasma by pheresis prior to CPB is employed by some centers; reinfusion following bypass may decrease bleeding and reduce transfusion requirements.

Cannulation

Placement of venous and arterial cannulas for CPB is a critical time. *After heparinization,* aortic cannulation is usually done first because of the hemodynamic problems frequently associated with venous cannulation and to allow convenient and rapid transfusion from the pump oxygenator. The inflow cannula is most often placed in the ascend-ing aorta. The small opening of most arterial cannu-las produces a jet stream that, when not positioned properly, can cause aortic dissection or preferential flow of blood to the innominate artery. The sys-temic arterial pressure is customarily reduced to 90–100 mm Hg systolic during placement of the aortic cannula to reduce the likelihood of dissection. Air bubbles should be absent from the arterial can-nula and inflow line, and adequacy of the connection between the arterial inflow line and the patient must be demonstrated before bypass is initiated. Failure to remove all air bubbles will result in air emboli, possibly into the coronary or cerebral circulations, whereas failure to enter the aorta may result in aor-tic dissection. Some clinicians routinely hand com-press the carotid arteries during aortic cannulation to decrease the likelihood of cerebral emboli, but the efficacy of this technique is doubtful.

One or two venous cannulas are placed in the right atrium, usually through the right atrial appendage. One cannula is usually adequate for most coronary artery bypass and aortic valve opera-tions. The single cannula used often has two por-tals (two-stage); when it is properly positioned, one opening is in the right atrium and the other is in the inferior vena cava.

Separate cannulas in the superior and inferior venae cavae are used for open-heart procedures. Hypotension from impaired ventricular filling may occur during manipulation of the venae cavae and the heart. Venous cannulation also fre-quently precipitates atrial or, less commonly, ventric-ular arrhythmias. Premature atrial contractions and transient bursts of a supraventricular tachycardia are common. Sustained paroxysmal atrial tachycardia or atrial fibrillation frequently leads to hemodynamic deterioration, which may be treated pharmacologi-cally, electrically, or by immediate initiation of bypass (provided that full anticoagulation has been con-firmed). Malpositioning of the venous cannulas can interfere with venous return or impede venous drainage from the head and neck (superior vena cava syndrome). Upon initiation of CPB, the former is manifested as inadequate volume in the venous reservoir, whereas the latter produces engorgement of the head and neck. Under these circumstances, central venous pressure may not increase if the tip of the central line is adjacent or very near the cannula.

3. Bypass Period

Initiation

Once the cannulas are properly placed and secured, the ACT is acceptable, and the perfusionist is ready, CPB is initiated. The clamps placed across the venous cannula(s) during insertion are removed, and the main CPB pump is started. Establishing the adequacy of venous return to the pump reservoir is critical. Normally, the reservoir level rises and CPB pump flow is gradually increased. If venous return is poor, as shown by a decreasing reservoir level, the pump prime will quickly empty and air can enter the pump circuit. When the venous reservoir falls the cannulas should be checked for proper placement and for forgotten clamps, kinks, or an air lock. Under these circumstances, pump flow should be slowed until the problem is resolved. Adding volume (blood or colloid) to the reservoir may be necessary. With full CPB and unimpeded venous drainage, the heart should empty; failure to empty or progressive distention implies malpositioning of the venous cannula or aortic regurgitation. In the rare case of severe aortic insufficiency that limits the extent of peripheral perfusion, immediate aortic cross-clamping (and cardioplegia) may be necessary.

Flow & Pressure

Systemic mean arterial pressure is closely monitored as pump flow is gradually increased to 2–2.5 L/min/m^2. At the onset of CPB, systemic arterial pressure usually decreases abruptly. Initial mean systemic arterial (radial) pressures of 30–40 mm Hg are not unusual. This decrease is usually attributed to abrupt hemodilution, which reduces blood viscosity and effectively lowers SVR. It is often treated with increased flow and vasopressors.

Persistent and excessive decreases (<30 mm Hg) should prompt a search for unrecognized aortic dissection. If dissection is present, CPB must be temporarily stopped until a cannula can be placed distally in the "true" aortic lumen. Other possible causes for hypotension include inadequate pump flow from poor venous return or a pump malfunction, or pressure transducer error. Factitious hypertension has been reported when the right radial artery is used for monitoring and the aortic cannula is directed toward the innominate artery.

The relationship between pump flow, SVR, and mean systemic arterial blood pressure may be conceptualized as follows:

Mean arterial pressure = Pump flow × SVR

Consequently, with a constant SVR, mean arterial pressure is proportional to pump flow. Similarly, at any given pump flow, mean arterial pressure is proportional to SVR. To maintain both adequate arterial pressures and blood flows one can manipulate pump flow and SVR. Most centers strive for blood flows of 2–2.5 L/min/m^2 (50–60 mL/kg/min) and mean arterial pressures between 50 and 80 mm Hg. Metabolic flow requirements generally decline with decreasing core body temperature. Evidence also suggests that during deep hypothermia (20–25°C), mean blood pressures as low as 30 mm Hg may still be consistent with adequate cerebral blood flow and cerebral oxygen delivery. SVR can be increased with phenylephrine, vasopressin, or norepinephrine.

Increased systemic arterial pressures (>150 mm Hg) are deleterious and may promote aortic dissection or cerebral hemorrhage. Generally, when mean arterial pressure exceeds 100 mm Hg, hypertension is said to exist and is treated by decreasing pump flow or increasing the concentration of a volatile agent to the oxygenator inflow gas. In the rare instance that the hypertension is refractory to these maneuvers or if pump flow is already low, a vasodilator such as clevidipine, nicardipine, or nitroprusside is used.

Monitoring

Additional monitoring during CPB includes the pump flow rate, venous reservoir level, arterial inflow line pressure (see above), blood (perfusate and venous) and myocardial temperatures, and in-line (arterial and venous) oxygen saturations. In-line pH, CO_2 tension, and oxygen tension sensors are also available. Blood gas tensions and pH should be

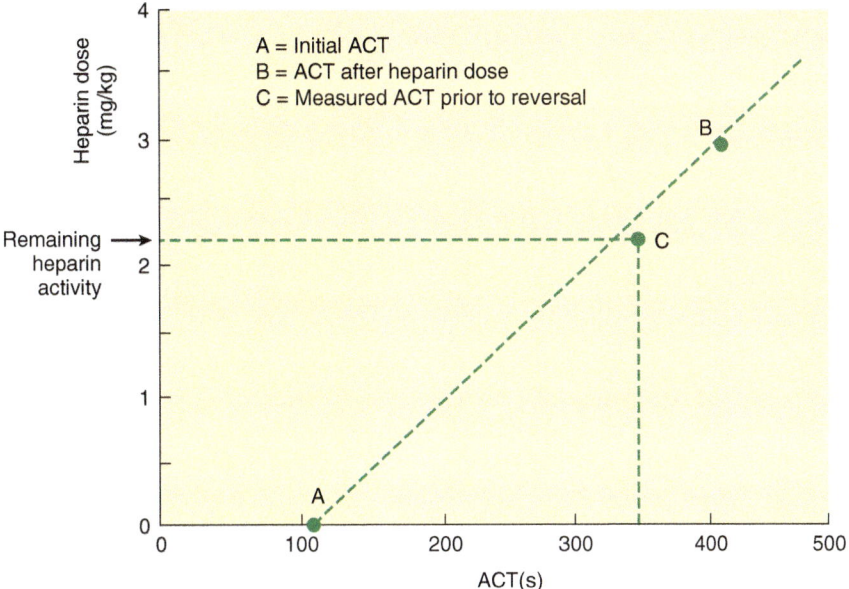

FIGURE 22–14 Heparin dose–response curve. Activated clotting time (ACT) in seconds versus total heparin dose in milligrams per kilogram. 1. Plot the initial ACT on the x-axis. 2. Plot the ACT after heparinization. 3. Draw the line defined by these two points. 4. If additional anticoagulation is needed, find the desired ACT on that line. The amount of additional heparin needed is the difference on the y-axis between the present ACT and the desired ACT. 5. If the third point does not lie on the original line, a new line is drawn originating from the baseline ACT and passing midway between the other two points. 6. For reversal of anticoagulation, the protamine dose is based on the remaining heparin activity, estimated to be the heparin dose corresponding to the latest ACT on the dose–response line.

confirmed by direct measurements (see below). In the absence of hypoxemia, low venous oxygen saturations (<70%), a progressive metabolic acidosis, or reduced urinary output may indicate inadequate flow rates.

During bypass, arterial inflow line pressure is almost always greater than the systemic arterial pressure recorded from a radial artery or even an aortic catheter. The difference in pressure represents the pressure drop across the arterial filter, the arterial tubing, and the narrow opening of the aortic cannula. Nonetheless, monitoring this pressure is important in detecting problems with an arterial inflow line. Inflow pressures should remain below 300 mm Hg; higher pressures may indicate a clogged arterial filter, obstruction of the arterial tubing or cannula, or aortic dissection.

Serial ACT, hematocrit, and potassium measurements are performed during CPB. Blood glucose should be checked even in patients without a history of diabetes. The ACT is measured immediately after bypass and then every 20–30 min thereafter. Cooling generally increases the half-life of heparin and prolongs its effect. Some centers calculate a heparin dose–response curve to guide calculation of heparin dosing and protamine reversal (Figure 22–14). The hematocrit is usually not allowed fall much below 20–25%. Red cell transfusions into the pump reservoir may be necessary. Marked increases in serum potassium concentrations (secondary to cardioplegia) are usually treated with a furosemide-induced diuresis.

Hypothermia & Cardioplegia

Moderate (26–32°C) or deep (20–25°C) hypothermia is used routinely for many procedures. The lower the temperature, the longer the time required for cooling and rewarming. Low temperatures, however, permit lower CPB flows to be used safely. At a temperature of 20°C, flows as low as 1.2 L/min/m² may be adequate.

Hypothermia produces characteristic changes in the ECG including the Osborne wave, a characteristic positive deflection between the QRS and ST segments. Ventricular fibrillation often occurs as the heart is cooled below 28–29°C. Cardioplegia should be established immediately, as fibrillation consumes high-energy phosphates at a greater rate than slower rhythms. Cardioplegia is achieved by cross-clamping the ascending aorta proximal to the aortic inflow cannula and (as previously described) infusing cardioplegia solution through a small catheter proximal to the cross-clamp or directly into the coronary ostia if the aorta is opened (eg, for aortic valve replacement). Many surgeons routinely employ retrograde cardioplegia via a catheter in the coronary sinus (see above). During aortocoronary bypass grafting, cardioplegia solution may also be given through the graft when the surgeon elects to perform the distal anastomosis first.

Ventilation

Ventilation of the lungs is discontinued when adequate pump flows are reached and the heart stops ejecting blood. Following institution of full CPB, ventricular ejection continues briefly until the left ventricular volume reaches a critically low level. Discontinuing ventilation prematurely when there is any remaining pulmonary blood flow acts as a right-to-left shunt that can promote hypoxemia. The importance of this mechanism depends on the relative ratio of remaining pulmonary blood flow to pump flow. At some centers, once ventilation is stopped, oxygen flow is continued in the anesthesia circuit with a small amount of continuous positive airway pressure (5 cm H_2O) in the hope of preventing postoperative pulmonary dysfunction. Most centers either stop all gas flow or continue a low flow of oxygen (1–2 L/min) in the anesthesia circuit. Ventilation is resumed at the conclusion of CPB in anticipation of the heart beginning to eject blood.

Management of Respiratory Gases

There formerly was controversy about whether to use temperature-corrected (pH stat) or uncorrected (α-stat) arterial blood gas tensions during hypothermic CPB in adults. The controversy stemmed from the fact that the solubility of a gas increases and the neutral pH (ie, the pH at which concentrations of H^+ and OH^- ions are the same) of water increases with hypothermia. As a result of the former effect, although total CO_2 content does not change (in a closed system), the partial pressure of CO_2 will decrease as blood temperature drops. The problem is most significant for arterial CO_2 tension because of its effect on arterial pH and cerebral blood flow. As the temperature decreases, the plasma bicarbonate concentration does not change, but the decrease in arterial CO_2 tension tends to increase pH and make blood alkalotic (by normothermic definitions). Blood with a CO_2 tension of 40 mm Hg and a pH of 7.40 at 37°C, when cooled to 25°C, will have a CO_2 tension of about 23 mm Hg and a pH of 7.60.

Normally—regardless of the patient's temperature—blood samples are heated to 37°C in blood gas analyzers before gas tensions are measured. If a temperature-corrected reading is desired, a table or a program in the blood gas machine can be used to estimate what would be the gas tension and pH if they had been measured at the patient's temperature. The practice of temperature correcting gas tensions with the goal of maintaining a constant CO_2 tension of 40 mm Hg and a constant pH of 7.40 during hypothermia is referred to as **pH-stat management**. During hypothermic CPB, pH-stat management, which may require adding CO_2 to the oxygenator gas inflow, increases total blood CO_2 content. Under these conditions, cerebral blood flow increases (due to increased CO_2 tension relative to α-stat management) more than is required based on oxygen consumption. Increased cerebral blood flow is useful to increase uniformity of brain cooling prior to deep hypothermic circulatory arrest (more often used in children than adults). On the other hand, increased cerebral blood flow can also direct a greater fraction of atheromatous arterial emboli to the brain—a greater concern than uniformity of brain cooling during cardiac surgery in adults.

The use of uncorrected gas tensions during hypothermia—**α-stat management**—is the rule in adults and is common in children when circulatory arrest will not be used. The basis of this approach is that preservation of normal protein function depends on maintaining a constant state of intracellular electroneutrality (the balance of charges on proteins). At physiological pH, these charges are primarily located on the imidazole rings of histidine residues (referred to as α residues). Moreover, as temperature decreases, K_w—the dissociation constant for water—also decreases (pK_w increases). Therefore, at lower temperatures, the electroneutrality of aqueous solutions, where $[H^+] = [OH^-]$, corresponds to a lower $[H^+]$ (a higher pH). Hypothermic "alkalosis" thus does not necessarily reflect $[OH^-] > [H^+]$ but rather an absolute decrease in both $[H^+]$ and $[OH^-]$. Hypothermic CPB with α-stat management does not require addition of CO_2 to the oxygenator: the total CO_2 content of blood and the electroneutrality are unchanged. In contrast to pH-stat management, α-stat management appears to preserve cerebral autoregulation of blood flow. Despite the theoretical and observed differences, in most studies comparisons between the two techniques fail to reveal appreciable differences in patient outcomes except in children undergoing circulatory arrest.

Anesthesia

[12] Hypothermia (<34°C) potentiates general anesthetic potency, but failure to give anesthetic agents, particularly during rewarming on CPB, may result in awareness and recall. With light anesthesia hypertension may be seen and, if muscle paralysis is also allowed to wear off, the patient may move. Consequently, additional doses of anesthetic agents may be necessary during CPB. Reduced concentrations of a volatile agent (eg, 0.5–0.75% isoflurane) via the oxygenator are frequently used. The volatile agent concentration may need to be reduced to a value that does not depress contractility immediately prior to termination of bypass if residual myocardial depression is apparent. Those relying on opioids and benzodiazepines for anesthesia during CPB may need to administer additional doses of these agents or commence a propofol infusion. Some clinicians routinely administer a benzodiazepine (eg, midazolam) or scopolamine (0.2–0.4 mg) when rewarming is initiated. Alternatively, a propofol, opioid, or ketamine–midazolam infusion may be continued throughout CPB. Sweating during rewarming is common and usually indicates a hypothalamic response to perfusion with warm blood (rather than "light" anesthesia). During rewarming, blood temperature should not exceed core temperature by more than 2°C.

Cerebral Protection

The incidence of neurobehavioral deficits after CPB varies widely, depending on how long after surgery the examination is performed and the criteria for diagnosis. In the first week after surgery the incidence may be as high as 80%. Fortunately, in most instances, these deficits are transient. Neurobehavioral deficits detectable 8 weeks or more (20–25%) after operation or strokes (2–6%) are less common. Factors that have been associated with neurological sequelae include increased numbers of cerebral emboli, combined intracardiac (valvular) and coronary procedures, advanced age, and preexisting cerebrovascular disease.

During open-heart procedures, deairing of cardiac chambers, assumption of a head-down position, and venting before and during initial cardiac ejection are important in preventing gas emboli. Some centers fill the surgical field with CO_2, a gas that if entrained and embolized will more rapidly be reabsorbed. TEE can detect residual air within the heart and the need for further deairing procedures. During coronary bypass procedures, minimizing the amount of aortic manipulation, the number of aortic clampings, and the number of graft sites on the surface of the aorta, and using sutureless proximal anastomotic devices may help reduce atheromatous emboli. Palpation of the aorta, TEE, and especially epiaortic echocardiography can help identify high-risk patients and guide management. Epiaortic echocardiography is the most sensitive and specific technique.

Although embolic phenomena appear responsible for most neurological deficits, the contribution of cerebral hypoperfusion remains unclear. The data are controversial and sparse that prophylactic drug infusions (eg, barbiturates or propofol to suppress electroencephalographic activity) immediately before and during intracardiac (open ventricle) procedures will decrease the incidence and severity of neurological deficits. Prior to circulatory arrest with very deep hypothermia, some clinicians administer a corticosteroid (methylprednisolone,

30 mg/kg, or the equivalent dose of dexamethasone) and mannitol (0.5 g/kg). The head is also covered with ice bags (avoiding the eyes). Surface cooling delays rewarming and may also facilitate adequacy of brain cooling. A long list of drugs has been tested and has failed to improve cerebral outcomes after heart surgery. Human studies during cardiac surgery have not shown improved neurobehavioral outcomes with prophylactic administration of calcium channel blockers (nimodipine), N-methyl-D-aspartate (NMDA) antagonists (remacemide), free radical scavengers (pegorgotein), sedative-hypnotics (thiopental, propofol, or clomethiazole), or lazaroids (tirilazad).

4. Termination of CPB

Discontinuation of bypass is accomplished by a series of necessary procedures and conditions:

1. Rewarming must be completed.

2. Air must be evacuated from the heart and any bypass grafts.

3. The aortic cross-clamp must be removed and the heart must beat.

4. Lung ventilation must be resumed.

The surgeon's decision about when to rewarm is important; adequate rewarming requires time, but rewarming too soon removes the protective effects of hypothermia. Rapid rewarming often results in large temperature gradients between well-perfused organs and peripheral vasoconstricted tissues; subsequent equilibration following separation from CPB decreases core temperature again. An excessive gradient between the infusate temperature and the patient's core temperature can result in deleterious brain hyperthermia. Infusion of a vasodilator drug (nitroprusside, isoflurane, or phentolamine [primarily in children]) by allowing higher pump flows often speeds the rewarming process and decreases large temperature gradients. Some believe that allowing some pulsatile flow (ventricular ejection) may also speed rewarming. Excessively rapid rewarming, however, can result in the formation of gas bubbles in the bloodstream as the solubility of gases rapidly decreases. If the heart fibrillates during rewarming, direct electrical defibrillation (5–10 J) may be

necessary. Administration of lidocaine, 100–200 mg, and magnesium sulfate, 1–2 g, prior to removal of aortic cross-clamping is a common protocol and may decrease the likelihood of fibrillation. Many clinicians advocate a head-down position while intracardiac air is being evacuated to decrease the likelihood of cerebral emboli. Lung inflation facilitates expulsion of (left-sided) intracardiac air by compressing pulmonary vessels and returning blood into the left heart. TEE is useful in detecting residual intracardiac air. Initial reinflation of the lungs requires greater than normal airway pressure and should generally be done under direct visualization of the surgical field because excessive lung expansion can interfere with internal mammary artery grafts.

General guidelines for separation from CPB include the following:

- The core body temperature should be at least 37°C.

- A stable rhythm must be present. Atrioventricular pacing is often used and confers the benefit of a properly timed atrial systole. Persistence of atrioventricular block should prompt measurement of serum potassium concentration. If hyperkalemia is present, it can be treated with calcium, $NaHCO_3$, furosemide, or glucose and insulin.

- The heart rate must be adequate (generally 80–100 beats/min). Slow heart rates are generally treated by pacing. Many inotropic agents will also increase heart rate. Supraventricular tachycardias generally require cardioversion.

- Laboratory values must be within acceptable limits. Significant acidosis (pH < 7.20), hypocalcemia (ionized), and hyperkalemia (>5.5 mEq/L) should be treated; ideally the hematocrit should exceed 22%; however, a hematocrit <22% should not by itself trigger transfusion of red blood cells at this time. When CPB reservoir volume and flow are adequate, ultrafiltration may be used to increase the hematocrit.

- Adequate ventilation with 100% oxygen must have been resumed.

- All monitors should be rechecked for proper function and recalibrated if necessary.

Weaning from CPB

CPB should be discontinued as systemic arterial pressure, ventricular volumes and filling pressures, and cardiac function (on TEE) are assessed. Central aortic pressure may be measured directly and should be compared with the radial artery pressure and cuff pressure (if there is a disparity). A reversal of the normal systolic pressure gradient, with aortic pressure being greater than radial pressure, is often seen immediately postbypass. This has been attributed to opening of arteriovenous connections in the hand as a consequence of rewarming. Central aortic root pressure can also be estimated by palpation by an experienced surgeon. Right ventricular volume and contractility can be estimated visually, whereas filling pressures are measured directly by central venous, pulmonary artery, or left atrial catheters. Cardiac output can be measured by thermodilution. TEE can define adequacy of end-diastolic volumes, right and left ventricular contractility, and valvular function.

Weaning is typically accomplished by progressively clamping the venous return line (tubing). As the beating heart fills, ventricular ejection resumes. Pump flow is gradually decreased as arterial pressure rises. Once the venous line is completely occluded and systolic arterial pressure is judged to be adequate (>80–90 mm Hg), pump flow is stopped and the patient is evaluated. **Some surgeons wean by clamping the venous line and then progressively "filling" the patient with arterial inflow.**

Most patients fall into one of four groups when coming off bypass (Table 22–2). Patients with good ventricular function are usually quick to develop good blood pressure and cardiac output and can be separated from CPB immediately. Hyperdynamic patients can also be rapidly weaned. These patients emerge from CPB with a very low SVR, demonstrating good contractility and adequate volume, but have low arterial pressure; their hematocrit is often reduced (<22%). Diuresis (off CPB) or red blood cell transfusions increase arterial blood pressure.

Hypovolemic patients include those with normal ventricular function and those with varying degrees of impairment. Those with preserved myocardial function quickly respond to 100-mL aliquots of pump blood infused via the aortic cannula. Blood pressure and cardiac output rise with each bolus,

TABLE 22–2 Post-CPB hemodynamic subgroups.[1]

	Group I: Vigorous	Group II: Hypovolemic	Group IIIA: LV Pump Failure	Group IIIB: RV Failure	Group IV: Vasodilated (Hyperdynamic)
Blood pressure	Normal	Low	Low	Low	Low
Central venous pressure	Normal	Low	Normal or high	High	Normal or low
Pulmonary wedge pressure	Normal	Low	High	Normal or high	Normal or low
TEE findings	Normal	Underfilled RV/LV	Reduced LV performance	Dilated RV	Normal or underfilled RV/LV
Cardiac output	Normal	Low	Low	Low	High
Systemic vascular resistance	Normal	Low, normal, or high	Low, normal or high	Normal or high	Low
Treatment	None	Volume	Inotrope; IABP, LVAD	Inotrope, pulmonary vasodilator; RVAD	Vasoconstrictor, volume

[1]CPB, cardiopulmonary bypass; LV, left ventricular; RV, right ventricular; IABP, intraaortic balloon pump; LVAD, left ventricular assist device; RVAD, right ventricular assist device; TEE, transesophageal echocardiography.

and the increase becomes progressively more sustained. Most of these patients maintain good blood pressure and cardiac output with a left ventricular filling pressure below 10–15 mm Hg. Ventricular impairment should be suspected (when definitive diagnosis using TEE is not available) in hypovolemic patients whose filling pressures rise during volume infusion without appreciable changes in blood pressure or cardiac output or in those who require filling pressures above 10–15 mm Hg. Ventricular dysfunction is easily diagnosed by TEE.

Patients with pump failure emerge from CPB with a sluggish, poorly contracting heart that progressively distends. In such cases, CPB may need to be reinstituted while inotropic therapy is initiated; alternatively, if the patient is less unstable, a positive inotrope (epinephrine, dopamine, dobutamine) can be administered while the patient is observed for improvement. If the patient does not respond to reasonable doses of one of these three agents, milrinone can be added. In patients with poor preoperative ventricular function milrinone may be administered as the first-line agent prior to separation from CPB. In the rare instance that SVR is increased, afterload reduction with nitroprusside or milrinone can be tried. The patient should be evaluated for unrecognized ischemia (kinked graft or coronary vasospasm), valvular dysfunction, shunting, or right ventricular failure (the distention is primarily right sided). TEE will facilitate the diagnosis in these cases.

If drug therapies fail, **intraaortic balloon pump** (IABP) counterpulsation should be initiated while the patient is "rested" on CPB. The efficacy of IABP depends on proper timing of inflation and deflation of the balloon (**Figure 22–15**). **The balloon should inflate just after the dicrotic notch is seen on the intraaortic pressure tracing to augment diastolic blood pressure and coronary flow after closure of the aortic valve**. Inflation too early increases afterload and exacerbates aortic regurgitation, whereas late inflation reduces diastolic augmentation. Balloon deflation should be timed just prior to left ventricular ejection to decrease its afterload. Early deflation makes diastolic augmentation and afterload reduction less effective. Use of a left or right ventricular assist device (LVAD or

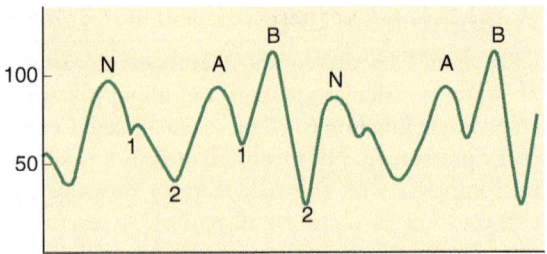

FIGURE 22–15   A central arterial waveform during 1:2 intraaortic balloon pump counterpulsation. Ideally the balloon, which is positioned in the descending aorta just distal to the left subclavian artery, should inflate at the dicrotic notch (1) and be completely deflated just as the left ventricle begins to eject (2). Note the lower end-diastolic pressures after balloon augmentation and slightly lower systolic pressure in the following beat. N, nonaugmented beat; A, augmented beat; B, balloon augmentation.

RVAD, respectively), may be necessary for patients with refractory pump failure. If myocardial stunning is a major contributor or there are areas of hibernating myocardium, a delayed improvement in contractile function may allow complete weaning from all drugs and support devices only after 12–48 h of therapy. Circulatory assist devices, such as the Abiomed and HeartMate, can be used as a bridge to cardiac transplantation; the former can be used for several days whereas the latter device can be left in place for months to years.

Many clinicians believe that positive inotropes should not routinely be used in patients coming off CPB because they increase myocardial oxygen demand. The routine use of calcium similarly may worsen ischemic injury and may contribute to coronary spasm (particularly in patients who were taking calcium channel blockers preoperatively). Nevertheless, there are centers that administer calcium salts or a positive inotrope (eg, dobutamine), or both, to every patient at the conclusion of CPB. Commonly used positive inotropes and vasopressors are listed in **Table 22–3**. Epinephrine, dopamine, and dobutamine are the most commonly used agents. Clinically, epinephrine is the most potent inotrope and is often effective in increasing both cardiac output and systemic blood pressure when others agents have failed. In lower doses, it

TABLE 22–3 Vasopressors and inotropic agents.[1]

| | Bolus | Infusion | Adrenergic Activity | | | Phosphodiesterase Inhibition |
			α	β	Indirect	
Epinephrine	2–10 mcg	0.01–0.03 mcg/kg/min	+	+++	0	0
		0.04–0.1 mcg/kg/min	++	+++	0	0
		>0.1 mcg/kg/min	+++	+++	0	0
Norepinephrine		0.01–0.1 mcg/kg/min	+++	++	0	0
Isoproterenol	1–4 mcg	0.01–0.1 mcg/kg/min	0	+++	0	0
Dobutamine		2–20 mcg/kg/min	0	++	0	0
Dopamine		2–10 mcg/kg/min	+	++	+	0
		10–20 mcg/kg/min	++	++	+	0
Ephedrine	5–25 mg		+	++	+	0
Phenylephrine	50–200 mcg	10–50 mcg/min	+++	0	0	0
Inamrinone	0.5–1.5 mg/kg	5–10 mcg/kg/min	0	0	0	+++
Milrinone	50 mcg/kg	0.375–0.75 mcg/kg/min	0	0	0	+++
Vasopressin	1–2 units	2–8 units/h	0	0	0	0

[1]+, mild activity; ++, moderate activity; +++, marked activity.

has predominantly β agonist activity. Dobutamine, unlike dopamine, does not increase filling pressures and *may* be associated with less tachycardia than dopamine; unfortunately, cardiac output often increases without significant changes in blood pressure. On the other hand, dopamine may improve renal blood flow (at reduced doses) and is often more effective in increasing blood pressure than in increasing cardiac output. Interestingly, when infused to increase cardiac output to similar extents, epinephrine is associated with no more increase (and perhaps less) in heart rate than dobutamine. Inamrinone and milrinone, both selective phosphodiesterase type III inhibitors, are inotropes with arterial and venous dilator properties; milrinone may be less likely than inamrinone to decrease the platelet count. In studies of patients with chronic heart failure these two inodilators, unlike other inotropes, did not appreciably increase myocardial

oxygen consumption. The combination of an inodilator (usually milrinone) and a β-adrenergic agonist results in at least additive (and possibly synergistic) inotropic effects. Norepinephrine is useful for increasing SVR but may compromise splanchnic and renal blood flow at increased doses. Some clinicians use norepinephrine in combination with phosphodiesterase inhibitors to prevent excessive reductions in systemic arterial pressure. Arginine vasopressin may be used in patients with refractory hypotension, a low SVR, and resistance to norepinephrine. Inhaled nitric oxide and prostaglandin E_1 may also be helpful for refractory pulmonary hypertension and right ventricular failure (Table 22–4); nitric oxide has the added advantage of not decreasing systemic arterial pressure. Studies have not confirmed outcome benefits to the use of nesiritide, a human B-type natriuretic peptide, thyroid hormone (T_3), or glucose–insulin–potassium

TABLE 22–4 Vasodilators.

Drug	Dosage
Clevidipine	1–16 mg/hr
Fenoldopam	0.03–0.6 mcg/kg/min
Nicardipine	2.5–10 mg/h
Nitric oxide	10–60 ppm (inhaled)
Nitroglycerin	0.5–10 mcg/kg/min
Nitroprusside	0.5–10 mcg/kg/min
Prostaglandin E$_1$	0.01–0.2 mcg/kg/min

infusions for vasoactive/inotropic support after CPB.

5. Postbypass Period

Following CPB, bleeding is controlled, bypass cannulas are removed, anticoagulation is reversed, and the chest is closed. Systolic arterial pressure is generally maintained at less than 140 mm Hg to minimize bleeding. Checking for bleeding, particularly from the posterior surface of the heart, requires lifting the heart, which can cause periods of precipitous hypotension. Some surgeons will need to be informed of the extent and duration of the hypotension; others have greater situational awareness. The atrial cannula(s) is removed before the aortic cannula in case the latter must be used to rapidly administer volume to the patient. Most patients need additional blood volume after termination of bypass. Administration of blood, colloids, and crystalloid is guided by filling pressures (and observation of the left ventricle on TEE), and the postbypass hematocrit. A final hematocrit of 25–30% is desirable, but is not mandatory. Blood remaining in the CPB reservoir can be transfused via the aortic cannula (while it remains in place) or washed and processed by a cell-saver device and given intravenously. Frequent ventricular ectopy may reflect electrolyte disturbances or residual ischemia and should be treated with amiodarone (or lidocaine or procainamide); hypokalemia or hypomagnesemia should be corrected. Ventricular

arrhythmias in this setting can rapidly deteriorate into ventricular tachycardia and fibrillation.

Reversal of Anticoagulation

Once hemostasis is judged acceptable and the patient continues to remain stable, heparin activity is reversed with protamine. **Protamine** is a highly positively charged protein that binds and effectively inactivates heparin (a highly negatively charged polysaccharide). Heparin–protamine complexes are then removed by the reticuloendothelial system. Protamine can be dosed in varying ways, but the results of all techniques should be checked for adequacy by repeating the ACT 3–5 min after completion of the protamine infusion. Additional incremental doses of protamine may be necessary.

One dosing technique bases the protamine dose on the amount of heparin initially required to produce the desired ACT; the protamine is then given in a ratio of 1–1.3 mg of protamine per 100 units of heparin. A still simpler approach is to give adult patients a defined dose (eg, 3–4 mg/kg) then check for adequacy of reversal. Another approach calculates the protamine dose based on the heparin dose–response curve (Figure 22–14). Automated heparin–protamine titration assays effectively measure residual heparin concentration and can also be used to calculate the protamine dose. The justification for using this methodology is the observation that when protamine is given in excess it may have anticoagulant activity, although this has never been demonstrated in humans. This approach also assumes that administered protamine remains in circulation for a prolonged time (which has been proven false in studies of patients undergoing cardiac surgery). To accomplish the heparin:protamine titration, premeasured amounts of protamine are added in varying quantities to several wells, each containing a blood sample. The well whose protamine concentration best matches the heparin concentration will clot first. Clotting will be prolonged in wells containing either too much or too little protamine. The protamine dose can then be estimated by multiplying the concentration in the tube that clots first by the patient's calculated blood volume. Supplemental protamine (50–100 mg) should be considered after administration of unwashed blood remaining in the pump reservoir after CPB because that blood contains heparin.

13 Protamine administration can result in a number of adverse hemodynamic effects, some of which are immunological in origin. Protamine given slowly (5–10 min) usually has few effects; when given more rapidly it produces a fairly consistent vasodilation that is easily treated with blood from the pump oxygenator and small doses of phenylephrine. Catastrophic protamine reactions often include myocardial depression and marked pulmonary hypertension. Diabetic patients previously maintained on protamine-containing insulin (such as NPH) may be at increased risk for adverse reactions to protamine.

Persistent Bleeding

14 Persistent bleeding often follows prolonged durations of bypass (>2 h) and in most instances has multiple causes. Inadequate surgical control of bleeding sites, incomplete reversal of heparin, thrombocytopenia, platelet dysfunction, hypothermia-induced coagulation defects, and undiagnosed preoperative hemostatic defects, or newly acquired factor deficiency or hypofibrinogenemia may be responsible. The absence (or loss) of clot formation may be noted in the surgical field. Normally, the ACT should return to baseline following administration of protamine; additional doses of protamine (25–50 mg) may be necessary. Reheparinization (heparin rebound) after apparent adequate reversal is poorly understood but often attributed to redistribution of peripherally bound heparin to the central compartment and to the exceedingly short persistence of protamine in blood. Hypothermia (<35°C) accentuates hemostatic defects and should be corrected. The administration of platelets and coagulation factors should be guided by additional coagulation studies, but empiric therapy may be necessary when such tests are not readily or promptly available as well as when treating massive transfusion. On the other hand, there can be abnormalities in multiple tests of coagulation whether or not there is bleeding, so the true diagnostic specificity and reliability of these tests is often overstated.

If diffuse oozing continues despite adequate surgical hemostasis and the ACT is normal or the heparin–protamine titration assay shows no residual heparin, thrombocytopenia or platelet dysfunction is most likely. Comparison of a conventional ACT with an ACT measured in the presence of heparinase (an enzyme that cleaves and inactivates heparin) can confirm that no residual heparin requiring protamine reversal remains present when both tests provide the same result. Platelet defects are recognized complications of CPB, which may necessitate platelet transfusion. Significant depletion of coagulation factors, particularly factors V and VIII, during CPB is less commonly responsible for bleeding but should be treated with fresh frozen plasma; both the prothrombin time and partial thromboplastin time are usually prolonged in such instances. Hypofibrinogenemia (fibrinogen level <100 mg/dL or a prolonged thrombin time without residual heparin) should be treated with cryoprecipitate. Desmopressin (DDAVP), 0.3 mcg/kg (intravenously over 20 min), can increase the activity of factors VIII and XII and the von Willebrand factor by releasing them from the vascular endothelium. DDAVP may be effective in reversing qualitative platelet defects in some patients but is not recommended for routine use. Accelerated fibrinolysis may occasionally be encountered following CPB and should be treated with ε-aminocaproic acid or tranexamic acid if one or the other of these agents has not already being given; the diagnosis should be confirmed by elevated fibrin degradation products (≥32 mg/mL), or evidence of clot lysis on thromboelastography. Increasingly, factor VII concentrate (at a cost of many thousands of dollars) is administered as a "last resort" in the setting of coagulopathic bleeding following cardiac surgery.

Anesthesia

Unless a continuous intravenous infusion technique is used, additional anesthetic agents are necessary following CPB; the choice may be determined by the hemodynamic response of the patient following CPB. Traditional teaching would have unstable patients receive small amounts of an opioid, benzodiazepine, or scopolamine, whereas anesthetic doses of a volatile agent might be recommended for hyperdynamic patients. Nevertheless, we have found that most patients tolerate modest doses of volatile agents or propofol infusion. Patients with hypertension that is unresponsive to adequate anesthesia with opioids and either a volatile agent or propofol (or both) should receive a vasodilator such as nitroglycerin, nitroprusside, clevidipine, or nicardipine (Table 22–4). Fenoldopam may be used and has the added benefit of increasing renal blood flow which might possibly improve kidney function in the early postoperative period.

It is common for an opioid (morphine or hydromorphone) and either propofol or dexmedetomidine to be given to provide analgesia and sedation during transfer to the ICU and analgesia (after discontinuation of the propofol or dexmedetomidine) during emergence.

Transportation

Transporting patients with critical illness from the operating room to the ICU is a consistently nerve-wracking and occasionally hazardous process that is complicated by the possibilities of monitor failure, overdosage or interruption of drug infusions, and hemodynamic instability en route. Portable monitoring equipment, infusion pumps, and a full oxygen cylinder with a self-inflating bag for ventilation should be readied prior to the end of the operation. Minimum monitoring during transportation includes the ECG, arterial blood pressure, and pulse oximetry. A spare endotracheal tube, laryngoscope, succinylcholine, and emergency resuscitation drugs should also accompany the patient. Upon arrival in the ICU, the patient should be attached to the ventilator, breath sounds should be checked, and an orderly transfer of monitors and infusions (one at a time) should follow. The ICU staff should be given a brief summary of the procedure, intraoperative problems, current drug therapy, and any expected difficulties. Many centers insist on a standard protocol for the "hand off."

6. Postoperative Period

Depending on the patient, the type of surgery, and local practices, most patients are mechanically ventilated for 1–12 h postoperatively. Sedation may be maintained by a propofol or dexmedetomidine infusion. The emphasis in the first few postoperative hours should be on maintaining hemodynamic stability and monitoring for excessive postoperative bleeding. Chest tube drainage in the first 2 h of more than 250–300 mL/h (10 mL/kg/h)—in the absence of a hemostatic defect—is excessive and may require surgical reexploration. Subsequent drainage that exceeds 100 mL/h is also worrisome. Intrathoracic bleeding at a site not adequately drained may cause cardiac tamponade, requiring immediate reopening of the chest.

Hypertension despite analgesia and sedation is a common postoperative problem and should generally be treated promptly so as not to exacerbate bleeding or myocardial ischemia. Nitroprusside, nitroglycerin, clevidipine, or nicardipine is generally used. β Blockade may be particularly useful for patients recovering from coronary artery surgery.

Fluid replacement may be guided by filling pressures, echocardiography, or by responses to treatment. Most patients present with relative hypovolemia for several hours following operation. Hypokalemia (from intraoperative diuretics) often develops and requires replacement. Postoperative hypomagnesemia is common in patients who receive no magnesium supplementation intraoperatively.

Extubation should be considered only when muscle paralysis has worn off (or been reversed) and the patient is hemodynamically stable. Caution should be exercised in obese and elderly patients and those with underlying pulmonary disease. Cardiothoracic procedures are typically associated with marked decreases in functional residual capacity and postoperative diaphragmatic dysfunction.

Off-Pump Coronary Artery Bypass Surgery

The development of advanced epicardial stabilizing devices, such as the Octopus (Figure 22–16), has facilitated coronary artery bypass grafting without the use of CPB, also known as off-pump coronary artery bypass (OPCAB). This type of retractor uses suction to stabilize and lift the anastomotic site rather than compress it down, which allows for

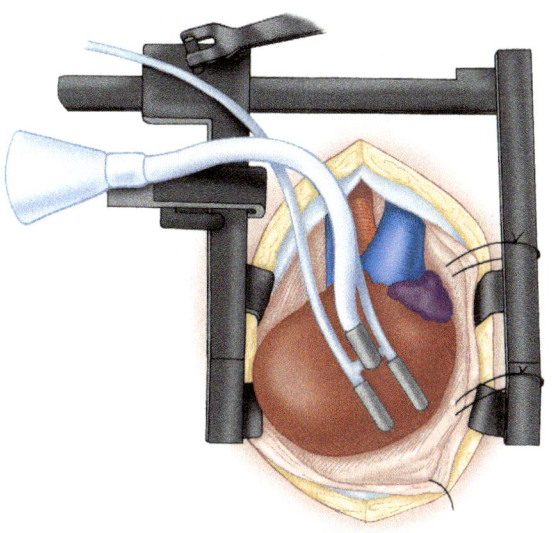

FIGURE 22–16 Schematic illustration of the Octopus retractor for off-pump coronary artery bypass surgery.

greater hemodynamic stability. Full (CPB) dose heparinization is usually given and the CPB machine is usually immediately available if needed.

Intravenous fluid loading together with intermittent or continuous infusion of a vasopressor may be necessary while the distal anastomoses are sewn. In contrast, a vasodilator may be required to reduce the systolic pressure to 90–100 mm Hg during partial clamping of the aorta for the proximal anastomosis. Intravenous nitroglycerin is often used because of its ability to ameliorate myocardial ischemia.

Although OPCAB was initially proposed for "simple" one- or two-vessel bypass grafting in patients with good left ventricular function, careful application of the technique has allowed it to be used routinely for multigraft surgery, redo operations, and patients with compromised left ventricular function (and it may be the "sicker" patients who benefit most from avoidance of CPB). Some surgeons use an intraluminal shunt to maintain coronary blood flow during sewing of distal anastomoses. Myocardial preconditioning, brief periods of coronary occlusion prior to the more prolonged occlusion, reduce areas of necrosis following prolonged periods of ischemia in animal studies, but the technique has found limited use in OPCAB. On the other hand, volatile

anesthetic agents and morphine provide myocardial protection during prolonged periods of ischemia. Maintenance of anesthesia with a volatile agent may therefore be desirable. When the surgeon is skillful, long-term graft patency may be comparable to procedures done with CPB. Patients with extensive coronary disease, particularly those with poor target vessels, may not be good candidates. OPCAB may decrease the incidence of postoperative neurological complications and the need for transfusion relative to conventional coronary bypass with CPB.

PEDIATRIC PATIENTS

Cardiovascular function in infants and young children differs from that in adults. Stroke volume is relatively fixed, so that cardiac output is primarily dependent on heart rate. The immature hearts of neonates and infants often are less forgiving of pressure or volume overload. Furthermore, the functions of both ventricles are more interdependent, so that failure of one ventricle often precipitates failure of the other (**biventricular heart failure**). Transition of the neonate from the fetal to the adult circulation is discussed in Chapter 40.

Preoperative Evaluation

The potentially complex nature of congenital heart defects and their operative repair require close communication among the anesthesiologist, cardiologist, and surgeon. The hemodynamic significance of the lesion and the planned surgical correction must be clearly understood. The patient's condition must be optimized. Congestive heart failure and pulmonary infections should be treated. Prostaglandin E_1 infusion (0.05–0.1 mcg/kg/min) is used preoperatively to prevent closure of the ductus arteriosus in infants dependent on ductal flow for survival.

Assessment of disease severity relies on both clinical and laboratory evaluation. Deterioration in infants may be manifested by increasing tachypnea, cyanosis, or sweating, particularly during feeding. Older children may complain of easy fatigability. In infants body weight is generally a good indication of disease severity, with the sickest children showing failure to thrive and reduced weight relative to expectations for age. Signs of congestive heart failure include failure to thrive, tachycardia, an S_3 gallop, weak pulses, tachypnea, pulmonary rales, and hepatomegaly. Cyanosis may be noted, but hypoxemia is best assessed by measurements of arterial blood gases and the hematocrit. In the absence of iron deficiency, the degree of polycythemia is related to the severity and duration of hypoxemia. Clubbing of the fingers is frequent in children with cyanotic defects. The evaluation should also search for other congenital abnormalities, which are present in up to 30% of patients with congenital heart disease.

The results of echocardiography, heart catheterization, electrocardiography, and chest radiography should be reviewed. Laboratory evaluation typically includes a complete blood count (with platelet count), coagulation studies, electrolytes, blood urea nitrogen, and serum creatinine. Measurements of ionized calcium and glucose are also useful in neonates and critically ill children.

Preinduction Period

A. Fasting

Fasting requirements vary according to the patient's age and current guidelines. A preoperative intravenous infusion that provides maintenance fluid requirements should be used in patients susceptible to dehydration, in those with severe polycythemia, and when excessive delays occur prior to surgery.

B. Premedication

Premedication varies according to age and cardiac and pulmonary reserves. Atropine, 0.02 mg/kg intramuscularly (minimum dose, 0.15 mg), has by tradition been given to pediatric cardiac patients to counteract enhanced vagal tone. Neonates and infants younger than 6 months of age may receive no premedication or given only atropine. Sedation is desirable in older patients, particularly those with cyanotic lesions (tetralogy of Fallot), as agitation and crying worsen right-to-left shunting. Patients older than 1 year may be given midazolam orally (0.5–0.6 mg/kg) or intramuscularly (0.08 mg/kg).

Induction of Anesthesia

A. Hemodynamic Anesthetic Goals

1. Obstructive lesions—Anesthetic management should strive to avoid hypovolemia, bradycardia, tachycardia, and myocardial depression. The optimal heart rate should be selected according to age; slow rates decrease cardiac output, whereas fast rates may impair ventricular filling. Mild cardiac depression may be desirable in some hyperdynamic patients, eg, those with coarctation of the aorta.

2. Shunts—A favorable ratio of pulmonary vascular resistance (PVR) to SVR should be maintained in the presence of shunting. Factors known to increase PVR such as acidosis, hypercapnia, hypoxia, enhanced sympathetic tone, and high mean airway pressures are to be avoided in patients with right-to-left shunting; hyperventilation (hypocapnia) with 100% oxygen is usually effective in lowering PVR. Specific pulmonary vasodilators are not available; alprostadil (prostaglandin E_1) or nitroglycerin may be tried but they often cause systemic hypotension. Systemic vasodilation also worsens right-to-left shunting and should be avoided; phenylephrine may be used to raise SVR. Inhaled nitric oxide has no effect on systemic arterial pressure. Conversely, patients with left-to-right shunting benefit from systemic vasodilation and increases in PVR, although specific hemodynamic manipulation is generally not attempted.

B. Monitoring

Standard intraoperative monitors are generally used until the patient is anesthetized, although they may be "added" during the course of an inhaled induction in some patients. A large discrepancy between end-tidal and arterial CO_2 tensions should be anticipated in patients with large right-to-left shunts because of increased dead space. Following induction, intraarterial and central venous pressure monitoring are employed for thoracotomies and all procedures employing CPB. A 22- or 24-gauge catheter is used to enter the radial artery; 24-gauge catheters may be more appropriate for small neonates and premature infants. A cutdown may be necessary in some instances. The internal jugular or subclavian vein is generally used for central venous cannulation; if this approach is unsuccessful, a right atrial catheter may be placed intraoperatively by the surgeon. Pulmonary artery catheterization is almost never used in pediatric patients. TEE is invaluable for assessing the surgical repair following CPB. Ever smaller probes are yielding better resolution as the technology advances. Probes are currently available for patients as small as 3 kg. Intraoperative epicardial echocardiography is commonly used either in addition to or instead of TEE.

C. Venous Access

Venous access is desirable but not always necessary for induction. Agitation and crying are particularly undesirable in patients with cyanotic lesions and can increase right-to-left shunting. Intravenous access can be established after induction but before intubation in most patients. Subsequently, at least two intravenous fluid infusion portals are required; one is typically via a central venous catheter. Caution is necessary to avoid even the smallest air bubbles. Shunting lesions allow the passage of venous air into the arterial circulation; paradoxical embolism can occur through the foramen ovale even in patients without obvious right-to-left shunting. Aspiration prior to each injection prevents dislodgment of any trapped air at stopcock injection ports.

D. Route of Induction

To a major extent, the effect of premedication and the presence of venous access determine the induction technique. Intubation is facilitated by a nondepolarizing agent (rocuronium, 1.2 mg/kg, or pancuronium, 0.1 mg/kg) or, much less commonly, succinylcholine, 1.5–2 mg/kg. Pancuronium's vagolytic effects are particularly useful in pediatric patients, but the agent itself is less often seen in North American hospitals.

1. Intravenous—Propofol (2–3 mg/kg), ketamine (1–2 mg/kg), fentanyl (25–50 mcg/kg), or sufentanil (5–15 mcg/kg) can be used for intravenous induction. High-dose opioids may be suitable for very small and critically ill patients when postoperative ventilation is planned. Intravenous agents' onset of action may be more rapid in patients with right-to-left shunting; drug boluses should be given slowly to avoid transiently high arterial blood levels. In contrast, recirculation in patients with large left-to-right shunts dilutes arterial blood concentration and can delay the appearance of intravenous agents' clinical effects.

2. Intramuscular—Ketamine, 4–10 mg/kg, is most commonly used, and onset of anesthesia is within 5 min. Coadministration with atropine helps prevent excessive secretions. Ketamine is a good choice for agitated and uncooperative patients as well as patients with decreased cardiac reserve. Its safety with cyanotic lesions (particularly in patients with Fallot's tetralogy) is well established. Ketamine does not appear to increase PVR in children.

3. Inhalation—Sevoflurane is the most commonly used volatile agent. The technique is the same as for noncardiac surgery, except for greater concerns about avoiding excessive anesthetic doses. Sevoflurane is particularly suitable for patients with good cardiac reserve. The safety of sevoflurane in patients with cyanotic heart disease and good cardiac reserve is now well established. Nitrous oxide may be used with inhalation inductions; its concentration should be limited to 50% in patients with cyanotic lesions. Nitrous oxide does not appear to increase PVR in pediatric patients. The uptake of inhalation agents may be slowed in patients with right-to-left shunts; in contrast, no significant effect on uptake is generally observed with left-to-right shunting.

Maintenance Anesthesia

Following induction, opioids or inhalation anesthetics are used for maintenance. Fentanyl and sufentanil are the most commonly used intravenous agents, and isoflurane and sevoflurane the most commonly used inhalation agents. Some clinicians choose the anesthetic according to the patient's hemodynamic responses. Isoflurane and sevoflurane may be more suitable than halothane (the most commonly used inhaled agent in years past) for most patients; in equivalent anesthetic doses, they cause less myocardial depression, less slowing of the heart rate, and more vasodilation than halothane. However, one can make a theoretical argument in favor of halothane over sevoflurane for patients with tetralogy of Fallot (and similarly obstructive lesions such as hypertrophic subaortic stenosis), where myocardial depression is much preferred over vasodilation.

Cardiopulmonary Bypass

The circuit and technique used are similar to those used for adults. Because the smallest circuit volume used is still about three times an infant's blood volume, blood is used to prime the circuit for neonates and infants to prevent excessive hemodilution. CPB may be complicated by intracardiac and extracardiac shunts and a very compliant arterial system (in very young patients); both tend to lower mean arterial pressure (20–50 mm Hg) and can impair systemic perfusion. High flow rates (up to 200 mL/kg/min) may be necessary to ensure adequate perfusion in very young patients. As noted previously, some evidence suggests that pH-stat management during CPB may be associated with better neurological outcome in children who will undergo circulatory arrest. Weaning from CPB is generally not a problem in pediatric patients if the surgical repair is adequate; primary pump failure is unusual. Difficulty in weaning should prompt the surgeon to check the repair and search for undiagnosed lesions. Intraoperative echocardiography, together with measurement of the pressure and oxygen saturation within the various chambers, may reveal the problem. Inotropic support may be provided by any of the agents used for adults. Calcium chloride is more often useful in critically ill young patients than in adults as children more often have impaired calcium homeostasis; ionized calcium measurements are invaluable in such cases. Close monitoring of glucose is required because both hyperglycemia and hypoglycemia may be observed. Dopamine and epinephrine are the most commonly used inotropes in pediatric patients. Addition of a phosphodiesterase inhibitor is also useful when PVR or SVR is increased. Hypocapnia, systemic alkalosis, and a high inspired oxygen concentration should also be used to decrease PVR in patients with pulmonary hypertension; additional pharmacological adjuncts may include prostaglandin E_1 (0.05–0.1 mcg/kg/min) or prostacyclin (1–40 mcg/kg/min). Inhalation nitric oxide may also be helpful for refractory pulmonary hypertension.

Children appear to have an intense inflammatory response during CPB that may be related to their blood being exposed to very large artificial surfaces relative to their size. Corticosteroids are often given to suppress this response. Many centers use modified ultrafiltration after weaning from CPB to partially correct the hemodilution but remove inflammatory vasoactive substances (cytokines); the technique takes blood from the aortic cannula and venous reservoir, passes it through an ultrafilter, and returns it to the right atrium.

Surgical correction of complex congenital lesions often requires a period of complete circulatory arrest under deep hypothermia (deep hypothermic circulatory arrest; DHCA). Following institution of CPB, cooling is accomplished by a combination of surface cooling and a cold perfusate. At a core temperature of 15°C, up to 60 min of complete circulatory arrest may be safe. Ice packing around the head is used to delay rewarming and for surface cooling of the brain. Pharmacological brain protection is often attempted with methylprednisolone, 30 mg/kg, and mannitol, 0.5 g/kg. Following the repair, CPB flow is restarted and rewarming takes place.

Postbypass Period

Because of the large priming volumes used (often 200–300% of the patient's blood volume), hemostatic defects from dilution of clotting factors and platelets are commonly seen after CPB in infants; in addition to heparin reversal, administration of fresh frozen plasma and platelets is often necessary.

Patients undergoing extensive or complicated procedures will generally remain intubated. Extubation may be considered for older, relatively healthy patients undergoing simple procedures such as closure of a patent ductus or atrial septal defect or repair of coarctation of the aorta.

Cardiac Transplantation

Preoperative Considerations

Cardiac transplantation is the treatment of choice for otherwise healthy patients with end-stage heart disease so severe that they are unlikely to survive the next 6–12 months. The procedure is generally associated with 80–90% postoperative survival at 1 year and 60–90% survival at 5 years. Transplantation improves the quality of life and most patients are able to resume a relatively normal lifestyle. Unfortunately, the number of cardiac transplants performed is limited by the supply of donor hearts, which are obtained from brain-dead patients, most commonly following intracranial hemorrhage or head trauma.

Patients with intractable heart failure have an ejection fraction of less than 20% and fall into NYHA functional class IV (see Chapter 21) and heart failure class D. For most patients, the primary diagnosis is cardiomyopathy. Intractable heart failure may be the result of a severe congenital lesion, ischemic cardiomyopathy, viral cardiomyopathy, peripartum cardiomyopathy, a failed prior transplantation, or valvular heart disease. Medical therapy should include the standard drugs used for heart failure, including angiotensin-converting enzyme inhibitors (or angiotensin receptor blockers, or both) and β blockade (usually with carvedilol). Other drugs may include diuretics, vasodilators, and even oral inotropes; oral anticoagulation with warfarin may also be necessary. Patients may not be able to survive without intravenous inotropes while awaiting transplantation. Intraaortic balloon counterpulsation, an LVAD, or even a total mechanical heart may also be necessary.

Transplant candidates must not have suffered extensive end-organ damage or have other major systemic illnesses. Reversible renal and hepatic dysfunction are common because of chronic hypoperfusion and venous congestion. PVR must be normal or at least responsive to oxygen or vasodilators. Irreversible pulmonary vascular disease is usually associated with a PVR of more than 6–8 Wood units (1 Wood unit = 80 dyn·s·cm⁻⁵), and is a contraindication to orthotopic cardiac transplantation because right ventricular failure is a major cause of early postoperative mortality. Patients with long-standing pulmonary hypertension may, however, be candidates for combined heart–lung transplantation.

Tissue cross-matching is generally not performed. Donor–recipient compatibility is based on size, ABO blood-group typing, and cytomegalovirus serology. Donor organs from patients with hepatitis B or C or HIV infections are excluded.

ANESTHETIC MANAGEMENT

Proper timing and coordination are necessary between the donor organ retrieval team and the transplant center. Premature induction of anesthesia unnecessarily prolongs the time under anesthesia for the recipient, whereas delayed induction may jeopardize graft function by prolonging the period of ischemia.

Patients may receive little advance warning of the availability of a suitable organ. Many—if not most—will have eaten a recent meal and should be considered to have a full stomach. Oral cyclosporine must be given preoperatively. Administration of a clear antacid (sodium citrate), a histamine H₂-receptor blocker, and metoclopramide should be considered. Any sedating premedication may be administered intravenously just prior to induction.

Monitoring is similar to that used for other cardiac procedures and is often established prior to induction. Strict asepsis should be observed during invasive procedures. Use of the right internal jugular vein for central access does not appear to compromise its future use for postoperative endomyocardial biopsies. A pulmonary artery catheter is used in many centers for postbypass management. It need not be placed in the pulmonary artery before CPB.

A rapid sequence induction may be performed. The principal objective of anesthetic management is to maintain organ perfusion until the patient is on CPB. Induction may be carried out with small doses of opioids (fentanyl, 5–10 mcg/kg) with or without etomidate (0.2–0.3 mg/kg). A low-dose ketamine-midazolam technique (above) may also be suitable. Sufentanil, 5 mcg/kg, followed by succinylcholine, 1.5 mg/kg, can be used as a rapid-sequence technique. Anesthesia is maintained in a similar fashion as for other cardiac operations. A TEE probe is placed following induction, and antirejection drugs are given.

Sternotomy and cannulation for CPB may be complicated by scarring from prior cardiac operations. Aminocaproic acid or tranexamic acid can be used to decrease postoperative bleeding. CPB is initiated following cannulation of the aorta and both cavae. If a pulmonary artery catheter was placed, it must be completely withdrawn from the heart with its tip in the superior vena cava. It must remain within its sterile, protective sheath if it is to be safely refloated again into the pulmonary artery following CPB. The recipient's heart is then excised, allowing the posterior wall of both atria (with the caval and pulmonary vein openings) to remain. The atria of the donor heart are anastomosed to the recipient's atrial remnants (left side first). The aorta and then the pulmonary artery are anastomosed end to end. The donor heart is then flushed with saline and intracardiac air is evacuated. Methylprednisolone is given before the aortic cross-clamp is released.

Inotropic support is usually started prior to separation from CPB to counteract bradycardia from sympathetic denervation. Prolonged graft ischemia may result in transient myocardial depression. Slow junctional rhythms are common and may require epicardial pacing. Although the transplanted heart is totally denervated and direct autonomic influences are absent, its response to circulating catecholamines is usually normal. The pulmonary artery catheter can be refloated into position after CPB and is used in conjunction with TEE to evaluate the patient. The most common post-CPB problem is right ventricular failure from pulmonary hypertension, which should be treated with hyperventilation, prostaglandin E_1 (0.025–0.2 mcg/kg/min), nitric oxide (10–60 ppm), and an RVAD, if necessary. Bleeding is a common problem because of extensive suture lines and preoperative hemostatic defects.

Patients will be extubated when they meet criteria, as with other major cardiac operations. The postoperative course may be complicated by acute rejection, renal and hepatic dysfunction, and infections.

PERICARDIAL DISEASE

The parietal pericardium is a fibrous membrane surrounding the heart, to which it normally is not adherent. The pericardium encompasses a relatively fixed intrapericardiac volume that includes a small volume of pericardial fluid (20–50 mL in adults), the heart, and blood. As a result, the pericardium normally limits acute dilation of the ventricles and promotes diastolic coupling of the two ventricles (distention of one ventricle interferes with filling of the other). The latter effect is also due to the interventricular septal wall they share. Moreover, diseases

of the pericardium or larger pericardial fluid collections can seriously impair cardiac output.

1. Cardiac Tamponade

Preoperative Considerations

Cardiac tamponade exists when increased pericardial pressure impairs diastolic filling of the heart. Cardiac filling is ultimately related to the diastolic transmural (distending) pressure across each chamber. Consequently, any increase in pericardial pressure relative to the pressure within the chamber reduces filling. Pressure is applied equally to each cardiac chamber when the problem is a pericardial fluid collection; or, it can be applied "selectively," as for example when an isolated pericardial blood clot compresses the left atrium. In general, the thin-walled atria and the right ventricle are more susceptible to pressure-induced abnormalities of filling than the left ventricle.

Pericardial pressure is normally similar to pleural pressure, varying with respiration between –4 and +4 mm Hg. Elevations in pericardial pressure are most commonly due to increases in pericardial fluid volume (as a consequence of effusions or bleeding). The magnitude of the increased pressure depends on both the volume of fluid and the rate of fluid accumulation; sudden increases exceeding 100–200 mL precipitously increase pericardial pressure, whereas very slow accumulations up to 1000 mL allow the pericardium to stretch with minimal increases in pericardial pressure.

The principal hemodynamic features of cardiac tamponade include decreased cardiac output from reduced stroke volume with an increase in central venous pressure. In the absence of severe left ventricular dysfunction, equalization of diastolic pressure occurs throughout the heart (right atrial pressure [RAP] = right ventricular end-diastolic pressure [RVEDP] = left atrial pressure [LAP] = left ventricular end-diastolic pressure [LVEDP]).

The central venous pressure waveform is characteristic in cardiac tamponade. Impairment of both diastolic filling and atrial emptying abolishes the y descent; the x descent (systolic atrial filling) is normal or even accentuated. Reflex sympathetic activation is a prominent compensatory response in cardiac tamponade. The resulting increases in heart rate and contractility help maintain cardiac output. Arterial vasoconstriction (increased SVR) supports systemic blood pressure, whereas sympathetic activation reduces vascular capacitance, having the effect of an autotransfusion. Because stroke volume remains relatively fixed, cardiac output becomes primarily dependent on heart rate.

Acute cardiac tamponade usually presents as sudden hypotension, tachycardia, and tachypnea. Physical signs include jugular venous distinction, a narrowed arterial pulse pressure, and muffled heart sounds. The patient may complain of an inability to lie flat. A friction rub may be audible. A prominent pulsus paradoxus (a cyclic inspiratory decrease in systolic blood pressure of more than 10 mm Hg) is typically present. The latter actually represents an exaggeration of a normal phenomenon related to inspiratory decreases in intrathoracic pressure. (A marked pulsus paradoxus may also be seen with severe airway obstruction or right ventricular infarction.) The heart may appear normal or enlarged on a chest radiograph. Electrocardiographic signs are generally nonspecific and are often limited to decreased voltage in all leads and nonspecific ST-segment and T-wave abnormalities. Electrical alternans (a cyclic alteration in magnitude of the P waves, QRS complex, and T waves) may be seen with large pericardial effusions and is thought to be due to pendular swinging of the heart within the pericardium. Generalized ST-segment elevation may also be seen in two or three limb leads as well as V_2 to V_6 in the early phase of pericarditis. Echocardiography is invaluable in diagnosing and measuring pericardial effusions and cardiac tamponade, and as a guide for accurate needle insertion for pericardiocentesis. Signs of tamponade include diastolic compression or collapse of the right atrium and right ventricle, leftward displacement of the ventricular septum, and an exaggerated increase in right ventricular size with a reciprocal decrease in left ventricular size during inspiration.

Pericardial effusions may be due to viral, bacterial, or fungal infections; malignancies; bleeding after cardiac surgery; trauma; uremia; myocardial infarction; aortic dissection; hypersensitivity or autoimmune disorders; drugs; or myxedema.

Anesthetic Considerations

Symptomatic cardiac tamponade requires evacuation of the pericardial fluid, either surgically or by pericardiocentesis. The latter is associated with a risk of lacerating the heart or coronary arteries and of pneumothorax. Traumatic postoperative (following thoracotomy) cardiac tamponade is nearly always treated surgically, whereas tamponade from other causes may more often be amenable to pericardiocentesis. Surgical treatment is also often undertaken for large recurrent pericardial effusions (infectious, malignant, autoimmune, uremic, or radiation induced) to prevent tamponade. Simple drainage of pericardial fluid may be achieved through a subxiphoid approach, whereas drainage combined with pericardial biopsy or pericardiectomy may be performed via a left anterior thoracotomy or median sternotomy. Drainage and biopsies can also be accomplished through left-sided thoracoscopy.

The anesthetic approach must be tailored to the patient. For the intubated postoperative cardiac patient in extremis, the chest may be reopened immediately in the ICU. For awake conscious patients who will undergo left thoracotomy or median sternotomy, general anesthesia and endotracheal intubation are necessary. Local anesthesia may be used for patients undergoing simple drainage through a subxiphoid approach or pericardiocentesis. Removal of even a small volume of fluid may be sufficient to greatly improve cardiac output and allow safe induction of general anesthesia. Small doses (10 mg intravenously at a time) of ketamine also provide excellent supplemental analgesia.

17 Induction of general anesthesia in patients with cardiac tamponade can precipitate severe hypotension and cardiac arrest. We find it useful to have an epinephrine infusion available and we sometimes initiate it before induction.

Large-bore intravenous access is mandatory. Monitoring of intraarterial pressure is useful, but placement of monitors should not delay pericardial drainage if the patient is unstable. The anesthetic technique should maintain a high sympathetic tone until the tamponade is relieved; in other words, "deep" anesthesia is not the object. Cardiac depression, vasodilation, and slowing of the heart rates should be avoided. Similarly, increases in mean airway pressures can seriously jeopardize venous return. Awake intubation with maintenance of spontaneous ventilation is theoretically desirable, but coughing, straining, hypoxemia, and respiratory acidosis are equally detrimental and should be avoided. Thoracoscopy requires one-lung anesthesia.

Ketamine is the agent of choice for induction and maintenance until the tamponade is relieved. Small doses of epinephrine (5–10 mcg) may be useful as a temporary inotrope and chronotrope. Generous intravenous fluid administration is useful in maintaining cardiac output.

2. Constrictive Pericarditis

Preoperative Considerations

Constrictive pericarditis may develop as a sequela of acute or recurrent pericarditis. Pathologically, the pericardium is thickened, fibrotic, and often calcified. The parietal pericardium is typically adherent to the visceral pericardium on the heart, often obliterating the pericardial space. The stiffened parietal pericardium limits diastolic filling of the heart to a fixed and reduced volume. In contrast to acute cardiac tamponade, filling during early diastole is typically accentuated and manifested by a prominent y descent on the central venous pressure waveform.

Patients with constrictive pericarditis display jugular venous distention, hepatomegaly, and often ascites. Liver function may be abnormal. In contrast to acute tamponade, constrictive pericarditis prevents respiratory fluctuations in pericardial pressure; because venous return to the heart does not increase during inspiration, a pulsus paradoxus is uncommon. In fact, venous pressure does not fall or may paradoxically rise during inspiration (Kussmaul's sign). The chest radiograph will often reveal pericardial calcification. Low QRS voltage and diffuse T-wave abnormalities are usually present on the ECG. Atrial fibrillation and conduction blocks may be present. Echocardiography may be helpful in making the diagnosis.

Anesthetic Considerations

Pericardiectomy is usually reserved for patients with moderate to severe disease. The procedure is usually performed through a median sternotomy. It is complicated by the necessity for extensive manipulations of the heart that interfere with cardiac filling and ejection, induce frequent arrhythmias, and risk cardiac perforation. CPB may be required.

Selection of specific anesthetic agents is less important than avoiding excessive cardiac depression, vasodilation, and bradycardia. Cardiac output is generally rate dependent. Adequate large-bore intravenous access and direct arterial and central venous pressure monitoring are usually employed. Although cardiac function usually improves immediately following pericardiectomy, some patients display a persistently low cardiac output and require temporary postoperative inotropic support.

Anesthetic Management of Vascular Surgery

ANESTHESIA FOR SURGERY ON THE AORTA

Preoperative Considerations

Surgery on the aorta represents one of the greatest challenges for anesthesiologists. Regardless of which part of the vessel is involved, the procedure is complicated by the need to cross-clamp the aorta and by the potential for large intraoperative blood losses. Aortic cross-clamping without CPB acutely increases left ventricular afterload and severely compromises organ perfusion distal to the point of occlusion. Severe hypertension, myocardial ischemia, left ventricular failure, or aortic valve regurgitation may be precipitated. Interruption of blood flow to the spinal cord, kidneys, and intestines can produce paraplegia, kidney failure, or intestinal infarction, respectively. Moreover, emergency aortic surgery is frequently necessary in critically ill patients who are acutely hypovolemic and have a high incidence of coexistent cardiac, renal, and pulmonary disease; hypertension; and diabetes.

Indications for aortic surgery include aortic dissections, aneurysms, occlusive disease, trauma, and coarctation. Lesions of the ascending aorta lie between the aortic valve and the innominate artery, whereas lesions of the aortic arch lie between the innominate and left subclavian arteries. Disease distal to the left subclavian artery but above the diaphragm involves the descending thoracic aorta; lesions below the diaphragm involve the abdominal aorta.

SPECIFIC LESIONS OF THE AORTA

Aortic Dissection

In an aortic dissection an intimal tear allows blood to track into the aortic wall (the media), creating a new pathway for blood flow. In many cases, a primary degenerative process called cystic medial necrosis predisposes for dissection to occur. Patients with hereditary connective tissue defects such as Marfan syndrome and Ehlers–Danlos syndrome eventually develop cystic medial necrosis and are at risk for aortic dissection. Propagation of the dissection is thought to occur as a result of hemodynamic shear forces acting on the intimal tear; indeed, hypertension is a common finding in patients with aortic dissection. Dissection can also occur from hemorrhage into an atheromatous plaque or at the aortic cannulation site following cardiac surgery.

Dissections may occlude the orifice of any artery arising directly from the aorta; they may extend into the aortic root, producing incompetence of the aortic valve; or may rupture into the pericardium or pleura, producing cardiac tamponade or hemothorax, respectively. TEE plays an important role in diagnosing and characterizing aortic dissections. Dissections are most commonly of the proximal type (Stanford type A, De Bakey types I and II) involving the ascending aorta. Type II dissections do not extend beyond the innominate artery. Distal dissections (Stanford type B, De Bakey type III) originate beyond the left subclavian artery and propagate only distally. Proximal dissections are nearly always treated surgically, whereas distal dissections may be treated medically. In either case, from the time the diagnosis is suspected, measures to reduce systolic blood pressure (usually to 90–120 mm Hg) and aortic wall stress are initiated. This usually includes intravenous vasodilators (nicardipine or nitroprusside) and β-adrenergic blockade (esmolol or a longer acting agent). The latter is important in reducing the shear forces related to the rate of rise of aortic pressure (dP/dt), which may actually increase with nitroprusside alone.

Aortic Aneurysms

Aneurysms more commonly occur in the abdominal than in the thoracic aorta. The vast majority of aortic aneurysms are due to atherosclerosis; cystic medial necrosis is also an important cause of thoracic aortic aneurysms. Syphilitic aneurysms characteristically involve the ascending aorta. Other etiologies include rheumatoid arthritis, spondyloarthropathies, and trauma. Dilation of the aortic root often produces aortic regurgitation. Expanding aneurysms of the upper thoracic aorta can also cause tracheal or bronchial compression or deviation, hemoptysis, and superior vena cava syndrome. Compression of the left recurrent laryngeal nerve produces hoarseness and left vocal cord paralysis. Distortion of the normal anatomy may also complicate endotracheal or endobronchial intubation or cannulation of the internal jugular and subclavian veins.

The greatest danger from untreated aortic aneurysms is rupture and exsanguination. A pseudoaneurysm forms when the intima and media are ruptured and only adventitia or blood clot forms the outer layer. Acute expansion (from leaking), manifested as sudden severe pain, may herald rupture. The likelihood of catastrophic rupture is related to size. The normal aorta in adults varies from 2 to 3 cm in width (it is wider cephalad). The data are clear for abdominal aortic aneurysms; rupture occurs in 50% of patients within 1 year when an aneurysm is 6 cm or greater in diameter. Elective treatment is generally performed in most patients with aneurysms 5 cm or greater. Most often this is accomplished with an intravascular stent; less often, open surgery and a prosthetic graft is used. The operative mortality rate is about 2–5% in good-risk patients and exceeds 50% if leaking or rupture has already occurred. The risks are much less with intravascular stenting, which has become the preferred procedure whenever the anatomy permits.

Occlusive Disease of the Aorta

Atherosclerotic obliteration of the aorta most commonly occurs near the aortic bifurcation (Leriche's syndrome). Occlusion results from a combination of atherosclerotic plaque and thrombosis. Atherosclerosis is usually generalized and affects other parts of the arterial system, including the cerebral, coronary, and renal arteries (see Chapters 21 and 28). Treatment may be accomplished by intravascular stenting or by open surgery with an aortobifemoral bypass graft; proximal thromboendarterectomy may also be necessary.

Aortic Trauma

Aortic trauma may be penetrating or nonpenetrating. Both types of injuries can result in massive hemorrhage and require immediate operation. Whereas penetrating injuries are usually obvious, blunt aortic trauma may be easily overlooked if not suspected and the appropriate diagnostic testing performed. Nonpenetrating aortic trauma typically results from sudden high-speed decelerations such as those caused by automobile accidents (eg, in which the driver's chest impacts the steering wheel) and falls. The injury can vary from a partial tear to a complete aortic transection. Because the aortic arch is relatively fixed whereas the descending aorta is relatively mobile, the shear forces are greatest and the site of injury most common just distal to the subclavian artery. The most consistent initial finding is a widened mediastinum on a chest radiograph. Definitive diagnosis can be accomplished with magnetic resonance or computed tomographic imaging or TEE.

Coarctation of the Aorta

This congenital heart defect may be classified according to the position of the narrowed segment relative to the position of the ductus arteriosus. In the *preductal* (infantile) type, the narrowing occurs proximal to the opening of the ductus. This lesion, which is often associated with other congenital heart defects, is recognized in infancy because of a marked difference in perfusion between the upper and lower halves of the body; the lower half is cyanotic. Perfusion to the upper body is derived from the aorta, whereas perfusion to the lower body is primarily from the pulmonary artery. *Postductal* coarctation of the aorta may not be recognized until adulthood. The symptoms and hemodynamic significance of this lesion depend on the severity of the narrowing and the extent of collateral circulation that develops to the lower body (internal mammary, subscapular, and lateral thoracic to intercostal arteries). Hypertension in the upper body, with or without left ventricular failure, is usually present. So-called "rib notching" may be present on the chest radiograph as a result of dilated collateral intercostal arteries.

ANESTHETIC MANAGEMENT

Surgery on the Ascending Aorta

Surgery on the ascending aorta routinely uses median sternotomy and CPB. The conduct of anesthesia is similar to that for cardiac operations involving CPB, but the intraoperative course may be complicated by long aortic cross-clamp times and large intraoperative blood losses. TEE is especially useful. Blood loss can be reduced by administration of ε-aminocaproic acid or tranexamic acid. Concomitant aortic valve replacement and coronary reimplantation are often necessary (Bentall procedure). The radial artery cannulation site should be guided by the possible need for clamping of either the subclavian or innominate arteries during the procedure. Nicardipine or nitroprusside may be used for precise blood pressure control. β-Adrenergic blockade should also be employed in the presence of an aortic dissection. On the other hand, bradycardia worsens aortic regurgitation and should be avoided. The arterial inflow cannula for CPB is placed in a femoral artery for patients with dissections. In the event that sternotomy may rupture an aneurysm, prior establishment of partial CPB (using the femoral artery and femoral vein) should be considered.

Surgery Involving the Aortic Arch

These procedures are usually performed through a median sternotomy with deep hypothermic circulatory arrest (following institution of CPB). Additional considerations focus on achieving optimal cerebral protection with systemic and topical hypothermia (above). Hypothermia to 15°C, barbiturate or propofol infusion to maintain a flat EEG, methylprednisolone or dexamethasone, mannitol, and phenytoin are also commonly administered (but there is vanishingly small evidence for efficacy of these drug treatments). The necessarily long rewarming periods probably contribute to the larger intraoperative blood losses commonly observed after CPB.

Surgery Involving the Descending Thoracic Aorta

Surgery limited to the descending thoracic aorta may be performed through a left thoracotomy without CPB, with or without (so-called "clamp-and–run" technique) a heparin-impregnated left ventricular apex to femoral artery shunt; or using partial right atrium to femoral artery bypass. A thoracoabdominal incision is necessary for lesions that also involve the abdominal aorta. One-lung anesthesia greatly facilitates surgical exposure. Correct positioning of the endobronchial tube (even with fiberoptic bronchoscopy) may be difficult because of distortion of the anatomy. A right-sided double-lumen tube or a regular endotracheal tube with a bronchial blocker may be necessary.

The aorta must be cross-clamped above and below the lesion. Acute hypertension develops above the clamp, with hypotension below when there is no shunt or partial bypass. Arterial blood pressure should be monitored from the right radial artery, as clamping of the left subclavian artery may be necessary. The sudden increase in left ventricular afterload after application of the aortic cross-clamp during aortic surgery may precipitate acute left ventricular failure and myocardial ischemia, particularly in patients with underlying ventricular dysfunction or coronary disease; it can also exacerbate preexisting aortic regurgitation. Cardiac output falls and left ventricular end-diastolic pressure and volume rise. The magnitude of these changes is inversely related to ventricular function. These effects can be ameliorated by the use of shunting or partial bypass. Moreover, the adverse effects of aortic clamping become less pronounced the more distal on the aorta that the clamp is applied. A vasodilator infusion is often needed to prevent excessive increases in blood pressure. In patients with good ventricular function, increasing anesthetic depth just prior to cross-clamping may also be helpful.

Excessive intraoperative bleeding may occur during these procedures. Prophylaxis with antifibrinolytic agents may be helpful. A blood scavenging device (cell saver) for autotransfusion is routinely used. Adequate venous access and intraoperative monitoring are critical. Multiple large-bore (14-gauge) intravenous catheters (preferably with blood warmers) are useful. Pulmonary artery catheterization and intraoperative TEE are often used. The period of greatest hemodynamic instability follows the release of the aortic cross-clamp; the abrupt decrease in afterload together with bleeding and the release of vasodilating acid metabolites from the ischemic lower body can precipitate severe systemic hypotension and less commonly hyperkalemia. Decreasing anesthetic depth, volume loading, and partial or slow release of the cross-clamp are helpful in avoiding severe hypotension. A bolus dose of a vasopressor may be necessary. Sodium bicarbonate is often used, particularly for persistent severe metabolic acidosis (pH < 7.20) in association with hypotension. Calcium chloride may be necessary when symptomatic hypocalcemia follows massive transfusion of citrated blood products.

A. Paraplegia

Spinal cord ischemia can complicate thoracic aortic cross-clamping. The incidence of transient postoperative deficits and postoperative paraplegia are 11% and 6%, respectively. Increased rates are associated with cross-clamping periods longer than 30 min, extensive surgical dissections, and emergency procedures. The classic deficit is an anterior spinal artery syndrome with loss of motor function and pinprick sensation but preservation of vibration and proprioception. Anatomic variations in spinal cord blood supply are responsible for the unpredictable occurrence and variable nature of deficits. The spinal cord receives its blood supply from the vertebral arteries and from the thoracic and abdominal aorta. One anterior and two posterior arteries descend along the cord. Intercostal arteries feed the anterior and posterior arteries in the upper thoracic aorta. Textbook descriptions suggest that in the lower thoracic and lumbar cord, the anterior spinal artery is supplied by the thoracolumbar artery of Adamkiewicz. The truth is that a single large feeding artery usually cannot be identified. When present, this artery has a variable origin from the aorta, arising between T5 and T8 in 15%, between T9 and T12 in 60%, and between L1 and L2 in 25% of individuals; it nearly always arises on the left side. It may be damaged during surgical dissection or occluded by the aortic cross-clamping. Monitoring motor and somatosensory evoked potentials may be useful in preventing paraplegia, but clearly surgical technique and speed are most important.

As noted earlier, use of a temporary heparin-coated shunt or partial CPB with hypothermia maintains distal perfusion and decreases the incidence of paraplegia, hypertension, and ventricular failure. Partial CPB has the disadvantage of requiring heparinization, which increases blood loss. Using a heparin-coated shunt precludes the need for heparinization. It is usually positioned proximally in the left ventricular apex and distally in a femoral artery. Other therapeutic measures that may be protective of the spinal cord include methylprednisolone, mild hypothermia, mannitol, and drainage of cerebrospinal fluid (CSF) to reduce the CSF pressure in the spine; magnesium is also protective in some animal models. The efficacy of mannitol appears to be related to its ability to lower CSF pressure by decreasing its production. Spinal cord perfusion pressure is mean arterial blood pressure minus CSF pressure; the rise in CSF pressure following experimental cross-clamping of the aorta may explain how a mannitol-induced decrease in CSF pressure could improve spinal cord perfusion pressure during cross-clamping. Any protective effect of drainage of CSF via a lumbar catheter may have a similar mechanism.

The excessive use of vasodilators to control the hypertensive response to cross-clamping may be a contributing factor in spinal cord ischemia, as drug actions also occur distal to the cross-clamp. Excessive reduction in blood pressure above the cross-clamp should therefore be avoided to prevent inadequate blood flow and excessive hypotension below it.

B. Kidney Failure

An increased incidence of kidney failure following aortic surgery is reported after emergency procedures, prolonged cross-clamping periods, and prolonged hypotension, particularly in patients with preexisting kidney disease. A variety of "cocktails" have been employed in the hope of reducing the risk of kidney failure, including infusion of mannitol (0.5 g/kg) prior to cross-clamping, furosemide, fenoldopam (or low-dose dopamine), etc. Low (renal)-dose dopamine or fenoldopam will increase renal blood flow and may be used as an adjunct for a persistently low urinary output after the cross-clamp is released, however there is no convincing evidence that these treatments alter renal outcomes.

Surgery on the Abdominal Aorta

Stents are most often placed via catheters inserted in a femoral artery. When an open technique is chosen, either an anterior transperitoneal or an anterolateral retroperitoneal approach can be used to access the abdominal aorta. Depending on the location of the lesion, the cross-clamp can be applied to the supraceliac, suprarenal, or infrarenal aorta. Heparin is usually administered prior to aortic clamping. Intraarterial blood pressure can be monitored from either upper extremity. In general, the more distally the clamp is applied to the aorta, the less the effect on left ventricular afterload. In fact, occlusion of the infrarenal aorta frequently results in minimal hemodynamic changes. In contrast, release of the clamp usually produces hypotension; the same techniques that were described earlier (see above) may be used. The large incision and extensive retroperitoneal surgical dissection increase fluid requirements beyond intraoperative blood loss. We recommend colloid to maintain intravascular volume and crystalloid for maintenance fluids. Fluid replacement may be guided by monitoring central venous pressure, noninvasive monitors of stroke volume, or TEE. Pulmonary artery catheters are rarely used.

Renal prophylaxis with mannitol should be considered, particularly in patients with preexisting renal impairment. Clamping of the infrarenal aorta has been shown to decrease renal blood flow, which may contribute to postoperative kidney failure. The decrease in renal blood flow is not prevented by epidural anesthesia or blockade of the renin–angiotensin system.

Some centers use continuous epidural anesthesia combined with general anesthesia for abdominal aortic surgery. This combined technique decreases the general anesthetic requirement and appears to suppress the release of stress hormones. It also provides an excellent route for administering postoperative epidural analgesia. Systemic heparinization during surgery introduces concern regarding the risk of paraplegia secondary to an epidural hematoma; however, all credible studies suggest that there when the catheter is placed well in advance of heparinization and removed after reversal of anticoagulation there is no increased risk of neuraxial hematomas as a consequence of epidural catheter placement.

Postoperative Considerations

Those undergoing stenting may not require intubation either during or after the procedure. Most patients undergoing open surgery on the ascending aorta, the arch, or the thoracic aorta will remain intubated and ventilated for 1–24 h postoperatively. As with cardiac surgery, the initial emphasis in their postoperative care should be on hemodynamic stability and monitoring for postoperative bleeding. Patients undergoing open abdominal aortic surgery may be extubated at the end of the procedure. These patients typically continue to require a marked increase in maintenance fluids for several hours postoperatively.

ANESTHESIA FOR CAROTID ARTERY SURGERY

Preoperative Considerations

Ischemic cerebrovascular disease accounts for 80% of strokes; the remaining 20% are due to hemorrhage. Ischemic strokes are usually the result of embolism or (less commonly) thrombosis in one of the blood vessels supplying the brain. Ischemic stroke may follow severe vasospasm after subarachnoid hemorrhage. By convention, a stroke is defined as a neurological deficit that lasts more than 24 h; its pathological correlate is typically focal infarction of brain. Transient ischemic attacks (TIAs), on the other hand, are neurological deficits that resolve within 24 h; they may be due to a low-flow state at a tightly stenotic lesion or to emboli that arise from an extracranial vessel or the heart. When a stroke is associated with progressive worsening of signs and symptoms, it is frequently termed a *stroke in evolution*. A second distinction is also often made between complete and incomplete strokes, based on whether the territory involved is completely affected or additional brain remains at risk for focal ischemia (eg, hemiplegia versus hemiparesis). The bifurcation of the common carotid artery (the origin of the internal carotid artery) is the most common site of atherosclerotic plaques that may lead to TIA or stroke. The mechanism may be embolization of platelet-fibrin or plaque material, stenosis, or complete occlusion. The last may be the result of thrombosis or hemorrhage into a plaque. Symptoms depend on the adequacy of collateral circulation. Emboli distal to regions lacking collateral blood flow are more likely to produce symptoms. Small emboli in the ophthalmic branches can cause transient monocular blindness (amaurosis fugax). Larger emboli usually enter the middle cerebral artery, producing contralateral motor and sensory deficits that primarily affect the arm and face. Aphasia also develops if the dominant hemisphere is affected. Emboli in the anterior cerebral artery territory typically result in contralateral motor and sensory deficits that are worse in the leg. It is common for TIAs or minor strokes to precede a major stroke.

Indications for open surgery or intravascular interventions include TIAs associated with ipsilateral severe carotid stenosis (>70% occlusion), severe ipsilateral stenosis in a patient with a minor (incomplete) stroke, and 30–70% occlusion in a patient with ipsilateral symptoms (usually an ulcerated plaque). In the past, carotid endarterectomy was recommended for asymptomatic but significantly stenotic lesions (>60%). Currently, stenting would often be the recommendation. Operative mortality for open surgery is 1–4% and is primarily due to cardiac complications (myocardial infarction). Perioperative morbidity is 4–10% and is principally neurological; patients with preexisting neurological deficits have the greatest risk of perioperative neurological events. **Studies suggest that age greater than 75 years,**

symptomatic lesions, uncontrolled hypertension, angina, carotid thrombus, and occlusions near the carotid siphon increase operative risk.

Preoperative Anesthetic Evaluation & Management

Most patients undergoing carotid endarterectomy are elderly and hypertensive, with generalized arteriosclerosis. Many are also diabetic. Preoperative evaluation and management should focus on defining preexisting neurological deficits as well as optimizing the patient's clinical status in terms of coexisting diseases. Most postoperative neurological deficits appear to be related to surgical technique. Uncontrolled perioperative hyperglycemia can increase morbidity by enhancing ischemic cerebral injury.

With the possible exception of diuretics, patients should receive their usual medications on schedule until the time of surgery. Blood pressure and the blood glucose concentration should be controlled. Angina should be stable and controlled, and signs of overt congestive heart failure should be absent. Because most patients are elderly, enhanced sensitivity to premedication should be expected.

General Anesthesia

19 The emphasis of anesthetic management during carotid surgery is on maintaining adequate perfusion to the brain and heart. Traditionally, this is accomplished by close regulation of arterial blood pressure and avoidance of tachycardia. Monitoring of intraarterial pressure is therefore nearly always done. Electrocardiographic monitoring should include the V_5 lead to detect ischemia. Continuous computerized ST-segment analysis is desirable. Carotid endarterectomy is not usually associated with significant blood loss or fluid shifts.

Regardless of the anesthetic agents selected, mean arterial blood pressure should be maintained at—or slightly above—the patient's usual range. Propofol and etomidate are popular choices for induction because they reduce cerebral metabolic rate proportionally more than cerebral blood flow. Small doses of an opioid or β-adrenergic blocker can be used to blunt the hypertensive response to endotracheal intubation. In theory, isoflurane may be the volatile agent of choice because it appears to provide the greatest protection against cerebral ischemia. Desflurane qualitatively has similar cerebral effects but may not be as effective as isoflurane; however, desflurane is very useful in accelerating awakening and allowing immediate neurological assessment in the operating room. We do not regard the differences in neuroprotection among inhaled agents as clinically important. Some clinicians also prefer remifentanil as the opioid for rapid emergence.

Intraoperative hypertension is common and generally necessitates the use of an intravenous vasodilator. Nitroglycerin is usually a good choice for mild to moderate hypertension because of its beneficial effects on the coronary circulation. Marked hypertension requires a more potent agent, such as nicardipine, nitroprusside, or clevidipine. β-Adrenergic blockade facilitates management of the hypertension and prevents reflex tachycardia from vasodilators, but should be used cautiously. Hypotension should be treated with vasopressors. Many clinicians consider phenylephrine the vasopressor of choice; if selected, it should be administered in small increments to prevent excessive hypertension.

Pronounced or sustained reflex bradycardia or heart block caused by manipulation of the carotid baroreceptor can be treated with atropine. To prevent this response, some surgeons infiltrate the area of the carotid sinus with lidocaine, but the infiltration itself can induce bradycardia. Arterial CO_2 tension should be maintained in the normal range because hypercapnia can induce intracerebral steal, whereas extreme hypocapnia decreases cerebral perfusion. Ventilation should be adjusted to maintain normocapnia. Maintenance intravenous fluids should consist of glucose-free solutions because of the potentially adverse effects of hyperglycemia. Heparin (5000–7500 units intravenously) is usually administered prior to occlusion of the carotid artery. Some clinicians routinely use a shunt (see below). Protamine, 50–150 mg, is usually given to reverse heparin prior to skin closure.

Rapid emergence from anesthesia is desirable because it allows immediate neurological assessment, but the clinician must be prepared to treat hypertension and tachycardia. **Postoperative hypertension may be related to surgical denervation of the ipsilateral carotid baroreceptor. Denervation of the carotid body blunts the ventilatory response to hypoxemia.** Following extubation, patients should be observed closely for the development of a wound hematoma. When an expanding wound hematoma compromises the airway, the initial treatment maneuver may require opening the wound to release the hematoma. Transient postoperative hoarseness and ipsilateral deviation of the tongue may be noted; they are due to intraoperative retraction of the recurrent laryngeal or hypoglossal nerves, respectively.

Monitoring Cerebral Function

Unless regional anesthesia is used (see below), indirect methods must be relied upon to assess the adequacy of cerebral perfusion during carotid cross-clamping. Some surgeons routinely use a shunt, but this practice may increase the incidence of postoperative neurological deficits; shunt insertion can dislodge emboli. Carotid stump pressure distal to the cross-clamp, EEG, somatosensory evoked potentials (SSEPs), and cerebral oximetry have been used in some centers to determine whether a shunt is needed. A distal stump pressure of less than 50 mm Hg has traditionally been used as an indication for a shunt. Electrophysiological signs of ischemia (or a marked decline in cerebral oxygen saturation) after cross-clamping dictate the use of a shunt; changes lasting more than 10 min may be associated with a new postoperative neurological deficit. Although multichannel recordings and computer processing can enhance the sensitivity of the EEG, neither EEG nor SSEP monitoring is sufficiently sensitive or specific to reliably predict the need for shunting or the occurrence of postoperative deficits (see Case Discussion in Chapter 26). Other techniques, including measurements of regional cerebral blood flow with radioactive xenon-133, transcranial Doppler measurement of middle cerebral artery flow velocity, cerebral oximetry, jugular venous oxygen saturation, and transconjunctival oxygen tension, are also not sufficiently reliable.

Regional Anesthesia

Carotid surgery may be performed under regional anesthesia. Blockade of the superficial cervical plexus effectively blocks the C2–C4 nerves and allows the patient to remain comfortably awake during surgery. Deep cervical plexus block is not required. A substantial fraction of patients will require administration of local anesthetic by the surgeon into the carotid sheath (whether or not a deep cervical block is performed). The principal advantage of regional anesthesia (and it is a tremendous advantage) is that the patient can be examined intraoperatively; thus, the need for a temporary shunt can be assessed and any new neurological deficits diagnosed immediately during surgery. In fact, intraoperative neurological examination may be the most reliable method for assessing the adequacy of cerebral perfusion during carotid cross-clamping. The examination minimally consists of level of consciousness, speech, and contralateral handgrip. Experienced clinicians use minimal sedation and "cocktail conversation" with the patient to monitor the neurological status. Some studies also suggest that when compared with general anesthesia, regional anesthesia results in more stable hemodynamics but outcomes appear similar. Regional anesthesia for carotid surgery requires the cooperation of the surgeon and patient.

CASE DISCUSSION

A Patient for Cardioversion

A 55-year-old man with new-onset atrial fibrillation is scheduled for elective cardioversion.

What are the indications for an elective cardioversion?

Direct current (DC) cardioversion may be used to terminate supraventricular and ventricular tachyarrhythmias caused by reentry. It is not effective for arrhythmias from enhanced automaticity (multifocal atrial tachycardia) or triggered activity (digitalis toxicity). By simultaneously depolarizing the entire myocardium and possibly prolonging the refractory period, DC cardioversion can terminate atrial fibrillation and flutter, atrioventricular nodal reentry, reciprocating tachycardias from pre-excitation syndromes, and ventricular tachycardia or fibrillation.

Specific indications for cardioversion of patients with atrial fibrillation include symptomatic fibrillation, recent onset, and no response to medications. Patients with long-standing fibrillation, a large atrium, chronic obstructive lung disease, congestive heart failure, or mitral regurgitation have a high recurrence rate. A TEE is usually performed shortly before cardioversion to rule out a left atrial blood clot. Such clots are typically located in the left atrial appendage and can be embolized by cardioversion or sinus rhythm.

Emergency cardioversion is indicated for any tachyarrhythmia associated with hypotension, congestive heart failure, or angina.

How is cardioversion performed?

Although the procedure is usually performed by cardiologists, the need for immediate cardioversion may arise in the operating room, ICU, or during cardiopulmonary resuscitation. Anesthesiologists must therefore be familiar with the technique. Following heavy sedation or light general anesthesia, DC shock is applied by either self-adhesive pads or 8- to 13-cm paddles. Larger paddles help reduce any shock-induced myocardial necrosis by distributing the current over a wider area. The energy output should be kept at the minimally effective level to prevent myocardial damage. Placement of the electrodes can be anterolateral or anteroposterior. In the first position, one electrode is placed on the right second intercostal space next to the sternum and the other is placed on the left fifth intercostal space in the midclavicular line. When pads are used for the anteroposterior technique, one is placed anteriorly over the ventricular apex in the fifth intercostal space and the other underneath the patient in the left infrascapular region.

For supraventricular tachycardias, with the notable exception of atrial fibrillation, energy levels of 25–50 J can successfully reestablish normal sinus rhythm. Synchronized shocks should be used for all tachyarrhythmias except ventricular

fibrillation. Synchronization times the delivery so that it is given during the QRS complex. If the shock occurs in the ST segment or the T wave (unsynchronized), it can precipitate a more serious arrhythmia, including ventricular fibrillation. All medical personnel should stand clear of the patient and the bed during the shock.

Atrial fibrillation usually requires a minimum of 50–100 J and larger energy levels are often used. Hemodynamically stable ventricular tachycardia can often be terminated with 25–50 J, but ventricular fibrillation and unstable ventricular tachycardia require 200–360 J. Regardless of the arrhythmia, a higher energy level is necessary when the first shock is ineffective.

The cardiologist wants to do the cardioversion in the postanesthesia care unit (PACU). Is this an appropriate place for cardioversion?

Elective cardioversion can be performed in any setting in which full provisions for cardiopulmonary resuscitation, including cardiac pacing capabilities, are immediately available. A physician skilled in airway management should be in attendance. Cardioversions are commonly performed in an ICU, emergency department, PACU, procedure room, or cardiac catheterization suite.

How would you evaluate this patient?

The patient should be fasted, evaluated, and treated as though he were receiving a general anesthetic in the operating room. An ECG is performed immediately before the procedure to confirm that the arrhythmia is still present; another is performed immediately afterward to confirm the new rhythm. Preoperative laboratory values should be within normal limits because metabolic disorders, particularly electrolyte and acid–base abnormalities, may contribute to the arrhythmia. If not corrected preoperatively, they can reinitiate the tachycardia following cardioversion. An antiarrhythmic agent is often started in patients with atrial fibrillation 1–2 days prior to the procedure to help maintain normal sinus rhythm. Patients may also be anticoagulated with warfarin for 1–2 weeks prior to cardioversion.

What are the minimum monitors and anesthetic equipment required?

Minimum monitoring consists of the ECG, blood pressure, and pulse oximetry. A precordial stethoscope is useful for monitoring breath sounds. Maintaining continuous verbal contact with the patient may the best method for assessing whether a sufficient amnestic dose of (usually) propofol has been given.

In addition to a DC defibrillator capable of delivering up to 400 J (synchronized or unsynchronized) and transcutaneous pacing, the minimum equipment should include the following:

- Reliable intravenous access.
- A functional bag-mask device capable of delivering 100% oxygen (see Chapter 3).
- An oxygen source from a wall outlet or a full tank.
- An airway kit with oral and nasal airways and appropriate laryngoscopes and endotracheal tubes.
- A functional suction apparatus.
- An anesthetic drug kit that includes at least one sedative-hypnotic as well as succinylcholine.
- A cart that includes all necessary drugs and equipment for cardiopulmonary resuscitation (see Chapter 55).

What anesthetic techniques would be appropriate?

Premedication is not necessary. Only very brief (1–2 min) amnesia or light general anesthesia is required. A short-acting agent such as propofol or a benzodiazepine (eg, midazolam, diazepam) can be used. Etomidate may be used but may be associated with phonation. Following preoxygenation with 60–100% oxygen for 3–5 min, the sedative-hypnotic is given in small increments) every 30–60 sec while maintaining verbal contact with the patient. The shock is delivered when the patient is no longer able to respond verbally; some clinicians use loss of the eyelid reflex as an end point. The shock usually arouses the patient. Transient airway obstruction or apnea may be observed, particularly if more than one shock is necessary.

What are the complications of cardioversion?

Complications include transient myocardial depression, postshock arrhythmias, and arterial embolism. Arrhythmias are usually due to inadequate synchronization, but even a properly timed cardioversion can occasionally result in ventricular fibrillation. Most arrhythmias are transient and resolve spontaneously. Although patients may develop ST-segment elevation, serum creatine phosphokinase levels (MB fraction) are usually normal. Embolism may be responsible for delayed awakening.

How should the patient be cared for following cardioversion?

Although recovery of consciousness is usually very rapid, patients should be treated like others receiving general anesthesia (see Chapter 56). Recovery also specifically includes monitoring for both recurrence of the arrhythmia and signs of cerebral embolism.

GUIDELINES

Hiratzka LF, Bakris GL, Beckman JA, et al: 2010 ACCF/AHA/AATS/ACR/ASA/SCA/SCAI/SIR/STS/SVM Guidelines for the diagnosis and management of patients with thoracic aortic disease: Executive summary: A report of the American College of Cardiology Foundation/American Heart Association Task Force on Practice Guidelines, American Association for Thoracic Surgery, American College of Radiology, American Stroke Association, Society of Cardiovascular Anesthesiologists, Society for Cardiovascular Angiography and Interventions, Society of Interventional Radiology, Society of Thoracic Surgeons, and Society for Vascular Medicine. Anesth Analg 2010;111:279.

See www.guidelines.gov for additional guidelines from multiple organizations related to these topics.

SUGGESTED READING

Augoustides JG, Andritsos M: Innovations in aortic disease: The ascending aorta and aortic arch. J Cardiothorac Vasc Anesth 2010;24:198.

Augoustides JG, Riha H: Recent progress in heart failure treatment and heart transplantation. J Cardiothorac Vasc Anesth 2009;23:738.

Chassot P-G, van der Linden P, Zaugg M, et al: Off-pump coronary artery bypass surgery: Physiology and anaesthetic management. Br J Anaesth 2004;92:400.

Grigore AM, Murray CF, Ramakrishna H, Djaiani G: A core review of temperature regimens and neuroprotection during cardiopulmonary bypass: Does rewarming rate matter? Anesth Analg 2009;109:1741.

Hogue CW Jr, Palin CA, Arrowsmith JE: Cardiopulmonary bypass management and neurologic outcomes: An evidence-based appraisal of current practices. Anesth Analg 2006;103:21.

Kam PCA, Egan MK: Platelet glycoprotein IIb/IIIa antagonists. Pharmacology and clinical developments. Anesthesiology 2002;96:1237.

Levy JH, Winkler AM: Heparin-induced thrombocytopenia and cardiac surgery. Curr Opin Anaesthesiol 2010;23:74.

Ling E, Arellano R: Systematic overview of the evidence supporting the use of cerebrospinal fluid drainage in the thoracoabdominal aneurysm surgery for prevention of paraplegia. Anesthesiology 2000;93:1115.

Murphy GS, Hessel EA 2nd, Groom RC: Optimal perfusion during cardiopulmonary bypass: An evidence-based approach. Anesth Analg 2009;108:1394.

Myles PS, Daly DJ, Djaiani G, et al: A systematic review of the safety and effectiveness of fast-track cardiac anesthesia. Anesthesiology 2003;99:982.

Priebe HJ: Triggers of perioperative myocardial ischaemia and infarction. Br J Anaesth 2004;93:9.

Royse AG, Royse CF: Epiaortic ultrasound assessment of the aorta in cardiac surgery. Best Pract Res Clin Anaesthesiol 2009;23:335.

Sellke FW, Chu LM, Cohn WE: Current state of surgical myocardial revascularization. Circ J 2010;74:1031.

Selnes OA, McKhann GM, Borowicz LM Jr, Grega MA: Cognitive and neurobehavioral dysfunction after cardiac bypass procedures. Neurol Clin 2006;24:133.

Shanewise JS, Ramsay JG: Off-pump coronary surgery: How do the anesthetic considerations differ? Anesth Clin North Am 2003;21:613.

Zaugg M, Schaub MC, Foëx P: Myocardial injury and its prevention in the perioperative setting. Br J Anaesth 2004;93:21.

Respiratory Physiology & Anesthesia

1. The trachea serves as a conduit for ventilation and the clearance of tracheal and bronchial secretions and has an average length of 10–13 cm. The trachea bifurcates at the carina into the right and left main stem bronchi. The right main stem bronchus lies in a more vertical orientation relative to the trachea, whereas the left main stem bronchus lies in a more horizontal orientation.

2. The periodic exchange of alveolar gas with the fresh gas from the upper airway reoxygenates desaturated blood and eliminates CO_2. This exchange is brought about by small cyclic pressure gradients established within the airways. During spontaneous ventilation, these gradients are secondary to variations in intrathoracic pressure; during mechanical ventilation, they are produced by intermittent positive pressure in the upper airway.

3. The lung volume at the end of a normal exhalation is called functional residual capacity (FRC). At this volume, the inward elastic recoil of the lung approximates the outward elastic recoil of the chest (including resting diaphragmatic tone).

4. Closing capacity is normally well below FRC, but it rises steadily with age. This increase is probably responsible for the normal age-related decline in arterial O_2 tension.

5. Whereas both forced expiratory volume in 1 sec (FEV_1) and forced vital capacity (FVC) are effort dependent, forced midexpiratory flow ($FEF_{25-75\%}$) is more effort independent and may be a more reliable measure of obstruction.

6. Changes in lung mechanics due to general anesthesia occur shortly after induction. The supine position reduces the FRC by 0.8–1.0 L, and induction of general anesthesia further reduces the FRC by 0.4–0.5 L. FRC reduction is a consequence of alveolar collapse and compression atelectasis due to loss of inspiratory muscle tone, change in chest wall rigidity, and upward shift of the diaphragm.

7. Local factors are more important than the autonomic system in influencing pulmonary vascular tone. Hypoxia is a powerful stimulus for pulmonary vasoconstriction (the opposite of its systemic effect).

8. Because alveolar ventilation ($\dot{V}_A$) is normally about 4 L/min and pulmonary capillary perfusion ($\dot{Q}$) is 5 L/min, the overall $\dot{V}/\dot{Q}$ ratio is about 0.8.

9. Shunting denotes the process whereby desaturated, mixed venous blood from the right heart returns to the left heart without being resaturated with O_2 in the lungs. The overall effect of shunting is to decrease (dilute) arterial O_2 content; this type of shunt is referred to as right-to-left.

—Continued next page

Continued—

10 General anesthesia commonly increases venous admixture to 5% to 10%, probably as a result of atelectasis and airway collapse in dependent areas of the lung.

11 Note that large increases in Pa_{CO_2} (>75 mm Hg) readily produce hypoxia (Pa_{O_2} <60 mm Hg) at room air, but not at high inspired O_2 concentrations.

12 The binding of O_2 to hemoglobin seems to be the principal rate-limiting factor in the transfer of O_2 from alveolar gas to blood.

13 The greater the shunt, the less likely the possibility that an increase in the fraction of inspired oxygen (F_{IO_2}) will prevent hypoxemia.

14 A rightward shift in the oxygen–hemoglobin dissociation curve lowers O_2 affinity, displaces O_2 from hemoglobin, and makes more O_2 available to tissues; a leftward shift increases hemoglobin's affinity for O_2, reducing its availability to tissues.

15 Bicarbonate represents the largest fraction of CO_2 in blood.

16 Central chemoreceptors are thought to lie on the anterolateral surface of the medulla and respond primarily to changes in cerebrospinal fluid (CSF) [H^+]. This mechanism is effective in regulating Pa_{CO_2}, because the blood–brain barrier is permeable to dissolved CO_2 but not to bicarbonate ions.

17 With increasing depth of anesthesia, the slope of the Pa_{CO_2}/minute ventilation curve decreases, and the apneic threshold increases.

The importance of pulmonary physiology to anesthetic practice is obvious. The most commonly used anesthetics—the inhalation agents—depend on the lungs for uptake and elimination. The most important side effects of both inhalation and intravenously administered anesthetics are primarily respiratory. Moreover, muscle paralysis, unusual positioning during surgery, and techniques such as one-lung anesthesia and cardiopulmonary bypass profoundly alter normal pulmonary physiology.

Much of modern anesthetic practice is based on a thorough understanding of pulmonary physiology and may be considered applied pulmonary physiology. This chapter reviews the basic pulmonary concepts necessary for understanding and applying anesthetic techniques. Although the pulmonary effects of each of the various anesthetic agents are discussed elsewhere in the book, this chapter also reviews the overall effects of general anesthesia on lung function.

FUNCTIONAL RESPIRATORY ANATOMY

1. Rib Cage & Muscles of Respiration

The rib cage contains the two lungs, each surrounded by its own pleura. The apex of the chest is small, allowing only for entry of the trachea, esophagus, and blood vessels, whereas the base is formed by the diaphragm. Contraction of the diaphragm—the principal pulmonary muscle—causes the base of the thoracic cavity to descend 1.5–7 cm and its contents (the lungs) to expand. Diaphragmatic movement normally accounts for 75% of the change in chest volume. Accessory respiratory muscles also increase chest volume (and lung expansion) by their action on the ribs. Each rib (except for the last two) articulates posteriorly with a vertebra and is angulated downward as it attaches anteriorly to the sternum. Upward and outward rib movement expands the chest.

During normal breathing, the diaphragm, and, to a lesser extent, the external intercostal muscles are responsible for inspiration; expiration is generally passive. With increasing effort, the sternocleidomastoid, scalene, and pectoralis muscles can be recruited during inspiration. The sternocleidomastoid muscles assist in elevating the rib cage, whereas the scalene muscles prevent inward displacement of the upper ribs during inspiration. The pectoralis muscles can assist chest expansion when the arms are placed on a fixed support. Expiration is normally passive in the supine position, but becomes active in the upright position and with increased effort. Exhalation may be facilitated by the abdominal muscles (rectus abdominis, external and internal oblique, and transversus) and perhaps the internal intercostal muscles—aiding the downward movement of the ribs.

Although not usually considered respiratory muscles, some pharyngeal muscles are important in maintaining the patency of the airway. Tonic and reflex inspiratory activity in the genioglossus keeps the tongue away from the posterior pharyngeal wall. Tonic activity in the levator palati, tensor palati, palatopharyngeus, and palatoglossus prevents the soft palate from falling back against the posterior pharynx, particularly in the supine position.

2. Tracheobronchial Tree

1 The trachea serves as a conduit for ventilation and the clearance of tracheal and bronchial secretions. The trachea begins at the lower border of the cricoid cartilage and extends to the level of the carina and has an average length of 10–13 cm. It is composed of C-shaped cartilaginous rings, which form the anterior and lateral walls of the trachea and are connected posteriorly by the membranous wall of the trachea. The external diameters of the trachea measure approximately 2.3 cm coronally and 1.8 cm sagitally in men, with corresponding values of 2.0 cm and 1.4 cm, respectively, in women. The cricoid cartilage is the narrowest part of the trachea, with an average diameter of 17 mm in men and 13 mm in women.

The trachea bifurcates at the carina into the right and left main stem bronchi. The tracheal lumen narrows slightly as it progresses toward the carina,

with the tracheal bifurcation located at the level of the sternal angle. The right main stem bronchus lies in a more vertical orientation relative to the trachea, whereas the left main stem bronchus lies in a more horizontal orientation. The right main stem bronchus continues as the bronchus intermedius after the take-off of the right upper lobe bronchus. The distance from the tracheal carina to the take-off of the right upper lobe bronchus is an average of 2.0 cm in men and approximately 1.5 cm in women. One in every 250 individuals in the general population may have an abnormal take-off of the right upper lobe bronchus emerging from above the tracheal carina on the right side. The left main stem bronchus is longer than the right main stem bronchus and measures an average of 5.0 cm in men and 4.5 cm in women. The left main stem bronchus divides into the left upper lobe bronchus and the left lower lobe bronchus.

Humidification and filtering of inspired air are functions of the upper airway (nose, mouth, and pharynx). The function of the tracheobronchial tree is to conduct gas flow to and from the alveoli. Dichotomous division (each branch dividing into two smaller branches), starting with the trachea and ending in alveolar sacs, is estimated to involve 23 divisions, or generations (**Figure 23–1**). With each generation, the number of airways is approximately doubled. Each alveolar sac contains, on average, 17 alveoli. An estimated 300 million alveoli provide an enormous membrane (50–100 m²) for gas exchange in the average adult.

With each successive division, the mucosal epithelium and supporting structures of the airways gradually change. The mucosa makes a gradual transition from ciliated columnar to cuboidal and finally to flat alveolar epithelium. Gas exchange can occur only across the flat epithelium, which begins to appear on respiratory bronchioles (generations 17–19). The wall of the airway gradually loses its cartilaginous support (at the bronchioles) and then its smooth muscle. Loss of cartilaginous support causes the patency of smaller airways to become dependent on radial traction by the elastic recoil of the surrounding tissue; as a corollary, airway diameter becomes dependent on total lung volume.

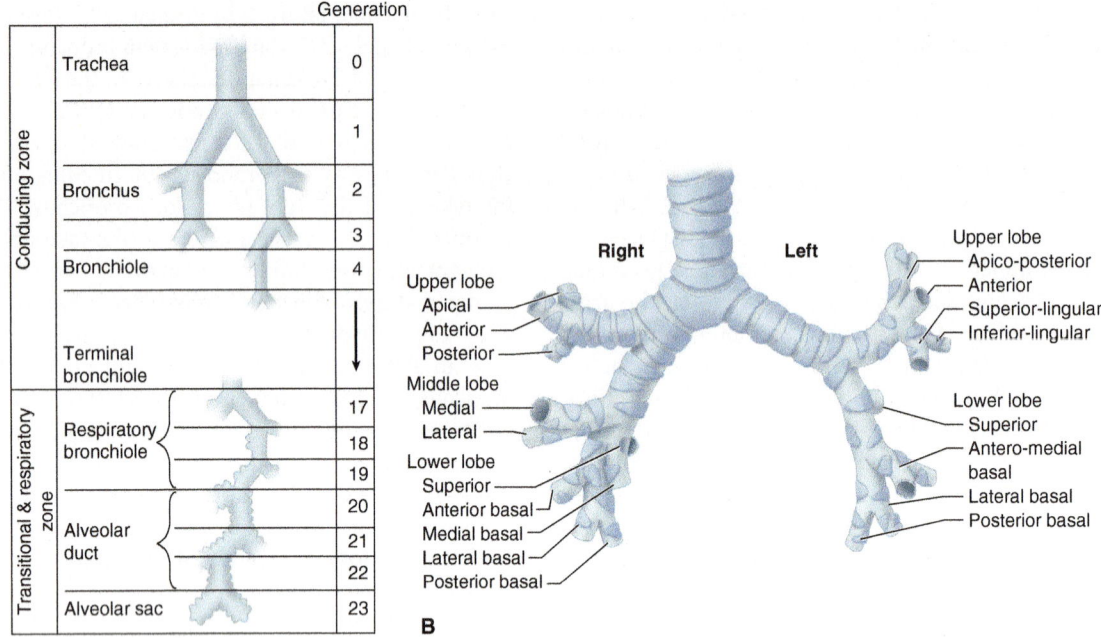

FIGURE 23–1 A: Dichotomous division of the airways. (Reproduced, with permission, from Guyton AC: *Textbook of Medical Physiology*, 7th ed. W.B. Saunders, 1986.) **B:** The segmental bronchi. (Reproduced, with permission, from Minnich DJ, Mathisen DJ: Anatomy of the trachea, carina, and bronchi. Thorac Surg Clin 2007 Nov;17(4):571-585.)

Cilia on the columnar and cuboidal epithelium normally beat in a synchronized fashion, such that the mucus produced by the secretory glands lining the airway (and any associated bacteria or debris) moves up toward the mouth.

Alveoli

Alveolar size is a function of both gravity and lung volume. The average diameter of an alveolus is thought to be 0.05–0.33 mm. In the upright position, the largest alveoli are at the pulmonary apex, whereas the smallest tend to be at the base. With inspiration, discrepancies in alveolar size diminish.

Each alveolus is in close contact with a network of pulmonary capillaries. The walls of each alveolus are asymmetrically arranged (**Figure 23–2**). On the thin side, where gas exchange occurs, the alveolar epithelium and capillary endothelium are separated only by their respective cellular and basement membranes; on the thick side, where fluid and solute exchange occurs, the pulmonary interstitial space separates alveolar epithelium from capillary endothelium. The pulmonary interstitial space contains mainly elastin, collagen, and perhaps nerve fibers. Gas exchange occurs primarily on the thin side of the alveolocapillary membrane, which is less than 0.4 μm thick. The thick side (1–2 μm) provides structural support for the alveolus.

The pulmonary epithelium contains at least two cell types. Type I pneumocytes are flat and form tight (1-nm) junctions with one another. These tight junctions are important in preventing the passage of large oncotically active molecules such as albumin into the alveolus. Type II pneumocytes, which are more numerous than type I pneumocytes (but because of their shape occupy less than 10% of the alveolar space), are round cells that contain prominent cytoplasmic inclusions (lamellar bodies). These inclusions contain surfactant, an important substance necessary for normal pulmonary mechanics (see below). Unlike type I cells, type II pneumocytes are capable of cell division and can produce type I

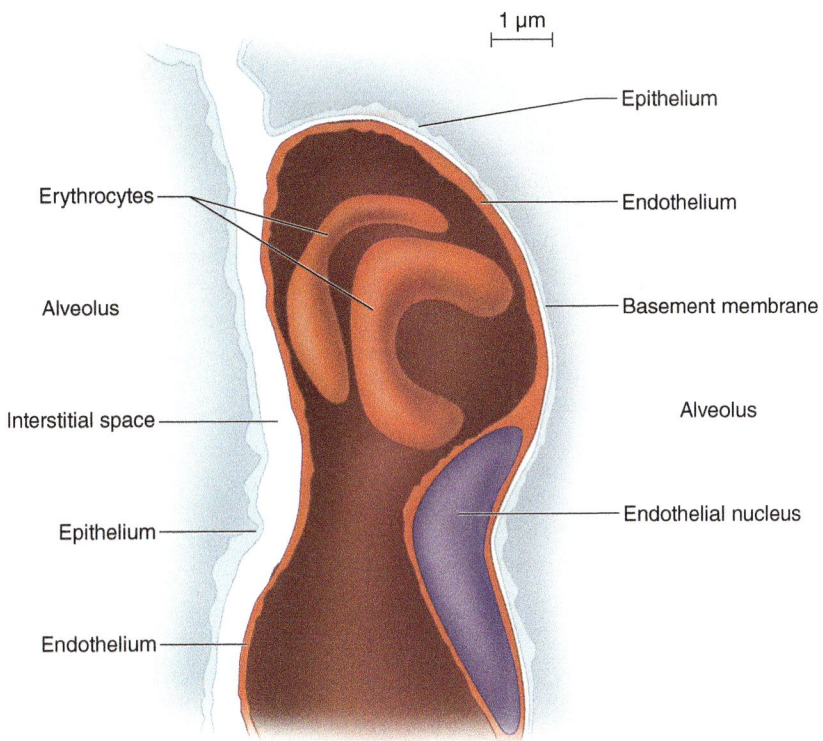

1 μm

Epithelium

Erythrocytes

Endothelium

Alveolus

Basement membrane

Alveolus

Interstitial space

Epithelium

Endothelial nucleus

Endothelium

FIGURE 23–2 The pulmonary interstitial space, with a capillary passing between the two alveoli. The capillary is incorporated into the thin (gas-exchanging) side of the alveolus on the right. The interstitial space is incorporated into the thick side of the alveolus on the left. (Reproduced, with permission, from Nunn JF: *Nunn's Applied Physiology*, 4th ed. Butterworth, 2000.)

pneumocytes if the latter are destroyed. They are also resistant to O_2 toxicity.

Other cell types present in the lower airways include pulmonary alveolar macrophages, mast cells, lymphocytes, and amino precursor uptake and decarboxylation (APUD) cells. Neutrophils are also typically present in smokers and patients with acute lung injury.

3. Pulmonary Circulation & Lymphatics

The lungs are supplied by two circulations, pulmonary and bronchial. The bronchial circulation arises from the left heart and sustains the metabolic needs of the tracheobronchial tree. The bronchial circulation provides a small amount of

blood flow (ie, less than 4% of the cardiac output). Branches of the bronchial artery supply the wall of the bronchi and follow the airways as far as the terminal bronchioles. Along their courses, the bronchial vessels anastomose with the pulmonary arterial circulation and continue as far as the alveolar duct. Below that level, lung tissue is supported by a combination of the alveolar gas and pulmonary circulation. Except for the main bronchi within the mediastinum, almost all the blood carried by the bronchial arteries enters the pulmonary circulation.

The pulmonary circulation normally receives the total output of the right heart via the pulmonary artery, which divides into right and left branches to supply each lung. Deoxygenated blood passes through the pulmonary capillaries, where O_2 is taken up and CO_2 is eliminated. The oxygenated blood is then returned to the left heart by four main pulmonary veins (two from each lung). Although flows through the systemic and pulmonary circulations are equal, the lower pulmonary vascular resistance results in pulmonary vascular pressures that are one-sixth of those in the systemic circulation; as a result, both pulmonary arteries and veins normally have thinner walls than systemic vessels with less smooth muscle.

There are connections between the bronchial and the pulmonary circulations. Direct pulmonary arteriovenous communications, bypassing the pulmonary capillaries, are normally insignificant but may become important in certain pathological states. The importance of the bronchial circulation in contributing to the normal venous admixture is discussed below.

Pulmonary Capillaries

Pulmonary capillaries are incorporated into the walls of alveoli. The average diameter of these capillaries (about 10 μm) is barely enough to allow passage of a single red cell. Because each capillary network supplies more than one alveolus, blood may pass through several alveoli before reaching the pulmonary veins. Because of the relatively low pressure in the pulmonary circulation, the amount of blood flowing through a given capillary network is affected by both gravity and alveolar size. Large alveoli have a smaller capillary cross-sectional area and consequently increased resistance to blood flow. In the upright position, apical capillaries tend to have reduced flows, whereas basal capillaries have higher flows.

The pulmonary capillary endothelium has relatively large junctions (5 nm wide), allowing the passage of large molecules such as albumin. As a result, pulmonary interstitial fluid is relatively rich in albumin. Circulating macrophages and neutrophils are able to pass through the endothelium, as well as the smaller alveolar epithelial junctions, with relative ease. Pulmonary macrophages are commonly seen in the interstitial space and inside alveoli; they serve to prevent bacterial infection and to scavenge foreign particles.

Pulmonary Lymphatics

Lymphatic channels in the lung originate in the interstitial spaces of large septa and are close to the bronchial arteries. Bronchial lymphatics return fluids, lost proteins, and various cells that have escaped in the peribronchovascular interstitium into the blood circulation, thus ensuring homeostasis and permitting lung function. Because of the large endothelial junctions, pulmonary lymph has a relatively high protein content, and total pulmonary lymph flow may be as much as 20 mL/hr. Large lymphatic vessels travel upward alongside the airways, forming the tracheobronchial chain of lymph nodes. Lymphatic drainage channels from both lungs communicate along the trachea.

4. Innervation

The diaphragm is innervated by the phrenic nerves, which arise from the C3–C5 nerve roots. Unilateral phrenic nerve block or palsy only modestly reduces most indices of pulmonary function (about 25%) in normal subjects. Although bilateral phrenic nerve palsies produce more severe impairment, accessory muscle activity may maintain adequate ventilation in some patients. Intercostal muscles are innervated by their respective thoracic nerve roots. Cervical cord injuries above C5 are incompatible with spontaneous ventilation because both phrenic and intercostal nerves are affected.

The vagus nerves provide sensory innervation to the tracheobronchial tree. Both sympathetic and parasympathetic autonomic innervation of bronchial smooth muscle and secretory glands is present. Vagal activity mediates bronchoconstriction and increases bronchial secretions via muscarinic receptors. Sympathetic activity (T1–T4) mediates bronchodilation and also decreases secretions via β_2-receptors. The nerve supply of the larynx is reviewed in Chapter 19.

Both α- and β-adrenergic receptors are present in the pulmonary vasculature, but the sympathetic system normally has little effect on pulmonary vascular tone. α_1-Activity causes vasoconstriction; β_2-activity mediates vasodilation. Parasympathetic vasodilatory activity seems to be mediated via the release of nitric oxide.

MECHANISMS OF BREATHING

② The periodic exchange of alveolar gas with the fresh gas from the upper airway reoxygenates desaturated blood and eliminates CO_2. This exchange is brought about by small cyclic pressure gradients established within the airways. During spontaneous ventilation, these gradients are secondary to variations in intrathoracic pressure; during mechanical ventilation, they are produced by intermittent positive pressure in the upper airway.

Spontaneous Ventilation

Normal pressure variations during spontaneous breathing are shown in **Figure 23–3**. The pressure within alveoli is always greater than the surrounding (intrathoracic) pressure unless the alveoli are collapsed. Alveolar pressure is normally atmospheric (zero for reference) at end-inspiration and end-expiration. By convention in pulmonary physiology, pleural pressure is used as a measure of intrathoracic pressure. Although it may not be entirely correct to refer to the pressure in a potential space, the concept allows the calculation of transpulmonary pressure. Transpulmonary pressure, or $P_{transpulmonary}$, is then defined as follows:

$$P_{transpulmonary} = P_{alveolar} - P_{intrapleural}$$

At end-expiration, intrapleural pressure normally averages about –5 cm H_2O, and because alveolar pressure is 0 (no flow), transpulmonary pressure is +5 cm H_2O.

Diaphragmatic and intercostal muscle activation during inspiration expands the chest and decreases intrapleural pressure from –5 cm H_2O to –8 or –9 cm H_2O. As a result, alveolar pressure also decreases (between –3 and –4 cm H_2O), and an alveolar–upper airway gradient is established; gas flows from the upper airway into alveoli. At end-inspiration (when gas inflow has ceased), alveolar pressure returns to zero, but intrapleural pressure remains decreased; the new transpulmonary pressure (5 cm H_2O) sustains lung expansion.

During expiration, diaphragmatic relaxation returns intrapleural pressure to –5 cm H_2O. Now the transpulmonary pressure does not support the new lung volume, and the elastic recoil of the lung causes a reversal of the previous alveolar–upper airway gradient; gas flows out of alveoli, and original lung volume is restored.

Mechanical Ventilation

Most forms of mechanical ventilation intermittently apply positive airway pressure at the upper airway. During inspiration, gas flows into alveoli until alveolar pressure reaches that in the upper airway. During the expiratory phase of the ventilator, the positive airway pressure is removed or decreased; the gradient reverses, allowing gas flow out of alveoli.

LUNG MECHANICS

The movement of the lungs is passive and determined by the impedance of the respiratory system, which can be divided into the elastic resistance of tissues and the gas–liquid interface and the nonelastic resistance to gas flow. Elastic resistance governs lung volume and the associated pressures under static conditions (no gas flow). Resistance to gas flow relates to frictional resistance to airflow and tissue deformation. The work necessary to overcome elastic resistance is stored as potential energy, but the work necessary to overcome nonelastic resistance is lost as heat.

1. Elastic Resistance

Both the lungs and the chest have elastic properties. The chest has a tendency to expand outward, whereas the lungs have a tendency to collapse. When the chest is exposed to atmospheric pressure (open pneumothorax), it usually expands about 1 L in adults. In contrast, when the lung is exposed to atmospheric pressure, it collapses completely and all the gas within it is expelled. The recoil properties of the chest are due to structural components that resist deformation and chest wall muscle tone. The elastic recoil of the lungs is due to their high content of elastin fibers, and, even more important, the surface tension forces acting at the air–fluid interface in alveoli.

Surface Tension Forces

The gas–fluid interface lining the alveoli causes them to behave as bubbles. Surface tension forces tend to

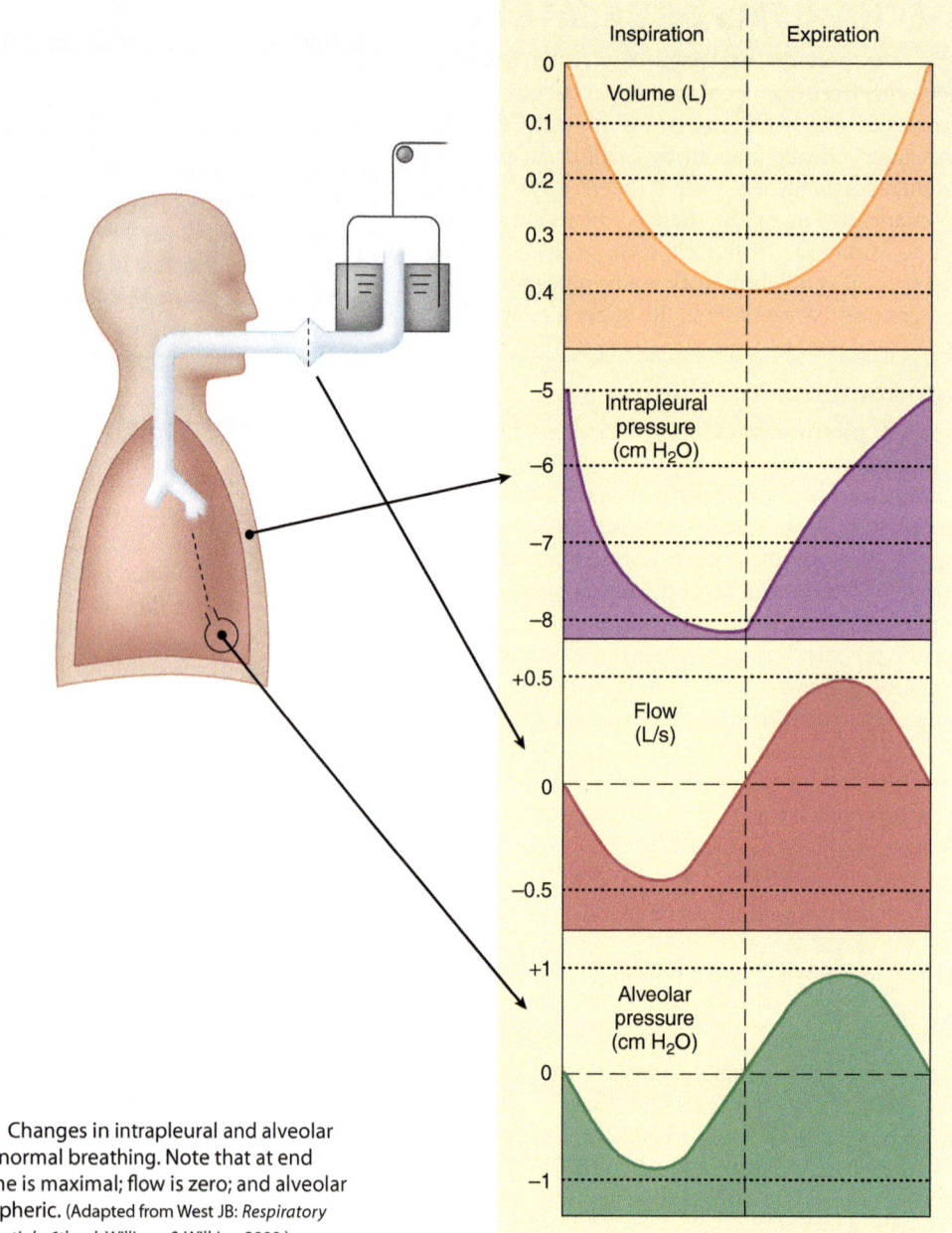

FIGURE 23–3 Changes in intrapleural and alveolar pressures during normal breathing. Note that at end inspiration, volume is maximal; flow is zero; and alveolar pressure is atmospheric. (Adapted from West JB: *Respiratory Physiology—The Essentials*, 6th ed. Williams & Wilkins, 2000.)

reduce the area of the interface and favor alveolar collapse. Laplace's law can be used to quantify these forces:

$$\text{Pressure} = \frac{2 \times \text{Surface tension}}{\text{Radius}}$$

The pressure derived from the equation is that within the alveolus. Alveolar collapse is therefore directly proportional to surface tension. **Fortunately, in contrast to a bubble, pulmonary surfactant decreases alveolar surface tension**. Moreover, the

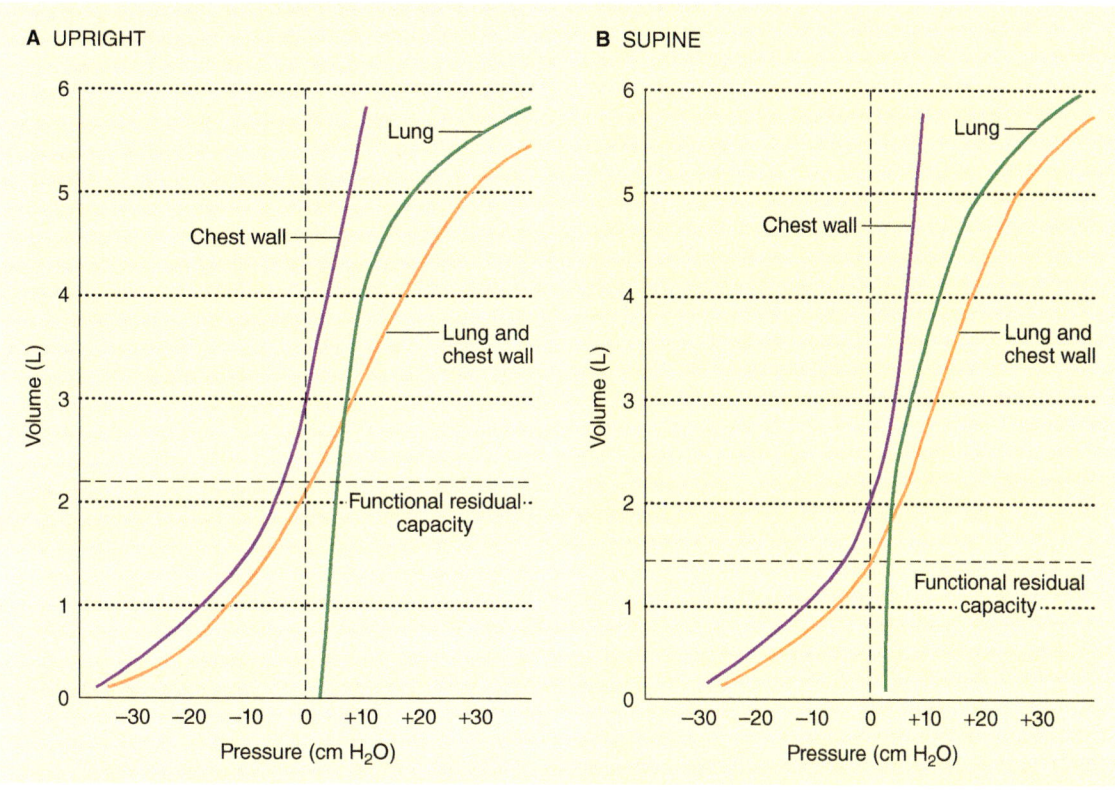

FIGURE 23-4 The pressure–volume relationship for the chest wall, lung, and both together in the upright (**A**) and supine (**B**) positions. (Modified and reproduced, with permission, from Scurr C, Feldman S: *Scientific Foundations of Anesthesia.* Heinemann, 1982.)

ability of the surfactant to lower surface tension is directly proportional to its concentration within the alveolus, resulting in lower intraalveolar pressure in smaller alveoli. As alveoli become smaller, the surfactant within becomes more concentrated, and surface tension is more effectively reduced. Conversely, when alveoli are overdistended, surfactant becomes less concentrated, and surface tension increases. The net effect is to stabilize alveoli; small alveoli are prevented from getting smaller, whereas large alveoli are prevented from getting larger.

Compliance

Elastic recoil is usually measured in terms of compliance (C), which is defined as the change in volume divided by the change in distending pressure. Compliance measurements can be obtained for either the chest, the lung, or both together (**Figure 23–4**).

In the supine position, chest wall compliance (C_W) is reduced because of the weight of the abdominal contents against the diaphragm. Measurements are usually obtained under static conditions, (ie, at equilibrium). (Dynamic lung compliance [$C_{dyn,L}$], which is measured during rhythmic breathing, is also dependent on airway resistance.) **Lung compliance (C_L)** is defined as

$$C_L = \frac{\text{Change in lung volume}}{\text{Change in transpulmonary pressure}}$$

C_L is normally 150–200 mL/cm H_2O. A variety of factors, including lung volume, pulmonary blood volume, extravascular lung water, and pathological processes (eg, inflammation and fibrosis) affect C_L

$$\text{Chest wall compliance} = \frac{\text{Change in chest volume}}{\text{Change in transthoracic pressure}}$$
$$(C_W)$$

where transthoracic pressure equals atmospheric pressure minus intrapleural pressure.

Normal chest wall compliance is 200 mL/cm H_2O. Total compliance (lung and chest wall together) is 100 mL/cm H_2O and is expressed by the following equation:

$$\frac{1}{C_{total}} = \frac{1}{C_W} + \frac{1}{C_L}$$

2. Lung Volumes

Lung volumes are important parameters in respiratory physiology and clinical practice (Table 23–1 and Figure 23–5). The sum of all of the named lung volumes equals the maximum to which the lung can be inflated. Lung capacities are clinically useful measurements that represent a combination of two or more volumes.

Functional Residual Capacity

3 The lung volume at the end of a normal exhalation is called functional residual capacity (FRC). At this volume, the inward elastic recoil of the lung approximates the outward elastic recoil of

TABLE 23–1 Lung volumes and capacities.

Measurement	Definition	Average Adult Values (mL)
Tidal volume (V_T)	Each normal breath	500
Inspiratory reserve volume (IRV)	Maximal additional volume that can be inspired above V_T	3000
Expiratory reserve volume (ERV)	Maximal volume that can be expired below V_T	1100
Residual volume (RV)	Volume remaining after maximal exhalation	1200
Total lung capacity (TLC)	$RV + ERV + V_T + IRV$	5800
Functional residual capacity (FRC)	$RV + ERV$	2300

the chest (including resting diaphragmatic tone). Thus, the elastic properties of both chest and lung define the point from which normal breathing takes place. Functional residual capacity can be measured by nitrogen washout or helium washin technique or

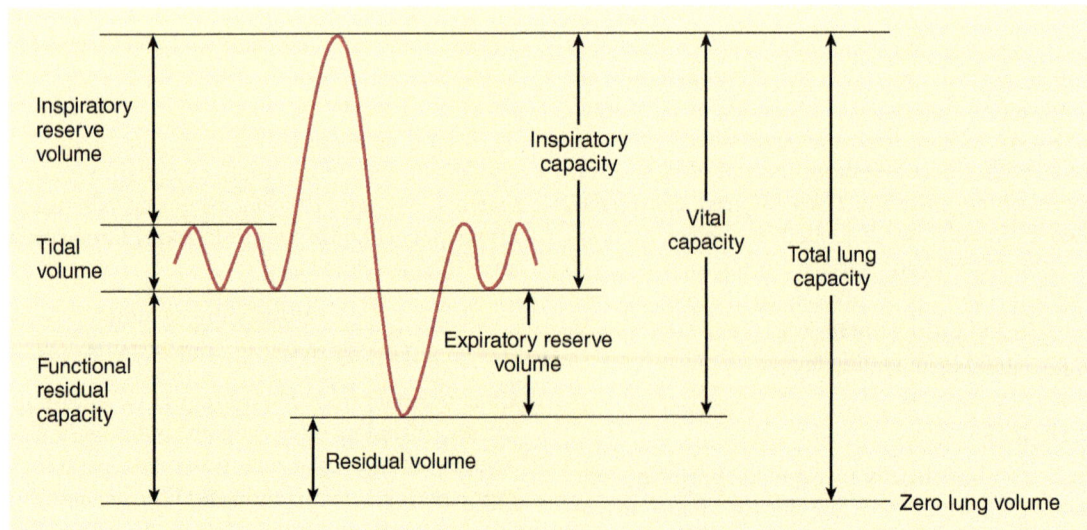

FIGURE 23–5 Spirogram showing static lung volumes. (Reproduced, with permission, from Nunn JF: *Nunn's Applied Physiology*, 4th ed. Butterworth, 2000.)

by body plethysmography. Factors known to alter the FRC include the following:

- **Body habitus:** FRC is directly proportional to height. Obesity, however, can markedly decrease FRC (primarily as a result of reduced chest compliance).

- **Sex:** FRC is reduced by about 10% in females compared with males.

- **Posture:** FRC decreases as a patient is moved from an upright to a supine or prone position. This is the result of reduced chest compliance as the abdominal contents push up against the diaphragm. The greatest change occurs between 0° and 60° of inclination. No further decrease is observed with a head-down position of up to 30°.

- **Lung disease:** Decreased compliance of the lung, chest, or both is characteristic of restrictive pulmonary disorders all of which are associated with a low FRC.

- **Diaphragmatic tone:** This normally contributes to FRC.

Closing Capacity

As described above (see the section on Functional Respiratory Anatomy), small airways lacking cartilaginous support depend on radial traction caused by the elastic recoil of surrounding tissue to keep them open; patency of these airways, particularly in basal areas of the lung, is highly dependent on lung volume. The volume at which these airways begin to close in dependent areas of the lung is called the **closing capacity**. At lower lung volumes, alveoli in dependent areas continue to be perfused but are no longer ventilated; **intrapulmonary shunting** of deoxygenated blood promotes hypoxemia (see below).

Closing capacity is usually measured using a tracer gas (xenon-133), which is inhaled near residual volume and then exhaled from total lung capacity.

4 Closing capacity is normally well below FRC (Figure 23–6), but rises steadily with age (Figure 23–7). This increase is probably responsible for the normal age-related decline in arterial O_2 tension. At an average age of 44 years, closing capacity

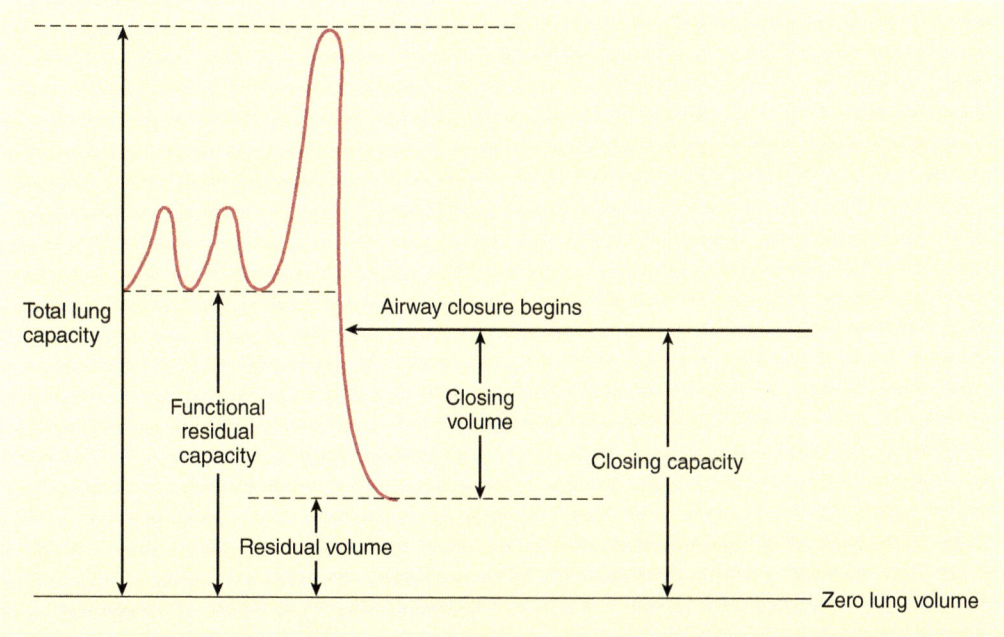

FIGURE 23–6 The relationship between functional residual capacity, closing volume, and closing capacity. (Reproduced, with permission, from Nunn JF: *Nunn's Applied Physiology*, 4th ed. Butterworth, 2000.)

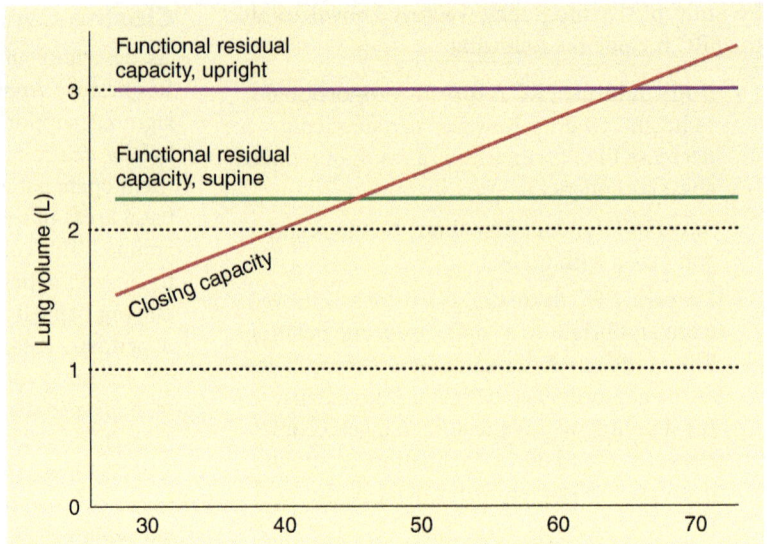

FIGURE 23–7 The effect of age on closing capacity and its relationship to functional residual capacity (FRC). Note that FRC does not change. (Reproduced, with permission, from Nunn JF: *Nunn's Applied Physiology*, 4th ed. Butterworth, 2000.)

equals FRC in the supine position; by age 66, closing capacity equals or exceeds FRC in the upright position in most individuals. Unlike FRC, closing capacity is unaffected by posture.

Vital Capacity

Vital capacity (VC) is the maximum volume of gas that can be exhaled following maximal inspiration. In addition to body habitus, VC is also dependent on respiratory muscle strength and chest–lung compliance. Normal VC is about 60–70 mL/kg.

3. Nonelastic Resistances

Airway Resistance to Gas Flow

Gas flow in the lung is a mixture of laminar and turbulent flow. Laminar flow can be thought of as consisting of concentric cylinders of gas flowing at different velocities; velocity is highest in the center and decreases toward the periphery. During laminar flow,

$$\text{Flow} = \frac{\text{Pressure gradient}}{R_{aw}}$$

where R_{aw} is airway resistance.

$$R_{aw} = \frac{8 \times \text{Length} \times \text{Gas viscosity}}{\pi \times (\text{Radius})^4}$$

Turbulent flow is characterized by random movement of the gas molecules down the air passages. Mathematical description of turbulent flow is considerably more complex:

$$\text{Pressure gradient} \approx \text{Flow}^2 \times \frac{\text{Gas density}}{\text{Radius}^5}$$

Resistance is not constant but increases in proportion to gas flow. Moreover, resistance is directly proportional to gas density and inversely proportional to the fifth power of the radius. As a result, turbulent gas flow is extremely sensitive to airway caliber.

Turbulence generally occurs at high gas flows, at sharp angles or branching points, and in response to abrupt changes in airway diameter. Whether turbulent or laminar flow occurs can be predicted by the Reynolds number, which results from the following equation:

$$\text{Reynolds number} = \frac{\text{Linear velocity} \times \text{Diameter} \times \text{Gas density}}{\text{Gas viscosity}}$$

A low Reynolds number (<1000) is associated with laminar flow, whereas a high value (>1500) produces turbulent flow. Laminar flow normally occurs only distal to small bronchioles (<1 mm). Flow in larger airways is probably turbulent. Of the

TABLE 23-2 Physical properties of several gas mixtures.[1]

Mixture	Viscosity[2]	Density[2]	Density/Viscosity[2]
Oxygen (100%)	1.11	1.11	1.00
N_2O/O_2	0.89	1.41	1.49
Helium/O_2 (80:20)	1.08	0.33	0.31

[1]Data from Nunn JF: *Nunn's Applied Physiology*, 4th ed. Butterworth, 2000.

[2]Viscosities and densities are expressed relative to air.

gases used clinically, only helium has a significantly lower density-to-viscosity ratio, making it useful clinically during severe turbulent flow (as caused by upper airway obstruction). A helium–O_2 mixture not only is less likely to cause turbulent flow but also reduces airway resistance when turbulent flow is present (Table 23–2).

Normal total airway resistance is about 0.5–2 cm H_2O/L/sec, with the largest contribution coming from medium-sized bronchi (before the seventh generation). Resistance in large bronchi is low because of their large diameters, whereas resistance in small bronchi is low because of their large total cross-sectional area. The most important causes of increased airway resistance include bronchospasm, secretions, and mucosal edema as well as volume-related and flow-related airway collapse.

A. Volume-Related Airway Collapse

At low lung volumes, loss of radial traction increases the contribution of small airways to total resistance; airway resistance becomes inversely proportional to lung volume (Figure 23–8). Increasing lung volume up to normal with positive end-expiratory pressure (PEEP) can reduce airway resistance.

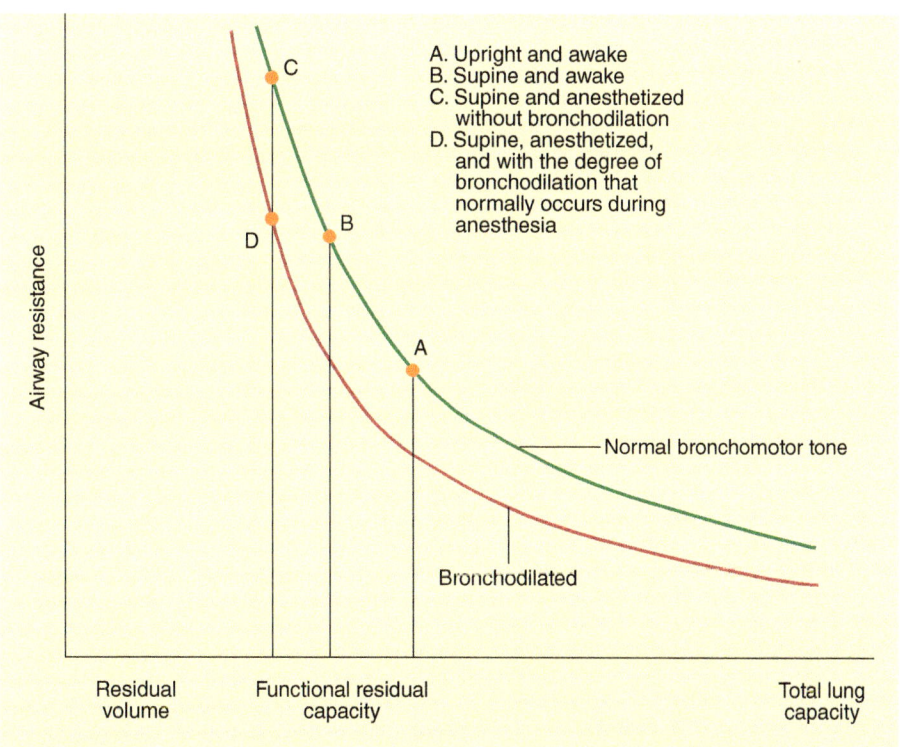

FIGURE 23-8 The relationship between airway resistance and lung volume. (Reproduced, with permission, from Nunn JF: *Nunn's Applied Physiology*, 4th ed. Butterworth, 2000.)

B. Flow-Related Airway Collapse

During forced exhalation, reversal of the normal transmural airway pressure can cause collapse of these airways (dynamic airway compression). Two contributing factors are responsible: generation of a positive pleural pressure and a large pressure drop across intrathoracic airways as a result of increased airway resistance. The latter is in turn due to high

(turbulent) gas flow and the reduced lung volume. The terminal portion of the flow/volume curve is therefore considered to be effort independent (Figure 23–9).

The point along the airways where dynamic compression occurs is called the equal pressure point. It is normally beyond the eleventh to thirteenth generation of bronchioles where cartilaginous support is

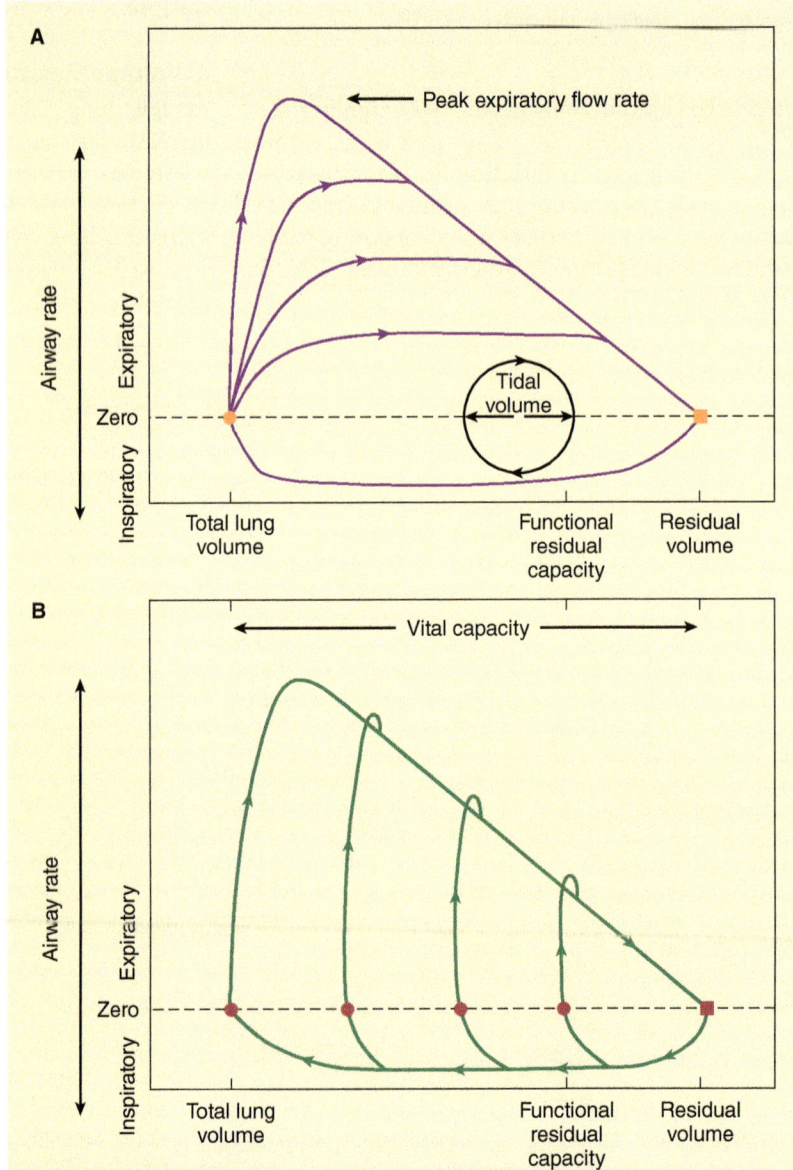

FIGURE 23–9 Gas flow (**A**) during forced exhalation from total lung capacity with varying effort and (**B**) with maximal effort from different lung volumes. Note that regardless of initial lung volume or effort, terminal expiratory flows are effort independent. (Reproduced, with permission, from Nunn JF: *Nunn's Applied Physiology,* 4th ed. Butterworth, 2000.)

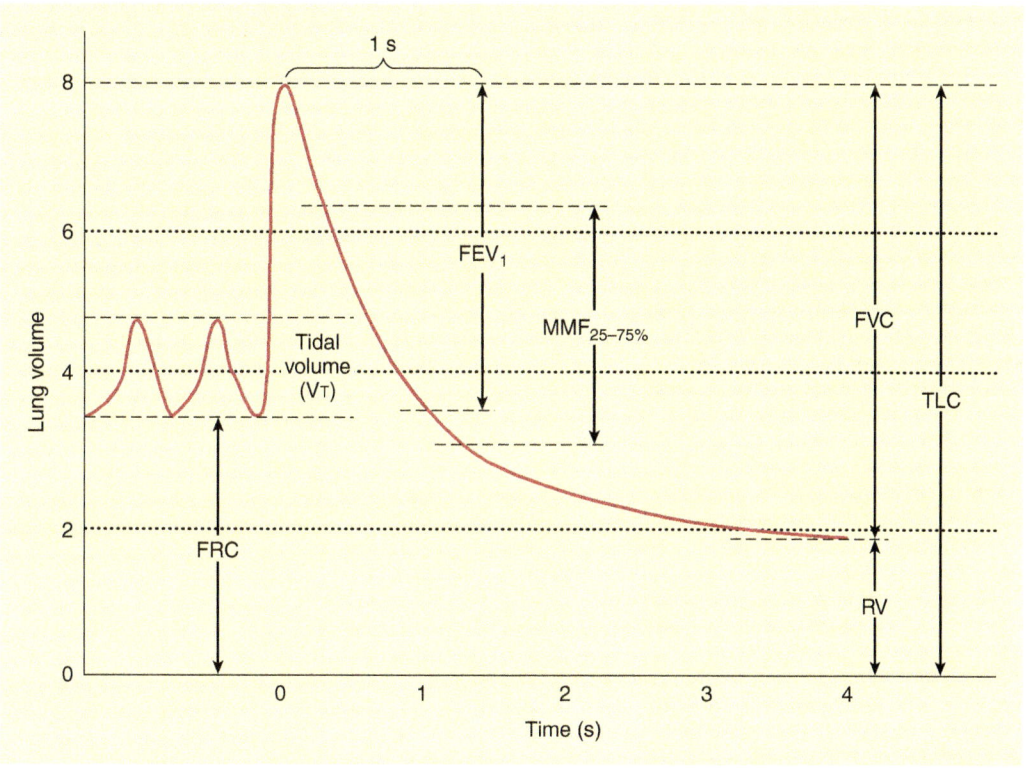

FIGURE 23–10 The normal forced exhalation curve. $FEF_{25-75\%}$ is also called the maximum midexpiratory flow rate ($MMF_{25-75\%}$). FRC, functional residual capacity; FEV_1, forced expiratory volume in 1 sec; FVC, forced vital capacity; RV, residual volume; TLC, total lung capacity.

absent (see above). The equal pressure point moves toward smaller airways as lung volume decreases. Emphysema or asthma predisposes patients to dynamic airway compression. Emphysema destroys the elastic tissues that normally support smaller airways. In patients with asthma, bronchoconstriction and mucosal edema intensify airway collapse and promote reversal of transmural pressure gradients across airways. Patients may terminate exhalation prematurely or purse their lips to increase expiratory resistance at the mouth. Premature termination of exhalation may increase FRC above normal, resulting in air trapping and auto-PEEP.

C. Forced Vital Capacity
Measuring vital capacity as an exhalation that is as forceful and rapid as possible (**Figure 23–10**)

provides important information about airway resistance. The ratio of the forced expiratory volume in the first second of exhalation (FEV_1) to the total forced vital capacity (FVC) is proportional to the degree of airway obstruction. Normally, FEV_1/FVC is ≥80%. Whereas both FEV_1 and FVC are effort dependent, forced midexpiratory flow ($FEF_{25-75\%}$) is more effort independent and may be a more reliable measurement of obstruction.

Tissue Resistance
This component of nonelastic resistance is generally underestimated and often overlooked, but may account for up to half of total airway resistance. It seems to be primarily due to viscoelastic (frictional) resistance of tissues to gas flow.

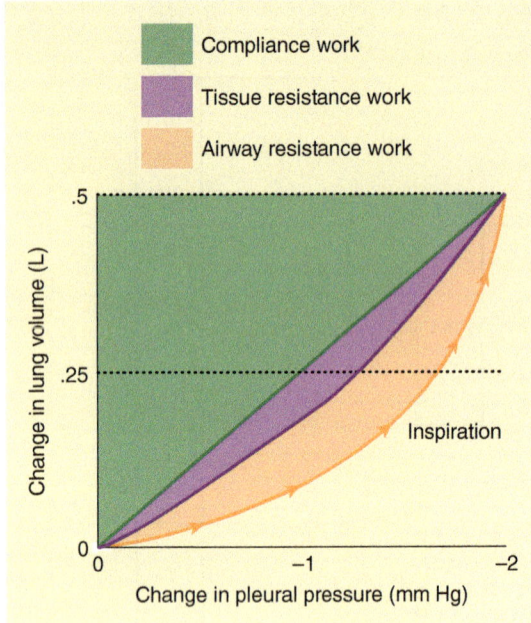

FIGURE 23–11 The work of breathing and its components during inspiration. (Reproduced, with permission, from Guyton AC: *Textbook of Medical Physiology*, 7th ed. W.B. Saunders, 1986.)

4. Work of Breathing

Because expiration is normally entirely passive, both the inspiratory and the expiratory work of breathing is performed by the inspiratory muscles (primarily the diaphragm). Three factors must be overcome during ventilation: the elastic recoil of the chest and lung, frictional resistance to gas flow in the airways, and tissue frictional resistance.

Respiratory work can be expressed as the product of volume and pressure (Figure 23–11). During inhalation, both inspiratory airway resistance and pulmonary elastic recoil must be overcome; nearly 50% of the energy expended is stored pulmonary elastic recoil. During exhalation, the stored potential energy is released and overcomes expiratory airway resistance. Increases in either inspiratory or expiratory resistance are compensated by increased inspiratory muscle effort. When expiratory resistance increases, the normal compensatory response is to increase lung volume such that V_T breathing occurs at an abnormally high FRC. The greater elastic recoil

energy stored at a higher lung volume overcomes the added expiratory resistance. Excessive amounts of expiratory resistance also activate expiratory muscles (see above).

Respiratory muscles normally account for only 2% to 3% of O_2 consumption but operate at about 10% efficiency. Ninety percent of the work is dissipated as heat (due to elastic and airflow resistance). In pathological conditions that increase the load on the diaphragm, muscle efficiency usually progressively decreases, and contraction may become uncoordinated with increasing ventilatory effort; moreover, a point may be reached whereby any increase in O_2 uptake (because of augmented ventilation) is consumed by the respiratory muscles themselves.

The work required to overcome elastic resistance increases as V_T increases, whereas the work required to overcome airflow resistance increases as respiratory rate (and, necessarily, expiratory flow) increases. Faced with either condition, patients minimize the work of breathing by altering the respiratory rate and V_T (Figure 23–12). **Patients with reduced compliance tend to have rapid, shallow breaths, whereas those with increased airflow resistance have a slow, deep breathing pattern.**

5. Effects of Anesthesia on Pulmonary Mechanics

The effects of anesthesia on breathing are complex and relate to changes both in position and anesthetic agent.

Effects on Lung Volumes & Compliance

⑥   Changes in lung mechanics due to general anesthesia occur shortly after induction. The supine position reduces the FRC by 0.8–1.0 L, and induction of general anesthesia further reduces the FRC by 0.4–0.5 L. FRC reduction is a consequence of alveolar collapse and compression atelectasis due to loss of inspiratory muscle tone, change in chest wall rigidity, and upward shift of the diaphragm. The mechanisms may be more complex; for example, only the dependent (dorsal) part of the diaphragm in the supine position moves cephalad. Other factors are likely due to a change in intrathoracic volume secondary to increased blood volume in the lung and changes in

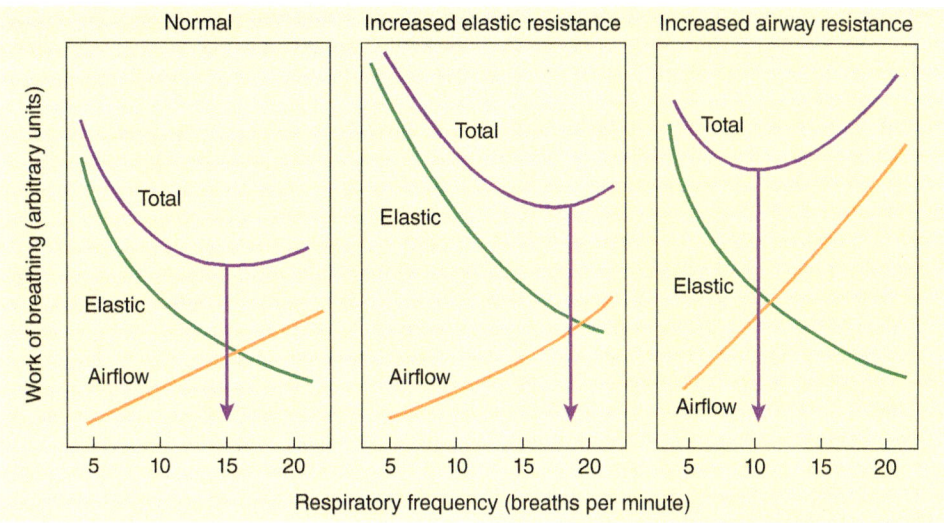

FIGURE 23–12 The work of breathing in relation to respiratory rate for normal individuals, patients with increased elastic resistance, and patients with increased airway resistance. (Reproduced, with permission, from Nunn JF: *Nunn's Applied Physiology*, 4th ed. Butterworth, 2000.)

chest wall shape (Figure 23–13). The higher position of the dorsal diaphragm and changes in the thoracic cavity itself decrease lung volumes. This decrease in FRC is not related to anesthetic depth and may persist for several hours or days after anesthesia. Steep head-down (Trendelenburg) position (>30°) may reduce FRC even further as intrathoracic blood volume increases. In contrast, induction of anesthesia in the sitting position seems to have little effect on FRC. Muscle paralysis does not seem to change FRC significantly when the patient is already anesthetized.

The effects of anesthesia on closing capacity are more variable. Both FRC and closing capacity, however, are generally reduced to the same extent under anesthesia. Thus, the risk of increased intrapulmonary shunting under anesthesia is similar to that in the conscious state; it is greatest in the elderly, in obese patients, and in those with underlying pulmonary disease.

Effects on Airway Resistance

The reduction in FRC associated with general anesthesia would be expected to increase airway resistance. Increases in airway resistance are not usually observed, however, because of the bronchodilating properties of the volatile inhalation anesthetics.

Awake

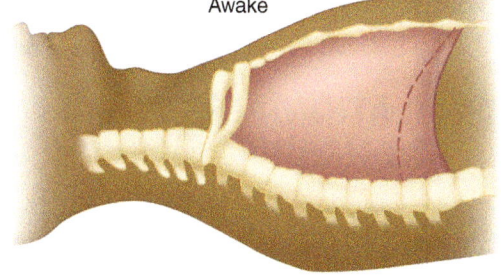

Anesthetized

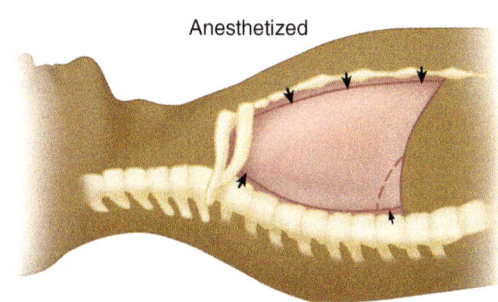

FIGURE 23–13 With induction of anesthesia in the supine position, the abdominal contents exert cephalad pressure on the diaphragm. At end-expiration, the dorsal portion of the diaphragm is more cephalad and the ventral portion is more caudal than when awake, the thoracic spine is more lordotic, and the rib cage moves inward, all secondary to loss of motor tone.

Increased airway resistance is more commonly due to pathological factors (posterior displacement of the tongue; laryngospasm; bronchoconstriction; or secretions, blood, or tumor in the airway) or equipment problems (small tracheal tubes or connectors, malfunction of valves, or obstruction of the breathing circuit).

Effects on the Work of Breathing

Increases in the work of breathing under anesthesia are most often secondary to reduced lung and chest wall compliance, and, less commonly, increases in airway resistance (see above). The problems of increased work of breathing are usually circumvented by controlled mechanical ventilation.

Effects on the Respiratory Pattern

Regardless of the agent used, light anesthesia often results in irregular breathing patterns; breath holding is common. Breaths become regular with deeper levels of anesthesia. Inhalation agents generally produce rapid, shallow breaths, whereas nitrous–opioid techniques result in slow, deep breaths.

VENTILATION/PERFUSION RELATIONSHIPS

1. Ventilation

Ventilation is usually measured as the sum of all exhaled gas volumes in 1 min (minute ventilation, or $\dot{V}$).

Minute ventilation = Respiratory rate × Tidal volume

For the average adult at rest, minute ventilation is about 5 L/min.

Not all of the inspired gas mixture reaches alveoli; some of it remains in the airways and is exhaled without being exchanged with alveolar gases. The part of the V_T not participating in alveolar gas exchange is known as dead space (V_D). Alveolar ventilation ($\dot{V}_A$) is the volume of inspired gases actually taking part in gas exchange in 1 min.

$$\dot{V}_A = \text{Respiratory rate} \times V_T - V_D$$

Dead space is actually composed of gases in nonrespiratory airways (**anatomic dead space**) and

TABLE 23–3 Factors affecting dead space.

Factor	Effect
Posture	
Upright	↑
Supine	↓
Position of airway	
Neck extension	↑
Neck flexion	↓
Age	↑
Artificial airway	↓
Positive-pressure ventilation	↑
Drugs—anticholinergic	↑
Pulmonary perfusion	
Pulmonary emboli	↑
Hypotension	↑
Pulmonary vascular disease	
Emphysema	↑

alveoli that are not perfused (**alveolar dead space**). The sum of the two components is referred to as **physiological dead space**. In the upright position, dead space is normally about 150 mL for most adults (approximately 2 mL/kg) and is nearly all anatomic. The weight of an individual in pounds is roughly equivalent to dead space in milliliters. Dead space can be affected by a variety of factors (Table 23–3).

Because V_T in the average adult is approximately 450 mL (6 mL/kg), V_D/V_T is normally 33%. This ratio can be derived by the Bohr equation:

$$\frac{V_D}{V_T} = \frac{P_{ACO_2} - P_{ECO_2}}{P_{ACO_2}}$$

where P_{ACO_2} is the alveolar CO_2 tension and P_{ECO_2} is the mixed expired CO_2 tension. This equation is useful clinically if arterial CO_2 tension (Pa_{CO_2}) is used to approximate the alveolar concentration and the CO_2 tension in expired air gases is the average measured over several minutes.

Distribution of Ventilation

Regardless of body position, alveolar ventilation is unevenly distributed in the lungs. The right lung receives more ventilation than the left lung

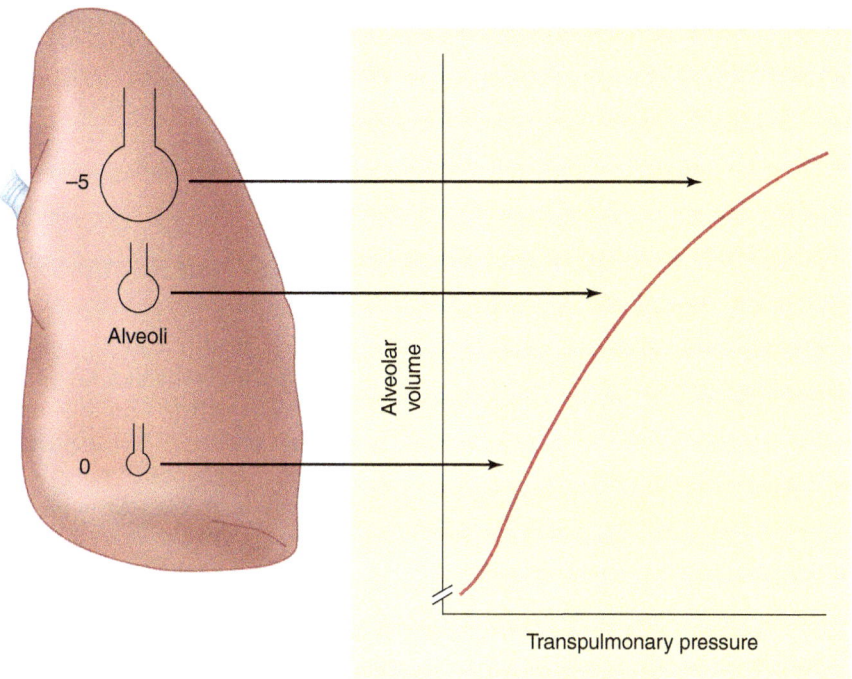

FIGURE 23–14 The effect of gravity on alveolar compliance in the upright position.

(53% vs 47%), and the lower (dependent) areas of both lungs tend to be better ventilated than do the upper areas because of a gravitationally induced gradient in intrapleural pressure (transpulmonary pressure). Pleural pressure decreases about 1 cm H_2O (becomes less negative) per 3-cm decrease in lung height. This difference places alveoli from different areas at different points on the pulmonary compliance curve (Figure 23–14). Because of a higher transpulmonary pressure, alveoli in upper lung areas are near-maximally inflated and relatively noncompliant, and they undergo little expansion during inspiration. In contrast, the smaller alveoli in dependent areas have a lower transpulmonary pressure, are more compliant, and undergo greater expansion during inspiration.

Airway resistance can also contribute to regional differences in pulmonary ventilation. Final alveolar inspiratory volume is solely dependent on compliance only if inspiratory time is unlimited. In reality, inspiratory time is necessarily limited by the respiratory rate and the time necessary for expiration; consequently,

an excessively short inspiratory time will prevent alveoli from reaching the expected change in volume. Moreover, alveolar filling follows an exponential function that is dependent on both compliance and airway resistance. Therefore, even with a normal inspiratory time, abnormalities in either compliance or resistance can prevent complete alveolar filling.

Time Constants

Lung inflation can be described mathematically by the time constant, τ.

$$\tau = \text{Total compliance} \times \text{Airway resistance}$$

Regional variations in resistance or compliance not only interfere with alveolar filling but can cause asynchrony in alveolar filling during inspiration; some alveolar units may continue to fill as others empty.

Variations in time constants within the normal lung can be demonstrated in normal individuals breathing spontaneously during abnormally high respiratory rates. Rapid shallow breathing reverses the normal distribution of ventilation, preferentially favoring upper (nondependent) areas of the lung over the lower areas.

2. Pulmonary Perfusion

Of the approximately 5 L/min of blood flowing through the lungs, only about 70–100 mL at any one time are within the pulmonary capillaries undergoing gas exchange. At the alveolar–capillary membrane, this small volume forms a 50–100 m²-sheet of blood approximately one red cell thick. Moreover, to ensure optimal gas exchange, each capillary perfuses more than one alveolus.

Although capillary volume remains relatively constant, total pulmonary blood volume can vary between 500 mL and 1000 mL. Large increases in either cardiac output or blood volume are tolerated with little change in pressure as a result of passive dilation of open vessels and perhaps some recruitment of collapsed pulmonary vessels. Small increases in pulmonary blood volume normally occur during cardiac systole and with each normal (spontaneous) inspiration. A shift in posture from supine to erect decreases pulmonary blood volume (up to 27%); Trendelenburg positioning has the opposite effect. Changes in systemic capacitance also influence pulmonary blood volume: systemic venoconstriction shifts blood from the systemic to the pulmonary circulation, whereas vasodilation causes a pulmonary-to-systemic redistribution. In this way, the lung acts as a reservoir for the systemic circulation.

7 Local factors are more important than the autonomic system in influencing pulmonary vascular tone (above). Hypoxia is a powerful stimulus for pulmonary vasoconstriction (the opposite of its systemic effect). Both pulmonary arterial (mixed venous) and alveolar hypoxia induce vasoconstriction, but the latter is a more powerful stimulus. This response seems to be due to either the direct effect of hypoxia on the pulmonary vasculature or increased production of leukotrienes relative to vasodilatory prostaglandins. Inhibition of nitric oxide production may also play a role. Hypoxic pulmonary vasoconstriction is an important physiological mechanism in reducing intrapulmonary shunting and preventing hypoxemia (see below). Hyperoxia has little effect on the pulmonary circulation in normal individuals. Hypercapnia and acidosis have a constrictor effect, whereas hypocapnia causes pulmonary vasodilation, the opposite of what occurs in the systemic circulation.

Distribution of Pulmonary Perfusion

Pulmonary blood flow is also not uniform. Regardless of body position, lower (dependent) areas of the lung receive greater blood flow than upper (nondependent) areas. This pattern is the result of a gravitational gradient of 1 cm H_2O/cm lung height. The normally low pressures in the pulmonary circulation allow gravity to exert a significant influence on blood flow. Also, in vivo perfusion scanning in normal individuals has shown an "onion-like" layering distribution of perfusion, with reduced flow at the periphery of the lung and increased perfusion toward the hilum.

Although the pulmonary perfusion pressure is not uniform across the lung, the alveolar distending pressure is relatively constant. The interplay of these pressures results in the dividing of the lung into four distinct zones (ie, the West Zones) (**Figure 23–15**). In zone 1 (PA > Pa > Pv), alveolar pressure (PA) is greater than both the arterial pulmonary pressure (Pa) and venous pulmonary pressure (Pv), resulting in obstruction of blood flow and creation of alveolar dead space. Zone 1 is fairly small in a spontaneously breathing individual, but can enlarge during positive pressure ventilation. In lower areas of the lungs, Pa progressively increases due to lower elevation above the heart. In zone 2 (Pa > PA > Pv), Pa is higher than PA, but Pv remains lower than both, resulting in blood flow that is dependent on the differential between Pa and PA. The bulk of the lung is described by zone 3 (Pa > Pv > PA), where both Pa and Pv are higher than PA, resulting in blood flow independent of the alveolar pressure. Zone 4, the most dependent part of the lung, is where atelectasis and/or interstitial pulmonary edema occur, resulting in blood flow that is dependent on the differential between Pa and pulmonary interstitial pressure.

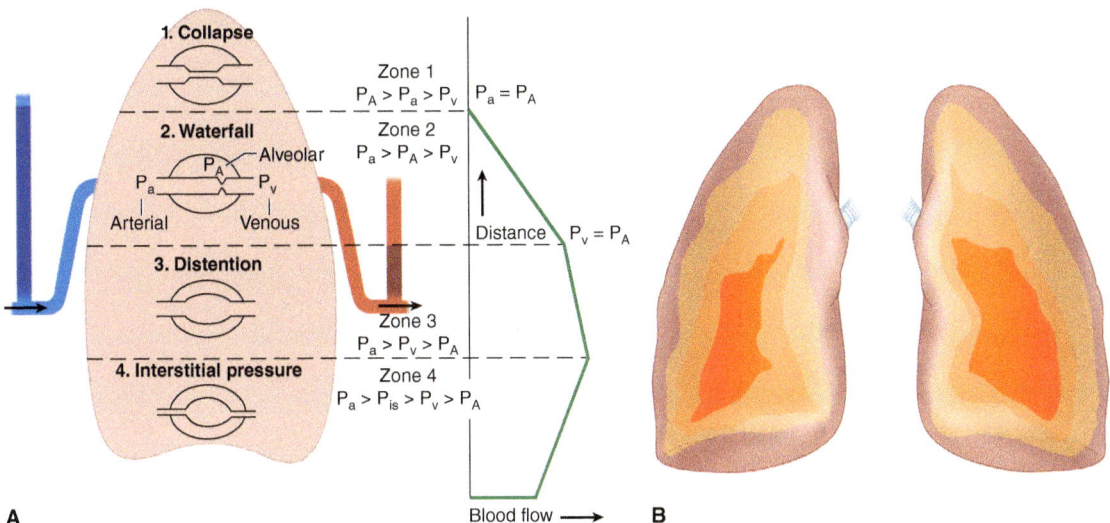

FIGURE 23–15 Pulmonary blood flow distribution relative to the alveolar pressure (P_A), the pulmonary arterial pressure (P_a), the pulmonary venous pressure (P_v), and the interstitial pressure (P_{is}) at various gravitation levels. **A**: Classic West Zones of blood flow distribution in the upright position. (Modified and reproduced, with permission, from West JB: *Respiratory Physiology: The Essentials*, 6th edition. Williams and Wilkins, 2000. p. 37.). **B**: In vivo perfusion scanning illustrating central-to-peripheral, in addition to gravitational blood flow distribution, in the upright position. (Reproduced, with permission, from Lohser J: Evidence based management of one lung ventilation. Anesthesiol Clin 2008;26:241.)

Ventilation/Perfusion Ratios

8 Because alveolar ventilation ($\dot{V}_A$) is normally about 4 L/min, and pulmonary capillary perfusion ($\dot{Q}$) is 5 L/min, the overall $\dot{V}/\dot{Q}$ ratio is about 0.8. $\dot{V}/\dot{Q}$ for individual lung units (each alveolus and its capillary) can range from 0 (no ventilation) to infinity (no perfusion); the former is referred to as intrapulmonary shunt, whereas the latter constitutes alveolar dead space. $\dot{V}/\dot{Q}$ normally ranges between 0.3 and 3.0; the majority of lung areas, however, are close to 1.0 (Figure 23–16A). Because perfusion increases at a greater rate than ventilation, nondependent (apical) areas tend to have higher $\dot{V}/\dot{Q}$ ratios than do dependent (basal) areas (Figure 23–16B).

The importance of $\dot{V}/\dot{Q}$ ratios relates to the efficiency with which lung units resaturate venous blood with O_2 and eliminate CO_2. **Pulmonary venous blood (the effluent) from areas with low $\dot{V}/\dot{Q}$ ratios has a low O_2 tension and high CO_2 tension—similar to systemic mixed venous blood.**

Blood from these units tends to depress arterial O_2 tension and elevate arterial CO_2 tension. Their effect on arterial O_2 tension is much more profound than that on CO_2 tension; in fact, arterial CO_2 tension often decreases from a hypoxemia-induced reflex increase in alveolar ventilation. An appreciable compensatory increase in O_2 uptake cannot take place in remaining areas where $\dot{V}/\dot{Q}$ is normal, because pulmonary end-capillary blood is usually already maximally saturated with O_2 (see below).

3. Shunts

9 Shunting denotes the process whereby desaturated, mixed venous blood from the right heart returns to the left heart without being resaturated with O_2 in the lungs (Figure 23–17). The overall effect of shunting is to decrease (dilute) arterial O_2 content; this type of shunt is referred to as right-to-left. Left-to-right shunts (in the absence of

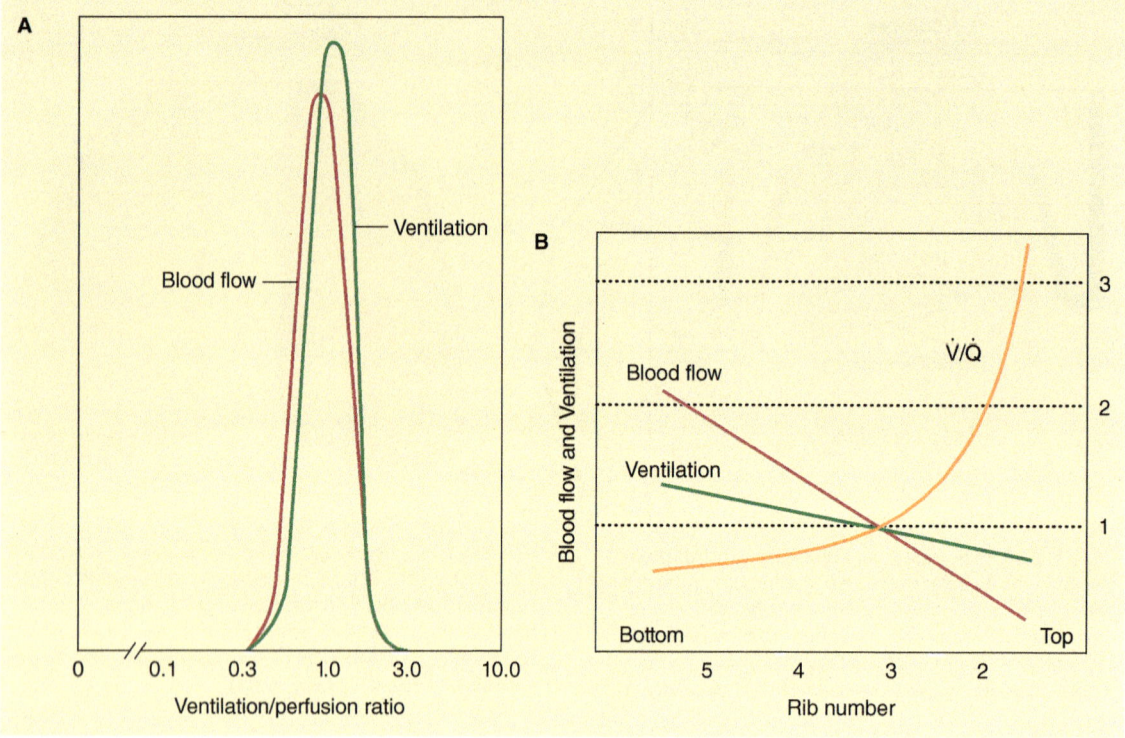

FIGURE 23–16 The distribution of $\dot{V}/\dot{Q}$ ratios for the whole lung (**A**) and according to height (**B**) in the upright position. Note that blood flow increases more rapidly than ventilation in dependent areas. (Reproduced, with permission, from West JB: *Ventilation/Blood Flow and Gas Exchange*, 3rd ed. Blackwell, 1977.)

pulmonary congestion), however, do not produce hypoxemia.

Intrapulmonary shunts are often classified as absolute or relative. Absolute shunt refers to anatomic shunts and lung units where $\dot{V}/\dot{Q}$ is zero. A relative shunt is an area of the lung with a low $\dot{V}/\dot{Q}$ ratio. Clinically, hypoxemia from a relative shunt can usually be partially corrected by increasing the inspired O_2 concentration; hypoxemia caused by an absolute shunt cannot.

Venous Admixture

Venous admixture refers to a concept rather than an actual physiological entity. **Venous admixture** is the amount of mixed venous blood that would have to be mixed with pulmonary end-capillary blood to account for the difference in O_2 tension between arterial and pulmonary end-capillary blood. Pulmonary end-capillary blood is considered to have the same

concentrations as alveolar gas. Venous admixture is usually expressed as a fraction of total cardiac output ($\dot{Q}s/\dot{Q}T$). The equation for $\dot{Q}s/\dot{Q}T$ may be derived with the law for the conservation of mass for O_2 across the pulmonary bed:

$$\dot{Q}T \times Ca_{O_2} = (\dot{Q}s \times C\overline{v}_{O_2}) + (\dot{Q}c' \times Cc'_{O_2})$$

where

$\dot{Q}s$ = blood flow through the physiologic shunt compartment

$\dot{Q}T$ = total cardiac output

$\dot{Q}c'$ = blood flow across normally ventilated pulmonary capillaries

$\dot{Q}T$ = $\dot{Q}c' + \dot{Q}s$

Cc'_{O_2} = oxygen content of ideal pulmonary end-capillary blood

Ca_{O_2} = arterial oxygen content

$C\overline{v}_{O_2}$ = mixed venous content

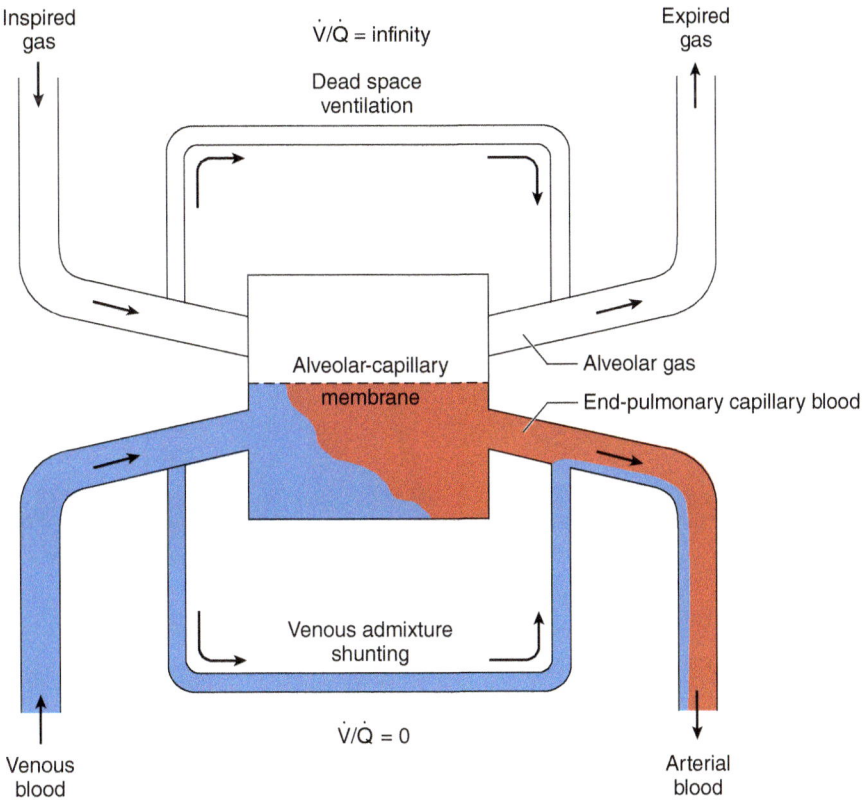

FIGURE 23-17 A three-compartment model of gas exchange in the lungs, showing dead space ventilation, normal alveolar–capillary exchange, and shunting (venous admixture). (Reproduced, with permission, from Nunn JF: *Nunn's Applied Physiology,* 4th ed. Butterworth, 2000.)

The simplified equation is

$$\dot{Q}s/\dot{Q}\text{T} = \frac{Cc'o_2 - Cao_2}{Cc'o_2 - C\overline{v}o_2}$$

The formula for calculating the O_2 content of blood is given below.

$\dot{Q}s/\dot{Q}\text{T}$ can be calculated clinically by obtaining mixed venous and arterial blood gas measurements; the former requires a pulmonary artery catheter. The alveolar gas equation is used to derive pulmonary end-capillary O_2 tension. Pulmonary capillary blood is usually assumed to be 100% saturated for an $FIO_2 \geq 0.21$.

The calculated venous admixture assumes that all shunting is intrapulmonary and due to absolute shunts ($\dot{V}/\dot{Q} = 0$). In reality, neither is ever the case; nonetheless, the concept is useful clinically. Normal $\dot{Q}s/\dot{Q}\text{T}$ is primarily due to communication between deep bronchial veins and pulmonary veins, the thebesian circulation in the heart, and areas of low $\dot{V}/\dot{Q}$ in the lungs (Figure 23–18). The venous admixture in normal individuals (physiological shunt) is typically less than 5%.

4. Effects of Anesthesia on Gas Exchange

Abnormalities in gas exchange during anesthesia are common. They include increased dead space, hypoventilation, and increased intrapulmonary shunting. There is increased scatter of $\dot{V}/\dot{Q}$ ratios. Increases in alveolar dead space are most commonly seen during controlled ventilation, but may also

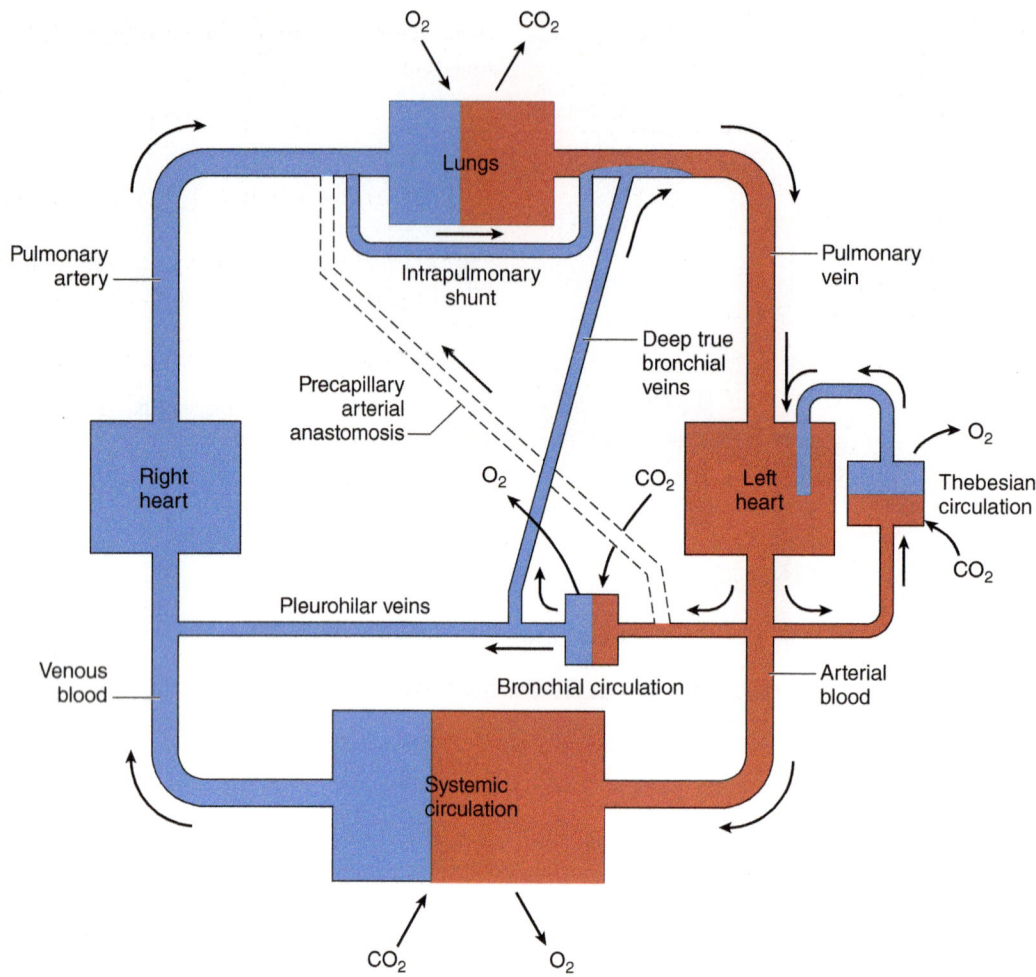

FIGURE 23–18 Components of the normal venous admixture. (Reproduced, with permission, from Nunn JF: *Nunn's Applied Physiology*, 4th ed. Butterworth, 2000.)

10 occur during spontaneous ventilation. General anesthesia commonly increases venous admixture to 5% to 10%, probably as a result of atelectasis and airway collapse in dependent areas of the lung. Inhalation agents, including nitrous oxide, also can inhibit **hypoxic pulmonary vasoconstriction** in high doses; for volatile agents, the ED_{50} is about 2 minimum alveolar concentration (MAC). Elderly patients seem to have the largest increases in $\dot{Q}s/\dot{Q}\text{T}$. Inspired O_2 tensions of 30% to 40% usually prevent hypoxemia, suggesting anesthesia increases relative shunt. PEEP is often effective in reducing venous

admixture and preventing hypoxemia during general anesthesia, as long as cardiac output is maintained. Prolonged administration of high inspired O_2 concentrations may be associated with atelectasis formation and increases in absolute shunt. Atelectasis in this situation is known as resorption atelectasis and appears in areas with a low $\dot{V}/\dot{Q}$ ratio ventilated at an O_2-inspired concentration close to 100%. Perfusion results in O_2 being transported out of the alveoli at a rate faster than it enters the alveoli, leading to an emptying of the alveoli and collapse.

ALVEOLAR, ARTERIAL, & VENOUS GAS TENSIONS

When dealing with gas mixtures, each gas is considered to contribute separately to total gas pressure, and its partial pressure is directly proportional to its concentration. Air has an O_2 concentration of approximately 21%; therefore, if the barometric pressure is 760 mm Hg (sea level), the partial pressure of O_2 (Po_2) in air is normally 159.6 mm Hg:

$$760 \text{ mm Hg} \times 0.21 = 159.6 \text{ mm Hg}$$

In its general form, the equation may be written as follows:

$$Pio_2 = Pb \times Fio_2$$

where Pb = barometric pressure and Fio_2 = the fraction of inspired O_2.

Two general rules can also be used:

- Partial pressure in millimeters of mercury approximates the percentage × 7
- Partial pressure in kilopascals is approximately the same as the percentage.

1. Oxygen

Alveolar Oxygen Tension

With every breath, the inspired gas mixture is humidified at 37°C in the upper airway. The inspired tension of O_2 (Pio_2) is therefore reduced by the added water vapor. Water vapor pressure is dependent only upon temperature and is 47 mm Hg at 37°C. In humidified air, the normal partial pressure of O_2 at sea level is 149.7 mm Hg:

$$(760 - 47) \times 0.21 = 149.1 \text{ mm Hg}$$

The general equation is

$$Pio_2 = (Pb - Ph_2o) \times Fio_2$$

where Ph_2o = the vapor pressure of water at body temperature.

In alveoli, the inspired gases are mixed with residual alveolar gas from previous breaths, O_2 is taken up, and CO_2 is added. The final alveolar O_2 tension (Pao_2) is therefore dependent on all of these factors and can be estimated by the following equation:

$$Pao_2 = Pio_2 - \frac{Paco_2}{RQ}$$

where $Paco_2$ = arterial CO_2 tension and RQ = respiratory quotient.

11 RQ is usually not measured. Note that large increases in $Paco_2$ (>75 mm Hg) readily produce hypoxia (Pao_2 < 60 mm Hg) at room air, but not at high inspired O_2 concentrations.

A yet simpler method of approximating Pao_2 in millimeters of mercury is to multiply the percentage of inspired O_2 concentration by 6. Thus, at 40%, Pao_2 is 6 × 40, or 240 mm Hg.

Pulmonary End-Capillary Oxygen Tension

For all practical purposes, pulmonary end-capillary O_2 tension ($Pc'o_2$) may be considered identical to Pao_2; the Pao_2–$Pc'o_2$ gradient is normally minute. $Pc'o_2$ is dependent on the rate of O_2 diffusion across the alveolar–capillary membrane, as well as on pulmonary capillary blood volume and transit time. The large capillary surface area in alveoli and the 0.4–0.5 μm thickness of the alveolar–capillary membrane greatly facilitate O_2 diffusion. Enhanced O_2 binding to hemoglobin at saturations above 80% also augments O_2 diffusion (see below). Capillary transit time can be estimated by dividing pulmonary capillary blood volume by cardiac output (pulmonary blood flow); thus, normal capillary transit time is 70 mL ÷ 5000 mL/min (0.8 s). Maximum $Pc'o_2$ is usually attained after only 0.3 sec, providing a large safety margin.

12 The binding of O_2 to hemoglobin seems to be the principal rate-limiting factor in the transfer of O_2 from alveolar gas to blood. Therefore, pulmonary diffusing capacity reflects not only the capacity and permeability of the alveolar–capillary membrane, but also pulmonary blood flow. Moreover, O_2 uptake is normally limited by pulmonary blood flow, not O_2 diffusion across the alveolar–capillary membrane; the latter may become significant during exercise in normal individuals at high altitudes and in patients with extensive destruction of the alveolar–capillary membrane.

O_2 transfer across the alveolar–capillary membrane is expressed as O_2 diffusing capacity (DL_{O_2}):

$$DL_{O_2} = \frac{\text{Oxygen uptake}}{PA_{O_2} - Pc'_{O_2}}$$

Because Pc'_{O_2} cannot be measured accurately, measurement of carbon monoxide diffusion capacity (DL_{CO}) is used instead to assess gas transfer across the alveolar–capillary membrane. Because carbon monoxide has a very high affinity for hemoglobin, there is little or no CO in pulmonary capillary blood, so that even when it is administered at low concentration, Pc'_{CO} can be considered zero. Therefore,

$$DL_{CO} = \frac{\text{Carbon monoxide uptake}}{PA_{CO}}$$

Reductions in DL_{CO} imply an impediment in gas transfer across the alveolar–capillary membrane. Such impediments may be due to abnormal $\dot{V}/\dot{Q}$ ratios, extensive destruction of the gas alveolar–capillary membrane, or very short capillary transit times. Abnormalities are accentuated by increases in O_2 consumption and cardiac output, such as occurs during exercise.

Arterial Oxygen Tension

Pa_{O_2} cannot be calculated like PA_{O_2} but must be measured at room air. The alveolar-to-arterial O_2 partial pressure gradient (A–a gradient) is normally less than 15 mm Hg, but progressively increases with age up to 20–30 mm Hg. Arterial O_2 tension can be approximated by the following formula (in mm Hg):

$$Pa_{O_2} = 120 - \frac{\text{Age}}{3}$$

The range is 60–100 mm Hg (8–13 kPa). Decreases are probably the result of a progressive increase in closing capacity relative to FRC (see above). Table 23–4 lists the mechanisms of hypoxemia (Pa_{O_2} <60 mm Hg).

The most common mechanism for hypoxemia is an increased alveolar–arterial gradient. The A–a gradient for O_2 depends on the amount of right-to-left shunting, the amount of $\dot{V}/\dot{Q}$ scatter, and the mixed venous O_2 tension (see below). The last

TABLE 23–4 **Mechanisms of hypoxemia.**

Low alveolar oxygen tension
  Low inspired oxygen tension
    Low fractional inspired concentration
    High altitude
  Alveolar hypoventilation
  Diffusion hypoxia
  Increased oxygen consumption

Increased alveolar–arterial gradient
  Right-to-left shunting
  Increased areas of low $\dot{V}/\dot{Q}$[1] ratios
  Low mixed venous oxygen tension
    Decreased cardiac output
    Increased oxygen consumption
    Decreased hemoglobin concentration

[1]$\dot{V}/\dot{Q}$, ventilation/perfusion.

depends on cardiac output, O_2 consumption, and hemoglobin concentration.

The A–a gradient for O_2 is directly proportional to shunt, but inversely proportional to mixed venous O_2 tension. The effect of each variable on Pa_{O_2} (and consequently the A–a gradient) can be determined only when the other variables are held constant. Figure 23–19 shows the effect of different degrees of shunting on Pa_{O_2}. It should also be noted that the greater the shunt, the less likely the possibility that an increase in FI_{O_2} will prevent hypoxemia. Moreover, isoshunt lines seem to be most useful for O_2 concentrations between 35% and 100%. Lower O_2 concentrations require modification of isoshunt lines to account for the effect of $\dot{V}/\dot{Q}$ scatter.

The effect of cardiac output on the A–a gradient (Figure 23–20) is due not only to its secondary effects on mixed venous O_2 tension but also to a direct relationship between cardiac output and intrapulmonary shunting. As can be seen, a low cardiac output tends to accentuate the effect of shunt on Pa_{O_2}. A reduction in venous admixture may be observed with low-normal cardiac outputs secondary to accentuated pulmonary vasoconstriction from a lower mixed venous O_2 tension. On the other hand, high cardiac outputs can increase venous admixture by elevating mixed venous O_2 tension, which in turn inhibits hypoxic pulmonary vasoconstriction.

O_2 consumption and hemoglobin concentration can also affect Pa_{O_2} through their secondary effects on mixed venous O_2 tension (below). High O_2

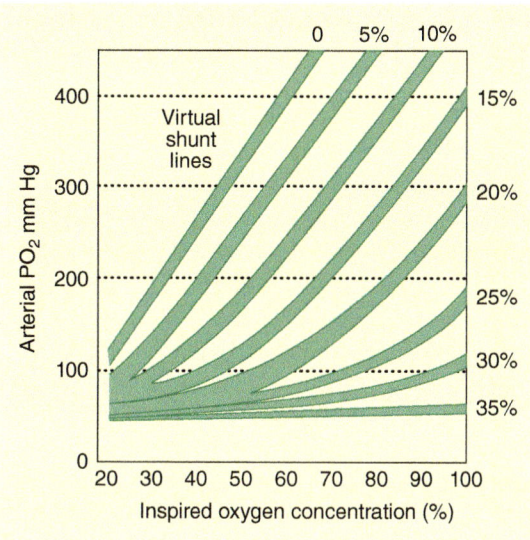

FIGURE 23–19 Isoshunt curves showing the effect of varying amounts of shunt on Pao_2. Note that there is little benefit in increasing inspired oxygen concentration in patients with very large shunts. (Modified and reproduced, with permission, from Benatar SR, Hewlett AM, Nunn JF: The use of isoshunt lines for control of oxygen therapy. Br J Anaesth 1973;45:711.)

consumption rates and low hemoglobin concentrations can increase the A–a gradient and depress Pao_2.

Mixed Venous Oxygen Tension

Normal mixed venous O_2 tension ($P\bar{v}o_2$) is about 40 mm Hg and represents the overall balance between O_2 consumption and O_2 delivery (Table 23–5). A true mixed venous blood sample contains venous drainage from the superior vena cava, the inferior vena cava, and the heart; it must therefore be obtained from a pulmonary artery catheter.

2. Carbon Dioxide

Carbon dioxide is a by-product of aerobic metabolism in mitochondria. There are therefore small continuous gradients for CO_2 tension from mitochondria to cell cytoplasm, extracellular fluid, venous blood, and alveoli, where the CO_2 is finally eliminated.

Mixed Venous Carbon Dioxide Tension

Normal mixed venous CO_2 tension ($P\bar{v}co_2$) is about 46 mm Hg and is the end result of mixing of blood from tissues of varying metabolic activity. Venous CO_2 tension is lower in tissues with low metabolic activity (eg, skin), but higher in blood from those with relatively high activity (eg, heart).

Alveolar Carbon Dioxide Tension

Alveolar CO_2 tension ($Paco_2$) is generally considered to represent the balance between total CO_2 production ($\dot{V}co_2$) and alveolar ventilation (elimination):

$$Paco_2 = \frac{\dot{V}co_2}{\dot{V}A}$$

where $\dot{V}A$ is alveolar ventilation (Figure 23–21). In reality, $Paco_2$ is related to CO_2 elimination rather than production. Although the two are equal in a steady state, an imbalance occurs during periods

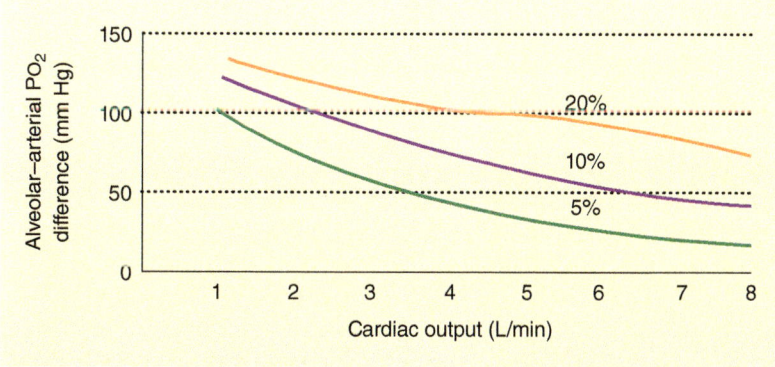

FIGURE 23–20 The effect of cardiac output on the alveolar–arterial Po_2 difference with varying degrees of shunting. $\dot{V}o_2$ = 200 mL/min and Pao_2 = 180 mm Hg.) (Reproduced, with permission, from Nunn JF: *Nunn's Applied Physiology*, 4th ed. Butterworth, 2000.)

TABLE 23–5 Alterations in mixed venous oxygen tension (and saturation).

Decreased $P\bar{v}_{O_2}$
  Increased O_2 consumption
    Fever
    Shivering
    Exercise
    Malignant hyperthermia
    Thyroid storm
  Decreased O_2 delivery
    Hypoxia
    Decreased cardiac output
    Decreased hemoglobin concentration
    Abnormal hemoglobin

Increased $P\bar{v}_{O_2}$
  Left-to-right shunting
  High cardiac output
  Impaired tissue uptake
    Cyanide poisoning
  Decreased oxygen consumption
    Hypothermia
  Combined mechanisms
    Sepsis
  Sampling error
    Wedged pulmonary artery catheter

of acute hypoventilation or hypoperfusion, and the excess CO_2 increases total body CO_2 content. Clinically, Pa_{CO_2} is more dependent on alveolar ventilation than is $\dot{V}_{CO_2}$, because CO_2 output does not vary appreciably under most circumstances. Moreover, the body's large capacity to store CO_2 (see below) buffers acute changes in $\dot{V}_{CO_2}$.

Pulmonary End-Capillary Carbon Dioxide Tension

Pulmonary end-capillary CO_2 tension (Pc'_{CO_2}) is virtually identical to Pa_{CO_2} for the same reasons as those discussed in the section about O_2. In addition, the diffusion rate for CO_2 across the alveolar–capillary membrane is 20 times that of O_2.

Arterial Carbon Dioxide Tension

Arterial CO_2 tension (Pa_{CO_2}), which is readily measurable, is identical to Pc'_{CO_2} and, necessarily, PA_{CO_2}. Normal Pa_{CO_2} is 38 ± 4 mm Hg (5.1 ± 0.5 kPa); in practice, 40 mm Hg is usually considered normal.

Although low $\dot{V}/\dot{Q}$ ratios tend to increase Pa_{CO_2}, whereas high $\dot{V}/\dot{Q}$ ratios tend to decrease it (in contrast to the case for O_2 [see above]), significant arterial-to-alveolar gradients for CO_2 develop only in the presence of marked $\dot{V}/\dot{Q}$ abnormalities (>30% venous admixture); even then the gradient is relatively small (2–3 mm Hg). Moreover, small increases in the gradient appreciably increase CO_2 output into alveoli with relatively normal $\dot{V}/\dot{Q}$. Even moderate to severe disturbances usually fail to appreciably alter arterial CO_2 because of a reflex increase in ventilation from concomitant hypoxemia.

End-Tidal Carbon Dioxide Tension

Because end-tidal gas is primarily alveolar gas and PA_{CO_2} is virtually identical to Pa_{CO_2}, end-tidal CO_2 tension (PET_{CO_2}) is used clinically as an estimate of Pa_{CO_2}. The Pa_{CO_2}–PET_{CO_2} gradient is normally less than 5 mm Hg and represents dilution of alveolar gas with CO_2-free gas from nonperfused alveoli (alveolar dead space).

TRANSPORT OF RESPIRATORY GASES IN BLOOD

1. Oxygen

O_2 is carried in blood in two forms: dissolved in solution and in reversible association with hemoglobin.

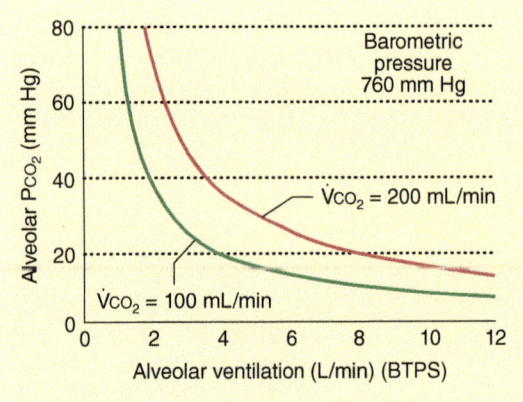

FIGURE 23–21 The effect of alveolar ventilation on alveolar P_{CO_2} at two rates of CO_2 production. (Reproduced, with permission, from Nunn JF: *Nunn's Applied Physiology*, 4th ed. Butterworth, 2000.)

Dissolved Oxygen

The amount of O_2 dissolved in blood can be derived from **Henry's law**, which states that the concentration of any gas in solution is proportional to its partial pressure. The mathematical expression is as follows:

$$\text{Gas concentration} = \alpha \times \text{Partial pressure}$$

where α = the gas solubility coefficient for a given solution at a given temperature.

The solubility coefficient for O_2 at normal body temperature is 0.003 mL/dL/mm Hg. Even with a Pao_2 of 100 mm Hg, the maximum amount of O_2 dissolved in blood is very small (0.3 mL/dL) compared with that bound to hemoglobin.

Hemoglobin

Hemoglobin is a complex molecule consisting of four heme and four protein subunits. Heme is an iron–porphyrin compound that is an essential part of the O_2-binding sites; only the divalent form (+2 charge) of iron can bind O_2. The normal hemoglobin molecule (hemoglobin A_1) consists of two α and two β chains (subunits); the four subunits are held together by weak bonds between the amino acid residues. Each gram of hemoglobin can theoretically carry up to 1.39 mL of O_2.

Hemoglobin Dissociation Curve

Each hemoglobin molecule binds up to four O_2 molecules. The complex interaction between the hemoglobin subunits results in nonlinear (an elongated S shape) binding with O_2 (**Figure 23–22**). Hemoglobin saturation is the amount of O_2 bound as a percentage of its total O_2-binding capacity. Four separate chemical reactions are involved in binding each of the four O_2 molecules. The change in molecular conformation induced by the binding of the first three molecules greatly accelerates binding of the fourth O_2 molecule. The last reaction is responsible for the accelerated binding between 25% and 100% saturation. At about 90% saturation, the decrease in available O_2 receptors flattens the curve until full saturation is reached.

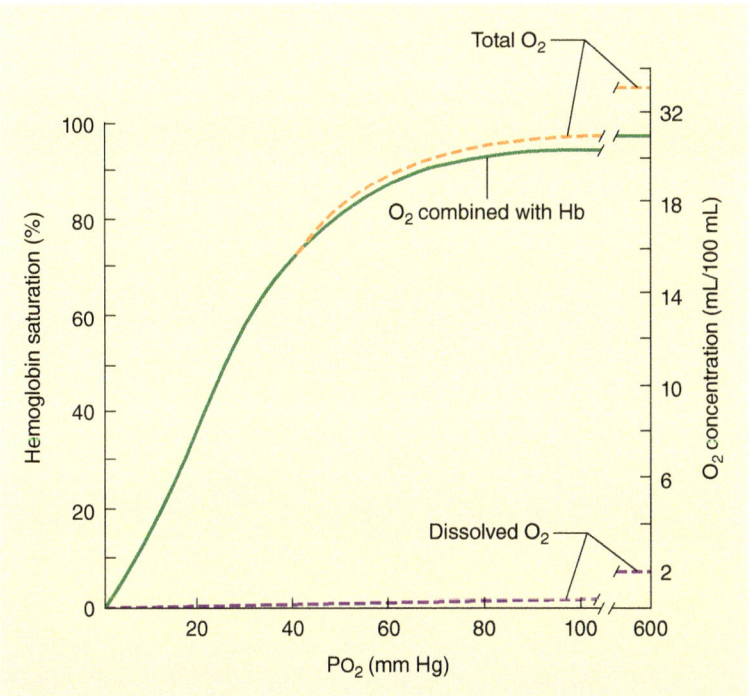

FIGURE 23–22 The normal adult hemoglobin–oxygen dissociation curve. (Modified and reproduced, with permission, from West JB: *Respiratory Physiology—The Essentials*, 6th ed. Williams & Wilkins, 2000.)

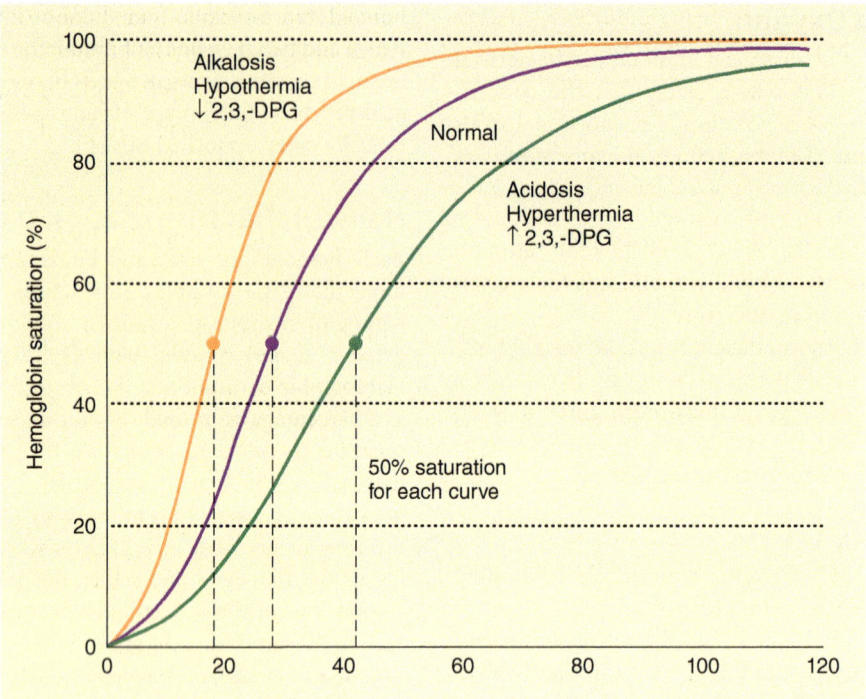

FIGURE 23–23 The effects of changes in acid–base status, body temperature, and 2,3-DPG concentration on the hemoglobin–oxygen dissociation curve.

Factors Influencing the Hemoglobin Dissociation Curve

Clinically important factors altering O_2 binding include hydrogen ion concentration, CO_2 tension, temperature, and 2,3-diphosphoglycerate (2,3-DPG) concentration. Their effect on hemoglobin–O_2 interaction can be expressed by P_{50}, the O_2 tension at which hemoglobin is 50% saturated (Figure 23–23). Each factor shifts the dissociation curve either to the right (increasing P_{50}) or to the left (decreasing P_{50}).

14 A rightward shift in the oxygen–hemoglobin dissociation curve lowers O_2 affinity, displaces O_2 from hemoglobin, and makes more O_2 available to tissues; a leftward shift increases hemoglobin's affinity for O_2, reducing its availability to tissues. The normal P_{50} in adults is 26.6 mm Hg (3.4 kPa).

An increase in blood hydrogen ion concentration reduces O_2 binding to hemoglobin (Bohr effect). Because of the shape of the **hemoglobin dissociation curve**, the effect is more important in

venous blood than arterial blood (Figure 23–23); the net result is facilitation of O_2 release to tissue with little impairment in O_2 uptake (unless severe hypoxia is present).

The influence of CO_2 tension on hemoglobin's affinity for O_2 is important physiologically and is secondary to the associated rise in hydrogen ion concentration when CO_2 tension increases. The high CO_2 content of venous capillary blood, by decreasing hemoglobin's affinity for O_2, facilitates the release of O_2 to tissues; conversely, the lower CO_2 content in pulmonary capillaries increases hemoglobin's affinity for O_2 again, facilitating O_2 uptake from alveoli.

2,3-DPG is a by-product of glycolysis (the Rapoport–Luebering shunt) and accumulates during anaerobic metabolism. Although its effects on hemoglobin under these conditions are theoretically beneficial, its physiological importance normally seems minor. 2,3-DPG levels may, however, play an important compensatory role in patients with chronic anemia and may significantly affect the O_2-carrying capacity of blood transfusions.

Abnormal Ligands & Abnormal Forms of Hemoglobins

Carbon monoxide, cyanide, nitric acid, and ammonia can combine with hemoglobin at O_2-binding sites. They can displace O_2 and shift the saturation curve to the left. Carbon monoxide is particularly potent, having 200–300 times the affinity of O_2 for hemoglobin, combining with it to form carboxyhemoglobin. Carbon monoxide decreases hemoglobin's O_2-carrying capacity and impairs the release of O_2 to tissues.

Methemoglobin results when the iron in heme is oxidized to its trivalent (+3) form. Nitrates, nitrites, sulfonamides, and other drugs can rarely result in significant methemoglobinemia. Methemoglobin cannot combine with O_2 unless reconverted by the enzyme methemoglobin reductase; methemoglobin also shifts the normal hemoglobin saturation curve to the left. Methemoglobinemia, like carbon monoxide poisoning, therefore decreases the O_2-carrying capacity and impairs the release of O_2. Reduction of methemoglobin to normal hemoglobin is facilitated by such agents as methylene blue or ascorbic acid.

Abnormal hemoglobins can also result from variations in the protein subunit composition. Each variant has its own O_2-saturation characteristics. These include fetal hemoglobin, hemoglobin A_2, and sickle hemoglobin.

Oxygen Content

The total O_2 content of blood is the sum of that in solution plus that carried by hemoglobin. In reality, O_2 binding to hemoglobin never achieves the theoretical maximum (see above), but is closer to 1.31 mL O_2/dL blood per mm Hg. Total O_2 content is expressed by the following equation:

$$O_2 \text{ content} = ([0.003 \text{ mL } O_2/\text{dL blood per mm Hg}] \times Po_2) + (So_2 \times Hb \times 1.31 \text{ mL/dL blood})$$

where Hb is hemoglobin concentration in g/dL blood, and So_2 is hemoglobin saturation at the given Po_2.

Using the above formula and a hemoglobin of 15 g/dL, the normal O_2 content for both arterial and mixed venous blood and the arteriovenous difference can be calculated as follows:

$$Cao_2 = (0.003 \times 100) + (0.975 \times 15 \times 1.39)$$
$$= 19.5 \text{ mL/dL blood}$$
$$C\bar{v}o_2 = (0.003 \times 40) + (0.75 \times 15 \times 1.31)$$
$$= 14.8 \text{ mL/dL blood}$$
$$Cao_2 - C\bar{v}o_2 = 4.7 \text{ mL/dL blood}$$

Oxygen Transport

O_2 transport is dependent on both respiratory and circulatory function. Total O_2 delivery ($\dot{D}o_2$) to tissues is the product of arterial O_2 content and cardiac output:

$$\dot{D}o_2 = Cao_2 \times \dot{Q}T$$

Note that arterial O_2 content is dependent on Pao_2 as well as hemoglobin concentration. **As a result, deficiencies in O_2 delivery may be due to a low Pao_2, a low hemoglobin concentration, or an inadequate cardiac output.** Normal O_2 delivery can be calculated as follows:

$$O_2 \text{ delivery} = 20 \text{ mL } O_2/\text{dL blood}$$
$$\times 50 \text{ dL per blood/min}$$
$$= 1000 \text{ mL } O_2/\text{min}$$

The Fick equation expresses the relationship between O_2 consumption, O_2 content, and cardiac output:

$$O_2 \text{ consumption} = \dot{V}o_2 = \dot{Q}T \times (Cao_2 - C\bar{v}o_2)$$

Rearranging the equation:

$$Cao_2 = \frac{\dot{V}o_2}{\dot{Q}T} + C\bar{v}o_2$$

Consequently, the arteriovenous difference is a good measure of the overall adequacy of O_2 delivery.

As calculated above, the arteriovenous difference ($Cao_2 - C\bar{v}o_2$) is about 5 mL O_2/dL blood (20 mL O_2/dL – 15 mL O_2/dL). Note that the normal extraction fraction for $O_2 [(Cao_2 - C\bar{v}o_2)/Cao_2]$ is 5 mL ÷ 20 mL, or 25%; thus, the body normally consumes only 25% of the O_2 carried on hemoglobin. When O_2 demand exceeds supply, the extraction fraction exceeds 25%. Conversely, if O_2 supply exceeds demand, the extraction fraction falls below 25%.

When $\dot{D}o_2$ is even moderately reduced, $\dot{V}o_2$ usually remains normal because of increased O_2 extraction (mixed venous O_2 saturation decreases); $\dot{V}o_2$ remains independent of delivery. With further reductions in $\dot{D}o_2$, however, a critical point is reached beyond which $\dot{V}o_2$ becomes directly proportional to $\dot{D}o_2$. **This state of supply-dependent O_2 is typically associated with progressive lactic acidosis caused by cellular hypoxia.**

Oxygen Stores

The concept of O_2 stores is important in anesthesia. When the normal flux of O_2 is interrupted by apnea, existing O_2 stores are consumed by cellular metabolism; if stores are depleted, hypoxia and eventual cell death follow. Theoretically, normal O_2 stores in adults are about 1500 mL. This amount includes the O_2 remaining in the lungs, that bound to hemoglobin (and myoglobin), and that dissolved in body fluids. Unfortunately, the high affinity of hemoglobin for O_2 (the affinity of myoglobin is even higher), and the very limited quantity of O_2 in solution, restrict the availability of these stores. The O_2 contained within the lungs at FRC (initial lung volume during apnea), therefore, becomes the most important source of O_2. Of that volume, however, probably only 80% is usable.

Apnea in a patient previously breathing room air leaves approximately 480 mL of O_2 in the lungs. (If $F_{IO_2} = 0.21$ and FRC = 2300 mL, O_2 content = $F_{IO_2} \times$ FRC.) The metabolic activity of tissues rapidly depletes this reservoir (presumably at a rate equivalent to $\dot{V}o_2$); severe hypoxemia usually occurs within 90 sec. The onset of hypoxemia can be delayed by increasing the F_{IO_2} prior to the apnea. Following ventilation with 100% O_2, FRC contains about 2300 mL of O_2; this delays hypoxemia following apnea for 4–5 min. This concept is the basis for preoxygenation prior to induction of anesthesia.

2. Carbon Dioxide

Carbon dioxide is transported in blood in three forms: dissolved in solution, as bicarbonate, and with proteins in the form of carbamino compounds (Table 23–6). The sum of all three forms is the total CO_2 content of blood (routinely reported with electrolyte measurements).

Dissolved Carbon Dioxide

Carbon dioxide is more soluble in blood than O_2, with a solubility coefficient of 0.031 mmol/L/mm Hg (0.067 mL/dL/mm Hg) at 37°C.

TABLE 23–6 Contributions to carbon dioxide transport in 1 L of whole blood.[1,2]

Form	Plasma	Erythrocytes	Combined	Contribution (%)
Mixed venous whole blood				
Dissolved CO_2	0.76	0.51	1.27	5.5
Bicarbonate	14.41	5.92	20.33	87.2
Carbamino CO_2	Negligible	1.70	1.70	7.3
Total CO_2	15.17	8.13	23.30	
Arterial whole blood				
Dissolved CO_2	0.66	0.44	1.10	5.1
Bicarbonate	13.42	5.88	19.30	89.9
Carbamino CO_2	Negligible	1.10	1.10	5.1
Total CO_2	14.08	7.42	21.50	

[1]Data from Nunn JF: *Nunn's Applied Physiology*, 4th ed. Butterworth, 2000.

[2]Values are expressed in millimoles, except where indicated otherwise.

Bicarbonate

In aqueous solutions, CO_2 slowly combines with water to form carbonic acid and bicarbonate, according to the following reaction:

$$H_2O + CO_2 \leftrightarrow H_2CO_3 \leftrightarrow H^+ + HCO_3^-$$

In plasma, although less than 1% of the dissolved CO_2 undergoes this reaction, the presence of the enzyme **carbonic anhydrase** within erythrocytes and endothelium greatly accelerates the reaction. As a result, bicarbonate represents the largest fraction of the CO_2 in blood (see Table 23–6). Administration of acetazolamide, a carbonic anhydrase inhibitor, can impair CO_2 transport between tissues and alveoli.

On the venous side of systemic capillaries, CO_2 enters red blood cells and is converted to bicarbonate, which diffuses out of red cells into plasma; chloride ions move from plasma into red cells to maintain electrical balance. In the pulmonary capillaries, the reverse occurs: chloride ions move out of red cells as bicarbonate ions reenter them for conversion back to CO_2, which diffuses out into alveoli. This sequence is referred to as the chloride or Hamburger shift.

Carbamino Compounds

Carbon dioxide can react with amino groups on proteins, as shown by the following equation:

$$R\text{-}NH_2 + CO_2 \rightarrow RNH - CO_2^- + H^+$$

At physiological pH, only a small amount of CO_2 is carried in this form, mainly as carbaminohemoglobin. Deoxygenated hemoglobin (deoxyhemoglobin) has a greater affinity (3.5 times) for CO_2 than does oxyhemoglobin. As a result, venous blood carries more CO_2 than does arterial blood (Haldane effect; see Table 23–6). P_{CO_2} normally has little effect on the fraction of CO_2 carried as carbaminohemoglobin.

Effects of Hemoglobin Buffering on Carbon Dioxide Transport

The buffering action of hemoglobin also accounts for part of the Haldane effect. Hemoglobin can act as a buffer at physiological pH because of its high content of histidine. Moreover, the acid–base behavior of hemoglobin is influenced by its oxygenation state:

$$H^+ + HbO_2 \rightarrow HbH^+ + O_2$$

Removal of O_2 from hemoglobin in tissue capillaries causes the hemoglobin molecule to behave more like a base; by taking up hydrogen ions, hemoglobin shifts the CO_2–bicarbonate equilibrium in favor of greater bicarbonate formation:

$$CO_2 + H_2O + HbO_2 \rightarrow HbH^+ + HCO_3^- + O_2$$

As a direct result, deoxyhemoglobin also increases the amount of CO_2 that is carried in venous blood as bicarbonate. As CO_2 is taken up from tissue and converted to bicarbonate, the total CO_2 content of blood increases (see Table 23–6).

In the lungs, the reverse is true. Oxygenation of hemoglobin favors its action as an acid, and the release of hydrogen ions shifts the equilibrium in favor of greater CO_2 formation:

$$O_2 + HCO_3^- + HbH^+ \rightarrow H_2O + CO_2 + HbO_2$$

Bicarbonate concentration decreases as CO_2 is formed and eliminated, so that the total CO_2 content of blood decreases in the lungs. Note that there is a difference between CO_2 content (concentration per liter) of whole blood (see Table 23–6) and plasma (Table 23–7).

Carbon Dioxide Dissociation Curve

A CO_2 dissociation curve can be constructed by plotting the total CO_2 content of blood against P_{CO_2}.

TABLE 23–7 Carbon dioxide content of plasma (mmol/L).[1,2]

	Arterial	Venous
Dissolved CO_2	1.2	1.4
Bicarbonate	24.4	26.2
Carbamino CO_2	Negligible	Negligible
Total CO_2	25.6	27.6

[1]Data from Nunn JF: *Nunn's Applied Physiology*, 4th ed. Butterworth, 2000.

[2]Values are expressed in millimoles, except where indicated otherwise.

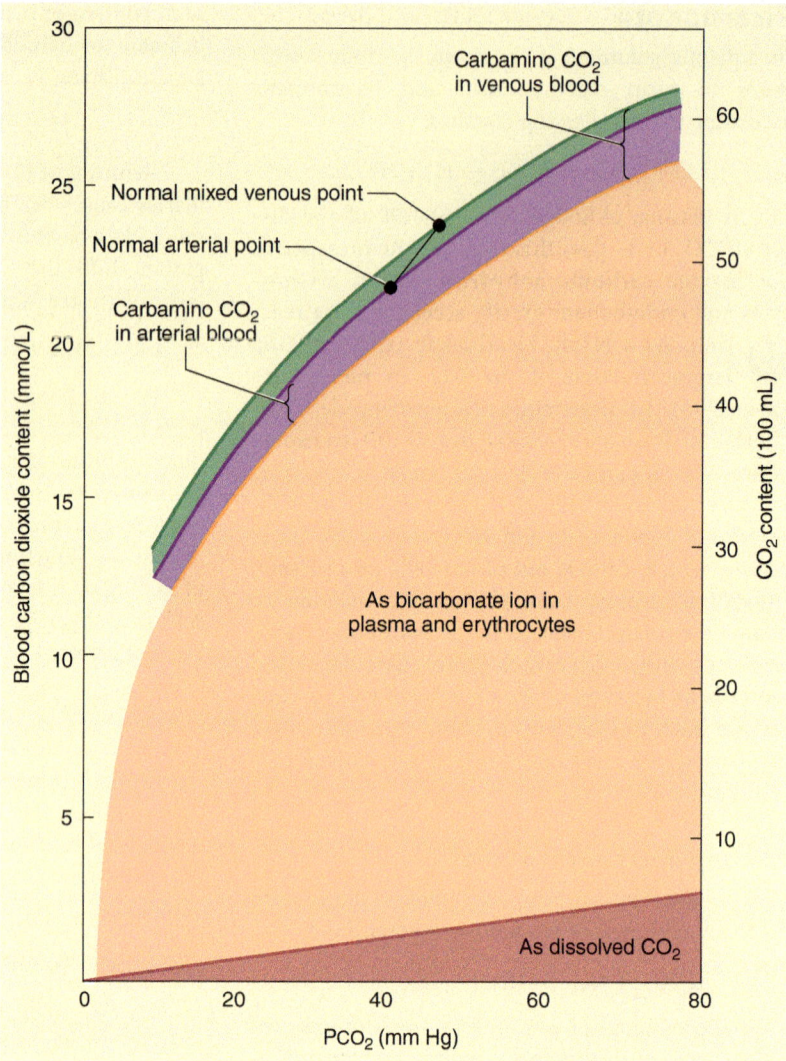

FIGURE 23–24 The CO_2 dissociation curve for whole blood. (Reproduced, with permission, from Nunn JF: *Nunn's Applied Physiology*, 4th ed. Butterworth, 2000.)

The contribution of each form of CO_2 can also be quantified in this manner (Figure 23–24).

Carbon Dioxide Stores

Carbon dioxide stores in the body are large (approximately 120 L in adults) and primarily in the form of dissolved CO_2 and bicarbonate. When an imbalance occurs between production and elimination, establishing a new CO_2 equilibrium requires 20–30 min (compared with less than 4–5 min for O_2; see above). Carbon dioxide is stored in the rapid-, intermediate-, and slow-equilibrating compartments. Because of the larger

capacity of the intermediate and slow compartments, the rate of rise in arterial CO_2 tension is generally slower than its fall following acute changes in ventilation.

CONTROL OF BREATHING

Spontaneous ventilation is the result of rhythmic neural activity in respiratory centers within the brainstem. This activity regulates respiratory muscles to maintain normal tensions of O_2 and CO_2 in the body. The basic neuronal activity is modified by inputs from other areas in the brain, volitional and autonomic, as well as various central and peripheral receptors (sensors).

1. Central Respiratory Centers

The basic breathing rhythm originates in the medulla. Two medullary groups of neurons are generally recognized: a dorsal respiratory group, which is primarily active during inspiration, and a ventral respiratory group, which is active during expiration. The close association of the dorsal respiratory group of neurons with the tractus solitarius may explain reflex changes in breathing from vagal or glossopharyngeal nerve stimulation.

Two pontine areas influence the dorsal (inspiratory) medullary center. A lower pontine (apneustic) center is excitatory, whereas an upper pontine (pneumotaxic) center is inhibitory. The pontine centers appear to fine-tune respiratory rate and rhythm.

2. Central Sensors

The most important of these sensors are chemoreceptors that respond to changes in hydrogen ion concentration. Central chemoreceptors are thought to lie on the anterolateral surface of the medulla and respond primarily to changes in cerebrospinal fluid (CSF) $[H^+]$. This mechanism is effective in regulating $Paco_2$, because the blood–brain barrier is permeable to dissolved CO_2, but not to bicarbonate ions. Acute changes in $Paco_2$, but not in arterial $[HCO_3^-]$, are reflected in CSF; thus, a change in CO_2 must result in a change in $[H^+]$:

$$CO_2 + H_2O \leftrightarrow H^+ + HCO_3^-$$

Over the course of a few days, CSF $[HCO_3^-]$ can compensate to match any change in arterial $[HCO_3^-]$.

Increases in $Paco_2$ elevate CSF hydrogen ion concentration and activate the chemoreceptors. Secondary stimulation of the adjacent respiratory medullary centers increases alveolar ventilation (Figure 23–25) and reduces $Paco_2$ back to normal. Conversely, decreases in CSF hydrogen ion concentration secondary to reductions in $Paco_2$ reduce alveolar ventilation and elevate $Paco_2$. Note that the relationship between $Paco_2$ and minute volume is nearly linear. Also note that very high arterial $Paco_2$ tensions depress the ventilatory response (CO_2 narcosis). The $Paco_2$ at which ventilation is zero (x-intercept) is known as the apneic threshold. Spontaneous

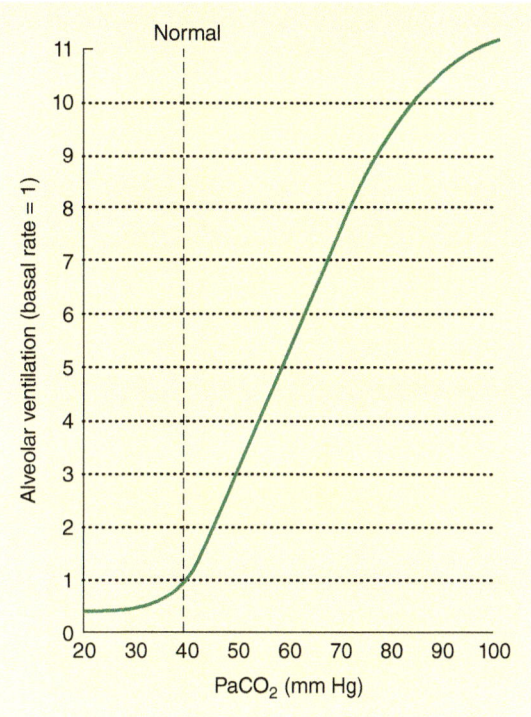

FIGURE 23–25 The normal relationship between $Paco_2$ and minute ventilation. (Reproduced, with permission, from Guyton AC: *Textbook of Medical Physiology*, 7th ed. W.B. Saunders, 1986.)

respirations are typically absent under anesthesia when $Paco_2$ falls below the apneic threshold. (In the awake state, cortical influences prevent apnea, so apneic thresholds are not ordinarily seen.) In contrast to peripheral chemoreceptors (see below), central chemoreceptor activity is depressed by hypoxia.

3. Peripheral Sensors

Peripheral Chemoreceptors

Peripheral chemoreceptors include the carotid bodies (at the bifurcation of the common carotid arteries) and the aortic bodies (surrounding the aortic arch). The carotid bodies are the principal peripheral chemoreceptors in humans and are sensitive to changes in Pao_2, $Paco_2$, pH, and arterial perfusion pressure. They interact with central respiratory centers via the glossopharyngeal nerves, producing reflex increases in alveolar ventilation in response to reductions in Pao_2, arterial perfusion, or elevations in $[H^+]$ and $Paco_2$. Peripheral chemoreceptors

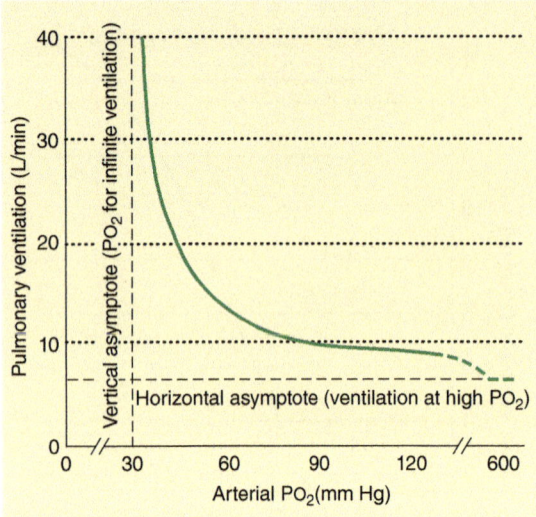

FIGURE 23–26 The relationship between Pa_{O_2} and minute ventilation at rest and with a normal Pa_{CO_2}. (Data from Weil JV, Byrne-Quinn E, Sodal IE, et al: Hypoxic ventilatory drive in normal man. J Clin Invest 1970;49:1061-1072; Dripps RD, Comroe JH: The effect of the inhalation of high and low oxygen concentration on respiration, pulse rate, ballistocardiogram and arterial oxygen saturation (oximeter) of normal individuals. Am J Physiol 1947;149:277-291; Cormac RS, Cunningham DJC, Gee JBL: The effect of carbon dioxide on the respiratory response to want of oxygen in man. Q J Exp Physiol 1957;42:303-316.)

are also stimulated by cyanide, doxapram, and large doses of nicotine. In contrast to central chemoreceptors, which respond primarily to Pa_{CO_2} (really [H^+]), the carotid bodies are most sensitive to Pa_{O_2} (Figure 23–26). Note that receptor activity does not appreciably increase until Pa_{O_2} decreases below 50 mm Hg. Cells of the carotid body (glomus cells) are thought to be primarily dopaminergic neurons. Anti-dopaminergic drugs (such as phenothiazines), most commonly used anesthetics, and bilateral carotid surgery abolish the peripheral ventilatory response to hypoxemia.

Lung Receptors

Impulses from these receptors are carried centrally by the vagus nerve. Stretch receptors are distributed in the smooth muscle of airways; they are responsible for inhibition of inspiration when the lung is inflated to excessive volumes (Hering–Breuer inflation reflex) and shortening of exhalation when the lung is deflated (deflation reflex). Stretch receptors normally play a minor role in humans. In fact, bilateral vagal nerve blocks have a minimal effect on the normal respiratory pattern.

Irritant receptors in the tracheobronchial mucosa react to noxious gases, smoke, dust, and cold gases; activation produces reflex increases in respiratory rate, bronchoconstriction, and coughing. J (juxta-capillary) receptors are located in the interstitial space within alveolar walls; these receptors induce dyspnea in response to expansion of interstitial space volume and various chemical mediators following tissue damage.

Other Receptors

These include various muscle and joint receptors on pulmonary muscles and the chest wall. Input from these sources is probably important during exercise and in pathological conditions associated with decreased lung or chest compliance.

4. Effects of Anesthesia on the Control of Breathing

The most important effect of most general anesthetics on breathing is a tendency to promote hypoventilation. The mechanism is probably dual: central depression of the chemoreceptor and depression of external intercostal muscle activity. The magnitude of the hypoventilation is generally proportional to anesthetic depth. With increasing depth of anesthesia, the slope of the Pa_{CO_2}/minute ventilation curve decreases, and the apneic threshold increases (Figure 23–27). This effect is at least partially reversed by surgical stimulation.

The peripheral response to hypoxemia is even more sensitive to anesthetics than the central CO_2 response and is nearly abolished by even subanesthetic doses of most inhalation agents (including nitrous oxide) and many intravenous agents.

NONRESPIRATORY FUNCTIONS OF THE LUNG

Filtration & Reservoir Function

A. Filtration

The unique in-series position of the pulmonary capillaries within the circulation allows them to act

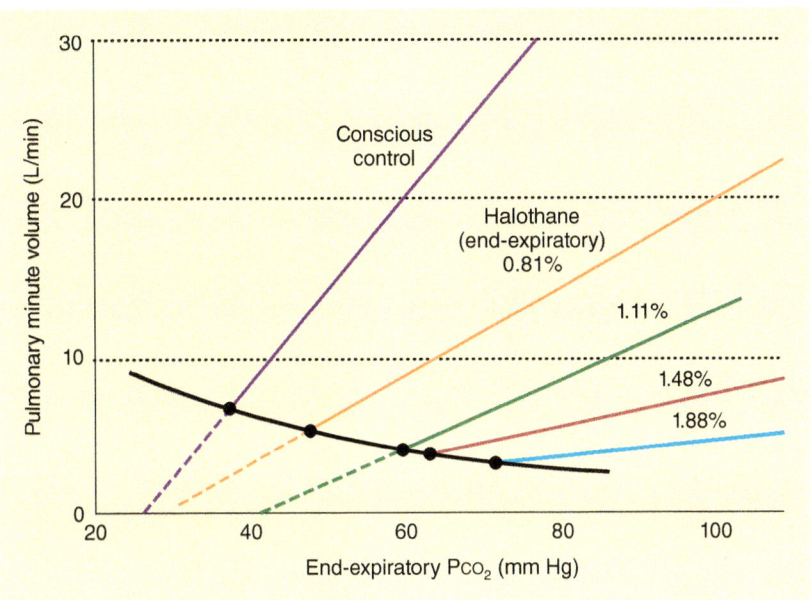

FIGURE 23–27 The effect of volatile agents (halothane) on the P_{ETCO_2}–ventilation response curve (see text). Data from Munson ES, Larson CP, Babad AA, et al: The effects of halothane, fluroxene and cyclopropane on ventilation: a comparative study in man. Anesthesiology 1966;27:716-728.

as a filter for debris in the bloodstream. The lungs' high content of heparin and plasminogen activator facilitates the breakdown of entrapped fibrin debris. Although pulmonary capillaries have an average diameter of 7 μm, larger particles have been shown to pass through to the left heart.

B. Reservoir Function

The role of the pulmonary circulation as a reservoir for the systemic circulation was discussed above.

Metabolism

The lungs are metabolically very active organs. In addition to surfactant synthesis, pneumocytes account for a major portion of extrahepatic mixed-function oxidation. Neutrophils and macrophages in the lung produce O_2-derived free radicals in response to infection. The pulmonary endothelium metabolizes a variety of vasoactive compounds, including norepinephrine, serotonin, bradykinin, and a variety of prostaglandins and leukotrienes. Histamine and epinephrine are generally not metabolized in the lungs; in fact the lungs can be a major site of histamine synthesis and release during allergic reactions.

The lungs are also responsible for converting angiotensin I to its physiologically active form, angiotensin II. The enzyme responsible, angiotensin-converting enzyme, is bound on the surface of the pulmonary endothelium.

CASE DISCUSSION

Unilaterally Diminished Breath Sounds During General Anesthesia

A 67-year-old man with carcinoma is undergoing colon resection under general anesthesia. His history includes an old anterior myocardial infarction and compensated congestive heart failure. Arterial and central venous catheters are placed preoperatively for monitoring during surgery. Following a smooth induction and an atraumatic intubation, anesthesia is maintained with 60% nitrous oxide in O_2, sevoflurane, and vecuronium. One-half hour into the operation, the surgeon asks for the Trendelenburg position to facilitate surgical exposure. The pulse oximeter, which had been reading 99% saturation, suddenly drops and remains at 93%. The pulse oximeter's signal strength and waveform are unchanged. Auscultation of the lungs reveals diminished breath sounds over the left lung.

What is the most likely explanation?

Unilaterally diminished breath sounds under anesthesia are most commonly caused by accidental placement or migration of the tracheal tube into one of the two main bronchi. As a result, only one lung is ventilated. Other causes of unilaterally diminished breath sounds (such as pneumothorax, a large mucus plug, lobar atelectasis, or undiagnosed bullae) are less easily diagnosed, but are fortunately less common during anesthesia.

The Trendelenburg (head-down) position typically causes the tip of the tracheal tube to advance 1–2 cm relative to the carina. In this case, the tube was apparently placed just above the carina with the patient in the supine position, but migrated into the right bronchus when the Trendelenburg position was imposed. The diagnosis is confirmed by drawing the tube back 1–2 cm at a time as the chest is auscultated. Breath sounds will become equal again when the tip of the tube reenters the trachea. Following initial placement, tracheal tubes should be routinely checked for correct positioning by auscultating the chest, ascertaining depth of tube insertion by the markings on the tube (normally 20–24 cm at the teeth for an adult), and feeling for the cuff in the suprasternal notch. Tube position relative to the carina can also be quickly confirmed with a flexible fiberoptic bronchoscope.

Are tracheal tubes just as likely to enter either main bronchus?

In most cases of unintentional bronchial intubation, the tracheal tube enters the right bronchus because the latter diverges away from the trachea at a less acute angle than does the left bronchus.

Why did hemoglobin saturation decrease?

Failure to ventilate one lung as it continues to be perfused creates a large intrapulmonary shunt.

Venous admixture increases and tends to depress Pa_{O_2} and hemoglobin saturation.

Does a saturation of 93% exclude bronchial intubation?

No; if both lungs continued to have equal blood flow, venous admixture should have theoretically increased to 50%, resulting in severe hypoxemia and very low hemoglobin saturation. Fortunately, hypoxic pulmonary vasoconstriction is a powerful compensatory response that tends to reduce flow to the hypoxic lung and reduces the expected venous admixture. In fact, if the patient has been receiving a higher inspired O_2 concentration (50% to 100%), the drop in arterial tension may not be detectable by the pulse oximeter due to the characteristics of the normal hemoglobin saturation curve. For example, bronchial intubation in a patient inspiring 50% O_2 might drop Pa_{O_2} from 250 mm Hg to 95 mm Hg; the resulting change in pulse oximeter readings (100–99 to 98–97) would hardly be noticeable.

Arterial and mixed venous blood gas tensions are obtained with the following results:

Pa_{O_2} = 69 mm Hg; Pa_{CO_2} = 42 mm Hg; Sa_{O_2} = 93%; $P\bar{v}_{O_2}$ = 40 mm Hg; and $S\bar{v}_{O_2}$ = 75%. Hemoglobin concentration is 15 g/dL.

What is the calculated venous admixture?

In this case, $Pc'_{O_2} = Pa_{O_2} = ([760 - 47] \times 0.4) - 42 = 243$ mm Hg. Therefore, $Cc'_{O_2} = (15 \times 1.31 \times 1.0) + (243 \times 0.003) = 20.4$ mL/dL.

$Ca_{O_2} = (15 \times 1.31 \times 0.93) + (69 \times 0.003) = 18.5$ mL/dL

$C\bar{v}_{O_2} = (15 \times 1.31 \times 0.75) + (40 \times 0.003) = 14.8$ mL/dL

$\dot{Q}s/\dot{Q}\tau = (20.4 - 18.5)/(20.4 - 14.8) = 34\%$

How does bronchial intubation affect arterial and end-tidal CO_2 tensions?

Pa_{CO_2} is typically not appreciably altered as long as the same minute ventilation is maintained (see One-Lung Anesthesia, Chapter 25). Clinically, the Pa_{CO_2}–Pet_{CO_2} gradient often widens, possibly because of increased alveolar dead space (overdistension of the ventilated lung). Thus, Pet_{CO_2} may decrease or remain unchanged.

SUGGESTED READING

Bruells C, Rossaint R: Physiology of gas exchange during anesthesia. Eur J Anaesthesiol 2011;29:570.

Campos J: Update on tracheobronchial anatomy and flexible fiberoptic bronchoscopy in thoracic anesthesia. Curr Opin Anaesthesiol 2009;22:4.

Lohser J: Evidence based management of one lung ventilation. Anesthesiol Clin 2008;26:241.

Minnich D, Mathisen D: Anatomy of the trachea, carina, and bronchi. Thorac Surg Clin 2007;17:571.

Warner DO: Diaphragm function during anesthesia: Still crazy after all these years. Anesthesiology 2002;97:295.

Anesthesia for Patients with Respiratory Disease

1 In a patient with an acute asthma attack, a normal or high Pa_{CO_2} indicates that the patient can no longer maintain the work of breathing and is often a sign of impending respiratory failure. A pulsus paradoxus and electrocardiographic signs of right ventricular strain (ST-segment changes, right axis deviation, and right bundle branch block) are also indicative of severe airway obstruction.

2 Asthmatic patients with active bronchospasm presenting for emergency surgery should be treated aggressively. Supplemental oxygen, aerosolized β_2-agonists, and intravenous glucocorticoids can dramatically improve lung function in a few hours.

3 Intraoperative bronchospasm is usually manifested as wheezing, increasing peak airway pressures (plateau pressure may remain unchanged), decreasing exhaled tidal volumes, or a slowly rising waveform on the capnograph.

4 Other causes, such as obstruction of the tracheal tube from kinking, secretions, or an overinflated balloon; bronchial intubation; active expiratory efforts (straining); pulmonary edema or embolism; and pneumothorax, can simulate bronchospasm.

5 Chronic obstructive pulmonary disease (COPD) is currently defined as a disease state characterized by airflow limitation that is not fully reversible. The chronic airflow limitation of this disease is due to a mixture of small and large airway disease (chronic bronchitis/bronchiolitis) and parenchymal destruction (emphysema), with the representation of these two components varying from patient to patient.

6 Cessation of smoking is the long-term intervention that has been shown to reduce the rate of decline in lung function.

7 Preoperative interventions in patients with COPD aimed at correcting hypoxemia, relieving bronchospasm, mobilizing and reducing secretions, and treating infections may decrease the incidence of postoperative pulmonary complications. Patients at greatest risk of complications are those with preoperative pulmonary function measurements less than 50% of predicted.

8 Restrictive pulmonary diseases are characterized by decreased lung compliance. Lung volumes are typically reduced, with preservation of normal expiratory flow rates. Thus, both forced expiratory volume in 1 sec (FEV_1) and forced vital capacity (FVC) are reduced, but the FEV_1/FVC ratio is normal.

9 Intraoperative pulmonary embolism usually presents as unexplained cardiovascular collapse, hypoxemia, or bronchospasm. A decrease in end-tidal CO_2 concentration is also suggestive of pulmonary embolism, but is not specific.

The impact of preexisting pulmonary disease on respiratory function during anesthesia and in the postoperative period is predictable: Greater degrees of preoperative pulmonary impairment are associated with more marked intraoperative alterations in respiratory function and higher rates of postoperative pulmonary complications. Failure to recognize patients who are at increased risk is a frequent contributory factor leading to complications, as patients may not receive appropriate preoperative and intraoperative care. This chapter examines pulmonary risk in general and then reviews the anesthetic approach in patients with the most common types of respiratory disease.

PULMONARY RISK FACTORS

Certain risk factors (Table 24–1) may predispose patients to postoperative pulmonary complications. The incidence of atelectasis, pneumonia, pulmonary embolism, and respiratory failure following surgery is quite high, but varies widely (from 6% to 60%), depending on the patient population studied and the surgical procedures performed. The two strongest predictors of complications seem to be operative site and a history of dyspnea, which correlate with the degree of preexisting pulmonary disease.

The association between smoking and respiratory disease is well established; abnormalities in maximal midexpiratory flow (MMEF) rates are often demonstrable well before symptoms of COPD appear. Although abnormalities can be demonstrated on pulmonary function tests (PFTs), because most patients who smoke do not have PFTs performed preoperatively, it is best to assume that such patients have some degree of pulmonary compromise. Even in normal individuals, advancing age is associated with an increasing prevalence of pulmonary disease and an increase in closing capacity. Obesity decreases functional residual capacity (FRC), increases the work of breathing, and predisposes patients to deep venous thrombosis.

Thoracic and upper abdominal surgical procedures can have marked effects on pulmonary function. Operations near the diaphragm often result in diaphragmatic dysfunction and a restrictive

TABLE 24–1   Risk factors for postoperative pulmonary complications.

Patient-related Factors[1]	Procedure-related Factors[1]
Supported by good evidence	
Advanced age	Aortic aneurysm repair
ASA class ≥2	Thoracic surgery
Congestive heart failure	Abdominal surgery
Functional dependency	Upper abdominal surgery
Chronic obstructive pulmonary disease	Neurosurgery
	Prolonged surgery
	Head and neck surgery
	Emergency surgery
	Vascular surgery
	Use of general anesthesia
Supported by fair evidence	
Weight loss	Perioperative transfusion
Impaired sensorium	
Cigarette use	
Alcohol use	
Abnormal chest exam	
Good evidence *against* being a risk factor	
Well-controlled asthma	Hip surgery
Obesity	Genitourinary/gynecologic surgery
Insufficient data	
Obstructive sleep apnea[2]	Esophageal surgery
Poor exercise capacity	

ASA, American Society of Anesthesiologists.

[1]Within each evidence category, risk factors are listed according to strength of evidence, with the first factor listed having the strongest evidence.

[2]Subsequent evidence indicates that this is a probable risk factor.

Data from Smetana GW, Lawrence VA, Cornell JE, et al: Preoperative pulmonary risk stratification for noncardiothoracic surgery: systematic review for the American College of Physicians, Ann Intern Med 2006;144(8):581-595.

ventilatory defect (see below). Upper abdominal procedures consistently decrease FRC (60% to 70%); the effect is maximal on the first postoperative day and usually lasts 7–10 days. Rapid shallow breathing with an ineffective cough caused by pain (splinting), a decrease in the number of sighs, and impaired mucociliary clearance lead to microatelectasis and loss of lung volume. Intrapulmonary shunting promotes hypoxemia. Residual anesthetic effects, the recumbent position, sedation from opioids, abdominal distention, and restrictive dressings may also be contributory. Complete relief of pain with regional

TABLE 24–2 Recommendations of the American College of Physicians to reduce perioperative pulmonary complications in patients undergoing noncardiothoracic surgery.

Recommendation 1:
- All patients undergoing noncardiothoracic surgery should be evaluated for the presence of the following significant risk factors for postoperative pulmonary complications in order to receive pre- and postoperative interventions to reduce pulmonary risk: chronic obstructive pulmonary disease, age older than 60 years, American Society of Anesthesiologists class of II or greater, functionally dependent, and congestive heart failure.
- The following are not significant risk factors for postoperative pulmonary complications: obesity and mild or moderate asthma.

Recommendation 2:
- Patients undergoing the following procedures are at higher risk for postoperative pulmonary complications and should be evaluated for other concomitant risk factors and receive pre- and postoperative interventions to reduce pulmonary complications: prolonged surgery (>3 hours), abdominal surgery, thoracic surgery, neurosurgery, head and neck surgery, vascular surgery, aortic aneurysm repair, emergency surgery, and general anesthesia.

Recommendation 3:
- A low serum albumin level (<35 g/L) is a powerful marker of increased risk for postoperative pulmonary complications and should be measured in all patients who are clinically suspected of having hypoalbuminemia; measurement should be considered in patients with one or more risk factors for perioperative pulmonary complications.

Recommendation 4:
- All patients who after preoperative evaluation are found to be at higher risk for postoperative pulmonary complications should receive the following postoperative procedures in order to reduce postoperative pulmonary complications: deep breathing exercises or incentive spirometry and the selective use of a nasogastric tube (as needed for postoperative nausea or vomiting, inability to tolerate oral intake, or symptomatic abdominal distention).

Recommendation 5:
- Preoperative spirometry and chest radiography should not be used routinely for predicting risk for postoperative pulmonary complications.
- Preoperative pulmonary function testing or chest radiography may be appropriate in patients with a previous diagnosis of chronic obstructive pulmonary disease or asthma.

Recommendation 6:
- The following procedures should not be used solely for reducing postoperative pulmonary complication risk: right heart catheterization and total parenteral nutrition or total enteral nutrition (for patients who are malnourished or have low serum albumin levels).

Data from Qaseem A, Snow V, Fitterman N, et al: Risk assessment for and strategies to reduce perioperative pulmonary complication for patients undergoing noncardiothoracic surgery: a guideline from the American College of Physicians. Ann Intern Med 2006;144:576.

anesthesia can decrease, but does not completely reverse these abnormalities. Persistent microatelectasis and retention of secretions favor the development of postoperative pneumonia.

Although many adverse effects of general anesthesia on pulmonary function have been described, the superiority of regional over general anesthesia in patients with pulmonary impairment is not firmly established.

Because of the prevalence of smoking and obesity, many patients may be at increased risk of developing postoperative pulmonary dysfunction. The risk of complications increases if the patient is having a thoracotomy or laparotomy, even if the patient has no risk factors. Patients with known disease should have their pulmonary function optimized preoperatively, with careful consideration given to the choice of general versus regional anesthesia.

The American College of Physicians has established guidelines to assist in the preoperative assessment of patients with pulmonary disease (see Table 24–2).

When patients with a history of dyspnea present without the benefit of a previous workup, the differential diagnosis can be quite broad and may include both primary pulmonary and cardiac pathologies. Diagnostic approaches to evaluating such patients are summarized in Figure 24–1.

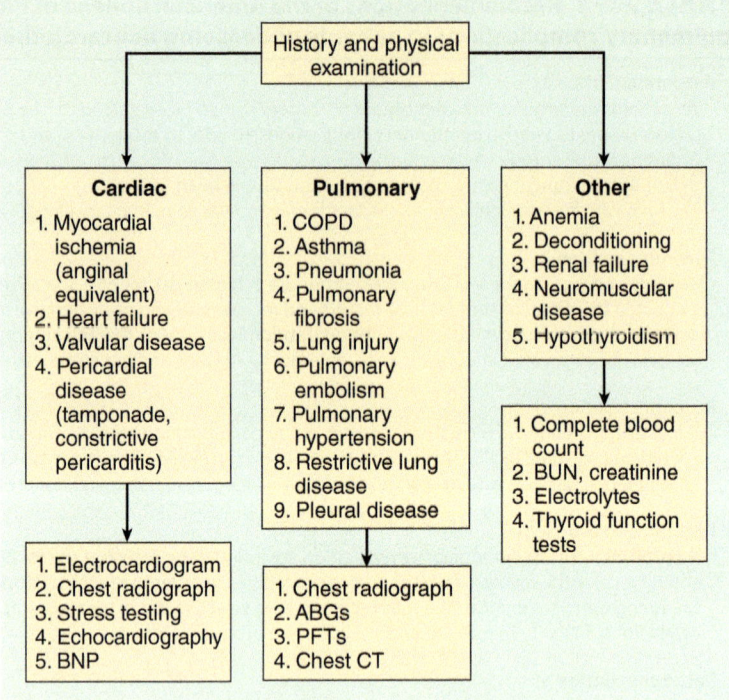

FIGURE 24–1 Evaluation of dyspnea. ABGs, arterial blood gases; BNP, brain natriuretic peptide; BUN, blood urea nitrogen; COPD, chronic obstructive pulmonary disease; CT, computed tomography; PFTs, pulmonary function tests. (Reproduced, with permission, from Sweitzer BJ, Smetana GW: Identification and evaluation of the patient with lung disease. Anesthesiol Clin 2009;27:673.)

Obstructive Pulmonary Disease

Obstructive and restrictive breathing are the two most common abnormal patterns, as determined by PFTs. Obstructive lung diseases are the most common form of pulmonary dysfunction. They include asthma, emphysema, chronic bronchitis, cystic fibrosis, bronchiectasis, and bronchiolitis. The primary characteristic of these disorders is resistance to airflow. An MMEF of <70% (forced expiratory flow [$FEF_{25-75\%}$]) is often the only abnormality early in the course of these disorders. Values for $FEF_{25-75\%}$ in adult males and females are normally >2.0 and >1.6 L/sec, respectively. As the disease progresses, both forced expiratory volume in 1 sec (FEV_1) and the FEV_1/FVC (forced vital capacity) ratio are less than 70% of the predicted values.

Elevated airway resistance and air trapping increase the work of breathing; respiratory gas exchange is impaired because of ventilation/perfusion ($\dot{V}/\dot{Q}$) imbalance. The predominance of expiratory airflow resistance results in air trapping; residual volume and total lung capacity (TLC) increase. Wheezing is a common finding and represents turbulent airflow. It is often absent with mild obstruction that may be manifested initially only by prolonged exhalation. Progressive obstruction typically results first in expiratory wheezing only, and then in both inspiratory and expiratory wheezing. With marked obstruction, wheezing may be absent when airflow has nearly ceased.

ASTHMA
Preoperative Considerations

Asthma is a common disorder, affecting 5% to 7% of the population. Its primary characteristic is airway (bronchiolar) inflammation and hyperreactivity in response to a variety of stimuli. Clinically, asthma is manifested by episodic attacks of dyspnea, cough, and wheezing. Airway obstruction, which is generally reversible, is the result of bronchial smooth muscle constriction, edema, and increased secretions.

Classically, the obstruction is precipitated by a variety of airborne substances, including pollens, animal dander, dusts, pollutants, and various chemicals. Some patients also develop bronchospasm following ingestion of aspirin, nonsteroidal antiinflammatory agents, sulfites, or tartrazine and other dyes. Exercise, emotional excitement, and viral infections also precipitate bronchospasm in many patients. Asthma is classified as acute or chronic. Chronic asthma is further classified as intermittent (mild) and mild, moderate, and severe persistent disease.

The terms extrinsic (allergic) asthma (attacks related to environmental exposures) and intrinsic (idiosyncratic) asthma (attacks usually occurring without provocation) were used in the past, but these classifications were imperfect; many patients show features of both forms. Moreover, overlap with chronic bronchitis (see below) is common.

A. Pathophysiology

The pathophysiology of asthma involves the local release of various chemical mediators in the airway, and, possibly, overactivity of the parasympathetic nervous system. Inhaled substances can initiate bronchospasm through both specific and nonspecific immune mechanisms by degranulating bronchial mast cells. In classic allergic asthma, antigen binding to immunoglobulin E (IgE) on the surface of mast cells causes degranulation. Bronchoconstriction is the result of the subsequent release of histamine; bradykinin; leukotrienes C, D, and E; platelet-activating factor; prostaglandins (PG) PGE_2, $PGF_2\alpha$, and PGD_2; and neutrophil and eosinophil chemotactic factors. The parasympathetic nervous system plays a major role in maintaining normal bronchial tone; a normal diurnal variation in tone is recognized in most individuals, with peak airway resistance occurring early in the morning (at about 6:00 AM). **Vagal afferents in the bronchi are sensitive to histamine and multiple noxious stimuli, including cold air, inhaled irritants, and instrumentation (eg, tracheal intubation).** Reflex vagal activation results in bronchoconstriction, which is mediated by an increase in intracellular cyclic guanosine monophosphate (cGMP).

During an asthma attack, bronchoconstriction, mucosal edema, and secretions increase resistance to gas flow at all levels of the lower airways. As an attack resolves, airway resistance normalizes first in the larger airways (main-stem, lobar, segmental, and subsegmental bronchi), and then in more peripheral airways. Consequently, expiratory flow rates are initially decreased throughout an entire forced exhalation, but during resolution of the attack, the expiratory flow rate is reduced only at low lung volumes. TLC, residual volume (RV), and FRC are all increased. In acutely ill patients, RV and FRC are often increased by more than 400% and 100%, respectively. Prolonged or severe attacks markedly increase the work of breathing and can fatigue respiratory muscles. The number of alveolar units with low ($\dot{V}/\dot{Q}$) ratios increases, resulting in hypoxemia. Tachypnea is likely due to stimulation of bronchial receptors and typically produces hypocapnia. A normal or high $Paco_2$ indicates that the patient can no longer maintain the work of breathing and is often a sign of impending respiratory failure. A pulsus paradoxus and electrocardiographic signs of right ventricular strain (ST-segment changes, right axis deviation, and right bundle branch block) are also indicative of severe airway obstruction.

B. Treatment

Drugs used to treat asthma include β-adrenergic agonists, methylxanthines, glucocorticoids, anticholinergics, leukotriene blockers, and mast cell–stabilizing agents; with the exception of the last, these drugs may be used for either acute or chronic treatment of asthma. Although devoid of any bronchodilating properties, cromolyn sodium and nedocromil are effective in preventing bronchospasm by blocking the degranulation of mast cells.

Sympathomimetic agents (Table 24–3) are the most commonly used for acute exacerbations. They produce bronchodilation via β₂-agonist activity. Activation of β₂-adrenergic receptors on bronchiolar smooth muscle stimulates the activity of adenylate cyclase, which results in the formation of intracellular cyclic adenosine monophosphate (cAMP). These agents are usually administered via a metered-dose inhaler or by aerosol. Use of more selective β₂-agonists, such as terbutaline or albuterol, may decrease the incidence of undesirable β₁

TABLE 24–3 A comparison of commonly used bronchodilators.[1]

Agent	Adrenergic Activity	
	β_1	β_2
Albuterol (Ventolin)	+	+++
Bitolterol (Tornalate)	+	++++
Epinephrine	++++	++
Fenoterol (Berotec)	+	+++
Formaterol (Foradil)	+	++++
Isoetharine (Bronkosol)	++	+++
Isoproterenol (Isuprel)	++++	—
Metaproterenol (Alupent)	+	+
Pirbuterol (Maxair)	+	++++
Salmeterol (Serevent)	+	++++
Terbutaline (Brethaire)	+	+++

[1]+ Indicates level of activity.

cardiac effects, but are often not particularly selective in high doses.

Traditionally, methylxanthines are thought to produce bronchodilation by inhibiting phosphodiesterase, the enzyme responsible for the breakdown of cAMP. Their pulmonary effects seem much more complex and include catecholamine release, blockade of histamine release, and diaphragmatic stimulation. Oral long-acting theophylline preparations are used for patients with nocturnal symptoms. Unfortunately, theophylline has a narrow therapeutic range; therapeutic blood levels are considered to be 10–20 mcg/mL. Lower levels, however, may be effective. Aminophylline is the only available intravenous theophylline preparation.

Glucocorticoids are used for both acute treatment and maintenance therapy of patients with asthma because of their antiinflammatory and membrane-stabilizing effects. Beclomethasone, triamcinolone, fluticasone, and budesonide are synthetic steroids commonly used in metered-dose inhalers for maintenance therapy. Although they are associated with a low incidence of undesirable

systemic effects, their use does not necessarily prevent adrenal suppression. Intravenous hydrocortisone or methylprednisolone is used acutely for severe attacks, followed by tapering doses of oral prednisone. Glucocorticoids usually require several hours to become effective.

Anticholinergic agents produce bronchodilation through their antimuscarinic action and may block reflex bronchoconstriction. Ipratropium, a congener of atropine that can be given by a metered-dose inhaler or aerosol, is a moderately effective bronchodilator without appreciable systemic anticholinergic effects.

Anesthetic Considerations

A. Preoperative Management

The emphasis in evaluating patients with asthma should be on determining the recent course of the disease and whether the patient has ever been hospitalized for an acute asthma attack, as well as on ascertaining that the patient is in optimal condition. Patients with poorly controlled asthma or wheezing at the time of anesthesia induction have a higher risk of perioperative complications. Conversely, well-controlled asthma has not been shown to be a risk factor for intraoperative or postoperative complications. A thorough history and physical examination are of critical importance. The patient should have no or minimal dyspnea, wheezing, or cough. Complete resolution of recent exacerbations should be confirmed by chest auscultation. Patients with frequent or chronic bronchospasm should be placed on an optimal bronchodilating regimen. A chest radiograph identifies air trapping; hyperinflation results in a flattened diaphragm, a small-appearing heart, and hyperlucent lung fields. PFTs—particularly expiratory airflow measurements such as FEV_1, FEV_1/FVC, $FEF_{25-75\%}$, and peak expiratory flow rate—help in assessing the severity of airway obstruction and reversibility after bronchodilator treatment. Comparisons with previous measurements are invaluable.

2 Asthmatic patients with active bronchospasm presenting for emergency surgery should be treated aggressively. Supplemental oxygen, aerosolized β_2-agonists, and intravenous glucocorticoids can dramatically improve lung function in a few hours. Arterial blood gases may be useful in managing severe cases. Hypoxemia and hypercapnia are typical of moderate and severe disease; even slight hypercapnia is indicative of severe air trapping and may be a sign of impending respiratory failure.

Some degree of preoperative sedation may be desirable in asthmatic patients presenting for elective surgery—particularly in patients whose disease has an emotional component. In general, benzodiazepines are the most satisfactory agents for premedication. Anticholinergic agents are not customarily given unless very copious secretions are present or if ketamine is to be used for induction of anesthesia. In typical intramuscular doses, anticholinergics are not effective in preventing reflex bronchospasm following intubation. The use of an H_2-blocking agent (such as cimetidine, ranitidine, or famotidine) is theoretically detrimental, since H_2-receptor activation normally produces bronchodilation; in the event of histamine release, unopposed H_1 activation with H_2 blockade may accentuate bronchoconstriction.

Bronchodilators should be continued up to the time of surgery; in order of effectiveness, they are β-agonists, inhaled glucocorticoids, leukotriene blockers, mast-cell stabilizers, theophyllines, and anticholinergics. Patients who receive chronic glucocorticoid therapy with more than 5 mg/day of prednisone (or its equivalent) should receive a graduated supplementation schedule based on the severity of the illness and complexity of the surgical procedure. Supplemental doses should be tapered to baseline within 1–2 days.

B. Intraoperative Management

The most critical time for asthmatic patients undergoing anesthesia is during instrumentation of the airway. General anesthesia by mask or regional anesthesia will circumvent this problem, but neither eliminates the possibility of bronchospasm. In fact, some clinicians believe that high spinal or epidural anesthesia may aggravate bronchoconstriction by blocking sympathetic tone to the lower airways (T1–T4) and allowing unopposed parasympathetic activity. Pain, emotional stress, or stimulation during light general anesthesia can precipitate bronchospasm. Drugs often associated with histamine release (eg, atracurium, morphine, and meperidine) should be avoided or given very slowly when used. The goal of any general anesthetic is a smooth induction and emergence, with anesthetic depth adjusted to stimulation.

The choice of induction agent is less important, if adequate depth of anesthesia is achieved before intubation or surgical stimulation. Thiopental may occasionally induce bronchospasm as a result of exaggerated histamine release. Propofol and etomidate are suitable induction agents; propofol may also produce bronchodilation. Ketamine has bronchodilating properties and is a good choice for patients with asthma who are also hemodynamically unstable. Ketamine should probably not be used in patients with high theophylline levels, as the combined actions of the two drugs can precipitate seizure activity. Halothane and sevoflurane usually provide the smoothest inhalation induction with bronchodilation in asthmatic children. Isoflurane and desflurane can provide equal bronchodilation, but are not normally used for inhalation induction. Desflurane is the most pungent of the volatile agents and may result in cough, laryngospasm, and bronchospasm.

Reflex bronchospasm can be blunted before intubation by an additional dose of the induction agent, ventilating the patient with a 2–3 minimum alveolar concentration (MAC) of a volatile agent for 5 min, or administering intravenous or intratracheal lidocaine (1–2 mg/kg). Note that intratracheal lidocaine itself can initiate bronchospasm if an inadequate dose of induction agent has been used. Administration of an anticholinergic agent may block reflex bronchospasm, but causes excessive tachycardia. Although succinylcholine may on occasion induce marked histamine release, it can generally be safely used in most asthmatic patients. In the absence of capnography, confirmation of correct tracheal placement by chest auscultation can be difficult in the presence of marked bronchospasm.

Volatile anesthetics are most often used for maintenance of anesthesia to take advantage of their potent bronchodilating properties. Ventilation should incorporate warmed humidified gases whenever possible. Airflow obstruction during expiration is apparent on capnography as a delayed rise of the end-tidal CO_2 value (Figure 24–2); the

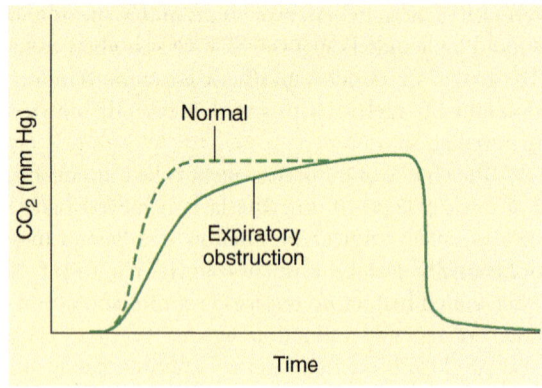

FIGURE 24–2 Capnograph of a patient with expiratory airway obstruction.

severity of obstruction is generally inversely related to the rate of rise in end-tidal CO_2. Severe bronchospasm is manifested by rising peak inspiratory pressures and incomplete exhalation. Tidal volumes of 6–8 mL/kg, with prolongation of the expiratory time, may allow more uniform distribution of gas flow to both lungs and may help avoid air trapping. The $Paco_2$ may increase, which is acceptable if there is no contraindication from a cardiovascular or neurologic perspective.

3 Intraoperative bronchospasm is usually manifested as wheezing, increasing peak airway pressures (plateau pressure may remain unchanged), decreasing exhaled tidal volumes, or a slowly rising waveform on the capnograph. Other causes **4** can simulate bronchospasm: obstruction of the tracheal tube from kinking, secretions, or an overinflated balloon; bronchial intubation; active expiratory efforts (straining); pulmonary edema or embolism; and pneumothorax. Bronchospasm should be treated by increasing the concentration of the volatile agent and administering an aerosolized bronchodilator. Infusion of low dose epinephrine may be needed if bronchospasm is refractory to other interventions.

Intravenous hydrocortisone can be given, particularly in patients with a history of glucocorticoid therapy.

At the completion of surgery, the patient should ideally be free of wheezing. Reversal of

nondepolarizing neuromuscular blocking agents with anticholinesterase agents does not precipitate bronchoconstriction, if preceded by the appropriate dose of an anticholinergic agent. Deep extubation (before airway reflexes return) reduces bronchospasm on emergence. Lidocaine as a bolus (1.5–2 mg/kg) may help obtund airway reflexes during emergence.

CHRONIC OBSTRUCTIVE PULMONARY DISEASE

Preoperative Considerations

COPD is the most common pulmonary disorder encountered in anesthetic practice, and its prevalence increases with age. The disorder is strongly associated with cigarette smoking and has a male **5** predominance. COPD is currently defined as a disease state characterized by airflow limitation that is not fully reversible. The chronic airflow limitation of this disease is due to a mixture of small and large airway disease (chronic bronchitis/bronchiolitis) and parenchymal destruction (emphysema), with representation of these two components varying from patient to patient.

Most patients with COPD are asymptomatic or only mildly symptomatic, but show expiratory airflow obstruction upon PFTs. In many patients, the obstruction has an element of reversibility, presumably from bronchospasm (as shown by improvement in response to administration of a bronchodilator). With advancing disease, maldistribution of both ventilation and pulmonary blood flow results in areas of low $(\dot{V}/\dot{Q})$ ratios (intrapulmonary shunt), as well as areas of high $(\dot{V}/\dot{Q})$ ratios (dead space).

A. Chronic Bronchitis

The clinical diagnosis of chronic bronchitis is defined by the presence of a productive cough on most days of 3 consecutive months for at least 2 consecutive years. In addition to cigarette smoking, air pollutants, occupational exposure to dusts, recurrent pulmonary infections, and familial factors may be responsible. Secretions from hypertrophied bronchial mucous glands and mucosal edema from inflammation of the airways produce airflow obstruction. The term "chronic asthmatic

TABLE 24–4 Signs and symptoms of chronic obstructive pulmonary disease.

Feature	Chronic Bronchitis	Emphysema
Cough	Frequent	With exertion
Sputum	Copious	Scant
Hematocrit	Elevated	Normal
$Paco_2$ (mm Hg)	Often elevated (>40)	Usually normal or <40
Chest radiograph	Increased lung markings	Hyperinflation
Elastic recoil	Normal	Decreased
Airway resistance	Increased	Normal to slightly increased
Cor pulmonale	Early	Late

bronchitis" may be used when bronchospasm is a major feature. Recurrent pulmonary infections (viral and bacterial) are common and often associated with bronchospasm. RV is increased, but TLC is often normal. Intrapulmonary shunting is prominent, and hypoxemia is common.

In patients with COPD, chronic hypoxemia leads to erythrocytosis, pulmonary hypertension, and eventually right ventricular failure (cor pulmonale); this combination of findings is often referred to as the blue bloater syndrome, but <5% of patients with COPD fit this description (Table 24–4). In the course of disease progression, patients gradually develop chronic CO_2 retention; the normal ventilatory drive becomes less sensitive to arterial CO_2 tension and may be depressed by oxygen administration (below).

B. Emphysema

Emphysema is a pathological disorder characterized by irreversible enlargement of the airways distal to terminal bronchioles and destruction of alveolar septa. The diagnosis can be reliably made with computed tomography (CT) of the chest. Mild apical emphysematous changes are a normal, but clinically insignificant, consequence of aging. Significant emphysema is more frequently related to cigarette smoking. Less commonly, emphysema occurs at an early age and is associated with a homozygous deficiency of α_1-antitrypsin. This is a protease inhibitor that prevents excessive activity of proteolytic enzymes (mainly elastase) in the lungs; these enzymes are produced by pulmonary neutrophils and macrophages in response to infection and pollutants. Emphysema associated with smoking may similarly be due to a relative imbalance between protease and antiprotease activities in susceptible individuals.

Emphysema may exist in a centrilobular or panlobular form. The centrilobular (or centriacinar) form results from dilatation or destruction of the respiratory bronchioles, is more closely associated with tobacco smoking, and has predominantly an upper lobe distribution. The panlobular (or panacinar) form results in a more even dilatation and destruction of the entire acinus, is associated with α_1-antitrypsin deficiency, and has predominantly a lower lobe distribution.

Loss of the elastic recoil that normally supports small airways by radial traction allows premature collapse during exhalation, leading to expiratory flow limitation with air trapping and hyperinflation. Patients characteristically have increases in RV, FRC, TLC, and the RV/TLC ratio. The FRC is shifted rightward along the compliance curve of the lungs, toward the flat portion of the curve, in detriment of the pulmonary mechanics.

Disruption of the alveolar–capillary structure and loss of the acinar structure leads to decreased diffusion lung capacity (DLCO), $\dot{V}/\dot{Q}$ mismatch, and impairment of gas exchange. Also, normal parenchyma may become compressed by the hyperinflated portions of the lung, resulting in a further increase in the $\dot{V}/\dot{Q}$ mismatch. Due to the higher diffusibility of CO_2, its elimination is well preserved until $\dot{V}/\dot{Q}$ abnormalities become severe. Chronic CO_2 retention occurs slowly and generally results in a compensated respiratory acidosis on blood gas analysis. Arterial oxygen tension is usually normal or slightly reduced. Acute CO_2 retention is a sign of impending respiratory failure.

Destruction of pulmonary capillaries in the alveolar septa leads to the development of pulmonary hypertension. However, the degree of pulmonary hypertension is usually low to moderate, rarely exceeding 35-40 mm Hg.

When dyspneic, patients with emphysema often purse their lips to delay closure of the small airways, which accounts for the term "pink puffers" that is often used (Table 24–4). However, as mentioned above, most patients diagnosed with COPD have a combination of bronchitis and emphysema.

C. Treatment

Treatment for COPD is primarily supportive. **(6)** Cessation of smoking is the long-term intervention that has been shown to reduce the rate of decline in lung function. Patients demonstrating a reversible element in airway obstruction (>15% improvement in FEV$_1$ following administration of a bronchodilator) should be started on long-term bronchodilator therapy. Inhaled β_2-adrenergic agonists, glucocorticoids, and ipratropium are very useful; ipratropium may play a more important role in the management of these patients than in patients with asthma. Even patients who do not show improvement in their PFTs from the use of bronchodilators may improve clinically with bronchodilator therapy. Treatment with systemic corticosteroids may be required in patients with acute exacerbations of COPD. However, systemic corticosteroids in patients with stable COPD is discouraged due to the lack of added benefit and the potential for systemic side effects. COPD exacerbations may be related to bouts of bronchitis, heralded by a change in sputum; frequent treatment with broad-spectrum antibiotics may be necessary. Hypoxemia should be treated carefully with supplemental oxygen. Patients with chronic hypoxemia (Pao$_2$ <55 mm Hg) and pulmonary hypertension require low-flow oxygen therapy (1–2 L/min). Oxygen treatment during acute COPD exacerbations to a Pao$_2$ above 60 mm Hg may lead to CO$_2$ retention, most likely due to an inhibition of the hypoxic vasoconstriction in areas with low $\dot{V}/\dot{Q}$ and the Haldane effect.

When cor pulmonale is present, diuretics are used to control peripheral edema; beneficial effects from vasodilators are inconsistent. Pulmonary rehabilitation may improve the functional status of the patient by improving physical symptoms and exercise capacity. Some studies suggest that the ability to increase oxygen consumption during exercise is inversely related to postoperative complications.

Anesthetic Considerations

A. Preoperative Management

Patients with COPD should be prepared prior to elective surgical procedures in the same way as patients with asthma (above). They should be questioned about recent changes in dyspnea, sputum, and wheezing. Patients with an FEV$_1$ less than 50% of predicted (1.2–1.5 L) usually have dyspnea on exertion, whereas those with an FEV$_1$ less than 25% (<1 L in men) typically have dyspnea with minimal activity. The latter finding, in patients with predominantly chronic bronchitis, is also often associated with CO$_2$ retention and pulmonary hypertension. PFTs, chest radiographs, and arterial blood gas measurements, if available, should be reviewed carefully. The presence of bullous changes on the radiograph should be noted. Many patients have concomitant cardiac disease and should also receive a careful cardiovascular evaluation.

In contrast to asthma, only limited improvement in respiratory function may be seen after a short period of intensive preoperative preparation. **(7)** Nonetheless, preoperative interventions in patients with COPD aimed at correcting hypoxemia, relieving bronchospasm, mobilizing and reducing secretions, and treating infections may decrease the incidence of postoperative pulmonary complications. Patients at greatest risk of complications are those with preoperative pulmonary function measurements less than 50% of predicted. The possibility that postoperative ventilation may be necessary in high-risk patients should be discussed with both the patient and the surgeon.

Smoking should be discontinued for at least 6–8 weeks before the operation to decrease secretions and to reduce pulmonary complications. Cigarette smoking increases mucus production and decreases clearance. Both gaseous and particulate phases of cigarette smoke can deplete glutathione and vitamin C and may promote oxidative injury to tissues. Cessation of smoking for as little as 24 hr has theoretical beneficial effects on the oxygen-carrying capacity of hemoglobin; acute inhalation of cigarette smoke releases carbon monoxide, which increases carboxyhemoglobin levels, as well as nitric oxide, and nitrogen dioxide, which can lead to formation of methemoglobin.

Long-acting bronchodilators and mucolytics should be continued, including on the day of surgery. COPD exacerbations should be treated aggressively.

Preoperative chest physiotherapy and lung expansion interventions with incentive spirometry, deep breathing exercises, cough, chest percussion, and postural drainage may be beneficial in decreasing postoperative pulmonary complications.

B. Intraoperative Management

Although regional anesthesia is often considered preferable to general anesthesia, high spinal or epidural anesthesia can decrease lung volumes, restrict the use of accessory respiratory muscles, and produce an ineffective cough, leading to dyspnea and retention of secretions. Loss of proprioception from the chest and positions such as lithotomy or lateral decubitus may accentuate dyspnea in awake patients.

Concerns about diaphragmatic paralysis may make interscalene blocks a less attractive option in the lung disease patient.

Preoxygenation prior to induction of general anesthesia prevents the rapid oxygen desaturation often seen in these patients. The selection of anesthetic agents and general intraoperative management must be tailored to the specific needs and goals of every patient. Unfortunately, the use of bronchodilating anesthetics improves only the reversible component of airflow obstruction; significant expiratory obstruction may still present, even under deep anesthesia. Expiratory airflow limitation, especially under positive pressure ventilation, may lead to air trapping, dynamic hyperinflation, and elevated intrinsic positive end-expiratory pressure (iPEEP). Dynamic hyperinflation may result in volutrauma to the lungs, hemodynamic instability, hypercapnia, and acidosis. Interventions to mitigate air trapping include: (1) allowing more time to exhale by decreasing both the respiratory rate and I:E ratio; (2) allowing permissive hypercapnia; (3) applying low levels of extrinsic PEEP; and (4) aggressively treating bronchospasm.

Intraoperative causes of hypotension include pneumothorax, and right heart failure due to hypercapnia and acidosis. A pneumothorax may manifest as hypoxemia, increased peak airway pressures, decreasing tidal volumes, and abrupt cardiovascular collapse unresponsive to fluid and vasopressor administration.

Nitrous oxide should be avoided in patients with bullae and pulmonary hypertension. Inhibition of hypoxic pulmonary vasoconstriction by inhalation anesthetics is usually not clinically significant at the usual doses. However, due to increased dead space, patients with severe COPD have unpredictable uptake and distribution of inhalational agents, and the end-tidal volatile anesthetic concentration is inaccurate.

Measurement of arterial blood gases is desirable for extensive intraabdominal and thoracic procedures. Although pulse oximetry accurately detects significant arterial desaturation, direct measurement of arterial oxygen tensions may be necessary to detect more subtle changes in intrapulmonary shunting. Moreover, arterial CO_2 measurements should be used to guide ventilation because increased dead space widens the normal arterial-to-end-tidal CO_2 gradient. Moderate hypercapnia with a $Paco_2$ of up to 70 mm Hg may be well tolerated in the short term, assuming a reasonable cardiovascular reserve. Hemodynamic support with inotropic agents may be required in more compromised patients. Hemodynamic monitoring should be dictated by any underlying cardiac dysfunction, as well as the extent of the surgery. In patients with pulmonary hypertension, measurements of central venous pressure reflect right ventricular function rather than intravascular volume.

At the end of surgery, the timing of extubation should balance the risk of bronchospasm with that of respiratory failure, but evidence suggests that early extubation (in the operating room) is beneficial. Successful extubation at the end of the procedure depends on multiple factors: adequate pain control, reversal of neuromuscular blockade, absence of significant bronchospasm and secretions, absence of significant hypercapnia and acidosis, and absence of respiratory depression due to residual anesthetic agents. Patients with an FEV_1 below 50% may require a period of postoperative ventilation, particularly following upper abdominal and thoracic operations.

Restrictive Pulmonary Disease

8 Restrictive pulmonary diseases are characterized by decreased lung compliance. Lung volumes are typically reduced, with preservation of normal expiratory flow rates. Thus, both FEV_1 and FVC are reduced, but the FEV_1/FVC ratio is normal.

Restrictive pulmonary diseases include many acute and chronic intrinsic pulmonary disorders, as well as extrinsic (extrapulmonary) disorders involving the pleura, chest wall, diaphragm, or neuromuscular function. Reduced lung compliance increases the work of breathing, resulting in a characteristic rapid, but shallow, breathing pattern. Respiratory gas exchange is usually maintained until the disease process is advanced.

ACUTE INTRINSIC PULMONARY DISORDERS

Acute intrinsic pulmonary disorders include pulmonary edema (including the acute respiratory distress syndrome [ARDS]), infectious pneumonia, and aspiration pneumonitis.

Preoperative Considerations

Reduced lung compliance in these disorders is primarily due to an increase in extravascular lung water, from either an increase in pulmonary capillary pressure or pulmonary capillary permeability. Increased pressure occurs with left ventricular failure, whereas fluid overload and increased permeability are present with ARDS. Localized or generalized increases in permeability also occur following aspiration or infectious pneumonitis.

Anesthetic Considerations

A. Preoperative Management

Patients with acute pulmonary disease should be spared elective surgery. In preparation for emergency procedures, oxygenation and ventilation should be optimized preoperatively to the greatest extent possible. Fluid overload should be treated with diuretics; heart failure may also require vasodilators and inotropes. Drainage of large pleural effusions should be considered. Similarly, massive abdominal distention should be relieved by nasogastric compression or drainage of ascites. Persistent hypoxemia may require mechanical ventilation.

B. Intraoperative Management

Selection of anesthetic agents should be tailored to each patient. Surgical patients with acute pulmonary disorders, such as ARDS, cardiogenic pulmonary edema, or pneumonia, are critically ill; anesthetic management should be a continuation of their preoperative intensive care. Anesthesia is most often provided with a combination of intravenous and inhalation agents, together with a neuromuscular blocking agent. High inspired oxygen concentrations and PEEP may be required. The decreased lung compliance results in high peak inspiratory pressures during positive-pressure ventilation and increases the risk of barotrauma and volutrauma. Tidal volumes for these patients should be reduced to 4–6 mL/kg, with a compensatory increase in the ventilatory rate (14–18 breaths/min), even if the result is an increase in end-tidal CO_2. Airway pressure should generally not exceed 30 cm H_2O. Airway pressure release ventilation may improve oxygenation in the ARDS patient. The ventilator on the anesthesia machine may prove inadequate for patients with severe ARDS because of its limited gas flow capabilities, low pressure-limiting settings, and the absence of certain ventilatory modes. A more sophisticated intensive care unit ventilator should be used in such instances. Aggressive hemodynamic monitoring is recommended.

CHRONIC INTRINSIC PULMONARY DISORDERS

Chronic intrinsic pulmonary disorders are also often referred to as interstitial lung diseases. Regardless of etiology, the disease process is generally characterized by an insidious onset, chronic inflammation of alveolar walls and perialveolar tissue, and progressive pulmonary fibrosis. The latter can eventually interfere with gas exchange and ventilatory function. The inflammatory process may be primarily confined to the lungs or may be part of a generalized multiorgan process. Causes include hypersensitivity pneumonitis from occupational and environmental pollutants, drug toxicity (bleomycin and nitrofu-rantoin), radiation pneumonitis, idiopathic pulmo-nary fibrosis, autoimmune diseases, and sarcoidosis. Chronic pulmonary aspiration, oxygen toxicity, and severe ARDS can also produce chronic fibrosis.

Preoperative Considerations

Patients typically present with dyspnea on exertion and sometimes a nonproductive cough. Symptoms of cor pulmonale are present only with advanced disease. Physical examination may reveal fine (dry) crackles over the lung bases, and, in late stages, evidence of right ventricular failure. The chest radiograph progresses from a "ground-glass" appearance to prominent reticulonodular markings, and, finally, to a "honeycomb" appearance. Arterial blood gases usually show mild hypoxemia with normocarbia. PFTs are typical of a restrictive ventilatory defect (see above), and carbon monoxide diffusing capacity is reduced.

Treatment is directed at abating the disease process and preventing further exposure to the causative agent (if known). Glucocorticoid and immunosuppressive therapy may be used for idiopathic pulmonary fibrosis, autoimmune disorders, and sarcoidosis. If the patient has chronic hypoxemia, oxygen therapy may be started to prevent, or attenuate, right ventricular failure.

Anesthetic Considerations

A. Preoperative Management

Preoperative evaluation should focus on determining the degree of pulmonary impairment as well as the underlying disease process. The latter is important in determining the potential involvement of other organs. A history of dyspnea on exertion (or at rest) should be evaluated further with PFTs and arterial blood gas analysis. A vital capacity of less than 15 mL/kg is indicative of severe dysfunction (normal is >70 mL/kg). A chest radiograph is helpful in assessing disease severity.

B. Intraoperative Management

The management of these patients is complicated by a predisposition to hypoxemia and the need to control ventilation to ensure optimum gas exchange;

anesthetic drug selection is generally not critical. The reduction in FRC (and oxygen stores) predisposes these patients to rapid hypoxemia following induction of anesthesia. Because these patients may be more susceptible to oxygen-induced toxicity, particularly patients who have received bleomycin, the inspired fractional concentration of oxygen should be kept to the minimum concentration compatible with acceptable oxygenation (Spo_2 of >88% to 92%). High peak inspiratory pressures during mechanical ventilation increase the risk of pneumothorax and should prompt adjustment of the ventilatory parameters. In patients with severe restrictive disease, using an I:E ratio of 1:1 (or even an inverse ratio ventilation) and dividing the minute ventilation to a higher respiratory rate (10–15 breaths/minute) may help to maximize the inspiratory time per tidal volume and minimize the peak and plateau ventilatory pressures.

EXTRINSIC RESTRICTIVE PULMONARY DISORDERS

Extrinsic restrictive pulmonary disorders alter gas exchange by interfering with normal lung expansion. They include pleural effusions, pneumothorax, mediastinal masses, kyphoscoliosis, pectus excavatum, neuromuscular disorders, and increased intraabdominal pressure from ascites, pregnancy, or bleeding. Marked obesity also produces a restrictive ventilatory defect. Anesthetic considerations are similar to those discussed for intrinsic restrictive disorders.

Pulmonary Embolism

Preoperative Considerations

Pulmonary embolism results from the entry of blood clots, fat, tumor cells, air, amniotic fluid, or foreign material into the venous system. Clots from the lower extremities, pelvic veins, or, less commonly, the right side of the heart are usually responsible. Venous stasis or hypercoagulability is often contributory in such cases (Table 24–5). Pulmonary embolism can also occur intraoperatively in normal individuals undergoing certain procedures.

TABLE 24–5 Factors associated with deep venous thrombosis and pulmonary embolism.

Prolonged bed rest
Postpartum state
Fracture of the lower extremities
Surgery on the lower extremities
Carcinoma
Heart failure
Obesity
Surgery lasting more than 30 min
Hypercoagulability
   Antithrombin III deficiency
   Protein C deficiency
   Protein S deficiency
   Plasminogen-activator deficiency

A. Pathophysiology

Embolic occlusions in the pulmonary circulation increase dead space, and, if minute ventilation does not change, this increase in dead space should theoretically increase $Paco_2$. However, in practice, hypoxemia is more often seen. Pulmonary emboli acutely increase pulmonary vascular resistance by reducing the cross-sectional area of the pulmonary vasculature, causing reflex and humoral vasoconstriction. Localized or generalized reflex bronchoconstriction further increases areas with low ($\dot{V}/\dot{Q}$) ratios. The net effect is an increase in $\dot{V}/\dot{Q}$ mismatch and hypoxemia. The affected area loses its surfactant within hours and may become atelectatic within 24–48 hr. Pulmonary infarction occurs if the embolus involves a large vessel and collateral blood flow from the bronchial circulation is insufficient for that part of the lung (incidence <10%). In previously healthy persons, occlusion of more than 50% of the pulmonary circulation (massive pulmonary embolism) is necessary before sustained pulmonary hypertension is seen. Patients with preexisting cardiac or pulmonary disease can develop acute pulmonary hypertension with occlusions of lesser magnitude. A sustained increase in right ventricular afterload can precipitate acute right ventricular failure. If the patient survives acute pulmonary thromboembolism, the thrombus usually begins to resolve within 1–2 weeks.

B. Diagnosis

Clinical manifestations of pulmonary embolism include sudden tachypnea, dyspnea, chest pain, or hemoptysis. The latter generally implies lung infarction. Symptoms are often absent or mild and nonspecific unless massive embolism has occurred. Wheezing may be present on auscultation. Arterial blood gas analysis typically shows mild hypoxemia with respiratory alkalosis (the latter due to an increase in ventilation). The chest radiograph is commonly normal, but may show an area of oligemia (radiolucency), a wedge-shaped density with an infarct, atelectasis with an elevated diaphragm, or an asymmetrically enlarged proximal pulmonary artery with acute pulmonary hypertension. Cardiac signs include tachycardia and wide fixed splitting of the S_2 heart sound; hypotension with elevated central venous pressure is usually indicative of right ventricular failure. The electrocardiogram frequently shows tachycardia and may show signs of acute cor pulmonale, such as new right axis deviation, right bundle branch block, and tall peaked T waves. Ultrasound studies of the lower extremities also may be helpful in demonstrating deep venous thrombosis. The diagnosis of embolism is more difficult to make intraoperatively (see below).

Pulmonary angiography is still the gold standard criterion for diagnosing a pulmonary embolism, but it is invasive and difficult to perform. Therefore, the less invasive spiral computed tomography angiography (CTA) is the initial imaging of choice in stable patients with suspected pulmonary embolism. Ventilation-perfusion ($\dot{V}/\dot{Q}$) scanning may also be used when CTA cannot be performed. High-, intermediate-, and low-probability criteria have been established for the diagnosis of pulmonary embolism by $\dot{V}/\dot{Q}$ scan.

C. Treatment and Prevention

The best treatment for pulmonary embolism is prevention. Heparin (unfractionated heparin 5000 U subcutaneously every 12 h begun preoperatively or immediately postoperatively in high-risk patients), enoxaparin or other related compounds, oral anticoagulation (warfarin), aspirin, or dextran therapy, together with early ambulation, can all be used to reduce the incidence of deep vein thrombosis. The use of high elastic stockings and pneumatic compression of the legs may also decrease the incidence of venous thrombosis in the legs, but not in the pelvis or the heart.

After a pulmonary embolism, systemic anticoagulation prevents the formation of new blood clots or the extension of existing clots. Heparin therapy is begun with the goal of achieving an activated partial thromboplastin time of 1.5–2.4 times normal. Low molecular-weight heparin (LMWH) is as effective and is given subcutaneously at a fixed dose (based on body weight) without laboratory monitoring. In high-risk patients, LMWH is started either 12 hr before surgery, 12–24 hr after surgery, or at 50% the usual dose 4–6 hr after surgery. All patients should start warfarin therapy concurrent with starting heparin therapy, and the two should overlap for 4–5 days. The international normalized ratio should be within the therapeutic range on two consecutive measurements, at least 24 hr apart, before the heparin is stopped. Warfarin should be continued for 3–12 months. Thrombolytic therapy with tissue plasminogen activator or streptokinase is indicated in patients with massive pulmonary embolism or circulatory collapse. Recent surgery and active bleeding are contraindications to anticoagulation and thrombolytic therapy. In these cases, an inferior vena cava umbrella filter may be placed to prevent recurrent pulmonary emboli. Pulmonary embolectomy may be indicated for patients with massive embolism in whom thrombolytic therapy is contraindicated.

Anesthetic Considerations

A. Preoperative Management

Patients with acute pulmonary embolism may present in the operating room for placement of an IVC filter, or, rarely, for pulmonary embolectomy. In most instances, the patient will have a history of pulmonary embolism and presents for unrelated surgery; in this group of patients, the risk of interrupting anticoagulant therapy perioperatively is unknown. If the acute episode is more than 1 year old, the risk of temporarily stopping anticoagulant therapy is probably small. Moreover, except in the case of chronic recurrent pulmonary emboli, pulmonary function has usually returned to normal. The emphasis in the perioperative management of these patients should be in preventing new episodes of embolism (see above).

B. Intraoperative Management

Vena cava filters are usually placed percutaneously under local anesthesia with sedation.

Patients presenting for pulmonary embolectomy are critically ill. They are usually already intubated, but tolerate positive-pressure ventilation poorly. Inotropic support is necessary until the clot is removed. They also tolerate all anesthetic agents very poorly. Small doses of an opioid, etomidate, or ketamine may be used, but the latter can theoretically increase pulmonary artery pressures. Cardiopulmonary bypass is required.

C. Intraoperative Pulmonary Embolism

Significant pulmonary embolism is a rare occurrence during anesthesia. Diagnosis requires a high index of suspicion. Air emboli are common, but are often overlooked unless large amounts are entrained. Fat embolism can occur during orthopedic procedures; amniotic fluid embolism is a rare, unpredictable, and often fatal, complication of obstetrical delivery. Thromboembolism may occur intraoperatively during prolonged procedures. The clot may have been present prior to surgery or may form intraoperatively; surgical manipulations or a change in the patient's position may then dislodge the venous thrombus. Manipulation of tumors with intravascular extension can similarly produce pulmonary embolism.

9 Intraoperative pulmonary embolism usually presents as sudden cardiovascular collapse, hypoxemia, or bronchospasm. A decrease in end-tidal CO_2 concentration is also suggestive of pulmonary embolism, but is not specific. Invasive monitoring may reveal elevated central venous and pulmonary arterial pressures. Depending on the type and location of an embolism, a transesophageal echocardiogram may be helpful. TEE may not reveal the embolus but will often demonstrate right heart distention and dysfunction. **If air is identified in the right atrium, or if it is suspected, emergent central vein cannulation and aspiration of the air may be lifesaving.** For all other emboli, treatment is supportive, with intravenous fluids and inotropes. Placement of a vena cava filter should be considered postoperatively.

CASE DISCUSSION

Laparoscopic Surgery

A 45-year-old woman is scheduled for a laparo-scopic cholecystectomy. Known medical prob-lems include obesity and a history of smoking.

What are the advantages of laparoscopic cholecystectomy compared with open cholecystectomy?

Laparoscopic techniques have rapidly increased in popularity because of the multiple benefits associated with much smaller incisions than with traditional open techniques. These ben-efits include decreased postoperative pain, less postoperative pulmonary impairment, a reduction in postoperative ileus, shorter hospital stays, earlier ambulation, and smaller surgical scars. Thus, lapa-roscopic surgery can provide substantial medical and economic advantages.

How does laparoscopic surgery affect intraoperative pulmonary function?

The hallmark of laparoscopy is the creation of a pneumoperitoneum with pressurized CO_2. The resulting increase in intraabdominal pres-sure displaces the diaphragm cephalad, causing a decrease in lung compliance and an increase in peak inspiratory pressure. **Atelectasis, dimin-ished FRC, ventilation/perfusion mismatch, and pulmonary shunting contribute to a decrease in arterial oxygenation.** These changes should be exaggerated in this obese patient with a long his-tory of tobacco use.

The high solubility of CO_2 increases systemic absorption by the vasculature of the peritoneum. This, combined with smaller tidal volumes because of poor lung compliance, leads to increased arterial CO_2 levels and decreased pH.

Why does patient position affect oxygenation?

A head-down (Trendelenburg) position is com-monly requested during insertion of the Veress needle and cannula. This position causes a cepha-lad shift in abdominal viscera and the diaphragm. FRC, total lung volume, and pulmonary compliance will be decreased. Although these changes are usually well tolerated by healthy patients, this patient's obesity and presumed preexisting lung disease increase the likelihood for hypoxemia. A head-down position also tends to shift the trachea upward, so that a tracheal tube anchored at the mouth may migrate into the right mainstem bron-chus. This tracheobronchial shift may be exacer-bated during insufflation of the abdomen.

After insufflation, the patient's position is usu-ally changed to a steep head-up position (reverse Trendelenburg) to facilitate surgical dissection. The respiratory effects of the head-up position are the opposite of the head-down position.

Does laparoscopic surgery affect cardiac function?

Moderate insufflation pressures usually leave heart rate, central venous pressure, and cardiac output unchanged or slightly elevated. This seems to result from increased effective cardiac fill-ing because blood tends to be forced out of the abdomen and into the chest. **Higher insufflation pressures (>25 cm H_2O or 18 mm Hg), however, tend to collapse the major abdominal veins (par-ticularly the inferior vena cava), which decreases venous return and leads to a drop in preload and cardiac output in some patients.**

Hypercarbia, if allowed to develop, will stimu-late the sympathetic nervous system and thus increase blood pressure, heart rate, and the risk of arrhythmias. Attempting to compensate by increasing the tidal volume or respiratory rate will increase the mean intrathoracic pressure, further hindering venous return and increasing mean pul-monary artery pressures. These effects can prove particularly challenging in patients with restrictive lung disease, impaired cardiac function, or intra-vascular volume depletion.

Although the Trendelenburg position increases preload, mean arterial pressure and cardiac out-put usually either remain unchanged or decrease. These seemingly paradoxical responses may be explained by carotid and aortic baroreceptor-mediated reflexes. The reverse Trendelenburg posi-tion decreases preload, cardiac output, and mean arterial pressure.

Describe the advantages and disadvantages of alternative anesthetic techniques for this patient.

Anesthetic approaches to laparoscopic surgery include infiltration of local anesthetic with an intravenous sedative, epidural or spinal anesthesia, or general anesthesia. Experience with local anesthesia has been largely limited to brief gynecologic procedures (laparoscopic tubal sterilization, intrafallopian transfers) in young, healthy, and motivated patients. Although postoperative recovery is rapid, patient discomfort and suboptimal visualization of intraabdominal organs preclude the use of this local anesthesia technique for laparoscopic cholecystectomy.

Epidural or spinal anesthesia represents another alternative for laparoscopic surgery. A high level is required for complete muscle relaxation and to prevent diaphragmatic irritation caused by gas insufflation and surgical manipulations. An obese patient with lung disease may not be able to increase spontaneous ventilation to maintain normocarbia in the face of a T2 level regional block during insufflation and a 20° Trendelenburg position. Another disadvantage of a regional technique is the occasional occurrence of referred shoulder pain from diaphragmatic irritation. General anesthesia would therefore be the preferred technique in this patient.

Does a general anesthetic technique require tracheal intubation?

Tracheal intubation with positive-pressure ventilation is usually favored for many reasons: the risk of regurgitation from increased intraabdominal pressure during insufflation; the necessity for controlled ventilation to prevent hypercapnia; the relatively high peak inspiratory pressures required because of the pneumoperitoneum; the need for neuromuscular blockade during surgery to allow lower insufflation pressures, provide better visualization, and prevent unexpected patient movement; and the placement of a nasogastric tube and gastric decompression to minimize the risk of visceral perforation during trocar introduction and optimize visualization. The obese patient presented here would benefit from intubation to decrease the likelihood of hypoxemia, hypercarbia, and aspiration.

What special monitoring should be considered for this patient?

Monitoring end-tidal CO_2 normally provides an adequate guide for determining the minute ventilation required to maintain normocarbia. This assumes a constant gradient between arterial CO_2 and end-tidal CO_2, which is generally valid in healthy patients undergoing laparoscopy. This assumption would not apply if alveolar dead space changes during surgery. For example, any significant reduction in lung perfusion increases alveolar dead space and therefore increases the gradient between arterial and end-tidal CO_2. This may occur during laparoscopy if cardiac output drops because of high inflation pressures, the reverse Trendelenburg position, or gas embolism. Furthermore, abdominal distention lowers pulmonary compliance. Large tidal volumes are usually avoided because they are associated with high peak inspiratory pressures and can cause considerable movement of the surgical field. The resulting choice of lower tidal volumes and higher respiratory rates may lead to poor alveolar gas sampling and erroneous end-tidal CO_2 measurements. In fact, end-tidal CO_2 values have been found to be particularly unreliable in patients with significant cardiac or pulmonary disease undergoing laparoscopy. Thus, placement of an arterial catheter should be considered in patients with cardiopulmonary disease.

What are some possible complications of laparoscopic surgery?

Surgical complications include hemorrhage, if a major abdominal vessel is lacerated, or peritonitis, if a viscus is perforated during trocar introduction. Significant intraoperative hemorrhage may go unrecognized because of the limitations of laparoscopic visualization. Fulguration has been associated with bowel burns and bowel gas explosions. The use of pressurized gas introduces the possibility of extravasation of CO_2 along tissue planes, resulting in subcutaneous emphysema, pneumomediastinum, or pneumothorax. Nitrous oxide should be discontinued and insufflating pressures decreased as much as possible. Patients with this complication may benefit from the continuation of mechanical ventilation into the immediate postoperative period.

Venous CO_2 embolism resulting from unintentional insufflation of gas into an open vein may lead to hypoxemia, pulmonary hypertension, pulmonary edema, and cardiovascular collapse. Unlike air embolism, end-tidal CO_2 may transiently increase during CO_2 gas embolism. Treatment includes immediate release of the pneumoperitoneum, discontinuation of nitrous oxide, insertion of a central venous catheter for gas aspiration, and placement of the patient in a head-down left lateral decubitus position.

Vagal stimulation during trocar insertion, peritoneal insufflation, or manipulation of viscera can result in bradycardia and even sinus arrest. Although this usually resolves spontaneously, elimination of the stimulus (eg, deflation of the peritoneum) and administration of a vagolytic drug (eg, atropine sulfate) should be considered. Intraoperative hypotension may be more common during laparoscopic cholecystectomy than during cholecystectomy by laparotomy. Preoperative fluid loading has been recommended to avoid this complication.

Even though laparoscopic procedures are associated with less muscle trauma and incisional pain than open surgery, pulmonary dysfunction can persist for at least 24 hr postoperatively. For example, forced expiratory volume, forced vital capacity, and forced expiratory flow are reduced by approximately 25% following laparoscopic cholecystectomy, compared with a 50% reduction following open cholecystectomy. The cause of this dysfunction may be related to diaphragmatic tension during the pneumoperitoneum.

Nausea and vomiting are common following laparoscopic procedures, despite routine emptying of the stomach with a nasogastric tube. Pharmacological prophylaxis is recommended.

GUIDELINES

Qaseem A, Snow V, Fitterman N, et al: Risk assessment for and strategies to reduce perioperative pulmonary complication for patients undergoing noncardiothoracic surgery: a guideline from the American College of Physicians. Ann Intern Med 2006;144:576.

See www.guidelines.gov for additional guidelines from multiple organizations on deep vein thrombosis prophylaxis and pulmonary embolism.

SUGGESTED READING

Hurford WE: The bronchospastic patient. Int Anesthesiol Clin 2000;38:77.

Reilly JJ Jr: Evidence-based preoperative evaluation candidates for thoracotomy. Chest 1999;116:474.

Smetana G. Postoperative pulmonary complications: an update on risk assessment and reduction. Cleveland Clin J Med 2009;76(S4):S60-S65.

Sweitzer B, Smetana G: Identification and evaluation of the patient with lung disease. Anesthesiol Clin 2009;27:673.

Anesthesia for Thoracic Surgery

KEY CONCEPTS

1 During one-lung ventilation, the mixing of unoxygenated blood from the collapsed upper lung with oxygenated blood from the still-ventilated dependent lung widens the alveolar-to-arterial (A-a) O_2 gradient and often results in hypoxemia.

2 There are certain clinical situations in which the use of a right-sided double-lumen tube is recommended: (1) distorted anatomy of the left main bronchus by an intrabronchial or extrabronchial mass; (2) compression of the left main bronchus due to a descending thoracic aortic aneurysm; (3) left-sided pneumonectomy; (4) left-sided single lung transplantation; and (5) left-sided sleeve resection.

3 If epidural opioids are to be used postoperatively, their intravenous use should be limited during surgery to prevent excessive postoperative respiratory depression.

4 Postoperative hemorrhage complicates about 3% of thoracotomies and may be associated with up to 20% mortality. Signs of hemorrhage include increased chest tube drainage (>200 mL/h), hypotension, tachycardia, and a falling hematocrit.

5 Bronchopleural fistula presents as a sudden large air leak from the chest tube that may be associated with an increasing pneumothorax and partial lung collapse.

6 Acute herniation of the heart into the operative hemithorax can occur through the pericardial defect that is left following a radical pneumonectomy.

7 Nitrous oxide is contraindicated in patients with cysts or bullae because it can expand the air space and cause rupture. The latter may be signaled by sudden hypotension, bronchospasm, or an abrupt rise in peak inflation pressure and requires immediate placement of a chest tube.

8 Following transplantation, peak inspiratory pressures should be maintained at the minimum pressure compatible with good lung expansion, and the inspired oxygen concentration should be maintained as close to room air as allowed by a Pao_2 >60 mm Hg.

9 Regardless of the procedure, a common anesthetic concern for patients with esophageal disease is the risk of pulmonary aspiration.

Indications and techniques for thoracic surgery continually evolve. Common indications now include thoracic malignancies (mainly of the lungs and esophagus), chest trauma, esophageal disease, and mediastinal tumors. Diagnostic procedures such as bronchoscopy, mediastinoscopy, and open-lung biopsies are also common. Anesthetic techniques for providing lung separation have allowed the refinement of surgical techniques to the point that many procedures are increasingly performed thoracoscopically.

Physiological Considerations During Thoracic Anesthesia

Thoracic surgery presents a unique set of physiological problems for the anesthesiologist. These include physiological derangements caused by placing the patient in the lateral decubitus position, opening the chest (**open pneumothorax**), and the need for one-lung ventilation.

THE LATERAL DECUBITUS POSITION

The lateral decubitus position provides optimal access for most operations on the lungs, pleura, esophagus, the great vessels, other mediastinal structures, and vertebrae. Unfortunately, this position may significantly alter the normal pulmonary ventilation/perfusion relationships. These derangements are further accentuated by induction of anesthesia, initiation of mechanical ventilation, neuromuscular blockade, opening the chest, and surgical retraction. Although perfusion continues to favor the dependent (lower) lung, ventilation progressively favors the less perfused upper lung. The resulting mismatch increases the risk of hypoxemia.

The Awake State

When a supine patient assumes the lateral decubitus position, ventilation/perfusion matching is preserved during spontaneous ventilation. The dependent (lower) lung receives more perfusion than does the upper lung due to gravitational influences on blood flow distribution in the pulmonary circulation. The dependent lung also receives more ventilation because: (1) contraction of the dependent hemidiaphragm is more efficient compared with the nondependent [upper] hemidiaphragm and (2) the dependent lung is on a more favorable part of the compliance curve (Figure 25–1).

Induction of Anesthesia

The decrease in functional residual capacity (FRC) with induction of general anesthesia moves the upper lung to a more favorable part of the compliance

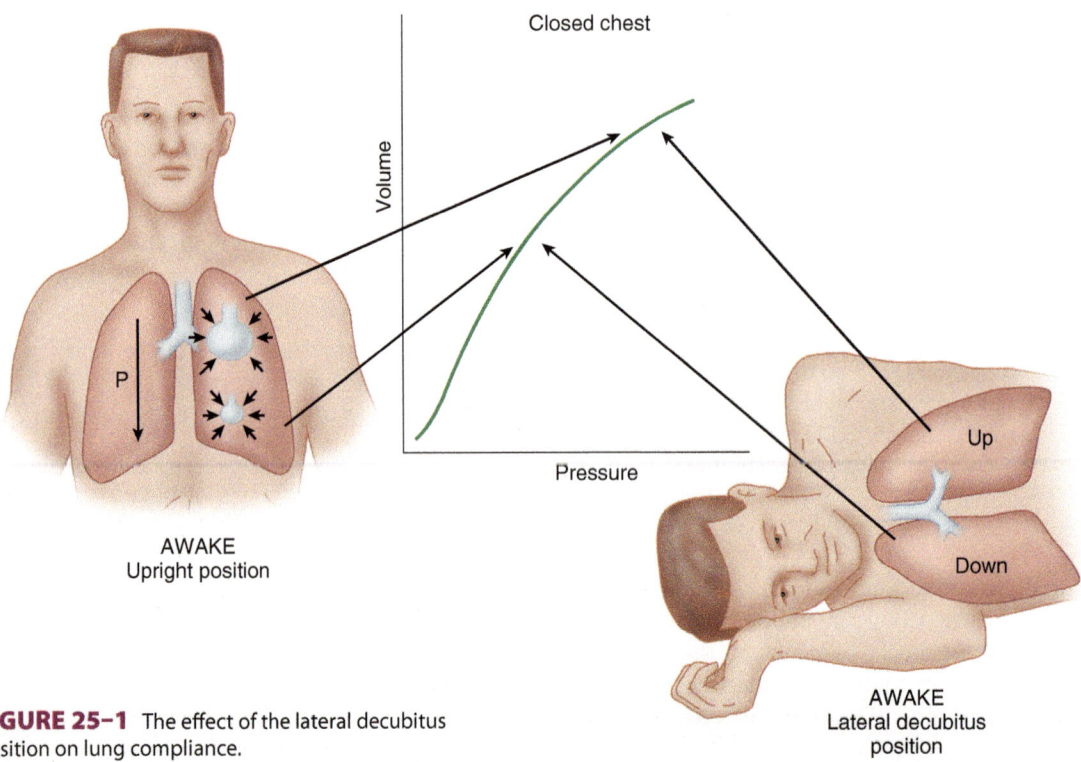

FIGURE 25–1 The effect of the lateral decubitus position on lung compliance.

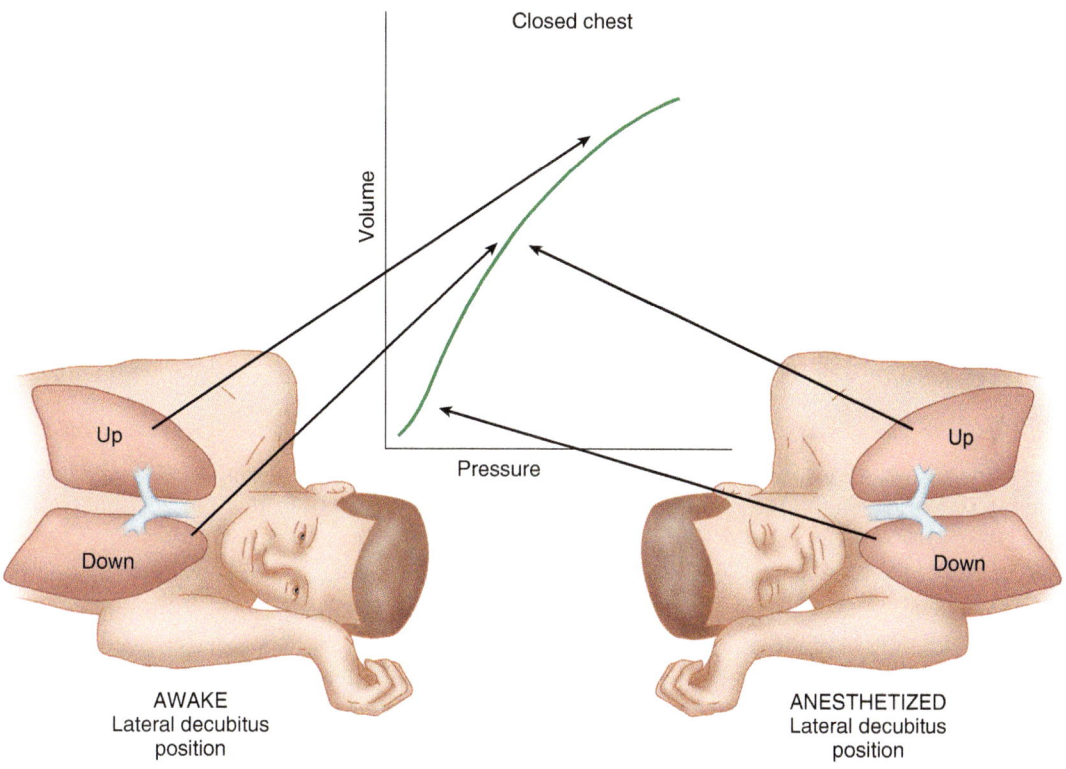

FIGURE 25–2 The effect of anesthesia on lung compliance in the lateral decubitus position. The upper lung assumes a more favorable position, and the lower lung becomes less compliant.

curve, but moves the lower lung to a less favorable-position (Figure 25–2). As a result, the upper lung is ventilated more than the dependent lower lung; ventilation/perfusion mismatching occurs because the dependent lung continues to have greater perfusion.

Positive-Pressure Ventilation

Controlled positive-pressure ventilation favors the upper lung in the lateral position because it is more compliant than the lower lung. Neuromuscular blockade enhances this effect by allowing the abdominal contents to rise up further against the dependent hemidiaphragm and impede ventilation of the lower lung. Using a rigid "bean bag" to maintain the patient in the lateral decubitus position further restricts movement of the dependent hemithorax. Finally, opening the nondependent side of the chest further accentuates differences in compliance between the two sides because the upper lung is now less restricted in movement. All of these effects

worsen ventilation/perfusion mismatching and predispose the patient to hypoxemia.

THE OPEN PNEUMOTHORAX

The lungs are normally kept expanded by a negative pleural pressure—the net result of the tendency of the lung to collapse and the chest wall to expand. When one side of the chest is opened, the negative pleural pressure is lost, and the elastic recoil of the lung on that side tends to collapse it. Spontaneous ventilation with an open pneumothorax in the lateral position results in paradoxical respirations and mediastinal shift. These two phenomena can cause progressive hypoxemia and hypercapnia, but, fortunately, their effects are overcome by the use of positive-pressure ventilation during general anesthesia and thoracotomy.

Mediastinal Shift

During spontaneous ventilation in the lateral position, inspiration causes pleural pressure to become

INSPIRATION

Pneumothorax

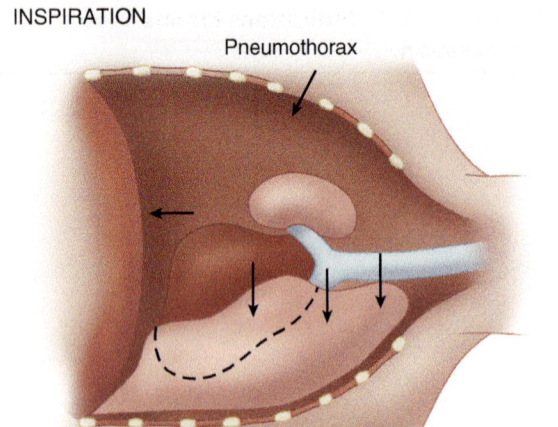

EXPIRATION

Pneumothorax

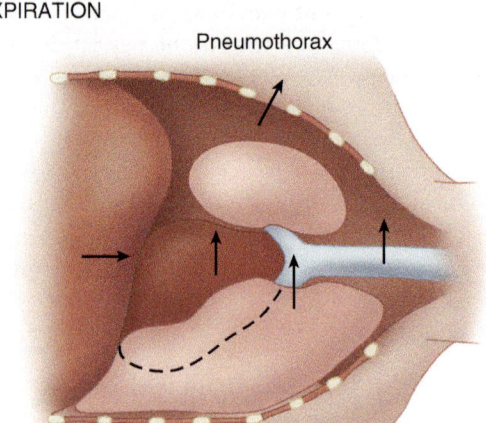

FIGURE 25–3 Mediastinal shift in a spontaneously breathing patient in the lateral decubitus position. (Reproduced, with permission, from Tarhan S, Moffitt EA: Principles of thoracic anesthesia. Surg Clin North Am 1973;53:813.)

more negative on the dependent side, but not on the side of the open pneumothorax. This results in a downward shift of the mediastinum during inspiration and an upward shift during expiration (Figure 25–3). The major effect of the mediastinal shift is to decrease the contribution of the dependent lung to the tidal volume.

Paradoxical Respiration

Spontaneous ventilation in a patient with an open pneumothorax also results in to-and-fro gas flow between the dependent and nondependent lung

(paradoxical respiration [pendeluft]). During inspiration, the pneumothorax increases, and gas flows from the upper lung across the carina to the dependent lung. During expiration, the gas flow reverses and moves from the dependent to the upper lung (Figure 25–4).

ONE-LUNG VENTILATION

Intentional collapse of the lung on the operative side facilitates most thoracic procedures, but greatly complicates anesthetic management. Because the

INSPIRATION

Pneumothorax

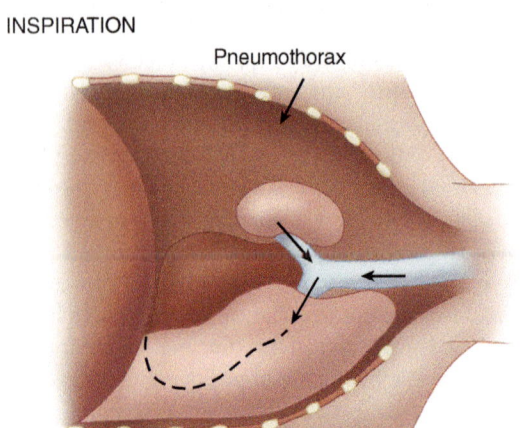

EXPIRATION

Pneumothorax

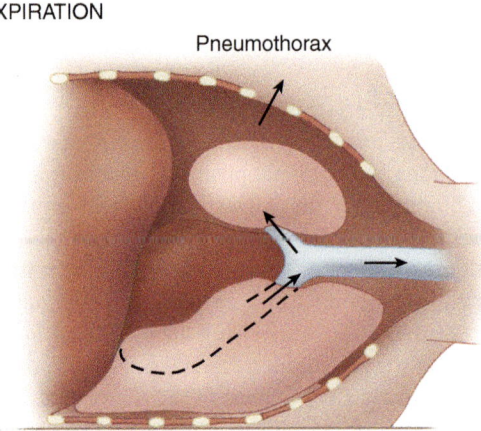

FIGURE 25–4 Paradoxical respiration in spontaneously breathing patients on their side. (Reproduced, with permission, from Tarhan S, Moffitt EA: Principles of thoracic anesthesia. Surg Clin North Am 1973;53:813.)

collapsed lung continues to be perfused and is deliberately no longer ventilated, the patient develops a large right-to-left intrapulmonary shunt (20% to 30%). During one-lung ventilation, the mixing of unoxygenated blood from the collapsed upper lung with oxygenated blood from the still-ventilated dependent lung widens the alveolar-to-arterial (A-a) O_2 gradient and often results in hypoxemia. Fortunately, blood flow to the nonventilated lung is decreased by hypoxic pulmonary vasoconstriction (HPV) and possibly surgical compression of the upper lung.

Factors known to inhibit HPV (increasing venous admixture), and thus worsen the right-to-left shunting, include (1) very high or very low pulmonary artery pressures; (2) hypocapnia; (3) high or very low mixed venous Po_2; (4) vasodilators such as nitroglycerin, nitroprusside, phosophodiesterase inhibitors (milrinone and inamrinone), β-adrenergic agonists, calcium channel blockers; (5) pulmonary infection; and (6) inhalation anesthetics.

Factors that decrease blood flow to the ventilated lung can be equally detrimental; they counteract the effect of HPV by indirectly increasing blood flow to the collapsed lung. Such factors include (1) high mean airway pressures in the ventilated lung due to high positive end-expiratory pressure (PEEP), hyperventilation, or high peak inspiratory pressures; (2) a low F_{IO_2}, which produces hypoxic pulmonary vasoconstriction in the ventilated lung; (3) vasoconstrictors that may have a greater effect on normoxic vessels than hypoxic ones; and (4) intrinsic PEEP that develops due to inadequate expiratory times.

Elimination of CO_2 is usually unchanged by one-lung ventilation, provided that minute ventilation is unchanged and that preexisting CO_2 retention was not present while ventilating both lungs; arterial CO_2 tension is usually not appreciably altered.

Techniques for One-Lung Ventilation

One-lung ventilation can also be utilized to isolate a lung or to facilitate ventilatory management under certain conditions (Table 25–1). Three techniques can be employed: (1) placement of a double-lumen

TABLE 25–1 Indications for one-lung ventilation.

Patient-related
Confine infection to one lung
Confine bleeding to one lung
Separate ventilation to each lung
Bronchopleural fistula
Tracheobronchial disruption
Large lung cyst or bulla
Severe hypoxemia due to unilateral lung disease
Procedure-related
Repair of thoracic aortic aneurysm
Lung resection
Pneumonectomy
Lobectomy
Segmental resection
Thoracoscopy
Esophageal surgery
Single-lung transplantation
Anterior approach to the thoracic spine
Bronchoalveolar lavage

bronchial tube; (2) use of a single-lumen tracheal tube in conjunction with a bronchial blocker; or (3) insertion of a conventional endotracheal tube into a mainstem bronchus. Double-lumen tubes are most often used.

DOUBLE-LUMEN BRONCHIAL TUBES

The principal advantages of double-lumen tubes are relative ease of placement, the ability to ventilate one or both lungs, and the ability to suction either lung.

All double-lumen tubes share the following characteristics:

- A longer bronchial lumen that enters either the right or left main bronchus and another shorter tracheal lumen that terminates in the lower trachea
- A preformed curve that when properly "aimed" allows preferential entry into a bronchus
- A bronchial cuff
- A tracheal cuff

Ventilation can be delivered to only one lung by clamping either the bronchial or tracheal lumen with both cuffs inflated; opening the port on the appropriate connector allows the ipsilateral lung to collapse. Because of differences in bronchial anatomy between the two sides, tubes are designed specifically for either the right or left bronchus. A right-sided double-lumen tube incorporates a modified cuff and a proximal portal on the endobronchial side for ventilation of the right upper lobe. The most commonly used double-lumen tube are available in several sizes: 35, 37, 39, and 41F.

Anatomic Considerations

On average, the adult trachea is 11–13 cm long. It begins at the level of the cricoid cartilage (C6) and bifurcates at the level of the carina behind the sternomanubrial joint (T5). Major differences between the right and left main bronchi are as follows: (1) the larger diameter right bronchus diverges away from the trachea at a less acute angle in relation to the trachea, whereas the left bronchus diverges at a more horizontal angle (Figure 25–5); (2) the

right bronchus has upper, middle, and lower lobe branches, whereas the left bronchus divides into only upper and lower lobe branches; and (3) the orifice of the right upper lobe bronchus is typically about 1–2.5 cm from the carina, whereas the bifurcation of the left main bronchus is typically about 5 cm distal to the carina. There is considerable anatomic variation: for example, the right upper lobe bronchus will occasionally arise from the trachea itself.

As previously noted, right-sided double-lumen tubes must have a portal through the bronchial cuff for ventilating the right upper lobe (Figure 25–6). Anatomic variations among individuals in the distance between the carina and the right upper lobe orifice will occasionally result in difficulty ventilating that lobe with right-sided tubes. A left-sided double-lumen tube can be used in most surgical procedures, **2** irrespective of the operative side. There are certain clinical situations in which the use of a right-sided double-lumen tube is recommended:

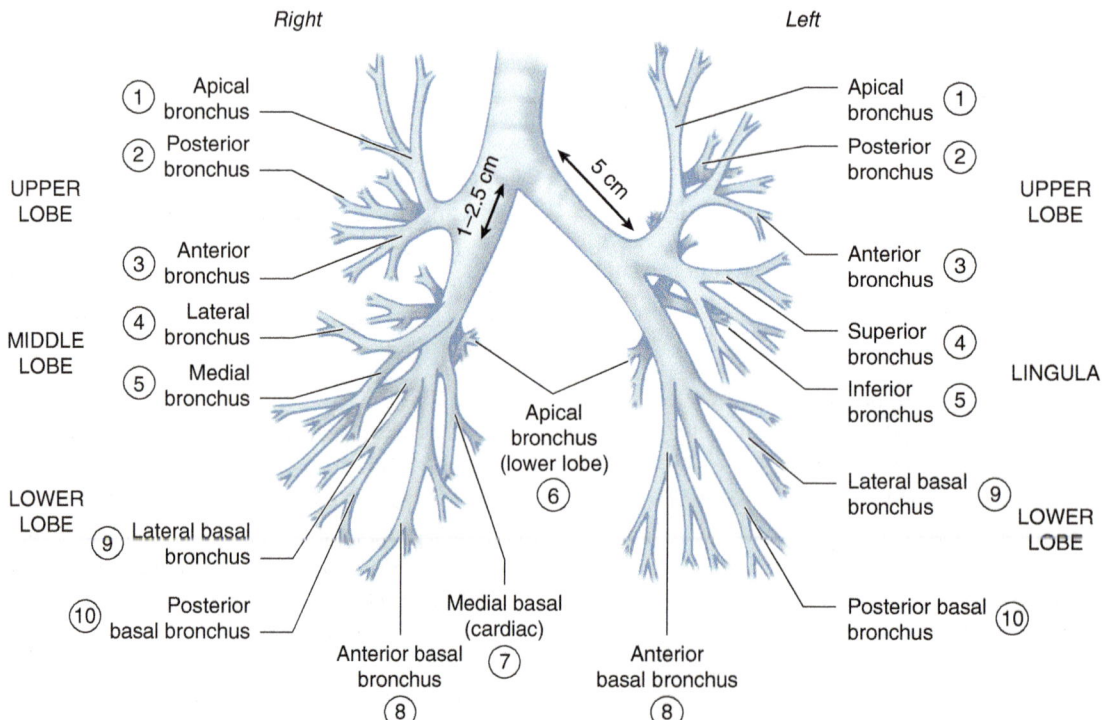

FIGURE 25–5 Anatomy of the tracheobronchial tree. Note bronchopulmonary segments (1–10) as numbered. (Adapted and reproduced, with permission, from Gothard JWW, Branthwaite MA: *Anesthesia for Thoracic Surgery.* Blackwell, 1982.)

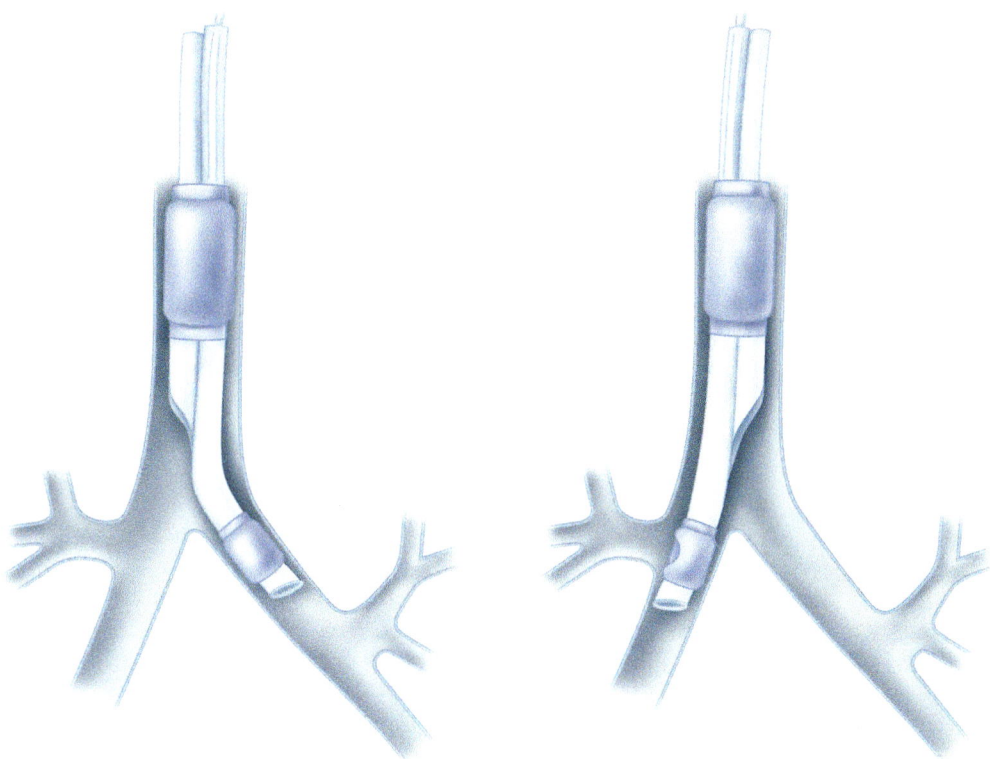

FIGURE 25–6 Correct position of a left- and right-sided double-lumen tube.

(1) distorted anatomy of the left main bronchus by an intrabronchial or extrabronchial mass; (2) compression of the left main bronchus due to a descending thoracic aortic aneurysm; (3) left-sided pneumonectomy; (4) left-sided single lung transplantation; and (5) left-sided sleeve resection. Finally, despite concerns about right upper lobe atelectasis and potentially difficult placement, studies have failed to detect differences in clinical performance of right- and left-sided double-lumen tubes when used clinically.

Placement of Double-Lumen Tubes

Laryngoscopy with a curved (MacIntosh) blade usually provides better intubating conditions than does a straight blade because the curved blade typically provides more room for manipulation of the large double-lumen tube. Video laryngoscopy can also be employed to facilitate tube placement. The double-lumen tube is passed with the distal curvature concave anteriorly and is rotated 90° (toward the side of the bronchus to be intubated) after the tip passes the vocal cords and enters the larynx (Figure 25–7). At this point, the operator has two options: the tube can be advanced until resistance is felt (the average depth of insertion is about 29 cm [at the teeth]), or alternatively, the fiberoptic bronchoscope can be inserted through the bronchial limb and advanced into the desired bronchus. The double-lumen tube can be advanced over the bronchoscope into the desired bronchus. Correct tube placement should be established using a preset protocol (Figure 25–8 and Table 25–2) and confirmed by flexible fiberoptic bronchoscopy. When problems are encountered in intubating the patient with the double-lumen tube, placement of a single-lumen endotracheal tube should be attempted; once positioned in the trachea, the latter can be exchanged for the double-lumen tube by using a specially designed catheter guide ("tube exchanger").

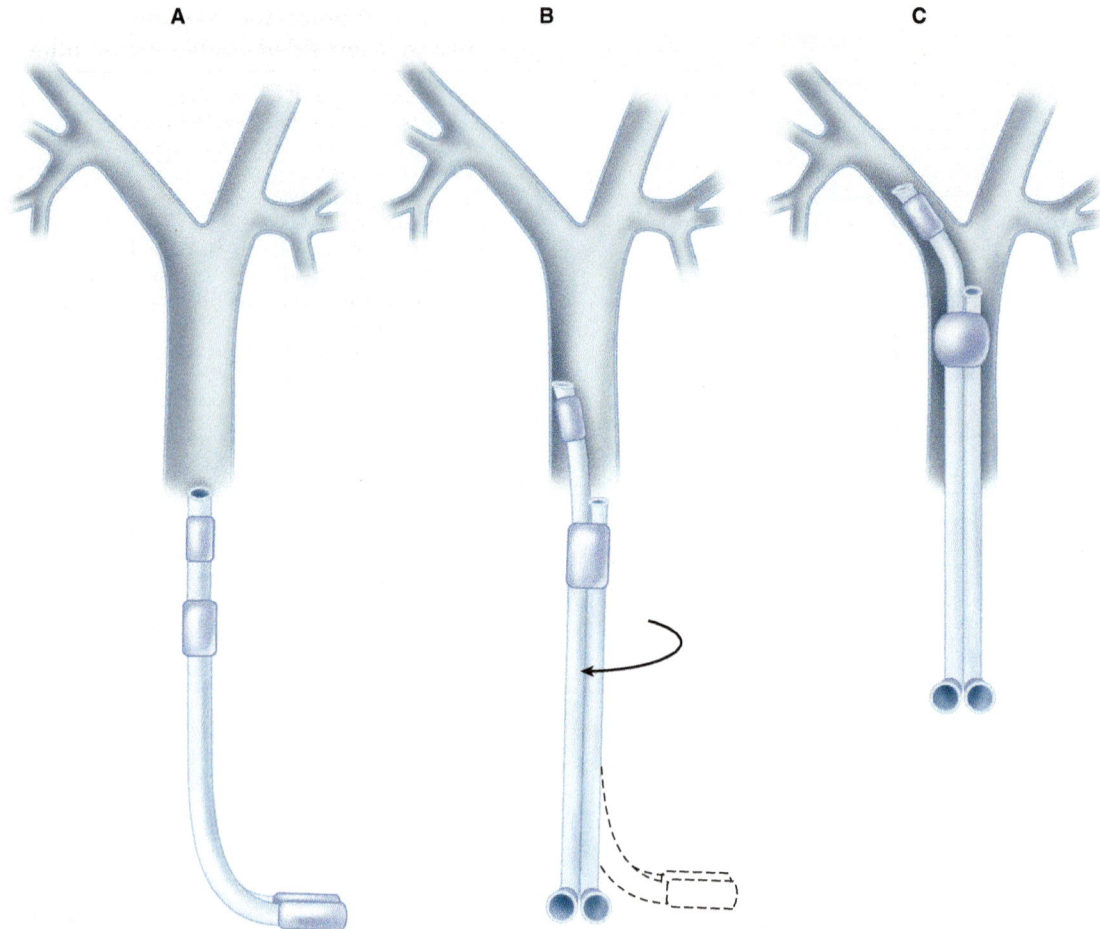

A

B

C

FIGURE 25–7 Placement of a left-sided double-lumen tube. Note that the tube is turned 90° as soon as it enters the larynx. **A**: Initial position. **B**: Rotated 90°. **C**: Final position.

Most double-lumen tubes easily accommodate bronchoscopes with a 3.6- to 4.2-mm outer diameter. When the bronchoscope is introduced into the tracheal lumen and advanced through the tracheal orifice, the carina should be visible (**Figure 25–9**), and the bronchial limb of the tube should be seen entering the respective bronchus; additionally, the top of the bronchial cuff (usually colored blue) should be visible, but should not extend above the carina. If the bronchial cuff of a left-sided double-lumen tube is not visible, the bronchial limb may have been inserted sufficiently far to allow the bronchial cuff to obstruct the orifice of the left upper or lower lobe; the tube should be withdrawn until the

cuff can be identified distal to the carina. The optimal position of a right-sided double-lumen tube is confirmed by placing the fiberoptic scope through the endobronchial lumen, which should show alignment of the endobronchial side portal with the opening of the right upper lobe bronchus. The bronchial cuff should be inflated only to the point at which the audible leak from the open tracheal lumen disappears while ventilating only through the bronchial lumen. Tube position should be reconfirmed after the patient is positioned for surgery because the tube may move relative to the carina as the patient is turned into the lateral decubitus position. Malpositioning of a double-lumen tube is usually

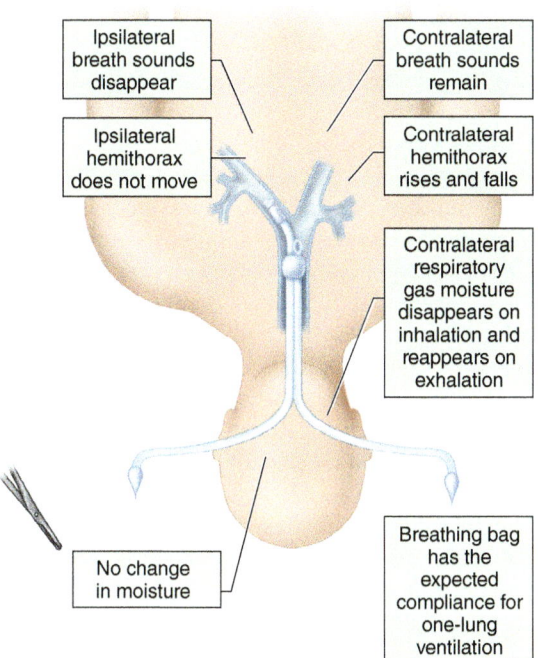

FIGURE 25–8 Results of unilateral clamping of the bronchial lumen tube when the double-lumen tube is in the correct position.

Ipsilateral breath sounds disappear

Ipsilateral hemithorax does not move

No change in moisture

Contralateral breath sounds remain

Contralateral hemithorax rises and falls

Contralateral respiratory gas moisture disappears on inhalation and reappears on exhalation

Breathing bag has the expected compliance for one-lung ventilation

TABLE 25–2   Protocol for checking placement of a left-sided double-lumen tube.

1. Inflate the tracheal cuff (5–10 mL of air).
2. Check for bilateral breath sounds. Unilateral breath sounds indicate that the tube is too far down (tracheal opening is bronchial).
3. Inflate the bronchial cuff (1–2 mL).
4. Clamp the tracheal lumen.
5. Check for unilateral left-sided breath sounds.
   a. Persistence of right-sided breath sounds indicates that the bronchial opening is still in the trachea (tube should be advanced).
   b. Unilateral right-sided breath sounds indicate incorrect entry of the tube in the right bronchus.
   c. Absence of breath sounds over the entire right lung and the left upper lobe indicates that the tube is too far down the left bronchus.
6. Unclamp the tracheal lumen and clamp the bronchial lumen.
7. Check for unilateral right-sided breath sounds. Absence or diminution of breath sounds indicates that the tube is not far enough down and that the bronchial cuff is occluding the distal trachea.

indicated by failure of the operative lung to collapse, poor lung compliance, and low exhaled tidal volume. Problems with left-sided double-lumen tubes are usually related to one of three possibilities: (1) the tube tip is too distal: (2) the tube tip is too proximal: or (3) the tube is in the right bronchus (the wrong side). If the tube tip is located too distally, the bronchial cuff can obstruct the left upper or the left lower lobe orifice, and the bronchial lumen can be inserted into the orifice of the left lower or left upper lobe bronchus, respectively. When the tube is not advanced distally enough, the inflated bronchial cuff may be above the carina and also occlude the tracheal lumen. In both instances, deflation of the bronchial cuff improves ventilation to the lung and helps to identify the problem. In some patients, the bronchial lumen may be within the left upper or left lower lobe bronchus but with the tracheal opening remaining above the carina; this situation is suggested by collapse of only one of the left lobes

when the bronchial lumen is clamped. In the same situation, if the surgical procedure is in the right thorax, clamping of the tracheal lumen will lead to ventilation of only the left upper or left lower lobe; hypoxia usually develops rapidly.

Right-sided double-lumen tubes can be accidentally inserted into the left main stem bronchus, inserted too distally or too proximally, or have

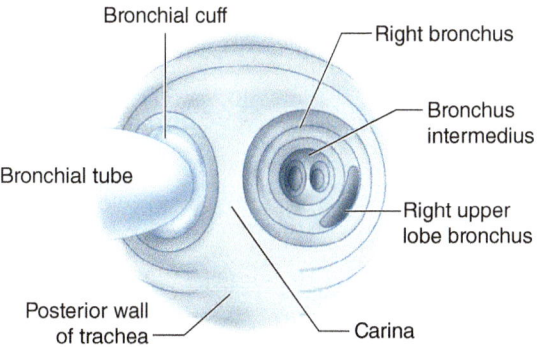

FIGURE 25–9 The view of the carina looking down the tracheal lumen of a properly positioned left double-lumen bronchial tube.

misalignment of the endobronchial side portal with the opening of the right upper lobe bronchus. If the tube inadvertently enters the wrong bronchus, the fiberoptic bronchoscope can be used to direct it into the correct side: (1) the bronchoscope is passed through the bronchial lumen to the tip of the tube; (2) under direct vision, the tube and the bronchoscope are withdrawn together into the trachea just above the carina; (3) the bronchoscope alone is then advanced into the correct bronchus; and (4) the double-lumen tube is gently advanced over the bronchoscope, which functions as a stylet to guide the bronchial lumen into the correct bronchus.

Complications of Double-Lumen Tubes

Major complications of double-lumen tubes include: (1) hypoxemia due to tube malplacement, tube occlusion, or excessive degrees of venous admixture with one-lung ventilation; (2) traumatic laryngitis; (3) tracheobronchial rupture resulting from traumatic placement or overinflation of the bronchial cuff; and (4) inadvertent suturing of the tube to a bronchus during surgery (detected as the inability to withdraw the tube during attempted extubation).

SINGLE-LUMEN TRACHEAL TUBES WITH A BRONCHIAL BLOCKER

Bronchial blockers are inflatable devices that are passed alongside or through a single-lumen tracheal tube to selectively occlude a bronchial orifice. A single-lumen tracheal tube with a built-in side channel for a retractable bronchial blocker is available. The tube is placed with the blocker fully retracted; its natural curve is such that turning the tube with the curve concave toward the right preferentially directs the bronchial blocker toward the right bronchus. Turning the tube with the curve concave toward the left usually directs the blocker toward the left bronchus. The bronchial blocker must be advanced, positioned, and inflated under direct visualization via a flexible bronchoscope.

The major advantage of a tube with an incorporated bronchial blocker is that, unlike a double-lumen tube, it does not need to be replaced with a conventional tracheal tube if the patient remains intubated postoperatively (below). Its major disadvantage is that the "blocked" lung collapses slowly (and sometimes incompletely) because of the small size of the channel within the blocker.

Another way to achieve lung separation is by using an independent bronchial blocker passed through a single-lumen endotracheal tube. There are several types of independent bronchial blockers. They come in different sizes (7Fr and 9Fr) and have a 1.4-mm diameter inner lumen. Bronchial blockers have a high-volume low-pressure cuff with either an elliptical or spherical shape. The spherical shape of the cuff facilitates adequate blockade of the right mainstem bronchus. The spherical or the elliptical cuff can be used for the left main stem bronchus. The inner lumen contains a nylon wire, which exits the distal end as a wireloop. The placement of the bronchial blocker involves inserting the endobronchial blocker through the endotracheal tube and using the fiberoptic bronchoscope and the distal loop of the guidewire to direct the blocker into a mainstem bronchus. The fiberoptic bronchoscope must be advanced beyond the bronchus opening so that the blocker enters the bronchus while it is being advanced. When the deflated cuff is beyond the entrance of the bronchus, the fiberoptic bronchoscope is withdrawn, and the blocker is secured in position. In order to obtain bronchial blockade, the cuff is fully inflated under fiberoptic visualization with 4 to 8 mL of air. The placement must be reconfirmed when the patient is placed in the lateral position. Bronchial blockers may be good choices for lung separation in intubated critically ill patients who require one-lung ventilation, patients who are difficult to intubate using direct laryngoscopy, patients with prior tracheostomies, and patients who may require postoperative mechanical ventilation. However, because bronchial blockers are more prone to dislodgement compared with double-lumen endotracheal tubes, and their small central lumens do not allow efficient suctioning of secretions or rapid collapse of the lung, some clinicians prefer not to use them.

In smaller children, an inflatable embolectomy (Fogarty) catheter can be used as a bronchial blocker in conjunction with a conventional tracheal tube (with the embolectomy catheter placed either inside or alongside the tracheal tube); a guidewire in the catheter can be used to facilitate placement. This technique is occasionally used to collapse one lung when other techniques do not work. As the embolectomy catheter does not have a communicating channel in the center, it also does not allow suctioning or ventilation of the isolated lung, and the catheter can be easily dislodged. Nonetheless, such bronchial blockers may be useful for one-lung anesthesia in pediatric patients and for tamponading bronchial bleeding in adult patients (see below).

Anesthesia for Lung Resection

PREOPERATIVE CONSIDERATIONS

Lung resections are usually carried out for the diagnosis and treatment of pulmonary tumors, and, less commonly, for complications of necrotizing pulmonary infections and bronchiectasis.

1. Tumors

Pulmonary tumors can be either benign or malignant, and, with the widespread use of bronchoscopic sampling, the diagnosis is usually available prior to surgery. Hamartomas account for 90% of benign pulmonary tumors; they are usually peripheral pulmonary lesions and represent disorganized normal pulmonary tissue. Bronchial adenomas are usually central pulmonary lesions that are typically benign, but occasionally may be locally invasive and rarely metastasize. These tumors include pulmonary carcinoids, cylindromas, and mucoepidermoid adenomas. They often obstruct the bronchial lumen and cause recurrent pneumonia distal to the obstruction in the same area. Primary pulmonary carcinoids may secrete multiple hormones, including adrenocorticotropic hormone (ACTH) and arginine vasopressin; however, manifestations of the carcinoid syndrome are uncommon and are more likely with metastases.

Malignant pulmonary tumors are divided into small ("oat") cell and non–small cell carcinomas. The latter group includes squamous cell (epidermoid) tumors, adenocarcinomas, and large cell (anaplastic) carcinomas. All types are more commonly encountered in smokers, but more "never smokers" die of lung cancer each year in the United States than the total number of people who die of ovarian cancer. Epidermoid and small cell carcinomas usually present as central masses with bronchial lesions; adenocarcinoma and large cell carcinomas are more typically peripheral lesions that often involve the pleura.

Clinical Manifestations

Symptoms may include cough, hemoptysis, wheezing, weight loss, productive sputum, dyspnea, or fever. Pleuritic chest pain or pleural effusion suggests pleural extension. Involvement of mediastinal structures is suggested by hoarseness that results from compression of the recurrent laryngeal nerve, Horner's syndrome caused by involvement of the sympathetic chain, an elevated hemidiaphragm caused by compression of the phrenic nerve, dysphagia caused by compression of the esophagus, or the superior vena cava syndrome caused by compression or invasion of the superior vena cava. Pericardial effusion or cardiomegaly suggests cardiac involvement. Extension of apical (superior sulcus) tumors can result in either shoulder or arm pain, or both, because of involvement of the C7–T2 roots of the brachial plexus (Pancoast syndrome). Distant metastases most commonly involve the brain, bone, liver, and adrenal glands.

Lung carcinomas—particularly small cell—can produce remote effects that are not related to malignant spread (paraneoplastic syndromes). Mechanisms include ectopic hormone production and immunologic cross-reactivity between the tumor and normal tissues. Cushing's syndrome, hyponatremia, and hypercalcemia may be encountered, resulting from secretion of ACTH, arginine vasopressin, and parathyroid hormone, respectively. Lambert–Eaton (myasthenic) syndrome is characterized by a proximal myopathy in which muscle strength increases with repeated effort (in contrast to myasthenia gravis). Other paraneoplastic syndromes include peripheral neuropathy and migratory thrombophlebitis.

Treatment

Surgery is the treatment of choice to reduce the tumor burden in nonmetastatic lung cancer. Various chemotherapy and radiation treatments are likewise employed, but there is wide variation among tissue types in their sensitivity to chemotherapy and radiation.

Resectability & Operability

Resectability is determined by the anatomic stage of the tumor, whereas operability is dependent on the interaction between the extent of the procedure required for cure and the physiological status of the patient. Anatomic staging is accomplished using chest radiography, computed tomography (CT) or magnetic resonance imaging (MRI), bronchoscopy, and (sometimes) mediastinoscopy. The extent of the surgery should maximize the chances for a cure but still allow for adequate residual pulmonary function postoperatively. Lobectomy via a posterior thoracotomy, through the fifth or sixth intercostal space, or thorough video assisted thoracoscopic surgery (VATS), is the procedure of choice for most lesions. Segmental or wedge resections may be performed in patients with small peripheral lesions and poor pulmonary reserve. Pneumonectomy is necessary for curative treatment of lesions involving the left or right main bronchus or when the tumor extends toward the hilum. A sleeve resection may be employed for patients with proximal lesions and limited pulmonary reserve as an alternative to pneumonectomy; in such instances, the involved lobar bronchus, together with part of the right or left main bronchus, is resected, and the distal bronchus is reanastomosed to the proximal bronchus or the trachea. Sleeve pneumonectomy may be considered for tumors involving the trachea.

The incidence of pulmonary complications after thoracotomy and lung resection is about 30% and is related not only to the amount of lung tissue resected, but also to the disruption of chest wall mechanics due to the thoracotomy. Postoperative pulmonary dysfunction seems to be less after VATS than "open" thoracotomy. The mortality rate for pneumonectomy is generally more than twice that of for a lobectomy. Mortality is greater for right-sided than left-sided pneumonectomy, possibly because of greater loss of lung tissue.

Evaluation for Lung Resection

A comprehensive preoperative pulmonary assessment is necessary to assess the operative risk, minimize perioperative complications, and achieve better outcomes. Preoperative assessment of respiratory function includes determinations of respiratory mechanics, gas exchange, and cardiorespiratory interaction.

Respiratory mechanics are assessed by pulmonary function tests. Of these parameters, the most useful is the predicted postoperative forced expiratory volume in one sec (FEV_1), which is calculated as follows:

$$\text{Postoperative } FEV_1 = \text{preoperative } FEV_1 \times (1 - \text{the percentage of functional lung tissue removed divided by } 100)$$

Removal of extensively diseased lung (nonventilated but perfused) does not necessarily adversely affect pulmonary function and may actually improve oxygenation. Mortality and morbidity are significantly increased if postoperative FEV_1 is less than 40% of normative FEV_1, and patients with predicted postoperative FEV_1 of less than 30% may need postoperative mechanical ventilatory support.

Gas exchange will sometimes be characterized by diffusion lung capacity for carbon monoxide (DLCO). DLCO correlates with the total functioning surface area of the alveolar–capillary interface. Predictive postoperative DLCO can be calculated in the same fashion as postoperative FEV_1. A predicted postoperative DLCO of less than 40% also correlates with increased postoperative respiratory and cardiac complications. Adequacy of gas exchange is more commonly assessed by arterial blood gas data such as $Pao_2 > 60$ mm Hg and a $Paco_2 < 45$ mm Hg.

Ventilation-perfusion ($\dot{V}/\dot{Q}$) scintigraphy provides the relative contribution of each lobe to overall pulmonary function and may further refine the assessment of predicted postoperative lung function, in patients where pneumonectomy is the indicated surgical procedure and there is concern whether a single lung will be adequate to support life.

Patients considered at greater risk of perioperative complications based on standard spirometry testing and calculation of postoperative function should undergo exercise testing for evaluation of

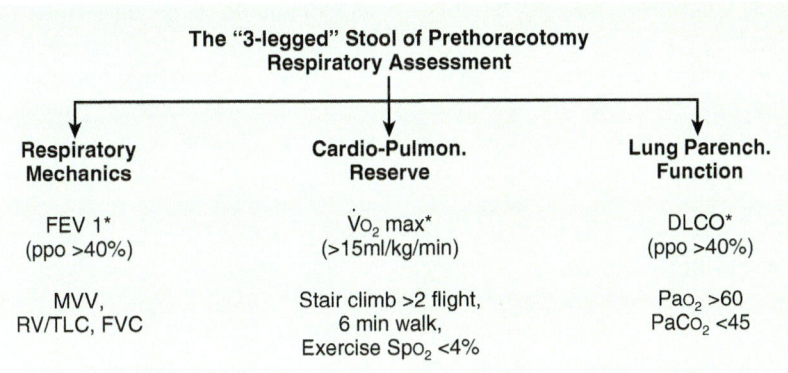

FIGURE 25-10 The "three-legged" stool of prethoracotomy respiratory assessment. *Most valid test. (Reproduced, with permission, from Slinger PD, Johnston MR: Preoperative assessment: an anesthesiologist's perspective. Thorac Surg Clin 2005;15:11.)

cardiopulmonary interaction. Stair climbing is the easiest way to assess exercise capacity and cardiopulmonary reserve. Patients capable of climbing two or three flights of stairs have decreased mortality and morbidity. On the other hand, the ability to climb less than two flights of stairs is associated with increased perioperative risk. The gold standard for evaluating cardiopulmonary interaction is by laboratory exercise testing and measurement of maximal minute oxygen consumption. A $\dot{V}o_2$ >20 mL/kg is not associated with a significant increase in perioperative mortality or morbidity, whereas a minute consumption of less than 10 mL/kg is associated with an increased perioperative risk.

A combination of tests to evaluate the three components of the respiratory function (ie, respiratory mechanics, gas exchange, and cardiopulmonary interaction) has been summarized in the so-called "three-legged" stool of respiratory assessment (Figure 25–10).

2. Infection

Pulmonary infections may present as a solitary nodule or cavitary lesion (necrotizing pneumonitis). An exploratory thoracotomy may be carried out to exclude malignancy and diagnose the infectious agent. Lung resection is also indicated for cavitary lesions that are refractory to antibiotic treatment, are associated with refractory empyema, or result in

massive hemoptysis. Responsible organisms include both bacteria and fungi.

3. Bronchiectasis

Bronchiectasis is a permanent dilation of bronchi. It is usually the end result of severe or recurrent inflammation and obstruction of bronchi. Causes include a variety of viral, bacterial, and fungal pathogens, as well as inhalation of toxic gases, aspiration of gastric acid, and defective mucociliary clearance (cystic fibrosis and disorders of ciliary dysfunction). Bronchial muscle and elastic tissue are typically replaced by very vascular fibrous tissue. The latter predisposes to bouts of hemoptysis. Pulmonary resection is usually indicated for massive hemoptysis when conservative measures have failed and the disease is localized. Patients with diffuse bronchiectasis have a chronic obstructive ventilatory defect.

ANESTHETIC CONSIDERATIONS

1. Preoperative Management

The majority of patients undergoing pulmonary resections have underlying lung disease. It should be emphasized that smoking is a risk factor for both chronic obstructive pulmonary disease and coronary artery disease; both disorders commonly coexist in patients presenting for thoracotomy.

Echocardiography is useful for assessing baseline cardiac function and may suggest evidence of cor pulmonale (right ventricular enlargement or hypertrophy) in patients with poor exercise tolerance. Stress echocardiography (exercise or dobutamine) may be useful in diagnosing coronary artery disease in patients with suggestive signs and symptoms.

Patients with tumors should be evaluated for complications related to local extension of the tumor and paraneoplastic syndromes (above). Preoperative chest radiographs and CT or MR images should be reviewed. Tracheal or bronchial deviation can make tracheal intubation and proper positioning of bronchial tubes much more difficult. Moreover, airway compression can lead to difficulty in ventilating the patient following induction of anesthesia. Pulmonary consolidation, atelectasis, and large pleural effusions predispose to hypoxemia. The location of any bullous cysts or abscesses should be noted.

Patients undergoing thoracic procedures are at increased risk of postoperative pulmonary and cardiac complications. Perioperative arrhythmias, particularly supraventricular tachycardias, are thought to result from surgical manipulations or distention of the right atrium following reduction of the pulmonary vascular bed. The incidence of arrhythmias increases with age and the amount of pulmonary resection.

2. Intraoperative Management

Preparation

As with anesthesia for cardiac surgery, optimal preparation may help to prevent potentially catastrophic problems. The frequent presence of poor pulmonary reserve, anatomic abnormalities, or compromise of the airways, and the need for one-lung ventilation predispose these patients to the rapid onset of hypoxemia. A well thought-out plan to deal with potential difficulties is necessary. Moreover, in addition to items for basic airway management, specialized and properly functioning equipment—such as multiple sizes of single- and double-lumen tubes, a flexible (pediatric) fiberoptic bronchoscope, a small-diameter "tube exchanger" of adequate length to accommodate a double lumen tube, a continuous positive airway pressure (CPAP) delivery system,

and an anesthesia circuit adapter for administering bronchodilators—should be immediately available.

Patients undergoing open-lung resections (segmentectomy, lobectomy, pneumonectomy) often receive postoperative thoracic epidural analgesia, unless there is a contraindication. However, patients are increasingly being treated with numerous antiplatelet and anticoagulant medications, which may preclude epidural catheter placement.

Venous Access

At least one large-bore (14- or 16-gauge) intravenous line is mandatory for all open thoracic surgical procedures. Central venous access (preferably on the side of the thoracotomy to avoid the risk of pneumothorax on the side that will be ventilated intraoperatively), a blood warmer, and a rapid infusion device are also desirable if extensive blood loss is anticipated.

Monitoring

Direct monitoring of arterial pressure is indicated for resections of large tumors (particularly those with mediastinal or chest wall extension), and any procedure performed in patients who have limited pulmonary reserve or significant cardiovascular disease. Central venous access with monitoring of central venous pressure (CVP) is desirable for pneumonectomies and resections of large tumors. Less invasive measures of cardiac output through use of pulse contour analysis and transpulmonary thermodilution provide better estimates of cardiac function and volume responsiveness (See Chapter 5). Pulmonary artery catheters are very rarely used. Measurement of pulmonary artery pressures may also not be accurate due to intrinsic and extrinsic PEEP, lateral decubitus, and open chest. In patients with significant coronary artery disease or pulmonary hypertension, intraoperative monitoring can be enhanced by the use of transesophageal echocardiography.

Induction of Anesthesia

After adequate preoxygenation, an intravenous anesthetic is used for induction of most patients. The selection of an induction agent should be based on the patient's preoperative status. Direct laryngoscopy should generally be performed only after adequate depth of anesthesia has been achieved to prevent reflex bronchospasm and to obtund the cardiovascular pressor response. This may be accomplished by incremental doses of the induction agent, an opioid, or deepening the anesthesia with a volatile inhalation agent (the latter is particularly useful in patients with reactive airways).

Tracheal intubation with a single-lumen tracheal tube (or with a laryngeal mask airway [LMA]) may be necessary, if the surgeon performs diagnostic bronchoscopy (below) prior to surgery. Once the bronchoscopy is completed, the single-lumen tracheal tube (or LMA) can be replaced with a double-lumen bronchial tube (above). Controlled positive-pressure ventilation helps prevent atelectasis, paradoxical breathing, and mediastinal shift; it also allows control of the operative field to facilitate the surgery.

Positioning

Following induction, intubation, and confirmation of correct tracheal or bronchial tube position, additional venous access and monitoring may be obtained before the patient is positioned for surgery. Most lung resections are performed with the patient in the lateral decubitus position. Proper positioning avoids injuries and facilitates surgical exposure. The lower arm is flexed and the upper arm is extended in front of the head, pulling the scapula away from the operative field (Figure 25–11). Pillows are placed between the arms and legs, and an axillary (chest) roll may be positioned just beneath the dependent axilla to reduce pressure on the inferior shoulder (it is assumed that this helps to protect the brachial plexus); care is taken to avoid pressure on the eyes and the dependent ear.

Maintenance of Anesthesia

All current anesthetic techniques have been successfully used for thoracic surgery, but the combination of a potent halogenated agent (isoflurane, sevoflurane, or desflurane) and an opioid is preferred by most clinicians. Advantages of the halogenated agents include: (1) potent dose-related bronchodilation; (2) depression of airway reflexes; (3) the ability to use a high inspired oxygen concentration (FiO_2), if necessary; (4) the ability to make relatively rapid adjustments in anesthetic depth; and (5) minimal effects on hypoxic pulmonary vasoconstriction (see below). Halogenated agents generally have minimal effects on HPV in doses <1 minimum alveolar concentration (MAC). Advantages of an opioid include: (1) generally minimal hemodynamic effects; (2) depression of airway reflexes; and (3) residual postoperative analgesia. If epidural opioids are used postoperatively, intravenous opioids should be limited during surgery to prevent excessive postoperative respiratory depression. Maintenance of neuromuscular blockade with a nondepolarizing neuromuscular blocker (NMB) during surgery facilitates rib spreading as well as anesthetic management. Intravenous fluids should generally be restricted in patients undergoing pulmonary resections. Excessive fluid administration in thoracic surgical patients has been associated with acute lung injury in the postoperative period. No fluid replacement for estimated "third space" losses should be administered during lung resection. Excessive fluid administration in the lateral decubitus position may promote a "lower lung syndrome" (ie, gravity-dependent transudation of fluid into the dependent lung). The latter increases intrapulmonary shunting and promotes hypoxemia, particularly

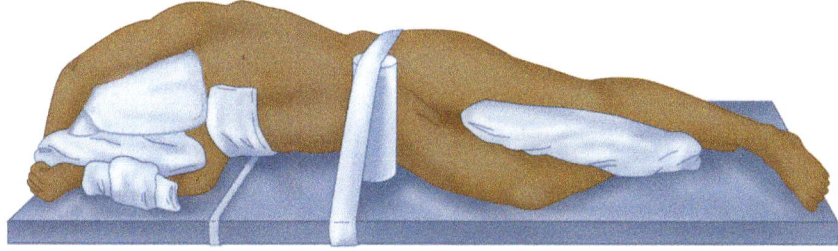

FIGURE 25–11 Proper positioning for a lateral thoracotomy. (Reproduced, with permission, from Gothard JWW, Branthwaite MA: *Anesthesia for Thoracic Surgery.* Blackwell, 1982.)

during one-lung ventilation. Moreover, the collapsed lung may be prone to acute lung injury due to surgical retraction during the procedure and possible ischemia–reperfusion injury. During lung resections, the bronchus (or remaining lung tissue) is usually divided with an automated stapling device. The bronchial stump is then tested for an air leak under water by transiently sustaining 30 cm of positive pressure to the airway. Prior to completion of chest closure, all remaining lung segments should be fully expanded manually under direct vision. Controlled mechanical ventilation is then resumed and continued until chest tubes are connected to suction.

Management of One-Lung Ventilation

Although still an intraoperative problem, hypoxemia has become less frequent due to better lung isolation methods, ventilation techniques, and the use of anesthetic agents with less detrimental effects on hypoxic pulmonary vasoconstriction. Attention has currently shifted toward avoidance of acute lung injury (ALI). Fortunately, ALI occurs infrequently, with an incidence of 2.5 % of all lung resections combined, and an incidence of 7.9% after pneumonectomy. However, when it occurs, ALI is associated with a risk of mortality or major morbidity of about 40%.

Based on current data, it seems that protective lung ventilation strategies may minimize the risk of acute lung injury *after* lung resection. This ventilatory strategy includes the use of lower tidal volumes (6–8 mL/kg), routine use of PEEP (5–10 cm H_2O), lower FIO_2 (50% to 80%), lower ventilatory pressures (plateau pressure <25 cm H_2O; peak airway pressure <35 cm H_2O) through the use of pressure-controlled ventilation and permissive hypercapnia. The use of lower tidal volumes may lead to lung derecruitment, atelectasis, and hypoxemia. Lung derecruitment may be avoided by application of external PEEP and frequent recruitment maneuvers. Although PEEP may prevent alveolar collapse and development of atelectasis, it may cause a decrease in Pao_2 due to diversion of blood flow away from the dependent, ventilated lung and an increase in total shunt. Thus, PEEP must be customized to the underlying disease of each patient, and a new application of PEEP will almost never be the appropriate way to treat hypoxemia that occurs immediately after the onset of one-lung ventilation. Patients with obstructive pathology may develop intrinsic PEEP. In these patients, the application of external PEEP may lead to unpredictable levels of total PEEP. Although the management of one-lung ventilation has long included the use of 100% oxygen, evidence of oxygen toxicity has accumulated both experimentally and clinically. Although there is no convincing evidence that outcomes are worsened with the use of 100% oxygen, some clinicians recommend titrating FIO_2 to maintain the oxygen saturation above 90%, especially in patients who have undergone adjuvant therapy and are at risk of developing ALI. Although there is no unequivocal evidence that one mode of ventilation may be more beneficial than the other, pressure-controlled ventilation may diminish the risk of barotrauma by limiting peak and plateau airway pressures, and the flow pattern results in a more homogenous distribution of the tidal volume and improved dead space ventilation.

At the end of the procedure, the operative lung is inflated gradually to a peak inspiratory pressure of less than 30 cm H_2O to prevent disruption of the staple line. During reinflation of the operative lung, it may be helpful to clamp the lumen serving the dependent lung to limit overdistension.

Periodic arterial blood gas analysis is helpful to ensure adequate ventilation. End-tidal CO_2 measurement may not be reliable due to increased dead-space and an unpredictable gradient between the arterial and end-tidal CO_2 partial pressure.

Management of Hypoxia

Hypoxemia during one-lung anesthesia requires one or more of the following interventions:

1. Adequate position of the bronchial tube (or bronchial blocker) must be confirmed, as its position relative to the carina can change as a result of surgical manipulations or traction; repeat fiberoptic bronchoscopy through the tracheal lumen can quickly detect this problem. Both lumens of the tube should also be suctioned to exclude excessive secretions or obstruction as a factor.

2. Increase FIO_2 to 1.0

3. Recruitment maneuvers on the dependent, ventilated lung may eliminate atelectasis and improve shunt.

4. Optimize PEEP to the dependent, nonoperative lung.

5. Ensure adequate cardiac output and adequate oxygen carrying capacity.

6. CPAP or blow-by oxygen to the operative lung will decrease shunting and improve oxygenation. However, inflation of the operative lung during VATS will make identification and visualization of the lung structures difficult for the surgeon; therefore, such maneuvers should be applied carefully and cautiously.

7. Two-lung ventilation should be instituted for severe hypoxemia. If possible, pulmonary artery clamp can also be placed during pneumonectomy to eliminate shunt.

8. In patients with chronic obstructive lung disease, one should always be suspicious of pneumothorax on the dependent, ventilated side as a cause of severe hypoxemia. This complication requires immediate detection and treatment by aborting the surgical procedure, reexpanding the operative lung, and immediately inserting a chest tube in the contralateral chest.

Alternatives to One-Lung Ventilation

Ventilation can be stopped for short periods if 100% oxygen is insufflated at a rate greater than oxygen consumption **(apneic oxygenation) into an unobstructed tracheal tube**. Adequate oxygenation can often be maintained for prolonged periods, but progressive respiratory acidosis limits the use of this technique to 10–20 min in most patients. Arterial P_{CO_2} rises 6 mm Hg in the first minute, followed by a rise of 3–4 mm Hg during each subsequent minute.

High-frequency positive-pressure ventilation and high-frequency jet ventilation have been used during thoracic procedures as alternatives to one-lung ventilation. A standard tracheal tube may be used with either technique. Small tidal volumes (<2 mL/kg) allow decreased lung excursion, which may facilitate the surgery but still allow ventilation of

both lungs. Unfortunately, mediastinal "bounce"— a to-and-fro movement—often interferes with the surgery.

3. Postoperative Management

General Care

Most patients are extubated shortly after surgery to decrease the risk of pulmonary barotrauma (particularly "blowout" [rupture] of the bronchial suture line). Patients with marginal pulmonary reserve should remain intubated until standard extubation criteria are met; if a double-lumen tube was used for one-lung ventilation, it should be replaced with a regular single-lumen tube at the end of surgery. A catheter guide ("tube exchanger") should be used if the original laryngoscopy was difficult (above).

Patients are observed in the postanesthesia care unit, and, in most instances, at least overnight or longer in an intensive care unit or intermediate care unit. Postoperative hypoxemia and respiratory acidosis are common. These effects are largely caused by atelectasis and "shallow breathing ('splinting')" due to incisional pain. Gravity-dependent transudation of fluid into the intraoperative dependent lung may also be contributory. Reexpansion edema of the collapsed nondependent lung can also occur.

4 Postoperative hemorrhage complicates about 3% of thoracotomies and may be associated with up to 20% mortality. Signs of hemorrhage include increased chest tube drainage (>200 mL/h), hypotension, tachycardia, and a falling hematocrit. Postoperative supraventricular tachyarrhythmias are common and usually require immediate treatment. Routine postoperative care should include maintenance of a semiupright (>30°) position, supplemental oxygen (40% to 50%), incentive spirometry, electrocardiographic and hemodynamic monitoring, a postoperative chest radiograph (to confirm proper position of all thoracostomy tube drains and central lines and to confirm expansion of both lung fields), and adequate pain relief.

Postoperative Analgesia

The importance of adequate pain management in the thoracic surgical patient cannot be overstated. Inadequate pain control in these high-risk patients will result in splinting; poor respiratory effort; and the inability to cough and clear secretions, with an end result of airway closure, atelectasis, shunting, and hypoxemia. Irrespective of the modality used, there must be a comprehensive plan for pain management.

A balance between comfort and respiratory depression in patients with marginal lung function is difficult to achieve with parenteral opioids alone. Patients who have undergone thoracotomy clearly benefit from the use of other techniques (described below) that may reduce the need for parenteral opioids. If parenteral opioids are used alone, they are best administered via a patient-controlled analgesia device.

In the absence of an epidural catheter, intercostal or paravertebral nerve blocks with long-acting local anesthetics may facilitate extubation, but have a limited duration of action, so alternative means of pain management must be employed. Alternatively, a cryoanalgesia probe may be used intraoperatively to freeze the intercostal nerves (cryoneurolysis) and produce long-lasting anesthesia; unfortunately, maximum analgesia may not be achieved until 24–48 hr after the cryoanalgesia procedure. Nerve regeneration is reported to occur approximately 1 month after the cryoneurolysis. Infusion of local anesthetic through a catheter placed in the surgical wound during closure will markedly reduce the requirement for parenteral opioids and improve the overall quality of analgesia relative to parenteral opioids alone.

Epidural analgesia is the current optimal method for acute pain control following thoracic surgical procedures. It provides excellent pain relief, continuous therapy, and avoidance of the side effects associated with administration of systemic opioids. On the other hand, epidural techniques require attention from the acute pain team for the duration of the infusion and subject the patient to the long list of epidural-related side effects and complications. However, there is still much debate over the level of placement of the epidural catheter (thoracic versus lumbar), type of medication administered (opioid and/or local anesthetic), and timing of medication administration (before surgical incision vs before end of surgery). Most practitioners use a combination of opioid (fentanyl, morphine, hydromorphone) and local anesthetic (bupivacaine or ropivacaine), with the epidural catheter placed at a thoracic level.

Postoperative Complications

Postoperative complications following thoracotomy are relatively common, but fortunately most are minor and resolve uneventfully. Blood clots and thick secretions may obstruct the airways and result in atelectasis; suctioning may be necessary. Atelectasis is suggested by tracheal deviation and shifting of the mediastinum to the operative side following segmental or lobar resections. Therapeutic bronchoscopy should be considered for persistent atelectasis, particularly when associated with thick secretions. Air leaks from the operative hemithorax are common following segmental and lobar resections. Most air leaks stop after a few days.

5 Bronchopleural fistulae present as a sudden large air leak from the chest tube that may be associated with an increasing pneumothorax and partial lung collapse. When they occur within the first 24–72 hr, they are usually the result of inadequate surgical closure of the bronchial stump. Delayed presentation is usually due to necrosis of the suture line associated with inadequate blood flow or infection.

Some complications are rare, but deserve special consideration because they can be life-threatening and require immediate exploratory thoracotomy. Postoperative bleeding was discussed above. Torsion of a lobe or segment can occur as the remaining lung on the operative side expands to occupy the hemithorax. The torsion usually occludes the pulmonary vein to that part of the lung, causing venous outflow obstruction. Hemoptysis and infarction can rapidly follow. The diagnosis is suggested by an enlarging homogeneous density on the chest radiograph and a closed lobar orifice on bronchoscopy.

6 Acute herniation of the heart into the operative hemithorax can occur through the pericardial defect that may remain following a pneumonectomy. A large pressure differential between the two hemithoraces is thought to trigger this catastrophic event. Cardiac herniation into the right hemithorax results in sudden severe hypotension with an elevated CVP because of torsion of the central veins. Cardiac herniation into the left hemithorax following left pneumonectomy results in sudden compression of the myocardium, resulting in hypotension, ischemia, and infarction. A chest radiograph shows a shift of the cardiac shadow into the operative hemithorax.

Extensive mediastinal dissections can injure the phrenic, vagus, and left recurrent laryngeal nerves. Postoperative phrenic nerve palsy presents as elevation of the ipsilateral hemidiaphragm together with difficulty in weaning the patient from the ventilator. Large chest wall resections may include part of the diaphragm, causing a similar problem, in addition to a flail chest. Paraplegia rarely follows thoracotomy for lung resection. There are reports of cellulose gauze and other debris migrating from the thoracic gutter into the spinal canal, resulting in spinal cord compression. If an epidural catheter has been placed, any loss of motor function or unexplained back pain should immediately trigger imaging to rule out epidural hematoma.

SPECIAL CONSIDERATIONS FOR PATIENTS UNDERGOING LUNG RESECTION

Massive Pulmonary Hemorrhage

Massive hemoptysis is usually defined as >500–600 mL of blood loss from the tracheobronchial tree within 24 hr. The etiology is usually tuberculosis, bronchiectasis, or a neoplasm, or complication of transbronchial biopsies. Emergency surgical management with lung resection is reserved for "potentially lethal" massive hemoptysis. In most cases, surgery is usually carried out on an urgent rather than on a true emergent basis whenever possible; even then, operative mortality may exceed 20% (compared with > 50% for medical management). Embolization of the involved bronchial arteries may be attempted. The most common cause of death is asphyxia secondary to blood in the airway. Patients may be brought to the operating room for rigid bronchoscopy when localization is not possible with fiberoptic flexible bronchoscopy. A bronchial blocker or Fogarty catheter (above) may be placed to tamponade the bleeding, or laser coagulation may be attempted.

Multiple large-bore intravenous catheters should be placed. Sedating drugs should not be given to awake, nonintubated, spontaneously ventilating patients because they are usually already hypoxic; 100% oxygen should be given continuously. If the patient is already intubated and has bronchial blockers in place, sedation is helpful to prevent coughing. The bronchial blocker should be left in position until the lung is resected. When the patient is not intubated, a rapid sequence induction (ketamine or etomidate with succinylcholine) is used. Patients usually swallow a large amount of blood and should be considered to have a full stomach. A large double-lumen bronchial tube is ideal for protecting the normal lung from blood and for suctioning each lung separately. If any difficulty is encountered in placing the double-lumen tube, or its relatively small lumens occlude easily, a large (>8.0-mm inner diameter) single-lumen tube may be used with a bronchial blocker to provide lung isolation.

Pulmonary Cyst & Bulla

Pulmonary cysts or bullae may be congenital or acquired as a result of emphysema. Large bullae can impair ventilation by compressing the surrounding lung. These air cavities often behave as if they have a one-way valve, predisposing them to progressively enlarge. Lung resection may be undertaken for progressive dyspnea or recurrent pneumothorax. The greatest risk of anesthesia is rupture of the air cavity during positive-pressure ventilation, resulting in tension pneumothorax; the latter may occur on either side prior to thoracotomy or on the nonoperative side during the lung resection. Induction of anesthesia with maintenance of spontaneous ventilation is desirable until the side with the cyst or bullae is isolated with a double-lumen tube, or until a chest tube is placed; most patients have a large increase in dead space, so assisted ventilation is necessary to avoid excessive hypercarbia. The use **7** of N_2O is contraindicated in patients with cysts or bullae because it can expand the air space and cause rupture. The latter may be signaled by sudden hypotension, bronchospasm, or an abrupt rise in peak inflation pressure and requires immediate placement of a chest tube.

Lung Abscess

Lung abscesses result from primary pulmonary infections, obstructing pulmonary neoplasms (above), or, rarely, hematogenous spread of systemic infections. The two lungs should be isolated to prevent contamination of the healthy lung. A rapid-sequence intravenous induction with tracheal intubation with a double-lumen tube is generally recommended, with the affected lung in a dependent position. As soon as the double-lumen tube is placed, both bronchial and tracheal cuffs should be inflated. The bronchial cuff should make a tight seal before the patient is turned into the lateral decubitus position, with the diseased lung in a nondependent position. The diseased lung should be frequently suctioned during the procedure to decrease the likelihood of contaminating the healthy lung.

Bronchopleural Fistula

Bronchopleural fistulas occur following lung resection (usually pneumonectomy), rupture of a pulmonary abscess into a pleural cavity, pulmonary barotrauma, or spontaneous rupture of bullae. The majority of patients are treated (and cured) conservatively; patients come to surgery when chest tube drainage has failed. **Anesthetic management may be complicated by the inability to effectively ventilate the patient with positive pressure because of a large air leak, the potential for a tension pneumothorax, and the risk of contaminating the other lung if an empyema is present.** The empyema is usually drained, prior to closure of the fistula.

A correctly placed double-lumen tube greatly simplifies anesthetic management by isolating the fistula and allowing one-lung ventilation to the normal lung. The patient should be extubated as soon as possible after the repair.

Anesthesia for Tracheal Resection

Preoperative Considerations

Tracheal resection is most commonly performed for tracheal stenosis, tumors, or, less commonly, congenital abnormalities. Tracheal stenosis can result from penetrating or blunt trauma, as well as tracheal intubation and tracheostomy. Squamous cell and adenoid cystic carcinomas account for the majority of tumors. Compromise of the tracheal lumen results in progressive dyspnea. Wheezing or stridor may be evident only with exertion. The dyspnea may be worse when the patient is lying down, with progressive airway obstruction. Hemoptysis can also complicate tracheal tumors. CT is valuable in localizing the lesion. **Measurement of flow–volume loops confirms the location of the obstruction and aids the clinician in evaluating the severity of the lesion** (Figure 25–12).

Anesthetic Considerations

Little premedication is given, as most patients presenting for tracheal resection have moderate to severe airway obstruction. Use of an anticholinergic agent to dry secretions is controversial because of the theoretical risk of inspissation. Monitoring should include direct arterial pressure measurements.

An inhalation induction (in 100% oxygen) is carried out in patients with severe obstruction. Sevoflurane is preferred because it is the potent anesthetic that is least irritating to the airway. Spontaneous ventilation is maintained throughout induction. NMBs are generally avoided because of the potential for complete airway obstruction following neuromuscular blockade. Laryngoscopy is performed only when the patient is judged to be under deep anesthesia. Intravenous lidocaine (1–2 mg/kg) can deepen the anesthesia without depressing respirations. The surgeon may then perform rigid bronchoscopy to evaluate and possibly dilate the lesion. Following bronchoscopy, the patient is intubated with a tracheal tube small enough to be passed distal to the obstruction whenever possible.

A collar incision is utilized for high tracheal lesions. The surgeon divides the trachea in the neck and advances a sterile armored tube into the distal trachea, passing off a sterile connecting breathing circuit to the anesthesiologist for ventilation during the resection. Following the resection and completion of the posterior part of the reanastomosis, the armored tube is removed, and the original tracheal tube is advanced distally, past the anastomosis (Figure 25–13). Alternatively, high-frequency jet ventilation may be employed during the anastomosis

A NORMAL

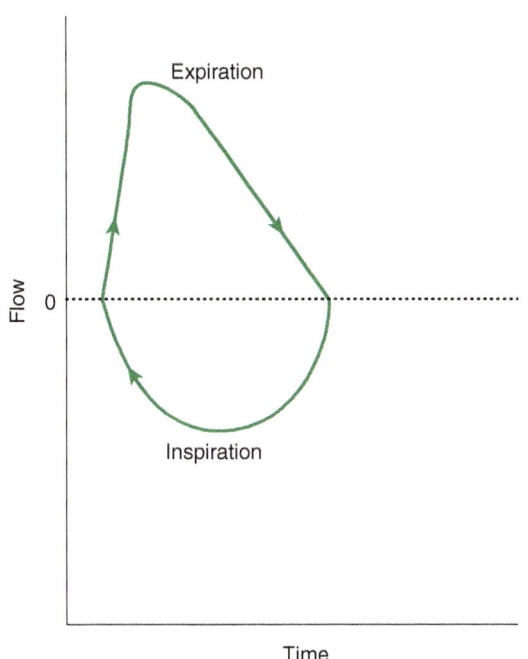

B VARIABLE EXTRATHORACIC OBSTRUCTION

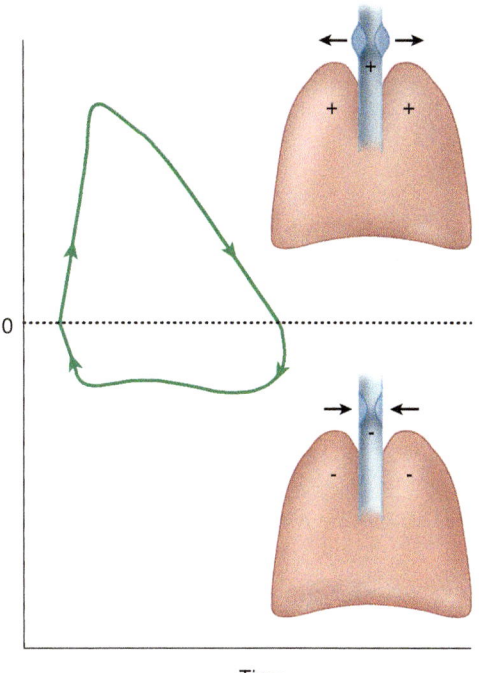

C VARIABLE INTRATHORACIC OBSTRUCTION

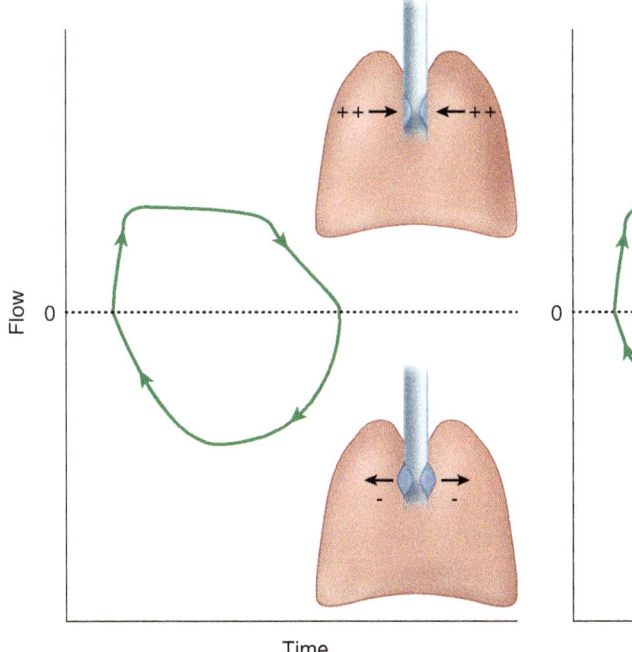

D FIXED LARGE AIRWAY OBSTRUCTION

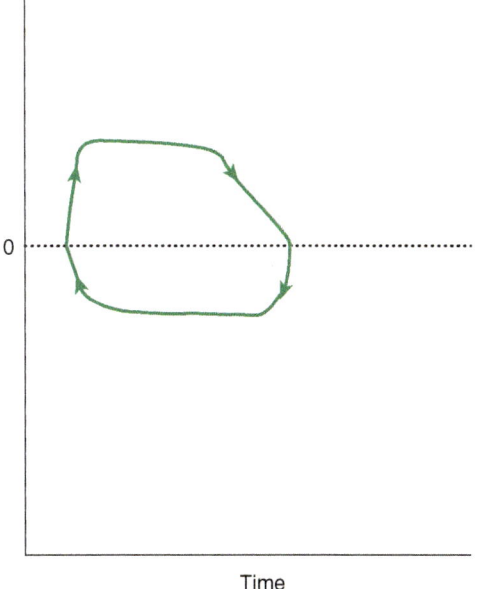

FIGURE 25–12 **A–D**: Flow–volume loops.

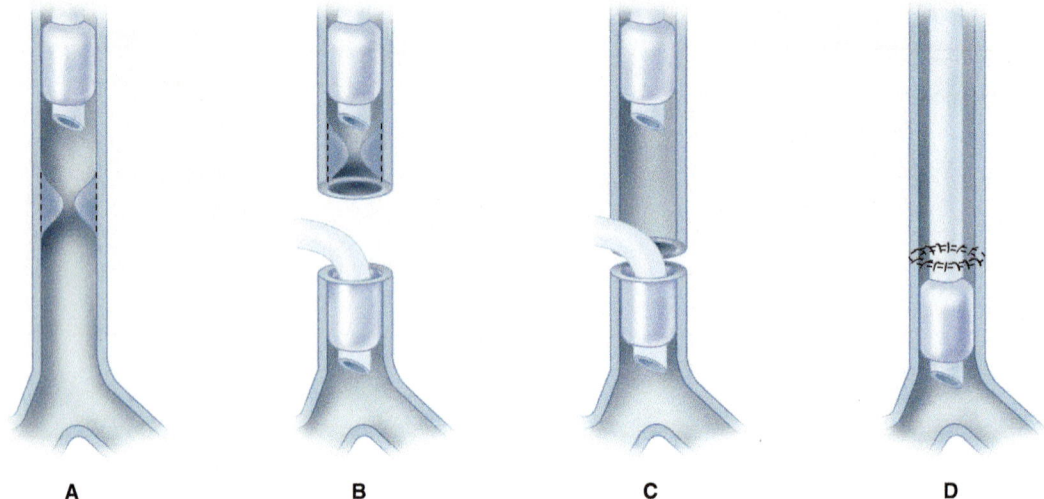

FIGURE 25–13 **A–D**: Airway management of a high tracheal lesion.

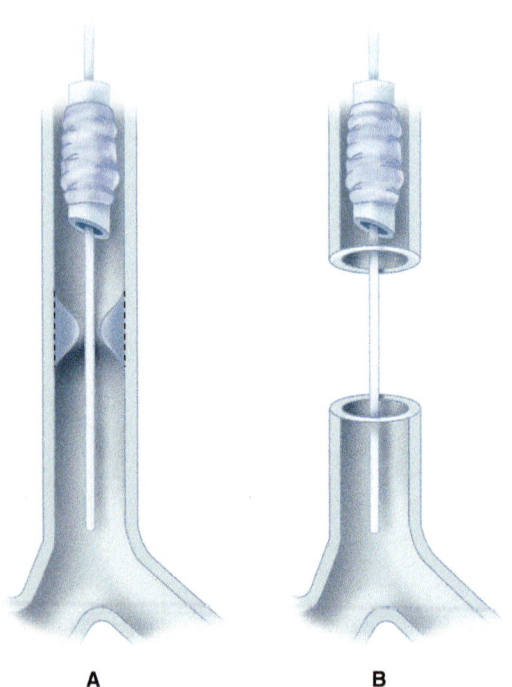

FIGURE 25–14 Tracheal resection using high-frequency jet ventilation. **A**: The catheter is advanced past the obstruction, and the cuff is deflated when jet ventilation is initiated. **B**: The catheter is advanced distally by the surgeon. Jet ventilation can be continued without interruption during resection and reanastomosis.

by passing the jet cannula past the obstruction and into the distal trachea (Figure 25–14). Return of spontaneous ventilation and early extubation at the end of the procedure are desirable. Patients should be positioned with the neck flexed immediately after the operation to minimize tension on the suture line (Figure 25–15).

Surgical management of low tracheal lesions requires a median sternotomy or right posterior thoracotomy. Anesthetic management is similar, but more regularly requires more complicated techniques, such as high-frequency ventilation or even cardiopulmonary bypass (CPB) in complex congenital cases.

Anesthesia for Video-Assisted Thoracoscopic Surgery (VATS)

VATS is now used for most lung resections that previously required open thoracotomy. The list of procedures that can be accomplished during VATS includes lung biopsy, segmental and lobar resections, pleurodesis, esophageal procedures, and pericardectomy. Most procedures are performed through three or more small incisions in the chest, with the patient in the lateral decubitus position.

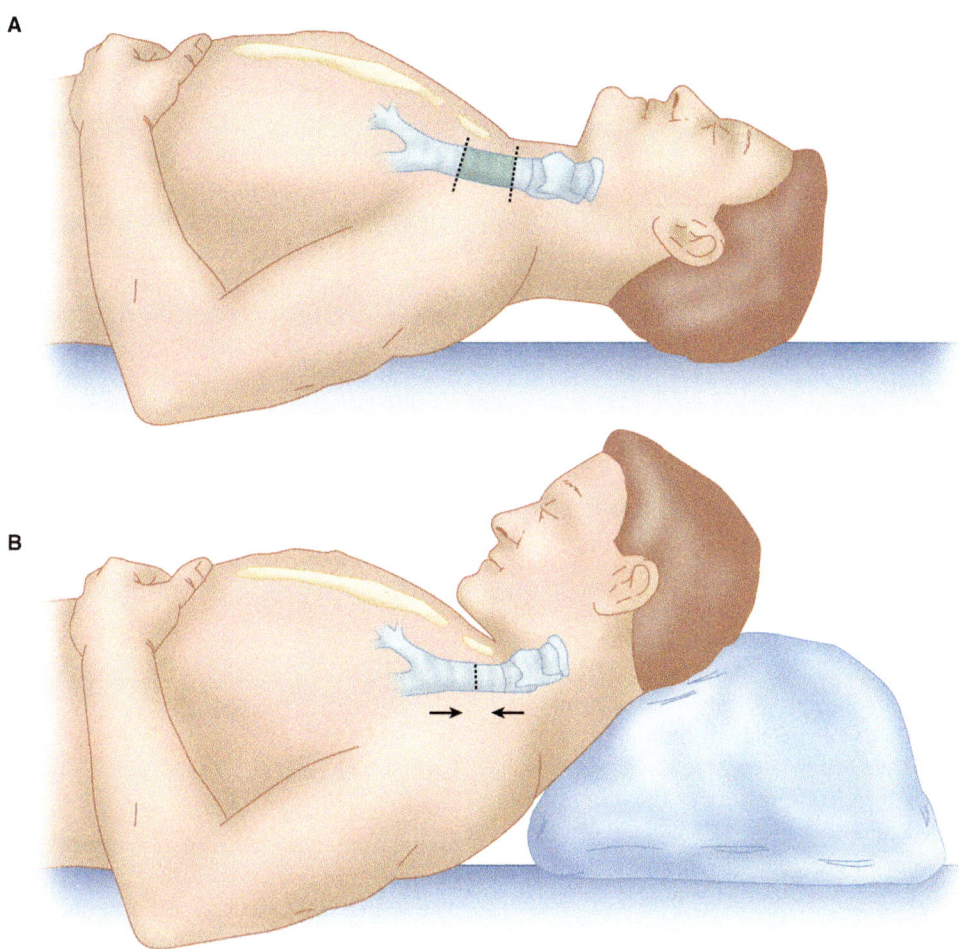

FIGURE 25–15 Position of the patient before (**A**) and after (**B**) tracheal resection and reanastomosis with the patient's neck flexed for the first 24–48 hr.

Anesthetic management is similar to that for open procedures, except that one-lung ventilation is required (as opposed to being desirable) for nearly all procedures.

Anesthesia for Diagnostic Thoracic Procedures

Bronchoscopy

Rigid bronchoscopy for removal of foreign bodies or tracheal dilatation is usually performed under general anesthesia. These procedures are complicated by the need to share the airway with the surgeon or pulmonologist; fortunately, they are often of short duration. After a standard intravenous induction, anesthesia is often maintained with total intravenous anesthesia, and a short- or intermediate-acting NMB. Brief airway procedures are among the few remaining indications for a succinylcholine infusion. One of three techniques can then be used during rigid bronchoscopy: (1) apneic oxygenation using a small catheter positioned alongside the bronchoscope to insufflate oxygen (above); (2) conventional ventilation through the side arm of a ventilating bronchoscope (when the proximal window of this instrument is opened for suctioning or biopsies, ventilation must be interrupted); or (3) jet ventilation through an injector-type bronchoscope.

Mediastinoscopy

Mediastinoscopy, much more commonly employed in the past than at present, provides access to the mediastinal lymph nodes and is used to establish either the diagnosis or the resectability of intrathoracic malignancies (above). Preoperative CT or MR imaging is useful for evaluating tracheal distortion or compression.

Mediastinoscopy is performed under general tracheal anesthesia with neuromuscular paralysis. Venous access with a large-bore (14- to 16-gauge) intravenous catheter is mandatory because of the risk of bleeding and the difficulty in controlling bleeding when it occurs. Because the innominate artery may be compressed during the procedure, blood pressure should be measured in the left arm.

Complications associated with mediastinoscopy include: (1) vagally mediated reflex bradycardia from compression of the trachea or the great vessels; (2) excessive hemorrhage (see above); (3) cerebral ischemia from compression of the innominate artery (detected with a right radial arterial line or pulse oximeter on the right hand); (4) pneumothorax (usually presents postoperatively); (5) air embolism (because of a 30° head elevation, the risk is greatest during spontaneous ventilation); (6) recurrent laryngeal nerve damage; and (7) phrenic nerve injury.

Bronchoalveolar Lavage

Bronchoalveolar lavage may be employed for patients with pulmonary alveolar proteinosis. These patients produce excessive quantities of surfactant and fail to clear it. They present with dyspnea and bilateral consolidation on the chest radiograph. In such patients, bronchoalveolar lavage may be indicated for severe hypoxemia or worsening dyspnea. Often, one lung is lavaged, allowing the patient to recover for a few days before the other lung is lavaged; the "sicker" lung is therefore lavaged first. Increasingly, both lungs are lavaged during the same procedure, creating unique challenges to ensure adequate oxygenation during lavage of the second lung.

Unilateral bronchoalveolar lavage is performed under general anesthesia with a double-lumen bronchial tube. The cuffs on the tube should be properly positioned and should make a watertight seal to prevent spillage of fluid into the other side. The procedure is normally done in the supine position; although lavage with the lung in a dependent position helps to minimize contamination of the other lung, this position can cause severe ventilation/perfusion mismatch. Warm normal saline is infused into the lung to be treated and is drained by gravity; treatment continues until the fluid returning is clear (about 10–20 L). At the end of the procedure, both lungs are well suctioned, and the double-lumen tracheal tube is replaced with a single-lumen tracheal tube.

Anesthesia for Lung Transplantation

PREOPERATIVE CONSIDERATIONS

Lung transplantation is indicated for end-stage pulmonary parenchymal disease or pulmonary hypertension. Candidates are functionally incapacitated by dyspnea and have a poor prognosis. Criteria vary according to the primary disease process. Common etiologies are listed in Table 25–3. Lung transplantation (as is true for all solid organ transplants) is limited by the availability of suitable organs, not by the availability of recipients. Patients typically have dyspnea at rest or with minimal activity and resting

TABLE 25–3 Indications for isolated lung transplantation.

Cystic fibrosis
Bronchiectasis
Obstructive
Chronic obstructive pulmonary disease
α_1-antitrypsin deficiency
Pulmonary lymphangiomatosis
Restrictive
Idiopathic pulmonary fibrosis
Primary pulmonary hypertension

hypoxemia (Pao_2 <50 mm Hg) with increasing oxygen requirements. Progressive CO_2 retention is also very common. Patients may be ventilator dependent. Cor pulmonale does not necessarily require combined heart–lung transplantation because right ventricular function may recover when pulmonary artery pressures normalize. Patients should have normal left ventricular function and be free of coronary artery disease, as well as other serious health problems.

Single-lung transplantation may be performed in selected patients with idiopathic pulmonary fibrosis, whereas double-lung transplantation is typically performed in patients with cystic fibrosis, bullous emphysema, or vascular diseases. Patients with Eisenmenger syndrome require combined heart–lung transplantation.

ANESTHETIC CONSIDERATIONS

1. Preoperative Management

Effective coordination between the organ-retrieval team and the transplant team minimizes graft ischemia time and avoids unnecessary prolongation of pretransplant anesthesia time. These procedures are performed on an emergency basis; therefore, patients may have little time to fast for surgery. Oral cyclosporine also may be given preoperatively. Administration of a clear antacid, an H_2 blocker, or metoclopramide should be considered. Patients are very sensitive to sedatives, so premedication is usually administered only in the operating room when the patient is directly attended. Immunosuppressants and antibiotics are also administered after induction and prior to surgical incision.

2. Intraoperative Management

Monitoring

Strict asepsis should be observed for invasive monitoring procedures. Central venous access might be accomplished only after induction of anesthesia because patients may not be able to lie flat while awake. Patients with a patent foramen ovale are at risk of paradoxical embolism because of high right atrial pressures.

Induction & Maintenance of Anesthesia

A rapid-sequence induction is utilized. Induction with ketamine, etomidate, an opioid, or a combination of these agents is employed, avoiding precipitous drops in blood pressure. An NMB is used to facilitate laryngoscopy. Hypoxemia and hypercarbia must be avoided to prevent further increases in pulmonary artery pressure. Hypotension should be treated with vasopressors instead of large fluid boluses (see below).

Anesthesia is usually maintained with total intravenous anesthesia or a volatile agent. Intraoperative difficulties in ventilation are not uncommon. Progressive retention of CO_2 can also be a problem intraoperatively. Ventilation should be adjusted to maintain a $Paco_2$ as close to the patient's baseline as possible. However, in the presence of a reasonable cardiovascular reserve and normal right heart function, higher levels of $Paco_2$ can be tolerated for short periods of time. Hypercarbia and acidosis may lead to pulmonary vasoconstriction and acute right heart failure, and hemodynamic support with inotropes may be required for these patients. Patients with cystic fibrosis have copious secretions and require frequent suctioning.

Single-Lung Transplantation

Single-lung transplantation is often attempted without CPB. The procedure is performed through a posterior thoracotomy. Whether to employ CPB during transplantation of one lung is based on the patient's response to collapsing the lung to be replaced and clamping its pulmonary artery. Persistent arterial hypoxemia (Spo_2 < 88%) or a sudden increase in pulmonary artery pressures necessitates CPB. Prostaglandin E_1, milrinone, nitroglycerin, and dobutamine may be utilized to reduce pulmonary hypertension and prevent right ventricular failure. Inotropic support may be necessary. After the recipient lung is removed, the pulmonary artery, left atrial cuff (with the pulmonary veins), and bronchus of the donor lung are anastomosed. Flexible bronchoscopy is used to examine the bronchial suture line after its completion.

Double-Lung Transplantation

A "clamshell" transverse sternotomy can be used for double-lung transplantation. The procedure is occasionally performed with CPB; sequential thoracotomies for double-lung transplantation can also be performed. Heart lung transplantation is performed through median sternotomy with CPB.

Posttransplantation Management

After anastomosis of the donor organ or organs, ventilation to both lungs is resumed. Following transplantation, peak inspiratory pressures should be maintained at the minimum pressure compatible with good lung expansion, and the inspired oxygen concentration should be maintained as close to room air as allowed by a PaO_2 >60 mm Hg. Methylprednisolone and mannitol are usually administered prior to the release of vascular clamps. Hyperkalemia may occur as the preservative fluid is washed out of the donor organ. If transplantation has been performed on CPB, the patient is separated from CPB. Pulmonary vasodilators, inhaled nitric oxide, and inotropes (above) may be necessary. Transesophageal echocardiography is helpful in differentiating right and left ventricular dysfunction, as well as in evaluating blood flow in the pulmonary vessels, particularly after transplantation.

Transplantation disrupts the neural innervation, lymphatic drainage, and bronchial circulation of the transplanted lung. The respiratory pattern is unaffected, but the cough reflex is abolished below the carina. Bronchial hyperreactivity is observed in some patients. Hypoxic pulmonary vasoconstriction remains normal. Loss of lymphatic drainage increases extravascular lung water and predisposes the transplanted lung to pulmonary edema. Intraoperative fluid replacement must therefore be kept to a minimum. Loss of the bronchial circulation predisposes to ischemic breakdown of the bronchial suture line.

3. Postoperative Management

Patients are extubated after surgery as soon as is feasible. A thoracic epidural catheter may be employed for postoperative analgesia when coagulation studies are normal. The postoperative course may be complicated by acute rejection, infections, and renal and hepatic dysfunction. Deteriorating lung function may result from rejection or reperfusion injury. Occasionally, temporary extracorporeal membrane oxygenation may be necessary. Frequent bronchoscopy with transbronchial biopsies and lavage are necessary to differentiate between rejection and infection. Nosocomial Gram-negative bacteria, cytomegalovirus, *Candida, Aspergillus,* and *Pneumocystis carinii* are common pathogens. Other postoperative surgical complications include damage to the phrenic, vagus, and left recurrent laryngeal nerves.

Anesthesia for Esophageal Surgery

PREOPERATIVE CONSIDERATIONS

Common indications for esophageal surgery include tumors, gastroesophageal reflux, and motility disorders (achalasia). Surgical procedures include simple endoscopy, esophageal dilatation, cervical esophagomyotomy, open or thoracoscopic distal esophagomyotomy, insertion or removal of esophageal stents, and esophagectomy. Squamous cell carcinomas account for the majority of esophageal tumors; adenocarcinomas are less common, whereas benign tumors (leiomyomas) are rare. Most tumors occur in the distal esophagus. Operative treatment may be palliative or curative. Although the prognosis is generally poor, surgical therapy offers the only hope of a cure. After esophageal resection, the stomach is pulled up into the thorax, or the esophagus is functionally replaced with part of the colon (interposition).

Gastroesophageal reflux is treated surgically when the esophagitis is refractory to medical management or results in complications such as stricture, recurrent pulmonary aspiration, or Barrett's esophagus (columnar epithelium). A variety of antireflux operations may be performed (Nissen, Belsey, Hill, or Collis–Nissen) via thoracic or abdominal approaches, often laparoscopically. They all involve wrapping part of the stomach around the esophagus.

Achalasia and systemic sclerosis (scleroderma) account for the majority of surgical procedures performed for motility disorders. The former usually occurs as an isolated finding, whereas the latter is part of a generalized collagen–vascular disorder. Cricopharyngeal muscle dysfunction can be associated with a variety of neurogenic or myogenic disorders and often results in a Zenker's diverticulum.

ANESTHETIC CONSIDERATIONS

9 Regardless of the procedure, a common anesthetic concern in patients with esophageal disease is the risk of pulmonary aspiration. This may result from obstruction, altered motility, or abnormal sphincter function. In fact, most patients typically complain of dysphagia, heartburn, regurgitation, coughing, and/or wheezing when lying flat. Dyspnea on exertion may also be prominent when chronic aspiration results in pulmonary fibrosis. Patients with malignancies may present with anemia and weight loss. Esophageal cancer patients usually have a history of cigarette smoking and alcohol consumption, so patients should be evaluated for coexisting chronic obstructive pulmonary disease, coronary artery disease, and liver dysfunction. Patients with systemic sclerosis (scleroderma) should be evaluated for involvement of other organs, particularly the kidneys, heart, and lungs; Raynaud's phenomena is also common.

In patients with reflux, consideration should be given to administering metoclopramide, an H_2-receptor blocker, or a proton-pump inhibitor preoperatively. In such patients, a rapid-sequence induction should be used. A double-lumen tube is used for procedures involving thoracoscopy or thoracotomy. The anesthesiologist may be asked to pass a large-diameter bougie into the esophagus as part of the surgical procedure; great caution must be exercised to help avoid pharyngeal or esophageal injury.

Transhiatal (blunt) and thoracic esophagectomies deserve special consideration. These procedures often involve considerable blood loss. The former requires an upper abdominal incision and a left cervical incision, whereas the latter requires posterolateral thoracotomy, an abdominal incision, and, finally, a left cervical incision. Parts of the procedure may be performed using laparoscopy or VATS.

Monitoring of arterial and central venous pressure is indicated. Multiple large-bore intravenous access, fluid warmers, and a forced-air body warmer are advisable. During the trans hiatal approach to esophagectomy, substernal and diaphragmatic retractors can interfere with cardiac function. Moreover, as the esophagus is freed up blindly from the posterior mediastinum by blunt dissection, the surgeon's hand transiently interferes with cardiac filling and produces profound hypotension. The dissection can also induce marked vagal stimulation.

Colonic interposition involves forming a pedicle graft of the colon and passing it through the posterior mediastinum up to the neck to take the place of the esophagus. This procedure is lengthy, and maintenance of an adequate blood pressure, cardiac output, and hemoglobin concentration is necessary to ensure graft viability. Graft ischemia may be heralded by a progressive metabolic acidosis.

Postoperative ventilation will often be used in patients undergoing esophagectomy, because so many of them will have coexisting cardiac and pulmonary disease. Postoperative surgical complications include damage to the phrenic, vagus, and left recurrent laryngeal nerves.

CASE DISCUSSION

Mediastinal Adenopathy

A 9-year-old boy with mediastinal lymphadenopathy seen on a chest radiograph presents for biopsy of a cervical lymph node.

What is the most important preoperative consideration?

Is there any evidence of airway compromise? Tracheal compression may produce dyspnea (proximal obstruction) or a nonproductive cough (distal obstruction).

Asymptomatic compression is also common and may be evident only as tracheal deviation on physical or radiographic examinations. A CT scan of the chest provides invaluable information about the presence, location, and severity of airway compression. Flow–volume loops will also detect subtle airway obstruction and provide important information regarding the location and functional importance of the obstruction (above).

Does the absence of any preoperative dyspnea make severe intraoperative respiratory compromise less likely?

No. Severe airway obstruction can occur following induction of anesthesia in these patients even in the absence of any preoperative symptoms. This mandates that the chest radiograph and CT scan be reviewed for evidence of asymptomatic airway obstruction. The point of obstruction is typically distal to the tip of the tracheal tube. Moreover, loss of spontaneous ventilation can precipitate complete airway obstruction.

What is the superior vena cava syndrome?

Superior vena cava syndrome is the result of progressive enlargement of a mediastinal mass and compression of mediastinal structures, particularly the vena cava. Lymphomas are most commonly responsible, but primary pulmonary or mediastinal neoplasms can also produce the syndrome. Superior vena cava syndrome is often associated with severe airway obstruction and cardiovascular collapse on induction of general anesthesia. The caval compression produces venous engorgement and edema of the head, neck, and arms. Direct mechanical compression, as well as mucosal edema, severely compromise airflow in the trachea. Most patients favor an upright posture, as recumbency worsens the airway obstruction. Cardiac output may be severely depressed due to impeded venous return from the upper body, direct mechanical compression of the heart, and (with malignancies) pericardial invasion. An echocardiogram is useful in evaluating cardiac function and detecting pericardial fluid.

What is the anesthetic of choice for a patient with superior vena cava syndrome?

The absence of signs or symptoms of airway compression or superior vena cava syndrome does not preclude potentially life-threatening complications following induction of general anesthesia. Therefore, biopsy of a peripheral node (usually cervical or scalene) under local anesthesia is safest whenever possible. Although establishing a diagnosis is of prime importance, the presence of significant airway compromise or the superior vena cava syndrome may dictate empiric treatment with corticosteroids prior to tissue diagnosis at surgery (cancer is the most common cause); preoperative radiation therapy or chemotherapy may also be considered. The patient can usually safely undergo surgery with general anesthesia once airway compromise and other manifestations of the superior vena cava syndrome are alleviated.

General anesthesia may be indicated for establishing a diagnosis in young or uncooperative patients who have no evidence of airway compromise or the superior vena cava syndrome, and, rarely, for patients unresponsive to steroids, radiation, and chemotherapy.

How does the presence of airway obstruction and the superior vena cava syndrome influence management of general anesthesia?

1. *Premedication*: Only an anticholinergic should be given. The patient should be transported to the operating room in a semiupright position with supplemental oxygen.
2. *Monitoring*: In addition to standard monitors, an arterial line is helpful, but it should be placed after induction in young patients. At least one large-bore intravenous catheter should be placed in a lower extremity, as venous drainage from the upper body may be unreliable.
3. *Airway management*: Difficulties with ventilation and intubation should be anticipated. Following preoxygenation, awake intubation with an armored tracheal tube may be safest in a cooperative patient. Use of a flexible bronchoscope is advantageous in the presence of airway distortion and will define the site and degree of obstruction. Coughing or straining, however, may precipitate complete airway obstruction because the resultant positive pleural pressure increases intrathoracic

tracheal compression. Passing the armored tube beyond the area of compression may obviate this problem. Uncooperative patients require a sevoflurane inhalation induction.

4. *Induction*: The goal should be a smooth induction maintaining spontaneous ventilation and hemodynamic stability. The ability to ventilate the patient with a good airway should be established prior to use of an NMB. Using 100% oxygen, one of three induction techniques can be used: (1) intravenous ketamine (because it results in greater hemodynamic stability in patients with reduced cardiac output); (2) inhalational induction with a volatile agent (usually sevoflurane); or (3) incremental small doses of propofol or etomidate.

   Positive-pressure ventilation can precipitate severe hypotension, and volume loading prior to induction may partly offset impaired ventricular filling secondary to caval obstruction.

5. *Maintenance of anesthesia*: The technique selected should be tailored to the patient's hemodynamic status. Following intubation, neuromuscular blockade prevents coughing or straining.

6. *Extubation*: At the end of the procedure, patients should be left intubated until the airway obstruction has resolved, as determined by flexible bronchoscopy or the presence of an air leak around the tracheal tube when the tracheal cuff is deflated.

SUGGESTED READING

Campos J: An update on bronchial blockers during lung separation techniques in adults. Anesth Analg 2003;97:1266.

Ehrenfeld JM, Walsh JL, Sandberg WS: Right- and left-sided Mallinckrodt double-lumen tubes have identical clinical performance. Anesth Analg 2008;106:1847.

Gothard J: Anesthetic considerations for patients with anterior mediastinal masses. Anesthesiol Clin 2008;26:305.

Grichnik K, Shaw A: Update on one lung ventilation: the use of continuous positive airway pressure ventilation and positive end expiratory pressure ventilation-clinical application. Curr Opin Anaesthesiol 2009;22:23.

Lohser J: Evidence based management of one lung ventilation. Anesthesiol Clin 2008;26:241.

Reilly JJ Jr: Evidence-based preoperative evaluation of candidates for thoracotomy. Chest 1999;116:474S.

Slinger P: Update on anesthetic management for pneumonectomy. Curr Opin Anaesthesiol 2009;22:31.

Slinger P, Johnston M: Preoperative assessment: an anesthesiologist's perspective. Thorac Surg Clin 2005;15:11.

Neurophysiology & Anesthesia

1. Cerebral perfusion pressure is the difference between mean arterial pressure and intracranial pressure (or central venous pressure, whichever is greater).

2. The cerebral autoregulation curve is shifted to the right in patients with chronic arterial hypertension.

3. The most important extrinsic influences on cerebral blood flow (CBF) are respiratory gas tensions—particularly Pa_{CO_2}. CBF is directly proportionate to Pa_{CO_2} between tensions of 20 and 80 mg Hg. Blood flow changes approximately 1–2 mL/100 g/min per mm Hg change in Pa_{CO_2}.

4. CBF changes 5% to 7% per 1°C change in temperature. Hypothermia decreases both cerebral metabolic rate and CBF, whereas pyrexia has the reverse effect.

5. The movement of a given substance across the blood–brain barrier is governed simultaneously by its size, charge, lipid solubility, and degree of protein binding in blood.

6. The blood–brain barrier may be disrupted by severe hypertension, tumors, trauma,

strokes, infection, marked hypercapnia, hypoxia, and sustained seizure activity.

7. The cranial vault is a rigid structure with a fixed total volume, consisting of brain (80%), blood (12%), and cerebrospinal fluid (8%). Any increase in one component must be offset by an equivalent decrease in another to prevent a rise in intracranial pressure.

8. With the exception of ketamine, all intravenous agents either have little effect on or reduce cerebral metabolic rate and CBF.

9. With normal autoregulation and an intact blood–brain barrier, vasopressors increase CBF only when mean arterial blood pressure is below 50–60 mm Hg or above 150–160 mm Hg.

10. The brain is very vulnerable to ischemic injury because of its relatively high oxygen consumption and near total dependence on aerobic glucose metabolism.

11. Hypothermia is the most effective method for protecting the brain during focal and global ischemia.

Anesthetic agents may have profound effects on cerebral metabolism, blood flow, cerebrospinal fluid (CSF) dynamics, and intracranial volume and pressure. In some instances, these alterations are deleterious, whereas in others they may be

beneficial. This chapter reviews important physiological concepts in anesthetic practice and discusses the effects of commonly used anesthetics on cerebral physiology.

Cerebral Physiology

CEREBRAL METABOLISM

The brain normally consumes 20% of total body oxygen. Most cerebral oxygen consumption (60%) is used to generate adenosine triphosphate (ATP) to support neuronal electrical activity (Figure 26–1). The cerebral metabolic rate (CMR) is usually expressed in terms of oxygen consumption (CMR_{O_2}) and averages 3–3.8 mL/100 g/min (50 mL/min) in adults. CMR_{O_2} is greatest in the gray matter of the cerebral cortex and generally parallels cortical electrical activity. Because of the relatively high oxygen consumption and the absence of significant oxygen reserves, interruption of cerebral perfusion usually results in unconsciousness within 10 sec, as oxygen tension rapidly drops below 30 mm Hg. If blood flow is not reestablished within 3–8 min under most conditions, ATP stores are depleted, and irreversible cellular injury begins to occur. The hippocampus and cerebellum seem to be most sensitive to hypoxic injury.

Neuronal cells normally utilize glucose as their primary energy source. Brain glucose consumption is approximately 5 mg/100 g/min, of which more than 90% is metabolized aerobically. CMR_{O_2} therefore normally parallels glucose consumption. This relationship is not maintained during starvation, when ketone bodies (acetoacetate and β-hydroxybutyrate) also become major energy substrates. Although the brain can also take up and metabolize lactate, cerebral function is normally dependent on a continuous supply of glucose. Acute sustained hypoglycemia is injurious to the brain. Paradoxically, hyperglycemia can exacerbate global and focal hypoxic brain injury by accelerating cerebral acidosis and cellular injury. Tight control of perioperative blood glucose concentration has been advocated in part because of adverse effects of hyperglycemia during ischemic episodes; however, overzealous blood glucose control can likewise produce injury through iatrogenic hypoglycemia.

CEREBRAL BLOOD FLOW

Cerebral blood flow (CBF) varies with metabolic activity. There are a variety of methods available to directly measure CBF. These methods include: positron emission tomography, xenon enhanced computed tomography, single photon emission computed tomography, and computed tomography perfusion scans. These methods do not lend themselves to bedside monitoring of CBF. Blood flow studies confirm that regional CBF parallels metabolic activity and can vary from 10–300 mL/100 g/min. For example, motor activity of a limb is associated with a rapid increase in regional CBF of the corresponding motor cortex. Similarly, visual activity is associated with an increase in regional CBF of the corresponding occipital visual cortex.

Although total CBF averages 50 mL/100 g/min, flow in gray matter is about 80 mL/100 g/min, whereas that in white matter is estimated to be 20 mL/100 g/min. Total CBF in adults averages 750 mL/min (15% to 20% of cardiac output). Flow rates below 20–25 mL/100 g/min are usually associated with cerebral impairment, as evidenced by slowing on the electroencephalogram (EEG). CBF rates between 15 and 20 mL/100 g/min typically produce a flat (isoelectric) EEG, whereas rates below 10 mL/100 g/min are usually associated with irreversible brain damage.

Indirect measures are often used to estimate the adequacy of CBF and brain tissue oxygen delivery in clinical settings. These methods include:

- The velocity of CBF can be measured using transcranial Doppler (TCD); see Chapters 5 and 6 for a discussion of the Doppler effect. An ultrasound probe (2 mHz, pulse wave Doppler) is placed in the temporal area above the

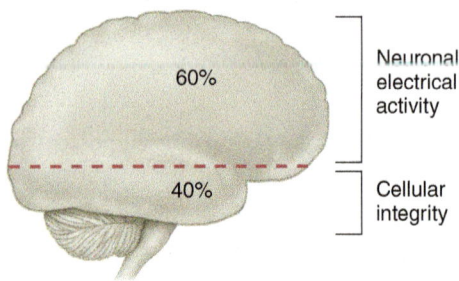

FIGURE 26–1 Normal brain oxygen requirements.

60% Neuronal electrical activity

40% Cellular integrity

zygomatic arch, which allows insonation of the middle cerebral artery. Normal velocity in the middle cerebral artery is approximately 55 cm/sec. Velocities greater than 120 cm/sec can indicate cerebral artery vasospasm following subarachnoid hemorrhage or hyperemic blood flow. Comparison between the velocities in the extracranial internal carotid artery and the middle cerebral artery (the Lindegaard ratio) can distinguish between these conditions. Middle cerebral artery velocity three times that of the velocity measured in the extracranial internal carotid artery more likely reflects cerebral artery vasospasm.

- Near infrared spectroscopy was discussed in Chapter 6. Decreased saturation is associated with impaired cerebral oxygen delivery, although near infrared spectroscopy primarily reflects cerebral venous oxygen saturation.

- Brain tissue oximetry measures the oxygen tension in brain tissue through placement of a bolt with a Clark electrode oxygen sensor. Brain tissue CO_2 tension can also be measured using a similarly placed infrared sensor. Normal brain tissue oxygen tension varies from 20–50 mm Hg. Brain tissue oxygen tensions less than 20 mm Hg warrant interventions, and values less than 10 mm Hg are indicative of brain ischemia.

- Intracerebral microdialysis can be used to measure changes in brain tissue chemistry that are indicative of ischemia and/or brain injury. Microdialysis can be used to measure cerebral lactate, neurotransmitters, markers of inflammation, and glucose concentration. Increases in the ratio of lactate/pyruvate have been associated with cerebral ischemia.

REGULATION OF CEREBRAL BLOOD FLOW

1. Cerebral Perfusion Pressure

 Cerebral perfusion pressure (CPP) is the difference between mean arterial pressure (MAP) and intracranial pressure (ICP) (or central venous

pressure [CVP], if it is greater than ICP). MAP – ICP (or CVP) = CPP. CPP is normally 80–100 mm Hg. Moreover, because ICP is normally less than 10 mm Hg, CPP is primarily dependent on MAP.

Moderate to severe increases in ICP (>30 mm Hg) can compromise CPP and CBF, even in the presence of a normal MAP. Patients with CPP values less than 50 mm Hg often show slowing on the EEG, whereas those with a CPP between 25 and 40 mm Hg typically have a flat EEG. Sustained perfusion pressures less than 25 mm Hg may result in irreversible brain damage.

2. Autoregulation

Much like the heart and kidneys, the brain normally tolerates a wide range of blood pressure, with little change in blood flow. The cerebral vasculature rapidly (10–60 s) adapts to changes in CPP. Decreases in CPP result in cerebral vasodilation, whereas elevations induce vasoconstriction. In normal individuals, CBF remains nearly constant between MAPs of about 60 and 160 mm Hg (**Figure 26–2**). Beyond these limits, blood flow becomes pressure dependent. Pressures above 150–160 mm Hg can disrupt the blood–brain barrier (see below) and may result in cerebral edema and hemorrhage.

2 The cerebral autoregulation curve (Figure 26–2) is shifted to the right in patients with chronic

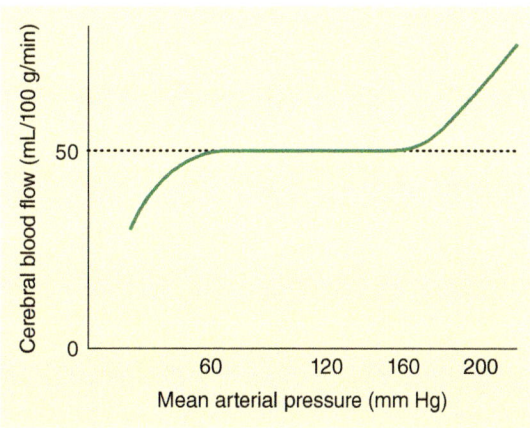

FIGURE 26–2 Normal cerebral autoregulation curve.

arterial hypertension. Both upper and lower limits are shifted. Flow becomes more pressure dependent at low "normal" arterial pressures in return for cerebral protection at higher arterial pressures. Studies suggest that long-term antihypertensive therapy can restore cerebral autoregulation limits toward normal.

Both myogenic and metabolic mechanisms may explain cerebral autoregulation. Myogenic mechanisms involve an intrinsic response of smooth muscle cells in cerebral arterioles to changes in MAP. Metabolic mechanisms indicate that cerebral metabolic demands determine arteriolar tone. Thus, when tissue demand exceeds blood flow, the release of tissue metabolites causes vasodilation and increases flow. Whereas hydrogen ions were once thought to mediate this response, other metabolites are likely involved.

3. Extrinsic Mechanisms

Respiratory Gas Tensions

3 The most important extrinsic influences on CBF are respiratory gas tensions—particularly $Paco_2$. CBF is directly proportionate to $Paco_2$ between tensions of 20 and 80 mm Hg (Figure 26–3). Blood flow changes approximately 1–2 mL/100 g/min per mm Hg change in $Paco_2$. This effect is almost immediate and is thought to

be secondary to changes in the pH of CSF and cerebral tissue. Because ions do not readily cross the blood–brain barrier (see below) but CO_2 does, acute changes in $Paco_2$ but not HCO_3^- affect CBF. Thus, acute metabolic acidosis has little effect on CBF because hydrogen ions (H^+) cannot readily cross the blood–brain barrier. After 24–48 hr, CSF HCO_3^- concentration adjusts to compensate for the change in $Paco_2$, so that the effects of hypocapnia and hypercapnia are diminished. Marked hyperventilation ($Paco_2$ < 20 mm Hg) shifts the oxygen–hemoglobin dissociation curve to the left, and, with changes in CBF, may result in EEG changes suggestive of cerebral impairment, even in normal individuals.

Only marked changes in Pao_2 alter CBF. Whereas hyperoxia may be associated with only minimal decreases (–10%) in CBF, severe hypoxemia (Pao_2 < 50 mm Hg) greatly increases CBF (Figure 26–3).

Temperature

4 CBF changes 5% to 7% per 1°C change in temperature. Hypothermia decreases both CMR and CBF, whereas hyperthermia has the reverse effect. Between 17°C and 37°C, the Q10 for humans is approximately 2—that is, for every 10° increase in temperature, the CMR doubles. Conversely, the CMR decreases by 50% if the temperature of the brain falls by 10°C (eg, from 37°C to 27°C) and another 50% if the temperature decreases from 27°C to 17°C. At 20°C, the EEG is isoelectric, but further decreases in temperature continue to reduce CMR throughout the brain. Hyperthermia (above 42°C) may result in neuronal cell injury.

Viscosity

The most important determinant of blood viscosity is hematocrit. A decrease in hematocrit decreases viscosity and can improve CBF; unfortunately, a reduction in hematocrit also decreases the oxygen-carrying capacity and thus can potentially impair oxygen delivery. Elevated hematocrit, as may be seen with marked polycythemia, increases blood viscosity and can reduce CBF. Some studies suggest

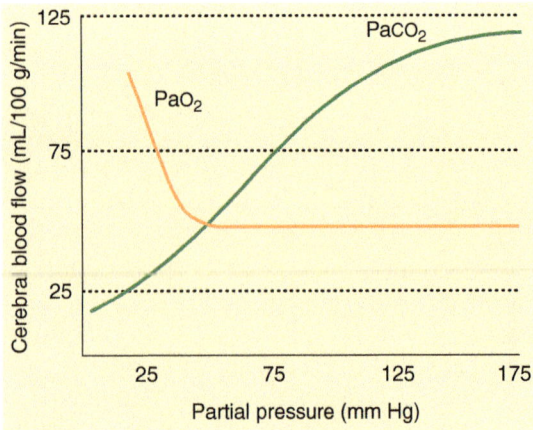

FIGURE 26–3 The relationship between cerebral blood flow and arterial respiratory gas tensions.

that optimal cerebral oxygen delivery may occur at hematocrits of approximately 30%.

Autonomic Influences

Intracranial vessels are innervated by the sympathetic (vasoconstrictive) and parasympathetic (vasodilatory) systems, Intense sympathetic stimulation induces vasoconstriction in these vessels, which can limit CBF. Autonomic innervation may also play an important role in cerebral vasospasm following brain injury and stroke.

BLOOD–BRAIN BARRIER

Cerebral blood vessels are unique in that the junctions between vascular endothelial cells are nearly fused. The paucity of pores is responsible for what is termed the blood–brain barrier. This lipid barrier allows the passage of lipid-soluble substances, but restricts the movement of those that are ionized or

5 have large molecular weights. Thus, the movement of a given substance across the blood–brain barrier is governed simultaneously by its size, charge, lipid solubility, and degree of protein binding in blood. Carbon dioxide, oxygen, and lipid-soluble molecules (such as most anesthetics) freely enter the brain, whereas most ions, proteins, and large substances (such as mannitol) penetrate poorly.

Water moves freely across the blood–brain barrier as a consequence of bulk flow, whereas movement of even small ions is impeded (the equilibration half-life of Na^+ is 2–4 h). As a result, rapid changes in plasma electrolyte concentrations (and, secondarily, osmolality) produce a transient osmotic gradient between plasma and the brain. Acute hypertonicity of plasma results in net movement of water out of the brain, whereas acute hypotonicity causes a net movement of water into the brain. These effects are short-lived, as equilibration eventually occurs, but, when marked, they can cause rapid fluid shifts in the brain. Mannitol, an osmotically active substance that does not normally cross the blood–brain barrier, causes a sustained decrease in brain water content and is often used to decrease brain volume.

6 The blood–brain barrier may be disrupted by severe hypertension, tumors, trauma, strokes, infection, marked hypercapnia, hypoxia, and sustained seizure activity. Under these conditions, fluid movement across the blood–brain barrier becomes dependent on hydrostatic pressure rather than osmotic gradients.

CEREBROSPINAL FLUID

CSF is found in the cerebral ventricles and cisterns and in the subarachnoid space surrounding the brain and spinal cord. Its major function is to protect the central nervous system (CNS) against trauma.

Most of the CSF is formed by the choroid plexuses of the cerebral (mainly lateral) ventricles. Smaller amounts are formed directly by the ventricles' ependymal cell linings, and yet smaller quantities are formed from fluid leaking into the perivascular spaces surrounding cerebral vessels (blood–brain barrier leakage). In adults, normal total CSF production is about 21 mL/hr (500 mL/d), yet total CSF volume is only about 150 mL. CSF flows from the lateral ventricles through the intraventricular foramina (of Monro) into the third ventricle, through the cerebral aqueduct (of Sylvius) into the fourth ventricle, and through the median aperture of the fourth ventricle (foramen of Magendie) and the lateral apertures of the fourth ventricle (foramina of Luschka) into the cerebellomedullary cistern (cisterna magna) (Figure 26–4). From the cerebellomedullary cistern, CSF enters the subarachnoid space, circulating around the brain and spinal cord before being absorbed in arachnoid granulations over the cerebral hemispheres.

CSF formation involves active secretion of sodium in the choroid plexuses. The resulting fluid is isotonic with plasma despite lower potassium, bicarbonate, and glucose concentrations. Its protein content is limited to the very small amounts that leak into perivascular fluid. Carbonic anhydrase inhibitors (acetazolamide), corticosteroids, spironolactone, furosemide, isoflurane, and vasoconstrictors decrease CSF production.

Absorption of CSF involves the translocation of fluid from the arachnoid granulations into the cerebral venous sinuses. Smaller amounts are absorbed at nerve root sleeves and by meningeal lymphatics.

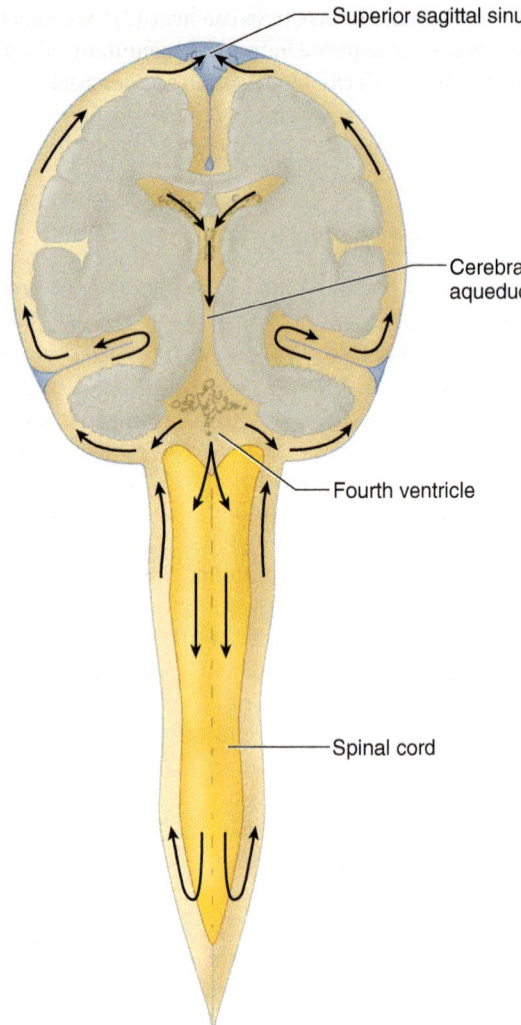

FIGURE 26–4 The flow of cerebrospinal fluid in the central nervous system. (Reproduced, with permission, from Waxman SG: *Correlative Neuroanatomy*, 24th ed. McGraw-Hill, 2000.)

Because the brain and spinal cord lack lymphatics, absorption of CSF is also the principal means by which perivascular and interstitial protein is returned to the blood.

INTRACRANIAL PRESSURE

7 The cranial vault is a rigid structure with a fixed total volume, consisting of brain (80%), blood (12%), and CSF (8%). Any increase in one

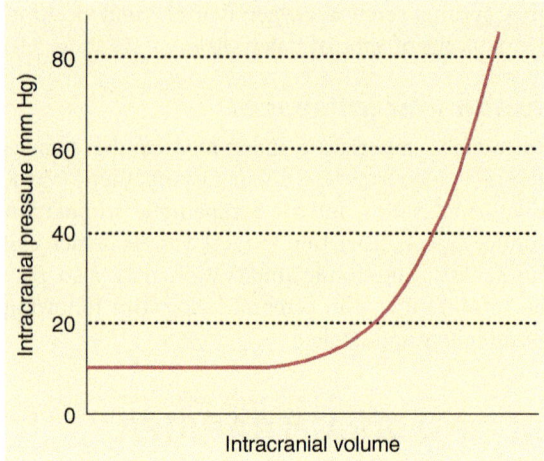

FIGURE 26–5 Normal intracranial elastance.

component must be offset by an equivalent decrease in another to prevent a rise in ICP. By convention, ICP means supratentorial CSF pressure measured in the lateral ventricles or over the cerebral cortex and is normally 10 mm Hg or less. Minor variations may occur, depending on the site measured, but, in the lateral recumbent position, lumbar CSF pressure normally approximates supratentorial pressure.

Intracranial elastance is determined by measuring the change in ICP in response to a change in intracranial volume. Normally, small increases in volume of one component are initially well compensated (Figure 26–5). A point is eventually reached, however, at which further increases produce precipitous rises in ICP. Major compensatory mechanisms include: (1) an initial displacement of CSF from the cranial to the spinal compartment, (2) an increase in CSF absorption, (3) a decrease in CSF production, and (4) a decrease in total cerebral blood volume (primarily venous).

The concept of total intracranial compliance is useful clinically, even though compliance probably varies in the different compartments of the brain and is affected by arterial blood pressure and $Paco_2$. Cerebral blood volume is estimated to increase 0.05 mL/100 g of brain per 1 mm Hg increase in $Paco_2$. Blood pressure effects upon cerebral blood volume are dependent on the autoregulation of CBF.

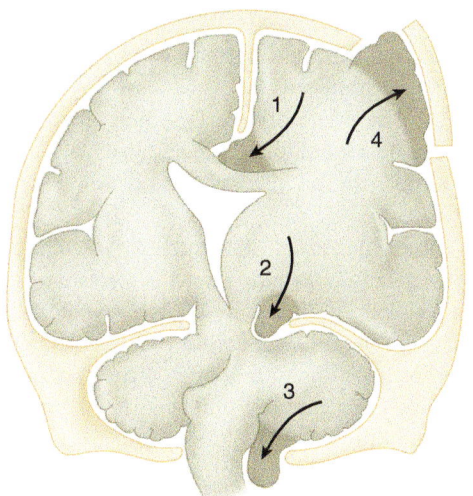

FIGURE 26–6 Potential sites of brain herniation. (Reproduced, with permission, from Fishman RA: Brain edema. N Engl J Med 1975;293:706.)

Sustained elevations in ICP can lead to catastrophic herniation of the brain. Herniation may occur at one of four sites (**Figure 26–6**): (1) the cingulate gyrus under the falx cerebri, (2) the uncinate gyrus through the tentorium cerebelli, (3) the cerebellar tonsils through the foramen magnum, or (4) any area beneath a defect in the skull (transcalvarial).

Effect of Anesthetic Agents on Cerebral Physiology

Overall, most general anesthetics have a favorable effect on the CNS by reducing electrical activity. Determination of the effects of the specific agents is complicated by the concomitant administration of other drugs, surgical stimulation, intracranial compliance, blood pressure, and CO_2 tension. For example, hypocapnia blunts the increases in CBF and ICP that usually occur with ketamine and volatile agents.

This section describes the changes generally associated with each drug when given alone. Table 26–1 summarizes and compares the effects of the various anesthetics. The effects of vasoactive agents and neuromuscular blocking agents are also discussed.

TABLE 26–1 Comparative effects of anesthetic agents on cerebral physiology.[1]

Agent	CMR	CBF	CSF Production	CSF Absorption	CBV	ICP
Halothane	↓↓	↑↑↑	↓	↓	↑↑	↑↑
Isoflurane	↓↓↓	↑	±	↑	↑↑	↑
Desflurane	↓↓↓	↑	↑	↓	↑	↑
Sevoflurane	↓↓↓	↑	?	?	↑	↑
Nitrous oxide	↓	↑	±	±	±	↑
Barbiturates	↓↓↓↓	↓↓↓	±	↑	↓↓	↓↓↓
Etomidate	↓↓↓	↓↓	±	↑	↓↓	↓↓
Propofol	↓↓↓	↓↓↓↓	?	?	↓↓	↓↓
Benzodiazepines	↓↓	↓	±	↑	↓	↓
Ketamine	±	↑↑	±	↓	↑↑	↑↑
Opioids	±	±	±	↑	±	±
Lidocaine	↓↓	↓↓	?	?	↓↓	↓↓

[1]↑, increase; ↓, decrease; ±, little or no change; ?, unknown; CMR, cerebral metabolic rate; CBF, cerebral blood flow; CSF, cerebrospinal fluid; CBV, cerebral blood volume; ICP, intracranial pressure.

EFFECT OF INHALATION AGENTS

1. Volatile Anesthetics

Cerebral Metabolic Rate

Halothane, desflurane, sevoflurane, and isoflurane produce dose-dependent decreases in CMR. Isoflurane produces the greatest maximal depression (up to 50% reduction), whereas halothane has the least effect (<25% reduction). The effects of desflurane and sevoflurane seem to be similar to that of isoflurane. No further reduction in CMR is produced by doses of anesthetics or other drugs greater than the doses that render the EEG isoelectric.

Cerebral Blood Flow & Volume

At normocarbia, volatile anesthetics dilate cerebral vessels and impair autoregulation in a dose-dependent manner (**Figure 26–7**). Halothane has the greatest effect on CBF; at concentrations greater than 1%, it nearly abolishes cerebral autoregulation. Moreover, the increase in blood flow is generalized throughout all parts of the brain. At an equivalent minimum alveolar concentration (MAC) and blood pressure, halothane increases CBF up to 200%,

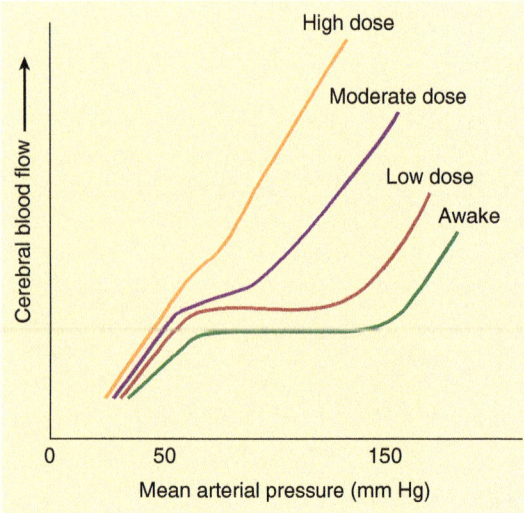

FIGURE 26–7 Dose-dependent depression of cerebral autoregulation by the volatile anesthetics.

compared with 20% for isoflurane. Qualitatively and quantitatively, desflurane may be closest to isoflurane. Sevoflurane produces the least cerebral vasodilation. The effect of volatile agents on CBF also seems to be time dependent, because, with continued administration (2–5 h), blood flow begins to return to normal.

The response of the cerebral vasculature to CO_2 is generally retained with all volatile agents. Hyperventilation (hypocapnia) can therefore abolish or blunt the initial effects of these agents on CBF. With halothane, the timing of the hyperventilation is important. Only if hyperventilation is initiated prior to the administration of halothane will halothane-induced increases in CBF be prevented. In contrast, simultaneous hyperventilation with administration of either isoflurane or sevoflurane can prevent increases in CBF and ICP.

Increases in cerebral blood volume (10% to 12%) generally parallel increases in CBF, but the relationship is not necessarily linear. Expansion of cerebral blood volume can markedly elevate ICP in patients with reduced intracranial compliance. Hypocapnia can blunt the increase in cerebral blood volume associated with volatile anesthetic administration.

Altered Coupling of Cerebral Metabolic Rate & Blood Flow

As is apparent from the discussion above, volatile agents alter, but do not uncouple, the normal relationship of CBF and CMR. The combination of a decrease in neuronal metabolic demand with an increase in CBF (metabolic supply) has been termed luxury perfusion. In contrast to this potentially beneficial effect during global ischemia, a detrimental **circulatory steal phenomenon** is possible with volatile anesthetics in the setting of focal ischemia. Volatile agents can increase blood flow in normal areas of the brain, but not in ischemic areas, where arterioles are already maximally vasodilated. The end result may be a redistribution ("steal") of blood flow away from ischemic to normal areas.

Cerebrospinal Fluid Dynamics

Volatile anesthetics affect both formation and absorption of CSF. Halothane impedes absorption of CSF, but only minimally retards formation. Isoflurane, on the other hand, facilitates absorption and is therefore an agent with favorable effects on CSF dynamics.

Intracranial Pressure

The net effect of volatile anesthetics on ICP is the result of immediate changes in cerebral blood volume, delayed alterations on CSF dynamics, and arterial CO$_2$ tension. Based on these factors, isoflurane and sevoflurane seem to be the volatile agents of choice in patients with decreased intracranial compliance.

2. Nitrous Oxide

The effects of nitrous oxide are influenced by other agents or changes in CO$_2$ tension. Thus, when combined with intravenous agents, nitrous oxide has minimal effects on CBF, CMR, and ICP. Adding this agent to a volatile anesthetic, however, can further increase CBF. When given alone, nitrous oxide causes mild cerebral vasodilation and can potentially increase ICP.

EFFECT OF INTRAVENOUS AGENTS

1. Induction Agents

⑧ With the exception of ketamine, all intravenous agents either have little effect on or reduce CMR and CBF. Moreover, with some exceptions, changes in blood flow generally parallel those in metabolic rate. Cerebral autoregulation and CO$_2$ responsiveness are preserved with all agents.

Barbiturates

Barbiturates have four major actions on the CNS: (1) hypnosis, (2) depression of CMR, (3) reduction of CBF due to increased cerebral vascular resistance, and (4) anticonvulsant activity. Barbiturates produce dose-dependent decreases in CMR and CBF until the EEG becomes isoelectric. At that point, maximum reductions of nearly 50% are observed; additional barbiturate dosing does not further reduce metabolic rate. Unlike isoflurane,

barbiturates reduce metabolic rate uniformly throughout the brain. CMR is depressed slightly more than CBF, such that metabolic supply exceeds metabolic demand (as long as CPP is maintained). Because barbiturate-induced cerebral vasoconstriction occurs only in normal areas, these agents tend to redistribute blood flow from normal to ischemic areas in the brain (Robin Hood, or reverse steal phenomenon). The cerebral vasculature in ischemic areas remains maximally dilated and is less affected by the barbiturate because of ischemic vasomotor paralysis.

Barbiturates also seem to facilitate absorption of CSF. The resultant reduction in CSF volume, combined with decreases in CBF and cerebral blood volume, makes barbiturates highly effective in lowering ICP. Their anticonvulsant properties are also advantageous in neurosurgical patients who are at increased risk of seizures.

Opioids

Opioids generally have minimal effects on CBF, CMR, and ICP, unless Paco$_2$ rises secondary to respiratory depression. Increases in ICP have been reported in some patients with intracranial tumors following administration of sufentanil and to a lesser degree, alfentanil. The mechanism seems to be a precipitous drop in blood pressure; reflex cerebral vasodilation likely increases intracranial blood volume and potentially ICP. Significant decreases in blood pressure can adversely affect CPP, regardless of the opioid selected. In addition, small doses of alfentanil (<50 mg/kg) can activate seizure foci in patients with epilepsy. Morphine is generally not considered optimal as a component of anesthesia for intracranial surgery. Morphine's poor lipid solubility results in slow CNS penetration and prolonged sedative effects. Normeperidine, a metabolite of meperidine, can induce seizures, particularly in patients with renal failure. The accumulation of normeperidine and the associated cardiac depression limit the use of meperidine, except in small doses to treat shivering.

Etomidate

Etomidate decreases the CMR, CBF, and ICP in much the same way as thiopental. Its effect on CMR is nonuniform, affecting the cortex more than the brainstem. Its limited effect on the brainstem may be responsible for greater hemodynamic stability during anesthesia induction, compared with that of barbiturates. Etomidate also decreases production and enhances absorption of CSF.

Induction with etomidate is associated with a relatively high incidence of myoclonic movements, but these movements are not associated with seizure activity on the EEG in normal individuals. The drug has been used to treat seizures, but reports of seizure activity following etomidate suggest that the drug is best avoided in patients with a history of epilepsy. In fact, small doses of etomidate can activate seizure foci in patients with epilepsy.

Propofol

Propofol reduces CBF and CMR, similar to barbiturates and etomidate; however, the decrease in CBF may exceed that in metabolic rate. Although it has been associated with dystonic and choreiform movements, propofol seems to have significant anticonvulsant activity. Moreover, its short elimination half-life makes it a useful agent for neuroanesthesia. Propofol infusion is commonly used for maintenance of anesthesia in patients with or at risk of intracranial hypertension. Propofol is by far the most common induction agent for neuroanesthesia.

Benzodiazepines

Benzodiazepines lower CBF and CMR, but to a lesser extent than barbiturates, etomidate, or propofol. Benzodiazepines also have useful anticonvulsant properties. Midazolam is the benzodiazepine of choice in neuroanesthesia because of its short half-life. Midazolam used as an induction agent frequently causes decreases in CPP in elderly and unstable patients and may result in prolonged emergence.

Ketamine

Ketamine is the only intravenous anesthetic that dilates the cerebral vasculature and increases CBF (50% to 60%). Selective activation of certain areas (limbic and reticular) is partially offset by depression of other areas (somatosensory and

auditory) such that total CMR does not change. Seizure activity in thalamic and limbic areas is also described. Ketamine may also impede absorption of CSF without affecting formation. Increases in CBF, cerebral blood volume, and CSF volume can potentially increase ICP markedly in patients with decreased intracranial compliance. However, ketamine administration does not increase ICP in neurologically impaired patients under controlled ventilation with concomitant administration of propofol or a benzodiazepine. Additionally, ketamine may offer neuroprotective effects, according to some investigations. Ketamine's blockade of the *N*-methyl-D-aspartate (NMDA) receptor during periods of increased glutamate concentrations, as occurs during brain injury, may be protective against neuronal cell death (**Figure 26–8**).

2. Anesthetic Adjuncts

Intravenous lidocaine decreases CMR, CBF, and ICP, but to a lesser degree than other agents. Its principal advantage is that it decreases CBF (by increasing cerebral vascular resistance) without causing other significant hemodynamic effects. Lidocaine may also have neuroprotective effects. Lidocaine infusions are used in some centers as a supplement to general anesthesia to reduce emergence delirium and the requirement for opioids.

Droperidol has little or no effect on CMR and minimally reduces CBF. When used in larger doses with an opioid as part of a neuroleptic technique, droperidol may sometimes cause undesirable prolonged sedation. Droperidol and narcotics were once mainstays of neuroanesthesia. Droperidol's prolongation of the QT interval and risk of fatal arrhythmia, as well as official warnings related to the drug, have retarded its use.

Reversal of opioids or benzodiazepines with naloxone or flumazenil, respectively, can reverse any beneficial reductions in CBF and CMR. Reversal of narcotics or benzodiazepines in chronic users can lead to symptoms of substance withdrawal.

3. Vasopressors

 With normal autoregulation and an intact blood–brain barrier, vasopressors increase

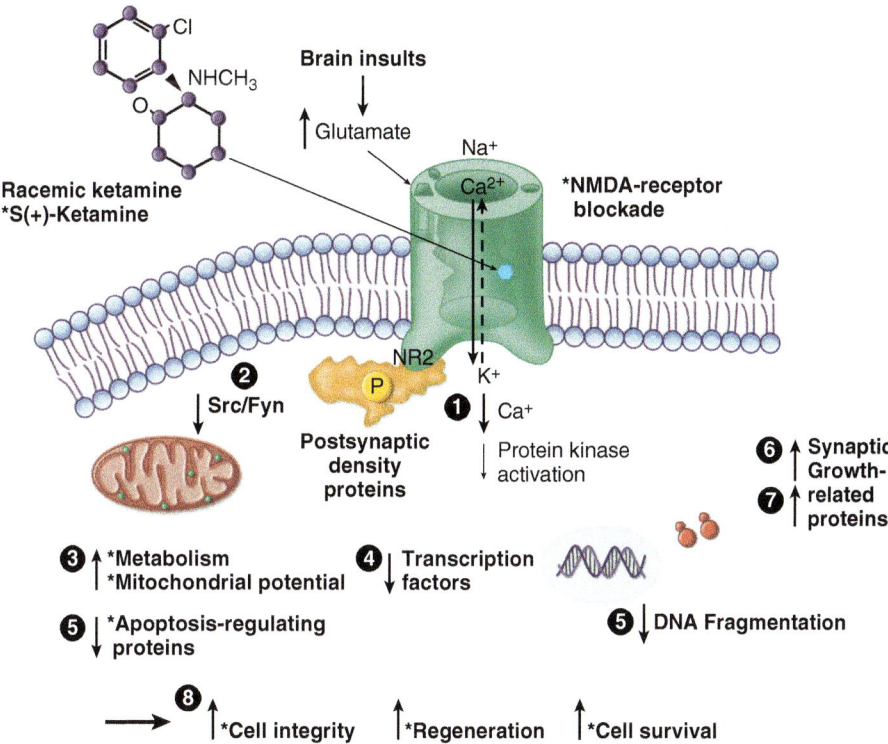

FIGURE 26–8 Pharmacological effects reported for racemic and S(+)-ketamine which are presumed to be relevant for neuroprotection. After onset of brain injury, blockade of excessive stimulation of *N*-methyl-D-aspartate (NMDA) receptors by ketamine reduces calcium influx through the receptor channel (1). This attenuates supraphysiological increases in the assembly and interaction of NMDA receptor subunits, postsynaptic density proteins, and other intracellular signaling systems such as protein kinases (2). Thus, several kinase transduction cascades become less activated. This improves preservation of metabolism and maintenance of the mitochondrial transmembrane potential (3). This, in turn, reduces pathological activation of transcription factors (4). Proteins involved in apoptosis are less activated, which is associated with less DNA fragmentation (5). A better preservation of synaptic proteins occurs, and the expression of growth proteins indicating regeneration in adult neurons is enhanced. The prevention of pathological amplification of NMDA receptor signaling finally results in increased cellular survival, preserved cellular and synaptic integrity, and regenerative efforts. *Superiority of effects induced by S(+)-ketamine, only. (Reproduced, with permission, from Himmelseher S, Durieux ME: Revising a dogma: ketamine for patients with neurological injury? Anesth Analg 2005:101:524.)

CBF only when mean arterial blood pressure is below 50–60 mm Hg or above 150–160 mm Hg. In the absence of autoregulation, vasopressors increase CBF by their effect on CPP. Changes in CMR generally parallel those in blood flow. β-Adrenergic agents seem to have a greater effect on the brain when the blood–brain barrier is disrupted; central β_1-receptor stimulation increases CMR and blood flow. β-Adrenergic blockers generally have no direct effect on CMR or CBF, whereas α_2-adrenergic agonists produce cerebral vasoconstriction. Excessive elevations in blood pressure with any agent can disrupt the blood–brain barrier.

4. Vasodilators

In the absence of hypotension, most vasodilators induce cerebral vasodilation and increase CBF in a dose-related fashion. When these agents decrease blood pressure, CBF is usually maintained and may even increase. The resultant increase in cerebral blood volume can significantly elevate ICP in patients with decreased intracranial compliance. Of this group of drugs, only the ganglionic blocker trimethaphan has little or no effect on CBF and cerebral blood volume. Trimethaphan is no longer available in the United States.

5. Neuromuscular Blocking Agents

Neuromuscular blockers (NMBs) lack direct action on the brain but can have important secondary effects. Hypertension and histamine-mediated cerebral vasodilation increase ICP, whereas systemic hypotension (from histamine release or ganglionic blockade) lowers CPP. Succinylcholine can increase ICP, possibly as a result of cerebral activation associated with enhanced muscle spindle activity, but the increase is generally minimal and clinically unimportant, if an adequate dose of propofol is given and hyperventilation is initiated at induction. Moreover, a small (defasciculating) dose of a nondepolarizing NMB seems to blunt the increase, at least partially. In the majority of instances, increases in ICP following administration of an NMB are the result of a hypertensive response due to light anesthesia during laryngoscopy and tracheal intubation. Acute elevations in ICP will also be seen, if hypercapnia or hypoxemia results from prolonged apnea.

Physiology of Brain Protection

PATHOPHYSIOLOGY OF CEREBRAL ISCHEMIA

10 The brain is very vulnerable to ischemic injury because of its relatively high oxygen consumption and near total dependence on aerobic glucose metabolism (above). Interruption of cerebral perfusion, metabolic substrate (glucose), or severe hypoxemia rapidly results in functional impairment; reduced perfusion also impairs clearance of potentially toxic metabolites. If normal oxygen tension, blood flow, and glucose supply are not reestablished within 3–8 min under most conditions, ATP stores are depleted, and irreversible neuronal injury begins. When CBF decreases below 10 mL/100 g/min, cell function is deranged, and ion pumps fail to maintain cellular vitality. The ratio of lactate to pyruvate is increased secondary to anaerobic metabolism. During ischemia, intracellular K^+ decreases, and intracellular Na^+ increases. More importantly, intracellular Ca^{2+} increases because of failure of ATP-dependent pumps to either extrude the ion extracellularly or into intracellular cisterns, increased intracellular Na^+ concentration, and release of the excitatory neurotransmitter glutamate. Glutamate acts at the NMDA receptor, further enhancing Ca^{2+} entry into the cell, hence the potential benefit of NMDA blockers for neuroprotection.

Sustained increases in intracellular Ca^{2+} activate lipases and proteases, which initiate and propagate structural damage to neurons. Increases in free fatty acid concentration and cyclooxygenase and lipoxygenase activities result in the formation of prostaglandins and leukotrienes, some of which are potent mediators of cellular injury. Accumulation of toxic metabolites, such as lactic acid, also impairs cellular function and interferes with repair mechanisms. Lastly, reperfusion of ischemic tissues can cause additional tissue damage due to the formation of oxygen-derived free radicals. Likewise, inflammation and edema can promote further neuronal damage, leading to cellular apoptosis.

STRATEGIES FOR BRAIN PROTECTION

Ischemic brain injury is usually classified as focal (incomplete) or global (complete). Global ischemia includes total circulatory arrest as well as global hypoxia. Cessation of perfusion may be caused by cardiac arrest or deliberate circulatory arrest, whereas global hypoxia may be caused by severe respiratory failure, drowning, and asphyxia (including anesthetic mishaps). Focal ischemia includes embolic, hemorrhagic, and atherosclerotic strokes, as well as blunt, penetrating, and surgical trauma.

In some instances, interventions aimed at restoring perfusion and oxygenation are possible; these include reestablishing effective circulation, normalizing arterial oxygenation and oxygen-carrying capacity, or reopening an occluded vessel. With focal ischemia, the brain tissue surrounding a severely damaged area may suffer marked functional impairment but still remain viable. Such areas are thought to have very marginal perfusion (<15 mL/100 g/min), but, if further injury can be limited and normal flow is rapidly restored, these areas (the "ischemic penumbra") may recover completely. When the above interventions are not applicable or available, the emphasis must be on limiting the extent of brain injury.

From a practical point of view, efforts aimed at preventing or limiting neuronal tissue damage are often the same whether the ischemia is focal or global. Clinical goals are usually to optimize CPP, decrease metabolic requirements (basal and electrical), and possibly block mediators of cellular injury. Clearly, the most effective strategy is prevention, because once injury has occurred, measures aimed at cerebral protection become less effective.

Hypothermia

11 Hypothermia is an effective method for protecting the brain during focal and global ischemia. Indeed, profound hypothermia is often used for up to 1 hr of total circulatory arrest. Unlike anesthetic agents, hypothermia decreases both basal and electrical metabolic requirements throughout the brain; metabolic requirements continue to decrease even after complete electrical silence. Additionally, hypothermia reduces free radicals and other mediators of ischemic injury. Induced hypothermia has shown benefit following cardiac arrest and is a routine part of most postarrest protocols for comatose patients.

Anesthetic Agents

Barbiturates, etomidate, propofol, and isoflurane can produce complete electrical silence of the brain and eliminate the metabolic cost of electrical activity; unfortunately, these agents have no effect on basal energy requirements. Furthermore, with the exception of barbiturates, their effects are nonuniform,

affecting different parts of the brain to variable extents.

Ketamine may also have a protective effect because of its ability to block the actions of glutamate at the NMDA) receptor.

No anesthetic agent has consistently been shown to be protective against global ischemia. The ever increasing number of studies highlighting the potential neurotoxicity of anesthetics (especially in infants) also questions the role of volatile anesthetics in neuroprotection.

Specific Adjuncts

Nimodipine plays a role in the in the treatment of vasospasm associated with subarachnoid hemorrhage. Studies are ongoing to discern the roles of various NMDA receptor antagonists, erythropoietin, Ca^{2+} antagonists, and free radical scavengers to mitigate ischemic neuronal injury.

General Measures

Maintenance of a satisfactory CPP is critical. Thus, arterial blood pressure should be normal or slightly elevated, and increases in venous and ICP should be avoided. Oxygen-carrying capacity should be maintained and normal arterial oxygen tension preserved. Hyperglycemia aggravates neurological injuries following either focal or global ischemia, and blood glucose should be maintained at less than 180 mg/dL. Normocarbia should be maintained, as both hypercarbia and hypocarbia have no beneficial effect in the setting of ischemia and could prove detrimental; hypocarbia-induced cerebral vasoconstriction may aggravate the ischemia, whereas hypercarbia may induce a steal phenomenon (with focal ischemia) or worsen intracellular acidosis.

EFFECT OF ANESTHESIA ON ELECTROPHYSIOLOGICAL MONITORING

Electrophysiological monitors are used to assess the functional integrity of the CNS. The most commonly used monitor for neurosurgical procedures is evoked potentials. EEG is much less commonly used. Proper application of these monitoring modalities

TABLE 26–2 Electroencephalographic changes during anesthesia.

Activation	Depression
Inhalational agents (subanesthetic)	Inhalation agents (1-2 MAC)
Barbiturates (small doses)	Barbiturates
Benzodiazepines (small doses)	Opioids
Etomidate (small doses)	Propofol
Nitrous oxide	Etomidate
Ketamine	Hypocapnia
Mild hypercapnia	Marked hypercapnia
Sensory stimulation	Hypothermia
Hypoxia (early)	Hypoxia (late) Ischemia

is critically dependent on monitoring the specific area at risk and recognizing anesthetic-induced changes. Both monitoring modalities are described in Chapter 6.

The effects of anesthetic agents on the EEG are summarized in Table 26–2.

ELECTROENCEPHALOGRAPHY

EEG monitoring is useful for assessing the adequacy of cerebral perfusion during carotid endarterectomy (CEA), as well as anesthetic depth (most often with processed EEG). EEG changes can be simplistically described as either activation or depression. EEG activation (a shift to predominantly high-frequency and low-voltage activity) is seen with light anesthesia and surgical stimulation, whereas EEG depression (a shift to predominantly low-frequency and high-voltage activity) occurs with deep anesthesia or cerebral compromise. **Most anesthetics produce an EEG consisting of an initial activation (at subanesthetic doses) followed by dose-dependent depression.**

Inhalation Anesthetics

Isoflurane can produce an isoelectric EEG at high clinical doses (1–2 MAC). **Desflurane and sevoflurane produce a burst suppression pattern at high doses (>1.2 and >1.5 MAC, respectively) but not electrical silence**. Nitrous oxide is also unusual in that it increases both frequency and amplitude (high-amplitude activation).

Intravenous Agents

Benzodiazepines can produce both activation and depression of the EEG. Barbiturates, etomidate, and propofol produce a similar pattern and are the only intravenous agents capable of producing burst suppression and electrical silence at high doses. In contrast, opioids characteristically produce only dose-dependent depression of the EEG. Lastly, ketamine produces an unusual activation consisting of rhythmic high-amplitude theta activity followed by very high-amplitude gamma and low-amplitude beta activities.

EVOKED POTENTIALS

Somatosensory evoked potentials test the integrity of the spinal dorsal columns and the sensory cortex and may be useful during resection of spinal tumors, instrumentation of the spine, CEA, and aortic surgery. The adequacy of perfusion of the spinal cord during aortic surgery is probably better assessed with motor evoked potentials (which assess the anterior part of the spinal cord). Brainstem auditory evoked potentials test the integrity of the eighth cranial nerve and the auditory pathways above the pons and are used for surgery in the posterior fossa. Visual evoked potentials may be used to monitor the optic nerve and occipital cortex during resections of large pituitary tumors.

Interpretation of evoked potentials is more complicated than that of the EEG. Evoked potentials have poststimulus latencies that are described as short, intermediate, and long. Short-latency evoked potentials arise from the nerve stimulated or the brain stem. Intermediate- and long-latency evoked potentials are primarily of cortical origin. In general, short-latency potentials are least affected by anesthetic agents, whereas long-latency potentials are affected by even subanesthetic levels of most agents. Visual evoked potentials are most affected by anesthetics, whereas brain stem auditory evoked potentials are least affected.

Intravenous agents in clinical doses generally have less marked effects on evoked potentials than do volatile agents, but, in high doses, can also decrease amplitude and increase latencies (see Chapter 6).

CASE DISCUSSION

Postoperative Hemiplegia

A 62-year-old man has undergone a right carotid endarterectomy (CEA). Immediately following surgery, in the recovery room, he is noted to be weak on the contralateral side.

How is a patient undergoing CEA evaluated preoperatively?

Patients with cerebrovascular disease, and, in particular, carotid stenosis are at very high risk of coronary artery and peripheral arterial disease. It would be unusual for a patient to have carotid stenosis who did not have evidence of atherosclerosis elsewhere. Patients undergoing CEA, therefore, require a preoperative cardiac evaluation, according to American College of Cardiology/American Heart Association guidelines.

With respect to patient risk factors, the guidelines provide algorithms for how patients should be evaluated and managed intraoperatively. As part of this patient's preoperative evaluation, a thorough neurological examination should have been performed with special attention paid to motor function. This patient may well have been weak on the left side prior to surgery, in which case the hemiparesis might be due to a preexisting condition. If this is a new finding, it requires aggressive management.

Is general or regional anesthesia the optimal anesthetic technique for managing patients undergoing CEA?

For the past several decades, the majority of patients undergoing CEAs in the United States have had general anesthesia. General anesthesia was chosen because many surgeons operating in the neck area felt more comfortable if the airway was controlled, and the patient was completely anesthetized should evidence of cerebral ischemia develop.

More recently, regional anesthesia has been advocated as providing an adequate surgical field, a comfortable and relaxed patient (if done with monitored anesthesia care), stable hemodynamics, and ideal monitoring of cerebral function during crossclamping because an awake patient provides the best evidence of adequate cerebral perfusion. The patient can indicate or be observed for evidence of aphasia, facial droop, or hemiparesis. Regional anesthesia is usually performed with superficial cervical plexus blocks.

How should cerebral function be monitored intraoperatively in this patient?

When the carotid is crossclamped, the ability to identify inadequate cerebral circulation in the ipsilateral hemisphere is critical, as there is a window of opportunity for immediate intervention and correction of any deficit.

Global and focal neurological status can continuously be assessed in awake patients, if the patient is mildly sedated when undergoing regional anesthesia. In such a situation, practical assessment consists of frequent (every 2–5 min) examination of strength using the contralateral handgrip and maintenance of constant verbal contact with the patient to assess level of consciousness.

In patients undergoing general anesthesia, indirect cerebral monitoring techniques have been used to assess the adequacy of the cerebral circulation. These techniques include stump bleeding, stump pressure, jugular venous oxygen saturation, EEG, a processed EEG (such as the bispectral index or evoked potentials), TCD, arteriography, and measurement of blood flow using xenon. Back bleeding of the distal carotid artery following crossclamp and incision of the artery suggests reasonable collateral circulation above the clamp. It is very subjective and nonquantitative.

To better qualify and quantify the adequacy of collateral perfusion (**Figure 26–9**), stump pressure measurements can be used. Some surgeons

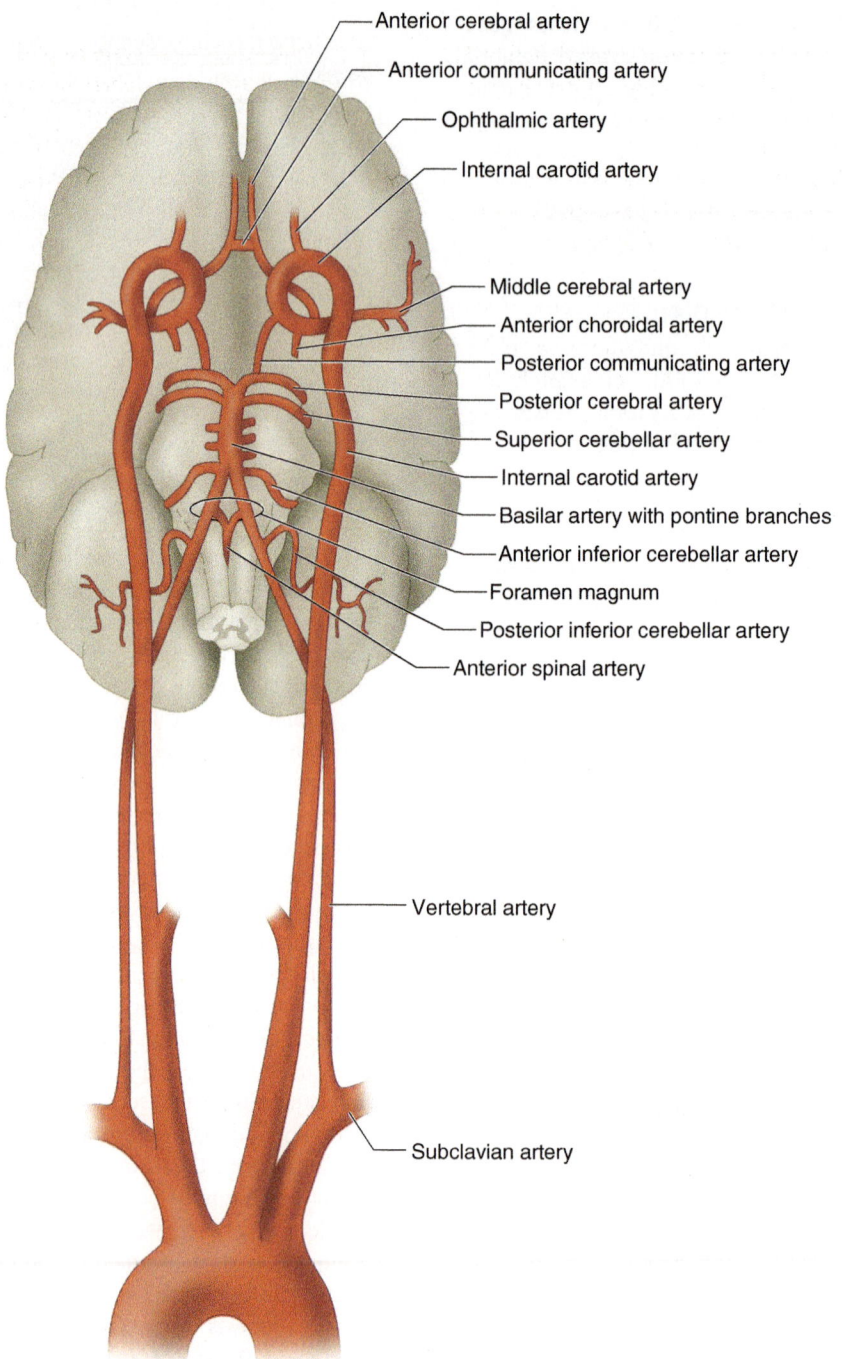

FIGURE 26–9 The cerebral circulation.

believe that a shunt should be used in all patients with a previous cerebrovascular accident, independent of stump pressure, and for any patient whose stump pressure is less than 25 mm Hg. However, this is controversial, as many neurosurgeons and vascular surgeons use 50 mm Hg as a cutoff.

The EEG is sometimes used for monitoring patients undergoing CEA under general anesthesia. In such a circumstance, inhalation or intravenous anesthesia can influence the EEG, but gross changes associated with carotid clamping can be detected. However, analyzing the EEG is labor and technology intensive and requires interpretation of the data.

For this reason, techniques that employ a processed EEG (eg, the bispectral index monitor) are being explored as a monitor for cerebral ischemia. Evoked potentials, such as auditory and visual evoked potentials, have also been examined, but do not seem to have significant clinical application.

Jugular venous oxygen saturation has been studied in an attempt to identify the acute onset of cerebral ischemia. Because it is a global measure, it does not reflect regional, or, in particular, focal cerebral ischemia and therefore is not used for routine clinical practice. TCD ultrasonography provides noninvasive assessment of blood flow in the middle cerebral artery.

How should hemodynamics be controlled intraoperatively?

During carotid clamping and immediately afterward in the recovery room, patients are often hemodynamically labile. **Bradycardia can develop during surgical manipulation of the carotid sinus because of the direct stimulation of the vagus nerve.** Tachycardia may develop as a result of stress or pain or as a direct result of manipulation of the carotid sinus with release of catecholamines into the circulation.

Hypotension is also observed because of the direct vasodilating and negative ionotropic effects of anesthetic agents. Hypotension following carotid unclamping is common, particularly in patients with more severe carotid stenosis. This could be due to a cerebral protective process. Cerebral autoregulation protects the brain from reperfusion by reducing cerebral production of renin, vasopressin, and norepinephrine, which results in hypotension. Hypertension is also a frequent finding in patients undergoing CEA. Many patients have hypertension as a comorbid condition, which is often further exacerbated by the surgical stress and manipulation of the carotid body, which causes release of catecholamines and sympathetic stimulation.

Invasive arterial pressure monitoring and suitable venous access to infuse vasoactive medications are necessary during carotid surgery.

What is the most likely etiology of this patient's findings?

This patient most likely has had a cerebrovascular accident due to an arterio-to-arterial embolus; more than 95% of patients will fit into this category. Weakness can also develop as a result of a hyperperfusion syndrome, which occurs in patients with severe carotid stenosis who have now reestablished flow to the affected cerebral hemisphere. Such patients usually have a greater than 95% carotid stenosis with a less than 1-mm channel in the affected carotid artery. Typically, the syndrome does not develop in the postoperative anesthesia care unit (PACU), but several hours afterward when the patient begins complaining of a headache, and, in severe cases, develops hemiparesis.

Because a cerebrovascular accident is most likely, when the anesthesiologist is called to see such a patient in the PACU, a thorough neurological examination quantifying any cranial nerve involvement and the degree of weakness on the contralateral side should be performed. Any hemodynamic changes need to be treated immediately, with assurance of adequate hemoglobin and oxygenation levels. Ultrasonic evaluation of the carotid artery is frequently required. The surgeon needs to be notified at once, as it may be necessary to return to the operating room to explore the carotid artery.

SUGGESTED READING

Chan M, Gin T, Goh K: Interventional neurophysiologic monitoring. Curr Opin Anaesthesiol 2004;17:389.

Dagal A, Lam A: Cerebral blood flow and the injured brain: how should we monitor and manipulate it? Curr Opin Anesthesiol 2011;24:131.

Drummond J, Sturaitis M: Brain tissue oxygenation during dexmedetomidine administration in surgical patients with neurovascular injuries. J Neurosurg Anesthesiol 2010;22:336.

Friedman D, Claassen J, Hirsch L: Continuous electroencephalogram monitoring in the intensive care unit. Anesth Analg 2009;109:506.

Gupta A, Azami J: Update on neuromonitoring. Current Anaesth Crit Care 2002;13:120.

Grocott H, Davie S, Fedorow C: Monitoring of brain function in anesthesia and intensive care. Curr Opin Anesthesiol 2010;23;759.

Himmelseher S, Durieux M: Revising a dogma: ketamine for patients with neurological injury. Anesth Analg 2005;101:524.

Rabinstein A: Elucidating the value of continuous brain oxygenation monitoring. Neurocrit Care 2010;12:144.

Saqqur M, Zygun D, Demchuk D: Role of transcranial Doppler in neurocritical care. Crit Care Med 2007;35:S216.

Anesthesia for Neurosurgery

1 Regardless of the cause, intracranial masses present according to growth rate, location, and intracranial pressure. Slowly growing masses are frequently asymptomatic for long periods (despite relatively large size), whereas rapidly growing ones may present when the mass remains relatively small.

2 Computed tomographic and magnetic resonance imaging scans should be reviewed for evidence of brain edema, a midline shift greater than 0.5 cm, and ventricular displacement or compression.

3 Operations in the posterior fossa can injure vital circulatory and respiratory brainstem centers, as well as cranial nerves or their nuclei.

4 Venous air embolism can occur when the pressure within an open vein is subatmospheric. These conditions may exist in any position (and during any procedure) whenever the wound is above the level of the heart.

5 Optimal recovery of air following venous air embolism is provided by a multiorificed catheter positioned at the junction between the right atrium and the superior vena cava. Confirmation of correct catheter positioning can be accomplished by intravascular electrocardiography, radiography, or transesophageal echocardiography.

6 In a patient with head trauma, correction of hypotension and control of any bleeding take precedence over radiographic studies and definitive neurosurgical treatment because systolic arterial blood pressures of less than 80 mm Hg predict a poor outcome.

7 Massive blood loss from injuries to the great vessels can occur intraoperatively with thoracic or lumbar spine procedures.

Anesthetic techniques must be modified in the presence of intracranial hypertension and marginal cerebral perfusion. In addition, many neurosurgical procedures require patient positions (eg, sitting, prone) that further complicate management. This chapter applies the principles developed in Chapter 26 to the anesthetic care of neurosurgical patients.

Intracranial Hypertension

Intracranial hypertension is defined as a sustained increase in intracranial pressure (ICP) above 15 mm Hg. Intracranial hypertension may result from an expanding tissue or fluid mass, a depressed skull fracture, interference with normal absorption of cerebrospinal fluid (CSF), excessive cerebral blood volume (CBV), or systemic disturbances promoting brain edema (see below). Multiple factors are often simultaneously present. For example, tumors in the posterior fossa usually are not only associated with some degree of brain edema and mass effect, but they also readily obstruct CSF outflow by compressing the fourth ventricle (obstructive hydrocephalus).

Although many patients with increased ICP are initially asymptomatic, they typically develop characteristic symptoms and signs, including headache, nausea, vomiting, papilledema, focal neurological deficits, and altered consciousness. When ICP exceeds 30 mm Hg, cerebral blood flow (CBF) progressively decreases, and a vicious circle is established: ischemia causes brain edema, which in turn, increases ICP, resulting in more ischemia. If left unchecked, this cycle continues until the patient dies of progressive neurological damage or catastrophic herniation. **Periodic increases in arterial blood pressure with reflex slowing of the heart rate (Cushing response) can be correlated with abrupt increases in ICP (plateau or A waves) lasting 1–15 min.** This phenomenon is the result of autoregulatory mechanisms periodically decreasing cerebral vascular resistance and increasing arterial blood pressure in response to cerebral ischemia; unfortunately, the latter further increases ICP as CBV increases. Eventually, severe ischemia and acidosis completely abolish autoregulation (vasomotor paralysis).

CEREBRAL EDEMA

An increase in brain water content can be produced by several mechanisms. Disruption of the blood–brain barrier (vasogenic edema) is most common and allows the entry of plasma-like fluid into the brain. Increases in blood pressure enhance the formation of this type of edema. Common causes of vasogenic edema include mechanical trauma, high altitudes, inflammatory lesions, brain tumors, hypertension, and infarction. Cerebral edema following metabolic insults (cytotoxic edema), such as hypoxemia or ischemia, results from failure of brain cells to actively extrude sodium causing progressive cellular swelling. Interstitial cerebral edema is the result of obstructive hydrocephalus and entry of CSF into brain interstitium. Cerebral edema can also be the result of intracellular movement of water secondary to acute decreases in serum osmolality (water intoxication).

TREATMENT

Treatment of intracranial hypertension and cerebral edema is ideally directed at the underlying cause. Metabolic disturbances are corrected, and operative intervention is undertaken whenever appropriate. Vasogenic edema—particularly that associated with tumors—often responds to corticosteroids (dexamethasone). Vasogenic edema from trauma typically does not respond to corticosteroids. Blood glucose should be monitored frequently and controlled with insulin infusions (if indicated) when steroids are used. Regardless of the cause, fluid restriction, osmotic agents, and loop diuretics are usually effective in temporarily decreasing brain edema and ICP until more definitive measures can be undertaken. Diuresis lowers ICP chiefly by removing intracellular water from normal brain tissue. Moderate hyperventilation ($Paco_2$ of 30–33 mm Hg) is often very helpful in reducing CBF, CBV, and ICP acutely, but may aggravate ischemia in patients with focal ischemia.

Mannitol, in doses of 0.25–0.5 g/kg, is particularly effective in rapidly decreasing intracranial fluid volume and ICP. Its efficacy is primarily related to its effect on serum osmolality. A serum osmolality of 300–315 mOsm/L is generally considered desirable. Mannitol can transiently decrease blood pressure by virtue of its weak vasodilating properties, but its principal disadvantage is a transient increase in intravascular volume, which can precipitate pulmonary edema in patients with borderline cardiac or renal function. Mannitol should generally not be used in patients with intracranial aneurysms, arteriovenous malformations (AVMs), or intracranial hemorrhage until the cranium is opened. Osmotic diuresis in such instances can expand a hematoma as the volume of the normal brain tissue around it decreases. Rapid osmotic diuresis in elderly patients can also occasionally cause a subdural hematoma due to rupture of fragile bridging veins entering the sagittal sinus. Rebound edema may follow the use of mannitol; thus, it is ideally used in procedures (such as a craniotomy for tumor resection) in which intracranial volume will be reduced.

Use of a loop diuretic (furosemide), although having a lesser maximal effect than mannitol and requiring up to 30 min, may have the additional advantage of directly decreasing formation of CSF. The combined use of mannitol and furosemide may be synergistic, but requires close monitoring of the serum potassium concentration.

Anesthesia & Craniotomy for Patients with Mass Lesions

Intracranial masses may be congenital, neoplastic (benign or malignant), infectious (abscess or cyst), or vascular (hematoma or arteriovenous malformation). Craniotomy is commonly undertaken for neoplasms of the brain. Primary tumors usually arise from glial cells (astrocytoma, oligodendroglioma, or glioblastoma), ependymal cells (ependymoma), or supporting tissues (meningioma, schwannoma, or choroidal papilloma). Childhood tumors include medulloblastoma, neuroblastoma, and astrocytoma.

1 Regardless of the cause, intracranial masses present according to growth rate, location, and ICP. Slowly growing masses are frequently asymptomatic for long periods (despite relatively large size), whereas rapidly growing ones may present when the mass remains relatively small. Common presentations include headache, seizures, a general decline in cognitive or specific neurological functions, and focal neurological deficits. Symptoms typical to supratentorial masses include seizures, hemiplegia, or aphasia, whereas symptoms typical of infratentorial may include cerebellar dysfunction (ataxia, nystagmus, and dysarthria) or brainstem compression (cranial nerve palsies, altered consciousness, or abnormal respiration). As ICP increases, signs of intracranial hypertension also develop (see above).

PREOPERATIVE MANAGEMENT

The preoperative evaluation for patients undergoing craniotomy should attempt to establish the presence

2 or absence of intracranial hypertension. Computed tomography (CT) and magnetic resonance imaging (MRI) scans should be reviewed for evidence of brain edema, a midline shift greater than 0.5 cm, and ventricular displacement or compression. The neurological examination should document mental status and any sensory or motor deficits. Medications should be reviewed with special reference to corticosteroid, diuretic, and anticonvulsant therapy. Laboratory evaluation should rule out corticosteroid-induced hyperglycemia, electrolyte disturbances due to diuretics, or abnormal secretion of antidiuretic hormone. Anticonvulsant blood concentrations may be measured, particularly when seizures are not well controlled.

Premedication

Sedative or opioid premedication is best avoided if intracranial hypertension is suspected. Hypercapnia secondary to respiratory depression increases ICP. Corticosteroids and anticonvulsant therapy should be continued until the time of surgery.

INTRAOPERATIVE MANAGEMENT

Monitoring

In addition to standard monitors, direct intraarterial pressure monitoring and bladder catheterization are used for most patients undergoing craniotomy. Rapid changes in blood pressure during anesthetic procedures, positioning, and surgical manipulation are best managed with guidance from continuous invasive monitoring of blood pressure. Moreover, arterial blood gas analyses are necessary to closely regulate $Paco_2$. Many neuroanesthesiologists zero the arterial pressure transducer at the level of the head (external auditory meatus)—instead of the right atrium—to facilitate calculation of cerebral perfusion pressure (CPP). End-tidal CO_2 measurements alone cannot be relied upon for precise regulation of ventilation; the arterial to end-tidal CO_2 gradient must be determined. Central venous access and pressure monitoring should be considered for patients requiring vasoactive drugs. Use of the internal jugular vein for access is theoretically problematic because of concern that the catheter might interfere with venous drainage from the brain. Some clinicians avoid this issue by passing a long catheter into the central circulation from the median basilic vein. The external jugular, subclavian, and femoral veins may be suitable alternatives for intraoperative use. A bladder catheter is necessary because of the use of diuretics, the long duration of most neurosurgical procedures, and its utility in guiding fluid therapy. Neuromuscular function should be monitored on the unaffected side in patients with hemiparesis because the twitch response is often abnormally resistant on the affected side. Monitoring visual evoked potentials may be useful in preventing optic nerve damage during resections of large pituitary tumors. Additional monitors for surgery in the posterior fossa are described below.

Management of patients with intracranial hypertension may be guided by monitoring ICP perioperatively. Various ventricular, intraparenchymal, and subdural devices can be placed by neurosurgeons to provide measurements of ICP. The transducer should be zeroed to the same reference level as the arterial pressure transducer (usually the external auditory meatus; see above). A ventriculostomy catheter provides the added advantage of allowing removal of CSF to decrease ICP.

Induction

Induction of anesthesia and tracheal intubation are critical periods for patients with compromised intracranial pressure to volume relationships, particularly if there is an elevated ICP. Intracranial elastance can be improved by osmotic diuresis, dexamethasone, or removal of small volumes of CSF via a ventriculostomy drain. The goal of any technique should be to induce anesthesia and intubate the trachea without increasing ICP or compromising CBF. Arterial hypertension during induction increases CBV and promotes cerebral edema. Sustained hypertension can lead to marked increases in ICP, decreasing CPP and risking herniation. Excessive decreases in arterial blood pressure can be equally detrimental by compromising CPP.

The most common induction technique employs propofol together with modest hyperventilation to reduce ICP and blunt the noxious effects of laryngoscopy and intubation. Cooperative patients can be asked to hyperventilate during preoxygenation. All patients receive controlled ventilation once the propofol has been injected. A neuromuscular blocker (NMB) is given to facilitate ventilation and prevent straining or coughing, both of which can abruptly increase ICP. An intravenous opioid given with propofol blunts the sympathetic response, particularly in young patients. Esmolol, 0.5–1.0 mcg/kg, is effective in preventing tachycardia associated with intubation in lightly anesthetized patients.

The actual induction technique can be varied according to individual patient responses and coexisting diseases). Succinylcholine may theoretically increase ICP, particularly if intubation is attempted prior to the establishment of deep anesthesia. Succinylcholine, however, remains the agent of choice for rapid sequence induction or when there are concerns about a potentially difficult airway, as hypoxemia and hypercarbia are much more detrimental than any effect of succinylcholine to the patient with intracranial hypertension.

Hypertension during induction can be treated with β_1-blockers or by deepening the anesthetic with additional propofol. Modest concentrations of volatile agents (eg, sevoflurane) may also be used, provided that hyperventilation is also used. Sevoflurane best preserves autoregulation of CBF and produces limited vasodilatation; it may be the preferred volatile agent in patients with elevated ICP. Because of their potentially deleterious effect on CBV and ICP, vasodilators (eg, nicardipine, nitroprusside, nitroglycerin, and hydralazine) are avoided until the dura is opened. Hypotension is generally treated with incremental doses of vasopressors (eg, phenylephrine).

Positioning

Frontal, temporal, and parietooccipital craniotomies are performed in the supine position. The head is elevated 15–30° to facilitate venous and CSF drainage of CSF. The head may also be turned to the side to facilitate exposure. Excessive flexion or rotation of the neck impedes jugular venous drainage and can increase ICP. Before and after positioning, the tracheal tube should be secured, and all breathing circuit connections checked. The risk of unrecognized disconnections may be increased because the patient's airway will not be easily assessed after surgical draping; moreover, the operating table is usually turned 90° or 180° away from the anesthesiologist.

Maintenance of Anesthesia

Anesthesia can be maintained with inhalation anesthesia, total intravenous anesthesia techniques (TIVA), or a combination of an opioid and intravenous hypnotic (most often propofol) and a low-dose inhalation agent. Even though periods of stimulation are few, neuromuscular blockade is recommended—unless neurophysiological monitoring contradicts its use—to prevent straining, bucking, or movement. Increased anesthetic requirements can be expected during the most stimulating periods: laryngoscopy–intubation, skin incision, dural opening, periosteal manipulations, including Mayfied pin placement and closure. TIVA with remifentanil and propofol facilitates rapid emergence and immediate neurological assessment. Likewise, the α_2-agonist dexmedetomidine can be employed during both asleep and awake craniotomies to similar effect.

Hyperventilation should be continued intraoperatively to maintain $Paco_2$ at roughly 30–35 mm Hg. Lower $Paco_2$ tensions provide little additional benefit and may be associated with cerebral ischemia and impaired oxygen dissociation from hemoglobin. Positive end-expiratory pressure (PEEP) and ventilatory patterns resulting in high mean airway pressures (a low rate with large tidal volumes) should be avoided because of a potentially adverse effect on ICP by increasing central venous pressure and the potential for lung injury. Hypoxic patients may require PEEP and increased mean airway pressures; in such patients, the effect of PEEP on ICP is variable.

Intravenous fluid replacement should be limited to glucose-free isotonic crystalloid or colloid solutions. Hyperglycemia is common in neurosurgical patients (corticosteroid effect) and has been implicated in increasing ischemic brain injury. Colloid solutions can be used to restore intravascular volume deficits, whereas isotonic crystalloid solutions are used for maintenance fluid requirements. Neurosurgical procedures are often associated with "occult" blood loss (underneath surgical drapes or on the floor).

Emergence

Most patients undergoing elective craniotomy can be extubated at the end of the procedure, provided that neurological function is intact. Patients who will remain intubated should be sedated to prevent agitation. Extubation in the operating room requires special handling during emergence. Straining or bucking on the tracheal tube may precipitate intracranial hemorrhage or worsen cerebral edema. As the skin is being closed, the patient should resume breathing spontaneously. Should the patient's head be secured in a Mayfield pin apparatus, care must be taken to avoid any patient motions (eg, "bucking on the tube"), which could promote neck or cranial injuries. After the head dressing is applied and full access to the patient is regained (the table is turned back to its original position as at induction), any anesthetic gases are completely discontinued, and the neuromuscular blockade is reversed. Rapid awakening facilitates immediate neurological assessment and can generally be expected following an appropriate anesthetic. Delayed awakening may be seen following opioid or sedative overdose, when the end-tidal concentration of the volatile agent remains >.2 minimum alveolar concentration (MAC), because of various metabolic derangements, or when there is a perioperative neurological injury. Patients may need to be transported to the CT scanner directly from the operating room for evaluation when they do not respond as predicted. Immediate reexploration may be required. Most patients are taken to the intensive care unit postoperatively for close monitoring of neurological function.

Anesthesia for Surgery in the Posterior Fossa

Craniotomy for a mass in the posterior fossa presents a unique set of potential problems: obstructive hydrocephalus, possible injury to vital brainstem centers, pneumocephalus, and, with unusual positioning, postural hypotension and **venous air embolism**.

Obstructive Hydrocephalus

Infratentorial masses can obstruct CSF flow through the fourth ventricle or the cerebral aqueduct of Sylvius. Small but critically located lesions can markedly increase ICP. In such cases, a ventriculostomy is often performed under local anesthesia to decrease ICP prior to induction of general anesthesia.

Brain Stem Injury

3 Operations in the posterior fossa can injure vital circulatory and respiratory brainstem centers and cranial nerves or their nuclei. Such injuries may occur as a result of direct surgical trauma or ischemia from retraction or other interruptions of the blood supply. Damage to respiratory centers is said to nearly always produce circulatory changes; therefore, abrupt changes in blood pressure, heart rate, or cardiac rhythm should alert the anesthesiologist to the possibility of such an injury. Such changes should be communicated to the surgeon. Isolated damage to respiratory centers may rarely occur without premonitory circulatory signs during operations in the floor of the fourth ventricle. Historically, some clinicians have employed spontaneous ventilation during these procedures as an additional monitor of brain function. At completion of the surgery, brainstem injuries may present as an abnormal respiratory pattern or an inability to maintain a patent airway following extubation. Monitoring brainstem auditory evoked potentials may be useful in preventing eighth nerve damage during resections of acoustic neuromas. Electromyography is also used to avoid injury to the facial nerve, but requires incomplete neuromuscular blockade intraoperatively.

Positioning

Although most explorations of the posterior fossa can be performed with the patient in either a modified lateral or prone position, the sitting position may be preferred by some surgeons.

The patient is actually semirecumbent in the standard sitting position (Figure 27–1); the back is elevated to 60°, and the legs are elevated with the knees flexed. The head is fixed in a three-point holder with the neck flexed; the arms remain at the sides with the hands resting on the lap.

Careful positioning and padding helps avoid injuries. Pressure points, such as the elbows, ischial spines, heels, and forehead, must be protected. Excessive neck flexion has been associated with swelling of the upper airway (due to venous

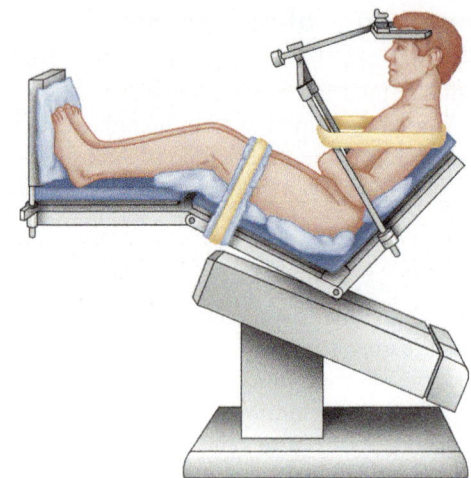

FIGURE 27–1 The sitting position for craniotomy.

obstruction), and, rarely, quadriplegia (due to compression of the cervical spinal cord). Preexisting cervical spinal stenosis probably predisposes patients to the latter injury.

Pneumocephalus

The sitting position increases the likelihood of pneumocephalus. In this position, air readily enters the subarachnoid space, as CSF is lost during surgery. In patients with cerebral atrophy, drainage of CSF is marked; air can replace CSF on the surface of the brain and in the lateral ventricles. Expansion of a pneumocephalus following dural closure can compress the brain. Postoperative pneumocephalus can cause delayed awakening and continued impairment of neurological function. Because of these concerns, nitrous oxide is rarely used for sitting craniotomies. (see also below).

Venous Air Embolism

4 Venous air embolism can occur when the pressure within an open vein is subatmospheric. These conditions may exist in any position (and during any procedure) whenever the wound is above the level of the heart. The incidence of venous air embolism is greater during sitting craniotomies (20% to 40%) than in craniotomies in any other position. Entry into large cerebral venous sinuses increases the risk.

The physiological consequences of venous air embolism depend on the volume and the rate of air entry and whether the patient has a right-to-left intracardiac shunt (eg, patent foramen ovale [10% to 25% incidence]). The latter are important because they can facilitate passage of air into the arterial circulation (**paradoxical air embolism**). Modest quantities of air bubbles entering the venous system ordinarily lodge in the pulmonary circulation, where they are eventually absorbed. Small quantities of embolized air are well tolerated by most patients. When the amount entrained exceeds the rate of pulmonary clearance, pulmonary artery pressure rises progressively. Eventually, cardiac output decreases in response to increases in right ventricular afterload. Preexisting cardiac or pulmonary disease enhances the effects of venous air embolism; relatively small amounts of air may produce marked hemodynamic changes. Nitrous oxide, by diffusing into the bubbles and increasing their volume, can markedly accentuate the effects of even small amounts of entrained air. The dose for lethal venous air embolism in animals receiving nitrous oxide anesthesia is one-third to one-half that of control animals not receiving nitrous oxide.

Definitive signs of venous air embolism are often not apparent until large volumes of air have been entrained. A decrease in end-tidal CO_2 or arterial oxygen saturation might be noticed prior to hemodynamic changes. Arterial blood gas values may show only slight increases in $Paco_2$ as a result of increased pulmonary dead space (areas with normal ventilation but decreased perfusion). Conversely, major hemodynamic manifestations, such as sudden hypotension, can occur well before hypoxemia is noted. Moreover, large amounts of intracardiac air impair tricuspid and pulmonic valve function and can produce sudden circulatory arrest by obstructing right ventricular outflow.

Paradoxic air embolism can result in a stroke or coronary occlusion, which may be apparent only postoperatively. Paradoxic air emboli are more likely to occur in patients with right-to-left intracardiac shunts, particularly when the normal transatrial (left > right) pressure gradient is reversed. Some studies suggest that a right > left

pressure gradient can develop at some time during the cardiac cycle, even when the overall mean gradient remains left > right.

A. Central Venous Catheterization

A properly positioned central venous catheter can be used to aspirate entrained air, but there is only limited evidence that this influences outcomes after venous air embolism. Some clinicians have considered right atrial catheterization mandatory for sitting craniotomies, but this is a minority viewpoint.

5 Optimal recovery of air following venous air embolism is provided by a multiorificed catheter positioned at the junction between the right atrium and the superior vena cava. Confirmation of correct catheter positioning can be accomplished by intravascular electrocardiography, radiography, or transesophageal echocardiography (TEE). Intravascular electrocardiography is accomplished by using the saline-filled catheter as a "V" lead. Correct high atrial position is indicated by the appearance of a biphasic P wave. If the catheter is advanced farther into the heart, the P wave changes from a biphasic to a undirectional deflection. A right ventricular or pulmonary artery waveform may also be observed when the catheter is connected to a pressure transducer and advanced too far.

B. Monitoring for Venous Air Embolism

The most sensitive monitors available should be used. Detecting even small amounts of venous air embolism is important because it allows surgical control of the entry site before additional air is entrained. Currently, the most sensitive intraoperative monitors are TEE and precordial Doppler sonography. These monitors can detect air bubbles as small as 0.25 mL. TEE has the added benefit of detecting the volume of the bubbles and any transatrial passage through a patent foramen ovale, as well as evaluating any effect venous air embolism may have on cardiac function. Doppler methods employ a probe over the right atrium (usually to the right of the sternum and between the third and sixth ribs). Interruption of the regular swishing of the Doppler signal by sporadic roaring sounds indicates venous air embolism. Changes in end-tidal respiratory gas concentrations are less sensitive but are important monitors that can also detect venous air embolism before overt clinical signs are present. Venous air embolism causes a sudden decrease in end-tidal CO_2 tension in proportion to the increase in pulmonary dead space; however, decreases can also be seen with hemodynamic changes unrelated to venous air embolism, such as decreased cardiac output. A reappearance (or increase) of nitrogen in expired gases may also be seen with venous air embolism. Changes in blood pressure and heart sounds ("mill wheel" murmur) are late manifestations of venous air embolism.

C. Treatment of Venous Air Embolism

1. The surgeon should be notified so that he or she can flood the surgical field with saline or pack it with wet gauzes and apply bone wax to the skull edges until the entry site is identified and occluded.

2. Nitrous oxide (if used) should be discontinued, and the inhalation anesthetic should be delivered in 100% oxygen.

3. If a central venous catheter is present, it should be aspirated in an attempt to retrieve the entrained air.

4. Intravascular volume infusion should be given to increase central venous pressure.

5. Vasopressors should be given to treat hypotension.

6. Bilateral jugular vein compression, by increasing cranial venous pressure, may slow air entrainment and cause back bleeding, which might help the surgeon identify the entry point of the embolus.

7. Some clinicians advocate PEEP to increase cerebral venous pressure; however, reversal of the normal transatrial pressure gradient may promote paradoxic embolism in a patient with incomplete closure of the foramen ovale.

8. If the above measures fail, the patient should be placed in a head-down position, and the wound should be closed quickly.

9. Persistent circulatory arrest necessitates the supine position and institution of resuscitation efforts using advanced cardiac life support algorithms.

Anesthesia for Stereotactic Surgery

Stereotaxis can be employed in treating involuntary movement disorders, intractable pain, and epilepsy and can also be used when diagnosing and treating tumors that are located deep within the brain.

These procedures are often performed under local anesthesia to allow evaluation of the patient. Propofol or dexmedetomidine infusions are routinely used for sedation and amnesia. Sedation should be omitted, however, if the patient already has increased ICP. The ability to rapidly provide controlled ventilation and general anesthesia for emergency craniotomy is mandatory, but is complicated by the platform and localizing frame that is attached to the patient's head for the procedure. Although mask ventilation or ventilation through a laryngeal mask airway (LMA) or orotracheal intubation might be readily accomplished in an emergency, awake intubation with a fiberoptic bronchoscope prior to positioning and surgery may be the safest approach when intubation is necessary for a patient whose head is already in a stereotactic head frame.

Functional neurosurgery is increasingly performed for removal of lesions adjacent to speech and other vital brain centers. Sometimes patients are managed with an asleep–awake–asleep technique, with or without instrumentation of the airway. Such operations require the patient to be awake to participate in cortical mapping to identify key speech centers, such as Broca's area. Patients sleep during the painful periods of surgery (ie, during opening and closure). LMAs are often employed to assist airway management during the asleep portions of these surgeries.

Patients undergo deep brain stimulator insertion for control of movement and other disorders. A stimulator electrode is placed via a burr hole using radiologic guidance to establish coordinates for electrode placement. A microelectrode recording (MER) is obtained to determine the correct placement of the stimulator in brain structures. The effect of stimulation upon the patient is noted. Sedative medications can adversely affect MER potentials, complicating the location of the correct depth of

TABLE 27–1 Advantages and disadvantages of drugs used for conscious sedation.

Agents	Advantages	Disadvantages
GABA receptor agonists		
Benzodiazepines	Anxiolysis	Large dose abolishes MER
		Alters the threshold for stimulation
		Induces dyskinesia
Propofol	Widely used	Abolish tremors
	Short acting	Attenuation of MER
	Predictable emergence profile	Unpredictable dosing in patients with
		Parkinson disease
		Induces dyskinesia
		Tendency to cause sneezing
Opioids		
Fentanyl	? Minimal effect on MER	Rigidity
Remifentanil	Short acting	Suppression of tremors
Alpha-2 agonist		
Dexmedetomidine	Non-GABA-mediated action	High doses can abolish MER
	Less effect on MER	Hypotension, bradycardia
	Anxiolysis and analgesic effects	
	Sedation—easily arousable	
	Does not ameliorate clinical signs of	
	Parkinsonism	
	Maintains hemodynamic stability	
	Preserves respiration	

MER, microelectrode recording; GABA, γ-aminobutyric acid.

Modified, with permission, from Venkatraghavan L, Luciano M, Manninen P: Anesthetic management of patients undergoing deep brain stimulator insertion. Anesth Analg 2010;110:1138.

stimulator placement. Dexmedetomidine has been used to provide sedation to these patients; however, during MER and stimulation testing, sedative infusions should be discontinued to facilitate patient participation in determining correct electrode placement (Table 27–1).

Anesthesia for Head Trauma

Head injuries are a contributory factor in up to 50% of deaths due to trauma. Most patients with head trauma are young, and many (10% to 40%) have associated intraabdominal or intrathoracic injuries, long bone fractures, and/or spinal injuries. The outcome from a head injury is dependent not only on the extent of the neuronal damage at the time of injury, but also on the occurrence of any secondary insults. These additional insults include: (1) systemic factors such as hypoxemia,

hypercapnia, or hypotension; (2) formation and expansion of an epidural, subdural, or intracerebral hematoma; and (3) sustained intracranial hypertension. Surgical and anesthetic management of these patients is directed at preventing these secondary insults. The **Glasgow Coma Scale (GCS) score** (Table 27–2) generally correlates well with the severity of injury and outcome. A GCS score of 8 or less on admission is associated with approximately 35% mortality. Evidence of greater than a 5-mm midline shift (on imaging) and ventricular compression on imaging are associated with substantially increased morbidity.

Specific lesions include skull fractures, subdural and epidural hematomas, brain contusions (including intracerebral hemorrhages), penetrating head injuries, and traumatic vascular occlusions and dissections. The presence of a skull fracture greatly increases the likelihood of an intracranial lesion. Linear skull fractures are commonly associated

TABLE 27–2 Glasgow coma scale.

Category	Score
Eye opening	
Spontaneous	4
To speech	3
To pain	2
Nil	1
Best motor response	
To verbal command	
Obeys	6
To pain	
Localizes	5
Withdraws	4
Decorticate flexion	3
Extensor response	2
Nil	1
Best verbal response	
Oriented	5
Confused conversation	4
Inappropriate words	3
Incomprehensible sounds	2
Nil	1

with subdural or epidural hematomas. Basilar skull fractures may be associated with CSF rhinorrhea, pneumocephalus, cranial nerve palsies, or even a cavernous sinus–carotid artery fistula. Depressed skull fractures often present with an underlying brain contusion. Contusions may be limited to the surface of the brain or may involve hemorrhage in deeper hemispheric structures or the brainstem. Deceleration injuries often produce both coup (frontal) and contrecoup (occipital) lesions. Epidural and subdural hematomas can occur as isolated lesions, as well as in association with cerebral contusions (more commonly with subdural than epidural lesions).

Operative treatment is usually elected for depressed skull fractures; evacuation of epidural, subdural, and some intracerebral hematomas; and debridement of penetrating injuries. Decompressive craniectomy is used to provide room for cerebral swelling. The cranium is subsequently reconstructed following resolution of cerebral edema.

ICP monitoring is usually indicated in patients with lesions associated with intracranial hypertension: large contusions, mass lesions, intracerebral

hemorrhage, or evidence of edema on imaging studies. ICP monitoring should also be considered in patients with signs of intracranial hypertension who are undergoing nonneurological procedures. Intracranial hypertension should be treated with moderate hyperventilation, mannitol, pentobarbital, or propofol Studies suggest that sustained increases in ICP of greater than 60 mm Hg result in severe disability or death. Unlike treatment following spinal cord trauma, multiple randomized trials have failed to detect the efficacy of early use of large doses of glucocorticoids in patients with head trauma.

PREOPERATIVE MANAGEMENT

Anesthetic care of patients with severe head trauma begins in the emergency department. Measures to ensure patency of the airway, adequacy of ventilation and oxygenation, and correction of systemic hypotension should go forward simultaneously with neurological and trauma surgical evaluation. Airway obstruction and hypoventilation are common. Up to 70% of such patients have hypoxemia, which may be complicated by pulmonary contusion, fat emboli, or neurogenic pulmonary edema. The latter is attributed to marked systemic and pulmonary hypertension secondary to intense sympathetic nervous system activity. Supplemental oxygen should be given to all patients while the airway and ventilation are evaluated. All patients must be assumed to have a cervical spine injury (up to 10% incidence) until the contrary is proven radiographically. Patients with obvious hypoventilation, an absent gag reflex, or a persistent score below 8 on the GCS (Table 27–2) require tracheal intubation and hyperventilation. All other patients should be carefully observed for deterioration.

Intubation

All patients should be regarded as having a full stomach and should have cricoid pressure applied during ventilation and tracheal intubation. In-line stabilization should be used during airway manipulation to maintain the head in a neutral position, unless radiographs confirm that there is no cervical spine injury. Following preoxygenation and hyperventilation by mask, the adverse effects of intubation on ICP are blunted by prior administration of propofol, 1.5–3.0 mg/kg, and a rapid-onset NMB. Succinylcholine may produce mild and transient increases in ICP in patients with closed head injury; however, the necessity for expeditious airway management trumps these concerns. Rocuronium is often used to facilitate intubation. Video laryngoscopy performed with in-line stabilization generally permits neutral position intubation of the trauma patient. An intubating bougie should be available to facilitate tube placement. If a difficult intubation is encountered with video laryngoscopy, fiberoptic or other techniques (eg, intubating LMA) can be attempted. If airway attempts are unsuccessful, a surgical airway should be obtained. Blind nasal intubation is contraindicated in the presence of a basilar skull fracture, which is suggested by CSF rhinorrhea or otorrhea, hemotympanum, or ecchymosis into periorbital tissues (raccoon sign) or behind the ear (Battle's sign).

Hypotension

Hypotension in the setting of head trauma is nearly always related to other associated injuries (often intraabdominal). Bleeding from scalp lacerations may be responsible in children. Hypotension may be seen with spinal cord injuries because of the sympathectomy associated with spinal shock. **6** In a patient with head trauma, correction of hypotension and control of any bleeding take precedence over radiographic studies and definitive neurosurgical treatment because systolic arterial blood pressures of less than 80 mm Hg predict a poor outcome. Glucose-containing or hypotonic solutions should not be used (see above). Otherwise, a mix of colloid, crystalloid, and blood products can be administered as necessary. Massive blood loss in the patient with multiple injuries should result in activation of a massive transfusion protocol to provide a steady supply of platelets, fresh frozen plasma, and packed red blood cells. Invasive monitoring of arterial pressure, central venous pressure, and ICP are valuable, but should not delay diagnosis and treatment. Arrhythmias

and electrocardiographic abnormalities in the T wave, U wave, ST segment, and QT interval are common following head injuries, but are not necessarily associated with cardiac injury; they likely represent altered autonomic function.

Diagnostic Studies

The choice between operative and medical management of head trauma is based on radiographic and clinical findings. Patients should be stabilized prior to any CT or other imaging studies. Critically ill patients should be closely monitored during such studies. Restless or uncooperative patients may additionally require general anesthesia. Sedation without control of the airway should generally be avoided because of the risk of further increases in ICP from hypercapnia or hypoxemia.

INTRAOPERATIVE MANAGEMENT

Anesthetic management is generally similar to that for other mass lesions associated with intracranial hypertension. Management of the airway is discussed above. Invasive monitoring should be established, if not already present, but should not delay surgical decompression in a rapidly deteriorating patient.

Anesthetic technique and agents are designed to preserve cerebral perfusion and mitigate increases in intracranial pressure. Hypotension may occur after induction of anesthesia as a result of the combined effects of vasodilation and hypovolemia and should be treated with an α-adrenergic agonist and volume infusion if necessary. Subsequent hypertension is common with surgical stimulation, but may also occur with acute elevations in ICP. The latter may be associated with bradycardia (Cushing reflex).

Hypertension can be treated with additional doses of the induction agent, with increased concentrations of an inhalation anesthetic or vasodilators. β-Adrenergic blockade is usually effective in controlling hypertension associated with tachycardia. CPP should be maintained between 70 and 110 mm Hg. Vasodilators should be avoided until the dura is opened. Hyperventilation to a $Paco_2$ <30 should be avoided in trauma patients to avoid excessive decreases in oxygen delivery.

Disseminated intravascular coagulation occasionally may be seen with severe head injuries. Such injuries cause the release of large amounts of brain thromboplastin and may also be associated with the acute respiratory distress syndrome. Pulmonary aspiration and neurogenic pulmonary edema may also be responsible for deteriorating lung function. PEEP can be applied on the ventilator. When PEEP is used, ICP monitoring can be useful to confirm an adequate CPP. Diabetes insipidus, characterized by excessive dilute urine, is frequently seen following injuries to the pituitary stalk. Other likely causes of polyuria should be excluded and the diagnosis confirmed by measurement of urine and serum osmolality prior to treatment with fluid restriction and vasopressin Gastrointestinal bleeding is common in patients not receiving prophylaxis; it is usually due to stress ulceration.

The decision whether to extubate the trachea at the conclusion of the surgical procedure depends on the severity of the injury, the presence of concomitant abdominal or thoracic injuries, preexisting illnesses, and the preoperative level of consciousness. Young patients who were conscious preoperatively may be extubated following the removal of a localized lesion, whereas patients with diffuse brain injury should remain intubated. Moreover, persistent intracranial hypertension requires continued paralysis, sedation, and hyperventilation.

Anesthesia & Craniotomy for Intracranial Aneurysms & Arteriovenous Malformations

Saccular aneurysms and AVMs are common causes of nontraumatic intracranial hemorrhages. Surgical or interventional neuroradiologic treatment may be undertaken either electively to prevent hemorrhage or emergently to prevent further complications once hemorrhage has taken place. Other nontraumatic hemorrhages (eg, from hypertension, sickle cell disease, or vasculitis) are usually treated medically.

CEREBRAL ANEURYSMS
Preoperative Considerations

Cerebral aneurysms typically occur at the bifurcation of the large arteries at the base of the brain; most are located in the anterior circle of Willis. Approximately 10% to 30% of patients have more than one aneurysm. The general incidence of saccular aneurysms in some estimates is reported to be 5%, but only a minority of those with aneurysms will have complications. Rupture of a saccular aneurysm is the most common cause of subarachnoid hemorrhage. The acute mortality following rupture is approximately 10%. Of those that survive the initial hemorrhage, about 25% die within 3 months from delayed complications. Moreover, up to 50% of survivors are left with neurological deficits. As a result, the emphasis in management is on prevention of rupture. Unfortunately, most patients present only after rupture has already occurred.

Unruptured Aneurysms

Patients may present with prodromal symptoms and signs suggesting progressive enlargement. The most common symptom is headache, and the most common physical sign is a third-nerve palsy. Other manifestations could include brainstem dysfunction, visual field defects, trigeminal nerve dysfunction, cavernous sinus syndrome, seizures, and hypothalamic–pituitary dysfunction. The most commonly used techniques to diagnose an aneurysm are MRI angiography, angiography, and helical CT angiography. Following diagnosis, patients are brought to the operating room, or more likely the radiology suite, for elective clipping or obliteration of the aneurysm. Most patients are in the 40- to 60-year-old age group and in otherwise good health.

Ruptured Aneurysms

Ruptured aneurysms usually present acutely as subarachnoid hemorrhage. Patients typically complain of a sudden severe headache without focal neurological deficits, but often associated with nausea and vomiting. Transient loss of consciousness may

TABLE 27–3 Hunt and Hess grading scale for SAH.

Grade	Clinical Description
I	Asymptomatic or minimal headache and slight nuchal rigidity
II	Moderate to severe headache, nuchal rigidity, no neurological deficit other than cranial nerve palsy
III	Drowsiness, confusion, or mild focal deficit
IV	Stupor, moderate to severe hemiparesis, and possibly early decerebrate rigidity and vegetative disturbances
V	Deep coma, decerebrate rigidity, and moribund appearance

Reproduced, with permission, from Priebe H-J: Aneurysmal subarachnoid haemorrhage and the anaesthetist. Br J Anaesth 2007;99:102.

TABLE 27–4 World Federation of Neurological Surgeons Grading scale for aneurismal SAH.

Grade	GCS score	Motor Deficit[1]
I	15	Absent
II	13 or 14	Absent
III	13 or 14	Present
IV	7-12	Present or absent
V	3-6	Present or absent

GCS, Glasgow Coma Scale.

[1]Excludes cranial neuropathies, but includes dysphasia.

Reproduced, with permission, from Priebe H-J: Aneurysmal subarachnoid haemorrhage and the anaesthetist. Br J Anaesth 2007;99:102.

occur and may result from a sudden rise in ICP and precipitous drop in CPP. If ICP does not decrease rapidly after the initial sudden increase, death usually follows. Large blood clots can cause focal neurological signs in some patients. Minor bleeding may cause only a mild headache, vomiting, and nuchal rigidity. Unfortunately, even minor bleeding in the subarachnoid space seems to predispose to delayed complications. The severity of subarachnoid hemorrhage (SAH) is graded according to the Hunt and Hess scale (Table 27–3), as well as the World Federation of Neurological Surgeons Grading Scale of SAH (Table 27–4). The Fisher grading scale, which uses CT to assess the amount of blood detected, gives the best indication of the likelihood of the development of cerebral vasospasm and patient outcome (Table 27–5).

Delayed complications include cerebral vasospasm, rerupture, and hydrocephalus. Cerebral vasospasm occurs in 30% of patients (usually after 4–14 days) and is a major cause of morbidity and mortality. Manifestations of vasospasm are due to cerebral ischemia and infarction and depend on the severity and distribution of the involved vessels. The Ca^{2+} channel antagonist nimodipine may antagonize vasospasm. Both transcranial Doppler and brain tissue oxygen monitoring can be used to guide vasospasm therapy (Figure 27–2). Increased velocity of flow >200cm/sec is indicative of severe spasm. The Lindegaard ratio compares the blood velocity of the cervical carotid artery with that of the middle cerebral artery. A ratio >3 is likewise indicative of severe spasm. Brain tissue oxygen tension less than 20 mm Hg is also worrisome. **In patients with symptomatic vasospasm with an inadequate response to nimodipine, intravascular volume expansion and induced hypertension ("triple H" therapy: hypervolemia, hemodilution, and hypertension) are added as part of the therapeutic regimen**. Refractory vasospasm may be treated with infusion of papaverine, infusion of nicardipine, or angioplasty. However, radiologic improvement in the vessel diameter does not necessarily correlate with an improvement in clinical status.

TABLE 27–5 Fisher grading scale of cranial computerized tomography (CCT).

Grade	Findings on CCT
1	No subarachnoid blood detected
2	Diffuse or vertical layers ≤ 1mm
3	Localized clot and/or vertical layer > 1mm
4	Intracerebral or intraventricular clot with diffuse or no subarachnoid haemorrhage

Reproduced, with permission, from Priebe H-J: Aneurysmal subarachnoid haemorrhage and the anaesthetist. Br J Anaesth 2007;99:102.

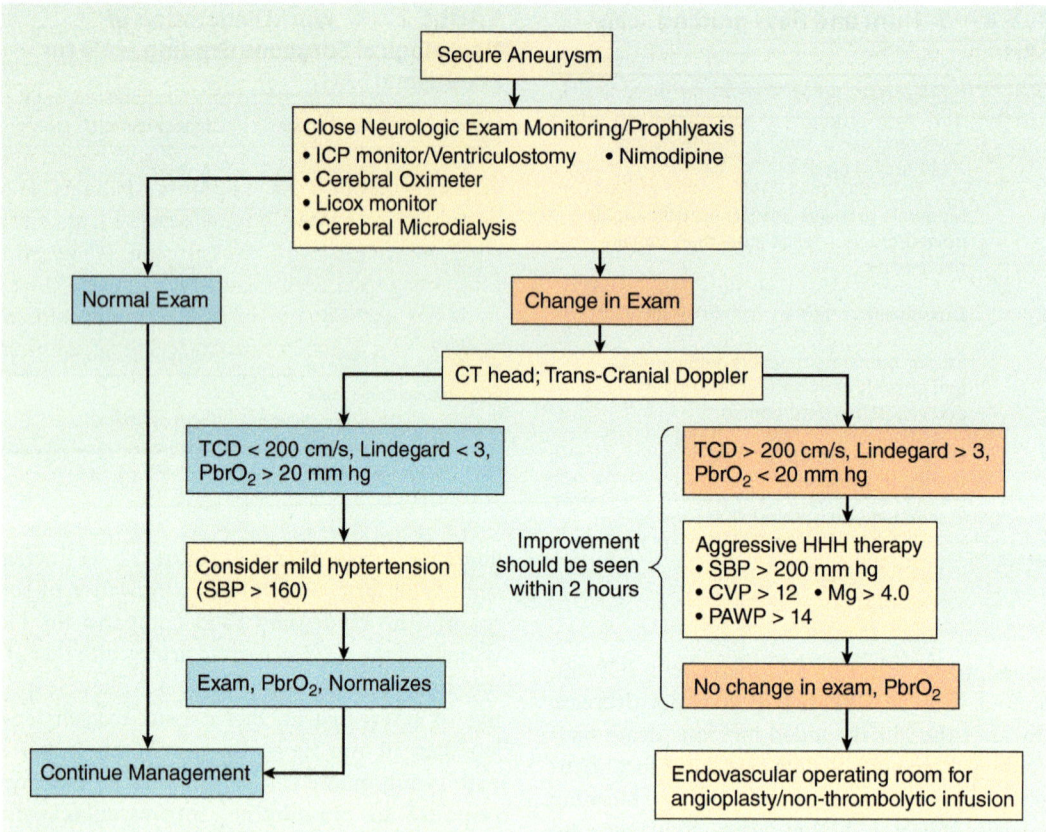

FIGURE 27–2 Schematic diagram of algorithm for management of vasospasm and delayed ischemic neurological deficit after aneurismal SAH. (Reproduced, with permission, from Bell RS, Vo AH, Veznedaroglu E, Armonda RA. The endovascular operating room as an extension of the intensive care unit: changing strategies in the management of neurovascular disease. Neurosurgery 2006;59:S3–56.)

PREOPERATIVE MANAGEMENT

In addition to assessing neurological findings, the preoperative evaluation should include a search for coexisting diseases, such as hypertension and renal, cardiac, or ischemic cerebrovascular disease. Electrocardiographic abnormalities are commonly seen in patients with subarachnoid hemorrhage, but do not necessarily reflect underlying heart disease. However, increases of cardiac troponin during SAH are associated with myocardial injury and may herald a poor outcome. Most conscious patients with normal ICP are sedated following rupture to prevent rebleeding; such sedation should be continued until induction of anesthesia. Patients with

persistent elevation in ICP should receive little or no premedication to avoid hypercapnia.

INTRAOPERATIVE MANAGEMENT

Aneurysm surgery can result in exsanguinating hemorrhage as a consequence of rupture or rebleeding. Blood should be available prior to the start of these operations.

Regardless of the anesthetic technique employed, anesthetic management should focus on preventing rupture (or rebleeding) and avoiding factors that promote cerebral ischemia or vasospasm.

Intraarterial and central venous pressure monitoring are useful. Sudden increases in blood pressure with tracheal intubation or surgical stimulation should be avoided. Judicious intravascular volume loading permits surgical levels of anesthesia without excessive decreases in blood pressure. Because calcium channel blockers, angiotensin receptor blockers, and ACE inhibitors cause systemic vasodilation and reduce systemic vascular resistance, patients receiving these agents preoperatively may be particularly prone to hypotension. Hyperventilation is unlikely to overcome ischemia-induced vasodilation. Once the dura is opened, mannitol is often given to facilitate surgical exposure and reduce the need for surgical retraction. Rapid decreases in ICP prior to dural opening may promote rebleeding by removing a tamponading effect on the aneurysm.

Elective (controlled) hypotension has been used in aneurysm surgery. Decreasing mean arterial blood pressure reduces the transmural tension across the aneurysm, making rupture (or rebleeding) less likely and facilitating surgical clipping. Controlled hypotension can also decrease blood loss and improve surgical visualization in the event of bleeding. The combination of a slightly head-up position with a volatile anesthetic enhances the effects of any of the commonly used hypotensive agents. Should accidental rupture of the aneurysm occur, the surgeon may request transient hypotension to facilitate control of the bleeding aneurysm.

Technical improvements in temporary vascular clips have enabled surgeons to use them more often to interrupt blood flow during aneurysm surgery; induced hypertension is often requested when temporary clips are applied. Neurophysiologic monitoring may be employed during aneurysm surgery to identify potential ischemia during temporary clip application.

Mild hypothermia has been used to protect the brain during periods of prolonged or excessive hypotension or vascular occlusion; however, its efficacy has been questioned. Rarely, hypothermic circulatory arrest is used for large basilar artery aneurysms.

Depending on neurological condition, most patients should be extubated at the end of surgery. Extubation should be handled similarly to other craniotomies (see above). A rapid awakening allows neurological evaluation in the operating room, prior to transfer to the intensive care unit.

The anesthetic concerns of patients taken for aneurysmal coiling in the neurointerventional suite are similar to those of surgical interventions. General anesthesia is employed. Patients require heparin anticoagulation and radiologic contrast. Communication with the surgeon or neuroradiologist as to the desired activated clotting time and need for protamine reversal is essential. Moreover, anesthesia staff in the neuroradiology suite must be prepared to manipulate and monitor the blood pressure, as with an open surgical procedure.

ARTERIOVENOUS MALFORMATIONS

AVMs cause intracerebral hemorrhage more often than subarachnoid hemorrhage. These lesions are developmental abnormalities that result in arteriovenous fistulas; they typically grow in size with time. AVMs may present at any age, but bleeding is most common between 10 and 30 years of age. Other common presentations include headache and seizures. The combination of high blood flow with low vascular resistance can rarely result in high-output cardiac failure. Acutely, neuroradiologists try to embolize AVMs. When neuroradiological interventions are not successful or available, surgical excision may be undertaken. Neuroradiological embolization employs various coils, glues, and balloons to obliterate the AVM. Risks include embolization into cerebral arteries feeding the normal brain, as well as systemic or pulmonary embolism.

Anesthetic management of patients undergoing surgical treatment of AVMs may be complicated by extensive blood loss. Venous access with multiple large-bore cannulas is necessary. Embolization may be carried out prior to surgery to reduce operative blood loss. Hyperventilation and mannitol may be used to facilitate surgical access. Hyperemia and swelling can develop following resection, possibly because of altered autoregulation in the remaining normal brain. Emergence hypertension is typically controlled using β_1-blockers to avoid any vasodilator induced increase in CBF.

Anesthesia for Surgery on the Spine

Spinal surgery is most often performed for symptomatic nerve root or cord compression secondary to trauma or degenerative disorders. Compression may occur from protrusion of an intervertebral disk or osteophytic bone (spondylosis) into the spinal canal or an intervertebral foramen. Prolapse of an intervertebral disk usually occurs at either the fourth or fifth lumbar or the fifth or sixth cervical levels in patients 30–50 years old. Spondylosis tends to affect the lower cervical spine more than the lumbar spine and typically afflicts older patients. Operations on the spinal column can help correct deformities (eg, scoliosis), decompress the cord, and fuse the spine if disrupted by trauma. Spinal surgery may also be performed to resect a tumor or vascular malformation or to drain an abscess or hematoma.

PREOPERATIVE MANAGEMENT

Preoperative evaluation should focus on any existing anatomic abnormalities and limited neck movements due to disease, traction, or braces that might complicate airway management and necessitate special techniques. Neurological deficits should be documented. Neck mobility should be assessed in all patients presenting for spine surgery at any level. Patients with unstable cervical spines can be managed with either awake fiberoptic intubation or asleep intubation with in-line stabilization.

INTRAOPERATIVE MANAGEMENT

For many of these procedures, anesthetic management is complicated by the use of the prone position. Spinal operations involving multiple levels, fusion, and instrumentation are also complicated by the potential for large intraoperative blood losses; a red cell salvage device is often used. Excessive distraction during spinal instrumentation (Harrington rod or pedicle screw fixation) can additionally injure the spinal cord. Transthoracic approaches to the spine require one-lung ventilation. Anterior/posterior approaches require the patient to be repositioned in the middle of surgery.

Positioning

Most spine surgical procedures are carried out in the prone position. The supine position may be used for an anterior approach to the cervical spine, making anesthetic management easier, but increasing the risk of injury to the trachea, esophagus, recurrent laryngeal nerve, sympathetic chain, carotid artery, or jugular vein. A sitting (for cervical spine procedures) or lateral decubitus (most commonly for lumbar spine procedures) position may occasionally be used.

Following induction of anesthesia and tracheal intubation in the supine position, the patient is turned to the prone position. Care must be taken to maintain the neck in a neutral position. Once in the prone position, the head may be turned to the side (not exceeding the patient's normal range of motion) or (more commonly) can remain face down on a cushioned holder. Caution is necessary to avoid corneal abrasions or retinal ischemia from pressure on either globe, or pressure injuries of the nose, ears, forehead, chin, breasts (females), or genitalia (males). The chest should rest on parallel rolls (of foam, gel, or other padding) or special supports—if a frame is used—to facilitate ventilation. The arms may be tucked by the sides in a comfortable position or extended with the elbows flexed (avoiding excessive abduction at the shoulder).

Turning the patient prone is a critical maneuver, sometimes complicated by hypotension. Abdominal compression, particularly in obese patients, may impede venous return and contribute to excessive intraoperative blood loss from engorgement of epidural veins. Prone positioning that permits the abdomen to hang freely can mitigate this increase in venous pressure. Deliberate hypotension has been advocated in the past to reduce bleeding associated with spine surgery. However, this should only be undertaken with a full understanding that controlled hypotension may increase the risk of perioperative vision loss (POVL).

POVL occurs secondary to:

- Ischemic optic neuropathy
- Perioperative glaucoma
- Cortical hypotension/embolism

Prolonged surgery in a head-down position, major blood loss, relative hypotension, diabetes, obesity, and smoking all put patients at greater risk of POVL following spine surgery.

Airway and facial edema can likewise develop after prolonged "head-down" positioning. Reintubation, if required, will likely present more difficulty than the intubation at the start of surgery.

When patients are placed in the prone position, the face must be checked periodically to determine that the eyes, nose, and ears are free of pressure. Even foam cushions can exert pressure over time on the chin, orbit, and maxilla. Turning the head is not easily accomplished when the head is positioned on a cushion; therefore, if prolonged procedures are planned, the head can be secured with pins keeping the face free from any pressure.

Monitoring

7 When major blood loss is anticipated or the patient has preexisting cardiac disease, intra-arterial and possibly central venous pressure monitors should be considered prior to "positioning" or "turning." Massive blood loss from injuries to the great vessels can occur intraoperatively with thoracic or lumbar spine procedures.

Instrumentation of the spine requires the ability to intraoperatively detect spinal cord injury. Intraoperative wake-up techniques employing nitrous oxide-narcotic or total intravenous anesthesia allow the testing of motor function following distraction. Once preservation of motor function is established, the patient's anesthetic can be deepened. Continuous monitoring of somatosensory evoked potentials and motor evoked potentials provides alternatives that avoid the need for intraoperative awakening. These monitoring techniques require substitution of propofol, opioid, and/or ketamine infusions for volatile anesthetics and avoidance of neuromuscular paralysis.

CASE DISCUSSION

Resection of a Pituitary Tumor

A 41-year-old woman presents to the operating room for resection of a 10-mm pituitary tumor. She had complained of amenorrhea and had started noticing some decrease in visual acuity.

What hormones does the pituitary gland normally secrete?

Functionally and anatomically, the pituitary is divided into two parts: anterior and posterior. The latter is part of the neurohypophysis, which also includes the pituitary stalk and the median eminence.

The anterior pituitary is composed of several cell types, each secreting a specific hormone. Anterior pituitary hormones include adrenocorticotropic hormone (ACTH), thyroid-stimulating hormone (TSH), growth hormone (GH), the gonadotropins (follicle-stimulating hormone [FSH] and luteinizing hormone [LH]), and prolactin (PRL). Secretion of each of these hormones is regulated by hypothalamic peptides (releasing hormones) that are transported to the adenohypophysis by a capillary portal system. The secretion of FSH, LH, ACTH, TSH, and their respective releasing hormones is also under negative feedback control by the products of their target organs. For example, an increase in circulating thyroid hormone inhibits the secretion of TSH-releasing factor and TSH.

The posterior pituitary secretes antidiuretic hormone (ADH, also called vasopressin) and oxytocin. These hormones are actually formed in supraoptic and paraventricular neurons, respectively, and are transported down axons that terminate in the posterior pituitary. Hypothalamic osmoreceptors, and, to a lesser extent, peripheral vascular stretch receptors, regulate secretion of ADH.

What is the function of these hormones?

ACTH stimulates the adrenal cortex to secrete glucocorticoids. Unlike production of mineralocorticoids, production of glucocorticoids is dependent on ACTH secretion. TSH accelerates the synthesis and release of thyroid hormone (thyroxine).

Normal thyroid function is dependent on production of TSH. The gonadotropins FSH and LH are necessary for normal production of testosterone and spermatogenesis in males and cyclic ovarian function in females. GH promotes tissue growth and increases protein synthesis as well as fatty acid mobilization. Its effects on carbohydrate metabolism are to decrease cellular glucose uptake and utilization and increase insulin secretion. PRL functions to support breast development during pregnancy. Dopamine receptor antagonists are known to increase secretion of PRL.

Through its effect on water permeability in renal collecting ducts, ADH regulates extracellular osmolarity and blood volume Oxytocin acts on areolar myoepithelial cells as part of the milk letdown reflex during suckling and enhances uterine activity during labor.

What factors determine the surgical approach in this patient?

The pituitary gland is attached to the brain by a stalk and extends downward to lie in the sella turcica of the sphenoid bone. Anteriorly, posteriorly, and inferiorly, it is bordered by bone. Laterally, it is bordered by the cavernous sinus, which contains cranial nerves III, IV, V_1, and VI, as well as the cavernous portion of the carotid artery. Superiorly, the diaphragma sella, a thick dural reflection, usually tightly encircles the stalk and forms the roof of the sella turcica. In close proximity to the stalk lie the optic nerves and chiasm. The hypothalamus lies contiguous and superior to the stalk.

Tumors less than 10 mm in diameter are usually approached via the transsphenoidal route, whereas tumors greater than 20 mm in diameter and with significant suprasellar extension are approached via a bifrontal craniotomy. With the use of prophylactic antibiotics, morbidity and mortality rates are significantly less with the transsphenoidal approach; the operation is carried out with the aid of a microscope through an incision in the gingival mucosa beneath the upper lip. The surgeon enters the nasal cavity, dissects through the nasal septum, and finally penetrates the roof of the sphenoid sinus to enter the floor of the sella turcica.

What are the major problems associated with the transsphenoidal approach?

Problems include (1) the need for mucosal injections of epinephrine-containing solution to reduce bleeding, (2) the accumulation of blood and tissue debris in the pharynx and stomach, (3) the risk of hemorrhage from inadvertent entry into the cavernous sinus or the internal carotid artery, (4) cranial nerve damage, and (5) pituitary hypofunction. Prophylactic administration of glucocorticoids is routinely used in most centers. Diabetes insipidus develops postoperatively in up to 40% of patients but is usually transient. Less commonly, the diabetes insipidus presents intraoperatively. The supine and slightly head-up position used for this procedure may also predispose to venous air embolism.

What type of tumor does this patient have?

Tumors in or around the sella turcica account for 10% to 15% of intracranial neoplasms. Pituitary adenomas are most common, followed by craniopharyngiomas and then parasellar meningiomas. Primary malignant pituitary and metastatic tumors are rare. Pituitary tumors that secrete hormones (functional tumors) usually present early, when they are still relatively small (<10 mm). Other tumors present late, with signs of increased ICP (headache, nausea, and vomiting) or compression of contiguous structures (visual disturbances or pituitary hypofunction). Compression of the optic chiasm classically results in bitemporal hemianopia. Compression of normal pituitary tissue produces progressive endocrine dysfunction. Failure of hormonal secretion usually progresses in the order of gonadotropins, GH, ACTH, and TSH. Diabetes insipidus can also be seen preoperatively. Rarely, hemorrhage into the pituitary results in acute panhypopituitarism (pituitary apoplexy) with signs of a rapidly expanding mass, hemodynamic instability, and hypoglycemia.

This patient has the most common type of secretory adenoma—that producing hyperprolactinemia. Women with this tumor typically have amenorrhea, galactorrhea, or both. Men with prolactin-secreting adenomas may have galactor-rhea or infertility, but more commonly present with symptoms of an expanding mass.

What other types of secretory hormones are seen?

Adenomas secreting ACTH (Cushing's disease) produce classic manifestations of Cushing's syndrome: truncal obesity, moon facies, abdominal striae, proximal muscle weakness, hypertension, and osteoporosis. Glucose tolerance is typically impaired, but frank diabetes is less common (<20%). Hirsutism, acne, and amenorrhea are also commonly seen in women.

Adenomas that secrete GH are often large and result in either gigantism (prepubertal patients) or acromegaly (adults). Excessive growth prior to epiphyseal fusion results in massive growth of the entire skeleton. After epiphyseal closure, the abnormal growth is limited to soft tissues and acral parts: hands, feet, nose, and mandible. Patients develop osteoarthritis, which often affects the temporomandibular joint and spine. Diabetes, myopathies, and neuropathies are common. Cardiovascular complications include hypertension, premature coronary disease, and cardiomyopathy in some patients. The most serious anesthetic problem encountered in these patients is difficulty in intubating the trachea.

Are any special monitors required for transsphenoidal surgery?

Monitoring should be carried out in somewhat the same way as for craniotomies. Visual evoked potentials may be employed with large tumors that involve the optic nerves. Precordial Doppler sonography may be used for detecting venous air embolism. Venous access with large bore catheters is desirable in the event of massive hemorrhage

What modifications, if any, are necessary in the anesthetic technique?

The same principles discussed for craniotomies apply, particularly if the patient has evidence of increased ICP. Intravenous antibiotic prophylaxis and glucocorticoid coverage (hydrocortisone, 100 mg) are usually given prior to induction. Many clinicians avoid nitrous oxide to prevent problems with a postoperative pneumocephalus (see above). Intense neuromuscular blockade is important to prevent movement while the surgeon is using the microscope. In some circumstances, the surgeon may request placement of a lumbar intrathecal catheter to drain CSF, thereby facilitating surgical exposure.

SUGGESTED READING

Bell R, Vo A, Vexnedaroglu E, et al: The endovascular operating room as an extension of the intensive care unit: changing strategies in the management of neurovascular disease. Neurosurgery 2006;59: S3-56.

Dinsmore J: Anaesthesia for elective neurosurgery. Br J Anaesth 2007;99:68.

Frost E, Booij L: Anesthesia in the patient for awake craniotomy. Curr Opin Anaesthesiol 2007;20:331.

Gonzalez A, Jeyanandarajan D, Hansen C, et al: Intraoperative neurophysiologic monitoring during spine surgery: a review. Neurosurg Focus 2009;27:1.

Gupta AK, Azami J: Update of neuromonitoring. Curr Anaesth Crit Care 2002;13:120.

Nadjat C, Ziv K, Osborn I: Anesthesia for carotid and cerebrovascular procedures in interventional neuroradiology. Int Anesthesiol Clin 2009;47:29.

Poon C, Irewin M: Anaesthesia for deep brain stimulation and in patients with implanted neurostimulator devices. Br J Anaesth 2009; 103:152.

Priebe H: Aneurysmal subarachnoid haemorrhage and the anaesthetist. Br J Anaesth 2007;99:102.

Rozet I: Anesthesia for functional neurosurgery: the role of dexmedetomidine. Curr Opin Anaesthesiol 2008;21:537.

Wang L, Paech M: Neuroanesthesia for the pregnant woman. Anesth Analg 2008;107:193.

Venkatraghavan L, Luciano M, Manninen P: Anesthetic management of patients undergoing deep brain stimulation insertion. Anesth Analg 2010;110:1138.

Anesthesia for Patients with Neurologic & Psychiatric Diseases

1. Induction of anesthesia in patients receiving long-term levodopa therapy may result in either marked hypotension or hypertension.

2. In patients with multiple sclerosis, increases in body temperature cause exacerbation of symptoms.

3. The major risk of anesthesia in patients with autonomic dysfunction is severe hypotension, compromising cerebral and coronary blood flow.

4. Autonomic hyperreflexia should be expected in patients with lesions above T6 and can be precipitated by surgical manipulations.

5. The most important interaction between anesthetic agents and tricyclic antidepressants is an exaggerated response to both indirect-acting vasopressors and sympathetic stimulation.

Patients with vascular and nonvascular neurologic diseases and/or psychiatric disorders are frequently encountered by anesthesia staff. Anesthesiologists must have a basic understanding of the major neurologic and psychiatric disorders and their drug therapy. Failure to recognize potential adverse anesthetic interactions may result in avoidable perioperative morbidity.

Cerebrovascular Disease

Preoperative Considerations

Patients with diagnosed cerebrovascular disease typically have a history of transient ischemic attacks (TIAs) or stroke. Patients with TIAs undergoing surgery for other indications have an increased risk of perioperative stroke. Asymptomatic carotid bruits occur in up to 4% of patients older than age 40 years, but do not necessarily indicate significant carotid artery obstruction. Fewer than 10% of patients with completely asymptomatic bruits have hemodynamically significant carotid artery lesions. An asymptomatic carotid bruit may not increase the risk of stroke following surgery, but increases the likelihood of coexisting coronary artery disease. Moreover, the absence of a bruit does not exclude significant carotid obstruction.

The risk of perioperative stroke increases with patient age and varies with the type of surgery. The overall risk of stroke associated with surgery is low, but is greater in patients undergoing cardiovascular surgery. Rates of stroke after general anesthesia and surgery range from 0.08% to 0.4%. Even in patients with known cerebrovascular disease, the risk is only 0.4% to 3.3%. Patients at greatest risk of postoperative stroke are those undergoing open heart procedures for valvular disease, coronary artery disease with ascending aortic atherosclerosis, and diseases of the thoracic aorta. Stroke following open heart surgery is usually due to embolism of air, clots, or atheromatous debris. In one study, 6.1% of patients experienced an adverse neurological outcome following cardiac surgery. Stroke following thoracic aortic surgery may be due to emboli or ischemia secondary to prolonged circulatory arrest or a clamp placed close to the origin of the carotid artery.

The pathophysiology of postoperative strokes following noncardiovascular surgery is less clear, but may involve severe sustained hypotension or hypertension. Hypotension with severe hypoperfusion can result in so-called "watershed" zone infarctions or thrombosis of cerebral arteries, whereas hypertension can result in intracerebral hemorrhage (hemorrhagic stroke). Sustained hypertension can disrupt the blood–brain barrier and promote cerebral edema. Widened pulse pressure (>80 mm Hg) can produce endothelial vessel injury, potentially resulting in cerebral hypoperfusion or embolism. Perioperative atrial fibrillation can likewise lead to atrial clot formation and cerebral embolism. The period of time during which anesthesia and surgery should best be avoided following a stroke has not been determined. Abnormalities in regional blood flow and metabolic rate usually resolve after 2 weeks, whereas alterations in CO_2 responsiveness and the blood–brain barrier may require more than 4 weeks. However, urgent surgery is performed for acute intracranial hemorrhage, symptomatic carotid disease, and cardiac sources of emboli.

Patients with TIAs have a history of transient (<24 h) impairment, and, by definition, no residual neurologic impairment. These attacks are thought to result from emboli of fibrin-platelet aggregates or atheromatous debris from plaques in extracranial vessels. Unilateral visual impairment, numbness or weakness of an extremity, or aphasia is suggestive of carotid disease, whereas bilateral visual impairment, dizziness, ataxia, dysarthria, bilateral weakness, or amnesia is suggestive of vertebral–basilar disease. Patients with TIAs have a 30% to 40% chance of developing a frank stroke within 5 years; 50% of these strokes occur within the first year. Patients with TIAs should not undergo any elective surgical procedure without an adequate medical evaluation that generally includes at least noninvasive (Doppler) flow and imaging studies. The presence of an ulcerative plaque of greater than 60% occlusion is generally an indication for carotid endarterectomy or endovascular intervention.

PREOPERATIVE MANAGEMENT

Preoperative assessment requires neurologic and cardiovascular evaluations. The type of stroke, the presence of neurologic deficits, and the extent of residual impairment should be determined. Thromboembolic strokes usually occur in patients with generalized atherosclerosis. Most patients are elderly and have comorbid conditions, such as hypertension, hyperlipidemia, and diabetes. Coexisting coronary artery disease and renal impairment are common. Following nonhemorrhagic strokes or TIAs, many patients are placed on long-term warfarin and/or antiplatelet therapy. Management of antiplatelet therapy and antithrombotic therapy should be reviewed by the anesthesia, primary care, and surgical teams to determine the risk/benefit of the discontinuation or maintenance of such therapy perioperatively. Other systemic diseases, such as diabetes, hypertension, coronary artery disease, heart failure, and chronic obstructive lung disease frequently manifest in the patient with cerebrovascular disease.

INTRAOPERATIVE MANAGEMENT

Patients may present for surgery following embolic, thrombotic, and hemorrhagic strokes.

Management of the patient following acute embolic stroke is directed toward the embolic source. Cardiac surgery is performed to remove atrial myxomas. Systemic emboli can also be produced from endocarditic vegetations, as well as from degenerated heart valves and intracardiac thrombus.

Patients with acute strokes secondary to carotid occlusive disease present for carotid endarterectomy and endovascular procedures. When an awake carotid endarterectomy is undertaken, the patient serves as a monitor of the adequacy of cerebral blood flow during application of vessel clamps to facilitate the surgical repair. When general anesthesia is used electroencephalography, evoked potentials, carotid stump pressure, cerebral infrared spectroscopy, transcranial Doppler, and surgeon subjective sense of collateral back flow are all used to estimate the adequacy of cerebral oxygen delivery during cross clamp. When monitors or lack of appropriate patient response indicate hypoperfusion, the surgeon places a shunt to deliver blood to the brain around the cross-clamped vessel. Even with adequate cerebral blood flow, perioperative stroke can occur during carotid surgery secondary to emboli.

Management of patients following thrombotic or hemorrhagic stroke for nonneurological surgery must be individualized. Cerebral autoregulation of blood flow may fail, leaving flow directly dependent upon cerebral perfusion pressure (Figure 28–1). The penumbra of potentially salvageable neurologic tissue may therefore be very sensitive to injury from the effects of both hypotension and hypertension (Figure 28–2).

Patients taken to surgery following administration of thrombolytic therapy are at risk of cerebral hemorrhage, and tighter blood pressure control may be indicated to mitigate the possibility of cerebral bleeding.

Patients with intracerebral hemorrhage or traumatic brain injury undergo evacuation of

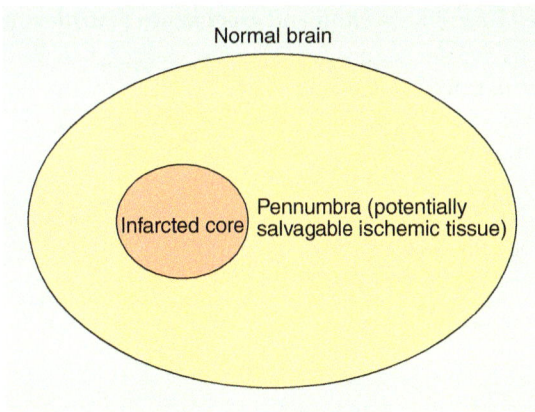

FIGURE 28–2 Penumbra. (Reproduced, with permission, from Shaikh S: Anesthesia consideration for the patient with acute ischemic stroke. Semin Cardiothorac Vasc Anesth 2010;14:62.)

hematoma and decompressive craniectomy. These patients usually require invasive arterial pressure monitoring to facilitate blood pressure management in settings where cerebral autoregulation is likely deranged (Figure 28–1). Hypertension is frequently treated with intravenous vasodilators and β-blockers. Subarachnoid hemorrhage is discussed in Chapter 27.

INTRACRANIAL MASS LESIONS

Patients with intracranial mass lesions present to surgery with both malignant and nonmalignant lesions. Such patients frequently present to their primary care physicians with complaints of headache, vision disturbance, or seizures. Radiologic studies confirm the presence of a lesion, and initial treatment is aimed at decreasing cerebral edema with dexamethasone. Electrolytes should be reviewed perioperatively in all patients undergoing cranial surgery, as both hyponatremia and hypernatremia can develop secondary to cerebral salt wasting, inappropriate antidiuretic hormone secretion, or central diabetes insipidus (Table 28–1). Patients with altered mentation preoperatively may likewise be dehydrated. Hyperglycemia secondary to steroid use is frequently seen.

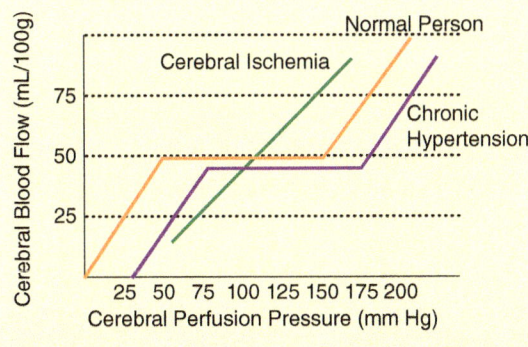

FIGURE 28–1 Cerebral autoregulation in a normal person, cerebral ischemia, and chronic hypertension. (Reproduced, with permission, from Shaikh S: Anesthesia consideration for the patient with acute ischemic stroke. Semin Cardiothorac Vasc Anesth 2010;14:62.)

TABLE 28–1 Fluid and electrolyte disorders associated with intracranial pathology.

Condition	Serum Sodium Concentration	Plasma Volume	Serum Osmolality	Urine Sodium Concentration	Urine Osmolality	Treatment
SIADH	Low	Normal or increased	Low	High	High	Fluid restriction
CSWS	Low	Decreased	Normal or high	High	Normal or high	Isotonic or hypertonic saline
DI	High	Decreased	High	Normal	Low	Hypotonic saline + vasopressin

CSWS, cerebral salt wasting; DI, diabetes insipidus; SIADH, syndrome of inappropriate antidiuretic hormone secretion.
Reproduced, with permission, from Reddy U, Amin Y: Preoperative assessment of neurosurgical patients. Anaesth Intensive Care Med 2010;11:357.

Seizure Disorders

Preoperative Considerations

Seizures represent abnormal synchronized electrical activity in the brain. They may be a manifestation of an underlying central nervous system disease, a systemic disorder, or idiopathic. Potential underlying mechanisms are thought to include (1) loss of inhibitory activity, (2) enhanced release of excitatory amino acids, and (3) enhanced neuronal firing due to abnormal voltage-mediated Ca^{2+} currents. Up to 2% of the population may experience a seizure in their lifetime. Epilepsy is a disorder characterized by recurrent paroxysmal seizure activity. Healthy individuals who experience an isolated nonrecurrent seizure are not considered to have epilepsy.

Seizure activity may be localized to a specific area in the brain or may be generalized. Moreover, initially localized (focal) seizures can subsequently spread, becoming generalized. A simple classification scheme is presented in Table 28–2. Partial

TABLE 28–2 Classification of seizures.

Partial (focal)
   Simple
   Complex
   Secondarily generalized tonic–clonic

Generalized
   Absence (petit mal)
   Myoclonic
   Clonic
   Tonic
   Tonic–clonic (grand mal)
   Atonic

seizures (also called focal) are clinically manifested by motor, sensory, autonomic, or psychiatric symptoms, depending on the cortical area affected. Focal seizures associated with impairment in consciousness are termed "complex partial" (psychomotor or temporal lobe) seizures. Generalized seizures characteristically produce bilaterally symmetric electrical activity without local onset. They result with or without abnormal motor activity, loss of consciousness, or both. Generalized activity resulting in isolated, transient lapses in consciousness are called absence (petit mal) seizures. Other generalized seizures are usually classified according to the type of motor activity. Tonic–clonic (grand mal) seizures are most common and are characterized by a loss of consciousness followed by clonic and then tonic motor activity.

PREOPERATIVE MANAGEMENT

Anesthetic evaluation should focus primarily on the underlying disorder and secondarily on the seizures. One should determine the cause and type of seizure activity and the drugs with which the patient is being treated. Seizures in adults are most commonly due to structural brain lesions (head trauma, tumor, degeneration, or stroke) or metabolic abnormalities (uremia, hepatic failure, hypoglycemia, hypocalcemia, drug toxicity, or drug/alcohol withdrawal). Idiopathic seizures occur most often in children, but may persist into adulthood. Characterization of the type of seizure is important in detecting such activity

TABLE 28–3 Commonly used antiepileptic drugs, mechanisms of action and common side effects.

Drug	Mechanism of Action	Major Side Effects	Comments
Phenytoin	Blocks voltage sensitive Na^+ channels	Dizziness, drowsiness, blurred vision, ataxia Fatigue Nausea and vomiting Constipation, abdominal pain, anorexia	Low therapeutic index Zero order kinetics Enzyme inducer Gingival hyperplasia Megaloblastic anaemia
Phenobarbital	Potentiates GABAergic inhibition AMPA receptor blockade	Sedation, dizziness, confusion, excitement	
Carbamazepine	Blocks voltage sensitive Na^+ channels	Allergic reactions	Introduced slowly
Oxycarbamazepine		Visual disturbance Enzyme induction Tetratogenic	Titrated to side effects
Valproic acid	Increases synthesis and release of GABA Reduces GHB Inhibits NMDA receptors	Sedation, tremor Weight gain Spina bifida Thrombocytopenia	Drug of choice in elderly Caution when combined with lamotrigine
Lamotrigine	Blocks voltage sensitive Na^+ channels	Allergic reactions	Non-sedative
Ethosuximide	Reduces low-threshold T-type Ca^{2+} currents in animals	Apathy, depression and drowsiness Nausea and vomiting	
Vigabatrine	Structural GABA analogue Irreversibly inhibits GABA-transaminase	Visual field defects	
Topiramate	Potentiates GABAergic inhibition	Allergic reactions Depression	Pulmonary embolism
Gabapentin	Unknown Reduces GABA	Somnolence, fatigue Ataxia	Used in intractable complex partial seizures

AMPA, α-amino-3-hydroxy-5-methyl-4-isoxazolepropionic acid; GABA, γ-amino butyric acid; GHB, γ-hydroxybutyric acid; NMDA, *N*-methyl-D-aspartate.
Adapted, with permission, from Veenith T, Burnstein RM. Management of patients with neurological and psychiatric disorders. Surgery 2010;28:441.

perioperatively. Seizures—particularly grand mal seizures—are serious complicating factors in surgical patients and should be treated promptly to prevent musculoskeletal injury, hypoventilation, hypoxemia, and aspiration of gastrointestinal content. Even partial seizures can progress to grand mal seizures. If a seizure occurs, maintaining an open airway and adequate oxygenation are the first priorities. Intravenous propofol (50–100 mg), phenytoin (500–1000 mg slowly), or a benzodiazepine such as diazepam (5–10 mg) or midazolam (1–5 mg) can be used to terminate the seizure.

Most patients with seizure disorders receive antiepileptic drugs preoperatively (Table 28–3). Antiseizure medications should be continued throughout the perioperative period to maintain therapeutic levels.

INTRAOPERATIVE MANAGEMENT

In selecting anesthetic agents, drugs with epileptogenic potential should be avoided, most notably the general anesthetic enflurane (now of only historic interest). Theoretically, ketamine and methohexital (in small doses) can precipitate seizure activity. Hypothetically, large doses of atracurium, cisatracurium, or meperidine may be relatively contraindicated because of the reported epileptogenic potential of their respective metabolites, laudanosine, and normeperidine. Hepatic microsomal enzyme induction should be expected from chronic antiseizure therapy. Enzyme induction may increase the dose requirement and frequency of intravenous anesthetics and nondepolarizing neuromuscular blockers (NMBs) and may increase the risk for hepatotoxicity from halothane.

Degenerative & Demyelinating Diseases

PARKINSON DISEASE

Preoperative Considerations

Parkinson disease (PD) is a common movement disorder that typically afflicts individuals aged 50–70 years; it has a prevalence of 3% in the United States and Canada. This neurodegenerative disease is characterized by bradykinesia, rigidity, postural instability, and resting (pill-rolling) tremor. Additional frequently occurring findings include facial masking, hypophonia, dysphagia, and gait disturbances. Increasing problems with freezing, rigidity, and tremor eventually result in physical incapacitation. Early in the course of the disease, intellectual function is usually preserved, but declines in intellectual function may be severe as the disease progresses. PD is caused by a progressive loss of dopamine in the nigrostriatum. The severity of loss of dopamine correlates with the severity of bradykinesia. Concurrent with the loss of dopamine, the activity of the gamma-aminobutyric acid (GABA) nuclei in the basal ganglia increases, leading to an inhibition of thalamic and brainstem nuclei. Thalamic inhibition, in turn, suppresses the motor system in the cortex, resulting in the characteristic signs and symptoms.

Medical treatment is directed at controlling the symptoms. A variety of drugs may be used for mild disease, including the anticholinergic agents

trihexyphenidyl, benztropine, and ethopropazine; the irreversible monoamine oxidase (MAO) inhibitors selegiline and rasagiline; and the antiviral drug, amantadine. Moderate to severe disease is typically treated pharmacologically with dopaminergic agents, either levodopa (a precursor of dopamine) or a dopamine-receptor agonist. Levodopa, which is given with a decarboxylase inhibitor to retard the peripheral breakdown of the drug (thereby increasing its central delivery and decreasing the dose of levodopa that is required to control symptoms), is the most effective therapy and is used to treat moderate to severe symptoms. Catechol methyltransferase inhibitors are also used to prevent the decarboxylation of levodopa. Levodopa is available in either an immediate or sustained-release formulation, with durations of action of 2–4 hr and 3–6 hr, respectively. Side effects include nausea, vomiting, dyskinesias, sudden sleepiness, cardiac irritability, and orthostatic hypotension. Dopamine receptor agonists include both ergot derivatives (bromocriptine, cabergoline, lisuride, and apomorphine) and nonergot derivatives (pramipexole and ropinirole). The nonergot derivatives have been shown to be beneficial when used as monotherapy in early PD; all dopamine receptor agonists are effective when given as combination therapy with levodopa in the treatment of moderate to severe PD. Side effects are similar to those found with the use of levodopa alone, and, in addition, include headache, confusion, and hallucinations. Pulmonary and retroperitoneal fibrosis, pleural effusion and thickening, Raynaud syndrome, and erythromyalgia are more common side effects with the use of ergot derivatives than with nonergot derivatives.

The surgical treatment of PD includes both ablative procedures (thalamotomy and pallidotomy), as well as electrical stimulation of the ventral intermediate nucleus of the thalamus, the globus pallidus internus, or the subthalamic nucleus. Pallidotomy is effective for treating the dyskinesia (70% to 90%), as well as the tremor, rigidity, bradykinesia, and gait symptoms (30% to 50%) of the disorder. Thalamotomy is most effective in treating the contralateral tremor, but not for the other symptoms of the disease, and has been largely replaced by the use of thalamic stimulation. The efficacy of deep brain stimulation of the thalamus is related to the effect on tremor; it has little to no effect on the other symptoms of PD. Subthalamic stimulation improves all of the primary symptoms of PD and decreases the amount of medication necessary for symptom relief. Bilateral stimulation has greater efficacy than unilateral stimulation. Some decrease in cognitive function may occur with this treatment, and, therefore, it should be used with caution in patients with cognitive impairment. The effects of globus pallidus internus stimulation are similar to those of pallidotomy with improvements in dyskinesia.

Anesthetic Considerations

Medications for PD should be continued perioperatively, including the morning of surgery. The half-life of levodopa is short. Abrupt withdrawal of levodopa can cause worsening of muscle rigidity and may interfere with ventilation. Phenothiazines, butyrophenones (droperidol), and metoclopramide can exacerbate symptoms as a consequence of their antidopaminergic activity and should be avoided. Anticholinergics (atropine) or antihistamines (diphenhydramine) may be used for acute exacerbation of symptoms. Diphenhydramine may be used for premedication and intraoperative sedation in patients with tremor. Induction of anesthesia **❶** in patients receiving long-term levodopa therapy may result in either marked hypotension or hypertension. Relative hypovolemia, catecholamine depletion, autonomic instability, and sensitization to catecholamines are probably contributory. Arterial blood pressure should be monitored carefully. Hypotension should be treated with small doses of a direct-acting vasopressor, such as phenylephrine, rather than ephedrine. The response to NMBs is generally normal, however, hyperkalemia may rarely follow succinylcholine. As mentioned previously, patients who fail medical treatment are candidates for surgical intervention—for example, an ablative therapy, such as a thalamotomy or pallidotomy or implantation of a deep brain stimulator of the subthalamic nucleus, the ventral intermediate nucleus, or the globus pallidus internus. Because general anesthesia alters the threshold for stimulation,

correct placement of the electrodes can be affected. Awake craniotomy has been the norm for epilepsy surgery, and is being used increasingly for deep brain stimulation procedures. Two techniques are advocated—a true awake craniotomy with heavy sedation (dexmedetomidine is often used) and an approach in which the patient receives a general anesthetic, usually a total intravenous anesthetic with propofol and remifentanil and a laryngeal mask airway for control of the airway. Following appropriate surgical exposure, the intravenous infusions are discontinued, and the laryngeal mask airway is removed. The patient can be reanesthetized once the implantation of leads is complete.

ALZHEIMER DISEASE
Preoperative Considerations

Neurodegenerative diseases often lead to dementia. Along with a loss of gray matter, elderly patients have altered pharmacokinetic and pharmacodynamic responses to many drugs that are used to induce and maintain anesthesia or sedation. Alzheimer disease (AD) is the most common neurodegenerative disease, causing approximately 40% to 80% of all cases of dementia, with a prevalence of approximately 20% in patients older than age 80 years. The disease is characterized by a slow decline in intellectual function. Progressive impairment of memory, judgment, and decision-making and emotional lability are hallmarks of the disease. Late in the course of the disease, severe extrapyramidal signs, apraxias, and aphasia are often present. Although some degree of brain atrophy is normal with advancing age, patients with AD usually show marked cortical atrophy with ventricular enlargement; the pathological hallmarks of AD seen at necropsy include neurofibrillary tangles that contain the phosphorylated microtubular protein tau and neuritic plaques composed of the peptide β-amyloid.

Anesthetic Considerations

Anesthetic management of patients with moderate to severe AD is often complicated by disorientation and uncooperativeness. New onset of temporary cognitive impairment is frequent in elderly patients and often persists for 1–3 days following surgery. Such patients require repeated reassurance and explanation. Legally incompetent patients cannot provide informed consent for anesthesia or surgery. Premedication is usually not given, and only small doses are used. Centrally acting anticholinergics, such as atropine and scopolamine, may contribute to postoperative confusion. Glycopyrrolate, which does not cross the blood–brain barrier, may be the preferred agent when an anticholinergic is required.

Laboratory studies have shown that anesthetic agents are increasingly associated with neuronal injury and cell death The outcome implications of general anesthesia in both the elderly and small children are currently the subject of much investigation and debate. Apoptotic neurodegeneration has been linked to the use of GABA receptor modulators and N-methyl-D-aspartic acid receptor antagonists, of which both mechanisms are used by common general anesthetics. Moreover, increased β-amyloid production is associated with both anesthetic exposure and AD. Consequently, there are concerns that anesthetic exposure may worsen dementia in the patient with AD; however, definitive conclusions regarding the risk of anesthetic toxicity in the patient with AD are not yet available.

MULTIPLE SCLEROSIS
Preoperative Considerations

Multiple sclerosis (MS) is characterized by reversible demyelination at random and multiple sites in the brain and spinal cord; chronic inflammation, however, eventually produces scarring (gliosis). The disease may be an autoimmune disorder that is initiated by a viral infection. It primarily affects patients between 20 and 40 years of age, with a 2:1 female predominance, and typically follows an unpredictable course of frequent attacks and remissions. With time, remissions become less complete, and the disease progresses to incapacitation; almost 50% of patients will require help with walking within 15 years of diagnosis. Clinical manifestations

depend on the sites affected, but frequently include sensory disturbances (paresthesias), visual problems (optic neuritis and diplopia), and motor weakness. Symptoms develop over the course of days and remit over weeks to months. Early diagnosis of exacerbations can often be confirmed by analysis of cerebrospinal fluid and magnetic resonance imaging. Remyelination is limited and often fails to occur. Moreover, axonal loss can develop. Changes in neurological function seem to be related to changes in axonal conduction. Conduction can occur across demyelinated axons, but seems to be affected by multiple factors, particularly temperature. Increases in body temperature cause exacerbation of symptoms.

The treatment of MS may be primarily symptomatic or used in an attempt to arrest the disease process. Diazepam, dantrolene, or baclofen, and, in refractory cases, an intrathecal delivery system for baclofen are used to control spasticity; bethanechol and other anticholinergics are useful for urinary retention. Painful dysesthesia may respond to carbamazepine, phenytoin, or antidepressants. Glucocorticoids may decrease the severity and duration of acute attacks. Corticosteroid-resistant relapses may respond to five to seven courses of plasma exchange offered on alternate days. Interferon has also been used to treat MS. Immunosuppression with azathioprine or cyclophosphamide may also be attempted to halt disease progression. Mitoxantrone is used for relapsing and progressive MS. The systemic effects of these therapies on coagulation and immunologic and cardiac function should be reviewed preoperatively.

Anesthetic Considerations

The effect of stress, anesthesia, and surgery on the course of MS is controversial. Overall, the effect of anesthesia is unpredictable. Elective surgery should be avoided during relapse, regardless of the anesthetic technique employed. The preoperative consent record should document counseling of the patient to the effect that the stress of surgery and anesthesia might worsen the symptoms. Spinal anesthesia has been associated with exacerbation of the disease; however, the entire surgery/delivery/

anesthetic process may likewise lead to exacerbations. Peripheral nerve blocks are less of a concern because MS is a disease of the central nervous system; however, patients may also have peripheral neuropathies. Epidural and other regional techniques seem to have no adverse effect on the course of the disease. No specific interactions with general anesthetics are recognized. Patients with advanced disease may have a labile cardiovascular system due to autonomic dysfunction. In the setting of paresis or paralysis, succinylcholine should be avoided because of hyperkalemia. Regardless of the anesthetic technique employed, increases in body temperature should be avoided. Irrespective of anesthetic technique, patients may experience a worsening of symptoms perioperatively and should be counseled accordingly.

AMYOTROPHIC LATERAL SCLEROSIS

Motor neuron disease is another common neurodegenerative disease, with amyotrophic lateral sclerosis (ALS) being the most prevalent. The cause of ALS is unknown, although small numbers of patients with the familial form of the disease have a defect in the superoxide dismutase-1 gene. ALS is a rapidly progressive disorder of both upper and lower motor neurons. Clinically, patients present in the fifth or sixth decade of life with muscular weakness, atrophy, fasciculation, and spasticity. The disease may initially be asymmetric, but over the course of 2–3 years becomes generalized, involving all skeletal and bulbar muscles. Progressive respiratory muscle weakness makes the patient susceptible to aspiration and eventually leads to death from ventilatory failure. Although the heart is unaffected, autonomic dysfunction can be seen. There is no specific treatment for ALS.

The primary emphasis in management is judicious respiratory care. As with other patients with lower motor neuron disease, succinylcholine is contraindicated because of the risk of hyperkalemia. Adequacy of ventilation should be carefully assessed both intraoperatively and postoperatively; an awake extubation is desirable. Difficulty in weaning patients from mechanical ventilation postoperatively is not uncommon in patients with moderate to advanced disease.

GUILLAIN–BARRÉ SYNDROME

Guillain–Barré syndrome (GBS), a relatively common disorder affecting one to four individuals per 100,000 population, is characterized by a sudden onset of ascending motor paralysis, areflexia, and variable paresthesias. Subtypes of GBS include acute inflammatory demyelinating polyneuropathy (about 75% of cases), acute motor axonal neuropathy (with antibodies against gangliosides), and acute motor sensory axonal neuropathy. Bulbar involvement, including respiratory muscle paralysis, is a frequent complication. Pathologically, the disease seems to be an immunologic reaction against the myelin sheath of peripheral nerves, particularly lower motor neurons. In most instances, the syndrome seems to follow viral respiratory or gastrointestinal infections; the disorder can also present as a paraneoplastic syndrome associated with Hodgkin's disease or as a complication of human immunodeficiency virus infection. Some patients respond to plasmapheresis. The prognosis is relatively good, with most patients recovering completely; unfortunately, however, approximately 10% of patients die of complications, and another 10% are left with long-term neurologic sequelae.

Anesthetic management is complicated by lability of the autonomic nervous system in addition to concerns about respiratory insufficiency. Exaggerated hypotensive and hypertensive responses during anesthesia may be seen. As with other lower motor neuron disorders, succinylcholine should not be used because of the risk of hyperkalemia. The use of regional anesthesia in these patients remains controversial, as it might worsen symptoms. As with all decisions, the risks and benefits of regional versus general anesthesia must be weighed on an individual basis. As damaged nerves are more susceptible to a second injury (the "double crush" effect), performance of neuraxial techniques in patients with preexistent neurologic dysfunction should be carefully considered.

AUTONOMIC DYSFUNCTION

Preoperative Considerations

Autonomic dysfunction, or dysautonomia, may be due to generalized or segmental disorders of the central or peripheral nervous system. Symptoms can be generalized, segmental, or focal. These disorders may be congenital, familial, or acquired. Common manifestations include impotence; bladder and gastrointestinal dysfunction; abnormal regulation of body fluids; decreased sweating, lacrimation, and salivation; and orthostatic hypotension. The latter can be the most serious manifestation of the disorder.

Acquired autonomic dysfunction can be isolated (pure autonomic failure), part of a more generalized degenerative process (Shy–Drager syndrome, PD, olivopontocerebellar atrophy), part of a segmental neurological process (MS, syringomyelia, reflex sympathetic dystrophy, or spinal cord injury), or a manifestation of disorders affecting peripheral nerves (GBS, diabetes, chronic alcoholism, amyloidosis, or porphyria).

Congenital or familial dysautonomia occurs most frequently in Ashkenazi Jewish children and is usually referred to as Riley–Day syndrome. Autonomic dysfunction is prominent and is associated with generalized diminished sensation and emotional lability. Moreover, patients are predisposed to dysautonomic crises triggered by stress and characterized by marked hypertension, tachycardia, abdominal pain, diaphoresis, and vomiting. Intravenous diazepam is effective in resolving such episodes. Hereditary dysautonomia associated with a deficiency of dopamine β-hydroxylase is described. Administration of α-dihydroxyphenylserine improves symptoms in these patients.

Anesthetic Considerations

3 The major risk of anesthesia in patients with autonomic dysfunction is severe hypotension, compromising cerebral and coronary blood flow. Marked hypertension can be equally deleterious. Most patients are chronically hypovolemic. The vasodilatory effects of spinal and epidural anesthesia are poorly tolerated. Similarly, the vasodilatory and cardiac depressant effects of most general anesthetic agents combined with positive airway pressure can be equally problematic. Continuous intraarterial blood pressure monitoring is useful. Hypotension should be treated with fluids and direct-acting vasopressors (in preference to indirect-acting agents). Enhanced sensitivity to vasopressors due to denervation sensitivity may be observed. Blood loss also is usually poorly tolerated. Body temperature should be monitored closely. Patients with anhidrosis are particularly susceptible to hyperpyrexia.

SYRINGOMYELIA

Syringomyelia results in progressive cavitation of the spinal cord. In many cases, obstruction of cerebrospinal fluid outflow from the fourth ventricle seems to be contributory. Many patients have craniovertebral abnormalities, particularly the Arnold–Chiari malformation. Increased pressure in the central canal of the spinal cord produces enlargement or diverticulation to the point of cavitation. Syringomyelia typically affects the cervical spine, producing sensory and motor deficits in the upper extremities, and, frequently, thoracic scoliosis. Extension upward into the medulla (syringobulbia) leads to cranial nerve deficits. Syringo-peritoneal shunting and other decompressive procedures have variable success in arresting the disease.

Anesthetic evaluation should focus on defining existing neurologic deficits and any pulmonary impairment due to scoliosis. Autonomic instability should be expected in patients with extensive lesions. Succinylcholine should be avoided when muscle wasting is present because of the risk of hyperkalemia. Adequacy of ventilation and reversal of nondepolarizing NMBs should be achieved prior to extubation. Neuraxial techniques in the setting of elevated intracranial pressure are contraindicated. Case reports of epidural anesthetics having been performed for labor analgesia in patients with Arnold Chiari malformations, with and without syringomyelia, can be found in the literature. Risks of cerebral herniation, worsening nerve injury, and infection must be weighed against potential benefits.

Spinal Cord Injury

Preoperative Considerations

Most spinal cord injuries are traumatic and may arise from partial or complete transection. The majority of injuries are due to fracture and dislocation of the vertebral column. The mechanism is usually either compression and flexion at the thoracic spine or extension at the cervical spine. Clinical manifestations depend on the level of the injury. Injuries above C3–5 (diaphragmatic innervation) require patients to receive ventilatory support to stay alive. Transections above T1 result in quadriplegia, whereas those above L4 result in paraplegia. The most common sites of injury are C5–6 and T12–L1. Acute spinal cord transection produces loss of sensation, flaccid paralysis, and loss of spinal reflexes below the level of injury. These findings characterize a period of spinal shock that typically lasts 1–3 weeks.

Over the course of the next few weeks, spinal reflexes gradually return, together with muscle spasms and signs of sympathetic overactivity. Injury in the low thoracic or lumbar spine may result in cauda equina (conus medullaris) syndrome. The latter usually consists of incomplete injury to nerve roots rather than the spinal cord.

Overactivity of the sympathetic nervous system is common with transections at T5 or above, but is unusual with injuries below T10. Interruption of normal descending inhibitory impulses in the cord results in autonomic hyperreflexia. Cutaneous or visceral stimulation below the level of injury can induce intense autonomic reflexes: sympathetic discharge produces hypertension and vasoconstriction below the transection and a baroreceptor-mediated reflex bradycardia and vasodilation above the transection. Cardiac arrhythmias are common.

Emergent surgical management is undertaken whenever there is reversible compression of the spinal cord due to dislocation of a vertebral body or bony fragment. Operative treatment is also indicated for spinal instability to prevent further injury.

Anesthetic Considerations

A. Acute Transection

Anesthetic management depends on the age of the injury. In the early care of acute injuries, the emphasis should be on preventing further spinal cord damage during patient movement, airway manipulation, and positioning. High-dose corticosteroid therapy (methylprednisolone) can be used for the first 24 hr following injury to improve neurologic outcome. Airway management of the patient with unstable cervical spine is discussed in Chapter 19. Patients with high transections often have impaired airway reflexes and are further predisposed to hypoxemia because of a decrease in functional residual capacity and atelectasis. Spinal shock can lead to hypotension and bradycardia prior to any anesthetic administration. Direct arterial pressure monitoring is helpful. An intravenous fluid bolus and the use of ketamine for anesthesia may help to prevent further decreases in blood pressure; vasopressors may also be required. Succinylcholine can be used safely in the first 24 hr, but should not be used thereafter because of the risk of hyperkalemia. The latter can occur within the first week following injury and is due to excessive release of potassium secondary to the proliferation of acetylcholine receptors outside of the neuromuscular synaptic cleft.

B. Chronic Transection

Anesthetic management of patients with nonacute transections is complicated by the possibility of autonomic hyperreflexia and the risk of hyperkalemia. Autonomic hyperreflexia should be expected in patients with lesions above T6 and can be precipitated by surgical manipulations. **Regional anesthesia and deep general anesthesia are effective in preventing hyperreflexia**. Many clinicians, however, are reluctant to administer spinal and epidural anesthesia in these patients because of the difficulties encountered in determining anesthetic level, exaggerated hypotension, and technical problems resulting from deformities. Severe hypertension can result in pulmonary edema, myocardial ischemia, or cerebral hemorrhage and should be treated promptly. Direct arterial vasodilators should be readily available. Nondepolarizing muscle relaxants may be used. Body temperature should be monitored carefully, particularly in patients with transections above T1, because chronic vasodilation and loss of normal reflex cutaneous vasoconstriction predispose to hypothermia.

Encephalitis

Various forms of encephalitis can present secondary to infectious or autoimmune mechanisms. Patients with encephalitis are managed with the normal care given any patient with potentially increased intracranial pressure at risk of cerebral hypoperfusion.

Psychiatric Disorders

DEPRESSION

Depression is a very common mood disorder characterized by sadness and pessimism. Its cause is multifactorial, but pharmacological treatment is based on the presumption that its manifestations are due to a brain deficiency of dopamine, norepinephrine, and serotonin or altered receptor activities. Up to 50% of patients with major depression hypersecrete cortisol and have abnormal circadian secretion. Current pharmacological therapy utilizes drugs that increase brain levels of these neurotransmitters: tricyclic antidepressants, selective serotonin reuptake inhibitors (SSRIs), MAO inhibitors, and atypical antidepressants. The mechanisms of action of these drugs result in some potentially serious anesthetic interactions. Electroconvulsive therapy (ECT) is increasingly used for refractory severe cases and may be continued prophylactically after the patient's mood recovers. The use of general anesthesia for ECT is largely responsible for its safety and widespread acceptance.

Tricyclic Antidepressants

Tricyclic antidepressants may be used for the treatment of depression and chronic pain syndromes. All tricyclic antidepressants work at nerve synapses by blocking neuronal reuptake of catecholamines, serotonin, or both. Desipramine and nortriptyline

are used because they are less sedating and tend to have fewer side effects. Other agents are generally more sedating and include amitriptyline imipramine, protriptyline, amoxapine, doxepin, and trimipramine. Clomipramine is used in the treatment of obsessive–compulsive disorders. Most tricyclic antidepressants also have significant anticholinergic (antimuscarinic) actions: dry mouth, blurred vision, prolonged gastric emptying, and urinary retention. Quinidine-like cardiac effects include tachycardia, T-wave flattening or inversion, and prolongation of the PR, QRS, and QT intervals. Amitriptyline has the most marked anticholinergic effects, whereas doxepin has the fewest cardiac effects.

St. John's wort is being used with increased frequency as an over-the-counter therapy for depression. Because it induces hepatic enzymes, blood levels of other drugs may decrease, sometimes with serious complications. During the preoperative evaluation, the use of all over-the-counter medications should be reviewed.

Antidepressant drugs are generally continued perioperatively. Increased anesthetic requirements, presumably from enhanced brain catecholamine activity, have been reported with these agents. Potentiation of centrally acting anticholinergic agents (atropine and scopolamine) may increase the likelihood of postoperative confusion and delirium.

5 The most important interaction between anesthetic agents and tricyclic antidepressants is an exaggerated response to both indirect-acting vasopressors and sympathetic stimulation. Pancuronium, ketamine, meperidine, and epinephrine-containing local anesthetic solutions should be avoided. Chronic therapy with tricyclic antidepressants is reported to deplete cardiac catecholamines, theoretically potentiating the cardiac depressant effects of anesthetics. If hypotension occurs, small doses of a direct-acting vasopressor should be used instead of an indirect-acting agent. Amitriptyline's anticholinergic action may occasionally contribute to postoperative delirium.

Monoamine Oxidase Inhibitors

MAO inhibitors block the oxidative deamination of naturally occurring amines. At least two MAO isoenzymes (types A and B) with differential substrate selectivities have been identified. MAO-A is selective for serotonin, dopamine, and norepinephrine, whereas MAO-B is selective for dopamine and phenylethylamine. Nonselective MAO inhibitors include phenelzine isocarboxazid, and tranylcypromine. Selective MAO-B inhibitors are useful in the treatment of PD. Additionally, unlike older nonreversible MAO inhibitors, reversible, MAO-A inhibitors have been developed. Side effects include orthostatic hypotension, agitation, tremor, seizures, muscle spasms, urinary retention, paresthesias, and jaundice. The most serious sequela is a hypertensive crisis that occurs following ingestion of tyramine-containing foods (cheeses and red wines), because tyramine is used to generate norepinephrine.

The practice of discontinuing MAO inhibitors at least 2 weeks prior to elective surgery is not recommended. Phenelzine can decrease plasma cholinesterase activity and prolong the duration of succinylcholine. Opioids should generally be used with caution in patients receiving MAO inhibitors, as rare but serious reactions to opioids have been reported. Most serious reactions are associated with meperidine, resulting in hyperthermia, seizures, and coma. Meperidine should not be administered to patients receiving MAO inhibitors. As with tricyclic antidepressants, exaggerated responses to vasopressors and sympathetic stimulation should be expected. If a vasopressor is necessary, a direct-acting agent in small doses should be employed. Drugs that enhance sympathetic activity, such as ketamine, pancuronium, and epinephrine (in local anesthetic solutions), should be avoided.

Atypical Antidepressants and Selective Serotonin Reuptake Inhibitors

SSRIs include fluoxetine, sertraline, and paroxetine, which some clinicians consider first-line agents of choice for depression. A surprisingly large fraction of patients undergoing elective surgery will be receiving one of these agents. These agents have little or no anticholinergic activity and do not generally affect cardiac conduction. Their principal side effects are headache, agitation, and insomnia. Other agents include the norepinephrine/dopamine reuptake inhibitors, the serotonin/norepinephrine reuptake inhibitors, selective serotonin reuptake enhancers, and

norepinephrine-dopamine disinhibitors. Patients taking St. John's wort are at increased risk of serotonin syndrome, as are those taking drugs with similar effects (eg, MAO inhibitors, meperidine). Serotonin syndrome manifestations include agitation, hypertension, hyperthermia, tremor, acidosis, and autonomic instability. Treatment is supportive, along with the administration of a 5-HT antagonist (eg, cyprohepatadine).

BIPOLAR DISEASE

Mania is a mood disorder characterized by elation, hyperactivity, and flight of ideas. Manic episodes may alternate with depression in patients with a bipolar (formerly manic–depressive) disorder. Mania is thought to be related to excessive norepinephrine activity in the brain. Lithium which interferes with Na^+ ion transport with effects on many signaling pathways in the brain affecting neurotransmitter release, and lamotrigine, which inhibits sodium channels and modulates release of excitatory amino acids, are the drugs of choice for treating acute manic episodes and preventing their recurrence, as well as suppressing episodes of depression. Concomitant administration of an antipsychotic (haloperidol) or a benzodiazepine (lorazepam) is usually necessary during acute mania. Alternative treatments include valproic acid, carbamazepine, and aripiprazole as well as ECT.

The mechanism of action of lithium is poorly understood. It has a narrow therapeutic range, with a desirable blood concentration between 0.8 and 1.0 mEq/L. Side effects include reversible T-wave changes, mild leukocytosis, and, on rare occasions, hypothyroidism or a vasopressin-resistant diabetes insipidus-like syndrome. Toxic blood concentrations produce confusion, sedation, muscle weakness, tremor, and slurred speech. Still higher concentrations result in widening of the QRS complex, atrioventricular block, hypotension, and seizures.

Although lithium is reported to decrease minimum alveolar concentration and prolong the duration of some NMBs, clinically these effects seem to be minor. Nonetheless, this is yet another reason why neuromuscular function should be monitored when NMBs are used. Blood levels should be checked perioperatively. Sodium depletion (secondary to loop or thiazide diuretics) decreases renal excretion of lithium and can lead to lithium toxicity. Fluid restriction and overdiuresis should be avoided. Lithium dilution cardiac output measurements are contraindicated in patients on lithium therapy.

SCHIZOPHRENIA

Patients with schizophrenia display disordered thinking, withdrawal, paranoid delusions, and auditory hallucinations. This disorder is thought to be related to an excess of dopaminergic activity in the brain.

The most commonly used antipsychotics include phenothiazines, thioxanthenes, phenylbutylpiperadines, dihydroindolones, dibenzapines, benzisoxazoles, and butyrophenones. There are numerous trade names for these drugs. Older antipsychotic medications had strong dopamine antagonistic effects, leading to extrapyramidal side effects (eg, muscle rigidity and progression to tardive dyskinesia). Other agents have less dopamine antagonism and occupy the D2 dopamine receptor to a lesser degree, thereby reducing extrapyramidal effects. The antipsychotic effect of these agents seems to be due to dopamine antagonist activity. Most are sedating and mildly anxiolytic. Mild α-adrenergic blockade and anticholinergic activity are also observed. Side effects include orthostatic hypotension, acute dystonic reactions, and parkinsonism-like manifestations. Risperidone and clozapine have little extrapyramidal activity, but the latter is associated with a significant incidence of granulocytopenia. T-wave flattening, ST segment depression, and prolongation of the PR and QT intervals may be seen, increasing the risk of les torsades des pointes.

Continuing antipsychotic medication perioperatively is desirable. Reduced anesthetic requirements may be observed in some patients, and some patients may experience perioperative hypotension.

NEUROLEPTIC MALIGNANT SYNDROME

Neuroleptic malignant syndrome is a rare complication of antipsychotic therapy that may occur hours or weeks after drug administration. Meperidine and metoclopramide can also precipitate the disorder. The mechanism is related to dopamine blockade in the basal ganglia and hypothalamus and impairment of thermoregulation. In its most severe form, the presentation is similar to that of malignant hyperthermia. Muscle rigidity, hyperthermia, rhabdomyolysis, autonomic instability, and altered consciousness are seen. Creatine kinase levels are often high. The mortality rate approaches 20% to 30%, with deaths occurring primarily as a result of renal failure or arrhythmias. Treatment with dantrolene seems to be effective; bromocriptine, a dopamine agonist, may also be effective. Differential diagnoses include malignant hyperthermia and serotonin syndrome.

SUBSTANCE ABUSE

Behavioral disorders from abuse of psychotropic (mind-altering) substances may involve a socially acceptable drug (alcohol), a medically prescribed drug (eg, diazepam), or an illegal substance (eg, cocaine). Characteristically, with chronic abuse, patients develop tolerance to the drug and varying degrees of psychological and physical dependence. Physical dependence is most often seen with opioids, barbiturates, alcohol, and benzodiazepines. Life-threatening complications primarily due to sympathetic overactivity can develop during abstention.

Knowledge of a patient's substance abuse preoperatively may prevent adverse drug interactions, predict tolerance to anesthetic agents, and facilitate the recognition of drug withdrawal. The history of substance abuse may be volunteered by the patient (usually only on direct questioning) or deliberately hidden.

Anesthetic requirements for substance abusers vary, depending on whether the drug exposure is acute or chronic (see Table 28–4). Elective procedures should be postponed for acutely intoxicated patients and those with signs of withdrawal. When surgery is deemed necessary in patients with physical dependence, perioperative doses of the abused substance should be provided, or specific agents should be given to prevent withdrawal. In the case of opioid dependence, any opioid can be used, whereas for alcohol, a benzodiazepine is usually substituted due to the reluctance of hospital pharmacies to dispense

TABLE 28–4 **Effect of acute and chronic substance abuse on anesthetic requirements.**[1]

Substance	Acute	Chronic
Opioids	↓	↑
Barbiturates	↓	↑
Alcohol	↓	↑
Marijuana	↓	0
Benzodiazepines	↓	↑
Amphetamines	↑[2]	↓
Cocaine	↑[2]	0
Phencyclidine	↓	?

[1]↓, decreases; ↑, increases; 0, no effect; ?, unknown.
[2]Associated with marked sympathetic stimulation.

alcohol-containing beverages to patients. Alcoholic patients should receive B vitamin/folate supplementation to prevent Korsakoff's syndrome. Tolerance to most anesthetic agents is often seen, but is not always predictable. For general anesthesia, a technique primarily relying on a volatile inhalation agent may be preferable so that anesthetic depth can be readily adjusted according to individual need. Awareness monitoring should be likewise considered. Opioids with mixed agonist–antagonist activity should be avoided in opioid-dependent patients because such agents can precipitate acute withdrawal. Clonidine is a useful adjuvant in the treatment of postoperative withdrawal syndromes.

Patients routinely present acutely intoxicated for emergency surgery following trauma related to substance abuse. Patients have often consumed more than one class of intoxicating agent. Acute cocaine intoxication may produce hypertension secondary to the increase in central neurotransmitters, such as norepinephrine and dopamine. Hypertension and arrhythmias can occur perioperatively. Chronic abusers deplete their sympathomimetic neurotransmitters, potentially developing hypotension. Amphetamine abusers have similar anesthetic concerns, as amphetamines also affect the sympathetic nervous system.

Patients on chronic prescribed opioid therapy, or those taking medications illicitly, have substantially increased opioid postoperative requirements. Multimodal approaches to pain control are useful perioperatively, and patients should be started on maintenance methadone as soon as possible.

Consultation with pain management and addiction specialists is often indicated.

CASE DISCUSSION

Anesthesia for Electroconvulsive Therapy

A 64-year-old man with depression refractory to drug therapy is scheduled for electroconvulsive therapy (ECT).

How is ECT administered?

The electroconvulsive shock is applied to one or both cerebral hemispheres to induce a seizure. Variables include stimulus pattern, amplitude, and duration. The goal is to produce a therapeutic generalized seizure 30–60 sec in duration. Electrical stimuli are usually administered until a therapeutic seizure is induced. A good therapeutic effect is generally not achieved until a total of 400–700 seizure seconds have been induced. Because only one treatment is given per day, patients are usually scheduled for a series of treatments, generally two or three a week. Progressive memory loss often occurs with an increasing number of treatments, particularly when electrodes are applied bilaterally.

Why is anesthesia necessary?

When the efficacy of ECT was discovered, enthusiasm was tempered in the medical community because drugs were not used to control the violent seizures caused by the procedure, thus engendering a relatively high incidence of musculoskeletal injuries. Moreover, when an NMB was used alone, patients sometimes recalled being paralyzed and awake just prior to the shock. The routine use of general anesthesia to ensure amnesia and neuromuscular blockade to prevent injuries has renewed interest in ECT. The current mortality rate for ECT is estimated to be one death per 10,000 treatments.

What are the physiological effects of ECT-induced seizures?

Seizure activity is characteristically associated with an initial parasympathetic discharge followed by a more sustained sympathetic discharge. The initial phase is characterized by bradycardia and increased secretions. Marked bradycardia (<30 beats/min) and even transient asystole (up to 6 s) are occasionally seen. The hypertension and tachycardia that follow are typically sustained for several minutes. Transient autonomic imbalance can produce arrhythmias and T-wave abnormalities on the electrocardiogram. Cerebral blood flow and ICP, intragastric pressure, and intraocular pressure all transiently increase.

Are there any contraindications to ECT?

Contraindications are a recent myocardial infarction (usually <3 months), a recent stroke (usually <1 month), an intracranial mass, or increased ICP from any cause. More relative contraindications include angina, poorly controlled heart failure, significant pulmonary disease, bone fractures, severe osteoporosis, pregnancy, glaucoma, and retinal detachment.

What are the important considerations in selecting anesthetic agents?

Amnesia is required only for the brief period (1–5 min) from when the NMB is given to when a therapeutic seizure has been successfully induced. The seizure itself usually results in a brief period of anterograde amnesia, somnolence, and often confusion. Consequently, only a short-acting induction agent is necessary. Moreover, because most induction agents (barbiturates, etomidate, benzodiazepines, and propofol) have anticonvulsant properties, small doses must be used. Seizure threshold is increased and **seizure duration** is decreased by all of these agents.

Following adequate preoxygenation, methohexital, 0.5–1 mg/kg, is most commonly employed. Propofol, 1–1.5 mg/kg, may be used, but higher doses reduce seizure duration. Benzodiazepines raise the seizure threshold and decrease duration. Ketamine increases seizure duration, but is generally not used

because it also increases the incidence of delayed awakening, nausea, and ataxia and is also associated with hallucinations during emergence. Use of etomidate also prolongs recovery. Short-acting opioids, such as alfentanil, are not given alone because they do not consistently produce amnesia. However, alfentanil (10–25 mg/kg) can be a useful adjunct when very small doses of methohexital (10–20 mg) are required in patients with a high seizure threshold. In very small doses, methohexital may actually enhance seizure activity. Increases in seizure threshold are often observed with each subsequent ECT.

Neuromuscular blockade is required from the time of electrical stimulation until the end of the seizure. A short-acting agent, such as succinylcholine (0.25–0.5 mg/kg), is most often selected. Controlled mask ventilation, using a self-inflating bag device or an anesthesia circle system, is required until spontaneous respirations resume.

Can seizure duration be increased without increasing the electrical stimulus?

Hyperventilation can increase seizure duration and is routinely employed in some centers. Intravenous caffeine, 125–250 mg (given slowly), has also been reported to increase seizure duration.

What monitors should be used during ECT?

Monitoring should be similar to what is appropriate with the use of any other general anesthetic. Seizure activity is sometimes monitored by an unprocessed electroencephalogram. It can also be monitored in an isolated limb: a tourniquet is inflated around one arm prior to injection of succinylcholine, preventing entry of the NMB and allowing observation of convulsive motor activity in that arm.

How can the adverse hemodynamic effects of the seizure be controlled in patients with limited cardiovascular reserve?

Exaggerated parasympathetic effects should be treated with atropine. In fact, premedication with glycopyrrolate is desirable both to prevent the profuse secretions associated with seizures and to attenuate bradycardia. Nitroglycerin, nifedipine, and α- and β-adrenergic blockers have all been employed successfully to control sympathetic manifestations. High doses of β-adrenergic blockers (esmolol, 200 mg), however, are reported to decrease seizure duration.

What if the patient has a pacemaker?

Patients with pacemakers may safely undergo electroconvulsive treatments, but a magnet should be readily available to convert the pacemaker to a fixed mode, if necessary.

SUGGESTED READING

Aronson S, Fontes M: Hypertension: a new look at an old problem. Curr Opin Anaesthesiol 2006;19:59.

Culley D, Xie Z, Crosby G: General anesthetic induced neurotoxicity: an emerging problem for the young and old. Curr Opin Anaesthesiol 2007;20:408.

Gregory T, Appleby I: Anaesthesia for interventional neuroradiology. Anaesth Intensive Care Med 2010;11:366.

Grocott H, White W, Morris R, et al: Genetic polymorphisms and the risk of stroke after cardiac surgery. Stroke 2005;36:1854.

Grunze H, Kasper S, Goodwin G, et al: The World Federation of Societies of Biological Psychiatry (WFSBP). Guidelines for the biological treatment of bipolar disorders, Part II: Treatment of mania. World J Biol Psychiatr 2003;4:5.

Hebl J, Horlocker T, Kopp S, et al: Neuraxial blockade in patients with preexisting spinal stenosis, lumbar disk disease, or prior spine surgery: efficacy and neurologic complications. Anesth Analg 2010;111:1511.

Horlocker TT: Complications of regional anesthesia and acute pain management. Anesthesiol Clin 2011;29:257.

Kumar R, Taylor C: Cervical spine disease and anaesthesia. Neurosurg Anaesth 2011;12:225.

Landau R, Giraud R, Delrue V, et al: Spinal anesthesia for cesarean delivery in a woman with a surgically corrected type 1 Arnold Chiari malformation. Anesth Analg 2003;97:253.

Lieb K, Selim M: Preoperative evaluation of patients with neurological disease. Semin Neurol 2008;28:603.

MRC Asymptomatic Carotid Surgery Trial (ACST) Collaborative Group: Prevention of disabling and fatal strokes by successful carotid endarterectomy in patients without recent neurological symptoms: randomised controlled trial. Lancet 2004;363:1491.

Nussbaum RL, Ellis CE: Alzheimer's disease and Parkinson's disease. N Engl J Med 2003;348:1356.

Pryzbylkowski P, Dunkman J, Liu R, et al: Anti-*N*-methyl–D-aspartate receptor encephalitis and its anesthetic implications. Anesth Analg 2011;113:1188.

Reide P, Yentis S: Anaesthesia for the obstetric patient with nonobstetric systemic disease. Best Pract Res Clin Obstet Gynaecol 2010;24:313.

Reddy U, Amin Y: Preoperative assessment of neurosurgical patients. Anaesth Intensive Care Med 2010;11:357.

Richards KJC, Cohen AT: Guillain–Barré syndrome. Br J Anaesth 2003;3:46.

Roach G, Kanchuger M, Mora Mangano C, et al: Adverse cerebral outcomes after coronary bypass surgery. N Eng J Med 1996;335:1857.

Sarang A, Dinsmore J: Anaesthesia for awake craniotomy—evolution of a technique that facilitates awake neurological testing. Br J Anaesth 2003;90:161.

Taheri S, Gasparovic C, Husia B, et al: Blood-brain barrier permeability abnormalities in vascular cognitive impairment. Stroke 2011;42:2158.

Veenith T, Burnstein RM: Management of patients with neurological and psychiatric disorders. Surgery 2010;28:441.

Renal Physiology
& Anesthesia

1 The combined blood flow through both kidneys normally accounts for 20–25% of total cardiac output.

2 Autoregulation of renal blood flow normally occurs between mean arterial blood pressures of 80 and 180 mm Hg and is principally due to intrinsic myogenic responses of the afferent glomerular arterioles to blood pressure changes.

3 Renal synthesis of vasodilating prostaglandins (PGD_2, PGE_2, and PGI_2) is an important protective mechanism during periods of systemic hypotension and renal ischemia.

4 Dopamine and fenoldopam dilate afferent and efferent arterioles via D_1-receptor activation. Fenoldopam and low-dose dopamine infusion can at least partially reverse norepinephrine-induced renal vasoconstriction.

5 Reversible decreases in renal blood flow, glomerular filtration rate, urinary flow, and sodium excretion occur during both regional and general anesthesia. Acute kidney injury is less likely if an adequate intravascular volume and a normal blood pressure are maintained.

6 The endocrine response to surgery and anesthesia is at least partly responsible for transient fluid retention seen postoperatively in many patients.

7 Compound A, a breakdown product of sevoflurane, has been shown to cause renal damage in laboratory animals. Its accumulation in the breathing circuit is favored by low flow rates. No clinical study has detected significant renal injury in humans during sevoflurane anesthesia; nonetheless, some regulatory authorities recommend fresh gas flow of at least 2 L/min with sevoflurane to prevent this theoretical problem.

8 The pneumoperitoneum produced during laparoscopy causes an abdominal compartment syndrome–like state. The increase in intraabdominal pressure typically produces oliguria (or anuria) that is generally proportional to the insufflation pressures. Mechanisms include central venous compression (renal vein and vena cava); renal parenchymal compression; decreased cardiac output; and increases in plasma levels of renin, aldosterone, and antidiuretic hormone.

The kidneys play a vital role in regulating the volume and composition of body fluids, eliminating toxins, and elaborating hormones, including renin, erythropoietin, and the active form of vitamin D. Factors directly and indirectly related to operative procedures and to anesthetic management frequently have a physiologically significant impact on renal physiology and renal function, and may lead to perioperative fluid overload, hypovolemia, renal insufficiency, and kidney failure, which are major causes of perioperative morbidity and mortality.

Diuretics are frequently used in the perioperative period. Diuretics are commonly administered on a chronic basis to patients with cardiovascular disease, including hypertension and chronic heart failure, and to patients with liver and kidney disease. Diuretics may be used intraoperatively, particularly during neurosurgical, cardiac, major vascular, ophthalmic, and urological procedures. Familiarity with the various types of diuretics, their mechanisms of action, side effects, and potential anesthetic interactions, is therefore essential.

The Nephron

Each kidney is made up of approximately 1 million functional units called nephrons. Anatomically, a nephron consists of a tortuous tubule with at least six specialized segments. At its proximal end (the *renal corpuscle*, composed of a glomerulus and a Bowman's capsule), an ultrafiltrate of blood is formed, and as this fluid passes through the nephron, its volume and composition are modified by both the reabsorption and the secretion of solutes. The final product is eliminated as urine.

Nephrons are classified as *cortical* or *juxtamedullary* (see below), and the renal corpuscles of all nephrons are located in the renal cortex. The six major anatomical and functional divisions of the nephron are the renal corpuscle, the proximal convoluted tubule, the loop of Henle, the distal renal tubule, the collecting tubule, and the juxtaglomerular apparatus (Figure 29–1 and Table 29–1).

The Renal Corpuscle

Each renal corpuscle contains a glomerulus, which is composed of tufts of capillaries that jut into

Bowman's capsule, providing a large surface area for the filtration of blood. Blood flow is provided by a single afferent arteriole and is drained by a single efferent arteriole (see below). Endothelial cells of the glomeruli are separated from the epithelial cells of Bowman's capsule only by their fused basement membranes. The endothelial cells are perforated with relatively large fenestrae (70–100 nm), but the epithelial cells interdigitate tightly with one another, leaving relatively small filtration slits (about 25 nm). The two cell types with their basement membranes provide an effective filtration barrier to cells and large-molecular-weight substances. This barrier has multiple anionic sites that give it a net negative charge, favoring filtration of cations relative to anions. A third cell type, called *intraglomerular mesangial cells*, is located between the basement membrane and epithelial cells near adjacent capillaries. These contractile cells regulate glomerular blood flow and also exhibit phagocytic activity. They secrete various substances, absorb immune complexes, and contain contractile proteins that respond to vasoactive substance. Mesangial cells contract, reducing glomerular filtration, in response to angiotensin II, vasopressin, norepinephrine, histamine, endothelins, thromboxane A_2, leukotrienes (C_4 and D_4), prostaglandin F_2, and platelet-activating factor. They relax, thereby increasing glomerular filtration, in response to atrial natriuretic peptide (ANP), prostaglandin E_2, and dopaminergic agonists.

Glomerular filtration pressure (about 60 mm Hg) is normally approximately 60% of mean arterial pressure and is opposed by both plasma oncotic pressure (about 25 mm Hg) and renal interstitial pressure (about 10 mm Hg). Afferent and efferent arteriolar tone are both important in determining glomerular filtration pressure: filtration pressure is directly proportional to efferent arteriolar tone but inversely proportional to afferent tone. Approximately 20% of plasma is normally filtered as blood passes through the glomerulus.

The Proximal Tubule

Of the ultrafiltrate formed in Bowman's capsule 65–75% is normally reabsorbed isotonically (proportional amounts of water and sodium) in the

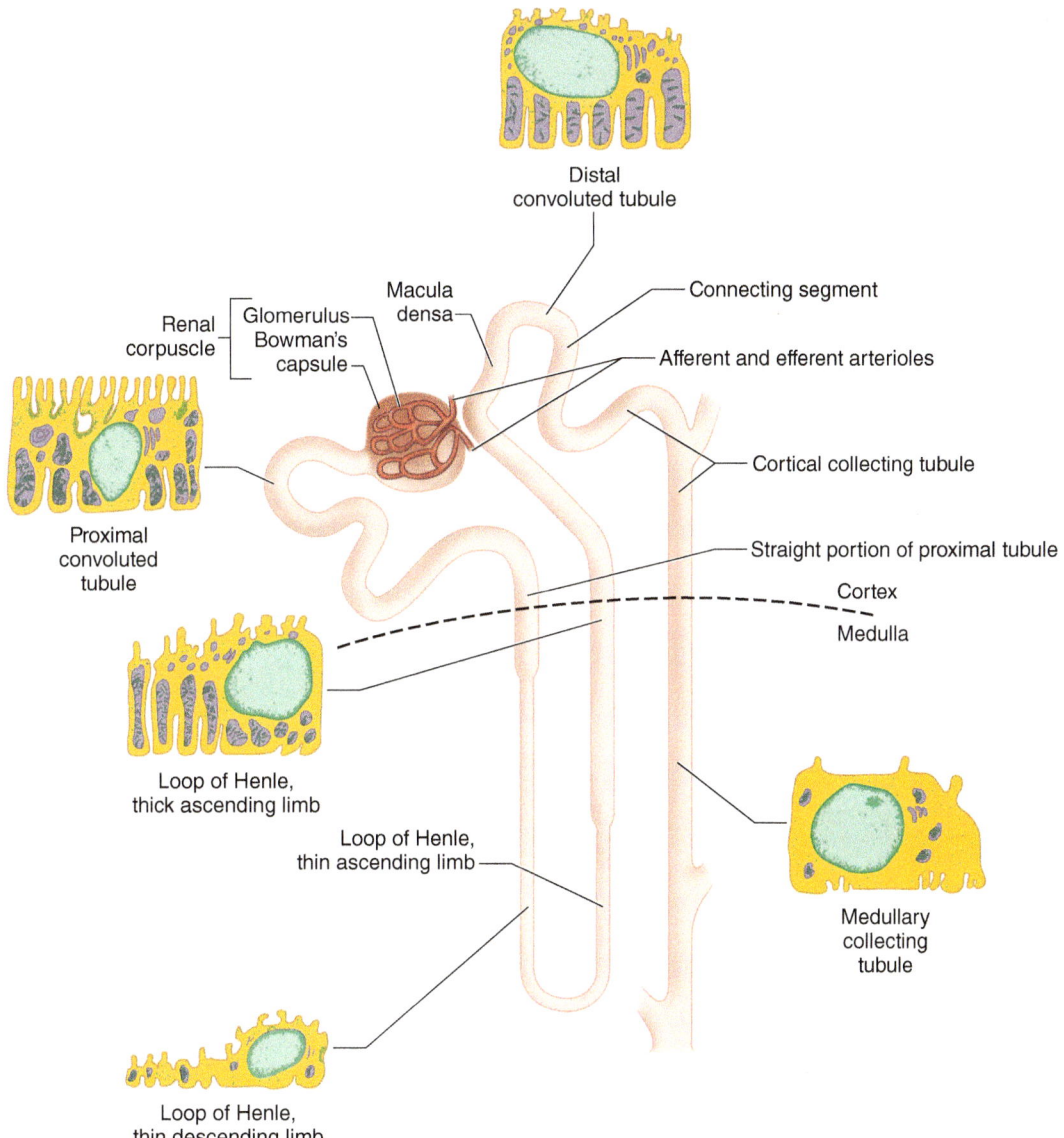

FIGURE 29–1 Major anatomic divisions of the nephron. (Reproduced, with permission, from Ganong WF: *Review of Medical Physiology*, 24th ed. McGraw-Hill, 2012.)

proximal renal tubules (Figure 29–2). To be reabsorbed, most substances must first traverse the tubular (apical) side of the cell membrane, and then cross the basolateral cell membrane into the renal interstitium before entering peritubular capillaries. The major function of the proximal tubule is Na^+ reabsorption. Sodium is actively transported out of proximal tubular cells at their capillary side by membrane-bound Na^+–K^+-adenosine triphosphatase (Na^+–K^+-ATPase) (Figure 29–3). The resulting low intracellular concentration of Na^+ allows passive movement of Na^+ down its gradient from tubular fluid into epithelial cells. Angiotensin II and norepinephrine enhance Na^+ reabsorption in the

TABLE 29–1 **Functional divisions of a nephron.**[1]

Segment	Function
Renal corpuscle (glomerulus, Bowman's capsule)	Ultrafiltration of blood

Proximal tubule	Reabsorption
	  Sodium[2] chloride
	  Water
	  Bicarbonate
	  Glucose, protein, amino acids
	  Potassium, magnesium, calcium
	  Phosphates,[3] uric acid, urea
	Secretion
	  Organic anions
	  Organic cations
	  Ammonia production

Loop of Henle	Reabsorption
	  Sodium, chloride
	  Water
	  Potassium, calcium, magnesium
	Countercurrent multiplier

Distal tubule	Reabsorption
	  Sodium[4] chloride
	  Water
	  Potassium
	  Calcium[5]
	  Bicarbonate
	Secretion
	  Hydrogen ion[4]
	  Potassium[4]
	  Calcium

Collecting tubule	Reabsorption
	  Sodium[4,6] chloride
	  Water[6,7]
	  Potassium
	  Bicarbonate
	Secretion
	  Potassium[4]
	  Hydrogen ion[4]
	  Ammonia production

Juxtaglomerular apparatus	Secretion of renin

[1]Adapted from Rose BD: *Clinical Physiology of Acid-Base and Electrolyte Disorders,* 3rd ed. McGraw-Hill, 1989.
[2]Partially augmented by angiotensin II.
[3]Inhibited by parathyroid hormone.
[4]At least partly aldosterone mediated.
[5]Augmented by parathyroid hormone.
[6]Inhibited by atrial natriuretic peptide.
[7]Antidiuretic hormone mediated.

early proximal tubule. In contrast, dopamine and fenoldopam decrease the proximal reabsorption of sodium via D_1-receptor activation.

Sodium reabsorption is coupled with the reabsorption of other solutes and the secretion of H^+ (Figure 29–3). Specific carrier proteins use the low concentration of Na^+ inside cells to transport phosphate, glucose, and amino acids. The net loss of intracellular positive charges, the result of Na^+–K^+-ATPase activity (exchanging $3Na^+$ for $2K^+$), favors the absorption of other cations (K^+, Ca^{2+}, and Mg^{2+}). Thus, the Na^+–K^+-ATPase at the basolateral side of the renal cells provides the energy for the reabsorption of most solutes. Sodium reabsorption at the luminal membrane is also coupled with countertransport (secretion) of H^+. The latter mechanism is responsible for reabsorption of 90% of the filtered bicarbonate ions (see Figure 50–3). Unlike other solutes, chloride can traverse the tight junctions between adjacent tubular epithelial cells, and accordingly, is passively resorbed via its concentration gradient. Active chloride reabsorption may also take place as a result of a K^+–Cl^- cotransporter that extrudes both ions at the capillary side of the cell membrane (Figure 29–3). Water moves passively out the proximal tubule along osmotic gradients. Apical membranes of epithelial cells contain specialized water channels, composed of a membrane protein called aquaporin-1, that facilitate water movement.

The proximal tubules are capable of secreting organic cations and anions. Organic cations such as creatinine, cimetidine, and quinidine may share the same pump mechanism and thus can compete for excretion with one another. Organic anions such as urate, ketoacids, penicillins, cephalosporins, diuretics, salicylates, and most radiocontrast dyes also share common secretory mechanisms. Both pumps probably play a major role in the elimination of many circulating toxins. Low-molecular-weight proteins, which are filtered by glomeruli, are normally reabsorbed by proximal tubular cells, to be metabolized intracellularly.

The Loop of Henle

The loop of Henle consists of *descending* and *ascending* portions. They are responsible for

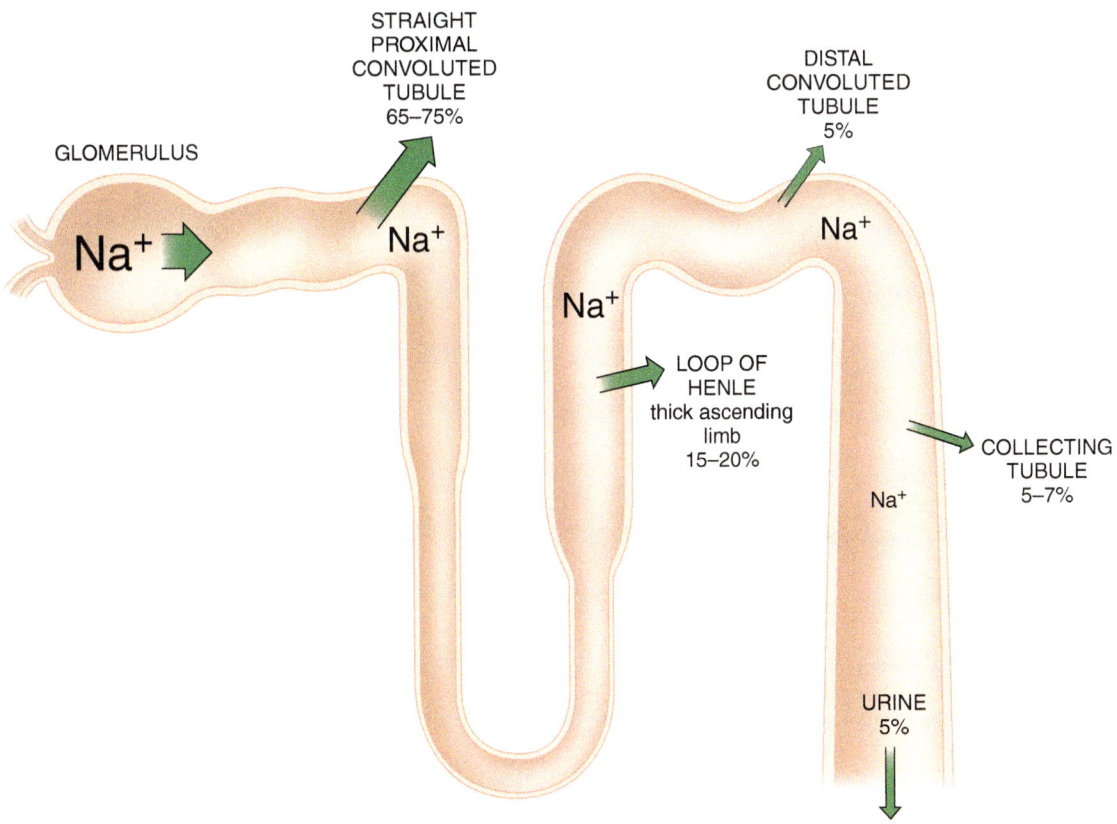

FIGURE 29–2 Sodium reabsorption in the nephron. Numbers represent the percentage of the filtered sodium reabsorbed at each site. (Reproduced, with permission, from Cogan MG: *Fluid and Electrolytes: Physiology and Pathophysiology.* Appleton & Lange, 1991.)

maintaining a hypertonic medullary interstitium and also indirectly provide the collecting tubules with the ability to concentrate urine. The thin descending segment is a continuation of the proximal tubule and descends from the renal cortex into the renal medulla. In the medulla, the descending portion acutely turns back upon itself and rises back up toward the cortex as the ascending portion. The ascending portion consists of a functionally distinct, thin ascending limb, a medullary thick ascending limb, and a cortical thick ascending limb (Figure 29–1). *Cortical* nephrons have relatively short loops of Henle which extend only into the more superficial regions of the renal medulla and often lack a thin ascending limb. *Juxtamedullary* nephrons, which have renal corpuscles located near the renal medulla, possess loops of Henle

that project deeply into the renal medulla. Cortical nephrons outnumber juxtamedullary nephrons by approximately 7:1.

Only 25–35% of the ultrafiltrate formed in Bowman's capsule normally reaches the loop of Henle. Once there, 15–20% of the filtered sodium load is normally reabsorbed in the loop of Henle. With the notable exception of the ascending thick segments, solute and water reabsorption in the loop of Henle is passive and follows concentration and osmotic gradients, respectively. In the ascending thick segment, however, Na^+ and Cl^- are reabsorbed in excess of water; moreover, Na^+ reabsorption in this part of the nephron is directly coupled to both K^+ and Cl^- reabsorption (Figure 29–4), and $[Cl^-]$ in tubular fluid appears to be the rate-limiting factor. Active Na^+ reabsorption still results from

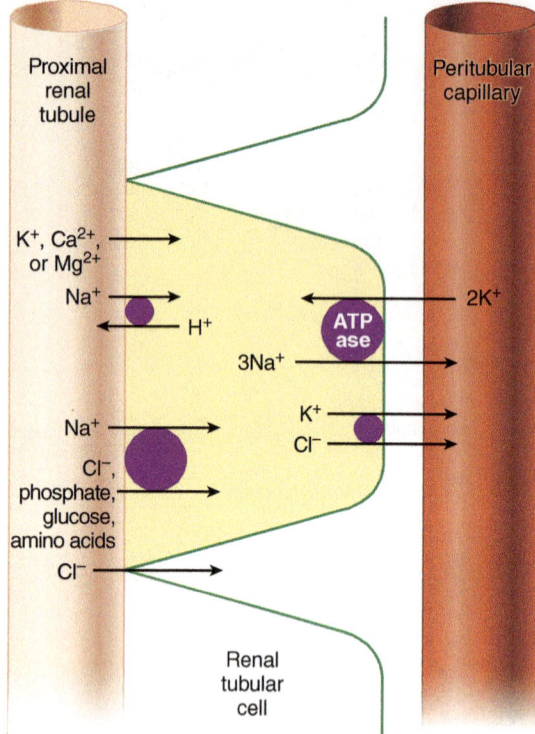

FIGURE 29–3 Reabsorption of solutes in proximal tubules. Note that Na⁺–K⁺-ATPase supplies the energy for reabsorption of most solutes by maintaining a low intracellular concentration of sodium.

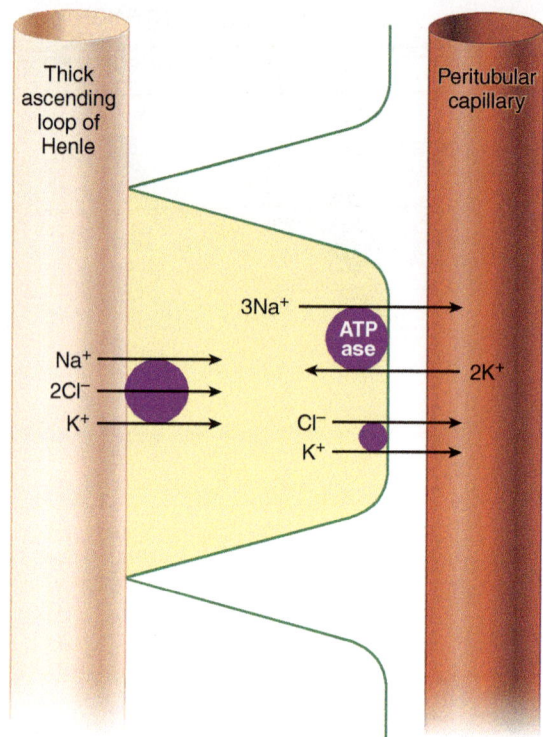

FIGURE 29–4 Sodium and chloride reabsorption in the thick ascending loop of Henle. All four sites on the luminal carrier protein must be occupied for transport to occur. The rate-limiting factor appears to be chloride concentration in tubular fluid.

Na^+–K^+-ATPase activity on the capillary side of epithelial cells.

Unlike the descending limb and the thin ascending limb, the thick parts of the ascending limb are impermeable to water. As a result, tubular fluid flowing out of the loop of Henle is hypotonic (100–200 mOsm/L) and the interstitium surrounding the loop of Henle is therefore hypertonic. A *countercurrent multiplier mechanism* is established such that both the tubular fluid and medullary interstitium become increasingly hypertonic with increasing depth into the medulla (Figure 29–5). Urea concentrations also increase within the medulla and contribute to the hypertonicity. The countercurrent mechanism includes the loop of Henle, the cortical and medullary collecting tubules, and their respective capillaries (vasarecta).

The thick ascending loop of Henle is also an important site for calcium and magnesium reabsorption, and parathyroid hormone may augment calcium reabsorption at this location.

The Distal Tubule

The distal tubule receives hypotonic fluid from the loop of Henle and is normally responsible for only minor modifications of tubular fluid. In contrast to more proximal portions, the distal nephron has very tight junctions between tubular cells and is relatively impermeable to water and sodium. It can therefore maintain the gradients generated by the loop of Henle. Sodium reabsorption in the distal tubule normally accounts for only about 5% of the filtered sodium load. As in other parts of the nephron, the energy is derived from Na^+–K^+-ATPase activity on the capillary side, but on the luminal side Na^+ is reabsorbed by an Na^+–Cl^- carrier. Sodium reabsorption in this segment is directly proportional to Na^+

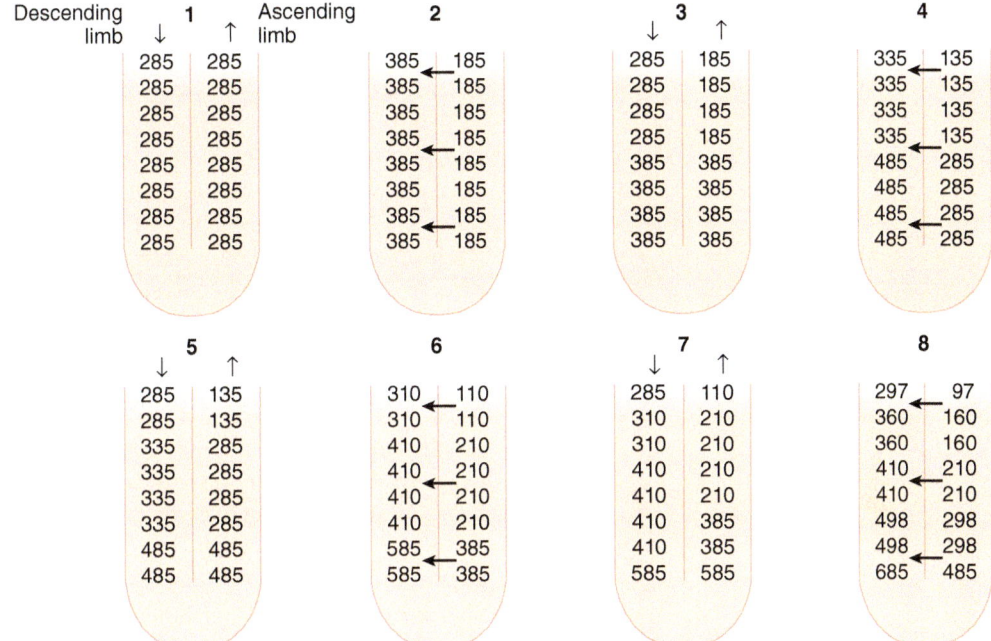

FIGURE 29–5 The countercurrent multiplier mechanism. This mechanism is dependent on differential permeability and transport characteristics between the descending and ascending limbs. The descending limb and the thin ascending limb are permeable to water, Na^+, Cl^-, and urea. The thick ascending limb is impermeable to water and urea, actively reabsorbs Na^+ and Cl^-, and therefore can generate an osmotic gradient. This figure depicts from "time zero," a progressive 200-mOsm/kg gradient between the descending and ascending limbs. Note that as urine flows, the gradient remains unchanged but the osmolality progressively increases at the bottom of the loop. (Reproduced, with permission, from Pitts RF: *Physiology of the Kidney and Body Fluids,* 3rd ed. Year Book, 1974.)

delivery. The distal tubule is the major site of parathyroid hormone–and vitamin D–mediated calcium reabsorption.

The latter portion of the distal tubule is referred to as the *connecting segment*. Although it is also involved in hormone-mediated calcium reabsorption, unlike more proximal portions, it participates in aldosterone-mediated Na^+ reabsorption.

The Collecting Tubule

The collecting tubule can be divided into cortical and medullary portions. Together, they normally account for the reabsorption of 5–7% of the filtered sodium load.

A. Cortical Collecting Tubule

This part of the nephron consists of two cell types: (1) principal cells (P cells), which primarily secrete potassium and participate in aldosterone-stimulated

Na^+ reabsorption, and (2) intercalated cells (I cells), which are responsible for acid–base regulation. Because P cells reabsorb Na^+ via an electrogenic pump, either Cl^- must also be reabsorbed or K^+ must be secreted to maintain electroneutrality. Increased intracellular $[K^+]$ favors K^+ secretion. Aldosterone enhances Na^+-K^+-ATPase activity in this part of the nephron by increasing the number of open K^+ and Na^+ channels in the luminal membrane. Aldosterone also enhances the H^+-secreting ATPase on the luminal border of I cells (Figure 29–6). I cells additionally have a luminal K^+–H^+-ATPase pump, which reabsorbs K^+ and secretes H^+, and some I cells are capable of secreting bicarbonate ion in response to large alkaline loads.

B. Medullary Collecting Tubule

The medullary collecting tubule courses down from the cortex through the hypertonic medulla before

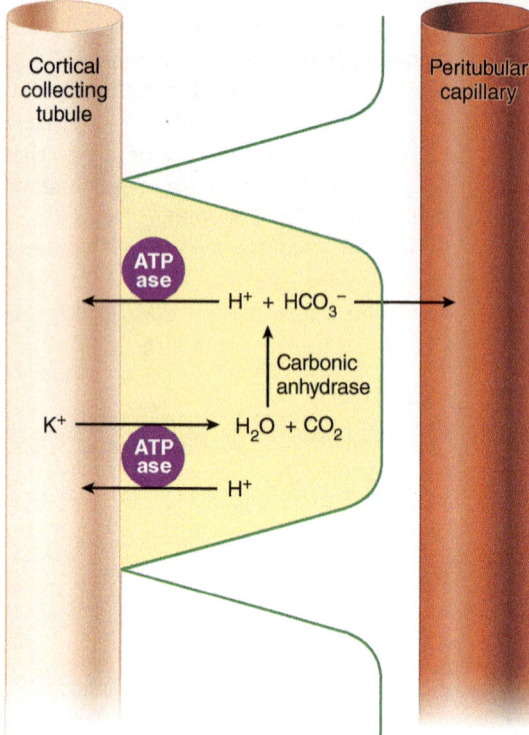

FIGURE 29–6 Secretion of hydrogen ions and reabsorption of bicarbonate and potassium in the cortical collecting tubule.

joining collecting tubules from other nephrons to form a single ureter in each kidney. This part of the collecting tubule is the principal site of action for antidiuretic hormone (ADH), also called arginine vasopressin (AVP). ADH stimulates the expression of a water channel protein, aquaporin-2, in the cell membrane. The permeability of the luminal membrane to water is entirely dependent on the presence of ADH (see Chapter 49). Dehydration increases ADH secretion, rendering the luminal membrane permeable to water. As a result, water is osmotically drawn out of the tubular fluid passing through the medulla, resulting in production of concentrated urine (up to 1400 mOsm/L). Conversely, adequate hydration suppresses ADH secretion, allowing fluid in the collecting tubules to pass through the medulla relatively unchanged and to remain hypotonic (100–200 mOsm/L). This part of the nephron is responsible for acidifying urine; the hydrogen ions

secreted are excreted in the form of titratable acids (phosphates) and ammonium ions (see Chapter 50).

C. Role of the Collecting Tubule in Maintaining a Hypertonic Medulla

Differences in permeability to urea in the cortical and medullary collecting tubules account for up to half the hypertonicity of the renal medulla. Cortical collecting tubules are freely permeable to urea, whereas medullary collecting tubules are normally impermeable. In the presence of ADH, the innermost part of the medullary collecting tubules becomes even more permeable to urea. Thus, when ADH is secreted, water moves out of the collecting tubules and the urea becomes highly concentrated. Urea can then diffuse out deeply into the medullary interstitium, increasing its tonicity.

The Juxtaglomerular Apparatus

This small organ within each nephron consists of a specialized segment of the afferent arteriole, containing juxtaglomerular cells within its wall, and the end of the thick, ascending cortical segment of the loop of Henle, the macula densa (Figure 29–7). Juxtaglomerular cells contain the enzyme renin and are innervated by the sympathetic nervous system. Release of renin depends on β_1-adrenergic sympathetic stimulation, changes in afferent arteriolar wall

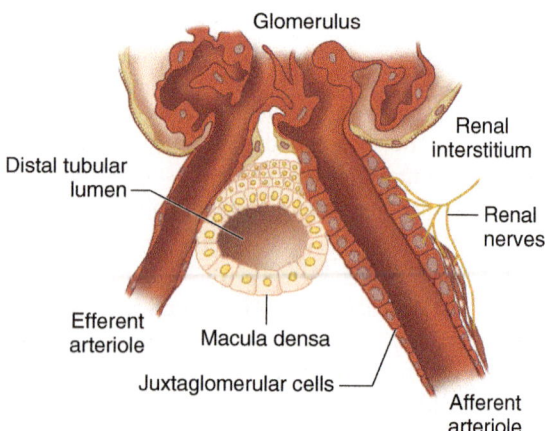

FIGURE 29–7 The juxtaglomerular apparatus.
(Reproduced, with permission, from Ganong WF: *Review of Medical Physiology,* 20th ed. McGraw-Hill, 2001.)

pressure (see Chapter 49), and changes in chloride flow past the macula densa. Renin released into the bloodstream catalyzes the conversion of angiotensinogen, a protein synthesized by the liver, to angiotensin I. This inert decapeptide is then rapidly converted, primarily in the lungs, by angiotensin-converting enzyme (ACE) to form the octapeptide angiotensin II. Angiotensin II plays a major role in blood pressure regulation (see Chapter 15) and aldosterone secretion (see Chapter 49). Proximal renal tubular cells have converting enzyme as well as angiotensin II receptors. Moreover, intrarenal formation of angiotensin II enhances sodium reabsorption in proximal tubules. Some extrarenal production of renin and angiotensin II also takes place in the vascular endothelium, the adrenal glands, and the brain.

The Renal Circulation

Renal function is intimately related to renal blood flow (RBF). In fact, the kidneys are the only organs for which oxygen consumption is determined by blood flow; the reverse is true in other organs. The combined blood flow through both kidneys normally accounts for 20–25% of total cardiac output. Approximately 80% of RBF normally goes to cortical nephrons, and only 10–15% goes to juxtamedullary nephrons. The renal cortex extracts relatively little oxygen, having an oxygen tension of about 50 mm Hg, because of the relatively high blood flow with a mostly filtration function. In contrast, the renal medulla maintains high metabolic activity because of solute reabsorption and requires low blood flow to maintain high osmotic gradients. The medulla has an oxygen tension of only about 15 mm Hg and is relatively vulnerable to ischemia.

Redistribution of RBF away from cortical nephrons with short loops of Henle to larger juxtamedullary nephrons with long loops occurs under certain conditions. Sympathetic stimulation, increased levels of catecholamines and angiotensin II, and heart failure can cause redistribution of RBF to the medulla and is associated with sodium retention.

In most individuals, each kidney is supplied by a single renal artery arising from the aorta. The renal artery then divides at the renal pelvis into interlobar arteries, which in turn give rise to arcuate arteries at the junction between the renal cortex and medulla (Figure 29–8). Arcuate arteries further divide into interlobular branches that eventually supply each nephron via a single afferent arteriole. Blood from each glomerular capillary tuft is drained via a single efferent arteriole and then travels alongside adjacent renal tubules in a second *peritubular* system of capillaries. In contrast to the glomerular capillaries, which favor filtration, peritubular capillaries are primarily "reabsorptive." Venules draining the second capillary plexus finally return blood to the inferior vena cava via a single renal vein on each side.

RENAL BLOOD FLOW & GLOMERULAR FILTRATION

Clearance

The concept of clearance is frequently used in measurements of RBF and the glomerular filtration rate (GFR). The renal clearance of a substance is defined as the volume of blood that is completely cleared of that substance per unit of time (usually, per minute).

Renal Blood Flow

Renal plasma flow (RPF) is most commonly measured by *p*-aminohippurate (PAH) clearance. PAH at low plasma concentrations can be assumed to be completely cleared from plasma by filtration and secretion in one passage through the kidneys. Consequently,

$$RPF = \text{Clearance of PAH} = \left(\frac{[PAH]_U}{[PAH]_P} \right) \times \text{Urine flow}$$

where $[PAH]_U$ = urinary concentration of PAH and $[PAH]_P$ = plasma PAH concentration.

If the hematocrit (measured as a decimal rather than as a percent) is known, then

$$RBF = \frac{RPF}{(1 - \text{Hematocrit})}$$

RPF and RBF are normally about 660 and 1200 mL/min, respectively.

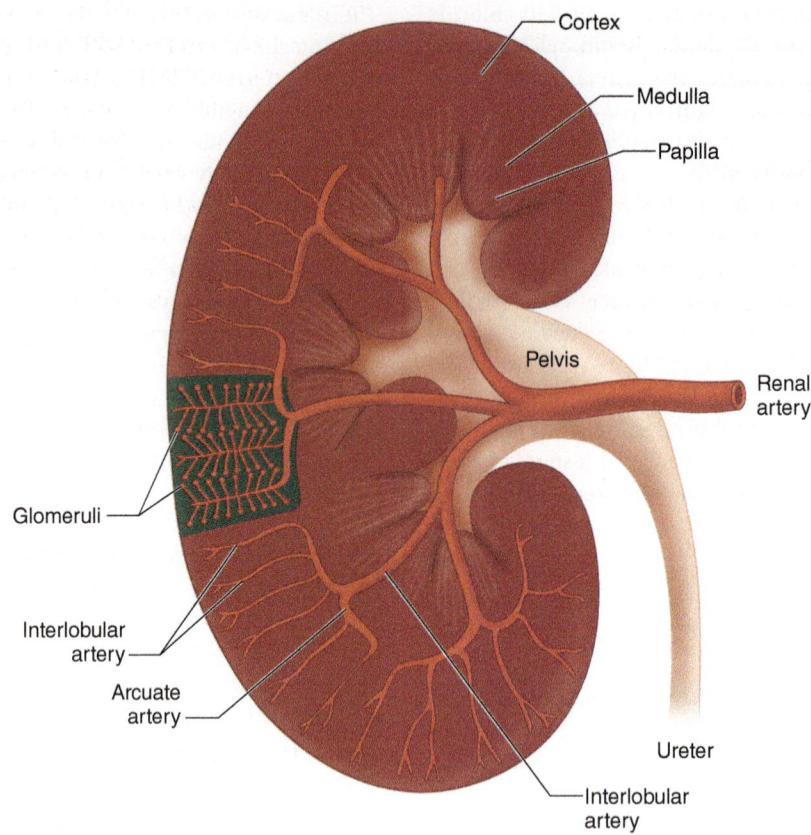

FIGURE 29–8 The renal circulation. (Reproduced, with permission, from Leaf A, Cotran RS: *Renal Pathophysiology.* Oxford University Press, 1976.)

Glomerular Filtration Rate

The GFR, the volume of fluid filtered from the glomerular capillaries into Bowman's capsule per unit time, is normally about 20% of RPF. Clearance of inulin, a fructose polysaccharide that is completely filtered but is neither secreted nor reabsorbed, is a good measure of GFR. Normal values for GFR are about 120 ± 25 mL/min in men and 95 ± 20 mL/min in women. Although less accurate than measuring inulin clearance, creatinine clearance is a much more practical measurement of GFR (see below). Creatinine clearance tends to overestimate GFR because some creatinine is normally secreted by renal tubules. Creatinine is a product of phosphocreatine breakdown in muscle. Creatinine clearance is calculated as follows:

$$\text{Creatinine clearance} = \frac{([\text{Creatinine}]_U \times \text{Urinary flow rate})}{[\text{Creatinine}]_P}$$

where $[\text{creatinine}]_U$ = creatinine concentration in urine and $[\text{creatinine}]_P$ = creatinine concentration in plasma.

The ratio of GFR to RPF is called the *filtration fraction* (FF) and is normally 20%. GFR is dependent on the relative tones of both the afferent and efferent arterioles (see above). Afferent arteriolar dilation or efferent arteriolar vasoconstriction can increase the FF and maintain GFR, even when RPF decreases. Afferent arteriolar tone appears to be responsible for maintaining a relatively constant GFR over a wide range of blood pressures.

Control Mechanisms

Regulation of RBF represents a complex interplay between intrinsic autoregulation, tubuloglomerular balance, and hormonal and neuronal influences.

A. Intrinsic Regulation

2 Autoregulation of RBF normally occurs between mean arterial blood pressures of 80 and 180 mm Hg and is principally due to intrinsic myogenic responses of the afferent glomerular arterioles to blood pressure changes. Within these limits, RBF (and GFR) can be kept relatively constant by afferent arteriolar vasoconstriction or vasodilation. Outside the autoregulation limits, RBF becomes pressure dependent. Glomerular filtration generally ceases when mean systemic arterial pressure is less than 40–50 mm Hg.

B. Tubuloglomerular Balance and Feedback

Tubuloglomerular feedback plays an important role in maintaining constant GFR over a wide range of perfusion pressures. Increased tubular flow tends to result in reduced GFR; conversely, decreased tubular flow tends to result in increased GFR. Although the mechanism is poorly understood, the macula densa appears to be responsible for tubuloglomerular feedback by inducing reflex changes in afferent arteriolar tone and possibly glomerular capillary permeability. Angiotensin II probably plays a permissive role in this mechanism. Local release of adenosine, which occurs in response to volume expansion, may inhibit renin release and dilate the afferent arteriole.

C. Hormonal Regulation

Increases in afferent glomerular arteriolar pressure stimulate renin release and formation of angiotensin II. Angiotensin II causes generalized arterial vasoconstriction and secondarily reduces RBF. Both afferent and efferent glomerular arterioles are constricted, but because the efferent arteriole is smaller, its resistance becomes greater than that of the afferent arteriole; GFR therefore tends to be relatively preserved. Very high levels of angiotensin II constrict both arterioles and can markedly decrease GFR. Adrenal catecholamines (epinephrine and norepinephrine) directly and preferentially increase afferent arteriolar tone but usually do not cause marked decreases in GFR because these agents also increase renin release and angiotensin II formation. Relative preservation of GFR during increased aldosterone or catecholamine secretion appears at least partly to be mediated by angiotensin-induced prostaglandin synthesis because it can be blocked by inhibitors of prostaglandin synthesis such as nonsteroidal antiinflammatory drugs (NSAIDs).

3 Renal synthesis of vasodilating prostaglandins (PGD_2, PGE_2, and PGI_2) is an important protective mechanism during periods of systemic hypotension and renal ischemia.

ANP is released from atrial myocytes in response to atrial distention. ANP is a direct smooth muscle dilator and antagonizes the vasoconstrictive action of norepinephrine and angiotensin II. It preferentially dilates the afferent glomerular arteriole, constricts the efferent glomerular arteriole, and relaxes mesangial cells, effectively increasing GFR (see Chapter 49). ANP also inhibits both the release of renin and angiotensin-induced secretion of aldosterone, and antagonizes the action of aldosterone in the distal and collecting tubules.

D. Neuronal and Paracrine Regulation

Sympathetic outflow from the spinal cord at the level of T4–L1 reaches the kidneys via the celiac and renal plexuses. Sympathetic nerves innervate the juxtaglomerular apparatus (β_1) as well as the renal vasculature (α_1). This innervation is largely responsible for stress-induced reductions in RBF (below). α_1-Adrenergic receptors enhance sodium reabsorption in proximal tubules, whereas α_2 receptors decrease such reabsorption and promote water excretion. Dopamine

4 and fenoldopam dilate afferent and efferent arterioles via D_1-receptor activation. Unlike dopamine, fenoldopam is selective for the D_1-receptor. Fenoldopam and low-dose dopamine infusion can at least partially reverse norepinephrine-induced renal vasoconstriction. Activation of D_2-receptors on presynaptic postganglionic sympathetic neurons can also vasodilate arterioles through inhibition of norepinephrine secretion (negative feedback). Dopamine is formed extraneuronally in the proximal tubule cells from circulating L-3,4-dihydroxyphenylalanine (L-dopa). Dopamine is released into the tubule where it can bind dopaminergic receptors to reduce proximal reabsorption of Na^+.

Effects of Anesthesia & Surgery on Renal Function

Acute kidney injury (AKI) is a common perioperative problem. It occurs in 1–5% of all hospitalized patients and is a major contributor to increased hospital length of stay, markedly increasing morbidity, mortality, and cost of care. Patients may develop AKI and kidney failure secondary to intrinsic kidney disease (Table 29–2). Risk factors for AKI in the perioperative setting include preexisting renal impairment, diabetes mellitus, cardiovascular disease, hypovolemia, and use of potentially nephrotoxic medication by elderly patients. The risk index in Table 29–3 identifies preoperative predictors of AKI following general surgery.

Clinical studies attempting to define the effects of anesthetic agents on renal function are complicated and difficult. However, several conclusions can be stated:

 1. Reversible decreases in RBF, GFR, urinary flow, and sodium excretion occur during both regional and general anesthesia.

TABLE 29–2 Causes of acute kidney injury secondary to intrinsic kidney disease.[1]

Vascular Effects	Renal Parenchymal Effects

Hemodynamic effects
  Acute kidney failure (eg, in elderly patients and
    those taking nonsteroidal antiinflammatory
    drugs [NSAIDs])
  Contrast agent–induced (producing renal
    vasoconstriction and avid sodium retention)
Hepatorenal syndrome
  Cirrhosis (producing intense renal
    vasoconstriction and sodium retention)
Impaired renal perfusion and autoregulation
  Angiotensin-converting enzyme inhibitors,
    NSAIDs
    plus
  Atherosclerotic renal vascular disease or
    hypovolemia
Abdominal compartment syndrome
  Postoperative abdominal exploration
  Tense ascites
Atheroembolism ("cholesterol embolism")
  Angiography
  Anticoagulation
  Thrombolysis
Renal embolism
  Endocarditis
  Cardiac thrombus
Renal vein thrombosis
  Malignancy
  Preexisting nephritis syndrome
	Glomerular diseases
	  Rapidly progressive glomerulonephritis (systemic vasculitis,
	    Goodpasture's disease, systemic lupus erythematosus,
	    other forms of glomerulonephritis)
	  Hemolytic uremic syndrome
	  Cryoglobulinemia
	Malignant hypertension
	  Untreated primary ("essential") hypertension
	  Chronic glomerulonephritis
	Acute tubular necrosis
	  Surgery (general, cardiac, vascular) Obstetric complications
	  Sepsis
	  Acute heart failure
	  Burns
	Rhabdomyolysis
	  Post–crush injury
	  Drug overdose
	  Status epilepticus
	Osmotic damage to proximal tubular cells
	  Sucrose-containing intravenous immunoglobulin solutions
	Acute pyelonephritis
	  Infection (eg, in patients with diabetes and partial obstruction
	    from papillary necrosis)
	Myeloma
	  Cast nephropathy
	  Light-chain deposition disease
	  Amyloidosis
	  Sepsis
	Interstitial nephropathy
	  Drug-induced (aminoglycosides, amphotericin, and many
	    other agents)
	  Acute interstitial nephritis
	Urate nephropathy
	  Chemotherapy for acute leukemia or lymphoma
	Hypercalcemia
	  Sarcoidosis
	  Milk-alkali syndrome

[1]Data from Armitage AJ, Tomson C: Acute renal failure. Medicine (UK ed. Abingdon) 2003;31:43.

TABLE 29–3 Acute kidney injury risk index for patients undergoing general surgery.[1,2]

Risk Factor
• Age ≥56 y
• Male sex
• Active congestive heart failure
• Ascites
• Hypertension
• Emergency surgery
• Intraperitoneal surgery
• Renal insufficiency—mild or moderate[3]
• Diabetes mellitus—oral or insulin therapy

[1]Reproduced, with permission, from Kheterpal S, Tremper KK, Heung M, et al: Development and validation of an acute kidney injury risk index for patients undergoing general surgery. Results from a national data set. Anesthesiology 2009;110:505.

[2]Risk Index classification is based on the number of risk factors present: class I (0–2 risk factors), class II (3 risk factors), class III (4 risk factors), class IV (5 risk factors), class V (≥6 risk factors).

[3]Preoperative serum creatinine >1.2 mg/dL.

2. Such changes are usually less pronounced during regional anesthesia.

3. Most of these changes are indirect and are mediated by autonomic and hormonal responses to surgery and anesthesia.

4. AKI is less likely when an adequate intravascular volume and a normal blood pressure are maintained.

5. There is no evidence that currently utilized vapor anesthetic agents cause AKI in patients. However, several studies have reported that compound A, a breakdown product of sevoflurane, produces renal toxicity when administered at low flow rates in laboratory animals.

INDIRECT EFFECTS

Cardiovascular

Most inhalation and intravenous anesthetics produce concentration-dependent cardiac depression or vasodilation; therefore they are capable of decreasing systemic blood pressure. Depending on the level of sympathetic blockade, spinal or epidural anesthesia may cause a drop in systemic blood pressure secondary to decreased cardiac output as a result of decreased sympathetic tone. This leads to increased pooling of blood and decreased systemic vascular resistance, decreased heart rate, and decreased cardiac output. Decreases in blood pressure below the limits of autoregulation reduce RBF, GFR, urinary flow, and sodium excretion, and this adverse impact on renal function can be reversed by administration of pressor agents and intravenous fluids.

Neurologic

Increased sympathetic tone commonly occurs in the perioperative period as a result of anxiety, pain, light anesthesia, and surgical stimulation. Heightened sympathetic activity increases renal vascular resistance and activates several hormonal systems (see below), reducing RBF, GFR, and urine output.

Endocrine

Endocrine changes during sedation and general anesthesia are a component of the stress response induced by factors that may include anxiety, pain, surgical stimulation, circulatory depression, hypoxia, acidosis, and hypothermia. Increases in epinephrine and norepinephrine, renin, angiotensin II, aldosterone, ADH, adrenocorticotropic hormone, and cortisol are common. Catecholamines, ADH, and angiotensin II all reduce RBF by inducing renal arterial constriction. Aldosterone enhances sodium reabsorption in the distal tubule and collecting tubule, resulting in sodium retention and expansion of the extracellular fluid compartment. Nonosmotic release of ADH also favors water retention and may result in hyponatremia. The endocrine response to surgery and anesthesia is at least partly responsible for transient fluid retention seen postoperatively in many patients.

DIRECT ANESTHETIC EFFECTS

The direct effects of anesthetics on renal function are minor compared with the secondary effects described above.

Volatile Agents

Halothane, sevoflurane, desflurane, and isoflurane decrease renal vascular resistance. As previously noted, compound A, a breakdown product of sevoflurane, has been shown to cause renal damage in laboratory animals. Its accumulation in the breathing circuit is favored by low flow rates. No clinical study has detected significant renal injury in humans during sevoflurane anesthesia; nonetheless, some regulatory authorities recommend fresh gas flow of at least 2 L/min with sevoflurane to prevent this theoretical problem.

Intravenous Agents

Opioids and propofol exhibit minor, if any, effects on the kidney when used alone. Ketamine minimally affects renal function and may, relative to other anesthetic agents, preserve renal function during hemorrhagic hypovolemia. Agents with α-adrenergic blocking activity may prevent catecholamine-induced redistribution of RBF. Drugs with antidopaminergic activity—such as metoclopramide, phenothiazines, and droperidol—may impair the renal response to dopamine. Inhibition of prostaglandin synthesis by NSAIDs such as ketorolac prevents renal production of vasodilatory prostaglandins in patients with high levels of angiotensin II and norepinephrine; attenuation of prostaglandin synthesis in this setting may result in AKI. ACE inhibitors block the protective effects of angiotensin II and may result in reductions in GFR during anesthesia.

Other Drugs

Many medications, including radiocontrast agents, used in the perioperative period can adversely affect renal function, particularly in the setting of preexisting renal dysfunction (Table 29–4). Mechanisms of injury include vasoconstriction, direct tubular injury, drug-induced immunological and inflammatory responses, and renal microvascular or tubular obstruction. In addition to intravenous hydration, pretreatment with *N*-acetylcysteine (600 mg orally every 12 h in four doses beginning prior to contrast administration) has been shown to decrease the risk of radiocontrast agent–induced AKI in patients with preexisting renal dysfunction. *N*-Acetylcysteine's protective action may be due to its free radical scavenging or sulfhydryl donor (reducing) properties. Fenoldopam, mannitol, loop diuretics, and low-dose dopamine infusion do not help maintain

TABLE 29–4 Drugs and toxins associated with acute kidney injury.[1]

Type of Injury	Drug or Toxin
Decreased renal perfusion	Nonsteroidal antiinflammatory drugs (NSAIDs), angiotensin-converting enzyme inhibitors, radiocontrast agents, amphotericin B, cyclosporine, tacrolimus
Direct tubular injury	Aminoglycosides, radiocontrast agents, amphotericin B, methotrexate, cisplatin, foscarnet, pentamidine, heavy metals, myoglobin, hemoglobin, intravenous immunoglobulin, HIV protease inhibitors
Intratubular obstruction	Radiocontrast agents, methotrexate, acyclovir, sulfonamides, ethylene glycol, uric acid, cocaine, lovastatin
Immunological–Inflammatory	Penicillin, cephalosporins, allopurinol, NSAIDs, sulfonamides, diuretics, rifampin, ciprofloxacin, cimetidine, proton pump inhibitors, tetracycline, phenytoin

[1]Reproduced, with permission, from Anderson RJ, Barry DW: Clinical and laboratory diagnosis of acute renal failure. Best Pract Res Clin Anaesthesiol 2004;18:1.

renal function or confer protection against AKI, and *N*-acetylcysteine has not been shown to be protective in the perioperative setting except in patients who receive radiocontrast dyes.

DIRECT SURGICAL EFFECTS

In addition to the physiological changes associated with the neuroendocrine stress response to surgery, certain surgical procedures can significantly alter renal physiology. The pneumoperitoneum produced during laparoscopy creates an abdominal compartment syndrome like state. The increase in intraabdominal pressure typically produces oliguria (or anuria) that is generally proportional to the insufflation pressures. Mechanisms include central venous compression (renal vein and vena cava); renal parenchymal compression; decreased cardiac output; and increases in plasma levels of renin, aldosterone, and ADH. Abdominal compartment syndrome can also be produced by severe intraabdominal tissue edema, with a similar adverse impact on renal function via the same mechanisms (see Chapter 39).

Other surgical procedures that can significantly impair renal function include cardiopulmonary bypass (see Chapter 22), cross-clamping of the aorta (see Chapter 22), and dissection near the renal arteries (see Chapter 31). The potential effects of neurosurgical procedures on ADH physiology are discussed in Chapters 27 and 49.

Diuretics

Diuretics increase urinary output by decreasing the reabsorption of Na^+ and water. Although classified according to their mechanism of action, many diuretics have more than one such mechanism; hence this classification system is imperfect. Only major mechanisms will be reviewed here.

The majority of diuretics exert their action on the luminal cell membrane from within the renal tubules. Because nearly all diuretics are highly protein bound, relatively little of the free drug enters the tubules by filtration. Most diuretics must therefore be secreted by the proximal tubule (usually via the organic anion pump) to exert their action. Impaired delivery into the renal tubules accounts for resistance to diuretics in patients with impaired renal function.

OSMOTIC DIURETICS (MANNITOL)

Osmotically active diuretics are filtered at the glomerulus and undergo limited or no reabsorption in the proximal tubule. Their presence in the proximal tubule limits the passive water reabsorption that normally follows active sodium reabsorption. Although their major effect is to increase water excretion, in large doses, osmotically active diuretics also increase electrolyte (sodium and potassium) excretion. The same mechanism also impairs water and solute reabsorption in the loop of Henle.

Mannitol is the most commonly used osmotic diuretic. It is a six-carbon sugar that normally undergoes little or no reabsorption. In addition

to its diuretic effect, mannitol appears to increase RBF. The latter can wash out some of the medullary hypertonicity and interfere with renal concentrating ability. Mannitol appears to activate the intrarenal synthesis of vasodilating prostaglandins. It also appears to be a free radical scavenger.

Uses

A. Prophylaxis Against Acute Kidney Injury in High-Risk Patients

Many clinicians continue to administer mannitol for renal protection and, less frequently, to convert oliguric acute kidney failure to nonoliguric kidney failure, with the goal of lowering associated morbidity and mortality. However, there is no evidence that such use of mannitol provides renal protection, lessens the severity of AKI, or lessens the morbidity or mortality associated with AKI when compared with correction of hypovolemia and preservation of adequate renal perfusion alone. In addition, high-dose mannitol can be nephrotoxic, especially in patients with renal insufficiency.

B. Evaluation of Acute Oliguria

Mannitol will augment urinary output in the setting of hypovolemia but will have little effect in the presence of severe glomerular or tubular injury. However, the optimal initial approach to evaluation of acute oliguria is to correct hypovolemia and optimize cardiac output and renal perfusion.

C. Acute Reduction of Intracranial Pressure & Cerebral Edema

See Chapter 27.

D. Acute Reduction of Intraocular Pressure in the Perioperative Period

See Chapter 36.

Intravenous Dosage

The intravenous dose for mannitol is 0.25–1 g/kg.

Side Effects

Mannitol solutions are hypertonic and acutely raise plasma and extracellular osmolality. A rapid intracellular to extracellular shift of water can transiently increase intravascular volume and precipitate cardiac decompensation and pulmonary edema in patients with limited cardiac reserve. Transient hyponatremia and reductions in hemoglobin concentration are also common and represent acute hemodilution resulting from rapid movement of water out of cells; a modest, transient increase in plasma potassium concentration may also be observed. It is also important to note that the initial hyponatremia does not represent hypoosmolality but reflects the presence of mannitol (see Chapter 49). If fluid and electrolyte losses are not replaced following diuresis, mannitol administration can result in hypovolemia, hypokalemia, and hypernatremia. The hypernatremia occurs because water is lost in excess of sodium. As noted above, high-dose mannitol can be nephrotoxic, especially in patients with renal insufficiency.

LOOP DIURETICS

The loop diuretics include furosemide (Lasix), bumetanide (Bumex), ethacrynic acid (Edecrin), and torsemide (Demadex). All loop diuretics inhibit Na^+ and Cl^- reabsorption in the thick ascending limb. Sodium reabsorption at that site requires that all four sites on the Na^+–K^+–$2Cl^-$ luminal carrier protein be occupied. Loop diuretics compete with Cl^- for its binding site on the carrier protein (see Figure 29–4). With a maximal effect, they can promote excretion of 15–20% of the filtered sodium load. Both urinary concentrating and urinary diluting capacities are impaired. The large amounts of Na^+ and Cl^- presented to the distal nephron overwhelm its limited reabsorptive capability. The resulting urine remains hypotonic, probably due to rapid urinary flow rates that prevent equilibration with the hypertonic renal medulla or due to interference with the action of ADH on the collecting tubules. A marked increase in diuresis may occur when a loop diuretic is combined with a thiazide diuretic, especially metolazone.

Loop diuretics also increase urinary calcium and magnesium excretion. Ethacrynic acid is the only loop diuretic that is not a sulfonamide derivative, and thus may be the diuretic of choice in patients allergic to sulfonamide drugs. Torsemide may have an antihypertensive action independent of its diuretic effect.

Uses

A. Edematous States (Sodium Overload)
These disorders include heart failure, cirrhosis, the nephrotic syndrome, and renal insufficiency. When given intravenously, these agents can rapidly reverse cardiac and pulmonary manifestations of fluid overload.

B. Hypertension
Loop diuretics may be used as adjuncts to other hypotensive agents, particularly when thiazides (below) alone are ineffective.

C. Evaluation of Acute Oliguria
The response to a small dose (10–20 mg) of furosemide may be useful in differentiating between oliguria resulting from hypovolemia and oliguria resulting from redistribution of RBF to juxtamedullary nephrons. Little or no response is seen with hypovolemia, whereas resumption of normal urinary output occurs with the latter. However, the optimal initial approach to evaluation of acute oliguria is to correct hypovolemia and optimize cardiac output and renal perfusion.

D. Conversion of Oliguric Kidney Failure to Nonoliguric Failure
As with mannitol, discussed earlier, many clinicians continue to administer loop diuretics for renal protection and to convert oliguric acute kidney failure to nonoliguric kidney failure, despite lack of evidence that such use provides renal protection, lessens the severity of AKI, or lessens the morbidity or mortality associated with AKI, when compared with correction of hypovolemia and preservation of adequate renal perfusion alone.

E. Treatment of Hypercalcemia
See Chapter 49.

F. Rapid Correction of Hyponatremia
See Chapter 49.

Intravenous Dosages

The intravenous doses are furosemide, 10–100 mg; bumetanide, 0.5–1 mg; ethacrynic acid, 50–100 mg; and torsemide 10–100 mg.

Side Effects

Increased delivery of Na^+ to the distal and collecting tubules increases K^+ and H^+ secretion at those sites and can result in hypokalemia and metabolic alkalosis. Marked Na^+ losses will also lead to hypovolemia and prerenal azotemia; secondary hyperaldosteronism often accentuates the hypokalemia and metabolic alkalosis. Urinary calcium and magnesium loss promoted by loop diuretics may result in hypocalcemia or hypomagnesemia, or both. Hypercalciuria can result in stone formation. Hyperuricemia may result from increased urate reabsorption and from competitive inhibition of urate secretion in the proximal tubule. Reversible and irreversible hearing loss has been reported with loop diuretics, especially furosemide and ethacrynic acid.

THIAZIDE & THIAZIDE-LIKE DIURETICS

This group of agents includes thiazides, containing a benzothiadiazine molecular structure, and also thiazide-like drugs with similar actions but without the benzothiadiazine structure, including chlorthalidone (Thalitone), quinethazone (Hydromox), metolazone (Zaroxolyn), and indapamide (Lozol). These diuretics act at the distal tubule, including the connecting segment, and inhibition of sodium reabsorption at this site impairs diluting but not concentrating ability. They compete for the Cl^- site on the luminal Na^+–Cl^- carrier protein. When given alone, thiazide and thiazide-like diuretics increase Na^+ excretion to only 3–5% of the filtered load because of enhanced compensatory Na^+ reabsorption in the collecting tubules. They also possess carbonic anhydrase–inhibiting activity in the proximal tubule, which is usually masked by sodium reabsorption in the loop of Henle and which is probably responsible for the marked diuresis often seen when they are combined with loop diuretics. In contrast to their effects on sodium excretion, thiazide and thiazide-like diuretics augment Ca^{2+} reabsorption in the distal tubule. Indapamide has some vasodilating properties and is the only thiazide or thiazide-like diuretic with significant hepatic excretion.

Uses

A. Hypertension

Thiazide and thiazide-like diuretics are often selected as first-line agents in the treatment of hypertension (see Chapter 21), and they have been shown to improve long-term outcomes in this disorder.

B. Edematous Disorders (Sodium Overload)

These drugs are used to treat mild to moderate edema and congestive heart failure related to mild to moderate sodium overload.

C. Hypercalciuria

Thiazide and thiazide-like diuretics are often used to decrease calcium excretion in patients with hypercalciuria who form renal stones.

D. Nephrogenic Diabetes Insipidus

The efficacy of these agents in this disorder reflects their ability to impair diluting capacity and increase urine osmolality (see Chapter 49).

Intravenous Dosages

These agents are only given orally.

Side Effects

Although thiazide and thiazide-like diuretics deliver less sodium to the collecting tubules than loop diuretics, the increase in sodium excretion is enough to enhance K^+ secretion and frequently results in hypokalemia. Enhanced H^+ secretion can also occur, resulting in metabolic alkalosis. Impairment of renal diluting capacity may produce hyponatremia. Hyperuricemia, hyperglycemia, hypercalcemia, and hyperlipidemia may also be seen.

POTASSIUM-SPARING DIURETICS

These are weak diuretic agents and characteristically do not increase potassium excretion. Potassium-sparing diuretics inhibit Na^+ reabsorption in the collecting tubules and therefore can maximally excrete only 1–2% of the filtered Na^+ load. They are usually used in conjunction with more potent diuretics for their potassium-sparing effect.

1. Aldosterone Antagonists (Spironolactone & Eplerenone)

Spironolactone (Aldactone) and eplerenone are direct aldosterone receptor antagonists in collecting tubules. They inhibit aldosterone-mediated Na^+ reabsorption and K^+ secretion. Both agents have been shown to improve survival in patients with chronic heart failure. Aldosterone may produce gynecomastia in male patients due to its antiandrogenic properties.

Uses

These agents may be used as adjuvants in the treatment of refractory edematous states associated with secondary hyperaldosteronism (see Chapter 49). Spironolactone is particularly effective in patients with ascites related to advanced liver disease. They have become part of the standard medical management of chronic heart failure.

Intravenous Dosage

These agents are only given orally.

Side Effects

These agents can result in hyperkalemia in patients with high potassium intake or renal insufficiency and in those receiving β blockers or ACE inhibitors. Metabolic acidosis may also be seen. Eplerenone lacks spironolactone's side effects of gynecomastia and sexual dysfunction.

2. Noncompetitive Potassium-Sparing Diuretics

Triamterene (Dyrenium) and amiloride (Midamor) are not dependent on aldosterone activity in the collecting tubule. They inhibit Na^+ reabsorption and K^+ secretion by decreasing the number of open sodium channels in the luminal membrane of collecting tubules. Amiloride may also inhibit Na^+–K^+-ATPase activity in the collecting tubule.

Uses

In patients with hypertension, these agents are often combined with a thiazide or similar diuretic to minimize hypokalemia produced by the other agent. They have been added to more potent loop diuretics in congestive heart failure patients with marked potassium wasting.

Intravenous Dosages

These agents are only given orally.

Side Effects

Amiloride and triamterene can cause hyperkalemia and metabolic acidosis similar to that seen with spironolactone (see above). Both can also cause nausea, vomiting, and diarrhea. Amiloride is generally associated with fewer side effects, but paresthesias, depression, muscle weakness, and cramping may occasionally be seen. Triamterene on rare occasions has resulted in renal stones and is potentially nephrotoxic, particularly when combined with nonsteroidal antiinflammatory agents.

CARBONIC ANHYDRASE INHIBITORS

Carbonic anhydrase inhibitors such as acetazolamide (Diamox) interfere with Na^+ reabsorption and H^+ secretion in proximal tubules. They are weak diuretics because the former effect is limited by the reabsorptive capacities of more distal segments of nephrons. Nonetheless, these agents significantly interfere with H^+ secretion in the proximal tubule and impair HCO_3^- reabsorption.

Uses

A. Correction of Metabolic Alkalosis in Edematous Patients

Carbonic anhydrase inhibitors often potentiate the effects of other diuretics.

B. Alkalinization of Urine

Alkalinization enhances urinary excretion of weakly acidic compounds such as uric acid.

C. Reduction of Intraocular Pressure

Inhibition of carbonic anhydrase in the ciliary processes reduces the formation of aqueous humor and, secondarily, intraocular pressure. Carbonic anhydrase inhibitors, including oral or intravenous acetazolamide, oral methazolamide (Neptazane), and ophthalmic topical brinzolamide (Azopt) and dorzolamide (Trusopt) are often used to treat glaucoma.

Intravenous Dosage

For acetazolamide, the intravenous dose is 250–500 mg.

Side Effects

Carbonic anhydrase inhibitors generally produce only a mild hyperchloremic metabolic acidosis because of an apparently limited effect on the distal nephron. Large doses of acetazolamide have been reported to cause drowsiness, paresthesias, and confusion. Alkalinization of the urine can interfere with the excretion of amine drugs, such as quinidine. Acetazolamide is frequently used for prophylaxis against mountain sickness.

OTHER "DIURETICS"

These agents may increase GFR by elevating cardiac output or arterial blood pressure, thereby increasing RBF. Drugs in this category are not primarily classified as diuretics because of their other major actions. They include methylxanthines (theophylline), cardiac glycosides (digitalis), fenoldopam (Corlopam), inotropes (dopamine, dobutamine), and intravenous crystalloid and colloid infusions. Methylxanthines also appear to decrease sodium reabsorption in both the proximal and distal renal tubules.

CASE DISCUSSION

Intraoperative Oliguria

A 58-year-old woman is undergoing radical hysterectomy under general anesthesia. She was in good health prior to the diagnosis of uterine carcinoma. An indwelling urinary catheter is placed following induction of general anesthesia. Total urinary output was 60 mL for the first 2 h of surgery. After the third hour of surgery, only 5 mL of urine is noted in the drainage reservoir.

Should the anesthesia provider be concerned?

Decreases in urinary output during anesthesia are very common. Although decreases may be expected owing to the physiological effects of surgery and anesthesia, a urinary output of less than 20 mL/h in adults generally requires evaluation.

What issues should be addressed?

The following questions should be answered:

1. Is there a problem with the urinary catheter and drainage system?
2. Are hemodynamic parameters compatible with adequate renal function?
3. Could the decrease in urinary output be directly related to surgical manipulations?

How can the urinary catheter and drainage system be evaluated intraoperatively?

Incorrect catheter placement is not uncommon and should be suspected if there has been a total absence of urine flow since the time of catheter insertion. The catheter may be inadvertently placed and inflated in the urethra in men or the vagina in women. Catheter displacement, kinking, obstruction, or disconnection from the reservoir tubing can all present with features similar to this case, with complete or near-complete cessation of urinary flow. The diagnosis of such mechanical problems requires retracing and inspecting the path of urine (often under the surgical drapes) from the catheter to the collection reservoir. Obstruction of the catheter can be confirmed by an inability to irrigate the bladder with saline through the catheter.

What hemodynamic parameters should be evaluated?

Decreased urinary output during surgery is most commonly the result of hormonal and hemodynamic changes. In many instances, a decrease in intravascular volume (hypovolemia), cardiac output, or mean arterial blood pressure is responsible. Redistribution of renal blood flow from the renal cortex to the medulla may also play a role.

Intravascular volume depletion can rapidly develop when intravenous fluid replacement does not match intraoperative blood loss and insensible fluid loss. Oliguria requires careful assessment of intravascular volume to exclude hypovolemia. An increase in urinary output following an intravenous fluid bolus is highly suggestive of hypovolemia. In contrast, oliguria in patients with a history of congestive heart failure may require inotropes, vasodilators, or diuretics. Intravascular volume status is often difficult to optimize, and goal-directed hemodynamic and fluid therapy utilizing arterial pulse contour analysis (eg, LIDCO Rapid, Vigileo FloTrak), esophageal Doppler, or transesophageal echocardiography should be considered when accurate determination of hemodynamic and fluid volume status is critically important, as in patients with underlying heart, kidney, or advanced liver disease (see Chapter 5). In addition to providing more accurate assessment of the patient's volume and hemodynamic status than that obtained with central venous pressure monitoring, these modalities avoid the risks associated with central venous access procedures and with pulmonary artery catheter placement and use.

When mean arterial blood pressure drops below the lower limit of renal autoregulation (80 mm Hg), urinary flow may become blood pressure dependent. The latter may be particularly true in patients with chronic systemic hypertension, in whom renal autoregulation occurs at higher mean arterial blood pressures. Reductions in anesthetic depth, intravenous fluid boluses, or the administration of a vasopressor or inotrope may increase blood pressure and urinary output in such instances.

Otherwise normal patients may exhibit decreased urinary output in spite of normal intravascular volume, cardiac output, and mean arterial blood pressure. A small dose of a loop diuretic (eg, furosemide, 5–10 mg) usually restores normal urinary flow in such instances—although such therapy does not convey protection against acute kidney injury.

How can surgical manipulations influence urinary output?

In addition to the neuroendocrine response to surgery, mechanical factors related to the surgery itself can alter urinary output. This is particularly true during pelvic surgery, when compression of the bladder by retractors, unintentional cystotomy, and ligation or severing of one or both ureters can dramatically affect urinary output. Retractor compression combined with a head-down

(Trendelenburg) position commonly impedes emptying of the bladder. Excessive pressure on the bladder will often produce hematuria.

When mechanical problems with the urinary catheter drainage system and hemodynamic factors are excluded (see above), a surgical explanation should be sought. The surgeon should be notified so that the position of the retractors can be checked, the ureters identified, and their path retraced in the operative area. Intravenous methylene blue or indigo carmine dyes (excreted in urine) are useful in identifying the site of an unintentional cystotomy or the end of a severed ureter. Note that the appearance of dye in the urinary drainage reservoir does not exclude unilateral ligation of one ureter. Methylene blue and, to a much lesser extent, indigo carmine, can transiently give falsely low pulse oximeter readings (see Chapter 6). Excessive insufflation pressure during laparoscopic procedures can result in abdominal compartment syndrome, reducing renal blood flow.

What was the outcome?

After the integrity of the urinary catheter and drainage system was checked, 2 L of lactated Ringer's solution along with 250 mL of 5% albumin and 10 mg of furosemide were administered intravenously, but failed to increase urinary output. Indigo carmine was given intravenously, and the proximal end of a severed left ureter was subsequently identified. A urologist was called and the ureter was reanastomosed.

SUGGESTED READING

Bellomo R: Acute renal failure. Semin Respir Crit Care Med 2011;32:639.

Bellomo R, Ronco C, Kellum JA, et al: Acute renal failure—definition, outcome measures, animal models, fluid therapy and information technology needs: The Second International Consensus Conference of the Acute Dialysis Quality Initiative (ADQI) Group. Crit Care 2004;8:R204.

Brienza N, Giglio MT, Marucci M, Fiore T: Does perioperative hemodynamic optimization protect renal function in surgical patients? A meta-analytic study. Crit Care Med. 2009;37:2079.

Craig RG, Hunter JM: Recent developments in the perioperative management of adult patients with chronic kidney disease. Br J Anaesth. 2008; 101:296.

Devarajan P: Biomarkers for the early detection of acute kidney injury. Curr Opin Pediatr 2011;23:194.

Ford DJ, Cullis B, Denton M: Dopaminergic and pressor agents in acute renal failure. In: Wilcox CS (editor): *Therapy in Nephrology & Hypertension,* 3rd ed. Saunders, 2008;13.

Goldstein SL, Chawla LS: Renal angina. Clin J Am Soc Nephrol 2010;5:943.

House AA, Haapio M, Lassus J, et al: Pharmacological management of cardiorenal syndromes. Int J Nephrol 2011;2011:630.

Kheterpal S, Tremper KK, Heung M, et al: Development and validation of an acute kidney injury risk index for patients undergoing general surgery. Results from a national data set. Anesthesiology 2009;110:505.

Kim IB, Prowle J, Baldwin I, et al: Incidence, risk factors and outcome associations of intra-abdominal hypertension in critically ill patients. Anaesth Intensive Care 2012;40:79.

Mandelbaum T, Scott DJ, Lee J, et al: Outcome of critically ill patients with acute kidney injury using the Acute Injury Network criteria. Crit Care Med 2011;39:2659.

McCullough PA: Radiocontrast-induced acute kidney injury. Nephron Physiol 2008;109:61.

Mehta RL, Kellum JA, Shah SV, et al: Acute Kidney Injury Network: Report of an initiative to improve outcomes in acute kidney injury. Crit Care 2007;11:R31.

Mohmand H, Goldfarb S: Renal dysfunction associated with intra-abdominal hypertension and the abdominal compartment syndrome. J Am Soc Nephrol 2011;22:615.

Noor S, Usami A: Postoperative renal failure. Clin Geriatric Med 2008;24:721.

Ricci Z, Cruz DN, Ronco C: Classification and staging of acute kidney injury: Beyond the RIFLE and AKIN criteria. Nature Rev Nephrol 2011;7:201.

Story DA: Postoperative mortality and complications. Best Pract Res Clin Anaesthesiol 2011;25:319.

Walbaum D, Kluth D: Clinical assessment of renal disease. Medicine (UK ed. Abingdon) 2007; 35:353.

Weisbord SD, Palevsky PM: Strategies for the prevention of contrast-induced acute kidney injury. Curr Opin Nephrol Hypertens 2010;19:539-549.

Anesthesia for Patients with Kidney Disease

30

1. The utility of serum creatinine measurement as an indicator of glomerular filtration rate (GFR) is limited in critical illness: the rate of creatinine production, and its volume of distribution, may be abnormal in the critically ill patient, and the serum creatinine concentration often does not accurately reflect GFR in the physiological disequilibrium of acute kidney injury (AKI).

2. Creatinine clearance measurement is the most accurate method available for clinically assessing overall renal function.

3. The accumulation of morphine and meperidine metabolites has been reported to prolong respiratory depression in patients with kidney failure.

4. Succinylcholine can be safely used in patients with kidney failure in the absence of hyperkalemia at the time of induction.

5. Extracellular fluid overload from sodium retention, in association with increased cardiac demand imposed by anemia and hypertension, makes patients with end-stage renal disease particularly prone to congestive heart failure and pulmonary edema.

6. Delayed gastric emptying secondary to autonomic neuropathy may predispose patients to aspiration perioperatively.

7. Controlled ventilation should be considered for patients with kidney failure. Inadequate

spontaneous or assisted ventilation with progressive hypercarbia under anesthesia can result in respiratory acidosis that may exacerbate preexisting acidemia, lead to potentially severe circulatory depression, and dangerously increase serum potassium concentration.

8. Correct anesthetic management of patients with renal insufficiency is as critical as management of those with frank kidney failure, especially during procedures associated with a relatively high incidence of postoperative kidney failure, such as cardiac and aortic reconstructive surgery.

9. Intravascular volume depletion, sepsis, obstructive jaundice, crush injuries, and renal toxins such as radiocontrast agents, certain antibiotics, angiotensin-converting enzyme inhibitors, and NSAIDs are major risk factors for acute deterioration in renal function.

10. Renal protection with adequate hydration and maintenance of renal blood flow is indicated for patients at high risk for AKI and kidney failure undergoing cardiac, major aortic reconstructive, and other surgical procedures associated with significant physiological trespass. The use of mannitol, low-dose dopamine infusion, loop diuretics, or fenoldopam for renal protection is controversial and without conclusive proof of efficacy.

Acute kidney injury (AKI) is a common problem, with an incidence of up to 5% in all hospitalized patients and up to 8% in critically ill patients. Postoperative AKI may occur in 1% or more of general surgery patients, and up to 30% of patients undergoing cardiothoracic and vascular procedures. Perioperative AKI greatly increases hospitalization costs, mortality rate, and perioperative morbidity, including fluid and electrolyte derangements, major cardiovascular events, infection and sepsis, and gastrointestinal hemorrhage. Preoperative risk factors for perioperative AKI include preexisting kidney disease, hypertension, diabetes mellitus, liver disease, sepsis, trauma, hypovolemia, multiple myeloma, and age greater than 55 years. The risk of perioperative AKI is also increased by exposure to nephrotoxic agents such as nonsteroidal antiinflammatory drugs (NSAIDs), radiocontrast agents, and antibiotics (see Table 29–4). When addressing abnormalities in renal function, the clinician must possess a thorough understanding of the differential diagnosis of AKI (**Figure 30–1**).

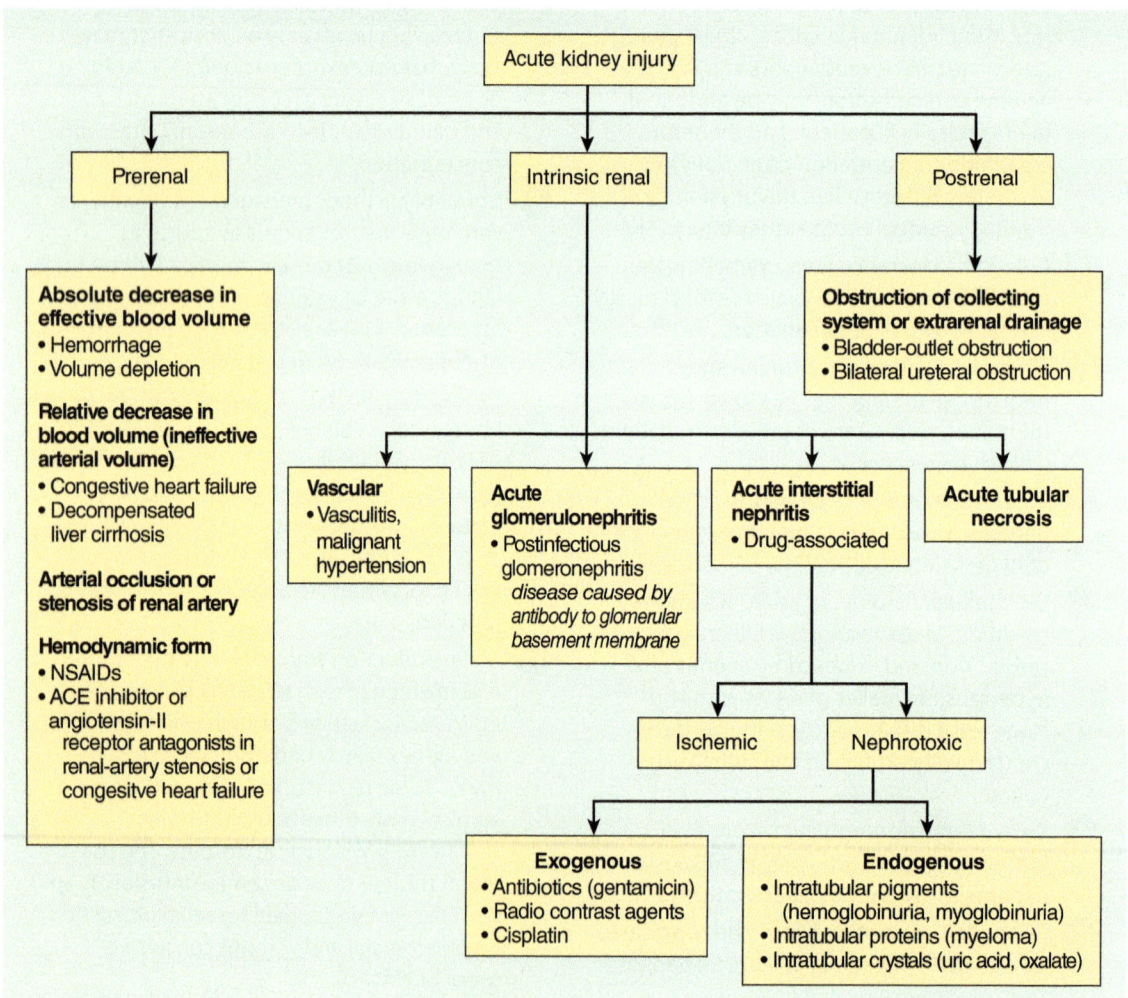

FIGURE 30–1 Differential diagnosis of acute kidney injury. ACE, angiotensin-converting enzyme; NSAID, nonsteroidal antiinflammatory drug. (Reproduced, with permission, from Lameire N, Van Biesen W, Vanholder R: Acute renal failure. Lancet 2005;29:417.)

Evaluating Renal Function

Renal impairment can be due to glomerular dysfunction, tubular dysfunction, or obstruction of the urinary tract. Because abnormalities of glomerular function cause the greatest derangements and are most readily detectable, the most useful laboratory tests utilized currently are those related to assessment of glomerular filtration rate (GFR). Accurate clinical assessment of renal function is often difficult and relies heavily on laboratory determinations such as the creatinine clearance (Table 30–1). Two systems for classification of AKI are helpful in defining and staging the degree of renal dysfunction; these are the Acute Dialysis Quality Initiative RIFLE criteria (Figure 30–2) and the Acute Kidney Injury Network (AKIN) staging system (Table 30–2). A great deal of research is currently evaluating plasma and urine biomarkers associated with AKI, such as cystatin C, neutrophil gelatinase–associated lipocalin, interleukin-18, and kidney injury molecule-1. It is likely that biomarkers will play a prominent role in the near future for diagnosis, staging, and prognostic assessment of AKI.

TABLE 30–1 Severity of kidney injury according to glomerular function.

	Creatinine Clearance (mL/min)
Normal	100–120
Decreased renal reserve	60–100
Mild renal impairment	40–60
Moderate renal insufficiency	25–40
Kidney failure	<25
End-stage renal disease[1]	<10

[1]This term applies to patients with chronic kidney failure.

BLOOD UREA NITROGEN

The primary source of urea in the body is the liver. During protein catabolism, ammonia is produced from the deamination of amino acids. Hepatic conversion of ammonia to urea prevents the buildup of toxic ammonia levels:

$$2NH_3 + CO_2 \rightarrow H_2N - CO - NH_2 + H_2O$$

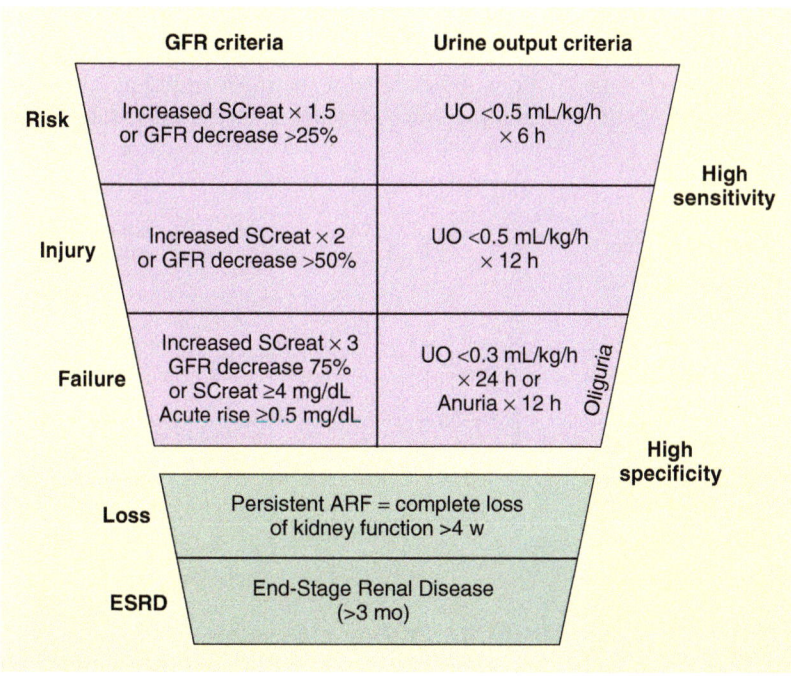

FIGURE 30–2 RIFLE criteria for acute kidney injury. ARF, acute renal failure; GFR, glomerular filtration rate; SCreat, serum creatinine concentration; UO, urine output. (Reproduced, with permission, from Bellomo R, Ronco C, Kellum JA, et al: Acute renal failure—definition, outcome measures, animal models, fluid therapy and information technology needs: The Second International Consensus Conference of the Acute Dialysis Quality Initiative (ADQI) Group. Crit Care 2004;8:R204.)

TABLE 30–2 Acute kidney injury network (AKIN) staging system for acute kidney injury.[1]

Stage	Serum Creatinine Criteria	Urine Output Criteria
1	Increase in serum creatinine of ≥0.3 mg/dL (≥26.4 µmol/L) or increase to ≥150–200% (1.5- to 2-fold) from baseline	Less than 0.5 mL/kg/h for more than 6 h
2	Increase in serum creatinine ≥200–300% (>2- to 3-fold) from baseline	Less than 0.5 mL/kg/h for more than 12 h
3	Increase in serum creatinine to >300% (>3-fold) from baseline (or serum creatinine of ≥4.0 mg/dL [≥354 µmol/L] with an acute increase of at least 0.5 mg/dL [44 µmol/L])	Less than 0.3 mL/kg/h for 24 h or anuria for 12 h

[1]Reproduced, with permission, from Mehta RL, Kellum JA, Shah SV, et al: Acute Kidney Injury Network: Report of an initiative to improve outcomes in acute kidney injury. Crit Care 2007;11:R31.

Blood urea nitrogen (BUN) is therefore directly related to protein catabolism and inversely related to glomerular filtration. As a result, BUN is not a reliable indicator of the GFR unless protein catabolism is normal and constant. Moreover, 40–50% of the urea filtrate is normally reabsorbed passively by the renal tubules; hypovolemia increases this fraction.

The normal BUN concentration is 10–20 mg/dL. Lower values can be seen with starvation or liver disease; elevations usually result from decreases in GFR or increases in protein catabolism. The latter may be due to a high catabolic state (trauma or sepsis), degradation of blood either in the gastrointestinal tract or in a large hematoma, or a high-protein diet. BUN concentrations greater than 50 mg/dL are generally associated with impairment of renal function.

SERUM CREATININE

Creatine is a product of muscle metabolism that is nonenzymatically converted to creatinine. Creatinine production in most people is relatively constant and related to muscle mass, averaging 20–25 mg/kg in men and 15–20 mg/kg in women. Creatinine is then filtered (and to a minor extent secreted) but not reabsorbed in the kidneys. Serum creatinine concentration is therefore directly related to body muscle mass but inversely related to glomerular filtration (Figure 30–3). Because body muscle mass is usually relatively constant, serum creatinine measurements are generally reliable indices of GFR in the healthy patient. However, the utility of a single serum creatinine measurement as an indicator of

GFR is limited in critical illness: the rate of creatinine production, and its volume of distribution, may be abnormal in the critically ill patient, and a single serum creatinine measurement often will not accurately reflect GFR in the physiological disequilibrium of AKI.

The normal serum creatinine concentration is 0.8–1.3 mg/dL in men and 0.6–1 mg/dL in women. Note from Figure 30–3 that each doubling of the serum creatinine represents a 50% reduction in GFR. Large meat meals, cimetidine therapy, and increases in acetoacetate (as during ketoacidosis) can increase serum creatinine measurements without a change in GFR. Meat meals increase the creatinine load, and high acetoacetate concentrations interfere with the most common laboratory method for measuring creatinine. Cimetidine

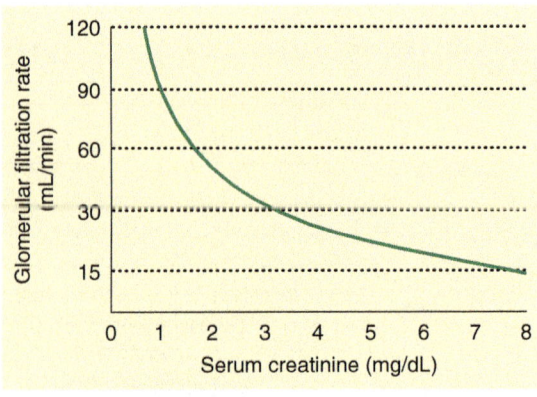

FIGURE 30–3 The relationship between the serum creatinine concentration and the glomerular filtration rate.

appears to inhibit creatinine secretion by the renal tubules.

GFR declines with increasing age in most individuals (5% per decade after age 20), but because muscle mass also declines, the serum creatinine remains relatively normal; creatinine production may decrease to 10 mg/kg. Thus, in elderly patients, small increases in serum creatinine may represent large changes in GFR. Using age and lean body weight (in kilograms), GFR can be estimated by the following formula for men:

$$\text{Creatinine clearance} = \frac{[(140 - \text{age}) \times \text{lean body weight}]}{(72 \times \text{plasma creatinine})}$$

For women, this equation must be multiplied by 0.85 to compensate for a smaller muscle mass.

The serum creatinine concentration requires 48–72 h to equilibrate at a new level following acute changes in GFR.

CREATININE CLEARANCE

2 Creatinine clearance measurement is the most accurate method available for clinically assessing overall renal function (actually, GFR). Although measurements are usually performed over 24 h, 2-h creatinine clearance determinations are reasonably accurate and easier to perform. Mild impairment of renal function generally results in creatinine clearances of 40–60 mL/min. Clearances between 25 and 40 mL/min produce moderate renal dysfunction and nearly always cause symptoms. Creatinine clearances less than 25 mL/min are indicative of overt kidney failure.

Progressive kidney disease enhances creatinine secretion in the proximal tubule. As a result, with declining renal function the creatinine clearance progressively overestimates the true GFR. Moreover, relative preservation of GFR may occur early in the course of progressive kidney disease due to compensatory hyperfiltration in the remaining nephrons and increases in glomerular filtration pressure. It is therefore important to look for other signs of deteriorating renal function such as hypertension, proteinuria, or other abnormalities in urine sediment.

BLOOD UREA NITROGEN: CREATININE RATIO

Low renal tubular flow rates enhance urea reabsorption but do not affect creatinine handling. As a result, the BUN to serum creatinine ratio increases above 10:1. Decreases in tubular flow can be caused by decreased renal perfusion or obstruction of the urinary tract. **BUN: creatinine ratios greater than 15:1 are therefore seen in volume depletion and in edematous disorders associated with decreased tubular flow (eg, congestive heart failure, cirrhosis, nephrotic syndrome) as well as in obstructive uropathies.** Increases in protein catabolism can also increase this ratio.

URINALYSIS

Urinalysis continues to be routinely performed for evaluating renal function. Although its utility for that purpose is justifiably questionable, urinalysis can be helpful in identifying some disorders of renal tubular dysfunction as well as some nonrenal disturbances. A routine urinalysis typically includes pH; specific gravity; detection and quantification of glucose, protein, and bilirubin content; and microscopic examination of the urinary sediment. Urinary pH is helpful only when arterial pH is also known. A urinary pH greater than 7.0 in the presence of systemic acidosis is suggestive of renal tubular acidosis (see Chapter 50). Specific gravity is related to urinary osmolality; 1.010 usually corresponds to 290 mOsm/kg. A specific gravity greater than 1.018 after an overnight fast is indicative of adequate renal concentrating ability. A lower specific gravity in the presence of hyperosmolality in plasma is consistent with diabetes insipidus.

Glycosuria is the result of either a low tubular threshold for glucose (normally 180 mg/dL) or hyperglycemia. Proteinuria detected by routine urinalysis should be evaluated by means of 24-h urine collection. Urinary protein excretions greater than 150 mg/d are significant. Elevated levels of bilirubin in the urine are seen with biliary obstruction.

Microscopic analysis of the urinary sediment detects the presence of red or white blood cells, bacteria, casts, and crystals. Red cells may be indicative of bleeding due to tumor, stones, infection, coagulopathy, or trauma. White cells and bacteria are generally associated with infection. Disease processes at the level of the nephron produce tubular casts. Crystals may be indicative of abnormalities in oxalic acid, uric acid, or cystine metabolism.

Altered Renal Function & the Effects of Anesthetic Agents

Most drugs commonly employed during anesthesia (other than volatile anesthetics) are at least partly dependent on renal excretion for elimination. In the presence of renal impairment, dosage modifications may be required to prevent accumulation of the drug or its active metabolites. Moreover, the systemic effects of AKI can potentiate the pharmacological actions of many of these agents. This latter observation may be the result of decreased protein binding of the drug, greater brain penetration due to some breach of the blood–brain barrier, or a synergistic effect with the toxins retained in kidney failure.

INTRAVENOUS AGENTS

Propofol & Etomidate

The pharmacokinetics of both propofol and etomidate are minimally affected by impaired renal function. Decreased protein binding of etomidate in patients with hypoalbuminemia may enhance its pharmacological effects.

Barbiturates

Patients with kidney disease often exhibit increased sensitivity to barbiturates during induction, even though pharmacokinetic profiles appear to be unchanged. The mechanism appears to be an increase in free circulating barbiturate as a result of decreased protein binding. Acidosis may also favor a more rapid entry of these agents into the brain by increasing the nonionized fraction of the drug (see Chapter 26).

Ketamine

Ketamine pharmacokinetics are minimally altered by kidney disease. Some active hepatic metabolites are dependent on renal excretion and can potentially accumulate in kidney failure.

Benzodiazepines

Benzodiazepines undergo hepatic metabolism and conjugation prior to elimination in urine. Because most are highly protein bound, increased sensitivity may be seen in patients with hypoalbuminemia. Diazepam and midazolam should be administered cautiously in the presence of renal impairment because of a potential for the accumulation of active metabolites.

Opioids

Most opioids currently in use in anesthetic management (morphine, meperidine, fentanyl, sufentanil, and alfentanil) are inactivated by the liver; some of these metabolites are then excreted in urine. Remifentanil pharmacokinetics are unaffected by renal function due to rapid ester hydrolysis in blood. With the exception of morphine and meperidine, significant accumulation of active metabolites generally does not occur with these agents. The accumulation of morphine (morphine-6-glucuronide) and meperidine (normeperidine) metabolites has been reported to prolong respiratory depression in patients with kidney failure, and increased levels of normeperidine has been associated with seizures. The pharmacokinetics of the most commonly used opioid agonist–antagonists (butorphanol, nalbuphine, and buprenorphine) are unaffected by kidney failure.

Anticholinergic Agents

In doses used for premedication, atropine and glycopyrrolate can generally be used safely in patients with renal impairment. Because up to 50% of these drugs and their active metabolites are normally excreted in urine, however, the potential for accumulation exists following repeated doses. Scopolamine is less dependent on renal excretion, but its central nervous system effects can be enhanced by the physiological alterations of renal insufficiency.

Phenothiazines, H₂ Blockers, & Related Agents

Most phenothiazines, such as promethazine, are metabolized to inactive compounds by the liver. Droperidol may be partly dependent on the kidneys for excretion. Although their pharmacokinetic profiles are not appreciably altered by renal impairment, potentiation of the central depressant effects of phenothiazines by the physiological milieu of renal insufficiency can occur.

All H₂-receptor blockers are dependent on renal excretion, and their dose must be reduced for patients with renal insufficiency. Proton pump inhibitor dosage does not need to be reduced for patients with renal insufficiency. Metoclopramide is partly excreted unchanged in urine and will accumulate in kidney failure. Although up to 50% of dolasetron is excreted in urine, no dosage adjustments are recommended for any of the 5-HT₃ blockers in patients with renal insufficiency.

INHALATION AGENTS

Volatile Agents

Volatile anesthetic agents are ideal for patients with kidney disease because of lack of dependence on the kidneys for elimination, ability to control blood pressure, and minimal direct effects on renal blood flow. Although patients with mild to moderate renal impairment do not exhibit altered uptake or distribution, accelerated induction and emergence may be seen in severely anemic patients (hemoglobin <5 g/dL) with chronic kidney failure; this observation may be explained by a decrease in the blood:gas partition coefficient or by a decrease in minimum alveolar concentration. Some clinicians avoid sevoflurane (with <2 L/min gas flows) for patients with kidney disease who undergo lengthy procedures (see Chapters 8 and 29).

Nitrous Oxide

Some clinicians omit entirely or limit the use of nitrous oxide to 50% concentration in severely anemic patients with end-stage renal disease in an attempt to increase arterial oxygen content. This may be justified

in patients with hemoglobin below 7 g/dL, in whom even a small increase in the dissolved oxygen content may represent a significant percentage of the arterial to venous oxygen difference (see Chapter 23).

MUSCLE RELAXANTS

Succinylcholine

4 Succinylcholine can be safely used in patients with kidney failure, in the absence of hyperkalemia at the time of induction. When the serum potassium is known to be increased or is in doubt, a nondepolarizing muscle relaxant should be substituted. Although decreased plasma cholinesterase levels have been reported in uremic patients following dialysis, significant prolongation of neuromuscular blockade is rarely seen.

Cisatracurium & Atracurium

Cisatracurium and atracurium are degraded by plasma ester hydrolysis and nonenzymatic Hofmann elimination. These agents are often the drugs of choice for muscle relaxation in patients with kidney failure, especially in clinical situations where neuromuscular function monitoring is difficult or impossible.

Vecuronium & Rocuronium

The elimination of vecuronium is primarily hepatic, but up to 20% of the drug is eliminated in urine. The effects of large doses of vecuronium (>0.1 mg/kg) are only modestly prolonged in patients with renal insufficiency. Rocuronium primarily undergoes hepatic elimination, but prolongation in patients with severe kidney disease has been reported. In general, with appropriate neuromuscular monitoring, these two agents can be used with few problems in patients with severe kidney disease.

Curare (d-Tubocurarine)

Elimination of d-tubocurarine is dependent on both renal and biliary excretion; 40–60% of a dose of curare is normally excreted in urine. Increasingly prolonged effects are observed following repeated doses in patients with renal insufficiency. Smaller doses and longer dosing intervals are therefore required for maintenance of optimal muscle relaxation. In the days before intermediate acting neuromuscular blockers, curare was the nondepolarizing paralytic of choice for patients with kidney disease.

Pancuronium

Pancuronium is primarily dependent on renal excretion (60–90%). Although pancuronium is metabolized by the liver into less active intermediates, its elimination half-life is still primarily dependent on renal excretion (60–80%). Neuromuscular function should be closely monitored if these agents are used in patients with abnormal renal function.

Reversal Agents

Renal excretion is the principal route of elimination for edrophonium, neostigmine, and pyridostigmine. The half-lives of these agents in patients with renal impairment are therefore prolonged at least as much as any of the above relaxants, and problems with inadequate reversal of neuromuscular blockade are usually related to other factors (see Chapter 11). In other words, "recurarization" due to inadequate duration of reversal agents is unlikely.

Anesthesia for Patients with Kidney Failure

PREOPERATIVE CONSIDERATIONS

Acute Kidney Failure

This syndrome is a rapid deterioration in renal function that results in retention of nitrogenous waste products (azotemia). These substances, many of which behave as toxins, are byproducts of protein and amino acid metabolism. Impaired renal metabolism of circulating proteins and peptides may contribute to widespread organ dysfunction.

Kidney failure can be classified as prerenal, renal, and postrenal, depending on its cause(s), and the initial therapeutic approach varies accordingly (see Figure 30–1 and Table 30–3). Prerenal kidney failure results from an acute decrease in renal

TABLE 30–3 **Management priorities in patients with acute kidney failure.[1]**

- Search for and correct prerenal and postrenal causes
- Review medications and patient-administered substances and stop any potential nephrotoxins
- Administer medications in doses appropriate for their clearance
- Optimize cardiac output and renal blood flow
- Monitor fluid intake and output; measure body weight daily
- Search for and treat acute complications (hyperkalemia, hyponatremia, acidosis, hyperphosphatemia, pulmonary edema)
- Search for and aggressively treat infections and sepsis
- Provide early nutritional support
- Provide expert supportive care (management of catheter and skin care; pressure sore and deep venous thromboembolic prophylaxis; psychological support).

[1]Reproduced, with permission, from Lameire N, Van Biesen W, Vanholder R: Acute renal failure. Lancet 2005;365:417.

perfusion; intrinsic kidney failure is usually due to underlying renal disease, renal ischemia, or nephrotoxins; and postrenal failure is the result of urinary tract obstruction or disruption. Both prerenal and postrenal forms of kidney failure are readily reversible in their initial stages but with time progress to intrinsic kidney failure. Most adult patients with kidney failure first develop oliguria. Nonoliguric patients (those with urinary outputs >400 mL/d) continue to form urine that is qualitatively poor; these patients tend to have greater preservation of GFR. Although glomerular filtration and tubular function are impaired in both cases, abnormalities tend to be less severe in nonoliguric kidney failure.

The course of intrinsic acute kidney failure varies widely, but the oliguria typically lasts for 2 weeks and is followed by a diuretic phase marked by a progressive increase in urinary output. This diuretic phase often results in very large urinary outputs and is usually absent in nonoliguric kidney failure. Urinary function improves over the course of several weeks, but may not return to normal for up to 1 year. The course of prerenal and postrenal kidney failure is dependent on correction of the causal condition.

End-Stage Renal Disease

The most common causes of end-stage renal disease (ESRD) are hypertensive nephrosclerosis, diabetic nephropathy, chronic glomerulonephritis, and

TABLE 30–4 Manifestations of uremia.

Neurological	**Metabolic**
Peripheral neuropathy	Metabolic acidosis
Autonomic neuropathy	Hyperkalemia
Muscle twitching	Hyponatremia
Encephalopathy	Hypermagnesemia
Asterixis	Hyperphosphatemia
Myoclonus	Hypocalcemia
Lethargy	Hyperuricemia
Confusion	Hypoalbuminemia
Seizures	**Hematological**
Coma	Anemia
Cardiovascular	Platelet dysfunction
Fluid overload	Leukocyte dysfunction
Congestive heart failure	**Endocrine**
Hypertension	Glucose intolerance
Pericarditis	Secondary
Arrhythmia	hyperparathyroidism
Conduction blocks	Hypertriglyceridemia
Vascular calcification	**Skeletal**
Accelerated	Osteodystrophy
atherosclerosis	Periarticular calcification
Pulmonary	**Skin**
Hyperventilation	Hyperpigmentation
Interstitial edema	Ecchymosis
Alveolar edema	Pruritus
Pleural effusion	
Gastrointestinal	
Anorexia	
Nausea and vomiting	
Delayed gastric emptying	
Hyperacidity	
Mucosal ulcerations	
Hemorrhage	
Adynamic ileus	

TABLE 30–5 Complications of hemodialysis.

Neurological
  Disequilibrium syndrome
  Dementia
Cardiovascular
  Intravascular volume depletion
  Hypotension
  Arrhythmia
Pulmonary
  Hypoxemia
Gastrointestinal
  Ascites
Hematological
  Anemia
  Transient neutropenia
  Residual anticoagulation
  Hypocomplementemia
Metabolic
  Hypokalemia
  Large protein losses
Skeletal
  Osteomalacia
  Arthropathy
  Myopathy
Infectious
  Peritonitis
  Transfusion-related hepatitis

polycystic kidney disease. The uncorrected manifestations of this syndrome (Table 30–4)—collectively referred to as **uremia**—are usually seen only after the GFR decreases below 25 mL/min. Patients with GFR below 10 mL/min are dependent on renal replacement therapy (RRT) for survival. RRT may take the form of hemodialysis, hemofiltration, peritoneal dialysis, or renal transplantation.

The generalized effects of uremia can usually be controlled by RRT. The majority of patients who do not undergo renal transplantation receive hemodialysis three times per week, and there are complications directly related to hemodialysis itself (Table 30–5). Hypotension, neutropenia, hypoxemia, and the disequilibrium syndrome are generally transient and resolve within hours after hemodialysis. Factors

contributing to hypotension during dialysis include the vasodilating effects of acetate dialysate solutions, autonomic neuropathy, and rapid removal of fluid. The interaction of white cells with cellophane-derived dialysis membranes can result in neutropenia and leukocyte-mediated pulmonary dysfunction leading to hypoxemia. Disequilibrium syndrome is characterized by transient neurological symptoms that appear to be related to a more rapid lowering of extracellular osmolality than intracellular osmolality.

Manifestations of Kidney Failure

A. Metabolic

Multiple metabolic abnormalities, including hyperkalemia, hyperphosphatemia, hypocalcemia, hypermagnesemia, hyperuricemia, and hypoalbuminemia, typically develop in patients with kidney failure. Water and sodium retention can result in worsening hyponatremia and extracellular fluid overload, respectively. Failure to excrete nonvolatile acids produces a high anion gap metabolic acidosis (see

Chapter 50). Hypernatremia and hypokalemia are uncommon complications.

Hyperkalemia is a potentially lethal consequence of kidney failure (see Chapter 49). It usually occurs in patients with creatinine clearances of less than 5 mL/min, but it can also develop rapidly in patients with higher clearances in the setting of large potassium loads (eg, trauma, hemolysis, infections, or potassium administration).

The hypermagnesemia is generally mild unless magnesium intake is increased (commonly from magnesium-containing antacids). Hypocalcemia is secondary to resistance to parathyroid hormone, decreased intestinal calcium absorption secondary to decreased renal synthesis of 1,25-dihydroxycholecalciferol, and hyperphosphatemia-associated calcium deposition into bone. Symptoms of hypocalcemia rarely develop unless patients are also alkalotic.

Patients with kidney failure also rapidly lose tissue protein and readily develop hypoalbuminemia. Anorexia, protein restriction, and dialysis are contributory.

B. Hematological

Anemia is nearly always present when the creatinine clearance is below 30 mL/min. Hemoglobin concentrations are generally 6–8 g/dL due to decreased erythropoietin production, decreased red cell production, and decreased red cell survival. Additional factors may include gastrointestinal blood loss, hemodilution, and bone marrow suppression from recurrent infections. Even with transfusions, it is often difficult to maintain hemoglobin concentrations greater than 9 g/dL. Erythropoietin administration may partially correct the anemia. Increased levels of 2,3-diphosphoglycerate (2,3-DPG), which facilitates the unloading of oxygen from hemoglobin (see Chapter 23), develop in response to the decrease in blood oxygen-carrying capacity. The metabolic acidosis associated with ESRD also favors a rightward shift in the hemoglobin–oxygen dissociation curve. In the absence of symptomatic heart disease, most ESRD patients tolerate anemia well.

Both platelet and white cell function are impaired in patients with kidney failure. Clinically, this is manifested as a prolonged bleeding time and increased susceptibility to infections, respectively. Most patients have decreased platelet factor III

activity as well as decreased platelet adhesiveness and aggregation. Patients who have recently undergone hemodialysis may also have residual anticoagulant effects from heparin.

C. Cardiovascular

Cardiac output increases in kidney failure to maintain oxygen delivery due to decreased blood oxygen-carrying capacity. Sodium retention and abnormalities in the renin–angiotensin system result in systemic arterial hypertension. Left ventricular hypertrophy is a common finding in ESRD. Extracellular fluid overload from sodium retention, in association with increased cardiac demand imposed by anemia and hypertension, makes ESRD patients prone to congestive heart failure and pulmonary edema. Increased permeability of the alveolar–capillary membrane may also be a predisposing factor for pulmonary edema associated with ESRD (see below). Arrhythmias, including conduction blocks, are common, and may be related to metabolic abnormalities and to deposition of calcium in the conduction system. Uremic pericarditis may develop in some patients, who may be asymptomatic, may present with chest pain, or may present with cardiac tamponade. Patients with ESRD also characteristically develop accelerated peripheral vascular and coronary artery atherosclerotic disease.

Intravascular volume depletion may occur in high-output acute kidney failure if fluid replacement is inadequate. Hypovolemia may occur secondary to excessive fluid removal during dialysis.

D. Pulmonary

Without RRT or bicarbonate therapy, ESRD patients may be dependent on increased minute ventilation as compensation for metabolic acidosis (see Chapter 50). Pulmonary extravascular water is often increased in the form of interstitial edema, resulting in a widening of the alveolar to arterial oxygen gradient and predisposing to hypoxemia. Increased permeability of the alveolar–capillary membrane in some patients can result in pulmonary edema even with normal pulmonary capillary pressures.

E. Endocrine

Abnormal glucose tolerance is common in ESRD, usually resulting from peripheral insulin resistance (indeed, type 2 diabetes mellitus is one of the most common causes of ESRD). Secondary hyperparathyroidism in patients with chronic kidney failure can produce metabolic bone disease, with osteopenia predisposing to fractures. Abnormalities in lipid metabolism frequently lead to hypertriglyceridemia and contribute to accelerated atherosclerosis. Increased circulating levels of proteins and polypeptides normally degraded by the kidneys are often present, including parathyroid hormone, insulin, glucagon, growth hormone, luteinizing hormone, and prolactin.

F. Gastrointestinal

Anorexia, nausea, vomiting, and adynamic ileus are commonly associated with uremia. Hypersecretion of gastric acid increases the incidence of peptic ulceration and gastrointestinal hemorrhage, which occurs in 10–30% of patients. Delayed gastric emptying secondary to autonomic neuropathy may predispose patients to perioperative aspiration. Patients with chronic kidney failure also have an increased incidence of hepatitis B and C, often with associated hepatic dysfunction.

G. Neurological

Asterixis, lethargy, confusion, seizures, and coma are manifestations of uremic encephalopathy, and symptoms usually correlate with the degree of azotemia. Autonomic and peripheral neuropathies are common in patients with ESRD. Peripheral neuropathies are typically sensory and involve the distal lower extremities.

Preoperative Evaluation

The systemic effects of kidney failure mandate a thorough evaluation of the patient. Most perioperative patients with acute kidney failure are critically ill, and their kidney failure is frequently associated with trauma or postoperative complications. Patients with acute kidney failure also tend to be in a catabolic metabolic state. Optimal perioperative management is dependent on dialysis. Hemodialysis is more effective than peritoneal dialysis and can be readily accomplished via a temporary internal jugular, subclavian, or femoral dialysis catheter. Continuous renal replacement therapy (CRRT) is

TABLE 30–6 Indications for dialysis.

Fluid overload
Hyperkalemia
Severe acidosis
Metabolic encephalopathy
Pericarditis
Coagulopathy
Refractory gastrointestinal symptoms
Drug toxicity

often used when patients are too hemodynamically unstable to tolerate intermittent hemodialysis. Indications for dialysis are listed in Table 30–6.

Patients with chronic kidney failure commonly present to the operating room for creation or revision of an arteriovenous dialysis fistula under local or regional anesthesia. However, regardless of the intended procedure or the anesthetic employed, one must be certain that the patient is in optimal medical condition; potentially reversible manifestations of uremia (see Table 30–4) should be addressed. Preoperative dialysis on the day of surgery or on the previous day is typical.

The history and physical examination should address both cardiac and respiratory function. Signs of fluid overload or hypovolemia should be sought. Patients are often relatively hypovolemic immediately following dialysis. A comparison of the patient's current weight with previous predialysis and postdialysis weights may be helpful. Hemodynamic data and a chest radiograph, if available, are useful in confirming clinical impressions. Arterial blood gas analysis is useful in evaluating oxygenation, ventilation, hemoglobin level, and acid–base status in patients with dyspnea or tachypnea. The electrocardiogram should be examined for signs of hyperkalemia or hypocalcemia (see Chapter 49) as well as ischemia, conduction block, and ventricular hypertrophy. Echocardiography can assess cardiac function, ventricular hypertrophy, wall motion abnormalities, and pericardial fluid. A friction rub may not be audible on auscultation of patients with a pericardial effusion.

Preoperative red blood cell transfusions are usually administered only for severe anemia as guided by the patient's clinical needs. A bleeding time and coagulation studies may be advisable, particularly if neuraxial anesthesia is being considered. Serum

TABLE 30–7 Drugs with a potential for significant accumulation in patients with renal impairment.

Muscle relaxants
  Pancuronium
	Antiarrhythmics
	  Bretylium

Anticholinergics
  Atropine
  Glycopyrrolate
	Disopyramide
	  Encainide (genetically
	    determined)
	  Procainamide

Metoclopramide	Tocainide

H$_2$-receptor antagonists
  Cimetidine
  Ranitidine
	Bronchodilators
	  Terbutaline

Digitalis	**Psychiatric** Lithium
Diuretics	

Calcium channel antagonists
  Diltiazem
  Nifedipine
	Antibiotics
	  Aminoglycosides
	  Cephalosporins
	  Penicillins

β-Adrenergic blockers
  Atenolol
  Nadolol
  Pindolol
  Propranolol
	Tetracycline
	  Vancomycin
	Anticonvulsants
	  Carbamazepine
	  Ethosuximide
	  Primidone

Antihypertensives
  Captopril
  Clonidine
  Enalapril
  Hydralazine
  Lisinopril
  Nitroprusside (thiocyanate)	

electrolyte, BUN, and creatinine measurements can assess the adequacy of dialysis. Glucose measurements guide the potential need for perioperative insulin therapy.

Drugs with significant renal elimination should be avoided if possible (Table 30–7). Dosage adjustments and measurements of blood levels (when available) are necessary to minimize the risk of drug toxicity.

Premedication

Alert patients who are stable can be given reduced doses of a benzodiazepine or an opioid, if needed. Aspiration prophylaxis with an H$_2$ blocker or proton pump inhibitor may be indicated in patients with nausea, vomiting, or gastrointestinal bleeding. Metoclopramide, 10 mg orally or slowly intravenously, may be useful in accelerating gastric emptying and decreasing the risk of aspiration. Preoperative medications—particularly

antihypertensive agents—should be continued until the time of surgery (see Chapter 21). The management of diabetic patients is discussed in Chapter 34.

INTRAOPERATIVE CONSIDERATIONS

Monitoring

Patients with renal insufficiency and kidney failure are at increased risk of perioperative complications, and their general medical condition and the planned operative procedure dictate monitoring requirements. Because of the risk of thrombosis, blood pressure should not be measured by a cuff on an arm with an arteriovenous fistula. Continuous intraarterial blood pressure monitoring may also be indicated in patients with poorly controlled hypertension, regardless of the procedure.

Induction

Patients with nausea, vomiting, or gastrointestinal bleeding should undergo rapid-sequence induction. The dose of the induction agent should be reduced for debilitated or critically ill patients, or for patients who have recently undergone hemodialysis (because of relative hypovolemia immediately following hemodialysis). Propofol, 1–2 mg/kg, or etomidate, 0.2–0.4 mg/kg, is often used. An opioid, β blocker (esmolol), or lidocaine may be used to blunt the hypertensive response to airway instrumentation and intubation. Succinylcholine, 1.5 mg/kg, can be used to facilitate endotracheal intubation in the absence of hyperkalemia. Vecuronium (0.1 mg/kg) or cisatracurium (0.15 mg/kg), or propofol–lidocaine induction without a relaxant, may be considered for intubation in patients with hyperkalemia.

Anesthesia Maintenance

The ideal anesthetic maintenance technique should control hypertension with minimal deleterious effect on cardiac output, because increased cardiac output is the principal compensatory mechanism for tissue oxygen delivery in anemia. Volatile anesthetics, propofol, fentanyl, sufentanil, alfentanil, and remifentanil are satisfactory maintenance agents. Nitrous oxide should be used cautiously in patients with poor ventricular function and should probably not be used for patients with very low hemoglobin concentrations (<7 g/dL) to allow the administration of 100% oxygen (see above). Meperidine is not an ideal choice because of the accumulation of its metabolite normeperidine. Morphine may be used, but some prolongation of its effects should be expected.

7 Controlled ventilation should be considered for patients with kidney failure. Inadequate spontaneous ventilation with progressive hypercarbia under anesthesia can result in respiratory acidosis that may exacerbate preexisting acidemia, lead to potentially severe circulatory depression, and dangerously increase serum potassium concentration (see Chapter 50). On the other hand, respiratory alkalosis may also be detrimental because it shifts the hemoglobin dissociation curve to the left, can exacerbate preexisting hypocalcemia, and may reduce cerebral blood flow.

Fluid Therapy

Superficial operations involving minimal tissue trauma require replacement of only insensible fluid losses. Procedures associated with major fluid losses require isotonic crystalloids, colloids, or both (see Chapter 51). Lactated Ringer's injection is best avoided in hyperkalemic patients when large volumes of fluid may be required, because it contains potassium (4 mEq/L); normal saline may be used instead. Glucose-free solutions should generally be used because of the glucose intolerance associated with uremia. Blood that is lost should generally be replaced with colloid or packed red blood cells as clinically indicated. Allogeneic blood transfusion may decrease the likelihood of rejection following renal transplantation because of associated immunosuppression.

Anesthesia for Patients with Mild to Moderate Renal Impairment

PREOPERATIVE CONSIDERATIONS

The kidney normally possesses large functional reserve. GFR, as determined by creatinine clearance, can decrease from 120 to 60 mL/min without any clinically perceptible change in renal function. Even patients with creatinine clearances of 40–60 mL/min usually are asymptomatic. These patients have only mild renal impairment but should still be thought of as having decreased renal reserve. The emphasis in the care of these patients is preservation of the remaining renal function, which is best accomplished by maintaining normovolemia and normal renal perfusion.

When creatinine clearance decreases to 25–40 mL/min, renal impairment is moderate, and patients are said to have renal insufficiency. Azotemia is always present, and hypertension and ane-
8 mia are common. Correct anesthetic management of this group of patients is as critical as management of those with frank kidney failure, especially during procedures associated with a relatively high incidence of postoperative kidney failure, such as cardiac and aortic recon-
9 structive surgery. Intravascular volume depletion, sepsis, obstructive jaundice, crush injuries, and renal toxins such as radiocontrast agents, certain antibiotics, angiotensin-converting enzyme inhibitors, and NSAIDs (see Table 29–4) are additional major risk factors for acute deterioration in renal function. Hypovolemia and decreased renal perfusion are particularly important causative factors in the development of acute postoperative kidney failure. The emphasis in management of these patients is on prevention, because the mortality rate of postoperative kidney failure may surpass 50%. The combination of diabetes and preexisting kidney disease markedly increases the perioperative risk of renal function deterioration and of kidney failure.

10 Renal protection with adequate hydration and maintenance of renal blood flow is indicated for patients at high risk for kidney injury and kidney failure undergoing cardiac, major aortic reconstructive, and other surgical procedures associated with significant physiological trespass. The use of mannitol, low-dose dopamine infusion, loop diuretics, or fenoldopam for renal protection is controversial and without conclusive proof of efficacy (see above). The value of renal protection with N-acetylcysteine prior to the administration of radiocontrast agents is reviewed in Chapter 29.

INTRAOPERATIVE CONSIDERATIONS

Monitoring

The American Society of Anesthesiologists' basic monitoring standards are used for procedures involving minimal fluid losses. For procedures associated with significant blood or fluid loss, close monitoring of hemodynamic performance and urinary output is useful (see Chapter 51). Although maintenance of urinary output does not ensure preservation of renal function, urinary outputs greater than 0.5 mL/kg/h are preferable. Continuous intraarterial blood pressure monitoring is also important if rapid changes in blood pressure are anticipated, such as in patients with poorly controlled hypertension and in those undergoing procedures associated with abrupt changes in sympathetic stimulation or in cardiac preload or afterload.

Induction

Selection of an induction agent is not as important as ensuring an adequate intravascular volume prior to induction; induction of anesthesia in hypovolemic patients with renal insufficiency frequently results in hypotension. Unless a vasopressor is administered, such hypotension typically resolves only following intubation or surgical stimulation. Renal perfusion, which may already be compromised by preexisting hypovolemia, may then deteriorate further, first as a result of hypotension, and subsequently from sympathetically or pharmacologically mediated renal vasoconstriction. If sustained, the decrease in renal perfusion may contribute to postoperative renal impairment or failure. Preoperative hydration usually prevents this sequence of events.

Maintenance of Anesthesia

All anesthetic maintenance agents are acceptable, with the possible exception of sevoflurane administered with low gas flows over a prolonged time period. Intraoperative deterioration in renal function may result from adverse effects of the operative procedure (hemorrhage, vascular occlusion, abdominal compartment syndrome, arterial emboli) or anesthetic (hypotension secondary to myocardial depression or vasodilation), from indirect hormonal effects (sympathoadrenal activation or antidiuretic hormone secretion), or from impeded venous return secondary to positive-pressure ventilation. Many of these effects are almost completely avoidable or reversible when adequate intravenous fluids are given to maintain a normal or slightly expanded intravascular volume. The administration of large doses of predominantly α-adrenergic vasopressors (phenylephrine and norepinephrine) may also be detrimental to preservation of renal function. Small, intermittent doses, or brief infusions, of vasoconstrictors may be useful in maintaining renal blood flow until other measures (eg, transfusion) are undertaken to correct hypotension.

Fluid Therapy

As reviewed above, appropriate fluid administration is important in managing patients with impaired renal function. Concern over fluid overload is justified, but problems are rarely encountered in such patients with normal urinary outputs if rational fluid administration guidelines and appropriate monitoring are employed (see Chapter 51). The adverse consequences of excessive fluid overload—namely, pulmonary congestion or edema—are far easier to treat than those of AKI and kidney failure.

CASE DISCUSSION

A Patient with Uncontrolled Hypertension

A 59-year-old man with a recent onset of hypertension is scheduled for reconstruction of a stenotic left renal artery. His preoperative blood pressure is 180/110 mm Hg.

What is the likely cause of this patient's hypertension?

Renovascular hypertension is one of the few surgically correctable forms of hypertension. Others include coarctation of the aorta, pheochromocytoma, Cushing's disease, and primary hyperaldosteronism.

Most studies suggest that renovascular hypertension accounts for 2–5% of all cases of hypertension. Characteristically it manifests as a relatively sudden onset of hypertension in persons younger than 35 years or older than 55 years of age. Renal artery stenosis can also be responsible for the development of accelerated or malignant hypertension in previously hypertensive persons of any age.

What is the pathophysiology of the hypertension?

Unilateral or bilateral stenosis of the renal artery decreases the perfusion pressure to the kidney(s) distal to the obstruction. Activation of the juxtaglomerular apparatus and release of renin increase circulating levels of angiotensin II and aldosterone, resulting in peripheral vascular constriction and sodium retention, respectively. The resulting systemic arterial hypertension is often severe.

In nearly two thirds of patients, the stenosis results from an atheromatous plaque in the proximal renal artery. These patients are typically men over the age of 55 years. In the remaining one third of patients, the stenosis is more distal and is due to malformations of the arterial wall, commonly referred to as *fibromuscular hyperplasia* (or, *dysplasia*). This latter lesion most commonly presents in women younger than 35 years. Bilateral renal artery stenosis is present in 30–50% of patients with renovascular hypertension. Less common causes of stenosis include dissecting aneurysms, emboli, polyarteritis nodosa, radiation, trauma, extrinsic compression from retroperitoneal fibrosis or tumors, and hypoplasia of the renal arteries.

What clinical manifestations other than hypertension may be present?

Signs of secondary hyperaldosteronism can be prominent. These include sodium retention in the form of edema, metabolic alkalosis, and hypokalemia. The latter can cause muscle weakness, polyuria, and even tetany.

How is the diagnosis made?

The diagnosis is suggested by the clinical presentation previously described. A midabdominal bruit may also be present, but the diagnosis requires laboratory and radiographic confirmation. A definitive diagnosis is made by renal arteriography, and percutaneous balloon angioplasty with stenting may be performed at the same time. The functional significance of the restrictive lesion(s) may be evaluated by selective catheterization of both renal veins and subsequent measurement of plasma renin activity in blood from each kidney. Restenosis rates following angioplasty are estimated to be <15% after 1 year. Patients who are not candidates for angioplasty and stenting are referred for surgery.

Should this patient undergo surgical correction given his present blood pressure?

Optimal medical therapy is important in preparing these patients for operation. Relative to patients with well-controlled hypertension, those with poorly controlled hypertension have a high incidence of intraoperative problems including marked hypertension, hypotension, myocardial ischemia, and arrhythmias. Ideally, arterial blood pressure should be well controlled prior to surgery. Patients should be evaluated for preexisting renal dysfunction, and metabolic disturbances such as hypokalemia should be corrected. Patients should also be evaluated as indicated for the presence and severity of coexisting atherosclerotic disease, according to current ACC/AHA guidelines (see Chapter 21).

What antihypertensive agents are most useful for controlling blood pressure perioperatively in these patients?

β-Adrenergic blocking drugs are frequently utilized for blood pressure control in the perioperative period. They are particularly effective because secretion of renin is partly mediated by β_1-adrenergic receptors. Although parenteral selective β_1-blocking agents such as metoprolol and esmolol would be expected to be most effective, nonselective agents such as propranolol appear equally effective. Esmolol may be the intraoperative β_1-blocking agent of choice because of its short half-life and titratability.

Direct vasodilators such as nitroprusside and nitroglycerin are also useful in controlling intraoperative hypertension.

ACE inhibitors and angiotensin converting enzyme receptor blockers are contraindicated in bilateral renal artery stenosis or in unilateral renal artery stenosis where there is only one functioning kidney because they can precipitate kidney failure.

What intraoperative considerations are important for the anesthesia provider?

Revascularization of a kidney is a major procedure, with the potential for major blood loss, fluid shifts, and hemodynamic changes. One of several procedures may be performed, including transaortic renal endarterectomy, aortorenal bypass (using a saphenous vein, synthetic graft, or segment of the hypogastric artery), a splenic to (left) renal artery bypass, a hepatic or gastroduodenal to (right) renal artery bypass, or excision of the stenotic segment with reanastomosis of the renal artery to the aorta. Rarely, nephrectomy may be performed. Regardless of the procedure, an extensive retroperitoneal dissection often necessitates relatively large volumes of intravenous fluid replacement. Large-bore intravenous access is mandatory because of the potential for extensive blood loss. Heparinization contributes to increased blood loss. Depending on the surgical technique, aortic cross-clamping, with its associated hemodynamic consequences, often complicates anesthetic management (see Chapter 22). Continuous intraarterial blood pressure monitoring is mandatory, and central venous pressure monitoring is often very helpful. Goal-directed hemodynamic and fluid therapy utilizing arterial pulse contour analysis, esophageal Doppler, or transesophageal echocardiography should be considered for patients with poor ventricular function, and may be advisable in most patients to guide fluid management (see Chapter 51). The choice of anesthetic technique is generally determined by the patient's cardiovascular function.

Urinary output should be followed carefully. Generous hydration and maintenance of adequate cardiac output and blood pressure are important to protect both the affected and the normal kidney against acute ischemic injury. Topical cooling of the affected kidney during the anastomosis may also be employed.

What postoperative considerations are important?

Although in most patients hypertension is ultimately cured or significantly improved, arterial blood pressure is often quite labile in the early postoperative period. Close hemodynamic monitoring should be continued well into the postoperative period. Reported operative mortality rates range from 1% to 6%, and most deaths are associated with myocardial infarction. The latter probably reflects the relatively high prevalence of coronary artery disease in older patients with renovascular hypertension.

SUGGESTED READING

Abi Antoun T, Palevsky PM: Selection of modality of renal replacement therapy. Semin Dial 2009;22:108.

Bagshaw SM, Wald R: Renal replacement therapy: When to start. Contrib Nephrol (Basel) 2011;174:232.

Bellomo R: Acute renal failure. Semin Respir Crit Care Med 2011;32:639.

Bellomo R, Ronco C, Kellum JA, et al: Acute renal failure—definition, outcome measures, animal models, fluid therapy and information technology needs: The Second International Consensus Conference of the Acute Dialysis Quality Initiative (ADQI) Group. Crit Care 2004;8:R204.

Brienza N, Giglio MT, Marucci M: Preventing acute kidney injury after noncardiac surgery. Curr Opin Crit Care 2010;16:353.

Chronopoulos A, Cruz DN, Ronco C: Hospital-acquired acute kidney injury in the elderly. Nat Rev Nephrol 2010;6:141.

Glassford NJ, Bellomo R: Acute kidney injury: How can we facilitate recovery? Curr Opin Crit Care 2011;17:562-568.

Harel Z, Chan CT: Predicting and preventing acute kidney injury after cardiac surgery. Curr Opin Nephrol Hypertens 2008;17:624.

Ho KM, Morgan DRJ: Meta-analysis of *N*-acetylcysteine to prevent acute renal failure after major surgery. Am J Kidney Dis 2009;53:33.

Hollmen M: Diagnostic test for early detection of acute kidney injury. Expert Rev Mol Diagn 2011;11:553.

House AA, Haapio M, Lassus J, et al: Pharmacological management of cardiorenal syndromes. Int J Nephrol 2011;2011:630.

Kim IB, Prowle J, Baldwin I, et al: Incidence, risk factors and outcome associations of intra-abdominal hypertension in critically ill patients. Anaesth Intensive Care 2012;40:79.

Mandelbaum T, Scott DJ, Lee J, et al: Outcome of critically ill patients with acute kidney injury using the Acute Injury Network criteria. Crit Care Med 2011;39:2659.

McCullough PA: Radiocontrast-induced acute kidney injury. Nephron Physiol 2008;109:61.

Mehta RL, Kellum JA, Shah SV, et al: Acute Kidney Injury Network: Report of an initiative to improve outcomes in acute kidney injury. Crit Care 2007;11:R31.

Mohmand H, Goldfarb S: Renal dysfunction associated with intra-abdominal hypertension and the abdominal compartment syndrome. J Am Soc Nephrol 2011;22:615.

Noor S, Usami A: Postoperative renal failure. Clin Geriatric Med 2008;24:721.

Ricci Z, Cruz DN, Ronco C: Classification and staging of acute kidney injury: Beyond the RIFLE and AKIN criteria. Nature Rev Nephrol 2011;7:201.

Trainor D, Borthwick E, Ferguson A: Perioperative management of the hemodialysis patient. Semin Dial 2011;24:314.

Weisbord SD, Palevsky PM: Strategies for the prevention of contrast-induced acute kidney injury. Curr Opin Nephrol Hypertens 2010;19:539.

Yilmaz R, Erdem Y: Acute kidney injury in the elderly population. Int Urol Nephrol 2010;42:259.

Anesthesia for Genitourinary Surgery

1 Next to the supine position, the lithotomy position is the most commonly used position for patients undergoing urological and gynecological procedures. Failure to properly position and pad the patient can result in pressure sores, nerve injuries, or compartment syndromes.

2 The lithotomy position is associated with major physiological alterations. Functional residual capacity decreases, predisposing patients to atelectasis and hypoxia. Elevation of the legs drains blood into the central circulation acutely. Mean blood pressure often increases, but cardiac output does not change significantly. Conversely, rapid lowering of the legs from the lithotomy or Trendelenburg position acutely decreases venous return and can result in hypotension. Blood pressure measurement should be taken immediately after the legs are lowered.

3 Because of the short duration (15–20 min) and outpatient setting of most cystoscopies, general anesthesia is often chosen, commonly employing a laryngeal mask airway.

4 Both epidural and spinal blockade with a T10 sensory level provide excellent anesthesia for cystoscopy.

5 Manifestations of TURP (transurethral resection of the prostate) syndrome are primarily those of circulatory fluid overload, water intoxication, and, occasionally, toxicity from the solute in the irrigating fluid.

6 Absorption of TURP irrigation fluid is dependent on the duration of the resection and the pressure of the irrigation fluid.

7 When compared with general anesthesia, regional anesthesia for TURP may reduce the incidence of postoperative venous thrombosis. It is also less likely to mask symptoms and signs of TURP syndrome or bladder perforation.

8 Patients with a history of cardiac arrhythmias and those with a pacemaker or internal cardiac defibrillator (ICD) may be at risk for developing arrhythmias induced by shock waves during extracorporeal shock wave lithotripsy (ESWL). Shock waves can damage the internal components of pacemaker and ICD devices.

9 Patients who are undergoing retroperitoneal lymph node dissection and who have received bleomycin preoperatively are at increased risk for developing postoperative pulmonary insufficiency. These patients may

—Continued next page

Continued—

be particularly at risk for oxygen toxicity and fluid overload, and for developing acute respiratory distress syndrome postoperatively.

10 For patients undergoing renal transplantation, the preoperative serum potassium concentration should be below 5.5 mEq/L and existing coagulopathies

should be corrected. Hyperkalemia has been reported after release of the vascular clamp following completion of the arterial anastomosis, particularly in pediatric and other small patients. Release of potassium contained in the preservative solution has been implicated as the cause of this phenomenon.

Urological procedures account for 10–20% of most anesthetic practices. Patients undergoing genitourinary procedures may be of any age, but many are elderly with coexisting medical illnesses, commonly renal dysfunction. The impact of anesthesia on renal function is discussed in Chapter 30. This chapter reviews the anesthetic management of common urological procedures. Use of the lithotomy and steep head-down (Trendelenburg) positions, the transurethral approach, and extracorporeal shock waves (lithotripsy) complicates many of these procedures. Moreover, advances in surgical technique and perioperative medical and surgical management allow more patients with coexisting disease to be considered acceptable candidates for renal transplantation and for extensive tumor debulking and reconstructive genitourinary procedures involving marked physiological trespass.

CYSTOSCOPY

Preoperative Considerations

Cystoscopy is the most commonly performed urological procedure, and indications for this investigative or therapeutic operation include hematuria, recurrent urinary infections, renal calculi, and urinary obstruction. Bladder biopsies, retrograde pyelograms, transurethral resection of bladder tumors, extraction or laser lithotripsy of renal stones, and placement or manipulation of ureteral catheters (stents) are also commonly performed through the cystoscope.

Anesthetic management varies with the age and gender of the patient and the purpose of the procedure. General anesthesia is usually necessary for children. Viscous lidocaine topical anesthesia with or without sedation is satisfactory for diagnostic studies in most women because of the short urethra. Operative cystoscopies involving biopsies, cauterization, or manipulation of ureteral catheters require regional or general anesthesia. Many men prefer regional or general anesthesia even for diagnostic cystoscopy.

Intraoperative Considerations

A. Lithotomy Position

1 Next to the supine position, the lithotomy position is the most commonly used position for patients undergoing urological and gynecological procedures. Failure to properly position and pad the patient can result in pressure sores, nerve injuries, or compartment syndromes. Two people are needed to safely move the patient's legs simultaneously up into, or down from, the lithotomy position. Straps around the ankles or special holders support the legs in lithotomy position (**Figure 31–1**). The leg supports should be padded wherever there is leg or foot contact, and straps must not impede circulation. When the patient's arms are tucked to the side, caution must be exercised to prevent the fingers from being caught between the mid and lower sections of the operating room table when the lower section is lowered and raised—many clinicians completely encase the patient's hands and fingers with

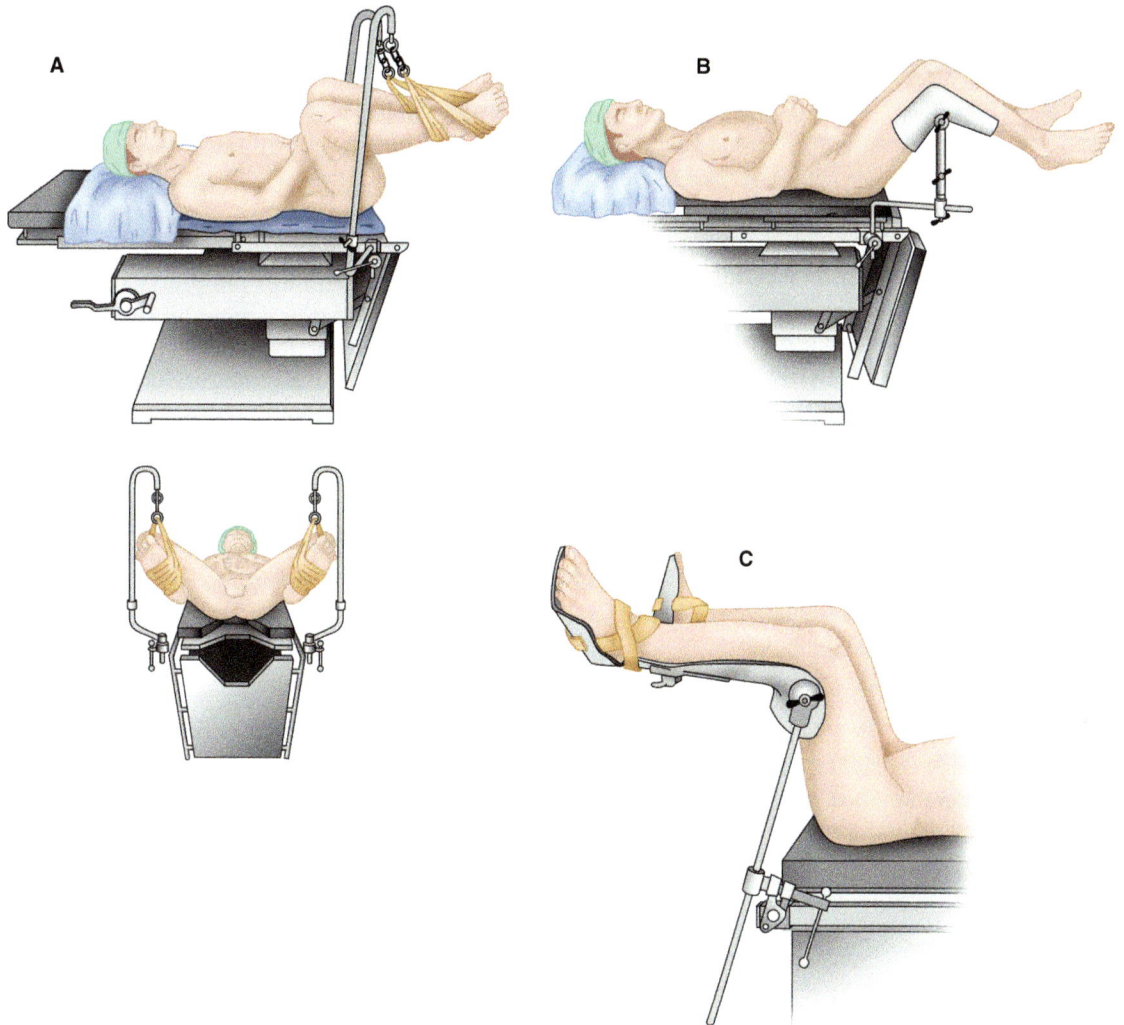

FIGURE 31–1 The lithotomy position. **A**: Strap stirrups. **B**: Bier–Hoff stirrups. **C**: Allen stirrups. (Reproduced, with permission, from Martin JT: *Positioning in Anesthesia*. W.B. Saunders, 1988.)

protective padding to minimize this risk. Injury to the tibial (common peroneal) nerve, resulting in loss of dorsiflexion of the foot, may result if the lateral knee rests against the strap support. If the legs are allowed to rest on medially placed strap supports, compression of the saphenous nerve can result in numbness along the medial calf. Excessive flexion of the thigh against the groin can injure the obturator and, less commonly, the femoral nerves. Extreme flexion at the thigh can also stretch the sciatic nerve. The most common nerve injuries directly associated

with the lithotomy position involve the lumbosacral plexus. Brachial plexus injuries can likewise occur if the upper extremities are inappropriately positioned (eg, hyperextension at the axilla). Compartment syndrome of the lower extremities with rhabdomyolysis has been reported with prolonged time in the lithotomy position, after which lower extremity nerve damage is also more likely.

2 The lithotomy position is associated with major physiological alterations. Functional residual capacity decreases, predisposing patients to atelectasis and hypoxia. This effect is amplified by steep Trendelenburg positioning (>30°), which is commonly utilized in combination with the lithotomy position. Elevation of the legs drains blood into the central circulation acutely and may thereby exacerbate congestive heart failure (or treat a relative hypovolemia). Mean blood pressure and cardiac output may increase. Conversely, rapid lowering of the legs from the lithotomy or Trendelenburg position acutely decreases venous return and can result in hypotension. Vasodilation from either general or regional anesthesia potentiates the hypotension in this situation, and for this reason, blood pressure measurement should be taken immediately after the legs are lowered.

B. Choice of Anesthesia

1. General anesthesia—Many patients are apprehensive about the procedure and prefer to be asleep. However, any anesthetic technique suitable for outpatients may be utilized. Because of the short duration (15–20 min) and outpatient setting of most cystoscopies, general anesthesia is often chosen, commonly employing a laryngeal mask airway. Oxygen saturation should be closely monitored when obese or elderly patients, or those with marginal pulmonary reserve, are placed in the lithotomy or Trendelenburg position.

2. Regional anesthesia—Both epidural and spinal blockade provide satisfactory anesthesia for cystoscopy. However, when regional anesthesia is chosen most anesthesiologists prefer spinal anesthesia because onset of satisfactory sensory blockade may require 15–20 min for epidural anesthesia compared with 5 min or less for spinal anesthesia. Some clinicians believe that the sensory level following injection of a hyperbaric spinal anesthetic solution should be well established ("fixed") before the patient is moved into the lithotomy position; however, studies fail to demonstrate that immediate elevation of the legs into lithotomy position following administration of hyperbaric spinal anesthesia either increases the dermatomal extent of anesthesia to a clinically significant degree or increases the likelihood of severe hypotension. A sensory level to T10 provides excellent anesthesia for essentially all cystoscopic procedures.

TRANSURETHRAL RESECTION OF THE PROSTATE

Preoperative Considerations

Benign prostatic hyperplasia (BPH) frequently leads to bladder outlet obstruction in men older than 60 years. Although increasingly being treated medically, some men require surgical intervention. Transurethral resection of the prostate (TURP) is the most common surgical procedure performed for bladder outlet obstruction due to BPH, and indications for TURP in this setting include obstructive uropathy, bladder calculi, and recurrent episodes of urinary retention, urinary tract infections, and hematuria. Patients with adenocarcinoma of the prostate may also benefit from TURP to relieve symptomatic urinary obstruction.

TURP requires regional or general anesthesia, and patients should be evaluated for coexistent major organ dysfunction. Despite advanced age (over half of TURP patients are older than 70 years) and prevalence of significant comorbidity in over two thirds of TURP patients, perioperative mortality and medical morbidity (most frequently myocardial infarction, pulmonary edema, and kidney failure) for this procedure are both less than 1%.

The most common surgical complications of TURP are clot retention, failure to void, uncontrolled hematuria requiring surgical revision, urinary tract infection, and chronic hematuria, although other, more rare, complications may include: TURP syndrome, bladder perforation, sepsis, hypothermia, and disseminated intravascular coagulation (DIC). A blood type and screen (see Chapter 51) is adequate for most patients, although crossmatched blood should be available for anemic patients and for patients with large glands in which extensive resection is contemplated. Prostatic bleeding can be difficult to control through the cystoscope.

Intraoperative Considerations

TURP is performed by passing a loop through a special cystoscope (resectoscope). Using continuous irrigation and direct visualization, prostatic tissue is resected by applying a cutting current to the loop. Because of the characteristics of the prostate and the large amounts of irrigation fluid often used, TURP

TABLE 31–1 Surgical complications associated with TURP.[1]

Most common
    Clot retention
    Failure to void
    Uncontrolled acute hematuria
    Urinary tract infection
    Chronic hematuria

Less common
    TURP syndrome
    Bladder perforation
    Hypothermia
    Sepsis
    Disseminated intravascular coagulation

[1]TURP, transurethral resection of the prostate.

TABLE 31–2 Manifestations of TURP syndrome.[1]

Hyponatremia
Hypoosmolality
Fluid overload
    Congestive heart failure
    Pulmonary edema
    Hypotension
Hemolysis
Solute toxicity
    Hyperglycinemia (glycine)
    Hyperammonemia (glycine)
    Hyperglycemia (sorbitol)
    Intravascular volume expansion (mannitol)

[1]TURP, transurethral resection of the prostate.

can be associated with a number of serious complications (Table 31–1).

A. TURP Syndrome

Transurethral prostatic resection often opens the extensive network of venous sinuses in the prostate, potentially allowing systemic absorption of the irrigating fluid. The absorption of large amounts of fluid (2 L or more) results in a constellation of symptoms and signs commonly referred to as the TURP syndrome (Table 31–2). This syndrome presents intraoperatively or postoperatively as headache, restlessness, confusion, cyanosis, dyspnea, arrhythmias, hypotension, or seizures, and it can be rapidly fatal. The manifestations are primarily those of circulatory fluid overload, water intoxication, and, occasionally, toxicity from the solute in the irrigating fluid. The incidence of TURP syndrome is less than 1%.

Electrolyte solutions cannot be used for irrigation during TURP because they disperse the electrocautery current. Water provides excellent visibility because its hypotonicity lyses red blood cells, but significant water absorption can readily result in acute water intoxication. Water irrigation is generally restricted to transurethral resection of bladder tumors only. For TURP, slightly hypotonic nonelectrolyte irrigating solutions such as glycine 1.5% (230 mOsm/L) or a mixture of sorbitol 2.7% and mannitol 0.54% (195 mOsm/L) are most commonly used. Less commonly used solutions include sorbitol 3.3%, mannitol 3%, dextrose 2.5–4%, and urea 1%.

Because all these fluids are still hypotonic, significant absorption of water can nevertheless occur. Solute absorption can also occur because the irrigation fluid is under pressure, and high irrigation pressures (bottle height) increase fluid absorption.

Absorption of TURP irrigation fluid is dependent on the duration of the resection and the pressure of the irrigation fluid. Most resections last 45–60 min, and, on average, 20 mL/min of the irrigating fluid is absorbed. Pulmonary congestion or florid pulmonary edema can readily result from the absorption of large amounts of irrigation fluid, particularly in patients with limited cardiac reserve. The hypotonicity of these fluids also results in acute hyponatremia and hypoosmolality, which can lead to serious neurological manifestations. Symptoms of hyponatremia usually do not develop until the serum sodium concentration decreases below 120 mEq/L. Marked hypotonicity in plasma ([Na$^+$] <100 mEq/L) may also result in acute intravascular hemolysis.

Toxicity may also arise from absorption of the solutes in these fluids. Marked **hyperglycinemia** has been reported with glycine solutions and may contribute to circulatory depression and central nervous system toxicity. Plasma glycine concentrations in excess of 1000 mg/L have been recorded (normal is 13–17 mg/L). Glycine is known to be an inhibitory neurotransmitter in the central nervous system and has also been implicated in rare instances of transient blindness following TURP. Hyperammonemia, presumably from the degradation of glycine, has also been documented in a few patients with marked central nervous system toxicity following TURP. Blood ammonia levels in some patients exceeded 500 μmol/L (normal is 5–50 μmol/L). The use of large amounts of sorbitol or dextrose irrigating solutions can lead to hyperglycemia, which can be marked in diabetic patients. Absorption of mannitol solutions causes intravascular volume expansion and exacerbates fluid overload.

Treatment of TURP syndrome depends on early recognition and should be based on the severity of the symptoms. The absorbed water must be eliminated, and hypoxemia and hypoperfusion treated. Most patients can be managed with fluid restriction and intravenous administration of furosemide. Symptomatic hyponatremia resulting in seizures or coma should be treated with hypertonic saline (see Chapter 49). Seizure activity can be terminated with small doses of midazolam (2–4 mg). Phenytoin, 10–20 mg/kg intravenously (no faster than 50 mg/min), should also be considered to provide more sustained anticonvulsant activity. Endotracheal intubation may be considered to prevent aspiration until the patient's mental status normalizes. The amount and rate of hypertonic saline solution (3% or 5%) needed to correct the hyponatremia to a safe level should be based on the patient's serum sodium concentration (see Chapter 49). The rate of hypertonic saline solution administration should be sufficiently slow as to not exacerbate circulatory fluid overload.

B. Hypothermia

Large volumes of irrigating fluids at room temperature can be a major source of heat loss in patients. Irrigating solutions should be warmed to body temperature prior to use to prevent hypothermia. Postoperative shivering associated with hypothermia may dislodge clots and promote postoperative bleeding, as well as add deleterious physiological stress to the patient with coexisting cardiopulmonary disease.

C. Bladder Perforation

The incidence of **bladder perforation** during TURP is less than 1%. Perforation may result from the resectoscope going through the bladder wall or from overdistention of the bladder with irrigation fluid.

Most bladder perforations are extraperitoneal and are signaled by poor return of the irrigating fluid. Awake patients will typically complain of nausea, diaphoresis, and retropubic or lower abdominal pain. Large extraperitoneal and most intraperitoneal perforations are usually even more obvious, presenting as sudden unexplained hypotension or hypertension, and with generalized abdominal pain in awake patients. Regardless of the anesthetic technique employed, perforation should be suspected in settings of sudden hypotension or hypertension, particularly with acute, vagally mediated bradycardia.

D. Coagulopathy

DIC has on rare occasion been reported following TURP and may result from the release of thromboplastins from prostate tissue into the circulation during the procedure. Up to 6% of patients may have evidence of subclinical DIC. A dilutional thrombocytopenia can also develop during surgery as part of the TURP syndrome from absorption of irrigation fluids. Rarely, patients with metastatic carcinoma of the prostate develop a coagulopathy from primary fibrinolysis due to secretion of a fibrinolytic enzyme. The diagnosis of coagulopathy may be suspected from diffuse, uncontrollable bleeding but must be confirmed by laboratory tests. Primary fibrinolysis should be treated with ε-aminocaproic acid (Amicar), 5 g followed by 1 g/h intravenously. Treatment of DIC in this setting may require heparin in addition to replacement of clotting factors and platelets, and consultation with a hematologist should be considered.

E. Septicemia

The prostate is often colonized with bacteria and may harbor chronic infection. Extensive surgical resection with the opening of venous sinuses can allow entry of organisms into the bloodstream. Bacteremia following transurethral surgery is common and can lead to septicemia or septic shock. Prophylactic antibiotic therapy (most commonly gentamicin, levofloxacin, or cefazolin) prior to TURP may decrease the likelihood of bacteremic and septic episodes.

F. Choice of Anesthesia

Either spinal or epidural anesthesia with a T10 sensory level, or general anesthesia, provides excellent anesthesia and good operating conditions for TURP. **7** When compared with general anesthesia, regional anesthesia may reduce the incidence of postoperative venous thrombosis. It is also less likely to mask symptoms and signs of TURP syndrome or bladder perforation. Clinical studies have failed to show any differences in blood loss, postoperative cognitive function, and mortality between regional and general anesthesia. The possibility of vertebral metastasis must be considered in patients with carcinoma, particularly those with back pain, as metastatic disease involving the lumbar spine is a relative contraindication to spinal or epidural anesthesia. Acute hyponatremia from TURP syndrome may delay or prevent emergence from general anesthesia.

G. Monitoring

Evaluation of mental status in the awake or moderately sedated patient is the best monitor for detection of early signs of TURP syndrome and bladder perforation. Tachycardia or decrease in arterial oxygen saturation may be an early sign of fluid overload. Perioperative ischemic electrocardiographic changes have been reported in up to 18% of patients. Temperature monitoring is standard of care for general anesthesia, and it should also be used in cases of lengthy resections under spinal or epidural anesthesia to detect hypothermia. Blood loss is particularly difficult to assess during TURP because of the use of irrigating solutions, so it is necessary to rely on clinical signs of hypovolemia (see Chapter 51). Blood loss averages approximately 3–5 mL/min of resection (usually 200–300 mL total) but is rarely life-threatening. Transient, postoperative decreases in hematocrit may simply reflect hemodilution from absorption of irrigation fluid. Less than 2% of patients require intraoperative blood transfusion; factors associated with need for transfusion include procedure duration longer than 90 min and resection of more than 45 g of prostate tissue.

LITHOTRIPSY

The treatment of kidney stones has evolved from primarily open surgical procedures to less invasive or entirely noninvasive techniques. Cystoscopic procedures, including flexible ureteroscopy with stone extraction, stent placement, and intracorporeal lithotripsy (laser or electrohydraulic), along with *medical expulsive therapy* (MET), have become first-line therapy. Extracorporeal shock wave lithotripsy (ESWL) is also utilized, primarily for 4-mm to 2-cm intrarenal stones, and percutaneous and laparoscopic nephrolithotomy for larger or impacted stones. MET has become the treatment of choice among many clinicians for acute episodes of urolithiasis: for stones up to 10 mm in diameter, administration of the α blockers tamsulosin (Flomax), doxazosin (Cardura), or terazosin (Hytrin) or the calcium channel blocker nifedipine (Procardia, Adalat) lessens the pain of acute urolithiasis and increases the rate of stone expulsion over a period of several days to several weeks.

During ESWL, repetitive high-energy shocks (sound waves) are generated and focused on the stone, causing it to fragment as tensile and shear forces develop inside the stone and cavitation occurs on its surface. Water or a conducting gel couples the generator to the patient. Because tissue has the same acoustic density as water, the waves travel through the body without damaging tissue. However, the change in acoustic impedance at the tissue–stone interface creates shear and tear forces on the stone. Subsequently, the stone is fragmented enough to allow its passage in small pieces down the urinary tract. Ureteral stents are often placed cystoscopically prior to the procedure. Tissue destruction can occur if the acoustic energy is inadvertently focused at air–tissue interfaces such as in the lung and intestine. The inability to position the patient so that lung and intestine are away from the sound wave focus is a contraindication to the procedure. Other contraindications include urinary obstruction below the stone, untreated infection, a bleeding diathesis, and pregnancy. The presence of a nearby aortic aneurysm or an orthopedic prosthetic device is considered a relative contraindication. Ecchymosis, bruising, or blistering of the skin over the treatment site is not uncommon. Rarely, a large perinephric hematoma can develop and may be responsible for a postoperative decrease in hematocrit.

Electrohydraulic, electromagnetic, or piezoelectric shock wave generators may be used for

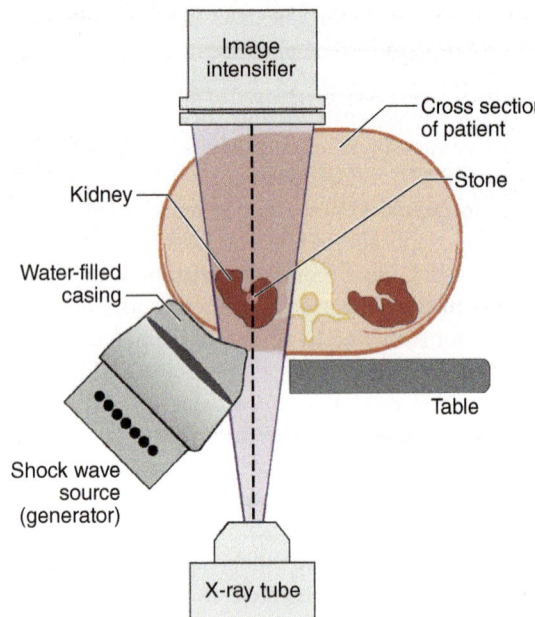

Image intensifier

Cross section of patient

Stone

Kidney

Water-filled casing

Table

Shock wave source (generator)

X-ray tube

FIGURE 31–2 Schematic representation of a newer tubless lithotripsy unit.

ESWL. With older electrohydraulic units, the patient is placed in a hydraulic chair and immersed in a heated water bath, which conducts the shock waves to the patient. Modern lithotriptors generate shock waves either electromagnetically or from piezoelectric crystals. The generator is enclosed in a water-filled casing and comes in contact with the patient via a conducting gel on a plastic membrane (Figure 31–2). Newer units allow both fluoroscopic and ultrasound localization. In the case of electromagnetic machines, the vibration of a metallic plate in front of an electromagnet produces the shock waves. With piezoelectric models, the waves are the result of changes in the external dimensions of ceramic crystals when electric current is applied.

Preoperative Considerations

⑧ Patients with a history of cardiac arrhythmias and those with a pacemaker or internal cardiac defibrillator (ICD) may be at risk for developing arrhythmias induced by shock waves during ESWL.

Synchronization of the shock waves with the electrocardiogram (ECG) R wave decreases the incidence of arrhythmias during ESWL. The shock waves are usually timed to be 20 ms after the R wave to correspond with the ventricular refractory period. Studies suggest that asynchronous delivery of shocks may be safe in patients without heart disease. Shock waves can damage the internal components of pacemaker and ICD devices. The manufacturer should be contacted as to the best method for managing the device (eg, reprogramming or applying a magnet).

Intraoperative Considerations

Anesthetic considerations for ureteroscopy, stone manipulation, and laser lithotripsy are similar to those for cystoscopic procedures. ESWL requires special considerations, particularly when older lithotriptors requiring the patient to be immersed in water are used.

A. Effects of Immersion During ESWL

Immersion into a heated water bath (36–37°C) initially results in vasodilation that can transiently lead to hypotension. Arterial blood pressure, however, subsequently rises as venous blood is redistributed centrally due to the hydrostatic pressure of water on the legs and abdomen. Systemic vascular resistance (SVR) rises and cardiac output often decreases. The sudden increase in intravascular volume and SVR can precipitate congestive heart failure in patients with marginal cardiac reserve. Moreover, the increase in intrathoracic blood volume reduces functional residual capacity 30–60% and may predispose some patients to hypoxemia.

B. Choice of Anesthesia

Pain during lithotripsy is from dissipation of a small amount of energy as shock waves enter the body through the skin. The pain is therefore localized to the skin and is proportionate to the shock wave intensity. Older water bath lithotripsy units require 1000–2400 relatively high-intensity shock waves, which most patients cannot tolerate without either regional or general anesthesia. In contrast, newer lithotripsy units that are coupled directly to the skin utilize 2000–3000 lower-intensity shock waves that usually require only light sedation.

C. Regional Anesthesia

Continuous epidural anesthesia is commonly employed when ESWL utilizes older water bath lithotriptors. Regional anesthesia with sedation greatly facilitates positioning and monitoring in this situation, and supplemental oxygen by face mask or nasal cannula is also useful in avoiding hypoxemia. A T6 sensory level ensures adequate anesthesia, as renal innervation is derived from T10 to L2. Supplementation of the block with epidural fentanyl (50–100 mcg) is often useful. When using the loss of resistance technique for placement of the epidural catheter, saline should be used instead of air during epidural catheter insertion; as air in the epidural space can dissipate shock waves and may promote injury to neural tissue. Foam tape should not be used to secure the epidural catheter as this type of tape has been shown to dissipate the energy of the shock waves when it is in their path. Spinal anesthesia can also be used satisfactorily but offers less control over the sensory level and an uncertain duration of surgery; for this reason, epidural anesthesia is usually preferred.

A major disadvantage of regional anesthesia or sedation is the inability to control diaphragmatic movement. Excessive diaphragmatic excursion during spontaneous ventilation can move the stone in and out of the wave focus and may prolong the procedure. This problem can be partially solved by asking the patient to breathe in a more rapid but shallow respiratory pattern. Bradycardia due to high sympathetic blockade also prolongs the procedure when shock waves are coupled to the ECG, and small doses of glycopyrrolate are often administered in this situation to accelerate the ESWL procedure.

D. General Anesthesia

General endotracheal anesthesia allows control of diaphragmatic excursion during lithotripsy using older water bath lithotriptors. The procedure is complicated by the inherent risks associated with placing a supine anesthetized patient in a chair, elevating and then lowering the chair into a water bath to shoulder depth, and then reversing the sequence at the end. A light general anesthetic technique in conjunction with a muscle relaxant is preferable. The muscle relaxant ensures patient immobility and control of diaphragmatic movement.

E. Monitored Anesthesia Care

Light intravenous sedation with midazolam and fentanyl is usually adequate for modern low-energy lithotripsy. Deeper sedation with low-dose propofol infusions with or without midazolam and opioid supplementation may also be used.

F. Monitoring

Standard anesthesia monitoring must be used for conscious or deep sedation, or for general anesthesia. **Even with R-wave synchronized shocks, supraventricular arrhythmias can occur.** With immersion lithotripsy, ECG pads should be attached securely with waterproof dressing. Changes in functional residual capacity with immersion mandate monitoring of oxygen saturation, particularly in patients at risk for developing hypoxemia. The temperature of the bath and the patient should be monitored to prevent hypothermia or hyperthermia.

G. Fluid Management

Intravenous fluid therapy is typically generous. Following an initial intravenous fluid bolus, an additional 1000–2000 mL of lactated Ringer's injection is often given with a small dose of furosemide to maintain brisk urinary flow and flush stone debris and blood clots. Patients with poor cardiac reserve require more conservative fluid therapy.

NONCANCER SURGERY OF THE UPPER URETER & KIDNEY

Laparoscopic urological procedures, including partial and total nephrectomy, live donor nephrectomy, nephrolithectomy, and pyeloplasty are increasingly utilized because of advantages that include relatively rapid recovery, shorter hospital stay, and less pain. Both transperitoneal and retroperitoneal approaches have been developed. A hand-assisted technique employs an additional larger incision that allows the surgeon to insert one hand for tactile sensation and facilitation of dissection. Anesthetic management is similar to that for any laparoscopic procedure.

Open procedures for kidney stones in the upper ureter and renal pelvis, and nephrectomies for nonmalignant disease, are often carried out in the "kidney rest position," more accurately described as the lateral flexed position. With the patient in a full lateral position, the dependent leg is flexed and the other leg is extended. An axillary roll is placed beneath the dependent upper chest to minimize the risk of brachial plexus injury. The operating table is then extended to achieve maximal separation between the iliac crest and the costal margin on the operative side, and the kidney rest (a bar in the groove where the table bends) is elevated to raise the nondependent iliac crest higher and increase surgical exposure.

The lateral flexed position is associated with adverse respiratory and circulatory effects. Functional residual capacity is reduced in the dependent lung but may increase in the nondependent lung. In the anesthetized patient receiving controlled ventilation, ventilation/perfusion mismatching occurs because the dependent lung receives greater blood flow than the nondependent lung, whereas the nondependent lung receives greater ventilation, predisposing the patient to atelectasis in the dependent lung and to shunt-induced hypoxemia. The arterial to end-tidal gradient for carbon dioxide progressively increases during general anesthesia in this position, indicating that dead space ventilation also increases in the nondependent lung. Moreover, elevation of the kidney rest can significantly decrease venous return to the heart in some patients by compressing the inferior vena cava. Venous pooling in the legs potentiates anesthesia-induced vasodilation.

Because of the potential for large blood loss and limited access to major vascular structures in the lateral flexed position, initial placement of at least one large-bore intravenous catheter is advisable. Arterial catheters are often utilized because of the need to closely monitor blood pressure and to frequently withdraw blood for laboratory analysis. Endotracheal tube placement may be altered during postinduction positioning of the patient for operation, and thus proper endotracheal tube placement must again be verified following final patient positioning prior to skin preparation and surgical draping. Intraoperative pneumothorax may occur as a result of surgical entry into the pleural space. Diagnosis requires a high index of suspicion. The pneumothorax may be subclinical intraoperatively but can be diagnosed postoperatively with a chest radiograph.

SURGERY FOR UROLOGICAL MALIGNANCIES

Demographic changes resulting in an increasingly elderly population, together with improved survival rates for patients with urological cancer following radical surgical resections, have resulted in an increase in the number of procedures performed for prostatic, bladder, testicular, and renal cancer. The desire for accelerated, less-complicated recovery with smaller, less painful incisions has prompted the development of laparoscopic pelvic and abdominal operations, including radical prostatectomy, cystectomy, pelvic lymph node dissection, nephrectomy, and adrenalectomy. Robotic-assisted technology has increasingly been applied to these procedures over the past decade.

Many urological procedures are carried out with the patient in a hyperextended supine position to facilitate exposure of the pelvis during pelvic lymph node dissection, retropubic prostatectomy, or cystectomy (**Figure 31–3**). The patient is positioned supine with the iliac crest over the break in the operating table, and the table is extended such that the distance between the iliac crest and the costal margin increases maximally. Care must be taken to avoid putting excessive strain on the patient's back. The operating room table is also tilted head-down to make the operative field horizontal. In the frog-leg position, a variation of the hyperextended supine position, the knees are also flexed and the hips are abducted and externally rotated.

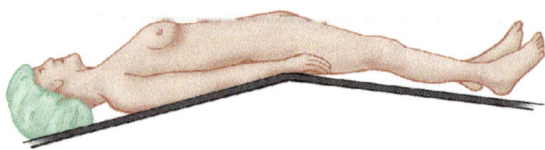

FIGURE 31–3 The hyperextended position. (Reproduced, with permission, from Skinner DG, Lieskovsky G: *Diagnosis and Management of Genitourinary Cancer.* W.B. Saunders, 1988.)

1. Prostate Cancer

Preoperative Considerations

Adenocarcinoma of the prostate is the most common nonskin cancer in men and is second only to lung cancer as the most common cause of cancer deaths in men older than 55 years. Approximately one in six men will be diagnosed with prostate cancer in their lifetime. Because of the tumor's wide spectrum of clinical behavior, management varies widely from surveillance to aggressive surgical therapy. Important variables include the grade and stage of the malignancy, the patient's age, and the presence of medical comorbidity. Transrectal ultrasound is used to evaluate tumor size and the presence or absence of extracapsular extension. Clinical staging is also based on the Gleason score of the biopsy, computed tomography (CT) scan or magnetic resonance imaging (MRI), and bone scan.

Intraoperative Considerations

Patients with prostate cancer may present to the operating room for laparoscopic or robotic prostatectomy with pelvic lymph node dissection, radical retropubic prostatectomy with lymph node dissection, salvage prostatectomy (following failure of radiation therapy), or bilateral orchiectomy for hormonal therapy.

A. Radical Retropubic Prostatectomy

Radical retropubic prostatectomy is usually performed with pelvic lymph node dissection through a lower midline abdominal incision. It may be curative for localized prostate cancer or occasionally used as a salvage procedure after failure of radiation. The prostate is removed en bloc with the seminal vesicles, ejaculatory ducts, and part of the bladder neck. A "nerve-sparing" technique may be used to help preserve sexual function. Following prostatectomy, the remaining bladder neck is anastomosed directly to the urethra over an indwelling urinary catheter. The surgeon may ask for intravenous administration of indigo carmine for visualization of the ureters, and this dye can be associated with hypertension or hypotension.

Radical retropubic prostatectomy may be accompanied by significant operative blood loss. Direct arterial blood pressure monitoring may be utilized. Routine placement of a central venous catheter for central venous pressure monitoring and as an additional route for administration of fluid and blood products has also been advocated, although many large cancer treatment centers routinely utilize just two large-bore peripheral intravenous catheters. Operative blood loss varies considerably from center to center, with mean values less than 500 mL common. Factors influencing blood loss include positioning, pelvic anatomy, prostate size, duration of operation, and the skill of the surgeon. Blood loss and operative morbidity and mortality are similar in patients receiving general anesthesia and those receiving regional anesthesia. Neuraxial anesthesia requires a T6 sensory level, but these patients typically do not tolerate regional anesthesia without deep sedation because of the hyperextended supine position. The combination of a prolonged Trendelenburg position together with administration of large amounts of intravenous fluids may rarely produce edema of the upper airway. The risk of hypothermia should be minimized by utilizing a forced-air warming blanket and an intravenous fluid warmer.

Postoperative complications include hemorrhage; deep venous thrombosis; pulmonary embolus; injuries to the obturator nerve, ureter, and rectum; and urinary incontinence and impotence. Extensive surgical dissection around the pelvic veins increases the risk of thromboembolic complications. Epidural analgesia is used in some centers following retropubic prostatectomy and may improve analgesia and accelerate recovery. Although epidural anesthesia may reduce the incidence of postoperative deep venous thrombosis following open prostatectomy, this beneficial effect may be negated by the routine use of warfarin or fractionated heparin prophylaxis postoperatively. The risk of epidural hematoma in the setting of anticoagulation therapy, particularly with fractionated heparin preparations, must be kept in mind when postoperative epidural analgesia is contemplated. Ketorolac can be used as an analgesic adjuvant and has been reported to decrease opioid requirements, improve analgesia, and promote earlier return of bowel function without increasing transfusion requirements. A multimodal approach to postoperative analgesia is often optimal.

B. Robot-Assisted Radical Prostatectomy

Laparoscopic radical prostatectomy with pelvic lymph node dissection differs from most other laparoscopic procedures by the frequent use of steep (>30°) Trendelenburg position for surgical exposure. Patient positioning, duration of procedure, need for abdominal distention, and desirability of increasing minute ventilation necessitate the use of general endotracheal anesthesia. Nitrous oxide is usually avoided to prevent bowel distention. Most laparoscopic prostatectomies are performed with robotic assistance, and the majority of radical prostatectomies in the United States are now performed via robot-assisted laparoscopy. When compared with open retropubic prostatectomy, laparoscopic robot-assisted prostatectomy is associated with a longer procedure time but may have a lower rate of complications. It is also associated with less blood loss and fewer blood transfusions, lower postoperative pain scores and lower opioid requirements, less postoperative nausea and vomiting, and shorter hospital length of stay. The steep Trendelenburg position can lead to head and neck tissue edema and to increased intraocular pressure. Complications reported to be associated with such positioning include upper airway edema and postextubation respiratory distress, postoperative visual loss involving ischemic optic neuropathy or retinal detachment, and brachial plexus injury. The surgeon should be routinely advised as to the length of time during which steep Trendelenburg positioning is maintained, and some centers have abandoned the routine use of this positioning entirely.

Most clinicians use a single large-bore intravenous catheter, and an arterial catheter may be used if clinically indicated. The risk of hypothermia should be minimized by utilizing a forced-air warming blanket and an intravenous fluid warmer. Adequate postoperative analgesia is provided initially by intravenous opioids with ketorolac and/or intravenous acetaminophen, and subsequently by oral analgesic preparations. Postoperative epidural analgesia is not warranted because of relatively low postoperative pain scores and because patients may be discharged less than 36 h after surgery.

C. Bilateral Orchiectomy

Bilateral orchiectomy is usually performed for hormonal control of metastatic adenocarcinoma of the prostate. The procedure is relatively short (20–45 min) and is performed through a single midline scrotal incision. Although bilateral orchiectomy can be performed under local anesthesia, most patients and many clinicians prefer general anesthesia (usually administered via a laryngeal mask airway) or spinal anesthesia.

2. Bladder Cancer

Preoperative Considerations

Bladder cancer occurs at an average patient age of 65 years with a 3:1 male to female ratio. Transitional cell carcinoma of the bladder is second to prostate adenocarcinoma as the most common malignancy of the male genitourinary tract. The association of cigarette smoking with bladder carcinoma results in coexistent coronary artery and chronic obstructive pulmonary disease in many of these patients. Underlying renal impairment, when present, may be age related or secondary to urinary tract obstruction. Staging includes cystoscopy and CT or MRI scans. Intravesical chemotherapy is used for superficial tumors, and transurethral resection of bladder tumors (TURBT) is carried out via cystoscopy for low-grade, noninvasive bladder tumors. Some patients may receive preoperative radiation to shrink the tumor before radical cystectomy. Urinary diversion is usually performed immediately following the cystectomy.

Intraoperative Considerations

A. Transurethral Bladder Resection

TURBT differs from TURP in that the surgical resection is not necessarily carried out in the midline. Bladder tumors may occur at various sites within the bladder. Unfortunately, laterally located tumors may lie in proximity to the obturator nerve. In such cases, if spinal anesthesia or general anesthesia without paralysis is administered, every use of the cautery resectoscope results in stimulation of the obturator nerve and adduction of the legs. Urologists rarely derive amusement from having their ear struck by the patient's knee; thus, in contrast to TURP, TURBT procedures are more commonly performed with general anesthesia and neuromuscular blockade. TURBT, unlike TURP, is rarely associated with absorption of significant amounts of irrigating solution.

B. Radical Cystectomy

Radical cystectomy is a major operation that is often associated with significant blood loss. It is usually performed through a midline incision but is increasingly performed as a robot-assisted laparoscopic procedure. All anterior pelvic organs including the bladder, prostate, and seminal vesicles are removed in males; the bladder, uterus, cervix, ovaries, and part of the anterior vaginal vault may be removed in females. Pelvic node dissection and urinary diversion are also carried out.

These procedures typically require 4–6 h and frequently are associated with blood transfusion. General endotracheal anesthesia with a muscle relaxant provides optimal operating conditions. Controlled hypotensive anesthesia may reduce intraoperative blood loss and transfusion requirements. Many surgeons also believe controlled hypotension improves surgical visualization. Supplementation of general anesthesia with spinal or continuous epidural anesthesia can facilitate the induced hypotension, decrease general anesthetic requirements, and provide highly effective postoperative analgesia.

Close monitoring of blood pressure, intravascular volume, and blood loss is always appropriate. Direct intraarterial pressure monitoring is indicated in most patients, and central venous catheters are often placed. Urinary output should be monitored and correlated with the progress of the operation, as the urinary path is interrupted at an early point during most of these procedures. As with all lengthy operative procedures, the risk of hypothermia should be minimized by utilizing a forced-air warming blanket and an intravenous fluid warmer.

C. Urinary Diversion

Urinary diversion is usually performed immediately following radical cystectomy. Many procedures are currently used, but all entail implanting the ureters into a segment of bowel. The selected bowel segment is either left in situ, such as in ureterosigmoidostomy, or divided with its mesenteric blood supply intact and attached to a cutaneous stoma or urethra. Moreover, the isolated bowel can either function as a conduit (eg, ileal conduit) or be reconstructed to form a continent reservoir (neobladder). Conduits may be formed from ileum, jejunum, or colon.

Major anesthetic goals for urinary diversion procedures include keeping the patient well hydrated and maintaining a brisk urinary output once the ureters are opened. Neuraxial anesthesia often produces unopposed parasympathetic activity due to sympathetic blockade, which results in a contracted, hyperactive bowel that makes construction of a continent ileal reservoir technically difficult. Papaverine (100–150 mg as a slow intravenous infusion over 2–3 h), a large dose of an anticholinergic (glycopyrrolate, 1 mg), or glucagon (1 mg) may alleviate this problem.

Prolonged contact of urine with bowel mucosa (slow urine flow) may produce significant metabolic disturbances. Hyponatremia, hypochloremia, hyperkalemia, and metabolic acidosis can occur following construction of jejunal conduits. In contrast, colonic and ileal conduits may be associated with hyperchloremic metabolic acidosis. The use of temporary ureteral stents and maintenance of high urinary flow help alleviate this problem in the early postoperative period.

3. Testicular Cancer

Preoperative Considerations

Testicular tumors are classified as either seminomas or nonseminomas. The initial treatment for all tumors is radical (inguinal) orchiectomy. Subsequent management depends on tumor histology. Nonseminomas include embryonal teratoma, choriocarcinoma, and mixed tumors. Retroperitoneal lymph node dissection (RPLND) plays a major role in the staging and management of patients with nonseminomatous germ cell tumors. Low-stage disease is managed with RPLND or in some instances by surveillance. High-stage disease is usually treated with chemotherapy followed by RPLND.

In contrast to nonseminomas, seminomas are very radiosensitive tumors that are primarily treated with retroperitoneal radiotherapy. Chemotherapy is used for patients who relapse after radiation. Patients with large bulky seminomas or those with increased α-fetoprotein levels (usually associated with nonseminomas) are treated primarily with chemotherapy. Chemotherapeutic agents commonly include cisplatin, vincristine, vinblastine, cyclophosphamide, dactinomycin, bleomycin, and etoposide. RPLND is usually undertaken for patients with residual tumor after chemotherapy.

Patients undergoing RPLND for testicular cancer are typically young (15–35 years old) but are at increased risk for morbidity from the residual effects of preoperative chemotherapy and radiation therapy. In addition to bone marrow suppression, specific organ toxicity may be encountered such as renal impairment following cisplatin, pulmonary fibrosis following bleomycin, and neuropathy following vincristine.

Intraoperative Considerations

A. Radical Orchiectomy

Inguinal orchiectomy can be carried out with regional or general anesthesia. Anesthetic management may be complicated by reflex bradycardia from traction on the spermatic cord.

B. Retroperitoneal Lymph Node Dissection

The retroperitoneum is usually accessed through a midline incision, but regardless of the surgical approach, all lymphatic tissue between the ureters from the renal vessels to the iliac bifurcation is removed. With the standard RPLND, all sympathetic fibers are disrupted, resulting in loss of normal ejaculation and infertility. A modified technique that may help preserve fertility limits the dissection below the inferior mesenteric artery to include lymphatic tissue only on the ipsilateral side of the testicular tumor.

9 Patients receiving bleomycin preoperatively may be particularly at risk for oxygen toxicity and fluid overload, and for developing pulmonary insufficiency or acute respiratory distress syndrome postoperatively. Excessive intravenous fluid administration may be contributory. Anesthetic management should include use of the lowest inspired concentration of oxygen compatible with oxygen saturation above 90%. Positive end-expiratory pressure (5–10 cm H_2O) may be helpful in optimizing oxygenation.

Evaporative and redistributive fluid losses ("third spacing") with open RPLND can be considerable as a result of the large wound and the extensive surgical dissection. Fluid replacement should be sufficient to maintain urinary output greater than 0.5 mL/kg/h; the combined use of both colloid and crystalloid solutions in a ratio of 1:2 or 1:3 may be more effective in preserving urinary output than crystalloid alone. Retraction of the inferior vena cava during surgery often results in transient arterial hypotension.

The postoperative pain associated with open RPLND incisions is severe, and aggressive postoperative analgesia is helpful. Continuous epidural analgesia, extended-release epidural morphine, or intrathecal morphine (or hydromorphone) should be considered. Because ligation of intercostal arteries during left-sided dissections has rarely resulted in paraplegia, it may be prudent to document normal motor function postoperatively prior to institution of epidural analgesia. The arteria radicularis magna (artery of Adamkiewicz), which is supplied by these vessels and is responsible for most of the arterial blood to the lower half of the spinal cord, arises on the left side in most individuals. It should be noted that unilateral sympathectomy following modified RPLND usually results in the ipsilateral leg being warmer than the contralateral one. Patients who have undergone RPLND frequently complain of severe bladder spasm pain in the postanesthesia care unit and postoperatively.

4. Renal Cancer

Preoperative Considerations

Renal cell carcinoma is frequently associated with paraneoplastic syndromes, such as erythrocytosis, hypercalcemia, hypertension, and nonmetastatic hepatic dysfunction. The classic triad of hematuria, flank pain, and palpable mass occurs in only 10% of patients, and the tumor often causes symptoms only after it has grown considerably in size. In fact, renal cell carcinoma is commonly discovered as an incidental finding in the course of working up a supposedly unrelated medical problem, such as in an MRI performed for evaluation of low back pain. This cancer has a peak incidence between the fifth and sixth decades of life, with 2:1 male to female ratio. Curative surgical treatment is undertaken for carcinomas confined to the kidney, but palliative surgical treatment may involve more extensive tumor debulking. In approximately 5–10% of patients, the tumor extends into the renal vein and inferior vena cava as a thrombus. Staging includes CT or MRI scans and an arteriogram. Preoperative arterial embolization may shrink the tumor mass and reduce operative blood loss.

Preoperative evaluation of the patient with renal carcinoma should focus on defining the degree of renal impairment, searching for the presence of coexisting systemic diseases, and planning the anesthetic management needs dictated by the scope of anticipated surgical resection. Preexisting renal impairment depends upon tumor size in the affected kidney as well as underlying systemic disorders such as hypertension and diabetes. Smoking is a well-established risk factor for renal carcinoma, and these patients have a high incidence of underlying coronary artery and chronic obstructive lung disease. Although some patients present with erythrocytosis, the majority are anemic. Preoperative blood transfusion to increase hemoglobin concentration above 10 g/dL should be considered when a large tumor mass is to be resected.

Intraoperative Considerations

A. Radical Nephrectomy

The operation may be carried out via an anterior subcostal, flank, or midline incision. Hand-assisted laparoscopic technique is often utilized for partial or total nephrectomy associated with a smaller tumor mass. Many centers prefer a thoracoabdominal approach for large tumors, particularly when a tumor thrombus is present. The kidney, adrenal gland, and perinephric fat are removed en bloc with the surrounding (Gerota's) fascia. General endotracheal anesthesia is used, often in combination with epidural anesthesia.

The operation has the potential for extensive blood loss because these tumors are very vascular and often very large. Direct arterial pressure monitoring should be used. Central venous cannulation is used for pressure monitoring and rapid transfusion. Transesophageal echocardiography should be strongly considered for all patients with extensive vena cava thrombus. Retraction of the inferior vena cava may be associated with transient arterial hypotension. Only brief periods of controlled hypotension should be used to reduce blood loss because of its potential to impair function in the contralateral kidney. Reflex renal vasoconstriction in the unaffected kidney can also result in postoperative renal dysfunction. Fluid replacement should be sufficient to maintain urinary output greater than 0.5 mL/kg/h.

If combined general–epidural anesthesia is employed, administration of epidural local anesthetic may be postponed until the risk of significant operative blood loss has passed as sympathectomy from epidural local anesthetic administration will potentiate the hypotensive effect of hemorrhage. As with all lengthy operative procedures, the risk of hypothermia should be minimized by utilizing a forced-air warming blanket and intravenous fluid warming. The postoperative course of open nephrectomy is extremely painful, and epidural analgesia is very useful in minimizing discomfort and accelerating acute postoperative convalescence.

B. Radical Nephrectomy with Excision of Tumor Thrombus

Some medical centers routinely perform complicated resections of renal cancers with tumor thrombus extending into the inferior vena cava. Because of the degree of physiological trespass and potential for major blood loss associated with this operation, the anesthetic management (as for nephrectomy) can be challenging. A thoracoabdominal approach allows the use of cardiopulmonary bypass when necessary.

The thrombus may extend only into the inferior vena cava but below the liver (level I), up to the liver but below the diaphragm (level II), or above the diaphragm into the right atrium (level III). Surgery can significantly prolong and improve quality of life in selected patients, and in some patients, metastases may regress after resection of the primary tumor. A preoperative ventilation-perfusion scan may detect preexisting pulmonary embolization of the thrombus. Intraoperative transesophageal echocardiography (TEE) is helpful in determining whether the uppermost margin of the tumor thrombus extends to the diaphragm, above the diaphragm, into the right atrium, or to the tricuspid valve. TEE can also be used to confirm the absence of tumor in the vena cava, right atrium, and right ventricle after successful surgery.

The presence of a large thrombus (level II or III) complicates anesthetic management. Invasive pressure monitoring and multiple large-bore intravenous catheters are necessary because transfusion requirements are commonly 10–15 units of packed red blood cells. Transfusion of platelets, fresh frozen plasma, and cryoprecipitate may also be required. Problems associated with massive blood transfusion should be anticipated (see Chapter 51). Central venous catheterization should be performed cautiously to prevent dislodgement and embolization of tumor thrombus. A high central venous pressure is typical in the setting of significant caval thrombus and reflects the degree of venous obstruction. Pulmonary artery catheters provide little information that cannot be obtained from a central line or TEE. Intraoperative TEE is preferable to a pulmonary catheter in every respect.

Complete obstruction of the inferior vena cava markedly increases operative blood loss because of dilated venous collaterals from the lower body that traverse the abdominal wall, retroperitoneum, and epidural space. Patients are also at significant risk for potentially catastrophic intraoperative pulmonary embolization of the tumor. Tumor embolization may be heralded by sudden supraventricular arrhythmias, arterial desaturation, and profound systemic hypotension. TEE is invaluable in this situation. Cardiopulmonary bypass may be used when the tumor occupies more than 40% of the right atrium and cannot be pulled back into the cava. Hypothermic circulatory arrest has been used in some centers. Heparinization and hypothermia greatly increase surgical blood loss.

RENAL TRANSPLANTATION

The success of renal transplantation, which is largely due to advances in immunosuppressive therapy, has greatly improved the quality of life for patients with end-stage renal disease. With modern immunosuppressive regimens, cadaveric transplants have achieved almost the same 80–90% 3-year graft survival rate as living-related donor grafts. In addition, restrictions on candidates for renal transplantation have gradually decreased. Infection and cancer are the only remaining absolute contraindications.

Preoperative Considerations

Current organ preservation techniques allow ample time (24–48 h) for preoperative dialysis of cadaveric recipients. Living-related transplants are performed electively with simultaneous donor and recipient operations. The recipient's serum potassium concentration should be below 5.5 mEq/L, and existing coagulopathies should be corrected.

Intraoperative Considerations

Renal transplantation is carried out by placing the donor kidney retroperitoneally in the iliac fossa and anastomosing the renal vessels to the iliac vessels and the ureter to the bladder. Heparin is administered prior to temporary clamping of the iliac vessels. Intravenous mannitol administered to the recipient helps establish an osmotic diuresis following reperfusion. Immunosuppression is initiated on the day of surgery with combination medications which may include corticosteroids, cyclosporine or tacrolimus, azathioprine or mycophenolate mofetil, antithymocyte globulin, monoclonal antibodies directed against specific subsets of T lymphocytes (OKT3), and interleukin-2 receptor antibodies (daclizumab or basiliximab). The anesthetist should discuss in advance with the surgery team the timing and dosage of any immunosuppressive agents which will need to be given perioperatively. Recipient nephrectomy (with a failed transplant) is performed for intractable hypertension or chronic infection.

A. Choice of Anesthesia

Most renal transplants are performed with general anesthesia, although spinal and epidural anesthesia are also utilized. All general anesthetic agents have been employed without any apparent detrimental effect on graft function. Cisatracurium and rocuronium may be the muscle relaxants of choice, as they are not dependent upon renal excretion for elimination. Vecuronium may be used with only modest prolongation of its effects.

B. Monitoring

Central venous cannulation may be useful for ensuring adequate hydration while avoiding fluid overload, particularly in patients with impaired cardiac status. Central lines are also useful portals for the various infusions that these patients require in the first few days after transplant. Normal saline is commonly used. A urinary catheter is placed preoperatively, and a brisk urine flow following the arterial anastomosis generally indicates good graft function. If the graft ischemic time was prolonged, an oliguric phase may precede the diuretic phase, in which case fluid therapy must be appropriately adjusted. Administration of furosemide or additional mannitol may be indicated in such cases. Hyperkalemia has been reported after release of the vascular clamp following completion of the arterial anastomosis, particularly in pediatric and other small patients, and release of potassium contained in the preservative solution has been implicated as the cause of this phenomenon. Donor kidney washout of the preservative solution with ice-cold lactated Ringer's solution just prior to the vascular anastomosis may help avoid this problem. Serum electrolyte concentrations should be monitored closely after completion of the anastomosis. Hyperkalemia may be suspected from peaking of the T wave on the ECG.

CASE DISCUSSION

Hypotension in the Recovery Room

A 69-year-old man with a history of an inferior myocardial infarction was admitted to the recovery room following TURP under general anesthesia. The procedure took 90 min and was reported to be uncomplicated. On admission, the patient is extubated but still unresponsive, and vital signs are stable. Twenty minutes later, he is noted to be awake but restless. He begins to shiver intensely, his blood pressure decreases to 80/35 mm Hg, and his respirations increase to 40 breaths/min. The bedside monitor shows a sinus tachycardia of 140 beats/min and an oxygen saturation of 92%.

What is the differential diagnosis?

The differential diagnosis of hypotension following TURP should always include (1) hemorrhage, (2) TURP syndrome, (3) bladder perforation, (4) myocardial infarction or ischemia, (5) septicemia, and (6) disseminated intravascular coagulation (DIC).

Other possibilities (see Chapter 56) are less likely in this setting but should always be considered, particularly when the patient fails to respond to appropriate measures (see below).

Based on the history, what is the most likely diagnosis?

A diagnosis cannot be made with reasonable certainty at this point, and the patient requires further evaluation. Nonetheless, the hypotension and shivering must be treated rapidly because of the history of coronary artery disease. The hypotension seriously compromises coronary perfusion, and the shivering markedly increases myocardial oxygen demand (see Chapter 21).

What diagnostic aids would be helpful?

A quick examination of the patient is extremely useful in narrowing down the possibilities. Hemorrhage from the prostate should be apparent from effluent of the continuous bladder irrigation system placed after the procedure. Relatively little blood in the urine makes it look pink or red; brisk hemorrhage is often apparent as grossly bloody drainage. Occasionally, the drainage may be scant because of clots blocking the drainage catheter; irrigation of the catheter is indicated in such cases.

Clinical signs of peripheral perfusion are invaluable. Hypovolemic patients have decreased peripheral pulses, and their extremities are usually cool and may be cyanotic. Poor perfusion is consistent with hemorrhage, bladder perforation, DIC, and severe myocardial ischemia or infarction. A full, bounding peripheral pulse with warm extremities is suggestive of, but not always present in, septicemia. Signs of fluid overload should be searched for, such as jugular venous distention, pulmonary crackles, and an S_3 gallop. Fluid overload is more consistent with TURP syndrome, but may also be seen in myocardial infarction or ischemia.

The abdomen should be examined for signs of perforation. A rigid and tender or distended abdomen is very suggestive of perforation and should prompt immediate surgical evaluation. When the abdomen is soft and nontender, perforation can reasonably be excluded.

Further evaluation requires laboratory measurements, an ECG, a chest radiograph, and consideration of a transthoracic echocardiogram. Blood should be immediately obtained for arterial blood gas analysis and measurements of hematocrit, hemoglobin, electrolytes, glucose, platelet count, and prothrombin and partial thromboplastin tests. If DIC is suggested by diffuse oozing, fibrinogen and fibrin split product measurements will confirm the diagnosis. A 12-lead ECG should be evaluated for evidence of ischemia, electrolyte abnormalities, or evolving myocardial infarction. A chest film should be obtained to search for evidence of pulmonary congestion, aspiration, pneumothorax, or cardiomegaly. An echocardiogram helps determine end-diastolic volume, systolic function (particularly the presence or absence of regional wall motion abnormalities), and can detect valvular abnormalities; comparison to prior studies would be invaluable.

While laboratory measurements are being performed, what therapeutic and diagnostic measures should be undertaken?

Immediate measures aimed at avoiding hypoxemia and hypoperfusion should be instituted. Supplemental oxygen should be administered, and endotracheal intubation is indicated if significant

hypoventilation or respiratory distress is present. Frequent blood pressure measurements should be obtained. If signs of fluid overload are absent, a diagnostic fluid challenge with 300–500 mL of crystalloid or 250 mL of colloid is helpful. A favorable response, as indicated by an increase in blood pressure and a decrease in heart rate, is suggestive of hypovolemia and may indicate the need for additional fluid boluses. Obvious bleeding in the setting of anemia and hypotension necessitates blood transfusion. The absence of a quick response to intravenous fluid volume challenge should prompt further evaluation. Administration of an inotrope, such as dopamine, is appropriate should ventricular dysfunction be detected by echocardiography. Direct intraarterial pressure measurement is invaluable in this setting.

If signs of fluid overload are present, intravenous furosemide in addition to an inotrope is indicated.

The patient's axillary temperature is 35.5°C. Does the absence of obvious fever exclude sepsis?

No. Anesthesia is commonly associated with altered temperature regulation. Moreover, correlation between axillary and core temperatures is quite variable (see Chapter 52). A high index of suspicion is therefore required to diagnose sepsis. Leukocytosis is common following surgery and is not a reliable indicator of sepsis in this setting.

The mechanism of shivering in patients recovering from anesthesia is poorly understood. Although shivering is common in patients who become hypothermic during surgery (and presumably functions to raise body temperature back to normal), its relation to body temperature is inconsistent. Anesthetics probably alter the normal behavior of hypothalamic thermoregulatory centers in the brain. In contrast, infectious agents, circulating toxins, or immune reactions cause the release of cytokines (interleukin-1 and tumor necrosis factor) that stimulate the hypothalamus to synthesize prostaglandin (PG) E_2. The latter, in turn, activates neurons responsible for heat production, resulting in intense shivering.

How can the shivering be stopped?

Regardless of its cause, shivering has the undesirable effects of markedly increasing metabolic oxygen demand (100–200%) and CO_2 production. Both cardiac output and minute ventilation must therefore increase, and these effects are often poorly tolerated by patients with limited cardiac or pulmonary reserve. Although the ultimate therapeutic goal is to correct the underlying problem, such as hypothermia or sepsis, additional measures are indicated in this patient. Supplemental oxygen therapy helps prevent hypoxemia. Unlike other opioid agonists, meperidine in small doses (25–50 mg intravenously) frequently terminates shivering regardless of the cause. Chlorpromazine, 10–25 mg, and butorphanol, 1–2 mg, may also be effective. These agents may have specific actions on temperature regulation centers in the hypothalamus. Shivering associated with sepsis and immune reactions can also be blocked by inhibitors of prostaglandin synthetase (aspirin, acetaminophen, and nonsteroidal antiinflammatory agents) as well as glucocorticoids. Intravenous acetaminophen is generally preferred perioperatively because it does not affect platelet function.

What was the outcome?

Examination of the patient reveals warm extremities with a good pulse, even with the low blood pressure. The abdomen is soft and nontender. The irrigation fluid from the bladder is only slightly pink. A diagnosis of probable sepsis is made. Blood cultures are obtained and antibiotic therapy is initiated to cover gram-negative organisms and enterococci, the most common pathogens. The patient receives empiric antibiotic coverage and a dopamine infusion is initiated. In settings of redistributive, vasodilatory shock, additional vasoconstrictors (eg, vasopressin) may be needed. The shivering ceases following administration of meperidine, 25 mg intravenously. The blood pressure increases to 110/60 mm Hg and the heart rate slows to 90 beats/min following a 1000 mL intravenous fluid bolus and initiation of a 5-mcg/kg/min dopamine infusion. The serum sodium concentration was found to be 130 mEq/L.

Four hours later, dopamine was no longer needed and was discontinued. The patient's subsequent recovery was uneventful.

SUGGESTED READING

American Society of Anesthesiologists: Practice advisory for the prevention of perioperative peripheral neuropathies: An updated report by the American Society of Anesthesiologists Task Force on Prevention of Perioperative Peripheral Neuropathies. Anesthesiology 2011;114:741.

Awad H, Santilli S, Ohr M, et al: The effects of steep Trendelenburg positioning on intraocular pressure during robotic radical prostatectomy. Anesth Analg 2009;109:473.

Bivalacqua TJ, Pierorazio PM, Su LM: Open, laparoscopic and robotic radical prostatectomy: Optimizing the surgical approach. Surg Oncol 2009; 18:233.

Brandina R, Berger A, Kamoi K, Gill IS: Critical appraisal of robotic-assisted radical prostatectomy. Curr Opin Urol 2009;19:290.

Chappell D, Jacob M: Influence of non-ventilatory options on postoperative outcome. Best Pract Res Clin Anaesthiol 2010;24:267.

Coelho RF, Rocco B, Patel MB, et al: Retropubic, laparoscopic, and robot-assisted radical prostatectomy: A critical review of outcomes reported by high-volume centers. J Endourol 2010; 24:2003.

Conacher ID, Soomro NA, Rix D: Anaesthesia for laparoscopic urological surgery. Br J Anaesthesia 2004;93;859.

Cousins J, Howard J, Borra P: Principles of anaesthesia in urological surgery. Br J Urol International 2005;96:223.

D'Alonzo RC, Gan TJ, Moul JW, et al: A retrospective comparison of anesthetic management of robot-assisted laparoscopic radical prostatectomy versus radical retropubic prostatectomy. J Clin Anesthesia 2009;21:322.

Ficarra V, Novara G, Artibani W, et al: Retropubic, laparoscopic, and robot-assisted radical prostatectomy: A systematic review and cumulative analysis of comparative studies. Eur Urol 2009;55:1037.

Fischer F, Engel N, Fehr JL, et al: Complications of robotic assisted radical prostatectomy. World J Urol 2008;26:595.

Gainsburg DM, Wax D, Reich DL, et al: Intraoperative management of robotic-assisted versus open radical prostatectomy. J Soc Laparoendoscop Surg 2010;14:1.

Hong JY, Kim JY, Choi YD, et al: Incidence of venous gas embolism during robotic-assisted laparoscopic radical prostatectomy is lower than that during radical retropubic prostatectomy. Br J Anaesthesia 2010;105:777.

Hong JY, Yang SC, Ahn S, et al: Preoperative comorbidities and relationship of comorbidities with postoperative complications in patients undergoing transurethral prostate resection. J Urol 2011;185:1374.

Jones DR, Lee HT: Perioperative renal protection. Best Pract Res Clin Anaesthesiol 2008;22:193.

Kakar PN, Das J, Roy PM, et al: Robotic invasion of operation theatre and associated anaesthetic issues: A review. Indian J Anaesth 2011;55:18.

Kauffman EC, Ng CK, Lee MM, et al: Critical analysis of complications after robotic-assisted radical cystectomy with identification of preoperative and operative risk factors. Br J Urol International 2010;105:520.

Park EY, Koo BN, Min KT, et al: The effect of pneumoperitoneum in the steep Trendelenburg position on cerebral oxygenation. Acta Anaesthesiol Scand 2009;53:895.

Valenza F, Chevallard G, Fossali T, et al: Management of mechanical ventilation during laparoscopic surgery. Best Pract Res Clin Anaesthesiol 2010;24:227.

Hepatic Physiology & Anesthesia

Michael Ramsay, MD, FRCA

1. The hepatic artery supplies 45% to 50% of the liver's oxygen requirements, and the portal vein supplies the remaining 50% to 55%.

2. All coagulation factors, with the exception of factor VIII and von Willebrand factor, are produced by the liver. Vitamin K is a necessary cofactor in the synthesis of prothrombin (factor II) and factors VII, IX, and X.

3. Many "liver function" tests, such as serum transaminase measurements, reflect hepatocellular integrity more than hepatic function. Liver tests that measure hepatic synthetic function include serum albumin, prothrombin time (PT, or international normalized ratio), cholesterol, and pseudocholinesterase.

4. Albumin values less than 2.5 g/dL are generally indicative of chronic liver disease, acute stress, or severe malnutrition. Increased losses of albumin in the urine

(nephrotic syndrome) or the gastrointestinal tract (protein-losing enteropathy) can also produce hypoalbuminemia.

5. The PT, which is normally 11–14 sec, depending on the control value, measures the activity of fibrinogen, prothrombin, and factors V, VII, and X.

6. The neuroendocrine stress response to surgery and trauma is characterized by elevated circulating levels of catecholamines, glucagon, and cortisol. Mobilization of carbohydrate stores and proteins results in hyperglycemia and a negative nitrogen balance (catabolism), respectively.

7. All opioids can potentially cause spasm of the sphincter of Oddi and increase biliary pressure.

8. When the results of liver tests are elevated postoperatively, the usual cause is underlying liver disease or the surgical procedure itself.

FUNCTIONAL ANATOMY

The liver is the heaviest organ in the body, weighing approximately 1500 g in adults. It is separated by the *falciform ligament* into right and left anatomic lobes; the larger right lobe has two additional smaller lobes at its posterior–inferior surface, the caudate and quadrate lobes. In contrast, surgical anatomy divides the liver based on its blood supply. Thus, the right and left surgical lobes are defined by the point of bifurcation of the hepatic artery and portal vein (*porta hepatis*); the falciform ligament therefore divides the left surgical lobe into medial and lateral segments. Surgical anatomy defines a total of eight segments.

The liver is made up of 50,000–100,000 discrete anatomic units called *lobules*. Each lobule is composed of plates of hepatocytes arranged cylindrically around a *centrilobular vein* (**Figure 32–1**). Four to

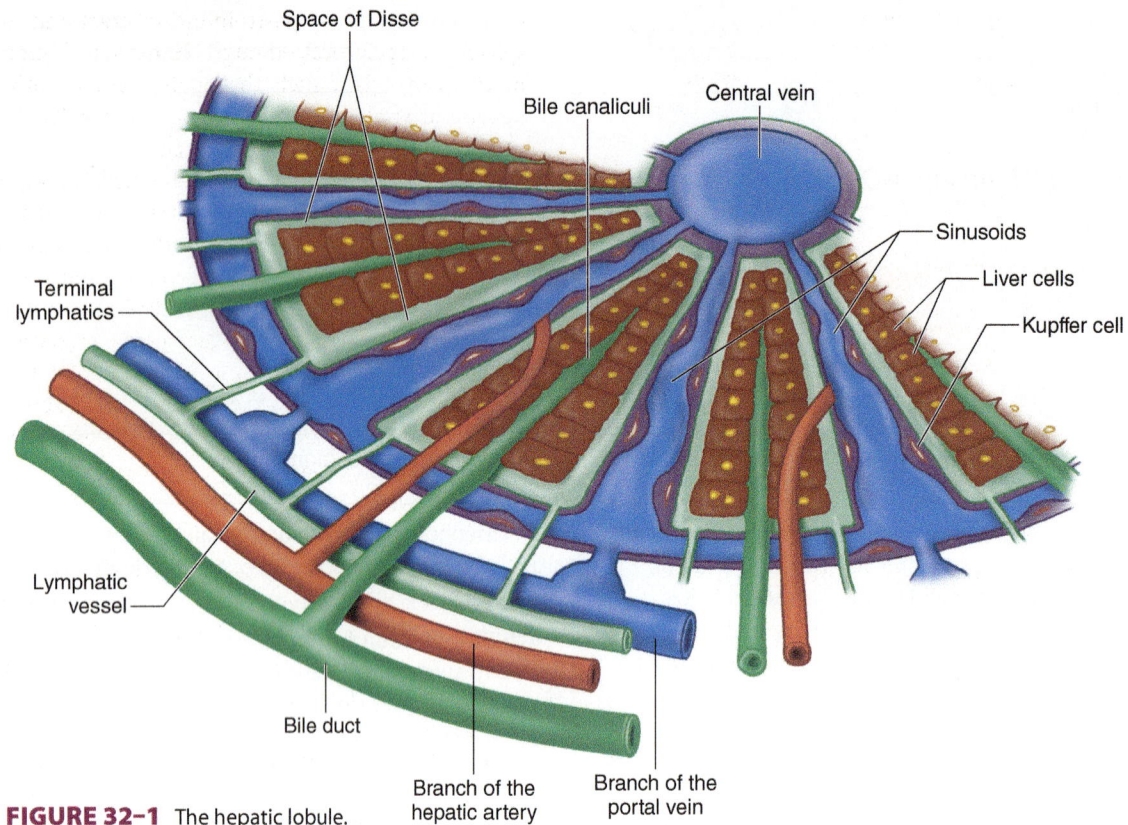

FIGURE 32–1 The hepatic lobule.

five portal tracts, composed of hepatic arterioles, portal venules, bile canaliculi, lymphatics, and nerves, surround each lobule.

In contrast to a lobule, an *acinus*, the functional unit of the liver, is defined by a portal tract in the middle and centrilobular veins at the periphery. Cells closest to the portal tract (zone 1) are well oxygenated; those closest to centrilobular veins (zone 3) receive the least oxygen and are most susceptible to injury.

Blood from hepatic arterioles and portal venules comingle in the sinusoidal channels, which lie between the cellular plates and serve as capillaries. These channels are lined by endothelial cells and by macrophages known as *Kupffer cells*. The Kupffer cells remove bacteria endotoxins, viruses, proteins and particulate matter from the blood. The *space of Disse* lies between the sinusoidal capillaries and the hepatocytes. Venous drainage from the central veins of hepatic lobules coalesces to form the hepatic veins (right, middle, and left), which empty into the

inferior vena cava (Figure 32–2). The caudate lobe is usually drained by its own set of veins.

Bile canaliculi originate between hepatocytes within each plate and join to form bile ducts. An extensive system of lymphatic channels also forms within the plates and is in direct communication with the space of Disse.

The liver is supplied by sympathetic nerve fibers (T6–T11), parasympathetic fibers (right and left vagus), and fibers from the right phrenic nerve. Some autonomic fibers synapse first in the celiac plexus, whereas others reach the liver directly via splanchnic nerves and vagal branches before forming the hepatic plexus. The majority of sensory afferent fibers travel with sympathetic fibers.

Hepatic Blood Flow

Normal hepatic blood flow is 25% to 30% of the cardiac output and is provided by the hepatic artery and portal vein. The hepatic artery supplies about 45% to 50% of the liver's oxygen requirements,

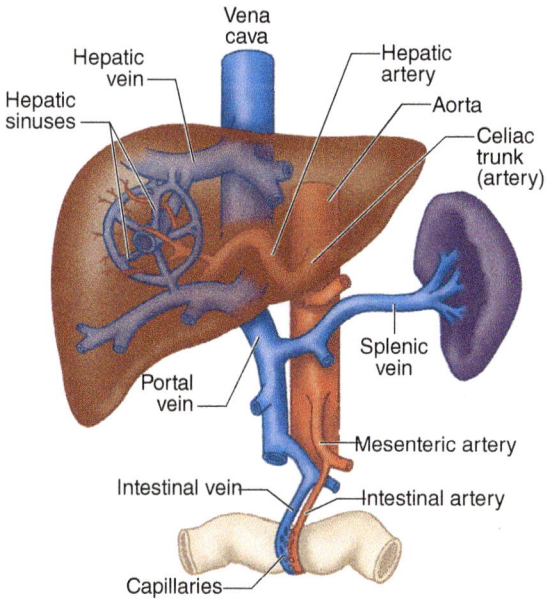

FIGURE 32–2 Hepatic blood flow. (Modified and reproduced, with permission, from Guyton AC: *Textbook of Medical Physiology*, 7th ed. W.B. Saunders, 1986.)

and the portal vein supplies the remaining 50% to 55% (Figure 32–2). Hepatic arterial flow seems to be dependent on metabolic demand (autoregulation), whereas flow through the portal vein is dependent

on blood flow to the gastrointestinal tract and the spleen. A reciprocal, though somewhat limited, mechanism exists, such that a decrease in either hepatic arterial or portal venous flow results in a compensatory increase in the other.

The hepatic artery has α_1-adrenergic vasoconstriction receptors as well as β_2-adrenergic, dopaminergic (D_1), and cholinergic vasodilator receptors. The portal vein has only α_1-adrenergic and dopaminergic (D_1) receptors. Sympathetic activation results in vasoconstriction of the hepatic artery and mesenteric vessels, decreasing hepatic blood flow. β-Adrenergic stimulation vasodilates the hepatic artery; β-blockers reduce blood flow, and, therefore, decrease portal pressure.

Reservoir Function

Portal vein pressure is normally only about 7–10 mm Hg, but the low resistance of the hepatic sinusoids allows relatively large blood flows through the portal vein. Small changes in hepatic venous tone and hepatic venous pressure thus can result in large changes in hepatic blood volume, allowing the liver to act as a blood reservoir (**Figure 32–3**). A decrease in hepatic venous pressure, as occurs during hemorrhage, shifts blood from hepatic veins and sinusoids into the central venous circulation and augments

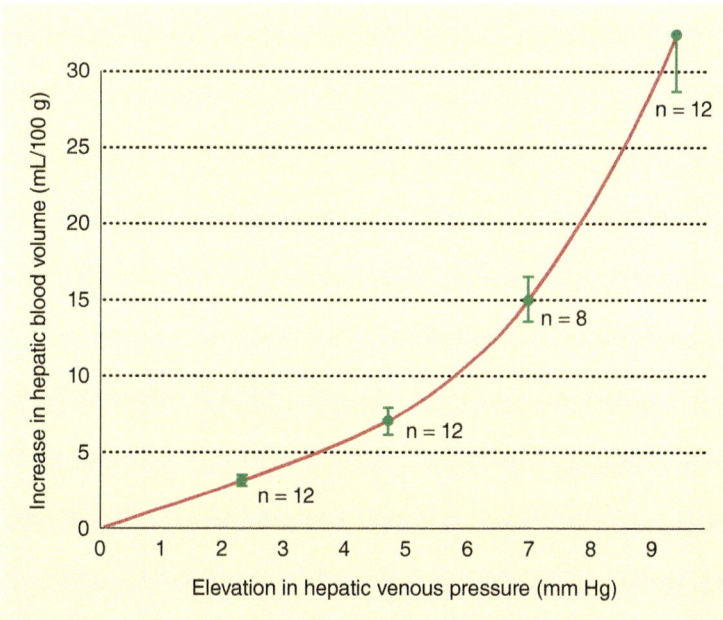

FIGURE 32–3 Hepatic venous compliance and the role of the liver as a blood reservoir. (Modified and reproduced, with permission, from Lautt WW, Greeway CV: *Am J Physiol* 1976;231:292.)

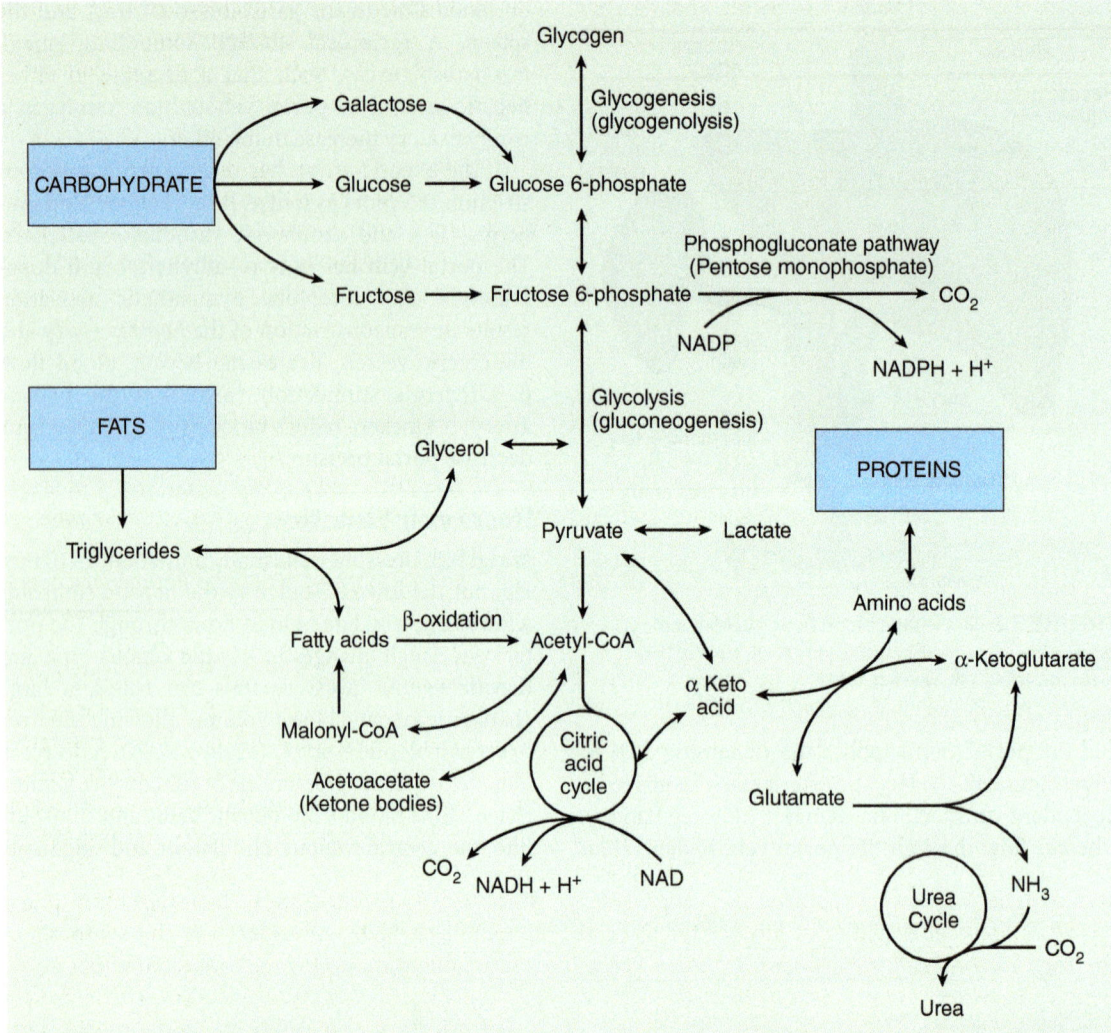

FIGURE 32–4 Important metabolic pathways in hepatocytes. Although small amounts of adenosine triphosphate (ATP) are derived directly from some intermediary reactions, the overwhelming majority of ATP produced is the result of oxidative phosphorylation of the reduced forms of nicotinamide adenine dinucleotide (NADH) and nicotinamide adenine dinucleotide phosphate (NADPH).

circulating blood volume. Blood loss can be reduced during liver surgery by lowering the central venous pressure, thereby reducing hepatic venous pressure and hepatic blood volume. In patients with congestive heart failure, the increase in central venous pressure is transmitted to the hepatic veins and causes congestion of the liver that can adversely affect liver function.

Metabolic Function

The abundance of enzymatic pathways in the liver allows it to play a key role in the metabolism of carbohydrates, fats, proteins, and other substances (see Figure 32–4 and Table 32–1). The final products of carbohydrate digestion are glucose, fructose, and galactose. With the exception of the large amount of fructose that is converted by the liver to lactate,

TABLE 32–1 Metabolic functions of the liver.

Creation and secretion of bile

Nutrient metabolism
  Amino acids
  Monosaccharides (sugars)
  Lipids (fatty acids, cholesterol, phospholipids,
    lipoproteins)
  Vitamins

Phase I and II biotransformation
  Toxins
  Drugs
  Hormones (steroids)

Synthesis
  Albumin, α_1-antitrypsin, proteases
  Clotting factors
  Acute phase proteins
  Plasma cholinesterase

Immune function
  Kupffer cells

hepatic conversion of fructose and galactose into glucose makes glucose metabolism the final common pathway for most carbohydrates.

All cells utilize glucose to produce energy in the form of adenosine triphosphate (ATP), either aerobically via the citric acid cycle or anaerobically via glycolysis. The liver and adipose tissue can also utilize the phosphogluconate pathway, which provides energy and fatty acid synthesis. Most of the glucose absorbed following a meal is normally stored as glycogen, which only the liver and muscle are able to store in significant amounts. When glycogen storage capacity is exceeded, excess glucose is converted into fat. Insulin enhances glycogen synthesis, and epinephrine and glucagon enhance glycogenolysis. Because glucose consumption averages 150 g/day, and hepatic glycogen stores are normally only about 70 g/day, glycogen stores are depleted after 24 hr of fasting. After this period of fasting, *gluconeogenesis*, the *de novo* synthesis of glucose, is necessary to provide an uninterrupted supply of glucose for other organs.

The liver and kidney are unique in their capacity to form glucose from lactate, pyruvate, amino acids (mainly alanine), and glycerol (derived from fat metabolism). Hepatic gluconeogenesis is vital in the maintenance of a normal blood glucose concentration. Glucocorticoids, catecholamines, glucagon, and thyroid hormone greatly enhance gluconeogenesis, whereas insulin inhibits it.

When carbohydrate stores are saturated, the liver converts the excess ingested carbohydrates and proteins into fat. The fatty acids thus formed can be used immediately for fuel or stored in adipose tissue or the liver for later consumption. Nearly all cells utilize fatty acids derived from ingested fats or synthesized from intermediary metabolites of carbohydrates and protein as an energy source—only red blood cells and the renal medulla are limited to glucose utilization. Neurons normally utilize only glucose, but, after a few days of starvation, they can switch to ketone bodies, the breakdown products of fatty acids that have been synthesized by the liver as an energy source.

To oxidize fatty acids, they are converted into acetylcoenzyme A (acetyl-CoA), which is then oxidized via the citric acid cycle to produce ATP. The liver is capable of high rates of fatty acid oxidation and can form acetoacetic acid (one of the ketone bodies) from excess acetyl-CoA. The acetoacetate released by hepatocytes serves as an alternative energy source for other cell types by reconversion into acetyl-CoA. Insulin inhibits hepatic ketone body production. Acetyl-CoA is also used by the liver for the production of cholesterol and phospholipids, which is necessary in the synthesis of cellular membranes throughout the body.

The liver performs a critical role in protein metabolism. Without this function, death usually occurs within several days. The steps involved in protein metabolism include: (1) deamination of amino acids, (2) formation of urea (to eliminate the ammonia produced from deamination), (3) interconversions between nonessential amino acids, and (4) formation of plasma proteins. Deamination is necessary for the conversion of excess amino acids into carbohydrates and fats. The enzymatic processes, most commonly transamination, convert amino acids into their respective keto acids and produce ammonia as a byproduct.

Ammonia formed from deamination (as well as that produced by colonic bacteria and absorbed through the gut) is highly toxic to tissues. Through a series of enzymatic steps, the liver combines two molecules of ammonia with CO_2 to form urea. The urea thus formed readily diffuses out of the liver and can then be excreted by the kidneys.

Nearly all plasma proteins, with the notable exception of immunoglobulins, are formed by the liver. These include albumin, α_1-antitrypsin and other proteases/elastases, and the coagulation factors. Albumin is responsible for maintaining a normal plasma oncotic pressure and is the principal binding and transport protein for fatty acids and a large number of hormones and drugs. Consequently, changes in albumin concentration can affect the concentration of the pharmacologically active, unbound fraction of many drugs.

2 All coagulation factors, with the exception of factor VIII and von Willebrand factor, are produced by the liver (see Table 32–2, Figure 32–5, and Chapter 51). Vascular endothelial cells synthesize factor VIII, levels of which are therefore usually maintained in chronic liver disease. Vitamin K is a necessary cofactor in the synthesis of prothrombin (factor II) and factors VII, IX, and X. The

TABLE 32–2 Coagulation factors.

	Factor	Approximate Half-Life (h)
I	Fibrinogen	100
II	Prothrombin	80
III	Tissue thromboplastin	—
IV	Calcium	—
V	Proaccelerin	18
VII	Proconvertin	6
VIII	Antihemophilic factor	10
IX	Christmas factor	24
X	Stuart factor	50
XI	Plasma thromboplastin antecedents	25
XII	Hageman factor	60
XIII	Fibrin-stabilizing factor	90

liver also produces plasma cholinesterase (pseudocholinesterase), an enzyme that hydrolyzes esters, including some local anesthetics and some muscle relaxants. Other important proteins formed by the liver include protease inhibitors (antithrombin III, α_2-antiplasmin, and α_1-antitrypsin), transport proteins (transferrin, haptoglobin, and ceruloplasmin), complement, α_1-acid glycoprotein, C-reactive protein, and serum amyloid A.

Drug Metabolism

Many exogenous substances, including most drugs, undergo hepatic biotransformation, and the end-products of these reactions are usually either inactivated or converted to more water-soluble substances that can be readily excreted in bile or urine. Hepatic biotransformations are often categorized as one of two types of reactions. *Phase I reactions* modify reactive chemical groups through mixed-function oxidases or the cytochrome P-450 enzyme systems, resulting in oxidation, reduction, deamination, sulfoxidation, dealkylation, or methylation. Barbiturates and benzodiazepines are inactivated by phase I reactions. *Phase II reactions*, which may or may not follow a phase I reaction, involve conjugation of the substance with glucuronide, sulfate, taurine, or glycine. The conjugated compound can then be readily eliminated in urine or bile.

Some enzyme systems, such as those of cytochrome P-450, can be induced by a few drugs, such as ethanol, barbiturates, ketamine, and perhaps benzodiazepines. This can result in increased tolerance to the drugs' effects. Conversely, some agents, such as cimetidine and chloramphenicol, can prolong the effects of other drugs by inhibiting these enzymes. Some drugs, including lidocaine, morphine, verapamil, labetalol, and propranolol, have very high rates of hepatic extraction from the circulation, and their metabolism is therefore highly dependent upon the rate of hepatic blood flow. As a result, a decrease in their metabolic clearance usually reflects decreased hepatic blood flow rather than hepatocellular dysfunction.

The liver plays a major role in hormone, vitamin, and mineral metabolism. It is an important site for the

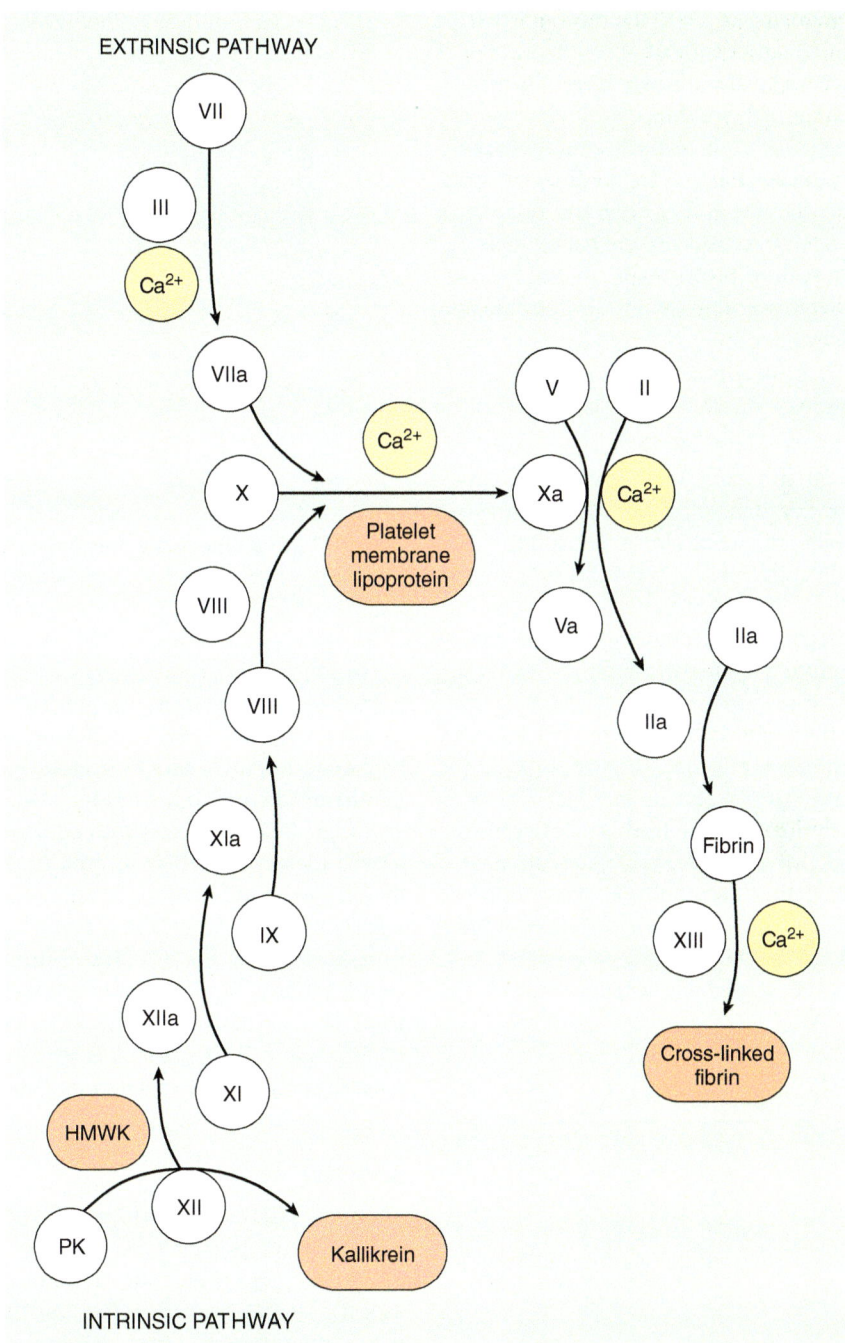

FIGURE 32–5 The intrinsic and extrinsic coagulation pathways.

conversion of thyroxine (T_4) into the more active tri-iodothyronine (T_3), and degradation of thyroid hormone is principally hepatic. The liver is also the major site of degradation for insulin, steroid hormones (estrogen, aldosterone, and cortisol), glucagon, and antidiuretic hormone. Hepatocytes are the principal storage sites for vitamins A, B_{12}, E, D, and K. Lastly, hepatic production of transferrin and haptoglobin is important because these proteins are involved in iron hemostasis, whereas ceruloplasmin is important in copper regulation.

Bile Formation

Bile (Table 32–3) plays an important role in absorption of fat and excretion of bilirubin, cholesterol, and many drugs. Hepatocytes continuously secrete bile salts, cholesterol, phospholipids, conjugated bilirubin, and other substances into bile canaliculi.

Bile ducts from hepatic lobules join and eventually form the right and left hepatic ducts. These ducts, in turn, combine to form the hepatic duct, which together with the cystic duct from the gallbladder becomes the common bile duct (Figure 32–6). The gallbladder serves as a reservoir for bile. The bile acids formed by hepatocytes from cholesterol are essential for emulsifying the insoluble components of bile and facilitating the intestinal absorption of lipids. Defects in the formation or secretion of bile salts interfere with the absorption of fats and fat-soluble vitamins (A, D, E, and K). Because of normally

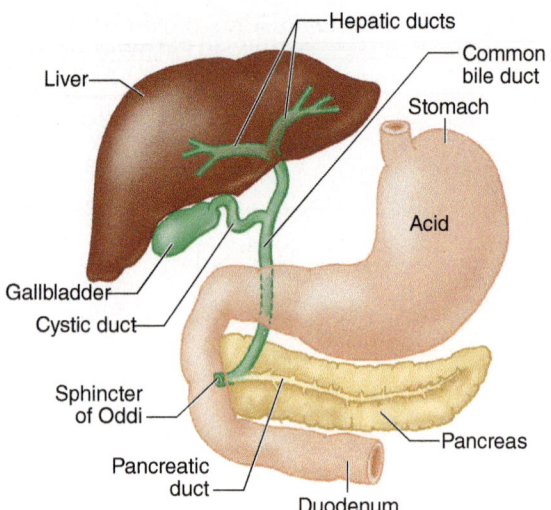

FIGURE 32–6 The biliary system. (Modified and reproduced, with permission, from Guyton AC: *Textbook of Medical Physiology*, 7th ed. W.B. Saunders, 1986.)

TABLE 32–3 Composition of bile.

97% water
<1% bile salts
Pigments
Inorganic salts
Lipids 　Cholesterol 　Fatty acids
Lecithin
Alkaline phosphatase

limited stores of vitamin K, a deficiency can develop in a few days. **Vitamin K deficiency is manifested as a coagulopathy due to impaired formation of prothrombin and of factors VII, IX, and X.**

Bilirubin is primarily the end-product of hemoglobin metabolism. It is formed from degradation of the heme ring in Kupffer cells. Bilirubin is then released into blood, where it readily binds to albumin. Hepatic uptake of bilirubin from the circulation is passive, but binding to intracellular proteins traps the bilirubin inside hepatocytes. Bilirubin is conjugated by the hepatocytes, primarily with glucuronide, and actively excreted into bile canaliculi.

LIVER TESTS

The most commonly performed liver tests are neither sensitive nor specific. No one test evaluates overall hepatic function, reflecting instead one aspect of hepatic function that must be interpreted in conjunction with other tests and clinical assessment of the patient.

3 Many "liver function" tests, such as serum transaminase measurements, reflect hepatocellular integrity more than hepatic function. Liver tests that measure hepatic synthetic function include

TABLE 32-4 Abnormalities in liver tests.[1,2,3]

	Parenchymal (Hepatocellular) Dysfunction	Biliary Obstruction or Cholestasis
AST (SGOT)	↑ to ↑↑↑	↑
ALT (SGPT)	↑ to ↑↑↑	↑
Albumin	0 to ↓↓↓	0
Prothrombin time	0 to ↑↑↑	0 to ↑↑[4]
Bilirubin	0 to ↑↑↑	0 to ↑↑↑
Alkaline phosphatase	↑	↑ to ↑↑↑
5'-Nucleotidase	0 to ↑	↑ to ↑↑↑
γ-Glutamyl transpeptidase	↑ to ↑↑↑	↑↑↑

[1]Adapted from Wilson JD et al. (eds): *Harrison's Principles of Internal Medicine*, 12th ed. McGraw-Hill, 1991.

[2]AST, aspartate aminotransferase; SGOT, serum glutamic-oxaloacetic transaminase; ALT, alanine aminotransferase; SGPT, serum glutamic pyruvic-transferase.

[3]↑, increases; 0, no change; ↓, decreases.

[4]Usually corrects with vitamin K.

serum albumin, prothrombin time (PT, or international normalized ratio [INR]), cholesterol, and pseudocholinesterase. Moreover, because of the liver's large functional reserve, substantial cirrhosis may be present with few or no laboratory abnormalities.

Liver abnormalities can often be divided into either parenchymal disorders or obstructive disorders based on laboratory tests (Table 32–4). Obstructive disorders primarily affect biliary excretion of substances, whereas parenchymal disorders result in generalized hepatocellular dysfunction.

Serum Bilirubin

The normal total bilirubin concentration, composed of conjugated (direct), water-soluble and unconjugated (indirect), lipid-soluble forms, is less than 1.5 mg/dL (<25 mmol/L) and reflects the balance between bilirubin production and excretion. Jaundice is usually clinically obvious when total bilirubin exceeds 3 mg/dL. A predominantly conjugated hyperbilirubinemia (>50%) is associated with increased urinary urobilinogen and may reflect hepatocellular dysfunction, congenital (Dubin–Johnson or Rotor syndrome) or acquired intrahepatic cholestasis, or extrahepatic biliary obstruction. Hyperbilirubinemia that is primarily unconjugated may be seen with hemolysis or with congenital (Gilbert or Crigler–Najjar syndrome) or acquired defects in bilirubin conjugation. Unconjugated bilirubin is neurotoxic, and high levels may produce encephalopathy.

Serum Aminotransferases (Transaminases)

These enzymes are released into the circulation as a result of hepatocellular injury or death. Two aminotransferases are most commonly measured: aspartate aminotransferase (AST), also known as serum glutamic-oxaloacetic transaminase (SGOT), and alanine aminotransferase (ALT), also known as serum glutamic pyruvic-transferase (SGPT).

Serum Alkaline Phosphatase

Alkaline phosphatase is produced by the liver, bone, small bowel, kidneys, and placenta and is excreted into bile. Normal serum alkaline phosphatase activity is generally 25–85 IU/L; children and adolescents have much higher levels, reflecting active growth. Most of the circulating enzyme is normally derived from bone; however, with biliary obstruction, more hepatic alkaline phosphatase is synthesized and released into the circulation.

Serum Albumin

The normal serum albumin concentration is 3.5–5.5 g/dL. Because its half-life is about 2–3 weeks, albumin concentration may initially be normal with acute liver disease. Albumin values less than 2.5 g/dL are generally indicative of chronic liver disease, acute stress, or severe malnutrition. Increased losses of albumin in the urine (nephrotic syndrome) or the gastrointestinal tract (protein-losing enteropathy) can also produce hypoalbuminemia.

Blood Ammonia

Significant elevations of blood ammonia levels usually reflect disruption of hepatic urea synthesis. Normal whole blood ammonia levels are 47–65 mmol/L (80–110 mg/dL). Marked elevations usually reflect severe hepatocellular damage and may cause encephalopathy.

Prothrombin Time

5 The PT, which normally ranges between 11–14 sec, depending on the control value, measures the activity of fibrinogen, prothrombin, and factors V, VII, and X. The relatively short half-life of factor VII (4–6 h) makes the PT useful in evaluating hepatic synthetic function of patients with acute or chronic liver disease. Prolongations of the PT greater than 3–4 sec from the control are considered significant and usually correspond to an INR >1.5. Because only 20% to 30% of normal factor activity is required for normal coagulation, prolongation of the PT usually reflects either severe liver disease or vitamin K deficiency. (See Table 32–5 for a list of coagulation test abnormalities.)

Point-of-Care Viscoelastic Coagulation Monitoring

This technology provides a "real time" assessment of the coagulation status and utilizes thromboelastography (TEG®), rotation thromboelastometry (ROTEM®), or Sonoclot® analysis to assess global coagulation via the viscoelastic properties of whole blood (Figure 32–7). A clear picture is provided of the global effect of imbalances between the procoagulant and anticoagulant systems and the profibrinolytic and antifibrinolytic systems and the resultant

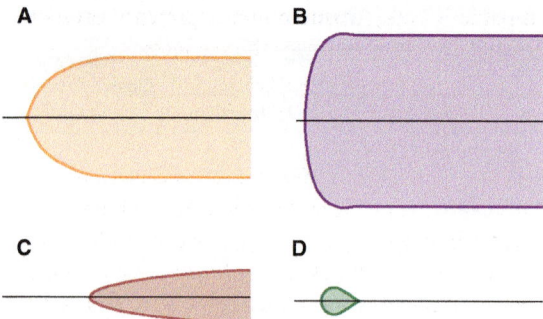

FIGURE 32–7 Examples of typical thromboelastograph tracings. **A:** Normal. **B:** Hypercoagulation. **C:** Hypocoagulation (eg, thrombocytopenia). **D:** Fibrinolysis. (Reproduced, with permission, from Johansson PI, Stissing T, Bochsen L, et al: Thrombelastography and thromboelastometry in assessing coagulopathy in trauma. Scand J Trauma Resusc Emerg Med 2009;17:45.)

clot tensile strength, allowing precise management of hemostatic therapy. The rate of clot formation, the strength of the clot, and the impact of any lysis can be observed. The presence of disseminated intravascular coagulation can be evaluated, as can the effect of heparin or heparinoid activity. In addition, platelet function can be assessed, including the effects of platelet inhibition.

EFFECT OF ANESTHESIA ON HEPATIC FUNCTION

Hepatic blood flow usually decreases during regional and general anesthesia, and multiple factors are responsible, including both direct and indirect effects of anesthetic agents, the type of ventilation employed, and the type of surgery being performed.

Decreases in cardiac output reduce hepatic blood flow via reflex sympathetic activation, which vasoconstricts both the arterial and the venous splanchnic vasculature.

The hemodynamic effects of ventilation can also have a significant impact on hepatic blood flow. Controlled positive-pressure ventilation with high mean airway pressures reduces venous return to the heart and decreases cardiac output; both mechanisms can compromise hepatic blood flow. The former increases hepatic venous pressure, whereas the latter can reduce blood pressure and increase

TABLE 32–5 Coagulation test abnormalities.[1]

	PT	PTT	TT	Fibrinogen
Advanced liver disease	↑	↑	N or ↑	N or ↓
DIC	↑	↑	↑	↓
Vitamin K deficiency	↑↑	↑	N	N
Warfarin therapy	↑↑	↑	N	N
Heparin therapy	↑	↑↑	↑	N

Hemophilia
  Factor VIII deficiency
  Factor IX deficiency
	N
	N
		↑
		↑
			N
			N
				N
				N

Factor VII deficiency	↑	N	N	N
Factor XIII deficiency	N	N	N	N

[1]PT, prothrombin time; PTT, partial thromboplastin time; TT, thrombin time; N, normal; DIC, disseminated intravascular coagulation.

sympathetic tone. Positive end-expiratory pressure (PEEP) further accentuates these effects.

Surgical procedures near the liver can reduce hepatic blood flow up to 60%. Although the mechanisms are not clear, they most likely involve sympathetic activation, local reflexes, and direct compression of vessels in the portal and hepatic circulations.

β-Adrenergic blockers, α$_1$-adrenergic agonists, H$_2$-receptor blockers, and vasopressin reduce hepatic blood flow. Low-dose dopamine infusions may increase liver blood flow.

Metabolic Functions

The effects of the various anesthetic agents on intermediary hepatic metabolism involving carbohydrate, fat, and protein are poorly defined. An endocrine stress response secondary to fasting and **6** surgical trauma is generally observed. The neuroendocrine stress response to surgery and trauma is characterized by elevated circulating levels of catecholamines, glucagon, and cortisol and results in the mobilization of carbohydrate stores and protein, causing hyperglycemia and negative nitrogen balance (catabolism). The neuroendocrine stress response may be at least partially blunted by regional anesthesia, deep general anesthesia and/or pharmacological blockade of the sympathetic system, with regional anesthesia having the most salutary effect **7** on catabolism. All opioids can potentially cause spasm of the sphincter of Oddi and increase biliary pressure. Naloxone and glucagon may relieve opioid-induced spasm.

Procedures in close proximity to the liver frequently result in modest elevations in lactate dehydrogenase and transaminase concentrations regardless of the anesthetic agent or technique employed. **8** When the results of liver function tests are elevated postoperatively, the usual cause is underlying liver disease or the surgical procedure itself. Persistent abnormalities in liver tests may be indicative of viral hepatitis (usually transfusion related), sepsis, idiosyncratic drug reactions, or surgical complications. **Postoperative jaundice can result from a variety of factors** (Table 32–6), **but the most common cause is overproduction of bilirubin because of resorption of a large hematoma or red cell breakdown following transfusion.** Nonetheless, all

TABLE 32–6 Causes of postoperative jaundice.

Prehepatic (increased bilirubin production)
Resorption of hematomas
Hemolytic anemia transfusion
Senescent red cell breakdown
Hemolytic reactions
Hepatic (hepatocellular dysfunction)
Preexisting liver disease
Ischemic or hypoxemic injury
Drug-induced
Gilbert's syndrome
Intrahepatic cholestasis
Halothane
Posthepatic (biliary obstruction)
Postoperative cholecystitis
Postoperative pancreatitis
Retained common bile duct stone
Bile duct injury
Miscellaneous

other causes should be considered. Correct diagnosis requires a careful review of preoperative liver function and of intraoperative and postoperative events, such as transfusions, sustained hypotension or hypoxemia, and drug exposure. Currently utilized volatile anesthetic agents have minimal, if any, direct adverse effect upon hepatocytes.

CASE DISCUSSION

Coagulopathy in a Patient with Liver Disease (also see Chapter 51)

A 52-year-old man with a long history of alcohol abuse presents for a splenorenal shunt after three major episodes of upper gastrointestinal hemorrhage from esophageal varices. Coagulation studies reveal a PT of 17 sec (control: 12 sec), INR of 1.7, and a partial PT of 43 sec (control: 29 sec). The platelet count is 75,000/μL.

What factors can contribute to excessive bleeding during and following surgery?

Hemostasis following trauma or surgery is dependent on three major processes: (1) vascular spasm, (2) formation of a platelet plug (primary hemostasis), and (3) coagulation of blood (secondary hemostasis) in addition to adequate surgical control of bleeding sites. The first two are nearly immediate (seconds), whereas the third is delayed (minutes). A defect in any of these processes can lead to a bleeding diathesis and increased blood loss.

Outline the mechanisms involved in primary hemostasis.

Injury to smaller blood vessels normally causes localized spasm as a result of the release of humoral factors from platelets and local myogenic reflexes. Sympathetic-mediated vasoconstriction is also operative in medium-sized vessels. Exposure of circulating platelets to the damaged endothelial surface causes them to undergo a series of changes that results in the formation of a platelet plug. If the break in a vessel is small, the plug itself can often completely stop bleeding. If the break is large, however, coagulation of blood is also necessary to stop the bleeding.

Formation of the platelet plug can be broken down into three stages: (1) adhesion, (2) release of platelet granules, and (3) aggregation. Following injury, circulating platelets adhere to subendothelial collagen via specific glycoprotein (GP) receptors on their membrane. This interaction is stabilized by a circulating GP called *von Willebrand factor* (vWF), which forms additional bridges between subendothelial collagen and platelets via GPIb. Collagen (as well as epinephrine and thrombin) activates platelet membrane-bound phospholipases A and C, which, in turn, results in the formation of thromboxane A_2 (TXA_2) and platelet degranulation. TXA_2 is a potent vasoconstrictor that also promotes platelet aggregation. Platelet granules contain a large number of substances, including adenosine diphosphate (ADP), factor V, vWF, fibrinogen, and fibronectin. These factors attract and activate additional platelets. ADP alters platelet membrane GPIIb/IIIa, which facilitates the binding of fibrinogen to activated platelets.

Describe the mechanisms involved in normal coagulation.

Coagulation, often referred to as secondary hemostasis, involves formation of a fibrin clot, which usually binds and strengthens a platelet plug. Fibrin can be formed via one of two pathways (*extrinsic* or *intrinsic*; Figure 32–5) that involve calcium and activation of soluble coagulation precursor proteins in blood (Table 32–2). Regardless of which pathway is activated, the coagulation cascade ends in the conversion of *fibrinogen* to *fibrin*. The extrinsic pathway of the coagulation cascade is triggered by the release of a tissue lipoprotein, *thromboplastin*, from the membranes of injured cells and is likely the more important pathway in humans. The intrinsic pathway can be triggered by the interaction between subendothelial collagen with circulating Hageman factor (XII), high-molecular-weight kininogen, and prekallikrein. The latter two substances are also involved in the formation of bradykinin.

Thrombin plays a central role in coagulation because it not only activates platelets, but also accelerates conversion of factors V, VIII, and XIII to their active forms. Conversion of prothrombin to thrombin is markedly accelerated by activated platelets. Thrombin then converts fibrinogen to soluble fibrin monomers that polymerize on the platelet plug. The cross-linking of fibrin polymers by factor XIII is necessary to form a strong, insoluble fibrin clot. Finally, retraction of the clot, which requires platelets, expresses fluid from the clot and helps pull the walls of the damaged blood vessel together.

What prevents coagulation of blood in normal tissues?

The coagulation process is limited to injured areas by localization of platelets to the injured area and by maintenance of normal blood flow in uninjured areas. Normal endothelium produces *prostacyclin* (prostaglandin I_2, PGI_2), which is a potent vasodilator that also inhibits platelet activation and helps to confine the primary hemostatic process to the injured area. Normal blood flow is important in clearing activated coagulation factors, which are taken up by the monocyte–macrophage scavenger system. Multiple inhibitors of coagulation are normally present in plasma, including antithrombin III, protein

C, protein S, and tissue factor pathway inhibitor. Antithrombin III complexes with and inactivates circulating coagulation factors (with the notable exception of factor VII), and protein C specifically inactivates factors V and VIII. *Heparin exerts its anticoagulant activity by augmenting the activity of antithrombin III.* Protein S enhances the activity of protein C, and deficiencies of protein C and protein S lead to hypercoagulability. Tissue factor pathway inhibitor antagonizes the action of activated factor VII.

What is the role of the fibrinolytic system in normal hemostasis?

The fibrinolytic system is normally activated simultaneously with the coagulation cascade and functions to maintain the fluidity of blood during coagulation. It is also responsible for clot lysis once tissue repair begins. When a clot is formed, a large amount of the protein *plasminogen* is incorporated. Plasminogen is then activated by tissue plasminogen activator (tPA), which is usually released by endothelial cells in response to thrombin, and by Hageman factor (XII). The resulting formation of *plasmin* degrades fibrin and fibrinogen, as well as other coagulation factors. Urokinase (found in urine) and streptokinase (a product of bacteria) are also potent activators of plasminogen to plasmin. The action of tPA is localized because (1) it is absorbed into the fibrin clot, (2) it activates plasminogen more effectively on the clot, (3) free plasmin is rapidly neutralized by a circulating α_2-antiplasmin, and (4) circulating tPA is cleared by the liver. Plasmin degrades fibrin and fibrinogen into small fragments. These fibrin degradation products possess anticoagulant activity because they compete with fibrinogen for thrombin; they are normally cleared by the monocyte–macrophage system. The drugs ε-aminocaproic acid (EACA) and tranexamic acid inhibit the conversion of plasminogen to plasmin. Endothelium also normally secretes a plasminogen activator inhibitor (PAI-1) that antagonizes tPA.

What hemostatic defects are likely to be present in this patient?

Multifactorial coagulopathy often develops in patients with advanced liver disease. Three major causes are usually responsible: (1) vitamin K deficiency due to dietary deficiency or to impaired absorption or storage, (2) impaired hepatic synthesis of coagulation factors, and (3) splenic sequestration of platelets resulting from hypersplenism. To complicate matters further, patients with cirrhosis typically have multiple potential bleeding sites (esophageal varices, gastritis, peptic ulcers, and hemorrhoids) and frequently require multiple blood transfusions. With severe liver disease, patients may also have decreased synthesis of coagulation inhibitors and may fail to clear activated coagulation factors and fibrin split products because of impaired Kupffer cell function; the resultant coagulation defect resembles, and becomes indistinguishable from, disseminated intravascular coagulation (DIC).

What is DIC?

In DIC, the coagulation cascade is activated by the release of endogenous tissue thromboplastin or thromboplastin-like substances, or by direct activation of factor XII by endotoxin or foreign surfaces. Widespread deposition of fibrin in the microcirculation results in consumption of coagulation factors, secondary fibrinolysis, thrombocytopenia, and a microangiopathic hemolytic anemia. Diffuse bleeding, and, in some cases, thromboembolic phenomena, usually follows. Treatment is generally aimed at the underlying cause. Supportive measures include transfusion of coagulation factors and platelets. Heparin therapy is controversial, but may benefit patients with thromboembolic phenomena.

What is primary fibrinolysis?

This bleeding disorder is due to uncontrolled fibrinolysis. Patients may have a deficiency of α_2-antiplasmin or impaired clearance of tPA. The latter may be common in patients with severe liver disease and during the anhepatic phase of liver transplantation. The disorder may occasionally be encountered in patients with carcinoma of the prostate. Diagnosis is often difficult, but is suggested by a bleeding diathesis with a low fibrinogen level but relatively normal coagulation tests and platelet count (below). Treatment includes fresh frozen plasma or cryoprecipitate and possibly either EACA or tranexamic acid.

How are coagulation tests helpful in evaluating inadequate hemostasis?

The diagnosis of coagulation abnormalities can be facilitated by measurement of the activated partial thromboplastin time (aPTT), PT, thrombin time (TT), fibrin degradation products (see below), and fibrinogen level (Table 32–5). The aPTT measures the intrinsic pathway (factors I, II, V, VIII, IX, X, XI, and XII). The whole blood clotting time and activated clotting time (ACT) also measure the intrinsic pathway. In contrast, the PT measures the extrinsic pathway (factors I, II, V, and VII). The TT specifically measures conversion of fibrinogen to fibrin (factors I and II). The normal plasma fibrinogen level is 200–400 mg/dL (5.9–11.7 μmol/L). Because heparin therapy primarily affects the intrinsic pathway, in low doses it usually prolongs the aPTT only. In high doses, heparin also prolongs the PT. In contrast, warfarin primarily affects vitamin K-dependent factors (II, VII, IX, and X), so the PT is prolonged at usual doses, and the aPTT is prolonged only at high doses. In vivo plasmin activity can be evaluated by measuring circulating levels of peptides cleaved from fibrin and fibrinogen by plasmin, namely *fibrin degradation products* (FDPs) and d-dimers. Patients with primary fibrinolysis usually have elevated FDPs, but normal d-dimer levels.

What tests are most helpful in evaluating inadequate primary hemostasis?

The most commonly performed tests include a platelet count and a bleeding time, but also include thromboelastography (TEG®), rotation thromboelastometry (ROTEM®), and Sonoclot® analysis (see Figure 32–7 and Chapter 51). Patients with normally-functioning platelets and platelet counts above 100,000/μL have normal primary hemostasis. The normal platelet count is 150,000–450,000/μL, and the bleeding time is generally not affected by the platelet count when the latter is greater than 100,000/μL. When the platelet count is 50,000/μL, excessive bleeding generally occurs only

with severe trauma or extensive surgery. In contrast, patients with platelet counts under 20,000/μL develop significant bleeding following even minor trauma. Thrombocytopenia usually results from one of three mechanisms: (1) decreased platelet production, (2) splenic sequestration of platelets, or (3) increased platelet destruction. The third mechanism may fall under one of two categories of destruction: immune or nonimmune. Nonimmune destruction includes vasculitis or DIC.

A prolonged bleeding time with a normal platelet count implies a qualitative platelet defect. Although the bleeding time is somewhat dependent on the technique employed, values longer than 10 min are generally considered abnormal. Significant intraoperative and postoperative bleeding may be expected when the bleeding time exceeds 15 min. Specialized testing is required to diagnose specific platelet functional defects.

What are the most common causes of qualitative platelet defects?

The most common platelet defect is due to inhibition of TXA_2 production by aspirin and other nonsteroidal antiinflammatory drugs (NSAIDs). In contrast to aspirin, which irreversibly acetylates and inactivates cyclooxygenase for the life of the platelet (up to 8 days), enzyme inhibition by other NSAIDs is reversible and generally lasts only 24 hr. Increasingly patients are treated with a variety of anti platelet agents such as clopidogrel which impair platelet function. Assays of platelet function are available to determine the degree to which platelet function is inhibited.

What is von Willebrand's disease?

The most common inherited bleeding disorder (1:800–1000 patients) is *von Willebrand's disease*. Patients with this disorder produce a defective vWF or low levels of a normal vWF (normal: 5–10 mg/L). Most patients are heterozygous and have relatively mild hemostatic defects that become apparent clinically only when they are subjected to major surgery or trauma or following ingestion of NSAIDs. In addition to helping link platelets, vWF serves as a carrier for coagulation factor VIII. As a result, these patients typically have a prolonged bleeding time, decreased plasma vWF concentration, and decreased factor VIII activity. Acquired forms of von Willebrand's disease may be encountered in patients with some immune disorders and those with tumors that absorb vWF onto their surface. At least three forms of the disease are recognized, ranging in severity from mild to severe.

Treatment with desmopressin (DDAVP) can raise vWF levels in some patients with mild von Willebrand's disease (as well as normal individuals). The drug is usually administered at a dose of 0.3 mcg/kg 30 min before surgery. Patients who do not respond to DDAVP should receive cryoprecipitate or factor VIII concentrates, both of which are rich in vWF; prophylactic infusions are generally recommended before and after surgery twice a day for 2–4 days to guarantee surgical hemostasis.

What other hereditary hemostatic defects may be encountered in anesthetic practice?

The most common inherited defect in secondary hemostasis is *factor VIII deficiency* (**hemophilia A**). This X-linked abnormality is estimated to affect 1:10,000 males. Disease severity is generally inversely related to factor VIII activity. Most symptomatic patients experience hemarthrosis, bleeding into deep tissues, and hematuria. Symptomatic patients generally have less than 5% of normal factor VIII activity. Classically, patients present with a prolonged aPTT, but a normal PT and bleeding time. The diagnosis is confirmed by measuring factor VIII activity in blood. Affected patients generally do not experience increased bleeding during surgery when factor VIII levels are more than 30%, but most clinicians recommend increasing factor VIII levels to more than 50% prior to surgery. Normal (fresh frozen) plasma, by definition, is considered to have 1 U of factor VIII activity per milliliter. In contrast, cryoprecipitate has 5–10 U/mL, whereas factor VIII concentrates have approximately 40 U/mL. Each unit of factor VIII transfused is estimated to raise factor VIII levels 2% per kilogram of body weight. Twice-a-day transfusions are generally recommended following surgery because of the relatively short half-life of factor VIII (8–12 h). Administration of DDAVP can raise factor VIII levels 2- to 3-fold in some patients. EACA or tranexamic acid may also be used as adjuncts.

Hemophilia B (also known as Christmas disease) is the result of an X-linked hereditary deficiency of factor IX. The disease is very similar to hemophilia A, but much less common (1:100,000 males). Measurement of factor IX levels establishes the diagnosis. Perioperative administration of fresh frozen plasma is generally recommended to maintain factor IX activity at more than 30% of normal. Recombinant or monoclonal purified factor IX is available.

Factor XIII deficiency is extremely rare, but notable in that the aPTT, PT, TT, and bleeding times are normal. The diagnosis requires measurement of factor XIII levels. Because only 1% of normal factor XIII activity is generally required, patients are treated by a single transfusion of fresh frozen plasma.

Do normal laboratory values exclude a hemostatic defect?

A bleeding diathesis may exist even in the absence of gross abnormalities on routine laboratory tests. Some hemostatic defects are often not detected by routine testing, but require additional specialized tests. A history of excessive bleeding after dental extractions, childbirth, minor surgery, minor trauma, or even during menstruation suggests a hemostatic defect. Conversely, there may be no excess bleeding despite abnormal laboratory testing. A family history of a bleeding diathesis may suggest an inherited coagulation defect, but such history is often absent because the increased bleeding is often minor and goes unnoticed.

Hemostatic defects can often be differentiated by their clinical presentation. Bleeding in patients with primary hemostatic defects usually immediately follows minor trauma, is confined to superficial sites (skin or mucosal surfaces), and often can be controlled by local compression. Small pinpoint hemorrhages from capillaries in the dermis (petechiae) are typically present on examination. Bleeding into subcutaneous tissues (ecchymosis) from small arterioles or venules is also common in patients with platelet disorders. In contrast, bleeding that results from secondary hemostatic defects is usually delayed following injury, is typically deep (subcutaneous tissues, joints, body cavities, or muscles), and is often difficult to stop even with compression. Hemorrhages may be palpable as hematomas or may go unnoticed when located deeper (retroperitoneal). Coagulation may be impaired by systemic hypothermic or subnormal temperature of the site of bleeding, even when coagulation test (PT, aPTT, bleeding time) results are normal and there is no history of hemostatic defects.

Anesthesia for Patients with Liver Disease

Michael Ramsay, MD, FRCA

KEY CONCEPTS

1 Because of the increased risk of perioperative morbidity and mortality, patients with acute hepatitis should have any elective surgery postponed until the acute hepatitis has resolved, as indicated by the normalization of liver tests.

2 Isoflurane and sevoflurane are the volatile agents of choice because they preserve hepatic blood flow and oxygen delivery. Factors known to reduce hepatic blood flow, such as hypotension, excessive sympathetic activation, and high mean airway pressures during controlled ventilation, should be avoided.

3 In evaluating patients for chronic hepatitis, laboratory test results may show only a mild elevation in serum aminotransferase activity and often correlate poorly with disease severity.

4 Approximately 10% of patients with cirrhosis also develop at least one episode of spontaneous bacterial peritonitis, and some patients may eventually develop hepatocellular carcinoma.

5 Massive bleeding from gastroesophageal varices is a major cause of morbidity and mortality, and, in addition to the cardiovascular effects of acute blood loss, the absorbed nitrogen load from the breakdown of blood in the intestinal tract can precipitate hepatic encephalopathy.

6 The cardiovascular changes observed in the patient with hepatic cirrhosis are usually that of a hyperdynamic circulation, although clinically significant cirrhotic cardiomyopathy is often present and not recognized.

7 The effects of hepatic cirrhosis on pulmonary vascular resistance vessels may result in chronic hypoxemia.

8 Hepatorenal syndrome is a functional renal defect in patients with cirrhosis that usually follows gastrointestinal bleeding, aggressive diuresis, sepsis, or major surgery. It is characterized by progressive oliguria with avid sodium retention, azotemia, intractable ascites, and a very high mortality rate.

9 Factors known to precipitate hepatic encephalopathy in patients with cirrhosis include gastrointestinal bleeding, increased dietary protein intake, hypokalemic alkalosis from vomiting or diuresis, infections, and worsening liver function.

10 Following the removal of large amounts of ascitic fluid, aggressive intravenous fluid replacement is often necessary to prevent profound hypotension and kidney failure.

The prevalence of liver disease is increasing in the United States. Cirrhosis, the terminal pathology in the majority of liver diseases, has a general population incidence as high as 5% in some autopsy series. It is a major cause of death in men in their fourth and fifth decades of life, and mortality rates are increasing. Ten percent of the patients with liver disease undergo operative procedures during the final 2 years of their lives. The liver has remarkable functional reserve, and thus overt clinical manifestations of hepatic disease are often absent until extensive damage has occurred. When patients with little hepatic reserve come to the operating room, effects from anesthesia and the surgical procedure can precipitate further hepatic decompensation, leading to frank hepatic failure.

COAGULATION IN LIVER DISEASE

In stable chronic liver disease, the causes of excessive bleeding primarily involve severe thrombocytopenia, endothelial dysfunction, portal hypertension, renal failure, and sepsis (see Chapters 32 and 51). However, the hemostatic changes that occur with liver disease may cause hypercoagulation and thrombosis, as well as an increased risk of bleeding.

Clot breakdown may be enhanced by an imbalance of the fibrinolytic system.

Chronic liver disease is characterized by the impaired synthesis of coagulation factors, resulting in prolongation of the prothrombin time (PT) and international normalized ratio (INR) (Table 33–1). However, the anticoagulant factors (protein C, antithrombin, and tissue factor pathway inhibitor) are also reduced and may balance out any effect of a prolonged PT. This may be confirmed by assessing thrombin generation in the presence of endothelial-produced thrombomodulin. Adequate thrombin production requires an adequate number of functioning platelets. If the platelet count is >60,000/μL, coagulation may well be normal in a patient with severe cirrhosis.

The patient with cirrhosis will typically have hyperfibrinolysis. However, there is a delicate balance between the activators and inactivators that regulate the conversion of plasminogen to plasmin, and, therefore, individual laboratory tests may not give a true picture of the state of fibrinolysis. The thromboelastography (TEG®), rotational thromboelastometry (ROTEM®), and Sonoclot® technologies are the optimal methods of demonstrating the global state of the coagulation system at a specific moment in time in any patient with liver disease (see Chapter 51).

TABLE 33–1 Coagulation test abnormalities.[1]

	PT	PTT	TT	Fibrinogen
Advanced liver disease	↑	↑	N or ↑	N or ↓
DIC	↑	↑	↑	↓
Vitamin K deficiency	↑↑	↑	N	N
Warfarin therapy	↑↑	↑	N	N
Heparin therapy	↑	↑↑	↑	N

Hemophilia
  Factor VIII deficiency
  Factor IX deficiency
	
	N
	N
		
		↑
		↑
			
			N
			N
				
				N
				N

Factor VII deficiency	↑	N	N	N
Factor XIII deficiency	N	N	N	N

[1]PT, prothrombin time; PTT, partial thromboplastin time; TT, thrombin time; N, normal; DIC, disseminated intravascular coagulation.

Hepatitis

ACUTE HEPATITIS

Acute hepatitis is usually the result of a viral infection, drug reaction, or exposure to a hepatotoxin. The illness represents acute hepatocellular injury with a variable degree of cellular necrosis. Clinical manifestations depend both on the severity of the inflammatory reaction, and, more importantly, on the degree of necrosis. Mild inflammatory reactions may present merely as asymptomatic elevations in the serum transaminases, whereas massive hepatic necrosis presents as acute fulminant hepatic failure.

Viral Hepatitis

Viral hepatitis is most commonly due to hepatitis A, hepatitis B, or hepatitis C viral infection. At least two other hepatitis viruses have also been identified: hepatitis D (delta virus) and hepatitis E (enteric non-A, non-B). Hepatitis types A and E are transmitted by the fecal-oral route, whereas hepatitis types B and C are transmitted primarily percutaneously and by contact with body fluids. Hepatitis D is unique in that it may be transmitted by either route and requires the presence of hepatitis B virus in the host to be infective. Other viruses may also cause hepatitis, including Epstein–Barr, herpes simplex, cytomegalovirus, and coxsackieviruses.

Patients with viral hepatitis often have a 1- to 2-week mild prodromal illness (fatigue, malaise, low-grade fever, or nausea and vomiting) that may or may not be followed by jaundice. The jaundice typically lasts 2–12 weeks, but complete recovery, as evidenced by serum transaminase measurements, usually takes 4 months. Because clinical manifestations overlap, serological testing is necessary to determine the causative viral agent. The clinical course tends to be more complicated and prolonged with hepatitis B and C viruses relative to other types of viral hepatitis. Cholestasis (see below) may be a major manifestation. Rarely, fulminant hepatic failure (massive hepatic necrosis) can develop.

The incidence of chronic active hepatitis (see below) is 3% to 10% following infection with hepatitis B virus and at least 50% following infection with hepatitis C virus. A small percentage of patients (mainly immunosuppressed patients and those on long-term hemodialysis regimens) become asymptomatic infectious carriers following infection with hepatitis B virus, and up to 30% of these patients remain infectious with the hepatitis B surface antigen (HBsAg) persisting in their blood. Most patients with chronic hepatitis C infection seem to have very low, intermittent, or absent circulating viral particles and are therefore not highly infective. Approximately 0.5% to 1% of patients with hepatitis C infection become asymptomatic infectious carriers, and infectivity correlates with the detection of hepatitis C viral RNA in peripheral blood. Such infectious carriers pose a major health hazard to operating room personnel.

In addition to "universal precautions" for avoiding direct contact with blood and secretions (gloves, mask, protective eyewear, and not recapping needles), immunization of healthcare personnel is highly effective against hepatitis B infection. A vaccine for hepatitis C is not available; moreover, unlike hepatitis B infection, hepatitis C infection does not seem to confer immunity to subsequent exposure. Postexposure prophylaxis with hyperimmune globulin is effective for hepatitis B, but not hepatitis C.

Drug-induced Hepatitis

Drug-induced hepatitis (Table 33–2) can result from direct, dose-dependent toxicity of a drug or drug metabolite, an idiosyncratic drug reaction, or a combination of these two causes. The clinical course often resembles viral hepatitis, making diagnosis difficult. Alcoholic hepatitis is probably the most common form of drug-induced hepatitis, but the etiology may not be obvious from the history. Chronic alcohol ingestion can also result in hepatomegaly from fatty infiltration of the liver, which reflects impaired fatty acid oxidation, increased uptake and esterification of fatty acids, and diminished lipoprotein synthesis and secretion. Acetaminophen ingestion of 25 g or more usually results in fatal fulminant hepatotoxicity. A few drugs, such as chlorpromazine and oral contraceptives, may cause cholestatic-type reactions (see below). Ingestion of potent hepatotoxins, such as carbon tetrachloride and certain species of

TABLE 33–2 Drugs and substances associated with hepatitis.

Toxic
  Alcohol
  Acetaminophen
  Salicylates
  Tetracyclines
  Trichloroethylene
  Vinyl chloride
  Carbon tetrachloride
  Yellow phosphorus
  Poisonous mushrooms (*Amanita, Galerina*)

Idiosyncratic
  Volatile anesthetics (halothane)
  Phenytoin
  Sulfonamides
  Rifampin
  Indomethacin

Toxic and idiosyncratic
  Methyldopa
  Isoniazid
  Sodium valproate
  Amiodarone

Primarily cholestatic
  Chlorpromazine
  Cyclosporine
  Oral contraceptives
  Anabolic steroids
  Erythromycin estolate
  Methimazole

mushrooms (*Amanita, Galerina*), also may result in fatal hepatotoxicity.

1 Because of the increased risk of perioperative morbidity and mortality, patients with acute hepatitis should have elective surgery postponed until the illness has resolved, as indicated by the normalization of liver tests. In addition, acute alcohol toxicity greatly complicates anesthetic management, and acute alcohol withdrawal during the perioperative period may be associated with a mortality rate as high as 50%. Only emergent surgery should be considered for patients presenting in acute alcohol withdrawal. Patients with hepatitis are at risk of deterioration of hepatic function and the development of complications from hepatic failure, such as encephalopathy, coagulopathy, or hepatorenal syndrome.

Laboratory evaluation of the patient with hepatitis should include blood urea nitrogen, serum electrolytes, creatinine, glucose, transaminases, bilirubin, alkaline phosphatase, and albumin, platelet count, and PT. Serum should also be checked for HBsAg whenever possible. A blood alcohol level is useful if the history or physical examination is compatible with ethanol intoxication. Hypokalemia and metabolic alkalosis are not uncommon and are usually due to vomiting. Concomitant hypomagnesemia may be present in chronic alcoholics and predisposes to cardiac arrhythmias. The elevation in serum transaminases does not necessarily correlate with the amount of hepatic necrosis. The serum alanine aminotransferase (ALT) is generally higher than the serum aspartate aminotransferase (AST), except in alcoholic hepatitis, where the reverse occurs. Bilirubin and alkaline phosphatase are usually only moderately elevated, except with the cholestatic variant of hepatitis. The PT is the best indicator of hepatic synthetic function. Persistent prolongation of longer than 3 sec (INR > 1.5) following administration of vitamin K is indicative of severe hepatic dysfunction. Hypoglycemia is not uncommon. Hypoalbuminemia is usually not present except in protracted cases, with severe malnutrition, or when chronic liver disease is present.

If a patient with acute hepatitis must undergo an emergent operation, the preanesthetic evaluation should focus on determining the cause and the degree of hepatic impairment. Information should be obtained regarding recent drug exposures, including alcohol intake, intravenous drug use, recent transfusions, and prior anesthetics. The presence of nausea or vomiting should be noted, and, if present, dehydration and electrolyte abnormalities should be anticipated and corrected. Changes in mental status may indicate severe hepatic impairment. Inappropriate behavior or obtundation in alcoholic patients may be signs of acute intoxication, whereas tremulousness and irritability usually reflect withdrawal. Hypertension and tachycardia are often also prominent with the latter. Fresh frozen plasma may be necessary to correct a coagulopathy. Premedication is generally not given, in an effort to minimize drug exposure and not confound hepatic encephalopathy in patients with advanced liver disease. However, benzodiazepines and thiamine are indicated in alcoholic patients with, or at risk for, acute withdrawal.

Intraoperative Considerations

The goal of intraoperative management is to preserve existing hepatic function and avoid factors that may be detrimental to the liver. Drug selection and dosage should be individualized. Some patients with viral hepatitis may exhibit increased central nervous system sensitivity to anesthetics, whereas alcoholic patients will often display cross-tolerance to both intravenous and volatile anesthetics. Alcoholic patients also require close cardiovascular monitoring, because the cardiac depressant effects of alcohol are additive to those of anesthetics; moreover, alcoholic cardiomyopathy is present in many alcoholic patients.

Inhalation anesthetics are generally preferable to intravenous agents because most of the latter are dependent on the liver for metabolism or elimination. Standard induction doses of intravenous induction agents can generally be used because their action is terminated by redistribution rather than metabolism or excretion. A prolonged duration of action, however, may be encountered with large or repeated doses of intravenous agents, particularly opioids. Isoflurane and sevoflurane are the **②** volatile agents of choice because they preserve hepatic blood flow and oxygen delivery. Factors known to reduce hepatic blood flow, such as hypotension, excessive sympathetic activation, and high mean airway pressures during controlled ventilation, should be avoided. Regional anesthesia, including major conduction blockade, may be employed in the absence of coagulopathy, provided hypotension is avoided.

CHRONIC HEPATITIS

Chronic hepatitis is defined as persistent hepatic inflammation for longer than 6 months, as evidenced by elevated serum aminotransferases. Patients can usually be classified as having one of three distinct syndromes based on a liver biopsy: chronic persistent hepatitis, chronic lobular hepatitis, or chronic active hepatitis. Patients with chronic active hepatitis have chronic hepatic inflammation with destruction of normal cellular architecture (piecemeal necrosis) on the biopsy. Evidence of cirrhosis is either present initially or eventually develops in 20% to 50% of patients. Although chronic active hepatitis seems to have many causes, it occurs most commonly as a sequela of hepatitis B or hepatitis C. Other causes include drugs (methyldopa, isoniazid, and nitrofurantoin) and autoimmune disorders. Both immunological factors and a genetic predisposition may be responsible in most cases. Patients usually present with a history of fatigue and recurrent jaundice; extrahepatic manifestations, such as arthritis and serositis, are not uncommon. Manifestations of cirrhosis eventually predominate in patients with progressive disease.

③ In evaluating patients for chronic hepatitis, laboratory test results may show only a mild elevation in serum aminotransferase activity and often correlate poorly with disease severity. Patients without chronic hepatitis B or C infection usually have a favorable response to immunosuppressants and are treated with long-term corticosteroid therapy with or without azathioprine.

Anesthetic Management

Patients with chronic persistent or chronic lobular hepatitis should be treated similarly to those with acute hepatitis. In contrast, those with chronic active hepatitis should be assumed to already have cirrhosis and should be treated accordingly (see below). Patients with autoimmune chronic active hepatitis may also present with problems related to other autoimmune manifestations (such as diabetes or thyroiditis) or long-term corticosteroid therapy that they have likely received.

Cirrhosis

Cirrhosis is a serious and progressive disease that eventually results in hepatic failure, and the most common cause of cirrhosis in the United States is chronic alcohol abuse. Other causes include chronic active hepatitis (postnecrotic cirrhosis), chronic biliary inflammation or obstruction (primary biliary cirrhosis, sclerosing cholangitis), chronic right-sided congestive heart failure (cardiac cirrhosis), autoimmune hepatitis, hemochromatosis, Wilson's disease, α_1-antitrypsin deficiency, nonalcoholic steatohepatitis, and cryptogenic cirrhosis. Regardless of the cause, hepatocyte necrosis is followed by fibrosis and nodular regeneration. Distortion of the liver's normal cellular and vascular architecture obstructs portal venous flow and leads to portal hypertension, whereas impairment of the liver's normal synthetic and other diverse metabolic functions results in multisystem disease. Clinically, signs and symptoms often do not correlate with disease severity. Manifestations are typically absent initially, but jaundice and ascites eventually develop in most patients. Other signs include spider angiomas, palmar erythema, gynecomastia, and splenomegaly. Moreover, cirrhosis is generally associated with the development of three major complications: (1) variceal hemorrhage from portal hypertension, (2) intractable fluid retention in the form of ascites and the hepatorenal syndrome, and (3) hepatic encephalopathy or coma. Approximately 10% of patients with cirrhosis also develop at least one episode of spontaneous bacterial peritonitis, and some patients eventually develop hepatocellular carcinoma.

A few diseases can produce hepatic fibrosis without hepatocellular necrosis or nodular regeneration, resulting in portal hypertension and its associated complications with hepatocellular function often preserved. These disorders include schistosomiasis, idiopathic portal fibrosis (Banti's syndrome), and congenital hepatic fibrosis. Obstruction of the hepatic veins or inferior vena cava (Budd–Chiari syndrome) can also cause portal hypertension. The latter may be the result of venous thrombosis (hypercoagulable state), a tumor thrombus (eg, renal carcinoma), or occlusive disease of the sublobular hepatic veins.

Preoperative Considerations

The detrimental effects of anesthesia and surgery on hepatic blood flow are discussed below. Patients with cirrhosis are at increased risk of deterioration of liver function because of their limited functional reserves. Successful anesthetic management of these patients is dependent on recognizing the multisystem nature of cirrhosis

TABLE 33–3 Manifestations of cirrhosis.

Gastrointestinal
  Portal hypertension
    Ascites
    Esophageal varices
    Hemorrhoids
    Gastrointestinal bleeding

Circulatory
  Hyperdynamic state (high cardiac output)
  Systemic arteriovenous shunts
  Low systemic vascular resistance
  Cirrhotic cardiomyopathy; pulmonary hypertension

Pulmonary
  Increased intrapulmonary shunting;
  hepatopulmonary syndrome
  Decreased functional residual capacity
  Pleural effusions
  Restrictive ventilatory defect
  Respiratory alkalosis

Renal
  Increased proximal reabsorption of sodium
  Increased distal reabsorption of sodium
  Impaired free water clearance
  Decreased renal perfusion
  Hepatorenal syndrome

Hematological
  Anemia
  Coagulopathy
  Hypersplenism
  Thrombocytopenia
  Leukopenia

Infectious
  Spontaneous bacterial peritonitis

Metabolic
  Hyponatremia and hypernatremia
  Hypokalemia and hypocalcemia
  Hypomagnesemia
  Hypoalbuminemia
  Hypoglycemia

Neurological
  Encephalopathy

(Table 33–3) and controlling or preventing its complications.

A. Gastrointestinal Manifestations

Portal hypertension leads to the development of extensive portosystemic venous collateral channels.

TABLE 33–4 Child's classification for evaluating hepatic reserve.[1]

Risk Group	A	B	C
Bilirubin (mg/dL)	<2.0	2.0–3.0	>3.0
Serum albumin (g/dL)	>3.5	3.0–3.5	<3.0
Ascites	None	Controlled	Poorly controlled
Encephalopathy	Absent	Minimal	Coma
Nutrition	Excellent	Good	Poor
Mortality rate (%)	2–5	10	50

[1]Adapted and reproduced, with permission, from Child CG: *The Liver and Portal Hypertension*. W.B. Saunders, 1964.

Four major collateral sites are generally recognized: gastroesophageal, hemorrhoidal, periumbilical, and retroperitoneal. Portal hypertension is often apparent preoperatively, as evidenced by dilated abdominal wall veins (*caput medusae*). Massive bleeding from gastroesophageal varices is a major cause of morbidity and mortality, and, in addition to the effects of acute blood loss, the absorbed nitrogen load from the breakdown of blood in the intestinal tract can precipitate hepatic encephalopathy.

The treatment of variceal bleeding is primarily supportive, but frequently involves endoscopic procedures for identification of the bleeding site(s) and therapeutic maneuvers, such as injection sclerosis of varices, monopolar and bipolar electrocoagulation, or application of hemoclips or bands. In addition to the risks posed by a patient who is physiologically fragile and acutely hypovolemic and hypotensive, anesthesia for such endoscopic procedures frequently involves the additional challenges of an encephalopathic and uncooperative patient and a stomach full of food and blood. Endoscopic unipolar electrocautery may adversely affect implanted cardiac pacing and defibrillator devices.

Blood loss should be replaced with intravenous fluids and blood products. Nonsurgical treatment includes vasopressin, somatostatin, propranolol, and balloon tamponade with a Sengstaken–Blakemore tube. Vasopressin, somatostatin, and propranolol reduce the rate of blood loss. High doses of vasopressin can result in congestive heart failure or myocardial ischemia; concomitant infusion of intravenous nitroglycerin may

reduce the likelihood of these complications and bleeding. Placement of a percutaneous transjugular intrahepatic portosystemic shunt (TIPS) can reduce portal hypertension and subsequent bleeding, but may increase the incidence of encephalopathy. When the bleeding fails to stop or recurs, emergency surgery may be indicated. Surgical risk has been shown to correlate with the degree of hepatic impairment, based on clinical and laboratory findings. Child's classification for evaluating hepatic reserve is shown in Table 33–4. Shunting procedures are generally performed on low-risk patients, whereas ablative surgery, esophageal transection, and gastric devascularization are reserved for high-risk patients.

B. Hematologic Manifestations

Anemia, thrombocytopenia, and, less commonly, leukopenia, may be present. The cause of the anemia is usually multifactorial and includes blood loss, increased red blood cell destruction, bone marrow suppression, and nutritional deficiencies. Congestive splenomegaly secondary to portal hypertension is largely responsible for the thrombocytopenia and leukopenia. Coagulation factor deficiencies arise as a result of decreased hepatic synthesis. Enhanced fibrinolysis secondary to decreased clearance of activators of the fibrinolytic system may also contribute to the coagulopathy.

The need for preoperative blood transfusions should be balanced against the obligatory increase in nitrogen load. Protein breakdown from excessive blood transfusions can precipitate encephalopathy.

However, coagulopathy should be corrected before surgery. Clotting factors should be replaced with appropriate blood products, such as fresh frozen plasma and cryoprecipitate. Platelet transfusions should be considered immediately prior to surgery for counts less than 75,000/μL.

C. Circulatory Manifestations

End-stage liver disease, and, in particular, cirrhosis of the liver, may be associated with disorders of all major organ systems (Tables 33–3 and 33–5). **6** The cardiovascular changes observed in the patient with hepatic cirrhosis are usually that of a hyperdynamic circulation, although clinically significant cirrhotic cardiomyopathy is often present and not recognized (Table 33–6). There may be a reduced cardiac contractile response to stress, altered diastolic relaxation, downregulation of β-adrenergic receptors, and electrophysiological changes as a result of cirrhotic cardiomyopathy.

Echocardiographic examination of cardiac function may initially be interpreted as normal because of significant afterload reduction caused by low systemic vascular resistance. However, both systolic and diastolic dysfunction are often found. Noninvasive stress imaging is frequently used to assess coronary artery disease in patients older than age 50 years and those with risk factors.

Hepatopulmonary Syndrome

7 The effects of hepatic cirrhosis on the pulmonary vascular resistance (PVR) vessels may result in chronic hypoxemia. *Hepatopulmonary syndrome* (Table 33–7) is found in approximately 30% of liver transplant candidates and is characterized

---

TABLE 33–6 **Hemodynamic and pathological changes in the typical cirrhotic patient.**

- Increased cardiac output
- Increased heart rate
- Decreased systemic vascular resistance
- Increased circulating volume
- Coronary artery disease
- Cirrhotic cardiomyopathy (often unrecognized)
- Low systemic vascular resistance conceals poor left ventricular function
- Reduced responsiveness to β-agonists

TABLE 33–5 **Differential diagnosis of cardiopulmonary dysfunction in chronic liver disease and portal hypertension.**

Primary cardiopulmonary disorders
- Chronic obstructive pulmonary disease
- Congestive heart failure
- Asthma
- Restrictive lung disease
- Pneumonia

Complications of cirrhosis
- Ascites
- Pleural effusions
- Muscle wasting

Cardiopulmonary/liver disease
- Alcoholic liver disease with alcoholic cardiomyopathy
- Hemochromatosis with iron overload cardiomyopathy
- A-1 antitrypsin deficiency with panacinar emphesema
- Primary biliary cirrhosis with fibrosing alveolitis

Pulmonary vascular disorders
- Hepatopulmonary syndrome
- Portopulmonary hypertension

TABLE 33–7 **Hepatopulmonary syndrome.**

Clinical features
- Cyanosis
- Digital clubbing
- Cutaneous telangiectasia
- Orthodeoxia – oxygen desaturation on sitting or standing
- Platypnea – breathing easier lying flat
- Dyspnea

Diagnostic criteria
- Presence of liver disease, usually with portal hypertension and cirrhosis
- An alveolar to arterial oxygen gradient of >15 mm Hg
- Pulmonary arteriovenous connections demonstrated by:
  - A delayed contrast-enhanced (agitated saline) echocardiogram showing contrast in the left heart chambers 4 to 6 heartbeats after contrast appears in the right heart chambers
  - Brain uptake >6% following technetium-99m macroaggregated albumin lung perfusion scan

Indications
- Liver transplantation is the only therapy that will cure hepatopulmonary syndrome

by pulmonary arteriolar endothelial dysfunction. The resultant intrapulmonary vascular dilatation causes intrapulmonary right-to-left shunting and an increase in the alveolar to arterial oxygen gradient.

Portopulmonary Hypertension

Pulmonary vascular remodeling may occur in association with chronic liver disease, involving vascular smooth muscle proliferation, vasoconstriction, intimal proliferation, and eventual fibrosis, all presenting as an obstructive pathology that causes an increased resistance to flow. This may result in pulmonary hypertension; if associated with portal hypertension, it is termed *portopulmonary hypertension* (POPH; Table 33–8).

The diagnostic criteria for POPH include a mean pulmonary artery pressure (mPAP) >25 mm Hg at rest, and a PVR > 240 dyn.s.cm^{-5}. The transpulmonary gradient of >12 mm Hg (mPAP – pulmonary arteriolar occlusion pressure [PAOP]) reflects the obstruction to flow and distinguishes the contribution of volume and resistance to the increase in mPAP.

POPH may be classified as mild (mPAP 25–35 mm Hg), moderate (mPAP > 35 and <45 mm Hg), and severe (mPAP > 45 mm Hg). Mild POPH is not associated with increased mortality at liver transplantation, although the immediate recovery period may be challenging if there is a significant increase in cardiac output after reperfusion of the new graft. Moderate and severe POPH are associated with significant mortality at transplantation. However, the key factor is not mPAP, but rather right ventricular (RV) function.

TABLE 33–8 Clinical features of portopulmonary hypertension.

- Increased pulmonary vascular resistance: vasoconstriction, structural vascular remodeling, and eventual fibrosis.
- Mean pulmonary artery pressure >25 mm Hg with normal pulmonary capillary wedge pressure
- Right ventricular overload
- Right heart failure
- Hepatic congestion
- Increased liver transplantation mortality risk, especially if mean pulmonary artery pressure is >35 mm Hg

The success of liver transplantation will depend on the right ventricle maintaining good function during and after the transplant procedure despite increases in cardiac output, volume, and PVR. If RV dysfunction or failure occurs, graft congestion with possible failure and serious morbidity, including mortality, may ensue. Assessment of the right ventricle using transesophageal echocardiography (TEE) is often helpful.

The role of liver transplantation in the management of POPH is not well defined. In some patients, pulmonary hypertension will reverse quickly after transplant; however, other patients may require months or years of ongoing vasodilator therapy. Other patients may continue to progress and eventually develop RV failure. Some patients will develop pulmonary hypertension after liver transplantation. Liver transplantation offers the best outcome in patients with POPH that is responsive to vasodilator therapy.

D. Respiratory Manifestations

Disturbances in pulmonary gas exchange and ventilatory mechanics are often present. Hyperventilation is common and results in a primary respiratory alkalosis. As noted above, hypoxemia is frequently present and is due to right-to-left shunting of up to 40% of cardiac output. Shunting is due to an increase in both pulmonary arteriovenous communications (absolute) and ventilation/perfusion mismatching (relative). Elevation of the diaphragm from ascites decreases lung volume, particularly functional residual capacity, and predisposes to atelectasis. Moreover, large amounts of ascites produce a restrictive ventilatory defect that increases the work of breathing.

Review of the chest radiograph and arterial blood gas measurements is useful preoperatively because atelectasis and hypoxemia are usually not evident on clinical examination. Paracentesis should be considered in patients with massive ascites and pulmonary compromise, but should be performed with caution because excessive fluid removal can lead to circulatory collapse.

E. Renal Manifestations and Fluid Balance

Derangements of fluid and electrolyte balance may manifest as ascites, edema, electrolyte disturbances, and hepatorenal syndrome. Important mechanisms responsible for ascites include (1) portal hypertension, which increases hydrostatic pressure and favors transudation of fluid across the intestine into the peritoneal cavity; (2) hypoalbuminemia, which decreases plasma oncotic pressure and favors fluid transudation; (3) seepage of protein-rich lymphatic fluid from the serosal surface of the liver secondary to distortion and obstruction of lymphatic channels in the liver; and (4) avid renal sodium and water retention.

Patients with cirrhosis and ascites have decreased renal perfusion, altered intrarenal hemodynamics, enhanced proximal and distal sodium reabsorption, and often an impairment of free water clearance. Hyponatremia and hypokalemia are common. The former is dilutional, whereas the latter is due to excessive urinary potassium losses (from secondary hyperaldosteronism or diuretics). The most severe expression of these abnormalities is seen with the development of hepatorenal syndrome. Patients with ascites have elevated levels of circulating catecholamines, probably due to enhanced sympathetic outflow. In addition to increased renin and angiotensin II, these patients are insensitive to circulating atrial natriuretic peptide.

8 **Hepatorenal syndrome** is a functional renal defect in patients with cirrhosis that usually follows gastrointestinal bleeding, aggressive diuresis, sepsis, or major surgery. It is characterized by progressive oliguria with avid sodium retention, azotemia, intractable ascites, and a very high mortality rate. Treatment is supportive and often unsuccessful unless liver transplantation is undertaken.

Judicious perioperative fluid management in patients with advanced liver disease is critical. The importance of preserving kidney function perioperatively cannot be overemphasized. Overzealous preoperative diuresis should be avoided, and acute intravascular fluid deficits should be corrected with colloid infusions. Diuresis of ascites and edema fluid should be accomplished over several days. Loop diuretics are administered only after measures such as bed rest, sodium restriction (<2 g NaCl/d), and spironolactone are deemed ineffective. Daily body weight measurements are useful in preventing intravascular volume depletion during diuresis.

In patients with both ascites and peripheral edema, no more than 1 kg/day should be lost during diuresis; in those with ascites alone, no more than 0.5 kg/day should be lost. Hyponatremia (serum $[Na^+] < 130$ mEq/L) also requires water restriction (<1.5 L/d), and potassium deficits should be replaced preoperatively.

F. Central Nervous System Manifestations

Hepatic encephalopathy is characterized by alterations in mental status with fluctuating neurological signs (asterixis, hyperreflexia, and/or inverted plantar reflex) and characteristic electroencephalographic changes (symmetric high-voltage, slow-wave activity). Some patients also have elevated intracranial pressure. Metabolic encephalopathy seems to be related to both the amount of hepatocellular damage present and the degree of shunting of portal blood away from the liver and directly into the systemic circulation. The accumulation of substances originating in the gastrointestinal tract (but normally metabolized by the liver) has been implicated.

9 Factors known to precipitate hepatic encephalopathy include gastrointestinal bleeding, increased dietary protein intake, hypokalemic alkalosis from vomiting or diuresis, infections, and worsening liver function.

Hepatic encephalopathy should be aggressively treated preoperatively. Precipitating causes should be corrected. Oral lactulose 30–50 mL every 8 hr or neomycin 500 mg every 6 hr is useful in reducing intestinal ammonia absorption. Lactulose acts as an osmotic laxative, and, like neomycin, likely inhibits ammonia production by intestinal bacteria. Sedatives should be avoided.

Intraoperative Considerations

Patients with postnecrotic cirrhosis due to hepatitis B or hepatitis C who are carriers of the virus may be infectious. Universal precautions are always indicated in preventing contact with blood and body fluids from all patients.

A. Drug Responses

The response to anesthetic agents is unpredictable in patients with cirrhosis. Changes in central nervous system sensitivity, volumes of distribution, protein binding, drug metabolism, and drug elimination are common. An increase in the volume of distribution for highly ionized drugs, such as neuromuscular blockers (NMBs), is due to the expanded extracellular fluid compartment; an apparent resistance may be observed, requiring larger than normal loading doses. However, smaller than normal maintenance doses of NMBs dependent on hepatic elimination (pancuronium, rocuronium, and vecuronium) are needed. The duration of action of succinylcholine may be prolonged because of reduced levels of pseudocholinesterase, but this is rarely of clinical consequence.

B. Anesthetic Technique

The cirrhotic liver is very dependent on hepatic arterial perfusion because of reduced portal venous blood flow. Preservation of hepatic arterial blood flow and avoidance of agents with potentially adverse effects on hepatic function are critical. Regional anesthesia may be used in patients without thrombocytopenia or coagulopathy, but hypotension must be avoided. A propofol induction followed by isoflurane or sevoflurane in oxygen or an oxygen–air mixture is commonly employed for general anesthesia. Opioid supplementation reduces the dose of the volatile agent required, but the half-lives of opioids are often significantly prolonged, which may cause prolonged postoperative respiratory depression. Cisatracurium may be the NMB of choice because of its nonhepatic metabolism.

Preoperative nausea, vomiting, upper gastrointestinal bleeding, and abdominal distention due to massive ascites require a well-planned anesthetic induction. Preoxygenation and a rapid-sequence induction with cricoid pressure are often performed. In unstable patients and those with active bleeding, either an awake intubation or a rapid-sequence induction using ketamine or etomidate and succinylcholine is suggested.

C. Monitoring

Pulse oximetry should be supplemented with arterial blood gas measurements to monitor acid–base status. Patients with large right-to-left intrapulmonary shunts may not tolerate the addition of nitrous oxide and may require positive end-expiratory pressure (PEEP) to treat ventilation/perfusion inequalities and subsequent hypoxemia. Patients receiving vasopressin infusions should be monitored for myocardial ischemia from coronary vasoconstriction.

Continuous intraarterial pressure monitoring is often used because hemodynamic instability frequently occurs as a result of excessive bleeding and surgical manipulations. Intravascular volume status is often difficult to optimize, and goal-directed hemodynamic and fluid therapy utilizing esophageal Doppler, arterial waveform analysis, or echocardiography should be considered. Such approaches may be helpful in preventing the hepatorenal syndrome. Urinary output must be followed closely; mannitol may be considered for persistently low urinary outputs despite adequate intravascular fluid replacement.

D. Fluid Replacement

Most patients are sodium-restricted preoperatively, but preservation of intravascular volume and urinary output takes priority intraoperatively. The use of predominantly colloid intravenous fluids (albumin) may be preferable to avoid sodium overload and to increase oncotic pressure. Intravenous fluid replacement should take into account the excessive bleeding and fluid shifts that often occur in these patients during abdominal procedures. Venous engorgement from portal hypertension, lysis of adhesions from previous surgery, and coagulopathy lead to excessive bleeding during surgical procedures, whereas evacuation of ascites and prolonged surgical procedures result in large fluid **10** shifts. Following the removal of large amounts of ascitic fluid, aggressive intravenous fluid replacement is often necessary to prevent profound hypotension and kidney failure.

Most preoperative patients are anemic and coagulopathic, and perioperative red blood cell transfusion may lead to hypocalcemia (citrate toxicity) because of elevated plasma citrate levels resulting from impaired citrate metabolism in the cirrhotic liver. Citrate, the anticoagulant in stored red blood cell preparations, binds with plasma calcium, producing hypocalcemia. Intravenous calcium is often necessary to reverse the negative inotropic effects of decreased blood ionized calcium concentration (see Chapter 51).

Hepatic Surgery

Common hepatic procedures include repair of lacerations, drainage of abscesses, and resection of primary or metastatic neoplasms, and up to 80% to 85% of the liver can be resected in many patients. In addition, liver transplantation is performed in many centers. The perioperative care of patients undergoing hepatic surgery is often challenging because of coexisting medical problems and debilitation found in many patients with intrinsic liver disease, and because of the potential for significant operative blood loss. Hepatitis and cirrhosis greatly complicate anesthetic management and increase perioperative mortality. Multiple large-bore intravenous catheters and fluid blood warmers are necessary; rapid infusion devices facilitate management when massive blood transfusion is anticipated. Continuous intraarterial pressure monitoring is typically utilized.

Hemodynamic optimization is often complicated by the conflict between the need to maintain sufficient intravascular volume to ensure adequate hepatic perfusion and the need to keep central venous pressure low to minimize liver engorgement and surgical bleeding." Central venous pressure measurement is not an accurate monitor of volume status, and, when this determination is important, the appropriate alternative modality is goal-directed therapy utilizing esophageal Doppler, arterial waveform analysis, or TEE. Care should be taken in placing an esophageal Doppler or TEE probe in a patient with esophageal variceal disease.

Some clinicians avoid hypotensive anesthesia because of its potentially deleterious effects on liver tissue, whereas others believe that it can reduce blood loss when used judiciously. Administration of antifibrinolytics, such as ε-aminocaproic acid or tranexamic acid, may reduce operative blood loss. Hypoglycemia, coagulopathy, and sepsis may occur following large liver resections. Drainage of an abscess or cyst may be complicated by peritoneal contamination. In the case of a hydatid cyst, spillage can cause anaphylaxis due to the release of *Echinococcus* antigens.

Postoperative complications include hepatic dysfunction, sepsis, and blood loss secondary to coagulopathy or surgical bleeding. Severe postoperative pain from the often extensive surgical incision may hinder postoperative mobilization and convalescence, but perioperative coagulopathy may limit the use of epidural analgesia. Infusion of local anesthetic into the surgical wound can reduce the need for opioids. Postoperative mechanical ventilation may be necessary in patients undergoing extensive resections.

Liver Transplantation

When a center opens a liver transplantation program, a credentialed director should be appointed to the anesthesia component. This individual should be an anesthesiologist with experience and training in liver transplantation anesthesia. A dedicated team of anesthesiologists should be assembled to manage the perioperative course of all liver transplantation patients. This team should have a thorough understanding of the indications for, and contraindications to, liver transplantation (Tables 33–9 and 33–10), as well as associated comorbidities (eg, coronary artery disease, cirrhotic cardiomyopathy, portopulmonary hypertension, hepatopulmonary syndrome, hepatorenal syndrome and hepatic encephalopathy and cerebral edema). It has been demonstrated that such an approach improves outcomes, as measured by

TABLE 33–9 Indications for liver transplantation.

Pediatric	Adult
Congenital hepatic fibrosis	Primary biliary cirrhosis
Alagille's disease	Primary sclerosing
Biliary atresia	cholangitis
α₁-antitrypsin deficiency	Autoimmune hepatitis
Byler's disease	Cryptogenic cirrhosis
Metabolic disorders	Viral hepatitis with cirrhosis
Wilson's disease	Alcoholic cirrhosis
Tyrosinemia	Primary hepatocellular
Glycogen storage diseases	malignancies
Crigler–Najjar disease	Nonalcoholic
Hemophilia	steatohepatitis
Lysosmal storage diseases	Fulminant hepatitis
Protoporpyria	Hepatic vein thrombosis
Familial	Familial amyloid
hypercholesterolemia	polyneuropathy
Primary hyperoxaluria	Chronic viral hepatitis

TABLE 33–10 Contraindications to liver transplantation.

Absolute	Relative
Active sepsis	Severe obesity
Active substance or alcohol abuse	Severe pulmonary hypertension
Advanced cardiac disease	
Extrahepatic malignancy	Severe cardiomyopathy
Metastatic malignancy	
Cholangiocarcinoma	High viral load HIV

reduced blood transfusions, the need for postoperative mechanical ventilation, and the duration of stay in the intensive care unit.

Preoperative Considerations

The **Model for End-stage Liver Disease (MELD)** score is used by the United Network for Organ Sharing (UNOS) to prioritize patients on the waiting list for a liver transplant. The score is based on the patient's serum bilirubin, serum creatinine, and INR, and is a predictor of survival time if the patient does not get a liver transplant. A score of 20 predicts a 19.6% risk of mortality at 3 months, whereas a score of 40 predicts a 71.3% risk of mortality at 3 months (Figure 33–1).

The MELD score
$$= 0.957 \times \log_e[\text{serum creatinine (mg/dL)}]$$
$$+ 0.378 \times \log_e[\text{total serum bilirubin (mg/dL)}]$$
$$+ 1.120 \times \log_e[\text{INR}]$$

Multiply the resulting value by 10, and round to nearest whole number. The minimum for all values is 1.0; the maximum value for creatinine is 4.0.

Most liver transplant candidates have high MELD scores and present with jaundice, renal failure, and coagulopathy. They may also be emaciated and have massive ascites, and some may have encephalopathy, hepatopulmonary syndrome, cirrhotic cardiomyopathy, and POPH. The typical hemodynamic finding is a high cardiac index and low systemic vascular resistance.

Significant blood loss may be anticipated, and large-bore intravenous catheters should be placed for access. A rapid infusion pump should be available. Routine hemodynamic monitoring should include intraarterial pressure monitoring and a central venous catheter. TEE is routinely utilized

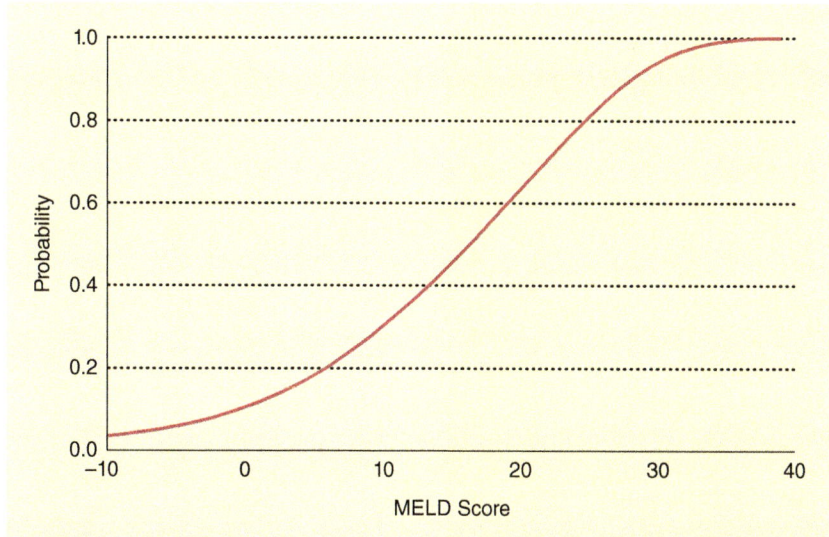

FIGURE 33–1 Relationship between Model for End-stage Liver Disease (MELD) score and 3-month mortality in patients with cirrhotic liver disease. (Reproduced, with permission, from Wiesner RH, McDiarmid SV, Kamath PS, et al: MELD and PELD: application of survival models to liver allocation. Liver Transpl 2001;7:567.)

in many centers. Pulmonary artery catheterization, once routine, has now been abandoned for liver transplant patients at many centers.

The immediate availability of intraoperative continuous venovenous hemodialysis (CVVHD) may be very helpful for volume management in the patient with marginal or no renal function. In patients with significant electrolyte abnormalities, serum sodium and potassium can be closely managed by adjusting the CVVHD dialysate solution.

Intraoperative Management

As noted above, hepatic disease causes endothelial dysfunction that impairs all organs of the body. The heart develops cirrhotic cardiomyopathy; the brain, encephalopathy and eventual cerebral edema; the kidneys, hepatorenal syndrome and eventual acute tubular necrosis; and the lungs, hepatopulmonary syndrome and/or portopulmonary hypertension. Therefore, each organ must be carefully managed throughout the operative procedure and the postoperative period.

Maintenance of cerebral perfusion pressure is particularly important in patients with cerebral edema, and many centers will temporarily correct the coagulopathy in order to place an intracranial transducer for monitoring intracranial pressure. Additional cerebral protective measures include head elevation of 20°, mild hypothermia, and mild hypocarbia with vasopressor support to maintain mean arterial pressure. When the patient's head is elevated, the arterial pressure transducer should be zeroed at the level of the external auditory meatus for accurate determination of cerebral perfusion pressure.

The coagulopathy is managed with the aid of a point-of-care viscoelastic coagulation assay device (TEG®, ROTEM®, or Sonoclot®) or frequent assessment of conventional tests of coagulation. Blood loss may be significant, and transfusions are targeted to maintain the hemoglobin level >7 g/dL.

Transfusions must be tempered to keep the central venous pressure (CVP) low during the liver dissection to reduce blood loss and minimize liver congestion, and at reperfusion and during the remainder of the procedure to prevent graft congestion and hepatic dysfunction. Most coagulopathies

will correct with the new liver if its function is good. Fibrinolysis, a low ionized calcium level, and hypothermia must be corrected, as these may promote bleeding. However, coagulation defects usually do not need to be treated preoperatively or intraoperatively unless bleeding is a problem. Intraoperative transfusion of platelets and fresh frozen plasma is associated with decreased long-term patient survival.

The liver transplantation surgical procedure is divided into three stages: dissection (preanhepatic), anhepatic, and neohepatic periods.

The dissection (preanhepatic) phase is highlighted by the management of hemodynamic changes related to blood loss and surgical compression of major vessels. Hyponatremia should be carefully managed without rapid serum sodium correction, because this may promote the development of central pontine myelinolysis. Hyperkalemia may require aggressive intervention with diuresis, transfusion of only washed packed red blood cells, or CVVHD. Citrate toxicity (hypocalcemia) will occur rapidly if blood is transfused; therefore, ionized calcium should be closely monitored, and calcium chloride administered as necessary. A low CVP is helpful to minimize blood loss while systemic arterial pressure is maintained.

The anhepatic phase begins with the vascular occlusion of the inflow to the liver and ends with reperfusion. Some centers utilize venovenous bypass to prevent congestion of the visceral organs and improve venous return. It *may* protect kidney function.

In the neohepatic phase, two pathophysiological events may occur on opening the portal vein and allowing reperfusion of the graft. The first is a reperfusion syndrome caused by the cold, acidotic, hyperkalemic solution that may contain emboli and vasoactive substances being flushed from the graft directly into the right heart. This may cause hypotension, right heart dysfunction, arrhythmias, and even cardiac arrest, and may be preempted to some extent by the prophylactic administration of calcium chloride and sodium bicarbonate. The second syndrome that may occur is ischemia/reperfusion injury. This may result from impaired reperfusion due to severe endothelial dysfunction, and, in rare cases, may lead to primary nonfunction of the graft.

Postoperative Management

Patients who undergo liver transplantation are often severely debilitated and malnourished and have multiorgan dysfunction; therefore, they will need careful support until they have recovered. Continuous monitoring of cardiovascular, pulmonary, renal, and neurological status is necessary. Early extubation is appropriate in selected patients if they are comfortable, cooperative, and not excessively coagulopathic. Immunosuppression must be precisely managed to minimize the risk of sepsis. A close watch on graft function must be maintained, with a low threshold for checking hepatic artery patency and flow. Postoperative bleeding, biliary leaks, and vascular thromboses may require surgical reexploration.

SPECIAL SITUATIONS

Patients with elevated intracranial pressure and those at risk of its development should have intracranial pressure (ICP) monitoring in place, if possible, to enable the appropriate management of cerebral perfusion pressure. The cerebral perfusion pressure should be maintained >50 mm Hg by adequate mean arterial pressure and a 20–25° head-up position. Mild hypothermia should be considered.

The management of patients who are at risk of or have elevated ICP should include the following:

- ICP < 20 mm Hg
- CPP > 50 mm Hg
- Mean arterial pressure >60 mm Hg
- Proper bed position (elevate the head of the bed by 20–25°)
- Controlled airway and ventilation
- Controlled sedation (eg, propofol)
- Vasopressor support (eg, vasopressin, norepinephrine) when necessary
- Controlled hypothermia (32–33°C)
- Glycemic control

- Aggressive treatment of metabolic acidosis and coagulopathy
- CVVHD

Pediatric Liver Transplantation

Selected pediatric centers report survival rates of 90% at one year. The use of reduced-size and living donor grafts has increased the organ availability in this patient population.

Living Donor Transplantation

The use of living donors has increased the pool of organs available for transplantation. However, this procedure does expose healthy individuals to morbidity and mortality risks. Informed consent from the donor must be obtained with the understanding that there is often a great deal of emotional pressure on family members to donate, and that consent must be freely given without coercion.

In most donor anesthesia protocols, maintenance of a CVP <5 cm H_2O is utilized to reduce intraoperative blood loss. Good postoperative analgesia is required so that comfortable donor patients may be extubated at the end of the procedure. Complications of this surgery for the donor patient include transient hepatic dysfunction, wound infection, postoperative bleeding, portal vein thrombosis, and biliary leaks. An increased incidence of perioperative nerve injury to the brachial plexus has been reported in donor patients.

CASE DISCUSSION

Liver Transplantation

A 23-year-old woman develops fulminant hepatic failure after ingesting wild mushrooms. She is not expected to survive without a liver transplant.

What are the indications for liver transplantation?

Orthotopic liver transplantation is usually performed in patients with end-stage liver disease who begin to experience life-threatening complications, especially when such complications become unresponsive to medical or nontransplant surgery. Transplantation is also carried out in patients with fulminant hepatic failure (from viral hepatitis or a hepatotoxin) when survival with medical management alone is judged unlikely. The Model for End-stage Liver Disease (MELD) score is used to assess urgency for transplantation.

The most common indications for liver transplantation in children, in order of decreasing frequency, are biliary atresia, inborn errors of metabolism (usually α_1-antitrypsin deficiency, Wilson's disease, tyrosinemia, and Crigler–Najjar type I syndrome), and postnecrotic cirrhosis.

The most common indications in adults are postnecrotic (nonalcoholic) cirrhosis, primary biliary cirrhosis, and sclerosing cholangitis, and, less commonly, primary malignant tumors in the liver.

What factors have contributed to the recent success of liver transplantation?

One-year survival rates for liver transplantations exceed 80% to 85% in some centers. Currently, 5-year survival rates are 50% to 60%. The success of this procedure owes much to the use of cyclosporine and tacrolimus for immunosuppressant therapy. These drugs selectively suppress the activities of helper T cells (CD4 lymphocytes) by inhibiting production of interleukin-2 (IL-2) and other cytokines. IL-2 is required for the generation and proliferation of cytotoxic T cells responsible for graft rejection and for activating B cells responsible for T cell-dependent humoral responses. Cyclosporine is usually initially combined with corticosteroids and other agents (eg, mycophenolate and azathioprine). Tacrolimus has proved effective in cyclosporine-resistant rejection and is the preferred alternative to cyclosporine as the primary immunosuppressant agent. The use of anti-OKT-3, a monoclonal antibody directed against lymphocytes, has been extremely useful in treating steroid-resistant acute rejection.

Additional factors influencing the improvement in liver transplantation outcome include a greater understanding and experience with transplantation, the safe use of venovenous bypass, and the introduction of rapid infusion devices that allow +transfusion of up to 2 L/min of warmed blood.

What are the three phases of the transplantation surgical procedure?

These procedures can be divided into three phases: A dissection (preanhepatic) phase, an anhepatic phase, and a neohepatic phase.
1. Dissection (preanhepatic) phase: Through a wide subcostal incision, the liver is dissected so that it remains attached only by the inferior vena cava, portal vein, hepatic artery, and common bile duct. Previous abdominal procedures greatly prolong the duration of, and increase the blood loss associated with, this phase.
2. Anhepatic phase: Once the liver is freed, the inferior vena cava is clamped above and below the liver, as are the hepatic artery, portal vein, and common bile duct. The liver is then completely excised. Venovenous bypass (see below) may or may not be employed during this phase. The donor liver is then anastomosed to the supra- and infrahepatic inferior venae cavae and the portal vein.
3. Revascularization and biliary reconstruction (neohepatic or postanhepatic) phase: Following completion of the venous anastomoses, venous clamps are removed and the circulation to the new liver is completed by anastomosing the hepatic artery. Lastly, the common bile duct of the donor liver is then usually connected to the recipient via a choledochocholedochostomy or Roux-en-Y choledochojejunostomy.

What major problems complicate anesthesia for liver transplantation?

Problems include the multisystem nature of cirrhosis, the often massive blood loss throughout the transplantation procedure, the hemodynamic consequences of clamping and unclamping the inferior vena cava and portal vein, the metabolic consequences of the anhepatic phase, and the risks of air embolism and hyperkalemia when circulation to the new liver is fully established.

Preoperative coagulation defects, thrombocytopenia, and previous abdominal surgery greatly increase blood loss. Extensive venous collaterals between the portal and systemic venous circulations also contribute to increased bleeding from the abdominal wall. Potential complications of massive blood transfusion include hypothermia, coagulopathies, hyperkalemia, citrate intoxication (hypocalcemia), and the potential transmission of infectious agents. Blood salvaging techniques can be extremely useful in reducing donor red blood cell transfusion.

What is adequate venous access for these procedures?

Bleeding is a recurring problem during each phase of liver transplantation. Adequate venous access is paramount in anesthetic management. Several large-bore (14-gauge or larger) intravenous catheters should be placed above the diaphragm. Specialized 8.5F catheters can be placed in antecubital veins and used in conjunction with rapid infusion devices. Efforts to minimize the risk of hypothermia should include the use of fluid warming and forced-air surface warming devices.

What monitoring techniques are most useful during surgery?

All patients require direct intraarterial pressure monitoring. A central venous catheter should be used to deliver fluid replacement. Goal-directed hemodynamic and fluid management utilizing arterial pulse wave analysis, esophageal Doppler, or TEE is becoming common. Urinary output should be monitored carefully throughout surgery via an indwelling urinary catheter.

Laboratory measurements constitute an important part of intraoperative monitoring. Serial hematocrit measurements are mandatory to guide red blood cell replacement. Similarly, frequent measurements of arterial blood gases, serum electrolytes, serum ionized calcium, and serum glucose are necessary to detect and appropriately treat metabolic derangements. Coagulation can be monitored by measuring PT, activated partial thromboplastin time, fibrinogen level, platelet counts, and by point-of-care viscoelastic coagulation analysis—TEG®, ROTEM®, or Sonoclot® analysis. These latter modalities not only assess overall clotting and platelet function, but can also detect fibrinolysis.

What anesthetic technique may be used for liver transplantation?

Most patients should be considered as having a "full stomach," often because of marked abdominal distention or recent upper gastrointestinal bleeding. General anesthesia is usually induced via a rapid sequence induction with cricoid pressure. The semiupright position during induction prevents rapid oxygen desaturation and facilitates ventilation until the abdomen is open. Hyperventilation should be avoided unless there is increased intracranial pressure. Anesthesia is generally maintained with a volatile agent (usually isoflurane or sevoflurane), and an intravenous opioid (usually fentanyl or sufentanil). The concentration of the volatile agent should be limited to less than 1 minimum alveolar concentration in patients with severe encephalopathy. Nitrous oxide is usually avoided. Many patients are routinely transferred to the intensive care unit intubated and mechanically ventilated at the end of the operative procedure. Immediate postoperative extubation may be considered if the patient is comfortable, cooperative, physiologically stable, and not hemorrhaging significantly.

What physiological derangements are associated with the anhepatic phase?

When the liver is removed, the large citrate load from blood products is no longer metabolized and results in hypocalcemia and secondary myocardial depression. Periodic calcium chloride administration (200–500 mg) is necessary, but should be guided by ionized calcium concentration measurements to avoid hypercalcemia. Progressive acidosis is also encountered because acid metabolites from the intestines and lower body are not cleared by the liver. Sodium bicarbonate therapy may be necessary and should similarly be guided by arterial blood gas analysis. Excessive administration of sodium bicarbonate results in hypernatremia, hyperosmolality, and accentuation of the metabolic alkalosis that typically follows massive blood transfusions. Tromethamine should be considered when large amounts of alkali therapy are necessary. Although hypoglycemia can occur during the anhepatic phase, hyperglycemia is a more common occurrence following reperfusion.

Pulmonary and systemic (paradoxic) air embolism can occur when the circulation is fully reestablished to the donor liver because air often enters hepatic sinusoids after harvesting. Systemic air embolism probably reflects the fact that many of these patients have extensive arteriovenous communications. The anhepatic phase ends when the three venous clamps are removed and the donor liver is perfused. Thromboembolic phenomena are also possible following reperfusion.

What problems may be anticipated during the revascularization phase?

Perfusion of the donor liver by the recipient's blood often results in transiently increased serum potassium concentration of up to 1–2 mEq/L and increased systemic acidosis. Reperfusion releases potassium from any remaining preservative solution (115–120 mEq/L of potassium) still within the liver, as well as potassium released from tissues distal to venous clamps. Unclamping may also release a large acid load from ischemic tissue in the lower body (particularly without venovenous bypass); preemptive administration of sodium bicarbonate is advocated by some.

When the circulation to the new liver is established, the sudden increase in blood volume, acidosis, and hyperkalemia can produce tachyarrhythmias, or, more commonly, bradyarrhythmias. In addition to calcium chloride and sodium bicarbonate, inotropic support is also often required. Hyperfibrinolysis is commonly present and seems to be due to a marked increase in tissue plasminogen activator and a decrease in plasminogen activator inhibitor and α_2-antiplasmin during the anhepatic phase. Fibrinolysis can be detected by point-of-care viscoelastic coagulation analysis. ε-Aminocaproic acid or tranexamic acid, which inhibit the formation of plasmin, may be indicated in those instances, but should not be used prophylactically.

What problems are encountered postoperatively?

Patients often have an uncomplicated postoperative course, and, after a sufficient period of observation in the postanesthesia care unit, may be transferred directly to the nursing unit designed for liver transplant patients. Problems to anticipate include persistent hemorrhage, fluid overload, metabolic abnormalities (particularly metabolic alkalosis and hypokalemia), respiratory failure, pleural effusions, acute kidney injury or failure, systemic infections, and surgical complications (eg, bile leaks or stricture, or thrombosis of the hepatic or portal vessels). The last two complications may be suspected during Doppler ultrasound and are confirmed by angiography. Neurological complications include seizures, intracranial hemorrhage, encephalopathy, central pontine myelinolysis from a sudden increase in serum sodium, and immunosuppressant-related neurotoxicity. Kidney dysfunction is often multifactorial in origin; contributory factors include periods of hypotension, impaired renal perfusion when the inferior vena cava is clamped (resulting in high pressures in the renal veins), and cyclosporine or antibiotic nephropathy. Measurement of immunosuppressant levels may be helpful in avoiding toxicity.

Prophylactic antibiotics and antifungal agents are routinely given in many centers because of a high incidence of infections.

Graft function is usually monitored by the PT, serum bilirubin, aminotransferase activity, and serum lactate measurements. Diagnosis requires liver biopsy.

SUGGESTED READING

Feltracco F, Ori C: Anesthetic management of living transplantation. Minerva Anestesiol 2010;76:525.

Ganter MT, Hofer CK: Coagulation monitoring: current techniques and clinical use of viscoelastic point-of-care coagulation devices. Anesth Analg 2008;106:1366.

Hammer GB, Krane EJ: Anaesthesia for liver transplantation in children. Paediatr Anaesth 2001;11:3.

Hevesi ZG, Lopukhin SY, Mezrich JD, et al: Designated liver transplant anesthesia team reduces blood transfusion, need for mechanical ventilation, and duration of intensive care. Liver Transpl 2009;15:460.

Johansson PI, Stissing T, Bochsen L, et al: Thromboelastography and thromboelastometry in assessing coagulopathy in trauma. Scand J Trauma Resusc Emerg Med 2009;17:45.

Kochar R, Nevah Rubin MI, Fallon MB: Pulmonary complications of cirrhosis. Curr Gastroenterol Rep 2011;13:34.

Muilenburg DJ, Singh A, Torzilli G, et al: Surgery in the patient with liver disease. Anesthesiol Clin 2009;27:721.

Ozier Y, Klinck JR: Anesthetic management of hepatic transplantation. Curr Opin Anaesthesiol 2008;21:391.

Sniecinski RM, Levy JH: Bleeding and management of coagulopathy. J Thorac Cardiovasc Surg 2011;142:662.

Anesthesia for Patients with Endocrine Disease

1. Diabetic autonomic neuropathy may limit the patient's ability to compensate (with tachycardia and increased peripheral resistance) for intravascular volume changes and may predispose the patient to cardiovascular instability (eg, postinduction hypotension) and even sudden cardiac death.

2. Temporomandibular joint and cervical spine mobility should be assessed preoperatively in diabetic patients to reduce the likelihood of unanticipated difficult intubation. Difficult intubation has been reported in as many as 30% of persons with type 1 diabetes.

3. Sulfonylureas and metformin have long half-lives and many clinicians will discontinue them 24–48 h before surgery. They can be started postoperatively when the patient resumes oral intake.

4. Incompletely treated hyperthyroid patients can be chronically hypovolemic and prone to an exaggerated hypotensive response during induction of anesthesia.

5. Clinically hypothyroid patients are more susceptible to the hypotensive effect of anesthetic agents because of their diminished cardiac output, blunted baroreceptor reflexes, and decreased intravascular volume.

6. Patients with glucocorticoid deficiency must receive adequate steroid replacement therapy during the perioperative period.

7. In patients with a pheochromocytoma, drugs or techniques that indirectly stimulate or promote the release of catecholamines (eg, ephedrine, hypoventilation, or bolus doses of ketamine), potentiate the arrhythmic effects of catecholamines (classically halothane), or consistently release histamine (eg, large doses of atracurium or morphine sulfate) may precipitate hypertension and are best avoided.

8. Obese patients may be difficult to intubate as a result of limited mobility of the temporomandibular and atlantooccipital joints, a narrowed upper airway, and a shortened distance between the mandible and sternal fat pads.

9. The key to anesthetic management of patients with carcinoid syndrome is to avoid anesthetic and surgical techniques or agents that could cause the tumor to release vasoactive substances.

The underproduction or overproduction of hormones can have dramatic physiological and pharmacological consequences. Therefore, it is not surprising that endocrinopathies affect anesthetic management. This chapter briefly reviews normal physiology and pathophysiology of four endocrine organs: the pancreas, the thyroid, the parathyroids, and the adrenal gland. It also considers obesity and carcinoid syndrome.

The Pancreas

Physiology

Adults normally secrete approximately 50 units of insulin each day from the β cells of the islets of Langerhans in the pancreas. The rate of insulin secretion is primarily determined by the plasma glucose concentration. Insulin, the most important anabolic hormone, has multiple metabolic effects, including facilitating glucose and potassium entry into adipose and muscle cells; increasing glycogen, protein, and fatty acid synthesis; and decreasing glycogenolysis, gluconeogenesis, ketogenesis, lipolysis, and protein catabolism.

In general, insulin stimulates anabolism, whereas lack of insulin is associated with catabolism and a negative nitrogen balance (Table 34–1).

DIABETES MELLITUS

Clinical Manifestations

Diabetes mellitus is characterized by impairment of carbohydrate metabolism caused by an absolute or relative deficiency of insulin or of insulin responsiveness, which leads to hyperglycemia and glycosuria. The diagnosis is based on an elevated fasting plasma glucose greater than 126 mg/dL or glycated hemoglobin (HbA_{1c}) of 6.5% or greater. Values are sometimes reported for blood glucose, which runs 12–15% lower than plasma glucose. Even when testing whole blood, newer glucose meters calculate and display plasma glucose.

Diabetes is classified in multiple ways (Table 34–2). Type 1 (insulin-requiring due to endogenous insulin deficiency) and type 2 (insulin-resistant) diabetes are the most common and well

TABLE 34–1 Effects of insulin.[1]

Effects on liver
Anabolic
Promotes glycogenesis
Increases synthesis of triglycerides, cholesterol, and VLDL[2]
Increases protein synthesis
Promotes glycolysis
Anticatabolic
Inhibits glycogenolysis
Inhibits ketogenesis
Inhibits gluconeogenesis
Effects on muscle
Anabolic
Increases amino acid transport
Increases protein synthesis
Anticatabolic
Increases glucose transport
Enhances activity of glycogen synthetase
Inhibits activity of glycogen phosphorylase
Effects on fat
Promotes triglyceride storage
Induces lipoprotein lipase, making fatty acids available for absorption into fat cells
Increases glucose transport into fat cells, thus increasing availability of α-glycerol phosphate for triglyceride synthesis
Inhibits intracellular lipolysis

[1]Reproduced, with permission, from Gardner DG, Shoback D (editors): *Greenspan's Basic & Clinical Endocrinology*, 9th edition, McGraw-Hill, 2011.
[2]VLDL, very low-density lipoprotein.

known. Diabetic ketoacidosis (DKA) is associated with type 1 diabetes mellitus, but rarely individuals with DKA appear phenotypically to have type 2 diabetes mellitus. Long-term complications of diabetes include retinopathy, kidney disease, hypertension, coronary artery disease, peripheral and cerebral vascular disease, and peripheral and autonomic neuropathies.

There are three life-threatening acute complications of diabetes and its treatment—DKA, hyperosmolar nonketotic coma, and hypoglycemia—in addition to other acute medical problems (such as sepsis) in which the presence of diabetes makes treatment more difficult. Decreased insulin activity allows the catabolism of free fatty acids into ketone bodies (acetoacetate and β-hydroxybutyrate), some of which are weak acids (see Chapter 50). Accumulation of these organic acids results in DKA,

TABLE 34–2 Diagnosis and classification of diabetes mellitus.

Diagnosis (based on blood glucose level)	
Fasting	126 mg/dL (7.0 mmol/L)
Glucose tolerance test	200 mg/dL (11.1 mmol/L)

Classification	
Type 1 (juvenile)	Absolute insulin deficiency secondary to immune-mediated or idiopathic causes
Type 2	Onset in childhood or adulthood secondary to insulin resistance (relative insulin insensitivity)
Gestational	Onset of disease during pregnancy; may or may not persist postpartum

an anion-gap metabolic acidosis. DKA can easily be distinguished from lactic acidosis, with which it can coexist; lactic acidosis is identified by elevated plasma lactate (>6 mmol/L) and the absence of urine and plasma ketones (although they can occur concurrently and starvation ketosis may occur with lactic acidosis). Alcoholic ketoacidosis can follow heavy alcohol consumption (binge drinking) in a nondiabetic patient and may include a normal or slightly elevated blood glucose level. Such patients may also have a disproportionate increase in β-hydroxybutyrate compared with acetoacetate, in contrast to those with DKA.

Infection is a common precipitating cause of DKA in a known diabetic patient, and DKA may be the reason that a previously undiagnosed person with type 1 diabetes presents for medical treatment. Clinical manifestations of DKA include tachypnea (respiratory compensation for the metabolic acidosis), abdominal pain, nausea and vomiting, and changes in sensorium. The treatment of DKA should include correcting the often substantial hypovolemia, the hyperglycemia, and the total body potassium deficit. This is typically accomplished with a continuous infusion of isotonic fluids and potassium and an insulin infusion.

The goal for decreasing blood glucose in ketoacidosis should be 75–100 mg/dL/h or 10%/h. Therapy generally begins with an intravenous insulin infusion at 0.1 units/kg/h. DKA patients may be resistant to insulin, and the insulin infusion rate may need to be increased if glucose concentrations do not decrease. As glucose moves intracellularly, so does potassium. Although this can quickly lead to a critical level of hypokalemia if not corrected, overaggressive potassium replacement can lead to an equally life-threatening hyperkalemia. Potassium and blood glucose should be monitored frequently during treatment of DKA.

Several liters of 0.9% saline (1–2 L the first hour, followed by 200–500 mL/h) may be required to correct dehydration in adult patients. When plasma glucose decreases to 250 mg/dL, an infusion of D_5W should be added to the insulin infusion to decrease the possibility of hypoglycemia and to provide a continuous source of glucose (with the infused insulin) for eventual normalization of intracellular metabolism. Patients may benefit from precise monitoring of urinary output during initial treatment of DKA.

Bicarbonate is rarely needed to correct severe acidosis (pH < 7.1) as the acidosis corrects with volume expansion and with normalization of the plasma glucose concentration.

Ketoacidosis is not a feature of **hyperosmolar nonketotic coma** possibly because enough insulin is available to prevent ketone body formation. Instead, a hyperglycemia-induced diuresis leads to dehydration and hyperosmolality. Severe dehydration may eventually lead to kidney failure, lactic acidosis, and a predisposition to form intravascular thromboses. Hyperosmolality (frequently exceeding 360 mOsm/L) induces dehydration of neurons, causing changes in mental status and seizures. Severe hyperglycemia causes a factitious hyponatremia: each 100 mg/dL increase in plasma glucose lowers plasma sodium concentration by 1.6 mEq/L. Treatment includes fluid resuscitation with normal saline, relatively small doses of insulin, and potassium supplementation.

Hypoglycemia in the diabetic patient is the result of an absolute or relative excess of insulin relative to carbohydrate intake and exercise. Furthermore, diabetic patients are incompletely able to counter hypoglycemia despite secreting glucagon or epinephrine (counterregulatory failure). The dependence of the brain on glucose as an energy source makes it the organ most susceptible to episodes of hypoglycemia. If hypoglycemia is not treated, mental status changes can progress from anxiety, lightheadedness, or confusion to convulsions and coma. Systemic manifestations of hypoglycemia result from catecholamine discharge and include diaphoresis, tachycardia, and nervousness. Most of the signs and symptoms of hypoglycemia will be masked by general anesthesia. Although the lower boundary of normal plasma glucose levels is ill-defined, medically important hypoglycemia is present when plasma glucose is less than 50 mg/dL. The treatment of hypoglycemia in anesthetized or critically ill patients consists of intravenous administration of 50% glucose (each milliliter of 50% glucose will raise the blood glucose of a 70-kg patient by approximately 2 mg/dL). Awake patients can be treated orally with fluids containing glucose or sucrose.

Anesthetic Considerations

A. Preoperative

Abnormally elevated hemoglobin A1c concentrations identify patients who have maintained poor control of blood glucose over time. These patients may be at greater risk for perioperative hyperglycemia, perioperative complications, and adverse outcomes. The perioperative morbidity of diabetic patients is related to their preexisting end-organ damage. Unfortunately, one third to one half of patients with type 2 diabetes mellitus may be unaware of their condition.

A preoperative chest radiograph in a diabetic patient is more likely to uncover cardiac enlargement, pulmonary vascular congestion, or pleural effusion, but is not routinely indicated. Diabetic patients also have an increased incidence of ST-segment and T-wave-segment abnormalities on preoperative electrocardiograms (ECGs). Myocardial ischemia or old infarction may be evident on an ECG despite a negative history. Diabetic patients with hypertension have a 50% likelihood of coexisting **diabetic autonomic neuropathy** (Table 34–3). Reflex dysfunction of the autonomic nervous system may be increased by old age, diabetes of longer than 10 years' duration, coronary artery disease, or β-adrenergic blockade. Diabetic autonomic neuropathy may limit the patient's ability to compensate (with tachycardia and increased peripheral resistance) for intravascular volume changes and may predispose the patient

TABLE 34–3 Clinical signs of diabetic autonomic neuropathy.

Hypertension
Painless myocardial ischemia
Orthostatic hypotension
Lack of heart rate variability[1]
Reduced heart rate response to atropine and propranolol
Resting tachycardia
Early satiety
Neurogenic bladder
Lack of sweating
Impotence

[1]Normal heart rate variability during voluntary deep breathing (6 breaths/min) should be >10 beats/min.

to cardiovascular instability (eg, postinduction hypotension) and even sudden cardiac death. The incidence of perioperative cardiovascular instability appears increased by the concomitant use of angiotensin-converting enzyme inhibitors or angiotensin receptor blockers. Autonomic dysfunction contributes to delayed gastric emptying (diabetic gastroparesis). Premedication with a nonparticulate antacid and metoclopramide is often used in an obese diabetic patient with signs of cardiac autonomic dysfunction. However, autonomic dysfunction can affect the gastrointestinal tract without any signs of cardiac involvement.

Diabetic renal dysfunction is manifested first by proteinuria and later by elevated serum creatinine. By these criteria, most patients with type 1 diabetes have evidence of kidney disease by 30 years of age. Because of an increased incidence of infections related to a compromised immune system, strict attention to aseptic technique, important for all patients, is especially important in those with diabetes.

Chronic hyperglycemia can lead to glycosylation of tissue proteins and limited mobility of joints. Temporomandibular joint and cervical spine mobility should be assessed preoperatively in diabetic patients to reduce the likelihood of unanticipated difficult intubations. Difficult intubation has been reported in as many as 30% of persons with type 1 diabetes.

B. Intraoperative

The goal of intraoperative blood glucose management is to avoid hypoglycemia while maintaining blood glucose below 180 mg/dL. Attempting to maintain strict euglycemia is imprudent; "loose" blood glucose control (>180 mg/dL) also carries risk. The exact range over which blood glucose should be maintained in critical illness has been the subject of several much-discussed clinical trials. Hyperglycemia has been associated with hyperosmolarity, infection, poor wound healing, and increased mortality. Severe hyperglycemia may worsen neurological outcome following an episode of cerebral ischemia and may compromise outcome following cardiac surgery or after an acute myocardial infarction. Unless severe hyperglycemia is treated aggressively in type 1 diabetic patients, metabolic control may be lost, particularly in association with major surgery or critical illness. Maintaining blood glucose control (<180 mg/dL) in patients undergoing cardiopulmonary bypass decreases infectious complications. A benefit of true "tight" control (<150 mg/dL) during surgery or critical illness has not yet been demonstrated convincingly and in some studies has been associated with worse outcome than "looser" control (<180 mg/dL).

Lack of consensus regarding the appropriate target for blood glucose has not prevented perioperative glucose management from becoming yet another indicator of so-called "quality" anesthetic care. Consequently, anesthesia staff should carefully review their current practices to ensure that their glucose management protocols are in line with institutional expectations.

Control of blood glucose in pregnant diabetic patients improves fetal outcome. Nonetheless, as noted earlier, the brain's dependence on glucose as an energy supply makes it essential that hypoglycemia be avoided.

There are several common perioperative management regimens for insulin-dependent diabetic patients. In the most time-honored (but not terribly effective) approach, the patient receives a fraction—usually half—of the total morning insulin dose in the form of intermediate-acting insulin (Table 34–4). To decrease the risk of hypoglycemia, insulin is administered *after* intravenous access has been established and the morning blood glucose level is checked. For example, a patient who normally takes 30 units of NPH (neutral protamine

TABLE 34–4 Two common techniques for perioperative insulin management in diabetes mellitus.

	Bolus Administration	Continuous Infusion
Preoperative	D₅W (1.5 mL/kg/h) NPH[1] insulin (half usual AM dose)	D₅W (1 mL/kg/h) Regular insulin: Units/h = Plasma glucose / 150
Intraoperative	Regular insulin (as per sliding scale)	Same as preoperative
Postoperative	Same as intraoperative	Same as preoperative

[1]NPH, neutral protamine Hagedorn.

Hagedorn; intermediate-acting) insulin and 10 units of regular or Lispro (short-acting) insulin or insulin analogue each morning and whose blood glucose is at least 150 mg/dL would receive 15 units (half the normal 30-unit morning dose) of NPH subcutaneously before surgery along with an infusion of 5% dextrose solution (1.5 mL/kg/h). Absorption of subcutaneous or intramuscular insulin depends on tissue blood flow, however, and can be unpredictable during surgery. Dedication of a small-gauge intravenous line for the dextrose infusion prevents interference with other intraoperative fluids and drugs. Supplemental dextrose can be administered if the patient becomes hypoglycemic (<100 mg/dL). However, intraoperative hyperglycemia (>150–180 mg/dL) is treated with intravenous regular insulin according to a sliding scale. One unit of regular insulin given to an adult usually lowers plasma glucose by 25–30 mg/dL. It must be stressed that these doses are approximations and do not apply to patients in catabolic states (eg, sepsis, hyperthermia).

An alternative method is to administer regular insulin as a continuous infusion. The advantage of this technique is more precise control of insulin delivery than can be achieved with a subcutaneous or intramuscular injection of NPH insulin, particularly in conditions associated with poor skin and muscle perfusion. Regular insulin can be added to normal saline in a concentration of 1 unit/mL and the infusion begun at 0.1 unit/kg/h. As blood glucose fluctuates, the regular insulin infusion can be adjusted up or down as required. The dose required may be approximated by the following formula:

$$\text{Unit per hour} = \frac{\text{Plasma glucose (mg/dL)}}{150}$$

A general target for the intraoperative maintenance of blood glucose is less than 180 mg/dL. The tighter control afforded by a continuous intravenous technique may be preferable in patients with type 1 diabetes.

When administering an intravenous insulin infusion to surgical patients, adding some (eg, 20 mEq) KCl to each liter of fluid may be useful, as insulin causes an intracellular potassium shift. Because individual insulin needs can vary dramatically, any formula should be considered as only a crude guideline.

3 If the patient is taking an oral hypoglycemic agent preoperatively rather than insulin, the drug can be continued until the day of surgery. However, sulfonylureas and metformin have long halflives and many clinicians will discontinue them 24–48 h before surgery. They can be started postoperatively when the patient resumes oral intake. Metformin is restarted if renal and hepatic function remain adequate. The effects of oral hypoglycemic drugs with a short duration of action can be prolonged in the presence of kidney failure. Many patients maintained on oral antidiabetic agents will require insulin treatment during the intraoperative and postoperative periods. The stress of surgery causes elevations in counterregulatory hormones (eg, catecholamines, glucocorticoids, growth hormone) and inflammatory mediators such as tumor necrosis factor and interleukins. Each of these contributes to stress hyperglycemia, which increases insulin requirements. In general, type 2 diabetic patients tolerate minor, brief surgical procedures without any exogenous insulin. However, many ostensibly "nondiabetic" patients show pronounced hyperglycemia during critical illness and require a period of insulin therapy.

The key to any management regimen is to monitor plasma glucose levels frequently. Patients receiving insulin infusions intraoperatively may need to have their glucose measured hourly. Those with type 2 diabetes vary in their ability to produce and respond to endogenous insulin, and measurement every 2 or 3 h may be sufficient. Likewise, insulin requirements vary with the extensiveness of the surgical procedure. Bedside glucose meters are capable of determining the glucose concentration in a drop of blood obtained from a finger stick (or withdrawn from a central or arterial line) within a minute. These devices measure the color conversion of a glucose oxidase–impregnated strip. Their accuracy depends, to a large extent, on adherence to the device's specific testing protocol. Monitoring urine glucose is of value only for detecting glycosuria.

Patients who take NPH or other protamine-containing insulin preparations have an increased risk of allergic reactions to protamine sulfate—including anaphylactoid reactions and death. Unfortunately, operations that require the use of heparin and subsequent reversal with protamine (eg, cardiopulmonary bypass) are more common in diabetic patients. The usefulness of a small protamine test dose of 1–5 mg over 5–10 min prior to the full reversal dose is unclear, although this is recommended by some clinicians.

Patients who use subcutaneous insulin infusion pumps for management of type 1 diabetes usually can leave the pump programmed to deliver "basal" amounts of regular insulin (or insulin glargine). This is the amount of insulin required during fasting. Such patients can safely undergo short outpatient surgery with the pump on the basal setting. If more extensive inpatient procedures are required, these patients will normally be managed with intravenous insulin infusions as described earlier.

C. Postoperative

Close monitoring of blood glucose must continue postoperatively. There is considerable patient-to-patient variation in onset and duration of action of insulin preparations (Table 34–5). For example, the onset of action of subcutaneous regular insulin is less than 1 h, but in rare patients its duration of action may continue for 6 h. NPH insulin typically has an onset of action within 2 h, but the action can last longer than 24 h. Another reason for close

TABLE 34–5 Summary of bioavailability characteristics of the insulins.[1]

	Insulin Type[2]	Onset	Peak Action	Duration
Short-acting	Lispro	10–20 min	30–90 min	4–6 h
	Regular	15–30 min	1–3 h	5–7 h
	Semilente, Semitard	30–60 min	4–6 h	12–16 h
Intermediate-acting	Lente, Lentard, NPH	2–4 h	8–10 h	18–24 h
Long-acting	Ultralente, Glargine, Insulatard	4–5 h	8–14 h	25–36 h

[1]There is considerable patient-to-patient variation. Not all formulations available in every country.
[2]NPH, neutral protamine Hagedorn; PZI, protamine zinc insulin.

monitoring is the progression of stress hyperglycemia in the recovery period.

The Thyroid

Physiology

Dietary iodine is absorbed by the gastrointestinal tract, converted to iodide ion, and actively transported into the thyroid gland. Once inside, iodide is oxidized back to iodine, which is bound to the amino acid tyrosine. The end result is two hormones—triiodothyronine (T_3) and thyroxine (T_4)—which are bound to proteins and stored within the thyroid. Although the gland releases more T_4 than T_3, the latter is more potent and less protein bound. Of all circulating T_3, most is formed peripherally from partial deiodination of T_4. An elaborate feedback mechanism controls thyroid hormone synthesis and involves the hypothalamus (thyrotropin-releasing factor [TRF] and thyrotropin-releasing hormone [TRH]), the anterior pituitary (thyroid-stimulating hormone [TSH]), autoregulation, and the adequacy of iodine intake.

Thyroid hormone (T_3) increases carbohydrate and fat metabolism and is an important factor in determining growth and metabolic rate. An increase in metabolic rate is accompanied by an increase in oxygen consumption and CO_2 production, indirectly increasing minute ventilation. Heart rate and contractility are also increased, presumably from an alteration in adrenergic-receptor physiology and other internal protein alterations, not from an increase in catecholamine concentrations.

HYPERTHYROIDISM

Clinical Manifestations

Excess thyroid hormone levels can be caused by Graves' disease, toxic multinodular goiter, TSH-secreting pituitary tumors, "toxic" or "hot" thyroid adenomas, or overdosage (accidental or intentional) of thyroid replacement hormone. Clinical manifestations of excess thyroid hormone concentrations include weight loss, heat intolerance, muscle weakness, diarrhea, hyperactive reflexes, and nervousness. A fine tremor, exophthalmos, or goiter may be noted, particularly when the cause is Graves' disease. New onset of atrial fibrillation is a classic presentation of hyperthyroidism, but cardiac signs also include sinus tachycardia and congestive heart failure. The diagnosis of hyperthyroidism is confirmed by abnormal thyroid function tests, which may include an elevation in serum T_4 and serum T_3 and a reduced TSH level.

Medical treatment of hyperthyroidism relies on drugs that inhibit thyroid hormone synthesis (eg, propylthiouracil, methimazole), prevent hormone release (eg, potassium, sodium iodide), or mask the signs of adrenergic overactivity (eg, propranolol). In addition, although β-adrenergic antagonists do not affect thyroid gland function, they do decrease the peripheral conversion of T_4 to T_3. Radioactive iodine destroys thyroid cell function and may result in hypothyroidism. Radioactive iodine is not recommended for pregnant patients. Subtotal thyroidectomy is rarely used as an alternative to medical therapy. Typically, it is reserved for patients with large toxic multinodular goiters or solitary toxic adenomas. Graves' disease is usually treated with so-called antithyroid drugs or radio-active iodine.

Anesthetic Considerations

A. Preoperative

All elective surgical procedures, including subto-tal thyroidectomy, should be postponed until the patient is rendered clinically and chemically euthy-roid with medical treatment. The patient should have normal T_3 and T_4 concentrations, and should not have resting tachycardia. Antithyroid medica-tions and β-adrenergic antagonists are continued through the morning of surgery. Administration of propylthiouracil and methimazole is particularly important because of their relatively short half-lives. If emergency surgery must proceed despite clinical hyperthyroidism, the hyperdynamic circu-lation can be controlled by titration of an esmolol infusion.

B. Intraoperative

Cardiovascular function and body temperature should be closely monitored in patients with a his-tory of hyperthyroidism. The exophthalmos of Graves' disease increases the risk of corneal abrasion or ulceration.

Ketamine, indirect-acting adrenergic agonists, and other drugs that stimulate the sympathetic ner-vous system or are unpredictable muscarinic antag-onists are best avoided in patients with current or recently corrected hyperthyroidism because of the possibility of exaggerated elevations in blood pres-sure and heart rate. Incompletely treated **4** hyperthyroid patients can be chronically hypovolemic and prone to an exaggerated hypoten-sive response during induction of anesthesia. Adequate anesthetic depth must be obtained, how-ever, before laryngoscopy or surgical stimulation to avoid tachycardia, hypertension, and ventricular arrhythmias.

Thyrotoxicosis is associated with an increased incidence of myopathies and myasthenia gravis; therefore, neuromuscular blocking agents (NMBs) should be administered cautiously. Hyperthyroidism does not increase anesthetic requirements; that is, there is no increase in minimum alveolar concentration.

C. Postoperative

The most serious threat to a hyperthyroid patient undergoing surgery is **thyroid storm**, which is characterized by hyperpyrexia, tachycardia, altered consciousness (eg, agitation, delirium, coma), and hypotension. The onset is usually 6–24 h after sur-gery but can occur intraoperatively, mimicking malignant hyperthermia. Unlike malignant hyper-thermia, however, thyroid storm is not associated with muscle rigidity, elevated creatine kinase, or a marked degree of metabolic (lactic) and respiratory acidosis. Treatment includes hydration and cool-ing, an esmolol infusion or another intravenous β blocker (with a target of maintaining heart rate <100/min), propylthiouracil (250–500 mg every 6 h orally or by nasogastric tube) followed by sodium iodide (1 g intravenously over 12 h), and correction of any precipitating cause (eg, infection). Cortisol (100–200 mg every 8 h) is recommended to prevent complications from coexisting adrenal gland sup-pression. Thyroid storm is a medical emergency that requires aggressive management and monitoring (see Case Discussion, Chapter 56).

Thyroidectomy is associated with several potential surgical complications. Recurrent laryn-geal nerve palsy will result in hoarseness (unilat-eral) or aphonia and stridor (bilateral). Vocal cord function can be evaluated by laryngoscopy imme-diately following "deep extubation", however, this is rarely necessary. Failure of one or both cords to move may require reintubation and exploration of the wound. Hematoma formation may cause airway compromise from collapse of the trachea, particu-larly in patients with tracheomalacia. Dissection of the hematoma into the compressible soft tissues of the neck may distort the airway anatomy and may make intubation difficult. Immediate treatment includes opening the neck wound and evacuating the clot, then reassessing the need for reintubation. Anesthesia staff in the postoperative setting must be prepared to open the surgical wound and relieve airway compression if the surgeon is for any reason unavailable.

Hypoparathyroidism from unintentional removal of all four parathyroid glands will cause acute hypo-calcemia within 12–72 h (see the section on Clin-ical Manifestations under Hypoparathyroidism).

Pneumothorax is an unusual complication of neck exploration.

HYPOTHYROIDISM
Clinical Manifestations

Hypothyroidism can be caused by autoimmune disease (eg, Hashimoto's thyroiditis), thyroidectomy, radioactive iodine, antithyroid medications, iodine deficiency, or failure of the hypothalamic–pituitary axis (secondary hypothyroidism). Hypothyroidism during neonatal development results in cretinism, a condition marked by physical and mental retardation. Clinical manifestations of hypothyroidism in the adult are usually subtle and include infertility, weight gain, cold intolerance, muscle fatigue, lethargy, constipation, hypoactive reflexes, dull facial expression, and depression. Heart rate, myocardial contractility, stroke volume, and cardiac output decrease, and extremities are cool and mottled because of peripheral vasoconstriction. Pleural, abdominal, and pericardial effusions are common. Hypothyroidism may be diagnosed by an elevated TSH concentration, or a reduced free (or total) T_3 level, or both. Primary hypothyroidism, the more common condition, is differentiated from secondary disease by an elevation in TSH in the former. Normal concentrations of TSH despite reduced T_3 concentrations (the so-called "euthyroid sick" syndrome) are often seen in critical illness. The treatment of hypothyroidism consists of oral replacement therapy with a thyroid hormone preparation, which takes several days to produce a physiological effect and several weeks to evoke clear-cut clinical improvement.

Myxedema coma results from extreme hypothyroidism and is characterized by impaired mentation, hypoventilation, hypothermia, hyponatremia (from inappropriate antidiuretic hormone secretion), and congestive heart failure. It is more common in elderly patients and may be precipitated by infection, surgery, or trauma. Myxedema coma is a life-threatening disease that can be treated with intravenous T_3. T_4 should not be used in this circumstance to avoid the need for peripheral conversion to T_3. The ECG should be monitored during therapy to detect myocardial ischemia or arrhythmias. Steroid replacement (eg, hydrocortisone, 100 mg intravenously every 8 h)

is routinely given due to frequent coexisting adrenal gland suppression. Some patients may require ventilatory support and external warming.

Anesthetic Considerations
A. Preoperative

Patients with uncorrected severe hypothyroidism or myxedema coma should not undergo elective surgery. Such patients should be treated with T_3 intravenously prior to emergency surgery. Although a euthyroid state is ideal, mild to moderate hypothyroidism does not appear to be an absolute contraindication to surgery, for example, urgent coronary bypass surgery.

Hypothyroid patients usually require minimal preoperative sedation and are very prone to drug-induced respiratory depression. In addition, they may fail to respond to hypoxia with increased minute ventilation. Patients who have been rendered euthyroid may receive their usual dose of thyroid medication on the morning of surgery; it must be remembered, however, that most commonly used preparations have long half-lives (the half-life of T_4 is about 8 days); therefore, omission of a single dose should have no medical importance.

B. Intraoperative

5 Clinically hypothyroid patients are more susceptible to the hypotensive effect of anesthetic agents because of their diminished cardiac output, blunted baroreceptor reflexes, and decreased intravascular volume. For these reasons, ketamine or etomidate can be recommended for induction of anesthesia. The possibility of coexistent primary adrenal insufficiency should be considered in cases of refractory hypotension. **Other potential coexisting conditions include hypoglycemia, anemia, hyponatremia, difficulty during intubation because of a large tongue, and hypothermia from a low basal metabolic rate.**

C. Postoperative

Recovery from general anesthesia may be delayed in hypothyroid patients by hypothermia, respiratory depression, or slowed drug biotransformation; thus these patients may require mechanical ventilation. Because hypothyroidism increases vulnerability to

TABLE 34–6   **Actions of major calcium-regulating hormones.**

	Bone	Kidney	Intestines
Parathyroid hormone (PTH)	Increases resorption of calcium and phosphate	Increases reabsorption of calcium; decreases reabsorption of phosphate; increases conversion of 25-OHD$_3$ to 1,25 (OH)$_2$ D$_3$;[1] decreases reabsorption of bicarbonate	No direct effects; increases renal production of vitamin D
Calcitonin	Inhibits osteoclastic resorption	Decreases reabsorption of calcium and phosphate	Inhibits reabsorption of phosphate; increases renal excretion of sodium and calcium
Vitamin D	Maintains Ca^{2+} homeostasis	Decreases reabsorption of calcium (probably less important than PTH)	Increases absorption of calcium

[1]25-OHD$_3$, 25-hydroxyvitamin D$_3$; 1,25 (OH)$_2$D$_3$, 1,25-dihydroxyvitamin D$_3$.

respiratory depression, a multimodal approach to postoperative pain management, rather than strict reliance on opioids would be appropriate.

The Parathyroid Glands

Physiology

Parathyroid hormone (PTH) is the principal regulator of calcium homeostasis. It increases serum calcium concentrations by promoting resorption of bone and teeth, limiting renal excretion of calcium, and indirectly enhancing gastrointestinal absorption by its effect on vitamin D metabolism. PTH decreases serum phosphate by increasing renal excretion. The effects of PTH on calcium serum levels are countered in lower animals by calcitonin, a hormone excreted by parafollicular C-cells in the thyroid, but a physiological calcium-lowering effect for calcitonin has not been demonstrated in humans (Table 34–6). Of total body calcium, 99% is in the skeleton. Of the calcium in the blood, 40% is bound to proteins and 60% is ionized or complexed to organic ions. Unbound ionized calcium is physiologically the most important fraction.

HYPERPARATHYROIDISM

Clinical Manifestations

Causes of primary hyperparathyroidism include parathyroid adenomas, hyperplasia of the parathyroid gland, and certain carcinomas. Secondary hyperparathyroidism is an adaptive response to hypocalcemia produced by conditions such as kidney failure or intestinal malabsorption syndromes. Ectopic hyperparathyroidism is due to production of PTH by rare tumors outside the parathyroid gland. Parathyroid hormone–related peptide may cause significant hypercalcemia when secreted by a carcinoma (eg, bronchogenic [lung] carcinoma or hepatoma). Bone invasion with osteolytic hypercalcemia may complicate multiple myeloma, lymphoma, or leukemia. Overall, the most common cause of hypercalcemia in hospitalized patients is malignancy. Nearly all clinical manifestations of hyperparathyroidism are due to hypercalcemia (Table 34–7). Rarer causes of hypercalcemia include bone metastases of solid organ tumors, vitamin D intoxication, milk-alkali syndrome, lithium therapy, sarcoidosis, and prolonged immobilization. The treatment of hyperparathyroidism depends on the cause, but surgical removal of all four glands is often required in the setting of parathyroid hyperplasia. When there is a single adenoma, its removal cures many patients with sporadic primary hyperparathyroidism.

Anesthetic Considerations

In patients with hypercalcemia due to hyperparathyroidism, hydration with normal saline and diuresis facilitated by furosemide will usually decrease serum calcium to acceptable values (<14 mg/dL, 7 mEq/L, or 3.5 mmol/L). More aggressive therapy with the intravenous bisphosphonates pamidronate (Aredia) or etidronate (Didronel) may be necessary for patients with hypercalcemia of malignancy.

TABLE 34–7 Effects of hyperparathyroidism.

Cardiovascular
Hypertension
Ventricular arrythmias
ECG[1] changes (shortened QT interval,[2] widened T wave)

Renal
Polyuria
Impaired renal concentrating ability
Kidney stones
Hyperchloremic metabolic acidosis
Dehydration
Polydipsia
Kidney failure

Gastrointestinal
Constipation
Nausea and vomiting
Anorexia
Pancreatitis
Peptic ulcer disease

Musculoskeletal
Muscle weakness
Osteoporosis

Neurological
Mental status change (eg, delirium, psychosis, coma)

[1]ECG, electrocardiogram.
[2]The QT interval may be prolonged at serum calcium concentrations >16 mg/dL.

TABLE 34–8 Effects of hypoparathyroidism.

Cardiovascular
ECG[1] changes (prolonged QT interval)
Hypotension
Congestive heart failure

Neurological
Neuromuscular irritability (eg, laryngospasm, inspiratory stridor, tetany, seizures)
Perioral paresthesia
Mental status changes (eg, dementia, depression, psychosis)

[1]ECG, electrocardiogram.

Plicamycin (Mithramycin), glucocorticoids, calcitonin, or dialysis may be necessary when intravenous bisphosphonates are not sufficient or are contraindicated. Hypoventilation should be avoided, as acidosis increases ionized calcium. Elevated calcium levels can cause cardiac arrhythmias. The response to NMBs may be altered in patients with preexisting muscle weakness caused by the effects of calcium at the neuromuscular junction. Osteoporosis worsened by hyperparathyroidism predisposes patients to vertebral compression and bone fractures during anesthetic procedures, positioning, and transport. The notable postoperative complications of parathyroidectomy are similar to those for subtotal thyroidectomy.

HYPOPARATHYROIDISM

Clinical Manifestations

Hypoparathyroidism is usually due to deficiency of PTH following parathyroidectomy. Clinical manifestations of hypoparathyroidism are a result of hypocalcemia (Table 34–8), which can also be caused by kidney failure, hypomagnesemia, vitamin D deficiency, and acute pancreatitis (see Chapter 49). Hypoalbuminemia decreases total serum calcium (a 1 g/dL drop in serum albumin causes a 0.8 mg/dL decrease in total serum calcium), but ionized calcium, the active entity, is unaltered. The archetypical presentation of hypocalcemia is tetany, classically diagnosed by Chvostek's sign (painful twitching of the facial musculature following tapping over the facial nerve) or Trousseau's sign (carpal spasm following inflation of an arm tourniquet above systolic blood pressure for 3 min). These signs are also occasionally present in nonhypocalcemic persons. Treatment of symptomatic hypocalcemia consists of intravenous administration of calcium salts.

Mild hypocalcemia is common following cardiopulmonary bypass or infusion of albumin solutions. In many adult patients this need not be treated as the response of the PTH–vitamin D axis will usually be sufficient to restore ionized calcium to normal values and mild hypocalcemia will usually have no hemodynamic consequences.

Anesthetic Considerations

Serum calcium should be normalized in any patient who presents with cardiac manifestations of severe hypocalcemia. Alkalosis from hyperventilation or sodium bicarbonate therapy will further decrease ionized calcium. Although citrate-containing blood products usually do not lower serum calcium significantly, they should be administered cautiously in patients with preexisting hypocalcemia. Other considerations include avoiding the use of albumin solutions (which bind and reduce ionized calcium concentrations) and being mindful of the possibility of coagulopathy.

The Adrenal Gland

Physiology

The adrenal gland is divided into the cortex and medulla. The adrenal cortex secretes androgens, mineralocorticoids (eg, aldosterone), and glucocorticoids (eg, cortisol). The adrenal medulla secretes catecholamines (primarily epinephrine, but also small amounts of norepinephrine and dopamine). The adrenal androgens have almost no relevance for anesthetic management and will not be considered further.

Aldosterone is primarily involved with fluid and electrolyte balance. Aldosterone secretion causes sodium to be reabsorbed in the distal renal tubule in exchange for potassium and hydrogen ions. The net effect is an expansion in extracellular fluid volume caused by fluid retention, a decrease in plasma potassium, and metabolic alkalosis. Aldosterone secretion is stimulated by the renin–angiotensin system (specifically, angiotensin II), pituitary adrenocorticotropic hormone (ACTH), and hyperkalemia. Hypovolemia, hypotension, congestive heart failure, and surgery result in an elevation of aldosterone concentrations. Blockade of the renin–angiotensin–aldosterone system with angiotensin-converting enzyme inhibitors or angiotensin receptor blockers, or both, is a cornerstone of therapy (and produces increased survival) in hypertension and chronic heart failure. Aldosterone receptor blockers (spironolactone or eplerenone) added to standard therapy prolong survival in patients with chronic heart failure.

Glucocorticoids are essential for life and have multiple physiological effects, including enhanced gluconeogenesis and inhibition of peripheral glucose utilization. These actions tend to raise blood glucose and worsen diabetic control. Glucocorticoids are required for vascular and bronchial smooth muscle to respond to catecholamines. Because glucocorticoids are structurally related to aldosterone, most tend to promote sodium retention and potassium excretion (a mineralocorticoid effect). ACTH released by the anterior pituitary is the principal regulator of glucocorticoid secretion. Basal secretion of ACTH and glucocorticoids exhibits a diurnal rhythm. Stressful conditions promote secretion of ACTH and cortisol, while circulating glucocorticoids inhibit ACTH and cortisol secretion. Endogenous production of cortisol, the most important endogenous glucocorticoid, averages 20 mg/d.

The structure, biosynthesis, physiological effects, and metabolism of catecholamines are discussed in Chapter 14. Epinephrine constitutes 80% of adrenal catecholamine output in humans. Catecholamine release is regulated mainly by sympathetic cholinergic preganglionic fibers that innervate the adrenal medulla. Stimuli include exercise, hemorrhage, surgery, hypotension, hypothermia, hypoglycemia, hypercapnia, hypoxemia, pain, and fear.

MINERALOCORTICOID EXCESS

Clinical Manifestations

Hypersecretion of aldosterone by the adrenal cortex (primary aldosteronism) can be due to a unilateral adenoma (aldosteronoma or Conn syndrome), bilateral hyperplasia, or in very rare cases carcinoma of the adrenal gland. Some disease states stimulate aldosterone secretion by affecting the renin–angiotensin system. For example, congestive heart failure, hepatic cirrhosis with ascites, nephrotic syndrome, and some forms of hypertension (eg, renal artery stenosis) can cause secondary aldosteronism. Although both primary and secondary aldosteronism are characterized by increased levels of aldosterone, only the latter is associated with increased renin activity. The usual clinical manifestations of mineralocorticoid excess include hypokalemia and hypertension, and an increased ratio of aldosterone–plasma renin activity has been noted in laboratory studies.

Anesthetic Considerations

Fluid and electrolyte disturbances can be corrected preoperatively using spironolactone. This aldosterone antagonist is a potassium-sparing diuretic with antihypertensive properties. Intravascular volume can be assessed preoperatively by testing for orthostatic hypotension.

MINERALOCORTICOID DEFICIENCY

Clinical Manifestations & Anesthetic Considerations

Atrophy or destruction of both adrenal glands results in a combined deficiency of mineralocorticoids and glucocorticoids (see the section on Glucocorticoid Deficiency). Isolated deficiency of mineralocorticoid activity almost never occurs.

GLUCOCORTICOID EXCESS

Clinical Manifestations

Glucocorticoid excess may be due to exogenous administration of steroid hormones, intrinsic hyperfunction of the adrenal cortex (eg, adrenocortical adenoma), ACTH production by a nonpituitary tumor (ectopic ACTH syndrome), or hypersecretion by a pituitary adenoma (Cushing's disease). Regardless of the cause, an excess of corticosteroids produces Cushing's syndrome, characterized by muscle wasting and weakness, osteoporosis, central obesity, abdominal striae, glucose intolerance, menstrual irregularity, hypertension, and mental status changes.

Anesthetic Considerations

Patients with Cushing's syndrome may be volume overloaded and have hypokalemic metabolic alkalosis resulting from the mineralocorticoid activity of glucocorticoids. These abnormalities should be corrected preoperatively in the manner previously described. Patients with osteoporosis are at risk for fracture during positioning. If the cause of Cushing's syndrome is exogenous glucocorticoids, the patient's adrenal glands may not be able to respond to perioperative stresses, and supplemental steroids are indicated (see the section on Glucocorticoid Deficiency). Likewise, patients undergoing adrenalectomy require intraoperative glucocorticoid replacement (in adults, intravenous hydrocortisone

succinate, 100 mg every 8 h). Other complications of adrenalectomy may include significant blood loss during resection of a highly vascularized tumor and unintentional pneumothorax. On the other hand, many adrenal tumors are removed uneventfully during laparoscopic surgery.

GLUCOCORTICOID DEFICIENCY

Clinical Manifestations

Primary adrenal insufficiency (Addison's disease) is caused by destruction of the adrenal gland, which results in a combined mineralocorticoid and glucocorticoid deficiency. Clinical manifestations are due to aldosterone deficiency (hyponatremia, hypovolemia, hypotension, hyperkalemia, and metabolic acidosis) and cortisol deficiency (weakness, fatigue, hypoglycemia, hypotension, and weight loss).

Secondary adrenal insufficiency is a result of inadequate ACTH secretion by the pituitary. The most common cause of secondary adrenal insufficiency is iatrogenic, the result of prior administration of exogenous glucocorticoids. Because mineralocorticoid secretion is usually adequate in secondary adrenal insufficiency, fluid and electrolyte disturbances are not present. Acute adrenal insufficiency (addisonian crisis), however, can be triggered in steroid-dependent patients who do not receive appropriate glucocorticoid doses during periods of stress (eg, infection, trauma, surgery), and in patients who receive infusions of etomidate. The clinical features of this medical emergency include fever, abdominal pain, orthostatic hypotension, and hypovolemia that may progress to circulatory shock unresponsive to resuscitation.

Anesthetic Considerations

6 Patients with glucocorticoid deficiency must receive adequate steroid replacement therapy during the perioperative period. All patients who have received potentially suppressive doses of steroids (eg, the daily equivalent of 5 mg of prednisone) by any route of administration (topical, inhalational, or oral) for a period of more than 2 weeks any time in the previous 12 months may be unable to respond appropriately to surgical stress and should receive perioperative glucocorticoid supplementation.

What represents adequate steroid coverage is controversial, and there are those who advocate variable dosing based on the extent of the surgery. Although adults normally secrete 20 mg of cortisol daily, this may increase to over 300 mg under conditions of maximal stress. Thus, a traditional recommendation was to administer 100 mg of hydrocortisone phosphate every 8 h beginning on the morning of surgery. An alternative low-dose regimen (25 mg of hydrocortisone at the time of induction followed by an infusion of 100 mg during the subsequent 24 h) maintains plasma cortisol levels equal to or higher than those reported in healthy patients undergoing similar elective surgery. This second regimen might be particularly appropriate for diabetic patients, in whom glucocorticoid administration often interferes with control of blood glucose.

CATECHOLAMINE EXCESS

Clinical Manifestations

Pheochromocytoma is a catecholamine-secreting tumor that consists of cells originating from the embryonic neural crest. This tumor accounts for 0.1% of all cases of hypertension. Although the tumor is usually localized in a single adrenal gland, 10–15% are bilateral or extraadrenal. Approximately 10% of tumors are malignant. The cardinal manifestations of pheochromocytoma are paroxysmal hypertension, headache, sweating, and palpitations. Unexpected intraoperative hypertension and tachycardia during manipulation of abdominal structures may occasionally be the first indications of an undiagnosed pheochromocytoma. The pathophysiology, diagnosis, and treatment of these tumors require an understanding of catecholamine metabolism and of the pharmacology of adrenergic agonists and antagonists. The Case Discussion in Chapter 14 examines these aspects of pheochromocytoma management.

Anesthetic Considerations

Preoperative assessment should focus on the adequacy of α-adrenergic blockade and volume replacement. Specifically, resting arterial blood pressure, orthostatic blood pressure and heart rate, ventricular ectopy, and electrocardiographic evidence of ischemia should be evaluated.

A decrease in plasma volume and red cell mass contributes to the severe chronic hypovolemia seen in these patients. The hematocrit may be normal or elevated, depending on the relative contribution of hypovolemia and anemia; thus neither hematocrit nor hemoglobin concentration reliably defines the adequacy of intravenous volume. Preoperative α-adrenergic blockade with phenoxybenzamine (a noncompetitive inhibitor) helps correct the volume deficit, in addition to correcting hypertension. β Blockade should not be initiated prior to initiation of α blockade but may be added if there is a need to control heart rate and to reduce arrhythmias provoked by excess catecholamine concentrations. A drop in hematocrit should accompany the expansion of circulatory volume, sometimes unmasking an underlying anemia.

Potentially life-threatening variations in blood pressure—particularly during induction and manipulation of the tumor—indicate the usefulness of invasive arterial pressure monitoring and of adequate intravenous access. Young patients with minimal or no heart disease may not need a central venous line. Patients with evidence of cardiac disease (or in whom cardiac disease is suspected) may benefit from having a central line (a convenient route of access for administering catecholamines, should they be required) and from intraoperative transesophageal echocardiography.

Intubation should not be attempted until a deep level of general anesthesia (possibly also including local anesthesia of the trachea) has been established. Intraoperative hypertension can be treated with phentolamine, nitroprusside, nicardipine, or clevidipine. Phentolamine specifically blocks α-adrenergic receptors and blocks the effects of excessive circulating catecholamines. Nitroprusside has a rapid onset of action, a short duration of action, and as a nitric oxide donor can be effective in cases where calcium channel blockers are ineffective. Nicardipine and clevidipine are being used more frequently preoperatively and intraoperatively. Drugs or techniques that indirectly stimulate or promote the release of catecholamines (eg, ephedrine, hypoventilation, or large bolus doses of ketamine), potentiate the arrhythmic effects of catecholamines (classically halothane), or consistently release histamine (eg, large doses of atracurium or morphine sulfate) are best avoided.

After ligation of the tumor's venous supply, the primary problem frequently becomes *hypotension* from hypovolemia, persistent adrenergic blockade, and tolerance to the high levels of endogenous catecholamines that have been abruptly withdrawn. Appropriate fluid resuscitation should reflect surgical bleeding and other sources of fluid loss. Assessment of intravascular volume can be guided by echocardiographic assessment of left ventricular filling using transesophageal echocardiography or other noninvasive measures of cardiac output and stroke volume. Infusions of adrenergic agonists, such as phenylephrine or norepinephrine, often prove necessary. Postoperative *hypertension* is rare and may indicate the presence of unresected occult tumors.

Obesity

Overweight and obesity are classified using the body mass index (BMI). Overweight is defined as a BMI of 24 kg/m² or higher, obesity as a BMI of 30 or higher, and extreme obesity (formerly termed "morbid obesity") as a BMI of more than 40. BMI is calculated by dividing the weight (in kilograms) by the height (in meters) squared. Health risks increase with the degree of obesity and with increased abdominal distribution of weight. Men with a waist measurement of 40 in. or more and women with a waist measurement of 35 in. or more are at increased health risk. For a patient 1.8 m tall and weighing 70 kg, the BMI would be as shown in the following formula:

$$BMI = \frac{\text{Weight (kg)}}{(\text{Height [meters]})^2} = \frac{70 \text{ kg}}{1.8^2} = \frac{70}{3.24}$$
$$= 21.6 \text{ kg/m}^2$$

Clinical Manifestations

Obesity is associated with many diseases, including type 2 diabetes mellitus, hypertension, coronary artery disease, obstructive sleep apnea, degenerative joint disease (osteoarthritis), and cholelithiasis. Even in the absence of obvious coexisting disease, however, extreme obesity has profound physiological consequences. Oxygen demand, CO_2 production, and alveolar ventilation are elevated because metabolic rate is proportional to body weight. Excessive adipose tissue over the thorax decreases chest wall compliance even though lung compliance may remain normal. Increased abdominal mass forces the diaphragm cephalad, yielding lung volumes suggestive of restrictive lung disease. Reductions in lung volumes are accentuated by the supine and Trendelenburg positions. In particular, functional residual capacity may fall below closing capacity. If this occurs, some alveoli will close during normal tidal volume ventilation, causing a ventilation/perfusion mismatch.

Whereas obese patients are often hypoxemic, only a few are hypercapnic, which should be a warning of impending complications. Obesity-hypoventilation syndrome, or obstructive sleep apnea (OSA), is a complication of extreme obesity characterized by hypercapnia, cyanosis-induced polycythemia, right-sided heart failure, and somnolence. These patients appear to have blunted respiratory drive and often suffer from loud snoring and upper-airway obstruction during sleep. OSA patients often report dry mouths and daytime somnolence; bed partners frequently describe apneic pauses. OSA has also been associated with increased perioperative complications including hypertension, hypoxia, arrhythmias, myocardial infarction, pulmonary edema, stroke, and death. The potential for difficult mask ventilation and difficult intubation, followed by upper airway obstruction during recovery, should be anticipated.

OSA patients are vulnerable during the postoperative period, particularly when sedatives or opioids have been given. When OSA patients are placed supine, the upper airway is even more prone to obstruction. For patients with known or suspected OSA, postoperative continuous positive airway pressure (CPAP) should be considered until the anesthesiologist can be sure that the patient can protect his or her airway and maintain spontaneous ventilation without evidence of obstruction. Both the American

Society of Anesthesiologists and the Society of Ambulatory Anesthesia offer guidelines on perioperative management of the patient with OSA.

An OSA patient's heart has an increased workload, as cardiac output and blood volume rise to perfuse additional fat stores. The elevation in cardiac output (0.1 L/min/kg of adipose tissue) is achieved through an increase in stroke volume—as opposed to heart rate. Arterial hypertension leads to left ventricular hypertrophy. Elevations in pulmonary blood flow and pulmonary artery vasoconstriction from persistent hypoxia can lead to pulmonary hypertension and cor pulmonale.

Obesity is also associated with gastrointestinal pathophysiology, including hiatal hernia, gastroesophageal reflux disease, delayed gastric emptying, and hyperacidic gastric fluid, as well as with an increased risk of gastric cancer. Fatty infiltration of the liver also occurs and may be associated with abnormal liver tests, but the extent of infiltration does not correlate well with the degree of liver test abnormality.

Anesthetic Considerations

A. Preoperative

For the reasons outlined above, obese patients are at an increased risk for developing aspiration pneumonia. Pretreatment with H_2 antagonists and metoclopramide should be considered. Premedication with respiratory depressant drugs must be avoided in patients with OSA.

Preoperative evaluation of extremely obese patients undergoing major surgery should attempt to assess cardiopulmonary reserve. Preoperative testing may include such items as chest radiograph, ECG, and arterial blood gas analysis. Physical signs of cardiac failure (eg, sacral edema) may be difficult to identify. Blood pressures must be taken with a cuff of the appropriate size. Potential sites for intravenous and intraarterial access should be checked in anticipation of technical difficulties. Obscured landmarks, difficult positioning, and extensive layers of adipose tissue may make regional anesthesia difficult with standard equipment and techniques. Obese patients may be difficult to intubate as a result of limited mobility of the temporomandibular and atlantooccipital joints, a narrowed upper airway, and a shortened distance between the mandible and sternal fat pads.

B. Intraoperative

Because of the risks of aspiration and hypoventilation, morbidly obese patients are usually intubated for all but short general anesthetics. If intubation appears likely to be difficult, the use of a fiberoptic bronchoscope or video laryngoscopy is recommended. Positioning the patient on an intubating ramp is helpful. Auscultation of breath sounds may prove difficult. Even controlled ventilation may require relatively increased inspired oxygen concentrations to prevent hypoxia, particularly in the lithotomy, Trendelenburg, or prone positions. Subdiaphragmatic abdominal laparotomy packs can cause further deterioration of pulmonary function and a reduction of arterial blood pressure by increasing the resistance to venous return. Volatile anesthetics may be metabolized more extensively in obese patients. Increased metabolism may explain the increased incidence of halothane hepatitis observed in obese patients. Obesity has little clinical effect on the rate of decline of alveolar anesthetic concentrations and wake-up time, even following long surgical procedures.

Theoretically, greater fat stores would increase the volume of distribution for lipid-soluble drugs (eg, benzodiazepines, opioids) relative to a lean person of the same body weight. However, the volume of distribution of, for example, fentanyl or sufentanil is so large that obesity has minimal influence. Water-soluble drugs (eg, NMBs) have a much smaller volume of distribution, which is minimally increased by body fat. Nonetheless, the dosing of water-soluble drugs should be based on ideal body weight to avoid overdosing. In reality, of course, clinical practice does not always validate these expectations.

Although dosage requirements for epidural and spinal anesthesia are difficult to predict, obese patients typically require 20–25% less local anesthetic per blocked segment because of epidural fat and distended epidural veins. Continuous epidural anesthesia has the advantage of providing pain relief and the potential for decreasing respiratory complications in the postoperative period. Regional nerve blocks, when appropriate for the surgery, have the additional advantages of not interfering with the postoperative deep vein thrombosis prophylaxis, rarely producing hypotension, and of reducing the need for opioids.

C. Postoperative

Respiratory failure is a major postoperative problem of morbidly obese patients. The risk of postoperative hypoxia is increased in patients with preoperative hypoxia, following surgery involving the thorax or upper abdomen (particularly vertical incisions). Extubation should be delayed until the effects of NMBs are completely reversed and the patient is awake. An obese patient should remain intubated until there is no doubt that an adequate airway and tidal volume will be maintained. This does *not* mean that all obese patients need be ventilated overnight in an intensive care unit. If the patient is extubated in the operating room, supplemental oxygen should be provided during transportation to the postanesthesia care unit. A 45° modified sitting position will improve ventilation and oxygenation. The risk of hypoxia extends for several days into the postoperative period, and providing supplemental oxygen or CPAP, or both, should be routinely considered. Other common postoperative complications in obese patients include wound infection, deep venous thrombosis, and pulmonary embolism. Morbidly obese and OSA patients may be candidates for outpatient surgery provided they are adequately monitored and assessed postoperatively before discharge to home, and provided the surgical procedure will not require large doses of opioids for postoperative pain control.

Carcinoid Syndrome

Carcinoid syndrome is the complex of symptoms and signs caused by the secretion of vasoactive substances (eg, serotonin, kallikrein, histamine) from enteroepinephrine tumors (carcinoid tumors). Because most of these tumors are located in the gastrointestinal tract, their metabolic products are released into the portal circulation and destroyed by the liver before they can cause systemic effects. However, the products of nonintestinal tumors (eg, pulmonary,

TABLE 34–9 Principal mediators of carcinoid syndrome and their clinical manifestations.

Mediator	Clinical Manifestations
Serotonin	Vasoconstriction (coronary artery spasm, hypertension), increased intestinal tone, water and electrolyte imbalance (diarrhea), tryptophan deficiency (hypoproteinemia, pellagra)
Kallikrein	Vasodilation (hypotension, flushing), bronchoconstriction
Histamine	Vasodilation (hypotension, flushing), arrhythmias, bronchoconstriction

ovarian) or hepatic metastases bypass the portal circulation and, therefore, can cause a variety of clinical manifestations. Many patients undergo surgery for resection of carcinoid tumors; most such patients have not experienced carcinoid syndrome.

Clinical Manifestations

The most common manifestations of carcinoid syndrome are cutaneous flushing, bronchospasm, profuse diarrhea, dramatic swings in arterial blood pressure (usually hypotension), and supraventricular arrhythmias (Table 34–9). **Carcinoid syndrome is associated with right-sided heart disease caused by valvular and myocardial plaque formation, and, in some cases, implantation of tumors on the tricuspid and pulmonary valves.** The diagnosis of carcinoid syndrome is confirmed by detection of serotonin metabolites in the urine (5-hydroxyindoleacetic acid) or suggested by elevated plasma levels of chromogranin A. Treatment varies depending on tumor location but may include surgical resection, symptomatic relief, or specific serotonin and histamine antagonists. Somatostatin, an inhibitory peptide, reduces the release of vasoactive tumor products.

Anesthetic Considerations

9 The key to perioperative management of patients with carcinoid syndrome is to avoid anesthetic and surgical techniques or agents that could cause the tumor to release vasoactive substances. Regional anesthesia may limit release of stress hormones perioperatively. Large bolus doses of histamine-releasing drugs (eg, morphine and atracurium) should be avoided. Surgical manipulation of the tumor can cause a massive release of hormones. Monitoring likely will include an arterial line. If there are concerns about hemodynamic instability or intrinsic heart disease caused by carcinoid syndrome, transesophageal echocardiography may be helpful. Alterations in carbohydrate metabolism may lead to unsuspected hypoglycemia or hyperglycemia. Consultation with an endocrinologist may help clarify the role of antihistamine, antiserotonin drugs (eg, methysergide), octreotide (a long-acting somatostatin analogue), or antikallikrein drugs (eg, corticosteroids) in specific patients.

CASE DISCUSSION

Multiple Endocrine Neoplasia

An isolated thyroid nodule is discovered during physical examination of a 36-year-old woman complaining of diarrhea and headaches. Workup of the tumor reveals hypercalcemia and an elevated calcitonin level, which leads to the diagnosis of medullary cancer of the thyroid and primary hyperparathyroidism. During induction of general anesthesia for total thyroidectomy, the patient's blood pressure rises to 240/140 mm Hg and her heart rate approaches 140 beats/min, with frequent premature ventricular contractions. The operation is canceled, an arterial line is inserted, and the patient is treated with intravenous esmolol and nicardipine.

What could be the cause of this patient's hypertensive crisis during induction of general anesthesia?

Multiple endocrine neoplasia (MEN) is characterized by tumor formation in several endocrine organs. MEN type 1 consists of pancreatic (gastrinomas, insulinomas), pituitary (chromophobes), and parathyroid tumors. MEN type 2 consists of medullary thyroid carcinoma, pheochromocytoma, and hyperparathyroidism (type 2a) or multiple mucosal neuromas (type 2b or type 3). The hypertensive episode in this case may be due to a previously undiagnosed pheochromocytoma. The pheochromocytoma in MEN may consist of small multiple tumors. These patients are typically young adults with strong family histories of MEN. If multiple surgeries are planned, pheochromocytoma resection will usually be scheduled first.

What is calcitonin, and why is it associated with medullary cancer?

Calcitonin is a polypeptide manufactured by the parafollicular cells (C cells) in the thyroid gland. It is secreted in response to increases in plasma ionic calcium and tends to lower calcium levels by affecting kidney and bone function. Therefore, it acts as an antagonist of parathyroid hormone (see Table 34–6).

Why is this patient hypercalcemic if calcitonin lowers serum calcium?

An excess or deficiency of calcitonin has minor effects in humans compared with the effects of parathyroid disorders. This patient's hypercalcemia is most likely due to coexisting primary hyperparathyroidism (MEN type 2a).

Are headache and diarrhea consistent with the diagnosis of MEN?

The history of headaches suggests the possibility of pheochromocytoma, whereas diarrhea may be due to calcitonin or one of the other peptides often produced by medullary thyroid carcinoma (eg, ACTH, somatostatin, β-endorphin).

What follow-up is required for this patient?

Because of the life-threatening hemodynamic changes associated with pheochromocytoma, this entity must be medically controlled before surgery can be considered (see Case Discussion, Chapter 14). Because MEN syndromes are hereditary, family members should be screened for early signs of pheochromocytoma, thyroid cancer, and hyperparathyroidism.

GUIDELINES

Gross JB, Bachenberg KL, Benumof JL, et al: Practice guidelines for the perioperative management of patients with obstructive sleep apnea: A report by the American Society of Anesthesiologists Task Force on Perioperative Management of patients with obstructive sleep apnea. Anesthesiology 2006;104:1081.

Society for Ambulatory Anesthesia Consensus Statement on Selection of Patients With Obstructive Sleep Apnea Undergoing Ambulatory Surgery. Available at: http://www.sambahq.org/main/clinical-practice-guidelines/(accessed July 18, 2012).

SUGGESTED READING

Adesanya AO, Lee W, Greilich NB, Joshi GP: Perioperative management of obstructive sleep apnea. Chest 2010;138:1489.

Arlt W, Allolio B: Adrenal insufficiency. Lancet 2003;361:1881.

Jones GC, Macklin JP, Alexander WD: Contraindications to the use of metformin. Evidence suggests that it is time to amend the list. BMJ 2003;326:4.

King DR, Velmahos GC: Difficulties in managing the surgical patient who is morbidly obese. Crit Care Med 2010;38:S478.

Kohl BA, Schwartz S: How to manage perioperative endocrine insufficiency. Anesthesiol Clin 2010;28:139.

NICE-SUGAR Study Investigators, Finfer S, Chittock DR, et al: Intensive versus conventional glucose control in critically ill patients. N Engl J Med 2009;360:1283.

Petri BJ, van Eijck CH, de Herder WW, et al: Phaeochromocytomas and sympathetic paragangliomas. Br J Surg 2009;96:1381.

Van den Berghe G, Schetz M, Vlasselaers D, et al: Clinical review: Intensive insulin therapy in critically ill patients: NICE-SUGAR or Leuven blood glucose target? J Clin Endocrinol Metab 2009;94:3163.

Zaghiyan KN, Murrell Z, Melmed GY, Fleshner PR: High-dose perioperative corticosteroids in steroid-treated patients undergoing major colorectal surgery: Necessary or overkill? Am J Surg 2012 Jun 28. [Epub ahead of print].

Anesthesia for Patients with Neuromuscular Disease

1 Weakness associated with myasthenia gravis is due to autoimmune destruction or inactivation of postsynaptic acetylcholine receptors at the neuromuscular junction, leading to reduced numbers of receptors and degradation of their function, and to complement-mediated damage to the postsynaptic membrane.

2 Patients who have myasthenia gravis with respiratory muscle or bulbar involvement are at increased risk for pulmonary aspiration.

3 Many patients with myasthenia gravis are exquisitely sensitive to nondepolarizing neuromuscular blockers (NMBs).

4 Patients who have myasthenia gravis are at risk for postoperative respiratory failure. Disease duration of more than 6 years, concomitant pulmonary disease, a peak inspiratory pressure of less than −25 cm H_2O (ie, −20 cm H_2O), a vital capacity less than 4 mL/kg, and a pyridostigmine dose greater than 750 mg/d are predictive of the need for postoperative ventilation following thymectomy.

5 Patients with Lambert–Eaton myasthenic syndrome and other paraneoplastic neuromuscular syndromes are very sensitive to both depolarizing and nondepolarizing NMBs.

6 Respiratory muscle degeneration in patients with muscular dystrophy interferes with an effective cough mechanism and leads to retention of secretions and frequent pulmonary infections.

7 Degeneration of cardiac muscle in patients with muscular dystrophy is also common, but results in dilated or hypertrophic cardiomyopathy in only 10% of patients.

8 Succinylcholine should be avoided in patients with Duchenne's or Becker's muscular dystrophies because of unpredictable response and the risk of inducing severe hyperkalemia or triggering malignant hyperthermia.

9 Anesthetic management in patients with periodic paralysis is directed toward preventing attacks. Intraoperative management should include frequent determinations of plasma potassium concentrations and careful electrocardiographic monitoring to detect arrhythmias.

10 In patients with periodic paralysis, the response to NMBs is unpredictable, and neuromuscular function should be carefully monitored during their use. Increased sensitivity to nondepolarizing NMBs is particularly apt to be encountered in patients with hypokalemic periodic paralysis.

Although neuromuscular diseases are relatively uncommon, patients with these conditions will present to the operating room and to non–operating room procedure areas for diagnostic studies, treatment of complications, or surgical management of related or unrelated disorders. Overall debility, with diminished respiratory muscle strength and increased sensitivity to neuromuscular blockers (NMBs), predisposes these patients to postoperative ventilatory failure and pulmonary aspiration, and may slow their post-procedure recovery because of difficulty with ambulation and increased risk of falling. A basic understanding of the major disorders and their potential interaction with anesthetic agents is necessary to minimize the risk of perioperative morbidity.

MYASTHENIA GRAVIS

Myasthenia gravis is an autoimmune disorder characterized by weakness and easy fatigability of skeletal muscle. It is classified according to disease distribution and severity (Table 35–1). The prevalence is estimated at 50–200 per million population. The incidence is highest in women during their third decade, and men exhibit two peaks, one in the third decade and another in the sixth decade.

1 Weakness associated with myasthenia gravis is due to autoimmune destruction or inactivation of postsynaptic acetylcholine receptors at the neuromuscular junction, leading to reduced numbers of receptors and degradation of their function, and to complement-mediated damage to the postsynaptic end plate. IgG antibodies against the nicotinic acetylcholine receptor in neuromuscular junctions are found in 85–90% of patients with generalized myasthenia gravis and up to 50–70% of patients with ocular myasthenia. Among patients with myasthenia, 10–15% percent develop thymoma, whereas approximately 70% exhibit histologic evidence of thymic lymphoid follicular hyperplasia. Other autoimmune-related disorders (hypothyroidism, hyperthyroidism, rheumatoid arthritis, and systemic lupus erythematosus) are also present in up to 10% of patients. The differential diagnosis of myasthenia gravis includes a number of other clinical conditions that may mimic its signs and symptoms

TABLE 35–1 Myasthenia Gravis Foundation of America clinical classification of myasthenia gravis.[1]

Class	Definition
I	Any ocular muscle weakness May have weakness of eye closure All other muscle strength is normal
II	Mild weakness affecting other than ocular muscles May also have ocular muscle weakness of any severity
IIa	Predominantly affecting limb, axial muscles, or both May also have lesser involvement of oropharyngeal muscles
IIb	Predominantly affecting oropharyngeal, respiratory muscles, or both May also have lesser or equal involvement of limb, axial muscles, or both
III	Moderate weakness affecting other than ocular muscles May also have ocular muscle weakness of any severity
IIIa	Predominantly affecting limb, axial muscles, or both May also have lesser involvement of oropharyngeal muscles
IIIb	Predominantly affecting oropharyngeal, respiratory muscles, or both May also have lesser or equal involvement of limb, axial muscles, or both
IV	Severe weakness affecting other than ocular muscles May also have ocular muscle weakness of any severity
IVa	Predominantly affecting limb and/or axial muscles May also have lesser involvement of oropharyngeal muscles
IVb	Predominantly affecting oropharyngeal, respiratory muscles, or both May also have lesser or equal involvement of limb, axial muscles, or both
V	Defined by intubation, with or without mechanical ventilation, except when employed during routine postoperative management. The use of a feeding tube without intubation places the patient in class IVb

[1]Reproduced, with permission, from Jaretzki III A, Barohn RJ: Myasthenia gravis: Recommendations for clinical research standards. Neurology 2000;55:16.

TABLE 35–2 Differential diagnosis of myasthenia gravis.[1]

Other neuromuscular disorders
  Congenital myasthenic syndromes
  Botulism
  Lambert–Eaton syndrome

Cranial nerve palsies
  Diabetes
  Intracranial aneurism
  Trauma (eg, orbital factures)
  Congenital (eg, Dwayne syndrome)
  Infections (eg, basilar meningitis)
  Inflammation (eg, cavernous sinus syndromes)
  Neoplasm (eg, basilar meningioma)
  Horner's syndrome

Muscle disease
  Myotonic muscular dystrophy
  Oculopharyngeal muscular dystrophy
  Mitochondrial myopathies (eg, chronic progressive
    external ophthalmoplegia)

Central nervous system pathology
  Stroke
  Demyelinating disease

Other
  Motor neuron disease
  Metabolic disease (eg, thyroid disease)

[1]Reproduced, with permission, from Mahadeva B, Phillips II L, Juel VC: Autoimmune disorders of neuromuscular transmission. Semin Neurol 2008;28:212.

TABLE 35–3 Drugs that may potentiate weakness in myasthenia gravis.[1]

Cardiovascular agents
  β-Blockers
  Lidocaine
  Procainamide
  Quinidine
  Verapamil

Antibiotics
  Ampicillin
  Azithromycin
  Ciprofloxacin
  Clarithromycin
  Erythromycin
  Gentamycin
  Neomycin
  Streptomycin
  Sulfonamides
  Tetracycline
  Tobramycin

Central nervous system drugs
  Chlorpromazine
  Lithium
  Phenytoin
  Trihexyphenidyl

Immunomodulators
  Corticosteroids
  Interferon-α

Rheumatological agents
  Chloroquine
  D-Penicillamine

Miscellanous
  Iodinated radiocontrast agents
  Magnesium
  Nondepolarizing neuromuscular blockers

[1]Data from Mahadeva B, Phillips II L, Juel VC: Autoimmune disorders of neuromuscular transmission. Semin Neurol 2008;28:212; and Matney S, Huff D: Diagnosis and treatment of myasthenia gravis. Consult Pharm 2007;22:239.

(Table 35–2). *Myasthenia gravis crisis* is an exacerbation requiring mechanical ventilation and should be suspected in any patient with respiratory failure of unclear etiology.

The course of myasthenia gravis is marked by exacerbations and remissions, which may be partial or complete. The weakness can be asymmetric, confined to one group of muscles, or generalized. Ocular muscles are most commonly affected, resulting in fluctuating ptosis and diplopia. With bulbar involvement, laryngeal and pharyngeal muscle weakness can result in dysarthria, difficulty in chewing and swallowing, problems clearing secretions, or pulmonary aspiration. Severe disease is usually also associated with proximal muscle weakness (primarily in the neck and shoulders) and involvement of respiratory muscles. Muscle strength characteristically improves with rest but deteriorates rapidly with exertion. Infection, stress, surgery, and pregnancy

have unpredictable effects on the disease but often lead to exacerbations. A number of medications may exacerbate the signs and symptoms of myasthenia gravis (Table 35–3).

Anticholinesterase drugs are used most commonly to treat the muscle weakness of this disorder. These drugs increase the amount of acetylcholine at the neuromuscular junction through inhibition of end plate acetylcholinesterase. Pyridostigmine is prescribed most often; when given orally, it has an effective duration of 2–4 h. Excessive administration of an anticholinesterase may precipitate *cholinergic crisis*, which is characterized by increased weakness and excessive muscarinic effects, including salivation, diarrhea, miosis, and bradycardia. An *edrophonium (Tensilon) test* may help differentiate a cholinergic from a myasthenic crisis. Increased weakness after administration of up to 10 mg of intravenous edrophonium indicates cholinergic crisis, whereas increasing strength implies myasthenic crisis. If this test is equivocal or if the patient clearly has manifestations of cholinergic hyperactivity, all cholinesterase drugs should be discontinued and the patient should be monitored in an intensive care unit or close-observation area. Anticholinesterase drugs are often the only agents used to treat patients with mild disease. Moderate to severe disease is treated with a combination of an anticholinesterase drug and immunomodulating therapy. Corticosteroids are usually tried first, followed by azathioprine, cyclosporine, cyclophosphamide, mycophenolate mofetil, and intravenous immunoglobulin. Plasmapheresis is reserved for patients with dysphagia or respiratory failure, or to normalize muscle strength preoperatively in patients undergoing a surgical procedure, including thymectomy. Up to 85% of patients younger than 55 years of age show clinical improvement following thymectomy even in the absence of a tumor, but improvement may be delayed up to several years.

Anesthetic Considerations

Patients with myasthenia gravis may present for thymectomy or for unrelated surgical or obstetric procedures, and medical management of their condition should be optimized prior to the intended procedure. Myasthenic patients with respiratory and oropharyngeal weakness should be treated preoperatively with intravenous immunoglobulin or plasmapheresis. If strength normalizes, the incidence of postoperative respiratory complications should be similar to that of a nonmyasthenic patient undergoing a similar surgical procedure. Patients scheduled for thymectomy may have deteriorating muscle strength, whereas those undergoing other elective procedures may be well controlled or in remission. Adjustments in anticholinesterase medication, immunosuppressants, or steroid therapy in the perioperative period may be necessary. Patients with advanced generalized disease may deteriorate significantly when anticholinesterase agents are withheld. These medications should be restarted when the patient resumes oral intake postoperatively. When necessary, cholinesterase inhibitors can also be given parenterally at $\frac{1}{30}$ the oral dose. Potential problems associated with management of anticholinesterase therapy in the postoperative period include altered patient requirements, increased vagal reflexes, and the possibility of disrupting bowel anastomoses secondary to hyperperistalsis. Moreover, because these agents also inhibit plasma cholinesterase, they could *theoretically* prolong the duration of ester-type local anesthetics and succinylcholine.

Preoperative evaluation should focus on the recent course of the disease, the muscle groups affected, drug therapy, and coexisting illnesses. **2** Patients who have myasthenia gravis with respiratory muscle or bulbar involvement are at increased risk for pulmonary aspiration. Premedication with metoclopramide or an H_2 blocker or proton pump inhibitor may decrease this risk. Because patients with myasthenia are often very sensitive to the respiratory depressant effect of opioids and benzodiazepines, premedication with these drugs should be done with caution, if at all.

With the exception of NMBs, standard anesthetic agents may be used in patients with myasthenia gravis. Marked respiratory depression, however, may be encountered following even moderate doses of propofol or opioids. When general anesthesia is required, a volatile agent–based anesthetic is frequently employed. Deep anesthesia with a volatile agent alone in patients with myasthenia may provide sufficient relaxation for tracheal intubation and most surgical procedures, and many clinicians routinely avoid NMBs entirely. The response to succinylcholine is said to be unpredictable, but we have not found this to be so in practice. Patients may manifest a relative resistance, or a moderately prolonged effect (see Chapter 11). The dose of succinylcholine may be increased to 2 mg/kg to overcome any resistance, expecting that the duration of paralysis could be increased by 5–10 min.

3 Many patients with myasthenia gravis are exquisitely sensitive to nondepolarizing NMBs. Even a defasciculating dose in some patients may result in nearly complete paralysis. If NMBs are necessary, small doses of a relatively short-acting nondepolarizing agent are preferred. We have not found nondepolarizing NMBs to be necessary during thymectomy with volatile anesthesia. Neuromuscular blockade should be monitored very closely with a nerve stimulator, and ventilatory function should be evaluated carefully prior to extubation.

4 Patients who have myasthenia gravis are at risk for postoperative respiratory failure. Disease duration of more than 6 years, concomitant pulmonary disease, peak inspiratory pressure of less than −25 cm H_2O (ie, −20 cm H_2O), vital capacity less than 4 mL/kg, and pyridostigmine dose greater than 750 mg/d are predictive of the need for postoperative ventilation following thymectomy.

Women with myasthenia can experience increased weakness in the last trimester of pregnancy and in the early postpartum period. Epidural anesthesia is generally preferable for these patients because it avoids potential problems with respiratory depression and NMBs related to general anesthesia. Excessively high levels of motor blockade, however, can also result in hypoventilation. Infants of myasthenic mothers may show transient myasthenia for 1–3 weeks following birth, induced by transplacental transfer of acetylcholine receptor antibodies, which may necessitate intubation and mechanical ventilation.

PARANEOPLASTIC NEUROMUSCULAR SYNDROMES

Paraneoplastic syndromes are immune-mediated diseases associated with an underlying cancer. Myasthenia gravis is often considered a paraneoplastic syndrome because it is an autoimmune disorder associated with thymic hyperplasia, including thymoma. Other neurological or neuromuscular paraneoplastic syndromes include Lambert–Eaton myasthenic syndrome, limbic encephalitis, neuromyotonia, stiff person syndrome, myotonic dystrophy, and polymyositis.

Lambert–Eaton Myasthenic Syndrome

The Lambert–Eaton myasthenic syndrome (LEMS) is a paraneoplastic syndrome characterized by proximal muscle weakness that typically begins in the lower extremities but may spread to involve upper limb, bulbar, and respiratory muscles. Dry mouth, male impotence, and other manifestations of autonomic dysfunction are also common. LEMS is usually associated with small cell carcinoma of the lung but may also be seen with other malignancies or as an idiopathic autoimmune disease. The disorder results from a presynaptic defect of neuromuscular transmission in which antibodies to voltage-gated calcium channels on the nerve terminal markedly reduce the quantal release of acetylcholine at the motor end plate. Small cell lung carcinoma cells express identical voltage-gated calcium channels, serving as a trigger for the autoimmune response in patients with paraneoplastic LEMS.

In contrast to myasthenia gravis, muscle weakness associated with LEMS improves with repeated effort and is improved less dramatically by anticholinesterase drugs. Guanidine hydrochloride and 3,4-diaminopyridine (DAP), which increase the presynaptic release of acetylcholine, often produce significant improvement in LEMS. Corticosteroid or other immunosuppressive medications, or plasmapheresis, may also be of benefit.

Limbic Encephalitis

Limbic encephalitis is a degenerative central nervous system disorder characterized by personality changes, hallucinations, seizures, autonomic dysfunction, varying degrees of dementia, and asymmetric loss of sensation in the extremities. It may involve the brain, brainstem, cerebellum, and spinal cord. In approximately 60% of cases, limbic encephalitis is paraneoplastic. There is a strong association with small cell lung carcinoma, and neurological dysfunction often precedes the cancer diagnosis. Therapy includes treatment of the underlying cancer, if present, and administration of immunosuppressive medications.

Neuromyotonia

Neuromyotonia is a condition of peripheral nerve hyperexcitability that is frequently associated with an underlying cancer but may also be inherited or associated with diabetic, drug- or toxin-induced, or other acquired neuropathies. Its features include *myokymia* (a continuous undulating movement of muscles described as being like a "bag of worms"), stiffness, impaired muscle relaxation, painful muscle cramping, hyperhidrosis, and muscle hypertrophy. Treatment includes immunoglobulin therapy, plasma exchange, and administration of anticonvulsants.

Stiff Person Syndrome

Stiff person syndrome is a progressive disorder characterized by axial stiffness and rigidity that may subsequently involve the proximal limb muscles. In advanced cases, paraspinal rigidity may cause marked spinal deformities, and the patient may have difficulty with ambulation and a history of frequently falling. Although stiff person syndrome is rare, when it occurs it is frequently associated with cancer. Therapy includes treatment of the underlying cancer, if present, and administration of immunoglobulin and benzodiazepines.

Myotonic Dystrophy

See next page.

Polymyositis

Polymyositis is an inflammatory myopathy of skeletal musculature, especially proximal limb muscles, characterized by weakness and easy fatigability. Patients are prone to aspiration and frequent pneumonias because of thoracic muscle weakness and dysphagia secondary to oropharyngeal muscle involvement. They may also exhibit cardiac dysrhythmias due to conduction defects. Therapy includes treatment of the underlying neoplasm, if present; plasma exchange; and administration of immunoglobulin, corticosteroids, and immunomodulators such as methotrexate, cyclosporine, and tumor necrosis factor-α inhibitors.

Anesthetic Considerations for Patients with Neuromuscular Paraneoplastic Syndromes

5 Patients with LEMS and other neuromuscular paraneoplastic syndromes are very sensitive to both depolarizing and nondepolarizing NMBs. Volatile agents alone are often sufficient to provide muscle relaxation for both intubation and most surgical procedures. NMBs should be given only in small increments and with careful neuromuscular monitoring. Because these patients frequently exhibit marked debility, benzodiazepines, opioids, and other medications with sedative effects should be administered with caution.

MUSCULAR DYSTROPHIES
Preoperative Considerations

Muscular dystrophies are a heterogeneous group of hereditary disorders characterized by muscle fiber necrosis and regeneration, leading to muscle degeneration and progressive weakness. Anticipated anesthetic risk is increased by the patient's overall debilitated status, which may impede clearance of secretions and postoperative ambulation, as well as by increased risk of respiratory failure and pulmonary aspiration. Duchenne's muscular dystrophy is the most common and most severe form of muscular dystrophy. Other muscular dystrophy variants include Becker's, myotonic, facioscapulohumeral, and limb-girdle dystrophies.

Duchenne's Muscular Dystrophy

An X-linked recessive disorder, Duchenne's muscular dystrophy affects males almost exclusively. It has an incidence of approximately one to three cases per 10,000 live male births and most commonly presents between 3 and 5 years of age. Affected individuals produce abnormal dystrophin, a protein found on the sarcolemma of muscle fibers. Patients characteristically develop symmetric proximal muscle weakness that is manifested as a gait disturbance. Fatty infiltration typically causes enlargement (pseudohypertrophy) of muscles, particularly the calves. Progressive weakness and contractures eventually result in kyphoscoliosis. Many patients are confined to wheelchairs by age 12. Disease progression may be delayed by up to 2–3 years with glucocorticoid therapy in some patients. Intellectual impairment is common but generally nonprogressive. Plasma creatine kinase (CK) levels are 10–100 times normal even early in the disease and may reflect an abnormal increase in the permeability of muscle cell membranes. Female genetic carriers often also have high plasma CK levels, variable degrees of muscle weakness, and, rarely, cardiac involvement. Plasma myoglobin concentration may also be elevated. The diagnosis is confirmed by muscle biopsy.

6 Respiratory muscle degeneration in patients with muscular dystrophy interferes with an effective cough mechanism and leads to retention of secretions and frequent pulmonary infections. The combination of marked kyphoscoliosis and muscle wasting may produce a severe restrictive ventilatory defect. Pulmonary hypertension is common with

7 disease progression. Degeneration of cardiac muscle in patients with muscular dystrophy is also common, but results in dilated or hypertrophic cardiomyopathy in only 10% of patients. Mitral regurgitation secondary to papillary muscle dysfunction is also found in up to 25% of patients. Electrocardiogram abnormalities include P–R interval prolongation, QRS and ST-segment abnormalities, and prominent R waves over the right precordium with deep Q waves over the left precordium. Atrial arrhythmias are common. Death at a relatively young age is usually due to recurrent pulmonary infections, respiratory failure, or cardiac failure.

Becker's Muscular Dystrophy

Becker's muscular dystrophy is, like Duchenne's, an X-linked recessive disorder but is less common (1:30,000 male births). Manifestations are nearly identical to those of Duchenne's muscular dystrophy except that they usually present later in life (adolescence) and progress more slowly. Mental retardation is less common. Patients often reach the fourth or fifth decade, although some may survive into their 80s. Death is usually from respiratory complications. Cardiomyopathy may occur in some cases and may precede severe skeletal weakness.

Myotonic Dystrophy

Myotonic dystrophy is a multisystem disorder that is the most common cause of *myotonia*, a slowing of relaxation after muscle contraction in response to electrical or percussive stimuli. The disease is autosomal dominant, with an incidence of 1:8000, and usually becomes clinically apparent in the second

to third decade of life, but it has also been reported as a paraneoplastic disorder in association with thymoma. Myotonia is the principal early manifestation; muscle weakness and atrophy become more prominent as the disease progresses. This weakness and atrophy usually affect cranial muscles (orbicularis oculi and oris, masseter, and sternocleidomastoid), and in contrast to most myopathies, distal muscles more than proximal muscles. Plasma CK levels are normal or slightly elevated.

Multiple organ systems are involved in myotonic dystrophy, as evidenced by presenile cataracts, premature frontal baldness, hypersomnolence with sleep apnea, and endocrine dysfunction leading to pancreatic, adrenal, thyroid, and gonadal insufficiency. Respiratory involvement leads to decreased vital capacity, and chronic hypoxemia may cause cor pulmonale. Gastrointestinal hypomotility may predispose patients to pulmonary aspiration. Uterine atony can prolong labor and increase the incidence of retained placenta. Cardiac manifestations, which are often present before other clinical symptoms appear, may include cardiomyopathy, atrial arrhythmias, and varying degrees of heart block.

The myotonia is usually described by patients as a "stiffness" that may lessen with continued activity—the so-called "warm-up" phenomenon. Patients often report that cold temperatures worsen stiffness. Antimyotonic treatment may include mexiletine, phenytoin, baclofen, dantrolene, or carbamazepine. A cardiac pacemaker may be placed in patients with significant conduction defect, even if they are asymptomatic.

Facioscapulohumeral Dystrophy

Facioscapulohumeral dystrophy, an autosomal dominant disorder with an incidence of approximately 1–3:100,000, affects both sexes, although more females than males are asymptomatic. Patients usually present in the second or third decade of life with weakness that is confined primarily to the muscles of the face and the shoulder girdle. Muscles in the lower extremities are less commonly affected, and respiratory muscles are usually spared. The disease is slowly progressive with a variable course. Plasma CK levels are usually normal or only slightly elevated. Cardiac involvement is rare, but loss of all atrial electrical activity with an inability to atrially pace the heart has been reported; ventricular pacing is still possible in these patients. Longevity is minimally affected.

Limb-Girdle Dystrophy

Limb-girdle muscular dystrophy is a heterogeneous group of genetic neuromuscular diseases. Limb-girdle syndromes include severe childhood autosomal recessive muscular dystrophy and other incompletely defined autosomal recessive syndromes such as Erb's (scapulohumeral type) and Leyden–Mobius (pelvifemoral type) dystrophies. Most patients present in childhood to the second or third decade of life with slowly progressive muscle weakness that may involve the shoulder girdle, the hip girdle, or both. Plasma CK levels are usually elevated. Cardiac involvement is relatively uncommon but may present as frequent arrhythmias or congestive heart failure. Respiratory complications, such as hypoventilation and recurrent respiratory infections, may occur.

Anesthetic Considerations

A. Duchenne's and Becker's Muscular Dystrophies

The anesthetic management of these patients is complicated not only by muscle weakness but also by cardiac and pulmonary manifestations. An association with malignant hyperthermia has been suggested but is unproven. Preoperative premedication with sedatives or opioids should be avoided because of increased aspiration risk due to respiratory muscle weakness, gastric hypomotility, or both. Intraoperative positioning may be complicated by kyphoscoliosis or by flexion contractures of the **8** extremities or neck. Succinylcholine should be avoided in patients with Duchenne's or Becker's muscular dystrophies because of unpredictable response and the risk of inducing severe hyperkalemia or triggering malignant hyperthermia. Although some patients exhibit a normal response to nondepolarizing NMBs, others may be very sensitive. Marked respiratory and circulatory depression may be seen with volatile anesthetics in patients with advanced disease, and regional or local anesthesia may be preferable in these patients.

Perioperative morbidity is usually due to respiratory complications. Patients with vital capacities less than 30% of predicted appear to be at greatest risk and often require temporary postoperative mechanical ventilation.

B. Myotonic Dystrophy

Patients with myotonic dystrophy are at increased risk for perioperative respiratory and cardiac complications. Most perioperative problems arise in patients with severe weakness and in those cases in which surgeons and anesthesiologists are unaware of the diagnosis. The diagnosis of myotonic dystrophy has been made in some patients in the course of investigating prolonged apnea following general anesthesia.

Patients with myotonic dystrophy have altered responses to a number of anesthetic medicines. They are often very sensitive to even small doses of opioids, sedatives, and inhalation and intravenous anesthetic agents, all of which may cause sudden and prolonged apnea. Premedication should therefore be avoided. Succinylcholine is relatively contraindicated because it may precipitate intense myotonic contractions, complicating orotracheal intubation. Myotonic contraction of respiratory, chest wall, or laryngeal muscles may make ventilation difficult or impossible. Other drugs that act on the motor end plate, such as decamethonium, neostigmine, and physostigmine, can aggravate myotonia. Regional anesthesia may be preferentially employed, but does not always prevent myotonic contractions.

The response to nondepolarizing NMBs is reported to be normal; however, they do not consistently prevent or relieve myotonic contractions. As reversal of nondepolarizing NMBs can induce myotonic contractions, the use of short-acting nondepolarizing agents is recommended. Postoperative shivering commonly associated with volatile agents, particularly when associated with decreased body temperature, can induce myotonic contractions in the recovery room. Small doses of meperidine can often prevent such shivering and may preempt myotonic contractions.

Induction of anesthesia without complications has been reported with a number of agents including inhalation agents and propofol. Neuromuscular blockade, if needed, should employ short-acting NMBs. An association between myotonic dystrophy and malignant hyperthermia has been suggested but not established. Nitrous oxide and inhalation agents can be used as maintenance anesthesia. Reversal with anticholinesterases should be avoided, if possible.

The principal postoperative complications of myotonic dystrophy are prolonged hypoventilation, atelectasis, aspiration, and pneumonia. Close postoperative monitoring should be accompanied by aggressive pulmonary hygiene with physical therapy and incentive spirometry. Aspiration prophylaxis is indicated. Patients undergoing upper abdominal surgery or those with severe proximal weakness are more likely to experience pulmonary complications. Perioperative cardiac conduction abnormalities are less likely to occur but still warrant close cardiovascular monitoring.

C. Other Forms of Muscular Dystrophy

Patients with facioscapulohumeral and limb-girdle muscular dystrophy generally have normal responses to anesthetic agents. Nevertheless, because of the great variability and overlap among the various forms of muscular dystrophy, sedative-hypnotics, opioids, and nondepolarizing NMBs should be used cautiously, and succinylcholine should be avoided.

MYOTONIAS

Myotonia Congenita & Paramyotonia Congenita

Myotonia congenita is a disorder manifested early in life with generalized myotonia. Both autosomal dominant (Thomsen's) and recessive (Becker's) forms exist. The disease is confined to skeletal muscle, and weakness is minimal or absent. Many patients have very well developed musculature due to near constant muscle contraction. Antimyotonic therapy includes phenytoin, mexiletine, quinine sulfate, or procainamide. Other medications that have been used include tocainide, dantrolene, prednisone, acetazolamide, and taurine. There is no cardiac involvement in myotonia congenita, and a normal life span is expected.

Paramyotonia congenita is a very rare autosomal dominant disorder characterized by transient stiffness (myotonia) and, occasionally, weakness after exposure to cold temperatures. The stiffness worsens with activity, in contrast to true myotonia, thus the term *paramyotonia*. Serum potassium concentration may rise following an attack similar to hyperkalemic periodic paralysis (see below). Medications that have been used to block the cold response include mexiletine and tocainide.

Anesthetic management of patients with myotonia congenita and paramyotonia is complicated by an abnormal response to succinylcholine, intraoperative myotonic contractions, and the need to avoid hypothermia. NMBs may paradoxically cause generalized muscle spasms, including trismus, leading to difficulty with intubation and ventilation.

Infiltration of muscles in the operative field with a dilute local anesthetic may alleviate refractory myotonic contraction. Among patients with these types of myotonia, none have been reported with positive in vitro tests for malignant hyperthermia. Excised muscle in these patients does, however, display a prolonged myotonic contraction when exposed to succinylcholine. Excessive muscle contraction during anesthesia, therefore, likely represents aggravation of myotonia and not malignant hyperthermia.

PERIODIC PARALYSIS

Periodic paralysis is a group of disorders characterized by spontaneous episodes of transient muscle weakness or paralysis. Symptoms usually begin in childhood, with episodes lasting a few hours and typically sparing respiratory muscle involvement. The weakness usually lasts less than 1 hour but can last several days, and frequent attacks may lead to progressive, long-term weakness in some patients. Hypothermia exacerbates the frequency and severity of episodes. Muscle strength and serum potassium concentrations are usually normal between attacks. The episodes of weakness are due to a loss of muscle fiber excitability secondary to partial depolarization of the resting potential. This partial depolarization prevents the generation of action potentials and thereby precipitates weakness.

Periodic paralysis is classified into primary genetic channelopathies and secondary acquired forms. The genetic types are due to dominantly inherited mutations in the voltage-gated sodium, calcium, or potassium ion channels. Classifications have been based on clinical differences, but these have not been shown to relate to specific ion channels. Different defects in the same channel can cause different clinical pictures, whereas mutations in different channels may have similar clinical pictures. However, the clinical classifications remain useful as guides to prognosis and therapy.

Hypokalemic periodic paralysis is typically associated with low serum potassium levels, and *hyperkalemic periodic paralysis* with elevated serum potassium levels, during episodes of weakness. In these defects, muscle membranes are inexcitable to both direct and indirect stimulation due to either decreased potassium conductance or increased sodium conductance, respectively. Both defects are associated with fluid and electrolyte shifts.

Thyrotoxicosis is associated with a secondary form of hypokalemic periodic paralysis. It resembles the primary form but is much more common in men than women, particularly in persons of Asian descent and in young adults. Once the thyroid condition is treated, the episodes usually cease. The disorder can develop in 10–25% of hyperthyroid Asian men. The metabolic sequelae and fluid and electrolyte shifts seen in the primary form are also seen in secondary hypokalemic periodic paralysis. Treatment involves management of the hyperthyroidism, avoidance of high carbohydrate and low potassium meals, and administration of potassium chloride for acute attacks.

Secondary hypokalemic paralysis can also develop if there are marked losses of potassium through the kidneys or the gastrointestinal tract. The associated weakness is, at times, episodic and potassium levels are much lower than in other variants of hypokalemic periodic paralysis. Management of the primary disease with potassium replacement, and treatment of acidosis or alkalosis, is important in preventing attacks.

Patients who consume large amounts of barium salts, which block potassium channels, can also develop hypokalemic periodic paralysis. This condition is treated by stopping the barium salts and administering oral potassium.

Potassium levels that exceed 7 mEq/L between episodes of weakness suggest a secondary form of hyperkalemic periodic paralysis. Treatment is targeted toward the primary disease and involves restriction of potassium.

Anesthetic Considerations

9 Anesthetic management of patients with periodic paralysis is directed toward preventing attacks. Intraoperative management should include frequent determinations of plasma potassium concentration and careful electrocardiographic monitoring to detect arrhythmias. Because of the potential for glucose-containing intravenous solutions to lower plasma potassium concentration, they should not be used in patients with hypokalemic paralysis, whereas they may benefit patients with hyperkalemic paralysis. **10** The response to NMBs is unpredictable, and neuromuscular function should be carefully monitored during their use. Increased sensitivity to nondepolarizing NMBs is particularly apt to be encountered in patients with hypokalemic periodic paralysis. Succinylcholine is contraindicated in hyperkalemic paralysis and perhaps other variants as well because of the risk of hyperkalemia. Intraoperative maintenance of core temperature is important because shivering and hypothermia may trigger or exacerbate episodes of periodic paralysis.

CASE DISCUSSION

Anesthesia for Muscle Biopsy

A 16-year-old boy with progressive proximal muscle weakness is suspected of having a primary myopathy and is scheduled for biopsy of the quadriceps muscle.

What other potential abnormalities should concern the anesthesiologist?

The diagnosis of myopathy can be difficult to make and the differential diagnosis may include any one of several hereditary, inflammatory, endocrine, metabolic, or toxic disorders. A muscle biopsy may be necessary to supplement clinical, laboratory, nerve conduction, and electromyographic findings and help establish the diagnosis. Although the cause of the myopathy in this case is not yet clear, the clinician must always consider potential problems that can be associated with primary myopathies.

Respiratory muscle involvement should always be suspected in patients with muscle weakness. Pulmonary reserve can be assessed clinically by asking about dyspnea and activity level. Pulmonary function tests are indicated if significant dyspnea on exertion is present. An increased risk of pulmonary aspiration is suggested by a history of dysphagia, regurgitation, recurrent pulmonary infections, or abdominal distention. Cardiac abnormalities may be manifested as arrhythmias, mitral valve prolapse, or cardiomyopathy. A 12-lead electrocardiogram is also helpful in excluding conduction abnormalities. A chest radiograph can evaluate inspiratory effort, the pulmonary parenchyma, and cardiac size; gastric distention secondary to smooth muscle or autonomic dysfunction may also be evident. Preoperative laboratory evaluation should have excluded a metabolic cause with measurement of serum sodium, potassium, magnesium, calcium, and phosphate concentrations. Similarly, thyroid, adrenal, and pituitary disorders should have been excluded. Plasma CK measurement may not be helpful, but very high levels (10 times normal) generally suggest a muscular dystrophy or polymyositis

What anesthetic technique should be used?

The choice of anesthesia should be based on both patient and surgical requirements. Most muscle biopsies can be performed under local or regional anesthesia with supplemental intravenous sedation, using small doses of midazolam. Spinal or epidural anesthesia may be utilized. A femoral nerve block can provide excellent anesthesia for biopsy of the quadriceps muscle; a separate injection may be necessary for the lateral femoral cutaneous nerve to anesthetize the anterolateral thigh. General anesthesia should be reserved for uncooperative patients or for times when local or regional anesthesia is inadequate. The anesthesiologist must therefore always be prepared with a plan for general anesthesia.

What agents may be safely used for general anesthesia?

Major goals include preventing pulmonary aspiration, avoiding excessive respiratory or circulatory depression, avoiding NMBs if possible, and perhaps avoiding agents known to trigger malignant hyperthermia. A normal response to a previous general anesthetic in the patient or a family member may be reassuring but does not guarantee the same response subsequently. General anesthesia may be induced and maintained with a combination of a benzodiazepine, propofol, or an opioid with or without nitrous oxide. Patients at increased risk for aspiration should be intubated. When an NMB is necessary, a short-acting nondepolarizing agent should be used. Succinylcholine should generally be avoided because of the unknown risk of an unusual response (myotonic contractions, prolonged duration, or phase II block), of inducing severe hyperkalemia, or of triggering malignant hyperthermia.

SUGGESTED READING

Díaz-Manera J, Rojas-García R, Illa I: Treatment strategies for myasthenia gravis. Expert Opin Pharmacother 2009;10:1329.

Farrugia ME, Vincent A: Autoimmune mediated neuromuscular junction defects. Curr Opin Neurol 2010;23:489.

Gold R, Schneider-Gold C: Current and future standards in treatment of myasthenia gravis. Neurotherapeutics 2008;5:535.

Jani-Acsadi A, Lisak RP: Myasthenic crisis: Guidelines for prevention and treatment. J Neurological Sci 2007;261:127.

Juel VC: Myasthenia gravis: Management of myasthenic crisis and perioperative care. Semin Neurol 2004;24:75.

Mahadeva B, Phillips II L, Juel VC: Autoimmune disorders of neuromuscular transmission. Semin Neurol 2008;28:212.

Skeie GO, Apostolski S, Evoli A, et al: Guidelines for treatment of autoimmune neuromuscular transmission disorders. Eur J Neurol 2010;17:893.

Toothaker TB, Rubin M: Paraneoplastic neurological syndromes: A review. The Neurologist 2009;15:21.

Tornoehlen LM, Pascuzzi RM: Thymoma, myasthenia gravis, and other paraneoplastic syndromes. Hematol Onc Clin N Am 2008;22:509.

Watanabe A, Watanabe T, Obama T, et al: Prognostic factors for myasthenic crisis after transsternal thymectomy in patients with myasthenia gravis. J Thorac Cardiovasc Surg 2004;127:868.

Wu JY, Kuo PH, Fan PC, et al: The role of non-invasive ventilation and factors predicting extubation outcome in myasthenic crisis. Neurocrit Care 2009;10:35.

Anesthesia for Ophthalmic Surgery

1. Any factor that increases intraocular pressure in the setting of an open globe may cause drainage of aqueous or extrusion of vitreous through the wound. The latter is a serious complication that can permanently worsen vision.

2. Succinylcholine increases intraocular pressure by 5–10 mm Hg for 5–10 min after administration, principally through prolonged contracture of the extraocular muscles. However, in studies of hundreds of patients with open eye injuries, no patient experienced extrusion of ocular contents after administration of succinylcholine.

3. Traction on extraocular muscles, pressure on the eyeball, administration of a retrobulbar block, and trauma to the eye can elicit a wide variety of cardiac dysrhythmias ranging from bradycardia and ventricular ectopy to sinus arrest or ventricular fibrillation.

4. Complications involving the intraocular expansion of gas bubbles injected by the ophthalmologist can be avoided by discontinuing nitrous oxide at least 15 min prior to the injection of air or sulfur hexafluoride, or by avoiding the use of nitrous oxide entirely.

5. Medications applied topically to the mucosa are absorbed systemically at a rate intermediate between absorption following intravenous and subcutaneous injection (the toxic subcutaneous dose of phenylephrine is 10 mg).

6. Echothiophate is an irreversible cholinesterase inhibitor used in the treatment of glaucoma. Topical application leads to systemic absorption and a reduction in plasma cholinesterase activity. Because succinylcholine is metabolized by this enzyme, echothiophate will prolong its duration of action.

7. The key to inducing anesthesia in a patient with an open eye injury is controlling intraocular pressure with a smooth induction. Coughing and gagging during intubation is avoided by first achieving a deep level of anesthesia and profound paralysis.

8. The postretrobulbar block apnea syndrome is probably due to injection of local anesthetic into the optic nerve sheath, with spread into the cerebrospinal fluid.

9. Regardless of the technique employed for intravenous sedation, ventilation and oxygenation must be monitored, and equipment to provide positive-pressure ventilation must be immediately available.

Ophthalmic surgery poses unique problems, including regulation of intraocular pressure, control of intraocular gas expansion, prevention of the oculocardiac reflex and management of its consequences, management of systemic effects of ophthalmic drugs, and frequent utilization of only mild to moderate sedation. A thorough understanding of potentially complicating issues, in addition to the mastery of general, regional, local, and sedation anesthesia techniques for ophthalmic surgery, will favorably influence perioperative outcome in these cases.

INTRAOCULAR PRESSURE DYNAMICS

Physiology of Intraocular Pressure

The eye can be considered a hollow sphere with a rigid wall. If the contents of the sphere increase, the **intraocular pressure** (normal: 12–20 mm Hg) must rise. For example, glaucoma is caused by an obstruction to aqueous humor outflow. Similarly, intraocular pressure will rise if the volume of blood within the globe is increased. A rise in venous pressure will increase intraocular pressure by decreasing aqueous drainage and increasing choroidal blood volume. Extreme changes in arterial blood pressure and ventilation can also affect intraocular pressure (Table 36–1). Any event that alters these parameters (eg, laryngoscopy, intubation, airway obstruction, coughing, Trendelenburg position) can affect intraocular pressure.

Alternatively, decreasing the size of the globe without a proportional change in the volume of its contents will increase intraocular pressure. Pressure on the eye from a tightly fitted mask, improper prone positioning, or retrobulbar hemorrhage can lead to a marked increase in intraocular pressure.

Intraocular pressure helps to maintain the shape, and therefore the optical properties, of the eye. Temporary variations in pressure are usually well tolerated in normal eyes. For example, blinking raises intraocular pressure by 5 mm Hg, and squinting (forced contraction of the orbicularis oculi muscles) may increase intraocular pressure greater than 50 mm Hg. However, even transient episodes of increased intraocular pressure in patients with underlying low ophthalmic artery pressure (eg,

TABLE 36–1 The effect of cardiac and respiratory variables on intraocular pressure (IOP).[1]

Variable	Effect on IOP
Central venous pressure	
Increase	↑↑↑
Decrease	↓↓↓
Arterial blood pressure	
Increase	↑
Decrease	↓
Pa_{CO_2}	
Increase (hypoventilation)	↑↑
Decrease (hyperventilation)	↓↓
Pa_{O_2}	
Increase	0
Decrease	↑

[1]↓, decrease (mild, moderate, marked); ↑, increase (mild, moderate, marked); 0, no effect.

deliberate hypotension, arteriosclerotic involvement of the retinal artery) may jeopardize retinal perfusion and cause retinal ischemia.

When the globe is open by surgical incision (Table 36–2) or traumatic perforation, intraocular pressure approaches atmospheric pressure. Any factor that increases intraocular pressure in the setting of an open globe may cause drainage of aqueous or extrusion of vitreous through the wound. The

TABLE 36–2 Open-eye surgical procedures.

Cataract extraction
Corneal laceration repair
Corneal transplant (penetrating keratoplasty)
Peripheral iridectomy
Removal of foreign body
Ruptured globe repair
Secondary intraocular lens implantation
Trabeculectomy (and other filtering procedures)
Vitrectomy (anterior and posterior)
Wound leak repair

TABLE 36–3 The effect of anesthetic agents on intraocular pressure (IOP).[1]

Drug	Effect on IOP
Inhaled anesthetics	
Volatile agents	↓↓
Nitrous oxide	↓
Intravenous anesthetics	
Propofol	↓↓
Benzodiazepines	↓↓
Ketamine	?
Opioids	↓
Muscle relaxants	
Succinylcholine	↑↑
Nondepolarizers	0/↓

[1]↓, decrease (mild, moderate); ↑, increase (mild, moderate); 0↓, no change or mild decrease; ?, conflicting reports.

latter is a serious complication that can permanently worsen vision.

Effect of Anesthetic Drugs on Intraocular Pressure

Most anesthetic drugs either lower intraocular pressure or have no effect (Table 36–3). Inhalational anesthetics decrease intraocular pressure in proportion to the depth of anesthesia. The decrease has multiple causes: a drop in blood pressure reduces choroidal volume, relaxation of the extraocular muscles lowers wall tension, and pupillary constriction facilitates aqueous outflow. Intravenous anesthetics also decrease intraocular pressure, with the exception of ketamine, which usually raises arterial blood pressure and does not relax extraocular muscles.

Topically administered anticholinergic drugs result in pupillary dilation (mydriasis), which may precipitate or worsen angle-closure glaucoma. Systemically administered atropine or glycopyrrolate for premedication are not associated with intraocular hypertension, even in patients with glaucoma.

2 Succinylcholine increases intraocular pressure by 5–10 mm Hg for 5–10 min after administration, principally through prolonged contracture of the extraocular muscles. However, in studies of hundreds of patients with open eye injuries, no patient experienced extrusion of ocular contents after administration of succinylcholine. Unlike other skeletal muscle, extraocular muscles contain myocytes with multiple neuromuscular junctions, and repeated depolarization of these cells by succinylcholine causes the prolonged contracture. The resulting increase in intraocular pressure may have several effects. It will cause spurious measurements of intraocular pressure during examinations under anesthesia in glaucoma patients, potentially leading to unnecessary surgery. Lastly, prolonged contracture of the extraocular muscles may result in an abnormal forced duction test, a maneuver utilized in strabismus surgery to evaluate the cause of extraocular muscle imbalance and determine the type of surgical correction. Nondepolarizing neuromuscular blockers (NMBs) do not increase intraocular pressure.

THE OCULOCARDIAC REFLEX

3 Traction on extraocular muscles, pressure on the eyeball, administration of a retrobulbar block, and trauma to the eye can elicit a wide variety of cardiac dysrhythmias ranging from bradycardia and ventricular ectopy to sinus arrest or ventricular fibrillation. This reflex consists of a trigeminal (V1) afferent and a vagal efferent pathway. The **oculocardiac reflex** is most commonly encountered in pediatric patients undergoing strabismus surgery, although it can be evoked in all age groups and during a variety of ocular procedures, including cataract extraction, enucleation, and retinal detachment repair. In awake patients, the oculocardiac reflex may be accompanied by nausea.

Routine prophylaxis for the oculocardiac reflex is controversial. Anticholinergic medication is often helpful in preventing the oculocardiac reflex, and intravenous atropine or glycopyrrolate immediately prior to surgery is more effective than intramuscular premedication. However, anticholinergic medication should be administered with caution to any patient who has, or may have, coronary artery disease, because of the potential for increase in heart rate sufficient to induce myocardial ischemia. Ventricular tachycardia and ventricular fibrillation following administration of anticholinergic medication has also been reported. Retrobulbar blockade or deep inhalational anesthesia may also be of value in preempting the oculocardiac reflex, although administration of a retrobulbar block may itself initiate the oculocardiac reflex.

Management of the oculocardiac reflex when it occurs includes: (1) immediate notification of the surgeon and temporary cessation of surgical stimulation until heart rate increases; (2) confirmation of adequate ventilation, oxygenation, and depth of anesthesia; (3) administration of intravenous atropine (10 mcg/kg) if bradycardia persists; and (4) in recalcitrant episodes, infiltration of the rectus muscles with local anesthetic. The reflex eventually fatigues (self-extinguishes) with repeated traction on the extraocular muscles.

INTRAOCULAR GAS EXPANSION

A gas bubble may be injected by the ophthalmologist into the posterior chamber during vitreous surgery. Intravitreal air injection will tend to flatten a detached retina and allow anatomically correct healing. The air bubble is absorbed within 5 days by gradual diffusion through adjacent tissue into the bloodstream. The bubble will increase in size if nitrous oxide is administered, because nitrous oxide is 35 times more soluble than nitrogen in blood (see Chapter 8). Thus, it tends to diffuse into an air bubble more rapidly than nitrogen (the major component of air) is absorbed by the bloodstream. If the bubble expands after the eye is closed, intraocular pressure will rise.

Sulfur hexafluoride is an inert gas that is less soluble in blood than is nitrogen—and much less soluble than nitrous oxide. Its longer duration of action (up to 10 days) compared with an air bubble can provide a therapeutic advantage. The bubble size doubles within 24 hr after injection, because nitrogen from inhaled air enters the bubble more rapidly than the sulfur hexafluoride diffuses into the bloodstream. Even so, unless high volumes of pure sulfur hexafluoride are injected, the slow bubble expansion does not typically raise intraocular pressure. If the patient is breathing nitrous oxide, however, the bubble will rapidly increase in size and may lead to intraocular hypertension. A 70% inspired nitrous oxide concentration will almost triple the size of a 1-mL bubble and may double the pressure in a closed eye within 30 min. Subsequent discontinuation of nitrous oxide

will lead to reabsorption of the bubble, which has become a mixture of nitrous oxide and sulfur hexafluoride. The consequent fall in intraocular pressure may precipitate another retinal detachment.

4 Complications involving the intraocular expansion of gas bubbles can be avoided by discontinuing nitrous oxide at least 15 min prior to the injection of air or sulfur hexafluoride, or by avoiding the use of nitrous oxide entirely. The amount of time required to eliminate nitrous oxide from the blood will depend on several factors, including fresh gas flow rate and adequacy of alveolar ventilation. Depth of anesthesia should be maintained by substituting other anesthetic agents. Nitrous oxide should be avoided until the bubble is absorbed (5 days after air and 10 days after sulfur hexafluoride injection). Many ophthalmologists routinely request that nitrous oxide not be used in their patients.

SYSTEMIC EFFECTS OF OPHTHALMIC DRUGS

Topically applied eye drops are systemically absorbed by vessels in the conjunctival sac and the nasolacrimal duct mucosa (see Case Discussion, Chapter 13). One drop (typically, approximately 1/20 mL) of 10% phenylephrine contains approximately 5 mg of drug. Compare this dose with the intravenous dose of phenylephrine (0.05–0.1 mg) used to treat an adult

5 patient with acute hypotension. Medications applied topically to mucosa are absorbed systemically at a rate intermediate between absorption following intravenous and subcutaneous injection (the toxic subcutaneous dose of phenylephrine is 10 mg). Children and the elderly are at particular risk of the toxic effects of topically applied medications and should receive at most a 2.5% phenylephrine solution (Table 36–4). Coincidentally, these patients are most apt to require eye surgery.

6 Echothiophate is an irreversible cholinesterase inhibitor used in the treatment of glaucoma. Topical application leads to systemic absorption and a reduction in plasma cholinesterase activity. **Because succinylcholine is metabolized by this enzyme, echothiophate will prolong its duration of action.** Paralysis usually does not exceed 20–30 min, however, and postoperative apnea is

TABLE 36–4 Systemic effects of ophthalmic medications.

Drug	Mechanism of Action	Effect
Acetylcholine	Cholinergic agonist (miosis)	Bronchospasm, bradycardia, hypotension
Acetazolamide	Carbonic anhydrase inhibitor (decreases IOP[1])	Diuresis, hypokalemic metabolic acidosis
Atropine	Anticholinergic (mydriasis)	Central anticholinergic syndrome[2]
Cyclopentolate	Anticholinergic (mydriasis)	Disorientation, psychosis, convulsions
Echothiophate	Cholinesterase inhibitor (miosis, decreases IOP)	Prolongation of succinylcholine and mivacurium paralysis, bronchospasm
Epinephrine	Sympathetic agonist (mydriasis, decreases IOP)	Hypertension, bradycardia, tachycardia, headache
Phenylephrine	α-Adrenergic agonist (mydriasis, vasoconstriction)	Hypertension, tachycardia, dysrhythmias
Scopolamine	Anticholinergic (mydriasis, vasoconstriction)	Central anticholinergic syndrome[2]
Timolol	β-Adrenergic blocking agent (decreases IOP)	Bradycardia, asthma, congestive heart failure

[1]IOP, intraocular pressure.
[2]See Case Discussion, Chapter 13.

unlikely. The inhibition of cholinesterase activity lasts for 3–7 weeks after discontinuation of echothiophate drops. Muscarinic side effects of echothiophate, such as bradycardia during induction, can be prevented with intravenous anticholinergic drugs (eg, atropine, glycopyrrolate).

Epinephrine eye drops can cause hypertension, tachycardia, and ventricular dysrhythmias; the dysrhythmogenic effects are potentiated by halothane. Direct instillation of epinephrine into the anterior chamber of the eye has not been associated with cardiovascular toxicity.

Timolol, a nonselective β-adrenergic antagonist, reduces intraocular pressure by decreasing production of aqueous humor. Topically-applied timolol eye drops, commonly used to treat glaucoma, will often result in reduced heart rate. In rare cases, it has been associated with atropine-resistant bradycardia, hypotension, and bronchospasm during general anesthesia.

General Anesthesia for Ophthalmic Surgery

The choice between general and local anesthesia should be made jointly by the patient, anesthesiologist, and surgeon. Patients may refuse to consider local anesthesia due to fear of being awake during the operation, fear of the eye block procedure, or unpleasant recall of a previous eye block or local eye procedure. General anesthesia is indicated in children and uncooperative patients, as even small head movements can prove disastrous during microsurgery.

PREMEDICATION

Patients undergoing eye surgery may be apprehensive, particularly if they have undergone multiple procedures or there is a possibility of permanent blindness. However, premedication must be administered with caution and only after careful consideration of the patient's medical status. Adult patients are often elderly, with myriad systemic illnesses, such as hypertension, diabetes mellitus, and coronary artery disease. Pediatric patients may have associated congenital disorders.

INDUCTION

The choice of induction technique for eye surgery usually depends more on the patient's other medical problems than on the patient's eye disease or the specific operation contemplated. One exception is the patient with a ruptured globe. The key to inducing anesthesia in a patient with an open eye injury is controlling intraocular pressure with a smooth induction. Specifically, coughing during intubation must be avoided by achieving a deep level of anesthesia and profound paralysis. The intraocular pressure response to laryngoscopy and endotracheal intubation can be moderated by prior administration of intravenous lidocaine (1.5 mg/kg) or an opioid (eg, remifentanil 0.5–1 mcg/kg or alfentanil 20 mcg/kg). A nondepolarizing muscle relaxant or succinylcholine may be used. Despite theoretical concerns, succinylcholine has not been shown to increase the likelihood of vitreous loss with open eye injuries. Many patients with open globe injuries have full stomachs and require a rapid-sequence induction technique because of the risk of aspiration (see Case Discussion below).

MONITORING & MAINTENANCE

Eye surgery necessitates positioning the anesthesia provider away from the patient's airway, making close monitoring of pulse oximetry and the capnograph particularly important. Endotracheal tube kinking, breathing circuit disconnection, and unintentional extubation may be more likely because of the surgeon working near the airway. Kinking and obstruction can be minimized by using a wire-reinforced or preformed oral RAE® (Ring-Adair-Elwyn) endotracheal tube (see **Figure 36–1**). The possibility of arrhythmias caused by the oculocardiac reflex increases the importance of constantly scrutinizing the electrocardiogram (ECG) and making sure that

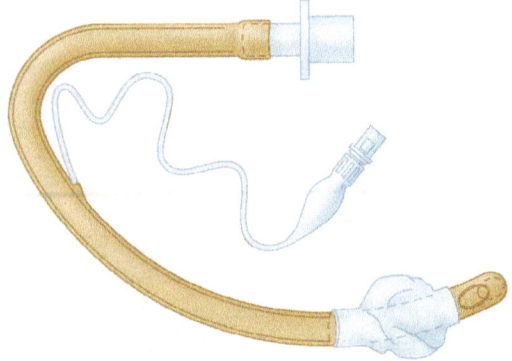

FIGURE 36–1 An oral RAE™ endotracheal tube has a preformed right-angle bend at the level of the teeth so that it exits the mouth away from the surgical field during ophthlamic or nasal surgery.

the pulse tone is audible. In contrast to most other types of pediatric surgery, infant body temperature may rise during ophthalmic surgery because of head-to-toe draping and insignificant body surface exposure. End-tidal CO_2 analysis helps to differentiate this phenomenon from malignant hyperthermia.

The pain and stress evoked by eye surgery are considerably less than during a major intraabdominal or intrathoracic procedure. A lighter level of anesthesia would be satisfactory if the consequences of patient movement were not so potentially catastrophic. The lack of cardiovascular stimulation inherent in most eye procedures combined with the need for adequate anesthetic depth can result in hypotension in elderly individuals. This problem is usually avoided by ensuring adequate intravenous hydration and administering small doses of ephedrine or phenylephrine. The practice of substituting muscle relaxation with nondepolarizing muscle relaxants for sufficient depth of anesthesia requires constant attention to the level of neuromuscular blockade to avoid patient movement, injury to the eye, and a malpractice claim.

Emesis caused by vagal stimulation is a common postoperative problem following eye surgery, particularly with strabismus repair. The Valsalva effect and the increase in central venous pressure that accompany vomiting can be detrimental to the surgical result and will increase the risk of aspiration. Intraoperative intravenous administration of a 5-HT_3 antagonist (eg, ondansetron) decreases the incidence of postoperative nausea and vomiting (PONV). Dexamethasone (8–10 mg in adults) should also be considered for patients with a strong history of PONV.

EXTUBATION & EMERGENCE

A smooth emergence from general anesthesia is very important in order to minimize the risk of postoperative wound dehiscence. Coughing or gagging due to stimulus from the endotracheal tube can be minimized by extubating the patient at a moderately deep level of anesthesia. As the end of the surgical procedure approaches, muscle relaxation is reversed, and spontaneous respiration is allowed to return. Anesthetic agents may be continued during gentle suction of the airway. Nitrous oxide, if used, is then discontinued, and intravenous lidocaine (1.5 mg/kg) can be given to blunt cough reflexes temporarily. Extubation proceeds 1–2 min after the lidocaine administration and during spontaneous respiration with 100% oxygen. Proper airway maintenance is crucial until the patient's cough and swallowing reflexes return. Obviously, this technique is not appropriate in patients at increased risk of aspiration (see Case Discussion at end of chapter).

Severe discomfort is unusual following eye surgery. Scleral buckling procedures, enucleation, and ruptured globe repair are the most painful operations. Modest incremental doses of intravenous opioid (eg, fentanyl 25 mcg or hydromorphone 0.25 mg for an adult) usually provide sufficient analgesia. The surgeon should be alerted if severe pain is noted following emergence from general anesthesia, as it may signal intraocular hypertension, corneal abrasion, or other surgical complications.

Regional Anesthesia for Ophthalmic Surgery

Options for local anesthesia for eye surgery include topical application of local anesthetic or placement of a **retrobulbar block** or the more commonly utilized **peribulbar or sub-Tenon's (episcleral) block.** All of these techniques are most commonly combined with intravenous sedation. Local anesthesia is preferred to general anesthesia for eye surgery because local anesthesia involves less physiologic trespass and is less likely to be associated with PONV. However, eye block procedures have potential complications and may not provide adequate akinesia or analgesia of the eye. Some patients may be unable to lie perfectly still for the duration of the surgery. For these reasons, appropriate equipment and qualified personnel required to treat the complications of local anesthesia and to induce general anesthesia must be readily available.

RETROBULBAR BLOCKADE

In this technique, local anesthetic is injected behind the eye into the cone formed by the extraocular muscles (**Figure 36–2**), and a facial nerve block is utilized to prevent blinking (**Figure 36–3**). A blunt-tipped 25-gauge needle penetrates the lower lid at the junction of the middle and lateral

FIGURE 36–2 A: During administration of a retrobulbar block, the patient looks supranasally as a needle is advanced 1.5 cm along the inferotemporal wall of the orbit. **B**: The needle is then redirected upward and nasally toward the apex of the orbit and advanced until its tip penetrates the muscle cone.

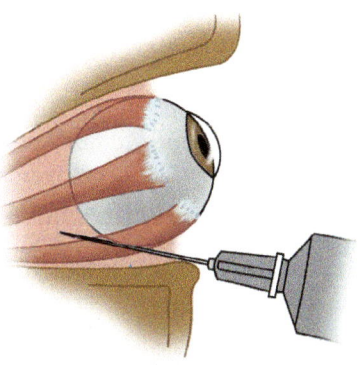

A   B

oculocephalic reflex (ie, a blocked eye does not move during head turning).

Complications of retrobulbar injection of local anesthetics include retrobulbar hemorrhage, perforation of the globe, optic nerve atrophy, intravascular injection with resultant convulsions, oculocardiac reflex, trigeminal nerve block, respiratory arrest, and, rarely, acute neurogenic pulmonary edema. Forceful injection of local anesthetic into the ophthalmic artery causes retrograde flow toward the brain and may result in an instantaneous seizure.

8 The postretrobulbar block apnea syndrome is probably due to injection of local anesthetic into the optic nerve sheath, with spread into the cerebrospinal fluid. The central nervous system is exposed to high concentrations of local anesthetic, leading to mental status changes that may include unconsciousness. Apnea occurs within 20 min and resolves within an hour. Treatment is supportive, with positive-pressure ventilation to prevent hypoxia, bradycardia, and cardiac arrest. Adequacy of ventilation must be constantly monitored in patients who have received retrobulbar anesthesia.

Retrobulbar injection is usually not performed in patients with bleeding disorders because of the risk of retrobulbar hemorrhage, extreme myopia because the elongated globe increases the risk of perforation, or an open eye injury because the pressure from injecting fluid behind the eye may cause extrusion of intraocular contents through the wound.

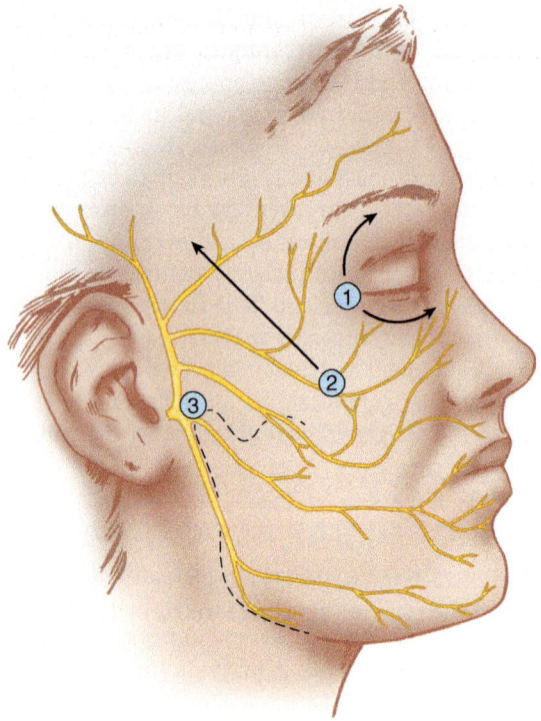

FIGURE 36–3 Facial nerve block techniques: van Lint (1), Atkinson (2), and O'Brien (3).

one-third of the orbit (usually 0.5 cm medial to the lateral canthus). Awake patients are instructed to stare supranasally as the needle is advanced 3.5 cm toward the apex of the muscle cone. Commonly, patients undergoing such eye blocks will receive a brief period of deep sedation during the block (using such agents as etomidate, propofol, and remifentanil). After aspiration to preclude intravascular injection, 2–5 mL of local anesthetic is injected, and the needle is removed. Choice of local anesthetic varies, but lidocaine 2% or bupivacaine 0.75% are most common. Ropivacaine may be used instead of bupivacaine. Addition of epinephrine (1:200,000 or 1:400,000) may reduce bleeding and prolong the anesthesia. Hyaluronidase (3–7 U/mL), a hydrolyzer of connective tissue polysaccharides, is frequently added to enhance the retrobulbar spread of the local anesthetic. A successful retrobulbar block is accompanied by anesthesia, akinesia, and abolishment of the

PERIBULBAR BLOCKADE

In contrast to retrobulbar blockade, in the peribulbar blockade technique, the needle does not penetrate the cone formed by the extraocular muscles. Advantages of the peribulbar technique include less risk of penetration of the globe, optic nerve, and artery, and less pain on injection. Disadvantages include a slower onset and an increased likelihood of ecchymosis. Both techniques will have equal success at producing akinesia of the eye.

The peribulbar block is performed with the patient supine and looking directly ahead (or possibly under a brief period of deep sedation). After topical anesthesia of the conjunctiva, one or two

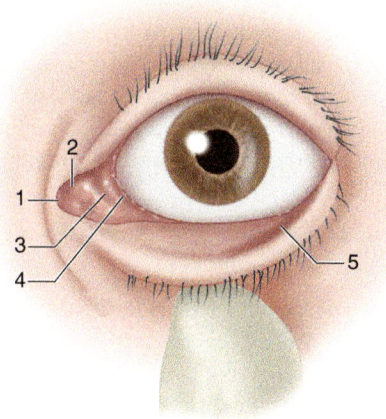

FIGURE 36–4 Anatomic landmarks for the introduction of a needle or catheter in most frequently employed eye blocks: (1) medial canthus peribulbar anesthesia, (2) lacrimal caruncle, (3) semilunaris fold of the conjunctiva, (4) medial canthus episcleral anesthesia, and (5) inferior and temporal peribulbar anesthesia.

transconjunctival injections are given (Figure 36–4). As the eyelid is retracted, an inferotemporal injection is given halfway between the lateral canthus and the lateral limbus. The needle is advanced under the globe, parallel to the orbital floor; when it passes the equator of the eye, it is directed slightly medial (20°) and cephalad (10°), and 5 mL of local anesthetic is injected. To ensure akinesia, a second 5-mL injection may be given through the conjunctiva on the nasal side, medial to the caruncle, and directed straight back parallel to the medial orbital wall, pointing slightly cephalad (20°).

Sub-Tenon's (Episcleral) Block

Tenon's fascia surrounds the globe and extraocular muscles. Local anesthetic injected beneath it into the episcleral space spreads circularly around the sclera and to the extraocular muscle sheaths (Figure 36–4). A special blunt 25-mm or 19-gauge curved cannula is used for a sub-Tenon block. After topical anesthesia, the conjunctiva is lifted along with Tenon's fascia in the inferonasal quadrant with forceps. A small nick is then made with blunt-tipped scissors, which are then slid underneath to create a path in Tenon's

fascia that follows the contour of the globe and extends past the equator. While the eye is still fixed with forceps, the cannula is inserted, and 3–4 mL of local anesthetic are injected. Complications with the sub-Tenon blocks are significantly less than with retrobulbar and peribulbar techniques. Globe perforation, hemorrhage, cellulitis, permanent visual loss, and local anesthetic spread into cerebrospinal fluid have been reported.

FACIAL NERVE BLOCK

A facial nerve block prevents squinting of the eyelids during surgery and allows placement of a lid speculum. There are several techniques of facial nerve block: van Lint, Atkinson, and O'Brien (Figure 36–3). The major complication of these blocks is subcutaneous hemorrhage. Another procedure, Nadbath's technique, blocks the facial nerve as it exits the stylomastoid foramen under the external auditory canal, in close proximity to the vagus and glossopharyngeal nerves. This block is not recommended because it has been associated with vocal cord paralysis, laryngospasm, dysphagia, and respiratory distress.

TOPICAL ANESTHESIA OF THE EYE

Simple topical local anesthetic techniques have evolved for anterior chamber (eg, cataract) and glaucoma operations, and, increasingly, the trend has been to eliminate local anesthetic injections entirely. A typical regimen for topical local anesthesia consists of application of 0.5% proparacaine (also known as proxymetacaine chlorhydrate) local anesthetic drops, repeated at 5-min intervals for five applications, followed by topical application of a local anesthetic gel (lidocaine chlorhydrate plus 2% methyl-cellulose) with a cotton swab to the inferior and superior conjunctival sacs. Ophthalmic 0.5% tetracaine may also be utilized. Topical anesthesia is not appropriate for posterior chamber surgery (eg, retinal detachment repair with a buckle), and it works best for faster surgeons with a gentle surgical technique that does not require akinesia of the eye.

INTRAVENOUS SEDATION

Many techniques of intravenous sedation are available for eye surgery, and the particular drug used is less important than the dose. Deep sedation, although sometimes used during placement of ophthalmic nerve blocks, is almost never used intraoperatively because of the risks of apnea, aspiration, and unintentional patient movement during surgery. An intraoperative light sedation regimen that includes midazolam (1–2 mg), with or without fentanyl (25–50 mcg) or sufentanil (2.5–5 mcg), is recommended. Doses vary considerably among patients, but should be administered in small increments. Concomitant use of more than one type of drug (benzodiazepine, hypnotic, and opioid) potentiates the effects of other agents, and doses must be reduced accordingly.

Administration of eye blocks can be quite uncomfortable, and many anesthesia providers will administer small incremental doses of etomidate or propofol to produce a brief state of unconsciousness during the regional block. Some will substitute a bolus of opioid (remifentanil 0.1–0.5 mcg/kg or alfentanil 375–500 mcg) to produce a brief period of intense analgesia during the eye block procedure.

Administration of an antiemetic should be considered if an opioid is used. Regardless of the technique employed, ventilation and oxygenation must be monitored, and equipment to provide positive-pressure ventilation must be immediately available.

oral intake before or after the injury should be established as accurately as possible. The patient must be considered to have a full stomach if the injury occurred within 8 hr after the last meal, even if the patient did not eat for several hours after the injury: gastric emptying is delayed by the pain and anxiety that follow trauma.

What is the significance of a full stomach in a patient with an open globe injury?

Managing patients who have sustained penetrating eye injuries provides a challenge to anesthesia providers because of the need to develop an anesthetic plan that is consistent with at least two conflicting objectives: (1) prevent further damage to the eye by avoiding increases in intraocular pressure and (2) prevent pulmonary aspiration in a patient with a full stomach.

Many of the common strategies used to achieve these objectives are in direct conflict with one another, however (Tables 36–5 and 36–6). For example, although regional anesthesia (eg, retrobulbar block) minimizes the risk of aspiration pneumonia, it is relatively contraindicated in patients with penetrating eye injuries because injecting local anesthetic behind the globe increases intraocular pressure and may lead to expulsion of intraocular contents. Therefore, these patients require general anesthesia—despite the increased risk of aspiration pneumonia.

CASE DISCUSSION

An Approach to a Patient with an Open Eye & a Full Stomach

A 12-year-old boy arrives at the emergency room after being shot in the eye with a pellet gun. A brief examination by the ophthalmologist reveals intraocular contents presenting at the wound. The boy is scheduled for emergency repair of the ruptured globe.

What should be stressed in the preoperative evaluation of this patient?

Aside from taking a routine history and performing a physical examination, the time of last

TABLE 36–5 Strategies to prevent increases in intraocular pressure (IOP).

| Avoid direct pressure on the globe |
| Patch eye with Fox shield |
| No retrobulbar or peribulbar injections |
| Careful face mask technique |

| Avoid increases in central venous pressure |
| Prevent coughing during induction and intubation |
| Ensure a deep level of anesthesia and relaxation prior to laryngoscopy[1] |
| Avoid head-down positions |
| Extubate under deep anesthesia[1] |

| Avoid pharmacological agents that increase IOP |

[1]These strategies are not recommended in patients with full stomachs.

TABLE 36–6 **Strategies to prevent aspiration pneumonia.**

Regional anesthesia with minimal sedation[1]

Premedication
   Metoclopramide
   Histamine H$_2$-receptor antagonists
   Nonparticulate antacids

Evacuation of gastric contents
   Nasogastric tube[1]

Rapid-sequence induction
   Cricoid pressure
   Rapid induction with rapid onset of paralysis
   Avoidance of positive-pressure ventilation via mask
   Intubation as soon as possible

Extubation awake

[1]These strategies are not recommended for patients with penetrating eye injuries.

What preoperative preparation should be considered in this patient?

The goal of preoperative preparation is to minimize the risk of aspiration pneumonia by decreasing gastric volume and acidity (see Case Discussion, Chapter 17). Aspiration in patients with eye injuries is prevented by proper selection of pharmacological agents and anesthetic techniques. Evacuation of gastric contents with a nasogastric tube may lead to coughing, retching, and other responses that can dramatically increase intraocular pressure.

Metoclopramide increases lower esophageal sphincter tone, speeds gastric emptying, lowers gastric fluid volume, and exerts an antiemetic effect. It should be given intravenously (10 mg) as soon as possible and repeated every 2–4 hr until surgery.

Ranitidine (50 mg intravenously), cimetidine (300 mg intravenously), and famotidine (20 mg intravenously) are H$_2$-histamine–receptor antagonists that inhibit gastric acid secretion. Because they have no effect on the pH of gastric secretions present in the stomach prior to their administration, they have limited value in patients presenting for emergency surgery.

Unlike H$_2$-receptor antagonists, antacids have an immediate effect. Unfortunately, they increase intragastric volume. Nonparticulate antacids (preparations of sodium citrate, potassium citrate, and citric acid) lose effectiveness within 30–60 min and should be given immediately prior to induction (15–30 mL orally).

Which induction agents are recommended in patients with penetrating eye injuries?

The ideal induction agent for patients with full stomachs would provide a rapid onset of action in order to minimize the risk of regurgitation. Ketamine, propofol, and etomidate have essentially equally rapid onsets of action (ie, one-arm-to-brain circulation time).

Furthermore, the ideal induction agent would not increase the risk of ocular expulsion by raising intraocular pressure. (In fact, most intravenous induction agents lower intraocular pressure.) Although investigations of the effects of ketamine on intraocular pressure have provided conflicting results, ketamine is not recommended in penetrating eye injuries, owing to the high rate of blepharospasm and nystagmus.

Although etomidate may prove valuable in some patients with cardiac disease, it is associated with an incidence of myoclonus ranging from 10% to 60%. An episode of severe myoclonus may have contributed to complete retinal detachment and vitreous prolapse in one patient with an open globe injury and limited cardiovascular reserve.

Propofol has a rapid onset of action and decreases intraocular pressure; however, it does not entirely prevent the hypertensive response to laryngoscopy and intubation or entirely prevent the increase in intraocular pressure that accompanies laryngoscopy and intubation. Prior administration of fentanyl (1–3 mcg/kg), remifentanil (0.5–1 mcg/kg), alfentanil (20 mcg/kg), esmolol (0.5–1 mg/kg), or lidocaine (1.5 mg/kg) attenuates this response with varying degrees of success.

How does the choice of muscle relaxant differ between these patients and other patients at risk of aspiration?

The choice of muscle relaxant in patients with penetrating eye injuries has been controversial. Succinylcholine definitely increases intraocular pressure. Although there is conflicting research, it is probably most prudent to conclude that this rise in pressure is not consistently and reliably prevented by pretreatment with a nondepolarizing agent, self-taming doses of succinylcholine, or lidocaine. Contradictory findings by various investigators using different regimens are probably due to differences in doses and timing of the pretreatment drugs.

Some anesthesiologists argue that the relatively small and transient rise in intraocular pressure caused by succinylcholine is insignificant when compared with changes caused by laryngoscopy and intubation. They claim that a slight rise in intraocular pressure is a small price to pay for two distinct advantages that succinylcholine offers: a rapid onset of action that decreases the risk of aspiration, and profound muscle relaxation that decreases the chance of a Valsalva response during intubation. Furthermore, advocates of succinylcholine usually point to the lack of case reports documenting further eye injury when succinylcholine has been used and to publications documenting safe use of succinylcholine with open eye injuries.

Nondepolarizing muscle relaxants do not increase intraocular pressure. Regardless of the muscle relaxant chosen, intubation should not be attempted until a level of paralysis is achieved that will definitely prevent coughing on the endotracheal tube.

How do induction strategies vary in pediatric patients without an intravenous line?

A hysterical child with a penetrating eye injury and a full stomach provides an anesthetic challenge for which there is no perfect solution. Once again, the dilemma is due to the need to avoid increases in intraocular pressure yet minimize the risk of aspiration. For example, screaming and crying can lead to tremendous increases in intraocular pressure. Attempting to sedate children with rectal suppositories or intramuscular injections, however, often heightens their state of agitation and may worsen the eye injury. Similarly, although preoperative sedation may increase the risk of aspiration by obtunding airway reflexes, it is often necessary

for establishing an intravenous line for a rapid-sequence induction. Although difficult to achieve, an ideal strategy would be to administer enough sedation painlessly to allow the placement of an intravenous line, yet maintain a level of consciousness adequate to protect airway reflexes. However, the most prudent strategy is to do everything reasonable to avoid aspiration—even at the cost of further eye damage.

Are there special considerations during extubation and emergence?

Patients at risk of aspiration during induction are also at risk during extubation and emergence. Therefore, extubation must be delayed until the patient is awake and has intact airway reflexes (eg, spontaneous swallowing and coughing on the endotracheal tube). Deep extubation increases the risk of vomiting and aspiration. Intraoperative administration of antiemetic medication and nasogastric or orogastric tube suctioning may decrease the incidence of emesis during emergence, but they do not guarantee an empty stomach.

SUGGESTED READING

Budd M, Brown JPR, Thomas J, et al: A comparison of sub-Tenon's with peribulbar anaesthesia in patients undergoing sequential bilateral cataract surgery. Anaesthesia 2009;64:19-22.

Clarke JP, Plummer J: Adverse events associated with regional ophthalmic anaesthesia in an Australian teaching hospital. Anaesth Intens Care 2011;39:61.

El-Hindy N, Johnston RL, Jaycock P, et al: The cataract national dataset electronic multi-centre audit of 55,567 operations: anaesthetic techniques and complications. Eye 2009;23:50.

Gayer S, Kumar CM: Ophthalmic regional anesthesia techniques. Minerva Anestesiol 2008;74:23.

Goldberg M: Complications of anesthesia for ocular surgery. Ophthalmol Clin N Am 2006;19:293.

Greenhalgh DL, Kumar CM: Sedation during ophthalmic surgery. Eur J Anaesthesiol 2008;25:701.

Kallio H, Rosenberg PH: Advances in ophthalmic regional anaesthesia. Best Pract Res Clin Anaesthesiol 2005;19:215.

Kumar C, Dowd T: Ophthalmic regional anaesthesia. Curr Opin Anaesthesiol 2008;21:632.

Kumar CM, Dowd TC: Complications of ophthalmic regional blocks: their treatment and prevention. Ophthalmologica 2006;220:73-82.

Lee LA, Posner KL, Cheney FW, et al: Complications associated with eye blocks and peripheral nerve blocks: an American Society of Anesthesiologists closed claims analysis. Reg Anesth Pain Med 2008;33:416.

Nouvellon E, Cuvillon P, Ripart J: Regional anesthesia and eye surgery. Anesthesiology 2010;113:1236.

Ripart J, Nouvellon E, Chaumeron A: Regional anesthesia for eye surgery. Reg Anesth Pain Med 2005;30:72.

Swetha V, Jeganathan E, Prajna Jeganathan V: Sub-Tenon's anaesthesia: a well tolerated and effective procedure for ophthalmic surgery. Curr Opin Ophthalmol 2009;20:205.

Vann MA, Ogunnaike BO, Joshi GP: Sedation and anesthesia care for ophthalmologic surgery during local/regional anesthesia. Anesthesiology 2007;107:502.

Warltier DC: Sedation and anesthesia care for ophthalmologic surgery during local/regional anesthesia. Anesthesiology 2007;107:502.

Woo JH, Au Eong KG, Kumar CM: Conscious sedation during ophthalmic surgery under local anesthesia. Minerva Anestesiol 2009;75:211.

Anesthesia for Otorhinolaryngologic Surgery

KEY CONCEPTS

1 The anesthetic goals for laryngeal endoscopy include profound muscle paralysis to provide masseter muscle relaxation for introduction of the suspension laryngoscope and an immobile surgical field, adequate oxygenation and ventilation during surgical manipulation of the airway, and cardiovascular stability during periods of rapidly varying surgical stimulation.

2 During jet ventilation, it is crucial to monitor chest wall motion and to allow sufficient time for exhalation in order to avoid air trapping and barotrauma.

3 The greatest concern during laser airway surgery is an endotracheal tube fire. This risk can be minimized by using a technique of ventilation that does not involve a flammable tube or catheter (eg, intermittent apnea or jet ventilation through the laryngoscope side port), or by using a laser-resistant endotracheal tube and lowering the fraction of inspired oxygen (ideally, as close to 21% as possible, consistent with adequate tissue oxygenation, as monitored by pulse oximetry) and not using nitrous oxide.

4 Techniques to minimize intraoperative blood loss include the use of cocaine or an epinephrine-containing local anesthetic for vasoconstriction, maintaining a slightly head-up position, and providing a mild degree of controlled hypotension.

5 As always, if there is serious preoperative concern regarding potential airway problems, an intravenous induction may be avoided in favor of awake direct or fiberoptic laryngoscopy (cooperative patient) or an inhalational induction while maintaining spontaneous ventilation (uncooperative patient). In any case, the appropriate equipment and qualified personnel required for an emergency tracheostomy must be immediately available.

6 The surgeon may request the omission of neuromuscular blockers during neck dissection or parotidectomy to identify nerves (eg, spinal accessory, facial nerves) by direct stimulation and to preserve them.

7 Manipulation of the carotid sinus and stellate ganglion during radical neck dissection (the right side more than the left) has been associated with wide swings in blood pressure, bradycardia, dysrhythmias, sinus arrest, and prolonged QT intervals. Infiltration of the carotid sheath with local anesthetic will usually ameliorate these problems. Bilateral neck dissection may result in postoperative hypertension and loss of hypoxic drive because of denervation of the carotid sinuses and bodies.

—Continued next page

Continued—

8 Patients undergoing maxillofacial reconstruction or orthognathic surgical procedures often pose the greatest airway challenges to the anesthesiologist. If there are any anticipated signs of problems with mask ventilation or tracheal intubation, the airway should be secured prior to induction of general anesthesia.

9 If there is a chance of postoperative edema involving structures that could obstruct the airway (eg, tongue), the patient should be carefully observed and perhaps should be left intubated.

10 Nitrous oxide is either entirely avoided during tympanoplasty or discontinued prior to graft placement.

In few other circumstances are cooperation and communication between surgeon and anesthesiologist more important than during airway surgery. Establishing, maintaining, and protecting an airway in the face of abnormal anatomy and simultaneous surgical intervention are demanding tasks. An understanding of airway anatomy (see Chapter 19) and an appreciation of common otorhinolaryngologic and maxillofacial procedures are invaluable in handling these anesthetic challenges.

ENDOSCOPY

Endoscopy includes laryngoscopy (diagnostic and operative), microlaryngoscopy (laryngoscopy aided by an operating microscope), esophagoscopy, and bronchoscopy (discussed in Chapter 25). Endoscopic procedures may be accompanied by laser surgery.

Preoperative Considerations

Patients presenting for endoscopic surgery are often being evaluated for voice disorders (often presenting as hoarseness), stridor, or hemoptysis. Possible diagnoses include foreign body aspiration, trauma to the aerodigestive tract, papillomas, tracheal stenosis, tumors, or vocal cord dysfunction. Thus, a preoperative medical history and physical examination, with particular attention to potential airway problems, must precede any decisions regarding the anesthetic plan. In some patients, flow–volume loops (Chapter 6) or radiographic, computed tomography, or magnetic resonance imaging studies may be available for review. Many patients will have undergone preoperative indirect laryngoscopy or fiberoptic nasopharyngoscopy, and the information gained from these procedures may be of critical importance.

Important initial questions that must be answered are whether the patient can be provided with positive-pressure ventilation with a face mask and rebreathing bag, and whether the patient can be intubated using conventional direct or video laryngoscopy. If the answer to either question is not "yes," the patient's airway should be secured prior to induction using an alternative technique (eg, use of a fiberoptic bronchoscope or a tracheostomy under local anesthesia; see Case Discussion, Chapter 19). However, even the initial securing of an airway with tracheostomy does not prevent intraoperative airway obstruction due to surgical manipulation and techniques.

Sedative premedication should be avoided in a patient with medically important upper airway obstruction. Glycopyrrolate (0.2–0.3 mg intramuscularly) 1 hr before surgery may prove helpful by minimizing secretions, thereby facilitating airway visualization.

Intraoperative Management

1 The anesthetic goals for laryngeal endoscopy include an immobile surgical field and adequate masseter muscle relaxation for introduction of the suspension laryngoscope (typically the result of profound muscle paralysis), adequate oxygenation and ventilation, and cardiovascular stability despite rapidly varying levels of surgical stimulation.

A. Muscle Relaxation

Intraoperative muscle relaxation can be achieved by intermittent boluses or infusion of intermediate-duration nondepolarizing neuromuscular blocking agents (NMBs) (eg, rocuronium, vecuronium, cisatracurium), or with a succinylcholine infusion. However, profound degrees of nondepolarizing block may prove difficult to reverse and may delay return of protective airway reflexes and extubation. Given that profound relaxation is often needed until the very end of the surgery, endoscopy remains one of the few remaining indications for succinylcholine infusions. Rapid recovery is important, as endoscopy is often an outpatient procedure.

B. Oxygenation & Ventilation

Several methods have successfully been used to provide oxygenation and ventilation during endoscopy, while simultaneously minimizing interference with the operative procedure. Most commonly, the patient is intubated with a small-diameter endotracheal tube through which conventional positive-pressure ventilation is administered. Standard tracheal tubes of smaller diameters, however, are designed for pediatric patients, and therefore are too short for the adult trachea and have a low-volume cuff that will exert high pressure against the tracheal mucosa. A 4.0-, 5.0-, or 6.0-mm specialized microlaryngeal tracheal tube (Mallinckrodt MLT®, Mallinckrodt Critical Care) is the same length as an adult tube, has a disproportionately large high-volume low-pressure cuff, and is stiffer and less prone to compression than is a conventional tracheal tube of the same diameter. The advantages of intubation in endoscopy include protection against aspiration and the ability to administer inhalational anesthetics and to continuously monitor end-tidal CO_2.

In some cases (eg, those involving the posterior commissure or vocal cords), intubation with a tracheal tube may interfere with the surgeon's visualization or performance of the procedure. A simple alternative is insufflation of high flows of oxygen through a small catheter placed in the trachea. Although oxygenation may be maintained in patients with good lung function, ventilation will be inadequate for longer procedures unless the patient is allowed to breathe spontaneously.

Another option is the intermittent apnea technique, in which ventilation with oxygen by face mask or endotracheal tube is alternated with periods of apnea, during which the surgical procedure is performed. The duration of apnea, usually 2–3 min, is determined by how well the patient maintains oxygen saturation, as measured by pulse oximetry. Risks of this technique include hypoventilation with hypercarbia, failure to reestablish the airway, and pulmonary aspiration.

Another attractive alternative approach involves connecting a manual jet ventilator to a side port of the laryngoscope. During inspiration (1–2 s), a high-pressure (30–50 psi) jet of oxygen is directed through the glottic opening and entrains a mixture of oxygen and room air into the lungs (Venturi effect). Expiration (4–6 s duration) is passive. It is crucial to monitor chest wall motion and to allow sufficient time for exhalation to avoid air trapping and barotrauma. This technique requires total intravenous anesthesia. A variation of this technique is high-frequency jet ventilation, which utilizes a small cannula or tube in the trachea, through which gas is injected 80–300 times per minute (see Chapter 57). Capnography will not provide an accurate estimate of end-tidal CO_2 during jet ventilation due to constant and sizable dilution of alveolar gases.

C. Cardiovascular Stability

Blood pressure and heart rate often fluctuate strikingly during endoscopic procedures for two reasons. First, some of these patients are elderly and have a long history of heavy tobacco and alcohol use that predisposes them to cardiovascular diseases. In addition, the procedure is, in essence, a series of physiologically stressful laryngoscopies and interventions, separated by varying periods of minimal surgical stimulation. Attempting to maintain a constant level of anesthesia invariably results in alternating intervals of hypertension and hypotension. Providing a modest baseline level of anesthesia allows supplementation with short-acting anesthetics (eg, propofol, remifentanil) or sympathetic antagonists (eg, esmolol), as needed, during periods of increased stimulation. Alternatively, some anesthesia providers use regional nerve block of the glossopharyngeal nerve and superior laryngeal nerve to help minimize intraoperative swings in blood pressure (see Case Discussion, Chapter 19).

Laser Precautions

Laser light differs from ordinary light in three ways: it is monochromatic (possesses one wavelength), coherent (oscillates in the same phase), and collimated (exists as a narrow parallel beam). These characteristics offer the surgeon excellent precision and hemostasis with minimal postoperative edema or pain. Unfortunately, lasers introduce several major hazards into the operating room environment.

The uses and side effects of a laser vary with its wavelength, which is determined by the medium in which the laser beam is generated. For example, a CO_2 laser produces a long wavelength (10,600 nm), whereas a yttrium–aluminum–garnet (YAG) laser produces a shorter wavelength (1064- or 1320-nm). As the wavelength increases, absorption by water increases, and tissue penetration decreases. Thus, the effects of the CO_2 laser are much more localized and superficial than are those of the YAG laser.

General laser precautions include the evacuation of toxic fumes (laser plume) from tissue vaporization; these have the potential to transmit microbiological diseases. When significant laser plume is generated, fitted respiratory filter masks compliant with Occupation Safety and Health Administration standards should be worn by all operating room personnel. In addition, during laser procedures, all operating room personnel should wear laser eye protection, and the patient's eyes should be taped shut.

③ The greatest risk of laser airway surgery (if an endotracheal tube is used) is an airway fire. This risk can be moderated by using a technique of ventilation that minimizes the fraction of inspired oxygen (FIO_2) and can be eliminated if there is no combustible material (eg, no flammable tube or catheter) in the airway. If an endotracheal tube is used, it must be relatively resistant to laser ignition (Table 37–1). These tubes not only resist laser beam strikes, but they also possess double cuffs that should be inflated with saline instead of air in order to better absorb thermal energy and reduce the risk of ignition. If the proximal cuff is struck by the laser

TABLE 37–1 Advantages and disadvantages of various tracheal tubes for laser airway surgery.

Type of Tube	Advantages	Disadvantages
Polyvinyl chloride	Inexpensive, nonreflective	Low melting point, highly combustible[1]
Red rubber	Puncture-resistant, maintains structure, nonreflective	Highly combustible[1]
Silicone rubber	Nonreflective	Combustible,[1] turns to toxic ash
Metal	Combustion-resistant,[1] kink-resistant	Thick-walled flammable cuff, transfers heat, reflects laser, cumbersome

[1]Combustibility depends on fraction of inspired oxygen and laser energy.

and the saline escapes, the distal cuff will continue to seal the airway. Alternatively, endotracheal tubes can be wrapped with a variety of metallic tapes; however, this is a suboptimal practice and should be avoided whenever use of a specialized, commercially available, flexible, stainless steel laser-resistant endotracheal tube is possible (Table 37–2).

Although specialized, laser-resistant endotracheal tubes may be used, it must be emphasized that no endotracheal tube or currently available endotracheal tube protection device is reliably laser-proof. Therefore, whenever laser airway surgery is being performed with an endotracheal tube in place, the following precautions should be observed:

- Inspired oxygen concentration should be as low as possible by utilizing air in the inspired gas mixture (many patients tolerate an FIO_2 of 21%).

TABLE 37–2 Disadvantages of wrapping a tracheal tube with metallic tape.

No cuff protection
Adds thickness to tube
Not a device approved by the US Food and Drug Administration
Protection varies with type of metal foil
Adhesive backing may ignite
May reflect laser onto nontargeted tissue
Rough edges may damage mucosal surfaces

TABLE 37–3 Airway fire protocol.

1. Stop ventilation and remove tracheal tube.
2. Turn off oxygen and disconnect circuit from machine.
3. Submerge tube in water.
4. Ventilate with face mask and reintubate.
5. Assess airway damage with bronchoscopy, serial chest x-rays, and arterial blood gases.
6. Consider bronchial lavage and steroids.

- Nitrous oxide supports combustion and should be avoided.
- The endotracheal tube cuffs should be filled with saline. Some practitioners add methylene blue to signal cuff rupture. A well-sealed cuffed tube will minimize oxygen concentration in the pharynx.
- Laser intensity and duration should be limited as much as possible.
- Saline-soaked pledgets (completely saturated) should be placed in the airway to limit risk of endotracheal tube ignition and damage to adjacent tissue.
- A source of water (eg, 60-mL syringe) should be immediately available in case of fire.

These precautions limit, but do not eliminate, the risk of an airway fire; anesthesia providers must proactively address the hazard of fire whenever laser or electrocautery is utilized near the airway (Table 37–3).

If an airway fire should occur, all air/oxygen should immediately be turned off at the anesthesia gas machine, and burning combustible material (eg, an endotracheal tube) should be removed from the airway. The fire can be extinguished with saline, and the patient's airway should be examined to be certain that all combustible fragments have been removed.

NASAL & SINUS SURGERY

Common nasal and sinus surgeries include polypectomy, endoscopic sinus surgery, maxillary sinusotomy (Caldwell–Luc procedure), rhinoplasty, and septoplasty.

Preoperative Considerations

Patients undergoing nasal or sinus surgery may have a considerable degree of preoperative nasal obstruction caused by polyps, a deviated septum, or mucosal congestion from infection. This may make face mask ventilation difficult, particularly if combined with other causes of difficult ventilation (eg, obesity, maxillofacial deformities).

Nasal polyps are often associated with allergic disorders, such as asthma. Patients who also have a history of allergic reactions to aspirin should not be given any nonsteroidal antiinflammatory drugs (including ketorolac) for postoperative analgesia. Nasal polyps are a common feature of cystic fibrosis.

Because of the rich vascular supply of the nasal mucosa, the preoperative interview should concentrate on questions concerning medication use (eg, aspirin, clopidogrel) and any history of bleeding problems.

Intraoperative Management

Many nasal procedures can be satisfactorily performed under local anesthesia with sedation. The anterior ethmoidal nerve and sphenopalatine nerves (Figure 19–3) provide sensory innervation to the nasal septum and lateral walls. Both can be blocked by packing the nose with gauze or cotton-tipped applicators soaked with local anesthetic. The topical anesthetic should be allowed to remain in place at least 10 min before instrumentation is attempted. Supplementation with submucosal injections of local anesthetic is often required. Use of an epinephrine-containing solution or cocaine (usually a 4% or 10% solution) will shrink the nasal mucosa and potentially decrease intraoperative blood loss. Intranasal cocaine (maximum dose, 3 mg/kg) is rapidly absorbed (reaching peak levels in 30 min) and may be associated with cardiovascular side effects (see Chapter 16).

General anesthesia is often preferred for nasal surgery because of the discomfort and incomplete block that may accompany topical anesthesia. Special considerations during and shortly following induction include using an oral airway during face mask ventilation to mitigate the effects of nasal obstruction; intubating with a reinforced or preformed Mallinckrodt oral RAE® (Ring–Adair–Elwyn)

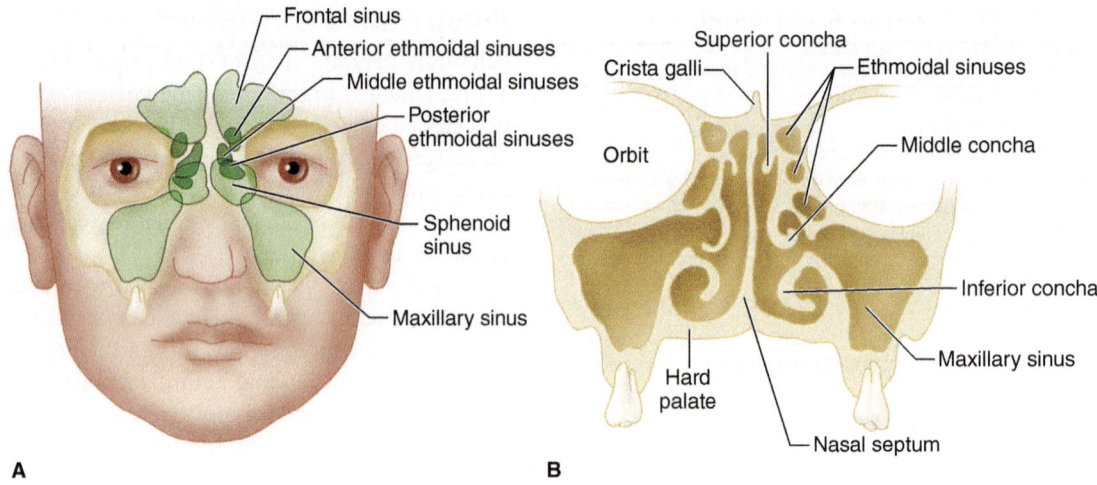

A
B

FIGURE 37–1   Orbital fracture is a risk of endoscopic sinus surgery because of the proximity of the sinuses to the orbit (**A**, frontal view; **B**, coronal section). (Reproduced and modified, with permission, from Snell RS, Katz J: *Clinical Anatomy for Anesthesiologists.* Appleton & Lange, 1988.)

endotracheal tube (Figure 36–1); and tucking the patient's padded arms, with protection of the fingers, to the side. Because of the proximity of the surgical field, it is important to tape the patient's eyes closed to avoid a corneal abrasion. One exception to this occurs during dissection in endoscopic sinus surgery, when the surgeon may wish to periodically check for eye movement because of the close proximity of the sinuses and orbit (Figure 37–1); nonetheless, the eyes should remain protected until the surgeon is ready to observe them. NMBs are often utilized because of the potential neurological or ophthalmic complications that might arise if the patient moves during sinus instrumentation.

4   Techniques to minimize intraoperative blood loss include supplementation with cocaine or an epinephrine-containing local anesthetic, maintaining a slightly head-up position, and providing a mild degree of controlled hypotension. A posterior pharyngeal pack is often placed to limit the risk of aspiration of blood. Despite these precautions, the anesthesiologist must be prepared for major blood loss, particularly during the resection of vascular tumors (eg, juvenile nasopharyngeal angiofibroma).

Coughing or straining during emergence from anesthesia and extubation should be avoided, as these events will increase venous pressure and increase postoperative bleeding. Unfortunately, relatively deep extubation strategies that are commonly and appropriately utilized to accomplish this goal also may increase the risk of aspiration.

HEAD & NECK CANCER SURGERY

Surgery for cancer of the head and neck includes laryngectomy, glossectomy, pharyngectomy, parotidectomy, hemimandibulectomy, and radical neck dissection. An endoscopic examination following induction of anesthesia often precedes these surgical procedures. Timing of a tracheostomy, if planned, depends upon the patient's preoperative airway compromise. Some procedures may include extensive reconstructive surgery, such as the transplantation of a free microvascular muscle flap.

Preoperative Considerations

The typical patient presenting for head and neck cancer surgery is older and often has had many years of heavy tobacco and alcohol use. Common coexisting medical conditions include chronic obstructive pulmonary disease, coronary artery disease, hypertension, diabetes, alcoholism, and malnutrition.

Airway management may be complicated by abnormal airway anatomy, an obstructing lesion, or by preoperative radiation therapy that has fibrosed, immobilized, and distorted the patient's airway structures. If there is concern regarding potential airway problems, intravenous induction may be avoided in favor of awake direct or fiberoptic laryngoscopy (cooperative patient) or direct or fiberoptic intubation following an inhalational induction, maintaining spontaneous ventilation (uncooperative patient). Elective tracheostomy under local anesthesia prior to induction of general anesthesia is often a prudent option. In any case, the appropriate equipment and qualified personnel required for an emergency tracheostomy must be *immediately* available.

Intraoperative Management

A. Monitoring

Because many of these procedures are lengthy and associated with substantial blood loss, and because of the prevalence of coexisting cardiopulmonary disease, arterial cannulation is often utilized for blood pressure monitoring and frequent laboratory analyses. If central venous access is deemed necessary, the surgeon should be consulted to ascertain that planned internal jugular or subclavian venous access will not interfere with the intended surgical procedures; in such cases, if both internal jugular and both subclavian veins are unavailable, antecubital or femoral veins are reasonable alternatives. Arterial lines and intravenous cannulas should not be placed in the operative arm if a radial forearm flap is planned. A minimum of two large-bore intravenous lines and a urinary catheter (preferably with temperature-monitoring capability) should be placed. A forced-air warming blanket should be positioned over the lower extremities to help maintain normal body temperature. Intraoperative hypothermia and consequent vasoconstriction can be detrimental to perfusion of a microvascular free flap.

Intraoperative nerve monitoring is increasingly utilized by surgeons in anterior neck operations to help preserve the superior laryngeal, recurrent laryngeal, and vagus nerves (Figure 37–2), and the anesthesia provider may be asked to place

a specialized nerve integrity monitor endotracheal tube (Medtronic Xomed NIM® endotracheal tube) to facilitate this process (Figure 37–3).

B. Tracheostomy

Head and neck cancer surgery often includes tracheostomy. Immediately prior to surgical entry into the trachea, the endotracheal tube and hypopharynx should be thoroughly suctioned to limit the risk of aspiration of blood and secretions. If electrocautery is used during the surgical dissection, the F_{IO_2} should be lowered to 30% or less, if possible, in order to minimize the risk of fire as the trachea is surgically entered. In any case, the easiest way to avoid an airway fire in this circumstance is for the surgeon NOT to use the cautery to enter the trachea. After dissection down to the trachea, the tracheal tube cuff is deflated to avoid perforation by the scalpel. When the tracheal wall is transected, the endotracheal tube is withdrawn so that its tip is immediately cephalad to the incision. Ventilation during this period is difficult because of the large leak through the tracheal incision. A sterile wire-reinforced endotracheal tube or L-shaped cuffed laryngectomy tube is placed in the trachea, the cuff is inflated, and the tube is connected to a sterile breathing circuit. As soon as correct position is confirmed by capnography and bilateral chest auscultation, the original endotracheal tube is removed. An increase in peak inspiratory pressure immediately after tracheostomy usually indicates a malpositioned endotracheal tube, bronchospasm, debris or secretions in the trachea, or, rarely, pneumothorax.

C. Maintenance of Anesthesia

The surgeon may request the omission of NMBs during neck dissection or parotidectomy to identify nerves (eg, spinal accessory, facial nerves) by direct stimulation and to preserve them. If a nerve integrity monitor endotracheal tube is utilized, succinylcholine (or propofol with no relaxant) may be used to facilitate intubation. Moderate controlled hypotension may be helpful in limiting blood loss; however, cerebral perfusion may be compromised with moderate hypotension when a tumor invades the carotid artery or jugular vein (the latter may increase cerebral venous pressure). If head-up

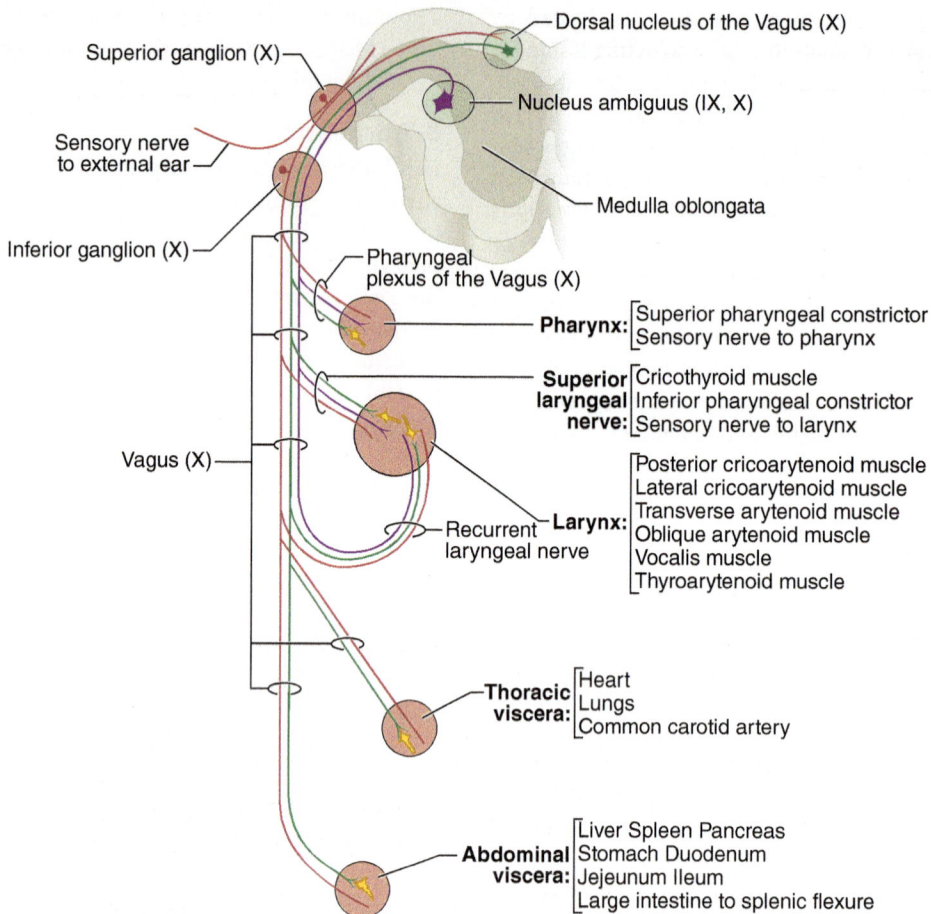

Dorsal nucleus of the Vagus (X)

Superior ganglion (X)

Nucleus ambiguus (IX, X)

Sensory nerve
to external ear

Medulla oblongata

Inferior ganglion (X)

Pharyngeal
plexus of the Vagus (X)

Pharynx: Superior pharyngeal constrictor / Sensory nerve to pharynx

Superior laryngeal nerve: Cricothyroid muscle / Inferior pharyngeal constrictor / Sensory nerve to larynx

Vagus (X)

Larynx: Posterior cricoarytenoid muscle / Lateral cricoarytenoid muscle / Transverse arytenoid muscle / Oblique arytenoid muscle / Vocalis muscle / Thyroarytenoid muscle

Recurrent
laryngeal nerve

Thoracic viscera: Heart / Lungs / Common carotid artery

Abdominal viscera: Liver Spleen Pancreas / Stomach Duodenum / Jejeunum Ileum / Large intestine to splenic flexure

FIGURE 37–2 The **vagus nerve** (cranial nerve X) originates in the medulla oblongata and then ramifies in the superior and inferior vagal ganglia in the neck. Its first major branch is the pharyngeal plexus of the vagus. The **superior laryngeal nerve** divides into the external and internal laryngeal nerves. The *internal branch* supplies sensory innervation of the laryngeal mucosa above the vocal cords, and the *external branch* innervates the inferior pharyngeal constrictor muscles and the cricothyroid muscle of the larynx. Cricothyroid muscle contraction increases the voice pitch by lengthening, tensing, and adducting the vocal folds. The superior laryngeal nerve is at risk of damage during operations of the anterior neck, especially thyroid surgery, and injury to this nerve may result in hoarseness and loss

of vocal volume. The next branch of the vagus is the **recurrent laryngeal nerve**, which innervates all of the muscles of the larynx except the cricothyroid, and is responsible for phonation and glottic opening. The recurrent laryngeal nerve runs immediately behind the thyroid gland and thus is the nerve of greatest risk for injury during thyroid surgery. Unilateral recurrent laryngeal nerve damage may result in vocal changes or hoarseness, and bilateral nerve damage may result in aphonia and respiratory distress. Inferior to this nerve, the vagus nerve provides autonomic motor and sensory nerve fibers to the thoracic and abdominal viscera. (Reproduced, with permission, from Dillon FX: Electromyographic (EMG) neuromonitoring in otolaryngology-head and neck surgery. Anesthesiol Clin 2010;28:423).

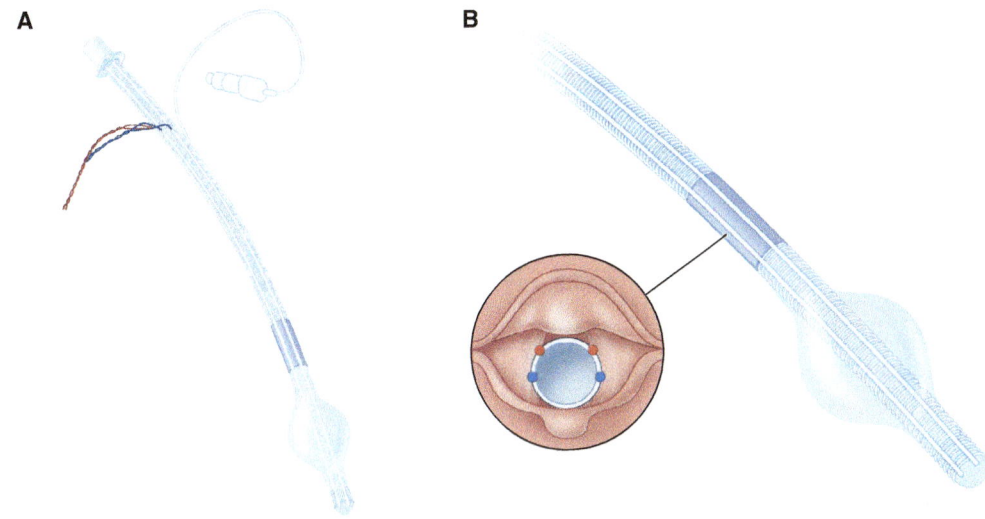

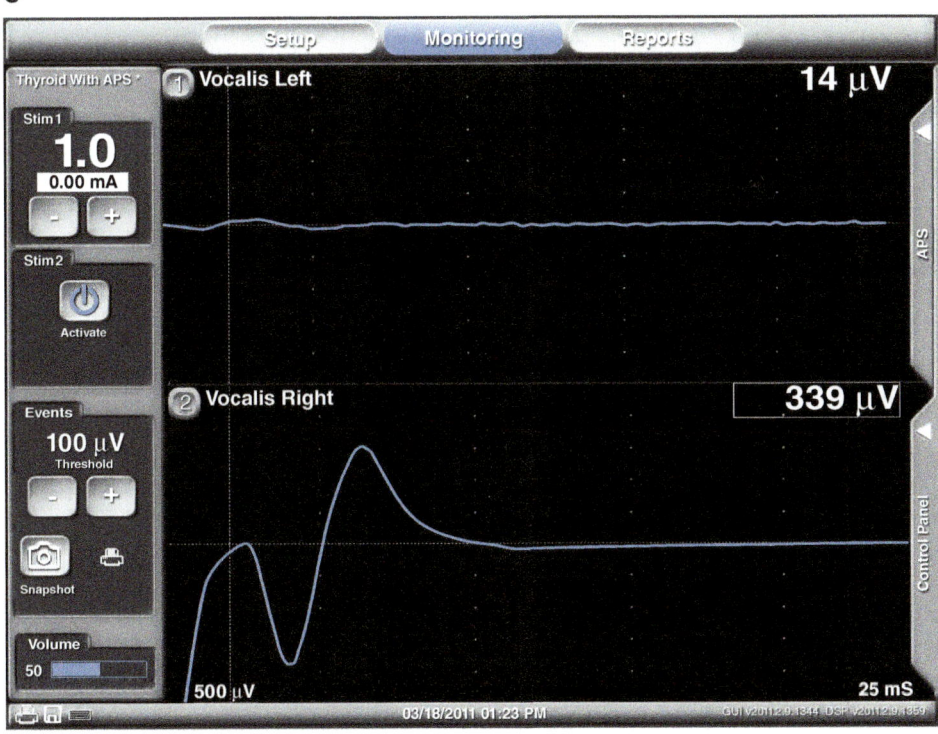

FIGURE 37–3 **A**: The Medtronic Xomed NIM® electromyographic (EMG) nerve integrity monitoring endotracheal tube. Succinylcholine (or no relaxant at all) should be used for intubation, and the tube should be secured in the midline. If lubricant is used, it must not contain local anesthetics. **B**: A slightly larger tube size should be used to facilitate mucosal contact with the electrodes, and the blue band of the NIM® tube must be positioned at the level of the vocal cords. **C**: Nerve integrity is continuously monitored via EMG activity (Medtronic Xomed NIM-Response® 3.0 Nerve Integrity Monitor). Nondepolarizing muscle relaxants are contraindicated because they preclude EMG monitoring. (Redrawn and reproduced, with permission, from Medtronic Xomed.)

tilt is utilized, it is important that the arterial blood pressure transducer be zeroed at the level of the brain (external auditory meatus) in order to most accurately determine cerebral perfusion pressure. In addition, head-up tilt may increase the chance of venous air embolism.

Following reanastomosis of a microvascular free flap, blood pressure should be maintained at the patient's baseline level. The use of vasoconstrictive agents (eg, phenylephrine) to maintain systemic blood pressure should be minimized because of potential decrease in flap perfusion due to vasoconstriction. Similarly, the use of vasodilators (eg, sodium nitroprusside or hydralazine) should be avoided in order to minimize any decrease in graft perfusion pressure.

D. Transfusion

Transfusion decisions must balance the patient's immediate surgical risks with the possibility of an increased cancer recurrence rate resulting from transfusion-induced immune suppression. Rheological factors make a relatively low hematocrit (eg, 27% to 30%) desirable when microvascular free flaps are performed. Excessive diuresis should be avoided during microvascular-free flap surgery in order to allow adequate graft perfusion in the postoperative period.

E. Cardiovascular Instability

7 Manipulation of the carotid sinus and stellate ganglion during radical neck dissection (the right side more than the left) has been associated with wide swings in blood pressure, bradycardia, arrhythmias, sinus arrest, and prolonged QT intervals. Infiltration of the carotid sheath with local anesthetic will usually moderate these problems. Bilateral neck dissection may result in postoperative hypertension and loss of hypoxic drive due to denervation of the carotid sinuses and carotid bodies.

MAXILLOFACIAL RECONSTRUCTION & ORTHOGNATHIC SURGERY

Maxillofacial reconstruction is often required to correct the effects of trauma (eg, LeFort fractures) or developmental malformations, for radical cancer surgeries (eg, maxillectomy or mandibulectomy), or for obstructive sleep apnea. Orthognathic procedures (eg, LeFort osteotomies, mandibular osteotomies) for skeletal malocclusion share many of the same surgical and anesthetic techniques.

Preoperative Considerations

8 Patients undergoing maxillofacial reconstruction or orthognathic surgical procedures often pose airway challenges. Particular attention should be focused on jaw opening, mask fit, neck mobility, micrognathia, retrognathia, maxillary protrusion (overbite), macroglossia, dental pathology, nasal patency, and the existence of any intraoral lesions or debris. If there are any anticipated signs of problems with mask ventilation or tracheal intubation, the airway should be secured prior to induction of general anesthesia. This may involve fiberoptic nasal intubation, fiberoptic oral intubation, or tracheostomy with local anesthesia facilitated with cautious sedation. Nasal intubation with a straight tube with a flexible angle connector (Figure 37–4A) or a preformed nasal RAE® (Figure 37–4B) tube is usually preferred in dental and oral surgery. The endotracheal tube can then be directed cephalad over the patient's forehead. With any nasal intubation, care should be taken to prevent the endotracheal tube from putting pressure on the tissues of the nasal opening, as this situation may result in local tissue pressure necrosis in the setting of a lengthy surgical procedure. Nasal intubation should be considered with caution in LeFort II and III fractures because of the possibility of a coexisting basilar skull fracture (Figure 37–5).

Intraoperative Management

Maxillofacial reconstructive and orthognathic surgeries can be lengthy and associated with substantial blood loss. An oropharyngeal ("throat") pack is often placed to minimize the amount of blood and other debris reaching the larynx and trachea. Strategies to minimize bleeding include a slight head-up position, controlled hypotension, and local infiltration with epinephrine solutions. Because the patient's arms are typically tucked at the side, two intravenous lines may be established prior to surgery. An arterial line may be placed. If head-up tilt is utilized,

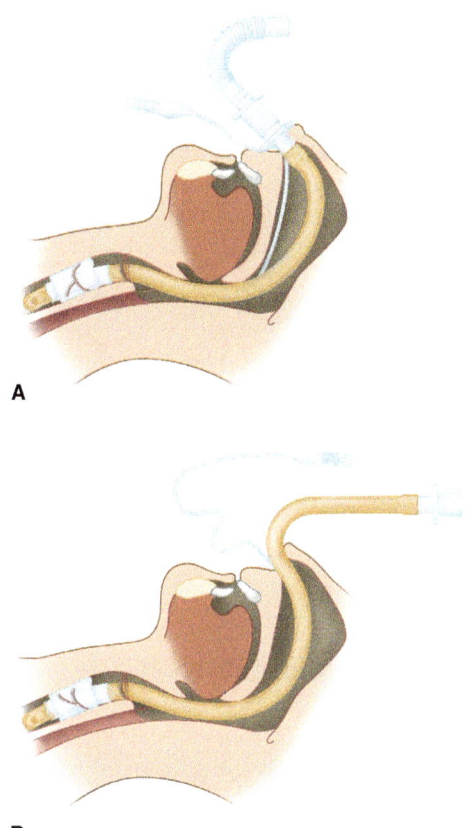

A

B

FIGURE 37–4 **A**: A regular straight endotracheal tube can be cut at the level of the nares, and a flexible connector attached. **B**: Alternatively, a nasal RAE™ tube has a preformed right-angle bend at the level of the nose so that the tube is directed over the forehead.

it is important that the arterial blood pressure transducer be zeroed at the level of the brain (external auditory meatus) in order to most accurately determine cerebral perfusion pressure. In addition, the anesthesia provider must be alert to the increased risk of venous air embolism in the setting of head-up tilt.

Because of the proximity of the airway to the surgical field, the anesthesiologist's location is more remote than usual. This increases the likelihood of serious intraoperative airway problems, such as endotracheal tube kinking, disconnection, or perforation by a surgical instrument. Monitoring of end-tidal CO_2, peak inspiratory pressures, and breath sounds via an esophageal stethoscope assume greater importance in such cases. If the operative procedure is near the airway, the use of electocautery or laser increases the risk of fire. At the end of surgery, the oropharyngeal pack must be removed and the pharynx suctioned. Bloody debris is typically found during initial suctioning, but should **9** diminish with repeat efforts. If there is a possibility of postoperative tissue edema involving structures that could potentially obstruct the airway (eg, tongue, pharynx), the patient should be carefully observed or left intubated. In such uncertain situations, extubation may be performed over an endotracheal tube exchanger (Cook Airway Exchange Catheter with Rapi-Fit® Adapter, Cook Medical), which can facilitate reintubation and provide oxygenation in the setting of immediate

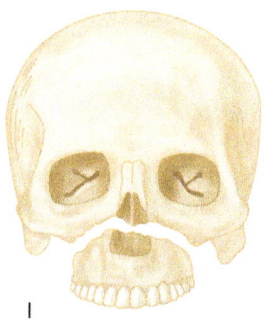

I

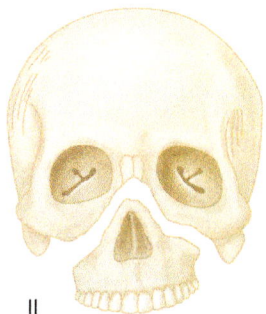

II

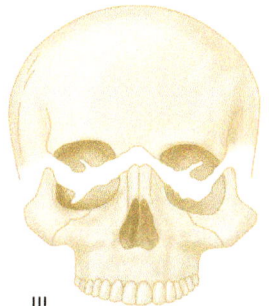

III

FIGURE 37–5 Diagrammatic representation of LeFort I, II, and III fractures. LeFort II and III fractures may coexist with a basilar skull fracture, a contraindication to nasal intubation.

postextubation respiratory obstruction. In addition, the operating team should be prepared for emergent tracheotomy or cricothyrotomy. Otherwise, extubation can be attempted once the patient is fully awake and there are no signs of continued bleeding. Patients with intermaxillary fixation (eg, maxillomandibular wiring) *must* have suction and appropriate wire cutting tools continuously at the bedside in case of vomiting or other airway emergencies. Extubating a patient whose jaws are wired shut and whose oropharyngeal pack has not been removed can lead to life threatening airway obstruction.

EAR SURGERY

Frequently performed ear surgeries include stapedectomy or stapedotomy, tympanoplasty, and mastoidectomy. Myringotomy with insertion of tympanostomy tubes is the most common pediatric surgical procedure and is discussed in Chapter 42.

Intraoperative Management

A. Nitrous Oxide

Nitrous oxide is not often used in anesthesia for ear surgery. Because nitrous oxide is more soluble than nitrogen in blood, it diffuses into air-containing cavities more rapidly than nitrogen (the major component of air) can be absorbed by the bloodstream (see Chapter 8). Normally, changes in middle ear pressures caused by nitrous oxide are well tolerated as a result of passive venting through the eustachian tube. However, patients with a history of chronic ear problems (eg, otitis media, sinusitis) often suffer from obstructed eustachian tubes and may, on rare occasion, experience hearing loss or tympanic membrane rupture from administration of nitrous oxide anesthesia.

During tympanoplasty, the middle ear is open to the atmosphere, and there is no pressure build-up. Once the surgeon has placed a tympanic membrane graft, the middle ear becomes a closed space. If nitrous oxide is allowed to diffuse into this space, middle ear pressure will rise, and the graft may be displaced. Conversely, discontinuing nitrous oxide after graft placement will create a negative middle ear pressure that could also cause graft dislodgment.

10 Therefore, nitrous oxide is either entirely avoided during tympanoplasty or discontinued prior to graft placement. Obviously, the exact amount of time required to wash out the nitrous oxide depends on many factors, including alveolar ventilation and fresh gas flows (see Chapter 8), but 15–30 min is usually recommended.

B. Hemostasis

As with any form of microsurgery, even small amounts of blood can obscure the operating field. Techniques to minimize blood loss during ear surgery include mild (15°) head elevation, infiltration or topical application of epinephrine (1:50,000–1:200,000), and moderate controlled hypotension. Because coughing on the endotracheal tube during emergence (particularly during head bandaging) will increase venous pressure and may cause bleeding (as well as increased middle ear pressure), deep extubation is often utilized.

C. Facial Nerve Identification

Preservation of the facial nerve is an important consideration during some types of ear surgery (eg, resection of a glomus tumor or acoustic neuroma). During these cases, intraoperative paralysis with NMBs may confuse the interpretation of facial nerve stimulation and should not be used unless requested by the surgeon.

D. Postoperative Vertigo, Nausea and Vomiting

Because the inner ear is intimately involved with the sense of balance, ear surgery may cause postoperative dizziness (vertigo) and postoperative nausea and vomiting (PONV). Induction and maintenance with propofol have been shown to decrease PONV in patients undergoing middle ear surgery. Prophylaxis with decadron prior to induction, and a 5-HT$_3$ blocker prior to emergence, should be considered. Patients undergoing ear surgery should be carefully assessed for vertigo postoperatively in order to minimize the risk of falling during ambulation secondary to an unsteady gait.

Oral Surgical Procedures

Most minor oral surgical procedures are performed in a clinic or office setting utilizing local anesthesia, augmented with varying degrees of oral or intravenous sedation. If intravenous sedation is employed, or if the procedure is complex, a qualified anesthesia provider should be present. Typically, a bite block and an oropharyngeal throat pack protect the airway. For light to moderate levels of sedation, the oropharyngeal pack prevents irrigating fluids and dental fragments from entering the airway. Deep sedation and general anesthesia require an increased level of airway control by the anesthesia provider. Regardless of whether deep sedation or general anesthesia is inadvertent or intended, appropriate equipment, supplies, and medications *must* be immediately available to help insure that any anticipated or unexpected anesthesia-related problem occurring in an office or clinic setting can be safely addressed with the same standard of care that is required in the hospital or ambulatory surgery center.

Minor oral surgical procedures, such as exodontias, typically last no more than 1 hr. The surgical field is amenable to a nerve block or infiltration by a local anesthetic. In adults, most oral surgeons use 2% lidocaine with 1/100,000 epinephrine or 0.5% bupivacaine with 1/200,000 epinephrine in quantities no greater than 12 mL and 8 mL, respectively. The anesthesia provider must be informed by the surgeon of the local anesthetic used and its concentration and volume injected so that the allowed dosage based on weight is not exceeded. Pediatric patients, in particular, are at risk of local anesthesia toxicity due to an actual overdose or an accidental intravascular injection.

Intravenous sedation during oral surgical procedures greatly increases the patient's comfort and facilitates surgery. A combination of fentanyl (1–3 mcg/kg) and midazolam (20–50 mcg/kg) is usually adequate prior to injection of the local anesthetic. The sedation can be further augmented by additional small dosages of fentanyl, midazolam, or propofol. Propofol (20–30 mg is a typical incremental dose for an adult) is a good standby drug, if the surgeon requires a brief episode of unconsciousness.

These techniques require a high level of cooperation and participation by both the surgeon and anesthesiologist. If there is the possibility of increased risk due to preexisting medical conditions, less than ideal airway, or extent of contemplated surgical procedure, it is safer to perform the procedure in a hospital or ambulatory surgery center setting with general endotracheal anesthesia.

CASE DISCUSSION

Bleeding Following Sinus Surgery

A 50-year-old man has a paroxysm of coughing in the recovery room while awakening following uneventful endoscopic sinus surgery. Immediately afterward, his respirations seem labored with a loud inspiratory stridor.

What is the differential diagnosis of inspiratory stridor?

The acute onset of inspiratory stridor in a postoperative patient may be due to laryngospasm, laryngeal edema, foreign body aspiration, or vocal cord dysfunction. Laryngospasm, an involuntary spasm of the laryngeal musculature, may be triggered by blood or secretions stimulating the superior laryngeal nerve (see Chapter 19). Laryngeal edema may be caused by an allergic drug reaction, hereditary or iatrogenic angioedema, or a traumatic intubation. Vocal cord dysfunction could be due to residual muscle relaxant effect, hypocalcemic alkalotic tetany, intubation trauma, or paradoxical vocal cord motion (ie, hysterical stridor).

Another paroxysm of coughing is accompanied by hemoptysis. What is your immediate management?

Bleeding after nose or throat surgery can be very serious. Patients who are not fully awake may continue to gag and cough on the secretions, increasing venous pressure and worsening the bleeding. Furthermore, they may aspirate blood and other secretions. Fortunately, because of its physiological pH, aspiration of blood is not as serious as aspiration of acidic gastric contents. Nonetheless, the airway should be immediately secured in the obtunded patient. This may be accomplished with an awake intubation or a rapid-sequence induction.

If the patient is awake and alert enough to cough and swallow and does not seem to be aspirating blood, the first priority should be to decrease the bleeding as quickly as possible. Immediate measures that should be considered include raising the head of the bed to decrease venous and arterial pressures at the site of bleeding and aggressively treating any degree of systolic hypertension with intravenous antihypertensive agents. Sedation should be avoided so that airway reflexes are not compromised.

Despite these measures, the bleeding continues, and surgical intervention seems to be necessary. Describe your strategy for induction of anesthesia in this patient.

Before induction of general anesthesia in a bleeding patient, hypovolemia should be corrected with isotonic crystalloid, or colloid if the patient does not respond to crystalloid. The degree of hypovolemia is difficult to assess because much of the blood may be swallowed, but it may be estimated by changes in vital signs, postural hypotension, and hematocrit. Cross-matched blood should be readily available, and a second large-bore intravenous line secured. It must be appreciated that from an anesthetic standpoint, this is an entirely different patient than the one who presented for surgery initially: the patient now has a full stomach, is hypovolemic, and may prove to be a more difficult intubation.

The preferred technique in this patient is a rapid-sequence induction with cricoid pressure. Drug choice (eg, ketamine, etomidate) and dosage should anticipate the possibility of hypotension from persistent hypovolemia. Qualified personnel and appropriate equipment for an emergency tracheostomy should be immediately available. An orogastric tube should be passed to decompress the stomach.

Which arteries supply blood to the nose?

The arterial supply of the nose is provided by the internal maxillary artery and the anterior ethmoid artery. These may have to be ligated in uncontrollable epistaxis.

Describe extubation.

Because this patient is still at risk of aspiration, extubation should not be attempted until the patient has fully awakened and regained airway reflexes. Although it is desirable to limit coughing and "bucking" on the endotracheal tube during emergence, this may be difficult to achieve in the awakening patient. Intravenous lidocaine (1.5 mg/kg) may be helpful in this situation.

SUGGESTED READING

Atkins JH, Mirza N: Anesthetic considerations and surgical caveats for awake airway surgery. Anesthesiol Clin 2010;28:555.

Biro P: Jet ventilation for surgical interventions in the upper airway. Anesthesiol Clin 2010;28:397.

Chi JJ, Mandel JE, Weinstein GS, et al: Anesthetic considerations for transoral robotic surgery. Anesthesiol Clin 2010;28:411.

Collins CE: Anesthesia for pediatric airway surgery: recommendations and review from a pediatric referral center. Anesthesiol Clin 2010;28:505.

Cordoba Amorocho MR, Sordillo A: Anesthesia for functional endoscopic sinus surgery: a review. Anesthesiol Clin 2010;28:497.

Dillon FX: Electromyographic (EMG) neuromonitoring in otolaryngology-head and neck surgery. Anesthesiol Clin 2010;28:423.

Dralle H, Sekulla C, Lorenz K, et al: Intraoperative monitoring of the recurrent laryngeal nerve in thyroid surgery. World J Surg 2008;32:1358.

Green JS, Tsui BCH: Applications of ultrasonography in ENT: airway assessment and nerve blockage. Anesthesiol Clin 2010;28:541.

Guay J: Regional anesthesia for carotid surgery. Curr Opin Anaesthesiol 2008;21:638.

Hillman DR, Platt PR, Eastwood PR: Anesthesia, sleep, and upper airway collapsibility. Anesthesiol Clin 2010;28:443.

Jourdy DN, Kacker A: Regional anesthesia for office-based procedures in otorhinolaryngology. Anesthesiol Clin 2010;28:457.

Liang S, Irwin MG: Review of anesthesia for middle ear surgery. Anesthesiol Clin 2010;28:519.

Lu I-C, Chu K-S, Tsai C-J, et al: Optimal depth of NIM EMG endotracheal tube for intraoperative neuromonitoring of the recurrent laryngeal nerve during thyroidectomy. World J Surg 2008;32:1935.

Mandel JE: Laryngeal mask airways in ear, nose, and throat procedures. Anesthesiol Clin 2010;28:469.

Mobley SR, Miller BT, Astor FC, et al: Prone positioning for head and neck reconstructive surgery. Head & Neck 2007;29:1041.

O'Neill JP, Fenton JE: The recurrent laryngeal nerve in thyroid surgery. Surgeon 2008;6:373.

Pandit JJ, Satya-Krishna R, Gration P: Superficial or deep cervical plexus block for carotid endarterectomy:

a systematic review of complications. Br J Anaesth 2007;99:159.

Sabour S, Manders E, Steward DL: The role of rapid PACU parathyroid hormone in reducing post-thyroidectomy hypocalcemia. Otolaryngol–Head Neck Surg 2009;141:727.

Sheinbein DS, Loeb RG: Laser surgery and fire hazards in ear, nose, and throat surgeries. Anesthesiol Clin. 2010;28:485.

Xiao P, Zhang X: Adult laryngotracheal surgery. Anesthesiol Clin 2010;28:529.

Anesthesia for Orthopedic Surgery

Edward R. Mariano, MD, MAS

1 Clinical manifestations of bone cement implantation syndrome include hypoxia (increased pulmonary shunt), hypotension, arrhythmias (including heart block and sinus arrest), pulmonary hypertension (increased pulmonary vascular resistance), and decreased cardiac output.

2 Use of a pneumatic tourniquet on an extremity creates a bloodless field that greatly facilitates the surgery. However, tourniquets can produce potential problems of their own, including hemodynamic changes, pain, metabolic alterations, arterial thromboembolism, and pulmonary embolism.

3 Fat embolism syndrome classically presents within 72 h following long-bone or pelvic fracture, with the triad of dyspnea, confusion, and petechiae.

4 Deep vein thrombosis and pulmonary embolism can cause morbidity and mortality following orthopedic operations on the pelvis and lower extremities.

5 Neuraxial anesthesia alone or combined with general anesthesia may reduce thromboembolic complications by several mechanisms, including sympathectomy-induced increases in lower extremity venous blood flow, systemic antiinflammatory effects of local anesthetics, decreased

platelet reactivity, attenuated postoperative increase in factor VIII and von Willebrand factor, attenuated postoperative decrease in antithrombin III, and alterations in stress hormone release.

6 For patients receiving prophylactic low-molecular-weight heparin once daily, neuraxial techniques may be performed (or neuraxial catheters removed) 10–12 h after the previous dose, with a 4-h delay before administering the next dose.

7 Flexion and extension lateral radiographs of the cervical spine should be obtained preoperatively in patients with rheumatoid arthritis severe enough to require steroids, immune therapy, or methotrexate. If atlantoaxial instability is present, intubation should be performed with inline stabilization utilizing video or fiberoptic laryngoscopy.

8 Effective communication between the anesthesiologist and surgeon is essential during bilateral hip arthroplasty. If major hemodynamic instability occurs during the first hip replacement procedure, the second arthroplasty should be postponed.

9 Adjuvants such as opioids, clonidine, ketorolac, and neostigmine when added to local anesthetic solutions for intraarticular

—*Continued next page*

Continued—

injection have been used in various combinations to extend the duration of analgesia following knee arthroscopy.

10 Effective postoperative analgesia facilitates early physical rehabilitation to maximize postoperative range of motion and prevent joint adhesions following knee replacement.

11 The interscalene brachial plexus block using ultrasound or electrical stimulation is ideally suited for shoulder procedures. Even when general anesthesia is employed, an interscalene block can supplement anesthesia and provide effective postoperative analgesia.

Orthopedic surgery challenges the anesthesia provider. The comorbidities of these patients vary widely based on age group. Patients may present as neonates with congenital limb deformities, as teenagers with sports-related injuries, as adults for procedures ranging from excision of minor soft-tissue mass to joint replacement, or at any age with bone cancer. This chapter focuses on perioperative care issues specific to patients undergoing common orthopedic surgical procedures. For example, patients with long bone fractures are predisposed to fat embolism syndrome. Patients are at increased risk for venous thromboembolism following pelvic, hip, and knee operations. Use of bone cement during arthroplasties can cause hemodynamic instability. Limb tourniquets limit blood loss but introduce additional risks.

Neuraxial and other regional anesthetic techniques play an important role in decreasing the incidence of perioperative thromboembolic complications, providing postoperative analgesia, and facilitating early rehabilitation and hospital discharge. Advances in surgical techniques, such as minimally invasive approaches to knee and hip replacement, are necessitating modifications in anesthetic and perioperative management to facilitate overnight or even same-day discharge of patients who formerly required days of hospitalization. It is impossible to cover the anesthetic implications of diverse orthopedic operations in one chapter; hence, the focus here on perioperative management considerations and strategies for the anesthetic management of patients undergoing select orthopedic surgical procedures. Anesthesia for surgery on the spine is discussed in Chapter 27.

PERIOPERATIVE MANAGEMENT CONSIDERATIONS IN ORTHOPEDIC SURGERY

Bone Cement

Bone cement, **polymethylmethacrylate**, is frequently required for joint arthroplasties. The cement interdigitates within the interstices of cancellous bone and strongly binds the prosthetic device to the patient's bone. Mixing polymerized methylmethacrylate powder with liquid methylmethacrylate monomer causes polymerization and cross-linking of the polymer chains. This exothermic reaction leads to hardening of the cement and expansion against the prosthetic components. The resultant intramedullary hypertension (>500 mm Hg) can cause embolization of fat, bone marrow, cement, and air into venous channels. Systemic absorption of residual methylmethacrylate monomer can produce vasodilation and a decrease in systemic vascular resistance. The release of tissue thromboplastin may trigger platelet aggregation, microthrombus formation in the lungs, and cardiovascular instability as a result of the circulation of vasoactive substances.

1 The clinical manifestations of bone cement implantation syndrome include hypoxia (increased pulmonary shunt), hypotension, arrhythmias (including heart block and sinus arrest), pulmonary hypertension (increased pulmonary vascular resistance), and decreased cardiac output. Emboli most frequently occur during insertion of a femoral prosthesis for hip arthroplasty. Treatment strategies for this complication include increasing inspired oxygen concentration prior to cementing, monitoring to maintain euvolemia, creating a vent hole in the distal femur to relieve intramedullary pressure, performing high-pressure lavage of the femoral shaft to remove debris (potential microemboli), or using a femoral component that does not require cement.

Another source of concern related to the use of cement is the potential for gradual loosening of the prosthesis over time. Newer cementless implants are made of a porous material that allows natural bone to grow into them. Cementless prostheses generally last longer and may be advantageous for younger, active patients; however, healthy active bone formation is required and recovery may be longer compared to cemented joint replacements. Therefore, cemented prostheses are preferred for older (>80 years) and less active patients who often have osteoporosis or thin cortical bone. Practices continue to evolve regarding selection of cemented versus cementless implants, depending on the joint affected, patient, and surgical technique.

Pneumatic Tourniquets

2 Use of a pneumatic tourniquet on an extremity creates a bloodless field that greatly facilitates surgery. However, tourniquets can produce potential problems of their own, including hemodynamic changes, pain, metabolic alterations, arterial thromboembolism, and pulmonary embolism. Inflation pressure is usually set approximately 100 mm Hg higher than the patient's baseline systolic blood pressure. Prolonged inflation (>2 h) routinely leads to transient muscle dysfunction from ischemia and may produce rhabdomyolysis or permanent peripheral nerve damage. Tourniquet inflation has also been associated with increases in body temperature in pediatric patients undergoing lower extremity surgery.

Exsanguination of a lower extremity and tourniquet inflation cause a rapid shift of blood volume into the central circulation. Although not usually clinically important, bilateral lower extremity exsanguination can cause an increase in central venous pressure and arterial blood pressure that may not be well tolerated in patients with noncompliant ventricles and diastolic dysfunction.

Awake patients predictably experience tourniquet pain with inflation pressures of 100 mm Hg above systolic blood pressure for more than a few minutes. The mechanism and neural pathways for this severe aching and burning sensation defy precise explanation. **Tourniquet pain gradually becomes so severe over time that patients may require substantial supplemental analgesia, if not general anesthesia, despite a regional block that is adequate for surgical anesthesia.** Even during general anesthesia, stimulus from tourniquet compression often manifests as a gradually increasing mean arterial blood pressure beginning approximately 1 h after cuff inflation. Signs of progressive sympathetic activation include marked hypertension, tachycardia, and diaphoresis. The likelihood of tourniquet pain and its accompanying hypertension may be influenced by many factors, including anesthetic technique (regional anesthesia versus general anesthesia), extent of dermatomal spread of regional anesthetic block, choice of local anesthetic and dose ("intensity" of block), and supplementation with adjuvants either intravenously or in combination with local anesthetic solutions when applicable.

Cuff deflation invariably and immediately relieves tourniquet pain and associated hypertension. In fact, cuff deflation may be accompanied by a precipitous decrease in central venous and arterial blood pressure. Heart rate usually increases and core temperature decreases. Washout of accumulated metabolic wastes in the ischemic extremity increases partial pressure of carbon dioxide in arterial blood (Pa_{CO_2}), end-tidal carbon dioxide (ET_{CO_2}), and serum lactate and potassium levels. **These metabolic alterations can cause an increase in minute ventilation in the spontaneously breathing patient and, rarely, arrhythmias.** Tourniquet-induced ischemia of a lower extremity may lead to the development of deep venous thrombosis. Transesophageal echocardiography can detect subclinical pulmonary embolism (miliary emboli in the right atrium and ventricle) following tourniquet deflation even in minor cases such as diagnostic knee arthroscopy. Rare episodes of massive pulmonary embolism during total knee arthroplasty have been reported during leg exsanguination, after tourniquet inflation, and following tourniquet deflation. Tourniquets have been safely used in patients with sickle cell disease, although particular attention should be paid to maintaining oxygenation, normocarbia or hypocarbia, hydration, and normothermia.

Fat Embolism Syndrome

Some degree of fat embolism probably occurs with all long-bone fractures. **Fat embolism syndrome** is less frequent but potentially fatal (10–20% mortality). It classically presents within 72 h following long-bone or pelvic fracture, with the triad of dyspnea, confusion, and petechiae. This syndrome can also be seen following cardiopulmonary resuscitation, parental feeding with lipid infusion, and liposuction. The most popular theory for its pathogenesis holds that fat globules are released by the disruption of fat cells in the fractured bone and enter the circulation through tears in medullary vessels. An alternative theory proposes that the fat globules are chylomicrons resulting from the aggregation of circulating free fatty acids caused by changes in fatty acid metabolism. Regardless of their source, the increased free fatty acid levels can have a toxic effect on the capillary–alveolar membrane leading to the release of vasoactive amines and prostaglandins and the development of acute respiratory distress syndrome (ARDS; see Chapter 57). Neurological manifestations (eg, agitation, confusion, stupor, or coma) are the probable result of capillary damage in the cerebral circulation and cerebral edema. These signs may be exacerbated by hypoxia.

The diagnosis of fat embolism syndrome is suggested by petechiae on the chest, upper extremities, axillae, and conjunctiva. Fat globules occasionally may be observed in the retina, urine, or sputum. Coagulation abnormalities such as thrombocytopenia or prolonged clotting times are occasionally present. Serum lipase activity may be elevated but does not predict disease severity. Pulmonary involvement typically progresses from mild hypoxia and a normal chest radiograph to severe hypoxia or respiratory failure with radiographic findings of diffuse pulmonary opacities. Most of the classic signs and symptoms of fat embolism syndrome occur 1–3 days after the precipitating event. During general anesthesia, signs may include a decline in E_{TCO_2} and

arterial oxygen saturation and a rise in pulmonary artery pressures. Electrocardiography may show ischemic-appearing ST-segment changes and a pattern of right-sided heart strain.

Management is two-fold: preventative and supportive. Early stabilization of the fracture decreases the incidence of fat embolism syndrome and, in particular, reduces the risk of pulmonary complications. Supportive treatment consists of oxygen therapy with continuous positive airway pressure ventilation to prevent hypoxia and with specific ventilator strategies in the event of ARDS. Systemic hypotension will require appropriate pressor support, and vasodilators may aid the management of pulmonary hypertension. High-dose corticosteroid therapy is not supported by randomized clinical trials.

Deep Venous Thrombosis & Thromboembolism

Deep vein thrombosis (DVT) and pulmonary embolism (PE) can cause morbidity and mortality following orthopedic operations on the pelvis and lower extremities. Risk factors include obesity, age greater than 60 years, procedures lasting more than 30 min, use of a tourniquet, lower extremity fracture, and immobilization for more than 4 days. Patients at greatest risk include those undergoing hip surgery and knee replacement or major operations for lower extremity trauma. Such patients will experience DVT rates of 40–80% without prophylaxis. The incidence of clinically important PE following hip surgery in some studies is reported to be as high as 20%, whereas that of fatal PE may be 1–3%. Underlying pathophysiological mechanisms include venous stasis with hypercoagulable state due to localized and systemic inflammatory responses to surgery.

Pharmacological prophylaxis and the routine use of mechanical devices such as intermittent pneumatic compression (IPC) have been shown to decrease the incidence of DVT and PE. While mechanical thromboprophylaxis should be considered for every patient, the use of pharmacological anticoagulants must be balanced against the risk of major bleeding. For patients at increased risk for DVT but having "normal" bleeding risk, low-dose subcutaneous unfractionated heparin (LUFH), warfarin, or low-molecular-weight heparin (LMWH) may be employed in addition to mechanical prophylaxis. Patients at significantly increased risk of bleeding may be managed with mechanical prophylaxis alone until bleeding risk decreases. In general, anticoagulants are started the day of surgery in patients without indwelling epidural catheters. Warfarin may be started the night before surgery depending on the particular orthopedic surgeon's routine.

5 Neuraxial anesthesia alone or combined with general anesthesia may reduce thromboembolic complications by several mechanisms. These include sympathectomy-induced increases in lower extremity venous blood flow, systemic antiinflammatory effects of local anesthetics, decreased platelet reactivity, attenuated postoperative increases in factor VIII and von Willebrand factor, attenuated postoperative decreases in antithrombin III, and alterations in stress hormone release.

According to the Third Edition of the American Society of Regional Anesthesia and Pain Medicine Evidence-Based Guidelines on regional anesthesia and anticoagulation, patients currently receiving antiplatelet agents (eg, ticlopidine, clopidogrel, and intravenous glycoprotein IIb/IIIa inhibitors), thrombolytics, fondaparinux, direct thrombin inhibitors, or therapeutic regimens of LMWH present an unacceptable risk for spinal or epidural hematoma following neuraxial anesthesia. Performance of neuraxial block (or removal of a neuraxial catheter) is not contraindicated with subcutaneous LUFH when the total daily dose is 10,000 units or less; there are no data on the safety of neuraxial anesthesia **6** when larger doses are given. For patients receiving prophylactic LMWH, the guidelines vary based on regimen. With once-daily dosing, neuraxial techniques may be performed (or neuraxial catheters removed) 10–12 h after the previous dose, with a 4-h delay before administering the next dose. With twice-daily dosing, neuraxial catheters should not be left in situ and should be removed 2 h before the first dose of LMWH. Patients on warfarin therapy should not receive a neuraxial block unless the international normalized ratio (INR) is normal, and catheters should be removed when the INR is 1.5 or lower. The Third Edition of the guidelines also suggests that these recommendations be applied to deep peripheral nerve and plexus blocks and catheters (see Suggested Reading). Revisions to these guidelines occur regularly.

Hip Surgery

Common hip procedures performed in adults include repair of hip fracture, total hip arthroplasty, and closed reduction of hip dislocation.

FRACTURE OF THE HIP
Preoperative Considerations

Most patients presenting for hip fractures are frail and elderly. An occasional young patient will have sustained major trauma to the femur or pelvis. Studies have reported mortality rates following hip fracture of up to 10% during the initial hospitalization and over 25% within 1 year. Many of these patients have concomitant diseases such as coronary artery disease, cerebrovascular disease, chronic obstructive pulmonary disease, or diabetes.

Patients presenting with hip fractures are frequently dehydrated from inadequate oral intake. Depending on the site of the hip fracture, occult blood loss may be significant, further compromising intravascular volume. In general, intracapsular (subcapital, transcervical) fractures are associated with less blood loss than extracapsular (base of the femoral neck, intertrochanteric, subtrochanteric) fractures (Figure 38–1). A normal or borderline-low preoperative hematocrit may be deceiving when hemoconcentration masks occult blood loss.

Another characteristic of hip fracture patients is the frequent presence of preoperative hypoxia that may, at least in part, be due to fat embolism; other factors can include bibasilar atelectasis from immobility, pulmonary congestion (and effusion) from congestive heart failure, or consolidation due to infection.

Intraoperative Management

The choice between regional (spinal or epidural) and general anesthesia has been extensively evaluated for hip fracture surgery. A meta-analysis of

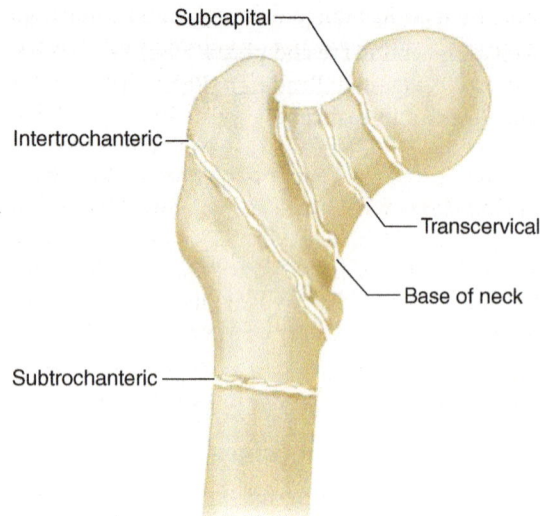

FIGURE 38–1 Blood loss from hip fracture depends on the location of the fracture (subtrochanteric, intertrochanteric > base of femoral neck > transcervical, subcapital) because the capsule restricts blood loss by acting like a tourniquet.

15 randomized clinical trials showed a decrease in postoperative DVT and 1-month mortality with regional anesthesia, but these advantages do not persist beyond 3 months. The incidence of postoperative delirium and cognitive dysfunction may be lower following regional anesthesia if intravenous sedation can be minimized.

A neuraxial anesthetic technique, with or without concomitant general anesthesia, provides the additional advantage of postoperative pain control. If a spinal anesthetic is planned, hypobaric or isobaric local anesthesia facilitates positioning since the patient can remain in the same position for both block placement and surgery. Intrathecal opioids such as morphine can extend postoperative analgesia but require close postoperative monitoring for delayed respiratory depression.

Consideration should also be given to the type of reduction and fixation to be used. This is dependent on the fracture site, degree of displacement, preoperative functional status of the patient, and surgeon preference. Undisplaced fractures of the proximal femur may be treated with percutaneous pinning

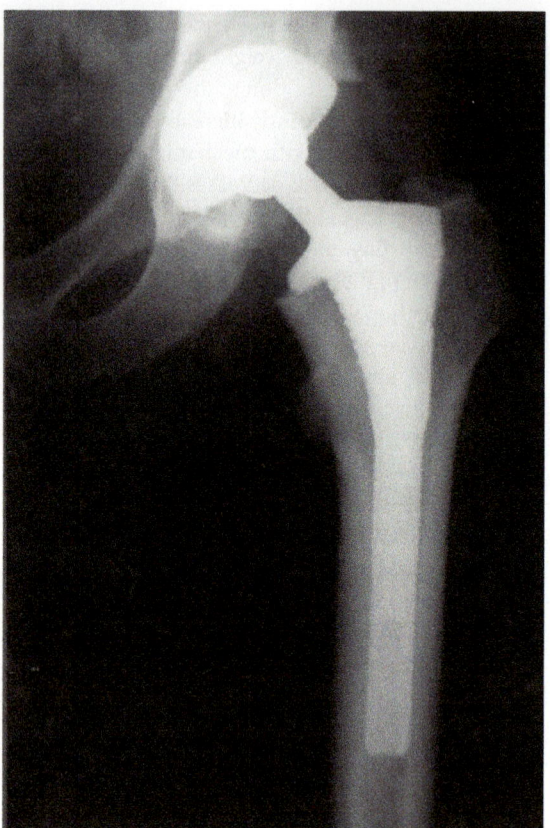

FIGURE 38–2 Uncemented total hip arthroplasty.

or cannulated screw fixation with the patient in the supine position. A hip compression screw and side plate are most often employed for intertrochanteric fractures. Displaced intracapsular fractures may require internal fixation, hemiarthroplasty, or total hip replacement (Figure 38–2). Surgical treatment of extracapsular hip fractures is accomplished with either an extramedullary implant (eg, sliding screw and plate) or intramedullary implant (eg, Gamma nail).

Hemiarthroplasty and total hip replacement are longer, more invasive operations than other procedures. They are usually performed with patients in the lateral decubitus position, are associated with greater blood loss, and, potentially, result in greater hemodynamic changes, particularly if cement is used. Therefore, one should secure sufficient venous access to permit rapid transfusion.

TOTAL HIP ARTHROPLASTY

Preoperative Considerations

Most patients undergoing total hip replacement suffer from osteoarthritis (degenerative joint disease), autoimmune conditions such as rheumatoid arthritis (RA), or avascular necrosis. Osteoarthritis is a degenerative disease affecting the articular surface of one or more joints (most commonly the hips and knees). The etiology of osteoarthritis appears to involve repetitive joint trauma. Because osteoarthritis may also involve the spine, neck manipulation during tracheal intubation should be minimized to avoid nerve root compression or disc protrusion.

RA is characterized by immune-mediated joint destruction with chronic and progressive inflammation of synovial membranes, as opposed to the articular wear and tear of osteoarthritis. RA is a systemic disease affecting multiple organ systems (Table 38–1). RA often affects the small joints of the hands, wrists, and feet causing severe deformity; when this occurs, intravenous and radial artery cannulation can be challenging.

Extreme cases of RA involve almost all synovial membranes, including those in the cervical spine and temporomandibular joint. Atlantoaxial subluxation, which can be diagnosed radiologically, may lead to

TABLE 38–1 Systemic manifestations of rheumatoid arthritis.

Organ System	Abnormalities
Cardiovascular	Pericardial thickening and effusion, myocarditis, coronary arteritis, conduction defects, vasculitis, cardiac valve fibrosis (aortic regurgitation)
Pulmonary	Pleural effusion, pulmonary nodules, interstitial pulmonary fibrosis
Hematopoietic	Anemia, eosinophilia, platelet dysfunction (from aspirin therapy), thrombocytopenia
Endocrine	Adrenal insufficiency (from glucocorticoid therapy), impaired immune system
Dermatological	Thin and atrophic skin from the disease and immunosuppressive drugs

protrusion of the odontoid process into the foramen magnum during intubation, compromising vertebral blood flow and compressing the spinal cord or brainstem (Figure 38–3). Flexion and extension lateral radiographs of the cervical spine should be obtained preoperatively in patients with RA severe enough to require steroids, immune therapy, or methotrexate. If atlantoaxial instability is present, tracheal intubation should be performed with inline stabilization utilizing video or fiberoptic laryngoscopy. Involvement of the temporomandibular joint can limit jaw mobility and range of motion to such a degree that conventional orotracheal intubation may be impossible. Hoarseness or inspiratory stridor may signal a narrowing of the glottic opening caused by cricoarytenoid arthritis. This condition may lead to postextubation airway obstruction even when a smaller diameter tracheal tube has been used.

Patients with RA or osteoarthritis commonly receive nonsteroidal antiinflammatory drugs (NSAIDs) for pain management. These drugs can have serious side effects such as gastrointestinal bleeding, renal toxicity, and platelet dysfunction.

Intraoperative Management

Total hip replacement (THR) involves several surgical steps, including positioning of the patient (usually in the lateral decubitus position), dislocation and removal of the femoral head, reaming of the acetabulum and insertion of a prosthetic acetabular cup (with or without cement), and reaming of the femur and insertion of a femoral component (femoral head and stem) into the femoral shaft (with or without cement). THR is also associated with three potentially life-threatening complications: bone cement implantation syndrome, intra- and postoperative hemorrhage, and venous thromboembolism. Thus, invasive arterial monitoring may be justified for select patients undergoing these procedures. Neuraxial administration of opioids such as morphine in the perioperative period extends the duration of postoperative analgesia.

A. Hip Resurfacing Arthroplasty

The increasing number of younger patients presenting for hip arthroplasty and of other patients who require revision of standard (metal-on-polyethylene) total

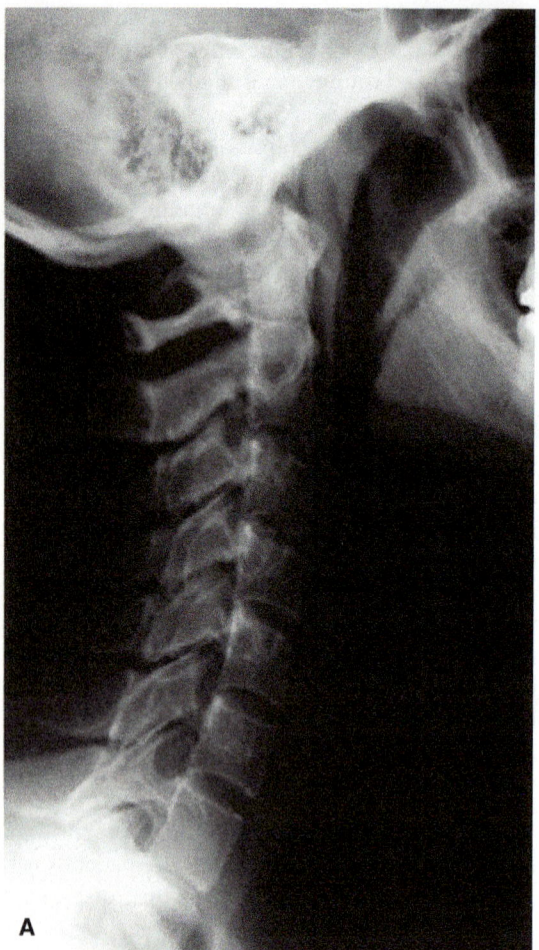

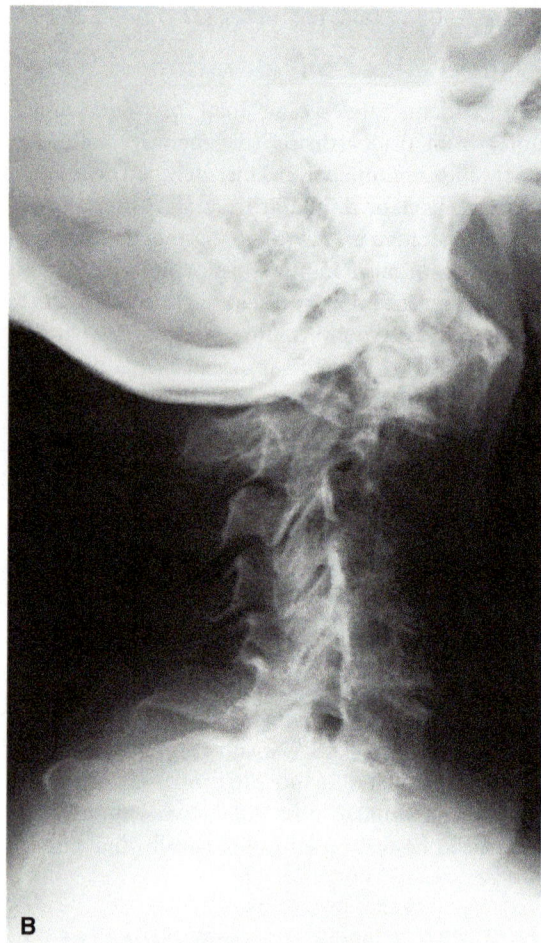

FIGURE 38–3 Because instability of the cervical spine may be asymptomatic, lateral radiographs are mandatory in patients with severe rheumatoid arthritis. **A**: Radiograph of a normal lateral cervical spine. **B**: Lateral cervical spine of a patient with rheumatoid arthritis; note the severe C1–C2 instability.

hip arthroplasty implants has led to redevelopment of hip resurfacing arthroplasty techniques. Compared with traditional hip arthroplasty implants, hip resurfacing maintains patients' native bone to a greater degree. Metal-on-metal hybrid implants are usually employed. Surgical approaches can be anterolateral or posterior, with the posterior approach theoretically providing greater preservation of the blood supply to the femoral head. With the posterior approach, patients are placed in the lateral decubitus position similar to traditional hip arthroplasty.

Outcomes data related to hip resurfacing versus traditional total hip arthroplasty are controversial.

Prospective studies have not shown a difference in gait or postural balance at 3 months postoperatively. A recent meta-analysis favored resurfacing in terms of functional outcome and blood loss despite comparable results for postoperative pain scores and patient satisfaction. Of particular concern is the finding that patients who undergo resurfacing are nearly twice as likely to require revision surgery as those receiving traditional hip arthroplasty. There is a higher incidence of aseptic component loosening (possibly from metal hypersensitivity) and femoral neck fracture, particularly in women. Finally, the presence of metal debris in the joint space (from metal-on-metal contact) has led to a marked narrowing of indications for the prostheses and the procedure.

B. Bilateral Arthroplasty

Bilateral hip arthroplasty can be safely performed in fit patients as a combined procedure, assuming the absence of significant pulmonary embolization after insertion of the first femoral component. Monitoring may include echocardiography. Effective communication between the anesthesia provider and surgeon is essential. If major hemodynamic instability occurs during the first hip replacement procedure, the second arthroplasty should be postponed.

C. Revision Arthroplasty

Revision of a prior hip arthroplasty may be associated with much greater blood loss than in the initial procedure. Blood loss depends on many factors, including the experience and skill of the surgeon. Some studies suggest that blood loss may be decreased during hip surgery if a regional anesthesia technique is used (eg, spinal or epidural anesthesia) compared with general anesthesia even at similar mean arterial blood pressures. The mechanism is unclear. Because the likelihood of perioperative blood transfusion is high, preoperative autologous blood donation and intraoperative blood salvage should be considered. Preoperative administration of vitamins (B_{12} and K) and iron can treat mild forms of chronic anemia. Alternatively (and more expensively), recombinant human erythropoietin (600 IU/kg subcutaneously weekly beginning 21 days before surgery and ending on the day of surgery) may also decrease the need for perioperative allogeneic blood transfusion. Erythropoietin increases red blood cell production by stimulating the division and differentiation of erythroid progenitors in the bone marrow. Maintaining normal body temperature during hip replacement surgery reduces blood loss.

D. Minimally Invasive Arthroplasty

Computer-assisted surgery (CAS) may improve surgical outcomes and promote early rehabilitation through minimally invasive techniques employing cementless implants. Computer software can accurately reconstruct three-dimensional images of bone and soft tissue based on radiographs, fluoroscopy, computed tomography, or magnetic resonance imaging. The computer matches preoperative images or planning information to the position of the patient on the operating room table. Tracking devices are attached to target bones (Figure 38–4) and instruments used during surgery, and the navigation system utilizes optical cameras and infrared light-emitting diodes to sense their positions. CAS thus allows accurate placement of implants through

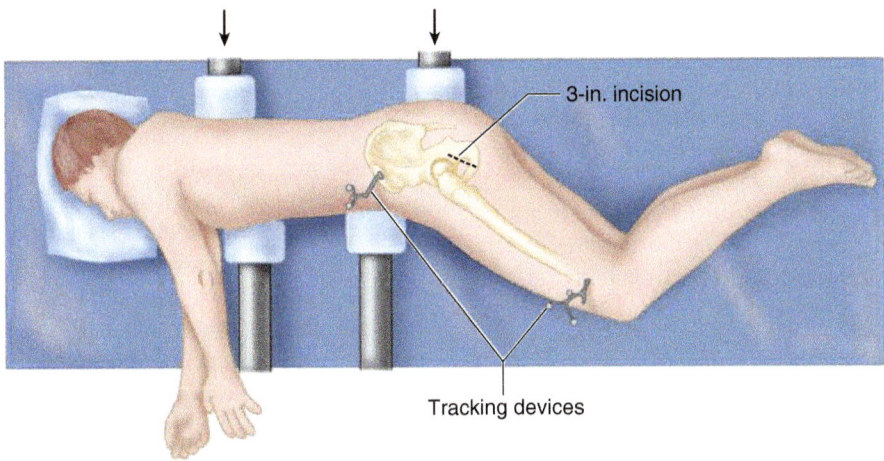

FIGURE 38–4 Minimally invasive total hip arthroplasty: lateral approach. Note the small 3-in. incision and tracking devices for the CAS navigation system.

small incisions, and the resulting reduction in tissue and muscle damage could lead to less pain and early rehabilitation. The lateral approach utilizes a single 3-in. incision with the patient in the lateral decubitus position (Figure 38–4); an anterior approach utilizes two separate 2-in. incisions (one for the acetabular component and another for the femoral component) with the patient supine. Minimally invasive techniques can reduce hospitalization to 24 h or less. Anesthetic techniques should promote rapid recovery and can include neuraxial regional anesthesia or total intravenous general anesthesia.

E. Hip Arthroscopy

In recent years, hip arthroscopy has increased in popularity as a minimally invasive alternative to open arthrotomy for a variety of surgical indications such as femoroacetabular impingement (FAI), acetabular labral tears, loose bodies, and osteoarthritis. At present, there is fair evidence in the published literature (small, randomized controlled trials) to support hip arthroscopy for FAI, but evidence is lacking for other indications.

CLOSED REDUCTION OF HIP DISLOCATION

There is a 3% incidence of hip dislocation following primary hip arthroplasty and a 20% incidence following total hip revision arthroplasty. Because less force is required to dislocate a prosthetic hip, patients with hip implants require special precautions during positioning for subsequent surgical procedures. Extremes of hip flexion, internal rotation, and adduction increase the risk of dislocation. Hip dislocations may be corrected with closed reduction facilitated by use of a brief general anesthetic. Temporary paralysis can be provided by succinylcholine, if necessary, to facilitate the reduction when the hip musculature is severely contracted. Successful reduction should be confirmed radiologically prior to the patient's emergence.

Knee Surgery

The two most frequently performed knee surgeries are arthroscopy and total or partial joint replacement.

KNEE ARTHROSCOPY
Preoperative Considerations

Arthroscopy has revolutionized surgery of many joints, including the hip, knee, shoulder, ankle, elbow, and wrist. Joint arthroscopies are usually performed as outpatient procedures. Although the typical patient undergoing knee arthroscopy is often thought of as being a healthy young athlete, knee arthroscopies are frequently performed in elderly patients with multiple medical problems.

Intraoperative Management

A bloodless field greatly facilitates arthroscopic surgery. Fortunately, knee surgery lends itself to the use of a pneumatic tourniquet. The surgery is performed as an outpatient procedure with the patient in a supine position under general anesthesia or neuraxial anesthesia. Alternative anesthetic techniques include peripheral nerve blocks, periarticular injections, or intraarticular injections employing local anesthetic solutions with or without adjuvants combined with intravenous sedation.

Comparing neuraxial anesthesia techniques, success and patient satisfaction appear to be equal between epidural and spinal anesthesia. However, for ambulatory surgery, time to discharge following neuraxial anesthesia may be prolonged compared with general anesthesia.

Postoperative Pain Management

Successful outpatient recovery depends on early ambulation, adequate pain relief, and minimal nausea and vomiting. Techniques that avoid large doses of systemic opioids have obvious appeal. Intraarticular local anesthetics (bupivacaine or ropivacaine) usually provide satisfactory analgesia for several hours postoperatively. Adjuvants such as opioids, clonidine, ketorolac, epinephrine, and neostigmine when added to local anesthetic solutions for intraarticular injection have been used in various combinations to extend the duration of analgesia. Other multimodal pain management strategies include systemic NSAIDs, gabapentin, and single or continuous peripheral nerve blocks for arthroscopic ligament reconstruction.

TOTAL KNEE REPLACEMENT

Preoperative Considerations

Patients presenting for total knee replacement (Figure 38–5) have similar comorbidities to those undergoing total hip replacement (eg, RA, osteoarthritis).

Intraoperative Management

During total knee arthroplasty, patients remain in a supine position, and intraoperative blood loss is limited by the use of a tourniquet. Cooperative patients usually tolerate a neuraxial anesthetic technique with intravenous sedation. Bone cement implantation syndrome following insertion of a femoral prosthesis is possible but is less likely than during hip arthroplasty. Subsequent release of emboli into the systemic circulation may exaggerate any tendency for hypotension following tourniquet release.

Preoperative placement of a lumbar epidural or perineural catheter can be very helpful in

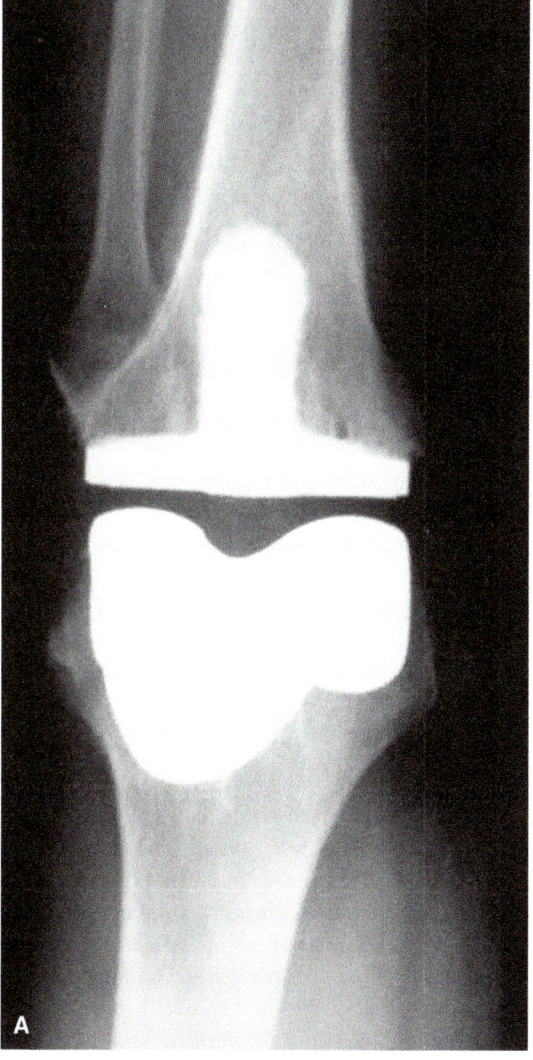

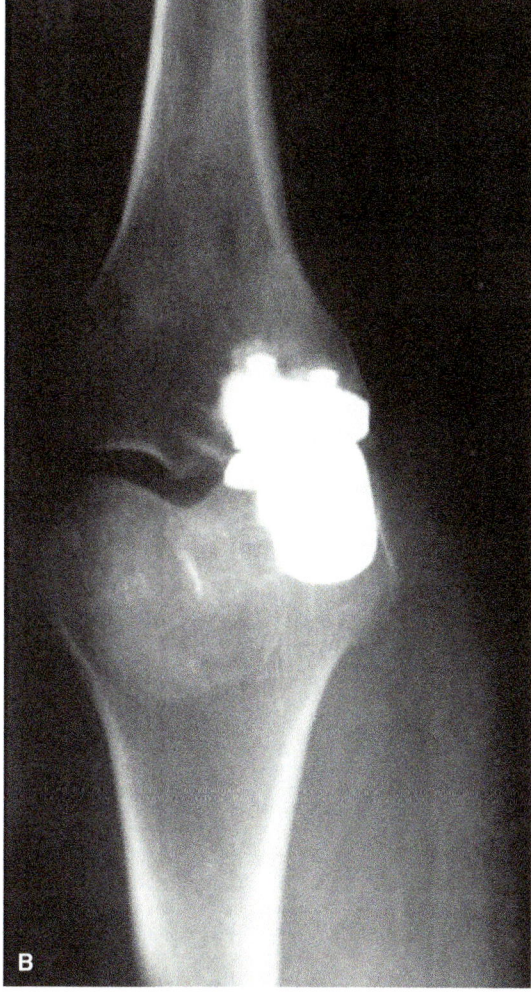

FIGURE 38–5 Total (**A**) and partial (**B**) knee replacement.

managing postoperative pain, which is typically more severe than pain following hip replacement **10** surgery. Effective postoperative analgesia facilitates early physical rehabilitation to maximize postoperative range of motion and prevent joint adhesions following knee replacement. It is important to balance pain control with the need for an alert and cooperative patient during physical therapy. Epidural analgesia is useful in bilateral knee replacements. **For unilateral knee replacement, lumbar epidural and femoral perineural catheters provide equivalent analgesia while femoral perineural catheters produce fewer side effects (eg, pruritus, nausea and vomiting, urinary retention, or orthostatic lightheadedness).** Preoperative placement in a "block room" can prevent operating room delays and ensure that patients receive this beneficial analgesic technique (**Figure 38–6**).

Partial knee replacement (unicompartmental or patellofemoral) and minimally invasive knee arthroplasty with muscle-sparing approaches have been described. With strict patient selection, these techniques may reduce quadriceps muscle damage, facilitating earlier achievement of range-of-motion

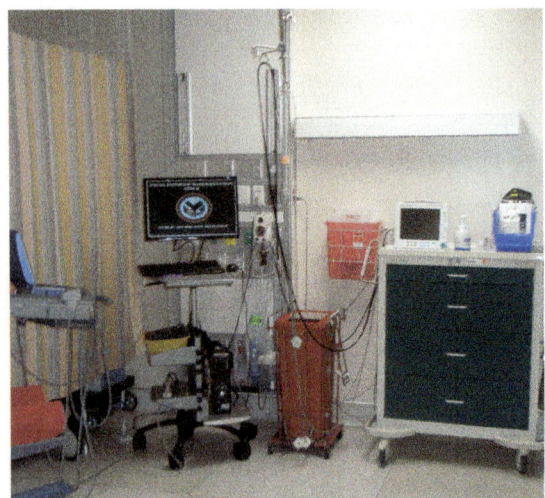

FIGURE 38–6 A "block room" can be located in a preoperative holding area, induction room, or postanesthesia care unit and should offer standard monitoring (as outlined by the American Society of Anesthesiologists) and ample storage for regional anesthesia supplies and equipment.

and ambulation goals, and may allow for discharge within 24 h following surgery if outpatient physical therapy is arranged. Anesthetic management and postoperative analgesia should accommodate and facilitate the accelerated recovery schedule. Single or continuous peripheral nerve blocks, alone or in combination, can provide target-specific pain control and facilitate early rehabilitation. **In randomized clinical trials, continuous peripheral nerve block catheters with subsequent perineural local anesthetic infusions have been shown to decrease time to meet discharge criteria for total knee arthroplasty.** The management of perineural catheters takes a hands-on team approach and can be incorporated into integrated clinical pathways involving surgery, nursing, and physical therapy. Among the complications of lower extremity perineural local anesthetic infusions, those involving patient falls are of greatest concern, and comprehensive fall prevention programs need to be in place wherever these techniques are employed.

Surgery on the Upper Extremity

Procedures on the upper extremities include those for disorders of the shoulder (eg, subacromial impingement or rotator cuff tears), traumatic fractures, nerve entrapment syndromes (eg, carpal tunnel syndrome), and joint arthroplasties (eg, rheumatoid arthritis).

SHOULDER SURGERY

Shoulder operations may be open or arthroscopic. These procedures are performed either in a sitting ("beach chair") or, less commonly, the lateral decubitus position. **The beach chair position may be associated with decreases in cerebral perfusion as measured by tissue oximetry; cases of blindness, stroke, and even brain death have been described, emphasizing the need to accurately measure blood pressure at the level of the brain.** When using noninvasive blood pressure monitoring, the cuff should be applied on the upper arm because systolic blood pressure readings from the calf can be 40 mm Hg higher than brachial readings on the same patient. If a surgeon requests controlled hypotension, an arterial catheter for invasive blood pressure monitoring is recommended, and the transducer should be positioned at least at the level of the heart or, preferably, the brainstem (external meatus of the ear).

11 The interscalene brachial plexus block using ultrasound or electrical stimulation is ideally suited for shoulder procedures. The supraclavicular approach also can be used. Even when general anesthesia is employed, an interscalene block can supplement anesthesia and provide effective postoperative analgesia. Intense muscle relaxation is usually required for major shoulder surgery during general anesthesia, particularly when not combined with a brachial plexus block.

Preoperative insertion of an indwelling perineural catheter with subsequent infusion of a dilute local anesthetic infusion solution allows postoperative analgesia for 48–72 h with most fixed-reservoir disposable pumps following arthroscopic or open shoulder operations (see Chapter 46). Alternatively, surgeons may insert a subacromial catheter to provide continuous infusion of local anesthetic for postoperative analgesia. Direct placement of intraarticular catheters into the glenohumeral joint with infusion of bupivacaine has been associated with postarthroscopic glenohumeral chondrolysis in retrospective human and prospective animal studies and is not currently recommended. Multimodal analgesia, including systemic NSAIDs (if no contraindications) and local anesthetic infusions in the perioperative period, can help reduce postoperative opioid requirements.

DISTAL UPPER EXTREMITY SURGERY

Distal upper extremity surgical procedures generally take place on an outpatient basis. Minor soft tissue operations of the hand (eg, carpal tunnel release) of short duration may be performed with local infiltration or with intravenous regional anesthesia (IVRA, or Bier block). The limiting factor with IVRA is tourniquet tolerance.

For operations lasting more than 1 h or more invasive procedures involving bones or joints, a brachial plexus block is the preferred regional anesthetic technique. Multiple approaches can be used to anesthetize the brachial plexus for distal upper extremity surgery (see Chapter 46). Selection of brachial plexus block technique should take into account the planned surgical site and location of the pneumatic tourniquet, if applicable. Continuous peripheral nerve blocks may be appropriate for inpatient and select outpatient procedures to extend the duration of analgesia further into the postoperative period or facilitate physical therapy. Brachial plexus blocks do not anesthetize the intercostobrachial nerve distribution (arising from the dorsal rami of T1 and sometimes T2); hence, subcutaneous infiltration of local anesthetic may be required for procedures involving the medial upper arm.

Anesthetic considerations for distal upper extremity surgery should include patient positioning and use of a pneumatic tourniquet. Most procedures can be performed with the patient supine; the operative arm abducted 90° and resting on a hand table; and the operating room table rotated 90° to position the operative arm in the center of the room. Exceptions to this rule often involve surgery around the elbow, and certain operations may require the patient be in lateral decubitus or even prone position. Because patients are often scheduled for same-day discharge, perioperative management should focus on ensuring rapid emergence and preventing severe postoperative pain and nausea (see Chapter 44).

CASE DISCUSSION

Managing Blood Loss in Jehovah's Witnesses

A 58-year-old Jehovah's Witness presents for hemipelvectomy to resect a malignant bone tumor (osteogenic sarcoma). The patient has received chemotherapy over the last 2 months with multiple drugs, including doxorubicin. The patient has no other medical problems, and the preoperative hematocrit is 47%.

How does the care of Jehovah's Witnesses particularly challenge the anesthesiologist?

Jehovah's Witnesses, a fellowship of more than 1 million Americans, object to the administration of blood for any indication. This objection stems from their interpretation of the Bible ("to keep abstaining from . . . blood," Acts 15:28,29) and not for medical reasons (eg, the fear of hepatitis). Physicians are obliged to honor the principle of autonomy, which upholds that patients have final authority over what is done to them. Witnesses typically sign a waiver releasing physicians of liability for any consequences of blood refusal.

Which intravenous fluids will Witnesses accept?

Witnesses abstain from blood and blood products (eg, packed red blood cells, fresh frozen plasma, platelets) but not non–blood-containing solutions. They accept crystalloids, hetastarch, and dextran replacement solutions. Witnesses often view albumin, erythropoietin (because of the use of albumin), immune globulins, and hemophiliac preparations as a gray area that requires a personal decision by the believer.

Do they allow the use of autologous blood?

According to their religion, any blood that is removed from the body should be discarded ("You should pour it out upon the ground as water," Deuteronomy 12:24) and not stored. Thus, the usual practice of autologous preoperative collection and storage would not be allowed. Techniques of acute normovolemic hemodilution and intraoperative blood salvage have been accepted by some Witnesses, however, as long as their blood maintains continuity with their circulatory systems at all times. For example, up to 4 units of blood could be drawn from the patient immediately before surgery and kept in anticoagulant-containing bags that maintain a constant link to the patient's body. The blood could be replaced by an acceptable colloid or crystalloid solution then reinfused as needed during surgery.

How would the inability to transfuse blood affect intraoperative monitoring decisions?

Hemipelvectomy involves radical resection that can lead to massive blood loss. This is particularly true for large tumors removed using the more invasive internal approach. Invasive arterial blood pressure and central venous pressure monitors would be indicated in most patients undergoing this procedure. Techniques that minimize intraoperative blood loss (eg, controlled hypotension, aprotinin) should be considered. In a Jehovah's Witness, the management of life-threatening anemia (Hb <5 g/dL) may be improved by monitoring cardiac output, oxygen delivery, and oxygen consumption. Continuous electrocardiographic ST-segment analysis may signal myocardial ischemia.

What physiological effects result from severe anemia?

Assuming the maintenance of normovolemia and the absence of preexisting major end-organ dysfunction, most patients tolerate severe anemia surprisingly well. Decreased blood viscosity and vasodilation lower systemic vascular resistance and increase blood flow. Augmentation of stroke volume increases cardiac output, allowing arterial blood pressure and heart rate to remain relatively unchanged. Coronary and cerebral blood flows increase in the absence of coronary artery disease and carotid artery stenosis. A decrease in venous oxygen saturation reflects an increase in tissue oxygen extraction. Oozing from surgical wounds as a result of dilutional coagulopathy may accompany extreme degrees of anemia.

What are some of the anesthetic implications of preoperative doxorubicin therapy?

This anthracycline chemotherapeutic agent has well-recognized cardiac side effects, ranging from transient arrhythmias and electrocardiographic changes (eg, ST-segment and T-wave abnormalities) to irreversible cardiomyopathy and congestive heart failure. The risk of cardiomyopathy appears to increase with a cumulative dose greater than 550 mg/m², prior radiotherapy, and concurrent cyclophosphamide treatment. Mild degrees of cardiomyopathy can be detected preoperatively with endomyocardial biopsy, echocardiography, or exercise radionuclide angiography. The other important toxicity of doxorubicin is myelosuppression manifesting as thrombocytopenia, leukopenia, and anemia.

Are there any special considerations regarding postoperative pain management in the Jehovah's Witness?

Witnesses generally refrain from any mind-altering drugs or medications, although opioids prescribed by a physician for severe pain are accepted by some believers. Insertion of an epidural catheter can provide pain relief with local anesthetics, with or without opioids.

GUIDELINES

Horlocker TT, Wedel DJ, Rowlingson JC, et al: Regional Anesthesia in the Patient Receiving Antithrombotic or Thrombolytic Therapy: American Society of Regional Anesthesia and Pain Medicine Evidence-Based Guidelines, 3rd ed. American Society of Regional Anesthesia, 2010. Available at: http://www.asra.com/publications-anticoagulation-3rd-edition-2010.php.

SUGGESTED READING

Amanatullah DF, Cheung Y, Di Cesare PE: Hip resurfacing arthroplasty: A review of the evidence for surgical technique, outcome, and complications. Orthop Clin North Am 2010;41:263.

Busfield BT, Romero DM: Pain pump use after shoulder arthroscopy as a cause of glenohumeral chondrolysis. Arthroscopy 2009;25:647.

Hebl JR, Dilger JA, Byer DE, et al: A preemptive multimodal pathway featuring peripheral nerve block improves perioperative outcomes after major orthopedic surgery. Reg Anesth Pain Med 2008;33:510.

Ilfeld BM, Enneking FK: Continuous peripheral nerve blocks at home: A review. Anesth Analg 2005;100:1822.

Ilfeld BM, Ball ST, Gearen PF, et al: Ambulatory continuous posterior lumbar plexus nerve blocks after hip arthroplasty: A dual-center, randomized, triple-masked, placebo-controlled trial. Anesthesiology 2008;109:491.

Ilfeld BM, Duke KB, Donohue MC: The association between lower extremity continuous peripheral nerve blocks and patient falls after knee and hip arthroplasty. Anesth Analg 2010;111:1552.

Ilfeld BM, Le LT, Meyer RS, et al: Ambulatory continuous femoral nerve blocks decrease time to discharge readiness after tricompartment total knee arthroplasty: A randomized, triple-masked, placebo-controlled study. Anesthesiology 2008;108:703.

Khanna A, Gougoulias N, Longo UG, et al: Minimally invasive total knee arthroplasty: A systematic review. Orthop Clin N Am 2009;40:479.

Lafont ND, Kalonji MK, Barre J, et al: Clinical features and echocardiography of embolism during cemented hip arthroplasty. Can J Anaesth. 1997;44:112.

Lisowska B, Rutkowska-Sak L, Maldyk P, et al: Anaesthesiological problems in patients with rheumatoid arthritis undergoing orthopaedic surgeries. Clin Rheumatol 2008;27:553.

Liu SS, Strodtbeck WM, Richman JM, Wu CL: A comparison of regional versus general anesthesia for ambulatory anesthesia: A meta-analysis of randomized controlled trials. Anesth Analg 2005;101:1634.

Mariano ER, Afra R, Loland VJ, et al: Continuous interscalene brachial plexus block via an ultrasound-guided posterior approach: A randomized, triple-masked, placebo-controlled study. Anesth Analg 2009;108:1688.

Mariano ER, Loland VJ, Sandhu NS, et al: A trainee-based randomized comparison of stimulating interscalene perineural catheters with a new technique using ultrasound guidance alone. J Ultrasound Med 2010;29:329.

Mason SE, Noel-Storr A, Ritchie CW: The impact of general and regional anesthesia on the incidence of post-operative cognitive dysfunction and post-operative delirium: A systematic review with meta-analysis. J Alzheimers Dis 2010;22(Suppl 3):67.

Neal JM, Gerancher JC, Hebl JR, et al: Upper extremity regional anesthesia: Essentials of our current understanding, 2008. Reg Anesth Pain Med 2009;34:134.

Pietak S, Holmes J, Matthews R, et al: Cardiovascular collapse after femoral prosthesis surgery for acute hip fracture. Can J Anaesth 1997;44:198.

Pohl A, Cullen DJ: Cerebral ischemia during shoulder surgery in the upright position: A case series. J Clin Anesth 2005;17:463.

Pollock JE, Mulroy MF, Bent E, et al: A comparison of two regional anesthetic techniques for outpatient knee arthroscopy. Anesth Analg 2003;97:397.

Rathmell JP, Pino CA, Taylor R, et al: Intrathecal morphine for postoperative analgesia: A randomized, controlled, dose-ranging study after hip and knee arthroplasty. Anesth Analg 2003;97:1452.

Schmied H, Schiferer A, Sessler DI, et al: The effects of red-cell scavenging, hemodilution, and active warming on allogenic blood requirements in patients undergoing hip or knee arthroplasty. Anesth Analg 1998;86:387.

Smith TO, Nichols R, Donell ST, et al: The clinical and radiological outcomes of hip resurfacing versus total hip arthroplasty: A meta-analysis and systematic review. Acta Orthop 2010;81:684.

Urwin SC, Parker MJ, Griffiths R: General versus regional anaesthesia for hip fracture surgery: A meta-analysis of randomized trials. Br J Anaesth 2000;84:450.

Zaric D, Boysen K, Christiansen C, et al: A comparison of epidural analgesia with combined continuous femoral-sciatic nerve blocks after total knee replacement. Anesth Analg 2006;102:1240.

Anesthesia for Trauma & Emergency Surgery

Brian P. McGlinch, MD

1. All trauma patients should be presumed to have "full" stomachs and an increased risk for pulmonary aspiration of gastric contents.

2. Cervical spine injury is presumed in any trauma patient complaining of neck pain, or with any significant head injury, neurological signs or symptoms suggestive of cervical spine injury, or intoxication or loss of consciousness.

3. In the multiple-injury patient, providers should maintain a high level of suspicion for pulmonary injury that could evolve into a tension pneumothorax when mechanical ventilation is initiated.

4. In up to 25% of major trauma patients, trauma-induced coagulopathy is present shortly after injury and before any resuscitative efforts have been initiated.

5. Administering blood products in equal ratios early in resuscitation has become an accepted approach to correction of trauma-induced coagulopathy. This balanced approach to transfusion, 1:1:1 (red blood cell:fresh frozen plasma:platelet), is termed *damage control resuscitation*.

6. Noninfectious transfusion reactions are now the leading complication of transfusion and represent a more than 10-fold greater risk than blood-borne infection. Transfusion-related acute lung injury is the leading cause of transfusion-related death.

7. The *assessment of blood consumption* (ABC) score is an attempt to predict which patients are likely to require a massive transfusion protocol. The ABC score assigns 1 point for the presence of each of four possible variables: (1) penetrating injury; (2) systolic blood pressure less than 90 mmHg; (3) heart rate greater than 120 beats per minute; and (4) positive results of a *focused assessment with sonography for trauma* evaluation. Patients with ABC scores of 2 or higher are likely to require massive transfusion.

8. Any trauma patient with altered level of consciousness must be considered to have a traumatic brain injury (TBI) until proven otherwise. The most reliable clinical assessment tool in determining the significance of TBI in a nonsedated, nonparalyzed patient is the Glasgow coma scale.

9. Acute subdural hematoma is the most common condition warranting emergency neurosurgery and is associated with the highest mortality.

10. Systemic hypotension (systolic blood pressures <90 mm Hg), hypoxemia (Pao_2 <60 mm Hg), hypercapnia ($Paco_2$ >50 mm Hg), and hyperthermia (temperature >38.0°C) have a negative impact on morbidity and mortality following head injuries, likely because of

—*Continued next page*

Continued—

their contributions to increasing cerebral edema and intracranial pressure (ICP).

11 Current guidelines recommend maintaining cerebral perfusion pressure between 50 and 70 mm Hg and ICP at less than 20 mm Hg for patients with severe head injury.

12 Maintaining supranormal mean arterial blood pressures to assure spinal cord perfusion in areas of reduced blood flow due to cord compression or vascular compromise is likely to be of more benefit than steroid administration.

13 Major burns (a second- or third-degree burn involving >20% total body surface area [TBSA]) induce a unique hemodynamic response. Cardiac output declines by up to 50% within 30 minutes in response to massive vasoconstriction, inducing a state of normovolemic hypoperfusion (*burn shock*).

14 In contrast to fluid management for blunt and penetrating trauma, which discourages use of crystalloid fluids, burn fluid resuscitation emphasizes the use of crystalloids, particularly lactated Ringer's solution, in preference to albumin, hydroxyethyl starch, hypertonic saline, and blood.

15 Carbon monoxide poisoning should be considered in all serious burn injury cases, as well as with lesser TBSA burns occurring in enclosed spaces. Unconsciousness or decreased levels of consciousness following burn injuries should be presumed to represent carbon monoxide poisoning.

16 Beyond 48 h after a major burn, succinylcholine administration is likely to produce potentially lethal elevation of serum potassium levels.

Trauma is a leading cause of morbidity and mortality in all age groups, and is the leading cause of death in the young. All aspects of trauma care, from that provided at the scene, through transport, resuscitation, surgery, intensive care, and rehabilitation, must be coordinated if the patient is to have the greatest chance for full recovery. The Advanced Trauma Life Support (ATLS) program developed by the American College of Surgeons' (ACS) Committee on Trauma has, over time, resulted in an increasingly consistent approach to trauma resuscitation. The development of criteria for level one trauma centers has also improved trauma care by directing severely injured patients to facilities with appropriate resources.

Although trauma anesthesia is sometimes thought of as a unique topic, many of the principles for managing trauma patients are relevant to any unstable or hemorrhaging patient. Thus, many common issues are addressed in this chapter.

PRIMARY SURVEY

Airway

Increasingly, emergency medical technician–paramedics and flight nurses are trained to intubate patients in the prehospital environment. More providers capable of airway management in the critically ill or injured patient are now available to intervene in the hospital setting as well. As a result, the anesthesiologist's role in providing initial trauma resuscitation has diminished in North America. This also means that when called upon to assist in airway management in the emergency department, anesthesia providers must expect a challenging airway, as routine airway management techniques likely have already proved unsuccessful.

There are three important aspects of airway management in the initial evaluation of a trauma patient: (1) the need for basic life support; (2) the presumed presence of a cervical spinal cord injury until proven otherwise; and (3) the potential for failed tracheal intubation. Effective basic life support prevents hypoxia and hypercapnia from contributing to the patient's depressed level of consciousness. When hypercarbia produces a depressed level of consciousness, basic airway interventions often lessen the need for endotracheal intubation as arterial carbon dioxide levels return to normal.

① Finally, all trauma patients should be presumed to have "full" stomachs and an increased risk for pulmonary aspiration of gastric contents. Assisted ventilation should be performed with volumes sufficient to provide chest rise. Some clinicians will apply cricoid pressure, although the efficacy of this maneuver is controversial.

② Cervical spine injury is presumed in any trauma patient complaining of neck pain, or with any significant head injury, neurological signs or symptoms suggestive of cervical spine injury, or intoxication or loss of consciousness. The application of a cervical collar ("C-collar") before transport to protect the cervical spinal cord will limit the degree of cervical extension that is ordinarily expected for direct laryngoscopy and tracheal intubation. Alternative devices (eg, videolaryngoscopes, fiberoptic bronchoscopes) should be immediately available. The front portion of the C-collar can be removed to facilitate tracheal intubation as long as the head and neck are maintained in neutral position by a designated assistant maintaining manual in-line stabilization.

Alternative devices for airway management (eg, esophageal–tracheal Combitube, King supralaryngeal device) may be used if direct laryngoscopy has failed, or in the prehospital environment. These devices, blindly placed into the airway, isolate the glottic opening between a large inflatable cuff positioned at the base of the tongue and a distal cuff that most likely rests in the proximal esophagus (**Figure 39–1**). The prolonged presence of these devices in the airway has been associated with glossal engorgement resulting from the large, proximal cuff obstructing venous outflow from the tongue, and in some cases, tongue engorgement has been sufficiently severe to warrant tracheostomy prior to their removal. There is limited evidence that prehospital airway management in trauma patients improves patient outcomes; however, failed tracheal intubation in the prehospital environment certainly exposes patients to significant morbidity.

Airway management of the trauma patient is uneventful in most circumstances, and

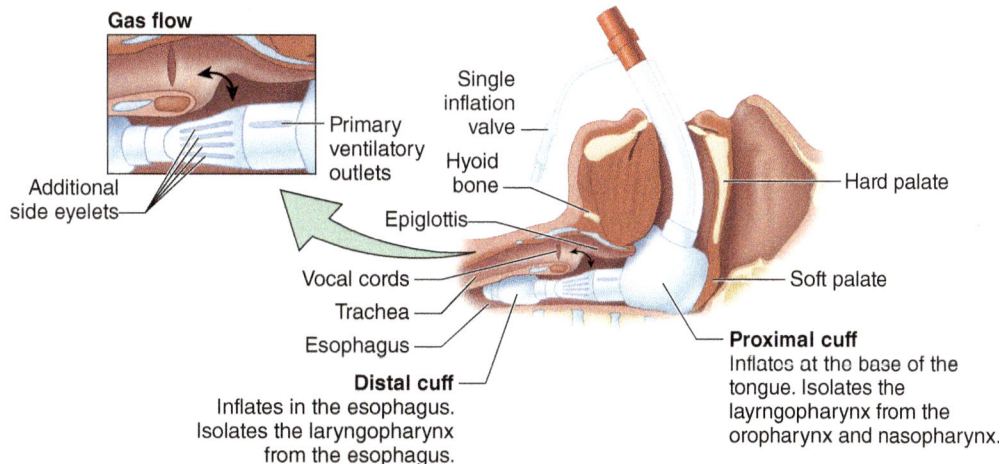

FIGURE 39–1 The King LT supralaryngeal device. The glottic opening lies between the large cuff positioned at the base of the tongue and the smaller balloon positioned in the proximal esophagus. The airway is not secured but rather isolated between the oropharynx and the proximal esophagus. (Reproduced, with permission, from King Systems Corporation, KLTD/KLTSD Disposable Supralaryngeal Airways Inservice Program, August 23, 2006, with permission.)

cricothyroidotomy or tracheostomy is rarely required to secure the trauma airway. When trauma significantly alters or distorts the facial or upper airway anatomy to the point of impeding adequate mask ventilation, or when hemorrhage into the airway precludes the patient from lying supine, elective cricothyroidotomy or tracheostomy should be considered before any attempts are made to anesthetize or administer neuromuscular blocking agents to the patient for orotracheal intubation.

Breathing

3 In the multiple-injury patient, providers should maintain a high level of suspicion for pulmonary injury that could evolve into a tension pneumothorax when mechanical ventilation is initiated. Attention must be paid to peak inspiratory pressure and tidal volumes throughout the initial resuscitation. Pulmonary injury may not be immediately apparent upon the patient's arrival at the hospital, and abrupt cardiovascular collapse shortly after instituting mechanical ventilation may announce the presence of a pneumothorax. This should be managed by disconnecting the patient from mechanical ventilation and performing bilateral needle thoracostomy (accomplished by inserting a 14-gauge intravenous catheter into the second interspace in the midclavicular line), and then by thoracostomy tube insertion. Inspired oxygen concentrations of 100% are used routinely in this early phase of resuscitation.

Circulation

During the primary trauma patient survey, signs of a pulse and blood pressure are sought. Unless the trauma patient arrives at the hospital other than by ambulance, the resuscitation team will likely have received information about the patient's vital signs from the prehospital personnel (emergency medical technicians, flight nurses). The absence of a pulse following trauma is associated with dismal chances of survival. The ACS Committee on Trauma no longer endorses the use of emergency thoracotomy in treating patients without blood pressure or palpable pulse following *blunt* trauma, even in the presence of organized cardiac activity, given the lack of evidence supporting survival following this intervention.

Retrospective review of emergency thoracotomy in Europe failed to demonstrate resuscitation benefit of this procedure following either blunt or penetrating trauma in the setting of cardiac arrest. In the setting of chest trauma without detectable blood pressure or palpable pulse, current practice supports reserving resuscitative thoracotomy for patients who experience *penetrating* trauma and have preserved, organized cardiac rhythms or other signs of life.

In light of these recommendations, prompt placement of bilateral chest tubes and administration of a 500–1000 mL fluid bolus should be implemented in the pulseless victim of penetrating trauma. If return of spontaneous circulation does not occur promptly, more aggressive interventions are not indicated and resuscitation efforts can be terminated.

Neurological Function

Once the presence of circulation is confirmed, a brief neurological examination is conducted. Level of consciousness, pupillary size and reaction, lateralizing signs suggesting intracranial or extracranial injuries, and indications of spinal cord injury are quickly evaluated. As noted earlier, hypercarbia often causes depressed neurological responsiveness following trauma; it is effectively corrected with basic life support interventions. Additional causes of depressed neurological function—eg, alcohol intoxication, effects of illicit or prescribed medications, hypoglycemia, hypoperfusion, or brain or spinal injury—must also be addressed. Mechanisms of injury must be considered as well as exclusion of other factors in determining the risk for central nervous system trauma. Persistently depressed levels of consciousness should be considered a result of central nervous system injury until disproved by diagnostic studies.

Injury Assessment: Minimizing Risks of Exposure

The patient must be fully exposed and examined in order to adequately assess the extent of injury, and this physical exposure increases the risk of hypothermia. The presence of shock and intravenous fluid therapy also place the trauma patient at great risk for developing hypothermia. As a result, the resuscitation bay must be maintained at near body temperature, all fluids should be warmed during administration, and the use of forced air patient warmers, either below or covering the patient, should be utilized.

RESUSCITATION

Hemorrhage

Certain trauma-related terminology must be understood and utilized in order to effectively communicate with surgeons during trauma resuscitations or surgeries in which blood loss is occurring. *Hemorrhage classifications I–IV, damage control resuscitation*, and *damage control surgery* are terms that quickly convey critical information between surgeons and anesthesia personnel, ensuring a common understanding of the various interventions that may be required to resuscitate a trauma or surgical patient experiencing bleeding. The ACS identifies four classes of hemorrhage. Understanding this classification scheme promotes more effective communication between surgeons and anesthesiologists.

Class I hemorrhage is the volume of blood that can be lost without hemodynamic consequence. The heart rate does not change and the blood pressure does not decrease in response to losing this volume of blood. In most circumstances, this volume represents less than 15% of circulating blood volume. The typical adult has a blood volume equivalent to 70 mL/kg. A 70-kg adult can be presumed to have nearly 5 L of circulating blood. Children are considered to have 80 mL/kg and infants, 90 mL/kg blood volume. Intravenous fluid is not required if the bleeding is controlled, as in brief, controlled bleeding encountered during an elective surgical procedure.

Class II hemorrhage is the volume of blood, that, when lost, prompts sympathetic responses to maintain perfusion; this usually represents 15–30% of circulating blood volume. The diastolic blood pressure will increase (a reflection of vasoconstriction) and the heart rate will increase to maintain cardiac output. Intravenous fluid or colloid is usually indicated for blood loss of this volume. Transfusions may be required if bleeding continues, suggesting progression to class III hemorrhage.

Class III hemorrhage represents the volume of blood loss (30–40% of circulating blood volume) that consistently results in decreased blood pressure. Compensatory mechanisms of vasoconstriction and tachycardia are not sufficient to maintain perfusion and meet the metabolic demands of the body. Metabolic acidosis will be detected on arterial blood gas analysis. Blood transfusions are necessary to restore tissue perfusion and provide oxygen to tissues. The patient may transiently respond to fluid boluses given in response to hemorrhage; however, if bleeding persists or given time for the fluid bolus to redistribute, the blood pressure will decline. Surgeons should be advised when this pattern persists, particularly during elective surgical cases where the development of shock is not expected. Class III hemorrhage may prompt an intervention such as a damage control procedure (see below).

Class IV hemorrhage represents life-threatening hemorrhage. When more than 40% of circulating blood volume is lost, the patient will be unresponsive and profoundly hypotensive. Rapid control of bleeding and aggressive blood-based resuscitation (ie, damage control resuscitation) will be required to prevent death. Patients experiencing this degree of hemorrhage will likely develop a trauma-induced coagulopathy, require massive blood transfusion, and experience a high likelihood of death.

Trauma-Induced Coagulopathy

Coagulation abnormalities are common following major trauma, and trauma-induced coagulopathy is

4 an independent risk factor for death. Recent prospective clinical studies suggest that in up to 25% of major trauma patients, trauma-induced coagulopathy is present shortly after injury and before any resuscitative efforts have been initiated. In one report, acute traumatic coagulopathy was only related to the presence of a severe metabolic acidosis (base deficit ≥6 mEq/L) and appeared to have a dose-dependent relationship with the degree of tissue hypoperfusion; 2% of patients with base deficits less than 6 mEq/L developed coagulopathy compared with 20% of patients with base deficits greater than 6 mEq/L. Although injury severity scores were likely high in those developing coagulopathy, only the

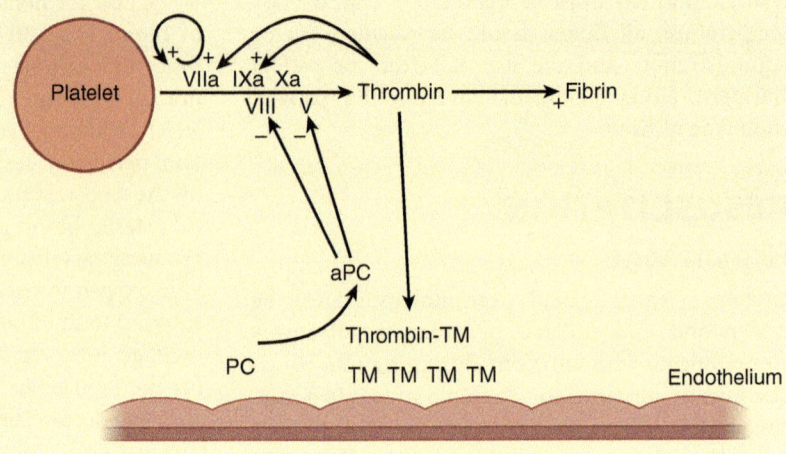

Thrombin is generated primarily via the 'extrinsic' pathway with multiple feed-forward loops. When thrombomodulin (TM) is presented by the endothelium, it complexes thrombin which is no longer available to cleave fibrinogen. This anticoagulent thrombin activates protein C which reduces further thrombin generation through inhibition of cofactors V and VIII.

FIGURE 39–2 Mechanism of trauma-induced coagulopathy. During periods of tissue hypoperfusion, thrombomodulin (TM) released by the endothelium complexes with thrombin. The thrombin–TM complexes prevent cleavage of fibrinogen to fibrin and also activate protein C (PC), reducing further thrombin generation through cofactors V and VIII. (Reproduced, with permission, from Brohi K, Cohen MJ, Davenport RA: Acute coagulopathy of trauma: mechanism, identification and effect. Curr Opin Crit Care 2007;13:680.)

presence of the metabolic acidosis correlated to developing trauma-induced coagulopathy.

Global tissue hypoperfusion appears to have a key role in the development of trauma-induced coagulopathy. During hypoperfusion, the endothelium releases thrombomodulin and activated protein C to prevent microcirculation thrombosis. Thrombomodulin binds thrombin, thereby preventing thrombin from cleaving fibrinogen to fibrin. The thrombomodulin–thrombin complex activates protein C, which then inhibits the extrinsic coagulation pathway through effects on cofactors V and VIII (Figure 39–2). Activated protein C also inhibits plasminogen activator inhibitor-1 proteins, which increases tissue plasminogen activator, resulting in hyperfibrinolysis (Figure 39–3). One prospective clinical study found the following effects of hypoperfusion on coagulation parameters: (1) progressive coagulopathy as base deficit increases; (2) increasing plasma thrombomodulin and falling protein C (indicating activation of the protein levels with increasing base deficit), supporting the argument that the anticoagulant effects of these proteins in the presence of hypoperfusion are related to the prolongation of prothrombin and partial thromboplastin times; and (3) an influence of early trauma-induced coagulopathy on mortality.

Trauma-induced coagulopathy is not solely related to impaired clot formation. Fibrinolysis is an equally important component as a result of plasmin activity on an existing clot. Tranexamic acid administration is associated with decreased bleeding during cardiac and orthopedic surgeries, presumably because of its antifibrinolytic properties. A randomized control study involving 20,000 trauma patients with or at risk of significant bleeding found a significantly reduced risk for death from hemorrhage when tranexamic acid therapy (loading dose, 1 g over 10 min followed by an infusion of 1 g over 8 h) was initiated within the first 3 h following major trauma. Figure 39–4 demonstrates the benefit of initiating this therapy in relation to the time of injury.

Hemostatic Resuscitation

Early coagulopathy of trauma is associated with increased mortality. Administering blood products in equal ratios early in resuscitation has become an accepted approach to correction of trauma-induced coagulopathy. This balanced approach to transfusion, 1:1:1 (red blood cell:fresh

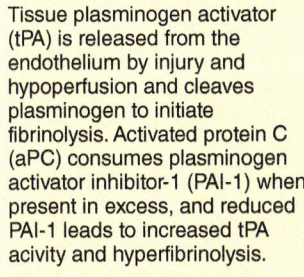
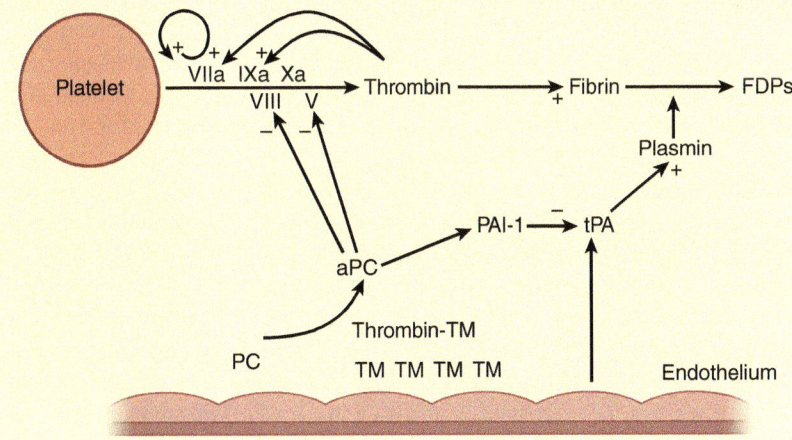

Tissue plasminogen activator (tPA) is released from the endothelium by injury and hypoperfusion and cleaves plasminogen to initiate fibrinolysis. Activated protein C (aPC) consumes plasminogen activator inhibitor-1 (PAI-1) when present in excess, and reduced PAI-1 leads to increased tPA acivity and hyperfibrinolysis.

FIGURE 39–3 Mechanism of hyperfibrinolysis in tissue hypoperfusion. Tissue plasminogen activator (tPA) released from the endothelium during hypoperfusion states cleaves plasminogen to initiate fibrinolysis. Activated protein C (aPC) consumes plasminogen activator inhibitor-1 (PAI-1) when present in excess, and reduced PAI-1 leads to increased tPA activity and hyperfibrinolysis. FDPs, fibrin degradation products; PC, protein C; TM, thrombomodulin. (Reproduced, with permission, from Brohi K, Cohen MJ, Davenport RA: Acute coagulopathy of trauma: Mechanism, identification and effect. Curr Opin Crit Care 2007;13:680.)

frozen plasma:platelet), is termed *damage control resuscitation.* Although the 1:1:1 combination attempts to replicate whole blood, it results in a pancytopenic solution with only a fraction of whole blood's hematocrit and coagulation factor concentration. Red blood cells will over time improve oxygen delivery to ischemic, hypoperfused tissues. Fresh frozen plasma provides clotting factors V and VIII along with fibrinogen, which improves clotting, possibly due to overwhelming of the thrombin–thrombomodulin complex. Platelets and cryoprecipitate, although included in the 1:1:1 massive

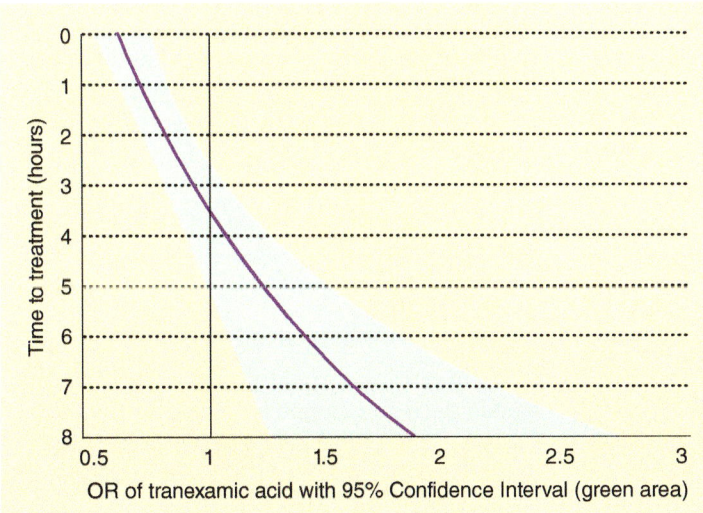

FIGURE 39–4 Influence of tranexamic acid in preventing death from bleeding. Outcomes ratios (OR) of tranexamic acid with 95% confidence interval (*green area*) on the *x*-axis and time (h) to treatment on the *y*-axis demonstrate improved survival if tranexamic acid therapy is initiated within 3 h of injury. The area of the curve to the left of OR 1.0 demonstrates the benefits of therapy, while that to the right demonstrates harm from intervention. (Reproduced, with permission, from Roberts I, Shakur H, Afolabi A, et al: The importance of early treatment with tranexamic acid in bleeding trauma patients: An exploratory analysis of the CRASH-2 randomised controlled trial. Lancet 2011;377:1096.)

transfusion protocol, are probably not necessary in the initial phase of resuscitation, given the normal platelet and fibrinogen levels noted in early coagulopathy. Additional platelet transfusions may be beneficial if the resuscitation is prolonged, as is typical for most major trauma resuscitations, or if a recalcitrant coagulopathy is noted with coagulation studies. The use of crystalloid fluids in early trauma resuscitation has markedly decreased with the increased emphasis upon early blood product administration.

Most trauma centers have early-release type O-negative blood available for immediate transfusion to patients with severe hemorrhage. Depending on the urgency of need for transfusion, administration of blood products typically progresses from O-negative to type-specific, then to crossmatched units as the acute need decreases. Patients administered uncrossmatched O-negative blood are those deemed at high risk of requiring massive transfusion. As the amount of uncrossmatched blood administered increases beyond 8 units, attempts to return to the patient's native blood type should not be pursued and type O blood should be continued until the patient is stabilized.

Military experience treating combat-wounded soldiers and civilians has provided great insight into trauma resuscitation and trauma-induced coagulopathy. As the use of blood and blood products has evolved, the 1:1:1 transfusion ratio has been uniformly adopted to address the frequent incidence of trauma-induced coagulopathy. Retrospective analysis of severely wounded solders found improved survival when this transfusion protocol was utilized. Consequently, hemostatic resuscitation has been rapidly adopted by civilian trauma centers, which have reported similar survival benefits for civilian patients with severe trauma. Nevertheless, using traditional definitions, this approach is not "evidence based" from randomized clinical trials.

Using hemostatic resuscitation (ie, damage control resuscitation), blood and blood products are administered preemptively to address a presumed coagulopathy. Often coagulation status is not assessed until the patient stabilizes. Although this treatment approach appears to be effective in controlling trauma-induced coagulopathy, patients

requiring this therapy may be exposed to unnecessary additional units of blood or blood products. An alternative approach that relies on thromboelastography (TEG) may allow more goal-directed transfusion of blood and blood products and is increasingly utilized in trauma resuscitations. The formation and stability of a clot represents interactions between the coagulation cascades, platelets, and the fibrinolytic system, all of which can be demonstrated with TEG (Figure 39–5). As TEG use during trauma resuscitation becomes more routine, the current 1:1:1 hemostatic resuscitation ratio will likely undergo modification to proportionately less fresh frozen plasma, and the use of antifibrinolytic therapy will likely increase.

Administration of blood products must be done with consideration for potential hazards that may result from transfusion. Although blood-borne diseases such as acquired immunodeficiency syndrome, hepatitis B, and hepatitis C are usually thought of as the highest transfusion-related risks, the incidence of such infections has decreased 10,000-fold due to better screening tests of donors and donated units (see Chapter 51). Noninfectious transfusion reactions are now the leading complication of transfusion and represent a more than 10-fold greater risk than blood-borne infection. Transfusion-related acute lung injury (TRALI) is the leading cause of transfusion-related death reported to the U.S. Food and Drug Administration. However, although the bleeding trauma patient is at risk for a transfusion-related reaction, that risk is minimal compared with the far greater likelihood of death from exsanguination. The most prudent approach for blood product utilization in the bleeding trauma patient is to administer the blood products that are necessary, based on laboratory studies, clinical evidence of significant bleeding, and the degree of hemodynamic instability that can be directly attributed to hemorrhage.

Massive Transfusion Protocols

Delay in obtaining blood products other than red blood cells is common in both civilian and military settings. Clinical evidence supports the need for, and benefit of, established massive transfusion protocols (MTPs), allowing the blood bank to assemble blood

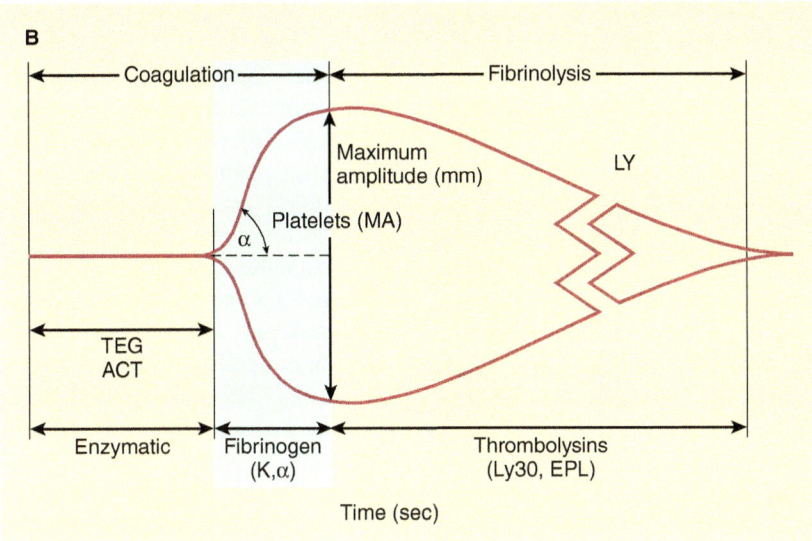

FIGURE 39–5 Thromboelastograph (TEG). The graph begins as a straight line until clot formation begins (the enzymatic stage of clotting). As a clot forms, increasing resistance develops on the strain gauge, creating a splaying of the graph. The pattern of the graph suggests the status of fibrinogen stores (α angle) and platelet function (maximum amplitude, MA). Eventually, fibrinolysis will occur as demonstrated by decreasing MA.

Deficiencies of various clotting components will affect each phase of the TEG whereas increased fibrinolysis will be demonstrated by an earlier decline in the maximum amplitude. ACT, activated clotting time; EPL, Ly30, K, R, values related to rate of clot breakdown. (Reproduced, with permission, from Kashuk JL, Moore EE, Sawyer M, et al: Postinjury coagulopathy management: Goal directed resuscitation via POC thrombelastography. Ann Surg 2010;251:604.)

products in prescribed ratios to support hemostatic resuscitation. With MTPs in place, hemostatic resuscitation can continue until the demand for blood products stops. An MTP-driven, blood-based resuscitation, rather than a crystalloid-based resuscitation, improves survival from trauma, reduces total blood product utilization in the first 24 h following injury, reduces acute infectious complications (severe sepsis, septic shock, and ventilator-associated pneumonia), and decreases postresuscitation organ dysfunction (an 80% decrease in odds of developing multisystem organ failure).

It is important to establish which personnel are empowered to invoke use of the MTP, given the expense and implications for the blood bank in terms of blood inventory, personnel training and availability, and disruption of routine blood bank duties. Establishing an MTP benefits both the patient, through improved survival and fewer complications, and the institution, through more efficient and effective processes for utilizing critical blood bank resources.

Initiating an MTP for all trauma patients is impractical; however, delaying request for an MTP until the patient has undergone a thorough trauma evaluation may increase the risk of morbidity and mortality. The *assessment of blood consumption* (ABC) score is an attempt to predict which patients are likely to require an MTP. The ABC score assigns 1 point for the presence of each of four possible variables: (1) penetrating injury; (2) systolic blood pressure less than 90 mmHg; (3) heart rate greater than 120 beats per minute; and (4) positive results of a *focused assessment with sonography for trauma* (FAST) evaluation. The FAST evaluation is a bedside ultrasonography screening examination performed by surgeons and emergency department physicians to assess the presence or absence of free fluid in the perihepatic and perisplenic spaces, pericardium, and pelvis.

Patients with ABC scores of 2 or higher are likely to require massive transfusion. This scoring system has been validated in multiple level 1 trauma centers and is now relatively commonplace in trauma evaluations.

DEFINITIVE TRAUMA INTERVENTIONS

The physical examination, emergency procedures, and evaluations used to determine the extent of injury, need for an MTP, and surgical intervention all occur outside the operating room. The decision to proceed to the operating room may be the first point in the trauma resuscitation process at which an anesthesiologist is involved. Key issues in the anesthetic management of trauma patients include the need to avoid vasopressors and minimize crystalloid infusions until bleeding is controlled. Blood products are the fluids of choice for trauma resuscitation.

Anesthetic Induction & Maintenance

Conscious and oriented trauma patients arriving for emergent surgery should have an abbreviated interview and examination, including emphasis on consent for blood transfusions and advice that intraoperative awareness may occur during emergency surgery. This discussion should be documented in the patient's record.

The operating room should be as warm as is practical. Intravenous fluid warmers and rapid infusion devices should be used. All patients arriving for trauma surgery should be presumed to have full stomachs and thus to be at increased risk for aspiration. As noted earlier, the presence of a C-collar may increase the difficulty of intubation. Accordingly, robust suction equipment and alternative airway devices (eg, fiberoptic bronchoscopes, videolaryngoscopes) should be immediately available for use.

Intravenous access is usually established in the prehospital setting or in the emergency department. If the existing peripheral intravenous lines are of sufficient caliber and quality for infusing blood under pressure (ie, a 16-gauge or 14-gauge catheter), a central line is usually not necessary for the initial surgical intervention. Patients may arrive in the operating room so profoundly hypotensive and hypovolemic

that peripheral intravenous access is impossible. In this circumstance, a subclavian or an intraosseous catheter should be inserted and blood-based resuscitation initiated. The subclavian vein is often preferred for central venous access in profoundly hypotensive patients owing to its position between the first rib and the clavicle, which tends to stent the vein open. An intraosseous catheter is usually seated into the bone marrow of the proximal tibia or humerus, a process that is facilitated by use of a bone drilling device. Use of intraosseous access requires that the bone distal to the intraosseous catheter to be intact; otherwise; extravasation of infused fluid through the fracture site, the path of least resistance, will occur. A pressure bag must be used for infusing any fluid through the intraosseous catheter due to resistance to passive flow from the bone marrow, although the intraosseous space is intimately connected with the venous system and transfused blood readily enters the central circulation via this route.

Major blood loss and hemodynamic instability create a dangerous situation for the conscious trauma patient and a challenging decision for the anesthesiologist planning the induction of general anesthesia. Trauma patients with severe injuries are poor candidates for induction with propofol, given the likelihood of profound hypotension following even modest doses (0.25–0.5 mg/kg intravenously). Etomidate preserves sympathetic tone, which makes it a modestly safer choice than propofol. Ketamine is also a reasonable choice, particularly if given in 10-mg intravenous boluses until the patient becomes unresponsive. Scopolamine, 0.4 mg intravenously, should be considered as an amnestic agent for the hemodynamically unstable but conscious patient at high risk for hemodynamic collapse on induction of anesthesia who arrives in the operating room for emergency surgery. What is most important is not the particular intravenous anesthetic induction agent chosen, but recognition that the hemodynamically unstable trauma patient will require significantly less anesthetic medication than in normal circumstances.

An arterial line will be helpful but insertion may prove difficult in the hypotensive, hypoperfused trauma patient. Attempts at placing invasive monitors can continue as the patient is prepped for surgery and the surgeon begins the operation. If halted, attention should focus on transfusion-related efforts.

Damage Control Surgery

If the trauma patient requires emergent laparotomy for intraabdominal hemorrhage, the trauma surgeon will perform an abbreviated procedure termed *damage control surgery* (DCS), which is intended to stop hemorrhage and limit gastrointestinal contamination of the abdominal compartment. After making a midline incision, the surgeon quickly searches for sources of bleeding through a quadrant-by-quadrant examination. Communication between the surgeon and the anesthesiologist is essential in DCS; the surgeon must know if the patient is becoming unstable, hypothermic, or coagulopathic in spite of ongoing resuscitation during the operative procedure. The surgeon will usually compress or pack the area of bleeding if the patient is hypotensive, an intervention that usually improves hemodynamics by slowing hemorrhage and allowing more rapid restoration of circulating blood volume. If direct compression of the hemorrhaging intraabdominal tissue fails to improve hemodynamic stability, the surgeon can also slow the rate of hemorrhage by compressing the aorta. Compression of the aorta also provides tactile information to the surgeon. Particularly in circumstances where invasive arterial monitoring was not accomplished, the surgeon's fingers on the aortic pulse can provide useful information regarding volume status: a soft, compressible aorta represents profound hypovolemia, whereas a firm, pulsatile aorta suggests more normal volume status.

Definitive repair of complex injuries is not part of DCS. Identification and control of injured blood vessels and solid organs, as well as inspection of injuries in areas relatively inaccessible to midline approaches (eg, deep liver lacerations, retroperitoneal hemorrhage) but potentially amenable to interventional radiology techniques, occurs during DCS laparotomy. Hollow viscus injuries are addressed with resection or stapling, or both, to prevent abdominal contamination, often leaving the intestines disconnected until the patient is more stable. At that later time, bowel continuity can be restored or colostomy can be performed. At any time during

DCS, if the patient becomes unstable or profoundly hypothermic, or if transfusions are insufficient in maintaining perfusion, the operation should be interrupted, the bleeding areas packed, and a decision should be made as to whether the patient can be transferred to the interventional radiology suite to treat bleeding from surgically inaccessible sites or transferred to the intensive care unit to allow warming, treatment of hemodynamic or hemostatic abnormalities, and continuation of resuscitation.

The interventional radiology suite is increasingly utilized as part of the DCS sequence, because interventional radiology techniques can reach essentially any bleeding vessel and deposit coils or foam to control hemorrhage. Most notably, liver, kidney, and retroperitoneal injuries, pelvic ring fractures, and major thoracic and abdominal vascular injuries are potentially controlled by interventional radiology procedures. Following DCS, trauma patients will frequently be transferred to the interventional radiology suite to assess blood flow and hemostasis of organs either injured by the initial trauma or potentially compromised as part of the DCS.

TRAUMATIC BRAIN INJURY

8 Any trauma patient with altered level of consciousness must be considered to have a traumatic brain injury (TBI) until proven otherwise (see Chapter 27). The presence or suspicion of a TBI mandates attention to maintaining cerebral perfusion and arterial oxygenation during all aspects of care. The most reliable clinical assessment tool in determining the significance of TBI in a nonsedated, nonparalyzed patient is the Glasgow coma scale (GCS, Table 27–2). A declining motor score is suggestive of progressing neurological deterioration, prompting urgent neurosurgical evaluation and possible surgical intervention. Although trauma patients frequently have head injuries, few head injuries require emergent neurosurgical intervention.

TBIs are categorized as either *primary* or *secondary*. Primary brain injuries are usually focal injuries directly related to trauma, disrupting normal anatomy or physiology, or both. Four categories of primary brain injury are seen: (1) subdural hematoma; (2) epidural hematoma; (3) intraparenchymal hemorrhage; and (4) nonfocal, diffuse neuronal injury disrupting axons of the central nervous system. These injuries potentially compromise cerebral blood flow and elevate intracranial pressure (ICP). Death occurring soon after significant head trauma is usually a result of the primary brain injury.

9 **Acute subdural hematoma** is the most common condition warranting emergency neurosurgery and is associated with the highest mortality. Small bridging veins between the skull and brain are disrupted in deceleration or blunt force injuries, resulting in blood accumulation and compression of brain tissue. The accumulation of blood raises ICP and compromises cerebral blood flow. Morbidity and mortality are related to the size of the hematoma and magnitude of the midline shift of intracranial contents. Midline shifts of intracranial contents may exceed the size of the hematoma, suggesting a significant contribution of cerebral edema. Acute subdural hematomas should be surgically evacuated, particularly in patients with elevated ICP.

Epidural hematoma occurs when the middle cerebral artery or other cranial vessels are disrupted, most often in association with a skull fracture. This injury accounts for less than 10% of neurosurgical emergencies and has a much better prognosis than acute subdural hematoma. The patient with an epidural hematoma may initially be consciousness, followed by progressive unresponsiveness and coma. Emergent surgical decompression is indicated when supratentorial lesions occupy more than 30 mL volume and infratentorial lesions occupy more than 10 mL volume (brainstem compression may occur at much lower hematoma volumes). A small epidural hematoma may not require immediate evacuation if the patient is neurologically intact, if close observation and repeated neurological examinations are possible, and if neurosurgical resources are available should emergent decompression become necessary.

Intraparenchymal injuries are caused by rapid deceleration of the brain within the skull, usually involving the tips of the frontal or temporal lobes. They represent nearly 20% of neurosurgical emergencies following trauma. These injuries tend to be associated with significant edema, necrosis, and infarcts in the tissue surrounding the damaged tissue. Intraparenchymal injury may coexist with a subdural hematoma. There is no consensus regarding the surgical interventions that should be performed for intraparenchymal hemorrhage, but surgical decompression may be necessary to reduce dangerously sustained increased ICP.

Diffuse neuronal injury results from events resulting in rapid deceleration or movement of the brain tissue of sufficient force to disrupt neurons and axons. This form of brain injury is more common in children than in adults. The extent of the injury may not be obvious in the period soon after injury but will become apparent with serial clinical and radiographic (magnetic resonance imaging) examinations. The greater the extent of diffuse neuronal injury following trauma, the higher will be the mortality and severe disability. Surgical interventions are not indicated for these injuries unless a decompressive craniectomy is required for relief of refractory elevated ICP (see below).

Secondary brain injuries are considered potentially preventable injuries. Systemic hypotension (systolic blood pressures <90 mm Hg), hypoxemia (Pao_2 <60 mm Hg), hypercapnia ($Paco_2$ >50 mm Hg), and hyperthermia (temperature >38.0°C) have a negative impact on morbidity and mortality following head injuries, likely because of their contributions to increasing cerebral edema and ICP. Hypotension and hypoxia are recognized as major contributors to poor neurological recovery from severe TBI. Hypoxia is the single most important parameter correlating to poor neurological outcomes following head trauma and should be corrected at the earliest possible opportunity. Hypotension (mean arterial blood pressure <60 mm Hg) should also be treated aggressively, using fluid or vasopressors, or both, to assure cerebral perfusion.

Management Considerations

A. Intracranial Pressure

In the absence of a clot requiring evacuation, medical interventions are the primary means of treating elevated ICP following head trauma.

Normal cerebral perfusion pressure (CPP), the difference between mean arterial pressure (MAP, discussed in Chapter 26) and ICP (ie, MAP − ICP = CPP), is approximately 80–100 mm Hg. ICP monitoring is not required for conscious and alert patients; in addition, patients who are intentionally anticoagulated or who have bleeding diathesis in response to trauma should not have ICP monitoring. However, an ICP monitor should be placed when serial neurological examinations and additional clinical assessments reveal impairment, or when there is an increased risk for elevated ICP (Table 39–1). Interventions to reduce ICP are indicated when readings are higher than 20–25 mm Hg. Although multiple studies have evaluated interventions aimed at improving CPP and managing ICP without finding obvious outcomes benefit for any treatment scheme, current Brain Trauma Foundation guidelines recommend maintaining CPP between 50 and 70 mm Hg and ICP at less than 20 mm Hg for patients with severe head injury.

TABLE 39–1 **Indications for intracranial ICP monitoring.**[1,2]

Severe head injury (defined as GCS score ≤8 after cardiopulmonary resuscitation) *plus*   (a) Abnormal admitting head CT scan *or*   (b) Normal CT scan plus ≥2 of: age >40 y, systolic blood pressure >90 mm Hg, decerebrate or decorticate position
Sedated patients; patient in induced coma after severe TBI
Multisystem injury with altered level of consciousness
Patient receiving treatment that increases risk of increased ICP, eg, high-volume IV fluids
Postoperatively after removal or intracranial mass
Abnormal values in noninvasive ICP monitoring, increased dynamics of simulated values, or abnormal shapes in transcranial Doppler blood flow velocity waveform (increased pulsatility) with exclusion of arterial hypotension and hypocapnia

[1]ICP, intracranial pressure; GCS, Glasgow Coma Scale; CT, computed tomographic; TBI, traumatic brain injury.

[2]Reproduced, with permission, from Li LM, Timofeev I, Czosnyka M, et al: Review article: The surgical approach to the management of increased intracranial pressure after traumatic brain injury. Anesth Analg 2010;111:736.

Cerebral blood flow is related to arterial carbon dioxide concentration in a dose-dependent relationship. As arterial carbon dioxide levels decrease, cerebral vasoconstriction occurs, reducing ICP. Conversely, as arterial carbon dioxide levels rise, cerebral vasodilation occurs, increasing ICP. Changes in arterial carbon dioxide levels exert a prompt cerebral blood flow and ICP response, making hyperventilation an effective intervention when brain herniation is suspected or proven. However, this intervention must be appreciated in the context of TBI: hyperventilation in the presence of systemic hypotension increases the risk of neurological ischemia and should be avoided in the early stages of resuscitation for patients with TBI.

Osmotic diuretic therapy is another commonly used and widely accepted method for reducing elevated ICP. Intravenous mannitol doses of 0.25–1.0 g/kg body weight are effective in drawing extravascular fluid from brain tissue into the vascular system. As extravascular fluid is drawn into the vascular system, brain edema and ICP will decrease. Because this intervention is very effective for inducing brisk diuresis, serum osmolarity and electrolytes (particularly potassium) must be monitored.

Barbiturate coma is an intervention that attempts to decrease cerebral metabolic rate, cerebral blood flow, and cerebral oxygen demand in order to reduce elevated ICP and suppress the metabolic rate of ischemic cells until cerebral perfusion improves. Hypotension is commonly associated with this therapy, which should limit its use in the hemodynamically unstable patient. Vasopressors may be used in order to maintain CPP between 50 and 70 mm Hg. The pentobarbital dose administered is based upon electroencephalographic evidence of burst suppression in order to maximally reduce the cerebral metabolic rate of oxygen.

B. Severe TBI & Multiple Trauma

The presence of a severe head injury in the presence of other major traumatic injuries and ongoing hemorrhage creates a situation in which patient management goals may conflict. As noted above, in the head-injured patient requiring emergent decompression, mean blood pressures must be maintained between 50 and 70 mmHg to assure adequate CPP and prevention of secondary ischemic neurological injuries. In patients without brain injury, hemorrhage is usually treated with a more hypotensive goal until bleeding is controlled. Deference is paid to the most life-threatening condition as the priority intervention with the expectation that CPP be maintained throughout, even if this approach results in greater transfusion requirements.

SPINAL CORD INJURY

The normal spine comprises three columns: anterior, middle, and posterior. The anterior column includes the anterior two thirds of the vertebral body and the anterior longitudinal ligament. The middle column includes the posterior third of the vertebral body, the posterior longitudinal ligament, and the posterior component of the annulus fibrosis. The posterior column includes the laminae and facets, the spinous processes, and the interspinous ligaments. Spine instability results when two or more of the three columns are disrupted. The trauma patient with a relevant mechanism of injury (typically blunt force involving acceleration–deceleration) must be approached with a high degree of suspicion for spine injury unless it has been ruled out radiographically.

A lateral radiograph of the cervical spine demonstrating the entire cervical spine to the top of the T1 vertebra will detect 85–90% of significant cervical spine abnormalities. Cervical spine radiographs should be examined for the appearance and alignment of the vertebral bodies, narrowing or widening of interspinous spaces and the central canal, alignment along the anterior and posterior ligament lines, and appearance of the spinolaminar line and posterior spinous processes of C2 through C7. The presence of one spinal fracture is associated with a 10–15% incidence of a second spinal fracture.

Thoracolumbar injuries most commonly involve the T11 through L3 vertebrae as a result of flexion forces. The presence of one thoracolumbar spinal injury is associated with a 40% chance of a second fracture caudal to the first, likely due to the force required to fracture the lower spine. Bilateral calcaneus fractures also warrant a thorough thoracolumbar spine evaluation due to the increased incidence of associated spinal fractures associated with this injury pattern.

Cervical spine injuries occurring above C2 are associated with apnea and death. Lesions of C3–5 impact phrenic nerve function, impairing diaphragmatic breathing. High spinal injuries are often accompanied by neurogenic shock due to loss of sympathetic tone. Neurogenic shock may be masked initially in major trauma because hypotension may be attributed to a hemorrhagic, rather than a neurologic, cause. The presence of profound bradycardia 24–48 h after a high thoracic spinal cord lesion likely represents compromise of the cardioaccelerator function found in the T1–4 region.

The principal therapeutic objectives following spinal cord injury are to prevent exacerbation of the primary structural injury and to minimize the risk of extending neurological injury from hypotension-related hypoperfusion of ischemic areas of the spinal cord. In patients with complete spinal cord transection, very few interventions will influence recovery. In patients with incomplete spinal cord lesions, careful management of hemodynamic parameters and surgical stabilization of the spine are critical in preventing extension of the existing injury.

Methylprednisolone is often administered for spinal cord injury to reduce spinal cord edema in the tight confines of the spinal canal, although there is scant evidence that this intervention improves outcomes following spinal cord injury in humans. While not considered a standard of care, it is included in the current clinical recommendations of the American Association of Neurological Surgeons as a treatment option. Maintaining supranormal mean arterial blood pressures to assure spinal cord perfusion in areas of reduced blood flow due to cord compression or vascular compromise is likely to be of more benefit than steroid administration. Hypotension must be avoided during induction of anesthesia and throughout surgical decompression and stabilization of a spinal injury.

Surgical decompression and stabilization of spinal fractures are indicated when a vertebral body loses more than 50% of its normal height or the spinal canal is narrowed by more than 30% of its normal diameter. Despite outcome studies from animal models of traumatic spinal cord injury demonstrating benefit from early surgical intervention or steroid therapy, or both, current human studies have failed to demonstrate significant benefit from either intervention. Currently, the presence of a decompressible lesion in the area of an incomplete spinal cord transection is not an indication for early operative intervention unless other, more life-threatening, conditions are present.

The elderly are at greater risk for spinal cord injury due to decreased mobility and flexibility, a higher incidence of spondylosis and osteophyte formation in the degenerative spine, and decreased intracanal space accommodating spinal cord edema following cord trauma. The incidence of spinal injury from falls in the elderly is rapidly approaching that of spinal cord injury from motor vehicle accidents in younger patients. Mortality following spinal cord injury in the elderly, particularly those over the age of 75 years, is higher than that in younger counterparts with similar injury.

The unique injury pattern of penetrating spinal cord injury warrants consideration. Unlike blunt spinal trauma, penetrating trauma of the spinal cord due to bullets and shrapnel is unlikely to induce an unstable spine. As a result, C-collar and longboard immobilization may not be indicated. In fact, C-collar placement in the presence of a cervical spine penetrating injury may hinder observation of soft tissue swelling, tracheal deviation, or other anatomic indications of imminent airway compromise. Unlike blunt trauma, penetrating injuries of the spinal cord induce damage at the moment of injury without risk of subsequent exacerbation of the injury. Like other spinal cord injuries, however, maintenance of spinal cord perfusion using supranormal mean arterial pressures is indicated until spinal cord function can be more fully evaluated.

BURNS

Burns represent a unique but common traumatic injury that is second only to motor vehicle accidents as the leading source of accidental death. Temperature and duration of heat contact determine the extent of burn injury. Children (because of a high body surface area to body mass ratio) and the elderly (whose thinner skin allows deeper burns from similar thermal insult) are at greater risk for major burn injury. The pathophysiological and hemodynamic responses to burn injuries are unique and warrant specialized burn care that can be optimally provided only at burn treatment centers, particularly when more than 20% of a patient's body surface area is involved in second- or third-degree burns. A basic understanding of burn pathophysiology and of resuscitation requirements, especially early initiation of therapies such as oxygen administration and aggressive fluid resuscitation, will improve patient survival.

Burns are classified as first, second, or third degree. *First-degree* burns are injuries that do not penetrate the epidermis (eg, sunburns and superficial thermal injuries). Fluid replacement for these burns is not necessary, and the area of first-degree burns should not be included in calculating fluid replacement requirements when extensive, more significant burns are also present. *Second-degree* burns are partial-thickness injuries (superficial or deep) that penetrate the epidermis, extend into the dermis for some depth, and are associated with blistering. Fluid replacement therapy is indicated for patients with second-degree burns when more than 20% of total body surface area (TBSA) is involved. Skin grafting also may be necessary in some cases of second-degree burns, depending upon size and location of the wounds. *Third-degree* burns are those in which the thermal injury penetrates the full thickness of the dermis. Nerves, blood vessels, lymphatic channels, and other deep structures may have been destroyed, creating a severe, but insensate, wound (although surrounding tissue may be very painful). Debridement and skin grafting are nearly always required for recovery of patients from third-degree burns.

13 Major burns (a second- or third-degree burn involving >20% TBSA) induce a unique hemodynamic response. Cardiac output declines by up to 50% within 30 minutes in response to massive vasoconstriction, inducing a state of normovolemic hypoperfusion (*burn shock*). Survival depends on restoration of circulating volume and infusion of crystalloid fluids according to recommended protocols (see below). This intense hemodynamic response may be poorly tolerated by patients with significant underlying medical conditions. If intravenous fluid therapy is provided, cardiac function returns to normal within 48 h of the injury, then typically progresses to a hyperdynamic physiology as the metabolic challenge of healing begins. Plasma volume and urine output are also reduced early on after major burn injuries.

(14) In contrast to fluid management for blunt and penetrating trauma, which discourages use of crystalloid fluids, burn fluid resuscitation emphasizes the use of crystalloids, particularly lactated Ringer's solution, in preference to albumin, hydroxyethyl starch, hypertonic saline, and blood. Following burn injuries, kidney failure is more common when hypertonic saline is used during initial fluid resuscitation, death is higher when blood is administered, and outcomes are unchanged when albumin is used in resuscitation.

Fluid resuscitation is continuous over the first 24 h following injury. Two formulas are commonly used to guide burn injury fluid resuscitation, the Parkland and the modified Brooke. Both require an understanding of the so-called *rule of nines* (**Figure 39–6**) to calculate resuscitation volumes. The (adult) *Parkland* protocol recommends 4 mL/kg/% TBSA burned to be given in the first 24 h, with half the volume given in the first 8 h and the remaining amount over the following 16 h. The (adult) *modified Brooke* protocol recommends 2 mL/kg/% TBSA, with administration of half the calculated volume beginning in the first 8 h and the remainder over the following 16 h. Both formulas use urine output as a reliable indicator of fluid resuscitation, targeting (adult) urine production of 0.5–1.0 mL/kg/h as indications of adequate circulating volume. If adult urine output exceeds 1.0 mL/kg/h, the infusion is slowed. In both protocols, an amount equal to half the volume administered in the first 24 h is infused in the second 24-h period following injury, with continued attention to maintaining adult urine output at 0.5–1.0 mL/kg/h. The formula for fluid resuscitation of children is the same as that for adults, but children weighing less than 30 kg should receive 5% dextrose in Ringer's lactate as their resuscitation fluid and target urine output should be 1.0 mL/kg/h. The target urine output for infants younger than 1 year of age is 1–2 mL/kg/h.

Management Considerations

The Parkland and modified Brooke protocols both use urine output as an indicator for adequate fluid resuscitation. However, circumstances may arise in which the volume of fluid administered exceeds the intended volumes. For example, initial fluid resuscitation volumes may be miscalculated if first-degree burns are mistakenly incorporated into the TBSA value. Prolonged use of sedatives and sedative infusions may also result in hypotension that is treated with additional fluids rather than vasoconstrictors. The phenomenon of *fluid creep* occurs when intravenous fluid therapy volumes are increased beyond intended calculations in response to various hemodynamic changes. Fluid creep is associated with abdominal compartment syndrome and pulmonary complications, which represent resuscitation morbidity.

A. Abdominal Compartment Syndrome

Abdominal compartment syndrome is a risk for pediatric patients, adults with circumferential abdominal burns, and patients receiving intravenous fluid volumes greater than 6 mL/kg/% TBSA. Intraabdominal pressure can be determined by measuring intraluminal bladder pressure using a Foley catheter. The transducer is connected to a 3-way stopcock at the point where the Foley catheter connects to the drainage tube. After the transducer is zeroed at the pelvic brim, 20 mL of fluid is instilled to distend the bladder. Intraabdominal pressure readings are taken 60 s after fluid installation, allowing the bladder to relax. Intraabdominal pressures exceeding 20 mmHg warrant abdominal cavity decompression. However, an abdominal surgical procedure places the burn patient at high risk for intraabdominal *Pseudomonas* infection, particularly if the laparotomy incision is near burned tissue.

B. Pulmonary Complications

Excessive resuscitative fluid volumes are associated with an increased incidence of pneumonia. Patients with severe burns frequently have pulmonary injury related to the burn. Decreased tracheal ciliary activity, the presence of resuscitation-induced pulmonary edema, reduced immunocompetence, and tracheal intubation predispose the burn patient to

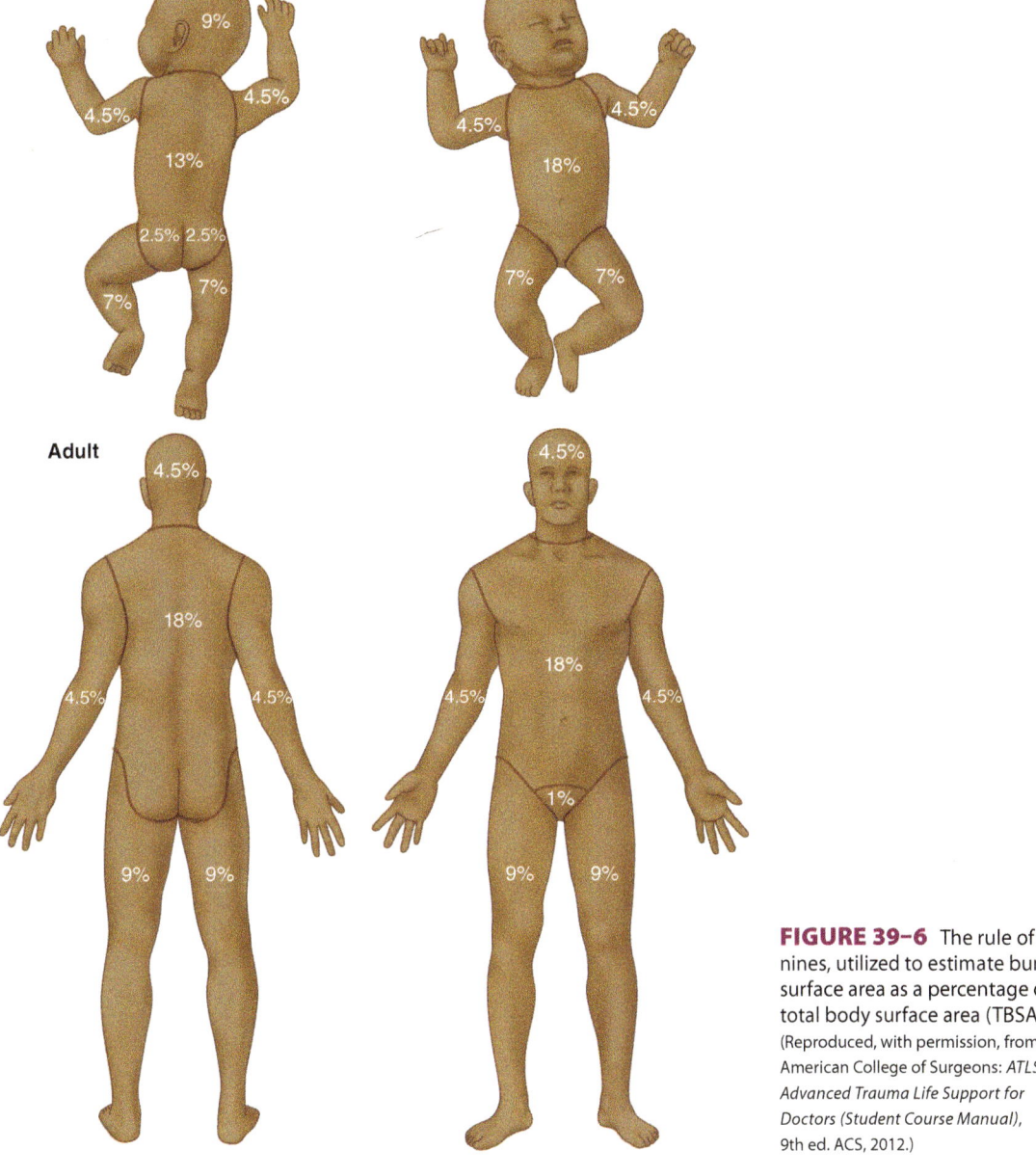

Pediatric

9%

4.5%

4.5%

13%

2.5% 2.5%

7%   7%

9%

4.5%   4.5%

18%

7%   7%

Adult

4.5%

18%

4.5%   4.5%

9%   9%

4.5%

4.5%   4.5%

18%

1%

9%   9%

FIGURE 39–6 The rule of nines, utilized to estimate burned surface area as a percentage of total body surface area (TBSA). (Reproduced, with permission, from American College of Surgeons: *ATLS: Advanced Trauma Life Support for Doctors (Student Course Manual)*, 9th ed. ACS, 2012.)

pneumonia. Abdominal compartment syndrome can have an adverse impact on pulmonary function. Intravenous fluid administration volumes must be monitored closely and documented to be consistent with American Burn Association recommendations (ie, the Parkland or modified Brooke protocol). Fluid administration that exceeds recommendations warrants careful review of the rationale for the increased fluid therapy volume, including assessment of possible causes for hypotension (eg, sepsis) or reduced urine output (eg, abdominal compartment syndrome).

C. Carbon Monoxide Poisoning

15 Carbon monoxide poisoning should be considered in all serious burn injury cases, as well as with lesser TBSA burns occurring in enclosed spaces. Unconsciousness or decreased levels of consciousness following burn injuries should be presumed to represent carbon monoxide poisoning, prompting endotracheal intubation and mechanical ventilation with high inspired concentration oxygen therapy. Carbon monoxide binds to hemoglobin with an affinity approximately 250 times that of oxygen. The resultant carboxyhemoglobin (HbCO) leaves less hemoglobin available to bind with oxygen (HbO_2) and shifts the O_2–Hb dissociation curve to the left; both of these processes result in impaired availability of oxygen molecules at the local tissue level. Pulse oximetry provides a falsely elevated indication of oxygen saturation in the setting of carbon monoxide exposure because of its inability to distinguish between HbO_2 and HbCO. If carbon monoxide poisoning is suspected, HbCO can be directly measured via arterial or venous blood gas analysis. HbCO concentrations below 10% are usually not clinically significant. However, with high inspired oxygen concentrations, HbCO levels of 20% correspond to a hemoglobin oxygen saturation of 80%; intubation and mechanical ventilation is indicated in such circumstances to improve local tissue oxygenation and enhance carbon monoxide elimination. Death from carbon monoxide poisoning occurs at HbCO levels of 60%.

Anesthetic Considerations

A primary characteristic of all burn patients is an inability to regulate temperature. The resuscitation environment must be maintained near body temperature through the use of radiant warming, forced air warming devices, and fluid warming devices.

Assessment of the patient begins with inspection of the airway. Although the face may be burned (singed facial hair, nasal vibrissae), facial burns are not an indication for tracheal intubation. The need for urgent airway management, mechanical ventilation, and oxygen therapy is indicated by hoarse voice, dyspnea, tachypnea, or altered level of consciousness. Arterial blood gases should be obtained early in the treatment process to assess HbCO levels.

Mechanical ventilation should be adjusted to afford adequate oxygenation at the lowest tidal volumes.

Tracheal intubation in the early period following burn injury (up to the first 48 h) can be facilitated with succinylcholine for paralysis. In patients with significant burns (>20% TBSA), injuries and disruption of neuromuscular end plates occur followed by upregulation of acetylcholine receptors. **16** Beyond 48 h after a major burn, succinylcholine administration is likely to produce potentially lethal elevation of serum potassium levels.

Analgesia for burn patients is challenging because of concerns about opioid tolerance and psychosocial complications. Multimodal approaches are often advantageous. Regional analgesia may provide benefit, although in the early postburn period this technique may mask the symptoms of compartment syndrome or other clinical signs and symptoms.

SUGGESTED READING

Beekley AC: Damage control resuscitation: A sensible approach to the exsanguinating surgical patient. Crit Care Med 2008;36:S267.

Bratton SL, Chestnut RM, Ghajar J, et al: Guidelines for the management of severe traumatic brain injury. IX. Cerebral perfusion thresholds. J Neurotrauma 2007;24:S59.

Brohi K, Cohen MJ, Davenport RA: Acute coagulopathy of trauma: Mechanism, identification and effect. Curr Opin Crit Care 2007;13:680.

Chi JH, Knudson MM, Vassar MJ, et al: Prehospital hypoxia affects outcome in patients with traumatic brain injury: A prospective multicenter study. J Trauma 2006;61:1134.

Cotton BA, Au BK, Nunez TC, et al: Predefined massive transfusion protocols are associated with a reduction in organ failure and postinjury complications. J Trauma 2009;66:41.

Cotton BA, Dossett LA, Haut ER, et al: Multicenter validation of a simplified score to predict massive transfusion in trauma. J Trauma 2010;69:S33.

Dimar JR, Carreon LY, Riina J, et al: Early versus late stabilization of the spine in the polytrauma patient. Spine 2010;35:S187.

Griffee MJ, DeLoughery TG, Thorborg PA: Coagulation management in massive bleeding. Curr Opin Anesthesiol 2010;23:263.

Hendrickson JE, Hillyer CD: Noninfectious serious hazards of transfusion. Anesth Analg 2009;108:759.

Holcomb JB: Damage control resuscitation. J Trauma 2007;62:S36.

Ipaktchi K, Arbabi S: Advances in burn critical care. Crit Care Med 2006;34:S239.

Kashuk JL, Moore EE, Sawyer M, et al: Postinjury coagulopathy management: Goal-directed resuscitation via POC thrombelastography. Ann Surg 2010;251:604.

Kortbeek JB, Al Turki SA, Ali J, et al: Advanced trauma life support, 8th edition, the evidence for change. J Trauma 2008;64:1638.

Li LM, Timofeev I, Czosnyka M, et al: The surgical approach to the management of increased intracranial pressure after traumatic brain injury. Anesth Analg 2010;111:736.

MacLeod JB, Lynn M, McKenney MG, et al: Early coagulopathy predicts mortality in trauma. J Trauma 2003;55:39.

Magnotti LJ, Zarzaur BL, Fischer PE, et al: Improved survival after hemostatic resuscitation: does the emperor have no clothes? J Trauma 2011;70:97.

Miko I, Gould R, Wolf S, Afifi S: Acute spinal cord injury. Int Anesthesiol Clinic 2009;47:37.

Perkins JG, Cap AP, Weiss BM, et al: Massive transfusion and nonsurgical hemostatic agents. Crit Care Med 2008;36:S325.

Pull ter Gunne AF, Skolasky RL, Cohen DB: Fracture characteristics predict patient mortality after blunt force cervical trauma. Eur J Emerg Med 2010;17:107.

Sihler KC, Napolitano LM: Complications of massive transfusion. Chest 2011;137:209.

Snyder CW, Weinberg JA, McGwin G, Jr., et al: The relationship of blood product ratio to mortality: Survival benefit or survival bias? J Trauma 2009;66:358.

Stuke LE, Pons PT, Guy JS, et al: Prehospital spine immobilization for penetrating trauma—review and recommendations from the prehospital trauma life support executive committee. J Trauma 2011;71:763.

Maternal & Fetal Physiology & Anesthesia

Michael A. Frölich, MD, MS

KEY CONCEPTS

1. The minimum alveolar concentration (MAC) progressively decreases during pregnancy—at term, by as much as 40%—for all general anesthetic agents; MAC returns to normal by the third day after delivery.

2. Pregnant patients display enhanced sensitivity to local anesthetics during regional anesthesia and analgesia, and neural blockade occurs at reduced concentrations of local anesthetics; dose requirements may be reduced as much as 30%.

3. Obstruction of the inferior vena cava by the enlarging uterus distends the epidural venous plexus and increases the risk of intravascular injection during epidural anesthesia.

4. Approximately 5% of women at term develop the supine hypotension syndrome, which is characterized by hypotension associated with pallor, sweating, or nausea and vomiting. The incidence of maternal hypotension syndrome may be higher in women receiving neuraxial analgesia.

5. The reduction in gastric motility and gastroesophageal sphincter tone place the parturient at high risk for regurgitation and pulmonary aspiration.

6. Ephedrine, which has considerable β-adrenergic activity, has traditionally been considered the vasopressor of choice for hypotension during pregnancy. However, clinical studies suggest that α-adrenergic agonists such as phenylephrine and metaraminol are just as effective in treating hypotension in pregnant patients and are associated with less fetal acidosis than ephedrine.

7. Volatile inhalational anesthetics decrease blood pressure and, potentially, uteroplacental blood flow. In concentrations of less than 1 MAC, however, their effects are generally minor, consisting of dose-dependent uterine relaxation and minor reductions in uterine blood flow.

8. The greatest strain on the parturient's heart occurs immediately after delivery, when intense uterine contraction and involution suddenly relieve inferior vena caval obstruction and increase cardiac output as much as 80% above late third trimester values.

9. Current techniques employing very dilute combinations of a local anesthetic (eg, bupivacaine, 0.125% or less) and an opioid (eg, fentanyl, 5 mcg/mL or less) for epidural or combined spinal–epidural (CSE) analgesia do not appear to prolong the first stage of labor or increase the likelihood of an operative delivery.

This chapter reviews the normal physiological changes associated with pregnancy, labor, and delivery. It concludes with a description of the physiological transition from fetal to neonatal life.

PHYSIOLOGICAL CHANGES DURING PREGNANCY

Pregnancy affects most organ systems (Table 40–1). Many of these physiological changes appear to be adaptive and useful to the mother in tolerating the stresses of pregnancy, labor, and delivery. Other changes lack obvious benefits but nonetheless require special consideration in caring for the parturient.

TABLE 40–1 **Average maximum physiological changes associated with pregnancy.**[1]

Parameter	Change
Neurological	
MAC	−40%
Respiratory	
Oxygen consumption	+20 to 50%
Airway resistance	−35%
FRC	−20%
Minute ventilation	+50%
Tidal volume	+40%
Respiratory rate	+15%
Pao_2	+10%
$Paco_2$	−15%
HCO_3	−15%
Cardiovascular	
Blood volume	+35%
Plasma volume	+55%
Cardiac output	+40%
Stroke volume	+30%
Heart rate	+20%
Systolic blood pressure	−5%
Diastolic blood pressure	−15%
Peripheral resistance	−15%
Pulmonary resistance	−30%
Hematologic	
Hemoglobin	−20%
Platelets	−10%
Clotting factors[2]	+30 to 250%
Renal	
GFR	+50%

[1]MAC, minimum alveolar concentration; FRC, functional residual capacity; GFR, glomerular filtration rate.

[2]Varies with each factor.

Central Nervous System Effects

1 The minimum alveolar concentration (MAC) progressively decreases during pregnancy—at term, by as much as 40%—for all general anesthetic agents; MAC returns to normal by the third day after delivery. Changes in maternal hormonal and endogenous opioid levels have been implicated. Progesterone, which is sedating when given in pharmacological doses, increases up to 20 times normal at term and is at least partly responsible for this observation. A surge in β-endorphin levels during labor and delivery also likely plays a major role.

2 Pregnant patients also display enhanced sensitivity to local anesthetics during regional anesthesia and analgesia, and neural blockade occurs at reduced concentrations of local anesthetics. The term *minimum local analgesic concentration* (MLAC) is used in obstetric anesthesia to compare the relative potencies of local anesthetics and the effects of additives; MLAC is defined as the local analgesic concentration leading to satisfactory analgesia in 50% of patients (EC_{50}). Local anesthetic dose requirements during epidural anesthesia may be reduced as much as 30%, a phenomenon that appears to be hormonally mediated but may also be related to engorgement of the epidural

3 venous plexus. Obstruction of the inferior vena cava by the enlarging uterus distends the epidural venous plexus and increases epidural blood volume. The latter has three major effects: (1) decreased spinal cerebrospinal fluid volume, (2) decreased potential volume of the epidural space, and (3) increased epidural (space) pressure. The first two effects enhance the cephalad spread of local anesthetic solutions during spinal and epidural anesthesia, respectively, whereas the last may complicate identification of the epidural space (see Chapter 45). Bearing down during labor further accentuates all these effects. Positive (rather than the usual negative) epidural pressures have been recorded in parturients. Engorgement of the epidural veins also increases the likelihood of placing an epidural needle or catheter in a vein, resulting in an unintentional intravascular injection. It is unclear whether pregnancy lowers the seizure threshold for local anesthetics.

Respiratory Effects

Oxygen consumption and minute ventilation progressively increase during pregnancy. Tidal volume and, to a lesser extent, respiratory rate and inspiratory reserve volume also increase. By term, both oxygen consumption and minute ventilation have increased up to 50%. $Paco_2$ decreases to 28–32 mm Hg; significant respiratory alkalosis is prevented by a compensatory decrease in plasma bicarbonate concentration. Hyperventilation may also increase Pao_2 slightly. Elevated levels of 2,3-diphosphoglycerate offset the effect of hyperventilation on hemoglobin's affinity for oxygen (see Chapter 23). The P_{50} for hemoglobin increases from 27 to 30 mm Hg; the combination of the latter with an increase in cardiac output (see section on Cardiovascular Effects below) enhances oxygen delivery to tissues.

The maternal respiratory pattern changes as the uterus enlarges. In the third trimester, elevation of the diaphragm is compensated by an increase in the anteroposterior diameter of the chest; diaphragmatic motion, however, is not restricted. Thoracic breathing is favored over abdominal breathing. Both vital capacity and closing capacity are minimally affected, but functional residual capacity (FRC) decreases up to 20% at term; FRC returns to normal within 48 h of delivery. This decrease is principally due to a reduction in expiratory reserve volume as a result of larger than normal tidal volumes. Flow–volume loops are unaffected, and airway resistance decreases. Physiological dead space decreases but intrapulmonary shunting increases toward term. A chest film may show prominent vascular markings due to increased pulmonary blood volume and an elevated diaphragm. Pulmonary vasodilation prevents pulmonary pressures from rising.

The combination of decreased FRC and increased oxygen consumption promotes rapid oxygen desaturation during periods of apnea. Preoxygenation (denitrogenation) prior to induction of general anesthesia is therefore mandatory to avoid hypoxemia in pregnant patients. Closing volume exceeds FRC in some pregnant women when they are supine at term. Under these conditions, atelectasis and hypoxemia readily occur. The decrease in FRC coupled with the increase in minute ventilation accelerates the uptake of all inhalational anesthetics. The reduction in dead space narrows the arterial end-tidal CO_2 gradient.

Capillary engorgement of the respiratory mucosa during pregnancy predisposes the upper airways to trauma, bleeding, and obstruction. Gentle laryngoscopy and smaller endotracheal tubes (6–6.5 mm) should be employed during general anesthesia.

Cardiovascular Effects

Cardiac output and blood volume increase to meet accelerated maternal and fetal metabolic demands. An increase (55%) in plasma volume in excess of an increase in red cell mass (45%) produces dilutional anemia and reduces blood viscosity. Hemoglobin concentration, however, usually remains greater than 11 g/dL. Moreover, in terms of tissue oxygen delivery, the reduction in hemoglobin concentration is offset by the increase in cardiac output and the rightward shift of the hemoglobin dissociation curve (see the section on Respiratory Effects). A decrease in systemic vascular resistance by the second trimester decreases both diastolic and, to a lesser degree, systolic blood pressure. The response to adrenergic agents and vasoconstrictors is blunted.

At term, blood volume has increased by 1000–1500 mL in most women, allowing them to easily tolerate the blood loss associated with delivery; total blood volume reaches 90 mL/kg. Average blood loss during vaginal delivery is 400–500 mL, compared with 800–1000 mL for a cesarean section. Blood volume does not return to normal until 1–2 weeks after delivery.

The increase in cardiac output (40% at term) is due to increases in both heart rate (20%) and stroke volume (30%). Cardiac chambers enlarge and myocardial hypertrophy is often noted on echocardiography. Pulmonary artery, central venous, and pulmonary artery wedge pressures remain unchanged. Most of these effects are observed in the first and, to a lesser extent, the second trimester. In the third trimester, cardiac output does not appreciably rise, except during labor. The greatest increases in cardiac output are seen during labor and immediately after delivery (see the section on Effect of Labor on Maternal Physiology). Cardiac output often does not return to normal until 2 weeks after delivery.

Decreases in cardiac output can occur in the supine position after week 20 of pregnancy. Such decreases have been shown to be secondary to impeded venous return to the heart as the enlarging uterus compresses the inferior vena cava. **(4)** Approximately 5% of women at term develop the supine hypotension syndrome (aortocaval compression), which is characterized by hypotension associated with pallor, sweating, or nausea and vomiting. The cause of this syndrome appears to be complete or near-complete occlusion of the inferior vena cava by the gravid uterus. When combined with the hypotensive effects of regional or general anesthesia, aortocaval compression can readily produce fetal asphyxia. Turning the patient on her side typically restores venous return from the lower body and corrects the hypotension in such instances. This maneuver is most readily accomplished by placing a wedge (>15°) under the right hip. The gravid uterus also compresses the aorta in most parturients when they are supine. This latter effect decreases blood flow to the lower extremities and, more importantly, to the uteroplacental circulation. Uterine contraction reduces caval compression but exacerbates aortic compression.

Chronic partial caval obstruction in the third trimester predisposes to venous stasis, phlebitis, and edema in the lower extremities. Moreover, compression of the inferior vena cava below the diaphragm distends and increases blood flow through the paravertebral venous plexus (including the epidural veins), and to a minor degree, the abdominal wall.

Lastly, elevation of the diaphragm shifts the heart's position in the chest, resulting in the appearance of an enlarged heart on a plain chest film and in left axis deviation and T wave changes on the electrocardiogram. Physical examination often reveals a systolic ejection flow murmur (grade I or II) and exaggerated splitting of the first heart sound (S_1); a third heart sound (S_3) may be audible. A few patients develop small, asymptomatic pericardial effusion.

Renal & Gastrointestinal Effects

Renal plasma flow and the glomerular filtration rate increase during pregnancy, and as a result serum creatinine and blood urea nitrogen may decrease to 0.5–0.6 mg/dL and 8–9 mg/dL,

respectively. A decreased renal tubular threshold for glucose and amino acids is common and often results in mild glycosuria (1–10 g/d) or proteinuria (<300 mg/d), or both. Plasma osmolality decreases by 8–10 mOsm/kg.

Gastroesophageal reflux and esophagitis are common during pregnancy. Gastric motility is reduced, and upward and anterior displacement of the stomach by the uterus promotes incompetence **(5)** of the gastroesophageal sphincter. These factors place the parturient at high risk for regurgitation and pulmonary aspiration. However, neither gastric acidity nor gastric volume changes significantly during pregnancy. Opioids and anticholinergics reduce lower esophageal sphincter pressure, may facilitate gastroesophageal reflux, and delay gastric emptying.

Hepatic Effects

Overall hepatic function and blood flow are unchanged; minor elevations in serum transaminases and lactic dehydrogenase levels may be observed in the third trimester. Mild elevations in serum alkaline phosphatase are due to its secretion by the placenta. A mild decrease in serum albumin is due to an expanded plasma volume, and as a result, colloid oncotic pressure is reduced. A 25–30% decrease in serum pseudocholinesterase activity is also present at term but rarely produces significant prolongation of succinylcholine's action. The breakdown of ester-type local anesthetics is not appreciably altered. Pseudocholinesterase activity may not return to normal until up to 6 weeks postpartum. High progesterone levels appear to inhibit the release of cholecystokinin, resulting in incomplete emptying of the gallbladder. The latter, together with altered bile acid composition, can predispose to the formation of cholesterol gallstones during pregnancy.

Hematological Effects

Pregnancy is associated with a hypercoagulable state that may be beneficial in limiting blood loss at delivery. Fibrinogen and concentrations of factors VII, VIII, IX, X, and XII all increase; only factor XI levels may decrease. Accelerated fibrinolysis can be observed late in the third trimester. In addition to the dilutional anemia (see the section on Cardiovascular

Effects), leukocytosis (up to 21,000/μL) and a 10% decrease in platelet count may be encountered during the third trimester. Because of fetal utilization, iron and folate deficiency anemias readily develop if supplements of these nutrients are not taken.

Metabolic Effects

Complex metabolic and hormonal changes occur during pregnancy. Altered carbohydrate, fat, and protein metabolism favors fetal growth and development. These changes resemble starvation, because blood glucose and amino acid levels are low whereas free fatty acids, ketones, and triglyceride levels are high. Nonetheless, pregnancy is a diabetogenic state; insulin levels steadily rise during pregnancy. Secretion of human placental lactogen, also called human chorionic somatomammotropin, by the placenta is probably responsible for the relative insulin resistance associated with pregnancy. Pancreatic beta cell hyperplasia occurs in response to an increased demand for insulin secretion.

Secretion of human chorionic gonadotropin and elevated levels of estrogens promote hypertrophy of the thyroid gland and increase thyroid-binding globulin; although T_4 and T_3 levels are elevated, free T_4, free T_3, and thyrotropin (thyroid-stimulating hormone) remain normal. Serum calcium levels decrease, but ionized calcium concentration remains normal.

Musculoskeletal Effects

Elevated levels of relaxin throughout pregnancy help prepare for delivery by softening the cervix, inhibiting uterine contractions, and relaxing the pubic symphysis and pelvic joints. Ligamentous laxity of the spine increases the risk of back injury. The latter may contribute to the relatively high incidence of back pain during pregnancy.

UTEROPLACENTAL CIRCULATION

A normal uteroplacental circulation (Figure 40–1) is critical in the development and maintenance of a healthy fetus. Uteroplacental insufficiency is an important cause of intrauterine fetal growth retardation, and when severe, can result in fetal demise. The integrity of this circulation is, in turn, dependent on both adequate uterine blood flow and normal placental function.

Uterine Blood Flow

At term, uterine blood flow represents about 10% of the cardiac output, or 600–700 mL/min (compared with 50 mL/min in the nonpregnant uterus). Eighty percent of uterine blood flow normally supplies the placenta; the remainder goes to the myometrium. Pregnancy maximally dilates the uterine vasculature, so that autoregulation is absent, but the uterine vasculature remains sensitive to α-adrenergic agonists. Uterine blood flow is not usually significantly affected by respiratory gas tensions, but extreme hypocapnia ($Paco_2$ <20 mm Hg) can reduce uterine blood flow and causes fetal hypoxemia and acidosis.

Blood flow is directly proportionate to the difference between uterine arterial and venous pressures but inversely proportionate to uterine vascular resistance. Although not under appreciable neural control, the uterine vasculature has α-adrenergic and possibly some β-adrenergic receptors.

Three major factors decrease uterine blood flow during pregnancy: (1) systemic hypotension, (2) uterine vasoconstriction, and (3) uterine contractions. Common causes of hypotension during pregnancy include aortocaval compression, hypovolemia, and sympathetic blockade following regional anesthesia. Stress-induced release of endogenous catecholamines (sympathoadrenal activation) during labor causes uterine arterial vasoconstriction. Any drug with α-adrenergic activity (eg, phenylephrine) potentially is capable of decreasing uterine blood flow by vasoconstriction. Ephedrine, which has considerable β-adrenergic activity, has traditionally been considered the vasopressor of choice for hypotension during pregnancy. However, clinical studies suggest that α-adrenergic agonists such as phenylephrine and metaraminol are just as effective in treating hypotension in pregnant patients and are associated with less fetal acidosis than ephedrine.

Paradoxically, hypertensive disorders are often associated with decreased uterine blood flow due to generalized vasoconstriction. **Uterine contractions decrease uterine blood flow by elevating uterine venous pressure and compressing arterial vessels as they traverse the myometrium.** Hypertonic

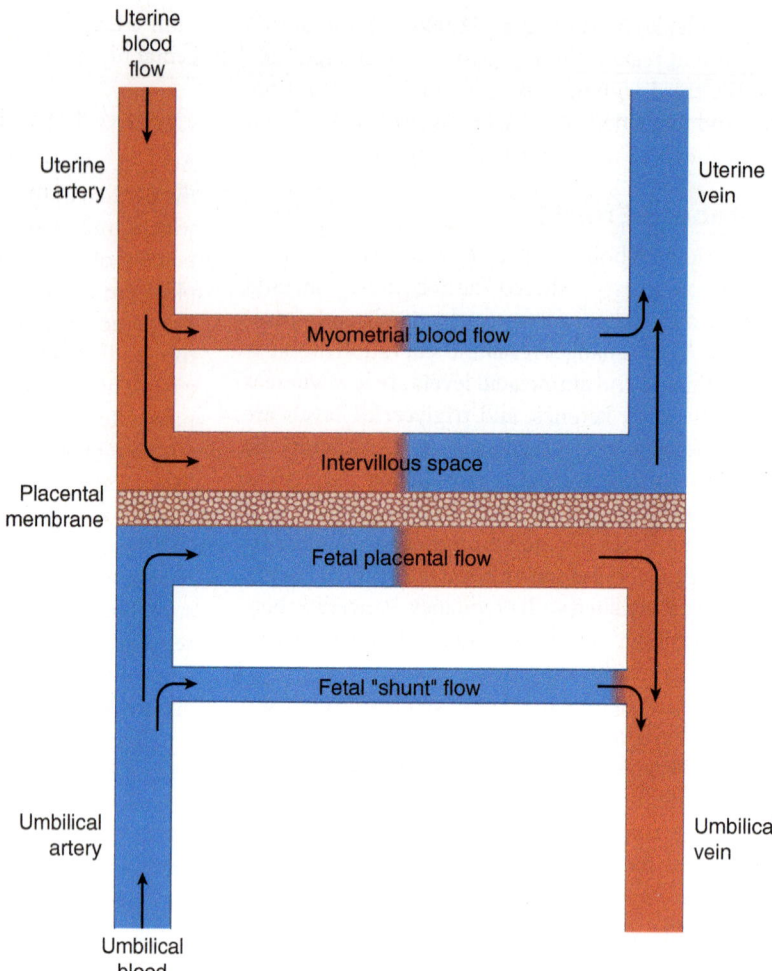

FIGURE 40–1 The uteroplacental circulation. (Reproduced, with permission, from Shnider S, Levinson G: *Anesthesia for Obstetrics*, 2nd ed. Williams & Wilkins, 1987.)

·contractions during labor or during oxytocin infusions can critically compromise uterine blood flow.

Placental Function

The fetus is dependent on the placenta for respiratory gas exchange, nutrition, and waste elimination. The placenta is formed by both maternal and fetal tissues and derives a blood supply from each. The resulting exchange membrane has a functional area of about 1.8 m².

A. Physiological Anatomy

The placenta (Figure 40–2) is composed of projections of fetal tissue (villi) that lie in maternal vascular spaces (intervillous spaces). As a result of this arrangement, the fetal capillaries within villi readily exchange substances with the maternal blood that bathes them. Maternal blood in the intervillous spaces is derived from spiral branches of the uterine artery and drains into the uterine veins. Fetal blood within villi is derived from the umbilical cord via two umbilical arteries and returns to the fetus via a single umbilical vein.

B. Placental Exchange

Placental exchange can occur by one of six mechanisms:

1. Diffusion—Respiratory gases and small ions are transported by diffusion. Most drugs used in

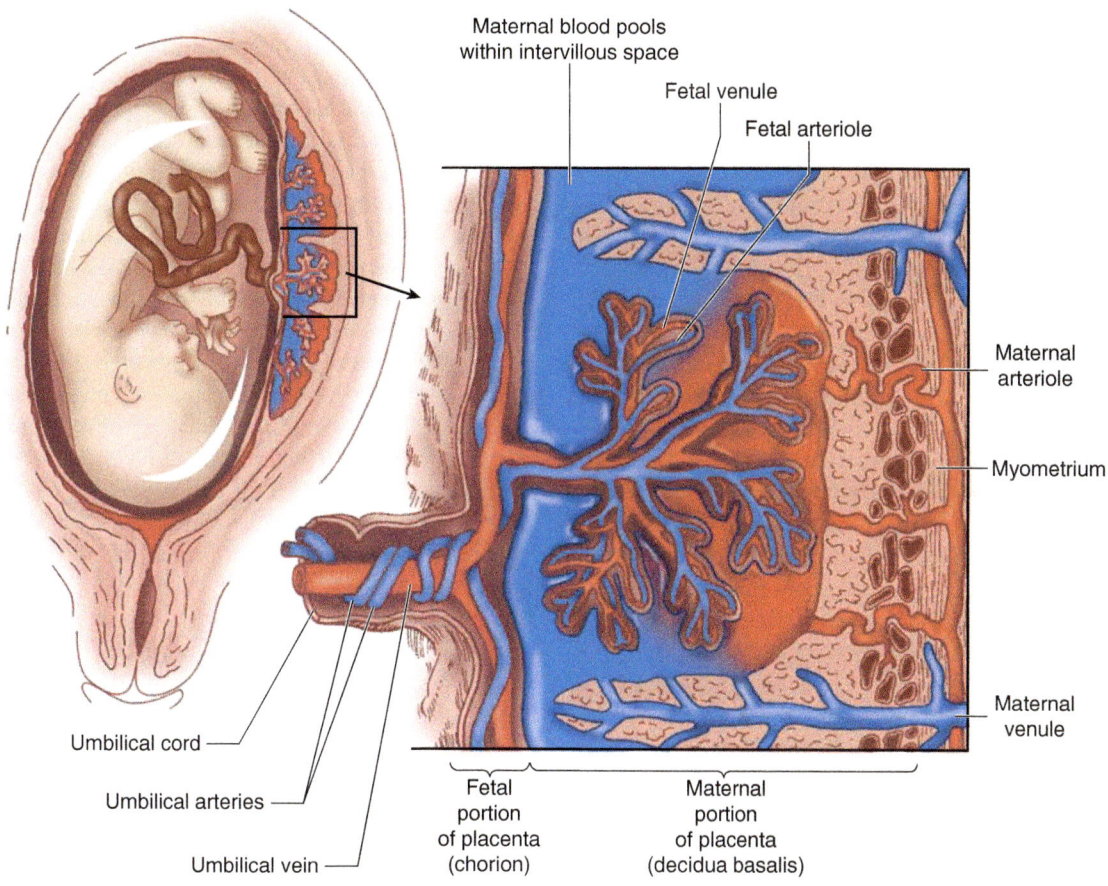

FIGURE 40–2 The placenta.

anesthesia have molecular weights well under 1000 and consequently can readily diffuse across the placenta.

2. Osmotic and hydrostatic pressure (bulk flow)— Water moves across by osmotic and hydrostatic pressures. Water enters the fetal circulation in quantities greater than any other substance.

3. Facilitated diffusion—Glucose enters the fetal circulation down the concentration gradient (no energy is consumed) facilitated by a specific transporter molecule.

4. Active transport—Amino acids, vitamin B_{12}, fatty acids, and some ions (calcium and phosphate) utilize this mechanism.

5. Vesicular transport—Large molecules, such as immunoglobulins, are transported by pinocytosis.

Iron enters the fetal circulation in this way, facilitated by ferritin and transferrin.

6. Breaks—Breaks in the placental membrane may permit mixing of maternal and fetal blood. This probably underlies Rh sensitization (see Chapter 51). Rh sensitization occurs most commonly during delivery.

Respiratory Gas Exchange

At term, fetal oxygen consumption averages about 7 mL/min per kilogram of fetal body weight. Fortunately, because of multiple adaptive mechanisms, the normal fetus at term can survive 10 min or longer instead of the expected 2 min in a state of total oxygen deprivation. Partial or complete oxygen deprivation can result from umbilical cord compression, umbilical cord prolapse, placental abruption, severe maternal hypoxemia, or hypotension. Compensatory fetal mechanisms include redistribution of blood flow primarily to the brain, heart, placenta, and adrenal gland; decreased oxygen consumption; and anaerobic metabolism.

Transfer of oxygen across the placenta is dependent on the ratio of maternal uterine blood flow to fetal umbilical blood flow. The reserve for oxygen transfer is small even during normal pregnancy. Normal fetal blood from the placenta has a Pao_2 of only 30–35 mm Hg. To aid oxygen transfer, the fetal hemoglobin oxygen dissociation curve is shifted to the left such that fetal hemoglobin has greater affinity for oxygen than does maternal hemoglobin (whose curve is already shifted to the right; see the section on Respiratory Effects). In addition, fetal hemoglobin concentration is usually 15 g/dL (compared with approximately 12 g/dL in the mother).

Carbon dioxide readily diffuses across the placenta. Maternal hyperventilation (see the section on Respiratory Effects) increases the gradient for the transfer of carbon dioxide from the fetus into the maternal circulation. Fetal hemoglobin has less affinity for carbon dioxide than do adult forms of hemoglobin. Carbon monoxide readily diffuses across the placenta, and fetal hemoglobin has greater affinity for carbon monoxide than do adult forms.

Placental Transfer of Anesthetic Agents

Transfer of a drug across the placenta is reflected by the ratio of its fetal umbilical vein to maternal venous concentrations (UV/MV), whereas its uptake by fetal tissues can be correlated with the ratio of its fetal umbilical artery to umbilical vein concentrations (UA/UV). Fetal effects of drugs administered to parturients depend on multiple factors, including route of administration (oral, intramuscular, intravenous, epidural, or intrathecal), dose, timing of administration (both relative to delivery as well as contractions), and maturity of the fetal organs (brain and liver). Thus, a drug given hours before delivery or as a single intravenous bolus during a uterine contraction just prior to delivery (when uterine blood flow is maximally reduced) is unlikely to produce high fetal levels. Fortunately, current anesthetic techniques for labor and delivery generally have minimal fetal effects despite significant placental transfer of anesthetic agents and adjuncts.

All inhalational agents and most intravenous agents freely cross the placenta. Inhalational agents generally produce little fetal depression when they are given in limited doses (<1 MAC) and delivery occurs within 10 min of induction. Ketamine, propofol, and benzodiazepines readily cross the placenta and can be detected in the fetal circulation. Fortunately, when these agents (with the exception of benzodiazepines) are administered in usual induction doses, drug distribution, metabolism, and possibly placental uptake may limit fetal effects. Although most opiates readily cross the placenta, their effects on neonates at delivery vary considerably. Newborns appear to be more sensitive to the respiratory depressant effect of morphine compared with other opioids. Although meperidine produces respiratory depression, peaking 1–3 h after administration, it produces less than morphine; butorphanol and nalbuphine produce even less respiratory depression but still may have significant neurobehavioral depressant effects. Although fentanyl readily crosses the placenta, it appears to have minimal neonatal effects unless larger intravenous doses (>1 mcg/kg) are given immediately before delivery. Epidural or intrathecal fentanyl, sufentanil, and, to a lesser extent, morphine, generally produce minimal neonatal effects. Alfentanil causes neonatal depression similar to meperidine. Remifentanil also readily crosses the placenta and has the potential to produce respiratory depression in newborns. Fetal blood concentrations of remifentanil are generally about half those of the mother just prior to delivery. The UA/UV ratio is about 30%, suggesting fairly rapid metabolism of remifentanil in the neonate. The highly ionized nature of muscle relaxants impedes placental transfer, resulting in minimal effects on the fetus.

Local anesthetics are weakly basic drugs that are principally bound to α_1-acid glycoprotein. Placental transfer depends on three factors: (1) pK_a (see Chapter 16), (2) maternal and fetal pH, and (3) degree of protein binding. Except for chloroprocaine, fetal acidosis increases fetal-to-maternal drug ratios because binding of hydrogen ions to the nonionized form causes trapping of the local anesthetic in the fetal circulation. Highly protein-bound agents diffuse slowly across the placenta; thus, greater protein binding of bupivacaine and ropivacaine, compared with that of lidocaine, likely accounts for their lower fetal blood levels. Chloroprocaine has the least placental transfer because it is rapidly broken down by plasma cholinesterase in the maternal circulation.

Most commonly used anesthetic adjuncts also readily cross the placenta. Thus, maternally administered ephedrine, β-adrenergic blockers (such as labetalol and esmolol), vasodilators, phenothiazines, antihistamines (H_1 and H_2), and metoclopramide are transferred to the fetus. Atropine and scopolamine, but not glycopyrrolate, cross the placenta; the latter's quaternary ammonium (ionized) structure results in only limited transfer.

Effect of Anesthetic Agents on Uteroplacental Blood Flow

Intravenous anesthetic agents have variable effects on uteroplacental blood flow. Propofol and barbiturates are typically associated with small reductions in uterine blood flow due to mild to moderate, dose-dependent decreases in maternal blood pressure. A small induction dose, however, can produce greater reductions in blood flow as a result of sympathoadrenal activation (due to light anesthesia). Ketamine in doses of less than 1.5 mg/kg does not appreciably alter uteroplacental blood flow; its hypertensive effect typically counteracts any vasoconstriction. Uterine hypertonus may occur with ketamine at doses of more than 2 mg/kg. Etomidate likely has minimal effects, but its actions on uteroplacental circulation have not been well-described.

7 Volatile inhalational anesthetics decrease blood pressure and, potentially, uteroplacental blood flow. In concentrations of less than 1 MAC, however, their effects are generally minor, consisting of dose-dependent uterine relaxation and minor reductions in uterine blood flow. Nitrous oxide has minimal effects on uterine blood flow when administered with a volatile agent. In animal studies, nitrous oxide alone can vasoconstrict the uterine arteries.

High blood levels of local anesthetics—particularly lidocaine—cause uterine arterial vasoconstriction. Such levels are seen only with unintentional intravascular injections and occasionally following paracervical blocks (in which the injection site is in close proximity to the uterine arteries), and local absorption or injection into these vessels cannot be ruled out). Spinal and epidural anesthesia typically do not decrease uterine blood flow except when arterial hypotension occurs. Moreover, uterine blood flow during labor may actually improve in preeclamptic patients following epidural anesthesia; a reduction in circulating endogenous catecholamines likely decreases uterine vasoconstriction. The addition of dilute concentrations of epinephrine to local anesthetic solutions does not appreciably alter uterine blood flow. Intravascular uptake of the epinephrine from the epidural space may result in only minor systemic β-adrenergic effects.

PHYSIOLOGY OF NORMAL LABOR

On average, labor commences 40 ± 2 weeks following the last menstrual period. The factors involved in the initiation of labor likely involve distention of the uterus, enhanced myometrial sensitivity to oxytocin, and altered prostaglandin synthesis by fetal membranes and decidual tissues. Although circulating oxytocin levels often do not increase at the beginning of labor, the number of myometrial oxytocin receptors rapidly increases. Several prodromal events usually precede true labor approximately 2–4 weeks prior to delivery: the fetal presenting part settles into the pelvis (lightening); patients develop uterine (Braxton Hicks) contractions that are characteristically irregular in frequency, duration, and intensity; and the cervix softens and thins out (cervical effacement). Approximately 1 week to 1 h before true labor, the cervical mucous plug (which is often bloody) breaks free (*bloody show*).

True labor begins when the sporadic Braxton Hicks contractions increase in strength (25–60 mm Hg), coordination, and frequency (15–20 min apart). Amniotic membranes may rupture spontaneously prior or subsequent to the onset of true labor. Following progressive cervical dilation, the contractions propel first the fetus and then the placenta through the pelvis and perineum. By convention, labor is divided into three stages. The first stage is defined by the onset of true labor and ends with

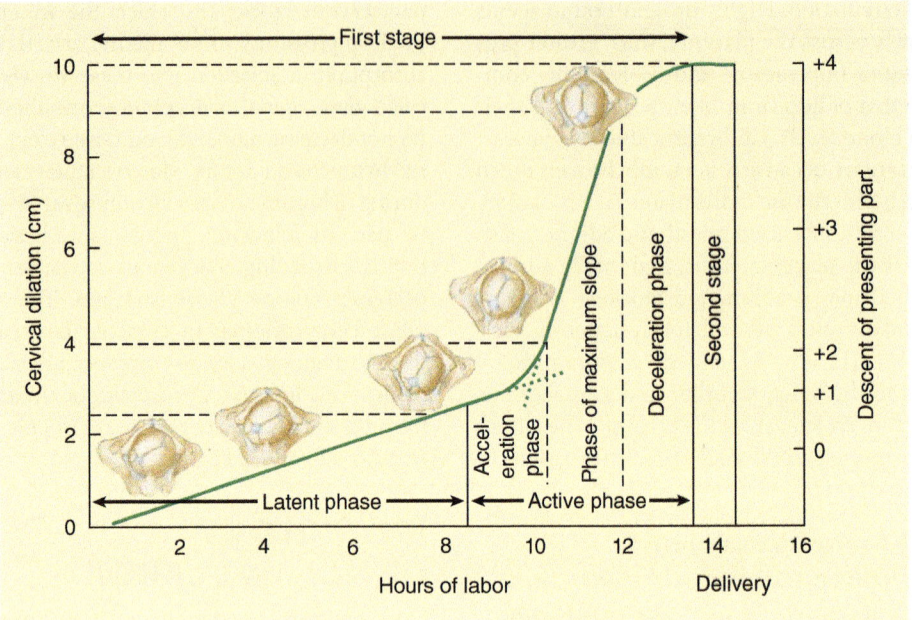

FIGURE 40–3 The course of normal labor. (Reproduced, with permission, from DeCherney AH, Pernoll ML [editors]: *Current Obstetric & Gynecologic Diagnosis & Treatment*, 9th ed. McGraw-Hill, 2001.)

complete cervical dilation. The second stage begins with full cervical dilation, is characterized by fetal descent, and ends with complete delivery of the fetus. Finally, the third stage extends from the birth of the baby to the delivery of the placenta.

Based on the rate of cervical dilation, the first stage is further divided into a slow latent phase followed by a faster active phase (Figure 40–3). The latent phase is characterized by progressive cervical effacement and minor dilation (2–4 cm). The subsequent active phase is characterized by more frequent contractions (3–5 min apart) and progressive cervical dilation up to 10 cm. The first stage usually lasts 8–12 h in nulliparous patients and about 5–8 h in multiparous patients.

Contractions during the second stage occur 1.5–2 min apart and last 1–1.5 min. Although contraction intensity does not appreciably change, the parturient, by bearing down, can greatly augment intrauterine pressure and facilitate expulsion of the fetus. The second stage usually lasts 15–120 min and the third stage typically 15–30 min.

The course of labor is monitored by uterine activity, cervical dilation, and fetal descent. Uterine

activity refers to the frequency and magnitude of uterine contractions. The latter may be measured directly, with a catheter inserted through the cervix, or indirectly, with a tocodynamometer applied externally around the abdomen. Cervical dilation and fetal descent are assessed by pelvic examination. Fetal station refers to the level of descent (in centimeters) of the presenting part relative to the ischial spines (eg, –1 or +1).

Effect of Labor on Maternal Physiology

During intense painful contractions, maternal minute ventilation may increase up to 300%. Oxygen consumption also increases by an additional 60% above third-trimester values. With excessive hyperventilation, $PaCO_2$ may decrease below 20 mm Hg. Marked hypocapnia can cause periods of hypoventilation and transient maternal and fetal hypoxemia between contractions. Excessive maternal hyperventilation also reduces uterine blood flow and promotes fetal acidosis.

Each contraction places an additional burden on the heart by displacing 300–500 mL of blood from the uterus into the central circulation (analogous to an autotransfusion). Cardiac output **8** rises 45% over third-trimester values. The greatest strain on the heart, however, occurs immediately after delivery, when intense uterine contraction and involution suddenly relieve inferior vena caval obstruction and increase cardiac output as much as 80% above late third trimester values.

Effect of Anesthetic Agents on Uterine Activity & Labor

A. Inhalational Agents

Sevoflurane, desflurane, isoflurane, and halothane depress uterine activity equally at equipotent doses; all cause dose-dependent uterine relaxation. Low doses (<0.75 MAC) of these agents, however, do not interfere with the effect of oxytocin on the uterus. Higher doses can result in uterine atony and increase blood loss at delivery. Nitrous oxide has minimal, if any, effects.

B. Parenteral Agents

Opioids minimally decrease the progression of labor; ketamine, in doses of less than 2 mg/kg, appears to have little effect.

C. Regional Anesthesia

The administration of epidural analgesia is usually based upon the patient's choice, and it is often utilized for patients with maternal or fetal factors that increase the likelihood of prolonged labor or cesar- **9** ean delivery (Table 40–2). Current evidence indicates that dilute combinations of a local anesthetic (eg, bupivacaine, 0.125% or less) and an opioid (eg, fentanyl, 5 mcg/mL or less) for epidural or combined spinal–epidural (CSE) analgesia do not prolong labor or increase the likelihood of operative delivery.

When greater concentrations of local anesthetic (eg, bupivacaine, 0.25%) are used for continuous epidural analgesia, the second stage of labor may be prolonged by approximately 15–30 min. Intense regional analgesia/anesthesia can remove the urge to bear down during the second stage (Ferguson reflex), and motor weakness can impair expulsive efforts, often prolonging the second stage of delivery. Use of dilute local anesthetic–opioid mixtures can preserve motor function and allow effective pushing. Intravenous fluid loading (crystalloid boluses) is often used to prevent or reduce the severity of hypotension following an epidural injection. So-called fluid loading does not reduce the incidence of hypotension and has been shown to reduce endogenous oxytocin secretion from the pituitary and transiently decrease uterine activity. Epinephrine-containing local anesthetic solutions could theoretically prolong the first stage of labor if absorption of epinephrine from the epidural space results in significant systemic β-adrenergic effects. Prolongation of labor is generally not clinically observed with very dilute (eg, 1:400,000) epinephrine-containing local anesthetics.

D. Vasopressors

Uterine muscle has both α and β receptors. α_1-Receptor stimulation causes uterine contraction, whereas β_2-receptor stimulation produces relaxation. Large doses of α-adrenergic agents, such as phenylephrine, in addition to causing uterine arterial constriction, can produce tetanic uterine contractions. Small doses of phenylephrine (40 mcg) may increase uterine blood flow in normal parturients by raising arterial blood pressure. In contrast, ephedrine has little effect on uterine contractions.

E. Oxytocin

Oxytocin (Pitocin) is usually administered intravenously to induce or augment uterine contractions or to maintain uterine tone postpartum. It has a half-life of 3–5 min. Induction doses for labor are 0.5–8 mU/min. **Complications include fetal distress due to hyperstimulation, uterine tetany, and, less commonly, maternal water retention**

TABLE 40–2 Factors that prolong labor, increase the likelihood of cesarean section, and often cause patients to request an epidural.

Primigravida
Prolonged labor
High parenteral analgesic requirements
Use of oxytocin
Large baby
Small pelvis
Fetal malpresentation

(antidiuretic effect). **Rapid intravenous infusion can cause transient systemic hypotension due to relaxation of vascular smooth muscle; reflex tachycardia may also be noted.**

Uterine atony is the most common cause of severe postpartum hemorrhage. Immediate administration of oxytocin after delivery is a standard measure to prevent this complication. Despite this practice, uterine atony complicates 4–6% of pregnancies. The concentration of volatile anesthetics should be reduced to 0.5 MAC in obstetric patients undergoing general anesthesia for cesarean delivery to avoid the uterine-relaxing effects of these drugs. Second-line oxytocics are methylergonovine (Methergine) and carboprost tromethamine (Hemabate).

F. Ergot Alkaloids

Methylergonovine (Methergine) causes intense and prolonged uterine contractions. It is therefore given only after delivery (postpartum) to treat uterine atony. Moreover, because it also constricts vascular smooth muscle and can cause severe hypertension if given as an intravenous bolus, it is usually administered only as a single 0.2 mg dose intramuscularly or in dilute form as an intravenous infusion over 10 minutes.

G. Prostaglandins

Carboprost tromethamine (Hemabate, prostaglandin $F_{2\alpha}$) is a synthetic analogue of prostaglandin F_2 that stimulates uterine contractions. It is often used to treat refractory postpartum hemorrhage. An initial dose of 0.25 mg intramuscularly may be repeated every 15–90 min to a maximum of 2 mg. Common side effects include nausea, vomiting, bronchoconstriction, and diarrhea. It is contraindicated in patients with bronchial asthma. Prostaglandin E_1 (Cytotec, rectal suppository) or E_2 (Dinoprostone, vaginal suppository) is sometimes administered and has no bronchoconstricting effect.

H. Magnesium

Magnesium is used in obstetrics both to stop premature labor (tocolysis) and to prevent eclamptic seizures. It is usually administered as a 4 g intravenous loading dose (over 20 min) followed by a 2 g/h infusion. Therapeutic serum levels are considered to be 6–8 mg/dL. Serious side effects include hypotension, heart block, muscle weakness, and sedation. Magnesium in these doses and concentrations intensifies neuromuscular blockade from nondepolarizing agents.

H. β₂ Agonists

The β_2-adrenergic agonists ritodrine and terbutaline inhibit uterine contractions and are used to treat premature labor.

FETAL PHYSIOLOGY

The placenta, which receives nearly half the fetal cardiac output, is responsible for respiratory gas exchange. As a result, the lungs receive little blood flow and the pulmonary and systemic circulations are parallel instead of in series, as in the adult (Figures 40–4 and 40–5). This arrangement is made possible by two cardiac shunts—the foramen ovale and the ductus arteriosus:

1. Well-oxygenated blood from the placenta (approximately 80% oxygen saturation) mixes with venous blood returning from the lower body (25% oxygen saturation) and flows via the inferior vena cava into the right atrium.

2. Right atrial anatomy preferentially directs blood flow from the inferior vena cava (67% oxygen saturation) through the foramen ovale into the left atrium.

3. Left atrial blood is then pumped by the left ventricle to the upper body (mainly the brain and the heart).

4. Poorly oxygenated blood from the upper body returns via the superior vena cava to the right atrium.

5. Right atrial anatomy preferentially directs flow from the superior vena cava into the right ventricle.

6. Right ventricular blood is pumped into the pulmonary artery.

7. Because of high pulmonary vascular resistance, 95% of the blood ejected from the right ventricle (60% oxygen saturation) is shunted across the ductus arteriosus, into the descending aorta, and back to the placenta and lower body.

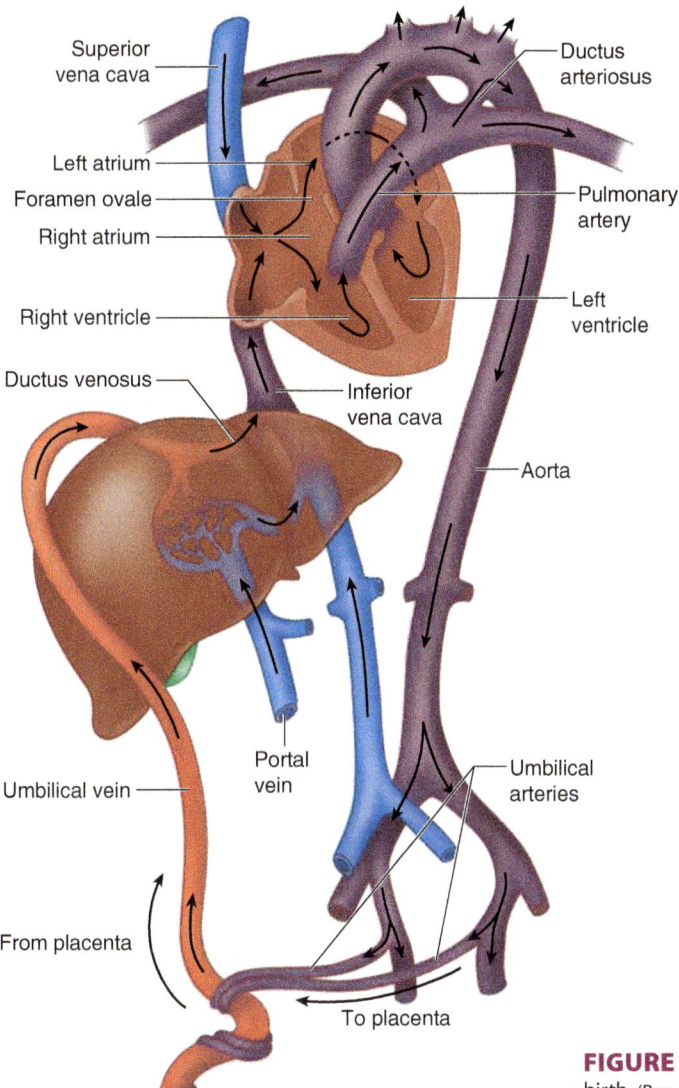

FIGURE 40–4 The fetal circulation before and after birth. (Reproduced, with permission, from Ganong WF: *Review of Medical Physiology*, 24th ed. McGraw-Hill, 2012.)

The parallel circulation results in unequal ventricular flows; the right ventricle ejects two thirds of the combined ventricular outputs, whereas the left ventricle ejects only one third.

Up to 50% of the well-oxygenated blood in the umbilical vein can pass directly to the heart via the ductus venosus, bypassing the liver. The remainder of the blood flow from the placenta mixes with blood from the portal vein (via the portal sinus) and passes through the liver before reaching the heart.

The latter may be important in allowing relatively rapid hepatic degradation of drugs (or toxins) that are absorbed from the maternal circulation.

In contrast to the fetal circulation, which is established very early during intrauterine life, maturation of the lungs lags behind. Extrauterine survival is not possible until after 24–25 weeks of gestation, when pulmonary capillaries are formed and come to lie in close approximation to an immature alveolar epithelium. At 30 weeks, the cuboidal alveolar epithelium

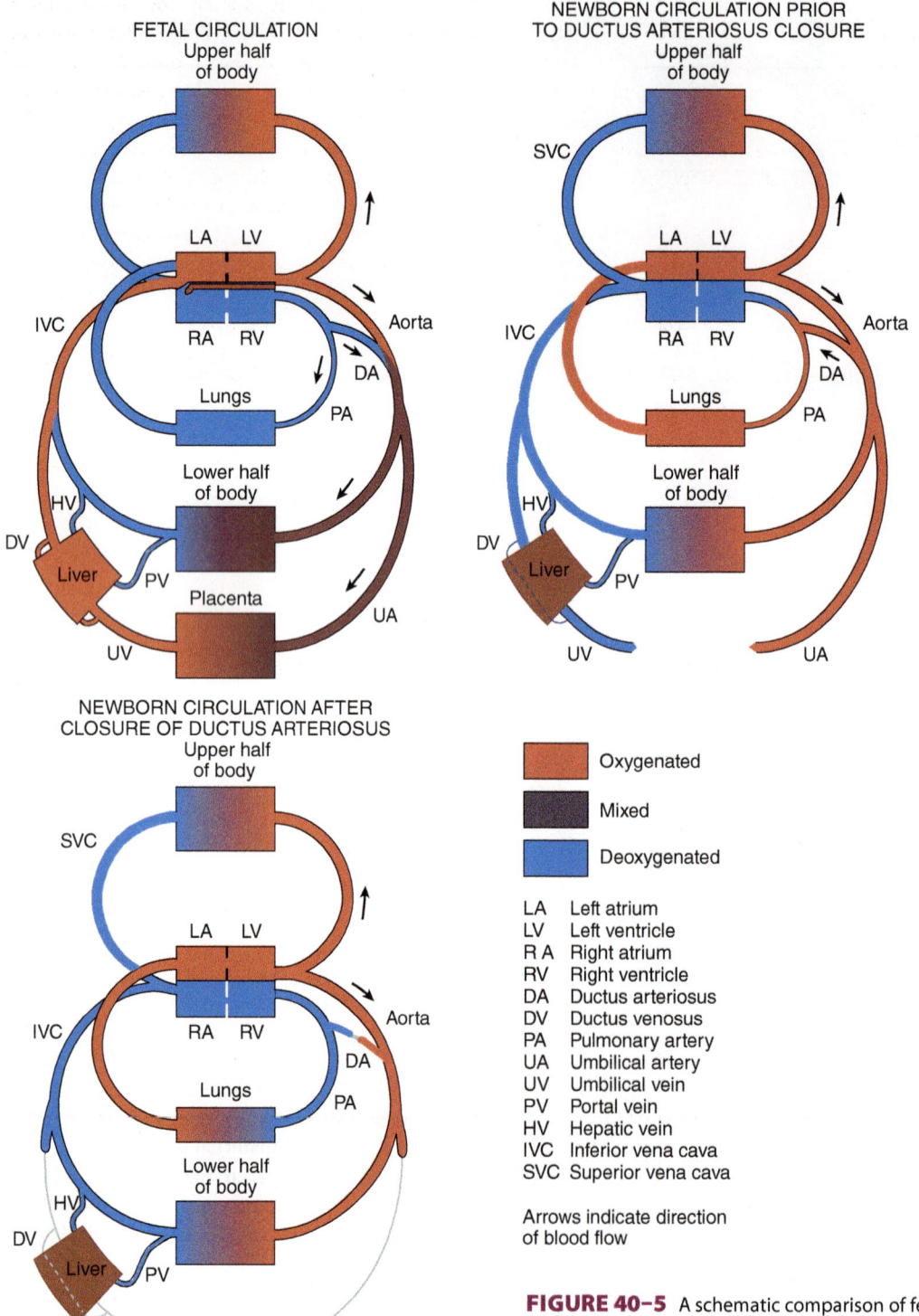

FETAL CIRCULATION
Upper half of body

NEWBORN CIRCULATION PRIOR TO DUCTUS ARTERIOSUS CLOSURE
Upper half of body

NEWBORN CIRCULATION AFTER CLOSURE OF DUCTUS ARTERIOSUS
Upper half of body

Oxygenated

Mixed

Deoxygenated

LA   Left atrium
LV   Left ventricle
R A   Right atrium
RV   Right ventricle
DA   Ductus arteriosus
DV   Ductus venosus
PA   Pulmonary artery
UA   Umbilical artery
UV   Umbilical vein
PV   Portal vein
HV   Hepatic vein
IVC   Inferior vena cava
SVC Superior vena cava

Arrows indicate direction of blood flow

FIGURE 40–5 A schematic comparison of fetal and neonatal circulation. (Reproduced, with permission, from Danforth DN, Scott JR: *Obstetrics and Gynecology*, 5th ed. Lippincott, 1986.)

flattens out and begins to produce pulmonary surfactant. This substance provides alveolar stability and is necessary to maintain normal lung expansion after birth (see Chapter 23). Sufficient pulmonary surfactant is usually present after 34 weeks of gestation. Administration of glucocorticoids to the mother may accelerate fetal surfactant production.

PHYSIOLOGICAL TRANSITION OF THE FETUS AT BIRTH

The most profound adaptive changes at birth involve the circulatory and respiratory systems. Failure to make this transition successfully results in fetal death or permanent neurological damage.

At term, the fetal lungs are developed but contain about 90 mL of a plasma ultrafiltrate. During expulsion of the fetus at delivery, this fluid is normally squeezed from the lungs by the forces of the pelvic muscles and the vagina acting on the baby (the vaginal squeeze). Any remaining fluid is reabsorbed by the pulmonary capillaries and lymphatics. Small (preterm) neonates and neonates delivered via cesarean section do not benefit from the vaginal squeeze and thus typically have greater difficulty in maintaining respirations (transient tachypnea of the newborn). Respiratory efforts are normally initiated within 30 s after birth and become sustained within 90 s. Mild hypoxia and acidosis as well as sensory stimulation—cord clamping, pain, touch, and noise—help initiate and sustain respirations, whereas the outward recoil of the chest at delivery aids in filling the lungs with air.

Lung expansion increases both alveolar and arterial oxygen tensions and decreases pulmonary vascular resistance. The increase in oxygen tension is a potent stimulus for pulmonary arterial vasodilation. The resultant increase in pulmonary blood flow and augmented flow to the left heart elevates left atrial pressure and functionally closes the foramen ovale. The increase in arterial oxygen tension also causes the ductus arteriosus to contract and functionally close. Other chemical mediators that may play a role in ductal closure include acetylcholine, bradykinin, and prostaglandins. The overall result is elimination of right-to-left shunting and establishment of the adult circulation (Figure 40–5). Anatomic closure of the ductus arteriosus does not usually occur until about 2–3 weeks, whereas closure of the foramen ovale takes months if it occurs at all.

Hypoxia or acidosis during the first few days of life can prevent or reverse these physiological changes, resulting in persistence of (or return to) the fetal circulation, or **persistent pulmonary hypertension of the newborn.** A vicious circle is established where the right-to-left shunting promotes hypoxemia and acidosis, which in turn promote more shunting (Figure 40–6). Right-to-left shunting may occur across the foramen ovale, the ductus arteriosus, or both. Unless this circle is broken, neonatal demise can occur rapidly.

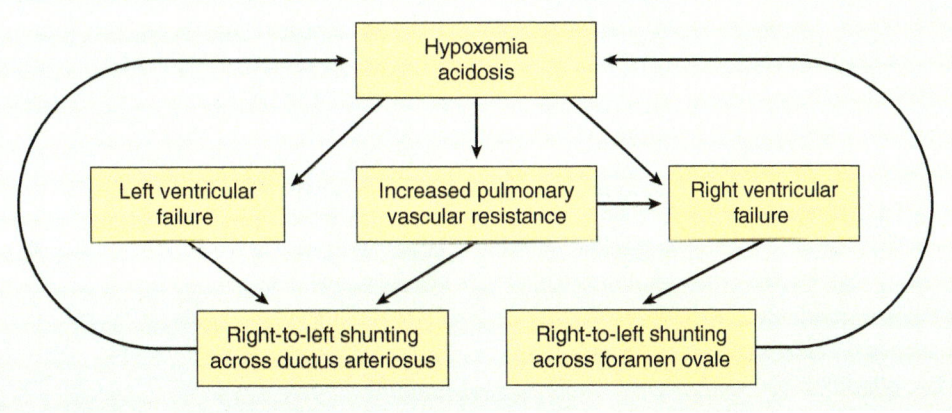

FIGURE 40–6 Pathophysiology of persistent pulmonary hypertension of the newborn (persistent fetal circulation). (Modified from Gregory GA: *Pediatric Anesthesia*, 2nd ed. Churchill Livingstone, 1989.)

CASE DISCUSSION

Postpartum Tubal Ligation

A 36-year-old woman is scheduled for bilateral tubal ligation 12 h after delivery of a healthy baby.

Is this patient still at increased risk for pulmonary aspiration?

Controversy exists over when the increased risk for pulmonary aspiration diminishes following pregnancy. Certainly, many factors contributing to delayed gastric emptying are alleviated shortly after delivery: mechanical distortion of the stomach is relieved, labor pains cease, and the circulating progesterone level rapidly declines. In addition, a period of 8–12 h of elective fasting is possible. Some studies suggest that the risk of pulmonary aspiration as judged by gastric volume and gastric fluid pH (see the section on Renal and Gastrointestinal Effects) normalizes within 24 h. Gastric volume and acidity usually do not differ in pregnant compared with nonpregnant women, although 30–60% of pregnant patients have a gastric volume greater than 25 mL or a gastric fluid pH less than 2.5. Therefore, most clinicians still consider the postpartum patient to be at increased risk for pulmonary aspiration and take appropriate precautions (see Chapters 17 and 41). It is not known when the risk returns to the level associated with elective surgical patients. Although some physiological changes associated with pregnancy may require up to 6 weeks for resolution, the increased risk of pulmonary aspiration probably returns to "normal" well before that time.

Other than aspiration risk, what factors determine the "optimal" time for postpartum sterilization?

The decision about when to perform postpartum tubal ligation (or laparoscopic fulguration) is complex and varies according to patient and obstetrician preferences as well as local practices. Factors influencing the decision include whether the patient had a vaginal or cesarean delivery and whether an anesthetic was administered for labor (epidural anesthesia) or delivery (epidural or general anesthesia).

Postpartum tubal ligation or fulguration may be (1) performed immediately following delivery of the baby and repair of the uterus during a cesarean section, (2) delayed 8–48 h following delivery to allow an elective fasting period, or (3) deferred until after the postpartum period (generally 6 weeks). Many obstetricians are reluctant to perform sterilizations immediately postpartum because the patient may change her mind later, particularly if something untoward happens to the baby. Furthermore, they want to ensure that the patient is stable, particularly after a complicated delivery. On the other hand, sterilization is technically much easier to perform in the immediate postpartum period because of the enlargement of the uterus and tubes. Postpartum sterilizations following natural vaginal delivery are generally performed within 48 h of delivery, because bacterial colonization of the reproductive tract thereafter is thought to increase the risk of postoperative infection.

What factors determine selection of an anesthetic technique for postpartum sterilization?

When continuous epidural anesthesia is administered for labor and vaginal delivery, the epidural catheter may be left in place up to 48 h for subsequent tubal ligation. The delay allows a period of elective fasting. A T4–5 sensory level with regional anesthesia is usually necessary to ensure a pain-free anesthetic experience. Lower sensory levels (as low as T10) may be adequate but sometimes fail to prevent pain during surgical traction on viscera.

When the patient has not had anesthesia for delivery, postpartum sterilization may be performed under either regional or general anesthesia. Because of the increased risk of pulmonary aspiration, regional anesthesia usually is preferred for bilateral tubal ligation via a minilaparotomy. Many clinicians prefer spinal over epidural anesthesia in this setting because of the risk of unintentional intravascular or intrathecal injections with the latter (see Chapter 45). Moreover, the risk of a precipitous decrease in blood pressure following spinal anesthesia may be significantly diminished following delivery (particularly when preceded by an intravenous fluid bolus). In addition, the incidence of postdural puncture headache is as low as 1% when a 25-gauge or smaller pencil-point needle is used. Dosage requirements for regional anesthesia generally return to normal within 24–36 h after delivery. Bupivacaine, 8–12 mg, or lidocaine, 60–75 mg, may be used for spinal anesthesia. For epidural anesthesia, 15–30 mL of lidocaine 1.5–2% or chloroprocaine 3% is most commonly used.

In contrast, when laparoscopic tubal fulguration is planned, general endotracheal anesthesia is usually preferred. Insufflation of gas during laparoscopy impairs pulmonary gas exchange and predisposes the patient to nausea, vomiting, and possibly pulmonary aspiration. Endotracheal intubation generally ensures adequate ventilation and protects the airway.

What considerations are important for postpartum patients undergoing general anesthesia?

Preoperative concerns include a decreased blood hemoglobin concentration and the persistent increased risk of pulmonary aspiration. Anemia is nearly always present as a result of the physiological effects of pregnancy combined with blood loss during and following delivery. Hemoglobin concentrations are usually greater than 9 g/dL, but levels as low as 7 g/dL are generally considered safe. Fortunately, sterilization procedures are rarely associated with significant blood loss.

The risk of pulmonary aspiration is diminished by a minimum of 8 h of fasting, premedication with an H_2 blocker (ranitidine), a clear antacid (sodium citrate), or metoclopramide (see Chapters 17 and 41). In addition, induction of anesthesia should employ a rapid-sequence technique with cricoid pressure prior to endotracheal intubation, and the patient should be extubated only when she is awake. Decreased plasma cholinesterase levels persist after delivery (see the section on Hepatic Effects), modestly prolonging the effect of succinylcholine. The duration of vecuronium but not atracurium (or cisatracurium) has also been reported to be prolonged in postpartum women. High concentrations of volatile agents should be avoided because of the at least theoretical risk of increasing uterine blood loss or inducing postpartum hemorrhage secondary to uterine relaxation. Intravenous opioids may be used to supplement inhalational agents. Intravenous drugs administered intraoperatively to mothers who are breast-feeding appear to have minimal if any effects on their neonates. Nonetheless, it may be prudent to avoid breast-feeding 12–24 h following general anesthesia. Mothers are advised by some anesthetists to "pump and dump" breast milk for 24 hours before resuming breast feeding.

SUGGESTED READING

Chestnut DH, Polley LS, Tsen LC, et al: *Chestnut's Obstetric Anesthesia: Principals and Practice*, 4th ed. Mosby, 2009.

Suresh M: *Shnider and Levinson's Anesthesia for Obstetrics*, 5th ed. Lippincott, Williams & Wilkins, 2012.

Obstetric Anesthesia

Michael A. Frölich, MD, MS

41

1 The most common morbidities encountered in obstetrics are severe hemorrhage and severe preeclampsia.

2 Regardless of the time of last oral intake, all obstetric patients are considered to have a full stomach and to be at risk for pulmonary aspiration.

3 Nearly all parenteral opioid analgesics and sedatives readily cross the placenta and can affect the fetus. Regional anesthetic techniques are preferred for management of labor pain.

4 Using a local anesthetic–opioid mixture for lumbar epidural analgesia during labor significantly reduces drug requirements, compared with using either agent alone.

5 Pain relief during labor requires neural blockade at the T10–L1 sensory level in the first stage of labor and at T10–S4 in the second stage.

6 Continuous lumbar epidural analgesia is the most versatile and most commonly employed technique, because it can be used for pain relief for the first stage of labor as well as analgesia/anesthesia for subsequent vaginal delivery or cesarean section, if necessary.

7 When dilute mixtures of a local anesthetic and an opioid are used, epidural analgesia has little if any effect on the progress of labor.

8 Even when aspiration does not yield blood or cerebrospinal fluid, unintentional intravascular or intrathecal placement of an epidural needle or catheter is possible.

9 Hypotension is a common side effect of regional anesthetic techniques and must be treated aggressively with phenylephrine or ephedrine, supplemental oxygen, left uterine displacement, and intravenous fluid boluses to prevent fetal compromise.

10 Techniques using combined spinal–epidural analgesia and anesthesia may particularly benefit patients with severe pain early in labor and those who receive analgesia/ anesthesia just prior to delivery.

11 Spinal or epidural anesthesia is preferred to general anesthesia for cesarean section because regional anesthesia is associated with lower maternal mortality.

12 Continuous epidural anesthesia allows better control over the sensory level than "single-shot" techniques. Conversely, spinal anesthesia has a more rapid, predictable onset; may produce a more dense (complete) block; and lacks the potential for serious systemic drug toxicity because of the smaller dose of local anesthetic employed.

13 Risk of systemic local anesthetic toxicity during epidural analgesia and anesthesia is minimized by slowly administering dilute solutions for labor pain and by fractionating the total dose administered for cesarean section into 5-mL increments.

—Continued next page

Continued—

14 Maternal hemorrhage is one of the most common severe morbidities complicating obstetric anesthesia. Causes include placenta previa, abruptio placentae, and uterine rupture.

15 Common causes of postpartum hemorrhage include uterine atony, a retained placenta, obstetric lacerations, uterine inversion, and use of tocolytic agents prior to delivery.

16 Intrauterine asphyxia during labor is the most common cause of neonatal depression. Fetal monitoring throughout labor is helpful in identifying which babies may be at risk, detecting fetal distress, and evaluating the effect of acute interventions.

This chapter focuses on the practice of obstetric anesthesia. Techniques for analgesia and anesthesia during labor, vaginal delivery, and cesarean section are presented. The chapter ends with a review of neonatal resuscitation.

ANESTHETIC RISK IN OBSTETRIC PATIENTS

Although the majority of women of childbearing age are healthy and would be considered to be at minimal operative risk, pregnancy, certain maternal–fetal factors, and preexisting medical conditions significantly increase surgical and obstetric risks.

Maternal Mortality

Maternal mortality is usually presented as the number of women who die while pregnant (or within 42 days of pregnancy termination) after excluding accidents and unrelated causes. This number is often indexed to the total number of live births. The maternal mortality index has decreased nearly 100-fold since 1900. Likely due to better reporting, it rose slightly in the United States to 21 deaths per 100,000 live births in 2010. The world average is 400 deaths per 100,000 live births. Of all maternal deaths worldwide, 99% occur in Africa, Asia, Latin America, and the Caribbean.

In the United States, overall mortality risk is greater for women older than 35 years of age, black women, and women who do not receive prenatal care. The leading causes of death associated with a live birth in 2010 were cardiovascular diseases (13.5%), cardiomyopathy (12.6%), hemorrhage (11.9%), noncardiovascular diseases (11.8%), hypertensive disorders of pregnancy (11.1%), infection/sepsis (11.1%), thrombotic pulmonary embolism (5.6%), amniotic fluid embolism (5.6%), cerebrovascular accidents (5.3%) and anesthesia complications (0.6%) Of all maternal deaths, only 34% of patients died within 24 h of delivery, whereas 55% died between 1 and 42 days, and another 11% died between 43 days and 1 year. Direct causes of maternal deaths are more clearly detailed from Canadian data, which show that, in addition to pulmonary embolism and preeclampsia/pregnancy-induced hypertension (PIH), amniotic fluid embolism and intracranial hemorrhage emerge as important additional causes of death.

Severe obstetric morbidity may be a more sensitive measure of outcome than maternal mortality. Data from the United Kingdom suggest that incidence of severe obstetric morbidity is 12 per 1000 deliveries, 100 times more common than mortality. Risk factors include age greater than 34 years, non-white ethnic group, multiple pregnancy, history of hypertension, previous postpartum hemorrhage, and emergency cesarean delivery. Table 41–1 lists the estimated incidence of the most common causes of severe morbidity; thromboembolic disease was deliberately excluded because of the difficulty in

1 making the diagnosis in nonfatal cases. By far the most common morbidities encountered in obstetrics are severe hemorrhage and severe preeclampsia.

TABLE 41–1 Incidence of severe obstetric morbidity.[1,3]

Morbidity	Incidence per 1000
Severe hemorrhage	6.7
Severe preeclampsia	3.9
HELLP syndrome[2]	0.5
Severe sepsis	0.4
Eclampsia	0.2
Uterine rupture	0.2

[1]Note thromboembolic disease was excluded.

[2]HELLP syndrome consists of hemolysis, elevated liver enzymes, and low platelet count.

[3]Data from Waterstone M, Bewley S, Wolfe C: Incidence and predictors of severe obstetric morbidity: Case-control study. BMJ 2001;322:1089.

Anesthetic Mortality

Anesthesia accidents and mishaps account for approximately 2–3% of maternal deaths. Data collected between 1985 and 1990 suggested a maternal mortality of 32 deaths per 1,000,000 live births due to general anesthesia and 1.9 deaths per 1,000,000 live births due to regional anesthesia. More recent data between 1998 and 2005 suggest a lower overall maternal mortality from anesthesia (about 1.2 % of live births), possibly due to greater use of regional anesthesia for labor and cesarean delivery. Most deaths occur during or after cesarean section. Moreover, the risk of an adverse outcome appears to be much greater with emergent than with elective cesarean sections.

Obstetric Anesthesia Closed Claims

Obstetric anesthesia care accounts for approximately 12% of the American Society of Anesthesiologists (ASA) Closed Claims database claims. A comparison of obstetric anesthesia claims from 1990 to 2003 or with pre-1990 claims shows a decrease in maternal deaths, as well as a decrease in respiratory-damaging events (aspiration, difficult intubation, esophageal intubation, and inadequate oxygenation/ventilation).

Although newborn deaths and brain damage also decreased over this period, they remained a leading cause of obstetric anesthesia malpractice claims. Maternal nerve injury was more common in claims reported after 1990 compared with earlier years.

General Approach to the Obstetric Patient

All patients entering the obstetric suite potentially require anesthesia services, whether planned or emergent. Patients requiring anesthetic care for labor or cesarean section should undergo a focused preanesthetic evaluation as early as possible. This should consist of a maternal health history, anesthesia and anesthesia-related obstetric history, blood pressure measurement, airway assessment, and back examination for regional anesthesia.

2 Regardless of the time of last oral intake, all patients are considered to have a full stomach and to be at risk for pulmonary aspiration. Because the duration of labor is often prolonged, guidelines usually allow small amounts of oral clear liquid for uncomplicated labor. The minimum fasting period for elective cesarean section remains controversial, but is recommended to be 6 h for light meals and 8 h for heavy meals. Prophylactic administration of a clear antacid (15–30 mL of 0.3 M sodium citrate orally) every 30 min prior to a cesarean section can help maintain gastric pH greater than 2.5 and may decrease the likelihood of severe aspiration pneumonitis. An H_2-blocking drug (ranitidine, 100–150 mg orally or 50 mg intravenously) or metoclopramide, 10 mg orally or intravenously, should also be considered in high-risk patients and in those expected to receive general anesthesia. H_2 blockers reduce both gastric volume and pH but have no effect on the gastric contents already present. Metoclopramide accelerates gastric emptying, decreases gastric volume, and increases lower esophageal sphincter tone. The supine position should be avoided unless a left uterine displacement device (>15° wedge) is placed under the right hip.

Anesthesia for Labor & Vaginal Delivery

PAIN PATHWAYS DURING LABOR

The pain of labor arises from contraction of the myometrium against the resistance of the cervix and perineum, progressive dilation of the cervix and lower uterine segment, and stretching and compression of pelvic and perineal structures.

Pain during the first stage of labor is primarily visceral pain resulting from uterine contractions and cervical dilation. It is usually initially confined to the T11–T12 dermatomes during the latent phase, but eventually involves the T10–L1 dermatomes as labor enters the active phase. The visceral afferent fibers responsible for labor pain travel with sympathetic nerve fibers first to the uterine and cervical plexuses, then through the hypogastric and aortic plexuses, before entering the spinal cord with the T10–L1 nerve roots. The pain is initially perceived in the lower abdomen but may increasingly be referred to the lumbosacral area, gluteal region, and thighs as labor progresses. Pain intensity also increases with progressive cervical dilation and with increasing intensity and frequency of uterine contractions. Nulliparous women and those with a history of dysmenorrhea appear to experience greater pain during the first stage of labor.

The onset of perineal pain at the end of the first stage signals the beginning of fetal descent and the second stage of labor. Stretching and compression of pelvic and perineal structures intensifies the pain. Sensory innervation of the perineum is provided by the pudendal nerve (S2–4) so pain during the second stage of labor involves the T10–S4 dermatomes.

PSYCHOLOGICAL & NONPHARMACOLOGICAL TECHNIQUES

Psychological and nonpharmacological techniques are based on the premise that the pain of labor can be suppressed by reorganizing one's thoughts. Patient education and positive conditioning about the birthing process are central to such techniques. Pain during labor tends to be accentuated by fear of the unknown or previous unpleasant experiences. Techniques include those of Bradley, Dick-Read, Lamaze, and LeBoyer. The Lamaze technique, one of the most popular, coaches the parturient to take a deep breath at the beginning of each contraction followed by rapid, shallow breathing for the duration of the contraction. The parturient also concentrates on an object in the room and attempts to focus her thoughts away from the pain. Less common nonpharmacological techniques include hypnosis, transcutaneous electrical nerve stimulation, biofeedback, and acupuncture. The success of all these techniques varies considerably from patient to patient, and many patients require additional forms of analgesia.

PARENTERAL AGENTS

3 Nearly all parenteral opioid analgesics and sedatives readily cross the placenta and can affect the fetus. Concern over fetal depression limits the use of these agents to the early stages of labor or to situations in which regional anesthetic techniques are not available or appropriate. Central nervous system depression in the neonate may be manifested by a prolonged time to sustain respirations, respiratory acidosis, or an abnormal neurobehavioral examination. Moreover, loss of beat-to-beat variability in the fetal heart rate (seen with most central nervous system depressants) and decreased fetal movements (due to sedation of the fetus) complicate the evaluation of fetal well-being during labor. Long-term fetal heart rate variability is affected more than short-term variability. The degree and significance of these effects depend on the specific agent, the dose, the time elapsed between its administration and delivery, and fetal maturity. Premature neonates exhibit the greatest sensitivity. In addition to maternal respiratory depression, opioids can also induce maternal nausea and vomiting and delay gastric emptying. Some clinicians have advocated use of opioids via patient-controlled analgesia (PCA) devices early in labor because this technique appears to reduce total opioid requirements.

Meperidine, a commonly used opioid, can be given in doses of 10–25 mg intravenously or

25–50 mg intramuscularly, usually up to a total of 100 mg. Maximal maternal and fetal respiratory depression is seen in 10–20 min following intravenous administration and in 1–3 h following intramuscular administration. Consequently, meperidine is usually administered early in labor when delivery is not expected for at least 4 h. Intravenous fentanyl, 25–100 mcg/h, has also been used for labor. Fentanyl in 25–100 mcg doses has a 3- to 10-min analgesic onset that initially lasts about 60 min, and lasts longer following multiple doses. However, maternal respiratory depression outlasts the analgesia. Lower doses of fentanyl may be associated with little or no neonatal respiratory depression and are reported to have no effect on Apgar scores. Morphine is not used because in equianalgesic doses it appears to cause greater respiratory depression in the fetus than meperidine and fentanyl. Agents with mixed agonist–antagonist activity (butorphanol, 1–2 mg, and nalbuphine, 10–20 mg intravenously or intramuscularly) are effective and are associated with little or no cumulative respiratory depression, but excessive sedation with repeat doses can be problematic.

Promethazine (25–50 mg intramuscularly) and hydroxyzine (50–100 mg intramuscularly) can be useful alone or in combination with meperidine. Both drugs reduce anxiety, opioid requirements, and the incidence of nausea, but do not add appreciably to neonatal depression. A significant disadvantage of hydroxyzine is pain at the injection site following intramuscular administration. Nonsteroidal antiinflammatory agents, such as ketorolac, are not recommended because they suppress uterine contractions and promote closure of the fetal ductus arteriosus.

Small doses (up to 2 mg) of midazolam (Versed) may be administered in combination with a small dose of fentanyl (up to 100 mcg) in healthy parturients at term to facilitate neuraxial blockade. At this dose, maternal amnesia has not been observed. Chronic administration of the longer acting benzodiazepine diazepam (Valium) has been associated with fetal depression.

Low-dose intravenous ketamine is a powerful analgesic. In doses of 10–15 mg intravenously, good analgesia can be obtained in 2–5 min without loss of consciousness. Unfortunately, fetal depression with low Apgar scores is associated with doses greater than 1 mg/kg. Large boluses of ketamine (>1 mg/kg) can be associated with hypertonic uterine contractions. Low-dose ketamine is most useful just prior to delivery or as an adjuvant to regional anesthesia. Some clinicians avoid use of ketamine because it may produce unpleasant psychotomimetic effects (see Chapter 9).

In the past, reduced concentrations of volatile anesthetic agents (eg, methoxyflurane) in oxygen were sometimes used for relief of milder labor pain. Inhalation of nitrous oxide–oxygen remains in common use for relief of mild labor pain in many countries. As previously noted, nitrous oxide has minimal effects on uterine blood flow or uterine contractions.

PUDENDAL NERVE BLOCK

Pudendal nerve blocks are often combined with perineal infiltration of local anesthetic to provide perineal anesthesia during the second stage of labor when other forms of anesthesia are not employed or prove to be inadequate. Paracervical plexus blocks are no longer used because of their association with a relatively high rate of fetal bradycardia; the close proximity of the injection site to the uterine artery may result in uterine arterial vasoconstriction, uteroplacental insufficiency, and increased levels of the local anesthetic in the fetal blood.

During a pudendal nerve block, a special needle (Koback) or guide (Iowa trumpet) is used to place the needle transvaginally underneath the ischial spine on each side (see Chapter 48); the needle is advanced 1–1.5 cm through the sacrospinous ligament, and 10 mL of 1% lidocaine or 2% chloroprocaine is injected following aspiration. The needle guide is used to limit the depth of injection and protect the fetus and vagina from the needle. Other potential complications include intravascular injection, retroperitoneal hematoma, and retropsoas or subgluteal abscess.

REGIONAL ANESTHETIC TECHNIQUES

Epidural or intrathecal techniques, alone or in combination, are currently the most popular methods of pain relief during labor and delivery. They can provide excellent analgesia while allowing the mother to be awake and cooperative during labor. Although spinal opioids or local anesthetics alone can provide satisfactory analgesia, techniques that combine the two have proved to be the most satisfactory in most parturients. Moreover, the synergy between opioids and local anesthetics decreases dose requirements and provides excellent analgesia with few maternal side effects and little or no neonatal depression.

1. Spinal Opioids Alone

Opioids may be given intrathecally as a single injection or intermittently via an epidural or intrathecal catheter (Table 41–2). Relatively large doses are required for analgesia during labor when epidural or intrathecal opioids are used alone. For example, the ED_{50} during labor is 124 mcg for epidural fentanyl and 21 mcg for epidural sufentanil. The higher doses may be associated with a high risk of side effects, most importantly respiratory depression. For that reason combinations of local anesthetics and opioids are most commonly used (see below). Pure opioid techniques are most useful for high-risk patients who may not tolerate the functional sympathectomy associated with spinal or epidural anesthesia (see Chapter 45). This group includes patients with hypovolemia or significant cardiovascular disease such as moderate to severe aortic stenosis, tetralogy of Fallot, Eisenmenger's syndrome, or pulmonary hypertension. With the exception of meperidine, which has local anesthetic properties, spinal opioids alone do not produce motor blockade or sympathectomy. Thus, they do not impair the ability of the parturient to "push." Disadvantages include

TABLE 41–2 Spinal opioid dosages for labor and delivery.

Agent	Intrathecal	Epidural
Morphine	0.1–0.5 mg	5 mg
Meperidine	10–15 mg	50–100 mg
Fentanyl	10–25 mcg	50–150 mcg
Sufentanil	3–10 mcg	10–20 mcg

less complete analgesia, lack of perineal relaxation, and side effects such as pruritus, nausea, vomiting, sedation, and respiratory depression. Side effects may be ameliorated with low doses of naloxone (0.1–0.2 mg/h intravenously).

Intrathecal Opioids

Intrathecal morphine in doses of 0.1–0.5 mg may produce satisfactory and prolonged (4–6 h) analgesia during the first stage of labor. Unfortunately, the onset of analgesia is slow (45–60 min), and these doses may not be sufficient in many patients. Higher doses are associated with a relatively high incidence of side effects. Morphine is therefore rarely used alone. The combination of morphine, 0.1–0.25 mg, and fentanyl, 12.5 mcg (or sufentanil, 5 mcg), may result in a more rapid onset of analgesia (5 min). Intermittent boluses of 10–15 mg of meperidine, 12.5–25 mcg of fentanyl, or 3–10 mcg of sufentanil via an intrathecal catheter can also provide satisfactory analgesia for labor. Early reports of fetal bradycardia following intrathecal opioid injections (eg, sufentanil) have not been confirmed by subsequent studies. Hypotension following administration of intrathecal opioids for labor is likely related to the resultant analgesia and decreased circulating catecholamine levels.

Epidural Opioids

Relatively large doses (≥7.5 mg) of epidural morphine are required for satisfactory labor analgesia, but doses larger than 5 mg are not recommended because of the increased risk of delayed respiratory depression and because the resultant analgesia is effective only in the early first stage of labor. Onset may take 30–60 min but analgesia lasts up to 12–24 h (as does the risk of delayed respiratory depression). Epidural meperidine, 50–100 mg, provides good, but relatively brief, analgesia (1–3 h). Epidural fentanyl, 50–150 mcg, or sufentanil, 10–20 mcg, usually produces analgesia within 5–10 min with few side effects, but it has a short duration (1–2 h). Although "single-shot" epidural opioids do not appear to cause significant neonatal depression, caution should be exercised following repeated administrations. Combinations of a lower dose of morphine, 2.5 mg, with fentanyl, 25–50 mcg (or sufentanil, 7.5–10 mcg), may result in a more rapid onset and prolongation of analgesia (4–5 h) with fewer side effects.

2. Local Anesthetic/Local Anesthetic–Opioid Mixtures

Epidural and spinal (intrathecal) analgesia more commonly utilizes local anesthetics either alone or **5** with opioids for labor and delivery. Analgesia during the first stage of labor requires neural blockade at the T10–L1 sensory level, whereas pain relief during the second stage of labor requires neural blockade at T10–S4. Continuous lumbar **6** epidural analgesia is the most versatile and most commonly-employed technique, because it can be used for pain relief for the first stage of labor as well as analgesia/anesthesia for subsequent vaginal delivery or cesarean section, if necessary. "Single-shot" epidural, spinal, or combined spinal epidural analgesia may be appropriate when pain relief is initiated just prior to vaginal delivery (the second stage). Obstetric caudal injections have largely been abandoned because of less versatility; although effective for perineal analgesia/anesthesia they require large volumes of local anesthetic to anesthetize upper lumbar and lower thoracic dermatomes. They have also been associated with early paralysis of the pelvic muscles that may interfere with normal rotation of the fetal head, and with a small risk of accidental puncture of the fetus.

Absolute contraindications to regional anesthesia include patient refusal, infection over the injection site, coagulopathy, marked hypovolemia, and true allergies to local anesthetics. The patient's inability to cooperate may prevent successful regional anesthesia. Neuraxial anesthesia and full anticoagulation is a dangerous combination. Regional anesthesia should generally not be performed within 6–8 h of a subcutaneous minidose of unfractionated heparin or within 12–24 h of administration of low-molecular-weight heparin (LMWH). Thrombocytopenia or concomitant administration of an antiplatelet agent increases the risk of spinal hematoma. A vaginal birth after cesarean (VBAC) delivery is not considered a contraindication to regional anesthesia during labor. Concern that the anesthesia may mask pain associated with uterine rupture during VBAC may not be justified, because dehiscence of a lower segment scar frequently does not cause pain even without epidural anesthesia; moreover, changes in uterine tone and contraction pattern may be more reliable signs.

Before performing any regional block, appropriate equipment and supplies for resuscitation should be checked and made immediately available. Minimum supplies include oxygen, suction, a mask with a positive-pressure device for ventilation, a functioning laryngoscope and blades, endotracheal tubes (6 or 6.5 mm), oral and nasal airways, intravenous fluids, ephedrine, atropine, propofol, and succinylcholine. The ability to frequently monitor blood pressure and heart rate is mandatory. A pulse oximeter and capnograph should be readily available.

Lumbar Epidural Analgesia

Epidural analgesia for labor may be administered in early labor after the patient has been evaluated by **7** her obstetrician. When dilute mixtures of a local anesthetic and an opioid are used, epidural analgesia has little if any effect on the progress of labor. Concerns that regional analgesia will increase the likelihood of oxytocin augmentation, operative (eg, forceps) delivery, or cesarean section, are unjustified. It is often advantageous to place an epidural catheter early, when the patient is less uncomfortable and can be positioned more easily. Moreover, should an urgent or emergent cesarean section become necessary, the presence of a well-functioning epidural catheter makes it possible to avoid general anesthesia.

A. Technique

Parturients may be positioned on their sides or in the sitting position for the procedure. The sitting position often makes it easier to identify the midline and spine in obese patients. When epidural anesthesia is being given for vaginal delivery (second stage), the sitting position helps ensure good sacral spread.

Because the lumbar epidural space pressure may be positive in some parturients, correct identification of the epidural space may be difficult. Unintentional dural puncture will occur even in experienced hands; the incidence of "wet taps" in obstetric patients is 0.25–9%, depending on clinician

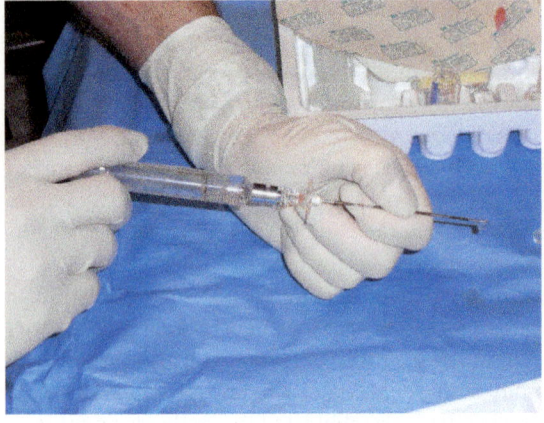

A

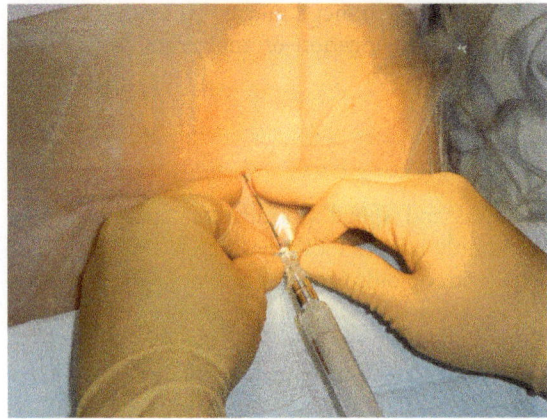

B

FIGURE 41–1 **A:** One-handed needle advancement; continuous pressure technique. The operator applies continuous pressure to the plunger of a loss-of-resistance syringe filled with saline and an air bubble while advancing the needle with the left hand braced against the patient's back. **B:** Bimanual needle advancement; intermittent pressure technique. The operator advances the loss-of-resistance syringe with both hands 2–3 mm at a time while appreciating the resistance encountered by the needle. **C:** In between bimanual advancements of the needle, the operator tests the tissue resistance of the needle tip by bouncing the plunger of the air-filled loss-of-resistance syringe. Many practitioners add a compressible air bubble to a saline-filled syringe and bounce the plunger to ensure that the plunger is moving freely and not sticking to the syringe barrel wall.

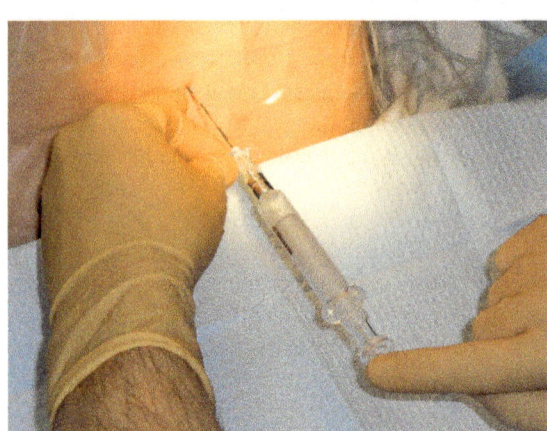

C

experience. Many practitioners add a compressible air bubble to the saline syringe and bounce the plunger to ensure that it moves freely and does not stick to the syringe wall (Figure 41–1A and C). Most clinicians advocate the midline approach, whereas a minority favors the paramedian approach. For the placement of a lumbar epidural catheter in the obstetric patient, most anesthesiologists advance the epidural needle with the left hand, which is braced against the patient's back, while applying continuous pressure to a glass syringe filled with sterile saline (Figure 41–1A and C). Alternatively, some make use of the "wings" of the Weiss epidural needle by advancing it with both hands few millimeters at a time (Figure 41–1B). A change of tissue resistance is then tested continuously using tactile feedback

when advancing the needle and by intermittently applying pressure to the air-filled loss-of resistance syringe. The later technique allows for precise control of needle advancement and may allow a better distinction of various tissue densities. If air is used for detecting loss of resistance, the amount injected should be limited; injection of larger volumes of air (>2–3 mL) in the epidural space has been associated with patchy or unilateral analgesia and headache. The average depth of the lumbar epidural space in obstetric patients is reported to be 5 cm from the skin. Placement of the epidural catheter at the L3–4 or L4–5 interspace is generally optimal for achieving a T10–S5 neural blockade. Ultrasound guidance has recently been offered as tool in assisting with the placement of an epidural catheter. This technique allows the practitioner to judge the depth of the epidural space and estimate the best angle of needle insertion. The potential benefit of this technique is most obvious in obese patients with poor anatomic landmarks. However, the technique is highly user-dependent, and few practitioners have adopted it.

If unintentional dural puncture occurs, the anesthetist has two choices: (1) place the epidural catheter in the subarachnoid space for continuous spinal (intrathecal) analgesia and anesthesia (see below), or (2) remove the needle and attempt placement at a higher spinal level. The intrathecally-placed epidural catheter may be used as continuous spinal anesthetic, possibly reducing the incidence of post–dural puncture headache. If used in this fashion, an infusion of 0.0625–0.125% bupivacaine with fentanyl, 2–3 mcg/mL starting at 1–3 mL/h, is a reasonable choice.

B. Choice of Epidural Catheter

Many clinicians advocate use of a multiholed catheter instead of a single-holed catheter for obstetric anesthesia. Use of a multiholed catheter may be associated with fewer unilateral blocks and greatly reduces the incidence of false-negative aspiration when assessing for intravascular or intrathecal catheter placement. Advancing a multiholed catheter 4–6 cm into the epidural space appears to be optimal for obtaining adequate sensory levels. A single-hole catheter need only be advanced 3–5 cm into the epidural space. Shorter insertion depths (<5 cm), however, may favor dislodgment of the catheter out of the epidural space in obese patients following flexion/extension movements of the spine. Spiral wire-reinforced catheters are very resistant to kinking. A spiral or spring tip, particularly when used without a stylet, is associated with fewer, less intense paresthesias and may also be associated with a lower incidence of accidental intravascular insertion.

C. Choice of Local Anesthetic Solutions

The addition of opioids to local anesthetic solutions for epidural anesthesia has dramatically changed the practice of obstetric anesthesia. The synergy between epidural opioids and local anesthetic solutions reflects separate sites of action, namely, opiate receptors and neuronal axons, respectively. When the two are combined, very low concentrations of both local anesthetic and opioid can be used. More importantly, the incidence of adverse side effects, such as hypotension and drug toxicity, is likely reduced. Although local anesthetics can be used alone, there is rarely a reason to do so. Moreover, when an opioid is omitted, the higher concentration of local anesthetic required (eg, bupivacaine, 0.25%, and ropivacaine, 0.2%) for adequate analgesia can impair the parturient's ability to push effectively as labor progresses. Bupivacaine or ropivacaine in concentrations of 0.0625–0.125% with either fentanyl, 2–3 mcg/mL, or sufentanil, 0.3–0.5 mcg/mL, is most often used. In general, the lower the concentration of the local anesthetic the greater the concentration of opioid that is required. Very dilute local anesthetic mixtures (0.0625%) generally do not produce motor blockade and may allow some patients to ambulate ("walking" or "mobile" epidural). The long duration of action of bupivacaine makes it a popular agent for labor. Ropivacaine may be preferable because of its reduced potential for cardiotoxicity (see Chapter 16). At equi-analgesic doses, ropivacaine and bupivacaine appear to produce the same degree of motor block.

The effect of epinephrine-containing solutions on the course of labor is somewhat controversial. Many clinicians use epinephrine-containing solutions only for intravascular test doses because of concern that the solutions may slow the progression of labor or adversely affect the fetus; others use only very dilute concentrations of epinephrine such as 1:800,000 or 1:400,000. Studies comparing these various agents have failed to find any differences in neonatal Apgar scores, acid–base status, or neurobehavioral evaluations.

D. Epidural Activation for the First Stage of Labor

Initial epidural injections may be done either before or after the catheter is placed. Administration through the needle can facilitate catheter placement, whereas administration through the catheter ensures proper function of the catheter. The following sequence is suggested for epidural activation:

1. Test for unintentional subarachnoid or intravascular placement of the needle or catheter with a 3-mL test dose of a local

anesthetic with 1:200,000 epinephrine (controversial; see the section on Prevention of Unintentional Intravascular and Intrathecal Injections). Many clinicians test with lidocaine 1.5% because of less toxicity following unintentional intravascular injection and a more rapid onset of spinal anesthesia than with bupivacaine and ropivacaine. The test dose should be injected between contractions to help reduce false positive signs of an intravascular injection (ie, tachycardia due to a painful contraction).

2. If after 5 min signs of intravascular or intrathecal injection are absent, with the patient supine and left uterine displacement, administer 10 mL of the local anesthetic–opioid mixture in 5-mL increments, waiting 1–2 min between doses, to achieve a T10–L1 sensory level. The initial bolus is usually composed of 0.1–0.2% ropivacaine or 0.0625–0.125% bupivacaine combined with either 50–100 mcg of fentanyl or 10–20 mcg of sufentanil.

3. Monitor with frequent blood pressure measurements for 20–30 min or until the patient is stable. Pulse oximetry should also be used. Oxygen is administered via face mask if there are any significant decreases in blood pressure or oxygen saturation readings.

4. Repeat steps 2 and 3 when pain recurs until the first stage of labor is completed. Alternatively, a continuous epidural infusion technique may be employed using bupivacaine or ropivacaine in concentrations of 0.0625–0.125% with either fentanyl, 1–5 mcg/mL, or sufentanil, 0.2–0.5 mcg/mL at a rate of 10 mL/h, which subsequently is adjusted to the patient's analgesic requirements (range: 5–15 mL/h). A third choice would be to use patient-controlled epidural analgesia (PCEA). Some studies suggest that total drug requirements may be less and patient satisfaction is greater with PCEA compared with other epidural techniques. PCEA settings are typically a 5-mL bolus dose with a 5–10 min lockout and 0–12 mL/h basal rate; a 1-h limit of 15–25 mL may used. Migration of the epidural catheter into a blood

vessel during a continuous infusion technique may be heralded by loss of effective analgesia; a high index of suspicion is required because overt signs of systemic toxicity may be absent. Erosion of the catheter through the dura results in a slowly progressive motor blockade of the lower extremities and a rising sensory level.

E. Epidural Administration During the Second Stage of Labor

Administration for the second stage of labor extends the block to include the S2–4 dermatomes. Whether a catheter is already in place or epidural anesthesia is just being initiated, the following steps should be undertaken:

1. If the patient does not already have a catheter in place, identify the epidural space while the patient is in a sitting position. A patient who already has an epidural catheter in place should be placed in a semiupright or sitting position prior to injection.

2. Give a 3-mL test dose of local anesthetic (eg, lidocaine 1.5%) with 1:200,000 epinephrine. Again, the injection should be completed between contractions.

3. If after 5 min signs of an intravascular or intrathecal injection are absent, give 10–15 mL of additional local anesthetic–opioid mixture at a rate not faster than 5 mL every 1–2 min.

4. Administer oxygen by face mask, lay the patient supine with left uterine displacement, and monitor blood pressure every 1–2 min for the first 15 min, then every 5 min thereafter.

F. Prevention of Unintentional Intravascular and Intrathecal Injections

Safe administration of epidural anesthesia is critically dependent on avoiding unintentional intrathecal or intravascular injection. Unintentional intravascular or intrathecal placement of an epidural needle or catheter is possible even when aspiration fails to yield blood or cerebrospinal fluid (CSF). The incidence of unintentional intravascular or intrathecal placement of an epidural catheter is 5–15% and 0.5–2.5%, respectively. Even a properly placed catheter can subsequently erode into an epidural vein or an intrathecal position. This possibility should be considered each time local anesthetic is injected through an epidural catheter.

Test doses of lidocaine, 45–60 mg, bupivacaine, 7.5–10 mg, ropivacaine, 6–8 mg, or chloroprocaine, 100 mg, can be given to exclude unintentional intrathecal placement. Signs of sensory and motor blockade usually become apparent within 2–3 min and 3–5 min, respectively, if the injection is intrathecal.

In patients not receiving β-adrenergic antagonists, the intravascular injection of a local anesthetic solution with 15–20 mcg of epinephrine consistently increases the heart rate by 20–30 beats/min within 30–60 s if the catheter (or epidural needle) is intravascular. This technique is not always reliable in parturients because they often have marked spontaneous baseline variations in heart rate with contractions. In fact, bradycardia has been reported in a parturient following intravenous injection of 15 mcg of epinephrine. Moreover, in animal studies, 15 mcg of epinephrine intravenously reduces uterine blood flow. Alternative methods of detecting unintentional intravascular catheter placement include eliciting tinnitus or perioral numbness following a 100-mg test dose of lidocaine or eliciting a chronotropic effect following injection of 5 mcg of isoproterenol. The use of dilute local anesthetic solutions and slow injection rates of no more than 5 mL at a time may also enhance detection of unintentional intravascular injections before catastrophic complications develop.

G. Management of Complications

9 **1. Hypotension**—Generally defined as a greater than 20% decrease in the patient's baseline blood pressure, or a systolic blood pressure less than 100 mm Hg, hypotension is a common side effect of neuraxial anesthesia. It is primarily due to decreased sympathetic tone and is greatly accentuated by aortocaval compression and an upright or semiupright position. Treatment should be aggressive in obstetric patients and consists of intravenous boluses of ephedrine (5–15 mg) or phenylephrine (25–50 mcg), supplemental oxygen, left uterine displacement, and an intravenous fluid bolus. Although the routine use of a crystalloid fluid bolus prior to dosing an epidural catheter is not effective in the prevention of hypotension, ensuring proper intravenous hydration of the pregnant patient is important.

Use of the head-down (Trendelenburg) position is controversial because of its potentially detrimental effects on pulmonary gas exchange.

2. Unintentional intravascular injection—Early recognition of intravascular injection, facilitated by the use of small, repeated doses of local anesthetic instead of a large bolus, may prevent more serious local anesthetic toxicity, such as seizures or cardiovascular collapse. Intravascular injections of toxic doses of lidocaine or chloroprocaine usually present as seizures. Propofol, 20–50 mg, will terminate seizure activity. Maintenance of a patent airway and adequate oxygenation are critical; however, immediate endotracheal intubation with succinylcholine and cricoid pressure is rarely necessary. Intravascular injections of bupivacaine can cause rapid and profound cardiovascular collapse as well as seizure activity. Cardiac resuscitation may be exceedingly difficult and is aggravated by acidosis and hypoxia. An immediate infusion of 20% Intralipid has shown efficacy in reversing bupivacaine-induced cardiac toxicity. Amiodarone is the agent of choice for treating local anesthetic–induced ventricular arrhythmias.

3. Unintentional intrathecal injection—Even when dural puncture is recognized immediately after injection of local anesthetic, attempted aspiration of the local anesthetic will usually be unsuccessful. The patient should be placed supine with left uterine displacement. Head elevation accentuates the adverse cerebral effects of hypotension and should be avoided. Hypotension should be treated with phenylephrine and intravenous fluids. A high spinal level can also result in diaphragmatic paralysis, which necessitates intubation and ventilation with 100% oxygen. Delayed onset of a very high and often patchy or unilateral block may be due to unrecognized subdural injection (see Chapter 45), which is managed similarly.

4. Postdural puncture headache (PDPH)—Headache frequently follows unintentional dural puncture in parturients. A self-limited headache may occur without dural puncture; in such instances, injection of significant amounts of air into the epidural space during a loss-of-resistance technique may be responsible. PDPH is due to decreased intracranial pressure with compensatory cerebral vasodilation (see Chapter 45). Bed rest, hydration, oral analgesics, and caffeine sodium benzoate (500 mg added to 1000 mL intravenous fluids administered at 200 mL/h) may be effective in patients with mild headaches and as temporary treatment. Patients with moderate to severe headaches usually require an epidural blood patch (10–20 mL) (see Chapter 45). Prophylactic epidural blood patches are not recommended; 25–50% of patients may not require a blood patch following dural puncture. Delaying a blood patch for 24 h increases its efficacy. Intracranial subdural hematoma has been reported as a rare complication 1–6 weeks following unintentional dural puncture in obstetric patients.

5. Maternal fever—Maternal fever is often interpreted as chorioamnionitis and may trigger an invasive evaluation for neonatal sepsis. There is no evidence that epidural anesthesia affects maternal temperature or that neonatal sepsis is increased with epidural analgesia. An elevation in maternal temperature is associated with a high body mass index and with nulliparity in women and prolonged labor.

Combined Spinal & Epidural (CSE) Analgesia

10 Techniques using CSE analgesia and anesthesia may particularly benefit patients with severe pain early in labor and those who receive analgesia/anesthesia just prior to delivery. Intrathecal opioid and local anesthetic are injected after which an epidural catheter is left in place. The intrathecal drugs provide nearly immediate pain control and have minimal effects on the early progress of labor, whereas the epidural catheter provides a route for subsequent analgesia for labor and delivery or anesthesia for cesarean section. Addition of small doses of local anesthetic agents to intrathecal opioid injection greatly potentiates their analgesia and can significantly reduce opioid requirements. Thus, many clinicians will inject 2.5 mg of preservative-free bupivacaine or 3–4 mg of ropivacaine with intrathecal opioids for analgesia in the first stage of labor. Intrathecal doses for CSE are fentanyl, 5–10 mcg, or sufentanil, 5 mcg. Some studies suggest that CSE techniques may be associated with greater patient satisfaction and lower incidence of PDPH than epidural analgesia alone. A 24- to 27-gauge pencil-point spinal needle (Whitacre, Sprotte, or Gertie Marx) is used to minimize the incidence of PDPH.

The spinal and epidural needles may be placed at separate interspaces, but most clinicians use a needle-through-needle technique at the same interspace. Use of saline for identification of the epidural space may potentially cause confusion of saline for CSF. With the needle-through-needle technique, the epidural needle is placed in the epidural space and a long spinal needle is then introduced through it and advanced farther into the subarachnoid space. A distinct pop is felt as the needle penetrates the dura. The needle-beside-needle technique typically employs a specially designed epidural needle that has a channel for the spinal needle. After the intrathecal injection and withdrawal of the spinal needle, the epidural catheter is threaded into position and the epidural needle is withdrawn. The risk of advancing the epidural catheter through the dural hole created by the spinal needle appears to be negligible when a 25-gauge or smaller needle is used. The epidural catheter, however, should be aspirated carefully and local anesthetic should always be given slowly and in small increments to avoid unintentional intrathecal injections. Moreover, epidural drugs should be titrated carefully because the dural hole may facilitate entry of epidural drugs into CSF and enhance their effects.

Spinal Anesthesia

Spinal anesthesia given just prior to delivery—also known as saddle block—provides profound anesthesia for operative vaginal delivery. Use of a 22-gauge or smaller, pencil-point spinal needle (Whitacre, Sprotte, or Gertie Marx) decreases the likelihood of PDPH. Hyperbaric tetracaine (3–4 mg), bupivacaine (2.5–5 mg), or lidocaine (20–40 mg) usually provides excellent perineal anesthesia. Addition of fentanyl (12.5–25 mcg) or sufentanil (5–7.5 mcg) significantly potentiates the block. A T10 sensory level can be obtained with slightly larger amounts of local anesthetic. Three minutes after injection, the patient is placed in the lithotomy position with left uterine displacement.

GENERAL ANESTHESIA

Because of the increased risk of aspiration, general anesthesia for vaginal delivery is avoided except for a true emergency. If an epidural catheter is already in

TABLE 41–3 Possible indications for general anesthesia during vaginal delivery.

Fetal distress during the second stage
Tetanic uterine contractions
Breech extraction
Version and extraction
Manual removal of a retained placenta
Replacement of an inverted uterus

TABLE 41–4 Major indications for cesarean section.

Labor unsafe for mother and fetus
Increased risk of uterine rupture
Previous classic cesarean section
Previous extensive myomectomy or uterine reconstruction
Increased risk of maternal hemorrhage
Central or partial placenta previa
Abruptio placentae
Previous vaginal reconstruction
Dystocia
Abnormal fetopelvic relations
Fetopelvic disproportion
Abnormal fetal presentation
Transverse or oblique lie
Breech presentation
Dysfunctional uterine activity
Immediate or emergent delivery necessary
Fetal distress
Umbilical cord prolapse with fetal bradycardia
Maternal hemorrhage
Genital herpes with ruptured membranes
Impending maternal death

place and time permits, rapid-onset regional anesthesia can be obtained with alkalinized lidocaine 2% or chloroprocaine 3%. Table 41–3 lists indications for general anesthesia during vaginal delivery. These indications are rare, and most share the need for uterine relaxation.

Anesthesia for Cesarean Section

Common indications for cesarean section are listed in Table 41–4. The choice of anesthesia for cesarean section is determined by multiple factors, including the indication for operative delivery, its urgency, patient and obstetrician preferences, and the skills of the anesthetist. In a given country, cesarean section rates may vary as much as two-fold between institutions. In some countries, cesarean delivery is seen as preferable to labor and rates are much greater than those in the United States (which generally vary between 15% and 35% from hospital to hospital). In the United States most elective cesarean sections are performed **11** under spinal anesthesia. Regional anesthesia has become the preferred technique because general anesthesia has been associated with a greater risk of maternal morbidity and mortality. Deaths associated with general anesthesia are generally related to airway problems, such as inability to intubate, inability to ventilate, or aspiration pneumonitis, whereas deaths associated with regional anesthesia are generally related to excessive dermatomal spread of blockade or to local anesthetic toxicity.

Other advantages of regional anesthesia include (1) less neonatal exposure to potentially depressant drugs, (2) a decreased risk of maternal pulmonary aspiration, (3) an awake mother at the birth of her child, and (4) the option of using spinal opioids for **12** postoperative pain relief. Continuous epidural anesthesia allows better continuing control over the sensory level than "single-shot" techniques. Conversely, spinal anesthesia has a more rapid, predictable onset; may produce a more dense (complete) block; and lacks the potential for serious systemic drug toxicity because of the smaller dose of local anesthetic employed. Regardless of the regional technique chosen, one must be prepared to administer a general anesthetic at any time during the procedure. Moreover, administration of a nonparticulate antacid within 30 min of surgery should be considered.

General anesthesia offers (1) a very rapid and reliable onset, (2) control over the airway and ventilation, (3) greater comfort for parturients who have morbid fears of needles or surgery, and (4) potentially less hypotension than regional anesthesia. General anesthesia also facilitates management in the event of severe hemorrhagic complications such as placenta accreta. Its principal disadvantages are the risk of pulmonary aspiration, the potential inability to intubate or ventilate the patient, and drug-induced fetal depression. Present anesthetic techniques, however, limit the dose of intravenous agents such that fetal depression is usually not clinically significant with general anesthesia when delivery occurs within 10 min of induction of anesthesia. Regardless of the type of anesthesia, neonates delivered more than 3 min after uterine incision have lower Apgar scores and pH values.

REGIONAL ANESTHESIA

Cesarean section requires that dermatomes up to and including T4 be anesthetized. Because of the associated sympathetic blockade, patients should receive an appropriate intravenous bolus of crystalloid such as lactated Ringer's (typically 1000–1500 mL) or colloid (typically 250–500 mL) solution at the time of neural blockade. Such boluses will not consistently prevent hypotension but can virtually eliminate preexisting hypovolemia. After the local anesthetic injection, phenylephrine may be titrated to maintain blood pressure within 20% of baseline. An approximate 10% decrease in blood pressure is expected. Administration of ephedrine (5–10 mg) may be necessary in the hypotensive patient with reduced heart rate. Some studies suggest that phenylephrine produces less neonatal acidosis compared with ephedrine.

After spinal anesthetic injection, the patient is placed supine with left uterine displacement; supplemental oxygen (40–50%) is given; and blood pressure is measured every 1–2 min until it stabilizes. Hypotension following epidural anesthesia typically has a slower onset. Slight Trendelenburg positioning facilitates achieving a T4 sensory level and may also help prevent severe hypotension. Extreme degrees of Trendelenburg may interfere with pulmonary gas exchange.

Spinal Anesthesia

The patient is usually placed in the lateral decubitus or sitting position, and a hyperbaric solution of lidocaine (50–60 mg) or bupivacaine (10–15 mg) is injected. Bupivacaine should be chosen if the

obstetrician will not likely complete the surgery in 45 minutes. Use of a 22-gauge or smaller, pencil-point spinal needle (Whitacre, Sprotte, or Gertie Marx) decreases the incidence of PDPH. Adding 10–25 mcg of fentanyl or 5–10 mcg of sufentanil to the local anesthetic solution enhances the intensity of the block and prolongs its duration without adversely affecting neonatal outcome. Addition of preservative-free morphine (0.1–0.3 mg) can prolong postoperative analgesia up to 24 h, but requires monitoring for delayed postoperative respiratory depression. Regardless of the anesthetic agents used, considerable variability in the maximal dermatomal extent of anesthesia should be expected (see Chapter 45). In obese patients, a standard 3.5-in. (9-cm) spinal needle may not be long enough to reach the subarachnoid space. In these cases, longer spinal needles of 4.75 in. (12 cm) to 6 in. (15.2 cm) may be required. To prevent these longer needles from bending, some anesthesiologists prefer larger diameter needles, such as the 22-gauge Sprotte needle. Alternatively, a 2.5-in. (6.3-cm) 20-gauge Quincke type spinal needle can be used as a long introducer and guide for a 25-gauge pencil-point spinal needle.

Continuous spinal anesthesia is also a reasonable option, especially for obese patients, following unintentional dural puncture sustained while attempting to place an epidural catheter for cesarean section. After the catheter is advanced 2–2.5 cm into the lumbar subarachnoid space and secured, it can be used to inject anesthetic agents; moreover, it allows later supplementation of anesthesia if necessary.

Epidural Anesthesia

Epidural anesthesia for cesarean section is typically performed using a catheter, which allows supplementation of anesthesia if necessary and provides an **13** excellent route for postoperative opioid administration. After negative aspiration and a negative test dose, a total of 15–25 mL of local anesthetic is injected slowly in 5-mL increments in order to minimize the risk of systemic local anesthetic toxicity. Lidocaine 2% (typically with 1:200,000 epinephrine) or chloroprocaine 3% are most commonly used in the United States. The addition of fentanyl,

50–100 mcg, or sufentanil, 10–20 mcg, greatly enhances the intensity of the analgesia and prolongs its duration without adversely affecting neonatal outcome. Some practitioners also add sodium bicarbonate (7.5% or 8.4% solution) to local anesthetic solutions (1 mEq/10 mL of lidocaine) to increase the concentration of the nonionized free base and produce a faster onset and more rapid spread of epidural anesthesia. If pain develops as the sensory level recedes, additional local anesthetic is administered in 5-mL increments to maintain a T4 sensory level. "Patchy" anesthesia prior to delivery of the baby can be treated with 10–20 mg of intravenous ketamine in combination with 1–2 mg of midazolam or 30% nitrous oxide. After delivery, intravenous opioid supplementation may also be used, provided excessive sedation and loss of consciousness are avoided. Pain that remains intolerable in spite of a seemingly adequate sensory level and that proves unresponsive to these measures necessitates general anesthesia with endotracheal intubation. Nausea can be treated intravenously with a 5-HT3-receptor antagonist such as ondansetron, 4 mg.

Epidural morphine (5 mg) at the end of surgery provides good to excellent pain relief postoperatively for 6–24 h. An increased incidence (3.5–30%) of recurrent herpes simplex labialis infection has been reported 2–5 days following epidural morphine administration in some studies. Postoperative analgesia can also be provided by continuous epidural infusions of fentanyl, 25–75 mcg/h, or sufentanil, 5–10 mcg/h, at a volume rate of approximately 10 mL/h. Epidural butorphanol, 2 mg, can also provide effective postoperative pain relief, but marked somnolence is often a side effect.

CSE Anesthesia

The technique for CSE is described in the earlier section on Combined Spinal & Epidural Analgesia for labor and vaginal delivery. For cesarean section, it combines the benefit of rapid, reliable, intense blockade of spinal anesthesia with the flexibility of an epidural catheter. The catheter also allows supplementation of anesthesia and can be used for postoperative analgesia. As mentioned previously, drugs given epidurally should be administered and titrated carefully because the dural hole created by the spinal needle may facilitate movement of epidural drugs into CSF and enhance their effects.

GENERAL ANESTHESIA

Pulmonary aspiration of gastric contents and failed endotracheal intubation are the major causes of maternal morbidity and mortality associated with general anesthesia. All patients should receive prophylaxis against aspiration pneumonia with 30 mL of 0.3 M sodium citrate 30–45 min prior to induction. Patients with additional risk factors predisposing them to aspiration should also receive intravenous ranitidine, 50 mg, or metoclopramide, 10 mg, or both, 1–2 h prior to induction; such factors include morbid obesity, symptoms of gastroesophageal reflux, a potentially difficult airway, or emergent surgical delivery without an elective fasting period. Premedication with oral omeprazole, 40 mg, at night and in the morning also appears to be highly effective in high-risk patients undergoing elective cesarean section. Although anticholinergics theoretically may reduce lower esophageal sphincter tone, premedication with glycopyrrolate (0.1 mg) helps reduce airway secretions and should be considered in patients with a potentially difficult airway.

Anticipation of a difficult endotracheal intubation may help reduce the incidence of failed intubations. Examination of the neck, mandible, dentition, and oropharynx often helps predict which patients may have problems. Useful predictors of a difficult intubation include Mallampati classification, short neck, receding mandible, prominent maxillary incisors, and history of difficult intubation (see Chapter 19). The higher incidence of failed intubations in pregnant patients compared with nonpregnant surgical patients may be due to airway edema, a full dentition, or large breasts that can obstruct the handle of the laryngoscope in patients with short necks. Proper positioning of the head and neck may facilitate endotracheal intubation in obese patients: elevation of the shoulders, flexion of the cervical spine, and extension of the atlantooccipital joint (Figure 41–2). A variety of laryngoscope blades, a short laryngoscope handle, at least one extra stiletted endotracheal tube (6 mm), Magill forceps (for nasal intubation), a laryngeal mask airway (LMA), an intubating LMA (Fastrach), a fiberoptic bronchoscope,

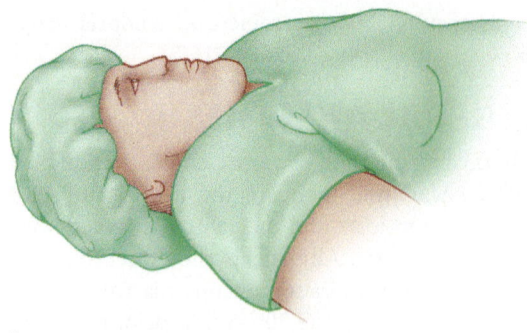

A

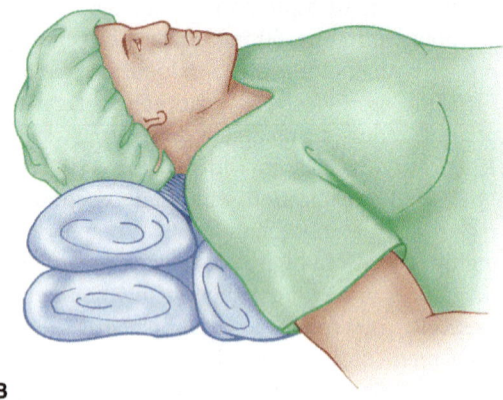

B

FIGURE 41–2 Optimal positioning for obese patients with a short neck. **A:** The normal supine position often prevents extension of the head and makes endotracheal intubation difficult. **B:** Elevation of the shoulder allows some neck flexion with more optimal extension of the head at the atlantooccipital joint, facilitating intubation.

a video-assisted laryngoscope (GlideScope or Stortz CMAC), the capability for transtracheal jet ventilation, and possibly an esophageal–tracheal Combitube should be readily available (see Chapter 19).

When potential difficulty in securing the airway is suspected, alternatives to the standard rapid-sequence induction with conventional laryngoscopy, such as regional anesthesia or awake fiberoptic techniques, should be considered. We have found that video-assisted laryngoscopy has greatly reduced the incidence of difficult or failed tracheal intubation at our institutions. Moreover, a clear plan should be formulated for a failed endotracheal intubation following induction of anesthesia (Figure 41–3). In the absence of fetal distress, the patient should be awakened, and an awake intubation, with regional

or local (infiltration) anesthesia, may be tried. In the presence of fetal distress, if spontaneous or positive-pressure ventilation (by mask or LMA) with cricoid pressure is possible, delivery of the fetus may be attempted. In such instances, a potent volatile agent with oxygen is employed for anesthesia, but once the fetus is delivered, nitrous oxide may be added to reduce the concentration of the volatile agent; sevoflurane may be the best volatile agent because it may be least likely to depress ventilation. The inability to ventilate the patient at any time may require immediate cricothyrotomy or tracheostomy.

Suggested Technique for Cesarean Section

1. The patient is placed supine with a wedge under the right hip for left uterine displacement.

2. Denitrogenation is accomplished with 100% oxygen for 3–5 min while monitors are applied.

3. The patient is prepared and draped for surgery.

4. When the surgeons are ready, a rapid-sequence induction with cricoid pressure is performed using propofol, 2 mg/kg, or ketamine, 1–2 mg/kg, and succinylcholine, 1.5 mg/kg. Ketamine is used instead of propofol in hypovolemic patients. Other agents, including methohexital and etomidate, offer little benefit in obstetric patients.

5. With few exceptions, surgery is begun only after proper placement of the endotracheal tube is confirmed. Excessive hyperventilation ($Paco_2 < 25$ mm Hg) should be avoided because it can reduce uterine blood flow and has been associated with fetal acidosis.

6. Fifty percent nitrous oxide in oxygen with up to 0.75 MAC of a low concentration of volatile agent (eg, 1% sevoflurane, 0.75% isoflurane, or 3% desflurane) is used for maintenance of anesthesia. The low dose of volatile agent helps ensure amnesia but is generally not enough to cause excessive uterine relaxation or prevent uterine contraction following oxytocin. A muscle relaxant of intermediate duration (atracurium, cisatracurium, or rocuronium) is used for relaxation, but may exhibit prolonged neuromuscular blockade in patients who are receiving magnesium sulfate.

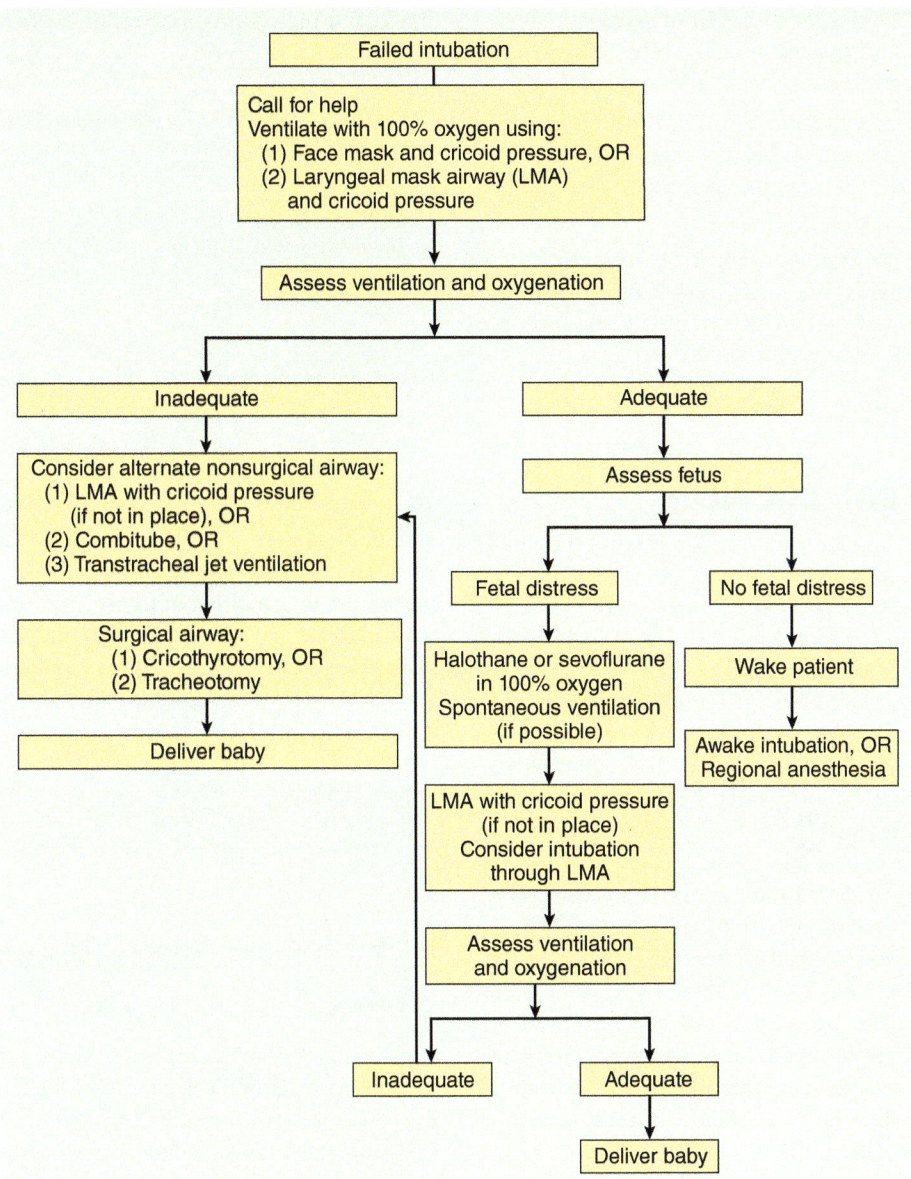

FIGURE 41–3 An algorithm for a difficult intubation in obstetric patients.

7. After the neonate and placenta are delivered, 20–80 units of oxytocin are added to the first liter of intravenous fluid, and another 20 units to the next. Additional intravenous agents, such as propofol, opioid, or benzodiazepine, can be given to ensure amnesia.

8. If the uterus does not contract readily, an opioid should be given, and the halogenated agent should be discontinued. Methylergonovine (Methergine), 0.2 mg intramuscularly or in 100-mL normal saline as slow intravenous infusion, may also be

given but can increase arterial blood pressure. 15-Methylprostaglandin $F_{2\alpha}$ (Hemabate), 0.25 mg intramuscularly, may also be used.

9. An attempt to aspirate gastric contents may be made via an oral gastric tube to decrease the likelihood of pulmonary aspiration on emergence.

10. At the end of surgery, muscle relaxants are completely reversed, the gastric tube (if placed) is removed, and the patient is extubated while awake to reduce the risk of aspiration.

ANESTHESIA FOR EMERGENCY CESAREAN SECTION

Indications for emergency cesarean section include massive bleeding (placenta previa or accreta, abruptio placentae, or uterine rupture), umbilical cord prolapse, and severe fetal distress. A distinction must be made between a true emergency requiring immediate delivery (previously referred to as "crash") and one in which some delay is possible. Close communication with the obstetrician is necessary to determine whether fetus, mother, or both are in immediate jeopardy.

The choice of anesthetic technique is determined by consideration for maternal safety (airway evaluation), technical issues, and the anesthesiologist's personal expertise. Criteria leading to the diagnosis of nonreassuring fetal status should be reviewed as the fetal evaluation may be based on criteria with poor predictive accuracy and the fetal status may change. This information is required to choose the anesthetic technique that will produce the best outcome for both mother and fetus. Rapid institution of regional anesthesia is an option in selected cases but is problematic in severely hypovolemic or hypotensive patients. If general anesthesia is chosen, adequate denitrogenation may be achieved rapidly with four maximal breaths of 100% oxygen while monitors are being applied. Ketamine, 1 mg/kg, may be substituted for propofol in hypotensive or hypovolemic patients.

Table 41–5 lists commonly accepted signs of fetal distress, an imprecise and poorly defined term. In most instances the diagnosis is primarily

TABLE 41–5 **Signs of fetal distress.**

Nonreassuring fetal heart rate pattern
Repetitive late decelerations
Loss of fetal beat-to-beat variability associated with late or deep decelerations
Sustained fetal heart rate <80 beats/min
Fetal scalp pH <7.20
Meconium-stained amniotic fluid
Intrauterine growth restriction

based on monitoring of fetal heart rate. Because worrisome fetal heart rate patterns have a relatively high incidence of false-positive results, careful interpretation of other parameters, such as fetal scalp pH or fetal pulse oximetry, may also be necessary. Moreover, continuation of fetal monitoring in the operating room may help avoid unnecessary induction of general anesthesia for fetal distress when additional time for use of regional anesthesia is possible. In selected instances where immediate delivery is not absolutely mandatory, epidural anesthesia (with 3% chloroprocaine or alkalinized 2% lidocaine) or spinal anesthesia may be appropriate.

Anesthesia for the Complicated Pregnancy

UMBILICAL CORD PROLAPSE

Prolapse of the umbilical cord complicates 0.2–0.6% of deliveries. Umbilical cord compression following prolapse can rapidly lead to fetal asphyxia. Predisposing factors include excessive cord length, malpresentation, low birth weight, grand parity (more than five pregnancies), multiple gestations, and artificial rupture of membranes. The diagnosis is suspected after sudden fetal bradycardia or profound decelerations and is confirmed by physical examination. Treatment includes immediate steep Trendelenburg or knee–chest position and manual pushing of the presenting fetal part back up into the pelvis until immediate cesarean section under general anesthesia can be performed. If the fetus is not viable, vaginal delivery is allowed to continue.

DYSTOCIA & ABNORMAL FETAL PRESENTATIONS & POSITIONS

Primary Dysfunctional Labor

A prolonged latent phase by definition exceeds 20 h in a nulliparous parturient and 14 h in a multiparous patient. The cervix usually remains at 4 cm or less but is completely effaced. The etiology is likely ineffective contractions without a dominant myometrial pacemaker. Arrest of dilation is present when the cervix undergoes no further change after 2 h in the active phase of labor. A protracted active phase refers to slower than normal cervical dilation, defined as less than 1.2 cm/h in a nulliparous patient and less than 1.5 cm/h in a multiparous parturient. A prolonged deceleration phase occurs when cervical dilation slows markedly after 8 cm. The cervix becomes very edematous and appears to lose effacement. A prolonged second stage (disorder of descent) is defined as a descent of less than 1 cm/h and 2 cm/h in nulliparous and multiparous parturients, respectively. Failure of the head to descend 1 cm in station after adequate pushing is referred to as arrest of descent.

Oxytocin is usually the treatment of choice for uterine contractile abnormalities. The drug is given intravenously at 1–6 mU/min and increased in increments of 1–6 mU/min every 15–40 min, depending on the protocol. Use of amniotomy is controversial. Treatment is usually expectant management, as long as the fetus and mother are tolerating the prolonged labor. When a trial of oxytocin is unsuccessful or when malpresentation or cephalopelvic disproportion is also present, operative vaginal delivery or cesarean section is indicated.

Breech Presentation

Breech presentations complicate 3–4% of deliveries and significantly increase both maternal and fetal morbidity and mortality rates. Breech presentations increase neonatal mortality and the incidence of cord prolapse more than 10-fold. External cephalic version may be attempted after 34 weeks of gestation and prior to the onset of labor; however, the fetus may spontaneously return to the breech presentation before the onset of labor. Some obstetricians may administer a tocolytic agent at the same time. External version can be facilitated, and its success rate improved, by providing epidural analgesia with 2% lidocaine and fentanyl. Although an external version is successful in 75% of patients, it can cause placental abruption and umbilical cord compression necessitating immediate cesarean section.

Because the shoulders or head can become trapped after vaginal delivery of the body, some obstetricians employ cesarean section for all breech presentations. Manual or forceps-assisted partial breech extraction is usually necessary during these vaginal deliveries. The need for breech extraction does not appear to be increased when epidural anesthesia is used for labor—if labor is well established prior to epidural activation. Moreover, epidural anesthesia may decrease the likelihood of a trapped head, because the former relaxes the perineum. Nonetheless, the fetal head can become trapped in the uterus even during cesarean section under regional anesthesia; rapid induction of general endotracheal anesthesia and administration of a volatile agent may be attempted in such instances to relax the uterus. Alternatively, nitroglycerin, 50–100 mcg intravenously, can be administered.

Abnormal Vertex Presentations

When the fetal occiput fails to spontaneously rotate anteriorly, a persistent occiput posterior presentation results in a more prolonged and painful labor. Manual, vacuum, or forceps rotation is usually necessary but increases the likelihood of maternal and fetal injuries. Regional anesthesia can be used to provide perineal analgesia and pelvic relaxation, allowing manual or forceps rotation followed by forceps delivery.

A face presentation occurs when the fetal head is hyperextended and generally requires cesarean section. A compound presentation occurs when an extremity enters the pelvis along with either the head or the buttocks. Vaginal delivery is usually still possible because the extremity often withdraws as the labor progresses.

Shoulder dystocia, or impaction of a shoulder against the pubic symphysis, complicates 0.2–2% of deliveries and is one of the major causes of birth injuries. The most important risk factor is fetal macrosomia. Shoulder dystocias are often difficult to predict. Several obstetric maneuvers can be used to relieve it, but a prolonged delay in the delivery could result in fetal asphyxia. Induction of general anesthesia may be necessary if an epidural catheter is not already in place.

MULTIPLE GESTATIONS

Multiple gestations account for approximately 1 in 150 births and are commonly associated with two complications: breech presentation and prematurity. Anesthesia may be necessary for version, extraction, or cesarean section. The second baby (and any subsequent ones) is often more depressed and asphyxiated than the first. Regional anesthesia provides effective pain relief during labor, minimizes the need for central nervous system depressants, and may shorten the interval between the birth of the first and second baby. Some studies suggest that the acid–base status of the second twin is better when epidural anesthesia is used. Patients with multiple gestations, however, are more prone to develop hypotension from aortocaval compression, particularly after regional anesthesia.

ANTEPARTUM HEMORRHAGE

(14) Maternal hemorrhage is one of the most common severe morbidities complicating obstetric anesthesia. Causes include uterine atony, placenta previa, abruptio placentae, and uterine rupture.

Placenta Previa

A placenta previa is present if the placenta implants in advance of the fetal presenting part. The incidence of placenta previa is 0.5% of pregnancies. Placenta previa often occurs in patients who have had a previous cesarean section or uterine myomectomy; other risk factors include multiparity, advanced maternal age, and a large placenta. An anterior-lying placenta previa increases the risk of excessive bleeding for cesarean section.

Placenta previa usually presents as painless vaginal bleeding. Although the bleeding often stops spontaneously, severe hemorrhage can occur at any time. When the gestation is less than 37 weeks in duration and the bleeding is mild to moderate, the patient is usually treated with bed rest and observation. After 37 weeks of gestation, delivery is usually accomplished via cesarean section. Patients with low-lying placenta may rarely be allowed to deliver vaginally if the bleeding is mild.

Active bleeding or an unstable patient requires immediate cesarean section under general anesthesia. The patient should have two large-bore intravenous catheters in place; intravascular volume deficits must be replaced, and blood must be available for transfusion. The bleeding can continue after delivery because the placental implantation site in the lower uterine segment often does not contract well (as does the rest of the uterus).

A history of a previous placenta previa or cesarean section increases the risk of abnormal placentation.

Abruptio Placentae

Premature separation of a normal placenta complicates approximately 1–2% of pregnancies. Most abruptions are mild (grade I), but up to 25% are severe (grade III). Risk factors include hypertension, trauma, a short umbilical cord, multiparity, prolonged premature rupture of membranes, alcohol abuse, cocaine use, and an abnormal uterus. Patients usually experience painful vaginal bleeding with uterine contraction and tenderness. An abdominal ultrasound can help in the diagnosis. The choice between regional and general anesthesia must factor in the urgency for delivery, maternal hemodynamic stability, and any coagulopathy. The bleeding may remain concealed inside the uterus and cause underestimation of blood loss. Severe abruptio placentae can cause coagulopathy, particularly following fetal demise. Fibrinogen levels are mildly reduced (150–250 mg/dL) with moderate abruptions but are typically less than 150 mg/dL with fetal demise. The coagulopathy is thought to be due to activation of circulating plasminogen (fibrinolysis) and the release of tissue thromboplastins that precipitate disseminated intravascular coagulation (DIC). Platelet count and factors V and VIII are low, and fibrin split products are elevated. Severe abruption is a life-threatening emergency that necessitates an emergency cesarean section. Massive blood transfusion, including replacement of coagulation factors and platelets, may be anticipated.

Uterine Rupture

Uterine rupture is relatively uncommon (1:1000–3000 deliveries) but can occur during labor as a result of (1) dehiscence of a scar from a previous (usually classic) cesarean section (VBAC), extensive myomectomy, or uterine reconstruction; (2) intrauterine manipulations or use of forceps (iatrogenic); or (3) spontaneous rupture following prolonged labor in patients with hypertonic contractions (particularly with oxytocin infusions), fetopelvic disproportion, or a very large, thin, and weakened uterus. Uterine rupture can present as frank hemorrhage, fetal distress, loss of uterine tone, or hypotension with occult bleeding into the abdomen. Even when epidural anesthesia is employed for labor, uterine rupture is often heralded by the abrupt onset of continuous abdominal pain and hypotension. Treatment requires volume resuscitation and immediate laparotomy, typically under general anesthesia. Ligation of the internal iliac (hypogastric) arteries, with or without hysterectomy, may be necessary to control intraoperative bleeding.

PREMATURE RUPTURE OF MEMBRANES & CHORIOAMNIONITIS

Premature rupture of membranes (PROM) is present when leakage of amniotic fluid occurs before the onset of labor. The pH of amniotic fluid causes Nitrazine paper to change color from blue to yellow. PROM complicates 10% of all pregnancies and up to 35% of premature deliveries. Predisposing factors include a short cervix, prior history of PROM or preterm delivery, infection, multiple gestations, polyhydramnios, and smoking. Spontaneous labor commences within 24 h of ruptured membranes in 90% of patients. Management of PROM balances the risk of infection with the risk of fetal prematurity. Delivery is usually indicated sometime after 34 weeks of gestation. Patients with a gestation of less than 34 weeks can be managed expectantly with prophylactic antibiotics and tocolytics for 5–7 days to allow some additional maturation of fetal organs. The longer the interval between rupture and the onset of labor, the higher the incidence of chorioamnionitis. PROM also predisposes to placental abruption and postpartum endometritis.

Chorioamnionitis represents infection of the chorionic and amnionic membranes, and may involve the placenta, uterus, umbilical cord, and fetus. It complicates up to 1–2% of pregnancies and is usually but not always associated with ruptured membranes. The contents of the amniotic cavity are normally sterile but become vulnerable to ascending bacterial infection from the vagina when the cervix dilates or the membranes rupture. Intraamniotic infections are less commonly caused by hematogenous spread of bacteria or retrograde seeding through the fallopian tubes. The principal maternal complications of chorioamnionitis are premature or dysfunctional labor, often leading to cesarean section, intraabdominal infection, septicemia, and postpartum hemorrhage. Fetal complications include acidosis, hypoxia, and septicemia.

Clinical signs of chorioamnionitis include fever (>38°C), maternal and fetal tachycardia, uterine tenderness, and foul-smelling or purulent amniotic fluid. Blood leukocyte count is useful only if markedly elevated because it normally increases during labor (normal average 15,000/μL). C-reactive protein levels are usually elevated (>2 mg/dL). Gram stain of amniotic fluid obtained by amniocentesis is helpful in ruling out infection.

The use of regional anesthesia in patients with chorioamnionitis is controversial because of the theoretical risk of promoting the development of meningitis or an epidural abscess. Available evidence suggests that this risk is very low and that concerns may be unjustified. Moreover, antepartum antibiotic therapy appears to reduce maternal and fetal morbidity. Nonetheless, concerns over hemodynamic stability following sympathectomy are justified, particularly in patients with chills, high fever, tachypnea, changes in mental status, or borderline hypotension. In the absence of overt signs of septicemia, thrombocytopenia, or coagulopathy, most clinicians offer regional anesthesia to those patients with chorioamnionitis who have received antibiotic therapy.

PRETERM LABOR

Preterm labor by definition occurs between 20 and 37 weeks of gestation and is the most common complication of the third trimester. Approximately 8% of live-born infants in the United States are delivered before term. Important contributory maternal factors include extremes of age, inadequate prenatal care, unusual body habitus, increased physical activity, infections, prior preterm labor, multiple gestation, and other medical illnesses or complications during pregnancy.

Because of their small size and incomplete development, preterm infants—particularly those less than 30 weeks of gestational age or weighing less than 1500 g—experience a greater number of complications than term infants. Premature rupture of membranes complicates one third of premature deliveries; the combination of premature rupture of membranes and premature labor increases the likelihood of umbilical cord compression resulting in fetal hypoxemia and asphyxia. Preterm infants with a breech presentation are particularly prone to prolapse of the umbilical cord during labor. Moreover, inadequate production of pulmonary surfactant frequently leads to the idiopathic respiratory distress syndrome (hyaline membrane disease) after delivery. Surfactant levels are generally adequate only after week 35 of gestation. Lastly, a soft, poorly calcified cranium predisposes these neonates to intracranial hemorrhage during vaginal delivery.

When preterm labor occurs before 35 weeks of gestation, bed rest and tocolytic therapy are usually initiated. Treatment is successful in 75% of patients. Labor is inhibited until the lungs mature and sufficient pulmonary surfactant is produced, as judged by amniocentesis. The risk of respiratory distress syndrome is markedly reduced when the amniotic fluid lecithin/sphingomyelin ratio is greater than 2. Glucocorticoid (betamethasone) may be given to induce production of pulmonary surfactant, which requires a minimum of 24–48 h. The most commonly used tocolytics are β_2-adrenergic agonists (ritodrine or terbutaline) and magnesium (6 g intravenously over 30 min followed by 2–4 g/h). Ritodrine (given intravenously as 100–350 mcg/min) and terbutaline (given orally as 2.5–5 mg every 4–6 h) also have some β_1-adrenergic receptor activity, which accounts for some of their side effects. Maternal side effects include tachycardia, arrhythmias, myocardial ischemia, mild hypotension, hyperglycemia, hypokalemia, and, rarely, pulmonary edema. Other tocolytic agents include calcium channel blockers (nifedipine), prostaglandin synthetase inhibitors,

oxytocin antagonists (atosiban), and possibly nitric oxide. Fetal ductal constriction can occur after 32 weeks of gestation with nonsteroidal antiinflammatory drugs such as indomethacin, but it is usually transient and resolves after discontinuation of the drug; renal impairment in the fetus may also cause oligohydramnios.

When tocolytic therapy fails to arrest labor, anesthesia often becomes necessary. The goal during vaginal delivery of a preterm fetus is a slow controlled delivery with minimal pushing by the mother. An episiotomy and low forceps are often employed. Spinal or epidural anesthesia allows complete pelvic relaxation. Cesarean section is performed for fetal distress, breech presentation, intrauterine growth retardation, or failure of labor to progress. Residual effects from β-adrenergic agonists may complicate general anesthesia. The half-life of ritodrine may be as long as 3 h. Ketamine and ephedrine (and halothane) should be used cautiously due to interaction with tocolytics. Hypokalemia is usually due to an intracellular uptake of potassium and rarely requires treatment; however, it may increase sensitivity to muscle relaxants. Magnesium therapy potentiates muscle relaxants and may predispose to hypotension (secondary to vasodilation). Residual effects from tocolytics interfere with uterine contraction following delivery. Lastly, preterm newborns are often depressed at delivery and frequently need resuscitation. Preparations for resuscitation should be completed prior to delivery.

HYPERTENSIVE DISORDERS

Hypertension during pregnancy can be classified as pregnancy-induced hypertension (PIH, often also referred to as preeclampsia), chronic hypertension that preceded pregnancy, or chronic hypertension with superimposed preeclampsia. **Preeclampsia is usually defined as a systolic blood pressure greater than 140 mm Hg or diastolic pressure greater than 90 mm Hg after the 20th week of gestation, accompanied by proteinuria (>300 mg/d) and resolving within 48 h after delivery.** When seizures occur, the syndrome is termed eclampsia. The HELLP syndrome describes preeclampsia associated with *h*emolysis, *e*levated *l*iver enzymes, and a *low* *p*latelet count. In the United States, preeclampsia complicates approximately 7–10% of pregnancies; eclampsia is much less common, occurring in one of 10,000–15,000 pregnancies. Severe preeclampsia causes or contributes to 20–40% of maternal deaths and 20% of perinatal deaths. Maternal deaths are usually due to stroke, pulmonary edema, and hepatic necrosis or rupture.

Pathophysiology & Manifestations

The pathophysiology of preeclampsia is probably related to a vascular dysfunction of the placenta that results in abnormal prostaglandin metabolism. Patients with preeclampsia have elevated production of thromboxane A_2 (TXA_2) and decreased production of prostacyclin (PGI_2). TXA_2 is a potent vasoconstrictor and promoter of platelet aggregation, whereas PGI_2 is a potent vasodilator and inhibitor of platelet aggregation. Endothelial dysfunction may reduce production of nitric oxide and increase production of endothelin-1. The latter is also a potent vasoconstrictor and activator of platelets. Marked vascular reactivity and endothelial injury reduce placental perfusion and can lead to widespread systemic manifestations.

Severe preeclampsia substantially increases both maternal and fetal morbidity and mortality, and is defined by a blood pressure greater than 160/110 mm Hg, proteinuria in excess of 5 g/d, oliguria (<500 mL/d), elevated serum creatinine, intrauterine growth restriction, pulmonary edema, central nervous system manifestations (headache, visual disturbances, seizures, or stroke), hepatic tenderness, or the HELLP syndrome (Table 41-6). Hepatic rupture may also occur in patients with the HELLP syndrome.

Patients with severe preeclampsia or eclampsia have widely differing hemodynamic profiles. Most patients have low-normal cardiac filling pressures with high systemic vascular resistance, but cardiac output may be low, normal, or high.

Treatment

Treatment of preeclampsia consists of bed rest, sedation, repeated doses of antihypertensive drugs (usually labetalol, 5–10 mg, or hydralazine, 5 mg intravenously), and magnesium sulfate (4 g intravenous loading, followed by 1–3 g/h) to treat hyperreflexia

TABLE 41-6 Complications of preeclampsia.

Neurological
  Headache
  Visual disturbances
  Hyperexcitability
  Seizures
  Intracranial hemorrhage
  Cerebral edema

Pulmonary
  Upper airway edema
  Pulmonary edema

Cardiovascular
  Decreased intravascular volume
  Increased arteriolar resistance
  Hypertension
  Heart failure

Hepatic
  Impaired function
  Elevated enzymes
  Hematoma
  Rupture

Renal
  Proteinuria
  Sodium retention
  Decreased glomerular filtration
  Renal failure

Hematological
  Coagulopathy
  Thrombocytopenia
  Platelet dysfunction
  Prolonged partial thromboplastin time
  Microangiopathic hemolysis

and prevent convulsions. Therapeutic magnesium levels are 4–6 mEq/L.

Invasive arterial and central venous monitoring are indicated in patients with severe hypertension, pulmonary edema, or refractory oliguria; an intravenous vasodilator infusion may be necessary. Definitive treatment of preeclampsia is delivery of the fetus and placenta.

Anesthetic Management

Patients with mild preeclampsia generally require only extra caution during anesthesia; standard anesthetic practices may be used. Spinal and epidural anesthesia are associated with similar decreases in arterial blood pressure in these patients. Patients with severe disease, however, are critically ill and require stabilization prior to administration of any anesthetic. Hypertension should be controlled and hypovolemia corrected before administration of anesthesia. In the absence of coagulopathy, continuous epidural anesthesia is the first choice for most patients with preeclampsia during labor, vaginal delivery, and cesarean section. Moreover, continuous epidural anesthesia avoids the increased risk of a failed intubation due to severe edema of the upper airway.

A platelet count and coagulation profile should be checked prior to the institution of regional anesthesia in patients with severe preeclampsia. It has been recommended that regional anesthesia be avoided if the platelet count is less than 100,000/µL, but a platelet count as low as 70,000/µL may be acceptable in selected cases, particularly when the count has been stable. Although some patients have a qualitative platelet defect, the usefulness of a bleeding time determination is questionable. Continuous epidural anesthesia has been shown to decrease catecholamine secretion and improve uteroplacental perfusion up to 75% in these patients, provided hypotension is avoided. Judicious fluid boluses with epidural activation may be required to correct the disease-related hypovolemia. Goal-directed hemodynamic and fluid therapy utilizing arterial pulse wave contour analysis (Virgileo/Flotrac, LiDCOrapid) or echocardiography may be employed to guide fluid replacement. Use of an epinephrine-containing test dose for epidural anesthesia is controversial because of questionable reliability (see earlier section Prevention of Unintentional Intravascular and Intrathecal Injection) and the risk of exacerbating hypertension. Hypotension should be treated with small doses of vasopressors because patients tend to be very sensitive to these agents. Recent evidence suggests that spinal anesthesia does not, as previously thought, result in a more severe reduction of maternal blood pressure. Therefore, this technique is a reasonable anesthetic choice for cesarean section in a preeclamptic patient.

Intraarterial blood pressure monitoring is indicated in patients with severe hypertension during both general and regional anesthesia. Intravenous vasodilator infusions may be necessary to control blood pressure during general anesthesia. Intravenous labetalol (5–10 mg increments) can also be effective in controlling the hypertensive response to intubation and does not appear to alter placental blood flow. Because magnesium potentiates muscle relaxants, doses of nondepolarizing muscle relaxants should be reduced in patients receiving magnesium therapy and should be guided by a peripheral nerve stimulator. The patient with suspected magnesium toxicity, manifested by hyporeflexia, excessive sedation, blurred vision, respiratory compromise and cardiac depression, can be treated with intravenous administration of calcium gluconate (1 g over 10 minutes).

HEART DISEASE

The marked cardiovascular changes associated with pregnancy, labor, and delivery often cause pregnant patients with heart disease (2% of parturients) to decompensate during this period. Although most pregnant patients with cardiac disease have rheumatic heart disease, an increasing number of parturients are presenting with corrected or palliated congenital lesions. Anesthetic management is directed toward employing techniques that minimize the added stresses of labor and delivery. Specific management of the various lesions is discussed elsewhere. Most patients can be divided into one of two groups. Patients in the first group benefit from the falls in systemic vascular resistance caused by neuraxial analgesia techniques, but usually not from overzealous fluid administration. These patients include those with mitral insufficiency, aortic insufficiency, chronic heart failure, or congenital lesions with left-to-right shunting. The induced sympathectomy from spinal or epidural techniques reduces both preload and afterload, relieves pulmonary congestion, and in some cases increases forward flow (cardiac output).

Patients in the second group do not benefit from a decrease in systemic vascular resistance. These patients include those with aortic stenosis, congenital lesions with right-to-left or bidirectional shunting, or primary pulmonary hypertension. Reductions in venous return (preload) or afterload are usually poorly tolerated. These patients are better managed with intraspinal opioids alone, systemic medications, pudendal nerve blocks, and, if necessary, general anesthesia.

AMNIOTIC FLUID EMBOLISM

Amniotic fluid embolism is a rare (1:20,000 deliveries) but often lethal complication (86% mortality rate in some series) that can occur during labor, delivery, cesarean section, or postpartum. Mortality may exceed 50% in the first hour. Entry of amniotic fluid into the maternal circulation can occur through any break in the uteroplacental membranes. Such breaks may occur during normal delivery or cesarean section or following placental abruption, placenta previa, or uterine rupture. In addition to fetal debris, amniotic fluid contains various prostaglandins and leukotrienes, which appear to play an important role in the genesis of this syndrome. The alternate term anaphylactoid syndrome of pregnancy has been suggested to emphasize the role of chemical mediators in this syndrome.

Patients typically present with sudden tachypnea, cyanosis, shock, and generalized bleeding. Three major pathophysiological manifestations are responsible: (1) acute pulmonary embolism, (2) disseminated intravascular coagulation (DIC), and (3) uterine atony. Mental status changes, including seizures, and pulmonary edema may develop; the latter has both cardiogenic and noncardiogenic components. Acute left ventricular dysfunction is common. Although the diagnosis can be firmly established only by demonstrating fetal elements in the maternal circulation (usually at autopsy or less commonly by aspirating amniotic fluid from a central venous catheter), amniotic fluid embolism should always be suggested by sudden respiratory distress and circulatory collapse. The presentation may initially mimic acute pulmonary thromboembolism, venous air embolism, overwhelming septicemia, or hepatic rupture or cerebral hemorrhage in a patient with toxemia.

Treatment consists of cardiopulmonary resuscitation and supportive care. When cardiac arrest occurs prior to delivery of the fetus, the efficacy of closed-chest compressions may be marginal at best. Aortocaval compression impairs resuscitation in the supine position, whereas chest compressions are less effective in a lateral tilt position. Moreover,

expeditious delivery appears to improve maternal and fetal outcome; immediate (cesarean) delivery should therefore be carried out. Once the patient is resuscitated, mechanical ventilation, fluid resuscitation, and inotropes are best provided under the guidance of invasive hemodynamic monitoring. Uterine atony is treated with oxytocin, methylergonovine, and prostaglandin $F_{2\alpha}$, whereas significant coagulopathies are treated with platelets and coagulation factors based on laboratory findings.

POSTPARTUM HEMORRHAGE

Postpartum hemorrhage is the leading cause of maternal mortality in developing countries. It is diagnosed when the postpartum blood loss exceeds 500 mL. Up to 4% of parturients may experience postpartum hemorrhage, which is often associated with a prolonged third stage of labor, preeclampsia, multiple gestations, and forceps delivery. Common causes include uterine atony, a retained placenta, obstetric lacerations, uterine inversion, and use of tocolytic agents prior to delivery. Atony is often associated with uterine overdistention (multiple gestation and polyhydramnios). Less commonly, a clotting defect may be responsible.

The anesthesiologist may be consulted to assist in venous access or fluid (and blood) resuscitation, as well as to provide anesthesia for careful examination of the vagina, cervix, and uterus. Perineal lacerations can usually be repaired with local anesthetic infiltration or pudendal nerve blocks. Residual anesthesia from prior epidural or spinal anesthesia facilitates examination of the patient; however, supplementation with an opioid, nitrous oxide, or both may be required. Induction of spinal or epidural anesthesia in the presence of hypovolemia is problematic. **General anesthesia is usually required for manual extraction of a retained placenta, reversion of an inverted uterus, or repair of a major laceration.** Uterine atony should be treated with oxytocin (20–30 units/L of intravenous fluid), methylergonovine (0.2 mg intramuscularly or in 100 mL of normal saline administered over 10 min intravenously), and prostaglandin $F_{2\alpha}$ (0.25 mg intramuscularly). Emergency laparotomy and hysterectomy may be necessary in rare instances. Early ligation of the internal iliac (hypogastric) arteries may help avoid hysterectomy or reduce blood loss.

Fetal & Neonatal Resuscitation

FETAL RESUSCITATION

Resuscitation of the neonate starts during labor. Any compromise of the uteroplacental circulation readily produces fetal asphyxia. Intrauterine asphyxia during labor is the most common cause of neonatal depression. Fetal monitoring throughout labor is helpful in identifying which babies may be at risk, detecting fetal distress, and evaluating the effect of acute interventions. These include correcting maternal hypotension with fluids or vasopressors, supplemental oxygen, and decreasing uterine contraction (stopping oxytocin or administering tocolytics). Some studies suggest that the normal fetus can compensate for up to 45 min of relative hypoxia, a period termed fetal stress; the latter is associated with a marked redistribution of blood flow primarily to the heart, brain, and adrenal glands. With time, however, progressive lactic acidosis and asphyxia produce increasing fetal distress that necessitates immediate delivery.

1. Fetal Heart Rate Monitoring

Monitoring of fetal heart rate (FHR) is presently the most useful technique in assessing fetal well-being, although alone it has a 35–50% false-positive rate of predicting fetal compromise. Because of this, the term *fetal distress* in the context of FHR monitoring has been largely replaced with *nonreassuring* FHR. Correct interpretation of heart rate patterns is crucial. Three parameters are evaluated: baseline heart rate, baseline variability, and the relationship to uterine contractions (deceleration patterns). Monitoring of heart rate is most accurate when fetal scalp electrodes are used, but this may require rupture of the membranes and is not without complications (eg, amnionitis or fetal injury).

Baseline Heart Rate

The mature fetus normally has a baseline heart rate of 110–160 beats/min. An increased baseline heart rate may be due to prematurity, mild fetal hypoxia, chorioamnionitis, maternal fever, maternally administered

drugs (anticholinergics or β agonists), or, rarely, hyperthyroidism. A decreased baseline heart rate may be due to a postterm pregnancy, fetal heart block, or fetal asphyxia.

Baseline Variability

The healthy mature fetus normally displays a baseline beat-to-beat (R wave to R wave) variability that can be classified as minimal (<5 beats/min), moderate (6–25 beats/min), or marked (>25 beats/min). Baseline variability, which is best assessed with scalp electrodes, has become an important sign of fetal well-being and represents a normally functioning autonomic system. **Sustained decreased baseline variability is a prominent sign of fetal asphyxia.** Central nervous system depressants (opioids, barbiturates, volatile anesthetics, benzodiazepines, or magnesium sulfate) and parasympatholytics (atropine) also decrease baseline variability, as do prematurity, fetal arrhythmias, and anencephaly. A sinusoidal pattern that resembles a smooth sine wave is associated with fetal depression (hypoxia, drugs, and anemia secondary to Rh isoimmunization).

Accelerations

Accelerations of FHR are defined as increases of 15 beats/min or more lasting for more than 15 s. Periodic accelerations in FHR reflect normal oxygenation and are usually related to fetal movements and to responses to uterine pressure. Such accelerations are generally considered reassuring. By 32 weeks, fetuses display periodic increases in baseline heart rate that are associated with fetal movements. Normal fetuses have 15–40 accelerations/h. The mechanism is thought to involve increases in catecholamine secretion with decreases in vagal tone. Accelerations diminish with fetal sleep, some drugs (opioids, magnesium, and atropine), as well as fetal hypoxia. Accelerations to fetal scalp or vibroacoustic stimulation are considered a reassuring sign of fetal well-being. The absence of both baseline variability and accelerations is nonreassuring and may be an important sign of fetal compromise.

Deceleration Patterns

A. Early (Type I) Decelerations

Early deceleration (usually 10–40 beats/min) (**Figure 41–4A**) is thought to be a vagal response

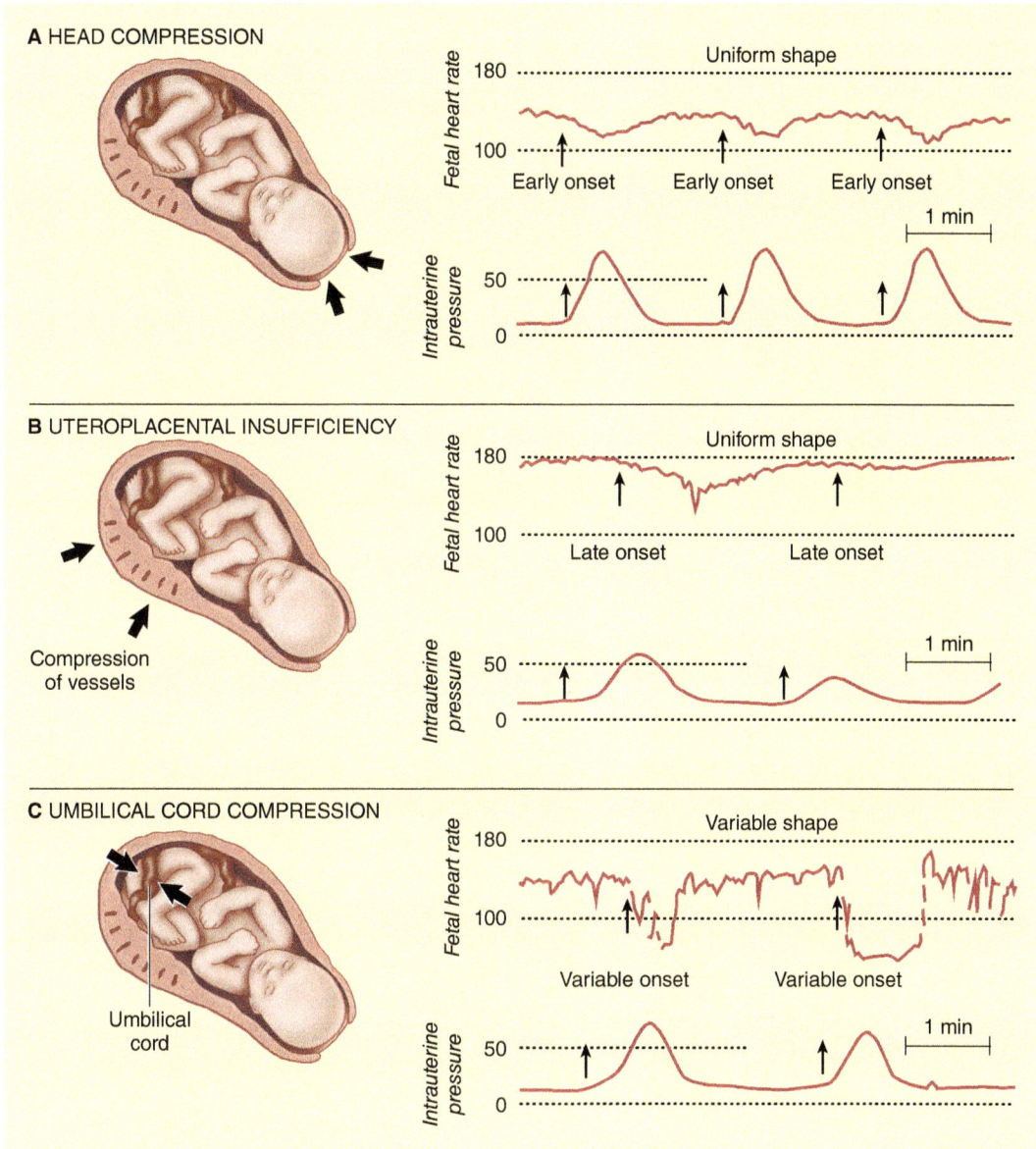

FIGURE 41–4 Periodic changes in fetal heart rate related to uterine contraction. **A:** Early (type I) decelerations. **B:** Late (type II) decelerations. **C:** Variable (type III) decelerations. (Reproduced, with permission, from Danforth DN, Scott JR: *Obstetrics and Gynecology*, 5th ed. Lippincott, 1986.)

to compression of the fetal head or stretching of the neck during uterine contractions. The heart rate forms a smooth mirror image of the contraction. Early decelerations are generally not associated with fetal distress and occur during descent of the head.

B. Late (Type II) Decelerations

Late decelerations (Figure 41–4B) are associated with fetal compromise and are characterized by a decrease in heart rate at or following the peak of uterine contractions. Late decelerations may be subtle (as few as 5 beats/min). They are thought to represent decreased arterial oxygen tension on atrial chemoreceptors. Late decelerations with normal variability may be observed following acute insults (maternal hypotension or hypoxemia) and are usually reversible with treatment. Late decelerations with decreased variability are associated with prolonged asphyxia and may be an indication for fetal scalp sampling (see Other Monitoring section below). Complete abolition of variability in this setting is an ominous sign signifying severe decompensation and the need for immediate delivery.

C. Variable (Type III) Decelerations

The most common type of decelerations are variable (Figure 41–4C). These decelerations are variable in onset, duration, and magnitude (often >30 beats/min). They are typically abrupt in onset and are thought to be related to umbilical cord compression and acute intermittent decreases in umbilical blood flow. Variable decelerations are typically associated with fetal asphyxia when fetal heart rate declines to less than 60 beats/min, last more than 60 s, or occur in a pattern that persists for more than 30 min.

2. Other Monitoring

Other less commonly used monitors include fetal scalp pH measurements, scalp lactate concentration, fetal pulse oximetry, and fetal ST-segment analysis. Clinical experience is limited with all except fetal scalp pH measurements. Unfortunately the latter is associated with a small but significant incidence of false negatives and false positives. Fetal blood can be obtained and analyzed via a small scalp puncture once the membranes are ruptured. A fetal scalp pH higher than 7.20 is usually associated with a vigorous neonate, whereas a pH less than 7.20 is often, but not always, associated with a depressed neonate and necessitates prompt (typically operative) delivery. Because of wide overlap, fetal blood sampling can be interpreted correctly only in conjunction with heart rate monitoring.

3. Treatment of the Fetus

Treatment of intrauterine fetal asphyxia is aimed at preventing fetal demise or permanent neurological damage. All interventions are directed at restoring an adequate uteroplacental circulation. Aortocaval compression, maternal hypoxemia or hypotension, or excessive uterine activity (during oxytocin infusions) must be corrected. Changes in maternal position, supplemental oxygen, and intravenous ephedrine or fluid, or adjustments in an oxytocin infusion often correct the problem. Failure to relieve fetal stress, as well as progressive fetal acidosis and asphyxia, necessitate immediate delivery.

NEONATAL RESUSCITATION

1. General Care of the Neonate

One healthcare provider whose sole responsibility is to care for the neonate and who is capable of providing resuscitation should attend every delivery. As the head is delivered, the nose, mouth, and pharynx are suctioned with a bulb syringe. After the remainder of the body is delivered, the skin is dried with a sterile towel. Once the umbilical cord stops pulsating or neonatal breathing is initiated, the cord is clamped and the neonate is placed in a radiant warmer with the bed tilted in a slight Trendelenburg position.

Neonatal evaluation and treatment are carried out simultaneously (Figure 41–5). If the neonate is obviously depressed, the cord is clamped early and resuscitation is initiated immediately. Breathing normally begins within 30 s and is sustained within 90 s. Respirations should be 30–60 breaths/min and the heart rate 120–160 beats/min. Respirations are assessed by auscultation of the chest, whereas heart rate is determined by palpation of the pulse at the base of the umbilical cord or auscultation of the precordium. It is critically important to keep the neonate warm.

In addition to respirations and heart rate, color, tone, and reflex irritability should be evaluated. The Apgar score (Table 41–7), recorded at 1 min and again at 5 min after delivery, remains the most valuable assessment of the neonate. The 1-min score correlates with survival, whereas the 5-min score has limited relationship to neurological outcome.

Neonates with Apgar scores of 8–10 are vigorous and may require only gentle stimulation (flicking the foot, rubbing the back, and additional drying). A catheter should first be gently passed

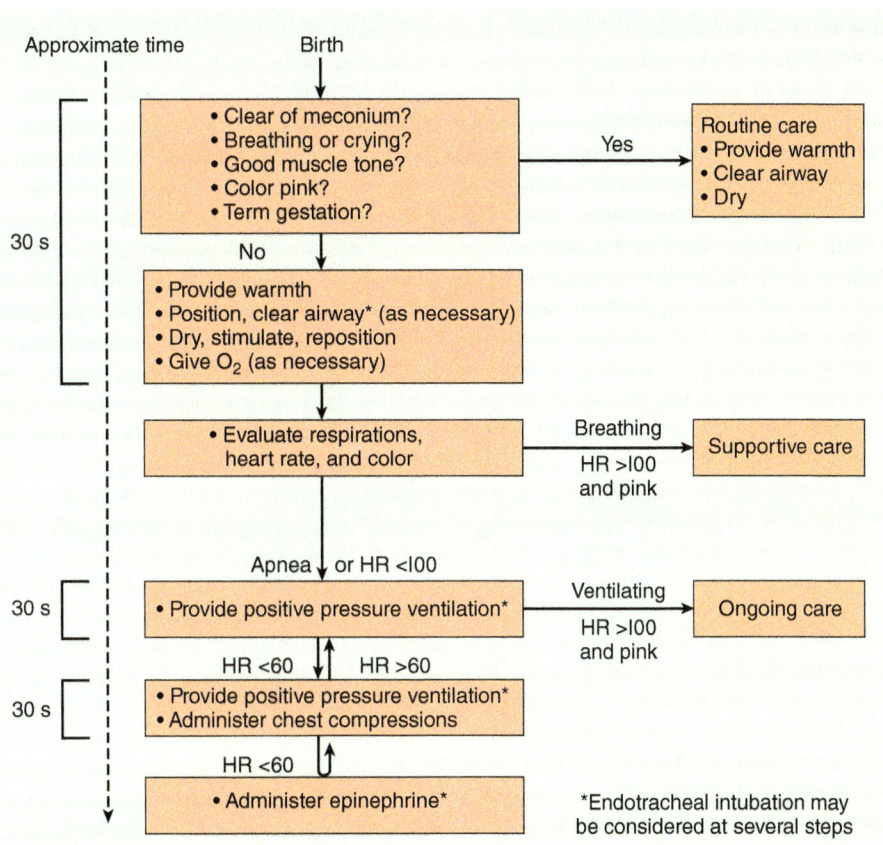

FIGURE 41–5 An algorithm for resuscitation of the newly born infant. (Reproduced, with permission, from ECC Committee, Subcommittees and Task Forces of the American Heart Association: 2005 American Heart Association Guidelines for Cardiopulmonary Resuscitation and Emergency Cardiovascular Care. Circulation 2005 Dec 13;112(24 Suppl):IV1-203.)

TABLE 41–7 Apgar score.

Sign	Points		
	0	1	2
Heart rate (beats/min)	Absent	<100	>100
Respiratory effort	Absent	Slow, irregular	Good, crying
Muscle tone	Flaccid	Some flexion	Active motion
Reflex irritability	No response	Grimace	Crying
Color	Blue or pale	Body pink, extremities blue	All pink

through each nostril to rule out choanal atresia, and then through the mouth to suction the stomach and rule out esophageal atresia.

2. Meconium-Stained Neonates

The presence or absence of meconium in the amniotic fluid (approximately 10–12% of deliveries) changes the immediate management of the neonate at birth. Fetal distress, particularly after 42 weeks of gestation, is often associated with release of thick meconium into the fluid. Fetal gasping during stress results in entry of a large amount of meconium-tainted amniotic fluid into the lungs. When the neonate initiates respiration at birth, the meconium moves from the trachea and large airways down toward the periphery of the lung. Thick or particulate meconium may obstruct small airways and cause severe respiratory distress in 15% of meconium-stained neonates. Moreover, these infants can develop persistent fetal circulation.

Unless the neonate has absent or depressed respirations, thin watery meconium does not require suctioning beyond careful bulb suctioning of the oropharynx when the head emerges from the perineum (or from the uterus at cesarean section). When thick "pea soup" meconium is present in the amniotic fluid, however, some clinicians intubate and suction the trachea immediately after delivery but before the first breath is taken. If the baby is not vigorous, tracheal suctioning is recommended when meconium is present. Tracheal suctioning of the thick meconium is accomplished by a special suctioning device attached to the endotracheal tube as the tube is withdrawn. If meconium is aspirated from the trachea, the procedure should be repeated until no meconium is obtained—but no more than three times, after which it is usually of no further benefit. The infant should then be given supplemental oxygen by face mask and observed closely. The stomach should also be suctioned to prevent passive regurgitation of any meconium. Newborns with meconium aspiration have an increased incidence of pneumothorax (10% compared with 1% for all vaginal deliveries).

3. Care of the Depressed Neonate

Approximately 6% of newborns, most of whom weigh less than 1500 g, require some form of advanced life support. Resuscitation of the depressed neonate requires two or more persons—one to manage the airway and ventilation and another to perform chest compressions, if necessary. A third person greatly facilitates the placement of intravascular catheters and the administration of fluids or drugs. The anesthesiologist caring for the mother can render only brief assistance and only when it does not jeopardize the mother; other personnel are, therefore, usually responsible for neonatal resuscitation.

Because the most common cause of neonatal depression is intrauterine asphyxia, the emphasis in resuscitation is on respiration. Hypovolemia

is also a contributing factor in a significant number of neonates. Factors associated with hypovolemia include early clamping of the umbilical cord, holding the neonate above the introitus prior to clamping, prematurity, maternal hemorrhage, placental transection during cesarean section, sepsis, and twin-to-twin transfusion.

Failure of the neonate to quickly respond to respiratory resuscitative efforts mandates vascular access and blood gas analysis; pneumothorax (1% incidence) and congenital anomalies of the airway, including tracheoesophageal fistula (1:3000–5000 live births), and congenital diaphragmatic hernia (1:2000–4000) should also be considered.

Grouping by the 1-min Apgar score greatly facilitates resuscitation: (1) mildly asphyxiated neonates (Apgar score of 5–7) usually need only stimulation while 100% oxygen is blown across the face; (2) moderately asphyxiated neonates (Apgar score of 3–4) require temporary assisted positive-pressure ventilation with mask and bag; and (3) severely depressed neonates (Apgar score of 0–2) should be immediately intubated, and chest compressions may be required.

Guidelines for Ventilation

Indications for positive-pressure ventilation include (1) apnea, (2) gasping respirations, (3) persistent central cyanosis with 100% oxygen, and (4) a persistent heart rate less than 100 beats/min. Excessive flexion or extension of the neck can cause airway obstruction. A 1-in.-high towel under the shoulders may be helpful in maintaining proper head position. Assisted ventilation by bag and mask should be at a rate of 30–60 breaths/min with 100% oxygen. Initial breaths may require peak pressures of up to 40 cm H_2O, but pressures should not exceed 30 cm H_2O thereafter. Adequacy of ventilation should be checked by auscultation and chest excursions. Gastric decompression with an 8F tube often facilitates ventilation. If after 30 s the heart rate is over 100 beats/min and spontaneous ventilations become adequate, assisted ventilation is no longer necessary. If the heart rate remains less than 60 beats/min or 60–80 beats/min without an increase in response to resuscitation, the neonate is intubated and chest compressions are started.

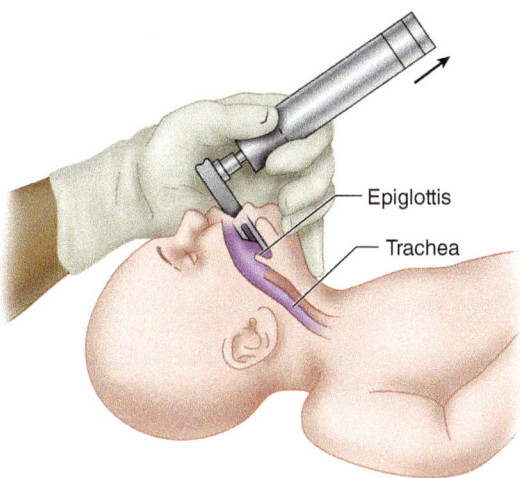

FIGURE 41–6 Intubation of the neonate. The head is placed in a neutral position, and the laryngoscope handle is held with the thumb and index finger as the chin is supported with the remaining fingers. Pressure applied over the hyoid bone with the little finger will bring the larynx into view. A straight blade such as a Miller 0 or 1 usually provides the best view.

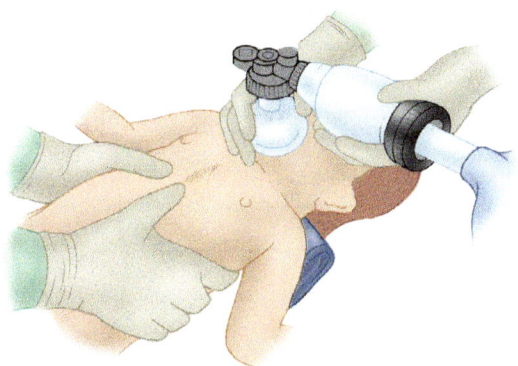

FIGURE 41–7 Chest compressions in the neonate. The neonate is held with both hands as each thumb is placed just beneath a line connecting the nipples and the remaining fingers encircle the chest. The sternum is compressed ⅓ to ¾ in. (1 cm) at a rate of 120/min. (Reproduced with permission from Rudolph CD, et al. *Rudolph's Pediatrics*. 22nd ed. McGraw-Hill; 2011.)

If the heart rate is 60–80 beats/min and increasing, assisted ventilation is continued and the neonate is observed. Failure of the heart rate to rise above 80 beats/min is an indication for chest compressions. Indications for endotracheal intubation include ineffective or prolonged mask ventilation and the need to administer medications.

Intubation (Figure 41–6) is performed with a Miller 00, 0, or 1 laryngoscope blade, using a 2.5-, 3-, or 3.5-mm endotracheal tube (for neonates <1 kg, 1–2 kg, and >2 kg, respectively). Correct endotracheal tube size is indicated by a small leak with 20 cm H_2O pressure. Right endobronchial intubation should be excluded by chest auscultation. The correct depth of the endotracheal tube ("tip to lip") is usually 6 cm plus the weight in kilograms. Oxygen saturation can usually be measured by a pulse oximeter probe applied to the palm. Capnography is also very useful in confirming endotracheal intubation. Transcutaneous oxygen sensors are useful for measuring tissue oxygenation but require time for initial equilibration. Use of a laryngeal mask airway (LMA#1) has been reported in neonates weighing more than 2.5 kg and may be useful if endotracheal intubation is difficult (eg, Pierre Robin syndrome).

Guidelines for Chest Compressions

Indications for chest compressions are a heart rate that is less than 60 beats/min or 60–80 beats/min and not rising after 30 s of adequate ventilation with 100% oxygen.

Cardiac compressions should be provided at a rate of 120/min. The two thumb/encircling hands technique (Figure 41–7) is generally preferred because it appears to generate higher peak systolic and coronary perfusion pressures. Alternatively, the two-finger technique can be used (Figure 41–8). The depth of compressions should be approximately one third of the anterior–posterior diameter of the chest and enough to generate a palpable pulse.

Compressions should be interposed with ventilation in a 3:1 ratio, such that 90 compressions and 30 ventilations are given per minute. The heart rate should be checked periodically. Chest compressions should be stopped when the spontaneous heart rate exceeds 80 beats/min.

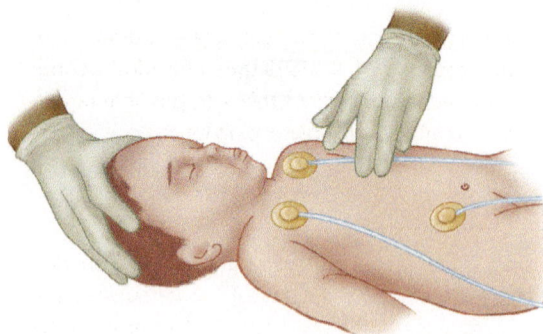

FIGURE 41–8 The alternative technique for neonatal chest compressions: two fingers are placed on the lower third of the sternum at right angles to the chest. The chest is compressed approximately 1 cm at a rate of 120/min.

Vascular Access

Cannulation of the umbilical vein with a 3.5F or 5F umbilical catheter is easiest and the preferred technique. The tip of the catheter should be just below skin level and allow free backflow of blood; further advancement may result in infusion of hypertonic solutions directly into the liver. A peripheral vein or even the endotracheal tube can be used as an alternate route for drug administration.

Cannulation of one of the two umbilical arteries allows measurement of blood pressure and facilitates blood gas measurements but may be more difficult. Specially designed umbilical artery catheters allow continuous Pao_2 or oxygen saturation monitoring as well as blood pressure. Care must be taken not to introduce any air into either the artery or the vein.

Volume Resuscitation

Some neonates at term and nearly two thirds of premature infants requiring resuscitation are hypovolemic at birth. Diagnosis is based on physical examination (low blood pressure and pallor) and a poor response to resuscitation. Neonatal blood pressure generally correlates with intravascular volume and should therefore routinely be measured. Normal blood pressure depends on birth weight and varies from 50/25 mm Hg for neonates weighing 1–2 kg to 70/40 mm Hg for those weighing over 3 kg. A low blood pressure suggests hypovolemia. Volume expansion may be accomplished with 10 mL/kg of lactated Ringer's injection, normal saline, or type O-negative blood cross-matched with maternal blood. Less common causes of hypotension include hypocalcemia, hypermagnesemia, and hypoglycemia.

Drug Therapy

A. Epinephrine

Epinephrine, 0.01–0.03 mg/kg (0.1–0.3 mL/kg of a 1:10,000 solution), should be given for asystole or a spontaneous heart rate of less than 60 beats/min in spite of adequate ventilation and chest compressions. It may be repeated every 3–5 min. Epinephrine may be given in 1 mL of saline via the endotracheal tube when venous access is not available.

B. Naloxone

Naloxone, 0.1 mg/kg intravenously or 0.2 mg/kg intramuscularly, is given to reverse the respiratory depressant effect of opioids given to the mother in the last 4 h of labor. Withdrawal symptoms may be precipitated in babies of mothers who chronically consume prescribed or illicit opioids.

C. Other Drugs

Other drugs may be indicated only in specific settings. Sodium bicarbonate (2 mEq/kg of a 0.5 mEq/mL 4.2% solution) should usually be given only for a severe metabolic acidosis documented by blood gas measurements and when ventilation is adequate. It may also be administered during prolonged resuscitation (>5 min)—particularly if blood gas measurements are not readily available. The infusion rate should not exceed 1 mEq/kg/min to avoid hypertonicity and intracranial hemorrhage. As noted above, in order to prevent hypertonicity-induced hepatic injury, the umbilical vein catheter tip should not be in the liver. Calcium gluconate 100 mg/kg ($CaCl_2$, 30 mg/kg) should be given only to neonates with documented hypocalcemia or those with suspected magnesium intoxication (from maternal magnesium therapy); these neonates are usually hypotensive, hypotonic, and appear vasodilated. Glucose (8 mg/kg/min of a 10% solution) is given only for documented hypoglycemia because hyperglycemia worsens hypoxic neurological deficits. Blood glucose should be measured because up to 10% of neonates may have hypoglycemia (glucose <35 mg/dL), particularly those delivered by cesarean section. Dopamine may be started at 5 mcg/kg/min to support arterial blood pressure. Lastly, surfactant may be given through the endotracheal tube to premature neonates with respiratory distress syndrome.

CASE DISCUSSION

Appendicitis in a Pregnant Woman

A 31-year-old woman with a 24-week gestation presents for an appendectomy.

How does pregnancy complicate the management of this patient?

Nearly 1–2% of pregnant patients require surgery during their pregnancy. The most common procedure during the first trimester is laparoscopy; appendectomy (1:1500 pregnancies) and cholecystectomy (1:2000–10,000 pregnancies) are the most commonly performed general surgical procedures. Cervical cerclage may be necessary in some patients for cervical incompetence. The physiological effects of pregnancy can alter the manifestations of disease process and make diagnosis difficult. Patients may therefore present with advanced or complicated disease. The physiological changes associated with pregnancy (see Chapter 40) further predispose the patient to increased morbidity and mortality. Moreover, both the operation and the anesthesia can adversely affect the fetus.

What are the potentially detrimental effects of surgery and anesthesia on the fetus?

The procedure can have both immediate and long-term undesirable effects on the fetus. Maternal hypotension, hypovolemia, severe anemia, hypoxemia, and marked increases in sympathetic tone can seriously compromise the transfer of oxygen and other nutrients across the uteroplacental circulation and promote intrauterine fetal asphyxia. The stress of the operative procedure and the underlying process may also precipitate preterm labor, which often follows intraabdominal surgery near the uterus. Laparoscopy may be safely performed although CO_2 insufflation has the potential to cause fetal respiratory acidosis. Mild to moderate maternal hyperventilation and limiting both insufflation pressure and duration of the procedure limit the degree of acidosis. Long-term detrimental effects relate to possible teratogenic effects on the developing fetus.

When is the fetus most sensitive to teratogenic influences?

Three stages of susceptibility are generally recognized. In the first 2 weeks of intrauterine life, teratogens have either a lethal effect or no effect on the embryo. The third to eighth weeks are the most critical period, when organogenesis takes place; drug exposure during this period can produce major developmental abnormalities. From the eighth week onward, organogenesis is complete, and organ growth takes place. Teratogen exposure during this last period usually results in only minor morphological abnormalities but can produce significant physiological abnormalities and growth retardation. Although the teratogenic influences of anesthetic agents have been extensively studied in animals, retrospective human studies have been inconclusive. Past concerns about possible teratogenic effects of nitrous oxide and benzodiazepines do not appear to be justified. Nonetheless, exposure to all anesthetic agents should be kept to a minimum in terms of the total number of agents, dosage, and duration of exposure. We tend to administer only those agents that are required—and in our practice, nitrous oxide is never required and benzodiazepines are only rarely needed—in a pregnant patient.

What would be the ideal anesthetic technique in this patient?

Toward the end of the second trimester (after 20–24 weeks of gestation), most of the major physiological changes associated with pregnancy have taken place. Regional anesthesia, when feasible, is preferable to general anesthesia in order to decrease the risks of pulmonary aspiration and failed intubation and to minimize drug exposure to the fetus. The patient should be maintained with left lateral uterine displacement when supine. Total drug exposure is least with spinal anesthesia. Moreover, spinal anesthesia may be preferable to epidural anesthesia because it is not associated with unintentional intravascular injection or the potential for accidental intrathecal injection of large epidural doses of local anesthetic. On the other hand, general anesthesia guarantees patient comfort and, when a volatile agent is used, may even suppress preterm labor (see Chapter 40). Nitrous oxide without concomitant administration of a halogenated anesthetic is reported to reduce uterine blood flow.

Although regional anesthesia is preferable in most instances, the choice between regional and general anesthesia must be individualized according to the patient, the anesthesiologist, and the type of surgery. Spinal anesthesia is usually satisfactory for open appendectomies, whereas general anesthesia is appropriate for laparoscopic procedures.

Are any special monitors indicated perioperatively?

In addition to standard monitors, fetal heart rate and uterine activity should be monitored with a Doppler and tocodynamometer immediately prior to surgery and during anesthesia recovery in a woman who is 24 weeks or more pregnant. When regular organized uterine activity is detected, early treatment with a β-adrenergic agonist such as ritodrine usually aborts the preterm labor. Magnesium sulfate and oral or rectal indomethacin may also be used as tocolytics.

When should elective operations be performed during pregnancy?

All elective operations should be postponed until 6 weeks after delivery. Only emergency procedures that pose an immediate threat to the mother or fetus should be routinely performed. The timing of semielective procedures, such as those for cancer, valvular heart disease, or intracranial aneurysms, must be individualized and must balance the threat to maternal health versus fetal well-being. Controlled (deliberate) hypotensive anesthesia has been utilized to reduce blood loss during extensive cancer operations; nitroprusside, nitroglycerin, and hydralazine have been used during pregnancy without apparent fetal compromise.

Nonetheless, large doses and prolonged infusions of nitroprusside should be avoided because the immature liver of the fetus may have a limited ability to metabolize the cyanide breakdown product. Cardiopulmonary bypass has been employed in pregnant patients successfully without adverse fetal outcome. Elective use of circulatory arrest during pregnancy is not recommended.

GUIDELINES

Kattwinkel J, Perlman JM, Aziz K, et al: Part 15: Neonatal resuscitation: 2010 American Heart Association Guidelines for Cardiopulmonary Resuscitation and Emergency Cardiovascular Care. Circulation 2010;122:S909. Erratum in: Circulation 2011;124:e406.

SUGGESTED READING

Ahmed A: New insights into the etiology of preeclampsia: Identification of key elusive factors for the vascular complications. Thromb Res 2011;127:S72.

Frölich MA, Esame A, Zhang K, et al: What factors affect intrapartum maternal temperature? A prospective cohort study: Maternal intrapartum temperature. Anesthesiology 2012;117:302.

Loubert C, Hinova A, Fernando R: Update on modern neuraxial analgesia in labour: A review of the literature of the last 5 years. Anaesthesia 2011;66:191.

MacKAy AP, Berg CJ, Liu X, et al: Changes in pregnancy mortality ascertainment: United States, 1999–2005. Obstet Gynecol 2011;118:104.

Ngan Kee WD: Prevention of maternal hypotension after regional anaesthesia for caesarean section. Curr Opin Anaesthesiol 2010;23:304.

Santos AC, Birnbach DJ: Spinal anesthesia in the parturient with severe preeclampsia: Time for reconsideration. Anesth Analg 2003;97:621.

Simmons SW, Cyna AM, Dennis AT, Hughes D: Combined spinal-epidural versus epidural analgesia in labour. Cochrane Database Syst Rev 2007;18:CD003401.

Toledo P: What's new in obstetric anesthesia: The 2011 Gerard W. Ostheimer lecture. Int J Obstet Anesth 2012;21:68.

Wong CA, Scavone BM, Peaceman AM, et al: The risk of cesarean delivery with neuraxial analgesia given early versus late in labor. N Engl J Med 2005;352:655.

Pediatric Anesthesia

1 Neonates and infants have fewer and smaller alveoli, reducing lung compliance; in contrast, their cartilaginous rib cage makes their chest wall very compliant. The combination of these two characteristics promotes chest wall collapse during inspiration and relatively low residual lung volumes at expiration. The resulting decrease in functional residual capacity (FRC) limits oxygen reserves during periods of apnea (eg, intubation attempts) and readily predisposes them to atelectasis and hypoxemia.

2 Compared with older children and adults, neonates and infants have a proportionately larger head and tongue, narrower nasal passages, an anterior and cephalad larynx, a longer epiglottis, and a shorter trachea and neck. These anatomic features make neonates and infants obligate nasal breathers until about 5 months of age. The cricoid cartilage is the narrowest point of the airway in children younger than 5 years of age.

3 Cardiac stroke volume is relatively fixed by a noncompliant and immature left ventricle in neonates and infants. The cardiac output is therefore very sensitive to changes in heart rate.

4 Thin skin, low fat content, and a greater surface area relative to weight promote greater heat loss to the environment in neonates. Heat loss is compounded by cold operating rooms, wound exposure, intravenous fluid administration, dry

anesthetic gases, and the direct effect of anesthetic agents on temperature regulation. Hypothermia has been associated with delayed awakening from anesthesia, cardiac irritability, respiratory depression, increased pulmonary vascular resistance, and altered drug responses.

5 Neonates, infants, and young children have relatively greater alveolar ventilation and reduced FRC compared with older children and adults even after adjustment for weight. This greater minute ventilation-to-FRC ratio with relatively greater blood flow to vessel-rich organs contributes to a rapid increase in alveolar anesthetic concentration and speeds inhalation induction.

6 Minimum alveolar concentration (MAC) for halogenated agents is greater in infants than in neonates and adults. Unlike other agents, sevoflurane has the same MAC in neonates and infants. Sevoflurane appears to have a greater therapeutic index than halothane and has become the preferred agent for inhaled induction in pediatric anesthesia.

7 Children are more susceptible than adults to cardiac arrhythmias, hyperkalemia, rhabdomyolysis, myoglobinemia, masseter spasm, and malignant hyperthermia associated with succinylcholine. When a child experiences cardiac arrest following administration of succinylcholine, immediate

—Continued next page

Continued—

treatment for hyperkalemia should be instituted.

8 Unlike adults, children may have profound bradycardia and sinus node arrest following the first dose of succinylcholine without atropine pretreatment.

9 A viral infection within 2–4 weeks before general anesthesia and endotracheal intubation appears to place the child at an increased risk for perioperative pulmonary complications, such as wheezing, laryngospasm, hypoxemia, and atelectasis.

10 Temperature must be closely monitored in pediatric patients because of their greater risk for malignant hyperthermia and the potential for both iatrogenic hypothermia and hyperthermia.

11 Meticulous attention to fluid intake and loss is required in younger pediatric patients

because these patients have limited margins of error. A programmable infusion pump or a buret with a microdrip chamber is useful for accurate measurements. Drugs can be flushed through low dead-space tubing to minimize unnecessary fluid administration.

12 Laryngospasm can usually be avoided by extubating the patient either while awake or while deeply anesthetized; both techniques have advocates. Extubation during the interval between these extremes, however, is generally recognized as more hazardous.

13 Patients with scoliosis due to muscular dystrophy are predisposed to malignant hypertension, cardiac arrhythmias, and untoward effects of succinylcholine (hyperkalemia, myoglobinuria, and sustained muscular contractures).

Pediatric anesthesia involves more than simply adjusting drug doses and equipment for smaller patients. Neonates (0–1 months), infants (1–12 months), toddlers (12–24 months), and young children (2–12 years of age) have differing anesthetic requirements. Safe anesthetic management depends on full appreciation of the physiological, anatomic, and pharmacological characteristics of each group (Table 42–1). Indeed infants are at much greater risk of anesthetic morbidity and mortality than older children; risk is generally inversely proportional to age. In addition, pediatric patients are prone to illnesses that require unique surgical and anesthetic strategies.

ANATOMIC & PHYSIOLOGICAL DEVELOPMENT

Respiratory System

The transition from fetal to neonatal physiology is reviewed in Chapter 40. Compared with older children and adults, neonates and infants have weaker

intercostal muscles and weaker diaphragms (due to a paucity of type I fibers) and less efficient ventilation, more horizontal and pliable ribs, and protuberant abdomens. Respiratory rate is increased in neonates and gradually falls to adult values by adolescence. Tidal volume and dead space per kilogram are nearly constant during development. The presence of fewer, smaller airways produces increased airway resistance. The alveoli are fully mature by late childhood (about 8 years of age). The work of breathing is increased and respiratory muscles easily fatigue.

1 Neonates and infants have fewer and smaller alveoli, reducing lung compliance; in contrast, their cartilaginous rib cage makes their chest wall very compliant. The combination of these two characteristics promotes chest wall collapse during inspiration and relatively low residual lung volumes at expiration. The resulting decrease in functional residual capacity (FRC) limits oxygen reserves during periods of apnea (eg, intubation attempts) and readily predisposes neonates and infants to atelectasis and hypoxemia. This may be exaggerated by their

TABLE 42–1 Characteristics of neonates and infants that differentiate them from adult patients.[1]

Physiological
Heart-rate-dependent cardiac output
Increased heart rate
Reduced blood pressure
Increased respiratory rate
Increased metabolic rate
Reduced lung compliance
Increased chest wall compliance
Reduced functional residual capacity
Increased ratio of body surface area to body weight
Increased total body water content

Anatomic
Noncompliant left ventricle
Residual fetal circulation
Difficult venous and arterial cannulation
Relatively larger head and tongue
Narrower nasal passages
Anterior and cephalad larynx
Relatively longer epiglottis
Shorter trachea and neck
More prominent adenoids and tonsils
Weaker intercostal and diaphragmatic muscles
Greater resistance to airflow

Pharmacological
Immature hepatic biotransformation
Decreased blood protein for drug binding
More rapid rise in FA/FI and more rapid induction and recovery from inhaled anesthetics
Increased minimum alveolar concentration
Relatively larger volume of distribution for water-soluble drugs
Immature neuromuscular junction

[1]FA/FI, Fractional alveolar concentration/fractional inspired concentration.

relatively higher rate of oxygen consumption. Moreover, hypoxic and hypercapnic ventilatory drives are not well developed in neonates and infants. In fact, unlike in adults, hypoxia and hypercapnia may depress respiration in these patients.

Neonates and infants have, compared with older children and adults, a proportionately larger head and tongue, narrower nasal passages, an anterior and cephalad larynx (the glottis is at a vertebral level of C4 versus C6 in adults), a longer epiglottis, and a shorter trachea and neck (Figure 42–1). These anatomic features make neonates and young infants obligate nasal breathers until about 5 months of age. **The cricoid cartilage is the narrowest point of the airway in children**

younger than 5 years of age; in adults, the narrowest point is the glottis. One millimeter of mucosal edema will have a proportionately greater effect on gas flow in children because of their smaller tracheal diameters.

Cardiovascular System

Cardiac stroke volume is relatively fixed by a noncompliant and immature left ventricle in neonates and infants. The cardiac output is therefore very sensitive to changes in heart rate (see Chapter 20). Although basal heart rate is greater than in adults (Table 42–2), activation of the parasympathetic nervous system, anesthetic overdose, or hypoxia can quickly trigger bradycardia and profound reductions in cardiac output. Sick infants undergoing emergency or prolonged surgical procedures appear particularly prone to episodes of bradycardia that can lead to hypotension, asystole, and intraoperative death. The sympathetic nervous system and baroreceptor reflexes are not fully mature. The infant cardiovascular system displays a blunted response to exogenous catecholamines. The immature heart is more sensitive to depression by volatile anesthetics and to opioid-induced bradycardia. The vascular tree is less able to respond to hypovolemia with compensatory vasoconstriction. Intravascular volume depletion in neonates and infants may be signaled by hypotension without tachycardia.

Metabolism & Temperature Regulation

Pediatric patients have a larger surface area per kilogram than adults (or a smaller body-mass index). Metabolism and its associated parameters (oxygen consumption, CO_2 production, cardiac output, and alveolar ventilation) correlate better with surface area than with weight.

Thin skin, low fat content, and a greater surface area relative to weight promote greater heat loss to the environment in neonates. This problem is compounded by inadequately warmed operating rooms, prolonged wound exposure, administration of room temperature intravenous or irrigation fluid, and dry anesthetic gases. Of course, there are also effects of anesthetic agents on temperature regulation (see Chapter 52). Even mild degrees of hypothermia can cause perioperative problems,

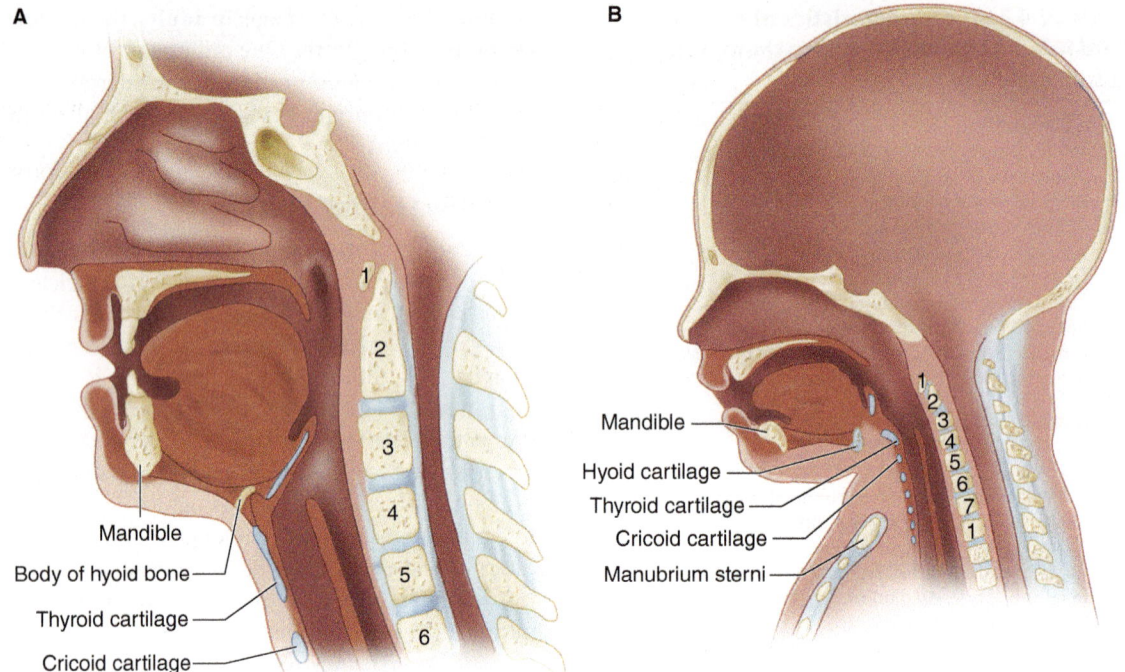

A

1
2
3
4
5
6

Mandible

Body of hyoid bone

Thyroid cartilage

Cricoid cartilage

B

1
2
3
4
5
6
7
1

Mandible

Hyoid cartilage

Thyroid cartilage

Cricoid cartilage

Manubrium sterni

FIGURE 42–1 Sagittal section of the adult (**A**) and infant (**B**) airway. (Reproduced, with permission, from Snell RS, Katz J: *Clinical Anatomy for Anesthesiologists*. Appleton & Lange, 1988.)

including delayed awakening from anesthesia, cardiac irritability, respiratory depression, increased pulmonary vascular resistance, and altered responses to anesthetics, neuromuscular blockers, and other agents. The more important mechanisms for heat production in neonates are nonshivering thermogenesis by metabolism of brown fat and shifting of hepatic oxidative phosphorylation to

a more thermogenic pathway. Yet, metabolism of brown fat is severely limited in premature infants and in sick neonates who are deficient in fat stores. Furthermore, volatile anesthetics inhibit thermogenesis in brown adipocytes.

Renal & Gastrointestinal Function

Kidney function approaches normal values (corrected for size) by 6 months of age, but this may be delayed until the child is 2 years old. Premature neonates often demonstrate multiple forms of renal immaturity, including decreased creatinine clearance; impaired sodium retention, impaired glucose excretion, and impaired bicarbonate reabsorption; and reduced diluting and concentrating ability. These abnormalities underscore the importance of appropriate fluid administration in the early days of life.

Neonates also have a relatively increased incidence of gastroesophageal reflux. The immature liver conjugates drugs and other molecules less readily early in life.

TABLE 42–2 **Age-related changes in vital signs.**[1]

Age	Respiratory Rate	Heart Rate	Arterial Blood Pressure	
			Systolic	Diastolic
Neonate	40	140	65	40
12 months	30	120	95	65
3 years	25	100	100	70
12 years	20	80	110	60

[1]Values are mean averages derived from numerous sources. Normal ranges may include measurements that deviate from these as much as 25–50%.

Glucose Homeostasis

Neonates have relatively reduced glycogen stores, predisposing them to hypoglycemia. Impaired glucose excretion by the kidneys may partially offset this tendency. In general, neonates at greatest risk for hypoglycemia are either premature or small for gestational age, receiving hyperalimentation, and the offspring of diabetic mothers.

PHARMACOLOGICAL DIFFERENCES

Pediatric drug dosing is typically adjusted on a per-kilogram basis for convenience (Table 42–3). In early childhood a patient's weight can be approximated based on age:

$$\text{50th percentile weight (kg)} = (\text{Age} \times 2) + 9$$

TABLE 42–3 Pediatric drug dosages.

Drug	Comment	Dosage	Drug	Comment	Dosage
Acetaminophen	Rectal	40 mg/kg	Ceftriaxone	IV	25–50 mg/kg
	PO	10–20 mg/kg	Cefuroxime	IV	25 mg/kg
	IV (age > 2 y)	15 mg/kg	Chloral hydrate	PO	25–100 mg/kg
	Maximum (per day)	60 mg/kg		Rectal	50 mg/kg
Adenosine	Rapid IV bolus	0.1 mg/kg	Cimetidine	IV or PO	5–10 mg/kg
	Repeat dose	0.2 mg/kg	Cisatracurium	Intubation (IV)	0.15 mg/kg
	Maximum dose	12 mg	Clindamycin	IV	20 mg/kg
Albuterol	Nebulized	1.25–2.5 mg in 2 mL saline	Dantrolene	Initial dose (IV)	2.5 mg/kg
Alfentanil	Anesthetic supplement (IV)	20–25 mcg/kg		Maximum dose	10 mg/kg
				Subsequent attempts	4 J/kg
	Maintenance infusion	1–3 mcg/kg/min	Desmopressin	IV	0.2–0.4 mcg/kg
			Dexamethasone	IV	0.1–0.5 mg/kg
Aminophylline	Loading dose administered over 20 min (IV)	5–6 mg/kg	Dextrose	$D_{25}W$ or $D_{50}W$ (IV)	0.5–1 g/kg
			Digoxin	IV	0.1–0.2 mg/kg
	Maintenance dose (therapeutic level: 10–20 mg/mL)	0.5–0.9 mg/kg/h		Three divided doses over 24 h (IV)	15–30 mcg/kg
			Diltiazem	IV over 2 min	0.25 mg/kg
			Diphenhydramine	IV, IM, or PO	1 mg/kg
Amiodarone	Loading dose (IV)	5 mg/kg	Dobutamine	Infusion	2–20 mcg/kg/min
	Repeat dose (slowly)	5 mg/kg	Dolasetron	IV	0.35 mg/kg
	Infusion	5–10 mcg/kg/min	Dopamine	Infusion	2–20 mcg/kg/min
			Droperidol	IV	50–75 mcg/kg
	Maximum dose	20 mg/kg/day	Edrophonium	Depends on degree of paralysis (IV)	0.5–1 mg/kg
Amoxicillin	PO	50 mg/kg	Ephedrine	IV	0.1–0.3 mg/kg
Ampicillin	IV	50 mg/kg	Epinephrine	IV bolus	10 mcg/kg
Ampicillin/ sulbactam	IV	25–50 mg/kg		Endotracheal dose	100 mcg/kg
				Infusion	0.05–1 mcg/kg/min
Atracurium	Intubation (IV)	0.5 mg/kg			
Atropine	IV	0.01–0.02 mg/kg	Epinephrine, 2.25% racemic	Nebulized	0.05 mL/kg in 3 mL saline
	IM	0.02 mg/kg	Esmolol	IV bolus	100–500 mcg/kg
	Minimum dose	0.1 mg		IV infusion	25–200 mcg/kg/min
	Premedication (PO)	0.03–0.05 mg/kg			
Bretylium	Loading dose (IV)	5 mg/kg	Famotidine	IV	0.15 mg/kg
Caffeine	IV	10 mg/kg	Fentanyl	Pain relief (IV)	1–2 mcg/kg
Calcium chloride	IV (slowly)	5–20 mg/kg		Pain relief (Intranasal)	2 mcg/kg
Calcium gluconate	IV (slowly)	15–100 mg/kg		Premedication (Actiq PO)	10–15 mcg/kg
Cefazolin	IV	25 mg/kg			
Cefotaxime	IV	25–50 mg/kg		Anesthetic adjunct (IV)	1–5 mcg/kg
Cefotetan	IV	20–40 mg/kg		Maintenance infusion	2–4 mcg/kg/h
Cefoxitin	IV	30–40 mg/kg		Main anesthetic (IV)	50–100 mcg/kg
Ceftazidime	IV	30–50 mg/kg			

(continued)

TABLE 42–3 Pediatric drug dosages. (continued)

Drug	Comment	Dosage	Drug	Comment	Dosage
Flumazenil	IV	0.01 mg/kg	Morphine	Pain relief (IV)	0.025–0.1 mg/kg
Fosphenytoin	IV	15–20 mg/kg		Premedication (IM)	0.1 mg/kg
Furosemide	IV	0.2–1 mg/kg	Naloxone	IV	0.01 mg/kg
Gentamicin	IV	2 mg/kg	Neostigmine	Depends on	0.04–0.07 mg/kg
Glucagon	IV	0.5–1 mg		degree of	
Glucose	IV	0.5–1 g/kg		paralysis (IV)	
Glycopyrrolate	IV	0.01 mg/kg	Nitroglycerin	IV	0.5–3 mcg/kg/min
Granisetron	IV	0.04 mg/kg	Nitroprusside	Infusion	0.5–4 mcg/kg/min
Heparin	IV (not for cardiac surgery)	100 units/kg	Norepinephrine	Infusion	0.05–2 mcg/kg/min
			Ondansetron	IV	0.1 mg/kg
	Cardiac surgery dose	300–400 units/kg	Oxacillin	IV	50 mg/kg
			Pancuronium	IV	0.1 mg/kg
Hydrocortisone	IV	1 mg/kg	Penicillin G	IV	50,000 units/kg
Hydromorphone	IV	15–20 mcg/kg	Pentobarbital	Premedication (IM)	1–2 mg/kg
Ibuprofen	PO	4–10 mg/kg	Phenobarbital	Anticonvulsant dose (IV)	5–20 mg/kg
Imipenem	IV	15–25 mg/kg			
Inamrinone	Loading (IV)	1.5 mg/kg	Phentolamine	IV	30 mcg/kg
	Maintenance	5–10 mcg/kg/min	Phenylephrine	IV	1–10 mcg/kg
Insulin	Infusion	0.02–0.1 units/kg/h	Phenytoin	Slowly IV	5–20 mg/kg
			Physostigmine	IV	0.01–0.03 mg/kg
Isoproterenol	Infusion	0.1–1 mcg/kg/min	Prednisone	PO	1 mg/kg
Ketamine	Induction (IV)	1–2 mg/kg	Procainamide	Loading dose (IV)	15 mg/kg
	Induction (IM)	6–10 mg/kg	Propofol	Induction (IV)	2–3 mg/kg
	Induction (per rectum)	10 mg/kg		Maintenance infusion	60–250 mcg/kg/min
	Maintenance infusion	25–75 mcg/kg/min	Propranolol	IV	10–25 mcg/kg
	Premedication (PO)	6–10 mg/kg	Prostaglandin E$_1$	Infusion	0.05–0.1 mcg/kg/min
	Sedation (IV)	0.5–1 mg/kg	Protamine	IV	1 mg/100 units heparin
Ketorolac	IV	0.5–0.75 mg/kg			
Labetalol	IV	0.25 mg/kg	Ranitidine	IV	0.25–1.0 mg/kg
Lidocaine	Loading	1 mg/kg	Remifentanil	IV bolus	0.25–1 mcg/kg
	Maintenance	20–50 mcg/kg/min		IV infusion	0.05–2 mcg/kg/min
Magnesium sulphate	IV (slowly)	25–50 mg/kg	Rocuronium	Intubation (IV)	0.6–1.2 mg/kg
	Maximum single dose	2 g	Sodium bicarbonate	IV	1 mEq/kg
			Succinylcholine	Intubation (IV)	1–2mg/kg
Mannitol	IV	0.25–1 g/kg		Intubation (IM)	4 mg/kg
Meperidine	Pain relief (IV)	0.2–0.5 mg/kg	Sufentanil	Premedication (Intranasal)	2 mcg/kg
Methohexital	Induction (IV)	1–2 mg/kg			
	Induction (per rectum)	25–30 mg/kg		Anesthetic adjunct (IV)	0.5–1 mcg/kg
	Induction (IM)	10 mg/kg		Maintenance infusion	0.5–2 mcg/kg/h
Methylprednisolone	IV	2–4 mg/kg		Main anesthetic (IV)	10–15 mcg/kg
Metoclopramide	IV	0.15 mg/kg			
Metronidazole	IV	7.5 mg/kg	Thiopental	Induction (IV)	5–6 mg/kg
Midazolam	Premedication (PO)	0.5 mg/kg			
	Maximum dose (PO)	20 mg	Trimethoprim/ sulfamethoxazole	IV	4–5 mg/kg
	Sedation (IM)	0.1–0.15 mg/kg			
	Sedation (IV)	0.05 mg/kg	Vancomycin	IV	20 mg/kg
Milrinone	Loading (IV)	50–75 mcg/kg	Vecuronium	IV	0.1 mg/kg
	Maintenance	0.375–0.75 mcg/kg/min	Verapamil	IV	0.1–0.3 mg/kg

Weight-adjustment of drug dosing is incompletely effective because it does not take into account the disproportionately larger pediatric intravascular and extracellular fluid compartments, the immaturity of hepatic biotransformation pathways, increased organ blood flow, decreased protein for drug binding, or higher metabolic rate.

Neonates and infants have a proportionately greater total water content (70–75%) than adults (50–60%). Total body water content decreases while fat and muscle content increase with age. As a direct result, the volume of distribution for most intravenous drugs is disproportionately greater in neonates, infants, and young children, and the optimal dose (per kilogram) is usually greater than in older children and adults. A disproportionately smaller muscle mass in neonates prolongs the clinical duration of action (by delaying redistribution to muscle) of drugs such as thiopental and fentanyl. Neonates also have a relatively decreased glomerular filtration rate, hepatic blood flow, and renal tubular function, and immature hepatic enzyme systems. Increased intraabdominal pressure and abdominal surgery further reduce hepatic blood flow. All these factors may impair renal drug handling, hepatic metabolism, or biliary excretion of drugs in neonates and young infants. Neonates also have decreased protein binding for some drugs, most notably thiopental, bupivacaine, and many antibiotics. In the case of thiopental, increased free drug enhances potency and reduces the induction dose in neonates compared with older children. An increase in free bupivacaine might increase the risk of systemic toxicity.

Inhalational Anesthetics

5 Neonates, infants, and young children have relatively greater alveolar ventilation and reduced FRC compared with older children and adults. This greater minute ventilation-to-FRC ratio with relatively greater blood flow to vessel-rich organs contributes to a rapid increase in alveolar anesthetic concentration and speeds inhalation induction. Furthermore, the blood/gas coefficients of volatile anesthetics are reduced in neonates compared with adults, resulting in even faster induction times and potentially increasing the risk of accidental overdosage.

TABLE 42–4 **Approximate MAC[1] values for pediatric patients reported in % of an atmosphere.[2]**

Agent	Neonates	Infants	Small Children	Adults
Halothane	0.90	1.1–1.2	0.9	0.75
Sevoflurane	3.2	3.2	2.5	2
Isoflurane	1.6	1.8–1.9	1.3–1.6	1.2
Desflurane	8–9	9–10	7–8	6

[1]MAC, minimum alveolar concentration.
[2]Values are derived from various sources.

6 The minimum alveolar concentration (MAC) for halogenated agents is greater in infants than in neonates and adults (Table 42–4). In contrast to other agents, no increase in sevoflurane MAC can be demonstrated in neonates and infants. Nitrous oxide does not appear to reduce the MAC of desflurane or sevoflurane in children to the same extent as it does for other agents.

The blood pressure of neonates and infants appears to be especially sensitive to volatile anesthetics. This clinical observation has been attributed to less-well-developed compensatory mechanisms (eg, vasoconstriction, tachycardia) and greater sensitivity of the immature myocardium to myocardial depressants. Halothane (now much less commonly used) sensitizes the heart to catecholamines. The maximum recommended dose of epinephrine in local anesthetic solutions during halothane anesthesia is 10 mcg/kg. Cardiovascular depression, bradycardia, and arrhythmias are less frequent with sevoflurane than with halothane. Halothane and sevoflurane are less likely than other volatile agents to irritate the airway or cause breath holding or laryngospasm during induction (see Chapter 8). In general, volatile anesthetics appear to depress ventilation more in infants than in older children. Sevoflurane appears to produce the least respiratory depression. The risk for halothane-induced hepatic dysfunction appears to be much reduced in prepubertal children compared with adults. There are no reported instances of renal toxicity attributed to inorganic fluoride production during sevoflurane anesthesia in children.

Overall, sevoflurane appears to have a greater therapeutic index than halothane and has become the preferred agent for inhaled induction in pediatric anesthesia.

Emergence is fastest following desflurane or sevoflurane, but both agents are associated with a greater incidence of agitation or delirium upon emergence, particularly in young children. Because of the latter, some clinicians switch to isoflurane for maintenance anesthesia following a sevoflurane induction (see below).

Nonvolatile Anesthetics

After weight-adjustment of dosing, infants and young children require larger doses of propofol because of a larger volume of distribution compared with adults. Children also have a shorter elimination half-life and higher plasma clearance for propofol. Recovery from a single bolus is not appreciably different from that in adults; however, recovery following a continuous infusion may be more rapid. For the same reasons, children may require increased weight-adjusted rates of infusion for maintenance of anesthesia (up to 250 mcg/kg/min). Propofol is not recommended for prolonged sedation of critically ill pediatric patients in the intensive care unit (ICU) due to an association with greater mortality than other agents. Although the "propofol infusion syndrome" has been reported more often in critically ill children, it has also been reported in adults undergoing long-term propofol infusion (>48 h) for sedation, particularly at increased doses (>5 mg/kg/h). Its essential features include rhabdomyolysis, metabolic acidosis, hemodynamic instability, hepatomegaly, and multiorgan failure.

Children require relatively larger doses of thiopental compared with adults. The elimination half-life is shorter and the plasma clearance is greater than in adults. In contrast, neonates, appear to be more sensitive to barbiturates. Neonates have less protein binding, a longer half-life, and impaired clearance. The thiopental induction dose for neonates is 3–4 mg/kg compared with 5–6 mg/kg for infants.

Opioids appear to be more potent in neonates than in older children and adults. Unproven (but popular) explanations include "easier entry" across the blood–brain barrier, decreased metabolic

capability, or increased sensitivity of the respiratory centers. Morphine sulfate, particularly in repeated doses, should be used with caution in neonates because hepatic conjugation is reduced and renal clearance of morphine metabolites is decreased. The cytochrome P-450 pathways mature at the end of the neonatal period. Older pediatric patients have relatively greater rates of biotransformation and elimination as a result of high hepatic blood flow. Sufentanil, alfentanil, and, possibly, fentanyl clearances may be greater in children than in adults. Remifentanil clearance is increased in neonates and infants but elimination half-life is unaltered compared with adults. Neonates and infants may be more resistant to the hypnotic effects of ketamine, requiring slightly higher doses than adults (but the "differences" are within the range of error in studies); pharmacokinetic values do not appear to be significantly different from those of adults. Etomidate has not been well-studied in pediatric patients younger than 10 years of age; its profile in older children is similar to that in adults. Midazolam has the fastest clearance of all the benzodiazepines; however, midazolam clearance is significantly reduced in neonates compared with older children. The combination of midazolam and fentanyl can cause hypotension in patients of all ages.

Muscle Relaxants

For a wide variety of reasons (including pharmacology, case mix, and convenience), muscle relaxants are less commonly used during induction of anesthesia in pediatric than in adult patients. Many children will have a laryngeal mask airway (LMA) or endotracheal tube placed after receiving a sevoflurane inhalation induction, placement of an intravenous catheter, and administration of various combinations of propofol, opioids, or lidocaine.

All muscle relaxants generally have a faster onset (up to 50% less delay) in pediatric patients because of shorter circulation times than adults. In both children and adults, intravenous succinylcholine (1–1.5 mg/kg) has the fastest onset (see Chapter 11). Infants require significantly larger doses of succinylcholine (2–3 mg/kg) than older children and adults because of the relatively larger volume of distribution. This discrepancy disappears

TABLE 42–5 Approximate ED_{95} for muscle relaxants in infants and children.[1]

Agents	Infants ED_{95} (mg/kg)	Children ED_{95} (mg/kg)
Succinylcholine	0.7	0.4
Atracurium	0.25	0.35
Cisatracurium	0.05	0.06
Rocuronium	0.25	0.4
Vecuronium	0.05	0.08
Pancuronium	0.07	0.09

[1]Average values during nitrous oxide/oxygen anesthesia.

if dosage is based on body surface area. Table 42–5 lists commonly used muscle relaxants and their ED_{95} (the dose that produces 95% depression of evoked twitches). With the notable exclusion of succinylcholine and possibly cisatracurium, infants require significantly smaller muscle relaxant doses than older children. Moreover, based on weight, older children require larger doses than adults for some neuromuscular blocking agents (eg, atracurium, see Chapter 11). As with adults, a more rapid intubation can be achieved with a muscle relaxant dose that is twice the ED_{95} dose at the expense of prolonging the duration of action.

The response of neonates to nondepolarizing muscle relaxants is variable. Popular (and unproven) explanations for this include "immaturity of the neuromuscular junction" (in premature neonates), tending to increase sensitivity (unproven), counterbalanced by a disproportionately larger extracellular compartment, reducing drug concentrations (proven). The relative immaturity of neonatal hepatic function prolongs the duration of action for drugs that depend primarily on hepatic metabolism (eg, pancuronium, vecuronium, and rocuronium). Atracurium and cisatracurium do not depend on hepatic biotransformation and reliably behave as intermediate-acting muscle relaxants.

7 Children are more susceptible than adults to cardiac arrhythmias, hyperkalemia, rhabdomyolysis, myoglobinemia, masseter spasm, and malignant hyperthermia (see Chapter 52) associated with succinylcholine. When a child experiences cardiac arrest following administration of succinylcholine, immediate treatment for hyperkalemia should be instituted. Prolonged, heroic (eg, potentially including cardiopulmonary bypass) resuscitative efforts may be required. For this reason, succinylcholine is avoided for routine, elective paralysis for intu-

8 bation in children and adolescents. Unlike adults, children may have profound bradycardia and sinus node arrest following the first dose of succinylcholine without atropine pretreatment. Atropine (0.1 mg minimum) must therefore always be administered prior to succinylcholine in children. Generally accepted indications for intravenous succinylcholine in children include rapid sequence induction with a "full" stomach and laryngospasm that does not respond to positive-pressure ventilation. When rapid muscle relaxation is required prior to intravenous access (eg, with inhaled inductions in patients with full stomachs), intramuscular succinylcholine (4–6 mg/kg) can be used. Intramuscular atropine (0.02 mg/kg) should be administered with intramuscular succinylcholine to reduce the likelihood of bradycardia. Some clinicians advocate intralingual administration (2 mg/kg in the midline to avoid hematoma formation) as an alternate emergency route for intramuscular succinylcholine.

Many clinicians consider rocuronium (0.6 mg/kg intravenously) to be the drug of choice (when a relaxant will be used) during routine intubation in pediatric patients with intravenous access because it has the fastest onset of nondepolarizing neuromuscular blocking agents (see Chapter 11). Larger doses of rocuronium (0.9–1.2 mg/kg) may be used for rapid sequence induction but a prolonged duration (up to 90 min) will likely follow. Rocuronium is the only nondepolarizing neuromuscular blocker that has been adequately studied for intramuscular administration (1.0–1.5 mg/kg), but this approach requires 3–4 min for onset.

Atracurium or cisatracurium may be preferred in young infants, particularly for short procedures, because these drugs consistently display short to intermediate duration.

As with adults, the effect of incremental doses of muscle relaxants (usually 25–30% of the initial dose) should be monitored with a peripheral nerve stimulator. Sensitivity can vary significantly between patients. Nondepolarizing blockade can be reversed with neostigmine (0.03–0.07 mg/kg) or edrophonium (0.5–1 mg/kg) along with an anticholinergic agent (glycopyrrolate, 0.01 mg/kg, or atropine, 0.01–0.02 mg/kg). Sugammadex, a specific antagonist for rocuronium and vecuronium, has yet to be released in the United States.

PEDIATRIC ANESTHETIC RISK

The Pediatric Perioperative Cardiac Arrest (POCA) Registry provides a useful database for assessing pediatric anesthetic risk. This registry includes reports derived from approximately one million pediatric anesthetics administered since 1994. Case records of children experiencing cardiac arrests or death during the administration of or recovery from anesthesia were investigated regarding any possible relationship with anesthesia. Nearly all patients received general anesthesia alone or combined with regional anesthesia. In a preliminary analysis that included 289 cases of cardiac arrest, anesthesia was judged to have contributed to 150 arrests. Thus the risk of cardiac arrest in pediatric anesthetic cases would appear to be approximately 1.4 in 10,000. Moreover, an overall mortality of 26% was reported following cardiac arrest. Approximately 6% suffered permanent injury, but the majority (68%) had either no or only temporary injury. Mortality was 4% in American Society of Anesthesiologists (ASA) physical status 1 and 2 patients compared with 37% in ASA physical status 3–5 patients. It is important to note that 33% of patients who suffered a cardiac arrest were ASA physical status 1–2. Infants accounted for 55% of all anesthesia-related arrests, with those younger than 1 month of age (ie, neonates) having the greatest risk. As with adults, two major predictors of mortality were ASA physical status 3–5 and emergency surgery.

Most (82%) arrests occurred during induction of anesthesia; bradycardia, hypotension, and a low SpO_2 frequently preceded arrest. The most common mechanism of cardiac arrest was judged to be medication related (**Figure 42–2**). Cardiovascular depression from halothane, alone or in combination with other drugs, was believed to be responsible in

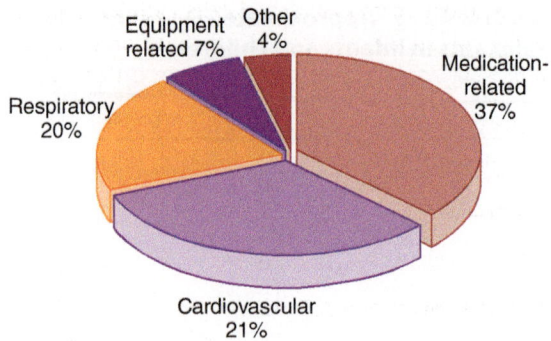

FIGURE 42–2 Mechanisms of cardiac arrest in pediatric patients, based on POCA Registry data.

66% of all medication-related arrests. Another 9% was due to intravascular injection of a local anesthetic, most often following a negative aspiration test during attempted caudal injection. Presumed cardiovascular mechanisms most often had no clear etiology; in more than 50% of those cases the patient had congenital heart disease. Where a cardiovascular mechanism could be identified, it was most often related to hemorrhage, transfusion, or inadequate or inappropriate fluid therapy.

Respiratory mechanisms included laryngospasm, airway obstruction, and difficult intubation (in decreasing order). In most cases the laryngospasm occurred during induction. Nearly all patients who had airway obstruction or were difficult to intubate had at least one other significant underlying disease.

The most common equipment-related mechanisms that led to a cardiac arrest were complications related to attempted central venous catheterization (eg, pneumothorax, hemothorax, or cardiac tamponade).

In recent years there has been increased concern and scientific interest in the possibility that general anesthesia and general anesthetic agents are toxic to the brains of small children. The experimental data in animals are consistently worrisome, but the clinical data are (currently) inconclusive as to the extent of the risk and whether one technique is safer than another. Progress in this area can be followed on the SmartTots web site (http://www.smarttots.org), maintained by the International Anesthesia Research Society.

Children are at greater risk than adults of developing malignant hyperthermia. This complex and important topic is covered in depth in Chapter 52.

PEDIATRIC ANESTHETIC TECHNIQUES

Preoperative Considerations

A. Preoperative Interview

Depending on age, past experiences, and maturity, children present with varying degrees of fright (even terror) when faced with the prospect of surgery. In contrast to adults, who are usually most concerned about the possibility of death, children are principally worried about pain and separation from their parents. Presurgical preparation programs—such as brochures, videos, or tours—can be very helpful in preparing many children and parents. Unfortunately, outpatient and morning-of-admission surgery together with a busy operating room schedule often make it nearly impossible for an anesthesiologist to break through the barriers presented by pediatric patients. For this reason, premedication (below) can be helpful. When time permits, one can demystify the process of anesthesia and surgery by explaining in age-appropriate terms what lies ahead. For example, the anesthesiologist might bring an anesthesia mask for the child to play with during the interview and describe it as like something the astronauts use. Alternatively, in some centers, someone the child trusts (eg, a parent, nurse, another physician) may be allowed to be in attendance during preanesthetic preparations and induction of anesthesia. This can have a particularly calming influence on children undergoing repeated procedures (eg, examination under anesthesia following glaucoma surgery). Some pediatric hospitals have induction rooms adjacent to their operating rooms to permit parental attendance and a quieter, less startling environment for anesthetic inductions.

B. Recent Upper Respiratory Tract Infection

Children frequently present for surgery with evidence—a runny nose with fever, cough, or sore throat—of a coincidental viral upper respiratory tract infection (URI). Attempts should be made to differentiate between an infectious cause of rhinorrhea and an allergic or vasomotor cause. A viral infection within 2–4 weeks before general anesthesia and endotracheal intubation appears to place the child at an increased risk for perioperative pulmonary complications, such as wheezing (10-fold), laryngospasm (5-fold), hypoxemia, and atelectasis. This is particularly likely if the child has a severe cough, high fever, or a family history of reactive airway disease. The decision to anesthetize children with URIs remains controversial and depends on the presence of other coexisting illnesses, the severity of URI symptoms, and the urgency of the surgery. When surgery will be performed in a child with a URI, one should consider giving anticholinergic premedication, avoiding intubation (if feasible), and humidifying inspired gases. In this circumstance one should anticipate that a longer-than-usual stay in the recovery room may be required.

C. Laboratory Tests

Few, if any, preoperative laboratory tests are cost effective. Some pediatric centers require *no* preoperative laboratory tests in *healthy* children undergoing *minor* procedures. Obviously, this places responsibility on the anesthesiologist, surgeon, and pediatrician to correctly identify those patients who should have preoperative testing for specific surgical procedures.

Most asymptomatic patients with cardiac murmurs do not have significant cardiac pathology. Innocent murmurs may occur in more than 30% of normal children. These are typically soft, short systolic ejection murmurs that are best heard along the left upper or left lower sternal border and that do not radiate. Innocent murmurs at the left upper sternal border typically are due to flow across the pulmonic valve (pulmonic ejection) whereas those at the lower left border typically are due to flow from the left ventricle to the aorta (Still's vibratory murmur). The pediatrician should carefully evaluate patients with a newly diagnosed murmur, particularly in infancy. Consultation with a pediatric cardiologist, echocardiography, or both, should be obtained if the patient is symptomatic (eg, poor feeding, failure to thrive, or easy fatigability); the murmur is harsh, loud, holosystolic, diastolic, or radiates widely; or pulses are either bounding or markedly diminished.

D. Preoperative Fasting

Because children are more prone to dehydration than adults, their preoperative fluid restriction has always been more lenient. Several studies, however, have documented low gastric pH (<2.5) and relatively high residual volumes in pediatric patients scheduled for surgery, suggesting that children may be at a greater risk for aspiration than was previously thought. The incidence of aspiration is reported to be approximately 1:1000. There is no convincing evidence that prolonged fasting decreases this risk. In fact, several studies have demonstrated lower residual volumes and higher gastric pH in pediatric patients who received clear fluids a few hours before induction (see Chapter 53). More specifically, infants are fed breast milk up to 4 h before induction, whereas formula or liquids and a "light" meal may be given up to 6 h before induction. Clear fluids are offered until 2–3 h before induction. These recommendations are for healthy neonates, infants, and children without risk factors for decreased gastric emptying or aspiration.

E. Premedication

There is great variation in the recommendations for premedication of pediatric patients. Sedative premedication is generally omitted for neonates and sick infants. Children who appear likely to exhibit uncontrollable separation anxiety should be given a sedative, such as midazolam (0.3–0.5 mg/kg, 15 mg maximum). The oral route is generally preferred because it is less traumatic than intramuscular injection, but it requires 20–45 min for effect. Smaller doses of midazolam have been used in combination with oral ketamine (4–6 mg/kg) for inpatients. For uncooperative patients, intramuscular midazolam (0.1–0.15 mg/kg, 10 mg maximum) or ketamine (2–3 mg/kg) with atropine (0.02 mg/kg) may be helpful. Rectal midazolam (0.5–1 mg/kg, 20 mg maximum) or rectal methohexital (25–30 mg/kg of 10% solution) may also be administered in such cases while the child is in the parent's arms. The nasal route can be used with some drugs but is unpleasant, and some concerns exist over potential neurotoxicity of nasal midazolam. Nasal dexmedetomidine has also been used by some clinicians. Fentanyl can also be administered as a lollipop (Actiq, 5–15 mcg/kg);

fentanyl levels continue to rise intraoperatively and can contribute to postoperative analgesia.

In the past anesthesiologists routinely premedicated young children with anticholinergic drugs (eg, atropine, 0.02 mg/kg intramuscularly) in hope of reducing the likelihood of bradycardia during induction. Atropine reduces the incidence of hypotension during induction in neonates and in infants younger than 3 months. Atropine can also prevent accumulation of secretions that can block small airways and endotracheal tubes. Secretions can be particularly problematic for patients with URIs or those who have been given ketamine. Atropine may be administered orally (0.05 mg/kg), intramuscularly, or occasionally rectally. In current practice, most anesthesiologists prefer to administer atropine intravenously at or shortly after induction.

Monitoring

Monitoring requirements for infants and children are generally similar to those for adults with some minor modifications. Alarm limits should be appropriately adjusted. Smaller electrocardiographic electrode pads may be necessary so that they do not encroach on sterile surgical areas. Blood pressure cuffs must be properly fitted. Noninvasive blood pressure monitors have proved to be reliable in infants and children. A precordial stethoscope provides an inexpensive means of monitoring heart rate, quality of heart sounds, and airway patency. Finally, monitors may sometimes need to be first attached (or reattached) following induction of anesthesia in less cooperative patients.

Small pediatric patients have a reduced margin for error. Pulse oximetry and capnography assume an even more important role in infants and small children because hypoxia from inadequate ventilation remains a common cause of perioperative morbidity and mortality. In neonates, the pulse oximeter probe should preferably be placed on the right hand or earlobe to measure preductal oxygen saturation. As in adult patients, end-tidal CO_2 analysis allows assessment of the adequacy of ventilation, confirmation of endotracheal tube placement, and early warning of malignant hyperthermia. Flow-through (mainstream) analyzers are usually less accurate in patients weighing less than 10 kg. Even with aspiration (sidestream) capnographs, the inspired (baseline) CO_2 can appear falsely elevated and the expired (peak) CO_2 can be falsely low. The degree of error depends on many factors but can be minimized by placing the sampling site as close as possible to the tip of the endotracheal tube, using a short length of sampling line, and lowering gas-sampling flow rates (100–150 mL/min). Furthermore, the size of some flow-through sensors may lead to kinking of the endotracheal tube or hypercapnia as a result of increased equipment dead space.

10 Temperature must be closely monitored in pediatric patients because of the greater risk for malignant hyperthermia and greater potential for intraoperative hypothermia or hyperthermia. The risk of hypothermia can be reduced by maintaining a warm operating room environment (26°C or warmer), by warming and humidifying inspired gases, by using a warming blanket and warming lights, and by warming all intravenous and irrigation fluids. The room temperature required for a neutral thermal environment varies with age; it is greatest in premature newborns. Note that care must be taken to prevent accidental burns and hyperthermia from overzealous warming efforts.

Invasive monitoring (eg, arterial cannulation, central venous catheterization) demands expertise and judgment. Air bubbles should be removed from pressure tubing and small volume flushes should be used to prevent air embolism, unintended heparinization, or fluid overload. The right radial artery is often chosen for cannulation in the neonate because its preductal location mirrors the oxygen content of the carotid and retinal arteries. A femoral artery catheter may be a suitable alternative in very small neonates, and left radial or right or left dorsalis pedis arteries are alternatives in infants. Critically ill neonates may retain an umbilical artery catheter. Internal jugular and subclavian approaches are often used for central lines. Ultrasonography should be used during placement of internal jugular catheters and provides useful information for arterial cannulation as well. Urinary output is an important (but neither sensitive nor specific) indicator of the adequacy of intravascular volume and cardiac output. Noninvasive monitors of stroke volume have only recently been tested in infants and young children.

Premature or small-for-gestational age neonates, and neonates who have received total parenteral nutrition or whose mothers are diabetic, are prone to hypoglycemia. These infants should have frequent blood glucose measurements: levels below 30 mg/dL in the neonate, below 40 mg/dL in infants, and below 60 mg/dL in children and adults indicate hypoglycemia requiring immediate treatment. Blood sampling for arterial blood gases, hemoglobin, potassium, and ionized calcium concentration can be invaluable in critically ill patients, particularly in those undergoing major surgery or who may be receiving transfusions.

Induction

General anesthesia is usually induced by an intravenous or inhalational technique. Induction with intramuscular ketamine (5–10 mg/kg) is reserved for specific situations, such as those involving combative, particularly mentally challenged, children and adults. Intravenous induction is usually preferred when the patient comes to the operating room with a functional intravenous catheter or will allow awake venous cannulation. Prior application of EMLA (eutectic mixture of local anesthetic) cream (see Chapter 16) may render intravenous cannulation less painful for the patient, and less stressful for the parent and anesthesiologist. EMLA cream is not a perfect solution. Some children become anxious at the sight of a needle, particularly those who have had multiple needle punctures in the past, with or without EMLA. Furthermore, it can be difficult to anticipate in which extremity intravenous cannulation will prove to be successful. Finally, to be effective, EMLA cream must remain in contact with the skin for at least 30–60 min. Awake or sedated-awake intubation with topical anesthesia should be considered for emergency procedures in neonates and small infants when they are critically ill or a potential difficult airway is present.

Intravenous Induction

The same induction sequence can be used as in adults: propofol (2–3 mg/kg) followed by a nondepolarizing muscle relaxant (eg, rocuronium, cisatracurium, atracurium) or succinylcholine. We recommend that atropine be given routinely prior to succinylcholine. The advantages of an intravenous technique include availability of intravenous access if emergency drugs need to be administered and rapidity of induction in the child at risk for aspiration. Alternatively (and very commonly in pediatric practice), intubation can be accomplished with the combination of propofol, lidocaine, and an opiate, with or without an inhaled agent, avoiding the need for a paralytic agent. Finally, paralytic agents are not needed for placement of LMAs, which are commonly used in pediatric anesthesia.

Inhalational Induction

Many children do not arrive in the operating room with an intravenous line in place and nearly all dread the prospect of being stuck with a needle. Fortunately, sevoflurane can render small children unconscious within minutes. We find this easier in children who have been sedated (most often with oral midazolam) prior to entering the operating room and who are sleepy enough to be anesthetized without ever knowing what has happened ("steal" induction). One can also insufflate the anesthetic gases over the face, place a drop of food flavoring on the inside of the mask (eg, oil of orange), and allow the child to sit during the early stages of induction. Specially contoured masks minimize dead space (see Figure 19–8).

There are many differences between adult and pediatric anatomy that influence mask ventilation and intubation. Equipment appropriate for age and size should be selected (Table 42–6). Neonates and most young infants are obligate nasal breathers and obstruct easily. Oral airways will help displace an oversized tongue; nasal airways, so useful in adults, can traumatize small nares or prominent adenoids in small children. Compression of submandibular soft tissues should be avoided during mask ventilation to prevent upper airway obstruction.

Typically, the child can be coaxed into breathing an odorless mixture of nitrous oxide (70%) and oxygen (30%). Sevoflurane (or halothane) can be added to the gas mixture in 0.5% increments every few breaths. As previously discussed, we favor sevoflurane in most situations. Desflurane and isoflurane are avoided for inhalation induction because they are pungent and associated with more coughing, breath-holding, and laryngospasm. We use a single (sometimes two) breath induction technique with sevoflurane (7–8% sevoflurane in 60% nitrous oxide) to speed the induction. After an adequate depth of anesthesia has been achieved, an intravenous line can be started and propofol and an opioid (or a muscle relaxant) administered to facilitate intubation. Patients typically pass through an excitement stage during which any stimulation can induce

TABLE 42–6 Sizing of airway equipment in children.

	Premature	Neonate	Infant	Toddler	Small Child	Large Child
Age	0–1 month	0–1 month	1–12 months	1–3 years	3–8 years	8–12 years
Weight (kg)	0.5–3	3–5	4–10	8–16	14–30	25–50
Tracheal (ET)[1] tube (mm i.d.)	2.5–3	3–3.5	3.5–4	4–4.5	4.5–5.5	5.5–6 (cuffed)
ET depth (cm at lips)	6–9	9–10	10–12	12–14	14–16	16–18
Suction catheter (F)	6	6	8	8	10	12
Laryngoscope blade	00	0	1	1.5	2	3
Mask size	00	0	0	1	2	3
Oral airway	000–00	00	0 (40 mm)	1 (50 mm)	2 (70 mm)	3 (80 mm)
Laryngeal mask airway (LMA#)	—	1	1	2	2.5	3

[1]ET, endotracheal tube.

laryngospasm. Breath-holding must be distinguished from laryngospasm. Steady application of 10 cm of positive end-expiratory pressure will usually overcome laryngospasm.

Alternatively, the anesthesiologist can deepen the level of anesthesia by increasing the concentration of volatile anesthetic, and place an LMA or intubate the patient under "deep" sevoflurane anesthesia. Because of the greater anesthetic depth required for tracheal intubation with the latter technique, the risk of cardiac depression, bradycardia, or laryngospasm occurring without intravenous access detracts from this technique. Intramuscular succinylcholine (4–6 mg/kg, not to exceed 150 mg) and atropine (0.02 mg/kg, not to exceed 0.4 mg) should be available if laryngospasm or bradycardia occurs before an intravenous line is established; intralingual succinylcholine may be an alterative route (see above).

Positive-pressure ventilation during mask induction and prior to intubation sometimes causes gastric distention, resulting in impairment of lung expansion. Suctioning with an orogastric or nasogastric tube will decompress the stomach, but it must be done without traumatizing fragile mucous membranes.

Intravenous Access

Intravenous cannulation in infants can be a vexing ordeal. This is particularly true for infants who have spent weeks in a neonatal intensive care unit and have few unpunctured veins left. Even healthy 1-year-old children can prove a challenge because of extensive subcutaneous fat. Venous cannulation usually becomes easier after 2 years of age. The saphenous vein has a consistent location at the ankle and an experienced practitioner can usually cannulate it even if it is not visible or palpable. Transillumination of the hands or ultrasonography will often reveal previously hidden cannulation sites. Twenty-four-gauge over-the-needle catheters are adequate in neonates and infants when blood transfusions are not anticipated. All air bubbles should be removed from the intravenous line, to reduce the risk of paradoxical air embolism from occult patent foramen ovale. In emergency situations where intravenous access is impossible, fluids can be effectively infused through an 18-gauge needle inserted into the medullary

sinusoids within the tibial bone. This intraosseous infusion can be used for all medications normally given intravenously, with almost as rapid results (see Chapter 55), and is considered part of the standard trauma resuscitation (ACLS) protocol when large-bore intravenous access cannot be obtained.

Tracheal Intubation

One hundred percent oxygen should be administered prior to intubation to increase patient safety during the obligatory period of apnea prior to and during intubation. The choice of muscle relaxant has been discussed earlier in the chapter. For awake intubations in neonates or infants, adequate preoxygenation and continued oxygen insufflation during laryngoscopy (eg, Oxyscope) may help prevent hypoxemia.

The infant's prominent occiput tends to place the head in a flexed position prior to intubation. This is easily corrected by slightly elevating the shoulders with towels and placing the head on a doughnut-shaped pillow. In older children, prominent tonsillar tissue can obstruct visualization of the larynx. Straight laryngoscope blades aid intubation of the anterior larynx in neonates, infants, and young children (Table 42–6). Endotracheal tubes that pass through the glottis may still impinge upon the cricoid cartilage, which is the narrowest point of the airway in children younger than 5 years of age. Mucosal trauma from trying to force a tube through the cricoid cartilage can cause postoperative edema, stridor, croup, and airway obstruction.

The appropriate diameter inside the endotracheal tube can be estimated by a formula based on age:

$$4 + Age/4 = \text{Tube diameter (in mm)}$$

For example, a 4-year-old child would be predicted to require a 5-mm tube. This formula provides only a rough guideline, however. Exceptions include premature neonates (2.5–3 mm tube) and full-term neonates (3–3.5 mm tube). Alternatively, the practitioner can remember that a newborn takes a 2.5- or 3-mm tube, and a 5-year-old takes a 5-mm tube. It should not be that difficult to identify which of the three sizes of tube between 3 and 5 mm is required in small children. In larger children, small (5–6 mm) cuffed tubes can be used either with or without the cuff inflated to minimize the need for precise sizing. Endotracheal tubes 0.5 mm larger and smaller than predicted should be readily available in or on the anesthetic cart. Uncuffed endotracheal tubes traditionally have been selected for children aged 5 years or younger to decrease the risk of postintubation croup, but many anesthesiologists no longer use size 4.0 or larger uncuffed tubes. The leak test will minimize the likelihood that an excessively large tube has been inserted. Correct tube size is confirmed by easy passage into the larynx and the development of a gas leak at 15–20 cm H_2O pressure for an uncuffed tube. No leak indicates an oversized tube that should be replaced to prevent postoperative edema, whereas an excessive leak may preclude adequate ventilation and contaminate the operating room with anesthetic gases. As noted above, many clinicians use a downsized cuffed tube with the cuff completely deflated in younger patients at high risk for aspiration; minimal inflation of the cuff can stop any air leak. There is also a formula to estimate endotracheal length:

$$12 + Age/2 = \text{Length of tube (in cm)}$$

Again, this formula provides only a guideline, and the result must be confirmed by auscultation and clinical judgment. To avoid endobronchial intubation, the tip of the endotracheal tube should pass only 1–2 cm beyond an infant's glottis. We favor an alternative approach: to intentionally place the tip of the endotracheal tube into the right mainstem bronchus and then withdraw it until breath sounds are equal over both lung fields.

Maintenance

Ventilation is almost always controlled during anesthesia of neonates and infants with a conventional semiclosed circle system. During spontaneous ventilation, even the low resistance of a circle system can become a significant obstacle for a sick neonate to overcome. Unidirectional valves, breathing tubes, and carbon dioxide absorbers account for most of this resistance. For patients weighing less than 10 kg, some anesthesiologists prefer the Mapleson D circuit or the Bain system because of their low resistance and light weight (see Chapter 3). Nonetheless, because breathing-circuit resistance is

easily overcome by positive-pressure ventilation, the circle system can be safely used in patients of all ages if ventilation is controlled. Monitoring of airway pressure may provide early evidence of obstruction from a kinked endotracheal tube or accidental advancement of the tube into a mainstem bronchus.

Many anesthesia ventilators on older machines are designed for adult patients and cannot reliably provide the reduced tidal volumes and rapid rates required by neonates and infants. Unintentional delivery of large tidal volumes to a small child can generate excessive peak airway pressures and cause barotrauma. The pressure-limited mode, which is found on nearly all newer anesthesia ventilators, should be used for neonates, infants, and toddlers. Small tidal volumes can also be manually delivered with greater ease with a 1-L breathing bag than with a 3-L adult bag. For children less than 10 kg, adequate tidal volumes are achieved with peak inspiratory pressures of 15–18 cm H_2O. For larger children the volume control ventilation may be used and tidal volumes may be set at 6–8 mL/kg. Many spirometers are less accurate at lower tidal volumes. In addition, the gas lost in long, compliant adult breathing circuits becomes large relative to a child's small tidal volume. For this reason, pediatric tubing is usually shorter, lighter, and stiffer (less compliant). Nevertheless, one should recall that the dead space contributed by the tube and circle system consists only of the volume of the distal limb of the Y-connector and that portion of the endotracheal tube that extends beyond the airway. In other words, the dead space is unchanged by switching from adult to pediatric tubing. Condenser humidifiers or heat and moisture exchangers (HMEs) can add considerable dead space; depending on the size of the patient, they either should not be used or an appropriately sized, pediatric HME should be employed.

Anesthesia can be maintained in pediatric patients with the same agents as in adults. Some clinicians switch to isoflurane following a sevoflurane induction in the hope of reducing the likelihood of emergence agitation or postoperative delirium (see above). If sevoflurane is continued for maintenance, administration of an opioid (eg, fentanyl, 1–1.5 mcg/kg) 15–20 min before the end of the procedure can reduce the incidence of emergence delirium and agitation if the surgical procedure is likely to produce postoperative pain. Although the MAC is greater in children than in adults (see Table 42–4), neonates may be particularly susceptible to the cardiodepressant effects of general anesthetics. Neonates and sick children may not tolerate increased concentrations of volatile agents required when the volatile agent alone is used to maintain good surgical operating conditions.

Perioperative Fluid Requirements

11 One must pay particular attention to fluid management in younger pediatric patients because these patients have limited margins for error. A programmable infusion pump or a buret with a microdrip chamber is useful for accurate measurements. Drugs can be flushed through low dead-space tubing to minimize unnecessary fluid administration. Fluid overload is diagnosed by prominent veins, flushed skin, increased blood pressure, decreased serum sodium, and a loss of the folds in the upper eyelids.

Fluid therapy can be divided into maintenance, deficit, and replacement requirements.

A. Maintenance Fluid Requirements

Maintenance requirements for pediatric patients can be determined by the "4:2:1 rule": 4 mL/kg/h for the first 10 kg of weight, 2 mL/kg/h for the second 10 kg, and 1 mL/kg/h for each remaining kilogram. The choice of maintenance fluid remains controversial. A solution such as $D_5\frac{1}{2}$ NS with 20 mEq/L of potassium chloride provides adequate dextrose and electrolytes at these maintenance infusion rates. $D_5\frac{1}{4}$ NS may be a better choice in neonates because of their limited ability to handle sodium loads. Children up to the age of 8 years require 6 mg/kg/min of glucose to maintain euglycemia (40–125 mg/dL); premature neonates require 6–8 mg/kg/min. Older children and adults require only 2 mg/kg/min and in these patients euglycemia is normally well maintained by hepatic glycogenolysis and gluconeogenesis. Both hypoglycemia and hyperglycemia should be avoided; however, the amount of hepatic glucose production is widely variable during major surgery and critical illness. Thus glucose infusion rates

during longer surgeries, particularly in neonates and infants, should be adjusted based on blood glucose measurements.

B. Deficits

In addition to a maintenance infusion, any preoperative fluid deficits must be replaced. For example, if a 5-kg infant has not received oral or intravenous fluids for 4 h prior to surgery, a deficit of 80 mL has accrued (5 kg × 4 mL/kg/h × 4 h). In contrast to adults, infants respond to dehydration with decreased blood pressure and without increased heart rate. Preoperative fluid deficits are often administered with hourly maintenance requirements in aliquots of 50% in the first hour and 25% in the second and third hours. In the example above, a total of 60 mL would be given in the first hour (80/2 + 20) and 40 mL in the second and third hours (80/4 + 20). Bolus administration of dextrose-containing solutions is avoided to prevent hyperglycemia. Preoperative fluid deficits are usually replaced with a balanced salt solution (eg, lactated Ringer's injection) or ½NS. In both cases, glucose is omitted to prevent hyperglycemia. Compared with lactated Ringer's injection, normal saline has the disadvantage of promoting hyperchloremic acidosis.

C. Replacement Requirements

Replacement can be subdivided into blood loss and third-space loss.

1. Blood loss—The blood volume of premature neonates (100 mL/kg), full-term neonates (85–90 mL/kg), and infants (80 mL/kg) is proportionately larger than that of adults (65–75 mL/kg). An initial hematocrit of 55% in the healthy full-term neonate gradually falls to as low as 30% in the 3-month-old infant before rising to 35% by 6 months. Hemoglobin (Hb) type is also changing during this period: from a 75% concentration of HbF (greater oxygen affinity, reduced Pao_2, poor tissue unloading) at birth to almost 100% HbA (reduced oxygen affinity, high Pao_2, good tissue unloading) by 6 months.

Blood loss has been typically replaced with non–glucose-containing crystalloid (eg, 3 mL of lactated Ringer's injection for each milliliter of blood lost) or colloid solutions (eg, 1 mL of 5% albumin for each milliliter of blood lost) until the patient's hematocrit reaches a predetermined lower limit. In recent years there has been increased emphasis on avoiding excessive fluid administration; thus blood loss is now commonly replaced by either colloid (eg, albumin) or packed red cells. In premature and sick neonates, the target hematocrit (for transfusion) may be as great as 40%, whereas in healthy older children a hematocrit of 20–26% is generally well tolerated. Because of their small intravascular volume, neonates and infants are at an increased risk for electrolyte disturbances (eg, hyperglycemia, hyperkalemia, and hypocalcemia) that can accompany rapid blood transfusion. Dosing of packed red blood cell transfusions is discussed in Chapter 51. Platelets and fresh frozen plasma, 10–15 mL/kg, should be given when blood loss exceeds 1–2 blood volumes. Recent practice, particularly with blood loss from trauma, favors "earlier" administration of plasma and platelets. One unit of platelets per 10 kg weight raises the platelet count by about 50,000/μL. The pediatric dose of cryoprecipitate is 1 unit/10 kg weight.

2. "Third-space" loss—These losses are impossible to measure and must be estimated by the extent of the surgical procedure. In recent years the third space has even been attributed to overzealous fluid administration during resuscitation.

One popular fluid administration guideline is 0–2 mL/kg/h for relatively atraumatic surgery (eg, strabismus correction where there should be *no* third-space loss) and up to 6–10 mL/kg/h for traumatic procedures (eg, abdominal abscess). Third-space loss is usually replaced with lactated Ringer's injection (see Chapter 49). It is safe to say that all issues relating to the third space have never been more controversial.

Regional Anesthesia and Analgesia

The primary uses of regional techniques in pediatric anesthesia have been to supplement and reduce general anesthetic requirements and to provide better postoperative pain relief. Blocks range in complexity from the relatively simple peripheral nerve blocks (eg, penile block, ilioinguinal block); to brachial plexus, sciatic nerve, and femoral nerve blocks; to major conduction blocks (eg, spinal or epidural techniques). Regional blocks in children (as in adults) are often facilitated by ultrasound guidance, sometimes with nerve stimulation.

Caudal blocks have proved useful following a variety of surgeries, including circumcision, inguinal herniorrhaphy, hypospadias repair, anal surgery, clubfoot repair, and other subumbilical procedures. Contraindications include infection around the sacral hiatus, coagulopathy, or anatomic abnormalities. The patient is usually lightly anesthetized or sedated and placed in the lateral position.

For pediatric caudal anesthesia, a short-bevel 22-gauge needle can be used. If the loss-of-resistance technique is used, the glass syringe should be filled with saline, not air, because of the latter's possible association with air embolism. After the characteristic pop that signals penetration of the sacrococcygeal membrane, the needle angle of approach is reduced and the needle is advanced only a few more millimeters to avoid entering the dural sac or the anterior body of the sacrum. Aspiration is used to check for blood or cerebrospinal fluid; local anesthetic can then be slowly injected; failure of a 2-mL test dose of local anesthetic with epinephrine (1:200,000) to produce tachycardia helps exclude intravascular placement.

Many anesthetic agents have been used for caudal anesthesia in pediatric patients, with 0.125–0.25% bupivacaine (up to 2.5 mg/kg) or 0.2% ropivacaine being most common. Ropivacaine, 0.2%, can provide analgesia similar to bupivacaine but with less motor blockade. Ropivacaine appears to have less cardiac toxicity than bupivacaine when compared milligram to milligram. Addition of epinephrine to caudal solutions tends to increase the degree of motor block. Clonidine, either by itself or combined with local anesthetics, has also been widely used. Morphine sulfate (25 mcg/kg) or hydromorphone (6 mcg/kg) may be added to the local anesthetic solution to prolong postoperative analgesia for inpatients, but it increases the risk of delayed postoperative respiratory depression. The volume of local anesthetic required depends on the level of blockade desired, ranging from 0.5 mL/kg for a sacral block to 1.25 mL/kg for a midthoracic block. Single-shot injections generally last 4–12 h. Placement of 20-gauge caudal catheters with continuous infusion of local anesthetic (eg, 0.125% bupivacaine or 0.1% ropivacaine at 0.2–0.4 mg/kg/h) or an opioid (eg, fentanyl, 2 mcg/mL at 0.6 mcg/kg/h) allows prolonged anesthesia and postoperative analgesia. Complications are rare but include local anesthetic toxicity from increased blood concentrations (eg, seizures, hypotension, arrhythmias), spinal blockade, and respiratory depression. Postoperative urinary retention does not appear to be a problem following single-dose caudal anesthesia.

Lumbar and thoracic epidural catheters can be placed in anesthetized children using the standard loss-of-resistance technique and either a midline or paramedian approach. In small children, caudal epidural catheters have been passed into a thoracic position with the tip localized radiographically.

Unilateral transversus abdominis plane (TAP) blocks are commonly used to provide analgesia after hernia repair. Bilateral TAP blocks can be used to provide effective postoperative analgesia after abdominal surgery with a lower midline incision. Rectus sheath blocks can be used for midline incision in the upper abdomen.

Spinal anesthesia has been used in some centers for infraumbilical procedures in neonates and infants. Infants and children typically have minimal hypotension from sympathectomy. Intravenous access can be established (conveniently in the foot) after the spinal anesthetic has been administered. This technique has become more widely used for neonates and infants as the potential neurotoxicity risks of general anesthesia in these patients have received greater attention.

Most children will not tolerate placement of nerve blocks or nerve block catheters while awake; however, most peripheral block techniques can be performed safely in anesthetized children. When the area of operation is the upper extremity we recommend those brachial plexus procedures that can most readily be performed using ultrasound guidance, specifically axillary, supraclavicular, and infraclavicular blocks. We suggest that interscalene block be performed only by those having experience and skill with ultrasound guidance and only for procedures where other block techniques would be inferior (eg, upper shoulder procedures) due to the reported rare occurrence of accidental intramedullary injections when interscalene blocks were performed in anesthetized adults. Single-shot and continuous femoral and sciatic blocks are easily performed using ultrasound guidance. The latter can be performed using either a gluteal or a popliteal approach.

A wide variety of other terminal nerve blocks (eg, digital nerve, median nerve, occipital nerve, etc) are easily performed to reduce postoperative pain in children.

Sedation for Procedures in and out of the Operating Room

Sedation is often requested for pediatric patients inside and outside the operating room for nonsurgical procedures. Cooperation and motionlessness may be required for imaging studies, bronchoscopy, gastrointestinal endoscopy, cardiac catheterization, dressing changes, and minor procedures (eg, casting and bone marrow aspiration). Requirements vary depending on the patient and the procedure, ranging from anxiolysis (minimal sedation), to conscious sedation (moderate sedation and analgesia), to deep sedation/analgesia, and finally to general anesthesia. Anesthesiologists are usually held to the same standards when they provide moderate or deep sedation as when they provide general anesthesia. This includes preoperative preparation (eg, fasting), assessment, monitoring, and postoperative care. Airway obstruction and hypoventilation are the most commonly encountered problems associated with moderate or deep sedation. With deep sedation and general anesthesia cardiovascular depression can also be a problem.

Table 42–3 includes doses of sedative-hypnotic drugs. One of the sedatives commonly used by nonanesthesia personnel in the past was chloral hydrate, 25–100 mg/kg orally or rectally. It has a slow onset of up to 60 min and a long half-life (8–11 h) that results in prolonged somnolence. Although it generally has little effect on ventilation, it can cause fatal airway obstruction in patients with sleep apnea. Overall, chloral hydrate is a poor choice given its propensity for producing cardiac arrhythmias when it is used in the larger doses needed for moderate sedation. Midazolam, 0.5 mg/kg orally or 0.1–0.15 mg/kg intravenously, is particularly useful because its effects can be readily reversed with flumazenil. Doses should be reduced whenever more than one agent is used because of the potential for synergistic respiratory and cardiovascular depression.

Propofol is by far the most useful sedative-hypnotic drug. Although the drug is not approved for sedation of pediatric ICU patients and is not approved for administration by anyone other than those trained in the administration of general anesthesia, it can be dosed safely for most procedures at infusion rates up to 200 mcg/kg/min. In countries other than the United States, propofol is often administered using the Diprifusor, a computer-controlled infusion pump that maintains a constant target site concentration. Supplemental oxygen and close monitoring of the airway, ventilation, and other vital signs are mandatory (as with other agents). An LMA is usually well tolerated at higher doses.

Emergence & Recovery

Pediatric patients are particularly vulnerable to two postanesthetic complications: laryngospasm and postintubation croup. As with adult patients, postoperative pain requires close, careful attention. Pediatric anesthesia practice varies widely, particularly in regard to extubation following a general anesthetic. In some pediatric hospitals, all children who will be extubated after a general anesthetic arrive in the postanesthesia care unit (PACU) with the tube still in place. They are subsequently extubated by the PACU nurse when defined criteria are reached. In other centers, nearly all children are extubated in the operating room before arriving in the PACU. High quality and safety are reported at centers following either protocol.

A. Laryngospasm

Laryngospasm is a forceful, involuntary spasm of the laryngeal musculature caused by stimulation of the superior laryngeal nerve (see Chapter 19). It may occur at induction, emergence, or any time in between without an endotracheal tube. Presumably it can also occur when a tube is in place, but its occurrence will not be recognized. Laryngospasm is more common in young pediatric patients (almost 1 in 50 anesthetics) than in adults, and is most common in infants 1–3 months old. Laryngospasm at the end of a procedure can usually be avoided by extubating the patient either while awake (opening the eyes) or while deeply anesthetized (spontaneously breathing but not swallowing or coughing); both techniques have advocates and despite strong opinions, evidence is lacking as to which is the better approach. Extubation during the interval between these extremes, however, is generally recognized as more hazardous. Recent URI or exposure to secondhand tobacco smoke predisposes children to laryngospasm on emergence. Treatment of laryngospasm includes gentle positive-pressure ventilation, forward jaw thrust, intravenous lidocaine (1–1.5 mg/kg), or paralysis with intravenous succinylcholine (0.5–1 mg/kg), or rocuronium (0.4 mg/kg) and controlled ventilation. Intramuscular succinylcholine (4–6 mg/kg) remains an acceptable alternative in patients without intravenous access and in whom conservative measures have failed. Laryngospasm is usually an immediate postoperative event but may occur in the recovery room as the patient wakes up and chokes on pharyngeal secretions. For this reason, recovering pediatric patients should be positioned in the lateral position so that oral secretions pool and drain away from the vocal cords. When the child begins to regain consciousness, having the parents at the bedside may reduce his or her anxiety.

B. Postintubation Croup

Croup is due to glottic or tracheal edema. Because the narrowest part of the pediatric airway is the cricoid cartilage, this is the most susceptible area. Croup is less common with endotracheal tubes that are small enough to allow a slight gas leak at 10–25 cm H_2O. Postintubation croup is associated with early childhood (age 1–4 years), repeated intubation attempts, overly large endotracheal tubes, prolonged surgery, head and neck procedures, and excessive movement of the tube (eg, coughing with the tube in place, moving the patient's head). Intravenous dexamethasone (0.25–0.5 mg/kg) may prevent formation of edema, and inhalation of nebulized racemic epinephrine (0.25–0.5 mL of a 2.25% solution in 2.5 mL normal saline) is an often effective treatment. Although postintubation croup is a complication that occurs later than laryngospasm, it will almost always appear within 3 h after extubation.

C. Postoperative Pain Management

Pain in pediatric patients has received considerable attention in recent years, and over that time the use of regional anesthetic and analgesic techniques (as described above) has greatly increased. Commonly used parenteral opioids include fentanyl (1–2 mcg/kg), morphine (0.05–0.1 mg/kg), hydromorphone (15 mcg/kg), and meperidine (0.5 mg/kg). A multimodal technique incorporating ketorolac (0.5–0.75 mg/kg) will reduce opioid requirements. Oral, rectal, or intravenous acetaminophen may also be a helpful substitute for ketorolac.

Patient-controlled analgesia (see Chapter 48) can also be successfully used in patients as young as 6–7 years old, depending on their maturity and on preoperative preparation. Commonly used opioids include morphine and hydromorphone. With a 10-min lockout interval, the recommended interval dose is either morphine, 20 mcg/kg, or hydromorphone, 5 mcg/kg. As with adults, continuous infusions increase the risk of respiratory depression; typical continuous infusion doses are morphine, 0–12 mcg/kg/h, or hydromorphone, 0–3 mcg/kg/h. The subcutaneous route may be used with morphine. Nurse-controlled and parent-controlled analgesia remain controversial but widely used techniques for pain control in children.

As with adults, epidural infusions for postoperative analgesia often consist of a local anesthetic combined with an opioid. Bupivacaine, 0.1–0.125%, or ropivacaine, 0.1–0.2%, are often combined with fentanyl, 2–2.5 mcg/mL (or equivalent concentrations of morphine or hydromorphone). Recommended infusion rates depend on the size of the patient, the final drug concentration, and the location of the epidural catheter, and range from 0.1 to 0.4 mL/kg/h. Local anesthetic infusions can also be used with continuous nerve block techniques, but this is less common than in adults.

Anesthetic Considerations in Specific Pediatric Conditions

PREMATURITY

Pathophysiology

Prematurity is defined as birth before 37 weeks of gestation. This is in contrast to *small for gestational age*, which describes an infant (full-term or premature) whose age-adjusted weight is less than the fifth percentile. The multiple medical problems of premature neonates are usually due to immaturity of major organ systems or to intrauterine asphyxia. Pulmonary complications include hyaline membrane disease, apneic spells, and bronchopulmonary dysplasia. Exogenous pulmonary surfactant has proved to be an effective treatment for respiratory distress syndrome in premature infants. A patent ductus arteriosus leads to shunting, and may possibly lead to pulmonary edema and congestive heart failure. Persistent hypoxia or shock may result in ischemic gut and necrotizing enterocolitis. Prematurity increases susceptibility to infection, hypothermia, intracranial hemorrhage, and kernicterus. Premature neonates also have an increased incidence of congenital anomalies.

Anesthetic Considerations

The small size (often <1000 g) and fragile medical condition of premature neonates demand that special attention be paid to airway control, fluid management, and temperature regulation. The problem of retinopathy of prematurity, a fibrovascular proliferation overlying the retina that may lead to progressive visual loss, deserves special consideration. While hyperoxia is associated with this blinding disease, the presence of fetal hemoglobin and treatment with vitamin E may be protective. Recent evidence suggests that fluctuating oxygen levels may be more damaging than increased oxygen tensions. Moreover, other major risk factors, such as respiratory distress, apnea, mechanical ventilation, hypoxia, hypercarbia, acidosis, heart disease, bradycardia, infection, parenteral nutrition, anemia, and multiple blood transfusions, must be present. Nonetheless, oxygenation should be continuously monitored with pulse oximetry or transcutaneous oxygen analysis, with particular attention given to infants younger than 44 weeks postconception. Normal PaO_2 is 60–80 mm Hg in neonates. Excessive inspired oxygen concentrations are avoided by blending oxygen with air. Excessive inspired oxygen tensions can also predispose to chronic lung disease.

Anesthetic requirements of premature neonates are reduced. Opioid-based anesthetics are often favored over pure volatile anesthetic-based techniques because of the perceived tendency of the latter to cause myocardial depression.

Premature infants whose age is less than 50 (some authorities would say 60) weeks postconception at the time of surgery are prone to postoperative episodes of obstructive and central apnea for up to 24 h. In fact, even term infants can experience rare apneic spells following general anesthesia. **Risk factors for postanesthetic apnea include a low gestational age at birth, anemia (<30%), hypothermia, sepsis, and neurological abnormalities**. The risk of postanesthetic apnea may be decreased by intravenous administration of caffeine (10 mg/kg) or aminophylline.

Thus, elective (particularly outpatient) procedures should be deferred until the preterm infant reaches the age of at least 50 weeks postconception. A 6-month symptom-free interval has been suggested for infants with a history of apneic episodes or bronchopulmonary dysplasia. If surgery must be performed earlier, monitoring with pulse oximetry for 12–24 h postoperatively is mandatory for infants less than 50 weeks postconception; infants between 50 and 60 weeks postconception should be closely observed in the postanesthesia recovery unit for at least 2 h.

Sick, premature neonates often receive multiple transfusions of blood during their stay in the intensive care nursery. Their immunocompromised status predisposes them to cytomegalovirus infection following transfusion. Signs of infection include generalized lymphadenopathy, fever, pneumonia, hepatitis, hemolytic anemia, and thrombocytopenia. Preventive measures include using cytomegalovirus-seronegative donor blood or, more commonly, leukocyte-reduced blood cells.

INTESTINAL MALROTATION & VOLVULUS

Pathophysiology

Malrotation of the intestines is a developmental abnormality that permits spontaneous abnormal rotation of the midgut around the mesentery (superior mesenteric artery). The incidence of malrotation is estimated to be about 1:500 live births. Most patients with malrotation of the midgut present during infancy with symptoms of bowel obstruction. Coiling of the duodenum with the ascending colon can produce complete or partial duodenal obstruction. The most serious complication of malrotation, a midgut volvulus, can rapidly compromise intestinal blood supply causing infarction. Midgut volvulus is a true surgical emergency that most commonly occurs in infancy, with up to one third occurring in the first week of life. The mortality rate is high (up to 25%). Typical symptoms are bilious vomiting, progressive abdominal distention and tenderness, metabolic acidosis, and hemodynamic instability. Bloody diarrhea may be indicative of bowel infarction. Abdominal ultrasonography or upper gastrointestinal imaging confirms the diagnosis.

Anesthetic Considerations

Surgery provides the only definitive treatment of malrotation and midgut volvulus. If obstruction is present but obvious volvulus has not yet occurred, preoperative preparation may include stabilization of any coexisting conditions, insertion of a nasogastric (or orogastric tube) to decompress the stomach, broad-spectrum antibiotics, fluid and electrolyte replacement, and prompt transport to the operating room.

These patients are at increased risk for pulmonary aspiration. Depending on the size of the patient, rapid sequence induction (or awake intubation) should be employed. Patients with volvulus are usually hypovolemic and acidotic, and may tolerate anesthesia poorly. Ketamine may be the preferred anesthetic induction agent. An opioid-based anesthetic can also be used as postoperative ventilation will often be necessary. Fluid resuscitation, likely including blood products, and sodium bicarbonate therapy are usually necessary. Arterial and central venous lines are helpful. Surgical treatment includes reducing the volvulus, freeing the obstruction, widening the base of mesenteric attachments, and resecting any obviously necrotic bowel. Bowel edema can complicate abdominal closure and has the potential to produce an abdominal compartment syndrome. The latter can impair ventilation, hinder venous return, and produce renal compromise; delayed fascial closure or temporary closure with a Silastic "silo" may be necessary. A second-look laparotomy may be required 24–48 h later to ensure viability of the remaining bowel.

CONGENITAL DIAPHRAGMATIC HERNIA
Pathophysiology

During fetal development, the gut can herniate into the thorax through one of three possible diaphragmatic defects: the left or right posterolateral foramen of Bochdalek or the anterior foramen of Morgagni. The reported incidence of diaphragmatic hernia is 1 in 3000–5000 live births. Left-sided herniation is the most common type (90%). Hallmarks of **diaphragmatic herniation** include hypoxia, a scaphoid abdomen, and evidence of bowel in the thorax by auscultation or radiography. Congenital diaphragmatic hernia is often diagnosed antenatally during a routine obstetric ultrasound examination. A reduction in alveoli and bronchioli (pulmonary hypoplasia) and malrotation of the intestines are almost always present. The ipsilateral lung is particularly impaired and the herniated gut can compress and retard the maturation of both lungs. Diaphragmatic hernia is often accompanied by marked pulmonary hypertension and is associated with 40–50% mortality. Cardiopulmonary compromise is primarily due to pulmonary hypoplasia and pulmonary hypertension rather than to the mass effect of the herniated viscera.

Treatment is aimed at immediate stabilization with sedation, paralysis, and moderate hyperventilation. Pressure-limited ventilation is used. Some centers employ permissive hypercapnia (postductal $Paco_2 < 65$ mm Hg) and accept mild hypoxemia (preductal $Spo_2 > 85\%$) in an effort to reduce pulmonary barotrauma. High-frequency oscillatory ventilation (HFOV) can improve ventilation and oxygenation with less barotrauma. Inhaled nitric oxide may be used to lower pulmonary artery pressures but does not appear to improve survival. If the pulmonary hypertension stabilizes and there is little right-to-left shunting, early surgical repair

may be undertaken. If the patient fails to stabilize, extracorporeal membrane oxygenation (ECMO) may be undertaken. When initiated in the critical care unit in a neonate, venoarterial ECMO usually involves pumping blood from the jugular vein through a membrane oxygenator and countercurrent heat exchanger before returning it to ipsilateral carotid artery. Timing of the repair following ECMO is controversial. Treatment with prenatal intrauterine surgery has not been shown to improve outcomes.

Anesthetic Considerations

Gastric distention must be minimized by placement of a nasogastric tube and avoidance of high levels of positive-pressure ventilation. The neonate is preoxygenated and intubated awake, or without the aid of muscle relaxants. Anesthesia is maintained with low concentrations of volatile agents or opioids, muscle relaxants, and air as tolerated. Hypoxia and expansion of air in the bowel contraindicate the use of nitrous oxide. If possible, peak inspiratory airway pressures should be less than 30 cm H_2O. **A sudden fall in lung compliance, blood pressure, or oxygenation may signal a contralateral (usually right-sided) pneumothorax and necessitate placement of a chest tube**. Arterial blood gases are preferably monitored by sampling a preductal artery if an umbilical artery catheter is not already in place. Surgical repair is performed via a subcostal incision of the affected side; the bowel is reduced into the abdomen and the diaphragm is closed. Aggressive attempts at expansion of the ipsilateral lung following surgical decompression are detrimental. Postoperative prognosis parallels the extent of pulmonary hypoplasia and the presence of other congenital defects.

TRACHEOESOPHAGEAL FISTULA
Pathophysiology

There are several types of tracheoesophageal fistula (Figure 42–3). The most common (type IIIB) is the combination of an upper esophagus that ends in a blind pouch and a lower esophagus that connects to

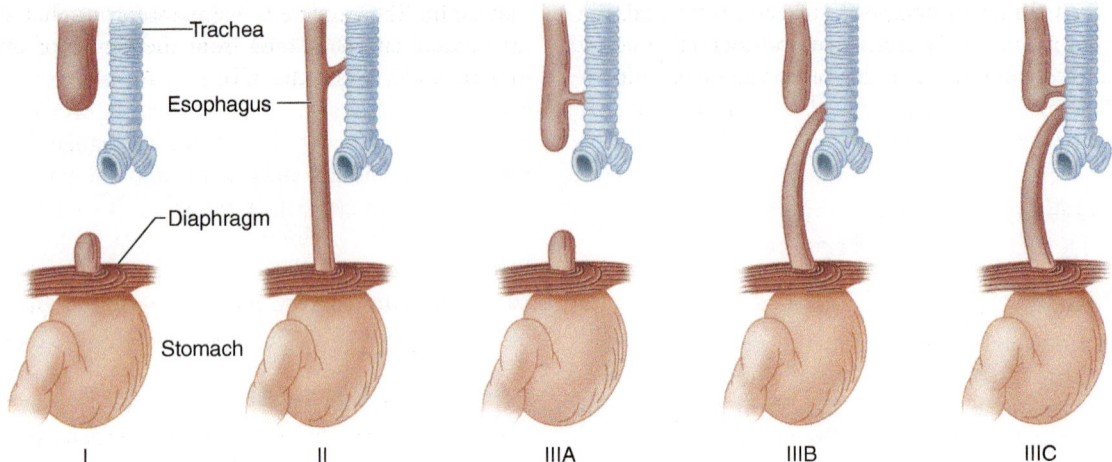

FIGURE 42–3 Of the five types of tracheoesophageal fistula, type IIIB represents 90% of cases.

the trachea. Breathing results in gastric distention, whereas feeding leads to choking, coughing, and cyanosis (three Cs). The diagnosis is suspected by failure to pass a catheter into the stomach and confirmed by visualization of the catheter coiled in a blind, upper esophageal pouch. Aspiration pneumonia and the coexistence of other congenital anomalies (eg, cardiac) are common. These may include the association of *v*ertebral defects, *a*nal atresia, *t*racheoesophageal fistula with *e*sophageal atresia, and *r*adial dysplasia, known as the VATER syndrome. The VACTERL variant also includes *c*ardiac and *l*imb anomalies. Preoperative management is directed at identifying all congenital anomalies and preventing aspiration pneumonia. This may include maintaining the patient in a head-up position, using an oral-esophageal tube, and avoiding feedings. In some instances gastrostomy may be performed under local anesthesia. Definitive surgical treatment is usually postponed until any pneumonia clears or improves with antibiotic therapy.

Anesthetic Considerations

These neonates tend to have copious pharyngeal secretions that require frequent suctioning before and during surgery. Positive-pressure ventilation is avoided prior to intubation, as the resulting gastric distention may interfere with lung expansion. Intubation is often performed awake and without

muscle relaxants. These neonates are often dehydrated and malnourished due to poor oral intake.

The key to successful management is correct endotracheal tube position. Ideally, the tip of the tube lies distal to the fistula and proximal to the carina, so that anesthetic gases pass into the lungs instead of the stomach. This is impossible if the fistula connects to the carina or a mainstem bronchus. In these situations, intermittent venting of a gastrostomy tube may permit positive-pressure ventilation without excessive gastric distention. Suctioning of the gastrostomy tube and upper esophageal pouch tube helps prevent aspiration pneumonia. Surgical division of the fistula and esophageal anastomosis is performed via a right extrapleural thoracotomy with the patient in the left lateral position. A precordial stethoscope should be placed in the dependent (left) axilla, since obstruction of the mainstem bronchus during surgical retraction is not uncommon. A drop in oxygen saturation indicates that the retracted lung needs to be reexpanded. Surgical retraction can also compress the great vessels, trachea, heart, and vagus nerve. Blood pressure should be continuously monitored with an arterial line. These infants often require ventilation with 100% oxygen. Blood should be immediately available for transfusion. Postoperative complications include gastroesophageal reflux, aspiration pneumonia, tracheal compression, and anastomotic leakage. Most patients must remain intubated and receive positive-pressure ventilation in the immediate postoperative period. Neck extension and instrumentation (eg, suctioning) of the esophagus may disrupt the surgical repair and should be avoided.

GASTROSCHISIS & OMPHALOCELE

Pathophysiology

Gastroschisis and omphalocele are congenital disorders characterized by defects in the abdominal wall that allow external herniation of viscera. Omphaloceles occur at the base of the umbilicus, have a hernia sac, and are often associated with other congenital anomalies such as trisomy 21, diaphragmatic hernia, and cardiac and bladder malformations. In contrast, the gastroschisis defect is usually lateral to the umbilicus, does not have a hernia sac, and is often an isolated finding. Antenatal diagnosis by ultrasound can be followed by elective cesarean section at 38 weeks and immediate surgical repair. Perioperative management centers around preventing hypothermia, infection, and dehydration. These problems are usually more serious in gastroschisis, as the protective hernial sac is absent.

Anesthetic Considerations

The stomach is decompressed with a nasogastric tube before induction. Intubation can be accomplished with the patient awake or asleep and with or without muscle relaxation. Nitrous oxide should be avoided to prevent further bowel distention. Muscle relaxation is required for replacing the bowel into the abdominal cavity. A one-stage closure (primary repair) is often not advisable, as it can cause an abdominal compartment syndrome. A staged closure with a temporary Silastic "silo" may be necessary, followed by a second procedure a few days later for complete closure. Suggested criteria for a staged closure include intragastric or intravesical pressure greater than 20 cm H_2O, peak inspiratory pressure greater than 35 cm H_2O, or an end-tidal CO_2 greater than 50 mm Hg. **Third-space fluid losses are replaced with a balanced salt solution and 5%**

albumin. The neonate remains intubated after the procedure and is weaned from the ventilator over the next 1–2 days in the ICU.

HYPERTROPHIC PYLORIC STENOSIS

Pathophysiology

Hypertrophic pyloric stenosis impedes emptying of gastric contents. **Persistent vomiting depletes potassium, chloride, hydrogen, and sodium ions, causing hypochloremic metabolic alkalosis**. Initially, the kidney tries to compensate for the alkalosis by excreting sodium bicarbonate in the urine. Later, as hyponatremia and dehydration worsen, the kidneys must conserve sodium even at the expense of hydrogen ion excretion (paradoxic aciduria). Correction of the volume and ion deficits and metabolic alkalosis requires hydration with a sodium chloride (rather than lactated Ringer's) solution supplemented with potassium chloride.

Anesthetic Considerations

Surgery should be delayed until fluid and electrolyte abnormalities have been corrected. Operation for correction of pyloric stenosis is never an emergency. The stomach should be emptied with a nasogastric or orogastric tube; the tube should be suctioned with the patient in the supine, lateral, and prone positions. Diagnosis often requires contrast radiography, and all contrast media will need to be suctioned from the stomach before induction. Techniques for intubation and induction vary, but in all cases the patient's increased risk of aspiration must be considered. Experienced clinicians have variously advocated awake intubation, rapid sequence intravenous induction, and even careful inhalation induction in selected patients. Pyloromyotomy is a short procedure that requires muscle relaxation. These neonates may be at increased risk for respiratory depression and hypoventilation in the recovery room because of persistent metabolic (measurable in arterial blood) or cerebrospinal fluid alkalosis (despite neutral arterial pH).

INFECTIOUS CROUP, FOREIGN BODY ASPIRATION, & ACUTE EPIGLOTTITIS

Pathophysiology

Croup is obstruction of the airway characterized by a barking cough. One type of croup, postintubation croup, has already been discussed. Another type is due to viral infection. **Infectious croup** usually follows a viral URI in children aged 3 months to 3 years. The airway *below* the epiglottis is involved (laryngotracheobronchitis). Infectious croup progresses slowly and rarely requires intubation. Foreign body aspiration is typically encountered in children aged 6 months to 5 years. Commonly aspirated objects include peanuts, coins, screws, nails, tacks, and small pieces of toys. Onset is typically acute and the obstruction may be supraglottic, glottic, or subglottic. Stridor is prominent with the first two, whereas wheezing is more common with the latter. A clear history of an aspiration may be absent. **Acute epiglottitis** is a bacterial infection (most commonly *Haemophilus influenzae* type B) classically affecting 2- to 6-year-old children but also occasionally appearing in older children and adults. It rapidly progresses from a sore throat to dysphagia and complete airway obstruction. The term *supraglottitis* has been suggested because the inflammation typically involves all supraglottic structures. Endotracheal intubation and antibiotic therapy can be lifesaving. Epiglottitis has increasingly become a disease of adults because of the widespread use of *H influenza* vaccines in children.

Anesthetic Considerations

Patients with croup are managed conservatively with oxygen and mist therapy. Nebulized racemic epinephrine (0.5 mL of a 2.25% solution in 2.5 mL normal saline) and intravenous dexamethasone (0.25–0.5 mg/kg) are used. Indications for intubation include progressive intercostal retractions, obvious respiratory fatigue, and central cyanosis.

Anesthetic management of a foreign body aspiration is challenging, particularly with supraglottic and glottic obstruction. Minor manipulation of the airway can convert partial into complete obstruction. Experts recommend careful inhalational induction for a supraglottic object and gentle upper airway endoscopy to remove the object, secure the airway, or both. When the object is subglottic, a rapid-sequence or inhalational induction is usually followed by rigid bronchoscopy by the surgeon or endotracheal intubation and flexible bronchoscopy. Surgical preferences may vary according to the size of the patient and the nature and location of the foreign body. Close cooperation between the surgeon and anesthesiologist is essential.

Children with impending airway obstruction from epiglottitis present in the operating room for definitive diagnosis by laryngoscopy followed by intubation. A preoperative lateral neck radiograph may show a characteristic thumblike epiglottic shadow, which is very specific but often absent. The radiograph is also helpful in revealing other causes of obstruction, such as foreign bodies. Stridor, drooling, hoarseness, rapid onset and progression, tachypnea, chest retractions, and a preference for the upright position are predictive of airway obstruction. Total obstruction can occur at any moment, and adequate preparations for a possible tracheostomy must be made prior to induction of general anesthesia. Laryngoscopy should not be performed before induction of anesthesia because of the possibility of laryngospasm. In most cases, an inhalational induction is performed with the patient in the sitting position, using a volatile anesthetic and oxygen. Oral intubation with an endotracheal tube one half to one size smaller than usual is attempted as soon as an adequate depth of anesthesia is established. The oral tube may be replaced with a well-secured nasal endotracheal tube at the end of the procedure, as the latter is better tolerated in the postoperative period. If intubation is impossible, rigid bronchoscopy or emergency tracheostomy must be performed.

TONSILLECTOMY & ADENOIDECTOMY

Pathophysiology

Lymphoid hyperplasia can lead to upper airway obstruction, obligate mouth breathing, and even pulmonary hypertension with cor pulmonale. Although these extremes of pathology are unusual, all children undergoing tonsillectomy or adenoidectomy should be considered to be at increased risk for perioperative airway problems.

Anesthetic Considerations

Surgery should be postponed if there is evidence of acute infection or suspicion of a clotting dysfunction (eg, recent aspirin ingestion). Administration of an anticholinergic agent will decrease pharyngeal secretions. A history of airway obstruction or apnea suggests an inhalational induction without paralysis until the ability to ventilate with positive pressure is established. A reinforced or preformed endotracheal tube (eg, RAE tube) may decrease the risk of kinking by the surgeon's self-retaining mouth gag. Blood transfusion is usually not necessary, but the anesthesiologist must be wary of occult blood loss. Gentle inspection and suctioning of the pharynx precede extubation. Although deep extubation decreases the chance of laryngospasm and may prevent blood clot dislodgment from coughing, most anesthesiologists prefer an awake extubation because of the risks of aspiration. Postoperative vomiting is common. The anesthesiologist must be alert in the recovery room for postoperative bleeding, which may be evidenced by restlessness, pallor, tachycardia, or hypotension. If reoperation is necessary to control bleeding, intravascular volume must first be restored. Evacuation of stomach contents with a nasogastric tube is followed by a rapid-sequence induction with cricoid pressure. Because of the possibility of bleeding and airway obstruction, children younger than 3 years old may be hospitalized for the first postoperative night. Sleep apnea and recent infection increase the risk of postoperative complications.

MYRINGOTOMY & INSERTION OF TYMPANOSTOMY TUBES

Pathophysiology

Children presenting for myringotomy and insertion of tympanostomy tubes have a long history of URIs that have spread through the eustachian tube, causing repeated episodes of otitis media. Causative organisms are usually bacterial and include *Pneumococcus, H influenza, Streptococcus,* and *Mycoplasma pneumoniae.* Myringotomy, a radial incision in the tympanic membrane, releases any fluid that has accumulated in the middle ear. Tympanostomy tubes provide long-term drainage. Because of the chronic and recurring nature of this illness, it is not surprising that these patients often have symptoms of a URI on the day of scheduled surgery.

Anesthetic Considerations

These are typically very short (10–15 min) outpatient procedures. Inhalational induction is a common technique. Unlike tympanoplasty surgery, nitrous oxide diffusion into the middle ear is not a problem during myringotomy because of the brief period of anesthetic exposure before the middle ear is vented. Because most of these patients are otherwise healthy and there is no blood loss, intravenous access is usually not necessary. Ventilation with a face mask or LMA minimizes the risk of perioperative respiratory complications (eg, laryngospasm) associated with intubation.

TRISOMY 21 SYNDROME (DOWN SYNDROME)

Pathophysiology

An additional chromosome 21—part or whole—results in the most common pattern of congenital human malformation: Down syndrome. Characteristic abnormalities of interest to the anesthesiologist include a short neck, irregular dentition, mental retardation, hypotonia, and a large tongue. Associated abnormalities include congenital heart disease in 40% of patients (particularly endocardial cushion defects and ventricular septal defect), subglottic stenosis, tracheoesophageal fistula, chronic pulmonary infections, and seizures. These neonates are often premature and small for their gestational age. Later in life many patients with Down syndrome undergo multiple procedures requiring general anesthesia.

Anesthetic Considerations

Because of anatomic differences, these patients often have difficult airways, particularly during infancy. The size of the endotracheal tube required is typically smaller than that predicted by age. Respiratory complications such as postoperative stridor and apnea are common. Neck flexion during laryngoscopy and intubation may result in atlantooccipital dislocation because of the congenital laxity of these ligaments. The possibility of associated congenital diseases must always be considered. As in all pediatric patients, care must be taken to avoid air bubbles in the intravenous line because of possible right-to-left shunts and paradoxical air emboli.

CYSTIC FIBROSIS

Pathophysiology

Cystic fibrosis is a genetic disease of the exocrine glands primarily affecting the pulmonary and gastrointestinal systems. Abnormally thick and viscous secretions coupled with decreased ciliary activity lead to pneumonia, wheezing, and bronchiectasis. Pulmonary function studies reveal increased residual volume and airway resistance with decreased vital capacity and expiratory flow rate. Malabsorption syndrome may lead to dehydration and electrolyte abnormalities.

Anesthetic Considerations

Premedication should not include respiratory depressants. Anticholinergic drugs have been used in large series without ill effects, and the choice either to use or not to use them appears to be inconsequential. Induction with inhalational anesthetics may be prolonged in patients with severe pulmonary disease. Intubation should not be performed until the patient is deeply anesthetized to avoid coughing and stimulation of mucus secretions. The patient's lungs should be suctioned during general anesthesia and before extubation to minimize the accumulation of secretions. Outcome is favorably influenced by preoperative and postoperative respiratory therapy that includes bronchodilators, incentive spirometry, postural drainage, and pathogen-specific antibiotic therapy.

SCOLIOSIS

Pathophysiology

Scoliosis is lateral rotation and curvature of the vertebrae and a deformity of the rib cage. It can have many etiologies, including idiopathic, congenital, neuromuscular, and traumatic. Scoliosis can affect cardiac and respiratory function. Elevated pulmonary vascular resistance from chronic hypoxia causes pulmonary hypertension and right ventricular hypertrophy. Respiratory abnormalities include reduced lung volumes and chest wall compliance. Pao_2 is reduced as a result of ventilation/perfusion mismatching, whereas an increased $Paco_2$ signals severe disease.

Anesthetic Considerations

Preoperative evaluation may include pulmonary function tests, arterial blood gases, and electrocardiography. Corrective surgery is complicated by the prone position, significant blood loss, and the possibility of paraplegia. Spinal cord function can be assessed by neurophysiological monitoring (somatosensory and motor evoked potentials, see Chapters 6 and 26) or by awakening the patient intraoperatively to test lower limb muscle strength. Patients with severe respiratory disease often **13** remain intubated postoperatively. Patients with scoliosis due to muscular dystrophy are predisposed to malignant hyperthermia, cardiac arrhythmias, and untoward effects of succinylcholine (hyperkalemia, myoglobinuria, and sustained muscular contractures).

WEB SITE & GUIDELINES

Smart Tots. http://www.smarttots.org/.

American Academy of Pediatrics—Section on Anesthesiology: Guidelines for the pediatric anesthesia environment. Pediatrics 1999;103:512.

American Society of Anesthesiologists Committee: Practice guidelines for preoperative fasting and the use of pharmacologic agents to reduce the risk of pulmonary aspiration: Application to healthy patients undergoing elective procedures: An updated report by the American Society of Anesthesiologists Committee on Standards and Practice Parameters. Anesthesiology 2011;114:495.

Smith I, Kranke P, Murat I, et al: Perioperative fasting in adults and children: Guidelines from the European Society of Anaesthesiology. Eur J Anaesthesiol 2011;28:556.

SUGGESTED READING

Butler MG, Hayes BG, Hathaway MM, Begleiter ML: Specific genetic diseases at risk for sedation/anesthesia complications. Anesth Analg 2000;91:837.

Cravero JP, Havidich JE: Pediatric sedation—evolution and revolution. Paediatr Anaesth 2011;21:800.

De Beer DAH, Thomas ML: Caudal additives in children—solutions or problems? Br J Anaesth 2003;90:487.

Fidkowski CW, Zheng H, Firth PG: The anesthetic considerations of tracheobronchial foreign bodies in children: A literature review of 12,979 cases. Anesth Analg 2010;111:1016.

Meretoja OA: Neuromuscular block and current treatment strategies for its reversal in children. Paediatr Anaesth 2010;20:591.

Morray JP: Cardiac arrest in anesthetized children: Recent advances and challenges for the future. Paediatr Anaesth 2011;21:722.

Tsui B, Suresh S: Ultrasound imaging for regional anesthesia in infants, children, and adolescents: A review of current literature and its application in the practice of extremity and trunk blocks. Anesthesiology 2010;112:473.

Geriatric Anesthesia

43

KEY CONCEPTS

1. In the absence of coexisting disease, resting systolic cardiac function seems to be preserved, even in octogenarians. Increased vagal tone and decreased sensitivity of adrenergic receptors lead to a decline in heart rate.

2. Elderly patients undergoing echocardiographic evaluation for surgery have an increased incidence of diastolic dysfunction compared with younger patients.

3. Diminished cardiac reserve in many elderly patients may be manifested as exaggerated drops in blood pressure during induction of general anesthesia. A prolonged circulation time delays the onset of intravenous drugs, but speeds induction with inhalational agents.

4. Aging decreases elasticity of lung tissue, allowing overdistention of alveoli and collapse of small airways. Residual volume and the functional residual capacity increase with aging. Airway collapse increases residual volume and closing capacity. Even in normal persons, closing capacity exceeds functional residual capacity at age 45 years in the supine position and age 65 years in the sitting position.

5. The neuroendocrine response to stress seems to be largely preserved, or, at most, only slightly decreased in healthy elderly patients. Aging is associated with a decreasing response to β-adrenergic agents.

6. Impairment of Na^+ handling, concentrating ability, and diluting capacity predispose elderly patients to both dehydration and fluid overload.

7. Liver mass and hepatic blood flow decline with aging. Hepatic function declines in proportion to the decrease in liver mass.

8. Dosage requirements for local and general (minimum alveolar concentration) anesthetics are reduced. Administration of a given volume of epidural local anesthetic tends to result in more extensive spread in elderly patients. A longer duration of action should be expected from a spinal anesthetic.

9. Aging produces both pharmacokinetic and pharmacodynamic changes. Disease-related changes and wide variations among individuals in similar populations prevent convenient generalizations.

10. Elderly patients display a lower dose requirement for propofol, etomidate, barbiturates, opioids, and benzodiazepines.

By the year 2040, persons aged 65 years or older are expected to comprise 24% of the population and account for 50% of health care expenditures. In Europe, persons aged 65 years or older are expected to comprise 30% of the population within the next 40 years. Of these individuals, many will require surgery. The elderly patient typically presents for surgery with multiple chronic medical conditions,

TABLE 43–1 **Similarities between elderly people and infants, compared with the general population.**

Decreased ability to increase heart rate in response to hypovolemia, hypotension, or hypoxia
Decreased lung compliance
Decreased arterial oxygen tension
Impaired ability to cough
Decreased renal tubular function
Increased susceptibility to hypothermia

in addition to the acute surgical illness. Age is not a contraindication to anesthesia and surgery; however, perioperative morbidity and mortality are greater in elderly than younger surgical patients.

As with pediatric patients, optimal anesthetic management of geriatric patients depends upon an understanding of the normal changes in physiology, anatomy, and response to pharmacological agents that accompany aging. In fact, there are many similarities between elderly and pediatric patients (Table 43–1). Individual genetic polymorphisms and lifestyle choices can modulate the inflammatory response, which contributes to the development of many systemic diseases. Consequently, chronologic age may not fully reflect an individual patient's true physical condition. The relatively high frequency of serious physiological abnormalities in elderly patients demands a particularly careful preoperative evaluation.

Elderly patients are frequently treated with β-blockers. β-Blockers should be continued perioperatively, if patients are taking such medications chronically, to avoid the effects of β-blocker withdrawal. A careful review of patients' often extensive medication lists can reveal the routine use of oral hypoglycemic agents, angiotensin-converting enzyme inhibitors or angiotensin receptor blockers, antiplatelet agents, statins, and anticoagulants. Because elderly patients frequently take multiple drugs for multiple conditions, they often benefit from an evaluation before the day of surgery, even when scheduled for outpatient surgery. Preoperative laboratory studies should be guided by patient condition and history. Patients who have cardiac stents requiring antiplatelet therapy present particularly

vexing problems. Their management should be closely coordinated between the surgeon, cardiologist, and anesthesiologist. At no time should the anesthesia staff discontinue antiplatelet therapy without discussing the plan with the patient's primary physicians.

Age-Related Anatomic & Physiological Changes

CARDIOVASCULAR SYSTEM

Cardiovascular diseases are more prevalent in the geriatric than general population. Still, it is important to distinguish between changes in physiology that normally accompany aging and the pathophysiology of diseases common in the geriatric population (Table 43–2). For example, atherosclerosis is pathological—it is not present in healthy elderly patients. On the other hand, a reduction in arterial elasticity caused by fibrosis of the media is part of the normal aging process. Changes in the cardiovascular system that accompany aging include decreased vascular and myocardial compliance and autonomic responsiveness. In addition to myocardial fibrosis, calcification of the valves can occur. Elderly patients with systolic murmurs should be suspected of having aortic stenosis. However, in the absence of co-existing disease, resting systolic cardiac function seems to be preserved, even in octogenarians. Functional capacity of less than 4 metabolic equivalents (METS) is associated with potential adverse outcomes (see Table 21–2). Increased vagal tone and decreased sensitivity of adrenergic receptors lead to a decline in heart rate; maximal heart rate declines by approximately one beat per minute per year of age over 50. Fibrosis of the conduction system and loss of sinoatrial node cells increase the incidence of dysrhythmias, particularly atrial fibrillation and flutter. Preoperative risk assessment and evaluation of the patient with cardiac disease were previously reviewed in this text (see Chapters 18, 20, & 21). Age *per se* does not mandate any particular battery of tests or evaluative tools, although there is a long tradition of routinely requesting tests such as 12-lead electrocardiography

TABLE 43–2 **Age-related physiological changes and common diseases of the elderly.**

Normal Physiological Changes	Common Pathophysiology
Cardiovascular	
Decreased arterial elasticity	Atherosclerosis
Elevated afterload	Coronary artery disease
Elevated systolic blood pressure	Essential hypertension
	Congestive heart failure
Left ventricular hypertrophy	Cardiac arrhythmias
Decreased adrenergic activity	Aortic stenosis
Decreased resting heart rate	
Decreased maximal heart rate	
Decreased baroreceptor reflex	
Respiratory	
Decreased pulmonary elasticity	Emphysema
Decreased alveolar surface area	Chronic bronchitis
Increased residual volume	Pneumonia
Increased closing capacity	
Ventilation/perfusion mismatching	
Decreased arterial oxygen tension	
Increased chest wall rigidity	
Decreased muscle strength	
Decreased cough	
Decreased maximal breathing capacity	
Blunted response to hypercapnia and hypoxia	
Renal	
Decreased renal blood flow	Diabetic nephropathy
Decreased renal plasma flow	Hypertensive nephropathy
Decreased glomerular filtration rate	Prostatic obstruction
Decreased renal mass	Congestive heart failure
Decreased tubular function	
Impaired sodium handling	
Decreased concentrating ability	
Decreased diluting capacity	
Impaired fluid handling	
Decreased drug excretion	
Decreased renin–aldosterone responsiveness	
Impaired potassium excretion	

(ECG) in patients who are older than a defined age. Nonetheless, elderly individuals are more likely to present for surgery with previously undetected conditions that require an intervention,

such as arrhythmias, congestive heart failure, or myocardial ischemia. Cardiovascular evaluation should be guided by American Heart Association guidelines.

2 Elderly patients undergoing echocardiographic evaluation for surgery have an increased incidence of diastolic dysfunction compared with younger patients. Diastolic dysfunction prevents the ventricle from relaxing and consequently inhibits diastolic ventricular filling at relatively low pressures. The ventricle becomes less compliant, and filling pressures are increased. Diastolic dysfunction is NOT equivalent to diastolic heart failure. In some patients, systolic ventricular function can be well preserved; however, the patient can have signs of congestion secondary to severe diastolic dysfunction. Diastolic heart failure most often coexists with systolic dysfunction.

Echocardiography is used to assess diastolic dysfunction. A ratio of greater than 15 between the peak E velocity of transmitral diastolic filling and the E′ tissue Doppler wave is associated with elevated left ventricular end-diastolic pressure and diastolic dysfunction. Conversely, a ratio of less than 8 is consistent with normal diastolic function (see **Figure 43–1**).

Marked diastolic dysfunction may be seen with systemic hypertension, coronary artery disease, cardiomyopathies, and valvular heart disease, particularly aortic stenosis. Patients may be asymptomatic or complain of exercise intolerance, dyspnea, cough, or fatigue. Diastolic dysfunction results in relatively large increases in ventricular end-diastolic pressure, with small changes of left ventricular volume; the atrial contribution to ventricular filling becomes even more important than in younger patients. Atrial enlargement predisposes patients to atrial fibrillation and flutter. Patients are at increased risk of developing congestive heart failure. The elderly patient with diastolic dysfunction may poorly tolerate perioperative fluid administration, resulting in elevated left ventricular end-diastolic pressure and pulmonary congestion.

3 Diminished cardiac reserve in many elderly patients may be manifested as exaggerated drops in blood pressure during induction of general anesthesia. A prolonged circulation time delays

A

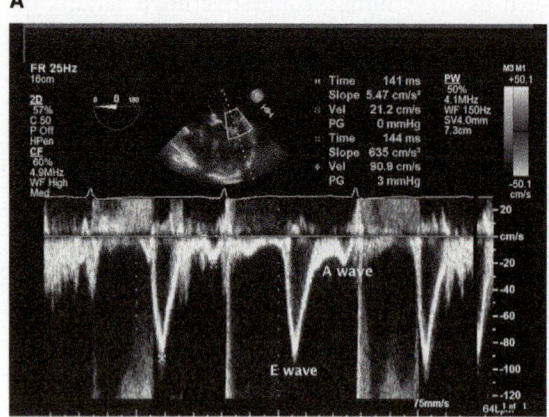

B

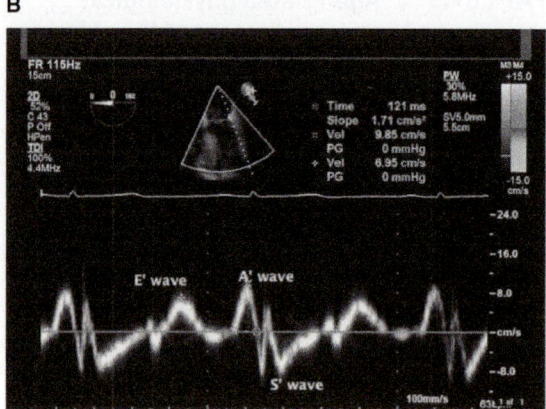

FIGURE 43–1 **A:** In this Doppler study of diastolic inflow, the E wave is seen with a peak velocity of 90.9 cm/sec. This Doppler study reflects the velocity of blood as it fills the left ventricle early in diastole. **B:** In tissue Doppler, the velocity of the movement of the lateral annulus of the mitral valve is measured. The E' wave in this image is 6.95 cm/sec. This corresponds to the movement of the myocardium during diastole. (Reproduced, with permission, from Wasnick J, Hillel Z, Kramer D, et al: *Cardiac Anesthesia & Transesophageal Echocardiography*, McGraw-Hill, 2011.)

the onset of intravenous drugs, but speeds induction with inhalational agents. Like infants, elderly patients have less ability to respond to hypovolemia, hypotension, or hypoxia with an increase in heart rate. Ultimately, cardiovascular diseases, including heart failure, stroke, arrhythmias, and hypertension contribute to an increased risk of morbidity, mortality, increased cost of care, and frailty in elderly patients.

Research is ongoing into the relationship between telomere biology and cardiovascular disease. Telomeres, which are located at the chromosome terminus, protect the DNA from degradation during cell division. With each cell division, there is progressive telomere loss. Cells with short telomeres undergo "replicative senescence" and apoptosis. Telomerase maintains telomere length, but has low activity in human cells. Indeed, telomere length varies among humans based upon inheritance and environmental factors. Telomerase activity is deficient in various early aging syndromes. Telomere shortening may be either a cause or a consequence of cardiovascular disease. Whatever the exact mechanism of cardiovascular aging, patient management should at all times be in accordance with American Heart Association/American College of Cardiology guidelines.

RESPIRATORY SYSTEM

④ Aging decreases the elasticity of lung tissue, allowing overdistention of alveoli and collapse of small airways. Residual volume and the functional residual capacity increase with aging. Airway collapse increases residual volume and closing capacity Even in normal persons, closing capacity exceeds functional residual capacity at age 45 years in the supine position and age 65 years in the sitting position. When this happens, some airways close during part of normal tidal breathing, resulting in a mismatch of ventilation and perfusion. The additive effect of these emphysema-like changes decreases arterial oxygen tension by an average rate of 0.35 mm Hg per year; however, there is a wide range of arterial oxygen tensions in elderly preoperative patients. Both anatomic and physiological dead space increase. Other pulmonary effects of aging are summarized in Table 43–2.

Decreased respiratory muscle function/mass, a less compliant chest wall, and intrinsic changes in lung function can increase the work of breathing and make it more difficult for elderly patients to muster a respiratory reserve in settings of acute illness (eg, infection). Many patients also present with obstructive or restrictive lung diseases. In patients who have no intrinsic pulmonary disease, gas exchange is unaffected by aging.

Measures to prevent perioperative hypoxia in elderly patients include a longer preoxygenation period prior to induction, increased inspired oxygen concentrations during anesthesia, positive end-expiratory pressure, and pulmonary toilet. Aspiration pneumonia is a common and potentially life-threatening complication in elderly patients, possibly as a consequence of a progressive decrease in protective laryngeal reflexes and immunocompetence with age. Ventilatory impairment in the recovery room is more common in elderly than younger patients. Factors associated with an increased risk of postoperative pulmonary complications include age older than 64 years, chronic obstructive pulmonary disease, sleep apnea, malnutrition, and abdominal or thoracic surgical incisions.

METABOLIC & ENDOCRINE FUNCTION

Basal and maximal oxygen consumption declines with age. After reaching peak weight at about age 60 years, most men and women begin losing weight; the average elderly man and woman weigh less than their younger counterparts. Heat production decreases, heat loss increases, and hypothalamic temperature-regulating centers may reset at a lower level.

Diabetes affects approximately 15% of patients older than age 70 years. Its impact on numerous organ systems can complicate perioperative management. Diabetic neuropathy and autonomic dysfunction are particular problems for the elderly.

Increasing insulin resistance leads to a progressive decrease in the ability to avoid hyperglycemia with glucose loads. Institutions typically have their own protocols on how to manage increased blood glucose perioperatively, and these protocols reflect the changing literature on "tight" control. Attempts to maintain blood glucose within a strictly normal range during surgery, anesthesia, and/or critical illness may lead to hypoglycemia and adverse outcomes. Anesthesia practitioners are advised to determine what the "acceptable" perioperative blood

glucose level is in their institution and to be aware of changing performance benchmarks related to this measure.

The neuroendocrine response to stress seems to be largely preserved, or, at most, only slightly **5** decreased in healthy elderly patients. Aging is associated with a decreasing response to β-adrenergic agents.

RENAL FUNCTION

Renal blood flow and kidney mass (eg, glomerular number and tubular length) decrease with age. Renal function, as determined by glomerular filtration rate and creatinine clearance, is reduced (Table 43–2). The serum creatinine level is unchanged because of a decrease in muscle mass and creatinine production, whereas blood urea nitrogen gradually **6** increases with aging. Impairment of Na+ handling, concentrating ability, and diluting capacity predispose elderly patients to both dehydration and fluid overload. The response to antidiuretic hormone and aldosterone is reduced. The ability to reabsorb glucose is decreased. The combination of reduced renal blood flow and decreased nephron mass in elderly patients increases the risk of acute renal failure in the postoperative period, particularly when they are exposed to nephrotoxic drugs and techniques.

As renal function declines, so does the kidney's ability to excrete drugs. The decreased capacity to handle water and electrolyte loads makes proper fluid management more critical; elderly patients are more predisposed to developing hypokalemia and hyperkalemia. This is further complicated by the common use of diuretics in the elderly population. The search is ongoing for drugs that might protect the kidney perioperatively, as well as for specific genetic profiles of patients at greater risk of perioperative kidney injury.

GASTROINTESTINAL FUNCTION

7 Liver mass and hepatic blood flow decline with aging. Hepatic function declines in proportion to the decrease in liver mass. Thus, the rate of biotransformation and albumin production decreases. Plasma cholinesterase levels are reduced in elderly men.

NERVOUS SYSTEM

Brain mass decreases with age; neuronal loss is prominent in the cerebral cortex, particularly the frontal lobes. Cerebral blood flow also decreases about 10% to 20% in proportion to neuronal losses. It remains tightly coupled to metabolic rate, and autoregulation is intact. Neurons lose complexity of their dendritic tree and the number of synapses. The synthesis of neurotransmitters, such as dopamine, and neurotransmitter receptors are reduced. Serotonergic, adrenergic, and gamma-aminobutyric acid (GABA) binding sites are also reduced. Astrocytes and microglial cells increase in number.

Aging is associated with an increasing threshold for nearly all sensory modalities, including touch, temperature sensation, proprioception, hearing, and **8** vision. Dosage requirements for local and general (minimum alveolar concentration [MAC]) anesthetics are reduced. Administration of a given volume of epidural local anesthetic tends to result in more extensive spread in elderly patients. A longer duration of action should be expected from a given dose of spinal local anesthetic.

Currently, much work is being done to determine whether surgery and anesthesia harm the brain in some manner. Postoperative cognitive dysfunction (POCD) is diagnosed by neurobehavioral testing. Unlike delirium, which is a clinical diagnosis, cognitive dysfunction must be sought by using evaluative techniques. Up to 30% of elderly patients can demonstrate abnormal neurobehavioral testing within the first week after an operation; however, such testing may identify dysfunction already present in these individuals prior to any surgery or anesthesia exposure.

Ultimately, the question arises as to whether general anesthetic agents result in neurotoxicity in the aged brain. Some current investigations are attempting to determine whether anesthetic agents produce POCD through a mechanism similar to that underlying Alzheimer's disease.

It is also possible that side effects of illness (eg, inflammation) and the neuroendocrine stress response contribute to perioperative brain injury in some manner, independent of anesthesia. Indeed, patients presenting for surgery may present with cognitive dysfunction. In one study, 20% of elderly patients presenting for elective total joint arthroplasty demonstrated preoperative cognitive impairment; furthermore, POCD was independent of type of anesthesia or surgery at 3 months postoperatively. Postoperative delirium is common in elderly patients, especially those with reduced preoperative neurocognitive test scores and reduced functional status. Preoperative frailty is also associated with postoperative delirium. Frailty is common in preoperative elderly patients awaiting surgery and predicts postoperative delirium. Delirium has a particularly frequent incidence following hip surgery. Factors associated with postoperative delirium in the elderly and ways to avoid it are presented in Tables 43–3 and 43–4.

Elderly patients often take more time to recover completely from the central nervous system effects of general anesthesia, especially if they were confused or disoriented preoperatively. This is important in geriatric outpatient surgery, where socioeconomic factors, such as the lack of a caretaker at home, necessitate that patients may need to assume a higher level of self care.

In the absence of disease, any perioperative decrease in cognitive function is normally modest. Short-term memory seems to be most affected. Continued physical and intellectual activity seems to have a positive effect on preservation of cognitive functions.

The etiology of POCD is likely multifactorial and includes drug effects, pain, underlying dysfunction, hypothermia, and metabolic disturbances. Elderly patients are particularly sensitive to centrally acting anticholinergic agents, such as scopolamine and atropine. Some patients suffer from prolonged or permanent POCD after surgery and anesthesia. Some studies suggest that POCD can be detected in 10% to 15% of patients older than age 60 years up to 3 months following major surgery. In some settings (eg, following cardiac and major orthopedic procedures), intraoperative arterial emboli may be contributory. Animal studies suggest that anesthesia without surgery can impair learning for weeks,

TABLE 43–3 Predisposing and precipitating factors for delirium after surgery.

Predisposing Factors, Preoperative	Precipitating Factors	
	Intraoperative	**Postoperative**
Demographics	Type of operation	Early complications of operation
Increasing age	Hip fracture	Low hematocrit
Male gender	Cardiac surgery	Cardiogenic shock
Comorbidities	Vascular surgery	Hypoxemia
Impaired cognition	Complexity of operation	Prolonged intubation
Dementia	Operation time	Sedation management
Mild cognitive impairment	Shock/hypotension	Pain
Preoperative memory complaint	Arrhythmia	Later complications of operation
Atherosclerosis	Decreased cardiac output	Low albumin
Intracranial stenosis	Emergency surgery	Abnormal electrolytes
Carotid stenosis	Operative factors	Latrogenic complications
Peripheral vascular disease	Intraoperative temperature	Pain
Prior stroke/transient ischemic attack	Benzodiazepine administration	Infection
Diabetes	Propofol administration	Liver failure
Hypertension	Blood transfusion	Renal failure
Atrial fibrillation	Anesthesia factors	Sleep-wake disturbance
Low albumin	Type of anesthesia	Alcohol withdrawal
Electrolyte abnormalities	Duration of anesthesia	
Psychiatric disease	Cognitively active medications	
Anxiety		
Depression		
Benzodiazepine use		
Function		
Impaired functional status		
Sensory impairment		
Lifestyle factors		
Alcohol use		
Sleep deprivation		
Smoking		

Reproduced, with permission, from Rudoph J, Marcantonio E: Postoperative delirium: acute change with long term implications. Anesth Analg 2011;112: 1202.

particularly in older animals. Elderly inpatients seem to have a significantly higher risk of POCD than elderly outpatients. Anesthetic neurotoxicity is also a potential risk for the developing brain. Progress in research in this area is documented on the Smart Tots™ website (see http://www.smarttots.org/).

MUSCULOSKELETAL

Muscle mass is reduced in elderly patients. Skin atrophies with age and is susceptible to trauma from removal of adhesive tape, electrocautery pads, and electrocardiographic electrodes. Veins are often frail and easily ruptured by intravenous infusions. Arthritic joints may interfere with positioning or regional anesthesia. Degenerative cervical spine disease can limit neck extension, potentially making intubation difficult.

Age-Related Pharmacological Changes

9 Aging produces both pharmacokinetic (the relationship between drug dose and plasma concentration) and pharmacodynamic (the relationship between plasma concentration and clinical effect) changes. Disease-related changes and wide variations among individuals in similar populations prevent generalizations.

TABLE 43–4 **Prevention of delirium after surgery.**

Module	Postoperative Intervention
Cognitive stimulation	Orientation (clock, calendar, orientation board) Avoid cognitively active medications
Improve sensory input	Glasses Hearing aids/amplifiers
Mobilization	Early mobilization and rehabilitation
Avoidance of psychoactive medication	Elimination of unnecessary medications Pain management protocol
Fluid and nutrition	Fluid management Electrolyte monitoring and repletion Adequate nutrition protocol
Avoidance of hospital complications	Bowel protocol Early removal of urinary catheters Adequate central nervous system O_2 delivery, including supplemental oxygen and transfusion for very low hematocrit Postoperative complication monitoring protocol

Reproduced, with permission, from Rudoph J, Marcantonio E: Postoperative delirium: acute change with long term implications. Anesth Analg 2011;112: 1202.

A progressive decrease in muscle mass and increase in body fat (particularly in older women) results in decreased total body water. The reduced volume of distribution for water-soluble drugs can lead to greater plasma concentrations; conversely, an increased volume of distribution for lipid-soluble drugs could theoretically reduce their plasma concentration. Any change in volume of distribution sufficient to significantly change concentrations will influence the elimination time. Because renal and hepatic functions decline with age, reductions in clearance prolong the duration of action of many drugs.

Distribution and elimination are also affected by altered plasma protein binding. Albumin, which binds acidic drugs (eg, barbiturates, benzodiazepines, opioid agonists), typically decreases with age. α_1-Acid glycoprotein, which binds basic drugs (eg, local anesthetics), is increased.

The principal pharmacodynamic change associated with aging is a reduced anesthetic requirement, represented by a reduced MAC. Careful titration of anesthetic agents helps to avoid adverse side effects and unexpected, prolonged duration; short-acting agents, such as propofol, desflurane, remifentanil, and succinylcholine, may be particularly useful in elderly patients. Drugs that are not significantly dependent on hepatic or renal function or blood flow, such as atracurium or cisatracurium, are useful.

INHALATIONAL ANESTHETICS

The MAC for inhalational agents is reduced by 4% per decade of age over 40 years. Onset of action is faster if cardiac output is depressed, whereas it is delayed if there is a significant ventilation/perfusion abnormality. Recovery from anesthesia with a volatile anesthetic may be prolonged because of an increased volume of distribution (increased body fat) and decreased pulmonary gas exchange. Decreased hepatic function is of less importance, even for halothane. Agents that are rapidly eliminated (eg, desflurane) are good choices for speeding emergence in the elderly patient.

NONVOLATILE ANESTHETIC AGENTS

10 In general, elderly patients display a lower dose requirement for propofol, etomidate, barbiturates, opioids, and benzodiazepines. The typical octogenarian will require a smaller induction dose of propofol than that required by a 20-year-old patient.

Although propofol may be close to an ideal induction agent in elderly patients because of its rapid elimination, it is more likely to cause apnea and hypotension than in younger patients. Both pharmacokinetic and pharmacodynamic factors are responsible for this enhanced sensitivity. Elderly patients require nearly 50% lower blood levels of propofol for anesthesia than do younger patients. Moreover, both the rapidly equilibrating peripheral compartment and systemic clearance for propofol are significantly reduced in elderly patients. The initial volume of distribution for etomidate significantly decreases with aging: lower doses are required to achieve the same electroencephalographic endpoint in elderly patients (compared with young patients).

Enhanced sensitivity to fentanyl, alfentanil, and sufentanil is primarily pharmacodynamic. Pharmacokinetics for these opioids are not significantly affected by age. Dose requirements for the same EEG endpoint using fentanyl and alfentanil are 50% lower in elderly patients. In contrast, the volume of the central compartment and clearance are reduced for remifentanil; thus, both pharmacodynamic and pharmacokinetic factors are important.

Use of sedative and antinausea agents with anticholinergic and antidopaminergic properties may produce adverse effects in patients with Parkinson's disease.

Aging increases the volume of distribution for all benzodiazepines, which effectively prolongs their elimination half-lives. Enhanced pharmacodynamic sensitivity to benzodiazepines is also observed. Midazolam requirements are generally 50% less in elderly patients, and its elimination half-life is prolonged by about 50%.

MUSCLE RELAXANTS

The response to succinylcholine and other neuromuscular blockers is unaltered by aging. Decreased cardiac output and slow muscle blood flow, however, may cause up to a 2-fold prolongation in the onset of neuromuscular blockade in elderly patients. Recovery from nondepolarizing muscle relaxants that depend on renal excretion (eg, pancuronium) may be delayed due to decreased drug clearance. Likewise, decreased hepatic excretion from a loss of liver mass prolongs the elimination half-life and duration of action of rocuronium and vecuronium. The pharmacological profile of atracurium is not significantly affected by age.

CASE DISCUSSION

The Elderly Patient with a Fractured Hip

An 86-year-old nursing home patient is scheduled for open reduction and internal fixation of a subtrochanteric fracture of the femur.

How should this patient be evaluated for the risk of perioperative morbidity?

Anesthetic risk correlates much better with the presence of coexisting disease than chronological age. Therefore, preanesthetic evaluation should concentrate on the identification of age-related diseases (Table 43–2) and an estimation of physiological reserve. There is a tremendous physiological difference between a patient who walks three blocks to a grocery store on a regular basis and one who is bedridden, even though both may be the same age. Obviously, any condition that may be amenable to preoperative therapy (eg, bronchodilator administration) must be identified and addressed. At the same time, lengthy delays may compromise surgical repair and increase overall morbidity.

What are some of the considerations in selection of premedication for this patient?

In general, elderly patients require lower doses of premedication. Nonetheless, hip fractures are painful, particularly during movement to the operating room. Unless contraindicated by severe concomitant disease, an opioid premedication may be valuable. Anticholinergic medication is rarely needed, as aging is accompanied by atrophy of the salivary glands. These patients may be at risk for aspiration, as opioid premedication and pain from the injury will decrease gastric emptying. Therefore, pretreatment with an H_2 antagonist or proton pump inhibitor should be considered.

What factors might influence the choice between regional and general anesthesia?

Advancing age is not a contraindication for either regional or general anesthesia. Each technique, however, has its advantages and disadvantages in the elderly population. For hip surgery, regional anesthesia can be achieved with a sub-arachnoid or epidural block extending to the T8 sensory level. Both of these blocks require patient cooperation and the ability to lie still for the duration of the surgery. A paramedian approach may be helpful when optimal positioning is not possible Unless regional anesthesia is accompanied by heavy sedation, postoperative confusion and disorientation are less troublesome than after general anesthesia. Cardiovascular changes are usually limited to a decrease in arterial blood pressure as sympathetic block is established. Although this decrease can be minimized by prophylactic fluid loading, a patient with borderline heart function may develop congestive heart failure when the block dissipates and sympathetic tone returns. Reduced afterload can result in profound hypotension and cardiac arrest in patients with aortic stenosis, a common valvular lesion in the elderly population. Patients with coronary artery disease may experience an increase in myocardial oxygen demand as a result of reflex tachycardia or a decrease in supply caused by lower coronary artery perfusion. Invasive arterial pressure monitoring is useful when taking the elderly patient to surgery. Monitors of hemodynamic function using pulse contour analysis that estimate stroke volume variation in addition to transesophageal echocardiography can all be employed to guide fluid therapy. The benefits of transesophageal echocardiography must be considered in the context of the risks of esophageal rupture and mediastinitis in the elderly.

Are there any specific advantages or disadvantages to a regional technique in elderly patients having hip surgery?

A major advantage in regional anesthesia—particularly for hip surgery—is a lower incidence of postoperative thromboembolism. This is presumably due to peripheral vasodilation and maintenance of venous blood flow in the lower extremities. In addition, local anesthetics inhibit platelet aggregation and stabilize endothelial cells. Many anesthesiologists believe that regional anesthesia maintains respiratory function better than general anesthesia. Unless the anesthetic level involves the intercostal musculature, ventilation and the cough reflex are well maintained.

Technical problems associated with regional anesthesia in the elderly include altered landmarks as a result of degeneration of the vertebral column and the difficulty of obtaining adequate patient positioning secondary to pain related to the fracture. To avoid having the patient lie on the fracture, a hypobaric or isobaric solution can be injected intrathecally. Postpuncture headache is less of a problem in the elderly population.

If the patient refuses regional anesthesia, is general anesthesia acceptable?

General anesthesia is an acceptable alternative to regional block. One advantage is that the patient can be induced in bed and moved to the operating room table after intubation, avoiding the pain of positioning. A disadvantage is that the patient is unable to provide feedback regarding pressure points on the unpadded orthopedic table.

What specific factors should be considered during induction and maintenance of general anesthesia with this patient?

It is important to remember that because a subtrochanteric fracture can be associated with more than 1 L of occult blood loss, induction with propofol may lead to an exaggerated decrease in arterial blood pressure. Initial hypotension may be replaced by hypertension and tachycardia during laryngoscopy and intubation. This rollercoaster volatility in blood pressure increases the risk of myocardial ischemia and can be avoided by preceding airway instrumentation with lidocaine (1.5 mg/kg), esmolol (0.3 mg/kg), or alfentanil (5–15mcg/kg). Elderly patients often have poor vascular compliance and wide pulse pressures, leading to dramatic swings in both systolic and diastolic blood pressure during anesthesia.

Intraoperative paralysis with a nondepolarizing muscle relaxant improves surgical conditions and allows maintenance of a lighter plane of anesthesia. Monitoring for anesthetic awareness is suggested if the patient's hemodynamics dictate reliance on muscle relaxants to prevent movement intraoperatively.

SUGGESTED READING

Bettelli G: Preoperative evaluation in geriatric surgery: comorbidity, functional status and pharmacological history. Minerva Anestesiol 2011;71:1.

Cheung C, Ponnusamy A, Anderton J: Management of acute renal failure in the elderly patient: a clinician's guide. Drugs Aging 2008;25:455.

Crosby G, Culley D, Patel P: At the sharp end of spines. Anesthiology 2010;112:521.

Evered L, Scott D, Silbert B, Maruff P: Postoperative cognitive dysfunction is independent of type of surgery and anesthetic. Anesth Analg 2011;112:1179.

Evered L, Silbert B, Scott D, et al: Preexisting cognitive impairment and mild cognitive impairment in subjects presenting for total hip joint replacement. Anesthiology 2011;114: 1297.

Fodale V, Santamaria L, Schifilliti D, Mandal P: Anaesthetics and postoperative cognitive dysfunction: a pathological mechanism mimicking Alzheimer's disease. Anaesthesia 2010;65:388.

Jankowski C, Trenerry M, Cook D, et al: Cognitive and functional predictors and sequelae of postoperative delirium in elderly patients undergoing elective joint arthroplasty. Anesth Analg 2011;112:1186-9.

Jin F, Chung F: Minimizing perioperative adverse events in the elderly. Br J Anaesth 2001;87:608.

Leung J, Tsai T, Sands L: Preoperative frailty in older surgical patients is associated with early postoperative delirium. Anesth Analg 2011;112:1199.

Levine W, Mehta V, Landesberg G: Anesthesia for the elderly: selected topics. Curr Opin Anaesthiol 2006;19:320.

Lin D, Feng C, Cao M, Zuo Z: Volatile anesthetics may not induce significant toxicity to human neuron like cells. Anesth Analg 2011;112:1194.

Rudoph J, Marcantonio E: Postoperative delirium: acute change with long term implications. Anesth Analg 2011;112:1202.

Samani N, van der Harst P: Biological aging and cardiovascular disease. Heart 2008;94:537.

Silvay G, Castillo J, Chikwe J, et al: Cardiac anesthesia and surgery in geriatric patients. Semin Cardiothorac Vasc Anesth 2008;12:18.

van Harten AE, Scheeren TW, Absalom AR: A review of postoperative cognitive dysfunction and neuroinflammation associated with cardiac surgery and anaesthesia. Anaesthesia 2012;67:280.

White PF, White LM, Monk T: Review article: perioperative care for the older outpatient undergoing ambulatory surgery. Anesth Analg 2012;114:1190.

Zaugg M, Lucchinetti E: Respiratory function in the elderly. Anesthesiol Clin North America 2000;18:47.

Zeleznik J: Normative aging of the respiratory system. Clin Geriatr Med 2003;19:1.

Ambulatory, Nonoperating Room, & Office-Based Anesthesia

44

Outpatient/ambulatory anesthesia is the subspecialty of anesthesiology that deals with the preoperative, intraoperative, and postoperative anesthetic care of patients undergoing elective, same-day surgical procedures. Patients undergoing ambulatory surgery rarely require admission to a hospital and are fit enough to be discharged from the surgical facility after the procedure.

Nonoperating room anesthesia (or out of the operating room anesthesia) refers to both inpatients and ambulatory surgery patients who undergo anesthesia in settings outside of a traditional operating room. These patients can vary greatly, ranging from claustrophobic individuals in need of anesthesia for

magnetic resonance imaging (MRI) procedures to critically ill septic patients undergoing endoscopic retrograde cholangiopancreatography in the gastrointestinal suite. **1** Out of the operating room anesthesia requires the anesthesia provider to work in remote locations in a hospital, where ease of access to the patient and anesthesia equipment is compromised; furthermore, the staff at these locations may be unfamiliar with the requirements for safe anesthetic delivery.

Office-based anesthesia refers to the delivery of anesthesia in a practitioner's office that has a procedural suite incorporated into its design. Office-based anesthesia is frequently administered to patients undergoing cosmetic surgery, and anesthesia for dental procedures is also routinely performed in an office-based setting.

Although treatment may be similar for inpatients, ambulatory surgery center patients, out of the operating room patients, and office-based anesthesia patients, there are nonetheless various guidelines and statements from the American Society of Anesthesiologists (ASA) that pertain to these different locations. All of these recommendations should be reviewed at the ASA website (www.asahq.org/For-Healthcare-Professionals/Standards-Guidelines-and-Statements.aspx), as they are subject to change and modification. In their guidelines and statements, the ASA reminds anesthesia staff that it is important that both the physical and operational infrastructure is in place at any location to ensure the safe conduct of anesthesia. In addition to the ASA guidelines, state regulatory guidelines, which include specific requirements for safety, governance, and emergency protocols for both office-based and free-standing ambulatory surgery centers, have also been established. Accreditation agencies, such as the Joint Commission, Accreditation Association for Ambulatory Healthcare, and American Association for the Accreditation of Ambulatory Surgical Facilities, engage in various inspections and reviews to ensure that facilities meet acceptable standards for the procedural services provided. Anesthesia staff should confirm that both the infrastructure and operational policies are consistent with acceptable anesthesia practice standards before providing anesthesia in such settings.

ADVANCES IN AMBULATORY ANESTHESIA AND SURGERY

Most patients are no longer admitted prior to the day of elective surgery. The trend for same-day admittance has been facilitated by advancements in surgical technique and technology (eg, laparoscopy), resulting in less invasive surgery, advancements in anesthesia care (eg, shorter acting medications) and improved postoperative pain and nausea management. The underlying reason for ambulatory anesthesia and surgery is that it is less

expensive and more convenient for the patient than inpatient admission. The transition from open cholecystectomy to a laparoscopic approach represents the type of development that permits a shortened postoperative course and ambulatory patient management. Consequently, a common procedure that once required hospital admission is now performed as outpatient surgery.

The use of short-acting anesthetic agents (eg, propofol, desflurane, and rocuronium) has likewise contributed to making ambulatory surgery easier; however, such cases were performed successfully using thiopental, isoflurane, and succinylcholine when the newer agents were not available. Although inhalational agents (eg, sevoflurane and desflurane) lead to prompt emergence, they also contribute to postoperative nausea and vomiting (PONV). Propofol, which may have antiemetic effects as a part of total intravenous anesthesia (TIVA), can potentially reduce PONV; however, TIVA may require more time for patients to meet discharge criteria. Regional and local anesthetic techniques are becoming increasingly popular in managing ambulatory orthopedic surgery. The use of ultrasound and nerve stimulation has improved regional block success rates. The use of regional techniques decreases postoperative opioid requirements, potentially reducing the likelihood of PONV. For example, paravertebral blocks are increasingly used to manage office-based breast augmentation surgery. Improved airway management using devices, such as the laryngeal mask airway (LMA) and video laryngoscopy, have likewise contributed to improved patient care. Consequently, anesthesia personnel working as solo providers in an office-based setting are better able to avoid airway catastrophes.

CANDIDATES FOR AMBULATORY AND OFFICE-BASED ANESTHESIA

With an aging and increasingly obese population, patients with significant comorbidities present for ambulatory surgery. Although age *per se* is not a factor in determining candidacy for ambulatory procedures, each patient must be considered in the context of his or her comorbidities, the type of surgery to be performed, and the expected response to anesthesia.

5 In general, ambulatory surgeries should be of a complexity and duration such that one could reasonably assume that the patient will make an expeditious recovery. ASA physical status and a thorough history and physical exam are crucial in the screening of patients selected for ambulatory or office-based surgery. ASA 4 and 5 patients normally would not be candidates for ambulatory surgery, whereas ASA 1 and 2 patients would be prime candidates for such surgery. ASA 3 patients with diabetes, hypertension, and stable coronary artery disease would not be precluded from an ambulatory procedure provided that their diseases are well controlled. Ultimately, the surgeon and anesthesia provider must identify patients for whom an ambulatory or office-based setting is likely to provide benefits (eg, convenience, reduced costs and charges) that outweigh risks (eg, the lack of immediate availability of all hospital services, such as a cardiac catheterization laboratory, emergency cardiovascular stents, assistance with airway rescue, rapid consultation).

6 Factors considered in selecting patients for ambulatory procedures include: systemic illnesses and their current management, airway management problems, sleep apnea, morbid obesity, previous adverse anesthesia outcomes (eg, malignant hyperthermia), allergies, and the patient's social network (eg, availability of someone to be responsive to the patient for 24 h).

Patients with known or likely difficult airways should probably not be candidates for office-based procedures; however, they may be appropriately cared for in a well equipped and fully staffed ambulatory surgery center. Important considerations for such patients include the availability of difficult airway equipment, such as an intubating LMA or videolaryngoscope, the availability of additional experienced anesthesia providers, and surgeons/anesthesiologists capable of performing emergency tracheostomy/cricothyroidotomy. If there are concerns regarding the ability to manage the airway in an ambulatory surgery setting, or if a surgical airway is thought to be a possibility, the patient may be better served in a hospital setting where immediate consultation and assistance is available.

Similarly, patients with unstable comorbid conditions, such as decompensated congestive heart failure or uncontrolled hypertension, may benefit more from having their procedure performed in a hospital than a free-standing facility. Indeed, many patients undergo ambulatory procedures in a hospital, as opposed to a free-standing surgery center or office. Such patients have the benefit of both the availability of a hospital's resources and the convenience of being an ambulatory patient. Should their condition warrant additional care, hospital admittance is possible; however, such flexibility comes with the costs associated with hospital care.

The anesthesiologist must know which preexisting medical conditions predict a specific intraoperative and/or postoperative adverse event (AE) for the patient in question. Likewise, procedures suitable for ambulatory surgery should have a minimal risk of perioperative hemorrhage, airway compromise, and no particular requirement for specialized postoperative care. Based on risk identification, the anesthesiologist should be able to mitigate unforeseen AEs and provide optimal care for patients in this type of setting. Although current evidence-based medicine can provide recommendations for some high-risk ambulatory issues, evidence is lacking for most such situations.

SPECIFIC PATIENT CONDITIONS AND AMBULATORY SURGERY

Obesity and Obstructive Sleep Apnea

Obesity is associated with many concomitant disease states, such as hypertension, diabetes, hyperlidipemia, and obstructive sleep apnea (OSA). The physiologic derangements that accompany these conditions include changes in oxygen demand, carbon dioxide production, alveolar ventilation, and cardiac output. Patients with obesity and OSA are at increased risk of postoperative respiratory complications, such as prolonged airway obstruction and apnea. Scores for predicting the probability of these complications can aid in the preoperative assessment and referral to a hospital setting (Tables 44–1 and 44–2). Although a sleep study is the standard way to

TABLE 44-1 Identification and assessment of obstructive sleep apnea: example.

A. Clinical signs and symptoms suggesting the possibility of OSA
1. Predisposing physical characteristics
   a. BMI 35 kg/m² [95th percentile for age and gender][1]
   b. Neck circumference 17 inches (men) or 16 inches (women)
   c. Craniofacial abnormalities affecting the airway
   d. Anatomical nasal obstruction
   e. Tonsils nearly touching or touching In the midline
2. History of apparent airway obstruction during sleep (two or more of the following are present; if patient lives alone or sleep is not observed by another person, then only one of the following needs to be present)
   a. Snoring (loud enough to be heard through closed door)
   b. Frequent snoring
   c. Observed pauses in breathing during sleep
   d. Awakens from sleep with choking sensation
   e. Frequent arousals from sleep
   f. [Intermittent vocalization during sleep][1]
   g. [Parental report of restless sleep, difficulty breathing, or struggling respiratory efforts during sleep][1]
3. Somnolence (one or more of the following is present)
   a. Frequent somnolence or fatigue despite adequate "sleep"
   b. Falls asleep easily in a nonstimulating environment (e.g., watching TV, reading, riding in or driving a car) despite adequate "sleep"
   c. [Parent or teacher comments that child appears sleepy during the day, is easily distracted, is overly aggressive, or has difficulty concentrating][1]
   d. [Child often difficult to arouse at usual awakening time][1]

If a patient has signs or symptoms in two or more of the above categories, there is a significant probability that he or she has OSA. The severity of OSA may be determined by sleep study (see below). If a sleep study is not available, such patients should be treated as though they have moderate sleep apnea unless one or more of the signs or symptoms above is severely abnormal (e.g., markedly increased BMI or neck circumference, respiratory pauses that are frightening to the observer, patient regularly falls asleep within minutes after being left unstimulated), in which case they should be treated as though they have severe sleep apnea.

B. If a sleep study has been done, the results should be used to determine the perioperative anesthetic management of a patient. However, because sleep laboratories differ in their criteria for detecting episodes of apnea and hypopnea, the Task Force believes that the sleep laboratory's assessment (none, mild, moderate, or severe) should take precedence over the actual AHI (the number of episodes of sleep-disordered breathing per hour). If the overall severity is not indicated, it may be determined by using the table below:

Severity of OSA	Adult AHI	Pediatric AHI
None	0–5	0
Mild OSA	6–20	1–5
Moderate OSA	21–40	6–10
Severe OSA	>40	>10

AHI, apnea-hypopnea index; BMI, body mass index; OSA, obstructive sleep apnea; TV, television.

[1]Items in brackets refer to pediatric patients.

Reproduced, with permission, from Gross JB, Bachenberg KL, Benumof JL, et al: Practice guidelines for the perioperative management of patients with obstructive sleep apnea: a report by the American Society of Anesthesiologists Task Force on Perioperative Management of patients with obstructive sleep apnea. Anesthesiology 2006;104:1081.

diagnose sleep apnea, many patients with OSA have never been identified as having OSA. Consequently, an anesthesiologist may be the first physician to detect the presence or risk of sleep apnea. The ASA has provided suggestions on the types of procedures and anesthetics that can safely be used in ambulatory patients with OSA (Table 44–3). In addition

to the usual discharge criteria, the ASA also recommends the following in patients with OSA:

- Return of room air oxygen saturation to baseline level

- No hypoxemic episodes or periods of airway obstruction when left alone

TABLE 44–2 Obstructive sleep apnea scoring system: example.

	Points
A. Severity of sleep apnea based on sleep study (or clinical indicators if sleep study not available). Point score _____ (0–3)[1-2]	
Severity of OSA (Table 44–1)	
None	0
Mild	1
Moderate	2
Severe	3
B. Invasiveness of surgery and anesthesia. Point score _____ (0–3)	
Type of surgery and anesthesia	
Superficial surgery under local or peripheral nerve block anesthesia without sedation	0
Superficial surgery with moderate sedation or general anesthesia	1
Peripheral surgery with spinal or epidural anesthesia (with no more than moderate sedation)	1
Peripheral surgery with general anesthesia	2
Airway surgery with moderate sedation	2
Major surgery, general anesthesia	3
Airway surgery, general anesthesia	3
C. Requirement for postoperative opioids. Point score _____ (0–3)	
Opioid requirement	
None	0
Low-dose oral opioids	1
High-dose oral opioids, parenteral or neuraxial opioids	3
D. Estimation of perioperative risk. Overall score = the score for A plus the greater of the score for either B or C. Point score _____ (0–6)[3]	

A scoring system similar to this table may be used to estimate whether a patient is at increased perioperative risk of complications from obstructive sleep apnea (OSA). This example, which has not been clinically validated, is meant only as a guide, and clinical judgment should be used to assess the risk of an individual patient.

[1]One point may be subtracted if a patient has been on continuous positive airway pressure (CPAP) or noninvasive positive-pressure ventilation (NIPPV) before surgery and will be using his or her appliance consistently during the postoperative period.

[2]One point should be added if a patient with mild or moderate OSA also has a resting arterial carbon dioxide tension ($Paco_2$) greater than 50 mm Hg.

[3]Patients with score of 4 may be at increased perioperative risk from OSA; patients with a score or 5 or 6 may be at significantly increased perioperative risk from OSA.

Reproduced, with permission, from Gross JB, Bachenberg KL, Benumof JL, et al: Practice guidelines for the perioperative management of patients with obstructive sleep apnea: a report by the American Society of Anesthesiologists Task Force on Perioperative Management of patients with obstructive sleep apnea. Anesthesiology 2006;104:1081.

TABLE 44–3 Consultant opinions regarding procedures that may be performed safely on an outpatient basis for patients at increased perioperative risk from obstructive sleep apnea.

Type of Surgery/Anesthesia	Consultant Opinion
Superficial surgery/local or regional anesthesia	Agree
Superficial surgery/general anesthesia	Equivocal
Airway surgery (adult, e.g., UPPP)	Disagree
Tonsillectomy in children less than 3 years old	Disagree
Tonsillectomy in children greater than 3 years old	Equivocal
Minor orthopedic surgery/local or regional anesthesia	Agree
Minor orthopedic surgery/general anesthesia	Equivocal
Gynecologic laparoscopy	Equivocal
Laparoscopic surgery, upper abdomen	Disagree
Lithotripsy	Agree

OSA, obstructive sleep apnea; UPPP, uvulopalatopharyngoplasty.
Reproduced, with permission, from Gross JB, Bachenberg KL, Benumof JL, et al: Practice guidelines for the perioperative management of patients with obstructive sleep apnea: a report by the American Society of Anesthesiologists Task Force on Perioperative Management of patients with obstructive sleep apnea. Anesthesiology 2006;104:1081.

- Monitoring for 3 hours longer prior to discharge than patients without OSA
- Monitoring for 7 hours following an episode of airway obstruction or hypoxemia while breathing room air in an unstimulating environment

According to the ASA Task Force on Obesity and OSA, these OSA patients can be managed safely as outpatients; however, they have an increased risk of postoperative complications requiring increased monitoring, availability of radiologic/laboratory services, and availability of continuous positive airway pressure and mechanical ventilation, thus making an office-based setting potentially inadequate for managing complications that may arise. Nonetheless, under certain conditions, anesthesia and surgery

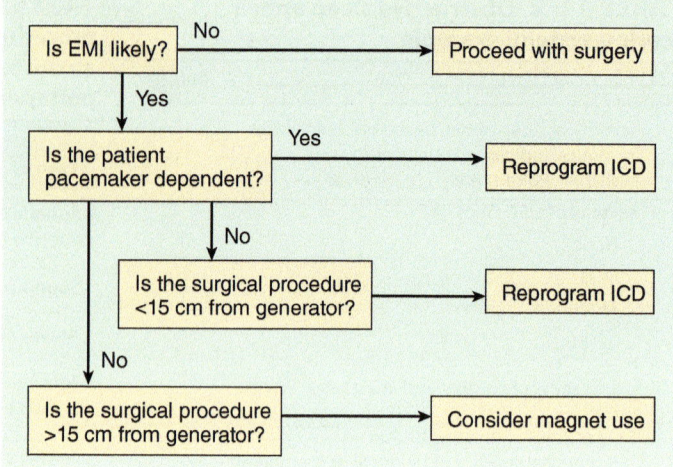

FIGURE 44–1 Preoperative considerations in a patient with an implanted cardioverter defibrillator. EMI, electromagnetic interference; ICD, implanted cardioverter defibrillator. (Reproduced, with permission, from Joshi GP: Perioperative management of outpatients with implantable cardioverter defibrillators. Curr Opin Anaesthesiol 2009;22:701.)

can be performed in an ambulatory surgery center or hospital outpatient facility.

Cardiac Conditions

Increasingly, patients present to ambulatory surgery with a variety of cardiac conditions treated both pharmacologically and mechanically (eg, cardiac resynchronization therapy, implantable cardioverter-defibrillators [ICDs], stents). It is therefore likely that anesthesia staff working in ambulatory settings will encounter increasing numbers of such patients, who, despite a cardiac history, have stable cardiac conditions. Patients previously treated with stents are likely to be on antiplatelet regimens. As always, these agents should not be discontinued unless a discussion has occurred between the patient, cardiologist, and surgeon regarding both the necessity of surgery and the discontinuation of antiplatelet therapy. Likewise, β-blockers should be continued perioperatively. Angiotensin-converting enzyme inhibitors and angiotensin receptor blockers may contribute to transient hypotension with anesthesia induction, but their continuation or discontinuation perioperatively seems to have minimal effects, as patients so treated likely will need to have intraoperative hypotension corrected in either case. The ASA guidelines recommend that patients presenting with a pacemaker or ICD should not leave a monitored setting until the device is interrogated, if electrocautery was employed; however, this ASA recommendation is controversial, as some argue that

if bipolar cautery is used at a distance of greater than 15 cm from the device, immediate interrogation of the device is not necessary prior to discharge from a monitored setting. Likewise, if an ICD is present, and there is anticipated electromagnetic interference the device's antitachycardia features should be inhibited perioperatively (see Figures 44–1 and 44–2).

Glucose Control

In a consensus statement on perioperative glucose control, the Society for Ambulatory Anesthesia found insufficient evidence to make strong recommendations about glucose management in ambulatory patients, and thus management suggestions parallel those of the inpatient population; however, the panel recommends a target intraoperative blood glucose concentration of <180 mg/dL.

Malignant Hyperthermia

Patients with a history of malignant hyperthermia can be safely given nontriggering anesthetics and discharged as ambulatory patients. Prophylactic dantrolene should not be administered.

INTRAOPERATIVE CONSIDERATIONS

Intraoperative management in the ambulatory patient undergoing surgery is aimed at providing rapid emergence, good analgesia, and minimal PONV while creating acceptable operating conditions. Often these

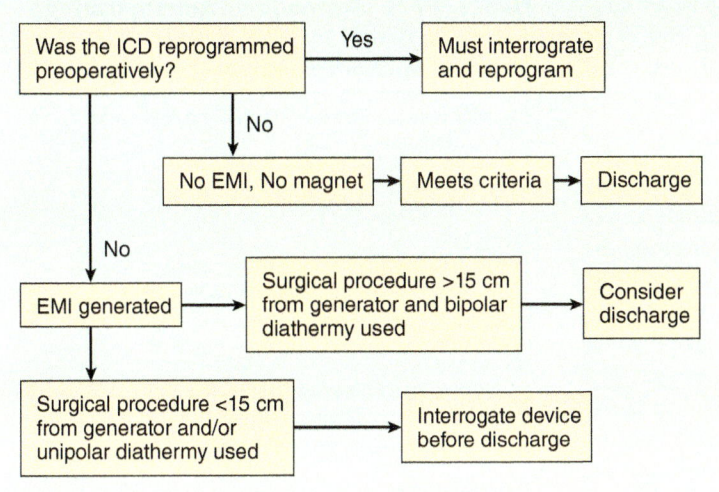

FIGURE 44–2 Postoperative considerations in a patient with an implanted cardioverter defibrillator. EMI, electromagnetic interference; ICD, implanted cardioverter defibrillator. (Reproduced, with permission, from Joshi GP: Perioperative management of outpatients with implantable cardioverter defibrillators. Curr Opin Anaesthesiol 2009;22:701.)

goals compete with one another. Although inhalational anesthesia with sevoflurane may speed emergence, compared with total intravenous anesthesia (TIVA), the likelihood of PONV may be greater, if an additional prophylactic drug is not administered. Numerous studies conducted by regional anesthesiologists have shown how regional anesthesia can speed discharge time, compared with general anesthetics, in the ambulatory population—in part, by potentially reducing the incidence of PONV. Nitrous oxide increases the likelihood of PONV, but this effect can be overcome by adding a prophylactic agent. Likewise, multimodal perioperative analgesia can be approached using a variety of drugs, including local anesthetics, acetaminophen, and nonsteroidal anti-inflammatory agents (NSAIDs) to reduce the use of opioids, which contribute to PONV risk.

Thromboembolism remains a risk after ambulatory and office-based surgery, as with inpatient surgery. Pneumatic compression devices and pharmacologic thromboprophylaxis should be used in patients at increased risk. During monitored anesthesia care, supplemental oxygen can contribute to operating room fires by creating an oxygen-rich environment that facilitates ignition by cautery devices. During head and neck surgery, anesthesia providers must be especially vigilant not to create an environment where fire becomes more likely. When oxygen is administered via a nasal cannula or face mask, the minimal amount of supplemental oxygen should be delivered, if any, and tenting of the drapes around the patient's head should be prevented.

POST ANESTHESIA RECOVERY AND DISCHARGE

Managing a patient's emergence, postoperative pain, and PONV is critical to expediting discharge. A plan to handle complications, such as postoperative pain and PONV, should be in place preoperatively to standardize and streamline management as much as possible.

The entire anesthetic experience of the ambulatory surgery patient should be focused on minimizing complications, especially postoperative pain and PONV. Multimodal approaches to both complications are advised; see Chapter 17 for a discussion of PONV management. Use of a combination of agents (eg, ondansetron, dexamethasone, and droperidol) has shown greater efficacy than monotherapy (eg, ondansetron alone) in patients at high risk of PONV. Likewise, analgesia regimens that minimize opioid use reduce PONV.

Pain management is centered on the combined use of regional techniques, opioids, and NSAIDSs (multimodal analgesia). Gabapentinoids (gabapentin, pregabalin) may have beneficial effects as part of a multimodal pain regimen. Likewise, oral, rectal, or intravenous acetaminophen or NSAIDs can be useful in the ambulatory setting. Cyclooxygenase-2 selective inhibitors have been used as part of multimodal pain management approaches, but their potential for prothrombotic effects has restricted their use.

DISCHARGE CRITERIA

Scoring systems have been devised to facilitate timely and safe PACU discharge and assess home readiness after ambulatory surgery. The Aldrete scoring system, which includes activity, respiration, circulation, consciousness, and oxygen saturation, helps guide recovery from the PACU in the ambulatory surgery unit. Scoring systems and guidelines that standardize patient discharge from the ambulatory surgery center to home are also available (see Tables 44–4, 44–5, 44–6, and 44–7).

Criteria for discharge generally require that the patient:

- Is alert and oriented to time and place
- Has stable vital signs
- Has pain controlled by oral analgesics or peripheral nerve block
- Has nausea or emesis controlled
- Is able to walk without dizziness
- Has no unexpected bleeding from the operative site
- Is able to take oral fluids and void
- Has discharge instructions and prescriptions from the surgeon and anesthesiologist
- Accepts readiness for discharge
- Has a responsible adult escort present

TABLE 44-4 Stages of recovery.

Stage of Recovery	Clinical Definition
Early recovery	Awakening and recovery of vital reflexes
Intermediate recovery	Immediate clinical recovery Home readiness
Late recovery	Full recovery Psychological recovery

Data from Steward DJ, Volgyesi G: Stabilometry: a new tool for measuring recovery following general anaesthesia. Can Anaesth Soc J 1978;25:4.

TABLE 44-5 The modified Aldrete scoring system for determining when patients are ready for discharge from the postanesthesia care unit.

Activity: able to move voluntarily or on command	
4 extremities	2
2 extremities	1
0 extremities	0
Respiration	
Able to deep breathe and cough freely	2
Dyspnea, shallow or limited breathing	1
Apneic	0
Circulation	
BP ± 20 mm of preanesthetic level	2
BP ± 20–50 mm of preanesthesia level	1
BP ± 50 mm of preanesthesia level	0
Consciousness	
Fully awake	2
Arousable on calling	1
Not responding	0
O_2 saturation	
Able to maintain O_2 saturation >92% on room air	2
Needs O_2 inhalation to maintain O_2 saturation >90%	1
O_2 saturation <90% even with O_2 supplementation	0

A score ≥9 was required for discharge.

BP, blood pressure.

Reproduced, with permission, from Aldrete AL: The post anesthesia recovery score revisited (letter). Clin Anesth 1995;7:89.

TABLE 44-6 Guidelines for safe discharge after ambulatory surgery.

Vital signs must have been stable for at least 1 h
The patient must be
Oriented to person, place, and time
Able to retain orally administered fluids
Able to void
Able to dress
Able to walk without assistance
The patient must not have
More than minimal nausea and vomiting
Excessive pain
Bleeding
The patient must be discharged by both the person who administered anaesthesia and the person who performed surgery, or by their designates. Written instructions for the postoperative period at home, including a contact place and person, must be reinforced.
The patient must have a responsible, "vested" adult escort them home and stay with them at home.

Reproduced, with permission, from Korttila K: Recovery from outpatient anaesthesia, factors affecting outcome. Anaesthesia 1995;50 (suppl)22-28.

TABLE 44–7 Postanesthesia discharge scoring system (PADS) for determining home-readiness.

Vital signs	
Vital signs must be stable and consistent with age and preoperative baseline	
BP and pulse within 20% of preoperative baseline	2
BP and pulse 20%–40% of preoperative baseline	1
BP and pulse >40% of preoperative baseline	0
Activity level	
Patient must be able to ambulate at preoperative level	
Steady gait, no dizziness, or meets preoperative level	2
Requires assistance	1
Unable to ambulate	0
Nausea and vomiting	
The patient should have minimal nausea and vomiting before discharge	
Minimal: successfully treated with PO medication	2
Moderate: successfully treated with IM medication	1
Severe: continues after repeated treatment	0
Pain	
The patient should have minimal or no pain before discharge	
The level of pain that the patient has should be acceptable to the patient	
Pain should be controllable by oral analgesics	
The location, type, and intensity of pain should be consistent with anticipated postoperative discomfort	
Acceptability	
Yes	2
No	1
Surgical bleeding	
Postoperative bleeding should be consistent with expected blood loss for the procedure	
Minimal: does not require dressing change	2
Moderate: up to two dressing changes required	1
Severe: more than three dressing changes required	0

Maximal score = 10; patients scoring ≥9 are fit for discharge.

Reproduced, with permission, from Marshall SI, Chung F: Assessment of "home readiness": discharge criteria and postdischarge complications. Curr Opin Anesthiol 1997;10:445.

Increasingly, patients are not being required to drink or void before discharge from ASCs. Such patients require plans and instructions for follow-up care to provide for possible rehydration and bladder catheterization, if required.

UNANTICIPATED HOSPITAL ADMISSION FOLLOWING AMBULATORY SURGERY

Various complications can occur that necessitate emergent transfer to a nearby hospital. Some surgical complications cannot be repaired in the ambulatory operating suite. Inadequately controlled pain and postoperative nausea and vomiting are the two most frequent causes of unplanned hospital admission from ASCs, with other causes less frequent. Accreditation agencies mandate that office based operating rooms have emergency equipment, drugs, and protocols for patient transfers. In addition to advanced cardiac life support medications, dantrolene and intravenous lipid emulsion should be available to treat malignant hyperthermia and local anesthetic-induced cardiotoxicity. Additionally, surgeons operating in an office-based practice must have admitting privileges at a nearby hospital or arrangements with an accepting physician to provide for patient transfer, if necessary in addition to a hospital transfer protocol in place. The American Association for Accreditation of Ambulatory Surgery Facilities reviewed 1,141,418 outpatient procedures from 2001 to 2006 in the facilities it accredits and noted 23 deaths. Pulmonary embolism following abdominoplasty was the leading cause of death in an office-based surgery facility (Figures 44–3 and 44–4).

NON-OPERATING ROOM ANESTHESIA

Off-site anesthesia (nonoperating room anesthesia) encompasses all sedation/anesthesia provided by anesthesiology services outside of the operating room environment. Over the past few decades, requests for these services in remote locations have been steadily increasing, and in many large hospitals today more anesthetics are routinely administered for procedures off-site than in the operating room suite. According to some estimates, nonoperating room anesthesia accounts for 12.4% of all anesthetic care in the United States. As a result, some clinical facilities have determined that is it safer and more cost-effective to assign anesthesia team(s) for

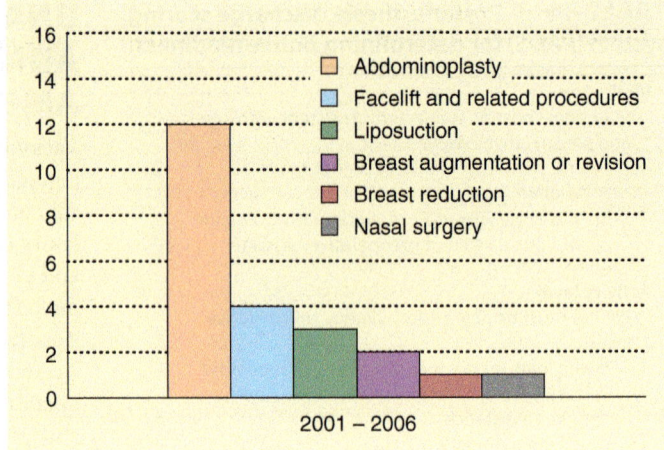

FIGURE 44–3 Bar chart showing the 23 deaths by procedure. (Reproduced, with permission, from Keyes GR, Singer R, Iverson RE, et al: Mortality in outpatient surgery. Plast Reconstr Surg 2008;122:245.)

scheduled blocks of times to provide care for such procedures, and some institutions are constructing procedural suites where bronchoscopy, gastrointestinal endoscopy, cardiac, and interventional radiology procedures can be performed in a centralized area for increased safety and efficiency. It is important to remember that the same basic standards for anesthesia care need to be met, regardless of the location. Furthermore, the challenges of unfamiliar environments that are far removed from the surgical suite, including anesthesia-naïve personnel, require advance planning for the off-site anesthesiologist.

Unlike patients undergoing office-based or ambulatory surgery center procedures, out of the operating room patients are frequently among the sickest of inpatients. Anesthesia staff are often called to work in the gastrointestinal suite, cardiac catheterization laboratory, electrophysiology laboratory, radiology suite, radiation oncology suite, and, occasionally, the critical care unit. Often these locations were constructed without anticipation that anesthesia would be provided there. Consequently, anesthesia work space is routinely constrained, and access to the patient is limited. Moreover, the procedure physicians and ancillary staff in these areas often fail to understand what is required to safely deliver anesthesia (hence the frequent request to "give them a squirt" of propofol) and do not know how to assist

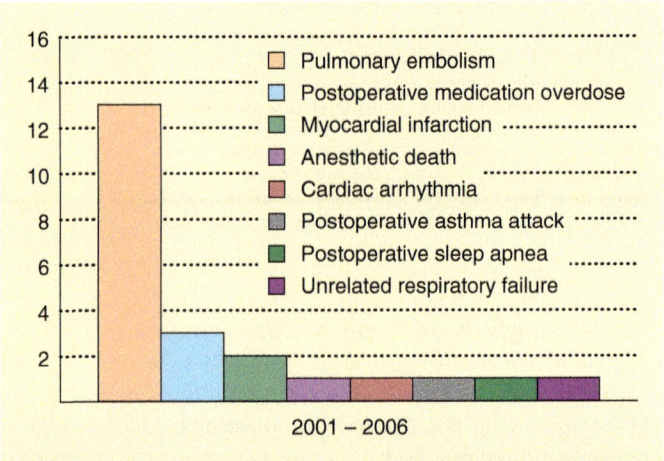

FIGURE 44–4 Bar chart showing the cause of death. (Reproduced, with permission, from Keyes GR, Singer R, Iverson RE, et al: Mortality in outpatient surgery. Plast Reconstr Surg 2008;122:245.)

TABLE 44–8 American Society of Anesthesiologists guidelines for nonoperating room anesthetizing locations.

Reliable O$_2$ source with backup	Sufficient space for anesthesia personnel, equipment
Suction apparatus	Emergency cart, defibrillator, drugs, etc.
Waste gas scavenging	Reliable means for two-way communication
Adequate monitoring equipment	Applicable facility, safety codes met
Safe electrical outlets	Appropriate post-anesthesia management
Adequate illumination, battery backup	

Data from American Society of Anesthesiologists guidelines for nonoperating room anesthetizing locations (2008). Committee of Origin: Standards and Practice Parameters (approved by the ASA House of Delegates on October 15, 2003 and amended on October 22, 2008.

TABLE 44–9 Specific conditions that warrant special care when providing anesthesia or sedation outside the operating room.

Patient unable to cooperate, e.g. severe intellectual disability
Severe gastroesophageal reflux
Medical conditions predisposing patients to reflux, e.g. gastroparesis secondary to diabetes mellitus
Orthopnea
Severe increased intracranial pressure
Decreased level of consciousness/depression of protective airway reflexes
Known difficult intubation especially when procedure is outside the operating room
Dental, oral, craniofacial, neck or thoracic abnormalities that could compromise the airway
Presence of respiratory tract infection or unexplained fever
Obstructive sleep apnea
Morbid obesity
Procedures limiting access to the airway
Lengthy, complex or painful procedures
Uncomfortable position
Prone position
Acute trauma
Extremes of age

Reproduced, with permission, from Robbertze R, Posner KL, Domino KB: Closed claims review of anesthesia for procedures outside the operating room. Curr Opin Anaesthesiol 2006;19:436.

TABLE 44–10 Personnel requirements for safe sedation and anesthesia outside the operating room.

Anesthesia staff
Trained in the clinical assessment of preanesthesia patients
Trained and experienced in airway management and cardiopulmonary resuscitation
Trained in the use of anesthetic and resuscitation drugs and equipment, and must ensure that the equipment is present and functional prior to induction
Dedicated to the continuous monitoring of the patient's physiologic parameters
Continuously present and vigilant
Nonanesthesia staff
Appropriately trained to help deal with a cardiopulmonary emergency
Assistant for the anesthesiologist—this person must be familiar with anesthetic procedures and equipment
Assistant to help with positioning
Staff trained in postprocedure observation and resuscitation

Reproduced, with permission, from Robbertze R, Posner KL, Domino KB: Closed claims review of anesthesia for procedures outside the operating room. Curr Opin Anaesthesiol 2006;19:436.

the anesthesia provider when difficulty arises. As noted in the ASA guidelines, the expectations for out of the operating room anesthesia are the same as in any practice location (Table 44–8).

Basic principles for nonoperating room anesthesia can be broadly classified into three categories: patient factors, environmental issues, and procedure-related aspects. Patient factors include comorbidity, airway assessment, fasting status, and monitoring. Environmental issues include anesthesia equipment, emergency equipment, and magnetic and radiation hazards. Procedure-related aspects include duration, level of discomfort, patient position, and surgical support.

The ASA Closed Claims Database has demonstrated that claims related to out of the operating room anesthesia care have a greater severity of injury than closed claims related to operating room anesthesia care. Monitored anesthesia care was the primary technique in more than half of the claims reviewed. Many of these closed claims arose from injuries related to inadequate oxygenation/ventilation during procedures in the gastrointestinal suite. Suggested requirements for the safe delivery of out of the operating room anesthesia are presented in Tables 44–9, 44–10, 44–11, and 44–12.

TABLE 44–11 Location/space requirements for nonoperating room anesthesia.

Adequate size with good access to the patient
Uncluttered floor space
An operating table, trolley or chair which can be readily tilted into Trendelenburg position
Adequate lighting including emergency lighting
Sufficient electrical outlets including clearly marked electrical outlets connected to an emergency back-up power source
Suitable clinical area for recovery of the patient which must include oxygen, suction, resuscitation drugs and equipment
Emergency back-up call system to summon assistance from the main operating room

Reproduced, with permission, from Robbertze R, Posner KL, Domino KB: Closed claims review of anesthesia for procedures outside the operating room. Curr Opin Anaesthesiol 2006;19:436.

TABLE 44–12 Equipment/monitoring requirements for nonoperating-room anesthesia.

Appropriate (for deep sedation, general anesthesia and a cardiorespiratory emergency)
Immediately available
Regularly serviced (service date indicated on the equipment)
Same standard as in the operating room (minimum pulse oximetry, end-tidal capnography, blood pressure, electrocardiogram, and temperature)
Alarms activated (with appropriate settings) and sufficiently audible
Airway gas with the recognized safety devices (e.g. indexed gas connection system, reserve supply of oxygen, oxygen analyzer, oxygen supply failure alarm, multiple gas analyzer, a volatile anesthetic agent monitor, a breathing system disconnection alarm and a scavenging system)
Anesthesia work cart stocked to operating-room standard (including appropriate anesthetic and resuscitation drugs, airway management equipment, a self-inflating hand resuscitator bag and a range of intravenous equipment)
Suction
Ready access to a defibrillator and a fully stocked emergency cart

Reproduced, with permission, from Robbertze R, Posner KL, Domino KB: Closed claims review of anesthesia for procedures outside the operating room. Curr Opin Anaesthesiol 2006;19:436.

Increasingly, nonanesthesia providers in the gastrointestinal lab and the emergency department provide sedation with a variety of agents, including propofol and ketamine. In fact, some reports indicate that nonanesthesia providers provide administer sedation and analgesia for almost 40% of the procedures performed in the United States. The ASA guidelines and the Joint Commission have described the continuum of depth of sedation, ranging from minimal sedation to general anesthesia (Table 44–13). Recently, the Centers for Medicare and Medicaid Services has mandated that all sedation in a hospital be under the direction of a physician—generally, the anesthesia service chief. Consequently, anesthesiologists must not only from time to time provide anesthesia in a nonoperating room setting, but must also develop policies and quality assurance review mechanisms for nonanesthesia providers to safely provide sedation. Such policies should be focused on assuring that the "sedationist" has the necessary skills to provide for patient rescue, should mild or moderate sedation become deep sedation or general anesthesia.

TABLE 44–13 Continuum of depth of sedation/analgesia/anesthesia.

Level	Type	Responsiveness	Airway	Spontaneous Ventilation	Cardiovascular Function
1	Minimal	Normal to verbal stimulation	Unaffected	Unaffected	Unaffected
2	Moderate	Purposeful response to verbal or tactile stimulation	No intervention required	Adequate	Usually maintained
3	Deep	Purposeful after repeated or painful stimulus	Intervention may be required	May be inadequate	Usually maintained
4	General Anesthesia	Unarousable to painful stimulus	Intervention often required	Often inadequate	May be impaired

Data from American Society of Anesthesiologists.

TABLE 44–14 Complications associated with sedation and analgesia.

Airway
Airway obstruction
Aspiration
Regurgitation
Dental/soft tissue injury

Respiratory
Respiratory depression
Hypoxemia
Hypercarbia
Apnea

Cardiovascular
Hypotension
Cardiac arrhythmias

Neurologic
Deeper level of sedation
Unresponsiveness

Other
Undesirable patient movement
Drug interactions
Adverse reactions
Unanticipated admission

Data from American Society of Anesthesiologists.

TABLE 44–15 Common locations for nonoperating room anesthesia.

- Radiology
  - Neurointerventional Radiology
  - Vascular Radiology
  - MRI/CT
  - PET Scan
- Endoscopy Suite
  - Gastrointestinal Suite
  - Bronchoscopy
- Intensive Care Unit
  - Tracheostomy, Percutaneous gastrostomy
  - Intracranial and other catheter placement
  - Abdominal/pelvic explorations
- Invasive Cardiology Suite
  - Cardiac Catheterization Lab
  - Cardioversion
  - Electrophysiology Suite
- Radiation Therapy
- Emergency Medicine Suite
- Psychiatry
  - Electroconvulsive Therapy suite
- Urology - Lithotripsy
- Dental Surgery

Data from American Society of Anesthesiologists.

Risks associated with sedation/analgesia are highlighted in Table 44–14. Sedation providers should know how to reverse benzodiazepines and opioids and provide bag/mask airway support and to be facile in the use of airway adjuvants. A mechanism to ensure the timely arrival of anesthesia personnel capable of airway rescue must likewise be incorporated into such policies.

SPECIAL CONSIDERATIONS IN OUT OF THE OPERATING ROOM LOCATIONS

Anesthesia services are requested at various locations throughout the hospital facility; some of these are delineated in Table 44–15. As noted throughout this chapter, routine anesthetic standards apply wherever the patient is anesthetized. Out of the operating room patients often present with a wide range of illnesses, unlike the elective patients generally found in an ambulatory setting. Furthermore,

disposition postprocedure (whether discharge or admission), needs appropriate coordination by the anesthesiologist for postanesthesia care and/or safe transport from the remote unit.

Patients presenting to the gastrointestinal endoscopy suite include healthy individuals for routine diagnostic screenings, as well as patients with fulminant cholangitis and sepsis or coexisting difficult airways. As always, the patient's condition, as well as the specific diagnostic/therapeutic procedure, determines both the anesthetic techniques (propofol deep sedation or general anesthesia vs. general anesthesia with LMA or endotracheal tube) and the monitoring required.

General anesthesia is usually required in patients undergoing endoscopic procedures for airway and pulmonary pathology; an added complexity may include the presence of a shared airway, and, in many patients, marginal pulmonary status.

Patients undergoing cardiac catheterization are routinely sedated by cardiologists without involvement of an anesthesiologist. Occasionally, a patient with significant comorbidities, (eg, morbid obesity) requires the presence of a qualified anesthesia provider. General anesthesia is often required for placement of aortic stents, which are increasingly being performed by cardiologists in the cardiac catheterization laboratory. Anesthesia staff should be prepared with arterial pressure monitoring and the necessary vascular access to facilitate resuscitation, should emergent open aneurysm repair be required.

Patients requiring electrophysiology procedures for catheter-mediated arrhythmia ablation often need general anesthesia. Such patients frequently have both systolic and diastolic heart failure, leading to potential hemodynamic difficulties perioperatively. Sudden hypotension can herald the development of pericardial tamponade secondary to catheter perforation of the heart. Other patients require sedation for the placement of ICDs. Once placed, the device will be tested by inducing ventricular fibrillation. During testing, deeper levels of sedation are required, as the defibrillation shock can be frightening and very uncomfortable. Likewise, anesthesia staff are called upon to provide anesthesia for cardioversion of patients in atrial fibrillation. These patients usually have associated cardiac diseases and require brief intravenous anesthetics to facilitate cardioversion. Oftentimes, a transesophageal echocardiogram must be performed prior to cardioversion to rule out clot in the left atrial appendage. In such cases, anesthesia staff may also provide sedation for this procedure. Determination as to whether a patient needs sedation or general anesthesia with or without intubation is dependent upon routine patient assessment.

Children and some adults (ie, those that are claustrophobic, developmentally disabled, or have conditions that prevent them to be still or to lie flat) require anesthesia or sedation for MRI and computed tomography (CT). Additionally, painful CT-guided biopsies may require anesthesia management. Anesthetic technique is dependent upon patient comorbidities.

MRI creates numerous problems for anesthesia staff. First, all ferromagnetic materials must be excluded from the area of the magnet. Most institutions have policies and training protocols to prevent

catastrophes (eg, oxygen tanks flying into the scanner). Second, all anesthetic equipment must be compatible with the magnet in use. Third, patients must be free of implants that could interact with the magnet, such as pacemakers, vascular clips, ICDs, and infusion pumps. As with all out of the operating room anesthesia, the exact choice of technique is dependent upon the patient's comorbidities. Both deep sedation and general anesthesia approaches with intubation or supraglottic airways can be used, depending on practitioner preference and patient requirements.

Patients usually require general anesthesia and tight blood pressure control to facilitate coiling and embolization of cerebral aneurysms or arteriovenous malformations. Patients taken to the radiology suite for relief of portal hypertension via creation of a transjugular intrahepatic portosystemic shunt (TIPS) are frequently hypovolemic, despite profound ascites, and at risk of esophageal variceal bleeding and aspiration. General anesthesia with intubation is preferred for management of the TIPS procedure.

Anesthesia for electroconvulsive therapy is often provided in a separate suite in the Psychiatry Unit or a monitored area in the hospital (eg, PACU). Patient comorbidity, drug interactions with various psychotropic medications, multiple anesthetic procedures, and effects of anesthetic agents on the quality of electroconvulsive therapy also need to be taken into account.

Anesthesia staff are at times called to provide anesthesia in the intensive care unit (ICU) for bedside tracheostomy or emergent chest and abdominal exploration in patients considered too critically ill to tolerate transport to the operating room. In most of these cases, the anesthesia staff generally employ ICU ventilator and monitors. Intravenous agents are typically used along with muscle relaxants. When performing anesthesia for bedside tracheostomy, it is important that the endotracheal tube not be withdrawn from the trachea until end tidal CO_2 is measured from the newly placed tracheostomy tube.

Pediatric patients deserve special mention; the (Table 44–16). Anesthesia considerations for nonoperating room anesthesia are summarized in Table 44–17.

TABLE 44–16 Goals of sedation in pediatric patients for diagnostic and therapeutic procedures.

Guard the patient's safety and welfare
Minimize physical discomfort and pain
Control anxiety, minimize psychological trauma, and maximize potential for amnesia
Control behavior and/or movement to allow safe completion of procedure
Return patient to a state in which safe discharge from medical supervision is possible

Data from American Society of Anesthesiologists.

TABLE 44–17 Basic considerations for nonoperating room anesthesia.

Patient
- ASA status, co-morbidity, emergent/elective
- Airway assessment
- Allergies – contrast
- Anesthesia plan – sedation/anesthesia
- Monitoring –
  - Basic/Standard: oxygenation, ventilation, circulation, temperature
  - Advanced: invasive hemodynamic, TEE, BIS

Environment
- Anesthesia equipment
- Anesthesia monitors
- Suction
- Resuscitation equipment
- Personnel
- Technical equipment
- Radiation hazard
- Magnetic fields
- Ambient temperature
- Warming blanket
- Portable transport monitors
- Oxygen cylinders

Procedure
- Diagnostic or therapeutic
- Duration
- Level of discomfort/pain
- Patient position
- Special requirements, e.g. monitoring
- Potential complications
- Surgical support

Data from American Society of Anesthesiologists.

CASE DISCUSSION

Acute Hypoxia after TIPS Procedure in the Radiology Suite

A 58-year-old Caucasian female with decompensated cryptogenic cirrhosis and refractory ascites, currently on the liver transplant list, is scheduled for an urgent TIPS procedure.

What does a TIPS procedure entail? What are its indications and contraindications?

TIPS (transjugular intrahepatic portosystemic shunt) involves the passage of a catheter, usually inserted through the internal jugular vein and directed into the liver, which creates a low-resistance conduit between a portal vein and a hepatic vein by deployment of an intrahepatic expandable stent. Hemodynamically, this allows immediate decompression of portal hypertension by partial or complete diversion of portal flow from hepatic sinusoids into the inferior vena cava and the systemic circulation.

Indications for the TIPS procedure include: variceal bleeding not controlled by endoscopic or medical therapy, intractable ascites, hepatic hydrothorax, Budd–Chiari syndrome, hepatorenal syndrome and hepatopulmonary syndrome, and bridge to liver transplantation. Some contraindications of TIPS are: primary prevention of variceal hemorrhage, congestive heart failure, severe pulmonary hypertension and tricuspid regurgitation, severe hepatic failure, hepatocellular carcinoma, active intrahepatic or systemic infection, and severe coagulopathy or thrombocytopenia.

What are the anesthetic strategies for TIPS? What are some preoperative and intraoperative concerns in these patients?

TIPS can be performed under moderate sedation, monitored anesthesia care, or general anesthesia. Given the usual need for long immobilization, potential risk of aspiration, and significant comorbidity, general anesthesia is often the recommended anesthetic plan.

Preoperative considerations include: risk of aspiration, gastrointestinal bleeding, decreased functional residual capacity from ascites, pleural effusions, coagulopathy, thrombocytopenia, and hepatic encephalopathy. Special intraoperative considerations should include careful hemodynamic monitoring (usually via arterial catheter), frequent performance of blood gases for electrolyte abnormalities and coagulation parameters, and testing to determine blood glucose and urine output levels. Altered pharmacokinetics of anesthetic agents should also be kept in mind.

Following informed consent and plan for general anesthesia, the patient is induced with etomidate, fentanyl, and succinylcholine, using rapid sequence induction; atraumatic intubation is accomplished uneventfully. Prior to placement of the TIPS, the radiologist evacuates approximately 8 L of ascitic fluid.

What are your concerns about this paracentesis? How would you balance these hemodynamic fluid shifts?

Large volume paracentesis is believed to be a relatively safe and effective procedure; however, it can lead to paracentesis-induced circulatory dysfunction (PICD), a frequently occurring silent complication. PICD is characterized by a marked activation of the renin–angiotensin axis, as well as accentuation of an already established arteriolar vasodilatation that may be combated with salt-free albumin as the plasma expander of choice, especially if at least 8 L are evacuated.

The TIPS procedure lasts about 2 hours; the patient is reversed appropriately with neostigmine and glycopyrrolate. She emerges smoothly and is transferred to the PACU on oxygen via a face mask at 6 L/min. Within 15 min of admission to the PACU, the patient complains of mild chest pain and shortness of breath. Bilateral wheezing is noted, followed by crackles at the bases.

What are some complications of TIPS procedure? How would you attempt to manage this patient?

Complications following TIPS are not insignificant; 3-month mortality has been reported to be approximately 32% to 45%. Complications can be broadly categorized as being associated with the anesthesia, patient comorbidity, and procedure. Patient- and anesthesia-related factors are similar to the ones described in the previous section. With regard to procedure-related factors, special note should be made of cardiopulmonary consequences resulting from a sudden increase in pulmonary artery pressures and systemic pressures, leading to pulmonary congestion.

GUIDELINES

Joshi G, Chung F, Vann M, et al: Society for Ambulatory Anesthesia consensus statement on perioperative blood glucose management in diabetic patients undergoing ambulatory surgery. Anesth Analg 2010;111:1378.

Lipp A, Hernon J: Day surgery guidelines. Surgery 2008;26:374.

Report by the American Society of Anesthesiologists Task Force on Perioperative Management of Patients with Obstructive Sleep Apnea. Practice guidelines for the perioperative management of patients with obstructive sleep apnea. Anesthesiology 2006;104:1081.

SUGGESTED READING

Chung S, Yuan H, Chung F: A systemic review of obstructive sleep apnea and its implications for anesthesiologists. Anesth Analg 2008;107:1543.

Desai M: Office based anesthesia: new frontiers, better outcomes, and emphasis on safety. Curr Opin Anaesthesiol 2008;21:699.

Elvir-Lazo O, White P: The role of multimodal analgesia in pain management after ambulatory surgery. Curr Opin Anesthesiol 2010;23:697.

Evron S, Tiberiu E: Organizational prerequisites for anesthesia outside of the operating room. Curr Opin Anaesthesiol 2009;22:514.

Joshi G: Perioperative management of outpatients with implantable cardioverter defibrillators. Curr Opin Anaesthesiol 2009;22:701.

Keyes G, Singer R, Iverson R, et al: Mortality in outpatient surgery. Plast Reconstr Surg 2008;122:245.

Kurrek M, Twersky R: Office based anesthesia. Can J Anesth 2010;57:256.

Lalwani K: Demographics and trends in nonoperating room anesthesia. Curr Opin Anaesthesiol 2006;19:430.

Marshall S, Chung F: Discharge criteria and complications after ambulatory surgery. Anesth Analg 1999;88:508.

Melloni C: Anesthesia and sedation outside the operating room: how to prevent risk and maintain good quality. Curr Opin Anaesthesiol 2007;20:513.

Metzner J, Domino K: Risks of anesthesia or sedation outside the operating room: the role of the anesthesia care provider. Curr Opin Anaesthesiol 2010;23:523.

Metzner J, Posner KL, Domino KB: The risk and safety of anesthesia at remote locations: the US closed claims analysis. Curr Opin Anaesthesiol 2009;22:502.

Owen AR, Stanley AJ, Vijayananthan A, Moss JG: The transjugular intrahepatic portosystemic shunt (TIPS). Clin Radiol 2009;64:664.

Robbertze R, Posner K, Domino K: Closed claims review of anesthesia for procedures outside of the operating room. Curr Opin Anaesthesiol 2006;19:436.

Schug S, Chong C: Pain management after ambulatory surgery. Curr Opin Anaesthesiol 2009;22:738.

Smith I, Jackson I: Beta blockers, calcium channel blockers, angiotensin converting enzyme inhibitors and angiotensin receptor blockers: should they be stopped or not before ambulatory anaesthesia? Curr Opin Anesthesiol 2010;23:687.

Souter KJ: Anesthesia provided at alternate sites. In: Barash PG, Cullen BF, Stoelting RK, Cahalan MK, Stock MC (eds). *Clinical Anesthesia*. Philadelphia: Lippincott, Williams & Wilkins, 2009; p 861.

Squizzato A, Venco A: Thromboprophylaxis in day surgery. Int J Surg 2008;8:S29.

White P, Tang J, Wender R, et al: The effects of oral ibuprofen and celecoxib in preventing pain, improving recovery outcomes and patient satisfaction after ambulatory surgery. Anesth Analg 2011;112:323.

Spinal, Epidural, & Caudal Blocks

KEY CONCEPTS

1 Neuraxial anesthesia greatly expands the anesthesiologists' armamentarium, providing alternatives to general anesthesia when appropriate. Neuraxial anesthesia may also be used simultaneously with general anesthesia or afterward for postoperative analgesia. Neuraxial blocks can be performed as a single injection or with a catheter to allow intermittent boluses or continuous infusions.

2 Performing a lumbar (subarachnoid) spinal puncture below L1 in an adult (L3 in a child) usually avoids potential needle trauma to the cord.

3 The mechanisms of spinal and epidural anesthesia remain speculative. The principal site of action for neuraxial blockade is believed to be the nerve root.

4 Differential blockade typically results in sympathetic blockade (judged by temperature sensitivity) that may be two segments or more cephalad than the sensory block (pain, light touch), which, in turn, is usually several segments more cephalad than the motor blockade.

5 Interruption of efferent autonomic transmission at the spinal nerve roots during neuraxial blocks produces sympathetic blockade.

6 Neuraxial blocks typically produce variable decreases in blood pressure that may be accompanied by a decrease in heart rate.

7 Deleterious cardiovascular effects should be anticipated and steps undertaken to minimize the degree of hypotension. However, volume loading with 10–20 mL/kg of intravenous fluid in a healthy patient before initiation of the block has been shown repeatedly to fail to prevent hypotension (in the absence of preexisting hypovolemia).

8 Excessive or symptomatic bradycardia should be treated with atropine, and hypotension should be treated with vasopressors.

9 Major contraindications to neuraxial anesthesia include patient refusal, bleeding diathesis, severe hypovolemia, elevated intracranial pressure, and infection at the site of injection.

10 For epidural anesthesia, a sudden loss of resistance (to injection of air or saline) is encountered as the needle passes through

—Continued next page

Continued—

the ligamentum flavum and enters the epidural space. For spinal anesthesia, the needle is advanced through the epidural space and penetrates the dura–subarachnoid membranes, as signaled by freely flowing cerebrospinal fluid.

11 Continuous epidural anesthesia is a neuraxial technique offering a range of applications wider than the typical all-or-nothing, single dose spinal anesthetic. An epidural block can be performed at the lumbar, thoracic, or cervical level.

12 Epidural techniques are widely used for surgical anesthesia, obstetric analgesia,

postoperative pain control, and chronic pain management.

13 Epidural anesthesia is slower in onset (10–20 min) and may not be as dense as spinal anesthesia.

14 The quantity (volume and concentration) of local anesthetic needed for epidural anesthesia is larger than that needed for spinal anesthesia. Toxic side effects are likely if a "full epidural dose" is injected intrathecally or intravascularly.

15 Caudal epidural anesthesia is a common regional technique in pediatric patients.

Spinal, caudal, and epidural blocks were first used for surgical procedures at the turn of the twentieth century. These central blocks were widely used worldwide until reports of permanent neurological injury appeared, most prominently in the United Kingdom. However, a large-scale epidemiological study conducted in the 1950s indicated that complications were rare when these blocks were performed skillfully, with attention to asepsis, and when newer, safer local anesthetics were used. Today, neuraxial blocks are widely used for labor analgesia, caesarian section, orthopedic procedures, perioperative analgesia, and chronic pain management. However, they are still associated with various complications, and much literature has examined the incidence of complications following neuraxial blocks associated with different disease states. Additionally, various organizations continue to issue "guidelines" related to the management of regional anesthesia.

1 Neuraxial anesthesia greatly expands the anesthesiologists' armamentarium, providing alternatives to general anesthesia when appropriate. Neuraxial anesthesia may be used simultaneously with general anesthesia or afterward for postoperative analgesia. Neuraxial blocks can be performed as a single injection or with a catheter to allow intermittent boluses or continuous infusions.

Neuraxial techniques have proved to be safe when well managed; however, there is still a risk of complications. Adverse reactions and complications range from self-limited back soreness to debilitating permanent neurological deficits and even death. The practitioner must therefore have a good understanding of the anatomy involved, be thoroughly familiar with the pharmacology and toxic dosages of the agents employed, diligently employ sterile techniques, and anticipate and quickly treat physiological derangements.

THE ROLE OF NEURAXIAL ANESTHESIA IN ANESTHETIC PRACTICE

Almost all operations at or below the neck have been performed under neuraxial anesthesia. Indeed, cardiac and thoracic surgeries have been performed in this manner. However, because intrathoracic, upper abdominal, and laparoscopic operations can significantly impair ventilation, general anesthesia with endotracheal intubation is usually necessary. So why perform a regional anesthetic for these cases, or for any other?

Some studies suggest that postoperative morbidity—and possibly mortality—may be reduced when neuraxial blockade is used either alone or in combination with general anesthesia. Neuraxial blocks may reduce the incidence of venous thrombosis and pulmonary embolism, cardiac complications in high-risk patients, bleeding and transfusion requirements, vascular graft occlusion, and pneumonia and respiratory depression following upper abdominal or thoracic surgery in patients with chronic lung disease. Neuraxial blocks may also allow earlier return of gastrointestinal function following surgery. Proposed mechanisms (in addition to avoidance of larger doses of anesthetics and opioids) include amelioration of the hypercoagulable state associated with surgery, sympathectomy-mediated increases in tissue blood flow, improved oxygenation from decreased splinting, enhanced peristalsis, and suppression of the neuroendocrine stress response to surgery. In patients with coronary artery disease, a decreased stress response may result in less perioperative ischemia and reduced morbidity and mortality. Reduction of parenteral opioid requirements may decrease the incidence of atelectasis, hypoventilation, and aspiration pneumonia and reduce the duration of ileus. Postoperative epidural analgesia may also significantly reduce both the time until extubation and the need for mechanical ventilation after major abdominal or thoracic surgery. Regional anesthesia may also preserve immunity perioperatively, reducing the risk of cancer spread according to some studies.

The Sick Elderly Patient

Anesthesiologists are all too familiar with situations in which a consultant "clears" a sick elderly patient with significant cardiac disease for surgery "under spinal anesthesia." But, is a spinal anesthetic really safer than general anesthesia in such a patient? A spinal anesthetic with no intravenous sedation may reduce the likelihood of postoperative delirium or cognitive dysfunction, which is sometimes seen in the elderly. Unfortunately, some, if not most, patients require some sedation during

the course of the procedure, either for comfort or to facilitate cooperation. Is spinal anesthesia always safer in a patient with severe coronary artery disease or a decreased ejection fraction? Ideally, an anesthetic technique in such a patient should not produce either hypotension (which decreases myocardial perfusion pressure) or hypertension and tachycardia (which increase myocardial oxygen consumption), and, also, should not require large fluid infusions (which can precipitate congestive heart failure). Spinal anesthesia can produce both hypotension and bradycardia, which may be rapid in onset and are sometimes profound. Moreover, treatment that includes rapid administration of intravenous fluid can cause fluid overload (when the vasodilatation wears off). The slower onset of hemodynamic responses to epidural anesthesia may give the anesthesiologist more time to correct these changes. General anesthesia, on the other hand, also poses potential problems for patients with cardiac compromise. Most general anesthetics are cardiac depressants, and many cause vasodilatation. Deep anesthesia can readily cause hypotension, whereas light anesthesia relative to the level of stimulation causes hypertension and tachycardia. Insertion of a laryngeal mask airway causes less of a stress response than does endotracheal intubation, but deeper levels of general anesthesia are still required to blunt the response to surgical stimulation.

Thus, arguments can be made for and against neuraxial and regional anesthesia in this setting. Perhaps then it is not the technique, *per se*, that is critical as much as the careful execution with appropriate monitoring and management of whatever anesthetic technique is planned.

The Obstetric Patient

Neuraxial anesthesia has had a great impact in obstetrics. Currently, epidural anesthesia is widely used for analgesia in women in labor and during vaginal delivery. Cesarean section is most commonly performed under epidural or spinal anesthesia. Both blocks allow a mother to remain awake and experience the birth of her child. Large population studies in Great Britain and the United States have shown that regional anesthesia for cesarean section is associated with less maternal morbidity and mortality than is general anesthesia. This may be largely due to a reduction in the incidence of pulmonary aspiration and failed intubation when neuraxial anesthesia is employed. Fortunately, the increased availability of video laryngoscopes may also reduce the incidence of adverse outcomes related to airway difficulties associated with general anesthesia for cesarean section.

Anatomy

THE VERTEBRAL COLUMN

The spine is composed of the vertebral bones and intervertebral disks (Figure 45–1). There are 7 cervical (C), 12 thoracic (T), and 5 lumbar (L) vertebrae (Figure 45–2). The sacrum is a fusion of 5 sacral (S)

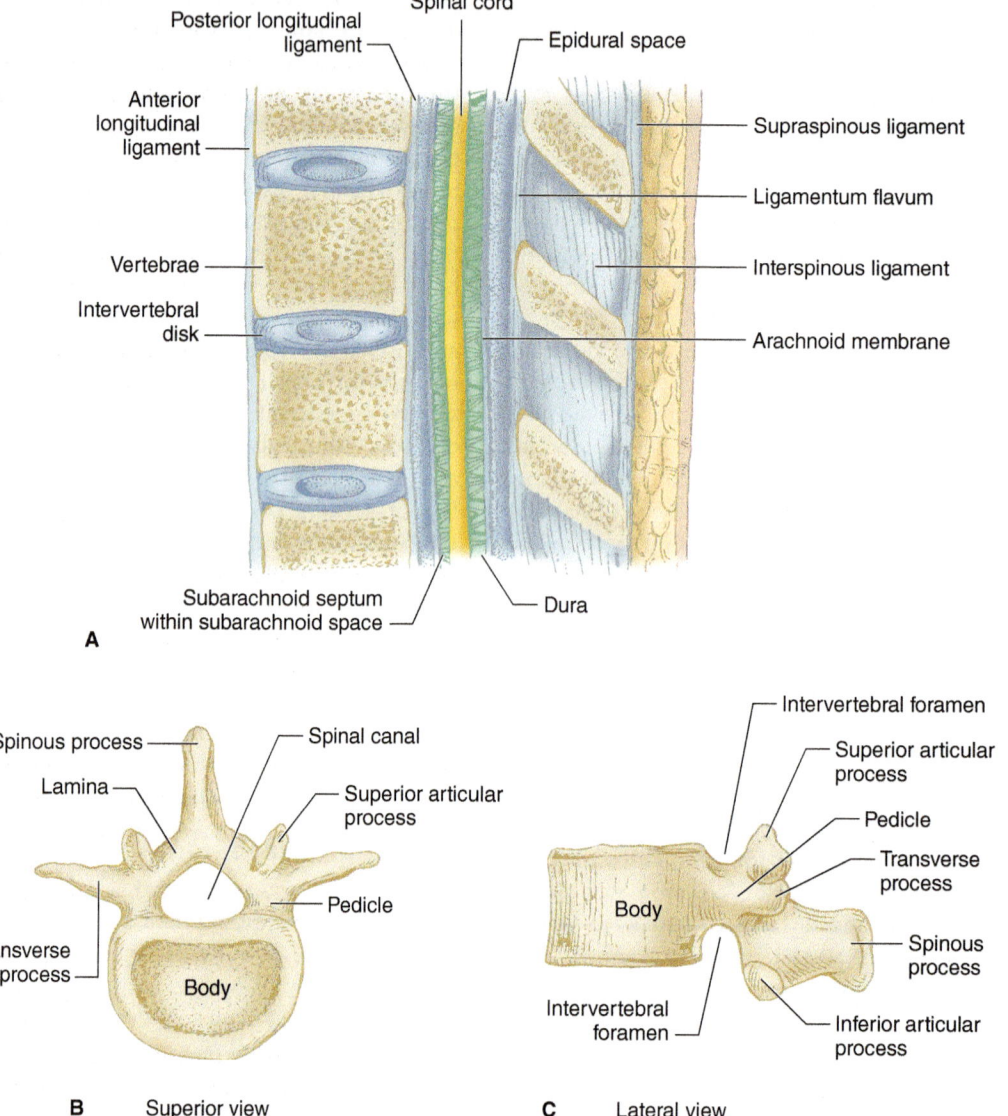

FIGURE 45–1 A: Sagittal section through lumbar vertebrae. B, C: Common features of vertebrae.

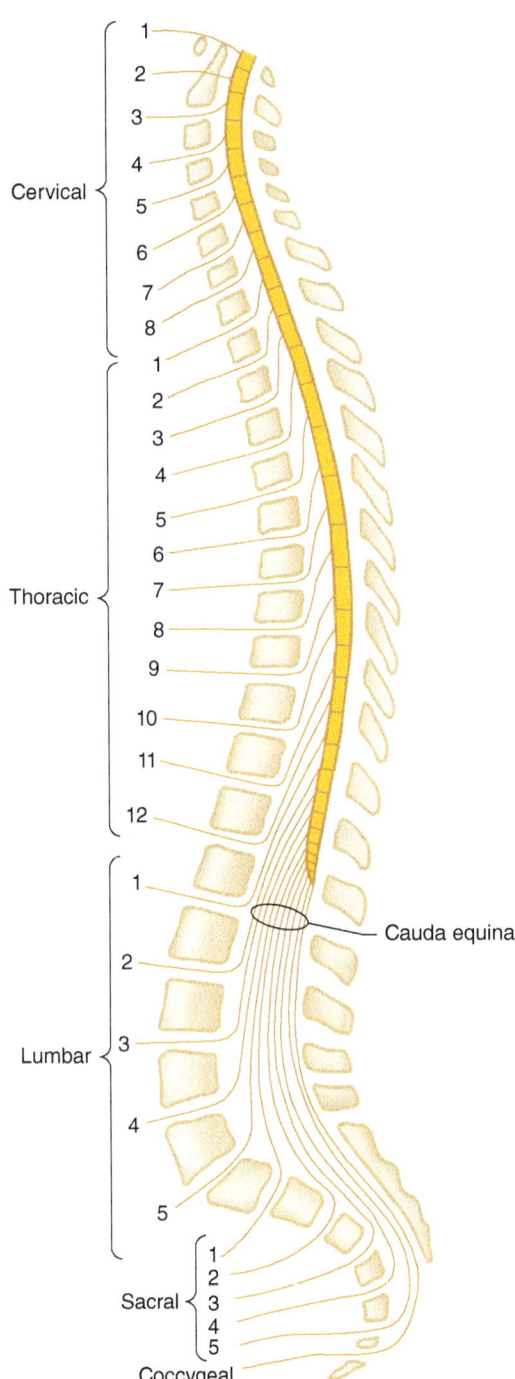

FIGURE 45–2 The vertebral column. (Adapted and reproduced, with permission, from Waxman SG: *Correlative Neuroanatomy*, 24th ed. McGraw-Hill, 2000.)

Cervical
1
2
3
4
5
6
7
8

Thoracic
1
2
3
4
5
6
7
8
9
10
11
12

Lumbar
1
2
3
4
5

Sacral
1
2
3
4
5

Coccygeal

Cauda equina

vertebrae, and there are small rudimentary coccygeal vertebrae. The spine as a whole provides structural support for the body and protection for the spinal cord and nerves and allows a degree of mobility in several spatial planes. At each vertebral level, paired spinal nerves exit the central nervous system (Figure 45–2).

Vertebrae differ in shape and size at the various levels. The first cervical vertebra, the atlas, lacks a body and has unique articulations with the base of the skull and the second vertebra. The second vertebra, called the axis, consequently has atypical articulating surfaces. All 12 thoracic vertebrae articulate with their corresponding rib. Lumbar vertebrae have a large anterior cylindrical vertebral body. A hollow ring is defined anteriorly by the vertebral body, laterally by the pedicles and transverse processes, and posteriorly by the lamina and spinous processes (Figure 45–1B and C). The laminae extend between the transverse processes and the spinous processes, and the pedicle extends between the vertebral body and the transverse processes. When stacked vertically, the hollow rings become the spinal canal in which the spinal cord and its coverings sit. The individual vertebral bodies are connected by the intervertebral disks. There are four small synovial joints at each vertebra, two articulating with the vertebra above it and two with the vertebra below. These are the facet joints, which are adjacent to the transverse processes (Figure 45–1C). The pedicles are notched superiorly and inferiorly, these notches forming the intervertebral foramina from which the spinal nerves exit. Sacral vertebrae normally fuse into one large bone, the sacrum, but each one retains discrete anterior and posterior intervertebral foramina. The laminae of S5 and all or part of S4 normally do not fuse, leaving a caudal opening to the spinal canal, the sacral hiatus (**Figure 45–3**).

The spinal column normally forms a double C, being convex anteriorly in the cervical and lumbar regions (Figure 45–2). Ligamentous elements provide structural support, and, together with supporting muscles, help to maintain the unique shape. Ventrally, the vertebral bodies and intervertebral disks are connected and supported by the anterior and posterior longitudinal ligaments (Figure 45–1A). Dorsally, the ligamentum flavum,

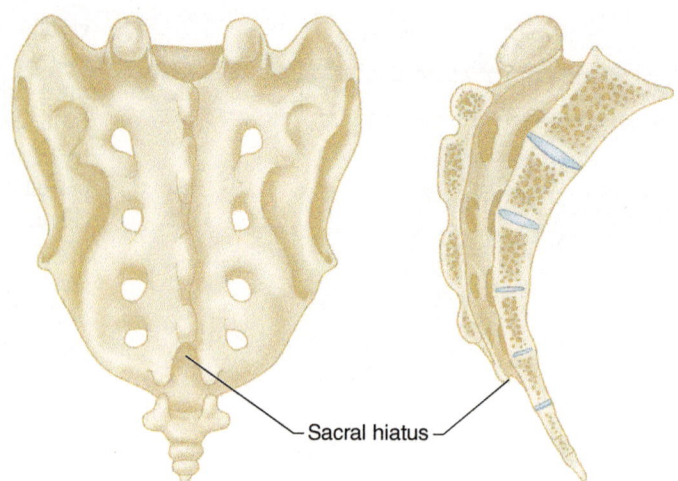

FIGURE 45–3 Posterior and sagittal views of the sacrum and coccyx.

interspinous ligament, and supraspinous ligament provide additional stability. Using the midline approach, a needle passes through these three dorsal ligaments and through an oval space between the bony lamina and spinous processes of adjacent vertebra (Figure 45–4).

THE SPINAL CORD

The spinal canal contains the spinal cord with its coverings (the meninges), fatty tissue, and a venous plexus (Figure 45–5). The meninges are composed of three layers: the pia mater, the arachnoid mater,

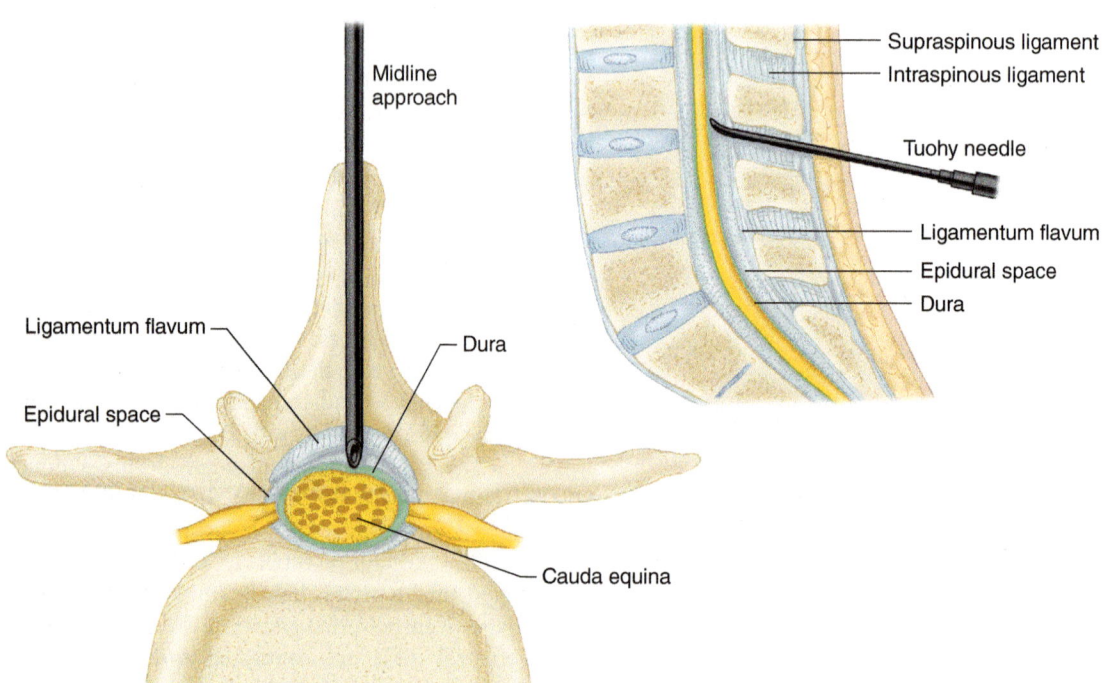

FIGURE 45–4 Lumbar epidural anesthesia; midline approach.

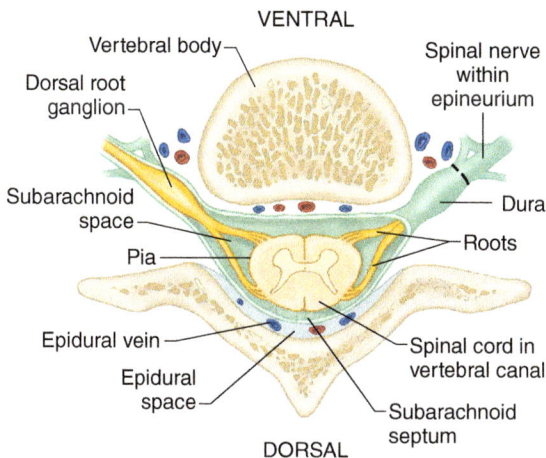

FIGURE 45–5 Exit of the spinal nerves. (Adapted and reproduced, with permission, from Waxman SG: *Correlative Neuroanatomy,* 24th ed. McGraw-Hill, 2000.)

and the dura mater; all are contiguous with their cranial counterparts (Figure 45–6). The pia mater is closely adherent to the spinal cord, whereas the arachnoid mater is usually closely adherent to the thicker and denser dura mater. Cerebrospinal fluid (CSF) is contained between the pia and arachnoid maters in the subarachnoid space. The spinal subdural space is generally a poorly demarcated, potential space that exists between the dura and arachnoid membranes. The epidural space is a better defined potential space within the spinal canal that is bounded by the dura and the ligamentum flavum (Figures 45–1 and 45–5).

The spinal cord normally extends from the foramen magnum to the level of L1 in adults (Figure 45–7). In children, the spinal cord ends at L3 and moves up with age. The anterior and posterior nerve roots at each spinal level join one another and exit the intervertebral foramina, forming spinal nerves from C1 to S5 (Figure 45–2). At the cervical level, the nerves arise above their respective vertebrae, but starting at T1, exit below their vertebrae. As a result, there are eight cervical nerve roots, but only seven cervical vertebrae. The cervical and upper thoracic nerve roots emerge from the spinal cord and exit the vertebral foramina nearly at the same level (Figure 45–2). But, because the spinal cord normally ends at L1, lower nerve roots course some

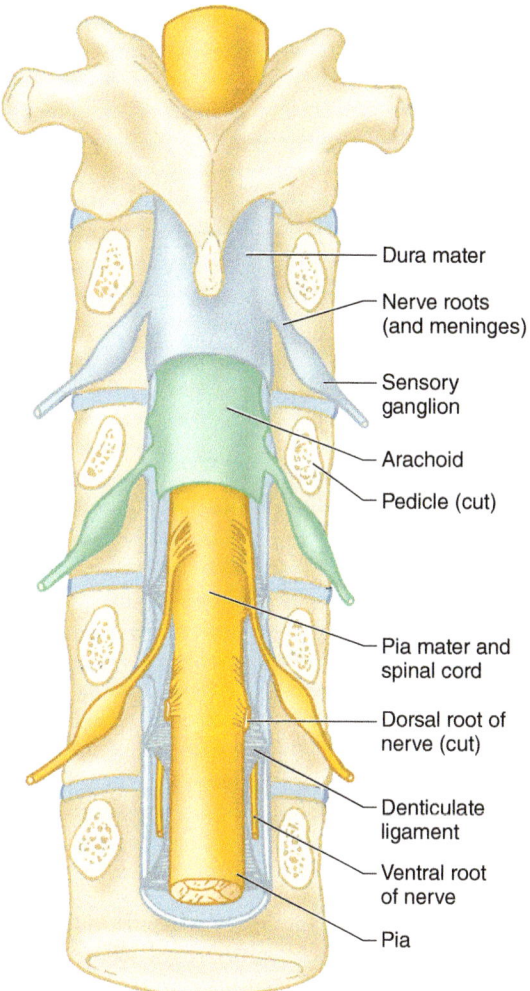

FIGURE 45–6 The spinal cord.

distance before exiting the intervertebral foramina. These lower spinal nerves form the *cauda equina* ("horse's tail"; Figure 45–2). Therefore, performing a lumbar (subarachnoid) puncture below L1 in an adult (L3 in a child) usually avoids potential needle trauma to the cord; damage to the *cauda equina* is unlikely, as these nerve roots float in the dural sac below L1 and tend to be pushed away (rather than pierced) by an advancing needle.

A dural sheath invests most nerve roots for a small distance, even after they exit the spinal canal (Figure 45–5). Nerve blocks close to the

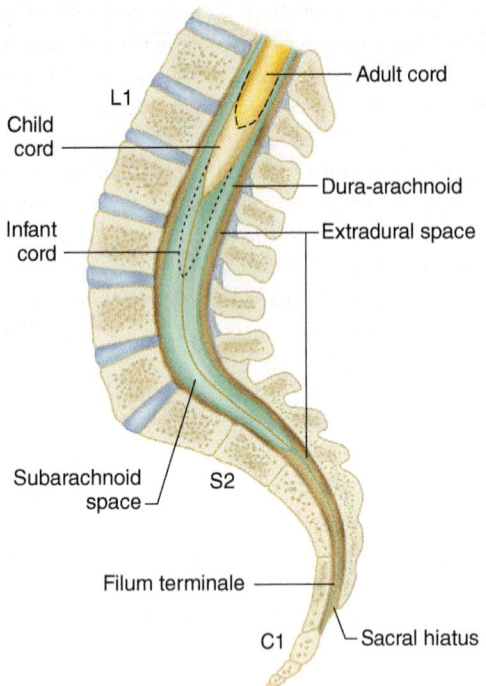

FIGURE 45–7 Sagittal view through the lumbar vertebrae and sacrum. Note the end of the spinal cord rises with development from approximately L3 to L1. The dural sac normally ends at S2.

intervertebral foramen therefore carry a risk of subdural or subarachnoid injection. The dural sac and the subarachnoid and subdural spaces usually extend to S2 in adults and often to S3 in children. Because of this fact and the smaller body size, caudal anesthesia carries a greater risk of subarachnoid injection in children than in adults. An extension of the pia mater, the filum terminale, penetrates the dura and attaches the terminal end of the spinal cord (conus medullaris) to the periosteum of the coccyx (Figure 45–7).

The blood supply to the spinal cord and nerve roots is derived from a single anterior spinal artery and paired posterior spinal arteries (Figure 45–8). The anterior spinal artery is formed from the vertebral artery at the base of the skull and courses down along the anterior surface of the cord. The anterior spinal artery supplies the anterior two-thirds of the cord, whereas the two posterior spinal arteries supply the posterior one-third. The posterior spinal

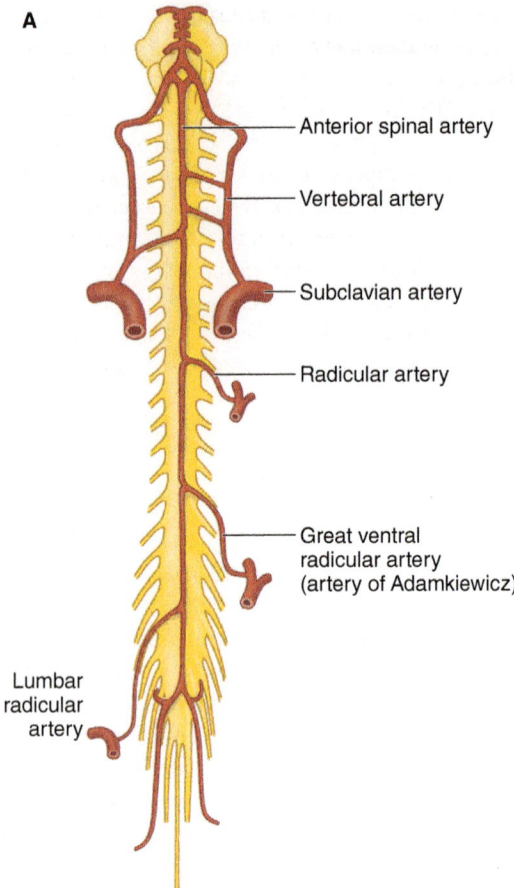

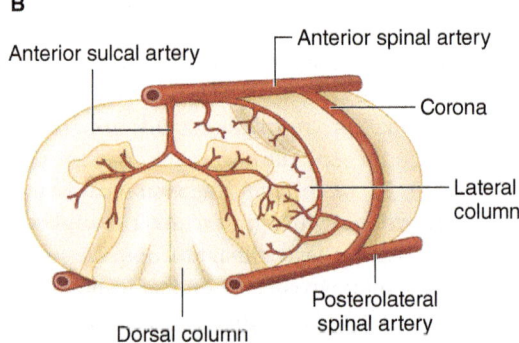

FIGURE 45–8 Arterial supply to the spinal cord. **A:** Anterior view showing principal sources of blood supply. **B:** Cross-sectional view through the spinal cord showing paired posterior spinal arteries and a single anterior spinal artery. (Adapted and reproduced, with permission, from Waxman SG: *Correlative Neuroanatomy*, 24th ed. McGraw-Hill, 2000.)

arteries arise from the posterior inferior cerebellar arteries and course down along the dorsal surface of the cord medial to the dorsal nerve roots. The anterior and posterior spinal arteries receive additional blood flow from the intercostal arteries in the thorax and the lumbar arteries in the abdomen. One of these radicular arteries is typically large, the artery of Adamkiewicz, or arteria radicularis magna, arising from the aorta (Figures 45–8A). It is typically unilateral and nearly always arises on the left side, providing the major blood supply to the anterior, lower two-thirds of the spinal cord. Injury to this artery can result in the anterior spinal artery syndrome.

Mechanism of Action

3 The mechanisms of spinal and epidural anesthesia remain speculative. The principal site of action for neuraxial blockade is believed to be the nerve root. Local anesthetic is injected into CSF (spinal anesthesia) or the epidural space (epidural and caudal anesthesia) and bathes the nerve root in the subarachnoid space or epidural space, respectively. Direct injection of local anesthetic into CSF for spinal anesthesia allows a relatively small dose and volume of local anesthetic to achieve dense sensory and motor blockade. In contrast, the same local anesthetic concentration is achieved within nerve roots only with much larger volumes and quantities of local anesthetic molecules during epidural and caudal anesthesia. Moreover, the injection site (level) for epidural anesthesia must generally be close to the nerve roots that must be anesthetized. Blockade of neural transmission (conduction) in the posterior nerve root fibers interrupts somatic and visceral sensation, whereas blockade of anterior nerve root fibers prevents efferent motor and autonomic outflow. Local anesthetics may also have actions on structures within the spinal cord during epidural and spinal anesthesia.

SOMATIC BLOCKADE

By interrupting the afferent transmission of painful stimuli and abolishing the efferent impulses responsible for skeletal muscle tone, neuraxial blocks can provide excellent operating conditions. Sensory blockade interrupts both somatic and visceral painful stimuli. The mechanism of action of local anesthetic agents is discussed in Chapter 16. The effect of local anesthetics on nerve fibers varies according to the size and characteristics of the nerve fiber, whether it is myelinated, the length of nerve that is bathed by the local anesthetic, and the concentration of the local anesthetic. Spinal nerve roots contain varying mixtures of these fiber types. Smaller and myelinated fibers are generally more easily blocked than larger and unmyelinated ones. The size and character of the fiber types, and the fact that the concentration of local anesthetic decreases with increasing distance from the level of injection, explains the phenomenon of differential blockade
4 during neuraxial anesthesia. Differential blockade typically results in sympathetic blockade (judged by temperature sensitivity) that may be two segments or more cephalad than the sensory block (pain, light touch), which, in turn, is usually several segments more cephalad than the motor blockade.

AUTONOMIC BLOCKADE

5 Interruption of efferent autonomic transmission at the spinal nerve roots during neuraxial blocks produces sympathetic blockade. Sympathetic outflow from the spinal cord may be described as thoracolumbar, whereas parasympathetic outflow is craniosacral. Sympathetic preganglionic nerve fibers (small, myelinated B fibers) exit the spinal cord with the spinal nerves from T1–L2 and may course many levels up or down the sympathetic chain before synapsing with a postganglionic cell in a sympathetic ganglion. In contrast, parasympathetic preganglionic fibers exit the spinal cord with the cranial and sacral nerves. Neuraxial anesthesia does not block the vagus nerve (tenth cranial nerve). The physiological responses of neuraxial blockade therefore result from decreased sympathetic tone and/or unopposed parasympathetic tone.

Cardiovascular Manifestations

6 Neuraxial blocks produce variable decreases in blood pressure that may be accompanied by a decrease in heart rate. These effects are generally proportional to the dermatomal level and extent of sympathectomy. Vasomotor tone is primarily determined by sympathetic fibers arising from T5–L1, innervating arterial and venous smooth muscle. Blocking these nerves causes vasodilation of the venous capacitance vessels and pooling of blood in the viscera and lower extremities, thereby decreasing the effective circulating blood volume and venous return to the heart. Arterial vasodilation may also decrease systemic vascular resistance. The effects of arterial vasodilation may be minimized by compensatory vasoconstriction above the level of the block, particularly when the extent of sensory anesthesia is limited to the lower thoracic dermatomes. A high sympathetic block not only prevents compensatory vasoconstriction, but may also block the sympathetic cardiac accelerator fibers that arise at T1–T4. Profound hypotension may result from arterial dilation and venous pooling combined with bradycardia (and possibly also milder degrees of decreased contractility). These effects are exaggerated if venous pooling is further augmented by a head-up position or the weight of a gravid uterus. Unopposed vagal tone may explain the sudden cardiac arrest sometimes seen with spinal anesthesia.

7 Deleterious cardiovascular effects should be anticipated and steps undertaken to minimize the degree of hypotension. However, volume loading with 10–20 mL/kg of intravenous fluid in a healthy patient before initiation of the block has been shown repeatedly to fail to prevent hypotension (in the absence of preexisting hypovolemia). Left uterine displacement in the third trimester of pregnancy helps to minimize physical obstruction to venous return. Despite these efforts, hypotension may still occur and should be treated promptly. Autotransfusion may be accomplished by placing the patient in a head-down position. A bolus of intravenous fluid (5–10 mL/kg) may be helpful in patients who have adequate cardiac and renal function to be able to "handle" the fluid load after the block wears off. Excessive or symptomatic **8** bradycardia should be treated with atropine, and hypotension should be treated with vasopressors. Direct α-adrenergic agonists (such as phenylephrine) primarily produce arteriolar constriction and may reflexively increase bradycardia, increasing systemic vascular resistance. The "mixed" agent

ephedrine has direct and indirect β-adrenergic effects that increase heart rate and contractility and indirect effects that also produce vasoconstriction. Much like ephedrine, small doses of epinephrine (2–5 mcg boluses) are particularly useful in treating spinal anesthesia induced hypotension. If profound hypotension and/or bradycardia persist, vasopressor infusions may be required.

Pulmonary Manifestations

Alterations in pulmonary physiology are usually minimal with neuraxial blocks because the diaphragm is innervated by the phrenic nerve, with fibers originating from C3–C5. Even with high thoracic levels, tidal volume is unchanged; there is only a small decrease in vital capacity, which results from a loss of the abdominal muscles' contribution to forced expiration.

Patients with severe chronic lung disease may rely upon accessory muscles of respiration (intercostal and abdominal muscles) to actively inspire or exhale. High levels of neural blockade will impair these muscles. Similarly, effective coughing and clearing of secretions require these muscles for expiration. For these reasons, neuraxial blocks should be used with caution in patients with limited respiratory reserve. These deleterious effects need to be weighed against the advantages of avoiding airway instrumentation and positive-pressure ventilation. For surgical procedures above the umbilicus, a pure regional technique may not be the best choice in patients with severe lung disease. On the other hand, these patients may benefit from the effects of thoracic epidural analgesia (with dilute local anesthetics and opioids) in the postoperative period, particularly following upper abdominal or thoracic surgery. Some evidence suggests that postoperative thoracic epidural analgesia in high-risk patients can improve pulmonary outcome by decreasing the incidence of pneumonia and respiratory failure, improving oxygenation, and decreasing the duration of mechanical ventilatory support.

Gastrointestinal Manifestations

Sympathetic outflow originates at the T5–L1 level. Neuraxial block-induced sympathectomy allows vagal tone dominance and results in a small, contracted gut with active peristalsis. This can improve operative conditions during laparoscopy when used as an adjunct to general anesthesia. Postoperative epidural analgesia with local anesthetics and minimal systemic opioids hastens the return of gastrointestinal function after open abdominal procedures.

Hepatic blood flow will decrease with reductions in mean arterial pressure from any anesthetic technique, including neuraxial anesthesia.

Urinary Tract Manifestations

Renal blood flow is maintained through autoregulation, and there is little effect of neuraxial anesthesia on renal function. Neuraxial anesthesia at the lumbar and sacral levels blocks both sympathetic and parasympathetic control of bladder function. Loss of autonomic bladder control results in urinary retention until the block wears off. If no urinary catheter is placed perioperatively, it is prudent to use the regional anesthetic of shortest duration sufficient for the surgical procedure and to administer the minimal safe volume of intravenous fluid. Patients with urinary retention should be checked for bladder distention after neuraxial anesthesia.

Metabolic & Endocrine Manifestations

Surgical trauma produces a systemic neuroendocrine response via activation of somatic and visceral afferent nerve fibers, in addition to a localized inflammatory response. This systemic response includes increased concentrations of adrenocorticotropic hormone, cortisol, epinephrine, norepinephrine, and vasopressin levels, as well as activation of the renin–angiotensin–aldosterone system. Clinical manifestations include intraoperative and postoperative hypertension, tachycardia, hyperglycemia, protein catabolism, suppressed immune responses, and altered renal function. Neuraxial blockade can partially suppress (during major invasive surgery) or totally block (during lower extremity surgery) the neuroendocrine stress response. To maximize this blunting of the neuroendocrine stress response, neuraxial block should precede incision and continue into the postoperative period.

Clinical Considerations Common to Spinal & Epidural Blocks

Indications

Neuraxial blocks may be used alone or in conjunction with general anesthesia for most procedures below the neck. Indeed, in some centers outside of North America, minimally invasive coronary artery surgery has been performed with thoracic epidural anesthesia alone. As a primary anesthetic, neuraxial blocks have proved most useful in lower abdominal, inguinal, urogenital, rectal, and lower extremity surgery. Lumbar spinal surgery may also be performed under spinal anesthesia. Upper abdominal procedures (eg, gastrectomy) have been performed with spinal or epidural anesthesia, but because it can be difficult to safely achieve a sensory level adequate for patient comfort, these techniques are not commonly used.

If a neuraxial anesthetic is being considered, the risks and benefits must be discussed with the patient, and informed consent should be obtained. The patient must be mentally prepared for neuraxial anesthesia, and neuraxial anesthesia must be appropriate for the type of surgery. Patients should understand that they will have little or no lower extremity motor function until the block resolves. Procedures that require maneuvers that might compromise respiratory function (eg, pneumoperitoneum or pneumothorax) or are unusually prolonged are typically performed with general anesthesia, with or without neuraxial blockade.

Contraindications

9 Major contraindications to neuraxial anesthesia include patient refusal, bleeding diathesis, severe hypovolemia, elevated intracranial pressure (particularly with an intracranial mass), and infection at the site of injection. Other relative contraindications include severe aortic or mitral stenosis and severe left ventricular outflow obstruction (hypertrophic obstructive cardiomyopathy); however, with close monitoring and control of the anesthetic level, neuraxial anesthesia can be performed safely in patients with valvular heart disease, particularly

TABLE 45–1 **Contraindications to neuraxial blockade.**

Absolute
Infection at the site of injection
Patient refusal
Coagulopathy or other bleeding diathesis
Severe hypovolemia
Increased intracranial pressure
Severe aortic stenosis
Severe mitral stenosis

Relative
Sepsis
Uncooperative patient
Preexisting neurological deficits
Demyelinating lesions
Stenotic valvular heart lesions
Left ventricular outflow obstruction (hypertrophic obstructive cardiomyopathy)
Severe spinal deformity

Controversial
Prior back surgery at the site of injection
Complicated surgery
Prolonged operation
Major blood loss
Maneuvers that compromise respiration

if extensive dermatomal spread of anesthesia is not required (eg, "saddle" block spinal anesthetics).

Relative and controversial contraindications are also shown in Table 45–1. Inspection and palpation of the back can reveal surgical scars, scoliosis, skin lesions, and whether the spinous processes can be identified. Although preoperative screening tests are not required in healthy patients undergoing neuraxial blockade, appropriate testing should be performed if the clinical history suggests a bleeding diathesis. Neuraxial anesthesia in the presence of sepsis or bacteremia could theoretically predispose patients to hematogenous spread of the infectious agents into the epidural or subarachnoid space, as has been shown for lumbar puncture in the presence of septicemia.

Patients with preexisting neurological deficits or demyelinating diseases may report worsening symptoms following a block. It may be impossible to discern effects or complications of the block from preexisting deficits or unrelated exacerbation of preexisting disease. For these reasons, some risk-averse

practitioners argue against neuraxial anesthesia in such patients. A preoperative neurological examination should thoroughly document any deficits. In a retrospective study examining the records of 567 patients with preexisting neuropathies, 2 of the patients developed new or worsening neuropathy following neuraxial anesthesia. Although this finding indicates a relatively low risk of further injury, study investigators suggest that an injured nerve is vulnerable to additional injury, increasing the likelihood of poor neurological outcomes.

Regional anesthesia requires at least some degree of patient cooperation. This may be difficult or impossible for patients with dementia, psychosis, or emotional instability. The decision must be individualized. Unsedated young children may not be suitable for pure regional techniques; however, regional anesthesia is frequently used with general anesthesia in children.

Neuraxial Blockade in the Setting of Anticoagulants & Antiplatelet Agents

Whether a block should be performed in the setting of anticoagulants and antiplatelet agents can be problematic. The American Society of Regional Anesthesia and Pain Medicine (ASRA) has issued several guidelines on this subject. Because guidelines are frequently revised and updated, practitioners are advised to seek the most recent edition. Although the incidence of epidural hematoma is reported to be quite low (1 in 150,000 epidurals), ASRA is concerned that the actual incidence may be somewhat higher. Moreover, the use of anticoagulant and antiplatelet medications continues to increase, placing an ever larger number of patients at potential risk of epidural hematomas. Because of the rarity of epidural hematomas, most guidelines are based on expert opinion and case series reviews, as clinical trials are not feasible.

A. Oral Anticoagulants

If neuraxial anesthesia is to be used in patients receiving warfarin therapy, a normal prothrombin time and international normalized ratio should be documented prior to the block. Anesthesia staff should always consult with the patient's primary physicians whenever considering the discontinuation of antiplatelet or antithrombotic therapy.

B. Antiplatelet Drugs

By themselves, aspirin and other nonsteroidal antiinflammatory drugs (NSAIDs) drugs do not increase the risk of spinal hematoma from neuraxial anesthesia procedures or epidural catheter removal. This assumes a normal patient with a normal coagulation profile who is not receiving other medications that might affect clotting mechanisms. In contrast, more potent agents should be stopped, and neuraxial blockade should generally be administered only after their effects have worn off. The waiting period depends on the specific agent: for ticlopidine (Ticlid), it is 14 days; clopidogrel (Plavix), 7 days; abciximab (Rheopro), 48 hr; and eptifibatide (Integrilin), 8 hr. In patients with a recently placed cardiac stent, discontinuation of antiplatelet therapy can result in stent thrombosis and acute ST-segment elevation myocardial infarction. Risks versus benefits of a neuraxial technique should be discussed with the patient and the patient's primary doctors.

C. Standard (Unfractionated) Heparin

"Minidose" subcutaneous heparin prophylaxis is not a contraindication to neuraxial anesthesia or epidural catheter removal. In patients who are to receive systemic heparin intraoperatively, blocks may be performed 1 hr or more before heparin administration. A bloody epidural or spinal does not necessarily require cancellation of surgery, but discussion of the risks with the surgeon and careful postoperative monitoring is needed. Removal of an epidural catheter should occur 1 hr prior to, or 4 hr following, subsequent heparin dosing.

Neuraxial anesthesia should be avoided in patients on therapeutic doses of heparin and with increased partial thromboplastin time. If the patient is started on heparin after the placement of an epidural catheter, the catheter should be removed only after discontinuation or interruption of heparin infusion and evaluation of the coagulation status. The risk of spinal hematoma (with or without neuraxial puncture) is unclear in the setting of full anticoagulation for cardiac surgery. Prompt diagnosis and evacuation of symptomatic epidural hematomas increase the likelihood that neuronal function will be preserved.

D. Low-Molecular-Weight Heparin (LMWH)

Many cases of spinal hematoma associated with neuraxial anesthesia followed the introduction of the "low-molecular weight heparin" (LMWH) enoxaparin (Lovenox) in the United States in 1993. **Many of these cases involved intraoperative or early postoperative LMWH use, and several patients were receiving concomitant antiplatelet medication**. If an unusually bloody needle or catheter placement occurs, LMWH should be delayed until 24 hr postoperatively, because this trauma may increase the risk of spinal hematoma. If postoperative LMWH thromboprophylaxis will be utilized, epidural catheters should be removed 2 hr prior to the first LMWH dose. If already present, the catheter should be removed at least 10 hr after a dose of LMWH, and subsequent dosing should not occur for another 2 hr.

E. Fibrinolytic or Thrombolytic Therapy

Neuraxial anesthesia should not be performed if a patient has received fibrinolytic or thrombolytic therapy.

Awake or Asleep?

Should lumbar neuraxial anesthesia, when used in conjunction with general anesthesia, be performed before or after induction of general anesthesia? This is controversial. The major arguments for having the patient asleep are that (1) most patients, if given a choice, would prefer to be asleep, and (2) the possibility of sudden patient movement causing injury is markedly diminished. The major argument for neuraxial blockade while the patient is still awake is that the patient can alert the clinician to paresthesias and pain on injection, both of which have been associated with postoperative neurological deficits. Although many clinicians are comfortable performing lumbar epidural or spinal puncture in anesthetized or deeply sedated adults, there is greater consensus that thoracic and cervical punctures should, except under unusual circumstances, only be performed in awake patients. Pediatric neuraxial blocks, particularly caudal and epidural blocks, are usually performed under general anesthesia.

Technical Considerations

Neuraxial blocks should be performed only in a facility in which all the equipment and drugs needed for intubation, resuscitation, and general anesthesia are immediately available. Regional anesthesia is greatly facilitated by adequate patient premedication.

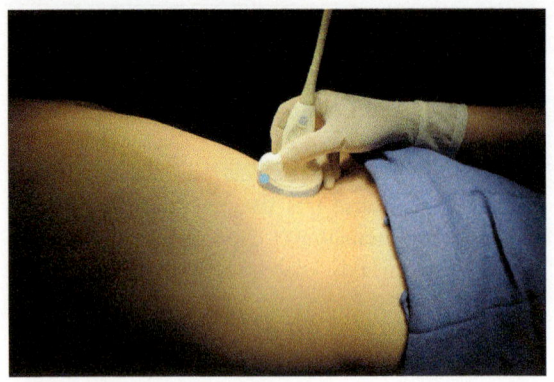

A

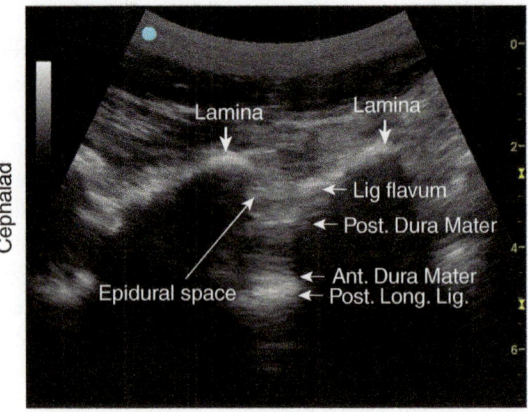

B

FIGURE 45–9 **A**: Transducer position to image paramedian epidural space at the lumbar spine, longitudinal view. **B**: Corresponding ultrasound image. Post. Long. Lig., Posterior Longitudinal Ligament; Lig. Flavum, Ligamentum Flavum; Ant. Dura Mater, Anterior

Dura Mater; Post. Dura Mater, Posterior Dura Mater. (Reproduced, with permission, from Hadzic, A: *Peripheral Nerve Blocks and Anatomy for Ultrasound-Guided Regional Anesthesia,* 2nd edition. McGraw-Hill, 2012.)

Nonpharmacologic patient preparation is also very helpful. The patient should be told what to expect so as to minimize anxiety. This is particularly important in situations in which premedication is not used, as is typically the case in obstetric anesthesia. Supplemental oxygen via a face mask or nasal cannula may be required to avoid hypoxemia when sedation is used. Minimum monitoring requirements include blood pressure and pulse oximetry for labor analgesia. Monitoring for blocks rendered in surgical anesthesia is the same as that in general anesthesia. Epidural steroid injections for management of pain (when little or no local anesthetic is injected) do not require continuous monitoring.

Surface Anatomy

Spinous processes are generally palpable and help to define the midline. Ultrasound can be used when landmarks are not palpable (Figure 45–9). The spinous processes of the cervical and lumbar spine are nearly horizontal, whereas those in the thoracic spine slant in a caudal direction and can overlap significantly (Figure 45–2). Therefore, when performing a lumbar or cervical epidural block (with maximum spinal flexion), the needle is directed with only a slight cephalad angle, whereas for a thoracic block, the needle must be angled significantly more cephalad to enter the thoracic epidural space. In the

cervical area, the first palpable spinous process is that of C2, but the most prominent one is that of C7 (vertebra prominens). With the arms at the side, the spinous process of T7 is usually at the same level as the inferior angle of the scapulae (Figure 45–10). A line drawn between the highest points of both iliac crests (Tuffier's line) usually crosses either the body of L4 or the L4–L5 interspace. Counting spinous processes up or down from these reference points identifies other spinal levels. A line connecting the posterior superior iliac spine crosses the S2 posterior foramina. In slender persons, the sacrum is easily palpable, and the sacral hiatus is felt as a depression just above or between the gluteal clefts and above the coccyx, defining the point of entry for caudal blocks.

Patient Positioning

A. Sitting Position

The anatomic midline is often easier to appreciate when the patient is sitting than when the patient is in the lateral decubitus position (Figure 45–11). This is particularly true with very obese patients. Patients sit with their elbows resting on their thighs or a bedside table, or they can hug a pillow. Flexion of the spine (arching the back "like a mad cat" maximizes the "target" area between adjacent spinous processes and brings the spine closer to the skin surface (Figure 45–12).

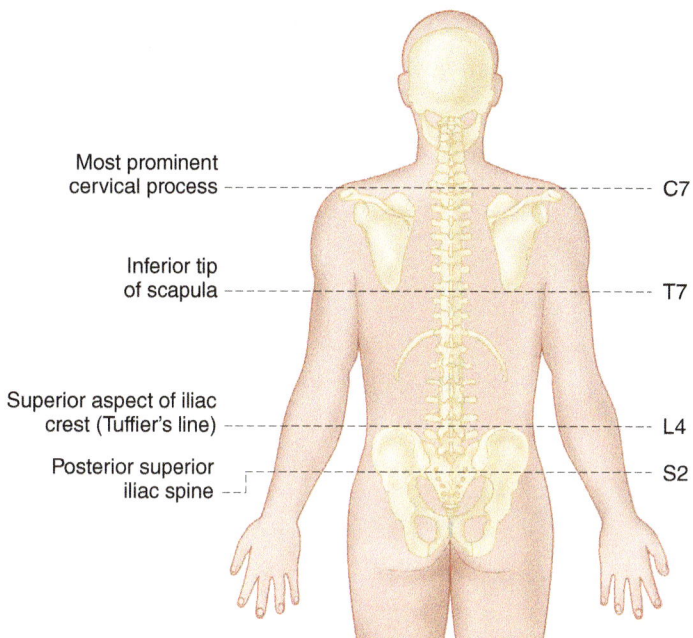

FIGURE 45–10 Surface landmarks for identifying spinal levels.

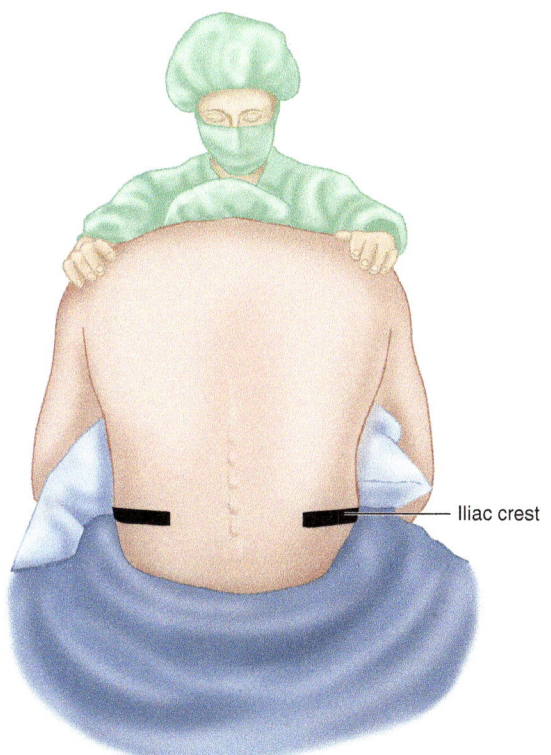

FIGURE 45–11 Sitting position for neuraxial blockade. Note an assistant helps in obtaining maximal spinal flexion.

B. Lateral Decubitus

Many clinicians prefer the lateral position for neuraxial blocks (Figure 45–13). Patients lie on their side with their knees flexed and pulled high against the abdomen or chest, assuming a "fetal position." An assistant can help the patient assume and hold this position.

C. Buie's (Jackknife) Position

This position may be used for anorectal procedures utilizing an isobaric or hypobaric anesthetic solution (see below). The advantage is that the block is done in the same position as the operative procedure, so that the patient does not have to be moved following the block. The disadvantage is that CSF will not freely flow through the needle, so that correct subarachnoid needle tip placement will need to be confirmed by CSF aspiration. A prone position is typically used when fluoroscopic guidance is required.

Anatomic Approach

A. Midline Approach

The spine is palpated, and the patient's body position is examined to ensure that the plane of the back is perpendicular to that of the floor. This ensures that a needle passed parallel to the floor will stay midline as it courses deeper (Figure 45–4). The depression

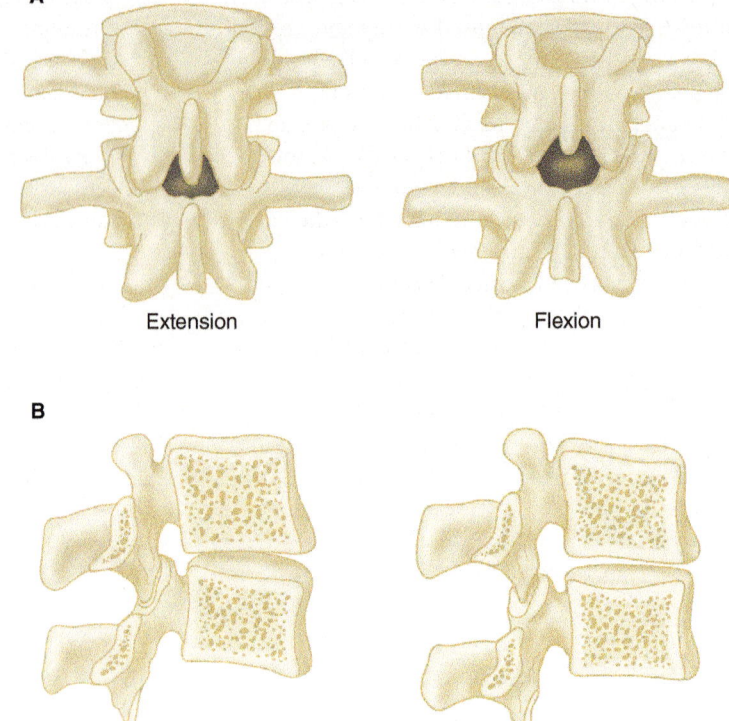

A

Extension

Flexion

B

Extension

Flexion

FIGURE 45–12 The effect of flexion on adjacent vertebrae. **A**: Posterior view. **B**: Lateral view. Note the target area (interlaminar foramen) for neuraxial blocks increases in size with flexion.

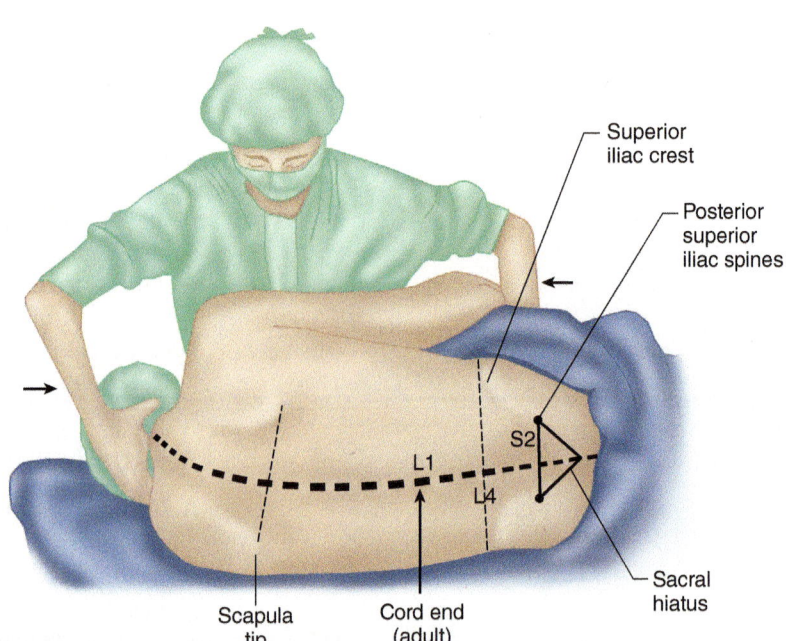

Superior
iliac crest

Posterior
superior
iliac spines

S2

L1

L4

Sacral
hiatus

Scapula
tip

Cord end
(adult)

FIGURE 45–13 Lateral decubitus position for neuraxial blockade. Note again the assistant helping to provide maximal spine flexion.

between the spinous processes of the vertebra above and below the level to be used is palpated; this will be the needle entry site. A sterile field is established with chlorhexidine or a similar solution. A fenestrated sterile drape is applied. After the preparation solution has dried, a skin wheal is raised at the level of the chosen interspace with local anesthetic using a small (25-gauge) needle. A longer needle can be used for deeper local anesthetic infiltration.

Next, the procedure needle is introduced in the midline. Remembering that the spinous processes course caudad from their origin at the spine, the needle will be directed slightly cephalad. The subcutaneous tissues offer little resistance to the needle. As the needle courses deeper, it will enter the supraspinous and interspinous ligaments, felt as an increase in tissue resistance. The needle also feels more firmly implanted in the back. If bone is contacted superficially, a midline needle is likely hitting the lower spinous process. Contact with bone at a deeper level usually indicates that the needle is in the midline and

hitting the upper spinous process, or that it is lateral to the midline and hitting a lamina. In either case, the needle must be redirected. As the needle penetrates the ligamentum flavum, an obvious increase in resistance is encountered. At this point, the procedures for spinal and epidural anesthesia differ.

10 For epidural anesthesia, a sudden loss of resistance (to injection of air or saline) is encountered as the needle passes through the ligamentum flavum and enters the epidural space. For spinal anesthesia, the needle is advanced through the epidural space and penetrates the dura–subarachnoid membranes, as signaled by freely flowing CSF.

B. Paramedian Approach

The paramedian technique may be selected if epidural or subarachnoid block is difficult, particularly in patients who cannot be positioned easily (eg, severe arthritis, kyphoscoliosis, or prior spine surgery) (Figure 45–14). Many clinicians routinely use the paramedian approach for thoracic epidural

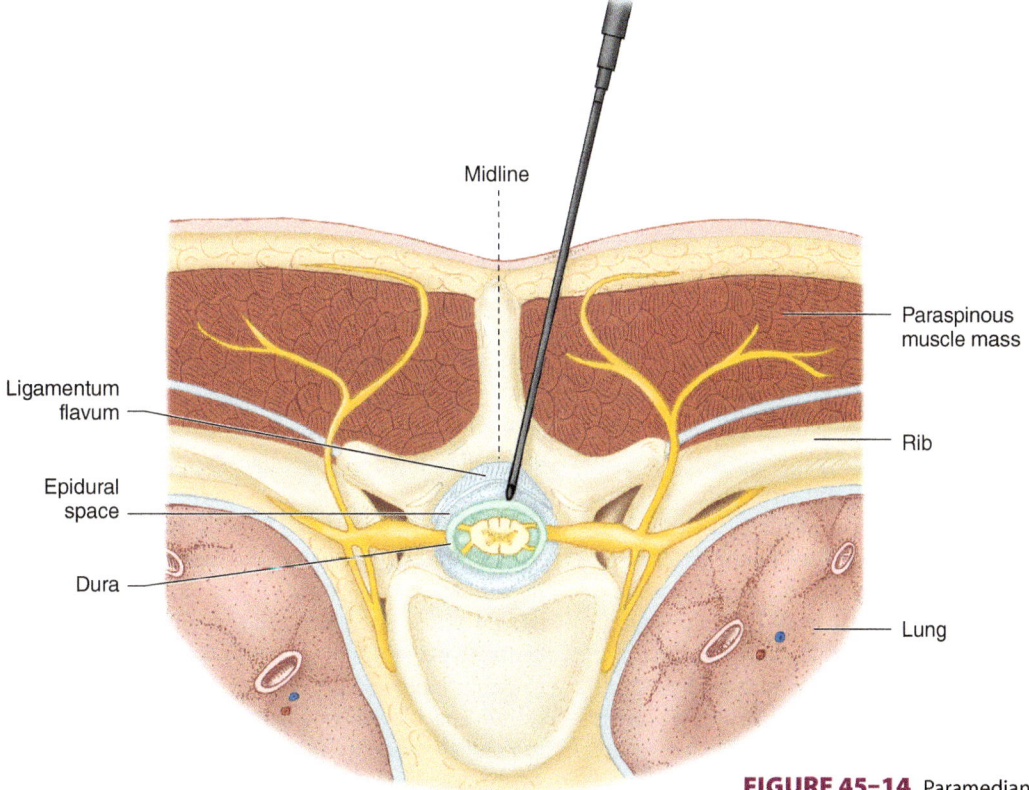

Midline

Paraspinous muscle mass

Ligamentum flavum

Rib

Epidural space

Dura

Lung

FIGURE 45–14 Paramedian approach.

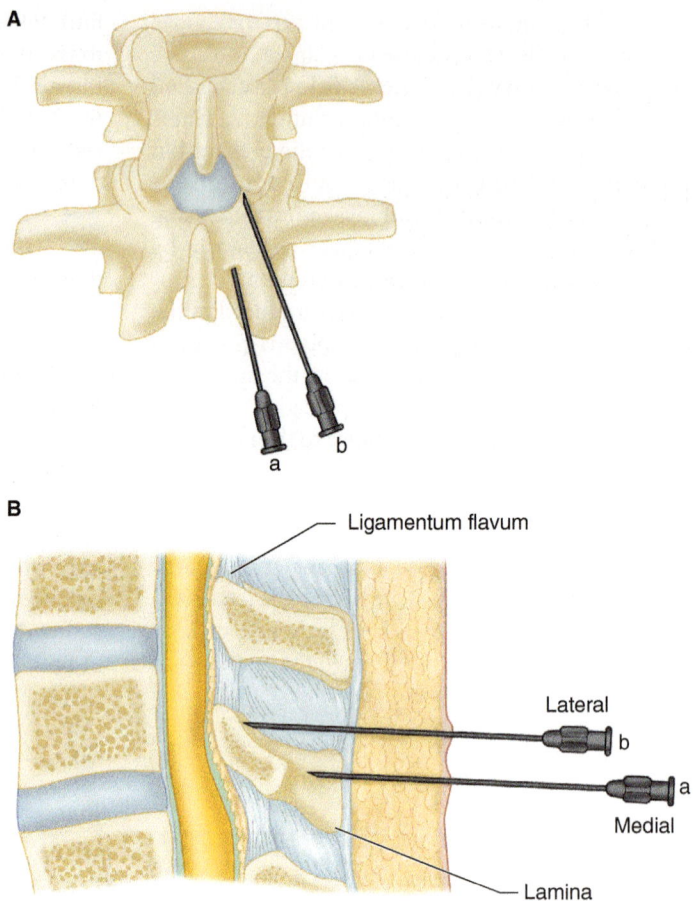

FIGURE 45–15 Paramedian approach. A needle that encounters bone at a shallow depth (a) is usually hitting the medial lamina, whereas one that encounters bone deeply (b) is farther lateral from the midline. **A:** Posterior view. **B:** Parasagittal view.

puncture. After skin preparation and sterile draping (as previously described), the skin wheal for a paramedian approach is raised 2 cm lateral to the inferior aspect of the superior spinous process of the desired level. Because this approach is lateral to most of the interspinous ligaments and penetrates the paraspinous muscles, the needle may encounter little resistance initially and may not seem to be in firm tissue. The needle is directed and advanced at a 10–25° angle toward the midline. If bone is encountered at a shallow depth with the paramedian approach, the needle is likely in contact with the medial part of the lower lamina and should be redirected mostly upward and perhaps slightly more laterally. On the other hand, if bone is encountered deeply, the needle is usually in contact with the lateral part of the lower lamina and should

be redirected only slightly craniad, more toward the midline (**Figure 45–15**).

C. Assessing Level of Blockade

With knowledge of the sensory dermatomes (see appendix), the extent of sensory block can be assessed by a blunted needle.

D. Ultrasound-Guided Neuraxial Blockade

Although it has not, as of yet, transformed the practice of neuraxial blockade in the same manner as it has for other procedures, ultrasound guidance can facilitate neuraxial blockade in patients with poorly palpable landmarks. As with other uses of ultrasound, specific training is required for practitioners to identify correctly the landmarks and interspaces necessary for neuraxial blockade.

Spinal Anesthesia

Initially after injection, spinal anesthetic solutions inhibit conduction in nerve roots as they course through the subarachnoid space. Over time, the local anesthetic permeates the spinal cord and likely interacts with other targets located therein. The spinal subarachnoid space extends from the foramen magnum to the S2 in adults and S3 in children. Injection of local anesthetic below L1 in adults and L3 (below the termination of the conus medullaris) in children helps to avoid direct trauma to the spinal cord. Spinal anesthesia is sometimes referred to a subarachnoid block, and it occurs as a result of an intrathecal injection.

Spinal Needles

Spinal needles are commercially available in an array of sizes lengths, and bevel and tip designs (Figure 45–16). All should have a tightly fitting removable stylet that completely occludes the lumen to avoid tracking epithelial cells into the subarachnoid space. Broadly, they can be divided into either sharp (cutting)-tipped or blunt-tipped needles. The Quincke needle is a cutting needle with end injection. The introduction of blunt tip (pencil-point) needles has markedly decreased the incidence of postdural puncture headache. The Whitacre and other pencil-point needles have rounded points and

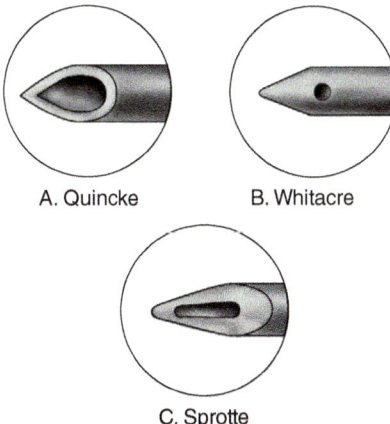

FIGURE 45–16 Spinal needles.

side injection. The Sprotte is a side-injection needle with a long opening. It has the advantage of more vigorous CSF flow compared with similar gauge needles. However, this can lead to a failed block if the distal part of the opening is subarachnoid (with free flow CSF), the proximal part is not past the dura, and the full dose of medication is not delivered. In general, the smaller the gauge needle, the lower the incidence of headache.

Spinal Catheters

Very small subarachnoid catheters are currently no longer approved by the US Food and Drug Administration. The withdrawal of these catheters was prompted by their association with cauda equina syndrome (CES). Larger catheters designed for epidural use are associated with relatively high complication rates when placed subarachnoid; however, they are frequently used for continuous spinal anesthesia following accidental dural puncture during performance of epidural anesthesia.

Specific Technique for Spinal Anesthesia

The midline, or paramedian, approaches, with the patient positioned in the lateral decubitus, sitting, or prone positions, can be used for spinal anesthesia. As previously discussed, the needle is advanced from skin through the deeper structures until two "pops" are felt. The first is penetration of the ligamentum flavum, and the second is penetration of the dura–arachnoid membrane. Successful dural puncture is confirmed by withdrawing the stylet to verify free flow of CSF. With small-gauge needles (<25 g), aspiration may be necessary to detect CSF. If free flow occurs initially, but CSF cannot be aspirated after attaching the syringe, the needle likely will have moved. Persistent paresthesias or pain with injection of drugs should alert the clinician to withdraw and redirect the needle.

Factors Influencing Level of Spinal Block

Table 45–2 lists factors that have been shown to affect the level of neural blockade following spinal anesthesia. The most important determinants are baricity of the local anesthetic solution, position of

TABLE 45–2 Factors affecting the dermatomal spread of spinal anesthesia.

Most important factors
  Baricity of anesthetic solution
  Position of the patient
    During injection
    Immediately after injection
  Drug dosage
  Site of injection

Other factors
  Age
  Cerebrospinal fluid
  Curvature of the spine
  Drug volume
  Intraabdominal pressure
  Needle direction
  Patient height
  Pregnancy

the patient during and immediately after injection, and drug dosage. In general, the larger the dosage or more cephalad the site of injection, the more cephalad the level of anesthesia that will be obtained. Moreover, migration of the local anesthetic cephalad in CSF depends on its density relative to CSF (baricity). CSF has a specific gravity of 1.003–1.008 at 37°C. Table 45–3 lists the specific gravity of anesthetic solutions. A hyperbaric solution of local anesthetic is denser (heavier) than CSF, whereas a

TABLE 45–3 Specific gravities of some spinal anesthetic agents.

Agent	Specific Gravity
Bupivacaine	
0.5% in 8.25% dextrose	1.0227–1.0278
0.5% plain	0.9990–1.0058
Lidocaine	
2% plain	1.0004–1.0066
5% in 7.5% dextrose	1.0262–1.0333
Procaine	
10% plain	1.0104
2.5% in water	0.9983
Tetracaine	
0.5% in water	0.9977–0.9997
0.5% in D$_5$W	1.0133–1.0203

hypobaric solution is less dense (lighter) than CSF. The local anesthetic solutions can be made hyperbaric by the addition of glucose or hypobaric by the addition of sterile water or fentanyl. Thus, with the patient in a head-down position, a hyperbaric solution spreads cephalad, and a hypobaric anesthetic solution moves caudad. A head-up position causes a hyperbaric solution to settle caudad and a hypobaric solution to ascend cephalad. Similarly, when a patient remains in a lateral position, a hyperbaric spinal solution will have a greater effect on the dependent (down) side, whereas a hypobaric solution will achieve a higher level on the nondependent (up) side. An isobaric solution tends to remain at the level of injection. Anesthetic agents are mixed with CSF (at least 1:1) to make their solutions isobaric. Other factors affecting the level of neural blockade include the level of injection and the patient's height and vertebral column anatomy. The direction of the needle bevel or injection port may also play a role; higher levels of anesthesia are achieved if the injection is directed cephalad than if the point of injection is oriented laterally or caudad.

Hyperbaric solutions tend to move to the most dependent area of the spine (normally T4–T8 in the supine position). With normal spinal anatomy, the apex of the thoracolumbar curvature is T4 (Figure 45–17). In the supine position, this should limit a hyperbaric solution to produce a level of anesthesia at or below T4. Abnormal curvatures of the spine, such as scoliosis and kyphoscoliosis, have multiple effects on spinal anesthesia. Placing the block becomes more difficult because of the rotation and angulation of the vertebral bodies and spinous processes. Finding the midline and the interlaminar space may be difficult. The paramedian approach to lumbar puncture may be preferable in patients with severe scoliosis and kyphoscoliosis. In the Taylor approach, a variant of the standard paramedian approach described previously, the needle enters 1 cm medial and 1 cm inferior to the posterior superior iliac spine and is directed cephalad and toward the midline. Reviewing radiographs of the spine before attempting the block may be useful. Spinal curvature affects the ultimate level by changing the contour of the subarachnoid space. Previous spinal surgery can similarly result in technical difficulties

A

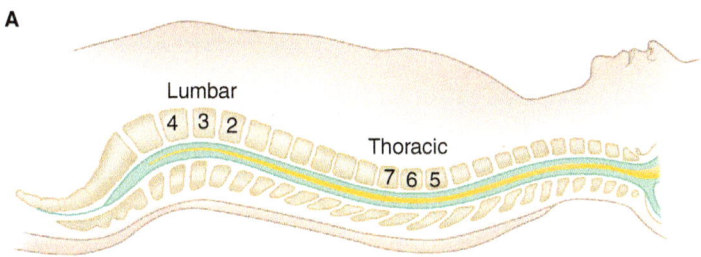

Lumbar

4 3 2

Thoracic

7 6 5

B

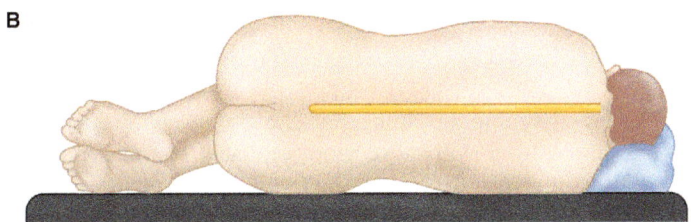

FIGURE 45–17 The position of the spinal canal in the supine position (**A**) and lateral decubitus position (**B**). Note the lowest point is usually between T5 and T7, where a hyperbaric solution tends to settle once the patient is placed supine.

in placing a block. Correctly identifying the interspinous and interlaminar spaces may be difficult at the levels of previous laminectomy or spinal fusion. The paramedian approach may be easier, or a level above the surgical site can be chosen. The block may be incomplete, or the level may be different than anticipated, due to postsurgical anatomic changes.

Lumbar CSF volume inversely correlates with the dermatomal spread of spinal anesthesia. Increased intraabdominal pressure or conditions that cause engorgement of the epidural veins, thus decreasing CSF volume, are associated with greater dermatomal spread for a given volume of injectate. This would include conditions such as pregnancy, ascites, and large abdominal tumors. In these clinical situations, higher levels of anesthesia are achieved with a given dose of local anesthetic than would otherwise be expected. For spinal anesthesia on a term parturient, some clinicians reduce the dosage of anesthetic by one-third compared with a nonpregnant patient, particularly when the block will be initiated with the patient in the lateral position. Age-related decreases in CSF volume are likely responsible for the higher anesthetic levels achieved in the elderly for a given dosage of spinal anesthetic. Severe kyphosis or kyphoscoliosis can also be associated with a decreased volume of CSF and often results in a higher

than expected level, particularly with a hypobaric technique or rapid injection. Tradition states that transient increases in CSF pressure from coughing or straining increase the spread of local anesthetic in the CSF, but data supporting this are lacking.

Spinal Anesthetic Agents

Many local anesthetics have been used for spinal anesthesia in the past, but only a few are currently in use (Table 45–4). Only preservative-free local anesthetic solutions are used. Addition of vasoconstrictors (α-adrenergic agonists, epinephrine (0.1–0.2 mg)) and opioids enhance the quality and/or prolong the duration of spinal anesthesia. Vasoconstrictors seem to delay the uptake of local anesthetics from CSF and may have weak spinal analgesic properties. Opioids and clonidine can likewise be added to spinal anesthetics to improve both the quality and duration of the subarachnoid block.

Hyperbaric bupivacaine and tetracaine are two of the most commonly used agents for spinal anesthesia. Both are relatively slow in onset (5–10 min) and have a prolonged duration (90–120 min). Although both agents produce similar sensory levels, spinal tetracaine more consistently produces motor blockade than does the equivalent dose of bupivacaine. Addition of epinephrine to spinal

TABLE 45–4 **Dosages and actions of commonly used spinal anesthetic agents.**

Drug	Preparation	Doses (mg)			Duration (min)	
		Perineum, Lower Limbs	Lower Abdomen	Upper Abdomen	Plain	Epinephrine
Procaine	10% solution	75	125	200	45	60
Bupivacaine	0.75% in 8.25% dextrose	4–10	12–14	12–18	90–120	100–150
Tetracaine	1% solution in 10% glucose	4–8	10–12	10–16	90–120	120–240
Lidocaine[1]	5% in 7.5% glucose	25–50	50–75	75–100	60–75	60–90

[1]No longer widely used for outpatients, particularly those undergoing surgery in the lithotomy position.

bupivacaine prolongs its duration only modestly. In contrast, epinephrine can prolong the duration of tetracaine by more than 50%. Phenylephrine also prolongs tetracaine anesthesia, but has no effect on bupivacaine spinal blocks. Ropivacaine has also been used for spinal anesthesia, but experience with it is more limited. Lidocaine and procaine have a relatively rapid onset (3–5 min) and short duration of action (60–90 min). Their duration is only modestly prolonged by vasoconstrictors. Although lidocaine spinal anesthesia has been used worldwide, some experts no longer use this agent because of the phenomenon of transient neurological symptoms and cauda equina syndrome (CES). **Repeat lidocaine doses following an initial "failed" block should be avoided**. Indeed, studies have shown that maldistribution of local anesthetic can lead to a failed spinal in spite of an adequate CSF concentration of local anesthetic. One alternative agent, 2-chloroprocaine, has been used in some centers with great success. Unfortunately, older formulations of this agent have produced cauda equine syndrome when accidentally injected intrathecally (in large doses) during attempted epidural anesthesia.

In North America, hyperbaric spinal anesthesia is more commonly used than hypobaric or isobaric techniques. The level of anesthesia is then dependent on the patient's position during and immediately following the injection. In the sitting position, "saddle block" can be achieved by keeping the patient sitting for 3–5 min following injection, so that only the lower lumbar nerves and sacral nerves are blocked. If the patient is moved from a sitting position to a supine position immediately after injection, the agent will move more cephalad to the dependent region defined by the thoracolumbar curve. Hyperbaric anesthetics injected intrathecally with the patient in a lateral decubitus position are useful for unilateral lower extremity procedures. The patient is placed laterally, with the extremity to be operated on in a dependent position. If the patient is kept in this position for about 5 min following injection, the block will tend to be denser and achieve a higher level on the operative dependent side.

If regional anesthesia is chosen for surgical procedures involving hip or lower extremity fracture, hypobaric or isobaric spinal anesthesia can be useful because the patient need not lie on the fractured extremity.

Epidural Anesthesia

11 Continuous epidural anesthesia is a neuraxial technique offering a range of applications wider than the typical all-or-nothing, single dose spinal anesthetic. An epidural block can be performed at the lumbar, thoracic, or cervical level. Sacral epidural anesthesia is referred to as a caudal

12 block and is described at the end of this chapter. Epidural techniques are widely used for surgical anesthesia, obstetric analgesia, postoperative pain control, and chronic pain management. Epidurals can be used as a single shot technique or with a catheter that allows intermittent boluses and/or continuous infusion. The motor block can range from none to complete. All of these variables are controlled by the choice of drug, concentration, dosage, and level of injection.

The epidural space surrounds the dura mater posteriorly, laterally, and anteriorly. Nerve roots travel in this space as they exit laterally through the foramen and course outward to become peripheral nerves. Other contents of the lumbar epidural space include fatty connective tissue, lymphatics, and a rich venous (Batson's) plexus. Fluoroscopic studies have suggested the presence of septa or connective tissue bands within the epidural space, possibly explaining the occasional one-sided epidural block.

13 Epidural anesthesia is slower in onset (10–20 min) and may not be as dense as spinal anesthesia. This can be manifested as a more pronounced differential block or a segmental block, a feature that can be useful clinically. For example, by using relatively dilute concentrations of a local anesthetic combined with an opioid, an epidural provides analgesia without motor block. This is commonly employed for labor and postoperative analgesia. Moreover, a segmental block is possible because the anesthetic can be confined close to the level at which it was injected. A segmental block is characterized by a well-defined band of anesthesia at certain nerve roots; leaving nerve roots above *and* below unblocked. This can be seen with a thoracic epidural that provides upper abdominal anesthesia while sparing cervical and lumbar nerve roots.

Epidural anesthesia and analgesia is most often performed in the lumbar region. The midline (Figure 45–4) or paramedian approach (Figure 45–14) can be used. Lumbar epidural anesthesia can be used for any procedure below the diaphragm. Because the spinal cord typically terminates at the L1 level, there is an extra measure of safety in performing the block in the lower lumbar interspaces, particularly if an accidental dural puncture occurs (see "Complications").

Thoracic epidural blocks are technically more difficult to accomplish than are lumbar blocks because of greater angulation and the overlapping of the spinous processes at the vertebral level (Figure 45–18). Moreover, the potential risk of spinal cord injury with accidental dural puncture, although exceedingly small with good technique, may be greater than that

at the lumbar level. Thoracic epidural blocks can be accomplished with either a midline or paramedian approach. Rarely used for primary anesthesia, the thoracic epidural technique is most commonly used for intraoperative and postoperative analgesia. Single shot or catheter techniques are used for the management of chronic pain. Infusions via an epidural catheter are useful for providing prolonged durations of analgesia and may obviate or shorten postoperative ventilation in patients with underlying lung disease and following chest surgery.

Cervical blocks are usually performed with the patient sitting, with the neck flexed, using the midline approach. Clinically, they are used primarily for the management of pain.

Epidural Needles

The standard epidural needle is typically 17–18 gauge, 3 or 3.5 inches long, and has a blunt bevel with a gentle curve of 15–30° at the tip. The Tuohy needle is most commonly used (Figure 45–19). The blunt, curved tip theoretically helps to push away the dura after passing through the ligamentum flavum instead of penetrating it. Straight needles without a curved tip (Crawford needles) may have a greater incidence of dural puncture, but facilitate passage of an epidural catheter. Needle modifications include winged tips and introducer devices set into the hub designed for guiding catheter placement.

Epidural Catheters

Placing a catheter into the epidural space allows for continuous infusion or intermittent bolus techniques. In addition to extending the duration of the block, it may allow a lower total dose of anesthetic to be used.

Epidural catheters are useful for intraoperative epidural anesthesia and/or postoperative analgesia. Typically, a 19- or 20-gauge catheter is introduced through a 17- or 18-gauge epidural needle. When using a curved tipped needle, the bevel opening is directed either cephalad or caudad, and the catheter is advanced 2–6 cm into the epidural space. The shorter the distance the catheter is advanced, the more likely it is to become dislodged. Conversely, the further the catheter is advanced, the greater chance of a unilateral block, due to the catheter tip

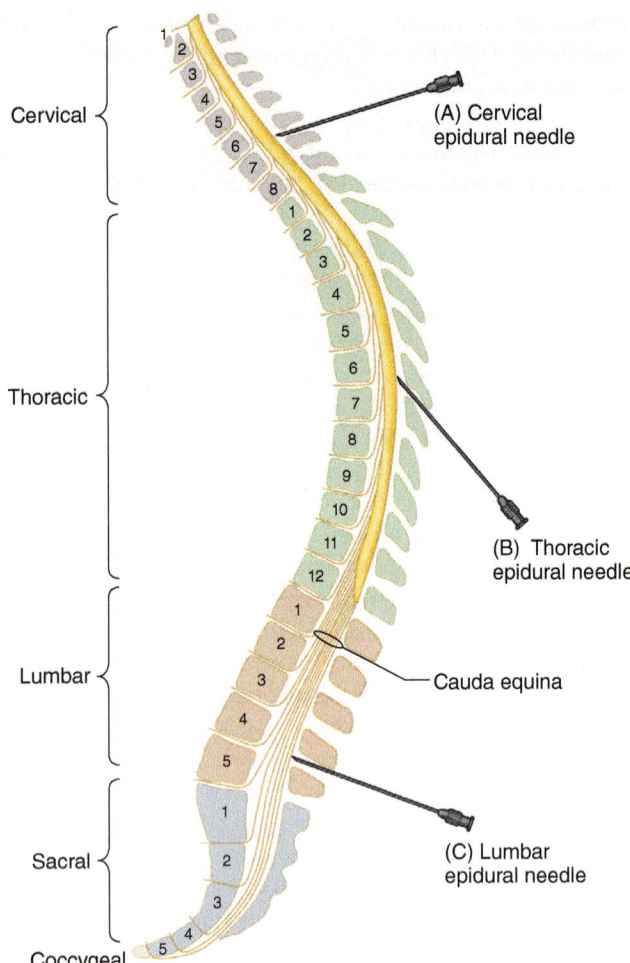

Cervical

(A) Cervical
epidural needle

Thoracic

(B) Thoracic
epidural needle

Lumbar

Cauda equina

FIGURE 45–18 Angulation of the epidural
needle at the cervical (**A**), thoracic (**B**), and lumbar
(**C**) levels. Note that an acute angulation (30–50°)
is required for a thoracic epidural block, whereas
only a slight cephalad orientation is usually
required for cervical and lumbar epidural blocks.

Sacral

(C) Lumbar
epidural needle

Coccygeal

either exiting the epidural space via an intervertebral
foramen or coursing into the anterolateral recesses
of the epidural space. After advancing the catheter
the desired depth, the needle is removed, leaving
the catheter in place. The catheter can be taped or
otherwise secured along the back. Catheters that will
remain in place for prolonged times (eg, >1 wk) may
be tunneled under the skin. Catheters have either a
single port at the distal end or multiple side ports
close to a closed tip. Some have a stylet for easier
insertion. Spiral wire-reinforced catheters are very
resistant to kinking. The spiral or spring tip is associated with fewer, less intense paresthesias and may
be associated with a lower incidence of inadvertent
intravascular insertion.

Specific Techniques for Epidural Anesthesia

Using the midline or paramedian approaches
detailed previously, the epidural needle is passed
through the skin and the ligamentum flavum. The
needle must stop short of piercing the dura. Two
techniques make it possible to determine when the
tip of the needle has entered the potential (epidural)
space: the "loss of resistance" and "hanging drop"
techniques.

The loss of resistance technique is preferred by
most clinicians. The needle is advanced through the
subcutaneous tissues with the stylet in place until
the interspinous ligament is entered, as noted by an

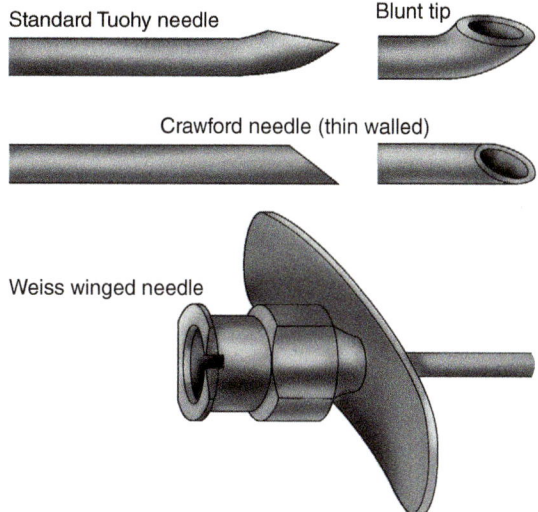

Standard Tuohy needle   Blunt tip

Crawford needle (thin walled)

Weiss winged needle

FIGURE 45–19 Epidural needles.

increase in tissue resistance. The stylet or introducer is removed, and a glass syringe filled with approximately 2 mL of saline or air is attached to the hub of the needle. If the tip of the needle is within the ligament, gentle attempts at injection are met with resistance, and injection is not possible. The needle is then slowly advanced, millimeter by millimeter, with either continuous or rapidly repeating attempts at injection. As the tip of the needle just enters the epidural space, there is a sudden loss of resistance, and injection is easy.

Once the interspinous ligament has been entered and the stylet has been removed, the hanging drop technique requires that the hub of the needle be filled with solution so that a drop hangs from its outside opening. The needle is then slowly advanced deeper. As long as the tip of the needle remains within the ligamentous structures, the drop remains "hanging." However, as the tip of the needle enters the epidural space, it creates negative pressure, and the drop of fluid is sucked into the needle. If the needle becomes plugged, the drop will not be drawn into the hub of the needle, and inadvertent dural puncture may occur. Some clinicians prefer to use this technique for the paramedian approach and cervical epidurals. Successful "epiduralists" rely on either the loss of resistance or hanging drop as

confirmation (rather than as the primary test) that the needle has entered the epidural space. Successful "epiduralists" will generally have sensed the "give" in their hands as the epidural needle tip passes through the ligamentum flavum.

Activating an Epidural

14 The quantity (volume and concentration) of local anesthetic needed for epidural anesthesia is larger than that needed for spinal anesthesia. Toxic side effects are likely if a "full epidural dose" is injected intrathecally or intravascularly. Safeguards against toxic epidural side effects include test and incremental dosing. These safeguards apply whether the injection is through the needle or an epidural catheter.

A test dose is designed to detect both subarachnoid and intravascular injection. The classic test dose combines local anesthetic and epinephrine, typically 3 mL of 1.5% lidocaine with 1:200,000 epinephrine (0.005 mg/mL). The 45 mg of lidocaine, if injected intrathecally, will produce spinal anesthesia that should be rapidly apparent. Some clinicians have suggested the use of lower doses of local anesthetic, as an unintended injection of 45 mg of intrathecal lidocaine can be difficult to manage in areas such as labor rooms. The 15 mcg dose of epinephrine, if injected intravascularly, should produce a noticeable increase in heart rate (20% or more), with or without hypertension. Unfortunately, epinephrine as a marker of intravenous injection is not ideal. False positives (a uterine contraction causing pain or an increase in heart rate coincident to test dosing) and false negatives (bradycardia and exaggerated hypertension in response to epinephrine in patients taking β-blockers) can occur. Simply aspirating prior to injection is insufficient to avoid inadvertent intravenous injection; most experienced practitioners have encountered false-negative aspirations through both a needle and a catheter.

Incremental dosing is a very effective method of avoiding serious complications. If aspiration is negative, a fraction of the total intended local anesthetic dose is injected, typically 5 mL. This dose should be large enough for mild symptoms of intravascular injection to occur, but small enough to avoid seizure or cardiovascular compromise. This is particularly important for labor epidurals that are to be used for cesarean section. If the initial labor epidural bolus was delivered through the needle, and the catheter was then inserted, it may be erroneously assumed that the catheter is well positioned because the patient is still comfortable from the initial bolus. If the catheter was inserted into a blood vessel, or after initial successful placement, has since migrated intravascularly, systemic toxicity will likely result if the full anesthetic dose is injected. Catheters can migrate intrathecally or intravascularly from an initially correct epidural position at any time after placement. Some cases of "catheter migration" may represent delayed recognition of an improperly positioned catheter.

If a clinician uses an initial test dose, is diligent about aspirating prior to each injection, and always uses incremental dosing, major systemic toxic side effects and/or total spinal anesthesia from accidental intrathecal injections will be rare. Rescue lipid emulsion (20% Intralipid 1.5 mL/kg) should be available whenever epidural blocks are performed, in the event of local anesthetic toxicity.

Factors Affecting Level of Block

Factors affecting the level of epidural anesthesia may not be as predictable as with spinal anesthesia. In adults, 1–2 mL of local anesthetic per segment to be blocked is a generally accepted guideline. For example, to achieve a T4 sensory level from an L4–L5 injection would require about 12–24 mL. For segmental or analgesic blocks, less volume is needed.

The dose required to achieve the same level of anesthesia decreases with age. This is probably a result of age-related decreases in the size or compliance of the epidural space. Although there is little correlation between body weight and epidural dosage requirements, patient height affects the extent of cephalad spread. Thus, shorter patients may require only 1 mL of local anesthetic per segment to be blocked, whereas taller patients generally require 2 mL per segment. Although less dramatic than with spinal anesthesia, spread of epidural local anesthetics tends to be partially affected by gravity. The lateral decubitus, Trendelenburg, and reverse Trendelenburg positions can be used to help achieve blockade in the desired dermatomes.

Additives to the local anesthetic, particularly opioids, tend to have a greater effect on the quality of epidural anesthesia than on the duration of the block. Epinephrine in concentrations of 5 mcg/mL prolongs the effect of epidural lidocaine, mepivacaine, and chloroprocaine more than that of bupivacaine, levobupivacaine, etidocaine, or ropivacaine. In addition to prolonging the duration and improving the quality of block, epinephrine delays vascular absorption and reduces peak systemic blood levels of all epidurally administered local anesthetics.

Epidural Anesthetic Agents

The epidural agent is chosen based on the desired clinical effect, whether it is to be used as a primary anesthetic, supplementation of general anesthesia, or analgesia. The anticipated duration of the procedure may call for a short- or long-acting single shot anesthetic or the insertion of a catheter (Table 45–5). Commonly used short- to intermediate-acting agents for surgical anesthesia include chloroprocaine, lidocaine, and mepivacaine. Longer acting agents include bupivacaine, levobupivacaine, and ropivacaine. Only preservative-free local anesthetic solutions or those specifically labeled for epidural or caudal use are employed.

Following the initial 1–2 mL per segment bolus (in fractionated doses), repeat doses delivered through an epidural catheter are either done on a fixed time interval, based on the practitioner's experience with the agent, or when the block demonstrates some degree of regression. Once some regression in sensory level has occurred, one-third to one-half of the initial activation dose can generally safely be reinjected in incremental doses.

It should be noted that chloroprocaine, an ester with rapid onset, short duration, and extremely low toxicity, may interfere with the analgesic effects of epidural opioids. Previous chloroprocaine formulations with preservatives, specifically bisulfite and ethylenediaminetetraacetic acid (EDTA), produced cauda equine syndrome when accidentally injected in a large volume intrathecally. Bisulfite preparations of chloroprocaine were believed to be associated with neurotoxicity, whereas EDTA formulations were associated with severe back pain (presumably due to localized hypocalcemia). Current preparations

TABLE 45–5 Agents for epidural anesthesia.

Agent	Concentration	Onset	Sensory Block	Motor Block
Chloroprocaine	2%	Fast	Analgesic	Mild to moderate
	3%	Fast	Dense	Dense
Lidocaine	≤1%	Intermediate	Analgesic	Minimal
	1.5%	Intermediate	Dense	Mild to moderate
	2%	Intermediate	Dense	Dense
Mepivacaine	1%	Intermediate	Analgesic	Minimal
	2–3%	Intermediate	Dense	Dense
Bupivacaine	≤0.25%	Slow	Analgesic	Minimal
	0.5%	Slow	Dense	Mild to moderate
	0.75%	Slow	Dense	Moderate to dense
Ropivacaine	0.2%	Slow	Analgesic	Minimal
	0.5%	Slow	Dense	Mild to moderate
	0.75–1.0%	Slow	Dense	Moderate to dense

of chloroprocaine are preservative-free and without these complications. Some experts believe that local anesthetics, when injected in very large doses intrathecally may have been at least partly responsible for neurotoxicity.

Surgical anesthesia is obtained with a 0.5% bupivacaine formulation. The 0.75% formulation of bupivacaine is no longer used in obstetrics, as its use in cesarean section has been associated with reports of cardiac arrest after accidental intravenous injection. Very dilute concentrations of bupivacaine (eg, 0.0625%) are commonly combined with fentanyl and used for analgesia for labor and postoperative pain. Compared with bupivacaine, ropivacaine may produce less motor block at similar concentrations while maintaining a good sensory block.

Local Anesthetic pH Adjustment

Local anesthetic solutions have an acidic pH for chemical stability and bacteriostasis. Local anesthetic solutions that are formulated with epinephrine by the manufacturer are more acidic than the "plain" solutions that do not contain epinephrine. Because they are weak bases, they exist primarily in the ionic form in commercial preparations. The onset of neural block requires permeation of lipid barriers by the uncharged form of the local anesthetic. Increasing the pH of the solutions increases the fraction of the uncharged form of the local anesthetic. Addition of sodium bicarbonate (1 mEq/10 mL of local anesthetic) immediately before injection may therefore accelerate the onset of the neural blockade. This approach is most useful for lidocaine, mepivacaine, and chloroprocaine. Sodium bicarbonate is typically not added to bupivacaine, which precipitates above a pH of 6.8.

Failed Epidural Blocks

Unlike spinal anesthesia, in which the endpoint is usually very clear (free flowing CSF) and the technique is associated with a very high success rate, epidural anesthesia is dependent on detection of a more subjective loss of resistance (or hanging drop). Also, the more variable anatomy of the epidural space and less predictable spread of local anesthetic make epidural anesthesia inherently less predictable than spinal anesthesia.

Misplaced injections of local anesthetic can occur in a number of situations. In some patients, the spinal ligaments are soft, and either good resistance is never appreciated or a false loss of resistance is encountered. Similarly, entry into the paraspinous muscles during an off-center midline approach may cause a false loss of resistance. Other causes of failed epidural anesthesia (such as intrathecal, subdural, and intravenous injection) are discussed in the section of this chapter on complications.

Even if an adequate concentration and volume of an anesthetic were delivered into the epidural space, and sufficient time was allowed for the block to take effect, some epidural blocks are not successful. A unilateral block can occur if the medication is delivered through a catheter that has either exited the epidural space or coursed laterally. The chance of this occurring increases as longer lengths of catheter are threaded into the epidural space. When unilateral block occurs, the problem may be overcome by withdrawing the catheter 1–2 cm and reinjecting it with the patient turned with the unblocked side down. Segmental sparing, which may be due to septations within the epidural space, may also be corrected by injecting additional local anesthetic with the unblocked segment down. The large size of the L5, S1, and S2 nerve roots may delay adequate penetration of local anesthetic and is thought to be responsible for sacral sparing. The latter is particularly a problem for surgery on the lower leg; in such cases, elevating the head of the bed and reinjecting the catheter with additional anesthetic solution can sometimes achieve a more intense block of these large nerve roots. Patients may complain of visceral pain, despite a seemingly good epidural block. In some cases (eg, traction on the inguinal ligament and spermatic cord), a high thoracic sensory level may alleviate the pain; in other cases (traction on the peritoneum), intravenous supplementation with opioids or other agents may be necessary. Visceral afferent fibers that travel with the vagus nerve may be responsible.

Caudal Anesthesia

15 Caudal epidural anesthesia is a common regional technique in pediatric patients. It may also be used for anorectal surgery in adults. The caudal space is the sacral portion of the epidural space. Caudal anesthesia involves needle and/or catheter penetration of the sacrococcygeal ligament covering the sacral hiatus that is created by the unfused S4 and S5 laminae. The hiatus may be felt as a groove or notch above the coccyx and between two bony prominences, the sacral cornua (Figure 45–3). Its anatomy is more easily appreciated in infants and children (Figure 45–20). The posterior superior iliac spines and the sacral hiatus define an equilateral triangle (Figure 45–13). Calcification of the sacrococcygeal ligament may make caudal anesthesia difficult or impossible in older adults. Within the sacral canal, the dural sac extends to the first sacral vertebra in adults and to about the third sacral vertebra in infants, making inadvertent intrathecal injection more common in infants.

In children, caudal anesthesia is typically combined with general anesthesia for intraoperative supplementation and postoperative analgesia. It is commonly used for procedures below the diaphragm, including urogenital, rectal, inguinal, and lower extremity surgery. Pediatric caudal blocks are most commonly performed after the induction of general anesthesia. The patient is placed in the lateral or prone position with one or both hips flexed, and the sacral hiatus is palpated. After sterile skin preparation, a needle or intravenous catheter

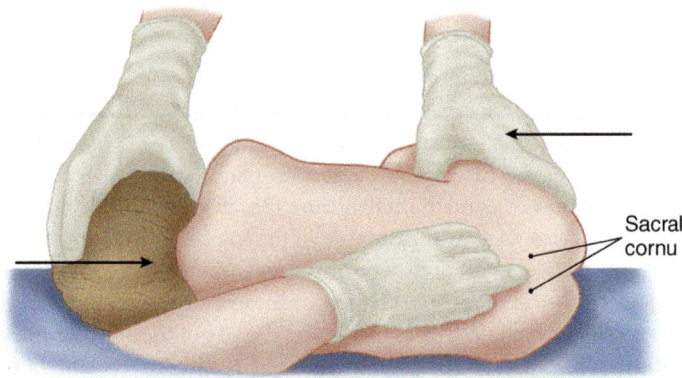

FIGURE 45–20 Positioning an anesthetized child for caudal block and palpation for the sacral hiatus. An assistant gently helps flex the spine.

Sacral cornu

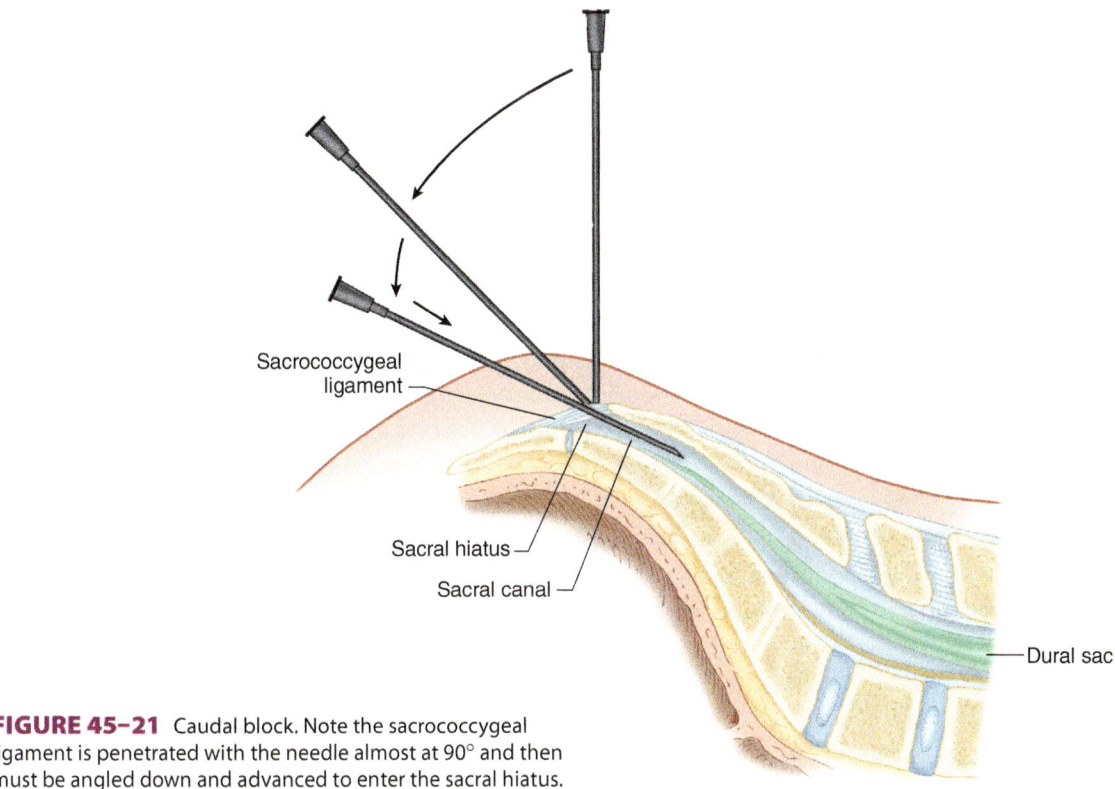

FIGURE 45–21 Caudal block. Note the sacrococcygeal ligament is penetrated with the needle almost at 90° and then must be angled down and advanced to enter the sacral hiatus.

(18–23 gauge) is advanced at a 45° angle cephalad until a pop is felt as the needle pierces the sacrococcygeal ligament. The angle of the needle is then flattened and advanced (Figure 45–21). Aspiration for blood and CSF is performed, and, if negative, injection can proceed. Some clinicians recommend test dosing as with other epidural techniques, although many simply rely on incremental dosing with frequent aspiration. Tachycardia (if epinephrine is used) and/or increasing size of the T waves on electrocardiography may indicate intravascular injection. Clinical data have shown that the complication rate for pediatric caudal blocks is low. Complications include total spinal and intravenous injection, causing seizure or cardiac arrest. Intraosseous injection has also been reported to cause systemic toxicity.

A dosage of 0.5–1.0 mL/kg of 0.125–0.25% bupivacaine (or ropivacaine), with or without epinephrine, can be used. Opioids may also be added (eg, 50–70 mcg/kg of morphine), although they are not recommended for outpatients because of the risk of delayed respiratory depression. Addition of epinephrine will tend to increase the degree of motor block. Clonidine is often added or substituted for local anesthetic. The analgesic effects of the block extend for hours into the postoperative period. Pediatric outpatients can safely be discharged home, even with mild residual motor block and without urinating, as most children will urinate within 8 hr.

Repeated injections can be accomplished via repeating the needle injection or via a catheter left in place and covered with an occlusive dressing after being connected to extension tubing. Higher dermatomal levels of epidural anesthesia/analgesia can be accomplished with epidural catheters threaded cephalad into the lumbar or even thoracic epidural space from the caudal approach in infants and children. Fluoroscopy can assist in catheter positioning. Smaller catheters are technically difficult to pass due to kinking. Catheters advanced into the thoracic

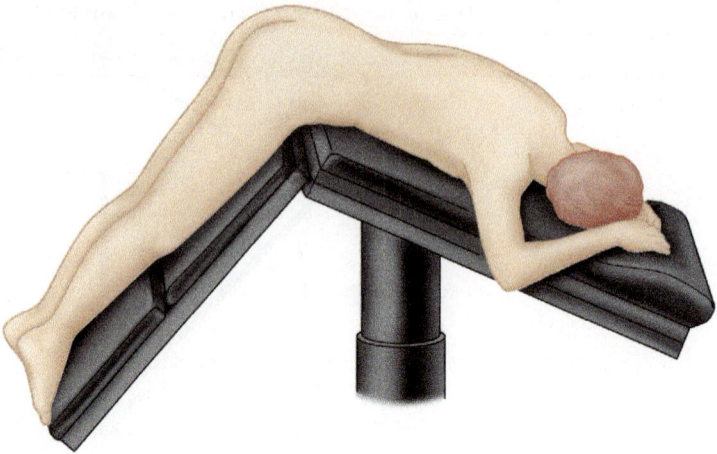

FIGURE 45–22 The prone jackknife position often used for anorectal surgery can also be used for caudal anesthesia in adults. (Reproduced, with permission, from Lambert DH, Covino BG: Hyperbaric, hypobaric, and isobaric spinal anesthesia. Res Staff Phys 1987;10:84.)

epidural space have been used to achieve T2–T4 blocks for ex-premature infants undergoing inguinal hernia repair. This is achieved using chloroprocaine (1 mL/kg) as an initial bolus and incremental doses of 0.3 mL/kg until the desired level is achieved.

In adults undergoing anorectal procedures, caudal anesthesia can provide dense sacral sensory blockade with limited cephalad spread. Furthermore, the injection can be given with the patient in the prone jackknife position, which is used for surgery (Figure 45–22). A dose of 15–20 mL of 1.5–2.0% lidocaine, with or without epinephrine, is usually effective. Fentanyl 50–100 mcg may also be added. This technique should be avoided in patients with pilonidal cysts because the needle may pass through the cyst track and can potentially introduce bacteria into the caudal epidural space. Although no longer commonly used for obstetric analgesia, a caudal block can be useful for the second stage of labor, in situations in which the epidural is not reaching the sacral nerves, or when repeated attempts at epidural blockade have been unsuccessful.

Complications of Neuraxial Blocks

The complications of epidural, spinal, or caudal anesthetics range from the bothersome to the crippling and life-threatening (Table 45–6). Broadly, the complications can be thought of as those resulting

TABLE 45–6 Complications of neuraxial anesthesia.

Adverse or exaggerated physiological responses
Urinary retention
High block
Total spinal anesthesia
Cardiac arrest
Anterior spinal artery syndrome
Horner's syndrome
Complications related to needle/catheter placement
Backache
Dural puncture/leak
Postdural puncture headache
Diplopia
Tinnitus
Neural injury
Nerve root damage
Spinal cord damage
Cauda equina syndrome
Bleeding
Intraspinal/epidural hematoma
Misplacement
No effect/inadequate anesthesia
Subdural block
Inadvertent subarachnoid block[1]
Inadvertent intravascular injection
Catheter shearing/retention
Inflammation
Arachnoiditis
Infection
Meningitis
Epidural abscess
Drug toxicity
Systemic local anesthetic toxicity
Transient neurological symptoms
Cauda equina syndrome

[1]For epidural block only.

TABLE 45–7 Incidence of serious complications from spinal and epidural anesthesia.[1]

Technique	Cardiac Arrest	Death	Seizure	Cauda Equina Syndrome	Paraplegia	Radiculopathy
Spinal (n = 40,640)	26	6	0	5	0	19
Epidural (n = 30,413)	3	0	4	0	1	5

[1]Data from Auroy Y, et al: Serious complications related to regional anesthesia, results of a prospective survey in France. Anesthesiology 1997;87:479.

from excessive effects of an appropriately injected drug, placement of the needle (or catheter), and systemic drug toxicity.

A very large survey of regional anesthesia from France provides an indication of the relatively low incidence of serious complications from spinal and epidural anesthesia (Table 45–7). The American Society of Anesthesiologists (ASA) Closed Claims Project helps to identify the most common causes of liability claims involving regional anesthesia in the operating room setting. In a 20-year period (1980–1999), regional anesthesia accounted for 18% of all liability claims. In the majority of these claims, the injuries were judged as temporary or nondisabling (64%). Serious injuries in the remaining claims included death (13%), permanent nerve injury (10%), permanent brain damage (8%), and other permanent injuries (4%). The majority of regional anesthesia claims involved either lumbar epidural anesthesia (42%) or spinal anesthesia (34%) and tended to occur mostly in obstetric patients. The latter may at least partly reflect the relatively higher use of neuraxial anesthesia compared with other regional techniques and its relatively very high utilization in obstetric patients. Of note is that caudal anesthesia was utilized in only 2% of claims.

Complications Associated with Excessive Responses to Appropriately Placed Drug

A. High Neural Blockade

Exaggerated dermatomal spread of neural blockade can occur readily with either spinal or epidural anesthesia. Administration of an excessive dose, failure to reduce standard doses in selected patients (eg, the elderly, pregnant, obese, or very short), or unusual sensitivity or spread of local anesthetic may be responsible. Patients may complain of dyspnea and have numbness or weakness in the upper extremities. Nausea often precedes hypotension. Once exaggerated spread of anesthesia is recognized, patients should be reassured, oxygen supplementation may be required, and bradycardia and hypotension should be treated.

Spinal anesthesia ascending into the cervical levels causes severe hypotension, bradycardia, and respiratory insufficiency. Unconsciousness, apnea, and hypotension resulting from high levels of spinal anesthesia are referred to as a "high spinal," or when the block extends to cranial nerves, as a "total spinal." These conditions can also occur following attempted epidural/caudal anesthesia if there is accidental intrathecal injection (see below). Apnea is more often the result of severe sustained hypotension and medullary hypoperfusion than a response to phrenic nerve paralysis from anesthesia of C3–C5 roots. Anterior spinal artery syndrome has been reported following neuraxial anesthesia, presumably due to prolonged severe hypotension together with an increase in intraspinal pressure.

Treatment of an excessively high neuraxial block involves maintaining an adequate airway and ventilation and supporting the circulation. When respiratory insufficiency becomes evident, in addition to supplemental oxygen, assisted ventilation, intubation, and mechanical ventilation may be necessary. Hypotension can be treated with rapid administration of intravenous fluids, a head-down position, and intravenous vasopressors. Bradycardia can be treated early with atropine. Ephedrine or epinephrine can also increase heart rate and arterial blood pressure. If respiratory and hemodynamic control can be readily achieved and maintained after high or total spinal anesthesia, surgery may proceed.

B. Cardiac Arrest During Spinal Anesthesia

Examination of data from the ASA Closed Claim Project identified several cases of cardiac arrest during spinal anesthesia. Because many of the reported cases predated the routine use of pulse oximetry, many physicians believed oversedation and unrecognized hypoventilation and hypoxia were the causes. However, large prospective studies continue to report a relatively high incidence (perhaps as high as 1:1500) of cardiac arrest in patients having received a spinal anesthetic, Many of the cardiac arrests were preceded by bradycardia, and many occurred in young healthy patients. Examination of this problem identified vagal responses and decreased preload as key factors and suggests that patients with high baseline vagal tone are at risk. To prevent this from occurring, hypovolemia should be corrected. Prompt drug treatment of hypotension and bradycardia are recommended. Many clinicians will not allow the heart rate to fall below 50 beats per minute during spinal anesthetic blockade.

C. Urinary Retention

Local anesthetic block of S2–S4 root fibers decreases urinary bladder tone and inhibits the voiding reflex. Epidural opioids can also interfere with normal voiding. These effects are most pronounced in male patients. Urinary bladder catheterization should be used for all but the shortest acting blocks. If a catheter is not present postoperatively, close observation for voiding is necessary. Persistent bladder dysfunction can also be a manifestation of serious neural injury, as discussed below.

Complications Associated with Needle or Catheter Insertion

A. Inadequate Anesthesia or Analgesia

As with other regional anesthesia techniques, neuraxial blocks are associated with a small, but measureable, failure rate that is usually inversely proportional to the clinician's experience. Failure may still occur, even when CSF is obtained during spinal anesthesia. Movement of the needle during injection, incomplete entry of the needle opening into the subarachnoid space, subdural injection, or loss of potency of the local anesthetic solution may be responsible. Causes for failed epidural blocks were discussed above (see "Failed Epidural Blocks").

B. Intravascular Injection

Accidental intravascular injection of the local anesthetic for epidural and caudal anesthesia can produce very high serum levels. Extremely high levels of local anesthetics affect the central nervous system (seizure and unconsciousness) and the cardiovascular system (hypotension, arrhythmias, and depressed contractility). Because the dosage of medication for spinal anesthesia is relatively small, this complication is seen after epidural and caudal (but not spinal) blocks. Local anesthetic may be injected directly into a vessel through a needle or later through a catheter that has entered a blood vessel (vein). The incidence of intravascular injection can be minimized by carefully aspirating the needle (or catheter) before every injection, using a test dose, always injecting local anesthetic in incremental doses, and close observation for early signs of intravascular injection (tinnitus, lingual sensations). Treatment is resuscitative, and lipid rescue should be employed.

The local anesthetics vary in their propensity to produce severe cardiac toxicity. The rank order of local anesthetic potency at producing seizures and cardiac toxicity is the same as the rank order for potency at nerve blocks. Chloroprocaine has relatively low potency and also is metabolized very rapidly; lidocaine and mepivacaine are intermediate in potency and toxicity; and levobupivacaine, ropivacaine, bupivacaine, and tetracaine are most potent and toxic.

C. Total Spinal Anesthesia

Total spinal anesthesia can occur following attempted epidural/caudal anesthesia if there is accidental intrathecal injection. Onset is usually rapid, because the amount of anesthetic required for epidural and caudal anesthesia is 5–10 times that required for spinal anesthesia. Careful aspiration, use of a test dose, and incremental injection techniques during epidural and caudal anesthesia can help avoid this complication.

D. Subdural Injection

As with accidental intravascular injection, and because of the larger amount of local anesthetic administered, accidental subdural injection of local anesthetic during attempted epidural anesthesia is much more serious than during attempted spinal anesthesia. A subdural injection of epidural doses of local anesthetic produces a clinical presentation similar to that of high spinal anesthesia, with the exception that the onset may be delayed for 15–30 min and the block may be "patchy". The spinal subdural space is a potential space between the dura and the arachnoid containing a small amount of serous fluid. Unlike the epidural space, the subdural space extends intracranially, so that anesthetic injected into the spinal subdural space can ascend to higher levels than epidural medications. As with high spinal anesthesia, treatment is supportive and may require intubation, mechanical ventilation, and cardiovascular support. The effects generally last from one to several hours.

E. Backache

As a needle passes through skin, subcutaneous tissues, muscle, and ligaments it causes varying degrees of tissue trauma. Bruising and a localized inflammatory response with or without reflex muscle spasm may be responsible for postoperative backache. One should remember that up to 25% to 30% of patients receiving general anesthesia also complain of backache postoperatively, and a significant percentage of the general population has chronic back pain. Postoperative back soreness or ache is usually mild and self-limited, although it may last for a number of weeks. If treatment is sought, acetaminophen, NSAIDs, and warm or cold compresses should suffice. Although backache is usually benign, it may be an important clinical sign of much more serious complications, such as epidural hematoma and abscess (see below).

F. Postdural Puncture Headache

Any breach of the dura may result in a postdural puncture headache (PDPH). This may follow a diagnostic lumbar puncture, a myelogram, a spinal anesthetic, or an epidural "wet tap" in which the epidural needle passed through the epidural space and entered the subarachnoid space. Similarly, an epidural catheter might puncture the dura at any time and result in PDPH. An epidural wet tap is usually immediately recognized as CSF pouring from the epidural needle or aspirated from an epidural catheter. However, PDPH can follow a seemingly uncomplicated epidural anesthetic and may

be the result of just the tip of the needle scratching through the dura. Typically, PDPH is bilateral, frontal or retroorbital, or occipital and extends into the neck. It may be throbbing or constant and associated with photophobia and nausea. The hallmark of PDPH is its association with body position. The pain is aggravated by sitting or standing and relieved or decreased by lying down flat. The onset of headache is usually 12–72 hr following the procedure; however, it may be seen almost immediately. Untreated, the pain may last weeks, and in rare instances, has required surgical repair.

PDPH is believed to result from leakage of CSF from a dural defect and intracranial hypotension. Loss of CSF at a rate faster than it can be produced causes traction on structures supporting the brain, particularly the meninges, dura, and tentorium. Increased traction on blood vessels and cranial nerves may also contribute to the pain. Traction on the cranial nerves may occasionally cause diplopia (usually the sixth cranial nerve) and tinnitus. The incidence of PDPH is strongly related to needle size, needle type, and patient population. The larger the needle, the greater the likelihood of PDPH. Cutting-point needles are associated with a higher incidence of PDPH than pencil-point needles of the same gauge. Factors that increase the risk of PDPH include young age, female sex, and pregnancy. The greatest risk, then, would be expected following an accidental wet tap with a large epidural needle in a young woman (perhaps as high as 20% to 50%). The lowest incidence would be expected in an elderly male using a 27-gauge pencil-point needle (<1%). Studies of obstetric patients undergoing spinal anesthesia for cesarean section with small-gauge pencil-point needles have shown rates as low as 3% or 4%.

Conservative treatment involves recumbent positioning, analgesics, intravenous or oral fluid administration, and caffeine. Keeping the patient supine will decrease the hydrostatic pressure driving fluid out of the dural hole and minimize the headache. Analgesic medication may range from acetaminophen to NSAIDs and opioids. Hydration and caffeine work to stimulate production of CSF. Caffeine further helps by vasoconstricting intracranial vessels. Stool softeners and soft diet are used to minimize Valsalva straining. Headache may persist for days, despite conservative therapy.

An epidural blood patch is an effective treatment for PDPH. It involves injecting 15–20 mL of autologous blood into the epidural space at, or one interspace below, the level of the dural puncture. It is believed to stop further leakage of CSF by either mass effect or coagulation. The effect is usually immediate but may take some hours as CSF production slowly builds intracranial pressure. Approximately 90% of patients will respond to a single blood patch, and 90% of initial nonresponders will obtain relief from a second injection. We do not recommend prophylactic blood patching through an epidural catheter that was placed after a wet tap. Not all patients will develop PDPH, and the tip of the catheter may be many levels away from the dural defect. Most practitioners either offer the epidural blood patch when PDPH becomes apparent or allow conservative therapy a trial of 12–24 hr.

When evaluating patients with presumed PDPH, other sources of headache, including meningeal infection and subarachnoid hemorrhage, should be considered in the differential diagnosis.

G. Neurological Injury

Perhaps no complication is more perplexing or distressing than persistent neurological deficits following an apparently routine neuraxial block. An epidural hematoma or abscess must be ruled out. Either nerve roots or spinal cord may be injured. The latter may be avoided if the neuraxial blockade is performed below the termination of the conus (L1 in adults and L3 in children). Postoperative peripheral neuropathies can be due to direct physical trauma to nerve roots. Although most resolve spontaneously, some are permanent. Some of these deficits have been associated with paresthesia from the needle or catheter or complaints of pain during injection. Some studies have suggested that multiple attempts during a technically difficult block are also a risk factor. Any sustained paresthesia should alert the clinician to redirect the needle. Injections should be immediately stopped and the needle withdrawn, if they are associated with pain. Direct injection into the spinal cord can cause paraplegia. Damage to the conus medullaris may cause isolated sacral

nerve dysfunction, including paralysis of the biceps femoris muscles; anesthesia in the posterior thigh, saddle area, or great toes; and loss of bowel or bladder function. Not all neurological deficits occurring after a regional anesthetic are the result of the block. Surveys of complications have reported many instances of postoperative neurological deficits that were attributed to regional anesthesia when, in fact, only general anesthesia was used. Postpartum deficits, including lateral femoral cutaneous neuropathy, foot drop, and paraplegia, were recognized before the modern era of anesthesia and still occur in the absence of anesthetics. Less clear are the postanesthetic cases complicated by concurrent conditions such as atherosclerosis, diabetes mellitus, intervertebral disk disease, and spinal disorders.

H. Spinal or Epidural Hematoma

Needle or catheter trauma to epidural veins often causes minor bleeding in the spinal canal, although this usually has no consequences. A clinically significant spinal hematoma can occur following spinal or epidural anesthesia, particularly in the presence of abnormal coagulation or a bleeding disorder. The incidence of such hematomas has been estimated to be about 1:150,000 for epidural blocks and 1:220,000 for spinal anesthetics. The vast majority of reported cases have occurred in patients with abnormal coagulation either secondary to disease or pharmacological therapies. Many hematomas have occurred immediately after removal of an epidural catheter. Thus, insertion and removal of an epidural catheter are risk factors.

The pathological insult to the spinal cord and nerves is due to the hematoma's mass effect, compressing neural tissue and causing direct pressure injury and ischemia. The diagnosis and treatment must be accomplished promptly, if permanent neurological sequelae are to be avoided. The onset of symptoms is typically more sudden than with epidural abscess. **Symptoms include sharp back and leg pain with a motor weakness and/or sphincter dysfunction**. When hematoma is suspected, neurological imaging (magnetic resonance imaging [MRI] or computed tomography [CT]) and neurosurgical consultation must be obtained immediately. In many cases, good neurological recovery has occurred in patients who have undergone surgical decompression within 8–12 hr.

Neuraxial anesthesia should be avoided in patients with coagulopathy, significant thrombocytopenia, platelet dysfunction, or those who have received fibrinolytic/thrombolytic therapy. Practice guidelines should be reviewed when considering neuraxial anesthesia in such patients, and the risk versus benefit of these techniques should be weighed and delineated in the informed consent process.

I. Meningitis and Arachnoiditis

Infection of the subarachnoid space can follow neuraxial blocks as the result of contamination of the equipment or injected solutions, or as a result of organisms tracked in from the skin. Indwelling catheters may become colonized with organisms that then track deep, causing infection. Fortunately, these are rare occurrences.

Arachnoiditis, another reported rare complication of neuraxial anesthesia, may be infectious or noninfectious. Clinically, it is marked by pain and other neurological symptoms, and, on radiographic imaging, is seen as a clumping of the nerve roots. Cases of arachnoiditis have been traced to detergent in a spinal procaine preparation. Lumbar arachnoiditis has been reported from subarachnoid steroid injection, but is more commonly seen following spinal surgery or trauma. Prior to of the wide availability of single-use disposable spinal anesthesia trays, caustic solutions used to clean reusable spinal needles caused chemical meningitis and severe neurological dysfunction. Strict sterile technique should be employed, and face masks should be worn by all individuals in the room where neuraxial blocks are to be placed. Careful attention is particularly warranted in the labor room where family members are often curious to see what is being done to mitigate the parturient's pain. Such individuals should be advised to avoid contaminating the tray, if hospital policy permits their presence during epidural placement. If permitted, family members should also wear a mask to prevent contamination of the epidural tray with oral flora.

J. Epidural Abscess

Spinal epidural abscess (EA) is a rare but potentially devastating complication of neuraxial anesthesia. The reported incidence varies widely, from 1:6500 to 1:500,000 epidurals. EA can occur in patients who did not receive regional anesthesia; risk factors in such cases include back trauma, injecting drug use, and neurosurgical procedures. Most reported anesthesia-related cases involve epidural catheters. In one reported series, there was a mean of 5 days from catheter insertion to the development of symptoms, although presentation can be delayed for weeks.

There are four classic clinical stages of EA, although progression and time course can vary. Initially, symptoms include back or vertebral pain that is intensified by percussion over the spine. Second, nerve root or radicular pain develops. The third stage is marked by motor and/or sensory deficits or sphincter dysfunction. Paraplegia or paralysis marks the fourth stage. Ideally, the diagnosis is made in the early stages. Prognosis has consistently been shown to correlate to the degree of neurological dysfunction at the time the diagnosis is made. Back pain and fever after epidural anesthesia should alert the clinician to consider EA. Radicular pain or neurological deficit heightens the urgency to investigate. Once EA is suspected, the catheter should be removed (if still present) and the tip cultured. The injection site is examined for evidence of infection; if pus is expressed, it is sent for culture. Blood cultures should be obtained. If suspicion is high and cultures have been obtained, anti-*Staphylococcus* coverage can be instituted, as the most common organisms causing EA are *Staphylococcus aureus* and *Staphylococcus epidermidis*. MRI or CT scanning should be performed to confirm or rule out the diagnosis. Early neurosurgical and infectious disease consultation is advisable. In addition to antibiotics, treatment of EA usually involves decompression (laminectomy), although percutaneous drainage with fluoroscopic or CT guidance has been reported. There are a few reports of patients with no neurological signs being treated with antibiotics alone.

Suggested strategies for guarding against the occurrence of EA include (1) minimizing catheter manipulations and maintaining a closed system when possible; (2) using a micropore (0.22-μm) bacterial filter; and (3) removing an epidural catheter or at least changing the catheter, filter, and solution after a defined time interval (eg, some clinicians replace or remove all epidurals after 4 days).

K. Sheering of an Epidural Catheter

There is a risk of neuraxial catheters sheering and breaking off inside of tissues if they are withdrawn through the needle. If a catheter must be withdrawn while the needle remains in situ, both must be carefully withdrawn *together*. If a catheter breaks off within the epidural space, many experts suggest leaving it and observing the patient. If, however, the breakage occurs in superficial tissues, the catheter should be surgically removed.

Complications Associated with Drug Toxicity

A. Systemic Toxicity

Absorption of excessive amounts of local anesthetics can produce toxic blood levels (see "Intravascular Injection"). Excessive absorption from epidural or caudal blocks is rare when appropriate doses of local anesthetic are used.

B. Transient Neurological Symptoms

First described in 1993, **transient neurological symptoms** (TNS), also referred to as transient radicular irritation, are characterized by back pain radiating to the legs without sensory or motor deficits, occurring after the resolution of spinal anesthesia and resolving spontaneously within several days. It is most commonly associated with hyperbaric lidocaine (incidence up to 11.9%), but has also been reported with tetracaine (1.6%), bupivacaine (1.3%), mepivacaine, prilocaine, procaine, and subarachnoid ropivacaine. There are also case reports of TNS following epidural anesthesia. The incidence of this syndrome is greatest among outpatients, particularly males undergoing surgery in the lithotomy position, and least among inpatients undergoing surgery in positions other than lithotomy. The pathogenesis of TNS is believed to represent concentration-dependent neurotoxicity of local anesthetics.

C. Lidocaine Neurotoxicity

CES was associated with the use of continuous spinal catheters (prior to their withdrawal) and 5% lidocaine (see "Spinal Catheters"). CES is characterized

by bowel and bladder dysfunction together with evidence of multiple nerve root injury. There is lower motor neuron type injury with paresis of the legs. Sensory deficits may be patchy, typically occurring in a peripheral nerve pattern. Pain may be similar to that of nerve root compromise. Animal studies suggest that pooling or "maldistribution" of hyperbaric solutions of lidocaine can damage the nerve roots of the cauda equina. However, there are reports of CES occurring after uneventful single shot lidocaine spinals. CES has also been reported following epidural anesthesia.

CASE DISCUSSION

Neuraxial Anesthesia for Lithotripsy

A 56-year-old male presents for cystoscopy and stent placement for a large kidney stone. The patient has a long history of spinal problems and has undergone fusion of the cervical spine (C3–C6) and laminectomy with fusion of the lower lumbar spine (L3–L5). On examination, he has no neck flexion or extension and has a Mallampati class IV airway.

What types of anesthesia are appropriate for this patient?

Cystoscopy and stent placement usually require general or neuraxial anesthesia. Selection of the type of anesthesia, as always, should be based on patient preference after informed consent. This patient presents potential difficulties for both general and regional anesthesia. The limited excursion of the cervical spine, together with the anatomy of a class IV airway, makes difficulty in intubation and possibly ventilation almost certain. Induction of general anesthesia would be safest after the airway is secured with an awake fiberoptic intubation.

Regional anesthesia also presents a problem in that the patient has had previous back surgery in the lumbar area, where neuraxial anesthesia is most commonly performed. Some clinicians consider prior back surgery to be a relative contraindication to neuraxial anesthesia. Postoperative distortion of the anatomy makes the block technically challenging and may increase the likelihood of a failure, inadvertent dural puncture during epidural anesthesia, paresthesias, and unpredictable spread of the local anesthetics. Most clinicians believe that the neuraxial blockade can be safely performed above or below the level of surgery. Indeed, lumbar laminectomy can facilitate spinal anesthesia at the level of the surgery.

If the patient chooses to have neuraxial anesthesia, would spinal or epidural anesthesia be more appropriate?

The associated sympathectomy and subsequent drop in blood pressure are more gradual after epidural anesthesia than that following spinal anesthesia. With either type of anesthesia, significant hypotension should be treated with vasoconstrictors and fluids; bradycardia should be treated.

After an explanation of the options, the patient seems to understand the risks of both types of anesthesia and desires epidural anesthesia. Placement of an epidural catheter is attempted at the L1–L2 interspace, but accidental dural puncture occurs: What options are now available?

Options include injecting a spinal dose of local anesthetic through the epidural needle to induce spinal anesthesia, passing an epidural catheter into the subarachnoid space to perform a continuous spinal anesthetic, or proceeding with an awake fiberoptic intubation in advance of general anesthesia. If a spinal dose of local anesthetic is to be injected, the syringe and needle should be kept in place for a few moments to prevent significant back leakage of anesthetic through the large dural hole. Threading an epidural catheter through the needle into the subarachnoid space allows subsequent redosing and may reduce the incidence of dural puncture headache. When a catheter is advanced in the subarachnoid space well below L2, it should not be advanced more than 2–3 cm to avoid injury to the cauda equina.

How might a dural puncture affect subsequent epidural or spinal anesthesia?

A potential hazard of epidural anesthesia at a level adjacent to a large dural puncture is the possibility that some local anesthetic might pass through the dural puncture into the subarachnoid space. This could result in a higher than expected level of sensory and motor blockade. Careful incremental injection of local anesthetic may help avoid this problem.

Conversely, a large dural puncture can theoretically diminish the effect of subsequent spinal anesthesia at an adjacent level. Because only a small amount is used, leakage of local anesthetic with CSF through dural puncture can theoretically limit the cephalad spread of the solution.

GUIDELINES

Hawkins J, Arens J, Bucklin B, et al: Practice guidelines for obstetric anesthesia. Anesth 2007;106:843.

Horlocker TT, Wedel DJ, Rowlingson JC, et al: Regional anesthesia in the patient receiving antithrombotic or thrombolytic therapy: American Society of Regional Anesthesia and Pain Medicine Evidence-Based Guidelines (Third Edition). Reg Anesth Pain Med 2010;35:64.

SUGGESTED READING

Auroy Y, Narchi P, Messiah A, et al: Serious complications related to regional anesthesia: results of a prospective survey in France. Anesthesiology 1997;87:479.

Auroy Y, Benhamou D, Bargues L, et al: Major complications of regional anesthesia in France. Anesthesiology 2002; 97:1274.

Apfel CC, Saxena A, Cakmakkaya O, et al: Prevention of postdural puncture headache after accidental dural puncture: a quantitative systematic review. Br J Anaesth 2010; 105: 255.

Arzola C, Davies S, Rofaeel A, et al: Ultrasound using the transverse approach to the lumbar spine provides reliable landmarks for labor epidurals. Anesth Analg 2007;104:1188.

Birnbach D, Ranasinghe J. Anesthesia complications in the birthplace; is the neuraxial block always to blame? Clin Perinatol 2008;35:35.

Broadman LM, Hannallah RS, Norden JM, McGill WA: "Kiddie caudals": experience with 1154 consecutive cases without complications. Anesth Analg 1987;66:S18.

Brookman CA, Rutledge ML: Epidural abscess: case report and literature review. Reg Anesth Pain Med 2000;25:428.

Chin KJ, Karmakar M, Peng P: Ultrasonography of the adult thoracic and lumbar spine for central neuraxial blockade. Anesthesiology 2011;114:1459.

Chin K J, Perlas A, Chan V, et al: Ultrasound imaging facilitates spinal anesthesia in adults with difficult surface anatomic landmarks. Anesthesiology 2011;115:94.

Choi S, Brull R. Neuraxial techniques in obstetric and nonobstetric patients with common bleeding diasthesis. Anesth Analg 2009;109:648.

Cook TM, Counsell D, Wildsmith JA. Major complications of central neuraxial block: report on the Third National Audit Project of the Royal College of Anaesthetists. Br J Anaesthes 2009;102:179.

Cousins MJ, Bridenbaugh PO, Carr DB, Horlocker TT: *Neural Blockade in Clinical Anesthesia and Pain Management*, 4th ed. Lippincott, Williams & Wilkins, 2008.

Dahlgren N, Tornebrandt K: Neurological complications after anaesthesia. A follow-up of 18,000 spinal and epidural anaesthetics performed over three years. Acta Anaesthesiol Scand 1995;39:872.

Dalens B: Some current controversies in paediatric regional anaesthesia. Curr Opin Anaesthesiol 2006;19:301.

Ecoffey C, Lacroiz F, Giaufre E, et al: Epidemiology and morbidity of regional anesthesia in children: a follow-up one year prospective survey of the French-Language Society of Paediatric Anaesthesiologists (ADARPEF). Pediatr Anesth 2010;20:1061.

Ellis H, Feldman S, Harrop-Griffiths W: *Anatomy for Anaesthetists*, 8th ed. Blackwell Publishing, 2004.

Grände P: Mechanisms behind postspinal headache and brain stem compression following lumbar dural puncture—a physiological approach. Acta Anaesthesiol Scand 2005;49:619.

Green L, Machin S: Managing anticoagulated patients during neuraxial anaesthesia. Br J Haematol 2010;149:195.

Hebl J, Horlocker T, Kopp S, et al: Neuraxial blockade in patients with preexisting spinal stenosis, lumbar disk disease, or prior spinae surgery: efficacy and neurologic complications. Anesth Analg 2010;111:1511.

Khalil S, Campos C, Farag AM, et al: Caudal block in children. Anesthesiology 1999;91:1279.

Lee LA, Posner KL, Domino KB, et al: Injuries associated with regional anesthesia in the 1980s and 1990s: a closed claims analysis. Anesthesiology 2004;101:143.

Liu SS, McDonald SB: Current issues in spinal anesthesia. Anesthesiology 2001;94:888.

Munnur U, Suresh S: Backache, headache, and neurological deficit after regional anesthesia. Anesthesiol Clin North Am 2003;21:71.

Peutrell JM, Lonnqvist P: Neuraxial blocks for anaesthesia and analgesia in children. Curr Opin Anaesthesiol 2003;16:461.

Pollard JB: Cardiac arrest during spinal anesthesia: common mechanisms and strategies for prevention. Anesth Analg 2001;92:252.

Reynolds F: Neurological infections after neuraxial anesthesia. Anesthesiol Clin 2008;26:23.

Rodgers A, Walker N, Schug S, et al: Reduction of postoperative mortality and morbidity with epidural or spinal anaesthesia: results from overview of randomised trials. BMJ 2000;321:1493.

Rukewe A, Alonge T, Fatiregun A: Spinal anesthesia in children: no longer an anathema. Pediatr Anesth 2010;20:1036.

Sarubbi FA, Vasquez JE: Spinal epidural abscess associated with the use of temporary epidural catheters: report of two cases and review. Clin Infect Dis 1997;25:1155.

Steiner L, Hauenstein L, Ruppen W, et al: Bupivacaine concentrations in lumbar cerebrospinal fluid in patients with failed spinal anaesthesia. Br J Anaesth 2009; 102:839.

Suresh S, Wheeler M: Practical pediatric regional anesthesia. Anesthesiol Clin North Am 2002; 20:83.

Vercauteren M, Heytens L: Anaesthetic considerations for patients with a pre-existing neurological deficit: are neuraxial techniques safe? Acta Anaesthesiol Scand 2007;51:831.

Wong CA: Nerve injuries after neuraxial anaesthesia and their medico legal implications. Best Pract Res Clin Obstet Gynaecol 2010;24:367.

Peripheral Nerve Blocks

Sarah J. Madison, MD and Brian M. Ilfeld, MD, MS

KEY CONCEPTS

1 In addition to potent analgesia, regional anesthesia may lead to reductions in the stress response, systemic analgesic requirements, opioid-related side effects, general anesthesia requirements, and possibly the incidence of chronic pain.

2 Regional anesthetics should be administered in an area where standard hemodynamic monitors, supplemental oxygen, and resuscitative medications and equipment are readily available.

3 Local anesthetic may be deposited at any point along the brachial plexus, depending on the desired block effects: interscalene for shoulder and proximal humerus surgical procedures; and supraclavicular, infraclavicular, and axillary for surgeries distal to the mid-humerus.

4 A properly performed interscalene block invariably blocks the ipsilateral phrenic nerve, so careful consideration should be given to patients with severe pulmonary disease or preexisting contralateral phrenic nerve palsy.

5 Brachial plexus block at the level of the cords provides excellent anesthesia for procedures at or distal to the elbow. The upper arm and shoulder are not anesthetized with this approach. As with other brachial plexus blocks, the intercostobrachial nerve (T2 dermatome) is spared.

6 The axillary, musculocutaneous, and medial brachial cutaneous nerves branch from the brachial plexus proximal to the location in which local anesthetic is deposited during an axillary nerve block, and thus are usually spared.

7 Often it is necessary to anesthetize a single terminal nerve, either for minor surgical procedures with a limited field or as a supplement to an incomplete brachial plexus block. Terminal nerves may be anesthetized anywhere along their course, but the elbow and the wrist are the two most favored sites.

8 Intravenous regional anesthesia, also called a Bier block, can provide intense surgical anesthesia for short surgical procedures (45–60 min) on an extremity.

9 A femoral nerve block alone will seldom provide surgical anesthesia, but it is often used to provide postoperative analgesia for hip, thigh, knee, and ankle procedures.

10 Posterior lumbar plexus blocks are useful for surgical procedures involving areas innervated by the femoral, lateral femoral cutaneous, and obturator nerves. Complete anesthesia of the knee can be attained with a proximal sciatic nerve block.

11 Blockade of the sciatic nerve may occur anywhere along its course and is indicated for surgical procedures involving the hip, thigh, knee, lower leg, and foot.

—Continued next page

Continued—

12 Popliteal nerve blocks provide excellent coverage for foot and ankle surgery, while sparing much of the hamstring muscles, allowing lifting of the foot with knee flexion, thus easing ambulation. All sciatic nerve blocks fail to provide complete anesthesia for the cutaneous medial leg and ankle joint capsule, but when a saphenous (or femoral) block is added, complete anesthesia below the knee is provided.

13 A complete ankle block requires a series of five nerve blocks, but the process may be streamlined to minimize needle insertions. All five injections are required to anesthetize the entire foot; however, many surgical procedures involve only a few terminal nerves, and only affected nerves should be blocked.

14 Intercostal blocks result in the highest blood levels of local anesthetic per volume injected of any block in the body, and care must be taken to avoid toxic levels of local anesthetic.

15 The thoracic paravertebral space is defined posteriorly by the superior costotransverse ligament, anterolaterally by the parietal pleura, medially by the vertebrae and the intervertebral foramina, and inferiorly and superiorly by the heads of the ribs.

16 The subcostal (T12), ilioinguinal (L1), and iliohypogastric (L1) nerves are targeted in the transversus abdominus plane block, providing anesthesia to the ipsilateral lower abdomen below the umbilicus.

An understanding of regional anesthesia anatomy and techniques is required of the well-rounded anesthesiologist. Although anatomic relationships have not changed over time, our ability to identify them has evolved. From the paresthesia-seeking techniques described by Winnie in the mid-twentieth century, to the popularization of the nerve stimulator, to the introduction of ultrasound guidance, anesthesiologists and their patients have benefitted from technology's evolution. The field of regional anesthesia has accordingly expanded to one that addresses not only the intraoperative concerns of the anesthesiologist, but also longer term perioperative pain management. **1** In addition to potent analgesia, regional anesthesia may lead to reductions in the stress response, systemic analgesic requirements, opioid-related side effects, general anesthesia requirements, and possibly the development of chronic pain.

PATIENT SELECTION

The selection of a regional anesthetic technique is a process that begins with a thorough history and physical examination. Although many patients are candidates for regional anesthesia/analgesia, as with any medical procedure a risk–benefit analysis must be performed. The risk–benefit ratio often favors regional anesthesia in patients with multiple comorbidities for whom a general anesthetic carries a greater risk. In addition, patients intolerant to systemic analgesics (eg, those with obstructive sleep apnea or at high risk for nausea) may benefit from the opioid-sparing effects of a regional analgesic. Patients with chronic pain and opioid tolerance may receive optimal analgesia with a continuous peripheral nerve block (so-called perineural local anesthetic infusion).

A comprehensive knowledge of anatomy and an understanding of the planned surgical procedure are important for selection of the appropriate regional anesthetic technique. If possible, discussion with the surgeon about various considerations (tourniquet placement, bone grafting, projected surgical duration) is ideal. Also, knowing the anticipated course of recovery and anticipated level of postoperative pain will often influence specific decisions regarding a regional anesthetic technique (eg, a single-injection versus continuous peripheral nerve block).

RISKS & CONTRAINDICATIONS

Patient cooperation and participation are key to the success and safety of every regional anesthetic procedure; patients who are unable to remain still for a procedure may be exposed to increased risk. Examples include younger pediatric patients and some developmentally delayed individuals, as well as patients with dementia or movement disorders. Bleeding disorders and pharmacological anticoagulation heighten the risk of local hematoma or hemorrhage, and this risk must be balanced against the possible benefits of regional block. Specific peripheral nerve block locations warranting the most concern are posterior lumbar plexus and paravertebral blocks owing to their relative proximity to the retroperitoneal space and neuraxis, respectively.

Placement of a block needle through a site of infection can theoretically track infectious material into the body, where it poses a risk to the target nerve tissue and surrounding structures. Therefore, the presence of a local infection is a relative contraindication to performing a peripheral nerve block. Indwelling perineural catheters can serve as a nidus of infection; however, the risk in patients with systemic infection remains unknown.

Although nerve injury is always a possibility with a regional anesthetic, some patients are at increased risk. Individuals with a preexisting condition (eg, peripheral neuropathy or previous nerve injury) may have a higher incidence of complications, including prolonged or permanent sensorimotor block. The precise mechanisms have yet to be clearly defined but may involve local ischemia from high injection pressure or vasoconstrictors, a neurotoxic effect of local anesthetics, or direct trauma to nerve tissue.

Other risks associated with regional anesthesia include local anesthetic toxicity from intravascular injection or perivascular absorption. In the event of a local anesthetic toxic reaction, seizure activity and cardiovascular collapse may occur. Supportive measures should begin immediately, including solicitation of assistance with a code blue, the initiation of cardiopulmonary resuscitation, lipid emulsion administration to sequester local anesthetic, and preparation for cardiopulmonary bypass.

Site-specific risks should also be considered for each individual patient. In a patient with severe pulmonary compromise or hemidiaphragmatic paralysis, for example, a contralateral interscalene or deep cervical plexus block with resultant phrenic nerve block could be disastrous.

CHOICE OF LOCAL ANESTHETIC

The decision about which local anesthetic to employ for a particular nerve block depends on the desired onset, duration, and relative blockade of sensory and motor fibers. Potential for toxicity should be considered, as well as site-specific risks. A detailed discussion of local anesthetics is provided elsewhere (see Chapter 16).

PREPARATION

2 Regional anesthetics should be administered in an area where standard hemodynamic monitors, supplemental oxygen, and resuscitative medications and equipment are readily available. Patients should be monitored with pulse oximetry, noninvasive blood pressure, and electrocardiography; measurement of end-tidal CO_2 and fraction of inspired oxygen (Fio_2) should also be available. Positioning should be ergonomically favorable for the practitioner and comfortable for the patient. Intravenous premedication should be employed to allay anxiety and minimize discomfort. A relatively short-acting benzodiazepine and opioid are most often used and should be titrated for comfort while ensuring that patients respond to verbal cues. Sterile technique should be strictly observed.

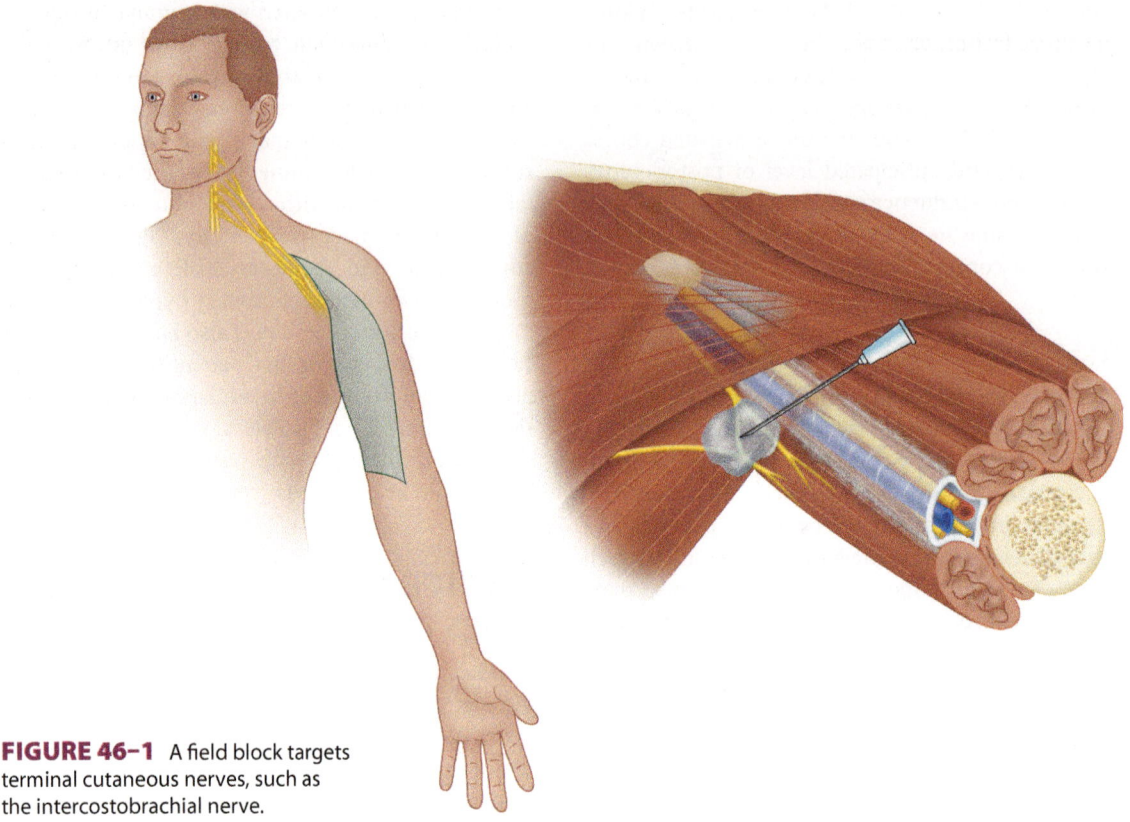

FIGURE 46–1 A field block targets terminal cutaneous nerves, such as the intercostobrachial nerve.

BLOCK TECHNIQUES

Field Block Technique

A *field block* is a local anesthetic injection that targets terminal cutaneous nerves (Figure 46–1). Field blocks are used commonly by surgeons to minimize incisional pain and may be used as a supplementary technique or as a sole anesthetic for minor, superficial procedures. Anesthesiologists often use field blocks to anesthetize the superficial cervical plexus for procedures involving the neck or shoulder; the intercostobrachial nerve for surgery involving the medial upper extremity proximal to the elbow (in combination with a brachial plexus nerve block); and the saphenous nerve for surgery involving the medial leg or ankle joint (in combination with a sciatic nerve block). Field blocks may be undesirable in cases where they obscure the operative anatomy, or where local tissue acidosis from infection prevents effective local anesthetic functioning.

Paresthesia Technique

Formerly the mainstay of regional anesthesia, this technique is now rarely used for nerve localization. Using known anatomic relationships and surface landmarks as a guide, a block needle is placed in proximity to the target nerve or plexus. When a needle makes direct contact with a sensory nerve, a paresthesia (abnormal sensation) is elicited in its area of sensory distribution.

Nerve Stimulation Technique

For this technique, an insulated needle concentrates electrical current at the needle tip, while a wire attached to the needle hub connects to a nerve stimulator—a battery-powered machine that emits a small amount (0–5 mA) of electric current at a set interval (usually 1 or 2 Hz). A grounding electrode is attached to the patient to complete the circuit (Figure 46–2). When the insulated needle is placed in

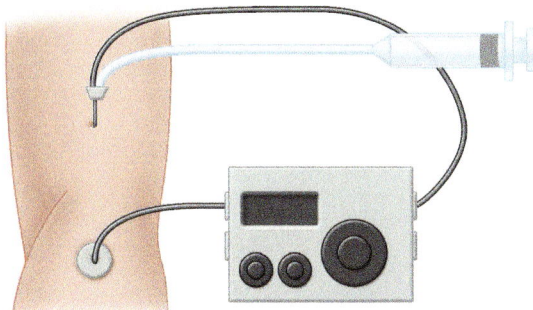

FIGURE 46–2 A nerve stimulator delivers a small amount of electric current to the block needle to facilitate nerve localization.

proximity to a motor nerve, muscle contractions are induced, and local anesthetic is injected. Although it is common to redirect the block needle until muscle contractions occur at a current less than 0.5 mA, there is scant evidence to support this specific current in all cases. Similarly, although some have suggested that muscle contraction with current less than 0.2 mA implies intraneural needle placement, there is little evidence to support this specific cutoff. Nonetheless, most practitioners inject local anesthetic when current between 0.2 and 0.5 mA results in a muscle response. For most blocks using this

technique, 30–40 mL of anesthetic is usually injected with gentle aspiration between divided doses.

Ultrasound Technique

Ultrasound for peripheral nerve localization is becoming increasingly popular; it may be used alone or combined with other modalities such as nerve stimulation. Ultrasound uses high-frequency (1–20 MHz) sound waves emitted from piezoelectric crystals that travel at different rates through tissues of different densities, returning a signal to the transducer. Depending on the amplitude of signal received, the crystals deform to create an electronic voltage that is converted into a two-dimensional grayscale image. The degree of efficiency with which sound passes through a substance determines its echogenicity. Structures and substances through which sound passes easily are described as *hypoechoic* and appear dark or black on the ultrasound screen. In contrast, structures reflecting more sound waves appear brighter—or white—on the ultrasound screen, and are termed *hyperechoic*.

The optimal transducer varies depending upon the depth of the target nerve and approach angle of the needle relative to the transducer (Figure 46–3). High-frequency transducers provide a high-resolution picture with a relatively clear image but

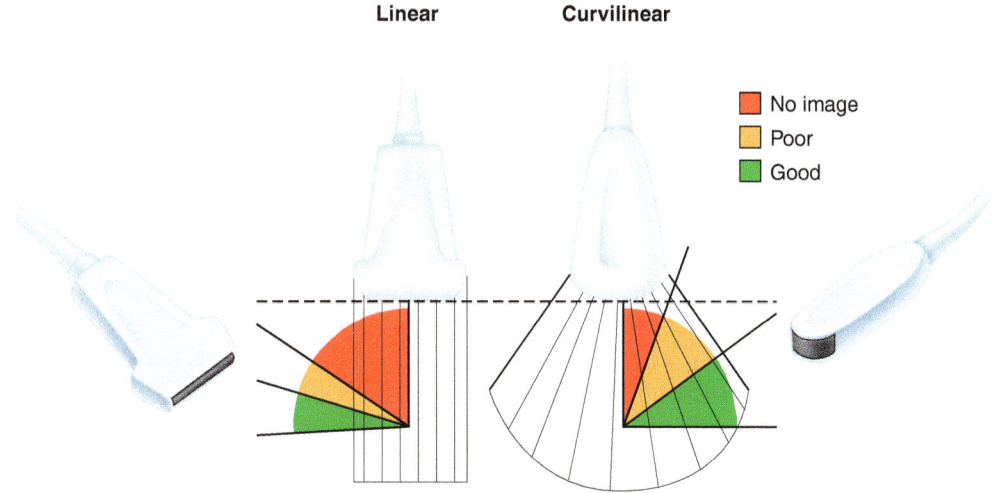

FIGURE 46–3 A linear probe offers higher resolution with less penetration. A curvilinear probe provides better penetration with lower resolution.

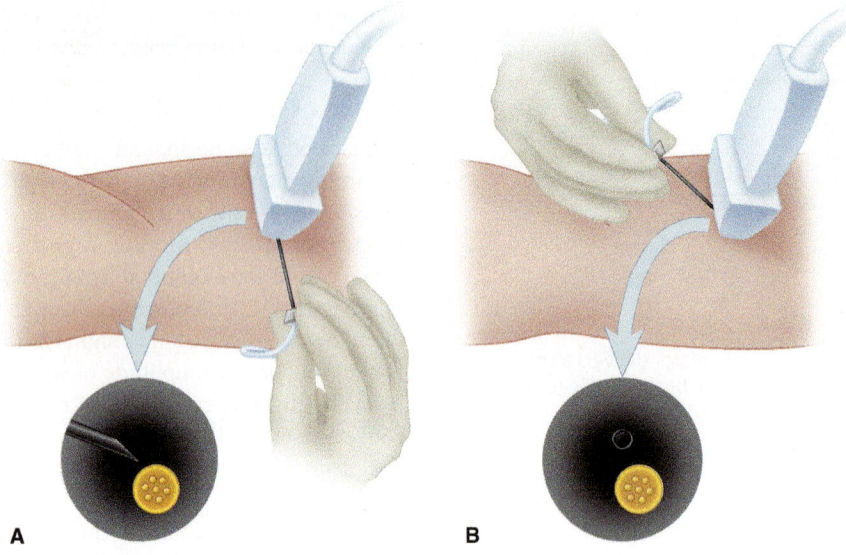

FIGURE 46–4   In-plane (**A**) and out-of-plane (**B**) ultrasound approaches.

offer poor tissue penetration and are therefore used predominantly for more superficial nerves. Low-frequency transducers provide an image of poorer quality but have better tissue penetration and are therefore used for deeper structures. Transducers with a linear array offer an undistorted image and are therefore often the first choice among practitioners. However, for deeper target nerves that require a more acute angle between the needle and long-axis of the transducer, a curved array (curvilinear) transducer will maximize returning ultrasound waves, providing the optimal needle image (Figure 46–3). Nerves are best imaged in cross-section, where they have a characteristic honeycomb appearance ("short axis"). Needle insertion can pass either parallel ("in plane") or not parallel ("out of plane") to the plane of the ultrasound waves (Figure 46–4). Unlike nerve stimulation alone, ultrasound guidance allows for a variable volume of local anesthetic to be injected, with the final amount determined by what is observed under direct vision. This technique usually results in a far lower injected volume of local anesthetic (10–30 mL).

Continuous Peripheral Nerve Blocks

Also termed *perineural local anesthetic infusion*, continuous peripheral nerve blocks involve the placement of a percutaneous catheter adjacent to a peripheral nerve, followed by local anesthetic administration to prolong a nerve block (Figure 46–5). Potential advantages appear to depend on successfully improving analgesia and include reductions in resting and dynamic pain, supplemental analgesic requirements, opioid-related side effects, and sleep disturbances. In some cases patient satisfaction, ambulation, and functioning may be improved; an accelerated resumption of passive joint range-of-motion realized; and reduced time until discharge-readiness as well as actual discharge from the hospital or rehabilitation center achieved.

There are many types of catheters, including nonstimulating and stimulating, flexible and more rigid, through-the-needle and over-the-needle. Currently, there is little evidence that a single design results in superior effects. Local anesthetic is the primary medication infused, as adjuvants do not add benefits to perineural infusions (unlike single-injection peripheral nerve blocks). Long-acting local anesthetics (eg, ropivacaine) are more commonly used as they provide a more favorable sensory-to-motor block ratio (optimizing analgesia while minimizing motor block). In an attempt to further minimize any induced motor block, dilute

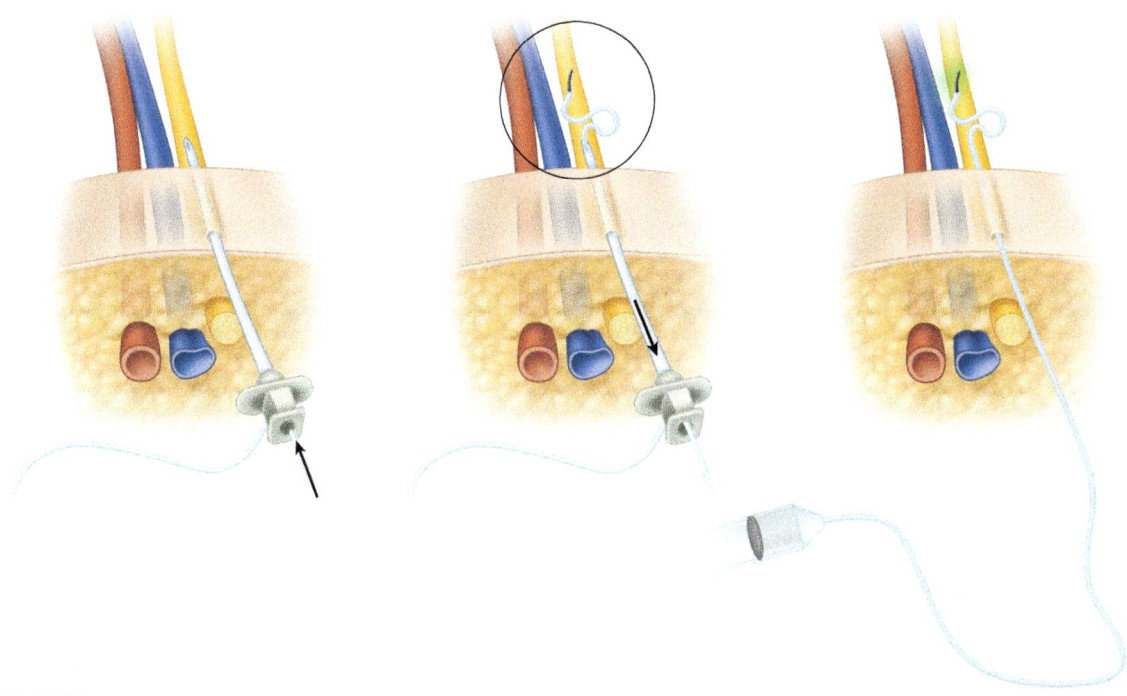

FIGURE 46–5 Placement of a percutaneous catheter adjacent to a peripheral nerve.

local anesthetic (0.1–0.2%) is often infused; however, recent evidence suggests that it is the total dose, and not concentration, that determines the majority of block effects. Unlike *single*-injection peripheral nerve blocks, no adjuvant added to a perineural local anesthetic *infusion* has been demonstrated to be of benefit. The local anesthetic may be administered exclusively as repeated bolus doses or a basal infusion, or as a combination of the two methods. Using a small, portable infusion pump (Figure 46–6), continuous peripheral nerve blocks may be provided on an ambulatory basis.

As with all medical procedures, there are potential risks associated with continuous peripheral nerve blocks. Therefore, these infusions are usually reserved for patients having procedures expected to result in postoperative pain that is difficult to control with oral analgesics and will not resolve in less time than the duration of a single-injection peripheral nerve block. Serious complications, which are relatively rare, include systemic local anesthetic toxicity, catheter retention, nerve injury, infection, and retroperitoneal hematoma

formation. In addition, a perineural infusion affecting the femoral nerve increases the risk of falling, although to what degree and by what specific mechanism (eg, sensory, motor, or proprioception deficits) remain unknown.

UPPER EXTREMITY PERIPHERAL NERVE BLOCKS

Brachial Plexus Anatomy

The brachial plexus is formed by the union of the anterior primary divisions (ventral rami) of the fifth through the eighth cervical nerves and the first thoracic nerves. Contributions from C4 and T2 are often minor or absent. As the nerve roots leave the intervertebral foramina, they converge, forming trunks, divisions, cords, branches, and then finally terminal nerves. The three distinct trunks formed between the anterior and middle scalene muscles are termed superior, middle, and inferior based on their vertical orientation. As the trunks pass over the lateral border of the first rib

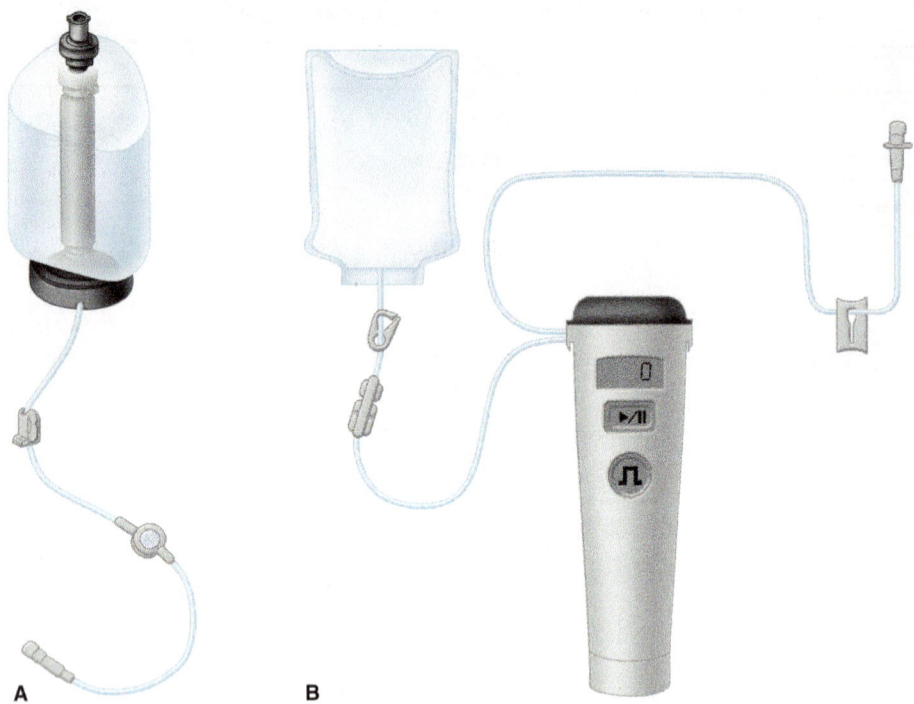

FIGURE 46–6   Elastomeric (**A**) and electronic (**B**) portable infusion pumps.

and under the clavicle, each trunk divides into anterior and posterior divisions. As the brachial plexus emerges below the clavicle, the fibers combine again to form three cords that are named according to their relationship to the axillary artery: lateral, medial, and posterior. At the lateral border of the pectoralis minor muscle, each cord gives off a large branch before ending as a major terminal nerve. The lateral cord gives off the lateral branch of the median nerve and terminates as the musculocutaneous nerve; the medial cord gives off the medial branch of the median nerve and terminates as the ulnar nerve; and the posterior cord gives off the axillary nerve and terminates as the ③ radial nerve. Local anesthetic may be deposited at any point along the brachial plexus, depending on the desired block effects (Figure 46–7): interscalene for shoulder and proximal humerus surgical procedures; and supraclavicular, infraclavicular, and axillary for surgeries distal to the mid-humerus.

Interscalene Block

An interscalene brachial plexus block is indicated for procedures involving the shoulder and upper arm (Figure 46–8). Roots C5–7 are most densely blocked with this approach; and the ulnar nerve originating from C8 and T1 may be spared. Therefore, interscalene blocks are not appropriate for surgery at or distal to the elbow. For complete surgical anesthesia of the shoulder, the C3 and C4 cutaneous branches may need to be supplemented with a superficial cervical plexus block or local infiltration.

Contraindications to an interscalene block include local infection, severe coagulopathy, local ④ anesthetic allergy, and patient refusal. A properly performed interscalene block invariably blocks the ipsilateral phrenic nerve (completely for nerve stimulation techniques; unclear for ultrasound-guided techniques), so careful consideration should be given to patients with severe pulmonary disease or preexisting contralateral phrenic nerve palsy. The hemidiaphragmatic paresis may result in

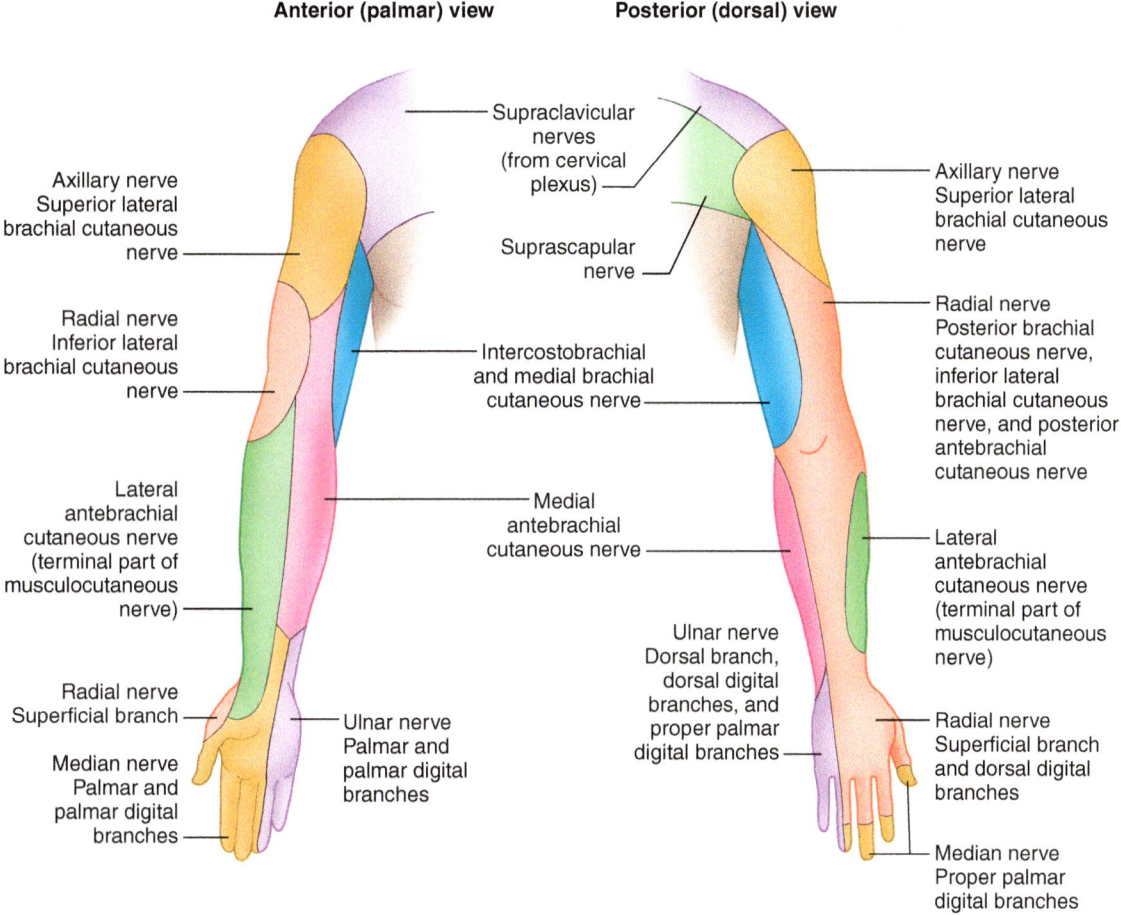

Anterior (palmar) view   **Posterior (dorsal) view**

Axillary nerve
Superior lateral
brachial cutaneous
nerve

Radial nerve
Inferior lateral
brachial cutaneous
nerve

Lateral
antebrachial
cutaneous nerve
(terminal part of
musculocutaneous
nerve)

Radial nerve
Superficial branch

Median nerve
Palmar and
palmar digital
branches

Supraclavicular
nerves
(from cervical
plexus)

Suprascapular
nerve

Intercostobrachial
and medial brachial
cutaneous nerve

Medial
antebrachial
cutaneous nerve

Ulnar nerve
Palmar and
palmar digital
branches

Axillary nerve
Superior lateral
brachial cutaneous
nerve

Radial nerve
Posterior brachial
cutaneous nerve,
inferior lateral
brachial cutaneous
nerve, and posterior
antebrachial
cutaneous nerve

Lateral
antebrachial
cutaneous nerve
(terminal part of
musculocutaneous
nerve)

Ulnar nerve
Dorsal branch,
dorsal digital
branches, and
proper palmar
digital branches

Radial nerve
Superficial branch
and dorsal digital
branches

Median nerve
Proper palmar
digital branches

FIGURE 46–7 The location of local anesthetic deposition along the brachial plexus depends on the desired effects of the block.

dyspnea, hypercapnia, and hypoxemia. A Horner's syndrome (myosis, ptosis, and anhidrosis) may result from proximal tracking of local anesthetic and blockade of sympathetic fibers to the cervicothoracic ganglion. Recurrent laryngeal nerve involvement often induces hoarseness. In a patient with contralateral vocal cord paralysis, respiratory distress may ensue. Other site-specific risks include vertebral artery injection (suspect if immediate seizure activity is observed), spinal or epidural injection, and pneumothorax. Even 1 mL of local anesthetic delivered into the vertebral artery may induce a seizure. Similarly, intrathecal, subdural, and epidural local anesthetic spread is possible.

Lastly, pneumothorax is possible due to the close proximity of the pleura.

The brachial plexus passes between the anterior and middle scalene muscles at the level of the cricoid cartilage, or C6 (Figure 46–9). Palpation of the interscalene groove is usually accomplished with the patient supine and the head rotated 30° or less to the contralateral side. The external jugular vein often crosses the interscalene groove at the level of the cricoid cartilage. The interscalene groove should not be confused with the groove between the sternocleidomastoid and the anterior scalene muscle, which lies further anterior. Having the patient lift and turn the head against resistance often helps delineate the

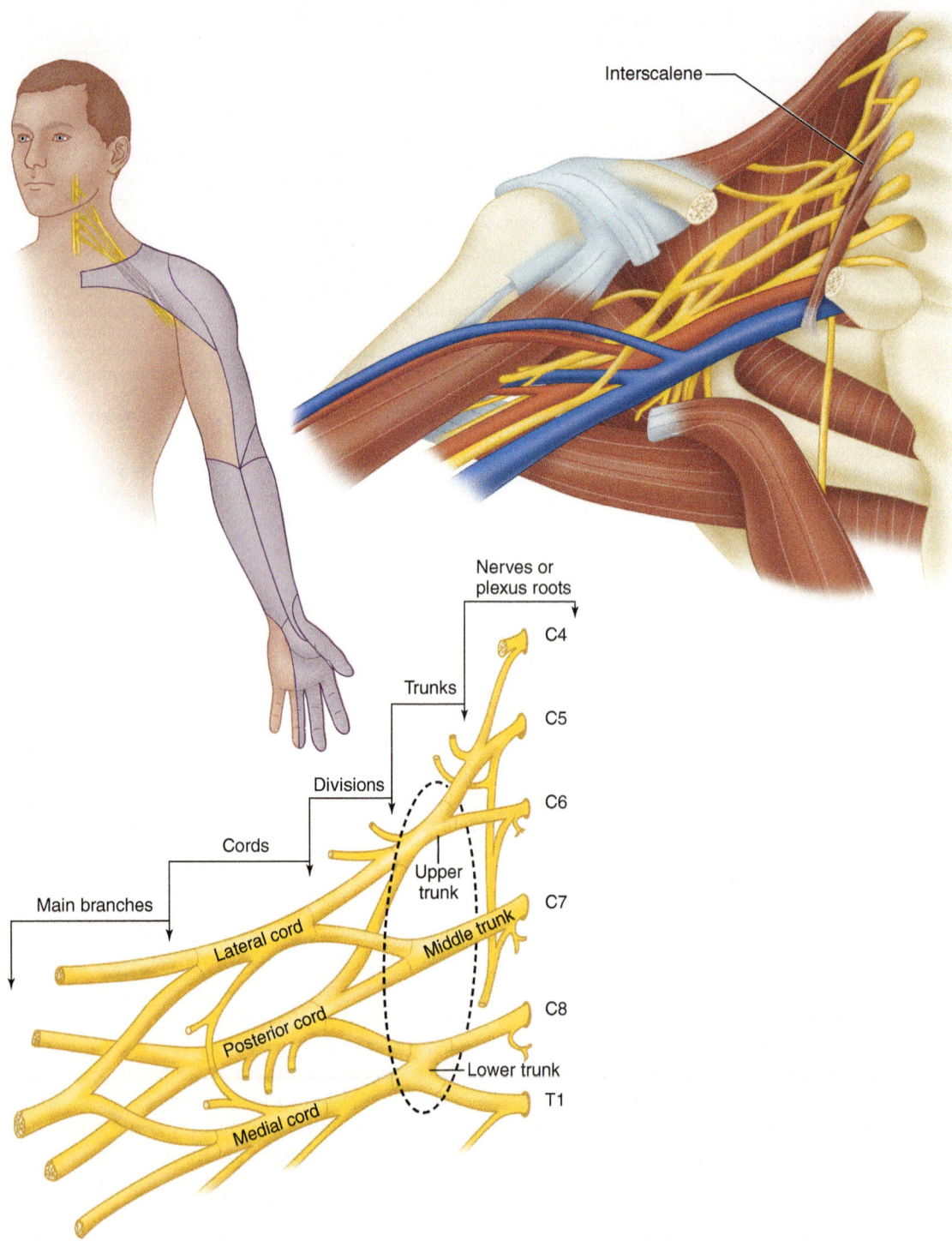

FIGURE 46–8 An interscalene block is appropriate for shoulder and proximal humerus procedures. The ventral rami of C5–C8 and T1 form the brachial plexus.

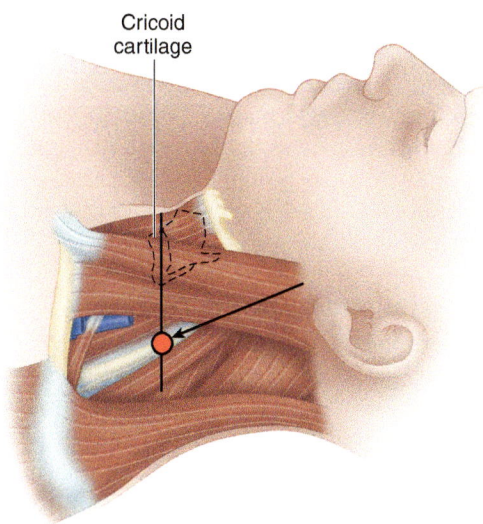

FIGURE 46–9 The brachial plexus passes between the anterior and middle scalene muscles at the level of the cricoid cartilage, or C6.

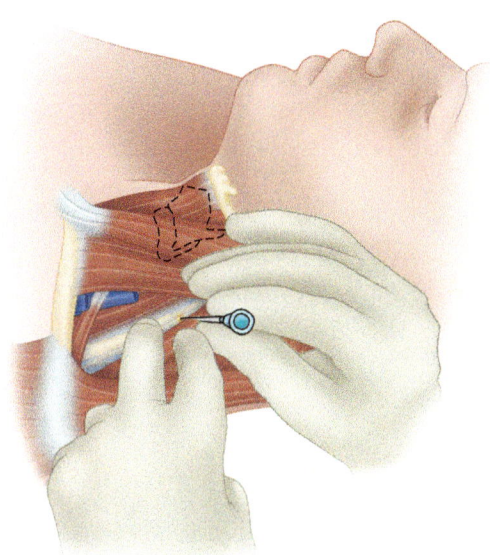

FIGURE 46–10 Interscalene block using nerve stimulation.

anatomy. If surgical anesthesia is desired for the entire shoulder, the intercostobrachial nerve must usually be targeted separately with a field block since it originates from T2 and is not affected with an interscalene block. Interscalene perineural infusions provide potent analgesia following shoulder surgery.

A. Nerve Stimulation

A relatively short (5-cm) insulated needle is usually employed. The interscalene groove is palpated using the nondominant hand, pressing firmly to stabilize the skin against the underlying structures (Figure 46–10). After the skin is anesthetized, the block needle is inserted at a slightly medial and caudad angle and advanced to optimally elicit a motor response of the deltoid or biceps muscles (suggesting stimulation of the superior trunk). A motor response of the diaphragm indicates that the needle is placed in too anterior a direction; a motor response of the trapezius or serratus anterior muscles indicates that the needle is placed in too posterior a direction. If bone (transverse process) is contacted, the needle should be redirected more anteriorly. Aspiration of arterial blood should raise concern for vertebral or carotid artery puncture; the needle should be

withdrawn, pressure held for 3–5 min, and landmarks reassessed.

B. Ultrasound

A needle in-plane or out-of-plane technique may be used, and an insulated needle attached to a nerve stimulator can be used to confirm the accuracy of the targeted structure. For both techniques, after identification of the sternocleidomastoid muscle and interscalene groove at the approximate level of C6, a high-frequency linear transducer is placed perpendicular to the course of the interscalene muscles (short axis; Figure 46–11). The brachial plexus and anterior and middle scalene muscles should be visualized in cross-section (Figure 46–12). The brachial plexus at this level appears as three to five hypoechoic circles. The carotid artery and internal jugular vein may be seen lying anterior to the anterior scalene muscle; the sternocleidomastoid is visible superficially as it tapers to form its lateral edge.

For an out-of-plane technique, the block needle is inserted just cephalad to the transducer and advanced in a caudal direction toward the visualized plexus. After careful aspiration for nonappearance of blood, local anesthetic (hypoechoic) spread

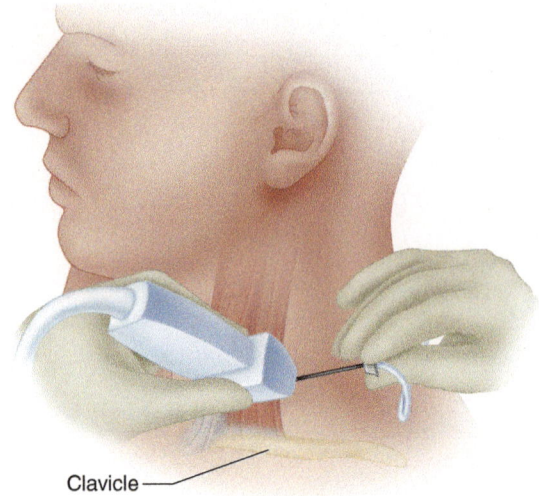

Clavicle

FIGURE 46–11 Ultrasound-guided interscalene block (in-plane technique).

should occur adjacent to (sometimes surrounding) the plexus.

For an in-plane technique, the needle is inserted just posterior to the ultrasound transducer in a direction exactly parallel to the ultrasound beam. A longer block needle (8 cm) is usually necessary. It may be helpful to have the patient turn slightly laterally with the affected side up to facilitate manipulation of the needle. The needle is advanced through the

middle scalene muscle until it has passed through the fascia anteriorly into the interscalene groove. The needle tip and shaft should be visualized during the entire block performance. Depending on visualized spread relative to the target nerve(s), a lower volume (10 mL) may be employed for postoperative analgesia, whereas a larger volume (20–30 mL) is commonly used for surgical anesthesia.

Supraclavicular Block

Once described as the "spinal of the arm," a supraclavicular block offers dense anesthesia of the brachial plexus for surgical procedures at or distal to the elbow (Figure 46–13). Historically, the supraclavicular block fell out of favor due to the high incidence of complications (namely, pneumothorax) that occurred with paresthesia and nerve stimulator techniques. It has seen a resurgence in recent years as the use of ultrasound guidance has theoretically improved safety. The supraclavicular block does not reliably anesthetize the axillary and suprascapular nerves, and thus is not ideal for shoulder surgery. Sparing of distal branches, particularly the ulnar nerve, may occur. Supraclavicular perineural catheters provide inferior analgesia compared with infraclavicular infusion and are often displaced due to a lack of muscle mass to aid catheter retention.

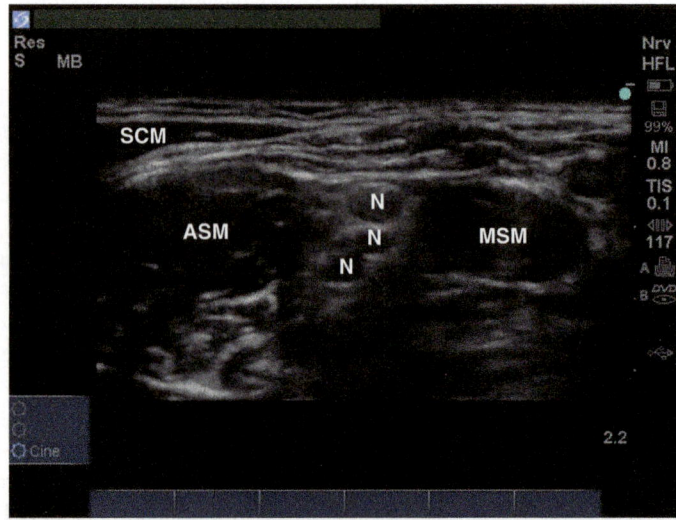

FIGURE 46–12 Interscalene block. Ultrasound image of the brachial plexus in the interscalene groove. ASM, anterior scalene muscle; MSM, middle scalene muscle; SCM, sternocleidomastoid; N, brachial plexus nerve roots in cross-section.

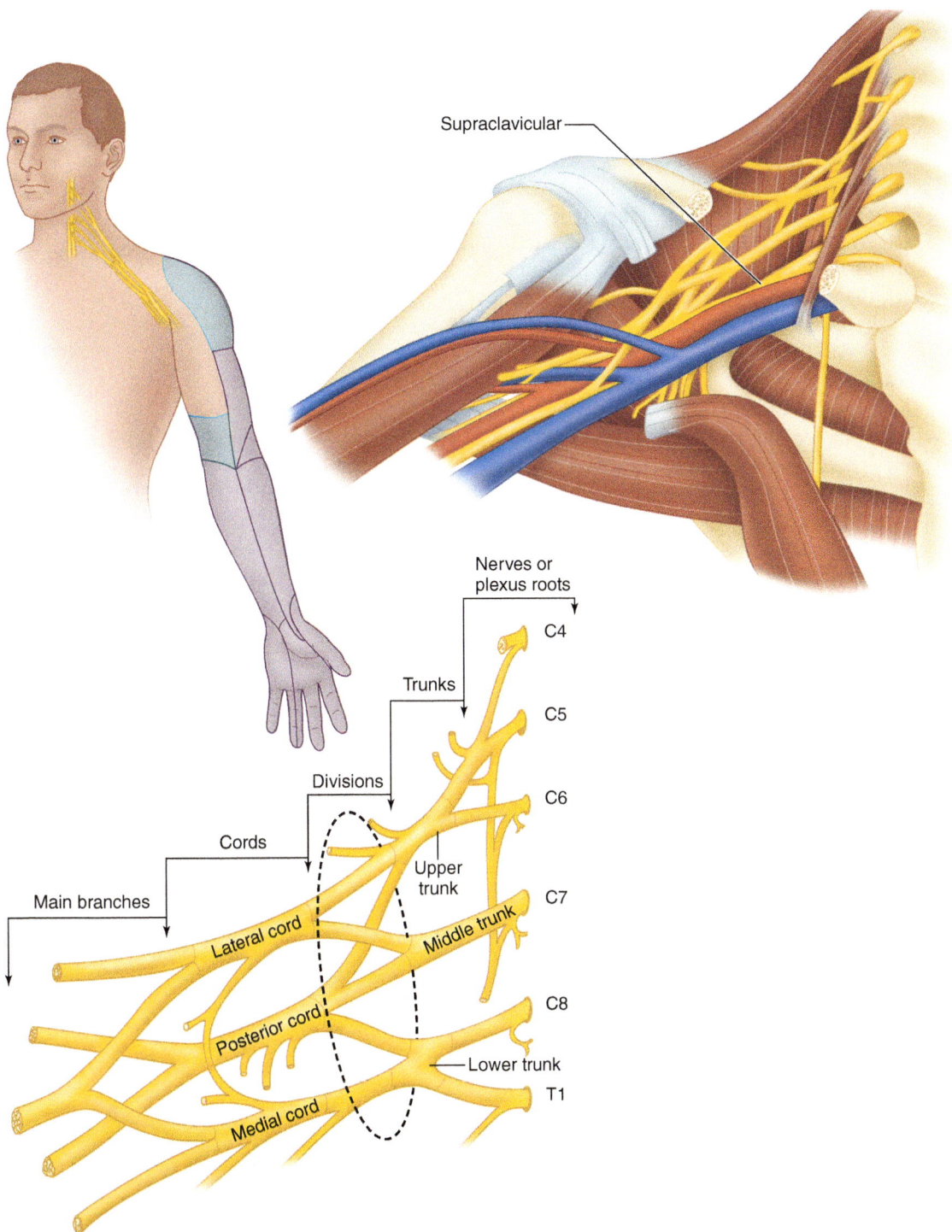

Supraclavicular

Nerves or
plexus roots

C4

C5

Trunks

C6

Divisions

Upper
trunk

C7

Cords

Lateral cord

Middle trunk

Main branches

Posterior cord

C8

Lower trunk

T1

Medial cord

FIGURE 46–13 A supraclavicular block can provide dense anesthesia for procedures at or distal to the elbow. Light blue shading indicates regions of variable blockade; purple shading indicates regions of more reliable blockade.

Many of the same precautions that are taken with patient selection for an interscalene block should be exercised with a supraclavicular block. Nearly half of patients undergoing supraclavicular block will experience ipsilateral phrenic nerve palsy, although this incidence may be decreased by using ultrasound guidance, allowing use of a minimal volume of local anesthetic. Horner's syndrome and recurrent laryngeal nerve palsy may also occur. Pneumothorax and subclavian artery puncture, although theoretically less likely under ultrasound guidance, remain potential risks.

A. Ultrasound

The patient should be supine with the head turned 30° toward the contralateral side. A linear, high-frequency transducer is placed in the supraclavicular fossa superior to the clavicle and angled slightly toward the thorax (**Figure 46–14**). The subclavian artery should be easily identified. The brachial plexus appears as multiple hypoechoic disks just superficial and lateral to the subclavian artery (**Figure 46–15**). The first rib should also be identified as a hyperechoic line just deep to the artery. Pleura may be identified adjacent to the rib, and can be distinguished from bone by its movement with breathing.

For an out-of-plane technique, a short, 22-gauge blunt-tipped needle is used. The skin is anesthetized, and the needle inserted just cephalad to the ultrasound transducer in a posterior and caudad

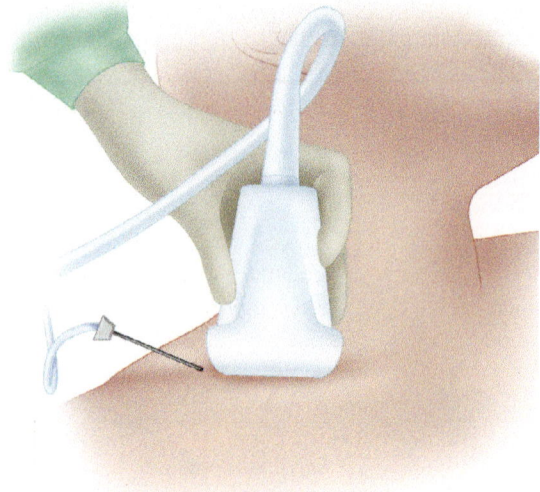

FIGURE 46–14 Ultrasound probe placement for supraclavicular block (in-plane technique).

direction. After careful aspiration for the nonappearance of blood, 30–40 mL of local anesthetic s injected in 5-mL increments while visualizing local anesthetic spread around the brachial plexus.

For an in-plane technique, a longer needle may be necessary. The needle is inserted lateral to the transducer in a direction parallel to the ultrasound beam. The needle is advanced medially toward the subclavian artery until the tip is visualized near the brachial plexus just lateral and superficial to the

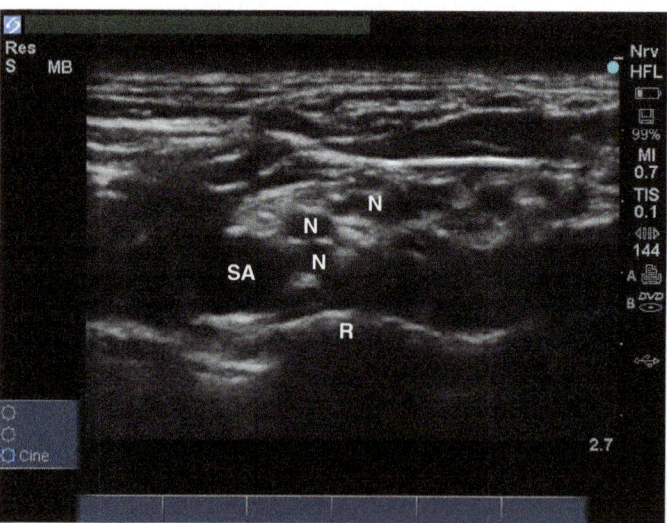

FIGURE 46–15 Supraclavicular block. Ultrasound image of the brachial plexus in the supraclavicular fossa. SA, subclavian artery; R, rib; N, brachial plexus in cross-section.

artery. Local anesthetic spread should be visualized surrounding the plexus after careful aspiration and incremental injection, which often requires injections in multiple locations and a highly variable volume (20–30 mL).

Infraclavicular Block

5 Brachial plexus block at the level of the cords provides excellent anesthesia for procedures at or distal to the elbow (Figure 46–16). The upper arm and shoulder are not anesthetized with this approach. As with other brachial plexus blocks, the intercostobrachial nerve (T2 dermatome) is spared. Site-specific risks of the infraclavicular approach include vascular puncture and pneumothorax (although less common than with supraclavicular block). It is often prudent to avoid this approach in patients with vascular catheters in the subclavian region, or patients with an ipsilateral pacemaker.

As the brachial plexus traverses beyond the first rib and into the axilla, the cords are arranged around the axillary artery according to their anatomic position: medial, lateral, and posterior.

A. Nerve Stimulation

The patient is positioned supine with the head turned to the contralateral side, and the coracoid process is identified (a bony prominence of the scapula that can be palpated between the acromioclavicular joint and the deltopectoral groove). The subclavian artery and brachial plexus run deep to the coracoid process and can be found approximately 2 cm medial and 2 cm caudad to it, about 4–5 cm deep in the average patient (Figure 46–17). A relatively long (8 cm) insulated needle is placed perpendicular to the skin and advanced directly posterior until a motor response is elicited. An acceptable motor response is finger flexion or extension at a current less than 0.5 mA, but not elbow flexion/extension.

B. Ultrasound

With the patient in the supine position, a small curvilinear transducer is placed in the parasagittal plane over the point 2 cm medial and 2 cm caudad to the coracoid process (Figure 46–18A). (Abducting the arm 90° improves axillary artery imaging.) A high-frequency linear transducer will often provide inadequate needle visualization due to the relatively acute needle-to-transducer angle. The axillary artery and vein are identified in cross-section (Figure 46–18B). The medial, lateral, and posterior cords appear as hyperechoic bundles positioned caudad, cephalad, and posterior to the artery, respectively. A relatively long needle is inserted 2–3 cm cephalad to the transducer. Optimal needle positioning is between the axillary artery and the posterior cord. Three randomized, controlled trials have demonstrated equivalent results with a single 30-mL injection adjacent to the posterior cord or divided among each of the cords. Insertion of a perineural catheter should always be in the same location posterior to the axillary artery, and infraclavicular infusion has been shown to provide superior analgesia to both supraclavicular and axillary catheters.

Axillary Block

At the lateral border of the pectoralis minor muscle, the cords of the brachial plexus form large terminal **6** branches. The axillary, musculocutaneous, and medial brachial cutaneous nerves branch from the brachial plexus proximal to the location in which local anesthetic is deposited during an axillary nerve block, and thus are usually spared (Figure 46–19). At this level, the major terminal nerves often are separated by fascia; therefore multiple injections (10-mL each) may be required to reliably produce anesthesia of the entire arm distal to the elbow (Figure 46–20).

There are few contraindications to axillary brachial plexus blocks. Local infection, neuropathy, and bleeding risk must be considered. Because the axilla is highly vascularized, there is a risk of local anesthetic uptake through small veins traumatized by needle placement. The axilla is also a suboptimal site for perineural catheter placement because of greatly inferior analgesia versus an infraclavicular infusion, as well as theoretically increased risks of infection and catheter dislodgement.

All of the numerous axillary block techniques require the patient to be positioned supine, with the arm abducted 90° and the head turned toward the contralateral side (Figure 46–20). The axillary artery pulse should be palpated and its location marked as a reference point.

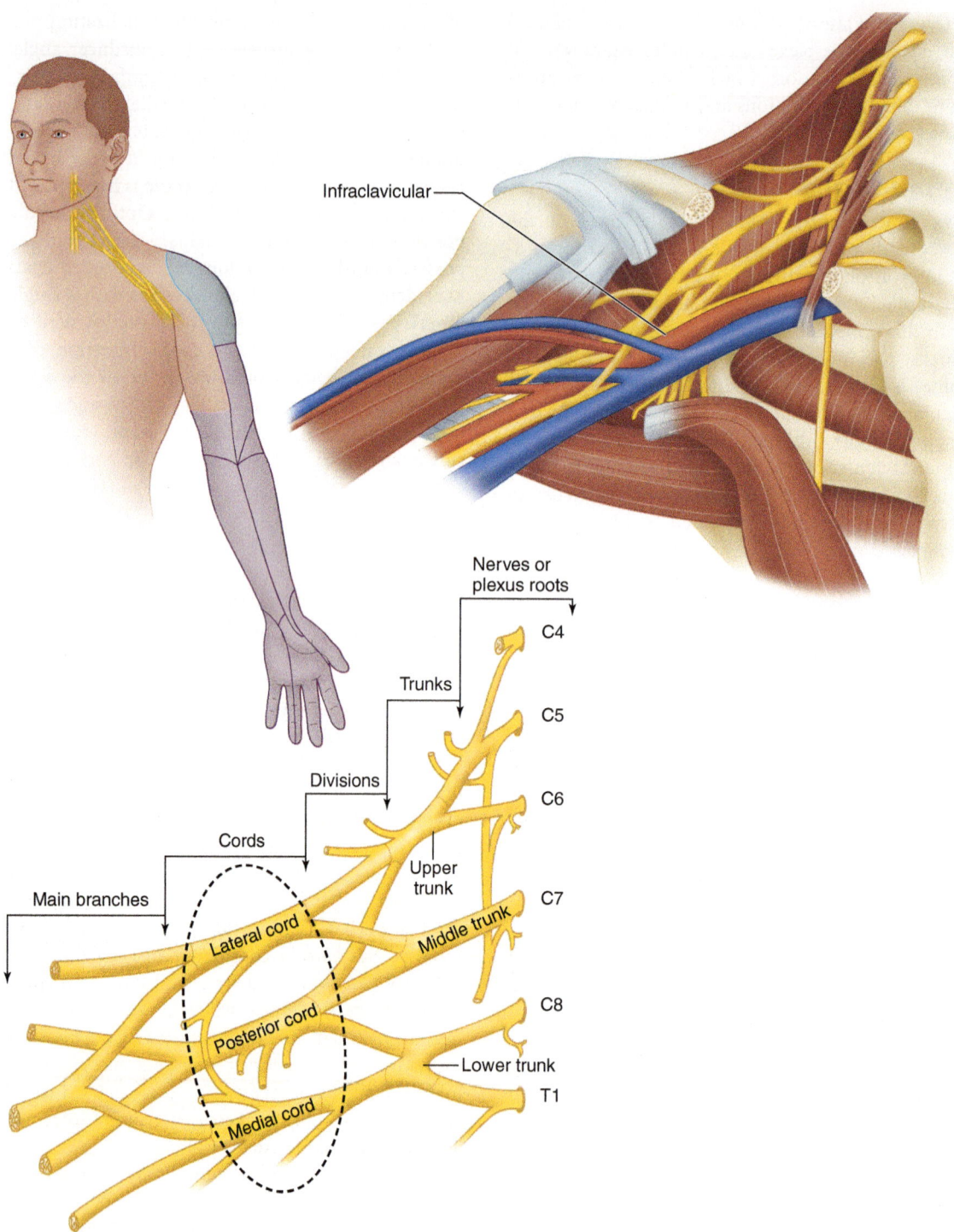

Infraclavicular

Nerves or plexus roots

C4

C5

C6

C7

C8

T1

Trunks

Divisions

Cords

Main branches

Upper trunk

Middle trunk

Lower trunk

Lateral cord

Posterior cord

Medial cord

FIGURE 46–16 Infraclavicular block coverage and anatomy. Light blue shading indicates regions of variable blockade; purple shading indicates regions of more reliable blockade.

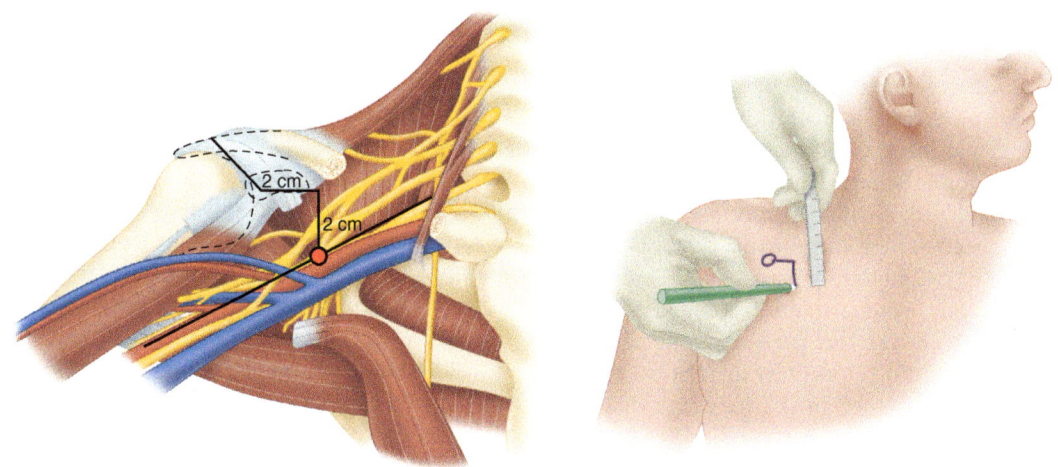

FIGURE 46–17 Infraclavicular block using nerve stimulation: coracoid technique.

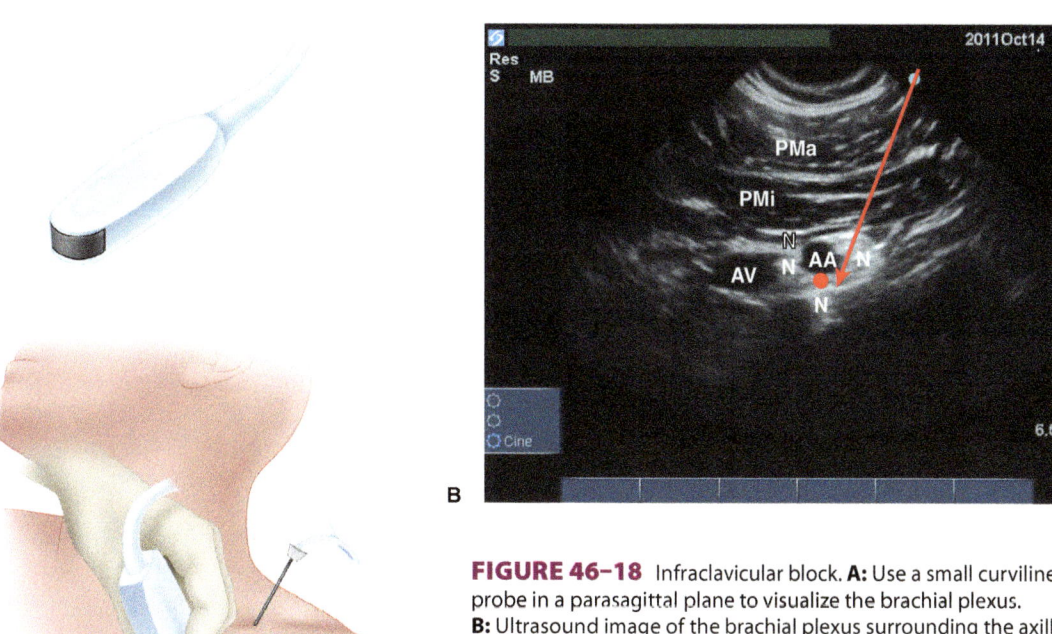

FIGURE 46–18 Infraclavicular block. **A:** Use a small curvilinear probe in a parasagittal plane to visualize the brachial plexus. **B:** Ultrasound image of the brachial plexus surrounding the axillary artery. AA, axillary artery; N, medial, lateral, and posterior cords of the brachial plexus; AV, axillary vein; PMa, pectoralis major muscle; PMi, pectoralis minor muscle. The red dot indicates the location of local anesthetic deposition.

A. Transarterial Technique

This technique has fallen out of favor due to the trauma of twice purposefully penetrating the axillary artery along with a theoretically increased risk of inadvertent intravascular local anesthetic injection. The nondominant hand is used to palpate and immobilize the axillary artery, and a 22-gauge needle is inserted high in the axilla (Figure 46–20) until bright red blood is aspirated. The needle is then slightly advanced until blood aspiration ceases. Injection can be performed posteriorly, anteriorly, or in both locations in relation to the artery. A total of 30–40 mL of local anesthetic is typically used.

B. Nerve Stimulation

Again the nondominant hand is used to palpate and immobilize the axillary artery. With the arm abducted and externally rotated, the terminal nerves usually lie in the following positions relative to the artery (Figure 46–21, although variations are common): median nerve superior (wrist flexion, thumb opposition, forearm pronation); ulnar nerve inferior (wrist flexion, thumb adduction, fourth/fifth digit flexion); and radial nerve inferior–posterior (digit/wrist/elbow extension, forearm supination). The musculocutaneous nerve (elbow flexion) is separate and deep within the coracobrachialis muscle, which is more superior (lateral) in this position and, as a consequence, is often not blocked with this procedure (Figure 46–21). A 2-in., 22-gauge insulated needle is inserted proximal to the palpating fingers to elicit muscle twitches in the hand. Once an acceptable muscle response is identified, and after reducing the stimulation to less than 0.5 mA, careful aspiration is performed and local anesthetic is injected. Although a single injection of 40 mL may be used, greater success will be seen with multiple nerve stimulations (ie, two or three nerves) and divided doses of local anesthetic.

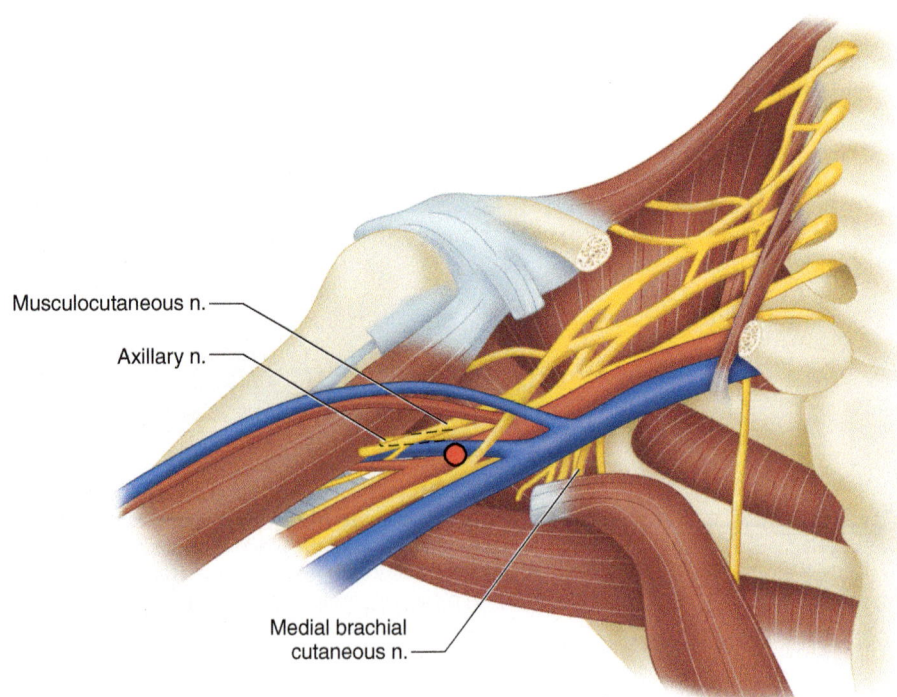

Musculocutaneous n.

Axillary n.

Medial brachial cutaneous n.

FIGURE 46–19   Axillary block. The axillary, musculocutaneous, and medial brachial cutaneous nerves are usually spared with an axillary approach.

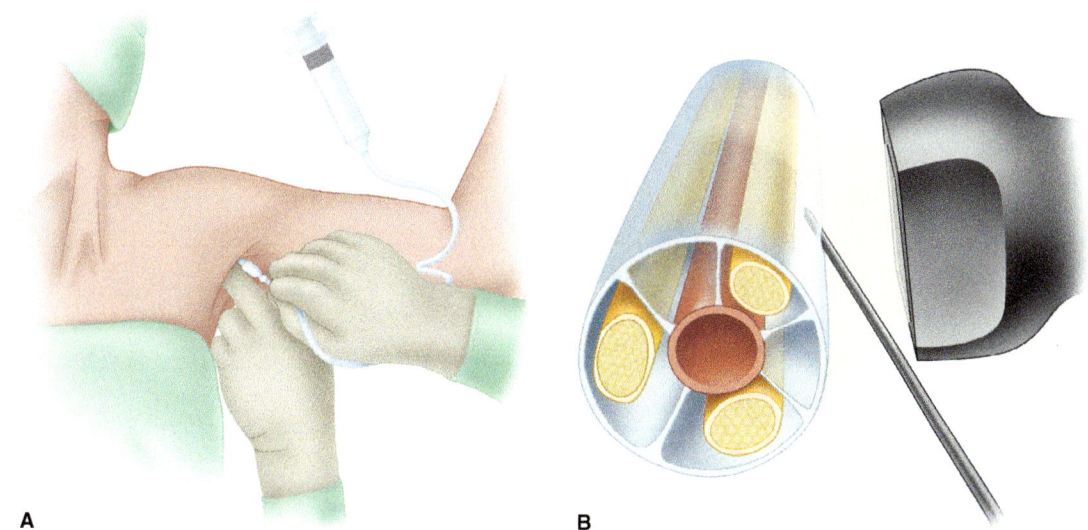

FIGURE 46–20 **A:** Patient positioning and needle angle for axillary brachial plexus block. **B:** A multiple injection technique is more effective because of fascial separation between nerves.

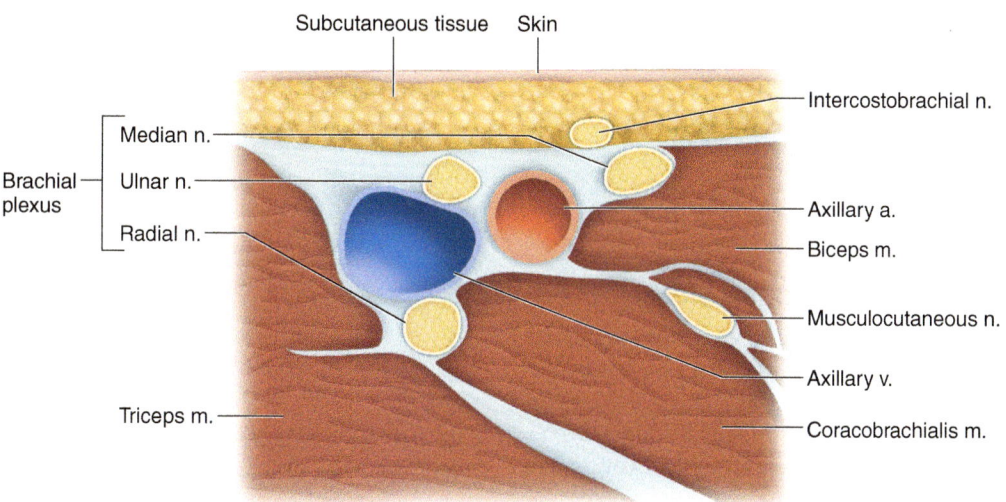

FIGURE 46–21 Positioning of terminal nerves about the axillary artery (variations are common).

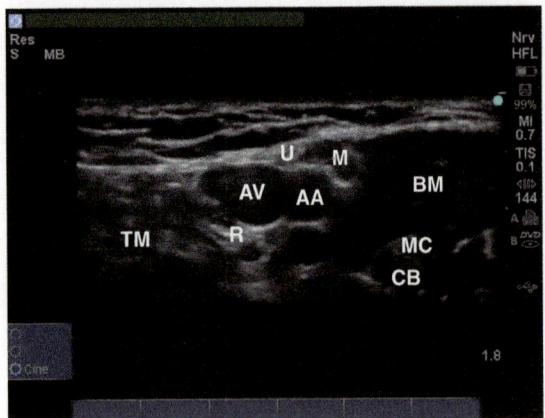

FIGURE 46–22 Ultrasound image of axillary brachial plexus block. AA, Axillary artery; AV, axillary vein; U, ulnar nerve; M, median nerve; MC, musculocutaneous nerve; R, radial nerve; CB, coracobrachialis muscle; TM, triceps muscle; BM, biceps muscle.

C. Ultrasound

Using a high-frequency linear array ultrasound transducer, the axillary artery and vein are visualized in cross-section. The brachial plexus can be identified surrounding the artery (Figure 46–22). The needle is inserted superior (lateral) to the transducer and advanced inferiorly (medially) toward the plexus under direct visualization. Ten milliliters of local anesthetic is then injected around each nerve (including the musculocutaneous, if indicated).

Blocks of the Terminal Nerves

7 Often it is necessary to anesthetize a single terminal nerve, either for minor surgical procedures with a limited field or as a supplement to an incomplete brachial plexus block. Terminal nerves may be anesthetized anywhere along their course, but the elbow and the wrist are the two most favored sites.

A. Median Nerve Block

The median nerve is derived from the lateral and medial cords of the brachial plexus. It enters the arm and runs just medial to the brachial artery

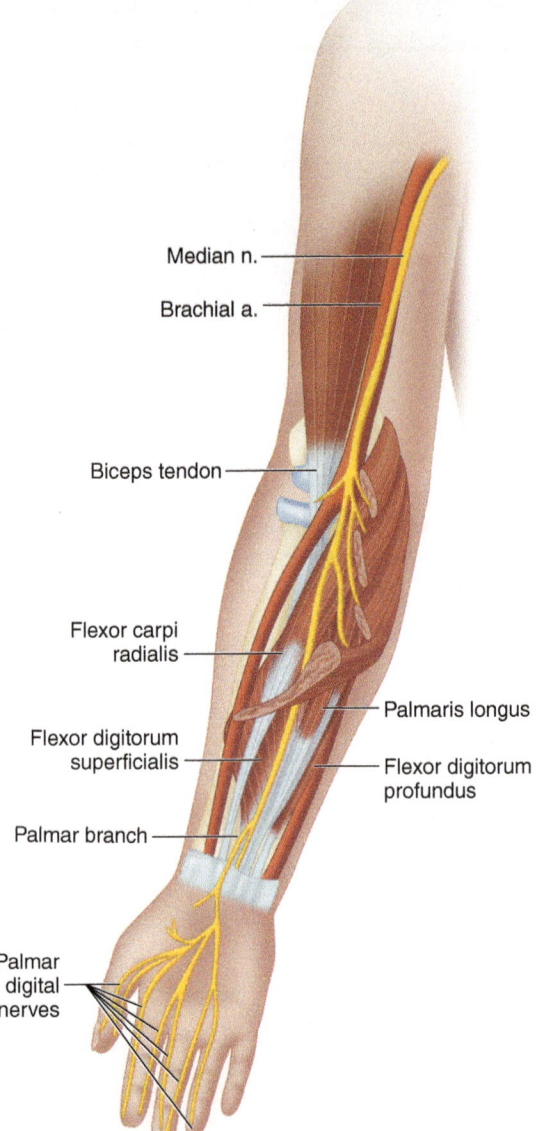

FIGURE 46–23 Median nerve course.

(Figure 46–23). As it enters the antecubital space, it lies medial to the brachial artery near the insertion of the biceps tendon. Just distal to this point, it gives off numerous motor branches to the wrist and finger flexors and follows the interosseous membrane to the wrist. At the level of the proximal wrist flexion crease, it lies directly behind the palmaris longus tendon in the carpal tunnel.

To block the median nerve at the elbow, the brachial artery is identified in the antecubital crease just medial to the biceps insertion. A short 22-gauge insulated needle is inserted just medial to the artery and directed toward the medial epicondyle until wrist flexion or thumb opposition is elicited (Figure 46–24); 3–5 mL of local anesthetic is then injected. If ultrasound is used, the median nerve may be identified in cross-section just medial to the brachial artery and local anesthetic injected to surround it (Figure 46–25).

To block the median nerve at the wrist, the palmaris longus tendon is first identified by asking the patient to flex the wrist against resistance. A short 22-gauge needle is inserted just medial and deep to the palmaris longus tendon, and 3–5 mL

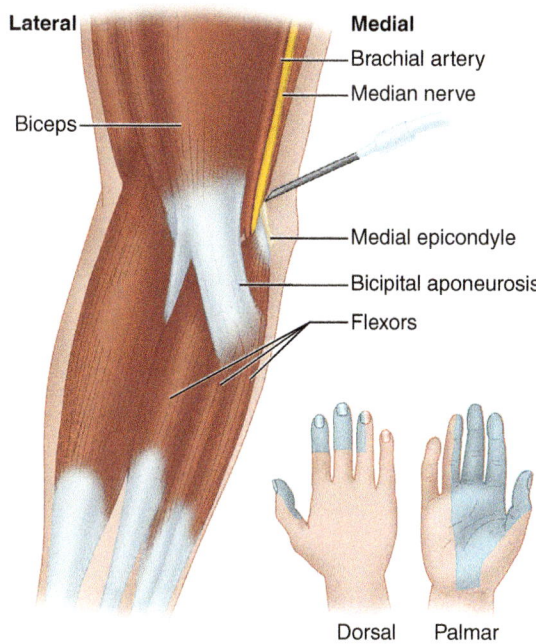

FIGURE 46–24 Median nerve block at the elbow.

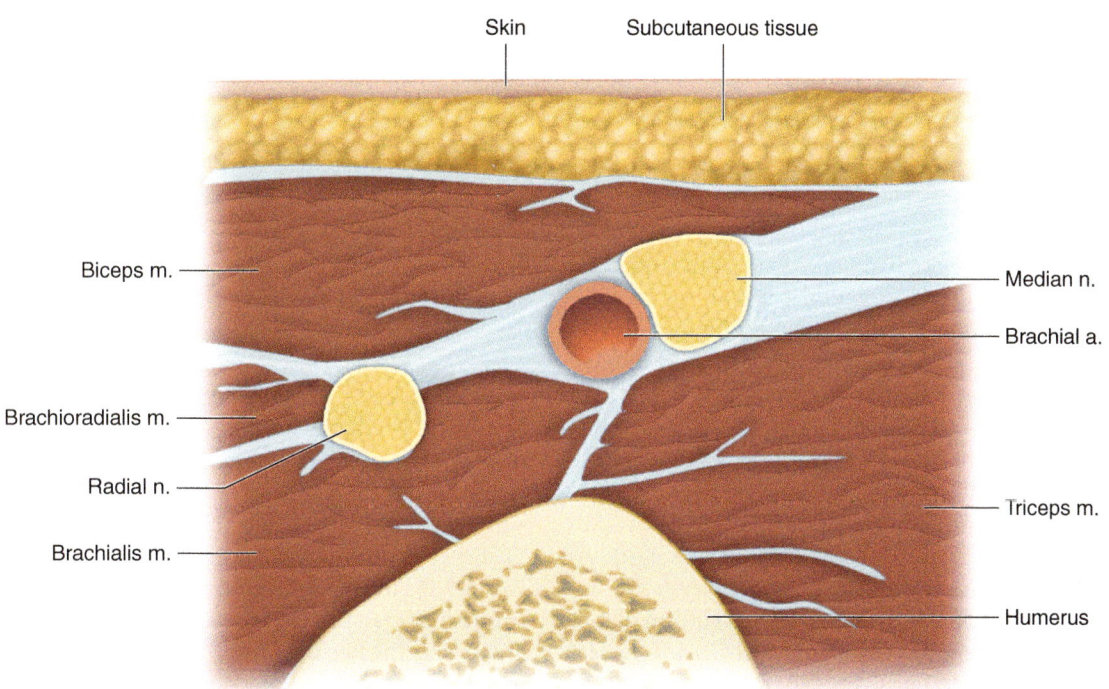

FIGURE 46–25 Cross-sectional anatomy of median nerve at the elbow.

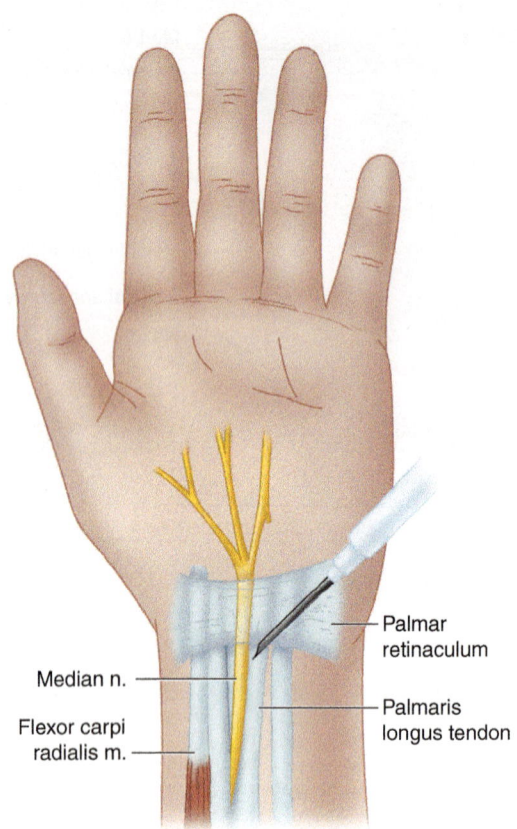

FIGURE 46–26 Median nerve block at the wrist.

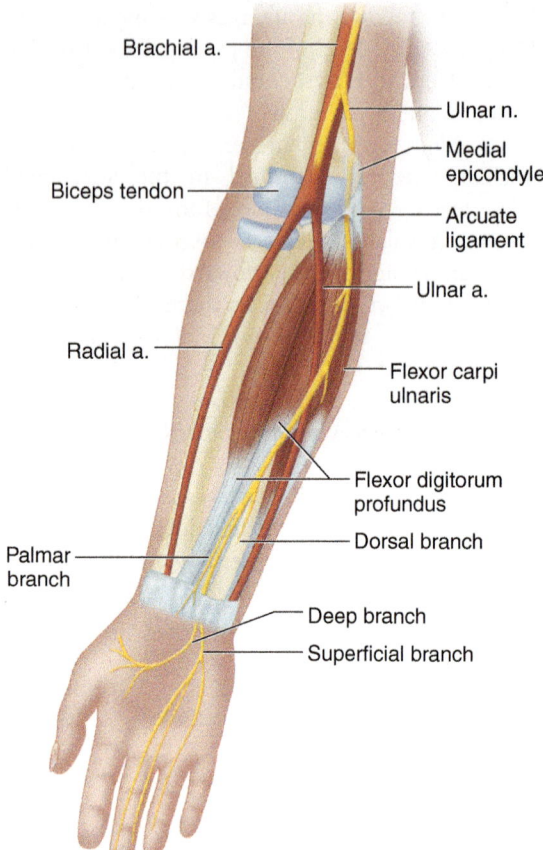

FIGURE 46–27 Ulnar nerve course.

of local anesthetic is injected (**Figure 46–26**). With ultrasound, the median nerve may be identified at the level of the mid-forearm between the muscle bellies of the flexor digitorum profundus, flexor digitorum superficialis, and flexor pollicis longus (transducer faces perpendicular to the trajectory of the nerves).

B. Ulnar Nerve Block

The ulnar nerve is the continuation of the medial cord of the brachial plexus and maintains a position medial to the axillary and brachial arteries in the upper arm (**Figure 46–27**). At the distal third of the humerus, the nerve moves more medially and passes under the arcuate ligament of the medial epicondyle. The nerve is frequently palpable just proximal to the medial epicondyle. In the mid-forearm, the nerve

lies between the flexor digitorum profundus and the flexor carpi ulnaris. At the wrist, it is lateral to the flexor carpi ulnaris tendon and medial to the ulnar artery.

To block the ulnar nerve at the level of the elbow, an insulated 22-gauge needle is inserted approximately one fingerbreadth proximal to the arcuate ligament (**Figure 46–28**), and advanced until fourth/fifth digit flexion or thumb adduction is elicited; 3–5 mL of local anesthetic is then injected. To block the ulnar nerve at the wrist, the ulnar artery pulse is palpated just lateral to the flexor carpi ulnaris tendon. The needle is inserted just medial to the artery (**Figure 46–29**) and 3–5 mL of local anesthetic is injected. If ultrasound is used, the ulnar nerve may be identified just medial to the ulnar artery.

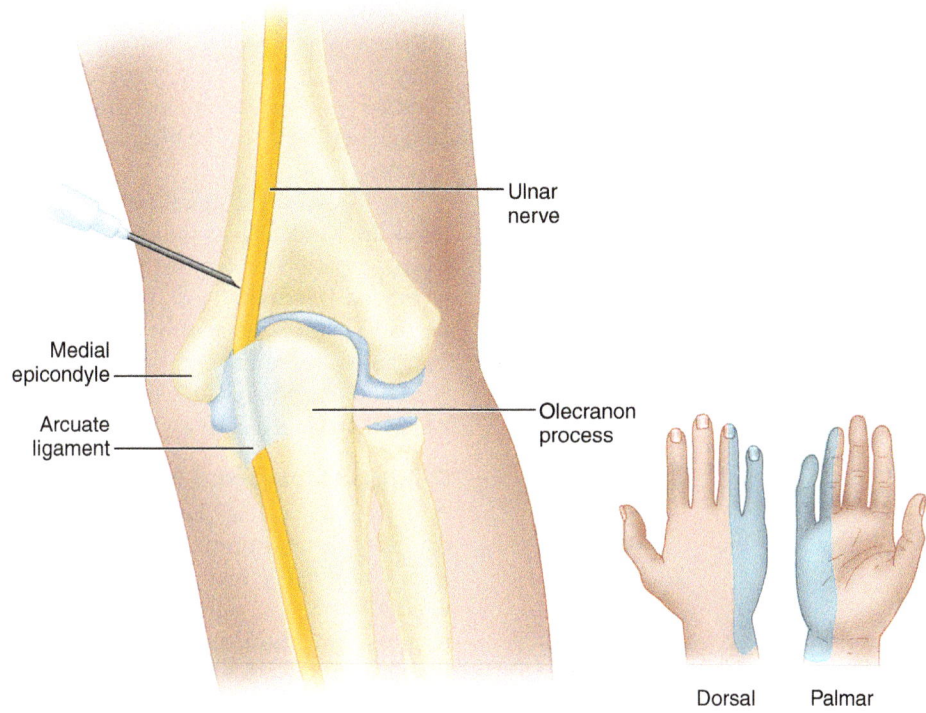

FIGURE 46–28 Ulnar nerve block at the elbow with region of anesthesia illustrated on the hand.

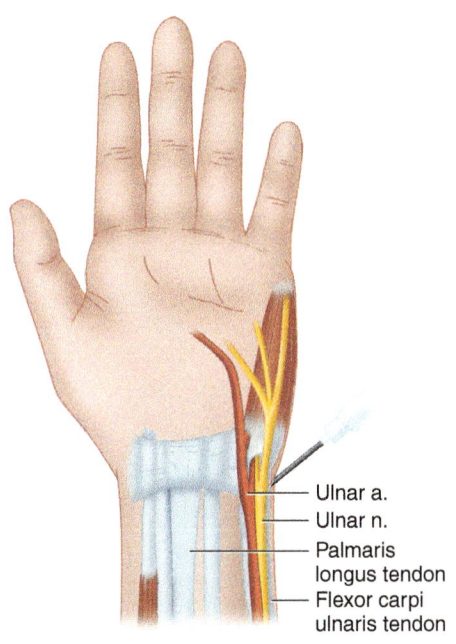

Ulnar a.
Ulnar n.
Palmaris longus tendon
Flexor carpi ulnaris tendon

FIGURE 46–29 Ulnar nerve block at the wrist.

C. Radial Nerve Block

The radial nerve—the terminal branch of the posterior cord of the brachial plexus—courses posterior to the humerus, innervating the triceps muscle, and enters the spiral groove of the humerus before it moves laterally at the elbow (Figure 46–30). Terminal sensory branches include the lateral cutaneous nerve of the arm and the posterior cutaneous nerve of the forearm. After exiting the spiral groove as it approaches the lateral epicondyle, the radial nerve separates into superficial and deep branches. The deep branch remains close to the periosteum and innervates the postaxial extensor group of the forearm. The superficial branch becomes superficial and follows the radial artery to innervate the radial aspects of the dorsal wrist and the dorsal aspect of the lateral three digits and half of the fourth.

To block the radial nerve at the elbow, the biceps tendon is identified in the antecubital fossa. A short 22-gauge insulated needle is inserted just lateral to the tendon and directed toward the lateral

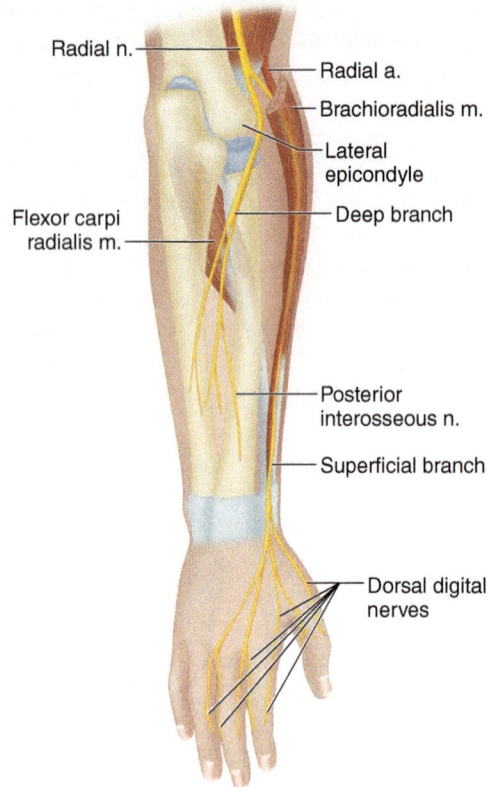

FIGURE 46–30   Radial nerve course.

epicondyle (**Figure 46–31**) until wrist or finger extension is elicited; 5 mL of local anesthetic is then injected. With ultrasound, the radial nerve can be identified in cross-section just proximal to the antecubital fossa between the biceps and brachioradialis muscles.

At the wrist, the superficial branch of the radial nerve lies just lateral to the radial artery, which can be easily palpated lateral to the flexor carpi radialis tendon (**Figure 46–32**). Using a short 22-gauge needle, 3–5 mL local anesthetic is injected lateral to the artery. Ultrasound may be used at the level of the wrist or mid-forearm to identify the radial nerve just lateral to the radial artery.

D. Musculocutaneous Nerve Block

A musculocutaneous nerve block is essential to complete the anesthesia for the forearm and wrist and is commonly included when performing the axillary block. The musculocutaneous nerve is the terminal branch of the lateral cord and the most proximal of the major nerves to emerge from the brachial plexus (**Figure 46–33**). This nerve innervates the biceps and brachialis muscles and distally terminates as the lateral antebrachial cutaneous nerve, supplying sensory input to the lateral aspect of the forearm and wrist.

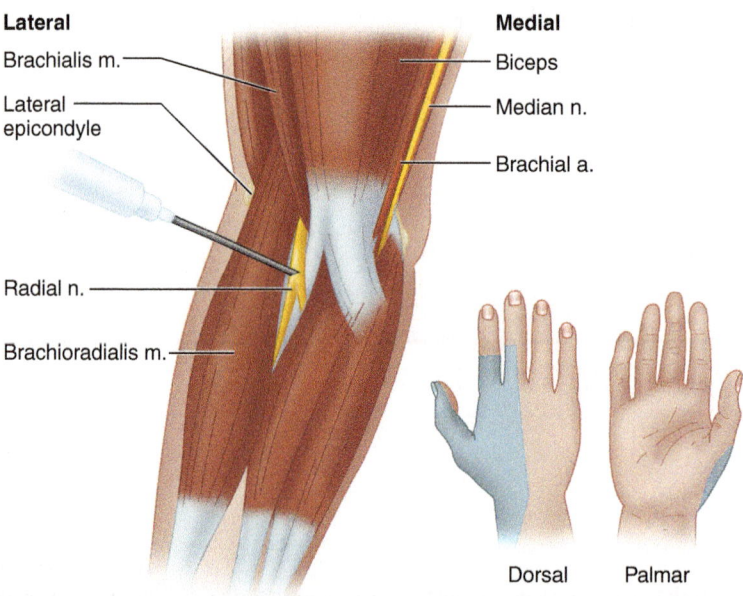

FIGURE 46–31   Radial nerve block at the elbow.

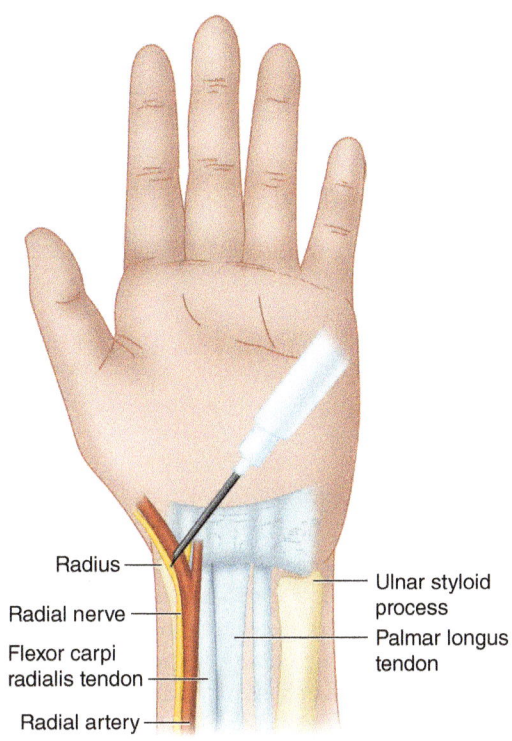

FIGURE 46–32 Radial nerve block at the wrist.

To target the musculocutaneous nerve following an axillary block, the needle is redirected superior and proximal to the artery (see Figure 46–21),

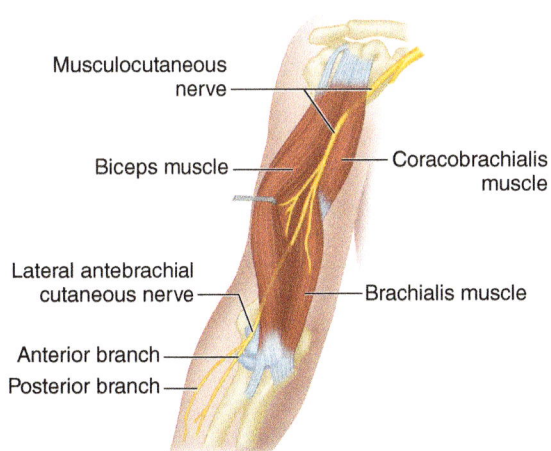

FIGURE 46–33 Musculocutaneous nerve course.

the coracobrachialis muscle is pierced, and 5–10 mL of local anesthetic is injected, with or without elicitation of elbow flexion. (Simple infiltration may be used, although the success rate using this technique is questionable.) Ultrasound may be used to confirm the location of the musculocutaneous nerve in the coracobrachialis muscle or between this muscle and the biceps (see Figure 46–22). Alternatively, the block can be performed at the elbow as the nerve courses superficially at the interepicondylar line. The insertion of the biceps tendon is identified, and a short 22-guage needle is inserted 1–2 cm laterally; 5–10 mL of local anesthetic is then injected as a field block.

E. Digital Nerve Blocks

Digital nerve blocks are used for minor operations on the fingers and to supplement incomplete brachial plexus and terminal nerve blocks. Sensory innervation of each finger is provided by four small digital nerves that enter each digit at its base in each of the four corners (Figure 46–34). A small-gauge needle is inserted at the medial and lateral aspects of the base of the selected digit, and 2–3 mL of local anesthetic

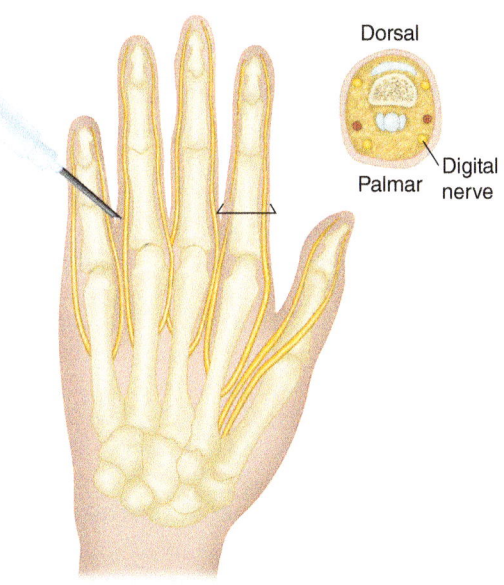

FIGURE 46–34 Sensory innervation of the fingers is provided by the digital nerves.

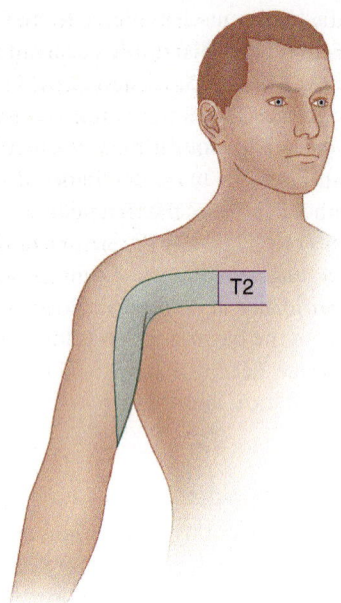

FIGURE 46–35 Intercostobrachial nerve cutaneous innervation.

is inserted *without* epinephrine. Addition of a vaso-constrictor (epinephrine) has been claimed to seri-ously compromise blood flow to the digit; however, there are no case reports involving lidocaine or other modern local anesthetics to confirm this claim.

F. Intercostobrachial Nerve Block

The intercostobrachial nerve originates in the upper thorax (T2) and becomes superficial on the medial upper arm. It supplies cutaneous innervation to the medial aspect of the proximal arm and is *not* anes-thetized with a brachial plexus block (Figure 46–35). The patient should be supine with the arm abducted and externally rotated. Starting at the deltoid promi-nence and proceeding inferiorly, a field block is performed in a linear fashion using 5 mL of local anesthetic, extending to the most inferior aspect of the medial arm (Figure 46–36).

Intravenous Regional Anesthesia

8 Intravenous regional anesthesia, also called a Bier block, can provide surgical anesthe-sia for short surgical procedures (45–60 min) on an extremity (eg, carpal tunnel release). An

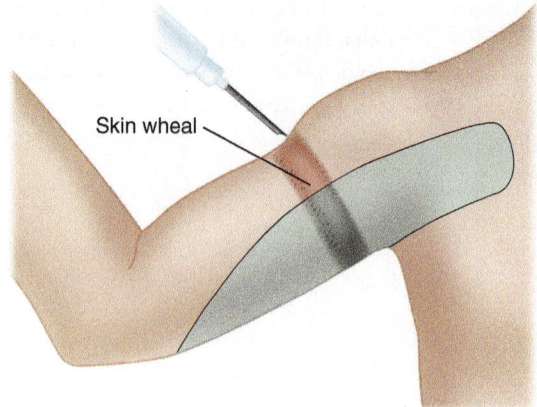

FIGURE 46–36 Intercostobrachial nerve block.

intravenous catheter is usually inserted on the dorsum of the hand (or foot) and a double pneu-matic tourniquet is placed on the arm or thigh. The extremity is elevated and exsanguinated by tightly wrapping an Esmarch elastic bandage from a distal to proximal direction. The proximal tourniquet is inflated, the Esmarch bandage removed, and 0.5% lidocaine (25 mL for a forearm, 50 mL for an arm, and 100 mL for a thigh tourniquet) injected over 2–3 min through the catheter, which is subsequently removed (Figure 46–37). Anesthesia is usually established after 5–10 min. Tourniquet pain usually develops after 20–30 min, at which time the distal tourniquet is inflated and the proximal tourniquet subsequently deflated. Patients usually tolerate the distal tourniquet for an additional 15–20 min because it is inflated over an anesthetized area. Even

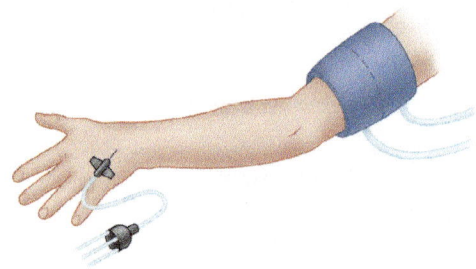

FIGURE 46–37 Intravenous regional anesthesia provides surgical anesthesia for procedures of short duration.

for surgical procedures of a very short duration, the tourniquet *must* be left inflated for a total of at least 15–20 min to avoid a rapid intravenous systemic bolus of local anesthetic resulting in toxicity. Slow deflation is also recommended to provide an additional margin of safety.

LOWER EXTREMITY PERIPHERAL NERVE BLOCKS

Lumbar & Sacral Plexus Anatomy

The lumbosacral plexus provides innervation to the lower extremities (**Figure 46–38**). The lumbar plexus is formed by the ventral rami of L1–4, with occasional contribution from T12. It lies within the psoas muscle with branches descending into the proximal thigh. Three major nerves from the lumbar plexus make contributions to the lower limb: the femoral (L2–4), lateral femoral cutaneous (L1–3), and obturator (L2–4). These provide motor and sensory innervation to the anterior portion of the thigh and sensory innervation to the medial leg. The sacral plexus arises from L4–5 and S1–4. The posterior thigh and most of the leg and foot are supplied by the tibial and peroneal portions of the sciatic nerve. The posterior femoral cutaneous nerve (S1–3), and not the sciatic nerve, provides sensory innervation to the posterior thigh; it travels with the sciatic nerve as it emerges around the piriformis muscle.

Femoral Nerve Block

The femoral nerve innervates the main hip flexors, knee extensors, and provides much of the sensory

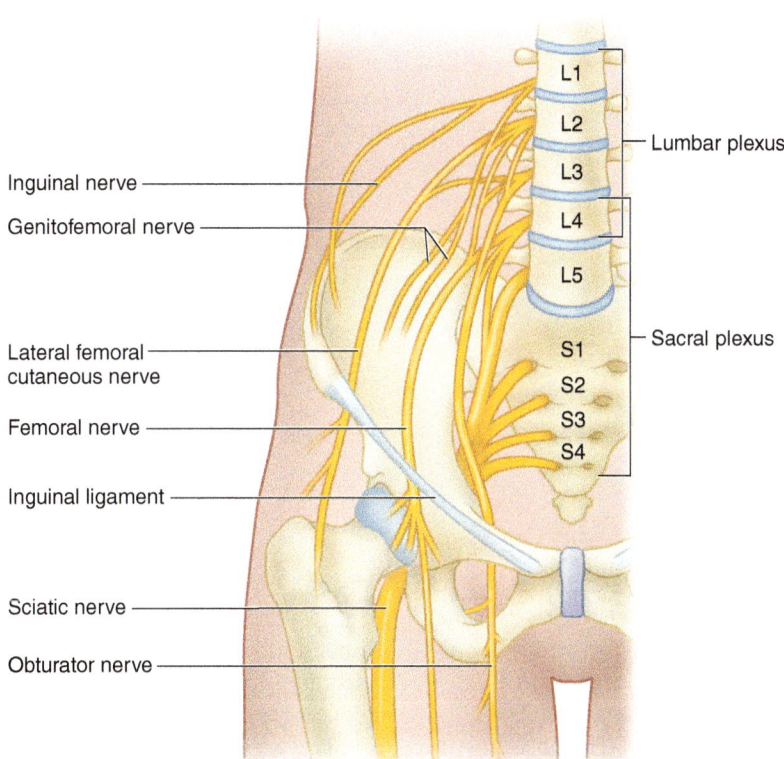

FIGURE 46–38 The ventral rami of L1–5 and S1–4 form the lumbosacral plexus, which provides innervation to the lower extremities.

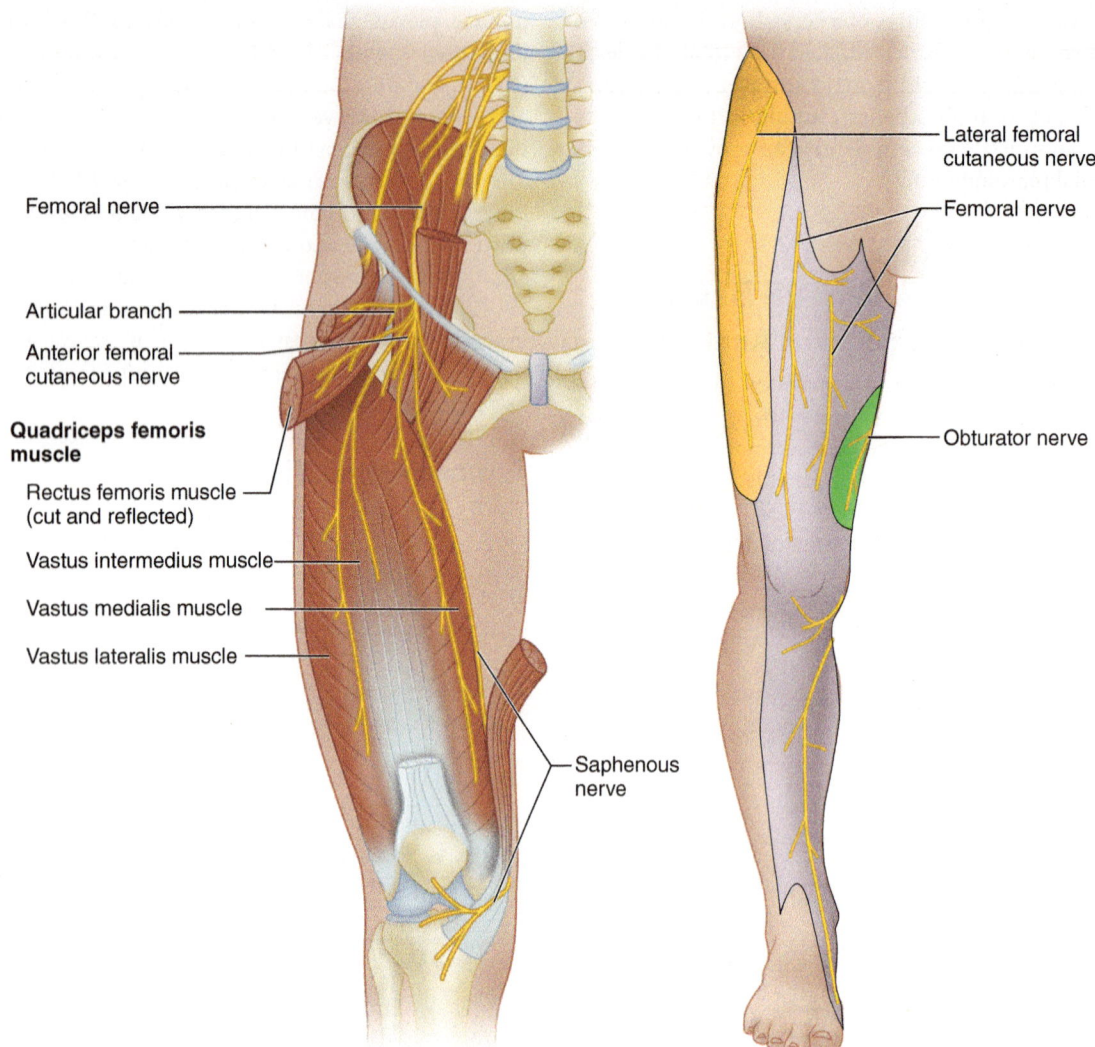

FIGURE 46–39 The femoral nerve provides sensory innervation to the hip and thigh, and to the medial leg via its terminal branch, the saphenous nerve.

innervation of the hip and thigh (Figure 46–39). Its most medial branch is the saphenous nerve, which innervates much of the skin of the medial leg and ankle joint. The term *3-in-1 block* refers to anesthetizing the femoral, lateral femoral cutaneous, and obturator nerves with a single injection below the inguinal ligament; this term has largely been abandoned as evidence accumulated demonstrating the failure of most single injections to consistently affect

9 all three nerves. A femoral nerve block alone will seldom provide surgical anesthesia, but it is often used to provide postoperative analgesia for hip, thigh, knee, and ankle (for the saphenous nerve) procedures. Femoral nerve blocks have a relatively low rate of complications and few contraindications. Local infection, previous vascular grafting, and local adenopathy should be carefully considered in patient selection.

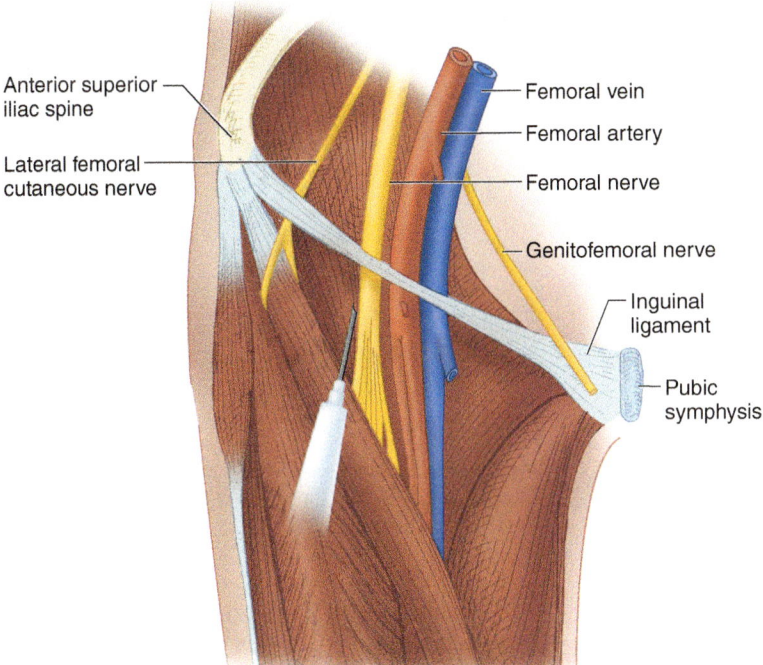

Anterior superior iliac spine

Lateral femoral cutaneous nerve

Femoral vein

Femoral artery

Femoral nerve

Genitofemoral nerve

Inguinal ligament

Pubic symphysis

FIGURE 46–40 Femoral block using nerve stimulation.

A. Nerve Stimulation

With the patient positioned supine, the femoral artery pulse is palpated at the level of the inguinal ligament. A short (5-cm) insulated needle is inserted at a 45° angle to the skin in a cephalad direction (Figure 46–40) until a clear quadriceps twitch is elicited at a current below 0.5 mA (look for patella motion).

B. Ultrasound

A high-frequency linear ultrasound transducer is placed over the area of the inguinal crease parallel to the crease itself, or slightly more transverse (Figure 46–41). The femoral artery and femoral vein are visualized in cross-section, with the overlying fascia iliaca. Just lateral to the artery and deep to the fascia iliaca, the femoral nerve appears in cross-section as a spindle-shaped structure with a "honeycomb" texture (Figure 46–42).

For an out-of-plane technique, the block needle is inserted just lateral to where the femoral nerve is seen, and directed cephalad at an angle approximately 45° to the skin. The needle is advanced until it is seen penetrating the fascia iliaca, or (if using concurrent electrical stimulation) until a motor response is elicited. Following careful aspiration for the nonappearance of blood, 30–40 mL of local anesthetic is injected.

For an in-plane technique, a longer needle may be used. The needle is inserted parallel to the ultrasound transducer just lateral to the outer edge. The needle is advanced through the sartorius muscle, deep to the fascia iliaca, until it is visualized just lateral to the femoral nerve. Local anesthetic is injected, visualizing its hypoechoic spread deep to the fascia iliaca and around the nerve.

C. Fascia Iliaca Technique

The goal of a fascia iliaca block is similar to that of a femoral nerve block, but the approach is slightly different. Without use of a nerve stimulator or ultrasound machine, a relatively reliable level of anesthesia may be attained simply with anatomic landmarks and tactile sensation. Once the inguinal ligament and femoral artery pulse are identified,

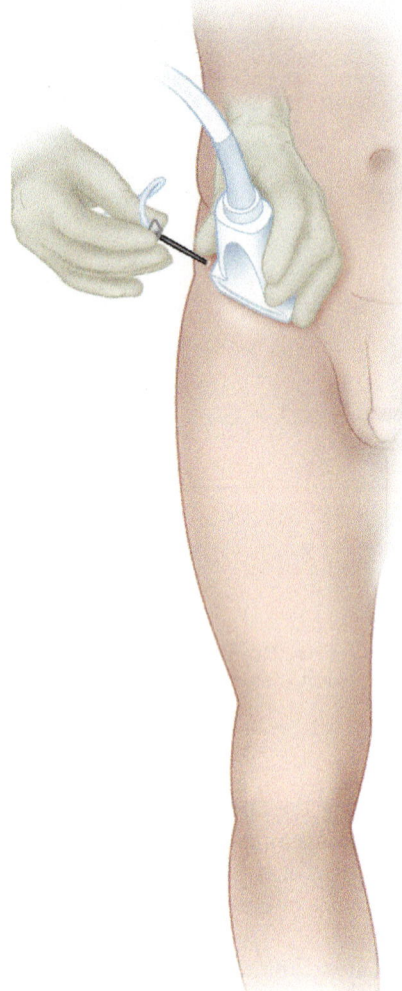

FIGURE 46–41 Ultrasound-guided femoral nerve block (in-plane technique).

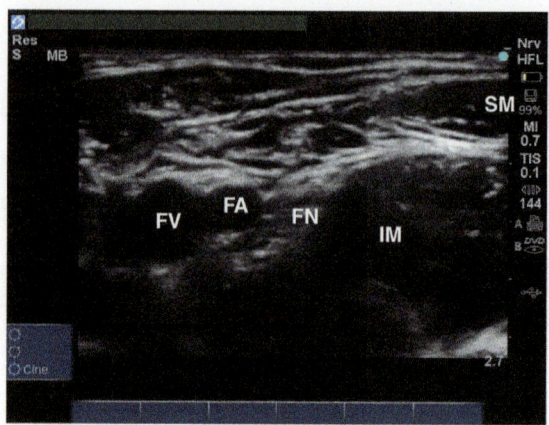

FIGURE 46–42 Femoral nerve block. Ultrasound image of the femoral nerve. FA, femoral artery; FV, femoral vein; FN, femoral nerve; SM, Sartorius muscle; IM, iliacus muscle.

local anesthetic is deposited under the fascia iliaca between the two nerves which run in the same plane between the fascia and underlying muscle.

Lateral Femoral Cutaneous Nerve Block

The lateral femoral cutaneous nerve provides sensory innervation to the lateral thigh (see Figure 46–39). It may be anesthetized as a supplement to a femoral nerve block or as an isolated block for limited anesthesia of the lateral thigh. As there are few vital structures in proximity to the lateral femoral cutaneous nerve, complications with this block are exceedingly rare. The lateral femoral cutaneous nerve (L2–3) departs from the lumbar plexus, traverses laterally from the psoas muscle, and courses anterolaterally along the iliacus muscle (see Figure 46–38). It emerges inferior and medial to the anterior superior iliac spine to supply the cutaneous sensory innervation of the lateral thigh.

The patient is positioned supine or lateral, and the point 2 cm medial and 2 cm distal to the anterior superior iliac spine is identified. A short 22-gauge block needle is inserted and directed laterally, observing for a "pop" as it passes through the fascia lata. A field block is performed with 10–15 mL of local anesthetic, which is deposited above and below the fascia (**Figure 46–44**).

the length of the inguinal ligament is divided into thirds (**Figure 46–43**). Two centimeters distal to the junction of the middle and outer thirds, a short, blunt-tipped needle is inserted in a slightly cephalad direction. As the needle passes through the two layers of fascia in this region (fascia lata and fascia iliaca), two "pops" will be felt. Once the needle has passed through the fascia iliaca, careful aspiration is performed and 30–40 mL of local anesthetic is injected. This block usually anesthetizes both the femoral nerve and lateral femoral cutaneous nerves, since the

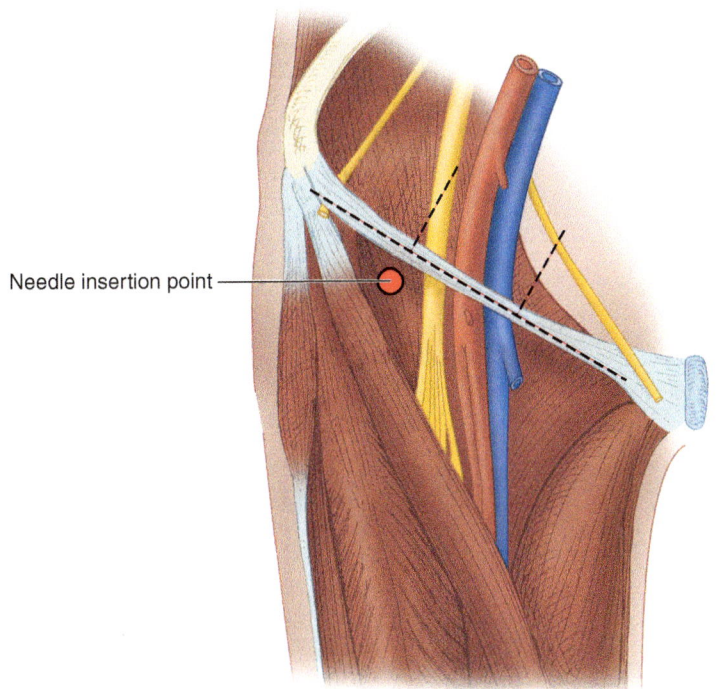

FIGURE 46–43 Fascia iliaca block.

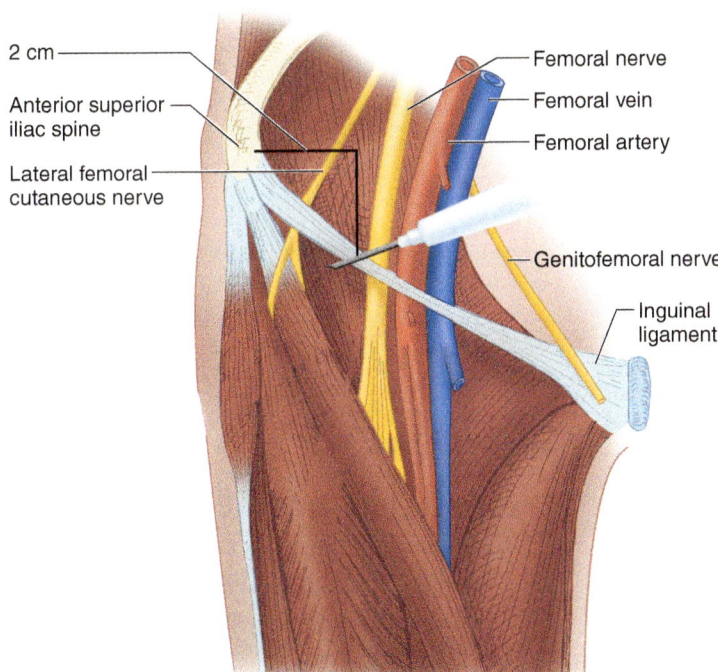

FIGURE 46–44 Lateral femoral cutaneous nerve block.

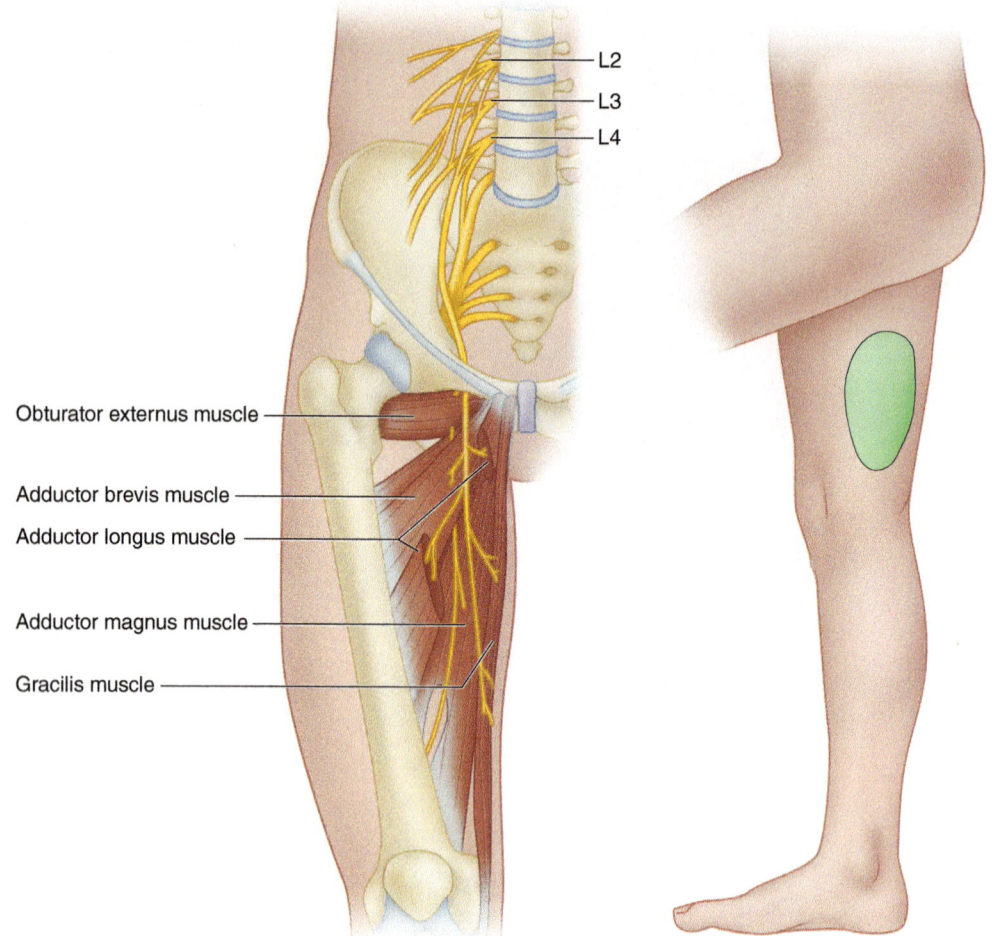

FIGURE 46–45 Obturator nerve innervation.

Obturator Nerve Block

A block of the obturator nerve is usually required for complete anesthesia of the knee and is most often performed in combination with femoral and sciatic nerve blocks for this purpose. The obturator nerve contributes sensory branches to the hip and knee joints, a variable degree of sensation to the medial thigh, and innervates the adductors of the hip (Figure 46–45). This nerve exits the pelvis and enters the medial thigh through the obturator foramen, which lies beneath the superior pubic ramus. After identification of the pubic tubercle, a long (10-cm) block needle is inserted 1.5 cm inferior and 1.5 cm lateral to the tubercle. The needle is advanced

posteriorly until bone is contacted (Figure 46–46). Redirecting laterally and caudally, the needle is advanced an additional 2–4 cm until a motor response (thigh adduction) is elicited and maintained below 0.5 mA. Following careful aspiration for the nonappearance of blood, 15–20 mL of local anesthetic is injected.

Posterior Lumbar Plexus (Psoas Compartment) Block

10 Posterior lumbar plexus blocks are useful for surgical procedures involving areas innervated by the femoral, lateral femoral cutaneous, and obturator nerves (Figure 46–47). These include

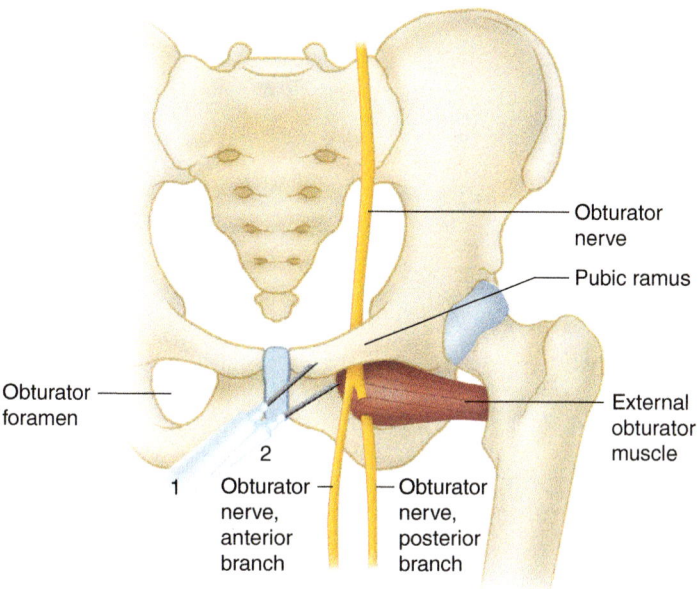

Obturator nerve

Pubic ramus

Obturator foramen

External obturator muscle

1   2   Obturator nerve, anterior branch   Obturator nerve, posterior branch

FIGURE 46–46 Obturator nerve block. Contact pubic tubercle (1), then redirect laterally and caudally (2) until a motor response is elicited.

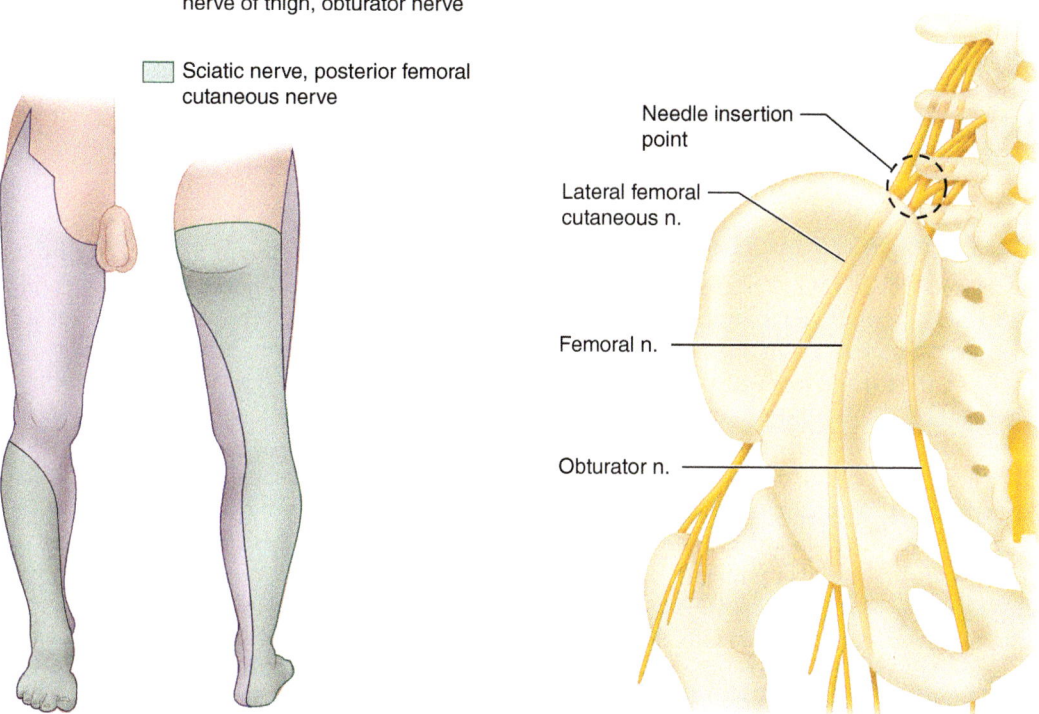

Femoral nerve, lateral cutaneous nerve of thigh, obturator nerve

Sciatic nerve, posterior femoral cutaneous nerve

Needle insertion point

Lateral femoral cutaneous n.

Femoral n.

Obturator n.

FIGURE 46–47 Lumbar plexus blocks provide anesthesia to the femoral, lateral femoral cutaneous, and obturator nerves.

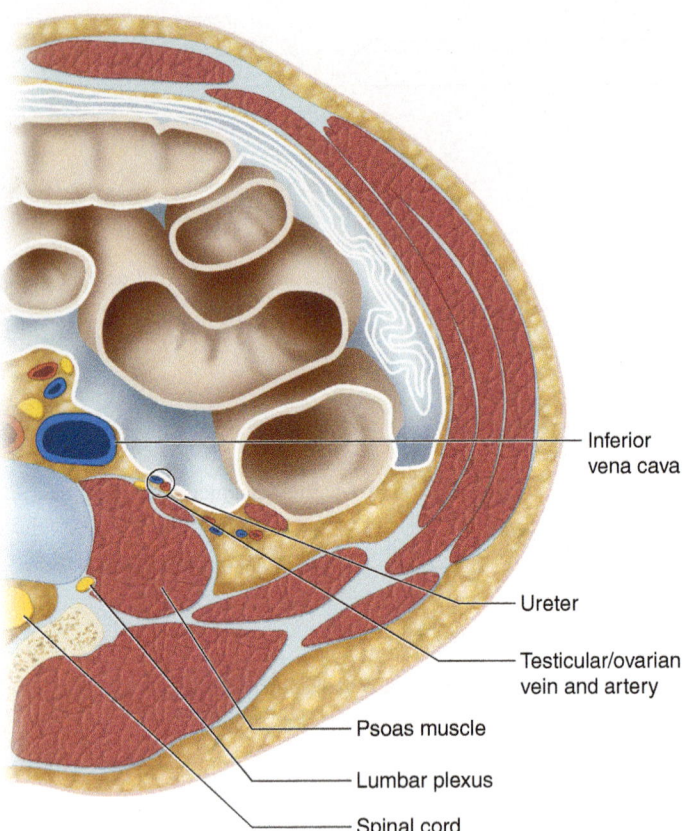

FIGURE 46–48 The lumbar plexus lies in close proximity to several important structures.

Labels on figure:
- Inferior vena cava
- Ureter
- Testicular/ovarian vein and artery
- Psoas muscle
- Lumbar plexus
- Spinal cord

procedures on the hip, knee, and anterior thigh. Complete anesthesia of the knee can be attained with a proximal sciatic nerve block. The lumbar plexus is relatively close to multiple sensitive structures (**Figure 46–48**) and reaching it requires a very long needle. Hence, the posterior lumbar plexus block has one of the highest complication rates of any peripheral nerve block; these include retroperitoneal hematoma, intravascular local anesthetic injection with toxicity, intrathecal and epidural injections, and renal capsular puncture with subsequent hematoma.

Lumbar nerve roots emerge into the body of the psoas muscle and travel within the muscle compartment before exiting as terminal nerves (see Figure 46–38). Modern posterior lumbar plexus blocks deposit local anesthetic within the body of the psoas muscle. The patient is positioned in lateral

decubitus with the side to be blocked in the nondependent position (**Figure 46–49**). The midline is palpated, identifying the spinous processes if possible. A line is first drawn through the lumbar spinous processes, and both iliac crests are identified and connected with a line to approximate the level of L4. The posterior superior iliac spine is then palpated and a line is drawn cephalad, parallel to the first line. If available, ultrasound imaging of the transverse process may be helpful to estimate lumbar plexus depth. A long (10- to 15-cm) insulated needle is inserted at the point of intersection between the transverse (intercristal) line and the intersection of the lateral and middle thirds of the two sagittal lines. The needle is advanced in an anterior direction until a femoral motor response is elicited (quadriceps contraction). If the transverse process is contacted, the needle should be withdrawn slightly

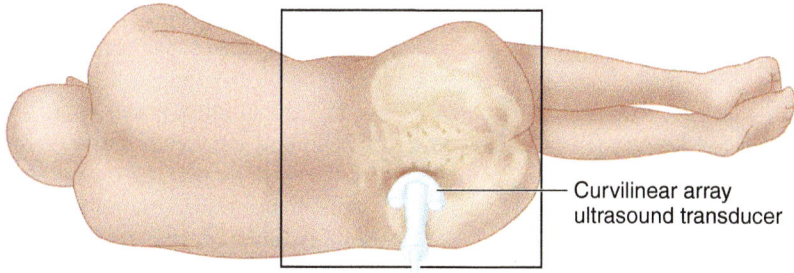

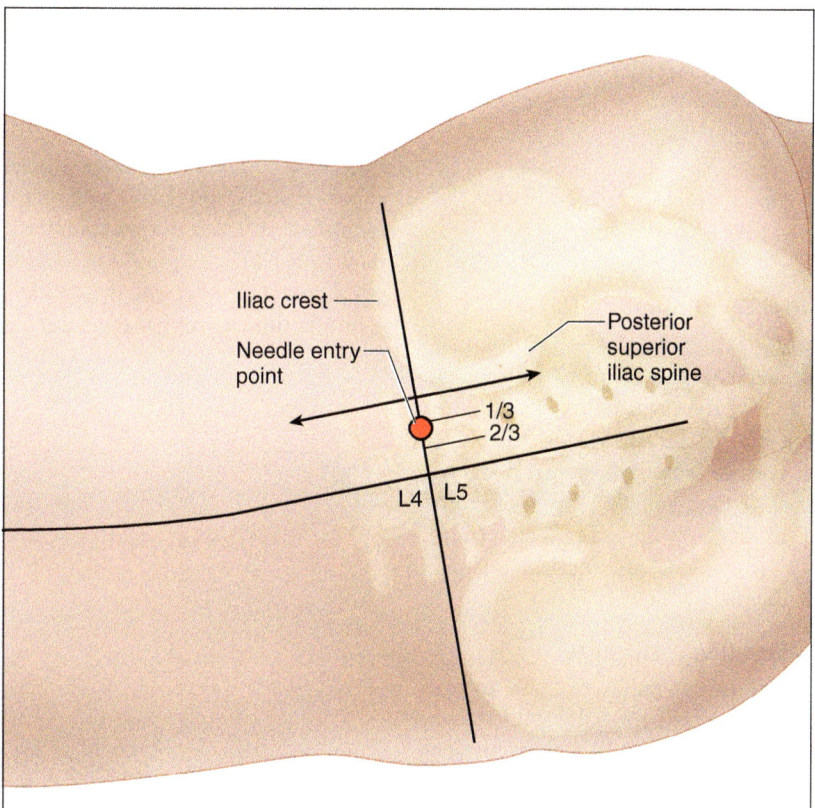

FIGURE 46–49 Patient positioning and surface landmarks for posterior lumbar plexus block.

and "walked off" the transverse process in a caudal direction, maintaining the needle in the parasagittal plane. The needle should never be inserted more than 3 cm past the depth at which the transverse process was contacted. Local anesthetic volumes greater than 20 mL will increase the risk of bilateral spread and contralateral limb involvement.

Saphenous Nerve Block

The saphenous nerve is the most medial branch of the femoral nerve and innervates the skin over the medial leg and the ankle joint (see Figure 46–39). Therefore, this block is used mainly in conjunction with a sciatic nerve block to provide complete anesthesia/analgesia below the knee.

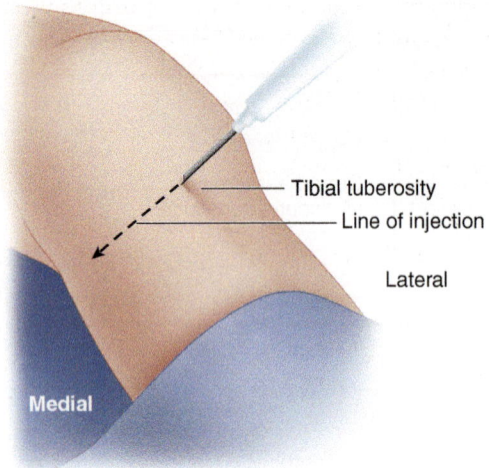

FIGURE 46–50 Proximal saphenous nerve block.

A. Trans-Sartorial Technique

The saphenous nerve may be accessed proximal to the knee, just deep to the sartorius muscle. A high-frequency linear probe is used to identify the junction between the sartorius, vastus medialis, and adductor muscles in cross-section just distal to the adductor canal. A long needle is inserted from medial to lateral (in-plane) or angled cephalad (out-of-plane) and 5–10 mL of local anesthetic deposited within this fascial plane.

B. Proximal Saphenous Technique

A short block needle is inserted 2 cm distal to the tibial tuberosity and directed medially, infiltrating 5–10 mL of local anesthetic as the needle passes toward the posterior aspect of the leg (Figure 46–50). Ultrasound may be used to identify the saphenous vein near the tibial tuberosity, facilitating a *perivascular technique* with infiltration about the vein.

C. Distal Saphenous Technique

The medial malleolus is identified, infiltrating 5 mL of local anesthetic in a line running anteriorly around the ankle (see Ankle Block below).

Sciatic Nerve Block

The sciatic nerve originates from the lumbosacral trunk and is composed of nerve roots L4–5 and S1–3

11 (see Figure 46–38). Blockade of the sciatic nerve may occur anywhere along its course and is indicated for surgical procedures involving the hip, thigh, knee, lower leg, and foot. The posterior femoral cutaneous nerve is variably anesthetized as well, depending on the approach. If sacral plexus or posterior femoral cutaneous nerve anesthesia is required, the parasacral approach is used (a technique that is beyond the scope of this chapter).

A. Posterior (Classic or Labat) Approach

The patient is positioned laterally with the side to be blocked in the nondependent position. The patient is asked to bend the knee of the affected leg and tilt the pelvis slightly forward (Sim's position; Figure 46–51). The greater trochanter, posterior superior iliac spine (PSIS), and sacral hiatus are then identified. A line is drawn from the greater trochanter to the PSIS, its midpoint identified, and a perpendicular line extended in a caudal direction. Next, a line is drawn from the greater trochanter to the

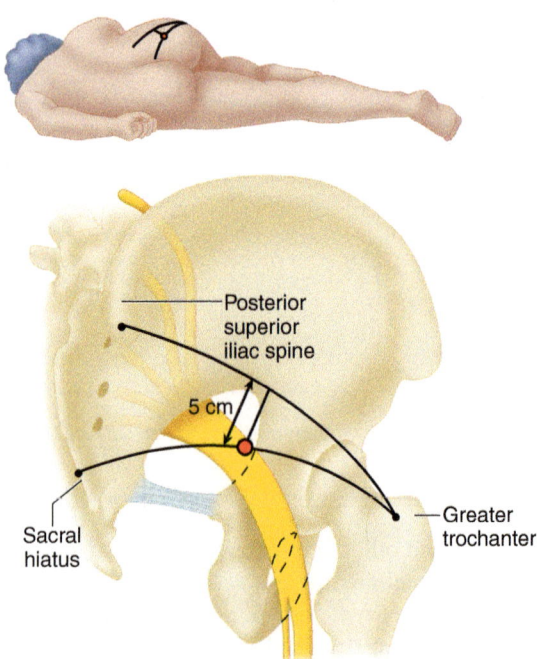

FIGURE 46–51 Patient positioning, surface landmarks, and needle positioning for proximal sciatic nerve block (classic approach).

sacral hiatus and the intersection point is marked; this is the initial needle insertion point. A long (10-cm) insulated needle is inserted at an angle perpendicular to all planes to the skin (Figure 46–51). The needle is advanced through the gluteal muscles (a motor response of these muscles may be encountered) until plantar- or dorsiflexion is elicited (plantarflexion or foot inversion is preferred for surgical anesthesia). A local anesthetic volume of 25 mL provides surgical anesthesia.

B. Anterior Approach

After leaving the sciatic notch, the sciatic nerve descends behind the lesser trochanter to a position posterior to the femur. It can be accessed from the anterior thigh just medial to the lesser trochanter. Lateral or prone positioning may present a challenge for some patients requiring a sciatic nerve block (ie, elderly patients, pediatric patients under general anesthesia). An anterior approach can be technically challenging but offers an alternative path to the sciatic nerve. Before proceeding with this block, which carries a risk of vascular puncture (femoral artery and vein), patient-specific risks should be considered (eg, coagulopathy and vascular grafting). In

addition, if combining this block with the femoral nerve block in an unanesthetized patient, performing the sciatic block first is recommended to avoid passing the block needle through a previously anesthetized femoral nerve. A local anesthetic volume of 25 mL provides surgical anesthesia.

1. Nerve stimulation—With the patient positioned supine, a line is drawn along the inguinal ligament, from the anterior superior iliac spine to the pubic tubercle (Figure 46–52). A second line is drawn parallel to the first that traverses the greater trochanter (intertrochanteric line). Next, these two lines are connected with a third line drawn from the point between the medial one third and lateral two thirds of the first line, at a 90° angle, and extended caudally to intersect with the intertrochanteric line. A long (10- to 15-cm) needle is inserted through this intersection and directly posterior until foot inversion or plantarflexion is elicited (dorsiflexion is acceptable for postoperative analgesia). Often with this approach, the femur is contacted before the needle reaches the sciatic nerve. When this occurs, the needle should be withdrawn 2–3 cm, the patient should be asked to internally rotate the leg, and then the needle should be advanced. If the femur is contacted

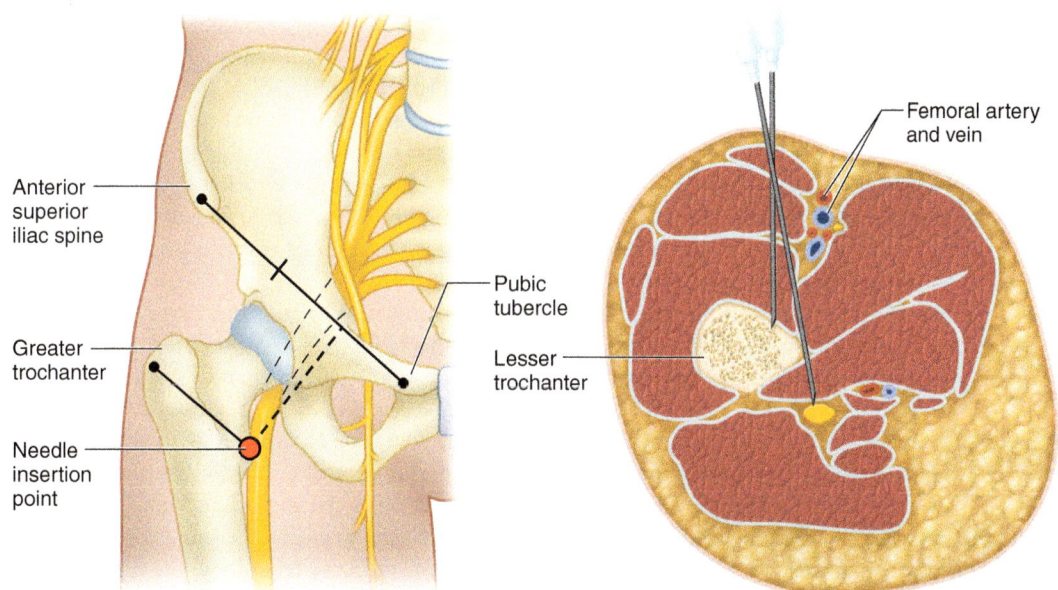

FIGURE 46–52 Anatomy and surface landmarks for anterior sciatic nerve block.

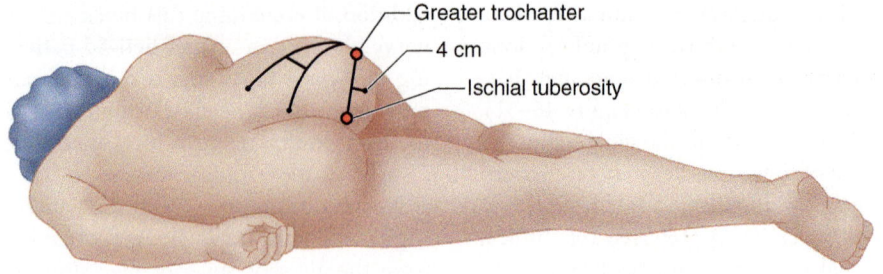

FIGURE 46–53 Patient positioning and surface landmarks for subgluteal sciatic block.

again, the landmarks may require reassessment. A local anesthetic volume of 25 mL provides surgical anesthesia.

2. Ultrasound—With the patient positioned supine and the leg externally rotated, a low-frequency curvilinear transducer is placed transversely over the medial thigh, approximately at the level of the lesser trochanter. The femur, femoral vessels, adductor muscles, and gluteus maximus are identified in cross-section. The elliptical, hyperechoic sciatic nerve is found in the fascial plane between adductors and gluteus muscles, posterior to the femur. Using a long (10-cm) needle, the nerve is approached in-plane (anterior to posterior) or out-of-plane (cephalad to caudad), taking care to avoid femoral vessels, until the needle tip lies in this muscle plane and a local anesthetic injection can be observed as hypoechoic spread surrounding the sciatic nerve.

C. Subgluteal Approach

A subgluteal approach to the sciatic nerve is a useful alternative to the traditional posterior approach. In many patients the landmarks are more easily identified, and less tissue is traversed. With the sciatic nerve at a more superficial location, the exclusive use of ultrasound becomes far more practical, as well. If sciatic nerve block is being combined with a femoral block and ambulation is desired within the local anesthetic duration, consider a popliteal approach (below) that will not affect the hamstring muscles to the same degree, allowing knee flexion to lift the foot with the use of crutches.

1. Nerve stimulation—With the patient in Sim's position, the greater trochanter and ischial

tuberosity are identified and a line drawn between them (**Figure 46–53**). From the midpoint of this line, a second line is drawn perpendicularly and extended caudally 4 cm. Through this point a long (10-cm) insulated needle is inserted directly slightly cephalad until foot plantarflexion or inversion is elicited (dorsiflexion is acceptable for analgesia). A local anesthetic volume of 25 mL provides surgical anesthesia.

2. Ultrasound—Using the same positioning and landmarks (Figure 46–53), a linear or low-frequency curvilinear (best) ultrasound transducer is placed over the midpoint between the ischial tuberosity and the greater trochanter in a transverse orientation. Both bony structures should be visible in the ultrasound field simultaneously. Gluteal muscles are identified superficially, along with the fascial layer defining their deep border. The triangular sciatic nerve should be visible in cross-section just deep to this layer in a location approximately midway between the ischial tuberosity and the greater trochanter, superficial to the quadratus femoris muscle.

For an out-of-plane ultrasound-guided sciatic block, the block needle is inserted just caudad to the ultrasound transducer and advanced in an anterior and cephalad direction. Once the needle passes through the gluteus muscles with the tip next to sciatic nerve, careful aspiration for the nonappearance of blood is performed and local anesthetic is injected, visualizing spread around the nerve.

For an in-plane technique, the block needle is inserted just lateral to the ultrasound transducer near the greater trochanter. It is advanced through

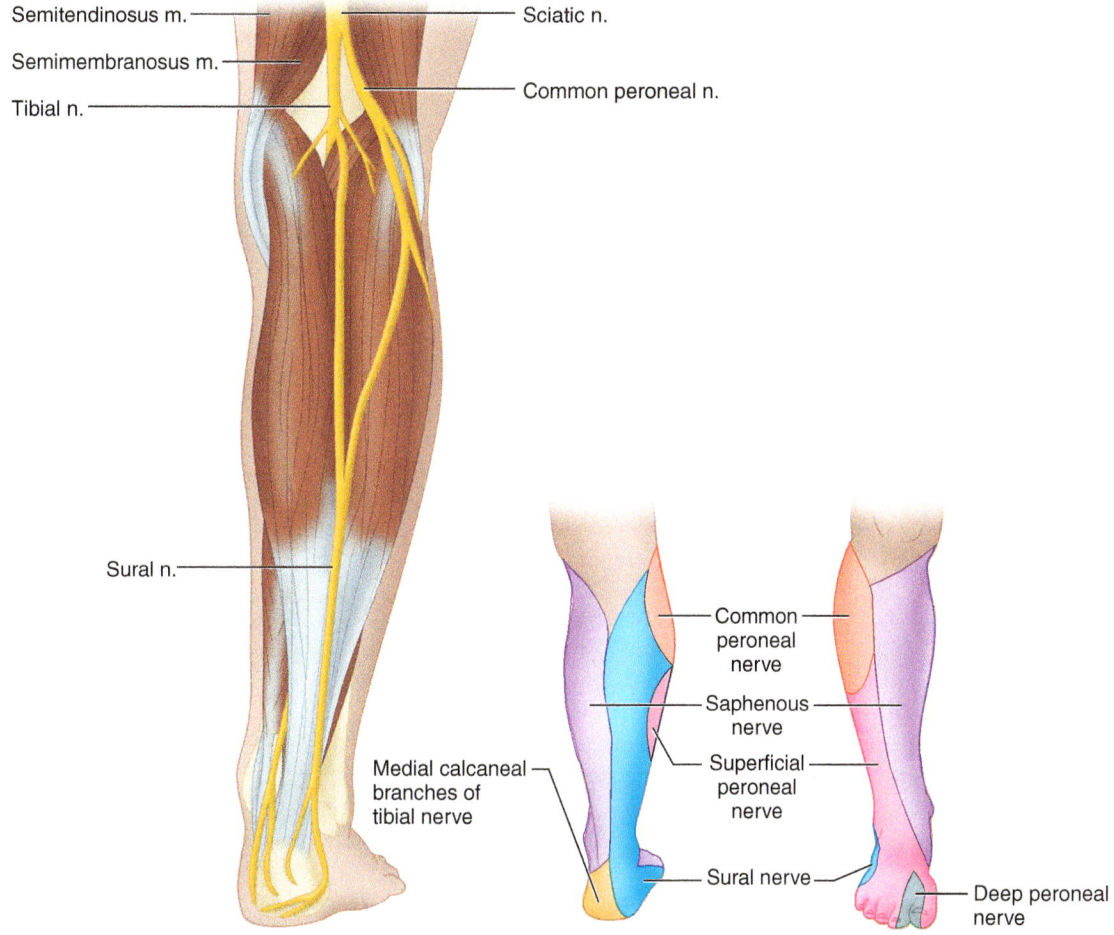

FIGURE 46–54 The sciatic nerve divides into tibial and peroneal branches just proximal to the popliteal fossa and provides sensory innervation to much of the lower leg.

the field of the ultrasound beam until the tip is visible deep to the gluteus maximus, next to the sciatic nerve. Again, local anesthetic spread around the nerve should be visualized.

D. Popliteal Approach

⑫ Popliteal nerve blocks provide excellent coverage for foot and ankle surgery, while sparing much of the hamstring muscles, allowing lifting of the foot with knee flexion, thus easing ambulation. All sciatic nerve blocks fail to provide complete anesthesia for the cutaneous medial leg and ankle joint capsule, but when a saphenous (or femoral)

block is added, complete anesthesia below the knee is provided. The major site-specific risk of a popliteal block is vascular puncture, owing to the sciatic nerve's proximity to the popliteal vessels at this location.

The sciatic nerve divides into the tibial and common peroneal nerves within or just proximal to the popliteal fossa (Figure 46–54). The upper popliteal fossa is bounded laterally by the biceps femoris tendon and medially by the semitendinosus and semimembranosus tendons. Cephalad to the flexion crease of the knee, the popliteal artery is immediately lateral to the semitendinosus tendon. The popliteal vein is lateral to the artery, and the tibial and common peroneal nerves are just lateral to the vein and medial to the biceps tendon, 2–6 cm deep to the skin. The tibial nerve continues deep behind the gastrocnemius muscle, and the common peroneal nerve leaves the popliteal fossa by passing between the head and neck of the fibula to supply the lower leg. The sciatic nerve is approached by either a posterior or a lateral approach. For posterior approaches, the patient is usually positioned prone with the knee slightly flexed by propping the ankle on pillows or towels. For lateral approaches, the patient may be in the lateral or supine position.

1. Nerve stimulation (posterior approach)—With the patient in the prone position, the apex of the popliteal fossa is identified. The hamstring muscles are palpated to locate the point where the biceps femoris (lateral) and the semimembranosus/semitendinosus complex (medial) join (**Figure 46–55**). Having the patient flex the knee against resistance facilitates recognition of these structures. The needle entry point is 1 cm caudad from the apex. An insulated needle (5–10 cm) is advanced until foot plantarflexion or inversion is elicited (dorsiflexion is acceptable for analgesia). A volume of 30–40 mL of local anesthetic is often required for single-injection popliteal–sciatic nerve block.

2. Nerve stimulation (lateral approach)—With the patient in the supine position and the knee fully extended, the intertendinous groove is palpated between the vastus lateralis and biceps femoris muscles approximately 10 cm proximal to the superior notch of the patella. A long (10-cm) insulated needle is inserted at this point and advanced at a 30° angle posteriorly until an appropriate motor response is elicited. If bone (femur) is contacted, the needle is withdrawn and redirected slightly posteriorly until an acceptable motor response is encountered.

3. Ultrasound—With the patient positioned prone, the apex of the popliteal fossa is identified, as described above. Using a high-frequency linear ultrasound transducer placed in a transverse orientation, the femur, biceps femoris muscle, popliteal vessels, and sciatic nerve or branches are identified in cross-section (Figure 46–55). The nerve is usually posterior and lateral (or immediately posterior) to the vessels and is often located in close

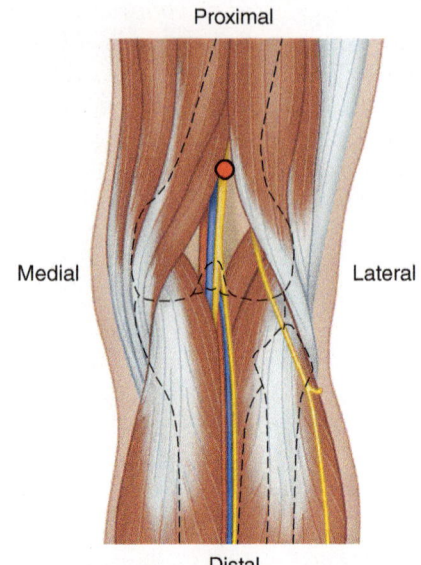

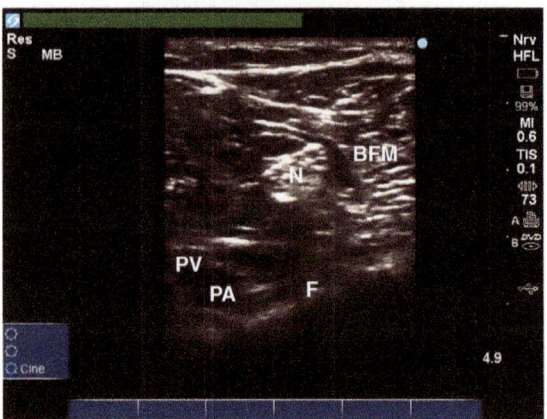

FIGURE 46–55 Anatomy and sonoanatomy of the sciatic nerve in the popliteal fossa. PA, popliteal artery; PV, popliteal vein; N, sciatic nerve; BFM, biceps femoris muscle; F, femur.

relationship to the biceps femoris muscle, just deep to its medial edge.

For an out-of-plane technique, the needle is inserted just caudad to the ultrasound transducer and directed anteriorly and slightly cephalad. When the needle is positioned in proximity to the sciatic nerve, and following careful aspiration, local anesthetic injected, observing for spread around the nerve.

For an in-plane technique, the block needle is inserted lateral to the ultrasound transducer, traversing—or just anterior to—the biceps femoris muscle (Figure 46–56). The needle is advanced in the ultrasound plane, while visualizing its approach either deep or superficial to the nerve.

If surgical anesthesia is desired, local anesthetic should be seen surrounding all sides of the nerve, which usually requires multiple needle tip placements with incremental injection. For analgesia alone, a single injection of local anesthetic is acceptable. Ultrasound-guided popliteal sciatic blocks may be performed with the patient in the lateral or supine positions (the latter with leg up-raised on several pillows). These maneuvers are often more technically challenging.

Ankle Block

For surgical procedures of the foot, an ankle block is a fast, low-technology, low-risk means of providing anesthesia. Excessive injectate volume and use of vasoconstrictors such as epinephrine must be avoided to minimize the risk of ischemic complications. Since this block includes five separate injections, it is often uncomfortable for patients and adequate premedication is required.

Five nerves supply sensation to the foot (Figure 46–57). The saphenous nerve is a terminal branch of the femoral nerve and the only innervation

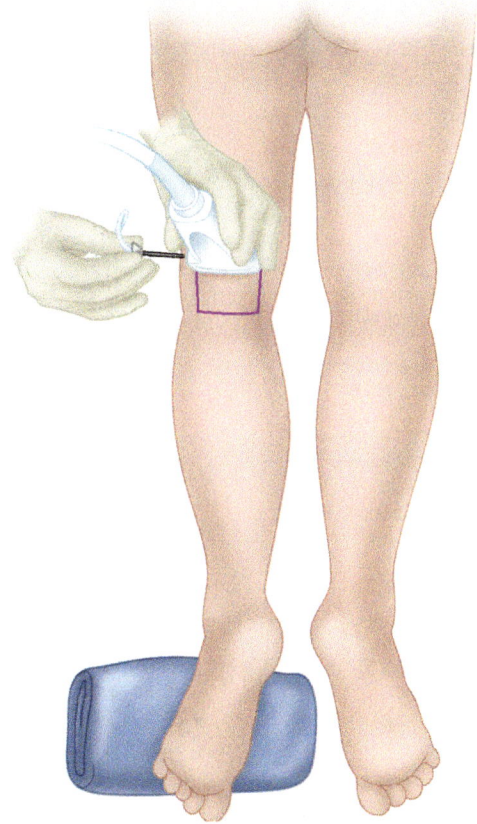

FIGURE 46–56 Patient positioning, probe, and needle orientation for popliteal block.

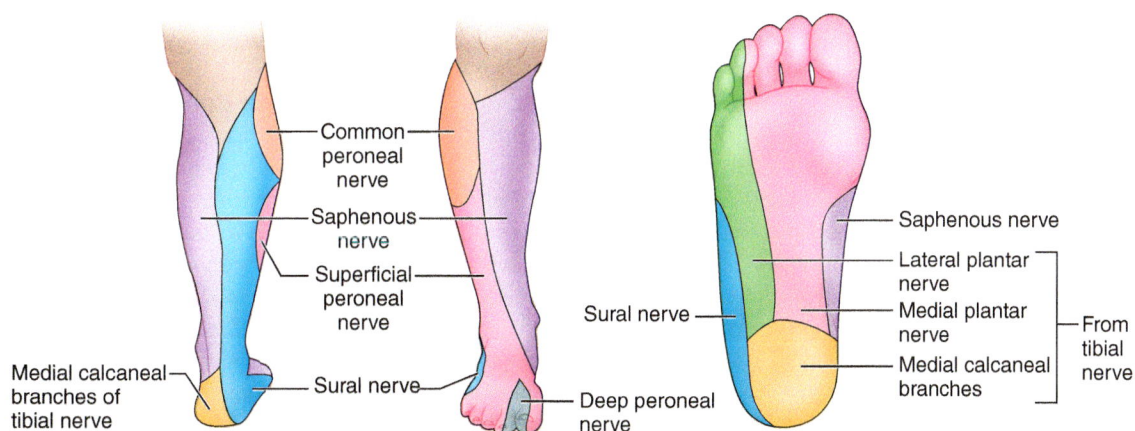

FIGURE 46–57 Cutaneous innervation of the foot.

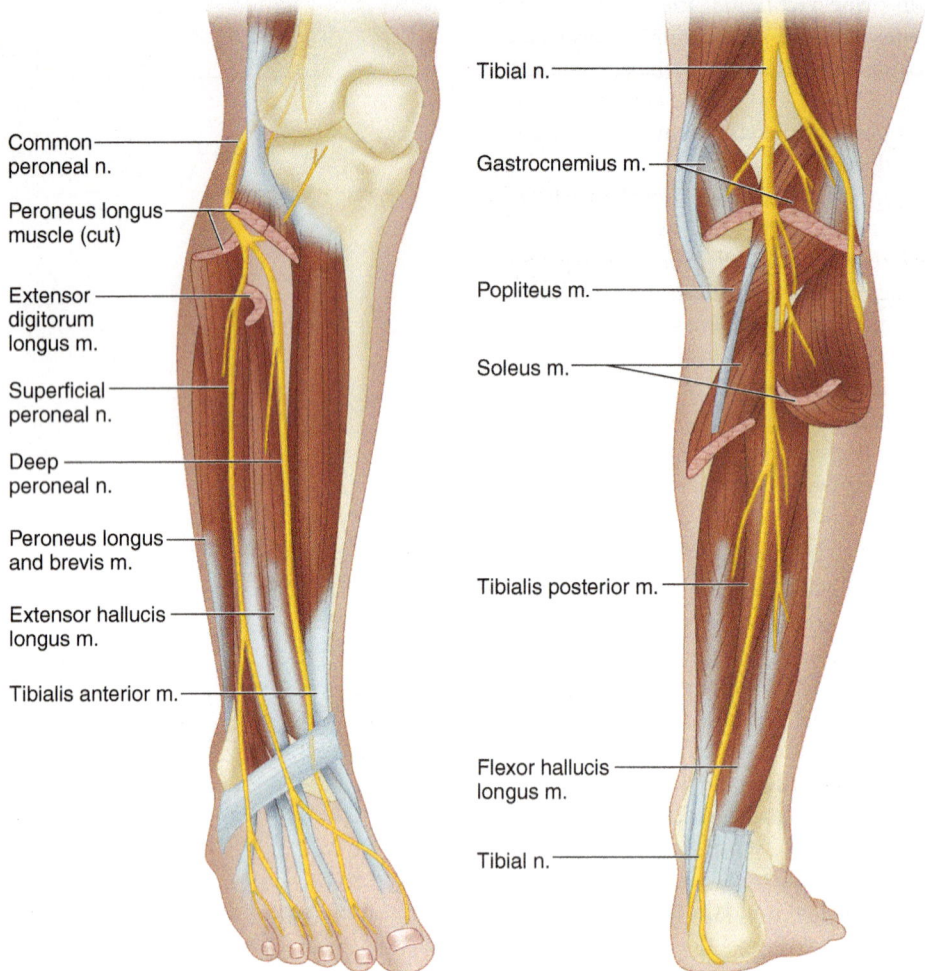

FIGURE 46–58 Tibial and common peroneal nerve courses.

of the foot not a part of the sciatic system. It supplies superficial sensation to the anteromedial foot and is most constantly located just anterior to the medial malleolus. The deep peroneal nerve runs in the anterior leg after branching off the common peroneal nerve, entering the ankle between the extensor hallucis longus and the extensor digitorum longus tendons (**Figure 46–58**), just lateral to the dorsalis pedis artery. It provides innervation to the toe extensors and sensation to the first dorsal webspace. The superficial peroneal nerve, also a branch of the common peroneal nerve, descends toward the ankle in the lateral compartment, giving motor branches to the muscles of eversion. It enters the ankle just lateral to the extensor digitorum longus and provides cutaneous sensation to the dorsum of the foot and toes. The posterior tibial nerve is a direct continuation of the tibial nerve and enters the foot posterior to the medial malleolus, branching into calcaneal, lateral plantar, and medial plantar nerves. It is located behind the posterior tibial artery at the level of the medial malleolus and provides sensory innervation to the heel, the medial sole, and part of the lateral sole of the foot, as well as the tips of the toes. The sural nerve is a branch of the tibial nerve and enters the foot between the Achilles tendon

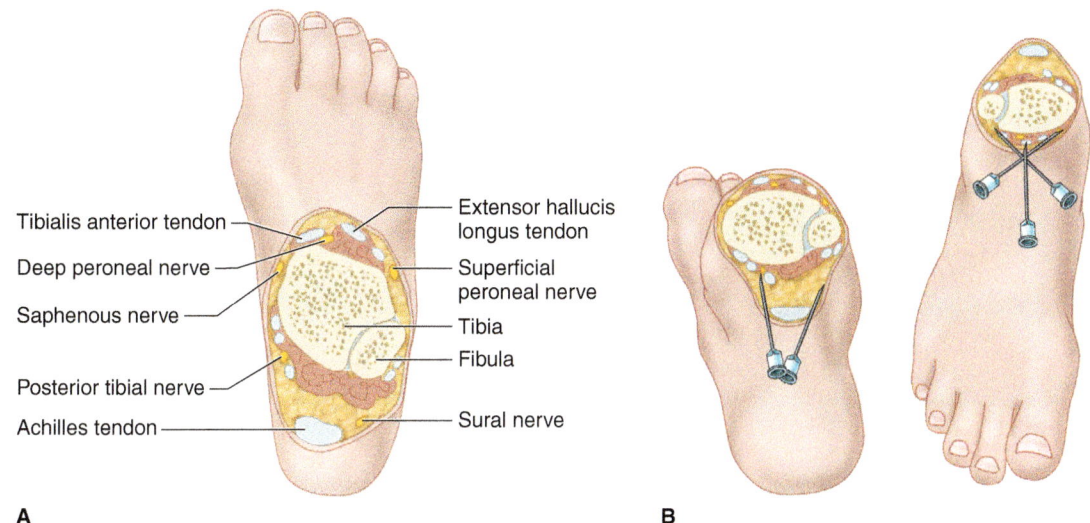

Tibialis anterior tendon

Deep peroneal nerve

Saphenous nerve

Posterior tibial nerve

Achilles tendon

Extensor hallucis longus tendon

Superficial peroneal nerve

Tibia

Fibula

Sural nerve

A

B

FIGURE 46–59 Needle placement for ankle block.

and the lateral malleolus to provide sensation to the lateral foot.

13 A complete ankle block requires a series of five nerve blocks, but the process may be streamlined to minimize needle insertions (Figure 46–59). All five injections are required to anesthetize the entire foot; however, many surgical procedures involve only a few terminal nerves, and only affected nerves should be blocked. In addition, unlike a sciatic nerve block, an ankle block provides no analgesia for (below-the-knee) tourniquet pain, nor does it allow for perineural catheter insertion. To block the deep peroneal nerve, the groove between the extensor hallucis longus and extensor digitorum longus tendons is identified. The dorsalis pedis pulse is often palpable here. A short, small-gauge block needle is inserted perpendicular to the skin just lateral to the pulse, bone is contacted, and 5 mL of local anesthetic is infiltrated as the needle is withdrawn. Continuing from this insertion site, a subcutaneous wheal of 5 mL of local anesthetic is extended toward the lateral malleolus to target the superficial peroneal nerve. The needle is withdrawn and redirected from the same location in a medial direction, infiltrating 5 mL of local anesthetic toward the medial malleolus to target the saphenous nerve. The posterior tibial nerve may be located by identifying the posterior tibial artery pulse behind the medial malleolus. A short, small-gauge block needle is inserted just posterior to the artery and 5 mL of local anesthetic is distributed in the pocket deep to the flexor retinaculum. To target the sural nerve, 5 mL of local anesthetic is injected subcutaneously posterior to the lateral malleolus.

PERIPHERAL NERVE BLOCKS OF THE TRUNK

Superficial Cervical Plexus Block

The superficial cervical plexus block provides cutaneous analgesia for surgical procedures on the neck, anterior shoulder, and clavicle. It is helpful to identify and avoid the external jugular vein. The cervical plexus is formed from the anterior rami of C1–4, which emerge from the platysma muscle posterior to the sternocleidomastoid (Figure 46–60). It supplies sensation to the jaw, neck, occiput, and areas of the chest and shoulder.

The patient is positioned supine with the head turned away from the side to be blocked. The sternocleidomastoid muscle is identified and its lateral edge marked. At the junction of the upper and middle thirds, a short (5-cm) block needle is inserted,

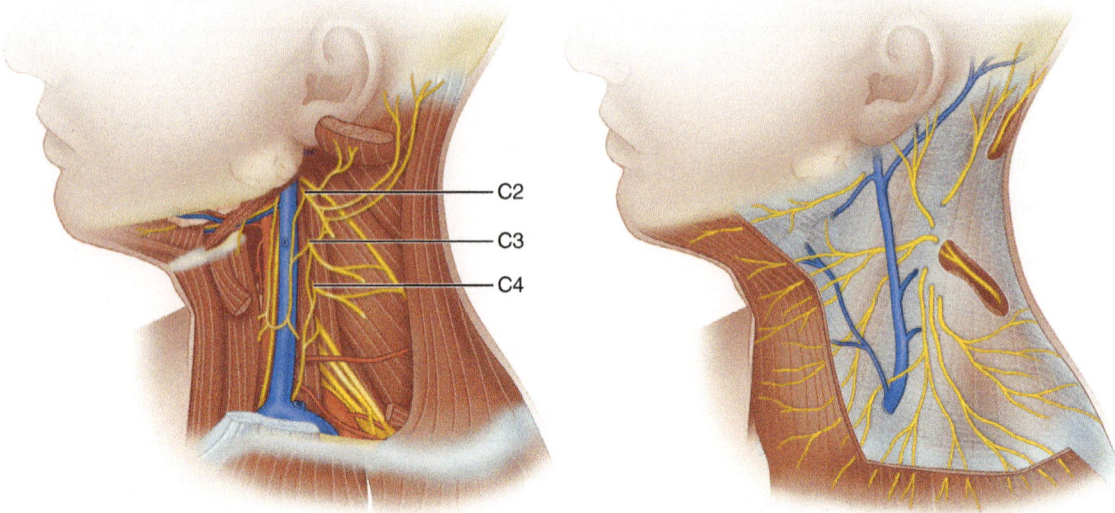

FIGURE 46–60 Distribution of the superficial cervical plexus.

directed cephalad toward the mastoid process, and 5 mL of local anesthetic is injected in a subcutaneous plane. The needle is turned to advance it in a caudad direction, maintaining a path along the posterior border of sternocleidomastoid. An additional 5 mL of local anesthetic is infiltrated subcutaneously.

Intercostal Block

Intercostal blocks provide analgesia following thoracic and upper abdominal surgery, and relief of pain associated with rib fractures, herpes zoster, and cancer. These blocks require individual injections delivered at the various vertebral levels that correspond to the area of body wall to be anesthetized. **14** Intercostal blocks result in the highest blood levels of local anesthetic per volume injected of any block in the body, and care must be taken to avoid toxic levels of local anesthetic. The intercostal block has one of the highest complication rates of any peripheral nerve block due to the close proximity of the intercostal artery and vein (intravascular local anesthetic injection), as well as underlying pleura (pneumothorax). In addition, duration is impressively short due to the high vascular flow, and

placement of a perineural catheter is tenuous, at best. With the advent of ultrasound guidance, the paravertebral approach is rapidly replacing the intercostal approach.

The intercostal nerves arise from the dorsal and ventral rami of the thoracic spinal nerves. They exit from the spine at the intervertebral foramen and enter a groove on the underside of the corresponding rib, running with the intercostal artery and vein; the nerve is generally the most inferior structure in the neurovascular bundle (Figure 46–61). Branches are given off for sensation in a single dermatome from the midline dorsally all the way to across the midline ventrally.

With the patient in the lateral decubitus or supine position, the level of each rib in the mid and posterior axillary line is palpated and marked. A small-gauge needle is inserted at the inferior edge of each of the selected ribs, bone is contacted, and the needle is then "walked off" inferiorly (Figure 46–61). The needle is redirected in a slightly cephalad direction and advanced approximately 0.25 cm. Following aspiration, observing for blood or air, 3–5 mL of local anesthetic is injected at each desired level.

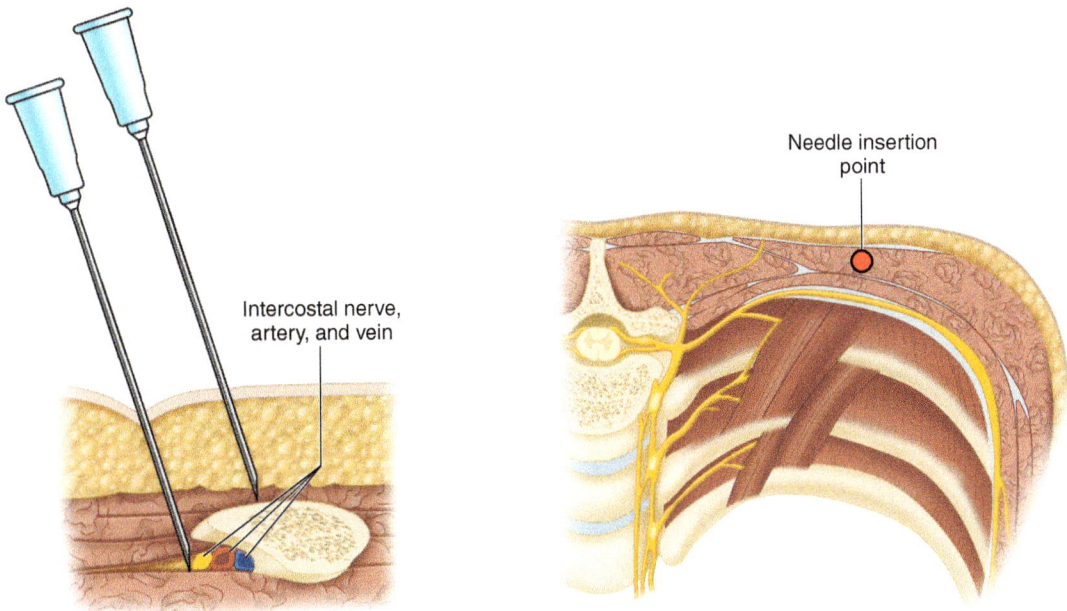

Needle insertion point

Intercostal nerve, artery, and vein

FIGURE 46–61 Anatomy and needle positioning for intercostal nerve block.

Paravertebral Block

Paravertebral blocks provide surgical anesthesia or postoperative analgesia for procedures involving the thoracic or abdominal wall, mastectomy, inguinal or abdominal hernia repair, and more invasive unilateral procedures such as open nephrectomy. Paravertebral blocks usually require individual injections delivered at the various vertebral levels that correspond to the area of body wall to be anesthetized. For example, a simple mastectomy would require blocks at levels T3–6; for axillary node dissection, additional injections should be made from C7 through T2. For inguinal hernia repair, blocks should be performed at T10 through L2. Ventral hernias require bilateral injections corresponding to the level of the surgical site. The major complication of thoracic injections is pneumothorax, whereas retroperitoneal structures may be at risk with lumbar-level injections. Hypotension secondary to sympathectomy can be observed with multilevel thoracic blocks. Unlike the intercostal approach, long-acting local anesthetic will have a nearly 24-hour duration, and perineural catheter insertion is a viable option (although local anesthetic spread from a single catheter to multiple levels is variable).

Each spinal nerve emerges from the intervertebral foramina and divides into two rami: a larger anterior ramus, which innervates the muscles and skin over the anterolateral body wall and limbs, and a smaller posterior ramus, which reflects posteriorly and innervates the skin and muscles of the back and neck (Figure 46–62). The thoracic para-vertebral space is defined posteriorly by the superior costotransverse ligament, anterolaterally by the parietal pleura, medially by the vertebrae and the intervertebral foramina, and inferiorly and superiorly by the heads of the ribs.

With the patient seated and vertebral column flexed, each spinous process is palpated, counting from the prominent C7 for thoracic blocks, and the iliac crests as a reference for lumbar levels. From the midpoint of the superior aspect of each spinous process, a point 2.5 cm laterally is measured and marked. In the thorax, the target nerve is located lateral to the spinous process *above* it, due to the steep

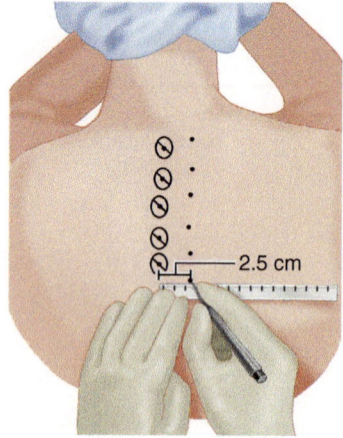

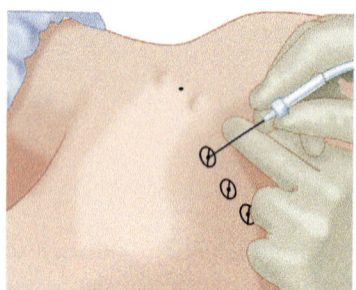

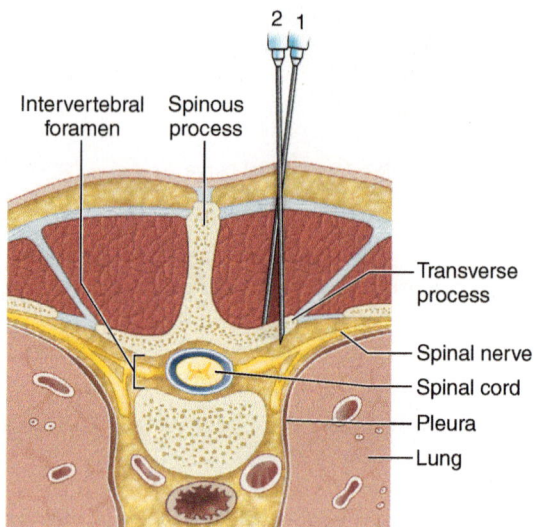

FIGURE 46–62 Paravertebral anatomy and traditional approach. Contact transverse process (1), then redirect the needle caudally (2) and advance 1 cm.

angulation of thoracic spinous processes (eg, the T4 nerve root is located lateral to the spinous process of T3).

A. Traditional Technique

A pediatric Tuohy needle (20 gauge) is inserted at each point and advanced perpendicular to the skin (Figure 46–62). Upon contact with the transverse process, the needle is withdrawn slightly and redirected caudally an additional 1 cm (0.5 cm for lumbar placement). A "pop" or loss of resistance may be felt as the needle passes through the costotransverse ligament. Some practitioners use a loss-of-resistance syringe to guide placement; others prefer use of a nerve stimulator with chest wall motion for the end point. Inject 5 mL of local anesthetic at each level. The difficulty with this technique is that the depth of the transverse process is simply estimated; thus the risk of pneumothorax is relatively high. Using ultrasound to gauge transverse process depth prior to needle insertion theoretically decreases the risk of pneumothorax.

B. Ultrasound

An ultrasound transducer with a curvilinear array is used, with the beam oriented in a parasagittal or transverse plane. The transverse process, head of the rib, costotransverse ligament, and pleura are identified. The paravertebral space may be approached from a caudal-to-cephalad direction (parasagittal) or a lateral-to-medial direction (transverse). It is helpful to visualize the needle in-plane as it passes through the costotransverse ligament and observe a downward displacement of the pleura as local anesthetic is injected. At each level 5 mL of local anesthetic is injected.

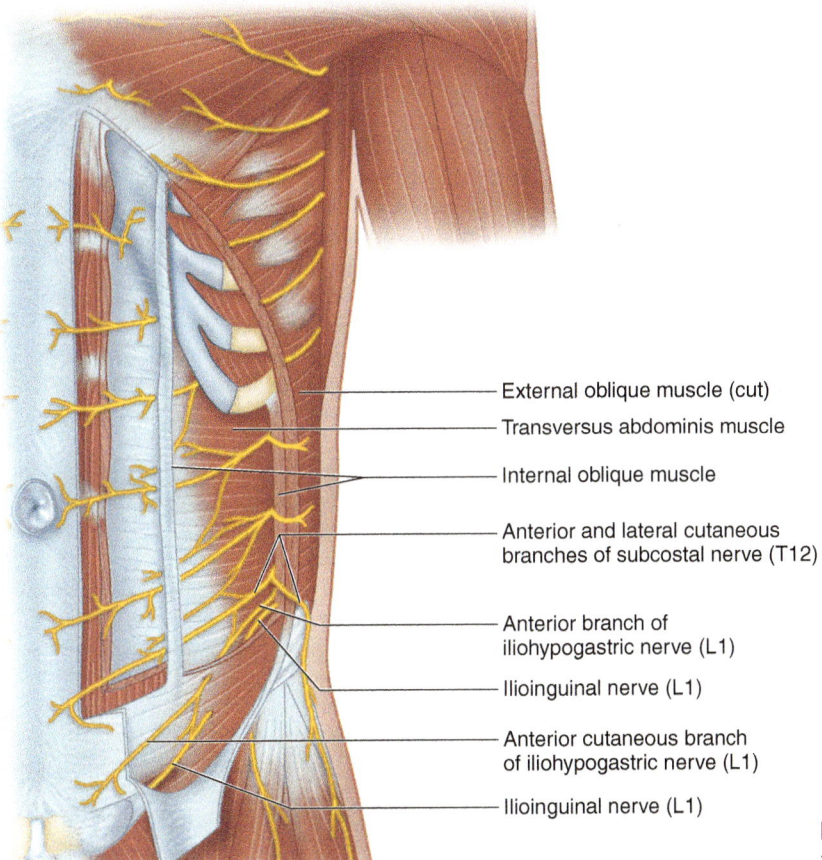

External oblique muscle (cut)

Transversus abdominis muscle

Internal oblique muscle

Anterior and lateral cutaneous
branches of subcostal nerve (T12)

Anterior branch of
iliohypogastric nerve (L1)

Ilioinguinal nerve (L1)

Anterior cutaneous branch
of iliohypogastric nerve (L1)

Ilioinguinal nerve (L1)

FIGURE 46–63 Transversus
abdominis plane (TAP)
anatomy.

Transversus Abdominis Plane Block

The transversus abdominis plane (TAP) block is most often used to provide surgical anesthesia for minor, superficial procedures on the lower abdominal wall, or postoperative analgesia for procedures below the umbilicus. For hernia surgeries, intravenous or local supplementation may be necessary to provide anesthesia during peritoneal traction. Potential complications include violation of the peritoneum with or without bowel perforation, and the use of ultrasound is highly recommended to minimize this risk.

16 The subcostal (T12), ilioinguinal (L1), and iliohypogastric (L1) nerves are targeted in the TAP block, providing anesthesia to the ipsilateral lower abdomen below the umbilicus (Figure 46–63). For part of their course, these three nerves travel in the muscle plane between the internal oblique and transversus abdominis muscles. Needle placement should be between the two fascial layers of these muscles, with local anesthetic filling the transversus abdominis plane. The patient is ideally positioned in lateral decubitus, but if mobility is limited the block may be performed in the supine position.

A. Ultrasound

With a linear or curvilinear array transducer oriented parallel to the inguinal ligament, the layers of the external oblique, internal oblique, and transversus abdominis muscles are identified just superior

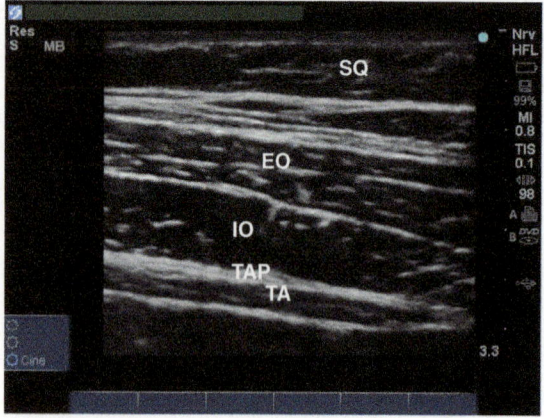

FIGURE 46–64 Ultrasound image of TAP block. SQ, subcutaneous tissue; EO, external oblique; IO, internal oblique; TA, transversus abdominis; TAP, transversus abdominis plane.

to the anterior superior iliac spine (Figure 46–64). Muscles appear as striated hypoechoic structures with hyperechoic layers of fascia at their borders. A long (10-cm) needle is inserted in-plane just lateral (posterior) to the transducer and advanced, noting tactile feedback from fascial planes, to the hyperechoic effacement of the deep border of internal oblique and the superficial border of transversus abdominis. Following careful aspiration for the nonappearance of blood, 20 mL of local anesthetic is injected, observing for an elliptical separation between the two fascial layers (Figure 46–64).

SUGGESTED READING

Capdevila X, Coimbra C, Choquet O: Approaches to the lumbar plexus: Success, risks, and outcome. Reg Anesth Pain Med 2005;30:150.

Hadzic A (editor): *Peripheral Nerve Blocks and Anatomy for Ultrasound-guided Regional Anesthesia, 2nd ed.* McGraw-Hill Medical, 2012.

Hebl JR, Lennon RL (editors): *Mayo Clinic Atlas of Regional Anesthesia and Ultrasound-Guided Nerve Blockade.* Oxford University Press, 2010.

Heil JW, Ilfeld BM, Loland VJ, et al: Ultrasound-guided transversus abdominis plane catheters and ambulatory perineural infusions for outpatient inguinal hernia repair. Reg Anesth Pain Med 2010;35:556.

Horn JL, Pitsch T, Salinas F, Benninger B: Anatomic basis to the ultrasound-guided approach for saphenous nerve blockade. Reg Anesth Pain Med 2009;34:486.

Ilfeld BM: Continuous peripheral nerve blocks: A review of the published evidence. Anesth Analg 2011;113:904.

Ilfeld BM, Fredrickson MJ, Mariano ER: Ultrasound-guided perineural catheter insertion: Three approaches, but little illuminating data. Reg Anesth Pain Med 2010;35:123.

Mariano ER, Loland VJ, Sandhu NS, et al: Ultrasound guidance versus electrical stimulation for femoral perineural catheter insertion. J Ultrasound Med 2009;28:1453.

Perlas A, Brull R, Chan VW, et al: Ultrasound guidance improves the success of sciatic nerve block at the popliteal fossa. Reg Anesth Pain Med. 2008;33:259.

Perlas A, Chan VW, Simons M: Brachial plexus examination and localization using ultrasound and electrical stimulation: A volunteer study. Anesthesiology 2003;99:429.

Sites BD, Brull R, Chan VW, et al: Artifacts and pitfall errors associated with ultrasound-guided regional anesthesia. Part I: Understanding the basic principles of ultrasound physics and machine operations. Reg Anesth Pain Med 2007;32: 412.

Sites BD, Brull R, Chan VW, et al: Artifacts and pitfall errors associated with ultrasound-guided regional anesthesia. Part II: A pictorial approach to understanding and avoidance. Reg Anesth Pain Med. 2007;32:419.

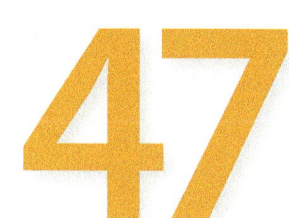
Chronic Pain Management

Richard W. Rosenquist, MD and Bruce M. Vrooman, MD

1 Pain may be classified according to pathophysiology (eg, nociceptive or neuropathic pain), etiology (eg, postoperative or cancer pain), or the affected area (eg, headache or low back pain).

2 Nociceptive pain is caused by activation or sensitization of peripheral nociceptors, specialized receptors that transduce noxious stimuli. Neuropathic pain is the result of injury or acquired abnormalities of peripheral or central neural structures.

3 Acute pain is caused by noxious stimulation due to injury, a disease process, or the abnormal function of muscle or viscera. It is nearly always nociceptive.

4 Chronic pain is pain that persists beyond the usual course of an acute disease or after a reasonable time for healing to occur; this healing period can vary from 1 to 6 months. Chronic pain may be nociceptive, neuropathic, or mixed.

5 Modulation of pain occurs peripherally at the nociceptor, in the spinal cord, or in supraspinal structures. This modulation can either inhibit (suppress) or facilitate (intensify) pain.

6 At least three mechanisms are responsible for central sensitization in the spinal cord: (1) wind-up and sensitization of second-order wide dynamic range neurons; (2) dorsal horn neuron receptor field expansion; and (3) hyperexitability of flexion reflexes.

7 Chronic pain may be caused by a combination of peripheral, central, and psychological mechanisms.

8 Moderate to severe acute pain, regardless of site, can affect the function of nearly every organ and may adversely influence perioperative morbidity and mortality.

9 The evaluation of any patient with pain should include several key components. Information about location, onset, and quality of pain, as well as alleviating and exacerbating factors, should be obtained along with a pain history that includes previous therapies and changes in symptoms over time.

10 Psychological evaluation is useful whenever medical evaluation fails to reveal an apparent cause for pain, pain intensity is disproportionate to disease or injury, or when depression or other psychological issues are apparent.

11 Myofascial pain syndromes are common disorders characterized by aching muscle pain, muscle spasm, stiffness, weakness, and, occasionally, autonomic dysfunction.

12 Ninety percent of disc herniations occur at L5–S1 or L4–L5. Symptoms usually develop following flexion injuries or heavy lifting and may be associated with bulging, protrusion, or extrusion of the disc.

13 Back pain caused by spinal stenosis usually radiates into the buttocks, thighs, and legs.

—Continued next page

Continued—

Termed *pseudoclaudication* or *neurogenic claudication,* the pain is characteristically worse with exercise and relieved by rest, particularly sitting with the spine flexed.

14. Diabetic neuropathy is the most common type of neuropathic pain.

15. Complex regional pain syndrome (CRPS) is a neuropathic pain disorder with significant autonomic features that is usually subdivided into two variants: CRPS 1, formerly known as *reflex sympathetic dystrophy* (RSD), and CRPS 2, formerly known as *causalgia.* The major difference between the two is the absence or presence, respectively, of documented nerve injury.

16. Trigeminal neuralgia (*tic douloureux*) is classically unilateral and usually located in the V2 or V3 distribution of the trigeminal nerve. It has an electric shock quality lasting from seconds to minutes at a time and is often provoked by contact with a discrete trigger.

17. Antidepressants are most useful for patients with neuropathic pain. These medications demonstrate an analgesic effect that occurs at a dose lower than needed for antidepressant activity.

18. Anticonvulsant medications are useful for patients with neuropathic pain, especially trigeminal neuralgia and diabetic neuropathy.

19. Patients who experience opioid tolerance require escalating doses of opioid to maintain the same analgesic effect. Physical dependence manifests in opioid withdrawal when the opioid medication is either abruptly discontinued or the dose is abruptly and significantly decreased. Psychological dependence, characterized by behavioral changes focusing on drug craving, is rare in cancer patients.

20. Complications of stellate block include intravascular and subarachnoid injection, hematoma, pneumothorax, epidural anesthesia, brachial plexus block, hoarseness due to blockade of the recurrent laryngeal nerve, and, rarely, osteomyelitis or mediastinitis.

21. Ganglion impar block is effective for patients with visceral or sympathetically maintained pain in the perineal area.

22. Neurolytic blocks are indicated for patients with severe, intractable cancer pain in whom more conventional therapy proves inadequate or conventional analgesic modalities are accompanied by unacceptable side effects.

23. Spinal cord stimulation may be most effective for neuropathic pain; accepted indications include sympathetically mediated pain, spinal cord lesions with localized segmental pain, phantom limb pain, ischemic lower extremity pain due to peripheral vascular disease, adhesive arachnoiditis, peripheral neuropathies, post-thoracotomy pain, intercostal neuralgia, postherpetic neuralgia, angina, visceral abdominal pain, and visceral pelvic pain.

24. Patients with pathological or osteoporotic vertebral compression fracture may benefit from vertebral augmentation with polymethylmethacrylate cement. Vertebroplasty involves injection of the cement through the trocar needle. Kyphoplasty involves inflation of a balloon inserted through a percutaneously placed trocar needle, with subsequent injection of cement.

25. Acupuncture can be a useful adjunct for patients with chronic pain, particularly that associated with chronic musculoskeletal disorders and headaches.

Pain—the most common symptom that brings patients to see a physician—is nearly always a manifestation of a pathological process. This symptom may have a wide variety of causes ranging from relatively benign conditions to acute injury, myocardial ischemia, degenerative changes, or malignancy. In most cases, after a diagnosis is made, conservative measures are prescribed and the patient responds successfully. In others, referral to a pain medicine specialist for evaluation and treatment improves outcomes and conserves health care resources. In still other situations, pain persists and patients develop chronic pain, the cause of which remains obscure after preliminary investigations have excluded serious and life-threatening illnesses and, if warranted, surgical intervention has either failed to relieve pain or has produced a new pain syndrome.

The term *pain management* in a general sense applies to the entire discipline of anesthesiology, but its modern usage more specifically involves management of pain throughout the perioperative period as well as nonsurgical pain in both inpatient and outpatient settings. Pain medicine practice may be broadly divided into acute and chronic pain management. The former primarily deals with patients recovering from surgery or with acute medical conditions in a hospital setting (see Chapter 48), whereas the latter includes diverse groups of patients almost always seen in the outpatient setting. Unfortunately, this distinction is artificial and considerable overlap exists; a good example is the patient with cancer who frequently requires short- and long-term pain management in both inpatient and outpatient settings.

The contemporary practice of pain management is not limited to anesthesiologists but often includes other physicians (physiatrists, surgeons, internists, oncologists, psychiatrists, and neurologists) and nonphysicians (psychologists, physical therapists, acupuncturists, and hypnotists). The most effective approaches are multidisciplinary, in which the patient is evaluated by one or more physicians who conduct an initial examination, make a diagnosis, and formulate a treatment plan, and where subsequent evaluation and use of the services and resources of other health care providers are readily available.

Anesthesiologists trained in pain management are in a unique position to coordinate multidisciplinary pain management centers because of their broad training in dealing with a wide variety of patients from surgical, obstetric, pediatric, and medical subspecialties and their expertise in clinical pharmacology and applied neuroanatomy, including the use of peripheral and central nerve blocks.

DEFINITIONS & CLASSIFICATION OF PAIN

Like other conscious sensations, normal pain perception depends on specialized neurons that function as receptors, detecting the stimulus, and then transducing and conducting it to the central nervous system. Sensation is often described as either protopathic (noxious) or epicritic (nonnoxious). Epicritic sensations (light touch, pressure, proprioception, and temperature discrimination) are characterized by low-threshold receptors and are generally conducted by large myelinated nerve fibers. In contrast, protopathic sensations (pain) are detected by high-threshold receptors and conducted by smaller, lightly myelinated ($A\delta$) and unmyelinated (C) nerve fibers.

What Is Pain?

Pain is not just a sensory modality but an experience. The International Association for the Study of Pain defines pain as "an unpleasant sensory and emotional experience associated with actual or potential tissue damage, or described in terms of such damage." This definition recognizes the interplay between the objective, physiological sensory aspects of pain and its subjective, emotional, and psychological components. The response to pain can be highly variable among different individuals as well as in the same person at different times.

The term *nociception* is derived from *noci* (Latin for harm or injury) and is used to describe neural responses to traumatic or noxious stimuli. All nociception produces pain, but not all pain results from nociception. Many patients experience pain in the absence of noxious stimuli. It is therefore clinically useful to divide pain into one of two

TABLE 47–1 Terms used in pain management.

Term	Description
Allodynia	Perception of an ordinarily nonnoxious stimulus as pain
Analgesia	Absence of pain perception
Anesthesia	Absence of all sensation
Anesthesia dolorosa	Pain in an area that lacks sensation
Dysesthesia	Unpleasant or abnormal sensation with or without a stimulus
Hypalgesia (hypoalgesia)	Diminished response to noxious stimulation (eg, pinprick)
Hyperalgesia	Increased response to noxious stimulation
Hyperesthesia	Increased response to mild stimulation
Hyperpathia	Presence of hyperesthesia, allodynia, and hyperalgesia usually associated with overreaction, and persistence of the sensation after the stimulus
Hypesthesia (hypoesthesia)	Reduced cutaneous sensation (eg, light touch, pressure, or temperature)
Neuralgia	Pain in the distribution of a nerve or a group of nerves
Paresthesia	Abnormal sensation perceived without an apparent stimulus
Radiculopathy	Functional abnormality of one or more nerve roots

categories: (1) acute pain, which is primarily due to nociception, and (2) chronic pain, which may be due to nociception, but in which psychological and behavioral factors often play a major role. Table 47–1 lists terms frequently used in describing pain.

① Pain may also be classified according to pathophysiology (eg, nociceptive or neuropathic pain), etiology (eg, arthritis or cancer pain), or the affected area (eg, headache or low back pain). Such classifications are useful in the selection of treatment modalities and drug therapy. Nociceptive pain **②** is caused by activation or sensitization of peripheral nociceptors, specialized receptors that

transduce noxious stimuli. Neuropathic pain is the result of injury or acquired abnormalities of peripheral or central neural structures.

There are differences in pain perception related to gender and age. Research has confirmed differences in pain experiences and coping strategies between genders, and there is ongoing investigation into exactly how this processing differs. Brain activation differs between genders, with men particularly influenced by the type and intensity of a noxious stimulus. Brain imaging patterns differ as well. Some of these differences decrease with age and may disappear after age 40.

A. Acute Pain

③ Acute pain is caused by noxious stimulation due to injury, a disease process, or the abnormal function of muscle or viscera. It is usually nociceptive. Nociceptive pain serves to detect, localize, and limit tissue damage. Four physiological processes are involved: transduction, transmission, modulation, and perception. This type of pain is typically associated with a neuroendocrine stress response that is proportional to the pain's intensity. Its most common forms include post-traumatic, postoperative, and obstetric pain as well as pain associated with acute medical illnesses, such as myocardial infarction, pancreatitis, and renal calculi. Most forms of acute pain are self-limited or resolve with treatment in a few days or weeks. When pain fails to resolve because of either abnormal healing or inadequate treatment, it becomes chronic (below). Two types of acute (nociceptive) pain—somatic and visceral—are differentiated based on origin and features.

1. Somatic pain—Somatic pain can be further classified as superficial or deep. Superficial somatic pain is due to nociceptive input arising from skin, subcutaneous tissues, and mucous membranes. It is characteristically well localized and described as a sharp, pricking, throbbing, or burning sensation.

Deep somatic pain arises from muscles, tendons, joints, or bones. In contrast to superficial somatic pain, it usually has a dull, aching quality and is less well localized. An additional feature is that both the intensity and duration of the stimulus affect the degree of localization. For example, pain following brief minor trauma to the elbow joint is localized to the elbow, but severe or sustained trauma often causes pain in the whole arm.

2. Visceral pain—Visceral acute pain is due to a disease process or abnormal function involving an internal organ or its covering (eg, parietal pleura, pericardium, or peritoneum). Four subtypes are described: (1) true localized visceral pain, (2) localized parietal pain, (3) referred visceral pain, and (4) referred parietal pain. True visceral pain is dull, diffuse, and usually midline. It is frequently associated with abnormal sympathetic or parasympathetic activity causing nausea, vomiting, sweating, and changes in blood pressure and heart rate. Parietal pain is typically sharp and often described as a stabbing sensation that is either localized to the area around the organ or referred to a distant site (Table 47–2). The phenomenon of visceral or parietal pain referred to cutaneous areas results from patterns of embryological development and migration of tissues, and the

convergence of visceral and somatic afferent input into the central nervous system. Thus, pain associated with disease processes involving the peritoneum or pleura over the central diaphragm is frequently referred to the neck and shoulder, whereas pain from disease processes affecting the parietal surfaces of the peripheral diaphragm is referred to the chest or upper abdominal wall.

B. Chronic Pain

Chronic pain is pain that persists beyond the usual course of an acute disease or after a reasonable time for healing to occur; this healing period typically can vary from 1 to 6 months. Chronic pain may be nociceptive, neuropathic, or mixed. A distinguishing feature is that psychological mechanisms or environmental factors frequently play a major role. Patients with chronic pain often have attenuated or absent neuroendocrine stress responses and have prominent sleep and affective (mood) disturbances. Neuropathic pain is classically paroxysmal and lancinating, has a burning quality, and is associated with hyperpathia. When it is also associated with loss of sensory input (eg, amputation) into the central nervous system, it is termed *deafferentation pain*. When the sympathetic system plays a major role, it is often termed *sympathetically maintained pain*.

The most common forms of chronic pain include those associated with musculoskeletal disorders, chronic visceral disorders, lesions of peripheral nerves, nerve roots, or dorsal root ganglia (including diabetic neuropathy, causalgia, phantom limb pain, and postherpetic neuralgia), lesions of the central nervous system (stroke, spinal cord injury, and multiple sclerosis), and cancer pain. The pain of most musculoskeletal disorders (eg, rheumatoid arthritis and osteoarthritis) is primarily nociceptive, whereas pain associated with peripheral or central neural disorders is primarily neuropathic. The pain associated with some disorders, eg, cancer and chronic back pain (particularly after surgery), is often mixed. Some clinicians use the term *chronic benign pain* when pain does not result from cancer. This terminology should be discouraged, however, because pain is never benign from the patient's point of view, regardless of its cause.

TABLE 47–2 Patterns of referred pain.

Location	Cutaneous Dermatome
Central diaphragm	C4
Lungs	T2–T6
Aorta	T1–L2
Heart	T1–T4
Esophagus	T3–T8
Pancreas and spleen	T5–T10
Stomach, liver, and gallbladder	T6–T9
Adrenals	T8–L1
Small intestine	T9–T11
Colon	T10–L1
Kidney, ovaries, and testes	T10–L1
Ureters	T10–T12
Uterus	T11–L2
Bladder and prostate	S2–S4
Urethra and rectum	S2–S4

Anatomy & Physiology of Nociception

PAIN PATHWAYS

Pain is conducted along three neuronal pathways that transmit noxious stimuli from the periphery to the cerebral cortex (**Figure 47–1**). The cell bodies of primary afferent neurons are located in the dorsal root ganglia, which lie in the vertebral foramina at each spinal cord level. Each neuron has a single axon that bifurcates, sending one end to the peripheral tissues it innervates and the other into the dorsal horn of the spinal cord. In the dorsal horn, the primary afferent neuron synapses with a second-order neuron whose axon crosses the midline and ascends in the contralateral spinothalamic tract to reach the thalamus. Second-order neurons synapse in thalamic nuclei with third-order neurons, which in turn send projections through the internal capsule and corona radiata to the postcentral gyrus of the cerebral cortex (**Figure 47–2**).

First-Order Neurons

The majority of first-order neurons send the proximal end of their axons into the spinal cord via the dorsal (sensory) spinal root at each cervical, thoracic, lumbar, and sacral level. Some unmyelinated afferent (C) fibers have been shown to enter the spinal cord via the ventral nerve (motor) root, accounting for observations that some patients continue to feel pain even after transection of the dorsal nerve root (rhizotomy) and report pain following ventral root stimulation. Once in the dorsal horn, in addition to synapsing with second-order neurons, the axons of first-order neurons may synapse with interneurons, sympathetic neurons, and ventral horn motor neurons.

Pain fibers originating from the head are carried by the trigeminal (V), facial (VII), glossopharyngeal (IX), and vagal (X) nerves. The gasserian ganglion contains the cell bodies of sensory fibers in the ophthalmic, maxillary, and mandibular divisions of the trigeminal nerve. Cell bodies of first-order afferent neurons of the facial nerve are located in the geniculate ganglion; those of the glossopharyngeal nerve lie in its superior and petrosal ganglia; and those of the vagal nerve are located in the jugular ganglion (somatic) and the ganglion nodosum (visceral). The

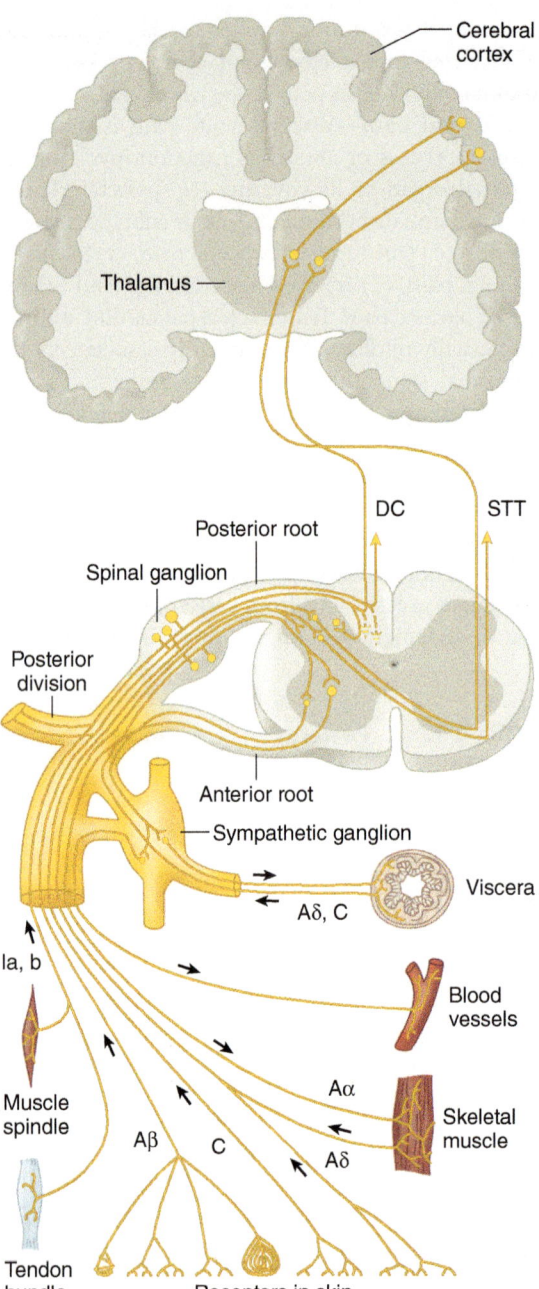

FIGURE 47–1 Pain pathways. DC, dorsal column; STT, spinothalamic tracts.

proximal axonal processes of the first-order neurons in these ganglia reach the brainstem nuclei via their respective cranial nerves, where they synapse with second-order neurons in brainstem nuclei.

A

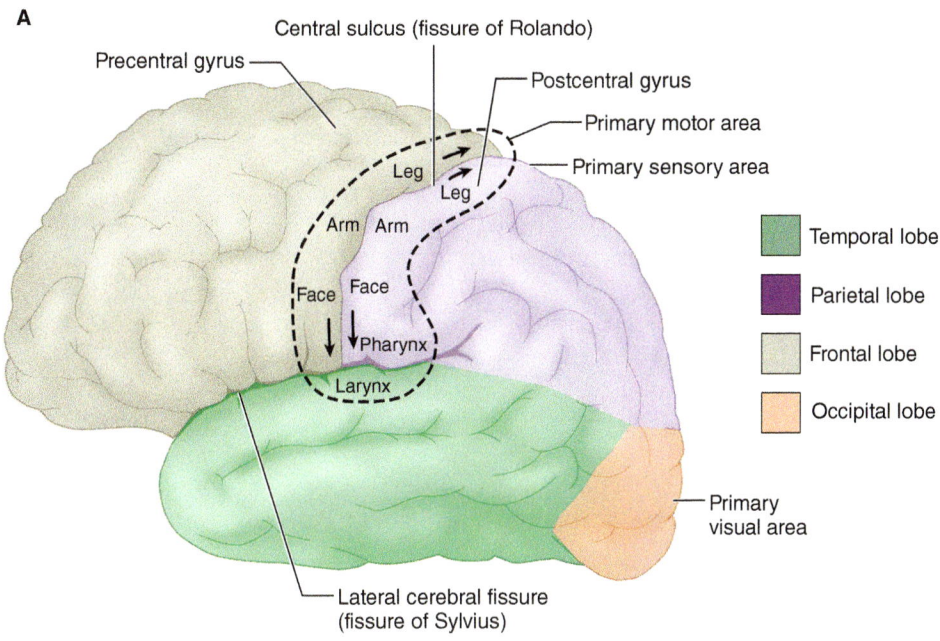

B

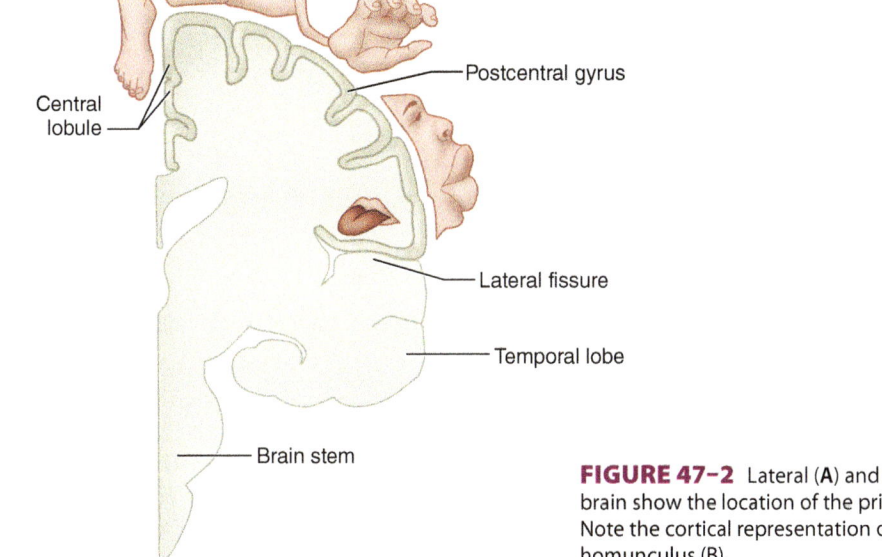

FIGURE 47–2 Lateral (**A**) and coronal (**B**) views of the brain show the location of the primary sensory cortex. Note the cortical representation of body parts, the sensory homunculus (B).

Second-Order Neurons

As afferent fibers enter the spinal cord, they segregate according to size, with large, myelinated fibers becoming medial, and small, unmyelinated fibers becoming lateral. Pain fibers may ascend or descend one to three spinal cord segments in Lissauer's tract before synapsing with second-order neurons in the gray matter of the ipsilateral dorsal horn. In many instances they communicate with second-order neurons through interneurons.

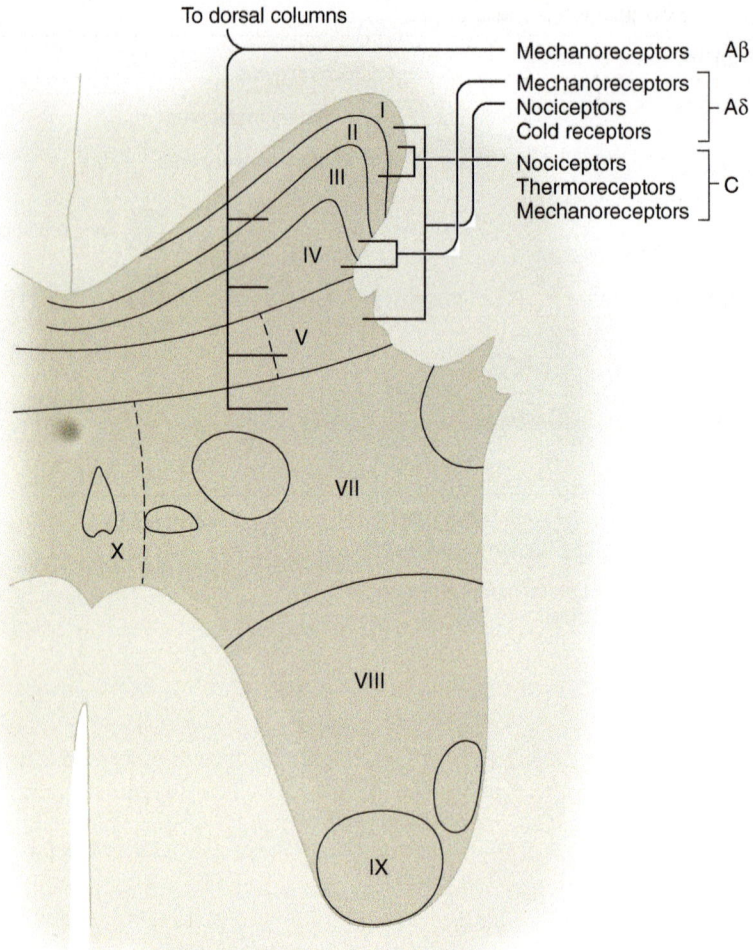

FIGURE 47–3 Rexed's spinal cord laminae. Note the termination of the different types of primary afferent neurons.

Spinal cord gray matter was divided by Rexed into 10 laminae (Figure 47–3 and Table 47–3). The first six laminae, which make up the dorsal horn, receive all afferent neural activity and represent the principal site of modulation of pain by ascending and descending neural pathways. Second-order neurons are either nociceptive-specific or wide dynamic range (WDR) neurons. Nociceptive-specific neurons serve only noxious stimuli, but WDR neurons also receive nonnoxious afferent input from Aβ, Aδ, and C fibers. Nociceptive-specific neurons are arranged somatotopically in lamina I and have discrete, somatic receptive fields; they are normally silent and respond only to high-threshold noxious stimulation, poorly encoding stimulus intensity. WDR neurons are the most prevalent cell type in the dorsal horn. Although they are found throughout the dorsal horn, WDR neurons are most abundant in lamina V. During repeated stimulation, WDR neurons characteristically increase their firing rate exponentially in a graded fashion ("wind-up"), even with the same stimulus intensity. They also have large receptive fields compared with nociceptive-specific neurons.

TABLE 47–3 Spinal cord lamina.

Lamina	Predominant Function	Input	Name
I	Somatic nociception thermoreception	Aδ, C	Marginal layer
II	Somatic nociception thermoreception	C, Aδ	Substantia gelatinosa
III	Somatic mechanoreception	Aβ, Aδ	Nucleus proprius
IV	Mechanoreception	Aβ, Aδ	Nucleus proprius
V	Visceral and somatic nociception and mechanoreception	Aβ, Aδ, (C)	Nucleus proprius WDR neurons[1]
VI	Mechanoreception	Aβ	Nucleus proprius
VII	Sympathetic		Intermediolateral column
VIII		Aβ	Motor horn
IX	Motor	Aβ	Motor horn
X		Aβ, (Aδ)	Central canal

[1]WDR, wide dynamic range.

Most nociceptive C fibers send collaterals to, or terminate on, second-order neurons in laminae I and II, and, to a lesser extent, in lamina V. In contrast, nociceptive Aδ fibers synapse mainly in laminae I and V, and, to a lesser degree, in lamina X. Lamina I responds primarily to noxious (nociceptive) stimuli from cutaneous and deep somatic tissues. Lamina II, also called the substantia gelatinosa, contains many interneurons and is believed to play a major role in processing and modulating nociceptive input from cutaneous nociceptors. It is also of special interest because it is believed to be a major site of action for opioids. Laminae III and IV primarily receive non-nociceptive sensory input. Laminae VIII and IX make up the anterior (motor) horn. Lamina VII is the intermediolateral column and contains the cell bodies of preganglionic sympathetic neurons.

Visceral afferents terminate primarily in lamina V, and, to a lesser extent, in lamina I. These two laminae represent points of central convergence between somatic and visceral inputs. Lamina V responds to both noxious and nonnoxious sensory input and receives both visceral and somatic pain afferents. The phenomenon of convergence between visceral and somatic sensory input is manifested clinically as referred pain (see Table 47–2). Compared with somatic fibers, visceral nociceptive fibers are fewer in number, more widely distributed, proportionately activate a larger number of spinal neurons, and are not organized somatotopically.

A. The Spinothalamic Tract

The axons of most second-order neurons cross the midline close to their dermatomal level of origin (at the anterior commissure) to the contralateral side of the spinal cord before they form the spinothalamic tract and send their fibers to the thalamus, the reticular formation, the nucleus raphe magnus, and the periaqueductal gray. The spinothalamic tract, which is classically considered the major pain pathway, lies anterolaterally in the white matter of the spinal cord (Figure 47–4). This ascending tract can be divided into a lateral and a medial tract. The lateral spinothalamic (neospinothalamic) tract projects mainly to the ventral posterolateral nucleus of the thalamus and carries discriminative aspects of pain, such as location, intensity, and duration. The medial spinothalamic (paleospinothalamic) tract projects to the medial thalamus and is responsible for mediating the autonomic and unpleasant emotional perceptions of pain. Some spinothalamic fibers also project to the periaqueductal gray and thus may be an

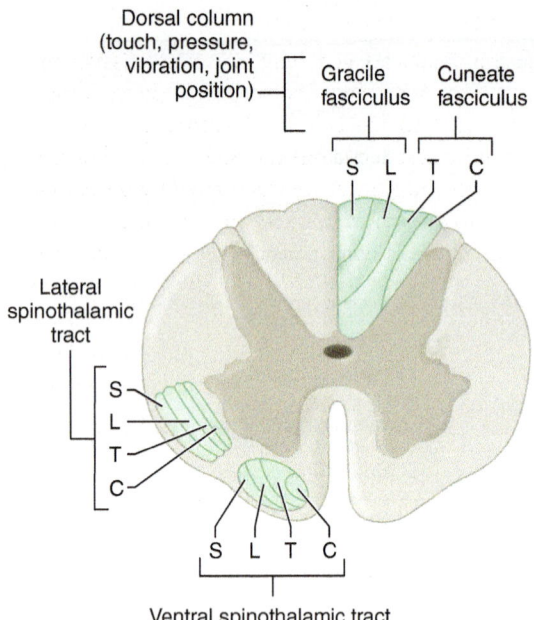

FIGURE 47–4 A cross section of the spinal cord showing the spinothalamic and other ascending sensory pathways. Note the spatial distribution of fibers from different spinal levels: cervical (C), thoracic (T), lumbar (L), and sacral (S).

important link between the ascending and descending pathways. Collateral fibers also project to the reticular activating system and the hypothalamus; these are likely responsible for the arousal response to pain.

B. Alternate Pain Pathways

As with epicritic sensation, pain fibers ascend diffusely, ipsilaterally, and contralaterally; some patients continue to perceive pain following ablation of the contralateral spinothalamic tract, and therefore other ascending pain pathways are also important. The spinoreticular tract is thought to mediate arousal and autonomic responses to pain. The spinomesencephalic tract may be important in activating antinociceptive, descending pathways, because it has some projections to the periaqueductal gray. The spinohypothalamic and spinotelencephalic tracts activate the hypothalamus and evoke emotional behavior. The spinocervical tract ascends uncrossed to the lateral cervical nucleus, which relays the fibers

to the contralateral thalamus; this tract is likely a major alternative pathway for pain. Lastly, some fibers in the dorsal columns (which mainly carry light touch and proprioception) are responsive to pain; they ascend medially and ipsilaterally.

C. Integration with the Sympathetic and Motor Systems

Somatic and visceral afferents are fully integrated with the skeletal motor and sympathetic systems in the spinal cord, brainstem, and higher centers. Afferent dorsal horn neurons synapse both directly and indirectly with anterior horn motor neurons. These synapses are responsible for the reflex muscle activity—whether normal or abnormal—that is associated with pain. In a similar fashion, synapses between afferent nociceptive neurons and sympathetic neurons in the intermediolateral column result in reflex sympathetically mediated vasoconstriction, smooth muscle spasm, and the release of catecholamines, both locally and from the adrenal medulla.

Third-Order Neurons

Third-order neurons are located in the thalamus and send fibers to somatosensory areas I and II in the postcentral gyrus of the parietal cortex and the superior wall of the sylvian fissure, respectively. Perception and discrete localization of pain take place in these cortical areas. Although most neurons from the lateral thalamic nuclei project to the primary somatosensory cortex, neurons from the intralaminar and medial nuclei project to the anterior cingulate gyrus and are likely involved in mediating the suffering and emotional components of pain.

PHYSIOLOGY OF NOCICEPTION

1. Nociceptors

Nociceptors are characterized by a high threshold for activation and encode the intensity of stimulation by increasing their discharge rates in a graded fashion. Following repeated stimulation, they characteristically display delayed adaptation, sensitization, and afterdischarges.

Noxious sensations can often be broken down into two components: a fast, sharp, and well-localized sensation ("first pain"), which is conducted with a short latency (0.1 s) by Aδ fibers (tested by pin-prick); and a slower onset, duller, and often poorly localized sensation ("second pain"), which is conducted by C fibers. In contrast to epicritic sensation, which may be transduced by specialized end organs on the afferent neuron (eg, pacinian corpuscle for touch), protopathic sensation is transduced mainly by free nerve endings.

Most nociceptors are free nerve endings that sense heat and mechanical and chemical tissue damage. Types include (1) mechanonociceptors, which respond to pinch and pinprick, (2) silent nociceptors, which respond only in the presence of inflammation, and (3) polymodal mechanoheat nociceptors. The last are most prevalent and respond to excessive pressure, extremes of temperature (>42°C and <40°C), and noxious substances such as bradykinin, histamine, serotonin (5-hydroxytrypta-mine or 5-HT), H^+, K^+, some prostaglandins, capsa-icin, and possibly adenosine triphosphate. At least two nociceptor receptors (containing ion channels in nerve endings) have been identified, TRPV1 and TRPV2. Both respond to high temperatures. Cap-saicin stimulates the TRPV1 receptor. Polymodal nociceptors are slow to adapt to strong pressure and display heat sensitization.

Cutaneous Nociceptors

Nociceptors are present in both somatic and visceral tissues. Primary afferent neurons reach tissues by traveling along spinal somatic, sympathetic, or para-sympathetic nerves. Somatic nociceptors include those in skin (cutaneous) and deep tissues (muscle, tendons, fascia, and bone), whereas visceral nociceptors include those in internal organs. The cornea and tooth pulp are unique in that they are almost exclusively innervated by nociceptive Aδ and C fibers.

Deep Somatic Nociceptors

Deep somatic nociceptors are less sensitive to noxious stimuli than cutaneous nociceptors but are easily sensitized by inflammation. The pain arising from them is characteristically dull and poorly localized. Specific nociceptors exist in muscles and joint capsules, and they respond to mechanical, thermal, and chemical stimuli.

Visceral Nociceptors

Visceral organs are generally insensitive tissues that mostly contain silent nociceptors. Some organs appear to have specific nociceptors, such as the heart, lung, testis, and bile ducts. Most other organs, such as the intestines, are innervated by polymodal nociceptors that respond to smooth muscle spasm, ischemia, and inflammation. These receptors generally do not respond to the cutting, burning, or crushing that occurs during surgery. A few organs, such as the brain, lack nociceptors altogether; however, the brain's meningeal coverings do contain nociceptors.

Like somatic nociceptors, those in the viscera are the free nerve endings of primary afferent neurons whose cell bodies lie in the dorsal horn. These afferent nerve fibers, however, frequently travel with efferent sympathetic nerve fibers to reach the viscera. Afferent activity from these neurons enters the spinal cord between T1 and L2. Nociceptive C fibers from the esophagus, larynx, and trachea travel with the vagus nerve to enter the nucleus solitarius in the brainstem. Afferent pain fibers from the bladder, prostate, rectum, cervix and urethra, and genitalia are transmitted into the spinal cord via parasympathetic nerves at the level of the S2–S4 nerve roots. Though relatively few compared with somatic pain fibers, fibers from primary visceral afferent neurons enter the cord and synapse more diffusely with single fibers, often synapsing with multiple dermatomal levels and often crossing to the contralateral dorsal horn.

2. Chemical Mediators of Pain

Several neuropeptides and excitatory amino acids function as neurotransmitters for afferent neurons subserving pain (Table 47–4). Many, if not most, of these neurons contain more than one neurotransmitter, which are simultaneously released. The most important of these peptides are substance P and calcitonin gene-related peptide (CGRP). Glutamate is the most important excitatory amino acid.

Substance P is an 11 amino acid peptide that is synthesized and released by first-order neurons both peripherally and in the dorsal horn. Also found in other parts of the nervous system and the intestines,

TABLE 47–4 Major neurotransmitters mediating or modulating pain.

Neurotransmitter	Receptor[1]	Effect on Nociception
Substance P	Neurokinin–1	Excitatory
Calcitonin gene-related peptide		Excitatory
Glutamate	NMDA, AMPA, kainate, quisqualate	Excitatory
Aspartate	NMDA, AMPA, kainate, quisqualate	Excitatory
Adenosine triphosphate (ATP)	P_1, P_2	Excitatory
Somatostatin		Inhibitory
Acetylcholine	Muscarinic	Inhibitory
Enkephalins	μ, δ, κ	Inhibitory
β-Endorphin	μ, δ, κ	Inhibitory
Norepinephrine	α_2	Inhibitory
Adenosine	A_1	Inhibitory
Serotonin	$5\text{-}HT_1$ $(5\text{-}HT_3)$	Inhibitory
γ-Aminobutyric acid (GABA)	A, B	Inhibitory
Glycine		Inhibitory

[1]NMDA, N-methyl-D-aspartate; AMPA, 2-(aminomethyl)phenylacetic acid; 5-HT, 5-hydroxytryptamine.

it facilitates transmission in pain pathways via neurokinin-1 receptor activation. In the periphery, substance P neurons send collaterals that are closely associated with blood vessels, sweat glands, hair follicles, and mast cells in the dermis. Substance P sensitizes nociceptors, degranulates histamine from mast cells and 5-HT from platelets, and is a potent vasodilator and chemoattractant for leukocytes. Substance P–releasing neurons also innervate the viscera and send collateral fibers to paravertebral sympathetic ganglia; intense stimulation of viscera, therefore, can cause direct postganglionic sympathetic discharge.

Both opioid and α_2-adrenergic receptors have been described on or near the terminals of unmyelinated peripheral nerves. Although their physiological role is not clear, the latter may explain the observed analgesia of peripherally applied opioids, particularly in the presence of inflammation.

3. Modulation of Pain

5 Modulation of pain occurs peripherally at the nociceptor, in the spinal cord, and in supraspinal structures. This modulation can either inhibit (suppress) or facilitate (intensify) pain.

Peripheral Modulation of Pain

Nociceptors and their neurons display sensitization following repeated stimulation. Sensitization may be manifested as an enhanced response to noxious stimulation or a newly acquired responsiveness to a wider range of stimuli, including nonnoxious stimuli.

A. Primary Hyperalgesia

Sensitization of nociceptors results in a decrease in threshold, an increase in the frequency response to the same stimulus intensity, a decrease in response latency, and spontaneous firing even after cessation

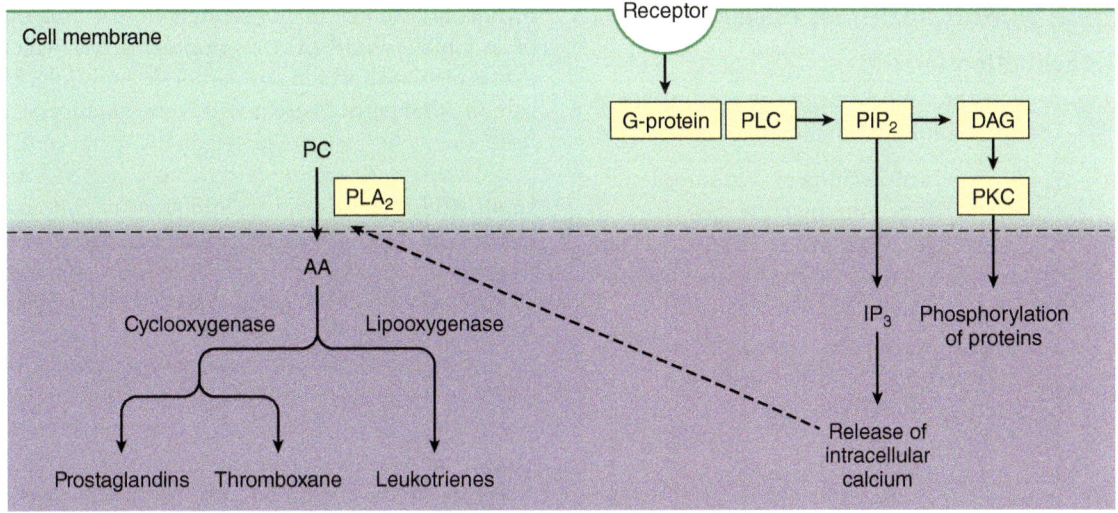

FIGURE 47–5 Phospholipase C (PLC) catalyzes the hydrolysis of phosphatidylinositol 4,5-bisphosphate (PIP$_2$) to produce inositol triphosphate (IP$_3$) and diacylglycerol (DAG). Protein kinase C (PKC) is also important. Phospholipase A$_2$ (PLA$_2$) catalyzes the conversion of phosphatidylcholine (PC) to arachidonic acid (AA).

of the stimulus (afterdischarges). Such sensitization commonly occurs with injury and following application of heat. Primary hyperalgesia is mediated by the release of noxious substances from damaged tissues. Histamine is released from mast cells, basophils, and platelets, whereas serotonin is released from mast cells and platelets. Bradykinin is released from tissues following activation of factor XII. Bradykinin activates free nerve endings via specific B1 and B2 receptors.

Prostaglandins are produced following tissue damage by the action of phospholipase A$_2$ on phospholipids released from cell membranes to form arachidonic acid (Figure 47–5). The cyclooxygenase (COX) pathway then converts the latter into endoperoxides, which in turn are transformed into prostacyclin and prostaglandin E$_2$ (PGE$_2$). PGE$_2$ directly activates free nerve endings, whereas prostacyclin potentiates the edema from bradykinin. The lipoxygenase pathway converts arachidonic acid into hydroperoxy compounds, which are subsequently converted into leukotrienes. The role of the latter is not well defined, but they appear to potentiate certain types of pain. Pharmacological agents such as acetylsalicylic acid (ASA, or aspirin), acetaminophen, and nonsteroidal antiinflammatory drugs (NSAIDs) produce analgesia by inhibition of COX. The analgesic effect of corticosteroids is likely the result of inhibition of prostaglandin production through blockade of phospholipase A$_2$ activation.

B. Secondary Hyperalgesia

Neurogenic inflammation, also called secondary hyperalgesia, plays an important role in peripheral sensitization following injury. It is manifested by the "triple response (of Lewis)" of a red flush around the site of injury (flare), local tissue edema, and sensitization to noxious stimuli. Secondary hyperalgesia is primarily due to antidromic release of substance P (and probably CGRP). Substance P degranulates histamine and 5-HT, vasodilates blood vessels, causes tissue edema, and induces the formation of leukotrienes. The neural origin of this response is supported by the following findings: (1) it can be produced by electrical stimulation of a sensory nerve, (2) it is not observed in denervated skin, and (3) it is diminished by injection of a local anesthetic. Capsaicin applied topically in a gel, cream, or patch depletes substance P and diminishes neurogenic inflammation, and is useful for some patients with postherpetic neuralgia.

Central Modulation of Pain

A. Facilitation

 At least three mechanisms are responsible for central sensitization in the spinal cord:

1. Wind-up and sensitization of second-order neurons. WDR neurons increase their frequency of discharge with the same repetitive stimuli and exhibit prolonged discharge, even after afferent C fiber input has stopped.

2. Receptor field expansion. Dorsal horn neurons increase their receptive fields such that adjacent neurons become responsive to stimuli (whether noxious or not) to which they were previously unresponsive.

3. Hyperexcitability of flexion reflexes. Enhancement of flexion reflexes is observed both ipsilaterally and contralaterally.

Neurochemical mediators of central sensitization include substance P, CGRP, vasoactive intestinal peptide (VIP), cholecystokinin (CCK), angiotensin, and galanin, as well as the excitatory amino acids L-glutamate and L-aspartate. These substances trigger changes in membrane excitability by interacting with G protein–coupled membrane receptors on neurons (Figure 47–5).

Glutamate and aspartate play important roles in wind-up, via activation of N-methyl-D-aspartate (NMDA) and other receptor mechanisms, and in the induction and maintenance of central sensitization. Activation of NMDA receptors also induces nitric oxide synthetase, increasing formation of nitric oxide. Both prostaglandins and nitric oxide facilitate the release of excitatory amino acids in the spinal cord. Thus, COX inhibitors such as ASA and NSAIDs have important analgesic actions in the spinal cord.

B. Inhibition

Transmission of nociceptive input in the spinal cord can be inhibited by segmental activity in the cord itself, as well as by descending neural activity from supraspinal centers.

1. Segmental inhibition—Activation of large afferent fibers subserving sensation inhibits WDR neuron and spinothalamic tract activity. Moreover, activation of noxious stimuli in noncontiguous parts of the body inhibits WDR neurons at other levels, which may explain why pain in one part of the body inhibits pain in other parts. These two phenomena support a "gate" theory for pain processing in the spinal cord.

Glycine and γ-aminobutyric acid (GABA) are amino acids that function as inhibitory neurotransmitters and likely play an important role in segmental inhibition of pain in the spinal cord. Antagonism of glycine and GABA results in powerful facilitation of WDR neurons and produces allodynia and hyperesthesia. There are two subtypes of GABA receptors: $GABA_A$, of which muscimol is an agonist, and $GABA_B$, of which baclofen is an agonist. Segmental inhibition appears to be mediated by $GABA_B$ receptor activity. The $GABA_A$ receptor functions as a Cl^- channel, and benzodiazepines activate this channel. Activation of glycine receptors also increases Cl^- conductance across neuronal cell membranes. The action of glycine is more complex than that of GABA, because the former also has a facilitatory (excitatory) effect on the NMDA receptor.

Adenosine also modulates nociceptive activity in the dorsal horn. At least two receptors are known: A_1, which inhibits adenyl cyclase, and A_2, which stimulates adenyl cyclase. The A_1 receptor mediates adenosine's antinociceptive action. Methylxanthines can reverse this effect through phosphodiesterase inhibition.

2. Supraspinal inhibition—Several supraspinal structures send fibers down the spinal cord to inhibit pain in the dorsal horn. Important sites of origin for these descending pathways include the periaqueductal gray, reticular formation, and nucleus raphe magnus (NRM). Stimulation of the periaqueductal gray area in the midbrain produces widespread analgesia in humans. Axons from these tracts act presynaptically on primary afferent neurons and postsynaptically on second-order neurons (or interneurons). These pathways mediate their antinociceptive action via α_2-adrenergic, serotonergic, and opiate (μ, δ, and κ) receptor mechanisms. The role of monoamines in pain inhibition explains the analgesic efficacy of antidepressants that block reuptake of catecholamines and serotonin.

Inhibitory adrenergic pathways originate primarily from the periaqueductal gray area and the reticular formation. Norepinephrine mediates this action via activation of presynaptic or postsynaptic α_2 receptors. At least part of the descending inhibition from the periaqueductal gray is relayed first to the NRM and medullary reticular formation; serotonergic fibers from the NRM then relay the inhibition to dorsal horn neurons via the dorsolateral funiculus.

The endogenous opiate system (primarily the NRM and reticular formation) acts via methionine enkephalin, leucine enkephalin, and β-endorphin, all of which are antagonized by naloxone. These opioids act presynaptically to hyperpolarize primary afferent neurons and inhibit the release of substance P; they also appear to cause some postsynaptic inhibition. Exogenous opioids preferentially act postsynaptically on the second-order neurons or interneurons in the substantia gelatinosa.

PATHOPHYSIOLOGY OF CHRONIC PAIN

7 Chronic pain may be caused by a combination of peripheral, central, and psychological mechanisms. Sensitization of nociceptors plays a major role in the origin of pain associated with peripheral mechanisms, such as chronic musculoskeletal and visceral disorders.

Neuropathic pain involves peripheral–central and central neural mechanisms that are complex and generally associated with partial or complete lesions of peripheral nerves, dorsal root ganglia, nerve roots, or more central structures (Table 47–5). Peripheral mechanisms include spontaneous discharges; sensitization of receptors to mechanical, thermal, and chemical stimuli; and up-regulation of adrenergic receptors. Neural inflammation may also be present. Systemic administration of local anesthetics and anticonvulsants has been shown to suppress the spontaneous firing of sensitized or traumatized neurons. This observation is supported by the efficacy of agents such as lidocaine, mexiletine, and carbamazepine in many patients with neuropathic pain. Central mechanisms include loss of segmental inhibition, wind-up of WDR neurons, spontaneous discharges in deafferentated neurons, and reorganization of neural connections.

TABLE 47–5 Mechanisms of neuropathic pain.

Spontaneous self-sustaining neuronal activity in the primary afferent neuron (such as a neuroma).

Marked mechanosensitivity associated with chronic nerve compression.

Short-circuits between pain fibers and other types of fibers following demyelination, resulting in activation of nociceptive fibers by nonnoxious stimuli at the site of injury (ephaptic transmission).

Functional reorganization of receptive fields in dorsal horn neurons such that sensory input from surrounding intact nerves emphasizes or intensifies any input from the area of injury.

Spontaneous electrical activity in dorsal horn cells or thalamic nuclei.

Release of segmental inhibition in the spinal cord.

Loss of descending inhibitory influences that are dependent on normal sensory input.

Lesions of the thalamus or other supraspinal structures.

The sympathetic nervous system appears to play a major role in some patients with chronic pain. The efficacy of sympathetic nerve blocks in some of these patients supports the concept of sympathetically maintained pain. Painful disorders that often respond to sympathetic blocks include complex regional pain syndrome, deafferentation syndromes due to nerve avulsion or amputations, and postherpetic neuralgia. However, the simplistic theory of heightened sympathetic activity resulting in vasoconstriction, edema, and hyperalgesia fails to account for the warm and erythematous phase observed in some patients. Similarly, clinical and experimental observations do not satisfactorily support the theory of ephaptic transmission between pain fibers and demyelinated sympathetic fibers.

Psychological mechanisms or environmental factors are rarely the sole mechanisms for chronic pain but are commonly seen in combination with other mechanisms (Table 47–6).

SYSTEMIC RESPONSES TO PAIN
Systemic Responses to Acute Pain

Acute pain is typically associated with a neuroendocrine stress response that is proportional to pain intensity. The pain pathways mediating the afferent limb of this response are discussed above. The

TABLE 47–6 **Psychological mechanisms or environmental factors associated with chronic pain.**

Psychophysiological mechanisms in which emotional factors act as the initiating cause (eg, tension headaches).
Learned or operant behavior in which chronic behavior patterns are rewarded (eg, by attention of a spouse) following an often minor injury.
Psychopathology such as major affective disorders (depression), schizophrenia, and somatization disorders (conversion hysteria) in which the patient has an abnormal preoccupation with bodily functions.
Pure psychogenic mechanisms (somatoform pain disorder), in which suffering is experienced despite absence of nociceptive input.

efferent limb is mediated by the sympathetic nervous and endocrine systems. Sympathetic activation increases efferent sympathetic tone to all viscera and releases catecholamines from the adrenal medulla. The hormonal response results from increased sympathetic tone and from hypothalamically mediated reflexes. Moderate to severe acute pain, regardless of site, can affect the function of nearly every organ and may adversely affect perioperative morbidity and mortality.

A. Cardiovascular Effects

Cardiovascular effects are often prominent and include hypertension, tachycardia, enhanced myocardial irritability, and increased systemic vascular resistance. Cardiac output increases in most normal patients but may decrease in patients with compromised ventricular function. Because of the increase in myocardial oxygen demand, pain can worsen or precipitate myocardial ischemia.

B. Respiratory Effects

An increase in total body oxygen consumption and carbon dioxide production necessitates a concomitant increase in minute ventilation. The latter increases the work of breathing, particularly in patients with underlying lung disease. Pain due to abdominal or thoracic incisions further compromises pulmonary function because of guarding (splinting). Decreased movement of the chest wall reduces tidal volume and functional residual capacity; this promotes atelectasis, intrapulmonary shunting, hypoxemia, and, less commonly, hypoventilation. Reductions in vital capacity impair coughing and clearing of secretions. Regardless of the pain's location, prolonged bed rest or immobilization can produce similar changes in pulmonary function.

C. Gastrointestinal and Urinary Effects

Enhanced sympathetic tone increases sphincter tone and decreases intestinal and urinary motility, promoting ileus and urinary retention, respectively. Hypersecretion of gastric acid can promote stress ulceration and worsen the consequences of pulmonary aspiration. Nausea, vomiting, and constipation are common.

D. Endocrine Effects

Stress increases catabolic hormones (catecholamines, cortisol, and glucagon) and decreases anabolic hormones (insulin and testosterone). Patients develop a negative nitrogen balance, carbohydrate intolerance, and increased lipolysis. The increase in cortisol, renin, angiotensin, aldosterone, and antidiuretic hormone results in sodium retention, water retention, and secondary expansion of the extracellular space.

E. Hematological Effects

Stress-mediated increases in platelet adhesiveness, reduced fibrinolysis, and hypercoagulability have been reported.

F. Immune Effects

The neuroendocrine stress response produces leukocytosis and has been reported to depress the reticuloendothelial system. The latter predisposes patients to infection. Stress-related immunodepression may also enhance tumor growth and metastasis.

G. Psychological Effects

Anxiety and sleep disturbances are common reactions to acute pain. With prolonged duration of the pain, depression is not unusual. Some patients react with frustration and anger that may be directed at family, friends, or the medical staff.

Systemic Responses to Chronic Pain

The neuroendocrine stress response is generally observed only in patients with severe recurring pain due to peripheral (nociceptive) mechanisms and in patients with prominent central mechanisms such as pain associated with paraplegia. It is attenuated or absent in most patients with chronic pain. Sleep and affective disturbances, particularly depression, are often prominent. Many patients also experience significant changes in appetite (increase or decrease) and stresses on social relationships.

Evaluation of the Patient with Chronic Pain

9 The evaluation of any patient with pain should include several key components. Information about location, onset, and quality of pain, as well as alleviating and exacerbating factors, should be obtained, along with a pain history that includes previous therapies and changes in symptoms over time. In addition to physical symptoms, chronic pain usually involves a psychological component that should be addressed as well. Questionnaires, diagrams, and pain scales are useful tools in helping patients adequately describe the characteristics of their pain and how it affects their quality of life. Information gathered during the physical examination can help distinguish pain location, type, and systemic sequelae, if any. Imaging studies such as plain radiographs, computed tomography (CT), magnetic resonance imaging (MRI), and bone scans can often suggest physiological causes. All components are necessary for a comprehensive evaluation of the pain patient prior to determining appropriate treatment options.

PAIN MEASUREMENT

Reliable quantitation of pain severity helps determine therapeutic interventions and evaluate the efficacy of treatments. This is a challenge, however, because pain is a subjective experience that is influenced by psychological, cultural, and other variables. Clear definitions are necessary, because pain may be described in terms of tissue destruction or bodily or emotional reaction.

The numerical rating scale, Wong-Baker FACES rating scale, visual analog scale (VAS), and McGill Pain Questionnaire (MPQ) are most commonly used. In the numerical scale, 0 corresponds to no pain and 10 is intended to reflect the worst possible pain. The

Wong-Baker FACES pain scale, designed for children 3 years of age and older, is useful in patients with whom communication may be difficult. The patient is asked to point to various facial expressions ranging from a smiling face (no pain) to an extremely unhappy one that expresses the worst possible pain. The VAS is a 10-cm horizontal line labeled "no pain" at one end and "worst pain imaginable" on the other end. The patient is asked to mark on this line where the intensity of the pain lies. The distance from "no pain" to the patient's mark numerically quantifies the pain. The VAS is a simple and efficient method that correlates well with other reliable methods.

The MPQ is a checklist of words describing symptoms. Unlike other pain rating methods that assume pain is one-dimensional and describe intensity but not quality, the MPQ attempts to define the pain in three major dimensions: (1) sensory–discriminative (nociceptive pathways), (2) motivational–affective (reticular and limbic structures), and (3) cognitive–evaluative (cerebral cortex). It contains 20 sets of descriptive words that are divided into four major groups: 10 sensory, 5 affective, 1 evaluative, and 4 miscellaneous. The patient selects the sets that apply to his or her pain and circles the words in each set that best describe the pain. The words in each class are given rank according to severity of pain. A pain rating index is derived based on the words chosen.

PSYCHOLOGICAL EVALUATION

10 Psychological evaluation is useful whenever medical evaluation fails to reveal an apparent cause for pain, when pain intensity, characteristics, or duration are disproportionate to disease or injury, or when depression or other psychological issues are apparent. These types of evaluations help define the role of psychological or behavioral factors. The most commonly used tests are the Minnesota Multiphasic Personality Inventory (MMPI) and Beck Depression Inventory.

The MMPI is a 566-item true–false questionnaire that attempts to define the patient's personality on 10 clinical scales. Three validity scales serve to identify patients deliberately trying to hide traits or alter the results. Cultural differences can affect scores.

Moreover, the test is lengthy and some patients find its questions insulting. The MMPI is used primarily to confirm clinical impressions about the role of psychological factors; it cannot reliably distinguish between "organic" and "functional" pain.

Depression is very common in patients with chronic pain. It is often difficult to determine the relative contribution of depression to the suffering associated with pain. The Beck Depression Inventory is a useful test for identifying patients with major depression.

Several tests have been developed to assess functional limitations or impairment (disability). These include the Multidimensional Pain Inventory (MPI), Medical Outcomes Survey 36-Item Short Form (SF-36), Pain Disability Index (PDI), and Oswestry Disability Index (ODI).

Emotional disorders are commonly associated with complaints of chronic pain, and chronic pain often results in varying degrees of psychological distress. Determination of which came first is often difficult. In either case, both the pain and emotional distress need to be treated. Table 47–7 lists emotional disorders in which treatment should be primarily directed at the emotional disorder.

TABLE 47–7 **Emotional and related disorders commonly associated with chronic pain.**

Disorder	Brief Description
Somatization disorder	Physical symptoms of a medical condition that cannot be explained, resulting in involuntary distress and physical impairment.
Conversion disorder	Symptoms of voluntary motor or sensory deficits that suggest a medical condition; symptoms cannot be medically explained but are associated with psychological factors and are not intentionally feigned.
Hypochondriasis	Prolonged (>6 months) preoccupation with the fear of having a serious illness despite adequate medical evaluation and reassurance.
Malingering	Intentional production of physical or psychological symptoms that is motivated by external incentives (eg, avoiding work or financial compensation).
Substance-related disorders	Habitual misuse of prescribed or illicit substances that often precedes and drives complaints of pain and drug-seeking behavior.

ELECTROMYOGRAPHY & NERVE CONDUCTION STUDIES

Electromyography and nerve conduction studies complement one another and are useful for confirming the diagnosis of entrapment syndromes, radicular syndromes, neural trauma, and polyneuropathies. They can often distinguish between neurogenic and myogenic disorders. Patterns of abnormalities can localize a lesion to the spinal cord, nerve root, limb plexus, or peripheral nerve. In addition, they may also be useful in excluding "organic" disorders when psychogenic pain or a "functional" syndrome is suspected.

Electromyography employs needle electrodes to record potentials in individual muscles. Muscle potentials are recorded first while the muscle is at rest and then as the patient is asked to move the muscle. A triphasic motor unit action potential is normally seen as the patient voluntarily moves the muscle. Abnormal findings suggestive of denervation include persistent insertion potentials, the presence of positive sharp waves, fibrillary activity, or fasciculation potentials. Abnormalities in muscles produce changes in amplitude and duration as well as polyphasic action potentials.

Peripheral nerve conduction studies employ supramaximal stimulations of motor or mixed sensorimotor nerve, whereas muscle potentials are recorded over the appropriate muscle. The time between the onset of the stimulation and the onset of the muscle potential (latency) is a measurement of the fastest conducting motor fibers in the nerve. The amplitude of the recorded potential indicates the number of functional motor units, whereas its duration reflects the range of conduction velocities in the nerve. Conduction velocity can be obtained by stimulating the nerve from two points and comparing the latencies. When a pure sensory nerve is evaluated, the nerve is stimulated while action potentials are recorded either proximally or distally (antidromic conduction).

Nerve conduction studies distinguish between mononeuropathies (due to trauma, compression, or entrapment) and polyneuropathies. The latter include systemic disorders that may produce abnormalities that are widespread and symmetrical or that are random (eg, mononeuropathy multiplex).

Selected Pain Syndromes

ENTRAPMENT SYNDROMES

Neural compression may occur wherever a nerve courses through an anatomically narrowed passage, and entrapment neuropathies can involve sensory, motor, or mixed nerves. Genetic factors and repetitive macrotrauma or microtrauma are likely involved, and adjacent tenosynovitis is often responsible. Table 47–8 lists the most commonly recognized entrapment syndromes. When a sensory nerve is involved, patients complain of pain and numbness in its distribution distal to the site of entrapment; occasionally, a patient may complain of pain referred proximal to the site of entrapment. Entrapment of the sciatic nerve can mimic a herniated intervertebral disc. Entrapment of a motor nerve produces weakness in the muscles it innervates. Even entrapments of "pure" motor nerves can produce a vague pain that may be mediated by

TABLE 47–8 Entrapment neuropathies.

Nerve	Entrapment Site	Location of Pain
Cranial nerves VII, IX, and X	Styloid process or stylohyoid ligament	Ipsilateral tonsil, base of tongue, temporomandibular joint, and ear (Eagle's syndrome)
Brachial plexus	Scalenus anticus muscle or a cervical rib	Ulnar side of arm and forearm (scalenus anticus syndrome)
Suprascapular nerve	Suprascapular notch	Posterior and lateral shoulder
Median nerve	Pronator teres muscle	Proximal forearm and palmar surface of the first three digits (pronator syndrome)
Median nerve	Carpal tunnel	Palmar surface of the first three digits (carpal tunnel syndrome)
Ulnar nerve	Cubital fossa (elbow)	Fourth and fifth digits of the hand (cubital tunnel syndrome)
Ulnar nerve	Guyon's canal (wrist)	Fourth and fifth digits of the hand
Lateral femoral cutaneous nerve	Anterior iliac spine under the inguinal ligament	Anterolateral thigh (meralgia paresthetica)
Obturator nerve	Obturator canal	Upper medial thigh
Saphenous nerve	Subsartorial tunnel (adductor canal)	Medial calf
Sciatic nerve	Sciatic notch	Buttock and leg (piriformis syndrome)
Common peroneal nerve	Fibular neck	Lateral distal leg and foot
Deep peroneal nerve	Anterior tarsal tunnel	Big toe or foot
Superficial peroneal nerve	Deep fascia above the ankle	Anterior ankle and dorsum of foot
Posterior tibial nerve	Posterior tarsal tunnel	Undersurface of foot (tarsal tunnel syndrome)
Interdigital nerve	Deep transverse tarsal ligament	Between toes and foot (Morton's neuroma)

afferent fibers from muscles and joints. The diagnosis can usually be confirmed by electromyography and nerve conduction studies. Neural blockade of the nerve with local anesthetic, with or without corticosteroid, may be diagnostic and can provide temporary pain relief. Treatment is generally symptomatic with oral analgesics and temporary immobilization, whenever appropriate. Development of complex regional pain syndrome may respond to sympathetic blocks. Refractory symptoms may require surgical decompression.

MYOFASCIAL PAIN

11 Myofascial pain syndromes are common disorders characterized by aching muscle pain, muscle spasm, stiffness, weakness, and, occasionally, autonomic dysfunction. Patients have discrete areas (trigger points) of marked tenderness in one or more muscles or the associated connective tissue. Palpation of the involved muscles may reveal tight, ropy bands over trigger points. Signs of autonomic dysfunction (vasoconstriction or piloerection) in the overlying muscles may be present. The pain characteristically radiates in a fixed pattern that does not follow dermatomes.

Gross trauma or repetitive microtrauma is thought to play a major role in initiating myofascial pain syndromes. Trigger points develop following acute injury; stimulation of these active trigger points produces pain, and the ensuing muscle spasm sustains the pain. When the acute episode subsides, the trigger points become latent (tender, but not pain producing) only to be reactivated at a later time by subsequent stress. The pathophysiology is poorly understood.

The diagnosis of a myofascial pain syndrome is suggested by the character of the pain and by palpation of discrete trigger points that reproduce it. Common syndromes produce trigger points in the levator scapulae, masseter, quadratus lumborum, and gluteus medius muscles. The latter two syndromes produce low back pain and should be considered in all patients with back pain; moreover, gluteal trigger points can mimic S_1 radiculopathy.

Although myofascial pain may spontaneously resolve without sequelae, many patients continue to have latent trigger points. When trigger points are active, treatment is directed at regaining muscle length and elasticity. Analgesia may be provided utilizing local anesthetic (1–3 mL) trigger point injections. Topical cooling with either an ethyl chloride or fluorocarbon (fluoromethane) spray can also induce reflex muscle relaxation, facilitating massage ("stretch and spray") and ultrasound therapy. Physical therapy is important in establishing and maintaining normal range of motion for affected muscles, and biofeedback may be helpful.

FIBROMYALGIA

The American College of Rheumatology recently identified three criteria that, if met, suggest the diagnosis of fibromyalgia:

1. Widespread Pain Index (WPI) score of 7 or higher, and Symptom Severity (SS) scale score of 5 or higher, or WPI of 3–6 and SS scale score of 9 or higher.

2. Symptoms present at a similar level for at least 3 months.

3. Absence of another disorder that would otherwise explain the pain.

Treatment of fibromyalgia includes cardiovascular conditioning, strength training, improving sleep hygiene, cognitive–behavioral therapy, patient education, and pharmacotherapy. Medications approved by the U.S. Food and Drug Administration (FDA) for the treatment of fibromyalgia include pregabalin (Lyrica), duloxetine (Cymbalta), and milnacipran (Savella).

LOW BACK PAIN & RELATED SYNDROMES

Back pain is an extremely common complaint and a major cause of work disability worldwide. Lumbosacral strain, degenerative disc disease, and myofascial syndromes are the most common causes. Low back pain, with or without associated leg pain, may also have congenital, traumatic, degenerative, inflammatory, infectious, metabolic, psychological, and neoplastic causes. Moreover, back pain can be due to disease processes in the abdomen and pelvis, particularly those affecting retroperitoneal structures (pancreas, kidneys, ureters, and aorta), the uterus and adnexa, the prostate, and the rectosigmoid colon. Disorders of the hip can also mimic back disorders. A positive Patrick's sign (or Patrick's test)—ie, the elicitation of pain in the hip or sacroiliac joint when the examiner places the ipsilateral heel of the supine patient on the contralateral knee and presses down on the ipsilateral knee—helps identify back pain due to hip or sacroiliac joint disorders. This sign is also referred to by an acronym, FABERE (sign), because the movement of the leg involves *f*lexion, *ab*duction, *e*xternal *r*otation, and *e*xtension.

1. Applied Anatomy of the Back

The back can be described in terms of *anterior* and *posterior* elements. The anterior elements consist of cylindrical vertebral bodies interconnected by intervertebral discs and supported by anterior and posterior longitudinal ligaments. The posterior elements are bony arches extending from each vertebral body, consisting of two pedicles, two transverse processes, two laminae, and a spinous process. The transverse and spinous processes provide points of attachment for the muscles that move and protect the spinal column. Adjacent vertebrae also articulate posteriorly by two gliding facet joints.

Spinal structures are innervated by the sinuvertebral branches and posterior rami of spinal nerves. The sinuvertebral nerve arises before each spinal nerve divides into anterior and posterior rami, and reenters the intervertebral foramen to innervate the posterior longitudinal ligament, the posterior annulus fibrosus, periosteum, dura, and epidural vessels. Paraspinal structures are supplied by the posterior primary ramus. Each facet joint is innervated by the medial branch of the posterior primary rami of the spinal nerves above and below the joint.

As lumbar spinal nerve roots exit the dural sac, they travel down 1–2 cm laterally before exiting through their respective intervertebral foramina; thus, for example, the L5 nerve root leaves the dural sac at the level of the L4–L5 disc (where it is more likely to be compressed) but leaves the spinal canal beneath the L5 pedicle opposite the L5–S1 disc.

2. Paravertebral Muscle & Lumbosacral Joint Sprain/Strain

Approximately 80–90% of low back pain is due to sprain or strain associated with lifting heavy objects, falls, or sudden abnormal movements of the spine. The term *sprain* is generally used when the pain is related to a well-defined acute injury, whereas *strain* is used when the pain is more chronic and is likely related to repetitive minor injuries.

Injury to paravertebral muscles and ligaments results in reflex muscle spasm, which may or may not be associated with trigger points. The pain is usually dull and aching, and occasionally radiates down the buttocks or hips. Sprain is a self-limited benign process that resolves in 1–2 weeks. Symptomatic treatment consists of rest and oral analgesics.

The sacroiliac joint is particularly vulnerable to rotational injuries. It is one of the largest joints in the body and functions to transfer weight from the upper body to the lower extremities. Acute or chronic injury can cause slippage, or subluxation, of the joint. Pain originating from this joint is characteristically located along the posterior ilium and radiates down the hips and posterior thigh to the knees. The diagnosis is suggested by tenderness on palpation, particularly on the medial aspect of the posterior superior iliac spine, and by compression of the joints. Pain relief following injection of the joint with local anesthetic (3 mL) is diagnostic and may also be therapeutic. Injection of intraarticular steroid medication may be considered. For potentially longer duration of analgesia, radiofrequency ablation may be performed at the dorsal ramus of L5 as well as the lateral branches of the S1, S2, and S3 nerves if the patient responded well to local anesthetic injections of the sacroiliac joint or to diagnostic injections of these nerves.

3. Buttock Pain

Buttock pain may be due to several different factors, and can be quite debilitating. Coccydynia (or, coccygodynia) may the result of trauma to the coccyx or surrounding ligaments. It may resolve by means of physical therapy, coccygeal nerve blocks to the lateral aspects of the coccyx, or ablative or neuromodulatory techniques. Piriformis syndrome presents as pain in the buttock, which can be accompanied by numbness and tingling in distribution of the sciatic nerve. The nerve may or may not be entrapped. Injection of local anesthetic into the belly of this muscle or into trigger points located at the origin and insertion of the muscle may help relieve the pain.

4. Degenerative Disc Disease

Intervertebral discs bear at least one third of the weight of the spinal column. Their central portion, the nucleus pulposus, is composed of gelatinous material early in life. This material degenerates and becomes fibrotic with advancing age and following trauma. The nucleus pulposus is ringed by the annulus fibrosus, which is thinnest posteriorly and bounded superiorly and inferiorly by cartilaginous plates. Disc (discogenic) pain may be due to one of two major mechanisms: (1) protrusion or extrusion of the nucleus pulposus posteriorly or (2) loss of disc height, resulting in the reactive formation of bony spurs (osteophytes) from the rims of the vertebral bodies above and below the disc. Degenerative disc disease most commonly affects the lumbar spine because it is subjected to the greatest motion and because the posterior longitudinal ligament is thinnest at L2–L5. Factors such as increased body weight and cigarette smoking may play a role in the development of lumbar disc disease. The role of the disc in producing chronic back pain is not clearly understood. In patients with persistent axial low back pain, the history and physical examination may provide clues. If the patient has pain when sitting or standing, or maintaining a certain position for an extended period of time, there may be an element of discogenic pain.

Discography is a procedure that is often used to try to provide some objective evidence of the role of a given disc in producing a patient's back pain. After a needle is inserted into the disc, the opening pressure can be assessed; a subsequent injection of radiocontrast material produces increased pressure that may reproduce the patient's pain and may provide radiographic identification of anatomic abnormalities within the disc (eg, a rent or tear). It the pain produced with injection is similar to that which the patient experiences on a daily basis, it is deemed

concordant pain. If not, it is deemed *discordant*. In some circumstances, the pressure in the disc following injection is not significantly higher than the opening pressure. This may be due to the presence of a fissure in the disc that tracks to the epidural space. Risks of discography include infection and discitis, which may be difficult to treat because the disc is relatively avascular.

Treatment options for discogenic pain include conservative therapy, steroid injections into the disc, intradiscal biacplasty, involving heating the posterior annulus of the disc by way of radiofrequency ablation, and surgical fusion with bone graft or hardware placement; each has shown mixed degrees of success. The evaluation and treatment of discogenic pain is an area of significant controversy and ongoing research.

Herniated (Prolapsed) Intervertebral Disc

Weakness and degeneration of the annulus fibrosus and posterior longitudinal ligament can cause herniation of the nucleus pulposus posteriorly into the spinal canal. Ninety percent of disc herniations occur at L5–S1 or L4–L5. Symptoms usually develop following flexion injuries or heavy lifting and may be associated with bulging, protrusion, or extrusion of the disc. Disc herniations usually occur posterolaterally and often result in compression of adjacent nerve roots, producing pain that radiates along that dermatome (radiculopathy). *Sciatica* describes pain along the sciatic nerve due to compression of the lower lumbar nerve roots. When disc material is extruded through the annulus fibrosus and posterior longitudinal ligament, free fragments can become wedged in the spinal canal or the intervertebral foramina. Less commonly a large disc bulges or large fragments extrude posteriorly, compressing the cauda equina in the dural sac; in these instances patients can experience bilateral pain, urinary retention, or, less commonly, fecal incontinence.

Pain associated with disc disease is aggravated by bending, lifting, prolonged sitting, or anything that increases intraabdominal pressure, such as sneezing, coughing, or straining. It is usually relieved by lying down. Numbness or weakness is indicative

TABLE 47-9 Lumbar disc radiculopathies.

	Disk Level		
	L3–L4 (L4 Nerve)	**L4–L5 (L5 Nerve)**	**L5–S1 (S1 Nerve)**
Pain distribution	Anterolateral thigh, anteromedial calf to the ankle	Lateral thigh, anterolateral calf, medial dorsum of foot, especially between the first and second toes	Gluteal region, posterior thigh, posterolateral calf, lateral dorsum and undersurface of the foot, particularly between fourth and fifth toes
Weakness	Quadriceps femoris	Dorsiflexion of the foot	Plantar flexion of foot
Reflex affected	Knee	None	Ankle

of radiculopathy (Table 47–9). Bulging of the disc through the posterior longitudinal ligament can also produce low back pain that radiates to the hips or buttocks. Straight leg-raising tests may be used to assess nerve root compression. With the patient supine and the knee fully extended, the leg on the affected side is raised and the angle at which the pain develops is noted; dorsiflexion of the ankle with the leg raised typically exacerbates the pain by further stretching the lumbosacral plexus. Pain while raising the contralateral leg is an even more reliable sign of nerve compression.

The use of MRI has increased dramatically in the past decade in association with a two- to three-fold increase in back surgeries, although this has not correlated with improved patient outcome. The American Pain Society's clinical practice guidelines for low back pain do not recommend routine imaging or other diagnostic tests for patients with nonspecific low back pain. Up to 30–40% of asymptomatic persons have abnormalities of spinal structures on CT or MRI. In addition, the patient's awareness of his or her imaging abnormalities may influence self-perception of health and functional ability.

Imaging studies and further tests should be acquired when severe or progressive neurological deficits are present, or when serious underlying conditions are suspected. CT myelography is the most sensitive test for evaluating subtle neural compression. Discography may be considered when the pain pattern does not match the clinical findings. A centrally herniated disc will usually cause pain at the lower level, and a laterally protruded disc will

cause pain at the same level as the disc. For example, a centrally located disc herniation at L4–L5 may compress the L5 nerve root whereas a laterally located disc herniation at this level may compress the L4 nerve root.

The natural course of herniated disc disorders is generally benign and the duration of pain is usually less than 2 months. Over 75% of patients treated nonsurgically, even those with radiculopathy, have complete or near-complete pain relief. The goals of treatment should therefore be to alleviate the pain and rehabilitate the patient to return to a functional quality of life. Acute back pain due to a herniated disc can be initially managed with modification of activity and with medications such as NSAIDs and acetaminophen. A short course of opioids may be considered for patients with severe pain. After the acute symptoms subside, the patient can be referred to a physical therapist for instruction on exercises to improve lower back health. Patients who smoke tobacco should be advised to stop smoking, not only for the obvious health benefits but also because nicotine further compromises blood flow to the relatively avascular intervertebral disc. Percutaneous disc decompression involving extraction of a small amount of nucleus pulposus may help to decompress the nerve root. For patients with acute-onset weakness correlating with the level of the disc herniation, surgical management should be considered.

When symptoms persist beyond 3 months, the pain may be considered chronic and may require a multidisciplinary approach. Physical therapy continues to be a very important component of rehabilitation. NSAIDs and antidepressants are also helpful, and percutaneous interventions may be considered. Of note, back supports should be discouraged because they may weaken paraspinal muscles.

Spinal Stenosis

Spinal stenosis is a disease of advancing age. Degeneration of the nucleus pulposus reduces disc height and leads to osteophyte formation (spondylosis) at the endplates of adjoining vertebral bodies. In conjunction with facet joint hypertrophy and with ligamentum flavum hypertrophy and calcification, this process leads to progressive narrowing of the neural foramina and spinal canal. Neural compression may cause radiculopathy that mimics a herniated disc. Extensive osteophyte formation may compress multiple nerve roots and cause bilateral pain. The back pain usually radiates into the buttocks, thighs, and legs. It is characteristically worse with exercise and relieved by rest, particularly sitting with the spine flexed (the "shopping cart sign"). The terms *pseudoclaudication* and *neurogenic claudication* are used to describe such pain that develops with prolonged standing or ambulation. The diagnosis is suggested by the clinical presentation and is confirmed by MRI, CT, or myelography. Electromyography and nerve conduction studies may be useful in evaluating neurological compromise.

Patients with mild to moderate stenosis and radicular symptoms may obtain benefit from epidural steroid injections via a transforaminal, interlaminar, or caudal approach. This may help these individuals tolerate physical therapy. Those with moderate to severe stenosis may be amenable to more recently developed procedures, such as the minimally invasive lumbar decompression (MILD) procedure, which involves percutaneously sculpting the lamina and ligamentum flavum to reduce central canal compression. Severe multilevel symptoms may warrant surgical decompression.

5. Facet Syndrome

Degenerative changes in the facet (zygapophyseal) joints may also produce back pain. Pain may be near the midline; may radiate to the gluteal region, thigh, and knee; and may be associated with muscle spasm. Hyperextension and lateral rotation of the spine usually exacerbate the pain. The diagnosis may be confirmed if pain relief is obtained following intraarticular injection of local anesthetic solution into affected joints or by blockade of the medial branch of the posterior division (ramus) of the spinal nerves that innervate them. Long-term studies suggest that medial branch nerve blocks are more effective than facet joint injections. Medial branch rhizotomy may provide long-term analgesia for patients with facet joint disease.

6. Cervical Pain

Although most spine-related pain due to disc disease, spinal stenosis, or degenerative changes in the zygapophyseal joints is felt in the low back and lower extremities, patients may have cervical pain attributed to these processes. A key anatomic difference is that the cervical nerve roots, unlike those in the thoracic and lumbar spine, exit the foramina above the vertebral bodies for which they are named. This occurs until the level of C7, where the extra cervical nerve roots, C8, exit below the pedicles of C7, thus transitioning to the nomenclature of the thoracic- and lumbar-level vertebral bodies and nerve root denominations. The clinical examination may help to identify the nerve root that is affected with confirmation by a selective nerve root block. Risks inherent with percutaneous cervical procedures include accidental intravascular injection of local anesthetic or steroid. Particulate steroid injections in the neck have been associated with devastating outcomes such as spinal cord injury and death and should be avoided.

For primarily axial pain in the neck with extension into the head or to the shoulders, cervical medial branch blocks may clarify the diagnosis. Long-term analgesia may be obtained with radiofrequency ablation of the medial branches innervating the zygapophyseal joints.

7. Congenital Abnormalities

Congenital abnormalities of the back are often asymptomatic and remain occult for many years. Abnormal spinal mechanics can make the patient prone to back pain, and in some instances, progressive deformities. Relatively common anomalies include sacralization of L5 (the vertebral body is fused to the sacrum), lumbarization of S1 (it functions as a sixth lumbar vertebra), spondylolysis (a disruption of the pars interarticularis), spondylolisthesis (displacement anteriorly of one vertebral body on the next due to disruption of the posterior elements, usually the pars), and spondyloptosis (subluxation of one vertebral body on another resulting in one body in front of the next). The diagnosis is made radiographically. Spinal fusion may be necessary in patients with progressive symptoms and spinal instability.

8. Tumors

Benign primary tumors of the spine include hemangiomas, osteomas, aneurysmal bone cysts, and eosinophilic granulomas. Malignant spine tumors include osteosarcomas, Ewing's sarcoma, and giant cell tumors. In addition, breast, lung, prostate, renal, gastrointestinal, and thyroid carcinomas, lymphomas, and multiple myelomas frequently metastasize to the lumbar spine. Pain is usually constant and may be associated with localized tenderness over involved vertebrae. Bony destruction, with or without neural or vascular compression, produces the pain. Intradural tumors such as meningiomas, schwannomas, ependymomas, and gliomas can present with a radiculopathy and may rapidly progress to flaccid paralysis. The primary site may be asymptomatic or difficult to localize, thus requiring imaging studies for diagnosis. Treatment options usually involve surgical decompression, chemotherapy, radiation therapy, and palliative symptom relief.

9. Infection

Bacterial infections of the spine usually begin as discitis before progressing to osteomyelitis, and can be due to pyogenic as well as tuberculous organisms. Patients may present with chronic back pain without fever or leukocytosis (eg, spinal tuberculosis). Those with acute discitis, osteomyelitis, or epidural abscess present with acute pain, fever, leukocytosis, elevated sedimentation rate, and elevated C-reactive protein, warranting immediate initiation of antibiotics. Urgent surgical intervention is indicated when the patient also suffers from acute weakness.

10. Arthritides

Ankylosing spondylitis is a familial disorder that is associated with histocompatibility antigen HLA-B27. It typically presents as low back pain associated with early morning stiffness in a young patient, usually male. The pain has an insidious onset and may initially improve with activity. After a few months to years, the pain gradually intensifies and is associated with progressively restricted movement of the spine. Diagnosis may be difficult early in the disease, but radiographic evidence of sacroiliitis is usually present. As the disease progresses, the spine develops a characteristic "bamboo-like" radiographic appearance. Some patients develop arthritis of the hips and shoulders, as well as extraarticular inflammatory manifestations. Treatment is primarily directed at functional preservation of posture. NSAIDs, particularly indomethacin, are effective analgesics that reduce the early morning stiffness. Anti–tumor necrosis factor-α agents have been shown to decrease the progression of ankylosing spondylitis when administered early in the course of therapy. These agents include infliximab (Remicaid), etanercept (Enbrel), adalimumab (Humira), and golimumab (Simponi). Although this treatment approach shows promise, patients may be at an increased risk for infection and the development of lymphoma.

Patients with Reiter's syndrome, psoriatic arthritis, or inflammatory bowel disease may also present with low back pain, but extraspinal manifestations are usually more prominent. Rheumatoid arthritis usually spares the spine except for the zygapophyseal joints of the cervical spine.

NEUROPATHIC PAIN

Neuropathic pain includes pain associated with diabetic neuropathy, causalgia, phantom limbs, postherpetic neuralgia, stroke, spinal cord injury, and multiple sclerosis. Cancer pain and chronic low back pain may have prominent neuropathic components. Neuropathic pain tends to be paroxysmal and sometimes lancinating with a burning quality, and is usually associated with hyperpathia. Mechanisms of neuropathic pain are reviewed earlier in this chapter.

Because neuropathic pain is often difficult to treat, multiple therapeutic modalities may be necessary. Treatment options include anticonvulsants (eg, gabapentin, pregabalin), antidepressants (tricyclic antidepressants or serotonin-norepinephrine reuptake inhibitors), antiarrhythmics (mexiletine), α_2-adrenergic agonists (clonidine), topical agents (lidocaine or capsaicin), and analgesics (NSAIDs and opioids). Of note, tricyclic antidepressants may have significant anticholinergic side effects that may limit their tolerability. Secondary amines, such as nortriptyline or desipramine, may have less severe or fewer anticholinergic side effects than tertiary amines such as amitriptyline or imipramine. Spinal opioids may be very effective for some patients. Sympathetic blocks are effective in selected disorders (see below). Spinal cord stimulation may be effective for patients who do not tolerate or respond to other treatments.

Diabetic Neuropathy

14 Diabetic neuropathy is the most common type of neuropathic pain encountered in practice and is a major cause of morbidity. Its pathophysiology is poorly understood but may be related to microangiopathy and to abnormal activation of metabolic (polyol) pathways and glycation of proteins as a consequence of chronic hyperglycemia. Diabetic neuropathy may be symmetric (generalized), focal, or multifocal, affecting peripheral (sensory or motor), cranial, or autonomic nerves.

The most common syndrome is peripheral polyneuropathy, which results in symmetric numbness ("stocking-and-glove" distribution), paresthesias, dysesthesias, and pain. The pain varies in intensity, may be severe, and is often worst at night. Loss of proprioception may lead to gait disturbances, and sensory deficits can lead to traumatic injuries. Isolated mononeuropathies affecting individual nerves may lead to wrist or foot drop or to cranial nerve palsy. Mononeuropathies typically have a sudden onset and are reversible, lasting a few weeks. Autonomic neuropathy typically affects the gastrointestinal tract, causing diarrhea, delayed

gastric emptying, and esophageal motility disorders. Orthostatic hypotension and other forms of autonomic dysfunction are common.

Treatment of diabetic neuropathy is symptomatic and directed at optimal glycemic control to slow progression. Acetaminophen and NSAIDs are usually ineffective for moderate to severe pain. Risks associated with opioids limit their use in the treatment of this condition. Adjuvant drugs play a major role. The combination of an antiepileptic drug and a tricyclic antidepressant may be particularly effective.

Sympathetically Maintained & Sympathetically Independent Pain

15 Complex regional pain syndrome (CRPS) is a neuropathic pain disorder with significant autonomic features that is usually subdivided into two variants: CRPS 1, formerly known as reflex sympathetic dystrophy (RSD), and CRPS 2, formerly known as causalgia. The major difference between the two is the absence or presence, respectively, of documented nerve injury. Signs, symptoms, pathophysiology, and response to treatment are quite similar. Previously, this condition was thought to represent sympathetically maintained pain, but there is recent evidence that in some cases the pain may be sympathetically independent.

CRPS is a largely underdiagnosed condition affecting at least 50,000 patients a year in the United States alone. It affects individuals from childhood to late adulthood and may occur more commonly in females. Patients frequently present with burning neuropathic pain having components of hyperalgesia and allodynia. The autonomic nervous system may be involved, exemplified by alterations in sweating (sudomotor changes), color, and skin temperature, and by trophic changes in the skin, hair, or nails. Decreases in strength and range of motion in the affected extremity may be present. CRPS may develop after minimal injury, although the most common initiating events are surgery, fractures, crush injuries, and sprains.

The pathophysiology of CRPS 1 and 2 is probably multifactorial, involving both the sympathetic nervous system and the central nervous system. There may be changes in the cutaneous innervation after a nerve injury, along with changes in central and peripheral sensitization. Genetic, inflammatory, and psychological factors may all play roles. Causalgia (which means burning pain), first identified in injured veterans of the American Civil War, typically follows gunshot injuries or other major trauma to large nerves. The pain often has an immediate onset and is associated with allodynia, hyperpathia, and vasomotor and sudomotor dysfunction. It is exacerbated by factors that increase sympathetic tone, such as fear, anxiety, light, noise, or touch. The syndrome has a variable duration that can range from days to months or may be permanent. Causalgia commonly affects the brachial plexus, particularly the median nerve, and the tibial division of the sciatic nerve in the lower extremity.

Patients with CRPS often respond to sympathetic blocks, but a multidisciplinary therapeutic approach must be utilized to avoid long-term functional and psychological disability. Some patients recover spontaneously, but if left untreated other patients can progress to severe and irreversible functional disability. Sympathetic blocks and intravenous regional sympatholytic blockade are equally effective; these blocks should be continued until either a cure is achieved or the response plateaus. The blocks facilitate physical therapy, which plays a central role and which typically consists of active movement without weights and of desensitization therapy. Many patients require a series of three to seven blocks. The likelihood of a cure is high (over 90%) if treatment is initiated within 1 month of symptom onset and appears to decrease over time with therapeutic delay.

Some patients benefit from transcutaneous electrical nerve stimulation (TENS) therapy. Spinal cord stimulation can be particularly effective in both acute and chronic settings. In the acute phase of treatment, there is increasing interest in placing tunneled epidural catheters for infusion therapy, or percutaneous electrodes for extended trials of spinal cord stimulation, in order to help patients tolerate physical therapy. Many patients benefit from surgical implantation of peripheral nerve stimulators placed directly on the larger injured nerves.

For sympathetically maintained pain, oral α-adrenergic blockers, such as the nonselective phenoxybenzamine or the α_1-selective prazosin, may be beneficial. Caution is advised because of the risk of orthostatic hypotension with these agents, and dosage should be increased gradually. Anticonvulsant and antidepressant medications may also be beneficial.

Surgical sympathectomy in patients with chronic symptoms is frequently disappointing, resulting in only transient relief and in some cases a new, alternate pain syndrome. Recent research suggests that patients with pain refractory to prior medical or procedural therapies may respond to intravenous infusions of ketamine in a monitored setting.

ACUTE HERPES ZOSTER & POSTHERPETIC NEURALGIA

During an initial childhood infection (chickenpox), the varicella-zoster virus (VZV) infects dorsal root ganglia, where it remains latent until reactivation. Acute herpes zoster, which represents VZV reactivation, manifests as an erythematous vesicular rash in a dermatomal distribution that is usually associated with severe pain. Dermatomes T3–L3 are most commonly affected. The pain often precedes the rash by 48–72 h, and the rash usually lasts 1–2 weeks. Herpes zoster is most common in elderly and immunocompromised patients but may occur at any age. It is typically a self-limited disorder in younger, healthy patients (<50 years old). Treatment is primarily supportive, consisting of oral analgesics and oral acyclovir, famciclovir, ganciclovir, or valacyclovir. Antiviral therapy reduces the duration of the rash and speeds healing. Immunocompromised patients with disseminated infection (nondermatomal distribution of vesicles) require intravenous acyclovir therapy. Epidural steroid injections have not been proven to prevent postherpetic neuralgia (PHN).

Older patients may continue to experience severe, radicular pain from PHN even after the rash resolves. The incidence of PHN following acute herpes zoster is estimated to be 50% in patients older than 50 years of age. Moreover, PHN is often very difficult to treat. An oral course of corticosteroids during acute zoster may decrease the incidence of

PHN but remains controversial and may increase the likelihood of viral dissemination in immunocompromised patients. Sympathetic blocks performed during the acute episode of herpes zoster often produce excellent analgesia and may decrease the incidence of PHN, although this is controversial. Some studies suggest that when sympathetic blocks are initiated within 2 months of the rash, PHN resolves in up to 80% of patients. Once the neuralgia is well established, however, sympathetic blocks, like other treatments, are generally ineffective. Antidepressants, anticonvulsants, opioids, and TENS may be useful in some patients. Tricyclic antidepressants may be particularly effective, though their use is often limited by anticholinergic side effects. Application of a transdermal lidocaine 5% patch (Lidoderm) over the most painful area may help relieve symptoms, presumably by decreasing peripheral sensitization of nerve endings and receptors. Application of capsaicin cream or a transdermal capsaicin 8% patch (Qutenza) may be helpful; however, Qutenza must be administered in a monitored setting. Administration of EMLA (*e*uctectic *m*ixture of *l*ocal *a*nesthetic) cream 1 h before application of the transdermal capsaicin patch may decrease the incidence and severity of pain from the capsaicin in the patch.

HEADACHE

Headache is a common complaint that affects nearly everyone at some time in life. In the vast majority of cases, headaches do not reflect a serious underlying disorder and are not of sufficient severity or frequency for the individual to seek medical attention. However, as with other complaints of pain, the possibility of a clinically significant underlying disorder should always be considered. The practitioner should solicit other associated symptoms or clinical findings that suggest serious underlying pathology. Table 47–10 lists important causes of headache. Disorders in which the primary complaint is headache are considered in the following discussion. As will become apparent, there is significant variability in clinical presentation and overlap in the symptoms of the major headache syndromes, particularly between tension and migraine headaches.

TABLE 47–10 Classification of headaches.

Classic headache syndromes
Migraine
Tension
Cluster
Vascular disorders
Temporal arteritis
Stroke
Venous thrombosis
Neuralgias
Trigeminal
Glossopharyngeal
Occipital
Intracranial pathology
Tumor
Cerebrospinal fluid leak
Pseudomotor cerebri
Meningitis
Aneurysm
Eye disorders
Glaucoma
Optic neuritis
Sinus disease
Allergic
Bacterial
Temporomandibular joint disease
Dental disorders
Drug-induced
Acute ingestion
Withdrawal (eg, caffeine and alcohol)
Systemic disorders
Infections
Viral (eg, influenza)
Bacterial
Fungal
Metabolic
Hypoglycemia
Hypoxemia
Hypercarbia
Trauma
Miscellaneous
Cold stimulus (swallowing cold liquid)

Tension Headache

Tension headaches are classically described as tight bandlike pain or discomfort that is often associated with tightness in the neck muscles. The headache may be frontal, temporal, or occipital, more often bilateral than unilateral. Intensity typically builds gradually and fluctuates, lasting hours to days. They may be associated with emotional stress or depression. Treatment is symptomatic and consists of NSAIDs.

Migraine Headache

Migraine headaches are typically described as throbbing or pounding and are often associated with photophobia, scotoma, nausea and vomiting, and localized transient neurological dysfunction (aura). The latter may be sensory, motor, visual, or olfactory. Classic migraines by definition are preceded by an aura, whereas common migraines are not. The pain is usually unilateral but can be bilateral with a frontotemporal location and lasts 4–72 h. Migraines primarily affect children (both sexes equally) and young adults (predominantly females). A family history is often present. Provocation by odors, certain foods (eg, red wine), menses, and sleep deprivation is common. Sleep characteristically relieves the headache. The mechanism is complex and may include vasomotor, autonomic (serotonergic brainstem systems), and trigeminal nucleus dysfunction. Treatment is both abortive and prophylactic. Rapid abortive treatment includes oxygen, sumatriptan (6 mg subcutaneously), dihydroergotamine (1 mg intramuscularly or subcutaneously), intravenous lidocaine (100 mg), nasal butorphanol (1–2 mg), and sphenopalatine ganglion block. Other abortive options include zolmitriptan nasal spray, dihydroergotamine nasal spray, or an oral serotonin 5-HT$_{1B/1D}$-receptor agonist (almotriptan, frovatriptan, naratriptan, rizatriptan, eletriptan, or sumatriptan). Prophylactic treatment may include β-adrenergic blockers, calcium channel blockers, valproic acid, amitriptyline, and onabotulinumtoxinA (Botox) injections.

Cluster Headache

Cluster headaches are classically unilateral and periorbital, occurring in clusters of one to three attacks a day over a 4- to 8-week period. The pain is described as a burning or drilling sensation that may awaken the patient from sleep. Each episode lasts 30–120 min. Remissions lasting a year at a time are common. Red eye, tearing, nasal stuffiness, ptosis, and Horner's syndrome are classic findings. The headaches are typically episodic but can become chronic without remissions. Cluster headaches primarily affect males (90%). Abortive treatments includes oxygen and sphenopalatine block. Lithium, a short course of steroid medication, and verapamil may be used for prophylaxis.

Temporal Arteritis

Temporal arteritis is an inflammatory disorder of extracranial arteries. The headache can be bilateral or unilateral and is located in the temporal area in at least 50% of patients. The pain develops over a few hours, is usually dull in quality but may be lancinating at times and worse at night and in cold weather. Scalp tenderness is usually present. Temporal arteritis is often accompanied by polymyalgia rheumatica, fever, and weight loss. It is a relatively common disorder of older patients (>55 years), with an incidence of about 1 in 10,000 per year and a slight female predominance. Early diagnosis and treatment with steroids is important because progression can lead to blindness through involvement of the ophthalmic artery.

Trigeminal Neuralgia

16 Trigeminal neuralgia (or *tic douloureux*) is classically unilateral and usually located in the V2 or V3 distribution of the trigeminal nerve. It has an electric shock quality lasting from seconds to minutes at a time and is often provoked by contact with a discrete trigger. Facial muscle spasm may be present. Patients are middle-aged and elderly, with a 2:1 female to male ratio. Common causes of trigeminal neuralgia include compression of the nerve by the superior cerebellar artery as it exits the brainstem, cerebellopontine angle tumor, or multiple sclerosis. The drug of choice for treatment is carbamazepine although it carries a risk of agranulocytosis. Phenytoin or baclofen may be added, particularly if patients do not tolerate the required doses of carbamazepine. More invasive treatments for patients who do not respond to drug therapy include glycerol injection, radiofrequency ablation, balloon compression of the gasserian ganglion, and microvascular decompression of the trigeminal nerve.

ABDOMINAL PAIN

Chronic abdominal pain can have a variety of causes, and it is useful to distinguish between somatosensory, visceral, and centralized pain symptoms. A differential epidural block may help in elucidating the primary source but is time consuming and may be difficult to interpret. A transversus abdominis plane (TAP) blockade with ultrasound guidance

TABLE 47–11 Selected oral nonopioid analgesics.

Analgesic	Onset (h)	Dose (mg)	Dosing Interval (h)	Maximum Daily Dosage (mg)
Salicylates				
Acetylsalicylic acid (aspirin)	0.5–1.0	500–1000	4	3600–6000
Diflunisal (Dolobid)	1–2	500–1000	8–12	1500
Choline magnesium trisalicylate (Trilisate)	1–2	500–1000	12	2000–3000
p-Aminophenols				
Acetaminophen (Tylenol, others)	0.5	500–1000	4	1200–4000
Proprionic acids				
Ibuprofen (Motrin, others)	0.5	400	4–6	3200
Naproxen (Naprosyn)	1	250–500	12	1500
Naproxen sodium (Anaprox)	1–2	275–550	6–8	1375
Indoles				
Indomethacin (Indocin)	0.5	25–50	8–12	150–200
Ketorolac (Toradol)	0.5–1	10	4–6	40
COX-2 Inhibitors				
Celecoxib (Celebrex)	3	100–200	12	400

may help treat somatosensory pain and thus may be potentially both diagnostic and therapeutic (see Chapter 46). The patient with pain of visceral origin may benefit from a celiac or splanchnic block.

CANCER-RELATED PAIN

Cancer-related pain may be due to the cancerous lesion itself, metastatic disease, complications such as neural compression or infection, or treatment such as chemotherapy or radiation therapy. In addition, the cancer patient may have acute or chronic pain that is entirely unrelated to the cancer. The pain manager must therefore have a thorough understanding of the nature of the cancer, its stage, the presence of metastatic disease, and treatments.

Cancer pain can be managed with oral analgesics in most patients. The World Health Organization recommends a progressive, three-step approach: (1) nonopioid analgesics such as aspirin, acetaminophen, or NSAID for mild pain, (2) "weak" oral opioids (codeine and oxycodone) for moderate pain, and (3) stronger opioids (morphine and hydromorphone) for severe pain (Tables 47–11 and 47–12). Parenteral therapy is necessary when patients have refractory pain, cannot take medication orally, or

have poor enteral absorption. Regardless of the agent selected, in most instances drug therapy should be provided on a fixed time schedule rather than as needed. Adjuvant drug therapy, particularly antidepressants, and other modalities should also be used liberally in patients with cancer-related pain (Table 47–13). Anticonvulsants may be useful (Table 47–14). Intrathecal drug delivery systems may improve analgesia and, via a drug-sparing effect, help decrease side effects associated with oral or intravenous agents. Numerous intrathecal agents have been studied, and opioids have been utilized both alone and in combination with other medications. Ziconotide is a direct-acting N-type calcium-channel blocker that may be helpful for refractory pain or as a first-line agent. It acts by decreasing the release of substance P from the presynaptic nerve terminal in the dorsal horn of the spinal cord. Side effects may be dose dependent and include auditory hallucinations and worsening of depression or psychosis. It does not lead to significant withdrawal conditions if abruptly discontinued.

Surgery, radiation therapy, and chemotherapy may prolong survivorship for patients with cancer. However, survivorship may be accompanied by therapy-related acute or chronic pain, including

TABLE 47–12 Oral opioids.

Opioid	Onset (h)	Relative Potency	Initial Dose (mg)	Dosing Interval (h)
Codeine	0.25–1.0	20	30–60	4
Hydromorphone (Dilaudid)	0.3–0.5	0.6	2–4	4
Hydrocodone[1]	0.5–1.0	3	5–7.5	4–6
Oxycodone[2] (OxyFast, Roxicodone)	0.5	3	5–10	6
Levorphanol (Levo-Dromoran)	1–2	0.4	4	6–8
Methadone (Dolophine)	0.5–1.0	1	20	6–8
Propoxyphene (Darvon)[3]	1–2	30	100	6
Tramadol (Rybix, Ryzolt, Ultram)	1–2	30	50	4–6
Morphine solution[4] (Roxanol)	0.5–1	1	10	3–4
Morphine sustained-release[4] (MS Contin, Oramorph SR)	1	1	15	8–12
(Kadian)	1	1	10–20	12–24
(Avinza)	1	1	30	24

[1]Preparations also contain acetaminophen (Hycet, Lorcet, Lortab, Norco, Vicodin, others).

[2]Preparations may contain acetaminophen (Percocet) or aspirin (Percodan).

[3]Some preparations contain acetaminophen (Darvocet).

[4]Used primarily for cancer pain.

radiation fibrosis or chemotherapy-induced peripheral neuropathy. Treatment of these pain conditions is an area of ongoing research.

Interventional Therapies

Interventional pain therapy may take the form of pharmacological treatment, nerve blocks with local anesthetics and steroid or a neurolytic solution, radiofrequency ablation, neuromodulatory techniques, or multidisciplinary treatment (psychological interventions, physical or occupational therapy, or modalities such as acupuncture).

PHARMACOLOGICAL INTERVENTIONS

Pharmacological interventions in pain management include acetaminophen, cyclooxygenase (COX) inhibitors, opioids, antidepressants, neuroleptic agents, anticonvulsants, corticosteroids, and systemic administration of local anesthetics.

Acetaminophen

Acetaminophen (paracetamol) is an oral analgesic and antipyretic agent that recently has become available in the United States as an intravenous preparation (Ofirmev) for inpatient use. It inhibits prostaglandin synthesis but lacks significant antiinflammatory activity. Acetaminophen has few side effects but is hepatotoxic at high doses. The recommended adult maximum daily limit is 3000 mg/d, reduced from a previously recommended limit of 4000 mg/d. Isoniazid, zidovudine, and barbiturates can potentiate acetaminophen toxicity.

Nonsteroidal Antiinflammatory Drugs (NSAIDs)

Nonopioid oral analgesics include salicylates, acetaminophen, and NSAIDs (see Table 47–11). NSAIDs inhibit prostaglandin synthesis (COX).

TABLE 47–13 Selected antidepressants.

Drug	Norepinephrine Reuptake Inhibition	Serotonin Reuptake Inhibition	Sedation	Antimuscarinic Activity	Orthostatic Hypotension	Half-Life (h)	Daily Dose (mg)
Amitriptyline (Elavil)	++	++++	High	High	Moderate	30–40	25–300
Bupropion (Wellbutrin)	+	+	Low	Low	Low	11–14	300–450
Citalopram (Celexa)	0	+++	Low	Low	Low	35	20–40
Clomipramine (Anafranil)	+++	+++	High	Moderate	Moderate	20–80	75–300
Desipramine (Norpramin)	+++	0	Low	Low	Low	12–50	50–300
Doxepin (Sinequan)	+	++	High	High	Moderate	8–24	75–400
Escitalopram	0	+++	Low	Low	Low	27–32	10–20
Fluoxetine (Prozac)	0	+++	Low	Low	Low	160–200	20–80
Imipramine (Tofranil)	++	+++	Moderate	Moderate	High	6–20	75–400
Nefazodone (Serzone)	0	+	Low	Low	Low	2–4	300–600
Nortriptyline (Pamelor)	++	+++	Moderate	Moderate	Low	15–90	40–150
Paroxetine (Paxil)	0	+++	Low	Low	Low	31	20–40
Sertraline (Zoloft)	0	+++	Low	Low	Low	26	50–200
Trazodone (Desyrel)	0	++	High	Low	Moderate	3–9	150–400
Venlafaxine (Effexor)	+	+++	Low	Low	Low	5–11	75–375

Prostaglandins sensitize and amplify nociceptive input, and blockade of their synthesis results in the analgesic, antipyretic, and antiinflammatory properties characteristic of NSAIDs. At least two types of COX are recognized. COX-1 is constitutive and widespread throughout the body, but COX-2 is expressed primarily with inflammation. Some types of pain, particularly pain that follows orthopedic and gynecological surgery, respond very well to COX inhibitors. COX inhibitors likely have important peripheral and central nervous system actions. Their analgesic action is limited by side effects and toxicity at higher doses. Selective COX-2 inhibitors, such as celecoxib, appear to have lower toxicity, particularly gastrointestinal side effects. Moreover, COX-2 inhibitors do not interfere with platelet aggregation. The COX-2 inhibitor rofecoxib increases the risk of cardiovascular complications; as a result, it has been taken off of the market in the United States.

All of the nonopioid oral analgesic agents are well absorbed enterally. Food delays absorption but otherwise has no effect on bioavailability. Because most of these agents are highly protein bound (>80%), they can displace other highly bound drugs such as warfarin. All undergo hepatic metabolism and are renally excreted. Dosages should therefore be reduced, or alternative medications selected, in patients with hepatic or renal impairment.

The most common side effects of aspirin (acetylsalicylic acid, ASA) and other NSAIDs are stomach upset, heartburn, nausea, and dyspepsia; some patients develop ulceration of the gastric mucosa, which appears to be due to inhibition of prostaglandin-mediated mucus and bicarbonate secretion. Diclofenac is available as both an oral preparation

TABLE 47–14 Anticonvulsants possibly useful in pain management.

Anticonvulsant	Half-Life (h)	Daily Dose (mg)	Therapeutic Level[1] (mcg/mL)
Carbamazepine (Tegretol)	10–20	200–1200	4–12
Clonazepam (Klonopin)	40–30	1–40	0.01–0.08
Gabapentin (Neurontin)	5–7	900–4000	>2
Lamotrigine (Lamictal)	24	25–400	2–20
Phenytoin (Dilantin)	22	200–600	10–20
Pregabalin (Lyrica)	6	150–600	2.8–8.2
Topiramate (Topamax)	20–30	25–200	Unknown
Valproic acid (Depakene)	6–16	750–1250	50–100

[1]Efficacy in pain management may not correlate with blood level.

and a topical gel or patch that may be less likely to contribute to gastric distress.

Other side effects of NSAIDs include dizziness, headache, and drowsiness. With the exception of selective COX-2 inhibitors, all other COX inhibitors induce platelet dysfunction. Aspirin irreversibly acetylates platelets, inhibiting platelet adhesiveness for 1–2 weeks, whereas the antiplatelet effect of other NSAIDs is reversible and lasts approximately five elimination half-lives (24–96 h). This antiplatelet effect does not appear to appreciably increase the incidence of postoperative hemorrhage following most outpatient procedures. NSAIDs can exacerbate bronchospasm in patients with the triad of nasal polyps, rhinitis, and asthma. ASA should not be used in children with varicella or influenza infections because it may precipitate Reye's syndrome. Lastly, NSAIDs can cause acute renal insufficiency and renal papillary necrosis, particularly in patients with underlying renal dysfunction.

Antidepressants

17 Antidepressants are most useful for patients with neuropathic pain. These medications demonstrate an analgesic effect that occurs at a dose lower than that needed for antidepressant activity,

and both of these actions are due to blockade of presynaptic reuptake of serotonin, norepinephrine, or both. Older tricyclic agents appear to be more effective analgesics than selective serotonin reuptake inhibitors (SSRIs). Serotonin and norepinephrine reuptake inhibitors (SNRIs) may provide the most favorable balance between analgesic efficacy and side effects. Antidepressants potentiate the action of opioids and frequently help normalize sleep patterns.

All antidepressant medications undergo extensive first-pass hepatic metabolism and are highly protein bound. Most are highly lipophilic and have large volumes of distribution. Elimination half-lives of most of these medications vary between 1 and 4 days, and many have active metabolites. Available agents differ in their side effects (see Table 47–13), which include antimuscarinic effects (dry mouth, impaired visual accommodation, urinary retention, and constipation), antihistaminic effects (sedation and increased gastric pH), α-adrenergic blockade (orthostatic hypotension), and a quinidine-like effect (atrioventricular block, QT prolongation, torsades de pointes).

Serotonin & Norepinephrine Reuptake Inhibitors (SNRIs)

Milnacipran, along with the SNRI duloxetine and the anticonvulsant pregabalin, has also been approved in the United States by the FDA for the treatment of fibromyalgia. It has an elimination half-life of 8 h, is minimally metabolized by the liver, and is primarily excreted unchanged in the urine.

Duloxetine (Cymbalta) is useful in the treatment of neuropathic pain, depression, and fibromyalgia. It has a half-life of 12 h, is metabolized by the liver, and most of its metabolites are excreted in the urine.

Absolute and relative contraindications for the use of SNRIs include known hypersensitivity, usage of other drugs that act on the central nervous system (including monoamine oxidase inhibitors), hepatic and renal impairment, uncontrolled narrow-angle glaucoma, and suicidal ideation. Common side effects include nausea, headache, dizziness, constipation, insomnia, hyperhydrosis, hot flashes, vomiting, palpitations, dry mouth, and hypertension.

Neuroleptics

Neuroleptic medications may occasionally be useful for patients with refractory neuropathic pain, and may be most helpful in patients with marked agitation or psychotic symptoms. The most commonly used agents are fluphenazine, haloperidol, chlorpromazine, and perphenazine. Their therapeutic action appears to be due to blockade of dopaminergic receptors in mesolimbic sites. Unfortunately, the same action in nigrostriatal pathways can produce undesirable extrapyramidal side effects, such as masklike facies, a festinating gait, cogwheel rigidity, and bradykinesia. Some patients also develop acute dystonic reactions such as oculogyric crisis and torticollis. Long-term side effects include akathisia (extreme restlessness) and tardive dyskinesia (involuntary choreoathetoid movements of the tongue, lip smacking, and truncal instability). Like antidepressants, many of these drugs also have antihistaminic, antimuscarinic, and α-adrenergic–blocking effects.

Antispasmodics & Muscle Relaxants

Antispasmodics may be helpful for patients with musculoskeletal sprain and pain associated with spasm or contractures. Tizanidine (Zanaflex) is a centrally acting α_2-adrenergic agonist used in the treatment of muscle spasm in conditions such as multiple sclerosis, low back pain, and spastic diplegia. Cyclobenzaprine (Flexeril) also may be effective for these conditions. Its precise mechanism of action is unknown.

Baclofen (Gablofen, Lioresal), a $GABA_B$ agonist, is particularly effective in the treatment of muscle spasm associated with multiple sclerosis or spinal cord injury when administered by continuous intrathecal drug infusion. Abrupt discontinuation of this medication has been associated with fever, altered mental status, pronounced muscle spasticity or rigidity, rhabdomyolysis, and death.

Corticosteroids

Glucocorticoids are extensively used in pain management for their antiinflammatory and possibly analgesic actions. They may be given topically, orally, or parenterally (intravenously, subcutaneously, intrabursally, intraarticularly, or epidurally). Table 47–15 lists the most commonly used agents, which differ in potency, relative glucocorticoid and mineralocorticoid activities, and duration or action. Large doses or prolonged administration result in significant side effects. Excess glucocorticoid activity can produce hypertension, hyperglycemia, increased susceptibility to infection, peptic ulcers, osteoporosis, aseptic necrosis of the femoral head, proximal myopathy, cataracts, and, rarely, psychosis. Patients with diabetes may have elevated blood glucose levels after corticosteroid injections. Patients can also develop the physical features characteristic of Cushing's syndrome. Excess mineralocorticoid

TABLE 47–15 Selected corticosteroids.[1]

Drug	Routes Given[2]	Glucocorticoid Activity	Mineralocorticoid Activity	Equivalent Dose (mg)	Half-Life (h)
Hydrocortisone	O, I, T	1	1	20	8–12
Prednisone	O	4	0.8	5	12–36
Prednisolone	O, I	4	0.8	5	12–36
Methylprednisolone (Depo-Medrol, Solu-Medrol)	O, I, T	5	0.5	4	12–36
Triamcinolone (Aristocort)	O, I, T	5	0.5	4	12–36
Betamethasone (Celestone)	O, I, T	25	0	0.75	36–72
Dexamethasone (Decadron)	O, I, T	25	0	0.75	36–72

[1]Data from Goodman LS, Gilman AG: *The Pharmacologic Basis of Therapeutics*, 8th ed. Pergamon, 1990.
[2]O, oral; I, injectable; T, topical.

activity causes sodium retention and hypokalemia, and can precipitate congestive heart failure.

Many corticosteroid preparations are suspensions, rather than solutions, and the relative particulate size of a given glucocorticoid suspension may affect the risk of neural damage due to arterial occlusion when accidental arterial injection occurs. Because of the relatively small size of its suspension particles, dexamethasone is becoming the preferred corticosteroid for injection procedures involving relatively vascular areas, such as the head and neck region.

Anticonvulsants

18 Anticonvulsant medications are useful for patients with neuropathic pain, especially trigeminal neuralgia and diabetic neuropathy. These agents block voltage-gated calcium or sodium channels and can suppress the spontaneous neural discharges that play a major role in these disorders. The most commonly utilized agents are phenytoin (Dilantin), carbamazepine (Tegretol), valproic acid (Depakene, Stavzor), clonazepam (Klonopin), and gabapentin (Neurontin) (Table 47–14). Pregabalin (Lyrica) is a newer agent that has been approved for the treatment of diabetic peripheral neuropathy and fibromyalgia but is widely prescribed for all forms of neuropathic pain. Lamotrigine (Lamictal) and topiramate (Topamax) may also be effective. All are highly protein bound and have relatively long half-lives. Carbamazepine (Carbatrol, Equetro, Tegretol) has a slow and unpredictable absorption, which requires monitoring of blood levels for optimal efficacy. Phenytoin may be effective, but there is a possible side effect of gum hyperplasia. Levetiracetam (Keppra) and oxcarbazepine (Trileptal) have been used as adjuvant pain therapies. Gabapentin and pregabalin may also be effective adjuvants for the treatment of acute postoperative pain.

Local Anesthetics

Systemic infusion of local anesthetic medication produces sedation and central analgesia and is occasionally used in the treatment of patients with neuropathic pain. The resultant analgesia may outlast the pharmacokinetic profile of the local anesthetic and break the "pain cycle." Lidocaine, procaine, and chloroprocaine are the most commonly used agents. They are given either as a slow bolus or by continuous infusion. Lidocaine is given by infusion over 5–30 min for a total of 1–5 mg/kg. Procaine, 200–400 mg, can be given intravenously over the course of 1–2 h, whereas chloroprocaine (1% solution) is infused at a rate of 1 mg/kg/min for a total of 10–20 mg/kg. Monitoring by qualified medical personnel should include electrocardiographic data, blood pressure, respiration, pulse oximetry, and mental status, and full resuscitation equipment should be immediately available. Signs of toxicity, such as tinnitus, slurring of speech, excessive sedation, or nystagmus, necessitate slowing or discontinuing the infusion to avoid the progression to seizures.

Patients who do not respond satisfactorily to anticonvulsants but respond to intravenous local anesthetics may benefit from chronic oral antiarrhythmic therapy. Mexiletine (150–300 mg every 6–8 h) is a class 1B antiarrhythmic that is commonly used and generally well tolerated.

A 5% lidocaine transdermal patch (Lidoderm) containing 700 mg of lidocaine has been approved for the treatment of PHN. One to three patches may be applied to dry, intact skin, alternating 12 h on, then 12 h off. Topical lidocaine preparations, in concentrations up to 5%, may be helpful in the treatment of some neuropathic pain conditions.

α_2-Adrenergic Agonists

The primary effect of α_2-adrenergic agonists is activation of descending inhibitory pathways in the dorsal horn. Epidural and intrathecal α_2-adrenergic agonists are particularly effective in the treatment of neuropathic pain and opioid tolerance. Clonidine (Catapres), a direct-acting α_2-adrenergic agonist, is effective as an adjunctive medication in the treatment of severe pain. When administered orally, the dosage is 0.1–0.3 mg twice daily; a transdermal patch (0.1–0.3 mg/d) is also available and is usually applied for 7 d. When used in combination with a local anesthetic or opioid in an epidural or intrathecal infusion, clonidine may contribute to a synergistic or prolonged analgesic effect, especially for neuropathic pain.

Opioids

The most commonly prescribed oral opioid agents are codeine, oxycodone, and hydrocodone. They are easily absorbed, but hepatic first-pass metabolism limits systemic delivery. Like other opioids, they undergo hepatic biotransformation and conjugation before renal elimination. Codeine is transformed by the liver into morphine. The side effects of orally administered opioids are similar to those of systemic opioids. When prescribed on a fixed schedule, stool softeners or laxatives are often indicated. Tramadol (Rybix, Ryzolt, Ultram) is a synthetic oral opioid that also blocks neuronal reuptake of norepinephrine and serotonin. It appears to have the same efficacy as the combination of codeine and acetaminophen but, unlike others, it is associated with significantly less respiratory depression and has little effect on gastric emptying.

Moderate to severe cancer pain is usually treated with an immediate-release morphine preparation (eg, liquid morphine, Roxanol, 10–30 mg every 1–4 h). These preparations have an effective half-life of 2–4 h. Once the patient's daily requirements are determined, the same dose can be given in the form of a sustained-release morphine preparation (MS Contin or Oramorph SR), which is dosed every 8–12 h. The immediate-release preparation is then used only for breakthrough pain (PRN). Oral transmucosal fentanyl lozenges (Actiq, 200–1600 mcg) can also be used for breakthrough pain. Excessive sedation can be treated with dextroamphetamine (Dexedrine, ProCentra) or methylphenidate (Ritalin), 5 mg in the morning and 5 mg the early afternoon. Most patients require a stool softener. Nausea may be treated with transdermal scopolamine, oral meclizine, or metoclopramide. Hydromorphone (Dilaudid) is an excellent alternative to morphine, particularly in elderly patients (because of fewer side effects) and in patients with impaired renal function. Methadone (Dolophine) is reported to have a half-life of 15–30 h, but clinical duration is shorter and quite variable (usually 6–8 h).

19 Patients who experience opioid tolerance require escalating doses of opioid to maintain the same analgesic effect. Physical dependence manifests in opioid withdrawal when the opioid medication is either abruptly discontinued or the dose is abruptly and significantly decreased. Psychological dependence, characterized by behavioral changes focusing on drug craving, is rare in cancer patients. The development of opioid tolerance is highly variable but results in some desirable effects such as decreased opioid-related sedation, nausea, and respiratory depression. Unfortunately, many patients continue to suffer from constipation. Physical dependence occurs in all patients receiving large doses of opioids for extended periods. Opioid withdrawal phenomena can be precipitated by the administration of opioid antagonists. Future concomitant use of peripheral opioid antagonists that do not cross the blood–brain barrier, such as methylnaltrexone (Relistor) and alvimopan (Entereg), may help reduce systemic side effects without significantly affecting analgesia.

Tapentadol (Nucynta), a μ-opioid receptor agonist that also has norepinephrine reuptake inhibition properties, has recently been introduced for the management of acute and chronic pain. This opioid may be associated with less nausea and vomiting and less constipation. It should not be used concomitantly with monoamine oxidase inhibitors due to potentially elevated levels of norepinephrine.

Propoxyphene with and without acetaminophen (Darvocet and Darvon) was withdrawn from the U.S. market in 2010 due to the risk of cardiac toxicity.

A. Parenteral Opioid Administration

Intravenous, intraspinal (epidural or intrathecal), or transdermal routes of opioid administration must be utilized when the patient fails to adequately respond to, or is unable to tolerate, oral regimens. However, when the patient's pain increases significantly, or changes markedly in quality, it is equally important to reevaluate the patient for adequacy of pain diagnosis and for the potential of disease progression. In patients with cancer, adjunctive treatments such as surgery, radiation, chemotherapy, hormonal therapy, and neurolysis may be helpful. Intramuscular opioid administration is rarely optimal because of variability in systemic absorption and resultant delay and variation in clinical effect.

B. Intravenous Opioid Therapy

Parenteral opioid therapy is usually best accomplished by intermittent or continuous intravenous infusion, or both, but can also be given subcutaneously. Modern portable infusion devices have

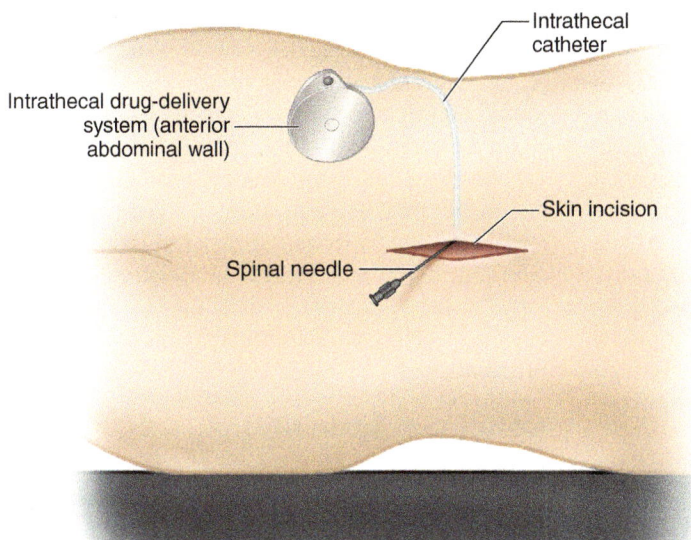

Intrathecal catheter

Intrathecal drug-delivery system (anterior abdominal wall)

Skin incision

Spinal needle

Lateral decubitus position

FIGURE 47–6 Placement of an implanted intrathecal drug delivery system. With the patient in right lateral decubitus position, access to the intrathecal space and to the anterior abdominal wall is optimized. After the posterior incision is made, a needle is advanced through the incision into the intrathecal space, and a catheter is advanced through the needle into the posterior intrathecal space. After the proximal catheter end is anchored, the distal end of the catheter is tunneled around the flank, beneath the costal margin to the anterolateral aspect of the abdominal wall.

patient-controlled analgesia (PCA) capability, allowing the patient to self-treat for breakthrough pain.

C. Spinal Opioid Therapy

The use of intraspinal opioids is an excellent alternative for patients obtaining poor relief with other analgesic techniques or who experience unacceptable side effects. Epidural and intrathecal opioids offer pain relief with substantially lower total doses of opioid and fewer side effects. Continuous infusion techniques reduce drug requirements (compared with intermittent boluses), minimize side effects, and decrease the likelihood of catheter occlusion. Myoclonic activity may be occasionally observed with intrathecal morphine or hydromorphone.

Epidural or intrathecal catheters can be placed percutaneously or implanted to provide long-term effective pain relief. Epidural catheters can be attached to lightweight external pumps that can be worn by ambulatory patients. A temporary catheter must be inserted first to assess the potential efficacy of the technique. Correct placement of the permanent catheter should be confirmed using fluoroscopy with contrast dye. Completely implantable intrathecal catheters with externally programmable pumps can also be used for continuous infusion (Figure 47–6). The reservoir of the implanted pump (Figure 47–7) is periodically

refilled percutaneously. Implantable systems are most appropriate for patients with a life expectancy of several months or longer, whereas tunneled epidural catheters are appropriate for patients expected to live only weeks. Formation of an inflammatory

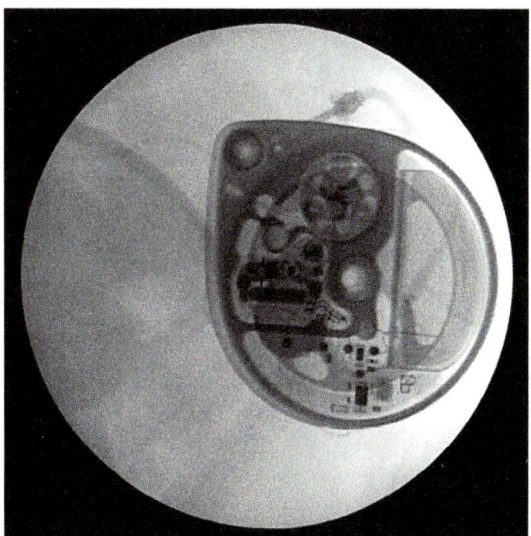

FIGURE 47–7 Fluoroscopic image showing an intrathecal drug pump implanted in the anterolateral abdomen wall. The catheter connecting the pump to the intrathecal space is tunneled around the flank.

mass (granuloma) at the tip of the intrathecal catheter can occur and may reduce efficacy.

The most frequently encountered problem associated with intrathecal opioids is tolerance. Generally a slow phenomenon, tolerance may develop rapidly in some patients. In such instances, adjuvant therapy must be used, including the intermittent use of local anesthetics or a mixture of opioids with local anesthetics (bupivacaine or ropivacaine 2–24 mg/d), clonidine (2–4 mcg/kg/h or 48–800 mcg/d, respectively), or the GABA agonist baclofen. Clonidine is particularly useful for neuropathic pain. In high doses, it is more likely to be associated with hypotension and bradycardia.

Complications of spinal opioid therapy include local skin infection, epidural abscess, meningitis, and death or permanent injury from pump programming or drug dilution errors. Superficial infections can be reduced by the use of a silver-impregnated cuff close to the exit site. Other complications of spinal opioid therapy include epidural hematoma, which may become clinically apparent either immediately following catheter placement or several days later, and respiratory depression. Respiratory depression secondary to spinal opioid overdose can be treated by decreasing the pump infusion rate to its lowest setting and initiating a naloxone intravenous infusion.

D. Transdermal Fentanyl

Transdermal fentanyl (Duragesic patch) is an alternative to sustained-release oral morphine and oxycodone preparations, particularly when oral medication is not possible. The currently available patches are constructed as a drug reservoir that is separated from the skin by a microporous rate-limiting membrane and an adhesive polymer. A very large quantity of fentanyl (10 mg) provides a large force for transdermal diffusion. Transdermal fentanyl patches are available in 25, 50, 75, and 100 mcg/h sizes that provide drug for 2–3 days. The largest patch is equivalent to 60 mg/d of intravenous morphine. The major obstacle to fentanyl absorption through the skin is the stratum corneum. Because the dermis acts as a secondary reservoir, fentanyl absorption continues for several hours after the patch is removed. The transdermal route avoids hepatic first-pass metabolism.

Major disadvantages of the transdermal route are its slow rate of drug delivery onset and the inability to rapidly change dosage in response to changing opioid requirements. Blood fentanyl levels rise and reach a plateau in 12–40 h, providing average concentrations of 1, 1.5, and 2 ng/mL for the 50, 75, and 100 mcg/h patches, respectively. Large inter-patient variability results in actual delivery rates ranging from 50 to 200 mcg/h. This formulation is popularly "diverted" for nonmedical uses and has been the cause of numerous deaths from "recreational" pharmacology.

Botulinum Toxin (Botox)

OnabotulinumtoxinA (Botox) injection has been increasingly utilized in the treatment of pain syndromes. Studies support its use in the treatment of conditions associated with involuntary muscle contraction (eg, focal dystonia and spasticity), and it is approved by the FDA for prophylactic treatment of chronic migraine headache. This toxin blocks acetylcholine released at the synapse in motor nerve endings but not sensory nerve fibers. Proposed mechanisms of analgesia include improved local blood flow, relief of muscle spasms, and release of muscular compression of nerve fibers

PROCEDURAL THERAPY

1. Diagnostic & Therapeutic Blocks

Local anesthetic nerve blocks are useful in delineating pain mechanisms, and they play a major role in the management of patients with acute or chronic pain. Pain relief following diagnostic nerve blockade often carries favorable prognostic implications for a subsequent therapeutic series of blocks. Although the utility of differential nerve blocks in distinguishing between somatic and sympathetic mechanisms has been questioned, this technique can identify patients exhibiting a placebo response and those with psychogenic mechanisms. In selected patients, "permanent" neurolytic nerve blocks may be appropriate.

The efficacy of nerve blocks is presumably due to interruption of afferent nociceptive activity. This is in addition to, or in combination with, blockade of afferent and efferent limbs of abnormal reflex activity involving sympathetic nerve fibers and skeletal muscle innervation. The pain relief frequently out-lasts (by hours up to several weeks) the known pharmacological duration of the agent employed. Selection of the type of block depends on the loca-tion of pain, its presumed mechanism, and the skills of the treating physician. Local anesthetic solutions may be applied locally (infiltration), or at a specific peripheral nerve, somatic plexus, sympathetic gan-glia, or nerve root. The local anesthetic may also be applied centrally in the neuraxis.

Ultrasound-Guided Procedures

The use of ultrasound in interventional pain medi-cine has increased over the past decade due to its utility in visualizing vascular, neural, and other ana-tomic structures; its role as an alternative to the use of fluoroscopy and iodine-based contrast agents; and progressive improvements in technology lead-ing to better visual images and greater simplicity of use. Most notably, ultrasound has become very useful for visualizing blood vessels and potentially decreasing the incidence of intravascular injection of particulate steroid medications. It may also be helpful in decreasing the risk of pneumothorax and of intraperitoneal injection. Procedures that may benefit from ultrasound guidance include trigger point injections, nerve blocks, and joint injections.

Fluoroscopy

Fluoroscopy is frequently used for interventional pain procedures. It is highly effective for visualizing bony structures and observing the spread of radiopaque contrast agents. Live fluoroscopy with contrast agent should be used to minimize the risk of intravascular injection of therapeutic agents. Care should be taken to avoid excessive use of fluoroscopy and to employ appropriate radiation shielding, given the risks of ionizing radiation to the patient and to the health care team members in the fluoroscopy suite.

2. Somatic Nerve Blocks

Trigeminal Nerve Block

A. Indications

The two principal indications for trigeminal nerve block are trigeminal neuralgia and intractable facial cancer pain. Depending on the site of pain, these blocks may be performed on the gasserian ganglion itself, on one of the major divisions (ophthalmic, maxillary, or mandibular), or on one of their smaller branches.

B. Anatomy

The rootlets of cranial nerve V arise from the brain-stem and join one another to form a crescent-shaped sensory (gasserian) ganglion in Meckel's cave. Most of the ganglion is invested with a dural sleeve. The three subdivisions of the trigeminal nerve arise from the ganglia and exit the cranium separately. (Figure 47–8A).

C. Technique

1. Gasserian ganglion block—Fluoroscopic guid-ance is mandatory for the performance of this pro-cedure (Figure 47–8B). An 8- to 10-cm 22-gauge needle is inserted approximately 3 cm lateral to the angle of the mouth at the level of the upper second molar. The needle is then advanced posteromedial-ly and angled superiorly to bring it into alignment with the pupil in the anterior plane and with the mid-zygomatic arch in the lateral plane. Without entering the mouth, the needle should pass be-tween the mandibular ramus and the maxilla, and lateral to the pterygoid process to enter the cra-nium through the foramen ovale. After a negative aspiration for cerebrospinal fluid and blood, local anesthetic is injected.

2. Blocks of the ophthalmic nerve and its branches—In this procedure, to avoid denerva-tion-related keratitis, only the supraorbital branch is blocked in most cases (Figure 47–8C); the oph-thalmic division itself is not blocked. The nerve is easily located and blocked with local anesthetic at the supraorbital notch, which is located on the su-praorbital ridge above the pupil. The supratrochlear branch can also be blocked with local anesthetic at the superior medial corner of the orbital ridge.

3. Blocks of the maxillary nerve and its branches—With the patient's mouth slightly opened, an 8- to 10-cm 22-gauge needle is inserted between the zygomatic arch and the notch of the mandible (Figure 47–8D). After contact with the lateral pter-ygoid plate at about 4-cm depth (position 1 in fig-ure), the needle is partially withdrawn and angled slightly superiorly and anteriorly to pass into the

A. Blocks of the trigeminal nerve

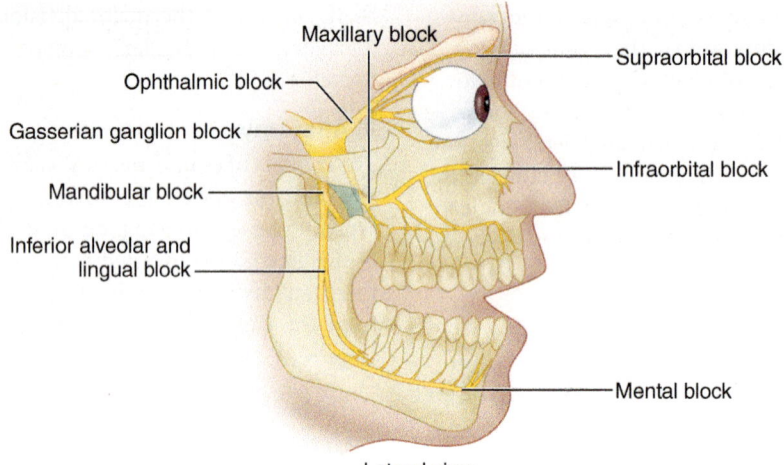

Lateral view

B. Gasserian ganglion block

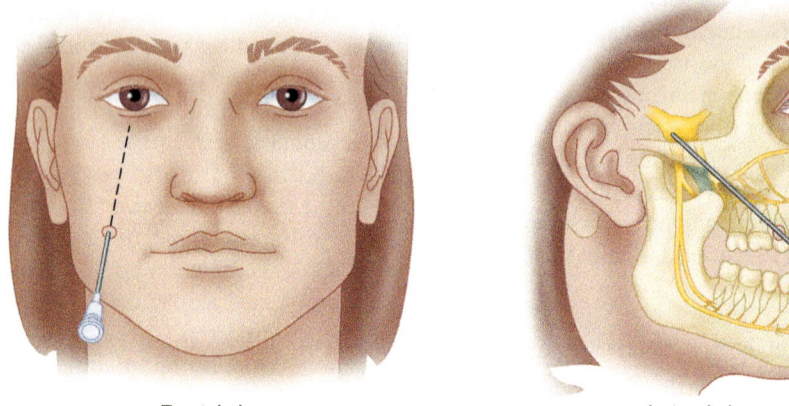

Frontal view   Lateral view

C. Supraorbital nerve block

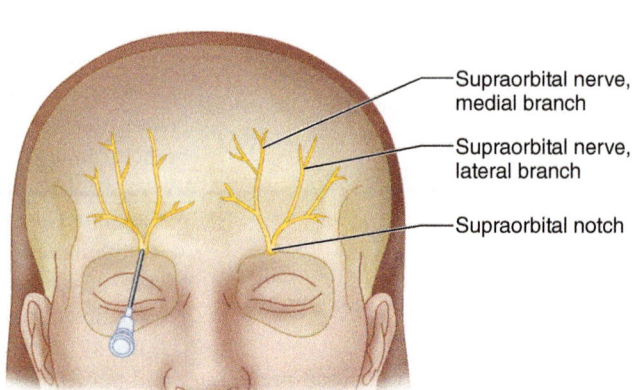

Frontal view

FIGURE 47–8 Trigeminal nerve blocks. (*continued*)

D. Maxillary nerve block

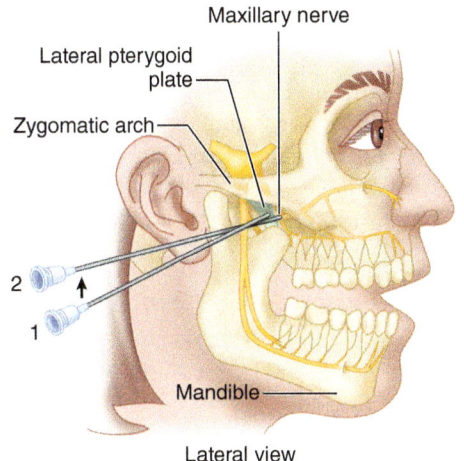

Maxillary nerve

Lateral pterygoid plate

Zygomatic arch

2

1

Mandible

Lateral view

E. Mandibular nerve block

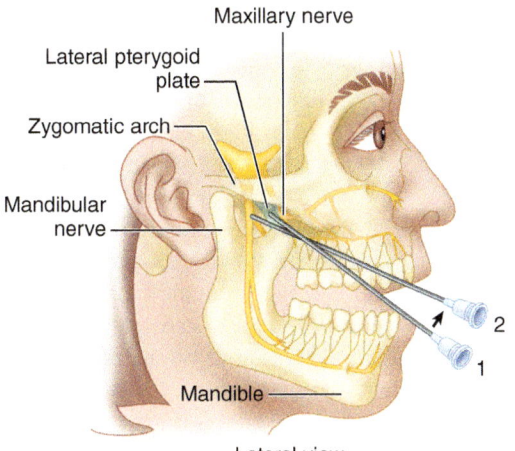

Maxillary nerve

Lateral pterygoid plate

Zygomatic arch

Mandibular nerve

2

1

Mandible

Lateral view

F. Lingual and inferior alveolar nerve block

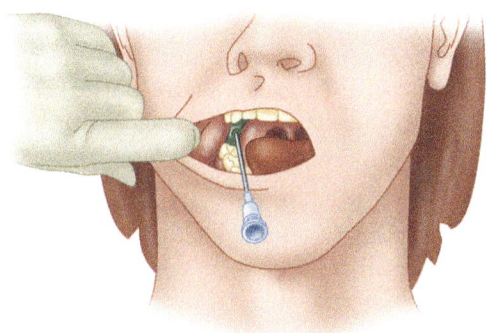

Frontal view

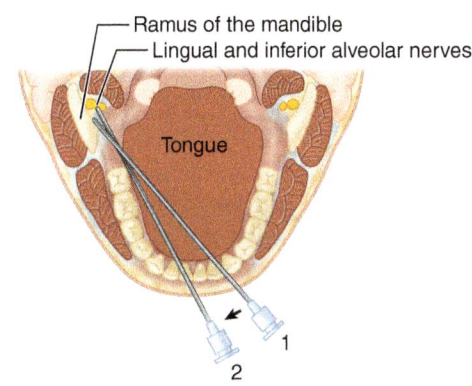

Ramus of the mandible

Lingual and inferior alveolar nerves

Tongue

1

2

Transverse view

FIGURE 47–8 (*continued*)

pterygopalatine fossa (position 2). Local anesthetic is injected once paresthesias are elicited. Both the maxillary nerve and the sphenopalatine (pterygopalatine) ganglia are usually anesthetized by this technique. The sphenopalatine ganglion (and anterior ethmoid nerves) can be anesthetized transmucosally with topical anesthetic applied through the nose; several cotton applicators soaked with local anesthetic (cocaine or lidocaine) are inserted along the medial wall of the nasal cavity into the area of the sphenopalatine recess. The sphenopalatine ganglion blockade may be helpful for patients with chronic nasal pain, cluster headache, or Sluder's neuralgia.

The infraorbital branch of cranial nerve V passes through the infraorbital foramen, where it can be blocked with local anesthetic. This foramen is approximately 1 cm below the orbit and is usually located with a needle inserted about 2 cm lateral to the nasal ala and directed superiorly, posteriorly, and slightly laterally.

4. Blocks of the mandibular nerve and its branches—With the patient's mouth slightly opened (Figure 47–8E), an 8 to10-cm 22-gauge needle is inserted between the zygomatic arch and the mandibular notch. After contact with the lateral pterygoid plate (position 1 in figure), the needle is partially withdrawn and angled slightly superiorly and posteriorly toward the ear (position 2). Local anesthetic is injected once paresthesias are elicited.

The lingual and inferior mandibular branches of the mandibular nerve may be blocked intraorally utilizing a 10-cm 22-gauge needle (Figure 47–8F). The patient is asked to open the mouth maximally and the coronoid notch is palpated with the index finger of the nonoperative hand. The needle is then introduced at the same level (approximately 1 cm above the surface of the last molar), medial to the finger but lateral to the pterygomandibular plica (position 1 in figure). It is advanced posteriorly 1.5–2 cm along the medial side of the mandibular ramus, making contact with the bone (position 2). Both nerves are usually blocked following injection of local anesthetic.

The terminal portion of the inferior alveolar nerve may be blocked as it emerges from the mental foramen at the mid-mandible just beneath the corner of the mouth. Local anesthetic is injected once paresthesias are elicited or the needle is felt to enter the foramen.

D. Complications

Complications of a gasserian ganglion block include accidental intravascular injection, subarachnoid injection, Horner's syndrome, and motor block of the muscles of mastication. The potential for serious hemorrhage is greatest for blockade of the maxillary nerve. The facial nerve may be unintentionally blocked during blocks of the mandibular division.

Facial Nerve Block

A. Indications

Blockade of the facial nerve is occasionally indicated to relieve spastic contraction of the facial muscles, to treat herpes zoster involving the facial nerve, and to facilitate certain surgical procedures involving the eye.

B. Anatomy

The facial nerve can be blocked where it exits the cranium through the stylomastoid foramen. A small sensory component supplies special sensation (taste) to the anterior two thirds of the tongue and general sensation to the tympanic membrane, the external auditory meatus, soft palate, and part of the pharynx.

C. Technique

The entry point is just anterior to the mastoid process, beneath the external auditory meatus, and at the midpoint of the mandibular ramus. The nerve is approximately 1–2 cm deep and is blocked with local anesthetic just below the stylomastoid process.

D. Complications

If the needle is inserted too deeply past the level of the styloid bone, the glossopharyngeal and vagal nerves may also be blocked. Careful aspiration is necessary because of the proximity of the facial nerve to the carotid artery and the internal jugular vein.

Glossopharyngeal Block

A. Indications

Glossopharyngeal nerve block may be used for patients with pain due to cancer involving the base of the tongue, the epiglottis, or the palatine tonsils. It can also be used to distinguish glossopharyngeal neuralgia from trigeminal and geniculate neuralgia.

B. Anatomy

The nerve exits from the cranium via the jugular foramen medial to the styloid process and courses anteromedially to supply the posterior third of the tongue, pharyngeal muscles, and mucosa. The vagus and spinal accessory nerves also exit the cranium via the jugular foramen and descend alongside the glossopharyngeal nerve in close proximity to the internal jugular vein.

C. Technique

The block is performed using a 5-cm 22-gauge needle inserted just posterior to the angle of the mandible (Figure 47–9). The nerve is approximately 3–4 cm deep; therefore, use of a nerve stimulator facilitates correct placement of the needle. An alternative approach is from a point over the styloid process, midway between the mastoid process and the angle of the mandible; the nerve is located just anteriorly.

D. Complications

Complications include dysphagia and vagal blockade resulting in ipsilateral vocal cord paralysis

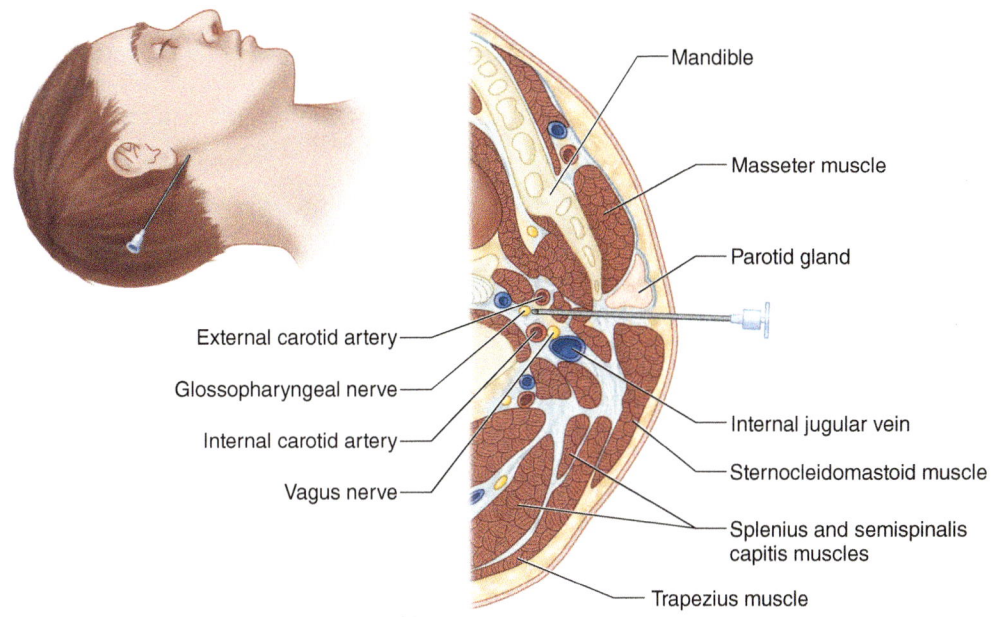

FIGURE 47–9 Glossopharyngeal nerve block.

and tachycardia. Block of the accessory nerve and hypoglossal nerves causes ipsilateral paralysis of the trapezius muscle and the tongue, respectively. Careful aspiration is necessary to prevent intravascular injection.

Occipital Nerve Block

A. Indications

Occipital nerve block is useful diagnostically and therapeutically in patients with occipital headaches and neuralgias.

B. Anatomy

The greater occipital nerve is derived from the dorsal primary rami of the C2 and C3 spinal nerves, whereas the lesser occipital nerve arises from the ventral rami of the same roots.

C. Technique

The greater occipital nerve is blocked approximately 3 cm lateral to the occipital prominence at the level of the superior nuchal line (Figure 47–10); the nerve is just medial to the occipital artery, which is often palpable. The lesser occipital nerve is blocked 2–3 cm more laterally along the nuchal ridge. Ultrasound

guidance may be employed to help identify the nerves and minimize the risk of inadvertent intravenous or intraarterial injection. For patients who have responded well but temporarily to occipital

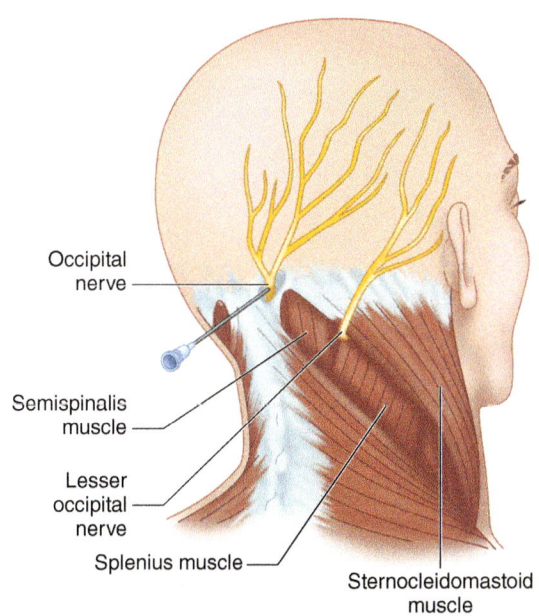

FIGURE 47–10 Occipital nerve blocks.

nerve blocks, implantation of an occipital nerve stimulator may provide prolonged relief.

D. Complications

Rarely, intravascular injections may occur.

Suprascapular Nerve Block

A. Indications

This block is useful for painful conditions arising from the shoulder (most commonly arthritis and bursitis).

B. Anatomy

The suprascapular nerve is the major sensory nerve of the shoulder joint. It arises from the brachial plexus (C4–C6) and passes over the upper border of the scapula in the suprascapular notch to enter the suprascapular fossa.

C. Technique

The nerve is blocked at the suprascapular notch, which is located at the junction of the lateral and middle thirds of the superior scapular border (**Figure 47–11**). Correct placement of the needle is determined by paresthesia, ultrasound, or the use of a nerve stimulator.

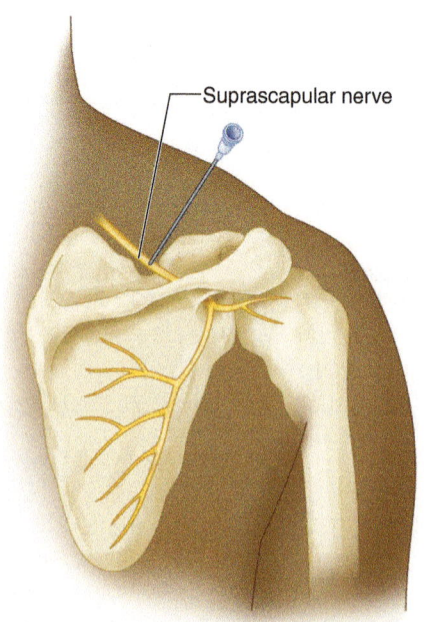

—Suprascapular nerve

FIGURE 47–11 Suprascapular nerve block.

D. Complications

Pneumothorax is possible if the needle is advanced too far anteriorly. Paralysis of the supraspinatus and infraspinatus muscles will result in impaired shoulder abduction.

Cervical Paravertebral Nerve Blocks

A. Indications

Cervical paravertebral nerve blocks can be useful diagnostically and therapeutically for patients with cervical disc displacement, cervical foraminal stenosis, or cancer-related pain originating from the cervical spine or shoulder.

B. Anatomy

The cervical spinal nerves lie in the sulcus of the transverse process of their respective vertebral levels. As noted earlier in this chapter, unlike thoracic and lumbar nerve roots, those in the cervical spine exit the foramina *above* the vertebral bodies for which they are named.

C. Technique

The lateral approach is most commonly used to block C2–C7 (**Figure 47–12**). Patients are asked to turn the head to the opposite side while in a sitting or supine position. A line is then drawn between the mastoid process and Chassaignac's tubercle (the tubercle of the C6 transverse process). A series of injections are made with a 5-cm 22-gauge needle along a second parallel line 0.5 cm posterior to the first line. In the case of diagnostic blocks, a smaller injectate volume may be helpful in order to minimize local anesthetic spread to adjacent structures and thereby increase block specificity. Because the transverse process of C2 is usually difficult to palpate, the injection for this level is placed 1.5 cm beneath the mastoid process. The other transverse processes are usually interspaced 1.5 cm apart and are 2.5–3 cm deep. Fluoroscopy is useful in identifying specific vertebral levels during diagnostic blocks. This procedure may also be performed with ultrasound guidance.

D. Complications

Unintentional intrathecal or epidural anesthesia at this level rapidly causes respiratory paralysis and hypotension. Injection of even small volumes of local anesthetic into the vertebral artery causes

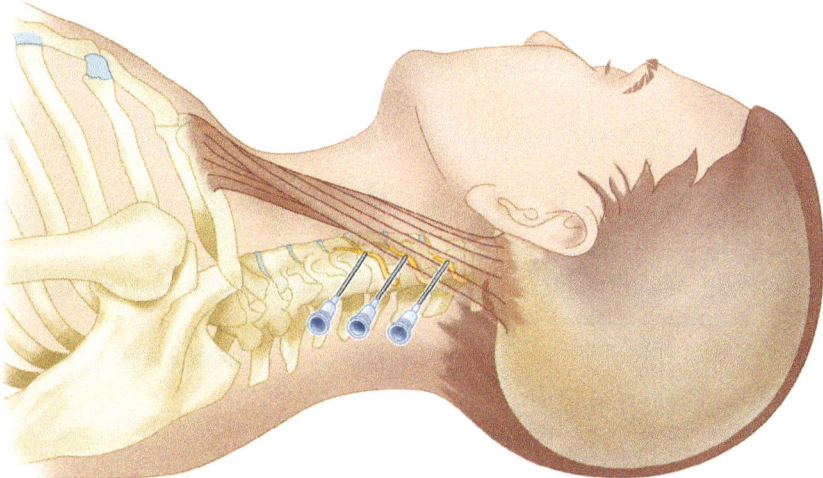

FIGURE 47–12 Cervical paravertebral nerve block.

unconsciousness and seizures. Other complications include Horner's syndrome, as well as blockade of the recurrent laryngeal and phrenic nerves.

Embolic cerebrovascular and spinal cord complications have resulted from injection of particulate steroid with this block. Particulate steroid should not be used with cervical paravertebral nerve blocks because of possible anomalous vertebral artery anatomy in this region.

Thoracic Paravertebral Nerve Block

A. Indications
This technique may be used to block the upper thoracic segments, because the scapula interferes with the intercostal technique at these levels. Unlike an intercostal nerve block, a thoracic paravertebral nerve block anesthetizes both the dorsal and ventral rami of spinal nerves. It is therefore useful in patients with pain originating from the thoracic spine, thoracic cage, or abdominal wall, including compression fractures, proximal rib fractures, and acute herpes zoster. This block is also frequently utilized for intraoperative anesthesia and for postoperative pain management in breast surgery.

B. Anatomy
Each thoracic nerve root exits from the spinal canal just inferior to the transverse process of its corresponding spinal segment.

C. Technique
This block may be performed with the patient prone, lateral, or seated position. A 5- to 8-cm 22-gauge spinal needle with an adjustable marker (bead or rubber stopper) is used. With the classic technique, the needle is inserted 4–5 cm lateral to the midline at the spinous process of the level above. The needle is directed anteriorly and medially using a 45° angle with the mid-sagittal plane, and advanced until it contacts the transverse process of the desired level. The needle is then partially withdrawn and redirected to pass just under the transverse process. The adjustable marker on the needle is used to mark the depth of the spinous process; when the needle is subsequently withdrawn and redirected, it should not be advanced more than 2 cm beyond this mark. An alternative technique that may decrease the risk of pneumothorax uses a more medial insertion point and a loss-of-resistance technique very similar to epidural anesthesia. The needle is inserted in a sagittal plane 1.5 cm lateral to the midline at the level of the spinous process above and advanced until it contacts the lateral edge of the lamina of the level to be blocked. It is then withdrawn to a subcutaneous position and reinserted 0.5 cm more laterally but still in a sagittal plane. As the needle is advanced, it engages the superior costotransverse ligament, just lateral to the lamina and inferior to the transverse process. The correct position may be identified by loss of resistance to injection of saline

when the needle penetrates the costotransverse ligament. Ultrasound guidance is helpful in performing this block (see Chapter 46).

D. Complications

The most common complication of paravertebral block is pneumothorax; accidental intrathecal, epidural, and intravascular injections may also occur. Sympathetic blockade and hypotension may be obtained if multiple segments are blocked or a large volume is injected at one level. A chest radiograph is mandatory if the patient exhibits signs or symptoms of pneumothorax.

Lumbar Paravertebral Nerve Blocks

A. Indications

Lumbar paravertebral nerve blocks may be useful in evaluating pain due to disorders involving the lumbar spine or spinal nerves.

B. Anatomy

The lumbar spinal nerves enter the psoas compartment as soon as they exit through the intervertebral foramina beneath the pedicles and transverse processes. This compartment is formed by the psoas fascia anteriorly, the quadratus lumborum fascia posteriorly, and the vertebral bodies medially.

C. Technique

The approach to lumbar spinal nerves is essentially the same as for thoracic paravertebral blockade (Figure 47–13). An 8-cm 22-gauge needle is usually used. Radiographic confirmation of the correct level is helpful. For diagnostic blocks, only 2 mL of local

anesthetic is injected at any one level, because larger volumes may block more than one level. Larger volumes of local anesthetic are used for therapeutic blocks, or to produce complete somatic and sympathetic block of the lumbar nerves.

D. Complications

Complications are primarily those of unintentional intrathecal or epidural anesthesia. Patients may experience paresthesias if inadvertent nerve injury occurs during needle placement. Some physicians advocate the use of a blunt-tipped needle to (theoretically) decrease the chance of accidental intraneural injection. Digital subtraction angiography with radiopaque contrast may lessen the risk of intravascular injection of local anesthetic or steroid.

Cervical, Thoracic, & Lumbar Medial Branch Blocks

A. Indications

These blocks may be utilized in patients with back pain to assess the contribution of lumbar facet (zygapophyseal) joint disease. Corticosteroids are commonly injected with the local anesthetic when the intraarticular technique is chosen. The cervical, thoracic, or lumbar facet joints may be injected for diagnostic and potentially therapeutic purposes.

B. Anatomy

Each facet joint is innervated by the medial branches of the posterior primary division of the spinal nerves above and below the joint (Figure 47–14). Thus,

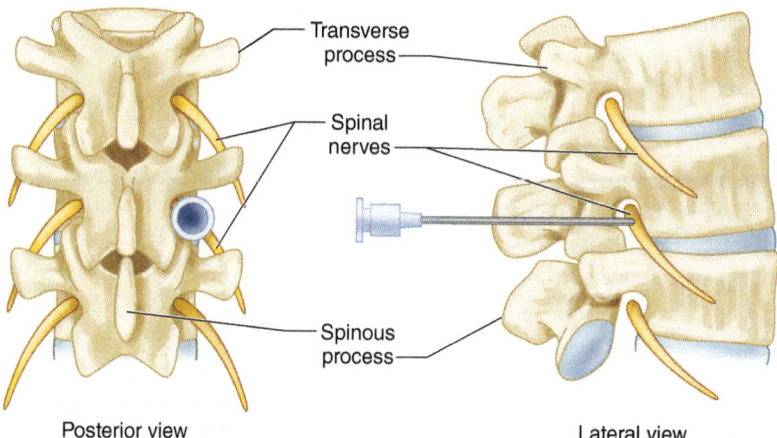

Transverse process

Spinal nerves

Spinal nerves

Transverse process

Spinous process

FIGURE 47–13 Lumbar paravertebral nerve blocks.   Posterior view   Lateral view

A

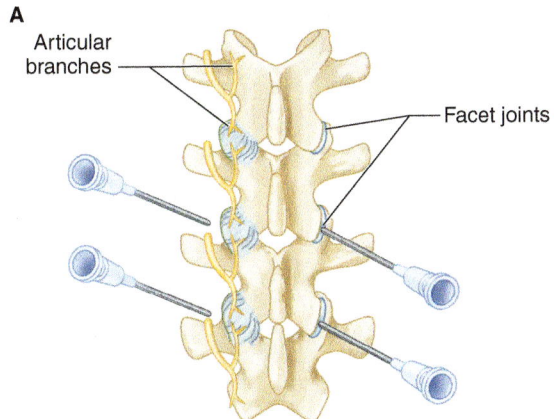

Articular branches

Facet joints

B

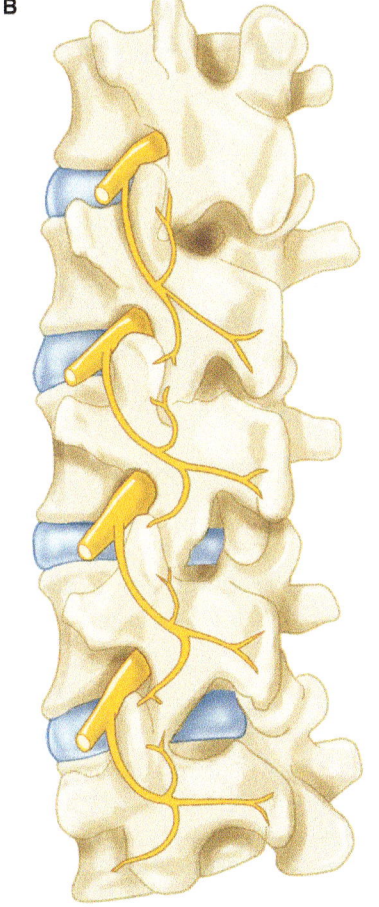

every joint is supplied by two or more adjacent spinal nerves. Each medial branch crosses the upper border of the lower transverse process running in a groove between the root of the transverse process and the superior articular process.

C. Technique

These blocks are performed under fluoroscopic guidance with the patient in a prone position, or in some cases, the lateral position for cervical procedures. A posterior–anterior view facilitates visualization of the spine for lumbar medial branch blocks. A 10-cm 22-gauge needle is inserted 3–4 cm lateral to the spinous process at the desired level and directed anteriorly toward the junction of the transverse process and the superior articular process to block the medial branch of the posterior division of the spinal nerve (Figures 47–15 through 47–17).

Alternatively, local anesthetic with or without corticosteroid may be directly injected into the facet joint. Positioning the patient prone and using an oblique fluoroscopic view facilitates identification of the joint space. Correct placement of the needle may be confirmed by injecting radiopaque contrast prior to injection of local anesthetic. Total injection volumes should ideally be limited to less than 1 mL in order to prevent rupture of the joint capsule.

D. Complications

Injection into a dural sleeve results in a subarachnoid block, whereas injection near the spinal nerve

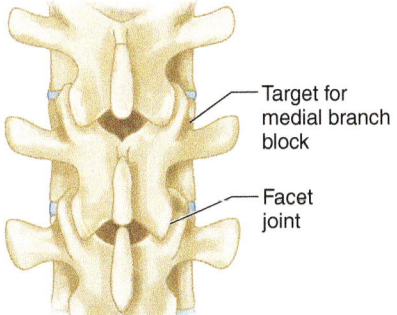

Target for medial branch block

Facet joint

FIGURE 47–14 Lumbar medial branch nerve and facet blocks. **A:** Posterior view; **B:** 30° oblique posterior view.

FIGURE 47–15 Anatomy of the lumbar facet joint and location for blocking the medial branch of the posterior primary division of the lumbar spinal nerves above and below the joint.

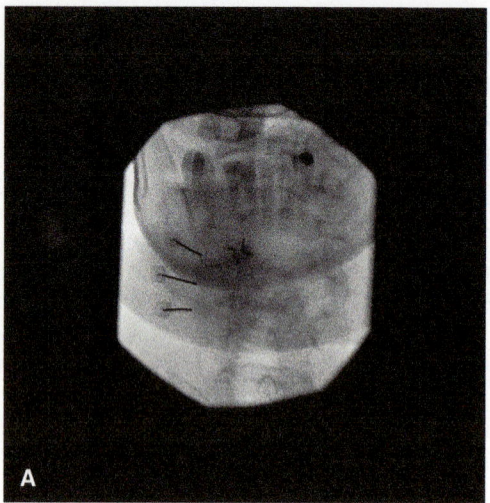

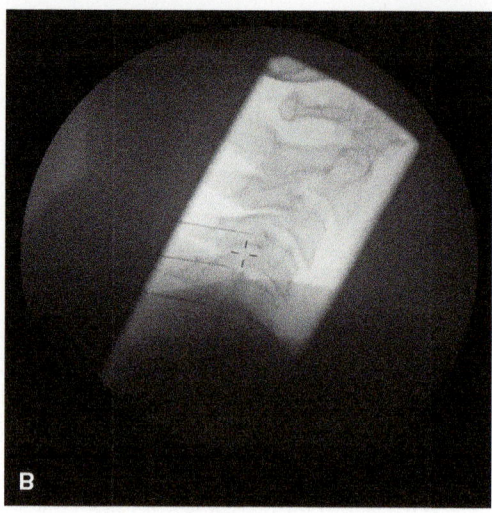

FIGURE 47–16 Fluoroscopic image of a cervical medial branch blockade. **A:** Anteroposterior view; **B:** Lateral view. The lateral view reveals the needles at C4, C5, and C6 advanced toward the trapezoid of the articular pillar at each level. Note the "waist" of the vertebrae. Spinal needles may be advanced to come into contact with the medial branch of the nerve.

root results in sensory and motor block at that level. Because the joint normally has a small volume, larger injections can cause rupture of the joint capsule.

If a patient achieves improved pain control after a diagnostic block, he or she may be considered for radiofrequency ablation of the medial branch. There is debate about whether a second, confirmatory diagnostic block should be performed prior to radiofrequency ablation. Injection of steroid may be considered before or after radiofrequency ablation to theoretically decrease the chance for postprocedural neuritis.

Trans-Sacral Nerve Block

A. Indications

This technique is useful in the diagnosis and treatment of pelvic and perineal pain. In addition, blockade of the S1 spinal root can help define its role in back pain.

B. Anatomy

The five paired sacral spinal nerves and one pair of coccygeal nerves descend in the sacral canal. Each nerve then travels through its respective intervertebral foramen. The S5 and coccygeal nerves exit through the sacral hiatus.

C. Technique

While the patient is prone, the sacral foramina are identified with a needle along a line drawn 1.5 cm medial to the posterior superior iliac spine and 1.5 cm

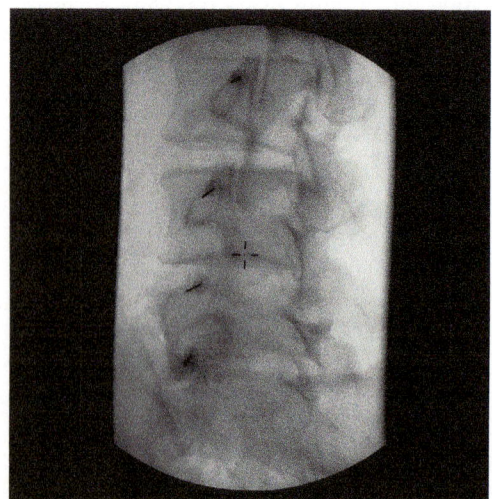

FIGURE 47–17 Left lumbar medial branch blockade, oblique view.

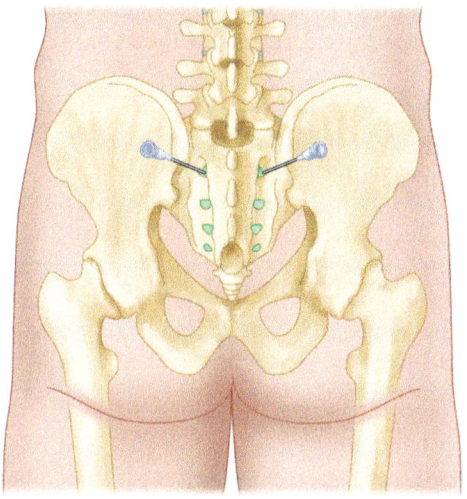

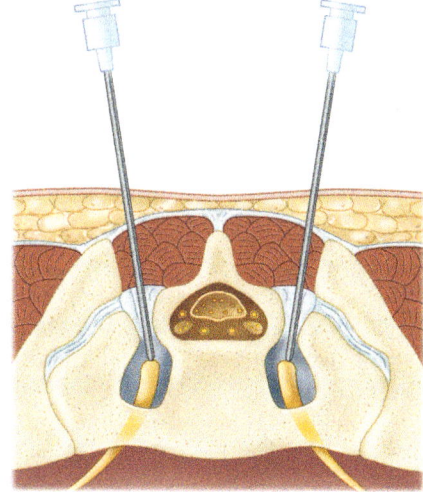

Posterior

Sagittal

FIGURE 47–18 Trans-sacral nerve block.

lateral to the ipsilateral sacral cornu (Figure 47–18). Correct positioning requires entry of the needle into the posterior sacral foramen and usually produces paresthesias. The S1 nerve root is usually 1.5 cm above the level of the posterior superior iliac spine along this imaginary line. Blockade of the S5 and coccygeal nerves can be accomplished by injection at the sacral hiatus.

D. Complications

Complications are rare but include nerve damage and intravascular injection.

Pudendal Nerve Block

A. Indications

Pudendal nerve block is useful in evaluating patients with perineal somatosensory pain.

B. Anatomy

The pudendal nerve arises from S2–S4 and courses between the sacrospinous and the sacrotuberous ligaments to reach the perineum.

C. Technique

This block is usually performed transperineally with the patient in the lithotomy position (Figure 47–19) although it may be performed via a posterior

approach in the prone position. Injection of anesthetic is carried out percutaneously just posterior to the ischial spine at the attachment of the sacrospinous ligament. The ischial spine can be palpated transrectally or transvaginally. Alternatively, this procedure may be performed in the prone position with a 22-gauge needle directed toward the base of

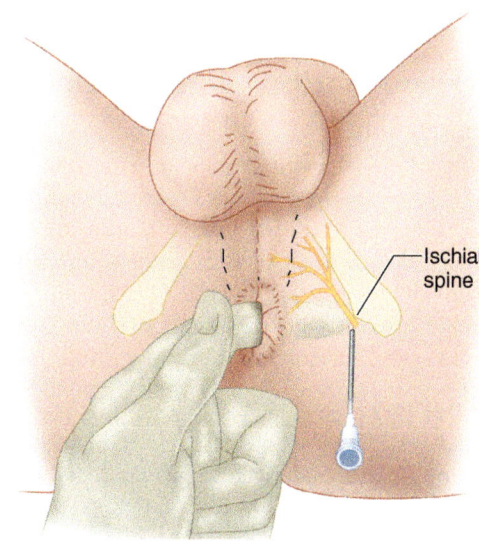

Ischial spine

FIGURE 47–19 Pudendal nerve block.

the ischial spine. Patients should be advised that they may have numbness of the genitalia for hours after this procedure is performed.

D. Complications

Potential complications include unintentional sciatic blockade and intravascular injection.

3. Sympathetic Nerve Blocks

Sympathetic blockade can be accomplished by a variety of techniques, including intrathecal, epidural, and paravertebral blocks. Unfortunately, these approaches usually block both somatic and sympathetic fibers. Problems with differential spinal and epidural techniques are discussed below. The following techniques specifically block sympathetic fibers and can be used to define the role of the sympathetic system in a patient's pain and possibly also provide long-term pain relief. The most common indications for sympathetic nerve blocks include reflex sympathetic dystrophy, visceral pain, acute herpetic neuralgia, postherpetic pain, and peripheral vascular disease. Isolated sympathetic blockade to a region is characterized by loss of sympathetic tone, as evidenced by increased cutaneous blood flow and cutaneous temperature, and by unaltered somatic sensation. Other tests include loss of the skin conductance (sympathogalvanic reflex) and sweat response (ninhydrin, cobalt blue, or starch tests) following a painful stimulus.

Cervicothoracic (Stellate) Block

A. Indications

This block is often used for patients with head, neck, arm, and upper chest pain. It is commonly referred to as a stellate block but usually blocks the upper thoracic as well as all cervical ganglia. Injection of larger volumes of anesthetic often extends the block to the T5 ganglia. Stellate blocks may also be used for vasospastic disorders of the upper extremity.

B. Anatomy

Sympathetic innervation of the head, neck, and most of the arm is derived from four cervical ganglia, the largest being the stellate ganglion. The latter usually represents a fusion of the lower cervical and first thoracic ganglia. Some sympathetic innervation

of the arm (T1) as well as innervation of all of the thoracic viscera derives from the five upper thoracic ganglia. The sympathetic supply to the arm in some persons may also originate from T2–T3 via anatomically distinct nerves (Kuntz's nerves) that join the brachial plexus high in the axilla. These nerves may be missed by a stellate block but not an axillary block. The point of injection is at the level of the stellate, which lies posterior to the origin of the vertebral artery from the subclavian artery, anterior to the longus colli muscle and the first rib, anterolateral to the prevertebral fascia, and medial to the scalene muscles.

C. Technique

The paratracheal technique is most commonly used (**Figure 47–20**), although an oblique or posterior approach may also be taken. With the patient's head extended, a 4- to 5-cm 22-gauge needle is inserted at the medial edge of the sternocleidomastoid muscle just below the level of the cricoid cartilage at the level of the transverse process of C6 (Chassaignac's tubercle) or C7 (3–5 cm above the clavicle). The nonoperative hand should be used to retract the muscle together with the carotid sheath prior to needle insertion. The needle is advanced to the transverse process and withdrawn 2–3 mm prior to injection. Aspiration must be carried out in two planes before a 1-mL test dose is used to exclude unintentional intravascular injection into the vertebral or subclavian arteries or subarachnoid injection into a dural sleeve. A total of 5–10 mL of local anesthetic may be injected. Although this procedure is often performed under fluoroscopy, ultrasound may also be used to visualize the anatomy and decrease the risk of inadvertent intravascular injection.

Correct placement of the needle is usually followed promptly by an increase in the skin temperature of the ipsilateral arm and the onset of Horner's syndrome. The latter consists of ipsilateral ptosis, meiosis, enophthalmos, nasal congestion, and anhydrosis of the neck and face. This may be considered a side effect of the block rather than a complication.

D. Complications

20 In addition to intravascular and subarachnoid injection, other complications of stellate block include hematoma, pneumothorax, epidural

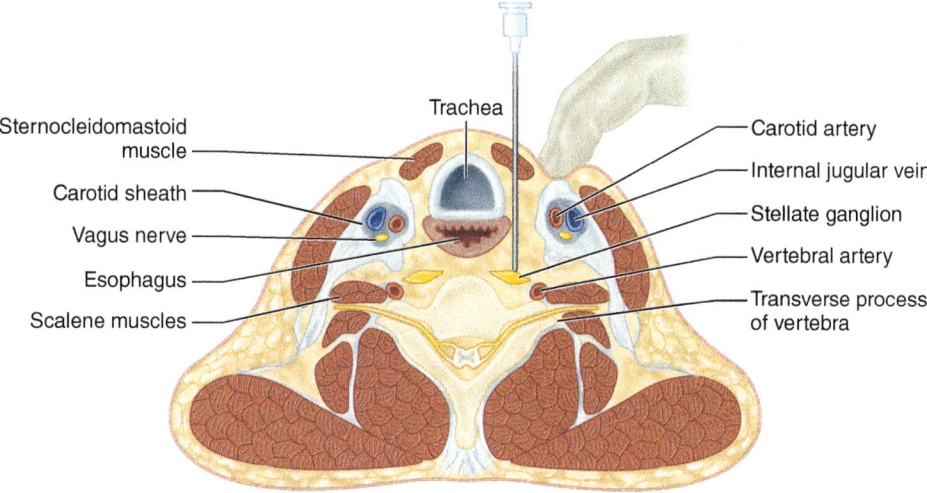

FIGURE 47–20 Stellate block.

anesthesia, brachial plexus block, hoarseness due to blockade of the recurrent laryngeal nerve, and, rarely, osteomyelitis or mediastinitis following esophageal puncture, particularly if a left-sided approach is taken. The posterior approach may have the highest incidence of pneumothorax.

Thoracic Sympathetic Chain Block

The thoracic sympathetic ganglia lie just lateral to the vertebral bodies and anterior to the spinal nerve roots, but this block is generally not used because of a significant risk of pneumothorax.

Splanchnic Nerve Block

Three groups of splanchnic nerves (greater, lesser, and least) arise from the lower seven thoracic sympathetic ganglia on each side and descend alongside the vertebral bodies to communicate with the celiac ganglia. Although similar to celiac plexus block, the splanchnic nerve block may be preferred because it is less likely to block the lumbar sympathetic chain and because it requires less anesthetic.

The needle is inserted 6–7 cm from the midline at the lower end of the T11 spinous process, and advanced under fluoroscopic guidance to the anterolateral surface of T12. Ten milliliters of local anesthetic is injected on each side. The needle should maintain contact with the vertebral body at all times

to avoid a pneumothorax. Other complications may include hypotension and possible injury to the azygos vein on the right or to the hemiazygos vein and the thoracic duct on the left.

If a patient's pain lessens after a splanchnic nerve block, the procedure may be repeated to ensure that this result was not due to placebo effect. In addition, if the patient obtained pain relief from the initial block, he or she may subsequently benefit from radiofrequency ablation of the splanchnic nerves at T11 and T12, with potentially longer duration of analgesia. Performing the procedure on one side initially, and then the other side on a subsequent day, is advised due to the risk of pneumothorax.

Celiac Plexus Block

A. Indications

A celiac plexus block is indicated for patients with pain arising from the abdominal viscera, particularly intraabdominal cancers.

B. Anatomy

The celiac ganglia vary in number (1–5), form, and position. They are generally clustered at the level of the body of L1, posterior to the vena cava on the right, just lateral to the aorta on the left, and posterior to the pancreas.

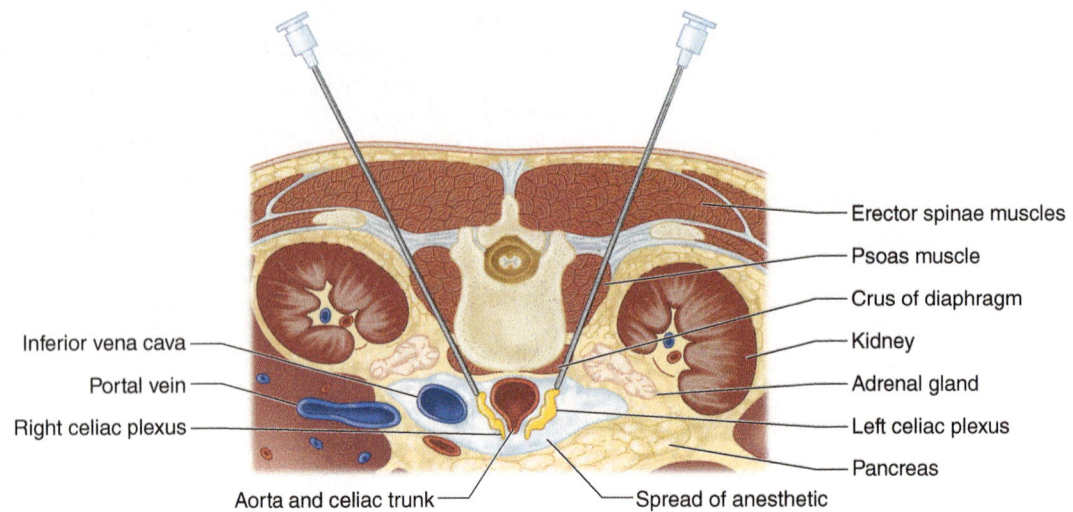

Inferior vena cava —
Portal vein —
Right celiac plexus —

Aorta and celiac trunk —

— Erector spinae muscles
— Psoas muscle
— Crus of diaphragm
— Kidney
— Adrenal gland
— Left celiac plexus
— Pancreas
— Spread of anesthetic

FIGURE 47–21 Celiac plexus block.

C. Technique

The patient is placed in a prone position and a 15-cm 22-gauge needle is used to inject 15–20 mL of local anesthetic (Figure 47–21). Under fluoroscopic guidance, each needle is inserted 7–8 cm from the midline at the inferior edge of the spinous process of L1. It is advanced under radiographic guidance toward the midline, making an approximately 10–45° angle. The needle passes under the edge of the twelfth rib and should be positioned anterior to the body of L1 in the lateral radiographic view and close to the midline overlying the same vertebral body in the anteroposterior view. When CT guidance is used, the tip of the needle should come to lie anterolateral to the aorta at a level between the celiac and superior mesenteric arteries.

The celiac plexus block may be performed from multiple approaches including a posterior retrocrural approach, a posterior anterocrural approach, a posterior transaortic approach, and an anterior approach. These blocks may be facilitated with the use of fluoroscopy, CT, or ultrasound guidance.

D. Complications

The most common complication is postural hypotension, from block of the visceral sympathetic innervation and resultant vasodilation. For this reason, patients should be adequately hydrated intravenously prior to this block. Accidental intravascular

injection into the vena cava is more likely to produce a severe systemic reaction than accidental intraaortic injection. Other, less common, complications include pneumothorax, retroperitoneal hemorrhage, injury to the kidneys or pancreas, sexual dysfunction, or, rarely, paraplegia (due to injury to the lumbar artery of Adamkiewicz). Blocking the sympathetic chain may result in relatively unopposed parasympathetic activity that may lead to increased gastrointestinal motility and diarrhea. Back pain is another common side effect of a celiac plexus block.

Lumbar Sympathetic Block

A. Indications

Lumbar sympathetic block may be indicated for painful conditions involving the pelvis or the lower extremities, and possibly for some patients with peripheral vascular disease.

B. Anatomy

The lumbar sympathetic chain contains three to five ganglia and is a continuation of the thoracic chain. It also supplies sympathetic fibers to the pelvic plexus and ganglia. The lumbar sympathetic chain ganglia are in a more anteromedial position to the vertebral bodies than the thoracic ganglia, and are anterior to the psoas muscle and fascia. The lumbar chain is usually posterior to the vena cava on the right but is just lateral to the aorta on the left.

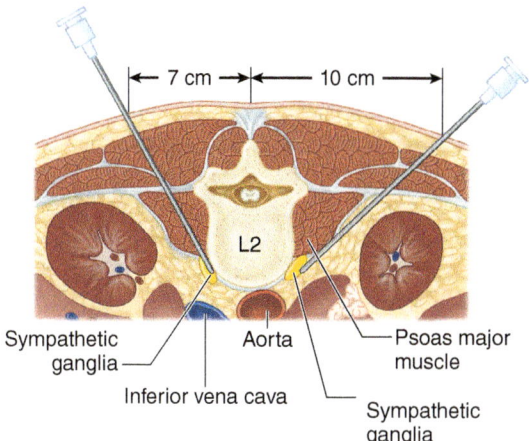

← 7 cm → |← 10 cm →

L2

Sympathetic ganglia

Aorta

Psoas major muscle

Inferior vena cava

Sympathetic ganglia

FIGURE 47–22 Lumbar sympathetic block.

C. Technique

A single-needle technique at the L3 level on either side is most commonly employed with the patient either prone or in a lateral position (Figure 47–22). The needle is inserted at the upper edge of the spinous process and is directed above or just lateral to the transverse process of the vertebrae (depending on the distance from the midline). Fluoroscopic guidance with injection of radiopaque contrast prior to local anesthetic injection is often used.

D. Complications

Complications include intravascular injection into the vena cava, aorta, or lumbar vessels and somatic nerve block of the lumbar plexus. In particular, the genitofemoral nerve may be blocked.

Superior Hypogastric Plexus Block

A. Indications

This procedure is indicated for pain that originates from the pelvis and is unresponsive to lumbar or caudal epidural blocks. The hypogastric plexus contains visceral sensory fibers that bypass the lower spinal cord. This block is usually appropriate for patients with cancer of the cervix, uterus, bladder, prostate, or rectum. It may also be effective in some women with chronic noncancer pelvic pain.

B. Anatomy

The hypogastric plexus contains not only postganglionic fibers derived from the lumbar sympathetic chain, but also visceral sensory fibers from the cervix, uterus, bladder, prostate, and rectum. The superior hypogastric plexus usually lies just to the left of the midline at the L5 vertebral body and beneath the bifurcation of the aorta. The fibers of this plexus divide into left and right branches and descend to the pelvic organs via the left and right inferior hypogastric and pelvic plexuses. The inferior hypogastric plexus additionally receives preganglionic parasympathetic fibers from the S2–S4 spinal nerve roots.

C. Technique

The patient is positioned prone, and a 15-cm needle is inserted approximately 7 cm lateral to the L4–L5 spinal interspace. The needle is directed medially and caudally under fluoroscopic guidance so that it passes by the transverse process of L5. In its final position, the needle should lie anterior to the intervertebral disc between L5 and S1 and within 1 cm of the vertebral bodies in the anteroposterior view. Injection of radiopaque contrast confirms correct position of the needle in the retroperitoneal space; 8–10 mL of local anesthetic is then injected. The superior hypogastric plexus block may also be performed using a transdiscal approach, though there is a risk of discitis associated with this procedure.

D. Complications

Complications include intravascular injection and transient bowel and bladder dysfunction.

Ganglion Impar Block

A. Indications

21 Ganglion impar block is effective for patients with visceral or sympathetically maintained pain in the perineal area.

B. Anatomy

The ganglion impar (ganglion of Walther) is the most caudal part of the sympathetic trunks. The two lowest pelvic sympathetic ganglia often fuse forming one ganglion in the midline just anterior to the coccyx.

C. Technique

The patient may be positioned in the prone, lateral decubitus, or lithotomy position. A 22-gauge needle is advanced through the sacrococcygeal ligament and the rudimentary disc into a position just anterior to the coccyx. This procedure can be facilitated with fluoroscopy or ultrasound. Radiofrequency ablation, or in some cases a neurolytic injection, may provide longer duration of analgesia for this sympathetically mediated pain.

D. Complications

Intravascular injection and transient bowel or bladder dysfunction are possible. Alternative approaches involve placement of the needle through the anococcygeal ligament, although these may have higher potential to perforate the rectum.

Intravenous Regional Block

A Bier block (see Chapter 46) utilizing local anesthetic solution with or without adjuvants can be used to interrupt sympathetic innervation to an extremity. A total volume of 50 mL of 0.5% lidocaine is typically injected, either alone or in combination with clonidine (150 mcg) and in some cases ketorolac (15–30 mg). A tourniquet is placed proximally on the extremity, which is then elevated and exsanguinated using an Esmarch bandage. The tourniquet is inflated to a pressure that is two times the systolic blood pressure, the Esmarch bandage is removed, and the limb is checked to be certain the pulse is absent and there is no evidence of blood flow. The solution is then injected and usually left in place for at least 30 min, after which the tourniquet is released incrementally and the patient is observed for any signs or symptoms of local anesthetic toxicity. Premature release of the tourniquet may result in seizure, hypotension, arrhythmia, edema, diarrhea, and nausea. Intravenous regional sympathetic block is a safe alternative to standard sympathetic blocks in patients with hemostatic defects.

4. Epidural Injections

Epidural steroid injections (Figure 47–23) are used for symptomatic relief of pain associated with nerve root compression (radiculopathy). Pathological studies often demonstrate inflammation following disc herniation. Clinical improvement appears to be correlated with the resolution of nerve root edema. Epidural steroid injections are clearly superior to local anesthetics alone. They are most effective when

given within 2 weeks of pain onset but appear to be of little benefit in the absence of neural compression or irritation. Long-term studies have failed to show any persistent benefit after 3 months, and these injections may change the time course of pain relief without changing long-term outcomes.

The two most commonly used agents are methylprednisolone acetate (40–80 mg) and triamcinolone diacetate (40–80 mg). Dexamethasone is being used with increased frequency due to its smaller particulate size (smaller than an erythrocyte). Intravascular injection of steroid suspension with larger particulate size may lead to embolic complications. The steroid may be injected with diluent (saline) or local anesthetic in volumes of 6–10 mL or 10–20 mL for lumbar and caudal injections, respectively. Simultaneous injection of opioids offers no added benefit and may significantly increase risks. The epidural needle should be cleared of the steroid prior to its withdrawal to prevent formation of a fistula tract or skin discoloration. Injection of local anesthetic along with the steroid can be helpful if the patient has significant muscle spasm, but it is associated with risks of intrathecal, subdural, and intravascular injection. The presenting pain is often transiently intensified following injection, and the local anesthetic provides immediate pain relief until the steroidal antiinflammatory effects take place, usually within 12–48 h.

Epidural steroid injections may be most effective when the injection is at the site of injury. Only a single injection is given if complete pain relief is achieved. If there is a good but temporary response, a second injection may be given 2–4 weeks later. Larger or more frequent doses increase the risk of adrenal suppression and systemic side effects. Most pain practitioners utilize fluoroscopy for epidural injection and confirm correct placement with injection of radiopaque contrast (Figures 47–24 through 47–26). A transforaminal epidural steroid injection may be more effective than the standard interlaminar epidural technique, especially for radicular pain. The needle is directed under fluoroscopic guidance into the foramen of the affected nerve root; contrast is then injected to confirm spread into the epidural space and absence of intravascular injection prior to steroid injection. This technique differs from a

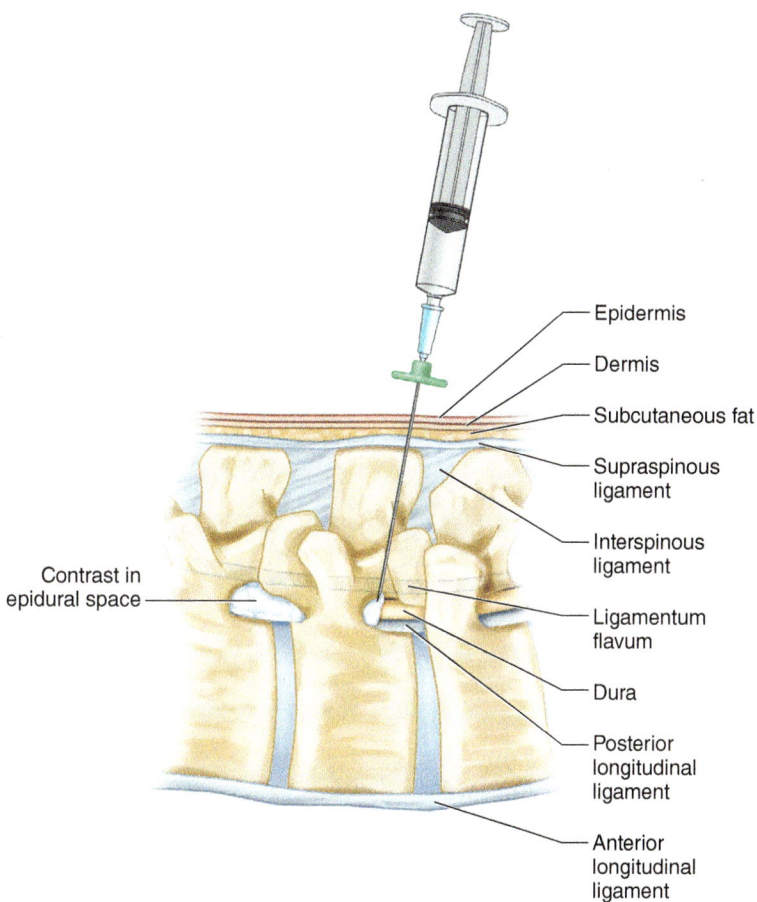

Epidermis

Dermis

Subcutaneous fat

Supraspinous
ligament

Interspinous
ligament

Ligamentum
flavum

Dura

Posterior
longitudinal
ligament

Anterior
longitudinal
ligament

Contrast in
epidural space

FIGURE 47–23 Epidural injection.

selective nerve root block (SNRB) in two important ways; with an SNRB, the needle does not enter the foramen and the injected solution tracks along the nerve but not into the epidural space. The SNRB may be helpful as a diagnostic procedure for the surgeon who is considering a foraminotomy at a particular affected level based upon imaging, clinical presentation, and the results of the SNRB.

Caudal injection may be used in patients with previous back surgery when scarring and anatomic distortion make lumbar epidural injections more difficult. Unfortunately, migration of the steroid to the site of injury may not be optimal. The use of a catheter to direct the injection within the sacral and epidural canal may improve outcome. However,

above the level of S2, there is a risk of thecal perforation with a stylet-guided catheter. Intrathecal steroid injections are not recommended because the ethylene glycol preservative in the suspension has been implicated in arachnoiditis following unintentional subarachnoid injections.

5. Radiofrequency Ablation & Cryoneurolysis

Percutaneous radiofrequency ablation (RFA) relies on the heat produced by current flow from an active electrode that is incorporated at the tip of a special needle. The needle is positioned using fluoroscopic guidance. Electrical stimulation (2 Hz for motor

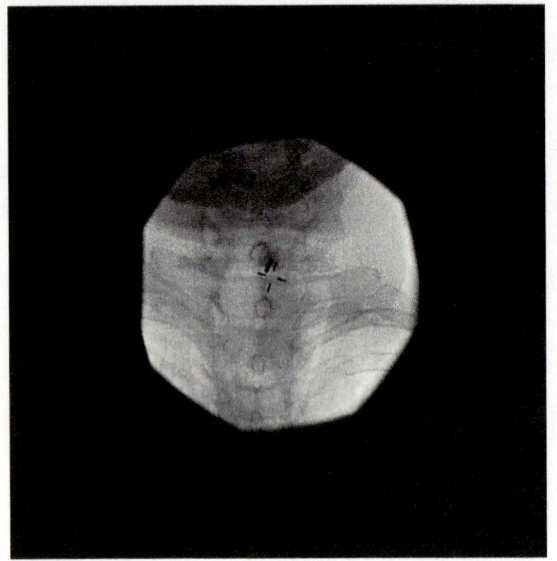

FIGURE 47–24 Fluoroscopic image of a C7–T1 epidural steroid injection; anteroposterior view. Note the Tuohy needle advanced just to the right of midline for treatment of degenerative disc disease and right radicular pain.

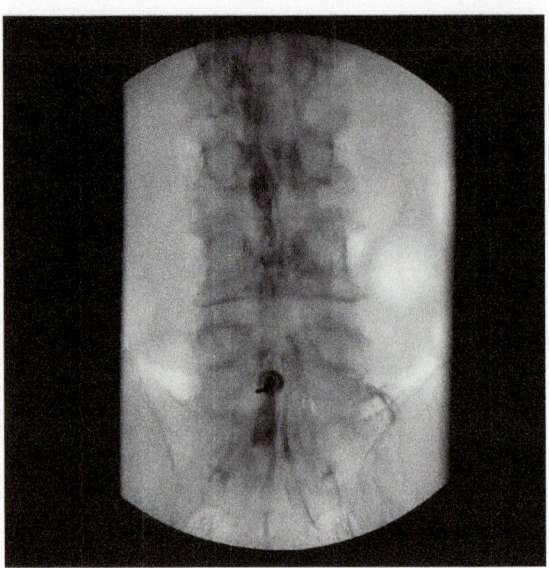

FIGURE 47–26 Lumbar epidural steroid injection, anteroposterior view. The epidural injection of contrast followed by local anesthetic and steroid solution results in spread at multiple levels of the epidural space and through the neuroforamen.

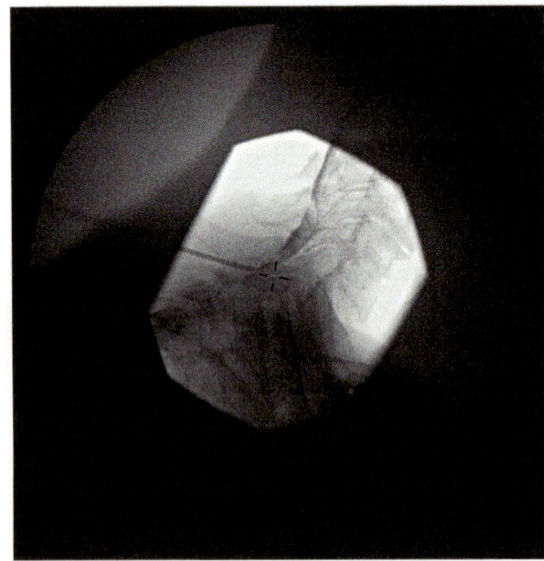

FIGURE 47–25 Fluoroscopic image of a C7–T1 epidural steroid injection with contrast; lateral view. Note radiopaque contrast confirmation of the needle in the epidural space. Live fluoroscopy is used to minimize the risk of inadvertent intravascular injection.

responses, 50 Hz for sensory responses) and impedance measurement via the electrode prior to ablation also help confirm correct electrode positioning. Depending on the location of the block, the heating temperature generated at the electrode is precisely controlled (60–90°C for 1–3 min) to ablate the nerve without causing excessive collateral tissue damage. RFA is commonly used for trigeminal rhizotomy and medial branch (facet) rhizotomy. It has also been used for dorsal root rhizotomy and lumbar sympathectomy. Pain relief is usually limited to 3–12 months due to nerve regeneration after RFA. This may be effective for medial branches of the spinal nerves that innervate facet joints. The lesion from thermal RFA is typically ovoid in shape and dependent upon factors such as the gauge of the needle, the temperature of the needle tip, and the duration of the heating procedure. Cooling the RFA needle with a sterile water system may decrease the charring associated with thermal lesioning and extend the spread of the lesion while heating at lower temperatures. Pulsed radiofrequency at 42°C is also being evaluated for various pain conditions.

Cryoanalgesia may produce temporary neurolysis for weeks to months by freezing and thawing tissue. The temperature at the tip of a cryoprobe rapidly drops as gas (carbon dioxide or nitrous oxide) at a high pressure is allowed to expand. The probe tip, which can achieve temperatures of –50°C to –70°C, is introduced via a 12- to 16-gauge catheter. Electrical stimulation (2–5 Hz for motor responses and 50–100 Hz for sensory responses) helps confirm correct positioning of the probe. Two or more 2-min cycles of freezing and thawing are usually administered. Cryoanalgesia is most commonly used to achieve long-term blockade of peripheral nerves. It may be particularly useful for post-thoracotomy pain. Patients often have neuropathic pain following thoracotomy or similar surgery. Diagnostic intercostal nerve blocks may be helpful to identify the nerve(s) that may be contributing to chronic thoracic or abdominal pain, and intercostal nerve blocks may also be utilized for longer term analgesia. The principal risks of intercostal nerve blocks are pneumothorax and local anesthetic toxicity. RFA of the intercostal nerves may be helpful as a palliative therapy for intercostal neuralgia, although there is a risk of deafferentation pain after this procedure.

6. Chemical Neurolysis

22 Neurolytic blocks are indicated for patients with severe, intractable cancer pain in whom more conventional therapy proves inadequate or conventional analgesic modalities are accompanied by unacceptable side effects. The most common chemical neurolytic techniques utilized for cancer patients are celiac plexus, lumbar sympathetic chain, hypogastric plexus, and ganglion impar blocks. Chemical neurolysis may also occasionally be used in patients with refractory benign neuralgia and, rarely, in patients with peripheral vascular disease. These blocks can be associated with considerable morbidity (loss of motor and sensory function), so patients must be selected carefully, and only after thorough consideration of alternative analgesic modalities. Moreover, although the initial result may be excellent, the original pain may recur, or new (deafferentation or central) pain will develop, in a majority of patients within weeks to months.

Temporary destruction of nerve fibers or ganglia can be accomplished by injection of alcohol or phenol. These neurolytic agents are not selective, affecting visceral, sensory, and motor fibers equally. Ethyl alcohol (50–100%) causes extraction of membrane phospholipids and precipitation of lipoproteins in axons and Schwann cells, whereas phenol (6–12%) appears to coagulate proteins. Alcohol causes severe pain on injection, thus local anesthetic is usually administered first. For peripheral nerve blocks, alcohol may be given undiluted, but for sympathetic blocks in which large volumes are injected, it is given in a 1:1 mixture with bupivacaine. Phenol is usually painless when injected either as an aqueous solution (6–8%) or in glycerol; a 12% phenol solution can be prepared in radiopaque contrast solution.

Neurolytic Techniques

Neurolytic celiac plexus or splanchnic nerve blocks may be effective for painful intraabdominal neoplasms, especially pancreatic cancer. Lumbar sympathetic, hypogastric plexus, or ganglion impar neurolytic blocks can be used for pain secondary to pelvic neoplasms. Neurolytic saddle block can provide pain relief for patients with refractory pain from pelvic malignancy; however, bowel and bladder dysfunction should be expected. Neurolytic intercostal blocks can be helpful for patients with painful rib metastases. Additional neurodestructive procedures, such as pituitary adenolysis and cordotomy, may be useful in end-of-life palliative care.

When considering any neurolytic technique, at least one diagnostic block with a local anesthetic solution alone should be used initially to confirm the pain pathway(s) involved and to assess the potential efficacy of the planned neurolysis. Local anesthetic solution should again be injected immediately prior to the neurolytic agent under fluoroscopic guidance. Following injection of any neurolytic agent, the needle must be cleared with air or saline prior to withdrawal to prevent damage to superficial structures.

Many clinicians prefer alcohol for celiac plexus block and phenol for lumbar sympathetic block. For subarachnoid neurolytic techniques, very small amounts of neurolytic agent (0.1 mL) are injected. Alcohol is hypobaric, whereas phenol in glycerin is hyperbaric; the patient undergoing subarachnoid neurolysis is carefully positioned so that the solution travels to the appropriate level and is confined to the dorsal horn region following subarachnoid administration.

Cancer patients frequently receive anticoagulation therapy if they are at elevated risk for venous thromboembolic phenomena. When such a patient has discontinued anticoagulant medication in preparation for a diagnostic local anesthetic block, it may be more practical to obtain consent for a neurolytic procedure in advance and to follow the diagnostic block immediately with chemical neurolysis if the diagnostic procedure has resulted in pain relief.

7. Differential Neural Blockade

Pharmacological or anatomic differential neural blockade has been advocated as a method of distinguishing somatic, sympathetic, and psychogenic pain mechanisms. The procedure is controversial owing to the challenges of interpreting the data and the inability to define exactly which nerve fibers or pathways are blocked. Theoretically, the pharmacological approach relies on the differential sensitivity of nerve fibers to local anesthetics. Preganglionic sympathetic (B) fibers are reported to be most sensitive, closely followed by pain (Aδ) fibers, somatosensory (Aβ) fibers, motor fibers (Aα), and finally C fibers. By using different concentrations of local anesthetic, it may be possible to selectively block certain types of fibers while preserving the function of others. The challenge is that the critical concentration needed to block sympathetic fibers can vary considerably between patients, and conduction block by local anesthetics is dependent not only on fiber size but also on the duration of contact and frequency of impulses conducted. Many clinicians have therefore abandoned the use of pharmacological differential neural blocks in favor of anatomic differential blockade.

Stellate ganglion blocks can be used to selectively block sympathetic fibers to the head, neck, and arm. Celiac plexus, hypogastric plexus, and lumbar paravertebral sympathetic blocks can be used for sympathetic blocks of the abdomen, pelvis, and leg, respectively. Selective nerve root, intercostal, cervical plexus, brachial plexus, or lumbosacral plexus blocks may be used for somatic nerve blockade.

TABLE 47–16 **Solutions for differential epidural blockade.**

Solution	Epidural[1]
Placebo	Saline
Sympatholytic	0.5% lidocaine
Somatic	1% lidocaine
All fibers	2% lidocaine

[1]Chloroprocaine may be used instead.

Differential epidural blocks may be used for thoracic pain when the techniques for sympathetic blockade carry a significant risk of pneumothorax (Table 47–16). After each epidural injection, the patient is evaluated for pain relief, signs of sympathetic blockade (a decrease in blood pressure), sensation to pinprick and light touch, and motor function. If the pain disappears after the saline injection, the patient either has psychogenic pain (usually a profound long-lasting effect) or is displaying a placebo effect (usually short lasting). If pain relief coincides with isolated signs of sympathetic blockade, it is likely mediated by sympathetic fibers. If pain relief only follows somatosensory blockade, it is likely mediated by somatic fibers. Lastly, if the pain persists even after signs of motor blockade, the pain is either central (supraspinal) or psychogenic.

The differential epidural block carries the risk of any neuraxial block, and the possibility of hypotension and blocking cardiac accelerator fibers at T1–T4. The level should not extend above the T5 dermatome due to these risks. Following catheter insertion, injections should be administered with the patient in a monitored setting for the rest of this procedure.

Although differential epidural blockade has limitations, it may be helpful to identify primarily centralized pain when a patient continues to have a significant level of pain despite multilevel dermatomal blockade over the painful region. It is unlikely that a subsequent nerve block would help to treat the painful condition.

When it is thought that a patient may have abdominal pain from the anterior abdominal wall, a transversus abdominis plane (TAP) block may be performed using ultrasound guidance. This may offer potential short- or long-term relief and can be considered as an alternative to differential epidural blockade. If no relief is obtained, the pain may have a visceral origin or a central cause. Visceral pain may best respond to a celiac or splanchnic nerve block and possibly to subsequent splanchnic RFA. Patients with pain that is primarily of a central origin may respond to multidisciplinary therapy, including counseling and biofeedback training.

8. Neuromodulation

Electrical stimulation of the nervous system can produce analgesia in patients with acute and chronic pain. Current may be applied transcutaneously, epidurally, or by electrodes implanted into the central nervous system.

Transcutaneous Electrical Nerve Stimulation

Transcutaneous electrical nerve stimulation (TENS) is thought to produce analgesia by stimulating large afferent fibers. It may have a role for patients with mild to moderate acute pain and those with chronic low back pain, arthritis, and neuropathic pain. The gate theory of pain processing suggests that the afferent input from large epicritic fibers competes with that from the smaller pain fibers. An alternative theory proposes that at high rates of stimulation, TENS causes conduction block in small afferent pain fibers. With conventional TENS, electrodes are applied to the same dermatome as the pain and are stimulated periodically by direct current from a generator (usually for 30 min several times a day). A current of 10–30 mA with a pulse width of 50–80 μs is applied at a frequency of 80–100 Hz. Some patients whose pain is refractory to conventional TENS respond to low-frequency TENS (acupuncture-like TENS), which employs stimuli with a pulse width greater than 200 μs at frequencies less than 10 Hz (for 5–15 min). Unlike conventional TENS, low-frequency stimulation is at least partly reversed by naloxone, suggesting a role for endogenous opioids. This technique is also called *dorsal column stimulation* because it was

thought to produce analgesia by directly stimulating large Aβ fibers in the dorsal columns of the spinal cord. Proposed mechanisms include activation of descending modulating systems and inhibition of sympathetic outflow.

Spinal Cord Stimulation

23 Spinal cord stimulation (SCS) may be effective for neuropathic pain; accepted indications include sympathetically mediated pain, spinal cord lesions with localized segmental pain, phantom limb pain, ischemic lower extremity pain due to peripheral vascular disease, adhesive arachnoiditis, peripheral neuropathies, post-thoracotomy pain, intercostal neuralgia, postherpetic neuralgia, angina, visceral abdominal pain, and visceral pelvic pain. Patients with persisting pain after back surgery, which is typically a mixed nociceptive–neuropathic disorder, also appear to benefit from SCS.

Temporary electrodes are initially placed in the posterior epidural space and connected to an external generator to evaluate efficacy in a 5- to 7-day trial (**Figures 47–27** and **47–28**). The trial may be extended, particularly if it allows a patient, such as one with CRPS, to tolerate more aggressive physical therapy. If a favorable response is obtained, a fully

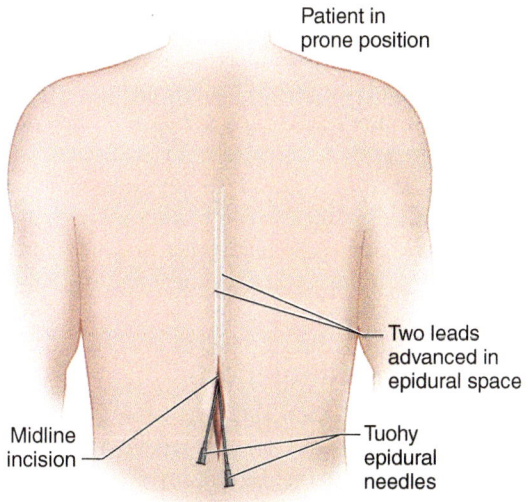

Patient in prone position

Two leads advanced in epidural space

Midline incision

Tuohy epidural needles

FIGURE 47–27 Patient positioning for insertion of a spinal cord stimulator.

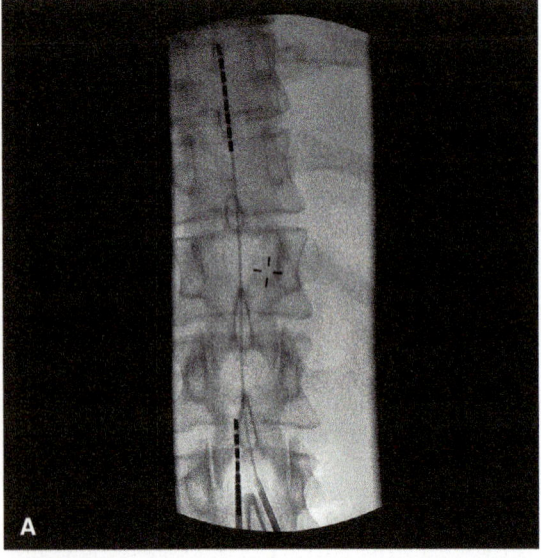

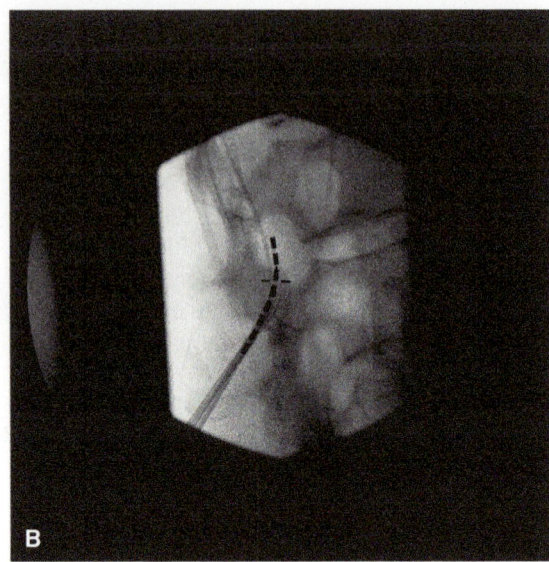

FIGURE 47–28 2-lead SCS placement.
A: Anteroposterior view. The right contact lead has been advanced to its final position at the top of T10. The left lead is advanced through the Tuohy needle. **B:** Lateral view. The first lead is in position, with the left lead entering the epidural space.

implantable system is inserted. Unfortunately, the effectiveness of the technique decreases with time in some patients. Complications include infection, lead migration, and lead breakage.

Peripheral Nerve Stimulation

Peripheral nerve stimulation (PNS) differs from SCS in that leads are placed in close anatomic proximity to an injured peripheral nerve. The leads may be placed percutaneously, with or without ultrasound guidance, or surgically under direct vision of the nerve. Occipital nerve stimulators are one form of peripheral nerve stimulator that may be helpful in treating occipital neuralgia and migraine headache (Figure 47–29).

Deep Brain Stimulation

Deep brain stimulation (DBS) is used for intractable cancer pain and for intractable nonmalignant neuropathic pain. Electrodes are implanted stereotactically into the periaqueductal and periventricular gray areas for nociceptive pain, usually in patients with cancer or chronic low back pain.

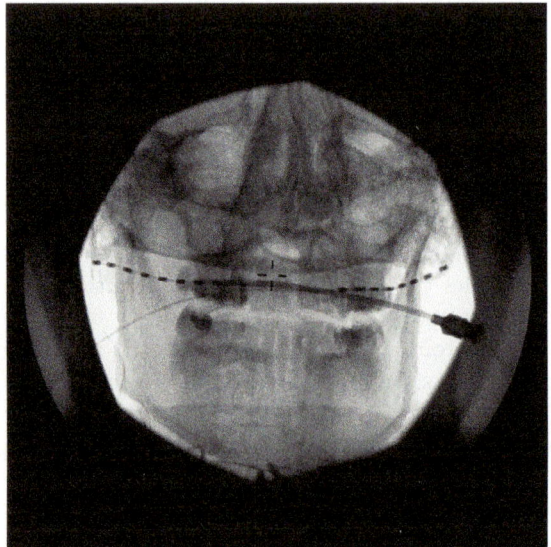

FIGURE 47–29 Occipital nerve stimulator placement, anteroposterior view. Following placement of right occipital nerve stimulator lead below the nuchal ridge, a left occipital nerve stimulator lead has been advanced through the introducer needle.

For neuropathic pain, the electrodes are frequently implanted into the ventral posterolateral and ventral posteromedial thalamic nuclei. DBS may also be helpful for patients with movement disorders, headache, and neuropsychiatric disorders. The most serious complications are intracranial hemorrhage and infection.

9. Vertebral Augmentation

24 Patients with pathological or osteoporotic vertebral compression fractures may benefit from vertebral augmentation with polymethylmethacrylate cement. Vertebroplasty involves injection of the cement through the trocar needle. Kyphoplasty involves inflation of a balloon inserted through a percutaneously placed trocar needle, with subsequent injection of cement. Anteroposterior and lateral fluoroscopic views facilitate optimal placement of the cement. For patients with a sacral insufficiency fracture, cement sacroplasty may help stabilize the fracture. Risks of vertebral augmentation include direct nerve injury (due to placement of the trocar needle), hemorrhage, cement extravasation, and embolic events.

MULTIDISCIPLINARY TREATMENT

Psychological Interventions

Psychological techniques, including cognitive therapy, behavioral therapy, biofeedback, relaxation techniques, and hypnosis, are most effective when employed by psychologists or psychiatrists. Cognitive interventions are based on the assumption that a patient's attitude toward pain can influence the perception of pain. Maladaptive attitudes contribute to suffering and disability. The patient is taught skills for coping with pain either individually or in group therapy. The most common techniques include attention diversion and imagery. Behavioral (operant) therapy is based on the premise that behavior in patients with chronic pain is determined by consequences of the behavior. Positive reinforcers (such as attention from a spouse) tend to enable or intensify the pain, whereas negative reinforcers reduce pain. The therapist's role is to guide behavior modification with the aid of family members and medical providers in order to nurture negative reinforcers and minimize positive reinforcers.

Relaxation techniques teach the patient to alter the arousal response and the increase in sympathetic tone associated with pain. The most commonly employed technique is a progressive muscle relaxation exercise. Biofeedback and hypnosis are closely related interventions. All forms of biofeedback are based on the principle that patients can be taught to control involuntary physiological parameters. Once proficient in the technique, the patient may be able induce a relaxation response and more effectively apply coping skills to control physiological factors (eg, muscle tension) that worsen pain. The most commonly utilized physiological parameters in biofeedback are muscle tension (electromyographic biofeedback) and temperature (thermal biofeedback). The effectiveness of hypnosis varies considerably among individuals. Hypnotic techniques teach patients to alter pain perception by having them focus on other sensations, localize the pain to another site, and dissociate themselves from a painful experience through imagery. Patients with chronic headaches and musculoskeletal disorders benefit most from these relaxation techniques.

Physical Therapy

Heat and cold can provide pain relief by alleviating muscle spasm. In addition, heat decreases joint stiffness and increases blood flow, and cold vasoconstricts and can reduce tissue edema. The analgesic action of heat and cold may at least partially be explained by the gate theory of pain processing.

Superficial heating modalities include conductive (hot packs, paraffin baths, fluidotherapy), convective (hydrotherapy), and radiant (infrared) techniques. Techniques for application of deep heat include ultrasound as well as shortwave and microwave diathermy. These modalities are more effective for pain involving deep joints and muscles. Cold is most effective for pain associated with acute injuries and edema. When applied selectively, cold can also relieve muscle spasm. Application may take the form of cold packs, ice massage, or vapocoolant sprays (ethyl chloride or fluoromethane).

Exercise should be part of any rehabilitation program for chronic pain. A graded exercise program prevents joint stiffness, muscle atrophy, and contractures, all of which can contribute to the patient's pain and functional disabilities. McKenzie exercises are particularly helpful for patients with lumbar disc displacement. Patients may state that physical therapy has not helped in the past. The efficacy of previous physical therapy techniques should be assessed, and the appropriateness of current physical therapy sessions and of the home exercise program should also be evaluated. By facilitating increased range of motion and providing constant resistance, aquatherapy may be particularly helpful for patients who may not be able to tolerate other forms of therapy.

Acupuncture

25   Acupuncture can be a useful adjunct for patients with chronic pain, particularly that associated with chronic musculoskeletal disorders and headaches. The technique involves insertion of needles into discrete anatomically defined points, called *meridians*. Stimulation of the needle after insertion takes the form of twirling or of application of a mild electrical current. Insertion points appear to be unrelated to the conventional anatomy of the nervous system. Although the scientific literature concerning the mechanism of action and role of acupuncture in pain management is controversial, some studies suggest that acupuncture stimulates the release of endogenous opioids, as its effects can be antagonized by naloxone.

GUIDELINES

American Society of Anesthesiologists Task Force on Chronic Pain Management; American Society of Regional Anesthesia and Pain Medicine: Practice guidelines for chronic pain management: An updated report by the American Society of Anesthesiologists Task Force on Chronic Pain Management and the American Society of Regional Anesthesia and Pain Medicine. Anesthesiology 2010;112:810.

Chou R, Qaseem A, Snow V, et al: Diagnosis and treatment of low back pain: A joint clinical practice guideline from the American College of Physicians and the American Pain Society. Ann Intern Med 2007;147:478.

Horlocker TT, Neal JM, Rathmell JP: 2011 Practice advisories by the American Society of Regional Anesthesia and Pain Medicine: Grading the evidence and making the grade. Reg Anesth Pain Med 2011;36:1.

SUGGESTED READING

Aeschbach A, Mekhail NA: Common nerve blocks in chronic pain management. Anesthesiol Clin N Am 2000;18:429.

Christo PJ: Opioid effectiveness and side effects in chronic pain. Anesthesiol Clin N Am 2003;21:699.

Bridges D, Thompson SWN, Rice ASC: Mechanisms of neuropathic pain. Br J Anaesth 2001;87:12.

Bruehl S: An update on the pathophysiology of complex regional pain syndrome. Anesthesiology 2010;113:713.

Chopko B, Caraway DL: MiDAS I (Mild Decompression Alternative to Open Surgery): A preliminary report of a prospective, multi-center clinical study. Pain Physician 2010;13:369.

Cohen SP, Liao W, Gupta A, et al: Ketamine in pain management. Adv Psychosom Med 2011;30:139.

Cohen SP, Rathmell JP: Tackling the technical challenges that hinder the success of facet joint radiofrequency treatment for spinal pain. Reg Anesth Pain Med 2010;35:327.

Deer TR, Kapural L: New image-guided ultra-minimally invasive lumbar decompression method: The MILD procedure. Pain Physician 2010;13:35.

Frey ME, Manchikanti L, Benyamin RM, et al: Spinal cord stimulation for patients with failed back surgery syndrome: A systematic review. Pain Physician 2009;12:379.

Guastella V, Mick G, Soriano C, et al: A prospective study of neuropathic pain induced by thoracotomy: Incidence, clinical description and diagnosis. Pain 2011;152:74.

Hollmann MW, Durieux ME: Local anesthetics and the inflammatory response: A new therapeutic indication? Anesthesiology 2000;93:858.

Huntoon MA, Burgherr AH: Ultrasound-guided permanent implantation of peripheral nerve stimulation (PNS) system for neuropathic pain of the extremities: Original cases and outcomes. Pain Medicine 2009;10:1369.

Kapural L, Narouze SN, Janicki TI, et al: Spinal cord stimulation is an effective treatment for the chronic intractable visceral pelvic pain. Pain Medicine 2006;7:440.

Manchikanti L, Singh V, Datta S, et al; American Society of Interventional Pain Physicians: Comprehensive review of epidemiology, scope, and impact of spinal pain. Pain Physician 2009;12:E35.

Mekhail NA, Cheng J, Narouze S, et al: Clinical applications of neurostimulation: Forty years later. Pain Pract 2010;10:103.

Narouze SN: Ultrasound-guided interventional procedures in pain management: Evidence-based medicine. Reg Anesth Pain Med 2010;35:S55.

Nguyen H, Garber JE, Hassenbusch SJ: Spinal analgesics. Anesthesiol Clin North Am 2003;21:805.

Pluijms W, Huygen F, Cheng J, et al: Evidence-based interventional pain medicine according to clinical diagnoses. 18. Painful diabetic polyneuropathy. Pain Pract 2011;11:191.

Raja SN, Grabow TS: Complex regional pain syndrome I (reflex sympathetic dystrophy). Anesthesiology 2002;96:1254.

Rathmell JP, Aprill C, Bogduk N: Cervical transforaminal injection of steroids. Anesthesiology 2004;100:1595.

Rathmell JP, Michna E, Fitzgibbon DR, et al: Injury and liability associated with cervical procedures for chronic pain. Anesthesiology 2011;114:918.

Soliman LM, Narouze SN: Ultrasound-guided transversus abdominis plane block for the management of abdominal pain: An alternative to the differential epidural block. Tech Reg Anesth Pain Manage 2009;13:117.

Tarver JM, Rathmell JP, Alsofrom GF: Lumbar discography. Reg Anesth Pain Med 2001;26:263.

Vad VB, Bhat AL, Lutz GE, et al: Transforaminal epidural steroid injections in lumbosacral radiculopathy—a prospective randomized study. Spine 2002;27:11.

van Eerd M, Patijn J, Lataster A, et al: 5. Cervical facet pain. Pain Pract 2010;10:113-123.

van Eijs F, Stanton-Hicks M, Van Zundert J, et al: Evidence-based interventional pain medicine according to clinical diagnoses. 16. Complex regional pain syndrome. Pain Practice 2011;11:70.

Wolfe F, Clauw DJ, Fitzcharles MA, et al: The American College of Rheumatology preliminary diagnostic criteria for fibromyalgia and measurement of symptom severity. Arthritis Care Res 2010;62:600.

Perioperative Pain Management & Enhanced Outcomes

48

Francesco Carli, MD, MPhil and Gabriele Baldini, MD, MSc

KEY CONCEPTS

1. A well-functioning enhanced recovery program (ERP) uses evidence-based practices to decrease variation in clinical management, minimize organ dysfunction, and accelerate convalescence; it requires adjustments in multiple aspects of care, including surgical and anesthetic techniques, nursing care, physiotherapy, and nutrition support.

2. Persistent postsurgical pain—chronic pain that continues beyond the typical healing period of 1–2 months following surgery, or well past the normal period for postoperative follow-up—is increasingly acknowledged as a common and significant problem following surgery.

3. The magnitude of the surgical stress response is related to the intensity of the surgical stimulus, can be amplified by other factors, including hypothermia and psychological stress, and can be moderated by perioperative interventions, including deeper planes of general anesthesia, neural blockade, and reduction in the degree of surgical invasiveness.

4. Neuraxial blockade of nociceptive stimuli by epidural and spinal local anesthetics has been shown to blunt the metabolic and neuroendocrine stress response to surgery. In major open abdominal and thoracic procedures, thoracic epidural blockade with local anesthetic provides excellent analgesia, facilitates mobilization and physical therapy, and decreases the incidence and severity of ileus.

5. By sparing opioid use and minimizing the incidence of systemic opioid-related side effects, epidural analgesia facilitates earlier mobilization and earlier resumption of oral nutrition, expediting exercise activity and attenuating loss of body mass.

6. Continuous peripheral nerve blocks with local anesthetics block afferent nociceptive pathways and are an excellent way to reduce the incidence of opioid-related side effects and facilitate recovery.

7. Lidocaine (intravenous bolus of 100 mg or 1.5–2 mg/kg, followed by continuous intravenous infusion of 1.5–3 mg/kg/h or 2–3 mg/min) has analgesic, antihyperalgesic, and antiinflammatory properties.

8. Multimodal analgesia combines different classes of medications, having different (multimodal) pharmacological mechanisms of action and additive or synergistic effects, to control multiple perioperative pathophysiological factors that lead to postoperative pain and its sequelae.

—Continued next page

Continued—

9 The addition of nonsteroidal antiinflammatory drugs (NSAIDs) to systemic opioids diminishes postoperative pain intensity, reduces the opioid requirement by approximately 30%, and decreases opioid-related side effects such as postoperative nausea and vomiting and sedation. However, NSAIDs may increase the risk of gastrointestinal and postoperative bleeding, decrease kidney function, and impair wound healing.

10 Opioid administration by patient-controlled analgesia provides better pain control, greater patient satisfaction, and fewer opioid side effects when compared with on-request parenteral opioid administration.

11 Single-shot and continuous peripheral nerve blockade is frequently utilized for fast-track ambulatory and inpatient orthopedic surgery, and can accelerate recovery from surgery and improve analgesia and patient satisfaction.

12 Postoperative ileus delays enteral feeding, causes patient discomfort, and is one of the most common causes of prolonged postoperative hospital stay. Nasogastric tubes should be discouraged whenever possible or used for only a very short period of time, even in gastric and hepatic surgery. Multimodal analgesia and nonopioid analgesia techniques shorten the duration of postoperative ileus.

13 Because either excessive, or excessively restricted, perioperative fluid therapy may increase the incidence and severity of postoperative ileus, a goal-directed fluid strategy should be selected to decrease postoperative morbidities and enhance recovery.

Evolution of Enhanced Recovery Programs

Despite increasing numbers of surgical patients who present with complex surgical problems and numerous medical comorbidities, major advances in surgical and anesthetic management have progressively decreased perioperative mortality and morbidity. Further improvement in perioperative outcomes, highlighted by accelerated postoperative convalescence and decreasing occurrence of perioperative complications, will depend on continued evolution of an integrated, multidisciplinary team approach to perioperative care that requires adjustments in multiple aspects of care, including surgical and anesthetic techniques, nursing care, physiotherapy, and nutrition support. The goal is to combine individual evidence-based elements of perioperative care, each of which may have modest benefits when used in isolation, into a tightly coordinated effort that has a synergistic, beneficial effect on surgical outcomes.

Such coordinated, multidisciplinary perioperative care programs are termed *enhanced recovery programs* (ERPs), *fast-track surgery*, or *enhanced recovery after surgery* (ERAS) (Figure 48–1). A well-functioning ERP uses evidence-based practices to decrease variation in clinical management, minimize organ dysfunction, and accelerate convalescence (Figure 48–2). Although many publications in the surgical literature have highlighted the positive impact of such programs on surgical outcomes, reports documenting the role of anesthesia and analgesia in these programs are few. Another challenge is determining how to assess the impact of anesthetic management on outcomes in an ERP. Hospital length of stay is the most commonly used measure of success, but in many systems timing of hospital discharge is more directly related to administrative and

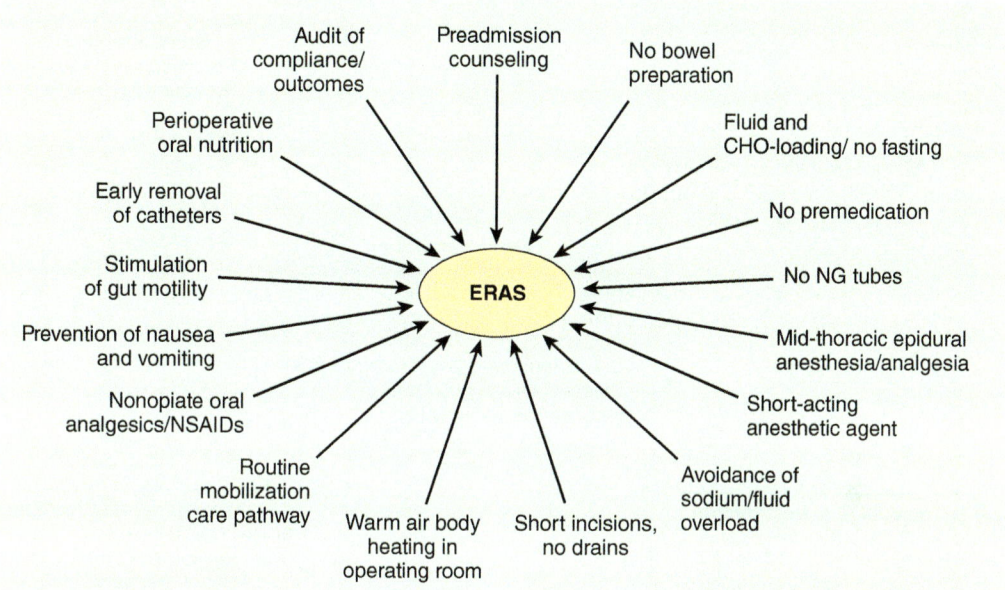

FIGURE 48–1 Perioperative elements contributing to enhanced recovery after surgery (ERAS). CHO, carbohydrate; NG, nasogastric; NSAID, nonsteroidal antiinflammatory drug. (Reproduced, with permission, from Fearon KC, Ljungqvist O, Von Meyenfeldt M, et al: Enhanced recovery after surgery: A consensus review of clinical care for patients undergoing colonic resection. Clin Nut 2005;24:466.)

organizational issues than to discrete milestones in the patient's postoperative recovery. Little research has been undertaken to define the process of postoperative recovery, and few outcome measures are currently available to confirm that postoperative recovery has been accomplished for a given surgical disease. Other measures of successful implementation of ERPs are reduced readmission and complication rates.

It is logical to assume that more effective anesthetic interventions will reduce pain, facilitate earlier postoperative mobilization, and allow earlier resumption of oral feeding. In this context, the role of the anesthesia provider must evolve from merely providing satisfactory anesthetic conditions throughout the operation to a focus on enhancing overall perioperative care through techniques that shorten postoperative convalescence and reduce the likelihood of perioperative complications. These goals can be achieved by optimizing the patient's preoperative condition, by ablating the adverse effects of the intraoperative neuroendocrine stress response, and by providing pain and symptom control to facilitate the postoperative recovery. In endeavoring to do so, the anesthesiologist must become a perioperative physician and an active participant in the surgical team.

2 The problem of **persistent postsurgical pain**, defined as chronic pain that continues beyond the typical healing period of 1–2 months following surgery—or well past the normal period for postoperative follow-up by anesthesia providers—is increasingly acknowledged as a common and significant issue following surgery. The incidence of persistent postsurgical pain may exceed 30% after some operations, especially amputations, thoracotomy, mastectomy, and inguinal herniorrhaphy. Although the cause is unclear, several risk factors have been identified (Figure 48–3), and aggressive, multimodal perioperative pain control is often suggested as a fundamental preemptive strategy.

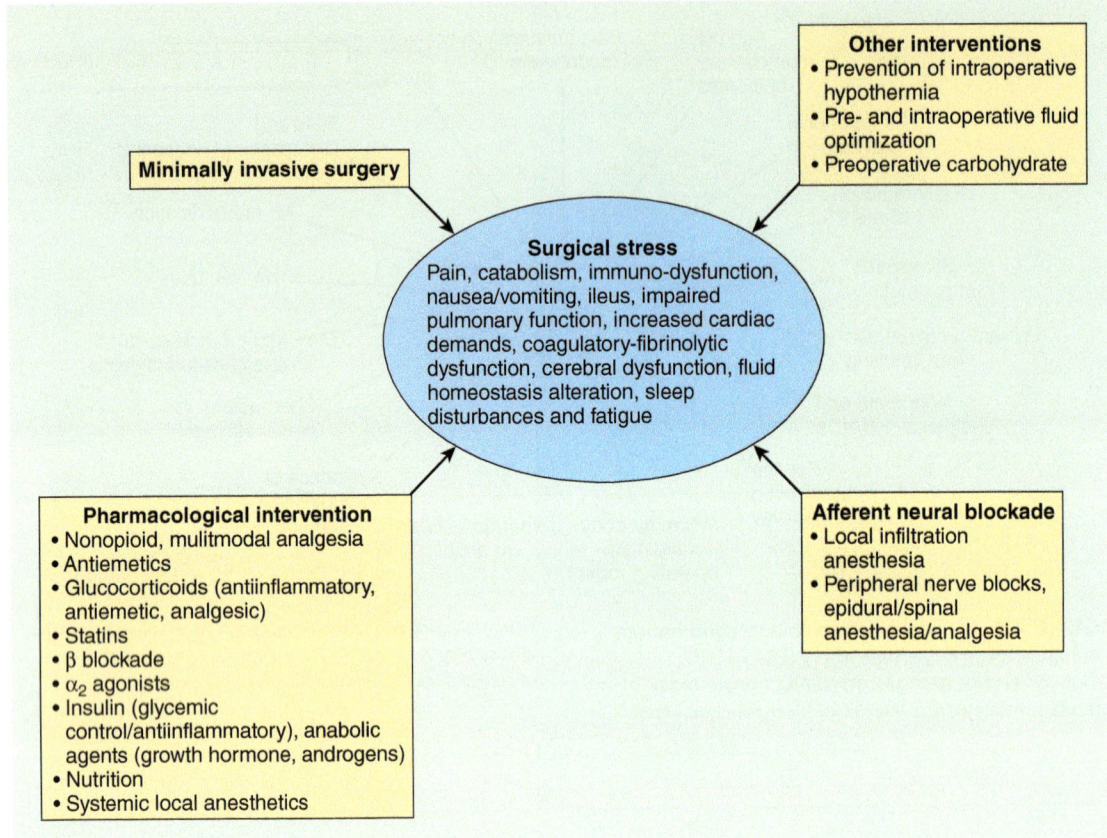

FIGURE 48–2 Multimodal interventions to attenuate the surgical stress response. (Reproduced, with permission, from Kehlet H, Wilmore DW: Evidence-based surgical care and the evolution of fast-track surgery. Ann Surg 2008;248:189.)

Anesthetic Management–Related Factors Contributing to Enhanced Recovery

PREOPERATIVE PERIOD

Patient Education

Cooperation from the patient and family is essential if an ERP is to be effectively implemented. Preoperative teaching must use plain language and avoid medical jargon. Well-designed printed materials, such as procedure-specific booklets can be given to patients and families with the advice to keep them at the bedside and utilize them during the hospitalization.

Preoperative Risk Assessment & Optimization of Functional Status

Identification of patients at risk for intraoperative and postoperative complications, along with preoperative efforts focusing on any comorbidities, can improve surgical recovery. Preoperative assessment is discussed in detail in Chapter 18. Although international guidelines evaluating the risk for developing cardiovascular, respiratory, or metabolic complications have been extensively reviewed and published, little attention has been given to assessment and optimization of preoperative functional and physiological status. Nonetheless, some recommendations can be made. For example, routine use of β blockers, especially in

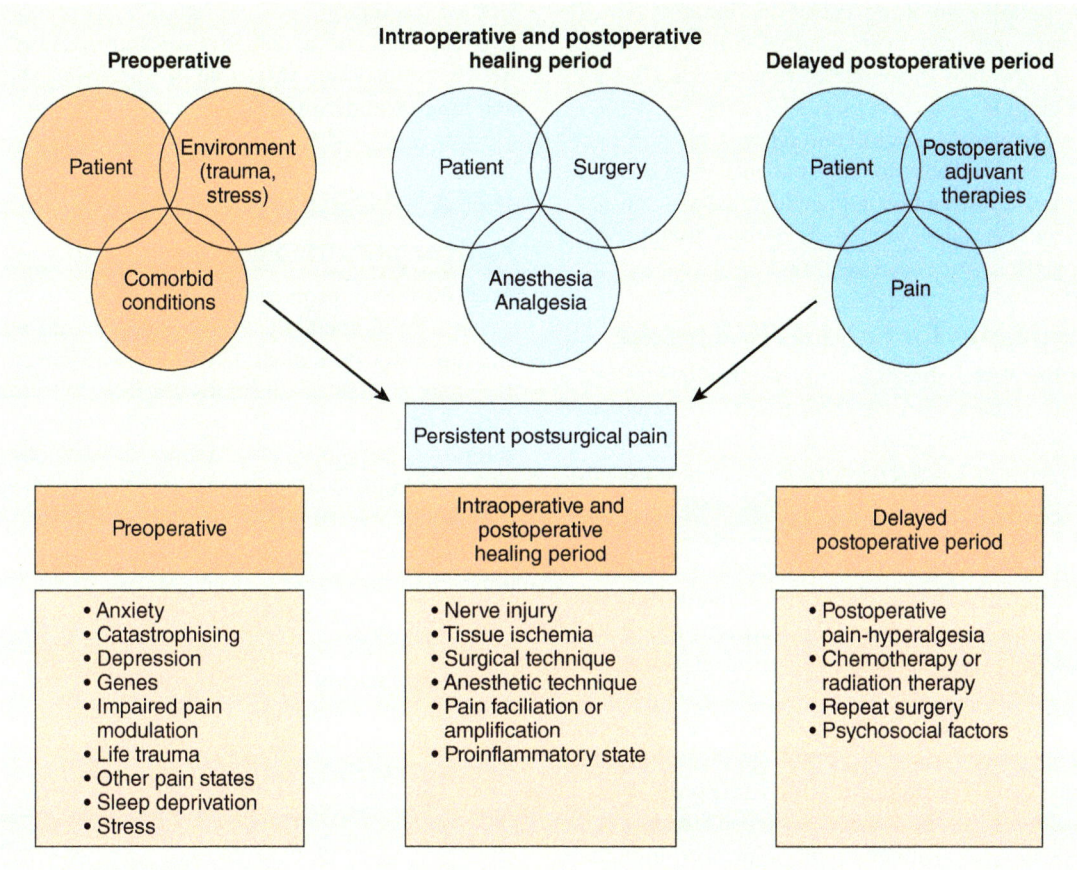

FIGURE 48–3 Risk factors for persistent postsurgical pain. (Reproduced, with permission, from Wu CL, Raja SN: Treatment of acute postoperative pain. Lancet 2011;377:2215.)

patients at low risk, has been associated with an increased risk of stroke; however, perioperative β blockers should be continued in patients already receiving this therapy. Perioperative statins appear to decrease postoperative cardiovascular complications and should not be abruptly discontinued perioperatively. Several procedure-specific scoring systems based on patient comorbidity, type of surgery, and biochemical data are being used to predict postoperative mortality and morbidity. In addition, risk-adjusted scoring systems, such as the American College of Surgeons' National Surgical Quality Improvement Program (NSQIP) and the Society of Thoracic Surgeons' National Database, can be used to compare outcomes among institutions.

Smoking & Alcohol Cessation

The preoperative period provides not only a time to evaluate surgical risk and optimize medical conditions, but also an opportunity to modify habits that can significantly affect a patient's short-term and long-term health and quality of life. Smoking, drug abuse, and excessive alcohol use are risk factors for the development of postoperative complications, and preoperative and postoperative interventions aimed at modifying these habits can improve surgical recovery. A recent meta-analysis found that preoperative smoking cessation, for any type of surgery, reduced postoperative complications by 41%, especially those related to wound healing and the lungs.

Many psychological and pharmacological strategies are available to help patients stop excessive alcohol consumption and reduce the risk of alcohol withdrawal. However, the optimal perioperative program has not been identified.

Guidelines for Food & Fluid Intake

Preoperative fasting and surgical stress induce insulin resistance. Furthermore, patients who are not allowed to drink fluids after an overnight fast and patients who receive a bowel preparation experience dehydration, which may increase discomfort and cause drowsiness and orthostatic lightheadedness. Although fasting has been advocated as a preoperative strategy to minimize the risk of pulmonary aspiration during induction of anesthesia, this benefit must be weighed against the detrimental aspects of this practice.

For instance, research suggests that avoiding preoperative fasting and ensuring adequate hydration and energy supply may moderate postoperative insulin resistance. All international fasting guidelines allow clear fluids up to 2 h prior to induction of anesthesia in patients at low risk for pulmonary aspiration (see Chapter 18). This practice has proved to be safe even in morbidly obese patients. Furthermore, recent studies have shown that preoperative administration of carbohydrate drinks (one 100-g dose administered the night before surgery and a second 50-g dose 2–3 h before induction of anesthesia) is safe; can reduce insulin resistance, hunger, fatigue, and postoperative nausea and vomiting (PONV); and positively influences immune status. Moreover, postoperative nitrogen loss and the loss of skeletal muscle mass are attenuated.

Magnetic resonance imaging studies in healthy volunteers have shown that the residual gastric volume 2 h after 400 mL of oral carbohydrate (12.5% maltodextrins) is minimal and similar to the residual volume after an overnight fast (mean volume of 21 mL). The safety of this practice has been tested in patients with uncomplicated type 2 diabetes mellitus, none of whom showed evidence of worsened risk of aspiration. Further studies of preoperative oral fluid and carbohydrate administration are needed to elaborate their role in improving short- and long-term perioperative outcomes.

INTRAOPERATIVE PERIOD
Antithrombotic Prophylaxis

Antithrombotic prophylaxis reduces perioperative venous thromboembolism and related morbidity and mortality. Both pneumatic compression devices and anticoagulant medications are now commonly used. Because neuraxial anesthesia techniques are commonly employed for many patients during major abdominal, vascular, thoracic and orthopedic surgery, appropriate timing and administration of antithrombotic agents in these cases is of critical importance in order to avoid the risk of epidural hematoma. International recommendations on the management of anticoagulated patients receiving regional anesthesia have been recently revised and published and are discussed in other chapters.

Antibiotic Prophylaxis

Appropriate selection and timing of preoperative antibiotic prophylaxis reduces the risk of surgical site infections. Antibiotics should be administered within 1 h before skin incision and, based on their plasma half-life, should be repeated during prolonged surgeries to ensure adequate tissue concentrations. Antibiotic prophylaxis of surgical site infections should be discontinued within 24 h after surgery (current guidelines permit cardiothoracic patients to receive antibiotics for 48 h following surgery).

Strategies to Minimize the Surgical Stress Response

The surgical stress response is characterized by neuroendocrine, metabolic, and inflammatory changes initiated by the surgical incision and subsequent procedures that can adversely affect organ function and perioperative outcomes, especially in elderly and physiologically compromised patients. These responses include a transient but reversible state of insulin resistance, characterized by decreased

peripheral glucose uptake and increased endogenous glucose production. The magnitude of
the surgical stress response is related to the
intensity of the surgical stimulus; can be amplified
by other factors, including hypothermia and psychological stress; and can be moderated by perioperative interventions, including deeper planes of
general anesthesia, neural blockade, and reduction
in the degree of surgical invasiveness. Much recent
effort has focused on developing surgical and anesthetic techniques that reduce the surgical stress
response, with the goal of lowering the risk of stress-
related organ dysfunction and perioperative complications. An overview of several techniques that have
proved effective in ERP protocols follows.

A. Minimally Invasive Surgery

Laparoscopic procedures are associated with a
reduced incidence of surgical complications, especially surgical site infections, compared with the
same procedures performed in "open" fashion.
Published data highlight the safety of minimally
invasive procedures in the hands of adequately
trained and experienced surgeons. Laparoscopic
cholecystectomy results in shorter length of hospital stay and fewer complications compared with
open cholecystectomy, and similar results have
been reported for colorectal surgery. A longer term

salutary impact is achieved when laparoscopic
techniques are included in ERPs. A laparoscopic
approach is also associated with less morbidity in
elderly surgical patients.

B. Regional Anesthesia/ Analgesia Techniques

A variety of fast-track surgical procedures have taken
advantage of the beneficial clinical and metabolic
effects of regional anesthesia/analgesia techniques
(Table 48–1). Neuraxial blockade of nociceptive stimuli by epidural and spinal local anesthetics has been shown to blunt the metabolic and
neuroendocrine stress response to surgery. To be
effective, the blockade must be established before
incision and continued postoperatively. In major
open abdominal and thoracic procedures, thoracic
epidural blockade with local anesthetic can be a recommended anesthetic component of a postoperative
ERP, providing excellent analgesia, facilitating mobilization and physical therapy, and decreasing the incidence and severity of ileus. However, the advantages
of neuraxial blockade are not as evident when minimally invasive surgical techniques are used. Lumbar
epidural anesthesia/analgesia should be discouraged
for abdominal surgery because it often does not provide adequate segmental analgesia for an abdominal
incision. In addition, it frequently causes urinary

TABLE 48–1 **Fast-track surgery programs that incorporate regional anesthesia/ analgesia techniques.[1]**

Type of Surgery	Incision	Regional Anesthesia /Analgesia Techniques	Length of Stay
Colorectal resection	Laparotomy, laparoscopy	TEA, wound infusion of ropivacaine, intraperitoneal local anesthetic, intravenous lidocaine	2–4 d
Hernia repair	Open	Local infiltration, INB, TAP	2-4 h
Thoracic surgery	Thoracotomy	TEA, ICB	1–4 d
Esophageal surgery	Laparotomy	TEA	3–5 d
Open aortic surgery	Laparotomy	TEA	3–5 d
Nephrectomy	Laparotomy, laparoscopy	TEA	2–4 d
Arthroplasty (hip, knee)	Open	CPNB (femoral and sciatic), periarticular infiltration	1–3 d

[1]TEA, thoracic epidural analgesia; ICB, intercostal block; INB, ilioinguinal nerve block; TAP, transversus abdominus plane block; CPNB, continuous peripheral nerve block.

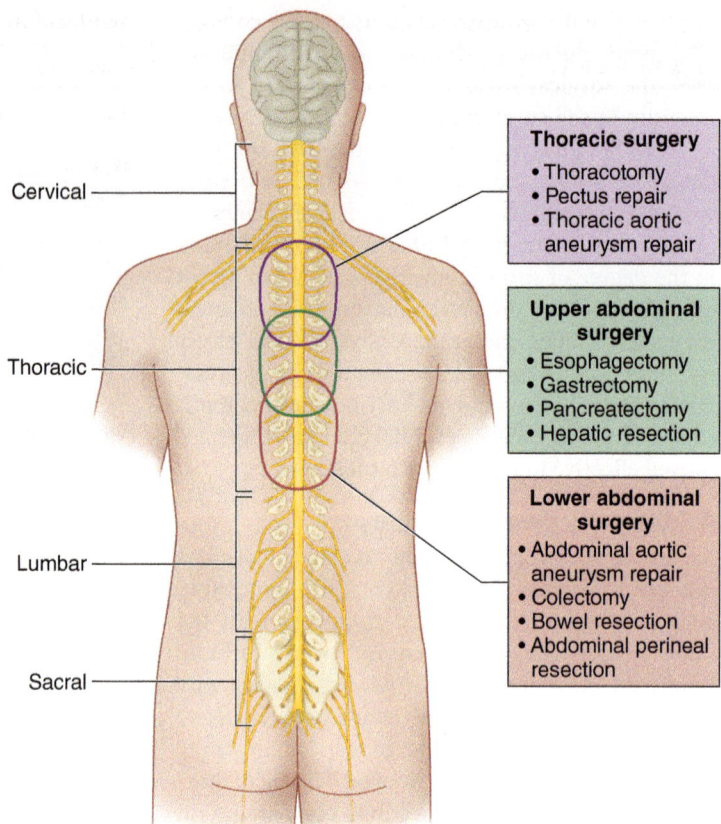

Cervical

Thoracic

Lumbar

Sacral

Thoracic surgery
- Thoracotomy
- Pectus repair
- Thoracic aortic aneurysm repair

Upper abdominal surgery
- Esophagectomy
- Gastrectomy
- Pancreatectomy
- Hepatic resection

Lower abdominal surgery
- Abdominal aortic aneurysm repair
- Colectomy
- Bowel resection
- Abdominal perineal resection

FIGURE 48–4 Optimal regions for placing an epidural catheter in the adult spine when administering epidural anesthesia/analgesia for thoracic and abdominal procedures. (Reproduced, with permission, from Manion SC, Brennan TJ: Thoracic epidural analgesia and acute pain management. Anesthesiology 2011;115:181.)

retention and lower limb sensory and motor blockade, increasing the need for urinary drainage catheters (with accompanying increased risk of urinary tract infection), delaying mobilization and recovery, and increasing the risk of falls.

Epidural blockade using a solution of local anesthetic and low-dose opioid provides better postoperative analgesia at rest and with movement than systemic opioids (Figure 48–4 and Table 48–2). **⑤** By sparing opioid use and minimizing the incidence of systemic opioid-related side effects, epidural analgesia facilitates earlier mobilization and earlier resumption of oral nutrition, expediting exercise activity and attenuating loss of body mass. Neural blockade minimizes postoperative insulin resistance, attenuating the postoperative hyperglycemic response and facilitating utilization of exogenous glucose, thereby preventing postoperative loss of amino acids and conserving lean body mass.

If spinal anesthesia is used for fast-track (and especially ambulatory) surgery, attention must be paid to delayed recovery due to prolonged motor blockade. The use of smaller doses of intrathecal local anesthetics (lidocaine, 30–40 mg; bupivacaine, 3–7 mg; or ropivacaine, 5–10 mg) with lipophilic intrathecal opioids (fentanyl, 10–25 mcg, or sufentanil, 5–10 mcg) can prolong postoperative analgesia and minimize the motor block without delaying recovery from anesthesia. The introduction of ultra-short-acting intrathecal agents such as 2-chloroprocaine (still controversial at present) may further speed the fast-track process. Spinal opioids are associated with side effects such as nausea, pruritus, and postoperative urinary retention. Adjuvants such as clonidine are effective alternatives to intrathecal opioids, with the goal of avoiding untoward side effects that may delay hospital discharge. For example, intrathecal clonidine added to spinal local anesthetic

TABLE 48–2 Options for composition of thoracic epidural infusion analgesia solutions.[1]

Local Anesthetic	Opioid	Advantages	Disadvantages
Bupivacaine, 0.125%	None	↓ Nausea/Vomiting ↓ Pruritus ↓ Sedation ↓ Respiratory depression	↑ Hypotension ↑ Motor blockage
Bupivacaine, 0.1%	Hydromorphone, 5–10 mcg/mL or Fentanyl, 2–5 mcg/mL	↓ Both hemodynamic and opioid side effects	—
Bupivacaine, 0.05%	Hydromorphone, 5–10 mcg/mL or Fentanyl, 2–5 mcg/mL	↓ Both hemodynamic and opioid side effects	—
Bupivacaine, 0.05%	Hydromorphone, 20 mcg/mL or Fentanyl, 5–10 mcg/mL	↓ Both hemodynamic and opioid side effects	—
None	Hydromorphone, 20–40 mcg/mL	↓ Hypotension ↓ Motor blockade	↑ Nausea/Vomiting ↑ Pruritus ↑ Sedation ↑ Respiratory depression

[1]Reproduced, with permission, from Manion SC, Brennan TJ. Thoracic epidural analgesia and acute pain management. Anesthesiology 2011;115:181.

provides effective analgesia with less urinary retention than intrathecal morphine. Further studies are needed to define the safety and efficacy of regional anesthesia techniques in fast-track cardiac surgery (and many clinicians avoid them due to concerns about neuraxial hematomas). Although some studies have shown that spinal analgesia with intrathecal morphine decreases extubation time, decreases length of stay in the intensive care unit, reduces pulmonary complications and arrhythmias, and provides analgesia with less respiratory depression, other studies have shown no benefit to this approach.

6 Continuous peripheral nerve blocks (CPNBs) with local anesthetics block afferent nociceptive pathways and are an excellent way to reduce the incidence of opioid-related side effects and facilitate recovery (see Chapter 46). The choice of local anesthetic, dosage, and concentration should be made with the goal of avoiding prolonged motor blockade and delayed mobilization and discharge. Ropivacaine, because of its lower toxicity relative to bupivacaine, is often preferred when high volumes of local anesthetic solution are needed. CPNB after knee arthroplasty facilitates earlier discharge and rehabilitation. Efforts must be made to minimize the motor

block of the quadriceps, which can be responsible for accidental falls. Administering a lumbar plexus block along with a sciatic nerve block decreases hospital length of stay, postoperative urinary retention, and ileus associated with lower extremity total joint replacement when compared with general or neuraxial anesthesia followed by intravenous opioids. The same benefits of fewer opioid side effects and accelerated discharge have been shown with regional anesthesia/analgesia for hand, shoulder, anorectal, and inguinal hernia repair surgery.

Advances in imaging techniques and peripheral catheter technology have generated interest in abdominal wall blockade, facilitating the selective localization of nerves and the direct deposition of local anesthetic in proximity to the compartments where the nerves are located. Transversus abdominis plane (TAP) block (see Chapter 46) has been used for abdominal surgery to facilitate postoperative analgesia and early return of bowel function. Rectus abdominis block can be used for midline incisions. These techniques are alternatives to epidural blockade when the latter is contraindicated.

The potential role of wound infusion of local anesthetic solution in providing analgesia for ERAS has not been determined; nevertheless, local anesthetic wound infusions are widely used to improve postoperative pain control and reduce the necessity for opioids.

C. Intravenous Lidocaine Infusion

(7) Lidocaine (intravenous bolus of 100 mg or 1.5–2 mg/kg, followed by continuous intravenous infusion of 1.5–3 mg/kg/h or 2–3 mg/min) has analgesic, antihyperalgesic, and antiinflammatory properties. In patients undergoing colorectal and radical retropubic prostate surgeries, intravenous lidocaine has been shown to reduce requirements for opioids and general anesthetic agents, to provide satisfactory analgesia, to facilitate early return of bowel function, and to accelerate hospital discharge. Although lidocaine infusion potentially may replace neuraxial blockade and regional anesthesia in some circumstances, more studies are needed to confirm the advantage of this technique in the context of ERPs. The most effective dose and duration of infusion for various surgical procedures remains to be determined; even short duration of lidocaine infusion may have benefit.

D. β-Blockade Therapy

β Blockers have been used to blunt the sympathetic response during laryngoscopy and intubation and to attenuate the surgical stress-induced increase in circulating catecholamines. They also have been shown to prevent perioperative cardiovascular events in at-risk patients undergoing noncardiac surgery and to help maintain hemodynamic stability during the intraoperative period and during emergence from anesthesia. β Blockers reduce the requirement of volatile anesthetic agents and decrease minimum alveolar concentration values; they may also have an opioid-sparing effect. They possess anticatabolic properties, which may be explained by reduced energy requirements associated with decreased adrenergic stimulation. A positive protein balance has been reported in critically ill patients when β blockade is combined with parenteral nutrition. In the context of ERPs, the anesthetic- and analgesic-sparing effects of β blockers may facilitate recovery by accelerating emergence from anesthesia and by reducing anesthetic- and analgesic-related postoperative side effects, including PONV.

E. Intravenous α₂-Agonist Therapy

Both clonidine and dexmedetomidine have anesthetic and analgesic properties. Clonidine decreases postoperative pain, reduces opioid consumption and opioid-related side effects, and prolongs neuraxial and peripheral nerve local anesthetic blockade. In patients undergoing cardiovascular fast-track surgery, spinal morphine with clonidine decreases extubation time, provides effective analgesia, and improves quality of recovery. Dexmedetomidine has not been extensively studied in ERP pathways.

Use of Short-Acting Intravenous & Inhalation Agents

A. Intravenous Anesthetics

Intravenous propofol is the deep sedation and general anesthesia induction agent of choice for many surgical procedures, and may reduce the risk of PONV.

B. Inhalational Anesthetics

Compared with other volatile anesthetic agents, desflurane and sevoflurane can shorten anesthesia emergence, reduce length of stay in the postanesthesia care unit, and decrease recovery-associated costs. When compared with propofol, all inhalation agents increase the risk of PONV. Nitrous oxide, because of its anesthetic- and analgesic-sparing effects, rapid pharmacokinetic profile, and low cost, is frequently administered with other inhalation agents. However, its use may increase the risk of PONV, and nitrous oxide is frequently avoided in patients with risk factors for PONV. Moreover, the use of nitrous oxide during laparoscopic surgery may distend the bowel and impair the surgeon's view of anatomic structures (see Chapter 8).

C. Opioids

Short-acting opioids such as fentanyl, alfentanil, and remifentanil are commonly used during fast-track surgery in combination with inhalation agents or propofol, and with regional analgesia techniques. However, intraoperative administration of remifentanil to patients who will experience extensive postoperative pain has been associated with opioid-induced hyperalgesia, acute opioid tolerance, and increased analgesic requirements during the postoperative period.

D. Muscle Relaxants

The short-acting muscle relaxant succinylcholine and intermediate-acting muscle relaxants such as rocuronium, atracurium, and cisatracurium are commonly used to minimize the risk of unplanned and prolonged muscle relaxation. They are chosen to facilitate tracheal extubation while decreasing the risk of residual blockade during anesthesia recovery.

Maintenance of Normothermia

The inhibitory effect of anesthetic agents on thermoregulation, exposure to the relatively cool surgical environment, and intraoperative loss of heat through the surgical field can lead to intraoperative hypothermia in all patients undergoing surgical procedures under general or regional anesthesia. The duration and extent of the surgical procedure directly correlate with hypothermia risk. Perioperative hypothermia, by increasing sympathetic discharge and inhibiting immune cellular response, increases cardiovascular morbidity and wound infection risk. A decrease in core body temperature of 1.9°C triples the incidence of surgical wound infection. The risk of bleeding and blood transfusion requirement are also increased with hypothermia. Furthermore, by impairing the metabolism of many anesthetic agents, hypothermia significantly prolongs anesthesia recovery. These issues are discussed in Chapter 52.

Maintenance of Adequate Tissue Oxygenation

Surgical stress leads to impaired pulmonary function and peripheral vasoconstriction, resulting in arterial and local tissue hypoxemia. Perioperative hypoxia can increase cardiovascular and cerebral complications, and many strategies should be adopted during the perioperative period to prevent its development.

Maintenance of adequate perioperative oxygenation by oxygen supplementation has been associated with the improvement of some clinically relevant outcomes without increasing the risk of postoperative complications. Ensuring complete recovery of neuromuscular blockade can reduce early postoperative hypoxemia. Intraoperative and postoperative (for 2 h) inspired oxygen concentration of 80% has been associated with increased arterial and subcutaneous oxygen tension, decreased rate of wound infection, and lower incidence of PONV, but without increasing potential complications associated with high oxygen fraction, such as atelectasis and hypercapnia. However, these advantages have not been confirmed in a large, randomized, multicenter trial of patients undergoing elective and emergent laparotomy. The use of regional anesthesia techniques, by decreasing systemic vascular resistance, can also improve superficial and deep peripheral tissue perfusion and oxygenation. Finally avoidance of bedrest, and encouraging early mobilization and physiotherapy, can also improve postoperative central and peripheral tissue oxygenation.

PONV Prophylaxis

Postoperative nausea and vomiting (PONV) is a frequent complication associated with anesthetic drugs that delay early feeding and recovery from surgery. Perioperative strategies for minimizing PONV are strongly advocated for any type of surgery, and consensus guidelines for prevention and management of PONV are available in the current literature. These issues are discussed in Chapters 17 and 56.

Goal-Directed Fluid & Hemodynamic Therapy

Intraoperative and postoperative fluids are commonly infused in excess of perioperative loss. Despite numerous studies seeking to define fluid strategy (amount and type of fluid administered, crystalloid versus colloid, etc), "liberal," "standard," or "restrictive" fluid regimens have failed to consistently improve postoperative outcomes. Liberal fluid administration and sodium excess lead to fluid overload, increase postoperative morbidity, and prolong hospitalization. Fluid overload, especially of crystalloid, has been associated with anastomotic leakage, pulmonary edema, pneumonia, wound infection, postoperative ileus, and reduced tissue oxygenation. Furthermore, excess fluids commonly increase body weight by 3–6 kg and may impair postoperative mobilization. On the other hand, restrictive fluid management does not offer any substantial, clinically relevant advantage, except possibly improving pulmonary function and reducing postoperative hypoxia. However, compared with liberal fluid management, restrictive fluid management increases the release of stress-related hormones such as aldosterone, renin, and angiotensin II. The amount of perioperative extracellular fluid losses can be minimized with limited preoperative fasting, avoidance of mechanical bowel preparation, minimally invasive surgical techniques such as laparoscopic and video-assisted thoracoscopic (VAT) surgery, and early postoperative enteral nutrition.

The concept of goal-directed fluid therapy is based on the optimization of hemodynamic measures such as heart rate, blood pressure, stroke volume, pulse pressure variation, and stroke volume variation obtained by noninvasive cardiac output devices such as pulse-contour arterial waveform analysis, transesophageal echocardiography, or esophageal Doppler (see Chapter 5). The type of fluid infused is also important: isotonic crystalloid should be used to replace extracellular losses, whereas iso-oncotic colloids are needed to replace intravascular volume (Table 48–3).

TABLE 48–3 **Physiologically based first-line fluid replacement for goal-directed therapy.[1]**

Physiological Requirement	Replace with	Amount
Extracellular		
Insensible perspiration	Crystalloids[2]	
Closed abdomen		0.5 mL/kg/h
Open abdomen		1 mL/kg/h
Urine production	Crystalloids	Measured output[4]
Intravascular		
Blood loss	Colloids[3]	Estimated losses
Further preload deficit	Colloids	According to clinical estimation[5]

[1]Reproduced, with permission, from Chappell D, Jacob M: Influence of non-ventilatory options on postoperative outcome. Best Pract Res Clin Anaesthesiol 2010;24:267.

[2]Crystalloids should be given in an isotonic balanced form.

[3]Colloids should be given in an iso-oncotic form in balanced solutions.

[4]First-line approach in healthy kidneys.

[5]If possible use extended monitoring (eg, PICCO system, esophageal Doppler, etc).

POSTOPERATIVE PERIOD
Immediate Postoperative Care

A. Strategies to Minimize Postoperative Shivering

The primary cause of postoperative shivering is perioperative hypothermia, although other, non-thermoregulatory, mechanisms may be involved. Postoperative shivering can greatly increase oxygen consumption, catecholamine release, cardiac output, heart rate and blood pressure, and intracerebral and intraocular pressure. It increases cardiovascular morbidity, especially in elderly patients, and increases length of stay in the postanesthesia care unit. Shivering is uncommon in elderly and hypoxic patients: the efficacy of thermoregulation decreases with aging, and hypoxia can directly inhibit shivering. Many drugs, notably meperidine, clonidine, and tramadol, can be used to reduce postoperative shivering; however, prevention of hypothermia is the most efficient strategy.

B. PONV Treatment

Pharmacological treatment of PONV should be promptly initiated once medical or surgical causes of PONV have been ruled out. PONV and its treatment are reviewed in Chapter 17.

C. Multimodal Analgesia

8 The scientific rationale for multimodal analgesia is to combine different classes of medications, having different (multimodal) pharmacological mechanisms of action and additive or synergistic effects, to control multiple perioperative pathophysiological factors that lead to postoperative pain and its sequelae. Such an approach may achieve desired analgesic effects while reducing analgesic dosage and associated side effects, and often includes utilization of regional analgesic techniques such as local anesthetic wound infusion, epidural or intrathecal analgesia, or single-shot or continuous peripheral nerve blockade. Multimodal analgesia is routinely utilized in ERPs to improve postoperative outcomes. Discussion here focuses on the principal analgesic interventions that can be used in perioperative multimodal analgesia regimens.

9 **1. NSAIDs**—The addition of nonsteroidal antiinflammatory drugs (NSAIDs) to systemic opioids diminishes postoperative pain intensity, reduces the opioid requirement by approximately 30%, and decreases opioid-related side effects such as PONV and sedation. However, NSAIDs may increase the risk of gastrointestinal and postoperative bleeding, decrease kidney function, increase the risk of anastomotic leakage after colorectal surgery, and impair wound healing.

Perioperative administration of cyclooxygenase-2 (COX-2) inhibitors likewise reduces postoperative pain and decreases both opioid consumption and opioid-related side effects, and while their use has reduced the incidence of NSAID-related platelet dysfunction and gastrointestinal bleeding, the adverse effects of COX-2 inhibitors on kidney function remain controversial. Concerns have also been raised regarding their safety for patients undergoing cardiovascular surgery; these have centered on rofecoxib and valdecoxib, specifically. Increased cardiovascular risk associated with the perioperative use of celecoxib or valdecoxib in patients with minimal cardiovascular risk factors and undergoing nonvascular surgery has not been proven. Further studies are needed to establish the analgesic efficacy and safety of COX-2 inhibitors and their clinical effect on postoperative outcomes.

2. Acetaminophen (paracetamol)—Oral, rectal, and parenteral acetaminophen is a common component of multimodal analgesia. Acetaminophen's analgesic effect is 20–30% less than that of NSAIDs, but its pharmacological profile is safer. Analgesic efficacy improves when the drug is administered together with NSAIDs, and it significantly reduces pain intensity and spares opioid consumption after orthopedic and abdominal surgery. However, acetaminophen may not reduce opioid-related side effects. Routine administration of acetaminophen in combination with regional anesthesia and analgesia techniques may allow NSAIDs and COX-2 inhibitors to be reserved for control of breakthrough pain, thus limiting the incidence of NSAID-related side effects.

3. Opioids—Despite the increasing use of new, nonopioid analgesic medications and adjuvants and of regional anesthesia and analgesia techniques intended to minimize opioid requirements and opioid-related side effects (Table 48–4), the use of systemic opioids remains a cornerstone in the management of surgical pain. Parenteral opioids are frequently prescribed in the postoperative period during the transitional phase **10** to oral analgesia. Opioid administration by patient-controlled analgesia (PCA) provides better pain control, greater patient satisfaction, and fewer opioid side effects when compared with on-request parenteral opioid administration. Oral administration of opioids, such as immediate-release and controlled-release oxycodone or hydromorphone, in combination with NSAIDs or acetaminophen, or both, is commonly used in the perioperative period. Preoperative administration of extended-release oxycodone in patients undergoing surgery of short duration provides adequate plasma concentration and analgesia following discontinuance of remifentanil infusion. Tramadol, a partial opioid agonist, has been associated with an increased incidence of PONV.

4. Epidural analgesia—In addition to providing excellent analgesia, epidural blockade blunts the stress response associated with surgery, decreases postoperative morbidity, attenuates catabolism, and accelerates postoperative functional recovery. Compared with systemic opioid analgesia, thoracic epidural analgesia provides better static and dynamic pain relief. Long-acting local anesthetics such as ropivacaine (0.2%), bupivacaine (0.1–0.125%), and levobupivacaine (0.1–0.125%) are commonly administered together with lipophilic opioids by continuous epidural infusion or by patient-controlled epidural analgesia (PCEA). Administering low doses of local anesthetic via thoracic epidural infusion avoids lower extremity motor blockade that may delay postoperative mobilization and recovery. Adding fentanyl or sufentanil to epidural local anesthetics improves the quality of postoperative analgesia without delaying recovery of bowel function.

High thoracic epidural analgesia has been introduced in patients undergoing cardiac surgery based on data from small randomized clinical trials that suggested beneficial effects on postoperative

TABLE 48–4 Analgesic adjuvants in the perioperative period.[1,2]

Adjuvant	Type of Surgery or Clinical Setting	Analgesic Efficacy as Adjuvant	Dosages Used (Boluses, CI)	Administration			Monitoring
				Route	Timing	Postoperative Duration	
Lidocaine	Tonsillectomy	–	1.5 mg/kg, *followed by* 1.5–2 mg/kg/h CI (Intra, until skin closure), *and then* 1 mg/kg/h CI (Post)	IV	Pre,[3] Intra, Peri	30 min–48 h	Signs of local anesthetic toxicity (CNS cardiovascular)
	Cardiac	+					
	Abdominal (laparotomy, laparoscopic)	+					
	Thoracotomy	+					
	Hysterectomy	+					
	Laparoscopic prostatectomy	+					
	Orthopedic	–					
Ketamine	Cardiac	+	0.5–1 mg/kg, *followed by* 2–10 mcg/kg/min CI	IV	Pre, Post (PCA[4]), Peri	4–72 h	CNS[5] (level of sedation, nystagmus hallucinations), cardiovascular
	Thoracotomy	+					
	Abdominal	+					
	Gynecological	–					
	Orthopedic	–					
	Spine	+/–					
	Chronic use of opioids	+					
	Preventing chronic pain	+/–					
	OIH	+/–					
Gabapentinoids							
Gabapentin	Cholecystectomy	–	300–1200 mg	PO	Pre,[6] Post		CNS[5] (level of sedation, somnolence, dizziness), leg edema
	Hysterectomy	+					
	Spine	+					
	Hip arthroplasty	–					
	Preventing chronic pain	+/–					
Pregabalin	Hysterectomy	+	75–300 mg	PO	Pre, Post		
	Laparoscopic cholecystectomy	–					
	Preventing chronic pain	+/–					

Agent	Surgery	Dose	Route	Timing	Side effects
MgSO$_4$	Cardiac + Cholecystectomy + Lower limb orthopedic + Gynecological + Ambulatory +	30–50 mg/kg, *followed by* 8–15 mg/kg/h CI	IV	Pre, Intra	CNS (somnolence), neuromuscular function, respiratory depression, cardiovascular (bradycardia)
Steroids	Hip arthroplasty + Breast + Laparoscopic cholecystectomy +	Dexamethasone: 8–16 mg Methylprednisolone: 125 mg	IV	Pre	Glycemia, GI bleeding, wound healing
α$_2$-Agonist Clonidine	PO Abdominal − Total knee arthroplasty + Hysterectomy + Prostatectomy − IV Cholecystectomy − Abdominal + Spine +	PO 3–5 mcg/kg IV 150 mcg	PO, IV	Pre,[7] Intra, Post (PCA[8])	CNS[5] (level of sedation), cardiovascular (hypotension, bradycardia)
Dexmedetomidine	Thoracotomy + Abdominal + Hysterectomy + Bariatric +	Loading dose 0.5–1 mcg/kg, *followed by* 0.2–0.4 mcg/kg/h CI	IV	Pre, Intra, Post (PCA[9])	

[1]Efficacy of these agents as adjuvant analgesics has been demonstrated by a reduction of pain or opioid consumption, or both; or opioid side effects; or all three.

[2]CI, continuous infusion; Intra, Intraoperative period; Post, postoperative period; Pre, preoperative period during induction; Peri, preoperative, intraoperative, and postoperative periods; CNS, central nervous system; PCA, patient-controlled analgesia; OIH, opioid-induced hyperalgesia; GI, gastrointestinal.

[3]Bolus, or 30 min before induction of anesthesia.

[4]As a 1-mg demand dose, lockout time 7 min.

[5]Psychotomimetic side effects are dose-dependent.

[6]Single dose, 1–2.5 h before surgery.

[7]Given PO 60–90 min before surgery.

[8]As a 20-mcg demand dose, lockout time 5 min.

[9]As a 5-mcg demand dose, lockout time 5 min.

outcomes. A recent meta-analysis of more than 2700 patients who underwent cardiac surgery and received high thoracic epidural analgesia showed an overall reduction of pulmonary complications (relative risk = 0.53) and supraventricular arrhythmias (relative risk = 0.68), but no reduction in incidence of myocardial infarction, stroke, or postoperative mortality. Due to concerns about the risk of epidural hematoma and its devastating neurological consequences in patients fully heparinized during cardiopulmonary bypass, the use of high thoracic epidural analgesia is understandably limited.

11   **5. Peripheral nerve block**—Single-shot and continuous peripheral nerve blockade is frequently utilized for fast-track ambulatory and inpatient orthopedic surgery, and can accelerate recovery from surgery and improve analgesia and patient satisfaction (see Chapter 46). The opioid-sparing effect of nerve blocks minimizes the risk of opioid-related side effects. Appropriate patient selection and strict adherence to institutional clinical pathways helps ensure the success of peripheral nerve blockade as a fast-track orthopedic analgesia technique. Peripheral nerve blockade has also been used as a component of multimodal analgesia for abdominal surgery; for example, transverseus abdominis plane (TAP) block in patients undergoing total abdominal hysterectomy provides effective analgesia and decreases morphine consumption and sedation when compared with patients receiving morphine alone via PCA.

6. Local anesthetic wound infusion—The analgesic efficacy of local anesthetic wound infusion has been established for multiple surgical procedures. Inconsistent results may be due to factors that include type, concentration, and dose of local anesthetic, catheter placement technique and type of catheter, mode of local anesthetic delivery, incision location, and dislodgment of the catheter during patient mobilization.

Strategies to Facilitate Recovery on the Surgical Unit

A. Organization of Multidisciplinary Surgical Care

The multidisciplinary aspect of postoperative care should bring together the surgeon, the nurse, the anesthesiologist, the nutritionist, and the physiotherapist in an effort to customize individual patient care based on standardized, procedure-specific protocols. Comfortable chairs and walkers need to be made readily available near each patient bed to encourage patients to sit, stand, and walk. The benefits of mobilization for cardiovascular homeostasis and bowel function have been shown repeatedly. Patients should be encouraged to sit the evening following surgery, with ambulation starting the next day for a minimum of 4–6 h each day. If patients cannot get out of bed, they should be encouraged to perform physical and deep breathing exercises.

B. Optimization of Analgesia to Facilitate Functional Recovery

A well-organized, well-trained, highly motivated acute pain service (APS) and surgical nursing workforce, utilizing procedure-specific clinical protocols to optimally manage analgesia and related side effects, is critically important for fast-track surgery. The quality of pain relief and symptom control heavily influences postoperative recovery; optimal mobilization and dietary intake depend upon adequate analgesia. The anesthesiologist, in coordination with the APS, must identify and employ the optimal analgesic techniques tailored to the specific surgical procedure, and the quality of analgesia and possible presence of side effects must be closely and continuously assessed. The patient must be comfortable ambulating and performing physiotherapy, with minimal side effects such as lightheadedness, sedation, nausea and vomiting, and leg weakness.

C. Strategies to Minimize Postoperative Ileus

12   Postoperative ileus delays enteral feeding, causes patient discomfort, and is one of the most common causes of prolonged postoperative hospital stay. Because early enteral nutrition is associated with decreased postoperative morbidity, interventions and strategies aimed at decreasing postoperative ileus are required for patients in an ERP. Three main mechanisms contribute to ileus: sympathetic inhibitory reflexes, local inflammation caused by surgery, and postoperative opioid analgesia. The nasogastric tube, frequently inserted after abdominal surgery, does not speed the recovery of bowel function and may increase pulmonary morbidity by increasing the incidence of aspiration. Therefore, nasogastric tubes should be discouraged whenever possible or used for only a very short period of time, even in gastric and hepatic surgery.

Multimodal analgesia and nonopioid analgesia techniques shorten the duration of postoperative ileus. Continuous epidural local anesthetic infusion improves the recovery of bowel function by suppressing the inhibitory sympathetic spinal cord reflexes. Thoracic epidural analgesia with local anesthetics and small doses of opioids reduces the incidence of ileus and improves postoperative pain relief. Minimally invasive surgery decreases surgical stress and inflammation, resulting in a faster return of bowel function. Any role of epidural analgesia in accelerating the recovery of bowel function after laparoscopic surgery remains controversial, at best. Laxatives, such as milk of magnesia and bisacodyl, reduce postoperative ileus duration. Prokinetic medications such as metoclopramide are ineffective. Neostigmine increases peristalsis but may also increase the incidence of PONV.

Excessive perioperative fluid administration commonly causes bowel mucosal edema and delays postoperative return of bowel function. However, results from a randomized double-blind study of liberal versus restricted fluid administration showed no differences with regard to recovery of bowel function in patients undergoing fast-track abdominal surgery. No studies have compared crystalloid versus colloid administration in terms of their effect ⑬ on the return of bowel function. Because either excessive, or excessively restricted, perioperative fluid therapy may increase the incidence and severity of postoperative ileus, a goal-directed fluid strategy (discussed earlier) should be selected to decrease postoperative morbidities and enhance recovery and should be utilized according to the type of surgery and patient comorbidities.

Postoperative chewing gum, by stimulating gastrointestinal reflexes, may decrease ileus duration. Although its effect has not been evaluated in ERP patients, postoperative chewing gum may be included in multimodal interventions to decrease postoperative ileus because of its safety and low cost. Peripheral opioid μ-receptor antagonists methylnaltrexone and alvimopan have been introduced to minimize the adverse effects of opioids on bowel function without antagonizing opioid analgesia. In patients receiving large-dose intravenous morphine analgesia, alvimopan decreases the duration of postoperative ileus by 16–18 h, the incidence of nasogastric tube reinsertion, postoperative morbidity, and hospital length of stay and readmission rates, especially in patients undergoing bowel resection. Nevertheless, the recovery of bowel function is slower when compared with patients receiving multimodal strategies in an ERP.

Issues in the Implementation of Enhanced Recovery Programs

The success of ERPs depends upon the capacity of multiple stakeholders to reach interdisciplinary consensus. Several aspects of perioperative care, such as use of drains, dietary and activity restrictions, fluid management, and bedrest, have been part of surgical "traditions" and must be significantly revised in ERPs. Patient involvement and patient and family expectations are critically important, but frequently overlooked, aspects of these programs. New surgical techniques, like transverse incisions or minimally invasive surgery, may require surgeons to acquire and perfect new skills. Similarly, the emphasis on thoracic epidural blockade or peripheral nerve blocks, pharmacological modulation of the neuroendocrine stress response to surgery, goal-directed fluid and hemodynamic therapy, and integral involvement of a well-organized and managed APS requires an expansion of the traditional role of anesthesia providers. Aggressive analgesia and symptom management, early ambulation and physiotherapy, early nutrition protocols, and early removal or total avoidance of urinary drainage catheters significantly change the way patients are cared for in the postanesthesia recovery unit and on the surgical unit and require a well-organized, highly trained, highly motivated nursing staff.

Although there are published studies of successful ERPs, there are no "off-the-shelf" protocols,

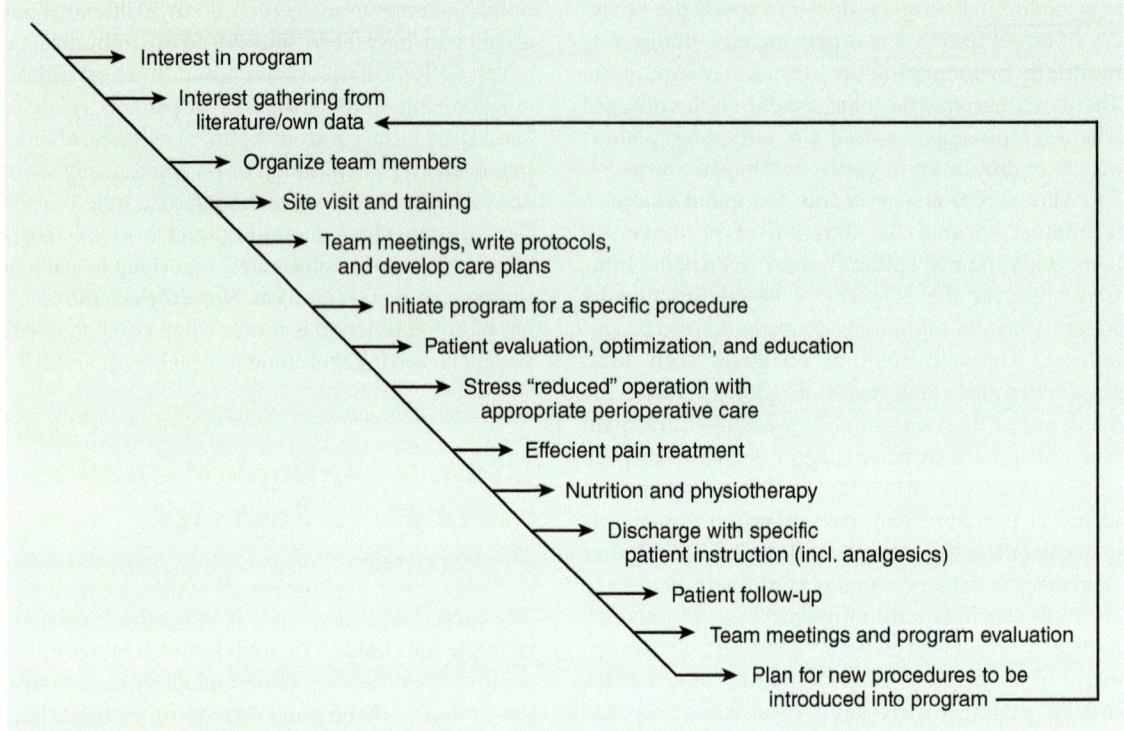

Interest in program

Interest gathering from
literature/own data

Organize team members

Site visit and training

Team meetings, write protocols,
and develop care plans

Initiate program for a specific procedure

Patient evaluation, optimization, and education

Stress "reduced" operation with
appropriate perioperative care

Effecient pain treatment

Nutrition and physiotherapy

Discharge with specific
patient instruction (incl. analgesics)

Patient follow-up

Team meetings and program evaluation

Plan for new procedures to be
introduced into program

FIGURE 48–5 Stepwise process for initiating and implementing an enhanced recovery program. (Reproduced, with permission, from Kehlet et al: Ann Surg 2008;248:189.)

and local differences in expertise, experience, and resources influence the development of such protocols for each institution. Each family of similar surgical procedures requires a standardized interdisciplinary clinical protocol or pathway, with specialized input from a team with experience in caring for those patients. Such an interdisciplinary team should include representatives from surgery, anesthesiology, nursing, pharmacy, physiotherapy, nutrition, and administration, and it should be responsible not only for the clinical protocol's creation, but also for continuously monitoring its efficacy and for instituting performance improvement-related protocol modifications and provider feedback as indicated by outcomes data (Figure 48–5).

The current era is one in which optimal surgical care requires the anesthesia provider to be part of the perioperative medicine team. The anesthesiologist's skill sets are essential for the success of ERPs and have potential benefits for surgical care delivery on a global basis, from preoperative evaluation and presurgical preparation to recovery and final dismissal from care. This opportunity must be seized.

GUIDELINES

Gustafsson UO, Scott MJ, Schwenk W, et al: Guidelines for perioperative care in elective colonic surgery: Enhanced Recovery After Surgery (ERAS) Society recommendations. Clin Nutr 2012;31:783.

Lassen K, Coolsen MM, Slim K, et al: Guidelines for perioperative care for pancreaticoduodenectomy: Enhanced Recovery After Surgery (ERAS) Society recommendations. Clin Nutr 2012;31:817.

Nygren J, Thacker J, Carli F, et al: Guidelines for perioperative care in elective rectal/pelvic surgery: Enhanced Recovery After Surgery (ERAS) Society recommendations. Clin Nutr 2012;31:801.

SUGGESTED READING

Aarts M-A, Okrainec A, Glicksman A, et al: Adoption of enhanced recovery after surgery (ERAS) strategies for colorectal surgery at academic teaching hospitals and impact on total length of hospital stay. Surg Endosc 2012;26:442.

Adamina M, Kehlet H, Tomlinson GA, et al: Enhanced recovery pathways optimize health outcomes and resource utilization: A meta-analysis of randomized controlled trials in colorectal surgery. Surgery 2011;149:830.

Baldini G, F Carli: Anesthetic adjunctive drugs for fast-track surgery. Curr Drug Targets 2009;10:667.

Carli F, Kehlet H, Baldini G, et al: Evidence basis for regional anesthesia in multidisciplinary fast-track surgical care pathways. Reg Anesth Pain Med 2011;36:63.

Chappell D, Jacob M: Influence of non-ventilatory options on postoperative outcome. Best Pract Res Clin Anaesthesiol 2010;24:267.

Chappell D, Jacob M, Hofmann-Kiefer K, et al: Rational approach to perioperative fluid management. Anesthesiology 2008;109:723.

Collard V, Mistraletti G, Taqi A, et al: Intraoperative esmolol infusion in the absence of opioids spares postoperative fentanyl in patients undergoing ambulatory laparoscopic cholecystectomy. Anesth Analg 2007;105:1255.

Coulter A, Ellins J: Effectiveness of strategies for informing, educating, and involving patients. Br Med J 2007;335:24.

Dunkelgrun M, Boersma E, Schouten O, et al: Dutch Echocardiographic Cardiac Risk Evaluation Applying Stress Echocardiography Study Group. Bisoprolol and fluvastatin for the reduction of perioperative cardiac mortality and myocardial infarction in intermediate-risk patients undergoing noncardiovascular surgery: A randomized controlled trial (DECREASE-IV). Ann Surg 2009;249:921.

Harvey KP, Adair JD, Mayyas I, et al: Can intravenous lidocaine decrease postsurgical ileus and shorten hospital stay in elective bowel surgery? A pilot study and literature review. Am J Surg 2009;198:231.

Kehlet H: Multimodal approach to postoperative recovery. Curr Opin Crit Care 2009;15:355.

Kehlet H, Wilmore DW: Evidence-based surgical care and the evolution of fast-track surgery. Ann Surg 2008;248:189.

Kelin J: Multimodal multidisciplinary standardization of perioperative care: Still a long way to go? Curr Opin Crit Care 2008;21:187.

Liu SS, Richman JM, Thirlby RC, et al: Efficacy of continuous wound catheters delivering local anesthetic for postoperative analgesia: A quantitative and qualitative systematic review of randomized controlled trials. J Am Coll Surg 2006;203:914.

Ljungqvist O: Preoperative fasting. Br J Surg 2003;90:400.

Lui F, Ng KF: Adjuvant analgesics in acute pain. Expert Opin Pharmacother 2011;12:363.

Manion, SC, Brennan TJ: Thoracic epidural anesthesia and acute pain management. Anesthesiology 2011;115:181.

Neugebaure EAM, Wilkinson RC, Kehlet H, et al: PROSPECT: A practical method for formulating evidence-based expert recommendations for the management of postoperative pain. Surg Endosc 2007;21:1047.

Pöpping DM, Elia N, Marret E, et al: Protective effects of epidural analgesia on pulmonary complications after abdominal and thoracic surgery: A meta-analysis. Arch Surg 2008;143:990.

Powell AE, Davies HTO, Bannister J, et al: Challenge of improving postoperative pain management: Case studies of three acute pain services in the UK National Health Service. Br J Anaesth 2009;102:824.

Tonnesen H, Nielsen PR, Lauritzen JB, et al: Smoking and alcohol intervention before surgery: Evidence for best practice. Br J Anaesth 2009;102:297.

Vigneault L, Turgeon AF, Côté D, et al: Perioperative intravenous lidocaine infusion for postoperative pain control: a meta-analysis of randomized controlled trials. Can J Anaesth 2011;58:22.

White PF, Kehlet H, Neal JM, et al: The role of the anesthesiologist in fast-track surgery: From multimodal analgesia to perioperative medical care. Anesth Analg 2007;104:1380.

Wu CI, Raja SN: Treatment of postoperative pain. Lancet 2011;377:2215.

Yardeni IZ, Beilin B, Mayburd E, et al: The effect of perioperative intravenous lidocaine on postoperative pain and immune function. Anesth Analg 2009,109:1464.

Management of Patients with Fluid & Electrolyte Disturbances

CHAPTER

49

KEY CONCEPTS

1 Osmotic pressure is generally dependent only on the number of nondiffusible solute particles. This is because the average kinetic energy of particles in solution is similar regardless of their mass.

2 Potassium is the most important determinant of intracellular osmotic pressure, whereas sodium is the most important determinant of extracellular osmotic pressure.

3 Fluid exchange between the intracellular and interstitial spaces is governed by the osmotic forces created by differences in nondiffusible solute concentrations.

4 Serious manifestations of hyponatremia are generally associated with plasma sodium concentrations <120 mEq/L.

5 Very rapid correction of hyponatremia has been associated with demyelinating lesions in the pons (central pontine myelinolysis), resulting in serious permanent neurological sequelae.

6 The major hazard of increases in extracellular volume is impaired gas exchange due to pulmonary interstitial edema, alveolar edema, or large collections of pleural or ascitic fluid.

7 Intravenous replacement of potassium chloride is usually reserved for patients

with, or at risk for, significant cardiac manifestations or severe muscle weakness.

8 Because of its lethal potential, hyperkalemia exceeding 6 mEq/L should always be corrected.

9 Symptomatic hypercalcemia requires rapid treatment. The most effective initial treatment is rehydration followed by a brisk diuresis (urinary output 200–300 mL/h) utilizing administration of intravenous saline infusion and a loop diuretic to accelerate calcium excretion.

10 Symptomatic hypocalcemia is a medical emergency and should be treated immediately with intravenous calcium chloride (3–5 mL of a 10% solution) or calcium gluconate (10–20 mL of a 10% solution).

11 Some patients with severe hypophosphatemia may require mechanical ventilation postoperatively because of muscle weakness.

12 Marked hypermagnesemia can lead to respiratory and cardiac arrest.

13 Isolated hypomagnesemia should be corrected prior to elective procedures because of its potential for causing cardiac arrhythmias.

Fluid and electrolyte disturbances are extremely common in the perioperative period. Large volumes of intravenous fluids are frequently required to correct fluid deficits and compensate for blood loss during surgery. Major disturbances in fluid and electrolyte balance can rapidly alter cardiovascular, neurological, and neuromuscular functions, and anesthesia providers must have a clear understanding of normal water and electrolyte physiology. This chapter examines the body's fluid compartments and common water and electrolyte derangements, their treatment, and anesthetic implications. Acid–base disorders and intravenous fluid therapy are discussed in other chapters.

Nomenclature of Solutions

The system of international units (SI) has still not gained universal acceptance in clinical practice, and many older expressions of concentration remain in common use. Thus, for example, the quantity of a solute in a solution may be expressed in grams, moles, or equivalents. To complicate matters further, the concentration of a solution may be expressed either as quantity of solute per volume of solution or quantity of solute per weight of solvent.

MOLARITY, MOLALITY, & EQUIVALENCY

One mole of a substance represents 6.02×10^{23} molecules. The weight of this quantity in grams is commonly referred to as gram-molecular weight. Molarity is the standard SI unit of concentration that expresses the number of moles of solute per *liter* of solution. Molality is an alternative term that expresses moles of solute per *kilogram* of solvent. Equivalency is also commonly used for substances that ionize: the number of equivalents of an ion in solution is the number of moles multiplied by its charge (valence). Thus, a 1 M solution of $MgCl_2$ yields 2 equivalents of magnesium per liter and 2 equivalents of chloride per liter.

OSMOLARITY, OSMOLALITY, & TONICITY

Osmosis is the net movement of water across a semipermeable membrane as a result of a difference in nondiffusible solute concentrations between the two sides. *Osmotic pressure* is the pressure that must be applied to the side with more solute to prevent a net movement of water across the membrane to dilute the solute.

1 Osmotic pressure is generally dependent only on the number of nondiffusible solute particles. This is because the average kinetic energy of particles in solution is similar regardless of their mass. One osmole equals 1 mol of nondissociable substances. For substances that ionize, however, each mole results in n Osm, where n is the number of ionic species produced. Thus, 1 mol of a highly ionized substance such as NaCl dissolved in solution should produce 2 Osm; in reality ionic interaction between the cation and anion reduces the effective activity of each such that NaCl behaves as if it is only 75% ionized. A difference of 1 mOsm/L between two solutions results in an osmotic pressure of 19.3 mm Hg. The osmolarity of a solution is equal to the number of osmoles per *liter* of solution, whereas its osmolality equals the number of osmoles per *kilogram* of solvent. *Tonicity,* a term that is often used interchangeably with osmolarity and osmolality, refers to the effect a solution has on cell volume. An *isotonic* solution has no effect on cell volume, whereas *hypotonic* and *hypertonic* solutions increase and decrease cell volume, respectively.

Fluid Compartments

Body water is distributed between two major fluid compartments separated by cell membranes: intracellular fluid (ICF) and extracellular fluid (ECF). The latter can be further subdivided into intravascular and interstitial compartments. The interstitium includes all fluid that is both outside cells and outside the vascular endothelium. The relative contributions of each compartment to total body water (TBW) and body weight are delineated in Table 49–1.

TABLE 49–1 Body fluid compartments (based on average 70-kg male).

Compartment	Fluid as Percent Body Weight (%)	Total Body Water (%)	Fluid Volume (L)
Intracellular	40	67	28
Extracellular			
Interstitial	15	25	10.5
Intravascular	5	8	3.5
Total	60	100	42

The volume of fluid (water) within a compartment is determined by its solute composition and concentrations (Table 49–2). Differences in solute concentrations are largely due to the characteristics of the physical barriers that separate compartments (see below). The osmotic forces created by "trapped" solutes govern the distribution of water between compartments and ultimately each compartment's volume.

INTRACELLULAR FLUID

The outer membrane of cells plays an important role in regulating intracellular volume and composition. A membrane-bound adenosine triphosphate (ATP)–dependent pump exchanges Na^+ for K^+ in a 3:2 ratio. Because cell membranes are relatively impermeable to sodium and (to a lesser extent) potassium ions, potassium is concentrated intracellularly, whereas sodium is concentrated extracellularly. As a result, potassium is the most important determinant of intracellular osmotic pressure, whereas sodium is the most important determinant of extracellular osmotic pressure.

The impermeability of cell membranes to most proteins results in a high intracellular protein concentration. Because proteins act as nondiffusible solutes (anions), the unequal exchange ratio of 3 Na^+ for 2 K^+ by the cell membrane pump is critical in preventing relative intracellular hyperosmolality. Interference with $Na^+–K^+$-ATPase activity, as occurs during ischemia or hypoxia, results in progressive swelling of cells.

EXTRACELLULAR FLUID

The principal function of ECF is to provide a medium for delivery of cell nutrients and electrolytes and for removal of cellular waste products. Maintenance of a normal extracellular volume—particularly the circulating component (intravascular volume)—is critical. For the reasons described

TABLE 49–2 The composition of fluid compartments.

	Gram-Molecular Weight	Intracellular (mEq/L)	Extracellular	
			Intravascular (mEq/L)	Interstitial (mEq/L)
Sodium	23.0	10	145	142
Potassium	39.1	140	4	4
Calcium	40.1	<1	3	3
Magnesium	24.3	50	2	2
Chloride	35.5	4	105	110
Bicarbonate	61.0	10	24	28
Phosphorus	31.0[1]	75	2	2
Protein (g/dL)		16	7	2

[1]PO_4^{3-} is 95 g.

above, sodium is quantitatively the most important extracellular cation and the major determinant of extracellular osmotic pressure and volume. Changes in ECF volume are therefore related to changes in total body sodium content. The latter is a function of sodium intake, renal sodium excretion, and extrarenal sodium losses (see below).

Interstitial Fluid

Very little interstitial fluid is normally in the form of free fluid. Most interstitial water is in chemical association with extracellular proteoglycans, forming a gel. Interstitial fluid pressure is generally thought to be negative (about −5 mm Hg). As interstitial fluid volume increases, interstitial pressure also rises and eventually becomes positive. When the latter occurs, the free fluid in the gel increases rapidly and appears clinically as edema.

Because only small quantities of plasma proteins can normally cross capillary clefts, the protein content of interstitial fluid is relatively low (2 g/dL). Protein entering the interstitial space is returned to the vascular system via the lymphatic system.

Intravascular Fluid

Intravascular fluid, commonly referred to as plasma, is restricted to the intravascular space by the vascular endothelium. Most electrolytes (small ions) freely pass between plasma and the interstitium, resulting in nearly identical electrolyte composition. However, the tight intercellular junctions between adjacent endothelial cells impede the passage of plasma proteins to outside the intravascular compartment. As a result, plasma proteins (mainly albumin) are the only osmotically active solutes in fluid not normally exchanged between plasma and interstitial fluid.

Increases in extracellular volume are normally proportionately reflected in intravascular and interstitial volume. However, when interstitial pressure becomes positive, continued increases in ECF result in expansion of only the interstitial fluid compartment (Figure 49–1). In this way, the interstitial compartment acts as an overflow reservoir for the intravascular compartment. This is seen clinically in the form of tissue edema.

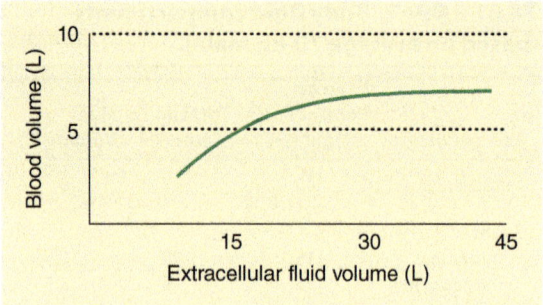

FIGURE 49–1 The relationship between blood volume and extracellular fluid volume. (Modified and reproduced, with permission, from Guyton AC: *Textbook of Medical Physiology*, 7th ed. W.B. Saunders, 1986.)

EXCHANGE BETWEEN FLUID COMPARTMENTS

Diffusion is the random movement of molecules due to their kinetic energy and is responsible for the majority of fluid and solute exchange between compartments. The rate of diffusion of a substance across a membrane depends upon (1) the permeability of that substance through that membrane, (2) the concentration difference for that substance between the two sides, (3) the pressure difference between either side because pressure imparts greater kinetic energy, and (4) the electrical potential across the membrane for charged substances.

Diffusion Through Cell Membranes

Diffusion between interstitial fluid and ICF may take place by one of several mechanisms: (1) directly through the lipid bilayer of the cell membrane, (2) through protein channels within the membrane, or (3) by reversible binding to a carrier protein that can traverse the membrane (facilitated diffusion). Oxygen, CO_2, water, and lipid-soluble molecules penetrate the cell membrane directly. Cations such as Na^+, K^+, and Ca^{2+} penetrate the membrane poorly because of the cell transmembrane voltage potential (which is positive to the outside) created by the Na^+–K^+ pump. Therefore, these cations can diffuse only through specific protein channels. Passage through these channels is dependent on membrane voltage and the binding of ligands (such as acetylcholine) to the membrane receptors. Glucose and amino acids diffuse with the help of membrane-bound carrier proteins.

③ Fluid exchange between the intracellular and interstitial spaces is governed by the osmotic forces created by differences in nondiffusible solute concentrations. Relative changes in osmolality between the intracellular and interstitial compartments result in a net water movement from the hypoosmolar to the hyperosmolar compartment.

Diffusion Through Capillary Endothelium

Capillary walls are typically 0.5 μm thick, consisting of a single layer of endothelial cells with their basement membrane. Intercellular clefts, 6–7 nm wide, separate each cell from its neighbors. Oxygen, CO_2, water, and lipid-soluble substances can penetrate directly through both sides of the endothelial cell membrane. Only low-molecular-weight water-soluble substances such as sodium, chloride, potassium, and glucose readily cross intercellular clefts. High-molecular-weight substances such as plasma proteins penetrate the endothelial clefts poorly (except in the liver and the lungs, where the clefts are larger).

Fluid exchange across capillaries differs from that across cell membranes in that it is governed by significant differences in hydrostatic pressures in addition to osmotic forces (**Figure 49–2**). These forces are operative on both arterial and venous ends of capillaries, with a tendency for fluid to move out of capillaries at the arterial end and back into capillaries at the venous end. Moreover, the magnitude of these forces differs between the various tissue beds. Arterial capillary pressure is determined by precapillary sphincter tone. Thus capillaries that require a high pressure such as glomeruli have low precapillary sphincter tone, whereas the normally low-pressure capillaries of muscle have high precapillary sphincter tone. Normally, all but 10% of the fluid filtered is reabsorbed back into capillaries. What is not reabsorbed (about 2 mL/min) enters the interstitial fluid and is then returned by lymphatic flow to the intravascular compartment.

Disorders of Water Balance

The human body at birth is approximately 75% water by weight. By 1 month this value decreases to 65%, and by adulthood to 60% for males and 50% for females. The higher fat content in females decreases water content. For the same reason, obesity and advanced age further decrease water content.

NORMAL WATER BALANCE

The normal adult daily water intake averages 2500 mL, which includes approximately 300 mL as a byproduct of the metabolism of energy substrates. Daily water loss averages 2500 mL and is typically accounted for by 1500 mL in urine, 400 mL in respiratory tract evaporation, 400 mL in skin evaporation, 100 mL in sweat, and 100 mL in feces. Evaporative loss is very important in thermoregulation because this mechanism normally accounts for 20–25% of heat loss.

Both ICF and ECF osmolalities are tightly regulated to maintain normal water content in tissues. Changes in water content and cell volume can induce serious impairment of function, particularly in the brain (see below).

RELATIONSHIP OF PLASMA SODIUM CONCENTRATION, EXTRACELLULAR OSMOLALITY, & INTRACELLULAR OSMOLALITY

The osmolality of ECF is equal to the sum of the concentrations of all dissolved solutes. Because Na^+ and its anions account for nearly 90% of these solutes, the following approximation is valid:

$$\text{Plasma osmolality} = 2 \times \text{Plasma sodium concentration}$$

Moreover, because ICF and ECF are in osmotic equilibrium, plasma sodium concentration $[Na^+]_{plasma}$ generally reflects total body osmolality:

$$\text{Total body osmolality} = \frac{\text{Extracellular solutes} + \text{intracellular solutes}}{\text{TBW}}$$

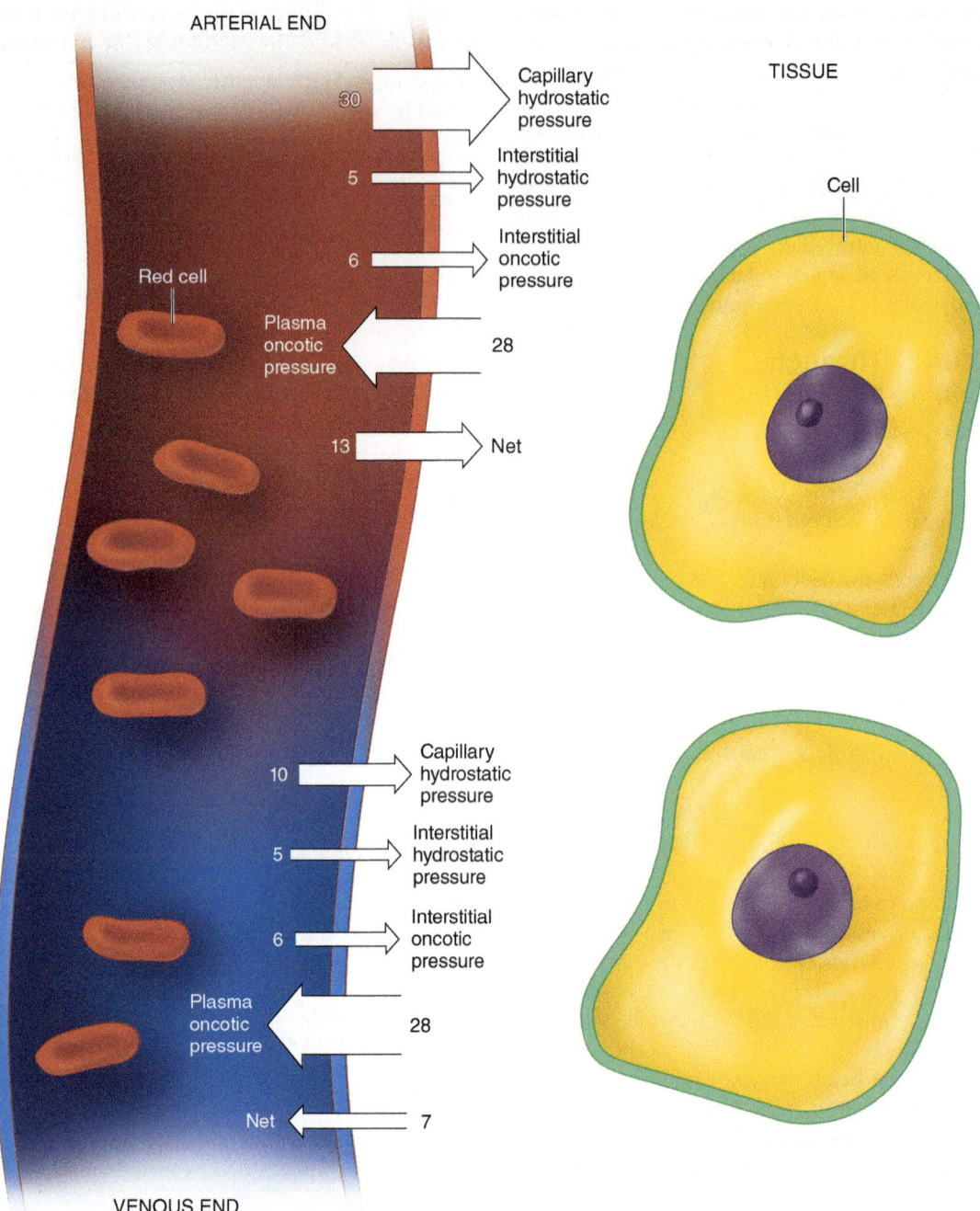

FIGURE 49–2 Capillary fluid exchange. The numbers in this figure are in mm Hg and indicate the pressure gradient for the respective pressures. "Net" refers to the net pressure at either end of the capillary, ie, 13 mm Hg at the arterial and 7 mm Hg at the venous end of the capillary.

Because sodium and potassium are the major intra- and extracellular solutes, respectively:

Total body osmolality

$$= \frac{(Na^+_{extracellular} \times 2) + (K^+_{intracellular\ solutes} \times 2)}{TBW}$$

Combining the two approximations:

$$[Na^+]_{plasma} \approx \frac{Na^+_{extracellular} + K^+_{intracellular}}{TBW}$$

Using these principles, the effect of isotonic, hypotonic, and hypertonic fluid loads on compartmental water content and plasma osmolality can be calculated (Table 49–3). The potential importance of intracellular potassium concentration is readily apparent from this equation. Thus significant potassium losses may contribute to hyponatremia.

In pathological states, glucose and—to a much lesser extent—urea can contribute significantly to extracellular osmolality. A more accurate approximation of plasma osmolality is therefore given by the following equation:

Plasma osmolality (mOsm/kg)

$$= [Na^+] \times 2 + \frac{BUN}{2.8} + \frac{glucose}{18}$$

where $[Na^+]$ is expressed as mEq/L and blood urea nitrogen (BUN) and glucose as mg/dL. Urea is an ineffective osmole because it readily permeates cell membranes and is therefore frequently omitted from this calculation:

$$\text{Effective plasma osmolality} = [Na^+] \times 2 + \frac{glucose}{18}$$

Plasma osmolality normally varies between 280 and 290 mOsm/L. Plasma sodium concentration decreases approximately 1 mEq/L for every 62 mg/dL increase in glucose concentration. A discrepancy between the measured and calculated osmolality is referred to as an *osmolal gap*. Significant osmolal gaps indicate a high concentration of an abnormal osmotically active molecule in plasma such as ethanol, mannitol, methanol, ethylene glycol, or isopropyl alcohol. Osmolal gaps may also be seen in patients with chronic kidney failure (attributed to retention of small solutes), patients with ketoacidosis (as a result of a high concentration of

TABLE 49–3 Effect of different fluid loads on extracellular and intracellular water contents.[1]

A. Normal
Total body solute = 280 mOsm/kg × 42 kg = 11,760 mOsm
Intracellular solute = 280 mOsm/kg × 25 kg = 7000 mOsm
Extracellular solute = 280 mOsm/kg × 17 kg = 4760 mOsm
Extracellular sodium concentration = 280 ÷ 2 = 140 mEq/L

	Intracellular	Extracellular
Osmolality	280	280
Volume (L)	25	17
Net water gain	0	0

B. Isotonic load: 2 L of Isotonic saline (NaCl)
Total body solute = 280 mOsm/kg × 44 kg = 12,320 mOsm
Intracellular solute = 280 mOsm/kg × 25 kg = 7000 mOsm
Extracellular solute = 280 mOsm/kg × 19 kg = 5320 mOsm

	Intracellular	Extracellular
Osmolality	280	280
Volume (L)	25	19
Net water gain	0	2

Net effect: Fluid remains in extracellular compartment.

C. Free water (hypotonic) load: 2 L water
New body water = 42 + 2 = 44 kg
New body osmolality = 11,760 mOsm ÷ 44 kg = 267 mOsm/kg
New intracellular volume = 7000 mOsm ÷ 267 mOsm/kg
= 26.2 kg
New extracellular sodium concentration = 267 ÷ 2 = 133 mEq/L

	Intracellular	Extracellular
Osmolality	267.0	267.0
Volume (L)	26.2	17.8
Net water gain	+1.2	+0.8

Net effect: Fluid distributes between both compartments.

D. Hypertonic load: 600 mEq NaCl (no water)
Total body solute = 11,760 + 600 = 12,360 mOsm/kg
New body osmolality = 12,360 mOsm/kg ÷ 42 kg
= 294 mOsm
New extracellular solute = 600 + 4760 = 5360 mOsm
New extracellular volume = 5360 mOsm ÷ 294 mOsm/kg
= 18.2 kg
New intracellular volume = 42 – 18.2 = 23.8 kg
New extracellular sodium concentration = 294 ÷ 2 = 147 mEq/L

	Intracellular	Extracellular
Osmolality	294.0	294.0
Volume (L)	23.8	18.2
Net water gain	–1.2	+1.2

Net effect: An intracellular to extracellular movement of water.

[1]Based on a 70-kg adult male.

ketone bodies), and those receiving large amounts of glycine (as during transurethral resection of the prostate). Lastly, osmolal gaps may also be present in patients with marked hyperlipidemia or hyperproteinemia. In such instances, the protein or lipid part of plasma contributes significantly to plasma volume; although plasma [Na^+] is decreased, [Na^+] in the water phase of plasma (true plasma osmolality) remains normal. The water phase of plasma is normally only 93% of its volume; the remaining 7% consists of plasma lipids and proteins.

CONTROL OF PLASMA OSMOLALITY

Plasma osmolality is closely regulated by osmoreceptors in the hypothalamus. These specialized neurons control both the secretion of antidiuretic hormone (ADH) and the thirst mechanism. Plasma osmolality is therefore maintained within relatively narrow limits by varying both water intake and water excretion.

Secretion of Antidiuretic Hormone

Specialized neurons in the supraoptic and paraventricular nuclei of the hypothalamus are very sensitive to changes in extracellular osmolality. When ECF osmolality increases, these cells shrink and release ADH from the posterior pituitary. ADH markedly increases water reabsorption in renal collecting tubules (see Chapter 29), which tends to reduce plasma osmolality back to normal. Conversely, a decrease in extracellular osmolality causes osmoreceptors to swell and suppresses the release of ADH. Decreased ADH secretion allows a water diuresis, which tends to increase osmolality to normal. Peak diuresis occurs once circulating ADH is metabolized (90–120 min). With complete suppression of ADH secretion, the kidneys can excrete up to 10–20 L of water per day.

Nonosmotic Release of Antidiuretic Hormone

The carotid baroreceptors and probably atrial stretch receptors can also stimulate ADH release following a 5–10% decrease in blood volume. Other nonosmotic stimuli include pain, emotional stress, and hypoxia.

Thirst

Osmoreceptors in the lateral preoptic area of the hypothalamus are also very sensitive to changes in extracellular osmolality. Activation of these neurons by increases in ECF osmolality induces thirst and causes the individual to drink water. Conversely, hypoosmolality suppresses thirst. Thirst is the major defense mechanism against hyperosmolality and hypernatremia, because it is the only mechanism that increases water intake.

HYPEROSMOLALITY & HYPERNATREMIA

Hyperosmolality occurs whenever total body solute content increases relative to TBW and is usually, but not always, associated with hypernatremia ([Na^+] > 145 mEq/L). Hyperosmolality without hypernatremia may be seen during marked hyperglycemia or following the accumulation of abnormal osmotically active substances in plasma (see above). In the latter two instances, plasma sodium concentration may actually decrease as water is drawn from the intracellular to the extracellular compartment. For every 100 mg/dL increase in plasma glucose concentration, plasma sodium decreases approximately 1.6 mEq/L.

Hypernatremia is nearly always the result of either a relative loss of water in excess of sodium (hypotonic fluid loss) or the retention of large quantities of sodium. Even when renal concentrating ability is impaired, thirst is normally highly effective in preventing hypernatremia. Hypernatremia is therefore most commonly seen in debilitated patients who are unable to drink, the very aged, the very young, and patients with altered consciousness. Patients with hypernatremia may have a low, normal, or high total body sodium content (Table 49–4).

Hypernatremia & Low Total Body Sodium Content

These patients have lost both sodium and water, but the water loss is in relative excess to that of the sodium loss. Hypotonic losses can be renal (osmotic diuresis) or extrarenal (diarrhea or sweat). In either case, patients usually manifest signs of hypovolemia (see Chapter 51). Urinary sodium concentration is generally greater than 20 mEq/L with renal losses and less than 10 mEq/L with extrarenal losses.

TABLE 49–4 Major causes of hypernatremia.

Impaired thirst
Coma
Essential hypernatremia

Solute diuresis
Osmotic diuresis: diabetic ketoacidosis, nonketotic hyperosmolar coma, mannitol administration

Excessive water losses
Renal
Neurogenic diabetes insipidus
Nephrogenic diabetes insipidus
Extrarenal
Sweating

Combined disorders
Coma plus hypertonic nasogastric feeding

Hypernatremia & Normal Total Body Sodium Content

This group of patients generally manifests signs of water loss without overt hypovolemia unless the water loss is massive. Total body sodium content is generally normal. Nearly pure water losses can occur via the skin, respiratory tract, or kidneys. Occasionally transient hypernatremia is observed with movement of water into cells following exercise, seizures, or rhabdomyolysis. The most common cause of hypernatremia in conscious patients with normal total body sodium content is **diabetes insipidus**. Diabetes insipidus is characterized by marked impairment in renal concentrating ability that is due either to decreased ADH secretion (central diabetes insipidus) or failure of the renal tubules to respond normally to circulating ADH (nephrogenic diabetes insipidus). Rarely, "essential hypernatremia" may be encountered in patients with central nervous system disorders. These patients appear to have "reset" osmoreceptors that function at a higher baseline osmolality.

A. Central Diabetes Insipidus

Lesions in or around the hypothalamus and the pituitary stalk frequently produce diabetes insipidus. Diabetes insipidus often develops with brain death. Transient diabetes insipidus is also commonly seen following neurosurgical procedures and

head trauma. The diagnosis is suggested by a history of polydipsia, polyuria (often >6 L/d), and the absence of hyperglycemia. In the perioperative setting, the diagnosis of diabetes insipidus is suggested by marked polyuria without glycosuria and a urinary osmolality lower than plasma osmolality. The absence of thirst in unconscious individuals leads to marked water losses and can rapidly produce hypovolemia. The diagnosis of central diabetes insipidus is confirmed by an increase in urinary osmolality following the administration of exogenous ADH. Aqueous vasopressin (5–10 units subcutaneously or intramuscularly every 4–6 h) is the treatment of choice for acute central diabetes insipidus. Vasopressin in oil (0.3 mL intramuscularly every day) is longer lasting but is more likely to cause water intoxication. Desmopressin (DDAVP), a synthetic analogue of ADH with a 12- to 24-h duration of action, is available as an intranasal preparation (10–40 mcg/d either as a single daily dose or divided into two doses) that can be used in both ambulatory and perioperative settings.

B. Nephrogenic Diabetes Insipidus

Nephrogenic diabetes insipidus can be congenital but is more commonly secondary to other disorders, including chronic kidney disease, hypokalemia and hypercalcemia, sickle cell disease, and hyperproteinemias. Nephrogenic diabetes insipidus can also be secondary to the side effects of some drugs (amphotericin B, lithium, demeclocycline, ifosfamide, mannitol). ADH secretion in nephrogenic diabetes insipidus is normal, but the kidneys fail to respond to ADH; urinary concentrating ability is therefore impaired. The mechanism may be either a decreased response to circulating ADH or interference with the renal countercurrent mechanism. The diagnosis is confirmed by failure of the kidneys to produce hypertonic urine following the administration of exogenous ADH. Treatment is generally directed at the underlying illness and ensuring an adequate fluid intake. Volume depletion by a thiazide diuretic can paradoxically decrease urinary output by reducing water delivery to collecting tubules. Sodium and protein restriction can similarly reduce urinary output.

Hypernatremia & Increased Total Body Sodium Content

This condition most commonly results from the administration of large quantities of hypertonic saline solutions (3% NaCl or 7.5% $NaHCO_3$). Patients with primary hyperaldosteronism and Cushing's syndrome may also have elevations in serum sodium concentration along with signs of increased sodium retention.

Clinical Manifestations of Hypernatremia

Neurological manifestations predominate in patients with hypernatremia and are generally thought to result from cellular dehydration. Restlessness, lethargy, and hyperreflexia can progress to seizures, coma, and ultimately death. Symptoms correlate more closely with the rate of movement of water out of brain cells than with the absolute level of hypernatremia. Rapid decreases in brain volume can rupture cerebral veins and result in focal intracerebral or subarachnoid hemorrhage. Seizures and serious neurological damage are common, particularly in children with acute hypernatremia when plasma $[Na^+]$ exceeds 158 mEq/L. Chronic hypernatremia is usually better tolerated than the acute form. After 24–48 h, intracellular osmolality begins to rise as a result of increases in intracellular inositol and amino

acid (glutamine and taurine) concentrations. As intracellular solute concentration increases, neuronal water content slowly returns to normal.

Treatment of Hypernatremia

The treatment of hypernatremia is aimed at restoring plasma osmolality to normal as well as correcting the underlying cause. Water deficits should generally be corrected over 48 h with a hypotonic solution such as 5% dextrose in water (see below). Abnormalities in extracellular volume must also be corrected (Figure 49–3). Hypernatremic patients with decreased total body sodium should be given isotonic fluids to restore plasma volume to normal *prior* to treatment with a hypotonic solution. Hypernatremic patients with increased total body sodium should be treated with a loop diuretic along with intravenous 5% dextrose in water. The treatment of diabetes insipidus is discussed above.

Rapid correction of hypernatremia can result in seizures, brain edema, permanent neurological damage, and even death. Serial Na^+ osmolalities should be obtained during treatment. In general, decreases in plasma sodium concentration should not proceed at a rate faster than 0.5 mEq/L/h.

Example

A 70-kg man is found to have a plasma $[Na^+]$ of 160 mEq/L. What is his water deficit?

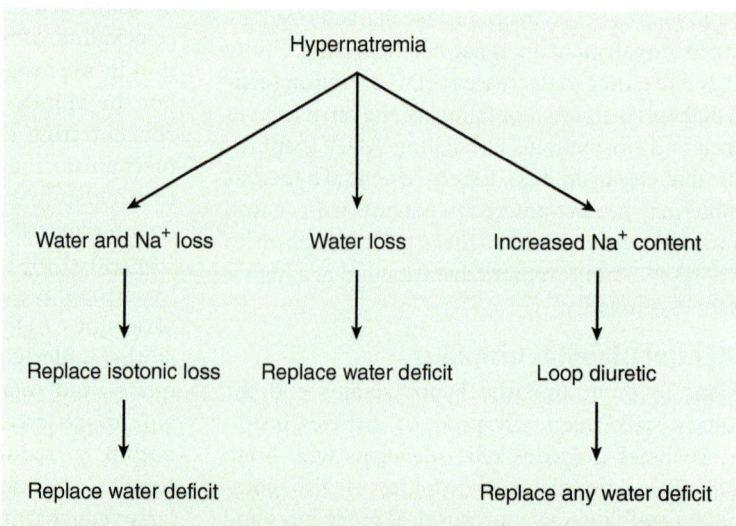

FIGURE 49–3 Algorithm for treatment of hypernatremia.

If one assumes that hypernatremia in this cases represents water loss only, then total body osmoles are unchanged. Thus, assuming a normal $[Na^+]$ of 140 mEq/L and TBW content that is 60% of body weight:

$$Normal\ TBW \times 140 = present\ TBW \times [Na^+]_{plasma}\ or$$

$$(70 \times 0.6) \times 140 = present\ TBW \times 160$$

Solving the equation:

$$Present\ TBW = 36.7\ L$$

$$Water\ deficit = normal\ TBW - present\ TBW\ or$$
$$(70 \times 0.6) - 36.7 = 5.3\ L$$

To replace this deficit over 48 h, it is necessary to give 5% dextrose in water intravenously, 5300 mL over 48 h, or 110 mL/h.

Note that this method ignores any coexisting isotonic fluid deficits, which if present should be replaced with an isotonic solution.

Anesthetic Considerations

Hypernatremia has been demonstrated to increase the minimum alveolar concentration for inhalation anesthetics in animal studies, but its clinical significance is more closely related to the associated fluid deficits. Hypovolemia accentuates any vasodilation or cardiac depression from anesthetic agents and predisposes to hypotension and hypoperfusion of tissues. Decreases in the volume of distribution for drugs necessitate dose reductions for most intravenous agents, whereas decreases in cardiac output enhance the uptake of inhalation anesthetics.

Elective surgery should be postponed in patients with significant hypernatremia (>150 mEq/L) until the cause is established and fluid deficits are corrected. Both water and isotonic fluid deficits should be corrected prior to elective surgery.

HYPOOSMOLALITY & HYPONATREMIA

Hypoosmolality is nearly always associated with hyponatremia ($[Na^+] < 135$ mEq/L). Table 49–5 lists rare instances in which hyponatremia does not necessarily reflect hypoosmolality (*pseudohyponatremia*). Routine measurement of plasma

TABLE 49–5 Causes of pseudohyponatremia.[1]

Hyponatremia with a normal plasma osmolality
Asymptomatic
Marked hyperlipidemia
Marked hyperproteinemia
Symptomatic
Marked glycine absorption during transurethral surgery
Hyponatremia with an elevated plasma osmolality
Hyperglycemia
Administration of mannitol

[1]Adapted from Rose RD: *Clinical Physiology of Acid-Base and Electrolyte Disorders*, 3rd ed. McGraw-Hill, 1989.

osmolality in hyponatremic patients rapidly excludes pseudohyponatremia.

Hyponatremia invariably reflects water retention from either an absolute increase in TBW or a loss of sodium in relative excess to loss of water. The kidneys' normal capacity to produce dilute urine with an osmolality as low as 40 mOsm/kg (specific gravity 1.001) allows them to excrete over 10 L of free water per day if necessary. Because of this tremendous reserve, hyponatremia is nearly always the result of a defect in urinary diluting capacity (urinary osmolality > 100 mOsm/kg or specific gravity > 1.003). Rare instances of hyponatremia without an abnormality in renal diluting capacity (urinary osmolality < 100 mOsm/kg) are generally attributed to primary polydipsia or reset osmoreceptors; the latter two conditions can be differentiated by water restriction.

Clinically, hyponatremia is best classified according to total body sodium content (Table 49–6). Hyponatremia associated with transurethral resection of the prostate is discussed in Chapter 31.

Hyponatremia & Low Total Body Sodium

Progressive losses of both sodium and water eventually lead to extracellular volume depletion. As the intravascular volume deficit reaches 5–10%, nonosmotic ADH secretion is activated (see above). With further volume depletion, the stimuli for nonosmotic ADH release overcome any hyponatremia-induced suppression of ADH. Preservation of circulatory volume takes place at the expense of plasma osmolality.

TABLE 49–6 Classification of hypoosmolal hyponatremia.

Decreased total sodium content
Renal
Diuretics
Mineralocorticoid deficiency
Salt-losing nephropathies
Osmotic diuresis (glucose, mannitol)
Renal tubular acidosis
Extrarenal
Vomiting
Diarrhea
Integumentary loss (sweating, burns)
"Third-spacing"
Normal total sodium content
Primary polydipsia
Syndrome of inappropriate antidiuretic hormone
Glucocorticoid deficiency
Hypothyroidism
Drug-induced
Increased total sodium content
Congestive heart failure
Cirrhosis
Nephrotic syndrome

Fluid losses resulting in hyponatremia may be renal or extrarenal in origin. Renal losses are most commonly related to thiazide diuretics and result in a urinary [Na$^+$] greater than 20 mEq/L. Extrarenal losses are typically gastrointestinal and usually produce a urinary [Na$^+$] of less than 10 mEq/L. A major exception to the latter is hyponatremia due to vomiting, which can result in a urinary [Na$^+$] greater than 20 mEq/L. In those instances, bicarbonaturia from the associated metabolic alkalosis obligates concomitant excretion of Na$^+$ with HCO$_3$ to maintain electrical neutrality in the urine; urinary chloride concentration, however, is usually less than 10 mEq/L.

Hyponatremia & Increased Total Body Sodium

Edematous disorders are characterized by an increase in both total body sodium and TBW. When the increase in water exceeds that in sodium, hyponatremia occurs. Edematous disorders include congestive heart failure, cirrhosis, kidney failure, and nephrotic syndrome. Hyponatremia in these settings results from progressive impairment of renal free water excretion and generally parallels underlying disease severity. Pathophysiological mechanisms include nonosmotic ADH release and decreased delivery of fluid to the distal diluting segment in nephrons (see Chapter 29). The "effective" circulating blood volume is reduced.

Hyponatremia with Normal Total Body Sodium

Hyponatremia in the absence of edema or hypovolemia may be seen with glucocorticoid insufficiency, hypothyroidism, drug therapy (chlorpropamide and cyclophosphamide), and the syndrome of inappropriate antidiuretic hormone secretion (SIADH). The hyponatremia associated with adrenal hypofunction may be due to cosecretion of ADH with corticotropin-releasing factor (CRF). Diagnosis of SIADH requires exclusion of other causes of hyponatremia and the absence of hypovolemia, edema, and adrenal, renal, or thyroid disease. Various malignant tumors, pulmonary diseases, and central nervous system disorders are commonly associated with SIADH. In most such instances, plasma ADH concentration is not elevated but is inadequately suppressed relative to the degree of hypoosmolality in plasma; urine osmolality is usually greater than 100 mOsm/kg and urine sodium concentration is greater than 40 mEq/L.

Clinical Manifestations of Hyponatremia

Symptoms of hyponatremia are primarily neurological and result from an increase in intracellular water. Their severity is generally related to the rapidity with which extracellular hypoosmolality develops. Patients with mild to moderate hyponatremia ([Na$^+$] > 125 mEq/L) are frequently asymptomatic. Early symptoms are typically nonspecific and may include anorexia, nausea, and weakness. Progressive cerebral edema, however, results in lethargy, confusion, seizures, coma, and finally death. **4** Serious manifestations of hyponatremia are generally associated with plasma sodium concentrations less than 120 mEq/L. Compared with

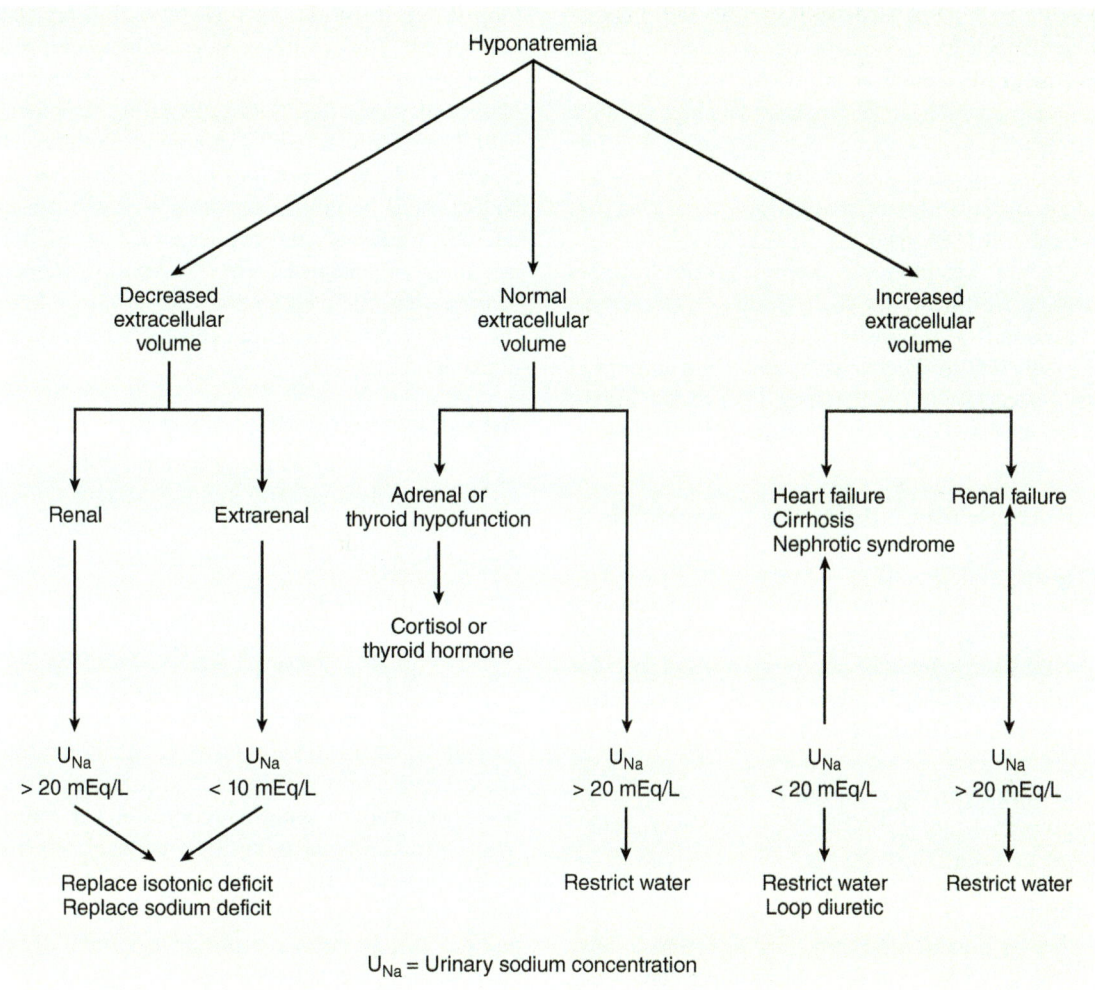

FIGURE 49–4 Algorithm for treatment of hyponatremia.

men, premenopausal women appear to be at greater risk of neurological impairment and damage from hyponatremia.

Patients with slowly developing or chronic hyponatremia are generally less symptomatic, probably because the gradual compensatory loss of intracellular solutes (primarily Na^+, K^+, and amino acids) restores cell volume to near normal. Neurological symptoms in patients with chronic hyponatremia may be related more closely to changes in cell membrane potential (due to a low extracellular $[Na^+]$) than to changes in cell volume.

Treatment of Hyponatremia

As with hypernatremia, the treatment of hyponatremia (Figure 49–4) is directed at correcting both the underlying disorder as well as the plasma $[Na^+]$. **Isotonic saline is generally the treatment of choice for hyponatremic patients with decreased total body sodium content.** Once the ECF deficit is corrected, spontaneous water diuresis returns plasma $[Na^+]$ to normal. Conversely, water restriction is the primary treatment for hyponatremic patients with normal or increased total body sodium. More specific treatments such as hormone replacement in patients with adrenal or thyroid hypofunction and measures aimed at improving cardiac output in patients with heart failure may also be indicated. Demeclocycline, a drug that antagonizes ADH activity at the renal tubules, has proved to be a useful adjunct to water restriction in the treatment of patients with SIADH.

Acute symptomatic hyponatremia requires prompt treatment. In such instances, correction of plasma [Na$^+$] to greater than 125 mEq/L is usually sufficient to alleviate symptoms. The amount of NaCl necessary to raise plasma [Na$^+$] to the desired value, the Na$^+$ deficit, can be estimated by the following formula:

$$Na^+ \text{ deficit} = TBW \times (\text{desired } [Na^+] - \text{present } [Na^+])$$

5 Excessively rapid correction of hyponatremia has been associated with demyelinating lesions in the pons (*central pontine myelinolysis*), resulting in permanent neurological sequelae. The rapidity with which hyponatremia is corrected should be tailored to the severity of symptoms. The following correction rates have been suggested: for mild symptoms, 0.5 mEq/L/h or less; for moderate symptoms, 1 mEq/L/h or less; and for severe symptoms, 1.5 mEq/L/h or less.

Example

An 80-kg woman is lethargic and is found to have plasma [Na$^+$] of 118 mEq/L. How much NaCl must be given to raise her plasma [Na$^+$] to 130 mEq/L?

$$Na^+ \text{ deficit} = TBW \times (130 - 118)$$

TBW is approximately 50% of body weight in females:

$$Na^+ \text{ deficit} = 80 \times 0.5 \times (130 - 118) = 480 \text{ mEq}$$

Because normal (isotonic) saline contains 154 mEq/L, the patient should receive 480 mEq ÷ 154 mEq/L, or 3.12 L of normal saline. For a correction rate of 0.5 mEq/L/h, this amount of saline should be given over 24 h (130 mL/h).

Note that this calculation does not take into account any coexisting isotonic fluid deficits, which, if present, should also be replaced. More rapid correction of hyponatremia can be achieved by giving a loop diuretic to induce water diuresis while replacing urinary Na$^+$ losses with isotonic saline. Even more rapid corrections can be achieved with intravenous hypertonic saline (3% NaCl). Hypertonic saline may be indicated in markedly symptomatic patients with plasma [Na$^+$] less than 110 mEq/L. Three percent NaCl should be given cautiously as it can precipitate pulmonary edema, hypokalemia, hyperchloremic metabolic acidosis, and transient hypotension; bleeding has been associated with prolongation of the prothrombin time and activated partial thromboplastin time.

Anesthetic Considerations

Hyponatremia is often a manifestation of a serious underlying disorder and requires careful preoperative evaluation. A plasma sodium concentration greater than 130 mEq/L is usually considered safe for patients undergoing general anesthesia. In most circumstances, plasma [Na$^+$] should be corrected to greater than 130 mEq/L for elective procedures, even in the absence of neurological symptoms. Lower concentrations may result in significant cerebral edema that can be manifested intraoperatively as a decrease in minimum alveolar concentration or postoperatively as agitation, confusion, or somnolence. Patients undergoing transurethral resection of the prostate can absorb signì cant amounts of water from irrigation fluids (as much as 20 mL/min) and are at high risk for rapid development of profound acute water intoxication.

Disorders of Sodium Balance

ECF volume is directly proportionate to total body sodium content. Variations in ECF volume result from changes in total body sodium content. A positive sodium balance increases ECF volume, whereas a negative sodium balance decreases ECF volume. It is important to reemphasize that *extracellular (plasma) Na$^+$ concentration is more indicative of water balance than total body sodium content.*

NORMAL SODIUM BALANCE

Net sodium balance is equal to total sodium intake (adults average 170 mEq/d) minus both renal sodium excretion and extrarenal sodium losses. (One gram of sodium yields 43 mEq of Na^+ ions, whereas 1 g of sodium chloride yields 17 mEq of Na^+ ions.) The kidneys' ability to vary urinary Na^+ excretion from less than 1 mEq/L to more than 100 mEq/L allows them to play a critical role in sodium balance (see Chapter 29).

REGULATION OF SODIUM BALANCE & EXTRACELLULAR FLUID VOLUME

Because of the relationship between ECF volume and total body sodium content, regulation of one is intimately tied to the other. This regulation is achieved via sensors (see below) that detect changes in the most important component of ECF, namely, the "effective" intravascular volume. The latter correlates more closely with the rate of perfusion in renal capillaries than with measurable intravascular fluid (plasma) volume. Indeed, with edematous disorders (heart failure, cirrhosis, and kidney failure), "effective" intravascular volume can be independent of the measurable plasma volume, ECF volume, and even cardiac output.

ECF volume and total body sodium content are ultimately controlled by appropriate adjustments in renal Na^+ excretion. In the absence of kidney disease, diuretic therapy, and selective renal ischemia, urinary Na^+ concentration reflects "effective" intravascular volume. A low urine Na^+ concentration (<10 mEq/L) is therefore generally indicative of a low "effective" intravascular fluid volume and reflects secondary retention of Na^+ by the kidneys.

Control Mechanisms

The multiple mechanisms involved in regulating ECF volume and sodium balance normally complement one another but can function independently. In addition to altering renal Na^+ excretion, some mechanisms also produce more rapid compensatory hemodynamic responses when "effective" intravascular volume is reduced.

A. Sensors of Volume

Baroreceptors are the principal volume receptors in the body. Because blood pressure is the product of

cardiac output and systemic vascular resistance (see Chapter 20), significant changes in intravascular volume (preload) not only affect cardiac output but also transiently affect arterial blood pressure. Thus, the baroreceptors at the carotid sinus and afferent renal arterioles (juxtaglomerular apparatus) indirectly function as sensors of intravascular volume. Changes in blood pressure at the carotid sinus modulate sympathetic nervous system activity and nonosmotic ADH secretion, whereas changes at the afferent renal arterioles modulate the renin–angiotensin–aldosterone system. Stretch receptors in both atria are affected by changes in intravascular volume, and the degree of atrial distention modulates the release of atrial natriuretic hormone and ADH.

B. Effectors of Volume Change

Regardless of the mechanism, effectors of volume change ultimately alter urinary Na^+ excretion. Decreases in "effective" intravascular volume decrease urinary Na^+ excretion, whereas increases in the "effective" intravascular volume increase urinary Na^+ excretion. These mechanisms include the following:

1. Renin–angiotensin–aldosterone—Renin secretion increases the formation of angiotensin II. The latter increases the secretion of aldosterone and has a direct effect in enhancing Na^+ reabsorption in the proximal renal tubules. Angiotensin II is also a potent direct vasoconstrictor and potentiates the actions of norepinephrine. Secretion of aldosterone enhances Na^+ reabsorption in the distal nephron (see Chapter 29) and is a major determinant of urinary Na^+ excretion.

2. Atrial natriuretic peptide (ANP)—This peptide is normally released from both right and left atrial cells following atrial distention. ANP appears to have two major actions: arterial vasodilation and increased urinary sodium and water excretion in the renal collecting tubules. Na^+-mediated afferent arteriolar dilation and efferent arteriolar constriction can also increase glomerular filtration rate (GFR). Other effects include the inhibition of both renin and aldosterone secretion and antagonism of ADH.

3. Brain natriuretic peptide (BNP)—ANP, BNP, and C-type natriuretic peptide are structurally related peptides. BNP is released by the ventricles in response to increased ventricular volume and pressure, and ventricular overdistention, and also by the brain in response to increased blood pressure. BNP levels are usually approximately 20% of ANP levels, but during an episode of acute congestive heart failure BNP levels may exceed those of ANP. BNP levels can be measured clinically, and a recombinant form of BNP, nesiritide (Natrecor), is available to treat acute decompensated congestive heart failure.

4. Sympathetic nervous system activity— Enhanced sympathetic activity increases Na⁺ reabsorption in the proximal renal tubules, resulting in Na⁺ retention, and increases renal vasoconstriction, which reduces renal blood flow (see Chapter 29). Conversely, stimulation of left atrial stretch receptors results in decreases in renal sympathetic tone and increases in renal blood flow (cardiorenal reflex) and glomerular filtration.

5. Glomerular filtration rate and plasma sodium concentration—The amount of Na⁺ filtered in the kidneys is directly proportionate to the product of the GFR and plasma Na⁺ concentration. Because GFR is usually proportionate to intravascular volume, intravascular volume expansion can increase Na⁺ excretion. Conversely, intravascular volume depletion decreases Na⁺ excretion. Similarly, even small elevations of blood pressure can result in a relatively large increase in urinary Na⁺ excretion because of the resultant increase in renal blood flow and glomerular filtration rate. Blood pressure–induced diuresis (*pressure natriuresis*) appears to be independent of any known humorally or neurally mediated mechanism.

6. Tubuloglomerular balance—Despite wide variations in the amount of Na⁺ filtered in nephrons, Na⁺ reabsorption in the proximal renal tubules is normally controlled within narrow limits. Factors considered to be responsible for tubuloglomerular balance include the rate of renal tubular flow and changes in peritubular capillary hydrostatic and oncotic pressures. Altered Na⁺ reabsorption in the proximal tubules can have a marked effect on renal Na⁺ excretion.

7. Antidiuretic hormone—Although ADH secretion has little effect on Na⁺ excretion, nonosmotic secretion of this hormone (see above) can play an important part in maintaining extracellular volume with moderate to severe decreases in the "effective" intravascular volume.

TABLE 49–7 Osmoregulation versus volume regulation.[1]

	Volume Regulation	Osmoregulation
Purpose	Control extracellular volume	Control extracellular osmolality
Mechanism	Vary renal Na⁺ excretion	Vary water intake Vary renal water excretion
Sensors	Afferent renal arterioles Carotid baroreceptors Atrial stretch receptors	Hypothalamic osmoreceptors
Effectors	Renin-angiotensin-aldosterone Sympathetic nervous system Tubuloglomerular balance Renal pressure natriuresis Atrial natriuretic peptide Antidiuretic hormone Brain natriuretic peptide	Thirst Antidiuretic hormone

[1]Adapted from Rose RD: *Clinical Physiology of Acid-Base and Electrolyte Disorders*, 3rd ed. McGraw-Hill, 1989.

Extracellular Osmoregulation versus Volume Regulation

Osmoregulation protects the normal ratio of solutes to water, whereas extracellular volume regulation preserves absolute solute and water content (Table 49–7). As noted previously, volume regulation generally takes precedence over osmoregulation.

Anesthetic Implications

Problems related to altered sodium balance result from its manifestations as well as the underlying disorder. Disorders of sodium balance present either as hypovolemia (sodium deficit) or hypervolemia (sodium excess). Both disturbances should be corrected prior to elective surgical procedures. Cardiac, liver, and renal function should also be carefully evaluated in the presence of sodium excess (generally manifested as tissue edema).

Hypovolemic patients are sensitive to the vasodilating and negative inotropic effects of vapor anesthetics, propofol, and agents associated with histamine release (morphine, meperidine). Dosage requirements for other drugs must also be reduced to compensate for decreases in their volume of distribution. Hypovolemic patients are particularly sensitive to sympathetic blockade from spinal or epidural anesthesia. If an anesthetic must be administered prior to adequate correction of hypovolemia, etomidate or ketamine may be the induction agents of choice for general anesthesia.

6 Hypervolemia should generally be corrected preoperatively with diuretics. The major hazard of increases in extracellular volume is impaired gas exchange due to pulmonary interstitial edema, alveolar edema, or large collections of pleural or ascitic fluid.

Disorders of Potassium Balance

Potassium plays a major role in the electrophysiology of cell membranes as well as in carbohydrate and protein synthesis (see below). The resting cell membrane potential is normally dependent on the ratio of intracellular to extracellular potassium concentrations. Intracellular potassium concentration is estimated to be 140 mEq/L, whereas extracellular potassium concentration is normally about 4 mEq/L. Under some conditions, a redistribution of K^+ between the ECF and ICF compartments can result in marked changes in extracellular $[K^+]$ without a change in total body potassium content.

NORMAL POTASSIUM BALANCE

Dietary potassium intake averages 80 mEq/d in adults (range, 40–140 mEq/d). About 70 mEq of that amount is normally excreted in urine, whereas the remaining 10 mEq is lost through the gastrointestinal tract.

Renal excretion of potassium can vary from as little as 5 mEq/L to over 100 mEq/L. Nearly all the potassium filtered in glomeruli is normally reabsorbed in the proximal tubule and the loop of Henle. The potassium excreted in urine is the result of distal tubular secretion. Potassium secretion in the distal tubules is coupled to aldosterone-mediated reabsorption of sodium (see Chapter 29).

REGULATION OF EXTRACELLULAR POTASSIUM CONCENTRATION

Extracellular potassium concentration is determined by cell membrane Na^+–K^+-ATPase activity and plasma $[K^+]$, and is influenced by the balance of potassium intake and excretion. Cell membrane Na^+–K^+-ATPase activity regulates the distribution of potassium between cells and ECF, whereas plasma $[K^+]$ is the major determinant of urinary potassium excretion.

INTERCOMPARTMENTAL SHIFTS OF POTASSIUM

Intercompartmental shifts of potassium are known to occur following changes in extracellular pH (see Chapter 50), circulating insulin levels, circulating catecholamine activity, plasma osmolality, and possibly hypothermia. Insulin and catecholamines are known to directly affect Na^+–K^+-ATPase activity and decrease plasma $[K^+]$. Exercise can also transiently increase plasma $[K^+]$ as a result of the release of K^+ by muscle cells; the increase in plasma $[K^+]$ (0.3–2 mEq/L) is proportionate to the intensity and duration of muscle activity. Intercompartmental potassium shifts are also thought to be responsible for changes in plasma $[K^+]$ in syndromes of periodic paralysis (see Chapter 35).

Because the ICF may buffer up to 60% of an acid load (see Chapter 50), changes in extracellular hydrogen ion concentration (pH) directly affect extracellular $[K^+]$. In the setting of acidosis, extracellular hydrogen ions enter cells, displacing intracellular potassium ions; the resultant movement of potassium ions out of cells maintains electrical balance but increases extracellular and plasma $[K^+]$. Conversely, during alkalosis, extracellular potassium ions move into cells to balance the movement of hydrogen ions out of cells; as a result, plasma $[K^+]$ decreases. Although the relationship is variable, a useful rule of thumb is that plasma potassium concentration changes approximately 0.6 mEq/L per 0.1 unit change in arterial pH (range 0.2–1.2 mEq/L per 0.1 unit).

Changes in circulating insulin levels can directly alter plasma [K$^+$] independent of that hormone's effect on glucose transport. Insulin enhances the activity of membrane-bound Na$^+$–K$^+$-ATPase, increasing cellular uptake of potassium in the liver and in skeletal muscle, and insulin secretion may play an important role in the basal control of plasma potassium concentration and in the physiological response to increased potassium loads.

Sympathetic stimulation also increases intracellular uptake of potassium by enhancing Na$^+$–K$^+$-ATPase activity. This effect is mediated through activation of β$_2$-adrenergic receptors. In contrast, α-adrenergic activity may impair the intracellular movement of K$^+$. Plasma [K$^+$] often decreases following the administration of β$_2$-adrenergic agonists as a result of uptake of potassium by muscle and the liver. Moreover, β-adrenergic blockade can impair the handling of a potassium load in some patients.

Acute increases in plasma osmolality (hypernatremia, hyperglycemia, or mannitol administration) may increase plasma [K$^+$] (about 0.6 mEq/L per 10 mOsm/L). In such instances, the movement of water out of cells (down its osmotic gradient) is accompanied by movement of K$^+$ out of cells. The latter may be the result of "solvent drag" or the increase in intracellular [K$^+$] that follows cellular dehydration.

Hypothermia has been reported to lower plasma [K$^+$] as a result of cellular uptake. Rewarming reverses this shift and may result in transient hyperkalemia if potassium was given during the hypothermia.

Urinary Excretion of Potassium

Urinary potassium excretion generally parallels its extracellular concentration. Potassium is secreted by tubular cells in the distal nephron. Extracellular [K$^+$] is a major determinant of aldosterone secretion from the adrenal gland. Hyperkalemia stimulates aldosterone secretion, whereas hypokalemia suppresses aldosterone secretion. Renal tubular flow in the distal nephron may also be an important determinant of urinary potassium excretion because high tubular flow rates (as during osmotic diuresis) increase potassium secretion by keeping the capillary to renal tubular gradient for potassium

secretion high. Conversely, slow tubular flow rates increase [K$^+$] in tubular fluid and decrease the gradient for K$^+$ secretion, thereby decreasing renal potassium excretion.

HYPOKALEMIA

Hypokalemia, defined as plasma [K$^+$] less than 3.5 mEq/L, can occur as a result of (1) an intercompartmental shift of K$^+$ (see above), (2) increased potassium loss, or (3) an inadequate potassium intake (Table 49–8). Plasma potassium concentration typically correlates poorly with the total potassium deficit. A decrease in plasma [K$^+$] from 4 mEq/L to 3 mEq/L usually represents a 100- to 200-mEq deficit, whereas plasma [K$^+$] below 3 mEq/L can represent a deficit anywhere between 200 mEq and 400 mEq.

TABLE 49–8 Major causes of hypokalemia.

Excess renal loss
  Mineralocorticoid excess
    Primary hyperaldosteronism (Conn's syndrome)
    Glucocorticoid-remediable hyperaldosteronism
  Renin excess
    Renovascular hypertension
  Bartter's syndrome
  Liddle's syndrome
  Diuresis
  Chronic metabolic alkalosis
  Antibiotics
    Carbenicillin
    Gentamicin
    Amphotericin B
  Renal tubular acidosis
    Distal, gradient-limited
    Proximal
    Ureterosigmoidostomy

Gastrointestinal losses
  Vomiting
  Diarrhea, particularly secretory diarrheas

ECF → ICF shifts
  Acute alkalosis
  Hypokalemic periodic paralysis
  Barium ingestion
  Insulin therapy
  Vitamin B$_{12}$ therapy
  Thyrotoxicosis (rarely)

Inadequate intake

Hypokalemia due to the Intracellular Movement of Potassium

Hypokalemia due to the intracellular movement of potassium occurs with alkalosis, insulin therapy, β_2-adrenergic agonists, and hypothermia and during attacks of hypokalemic periodic paralysis (see above). Hypokalemia may also be seen following transfusion of previously frozen red cells; these cells lose potassium in the preservation process and take up potassium following reinfusion. Cellular K^+ uptake by red blood cells (and platelets) also accounts for the hypokalemia seen in patients recently treated with folate or vitamin B_{12} for megaloblastic anemia.

Hypokalemia due to Increased Potassium Losses

Excessive potassium losses are usually either renal or gastrointestinal. Renal wasting of potassium is most commonly the result of diuresis or enhanced mineralocorticoid activity. Other renal causes include hypomagnesemia (see below), renal tubular acidosis (see Chapter 29), ketoacidosis, salt-wasting nephropathies, and some drug therapies (carbenicillin and amphotericin B). Increased gastrointestinal loss of potassium is most commonly due to nasogastric suctioning or to persistent vomiting or diarrhea. Other gastrointestinal causes include losses from fistulae, laxative abuse, villous adenomas, and pancreatic tumors secreting vasoactive intestinal peptide.

Chronic increased sweat formation occasionally causes hypokalemia, particularly when potassium intake is limited. Dialysis with a low-potassium-containing dialysate solution can also cause hypokalemia. Uremic patients may actually have a total body potassium deficit (primarily intracellular) despite a normal or even high plasma concentration; the absence of hypokalemia in these instances is probably due to an intercompartmental shift from the acidosis. Dialysis in these patients unmasks the total body potassium deficit and often results in hypokalemia.

Urinary $[K^+]$ less than 20 mEq/L is generally indicative of increased extrarenal losses, whereas concentrations greater than 20 mEq/L suggest renal wasting of K^+.

Hypokalemia due to Decreased Potassium Intake

Because of the kidney's ability to decrease urinary potassium excretion to as low as 5–20 mEq/L, marked reductions in potassium intake are required to produce hypokalemia. Low potassium intakes, however, often accentuate the effects of increased potassium losses.

Clinical Manifestations of Hypokalemia

Hypokalemia can produce widespread organ dysfunction (Table 49–9). Most patients are asymptomatic until plasma $[K^+]$ falls below 3 mEq/L. Cardiovascular effects are most prominent and include an abnormal ECG (Figure 49–5), arrhythmias, decreased cardiac contractility, and a labile arterial blood pressure due to autonomic dysfunction. Chronic hypokalemia has also been reported to cause myocardial fibrosis. **ECG manifestations are primarily due to delayed ventricular repolarization and include T-wave flattening and inversion, an increasingly prominent U wave, ST-segment depression, increased P-wave amplitude, and prolongation of the P–R interval.**

TABLE 49–9 Effects of hypokalemia.[1]

Cardiovascular
  Electrocardiographic changes/arrhythmias
  Myocardial dysfunction

Neuromuscular
  Skeletal muscle weakness
  Tetany
  Rhabdomyolysis
  Ileus

Renal
  Polyuria (nephrogenic diabetes insipidus)
  Increased ammonia production
  Increased bicarbonate reabsorption

Hormonal
  Decreased insulin secretion
  Decreased aldosterone secretion

Metabolic
  Negative nitrogen balance
  Encephalopathy in patients with liver disease

[1]Adapted from Schrier RW, ed: *Renal and Electrolyte Disorders*, 3rd ed. Little, Brown and Company, 1986.

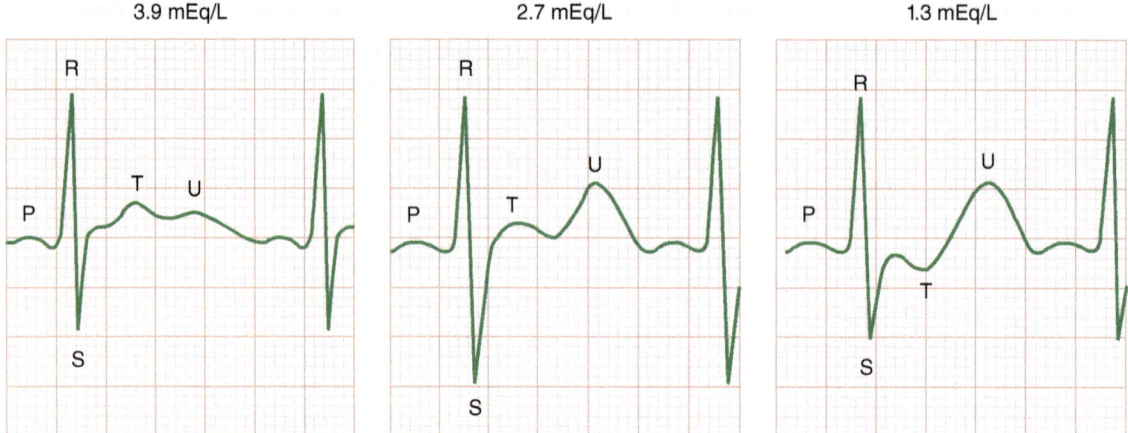

FIGURE 49–5 Electrocardiographic effects of acute hypokalemia. Note progressive flattening of the T wave, an increasingly prominent U wave, increased amplitude of the P wave, prolongation of the P–R interval, and ST-segment depression.

Increased myocardial cell automaticity and delayed repolarization promote both atrial and ventricular arrhythmias.

Neuromuscular effects of hypokalemia include skeletal muscle weakness, flaccid paralysis, hyporeflexia, muscle cramping, ileus, and, rarely, rhabdomyolysis. Hypokalemia induced by diuretics is often associated with metabolic alkalosis; as the kidneys absorb sodium to compensate for intravascular volume depletion and in the presence of diuretic-induced hypochloremia, bicarbonate is absorbed. The end result is hypokalemia and hypochloremic metabolic alkalosis. Renal dysfunction is seen due to impaired concentrating ability (resistance to ADH, resulting in polyuria) and increased production of ammonia resulting in impairment of urinary acidification. Increased ammonia production represents intracellular acidosis; hydrogen ions move intracellularly to compensate for intracellular potassium losses. The resulting metabolic alkalosis, together with increased ammonia production, can precipitate encephalopathy in patients with advanced liver disease. Chronic hypokalemia has been associated with renal fibrosis (tubulointerstitial nephropathy).

Treatment of Hypokalemia

The treatment of hypokalemia depends on the presence and severity of any associated organ dysfunction. Significant ECG changes such as ST-segment changes or arrhythmias mandate continuous ECG monitoring, particularly during intravenous K^+ replacement. Digoxin therapy—as well as the hypokalemia itself—sensitizes the heart to changes in potassium ion concentration. Muscle strength should also be periodically assessed in patients with weakness.

In most circumstances, the safest method by which to correct a potassium deficit is oral replacement over several days using a potassium chloride solution (60–80 mEq/d). Intravenous replacement of potassium chloride is usually be reserved for patients with, or at risk for, significant cardiac manifestations or severe muscle weakness. The goal of intravenous therapy is to remove the patient from immediate danger, not to correct the entire potassium deficit. Because of potassium's irritative effect on peripheral veins, peripheral intravenous replacement should not exceed 8 mEq/h. Dextrose-containing solutions should generally be avoided because the resulting hyperglycemia and secondary insulin secretion may actually worsen the low plasma $[K^+]$. More rapid intravenous potassium replacement (10–20 mEq/h) requires central venous administration and close monitoring of the ECG. Intravenous replacement should generally not exceed 240 mEq/d.

Potassium chloride is the preferred potassium salt when a metabolic alkalosis is also present because it also corrects the chloride deficit discussed above. Potassium bicarbonate or equivalent (K^+ acetate or K^+ citrate) is preferable for patients with metabolic acidosis. Potassium phosphate is a suitable alternative with concomitant hypophosphatemia (diabetic ketoacidosis).

Anesthetic Considerations

Hypokalemia is a common preoperative finding. The decision to proceed with elective surgery is often based on lower plasma $[K^+]$ limits somewhere between 3 and 3.5 mEq/L. The decision, however, should also be based on the rate at which the hypokalemia developed as well as the presence or absence of secondary organ dysfunction. In general, chronic mild hypokalemia (3–3.5 mEq/L) without ECG changes does not substantially increase anesthetic risk. The latter may not apply to patients receiving digoxin, who may be at increased risk of developing digoxin toxicity from the hypokalemia; plasma $[K^+]$ values above 4 mEq/L are desirable in such patients.

The intraoperative management of hypokalemia requires vigilant ECG monitoring. Intravenous potassium should be given if atrial or ventricular arrhythmias develop. Glucose-free intravenous solutions should be used and hyperventilation avoided to prevent further decreases in plasma $[K^+]$. Increased sensitivity to neuromuscular blockers (NMBs) may be seen; therefore dosages of NMBs should be reduced 25–50%, and a nerve stimulator should be used to follow both the degree of paralysis and the adequacy of reversal.

HYPERKALEMIA

Hyperkalemia exists when plasma $[K^+]$ exceeds 5.5 mEq/L. Hyperkalemia rarely occurs in normal individuals because of the kidney's capability to excrete large potassium loads. When potassium intake is increased slowly, the kidneys can excrete as much as 500 mEq of K^+ per day. The sympathetic nervous system and insulin secretion also play important roles in preventing acute increases in plasma $[K^+]$ following acquired potassium loads.

TABLE 49–10 Causes of hyperkalemia.

Pseudohyperkalemia
Red cell hemolysis
Marked leukocytosis/thrombocytosis
Intercompartmental shifts
Acidosis
Hypertonicity
Rhabdomyolysis
Excessive exercise
Periodic paralysis
Succinylcholine
Decreased renal potassium excretion
Renal failure
Decreased mineralocorticoid activity and impaired Na^+ reabsorption
Acquired immunodeficiency syndrome
Potassium-sparing diuretics
Spironolactone
Eplerenone
Amiloride
Triamterene
ACE^1 inhibitors
Nonsteroidal antiinflammatory drugs
Pentamidine
Trimethoprim
Enhanced Cl^- reabsorption
Gordon's syndrome
Cyclosporine
Increased potassium intake
Salt substitutes

[1]ACE, angiotensin-converting enzyme.

Hyperkalemia can result from (1) an intercompartmental shift of potassium ions, (2) decreased urinary excretion of potassium, or, rarely, (3) an increased potassium intake (Table 49–10). Measurements of plasma potassium concentration can be spuriously elevated if red cells hemolyze in a blood specimen. In vitro release of potassium from white cells in a blood specimen can also falsely indicate increased levels in the measured plasma $[K^+]$ when the leukocyte count exceeds $70,000 \times 10^9$/L. A similar release of potassium from platelets occurs when the platelet count exceeds $1,000,000 \times 10^9$/L.

Hyperkalemia due to Extracellular Movement of Potassium

Movement of K^+ out of cells can be seen with acidosis, cell lysis following chemotherapy, hemolysis, rhabdomyolysis, massive tissue trauma, hyperosmolality, digitalis overdoses, during episodes of hyperkalemic periodic paralysis, and with administration of succinylcholine, β_2-adrenergic blockers, and arginine hydrochloride. The average increase in plasma [K^+] of 0.5 mEq/L following succinylcholine administration can be exaggerated in patients with large burns or severe muscle trauma and in those with muscle denervation, and its use in these settings should be avoided.

β_2-Adrenergic blockade accentuates the increase in plasma [K^+] that occurs following exercise. Digoxin inhibits Na^+–K^+-ATPase in cell membranes, and digoxin overdose has been reported to cause hyperkalemia in some patients. Arginine hydrochloride, which is used to treat metabolic alkalosis, evaluate pituitary growth hormone reserve, and as a performance-enhancing supplement by athletes, can cause hyperkalemia as the cationic arginine ions enter cells and potassium ions move out to maintain electroneutrality.

Hyperkalemia due to Decreased Renal Excretion of Potassium

Decreased renal excretion of potassium can result from (1) marked reductions in glomerular filtration, (2) decreased aldosterone activity, or (3) a defect in potassium secretion in the distal nephron.

Glomerular filtration rates less than 5 mL/min are nearly always associated with hyperkalemia. Patients with lesser degrees of renal impairment can also readily develop hyperkalemia when faced with increased potassium loads (dietary, catabolic, or iatrogenic). Uremia may also impair Na^+–K^+-ATPase activity.

Hyperkalemia due to decreased aldosterone activity can result from a primary defect in adrenal hormone synthesis or a defect in the renin–aldosterone system. Patients with primary adrenal insufficiency (Addison's disease) and those with isolated 21-hydroxylase adrenal enzyme deficiency have marked impairment of aldosterone synthesis. Patients with the syndrome of isolated hypoaldosteronism (also called hyporeninemic hypoaldosteronism, or type IV renal tubular acidosis) are usually diabetics with some degree of renal impairment; they have an impaired ability to increase aldosterone

secretion in response to hyperkalemia. Although usually asymptomatic, these patients develop hyperkalemia when they increase their potassium intake or when given potassium-sparing diuretics. They also often have varying degrees of Na^+ wasting and a hyperchloremic metabolic acidosis. Similar findings have been reported in patients with AIDS who have relative adrenal insufficiency due to cytomegalovirus infection.

Drugs interfering with the renin–aldosterone system have the potential to cause hyperkalemia, particularly in the presence of any degree of renal impairment. Nonsteroidal antiinflammatory drugs (NSAIDs) inhibit prostaglandin-mediated renin release. Angiotensin-converting enzyme (ACE) inhibitors interfere with angiotensin II–mediated release of aldosterone. Large doses of heparin can interfere with aldosterone secretion. The potassium-sparing diuretic spironolactone directly antagonizes aldosterone activity at the kidneys.

Decreased renal excretion of potassium can also occur as a result of an intrinsic or acquired defect in the distal nephron's ability to secrete potassium. Such defects may occur even in the presence of normal renal function and are characteristically unresponsive to mineralocorticoid therapy. The kidneys of patients with pseudohypoaldosteronism display an intrinsic resistance to aldosterone. Acquired defects have been associated with systemic lupus erythematosus, sickle cell anemia, obstructive uropathies, and cyclosporine nephropathy in transplanted kidneys.

Hyperkalemia due to Increased Potassium Intake

Increased potassium loads rarely cause hyperkalemia in normal individuals unless large amounts are given rapidly and intravenously. Hyperkalemia, however, may be seen when potassium intake is increased in patients receiving β blockers or in patients with renal impairment. Unrecognized sources of potassium include potassium penicillin, sodium substitutes (primarily potassium salts), and transfusion of stored whole blood. The plasma [K^+] in a unit of whole blood can increase to 30 mEq/L after 21 days of storage. The risk of hyperkalemia from multiple transfusions is reduced, although not

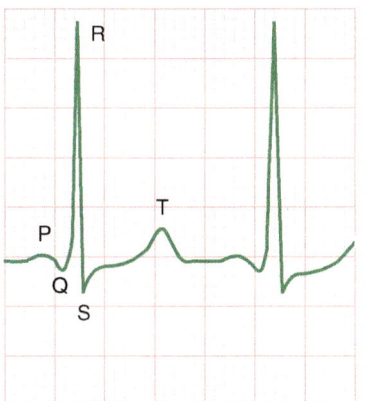 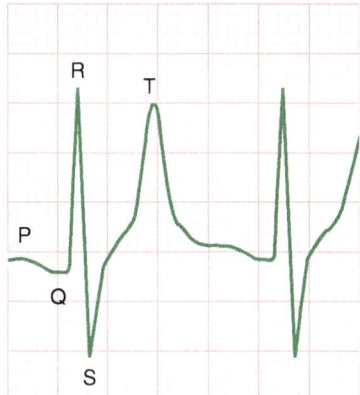 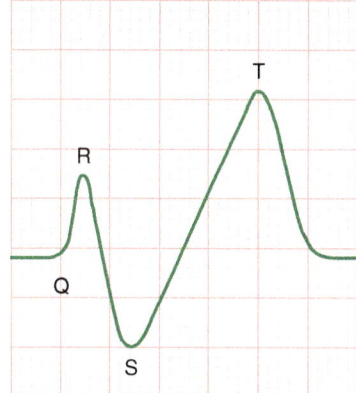

FIGURE 49–6 Electrocardiographic effects of hyperkalemia. Electrocardiographic changes characteristically progress from symmetrically peaked T waves, often with a shortened QT interval, to widening of the QRS complex, prolongation of the P–R interval, loss of the P wave, loss of R-wave amplitude, and ST-segment depression (occasionally elevation)—to an ECG that resembles a sine wave—before final progression into ventricular fibrillation or asystole.

eliminated, by minimizing the volume of plasma given through the use of packed red blood cell transfusions (see Chapter 51).

Clinical Manifestations of Hyperkalemia

The most important effects of hyperkalemia are on skeletal and cardiac muscle. Skeletal muscle weakness is generally not seen until plasma [K⁺] is greater than 8 mEq/L, and is due to sustained spontaneous depolarization and inactivation of Na⁺ channels of muscle membrane, eventually resulting in paralysis. Cardiac manifestations (Figure 49–6) are primarily due to delayed depolarization, and are consistently present when plasma [K⁺] is greater than 7 mEq/L. ECG changes characteristically progress sequentially from symmetrically peaked T waves (often with a shortened QT interval) → widening of the QRS complex → prolongation of the P–R interval → loss of the P wave → loss of R-wave amplitude → ST-segment depression (occasionally elevation) → an ECG that resembles a sine wave, before progression to ventricular fibrillation and asystole. Contractility may be relatively well preserved until late in the course of progressive hyperkalemia. Hypocalcemia, hyponatremia, and acidosis accentuate the cardiac effects of hyperkalemia.

Treatment of Hyperkalemia

8 Because of its lethal potential, hyperkalemia exceeding 6 mEq/L should always be corrected. Treatment is directed to reversal of cardiac manifestations and skeletal muscle weakness, and to restoration of normal plasma [K⁺]. Therapeutic modalities employed depend on the cause of hyperkalemia and the severity of manifestations. Hyperkalemia associated with hypoaldosteronism can be treated with mineralocorticoid replacement. Drugs contributing to hyperkalemia should be discontinued and sources of increased potassium intake reduced or stopped.

Calcium (5–10 mL of 10% calcium gluconate or 3–5 mL of 10% calcium chloride) partially antagonizes the cardiac effects of hyperkalemia and is useful in patients with marked hyperkalemia. Its effects are rapid but short lived. Care must be exercised in administering calcium to patients taking digoxin, as calcium potentiates digoxin toxicity.

When metabolic acidosis is present, intravenous sodium bicarbonate (usually 45 mEq) will promote cellular uptake of potassium and can decrease plasma [K⁺] within 15 min. β Agonists promote cellular uptake of potassium and may be useful in acute hyperkalemia associated with massive transfusions; low-dose epinephrine infusion often rapidly decreases plasma [K⁺] and provides inotropic support in this setting. An intravenous infusion of glucose and insulin (30–50 g of glucose with 10 units of insulin) is also effective in promoting cellular uptake of potassium and lowering plasma [K⁺], but may take up to 1 h for peak effect.

For patients with some renal function, furosemide is a useful adjunct in increasing urinary excretion of potassium. In the absence of renal function, elimination of excess potassium can be accomplished only with nonabsorbable cation-exchange resins such as oral or rectal sodium polystyrene sulfonate (Kayexalate). Each gram of resin binds up to 1 mEq of K⁺ and releases 1.5 mEq of Na⁺; the oral dose is 20 g in 100 mL of 20% sorbitol.

Dialysis is indicated in symptomatic patients with severe or refractory hyperkalemia. Hemodialysis is faster and more effective than peritoneal dialysis in decreasing plasma [K⁺]. Maximal potassium removal with hemodialysis approaches 50 mEq/h, compared with 10–15 mEq/h for peritoneal dialysis.

Anesthetic Considerations

Elective surgery should not be undertaken in patients with significant hyperkalemia. Anesthetic management of hyperkalemic surgical patients is directed at both lowering the plasma potassium concentration and preventing any further increases. The ECG should be carefully monitored. Succinylcholine is contraindicated, as is the use of any potassium-containing intravenous solutions such as lactated Ringer's injection. The avoidance of metabolic or respiratory acidosis is critical to prevent further increases in plasma [K⁺]. Ventilation should be controlled under general anesthesia, and mild hyperventilation may be desirable. Lastly, neuromuscular function should be monitored closely, as hyperkalemia can accentuate the effects of NMBs.

Disorders of Calcium Balance

Although 98% of total body calcium is in bone, maintenance of a normal extracellular calcium concentration is critical to homeostasis. Calcium ions are involved in nearly all essential biological functions, including muscle contraction, the release of neurotransmitters and hormones, blood coagulation, and bone metabolism, and abnormalities in calcium balance can result in profound physiological derangements.

NORMAL CALCIUM BALANCE

Calcium intake in adults averages 600–800 mg/d. Intestinal absorption of calcium occurs primarily in the proximal small bowel but is variable. Calcium is also secreted into the intestinal tract; moreover, this secretion appears to be constant and independent of absorption. Up to 80% of the daily calcium intake is normally lost in feces.

The kidneys are responsible for most calcium excretion. Renal calcium excretion averages 100 mg/d but may vary from as low as 50 mg/d to more than 300 mg/d. Normally, 98% of the filterable calcium is reabsorbed. Calcium reabsorption parallels that of sodium in the proximal renal tubules and the ascending loop of Henle. In the distal tubules, however, calcium reabsorption is dependent on parathyroid hormone (PTH) secretion, whereas sodium reabsorption is dependent on aldosterone secretion. Increased PTH levels enhance distal calcium reabsorption and thereby decrease urinary calcium excretion.

Plasma Calcium Concentration

The normal plasma calcium concentration is 8.5–10.5 mg/dL (2.1–2.6 mmol/L). Approximately 50% is in the free ionized form, 40% is protein bound (mainly to albumin), and 10% is complexed with anions such as citrate and amino acids. The free ionized calcium concentration ([Ca²⁺]) is physiologically most important. Plasma [Ca²⁺] is normally 4.75–5.3 mg/dL (2.38–2.66 mEq/L or 1.19–1.33 mmol/L). Changes in plasma albumin concentration affect total but not ionized calcium concentrations: for each increase or decrease of 1 g/dL in albumin, the total plasma calcium concentration increases or decreases approximately 0.8–1.0 mg/dL, respectively.

Changes in plasma pH directly affect the degree of protein binding and thus ionized calcium concentration. Ionized calcium increases approximately

0.16 mg/dL for each decrease of 0.1 unit in plasma pH and decreases by the same amount for each 0.1 unit increase in pH.

Regulation of Extracellular Ionized Calcium Concentration

Calcium normally enters ECF by either absorption from the intestinal tract or resorption of bone; only 0.5–1% of calcium in bone is exchangeable with ECF. In contrast, calcium normally leaves the extracellular compartment by (1) deposition into bone, (2) urinary excretion, (3) secretion into the intestinal tract, and (4) sweat formation. Extracellular [Ca^{2+}] is closely regulated by three hormones: parathyroid hormone (parathormone, PTH), vitamin D, and calcitonin. These hormones act primarily on bone, the distal renal tubules, and the small bowel.

PTH is the most important regulator of plasma [Ca^{2+}]. Decreases in plasma [Ca^{2+}] stimulate PTH secretion, while increases in plasma [Ca^{2+}] inhibit PTH secretion. The calcemic effect of PTH is due to (1) mobilization of calcium from bone, (2) enhancement of calcium reabsorption in the distal renal tubules, and (3) an indirect increase in intestinal absorption of calcium via acceleration of 1,25-dihydroxycholecalciferol synthesis in the kidneys (see below).

Vitamin D exists in several forms in the body, but 1,25-dihydroxycholecalciferol has the most important biological activity. It is the product of the metabolic conversion of (primarily endogenous) cholecalciferol, first by the liver to 25-cholecalciferol and then by the kidneys to 1,25-dihydroxycholecalciferol. The latter transformation is enhanced by secretion of PTH as well as hypophosphatemia. Vitamin D augments intestinal absorption of calcium, facilitates the action of PTH on bone, and appears to augment renal reabsorption of calcium in the distal tubules.

Calcitonin is a polypeptide hormone that is secreted by parafollicular cells in the thyroid gland. Its secretion is stimulated by hypercalcemia and inhibited by hypocalcemia. Calcitonin inhibits bone reabsorption and increases urinary calcium excretion.

TABLE 49–11 **Causes of hypercalcemia.**

Hyperparathyroidism
Malignancy
Excessive vitamin D intake
Paget's disease of bone
Granulomatous disorders (sarcoidosis, tuberculosis)
Chronic immobilization
Milk-alkali syndrome
Adrenal insufficiency
Drug-induced
Thiazide diuretics
Lithium

HYPERCALCEMIA

Hypercalcemia can occur as a result of a variety of disorders (Table 49–11). In *primary hyperparathyroidism*, secretion of PTH is increased and is independent of [Ca^{2+}]. In contrast, in *secondary hyperparathyroidism* (chronic renal failure or malabsorption), the elevated PTH levels are in response to chronic hypocalcemia. Prolonged secondary hyperparathyroidism, however, can occasionally result in autonomous secretion of PTH, resulting in a normal or elevated [Ca^{2+}] (*tertiary hyperparathyroidism*).

Patients with cancer can present with hypercalcemia whether or not bone metastases are present. Most often this is due to direct bony destruction, or secretion of humoral mediators of hypercalcemia (PTH-like substances, cytokines, or prostaglandins), or both. Hypercalcemia due to increased turnover of calcium from bone can also be encountered in patients with benign conditions such as Paget's disease and chronic immobilization. Increased gastrointestinal absorption of calcium can lead to hypercalcemia in patients with the *milk-alkali syndrome* (marked increase in calcium intake), hypervitaminosis D, or granulomatous diseases (enhanced sensitivity to vitamin D).

Clinical Manifestations of Hypercalcemia

Hypercalcemia often produces anorexia, nausea, vomiting, weakness, and polyuria. Ataxia, irritability, lethargy, or confusion can rapidly progress to coma. Hypertension is often present initially before hypovolemia supervenes. ECG signs include a shortened ST segment and a shortened QT interval. Hypercalcemia increases cardiac sensitivity to digitalis. Pancreatitis, peptic ulcer disease, and kidney failure may also complicate hypercalcemia.

Treatment of Hypercalcemia

9 Symptomatic hypercalcemia requires rapid treatment. The most effective initial treatment is rehydration followed by a brisk diuresis (urinary output 200–300 mL/h) utilizing intravenous saline infusion and a loop diuretic to accelerate calcium excretion. Premature diuretic therapy prior to rehydration may aggravate the hypercalcemia by exacerbating volume depletion. Renal loss of potassium and magnesium usually occurs during diuresis, and laboratory monitoring and intravenous replacement as necessary should be performed. Although hydration and diuresis may remove the potential risk of cardiovascular and neurological complications of hypercalcemia, the serum calcium level usually remains elevated above normal. Additional therapy with a bisphosphonate or calcitonin may be required to further lower the serum calcium level. Severe hypercalcemia (>15 mg/dL) usually requires additional therapy after saline hydration and furosemide calciuresis. Bisphosphonates or calcitonin are preferred agents. Intravenous administration of pamidronate (Aredia) or etidronate (Didronel) is often utilized in this setting. Dialysis is very effective in correcting severe hypercalcemia and may be necessary in the presence of kidney or heart failure. Additional treatment depends on the underlying cause of the hypercalcemia and may include glucocorticoids in the setting of vitamin D–induced hypercalcemia such as granulomatous disease states.

It is necessary to look for the underlying etiology and direct appropriate treatment toward the cause of the hypercalcemia once the initial threat of hypercalcemia has been removed. Approximately 90% of all hypercalcemia is due to either malignancy or hyperparathyroidism. The best laboratory test for discriminating between these two main categories of hypercalcemia is the PTH assay. The serum PTH concentration is usually suppressed in malignancy states and elevated in hyperparathyroidism.

Anesthetic Considerations

Significant hypercalcemia is a medical emergency and should be corrected, if possible, before administration of any anesthetic. Ionized calcium levels should be monitored closely. If surgery must be performed, saline diuresis should be continued intraoperatively with care to avoid hypovolemia; appropriate goal-directed hemodynamic and fluid management therapy (see Chapter 51) should be utilized, especially for patients with cardiac impairment. Serial measurements of $[K^+]$ and $[Mg^{2+}]$ are helpful in detecting iatrogenic hypokalemia and hypomagnesemia. Responses to anesthetic agents are not predictable. Ventilation should be controlled under general anesthesia. Acidosis should be avoided so as to not worsen the elevated plasma $[Ca^{2+}]$.

HYPOCALCEMIA

Hypocalcemia should be diagnosed only on the basis of the plasma ionized calcium concentration. When direct measurements of plasma $[Ca^{2+}]$ are not available, the total calcium concentration must be corrected for decreases in plasma albumin concentration (see above). The causes of hypocalcemia are listed in Table 49–12.

TABLE 49–12 Causes of hypocalcemia.

Hypoparathyroidism
Pseudohypoparathyroidism

Vitamin D deficiency
  Nutritional
  Malabsorption
    Postsurgical (gastrectomy, short bowel)
    Inflammatory bowel disease
  Altered vitamin D metabolism

Hyperphosphatemia

Precipitation of calcium
  Pancreatitis
  Rhabdomyolysis
  Fat embolism

Chelation of calcium
  Multiple rapid red blood transfusions or rapid infusion
  of large amounts of albumin

Hypocalcemia due to hypoparathyroidism is a relatively common cause of symptomatic hypocalcemia. Hypoparathyroidism may be surgical, idiopathic, part of multiple endocrine defects (most often with adrenal insufficiency), or associated with hypomagnesemia. Magnesium deficiency may impair the secretion of PTH and antagonize the effects of PTH on bone. Hypocalcemia during sepsis is also thought to be due to suppression of PTH release. Hyperphosphatemia (see below) is also a relatively common cause of hypocalcemia, particularly in patients with chronic renal failure. Hypocalcemia due to vitamin D deficiency may be the result of a markedly reduced intake (nutritional), vitamin D malabsorption, or abnormal vitamin D metabolism.

Chelation of calcium ions with the citrate ions in blood preservatives is an important cause of perioperative hypocalcemia in transfused patients; similar transient decreases in [Ca^{2+}] are also possible following rapid infusions of large volumes of albumin. Hypocalcemia following acute pancreatitis is thought to be due to precipitation of calcium with fats (soaps) following the release of lipolytic enzymes and fat necrosis; hypocalcemia following fat embolism may have a similar basis. Precipitation of calcium (in injured muscle) may also be seen following rhabdomyolysis.

Less common causes of hypocalcemia include calcitonin-secreting medullary carcinomas of the thyroid, osteoblastic metastatic disease (breast and prostate cancer), and pseudohypoparathyroidism (familial unresponsiveness to PTH). Transient hypocalcemia may be seen following heparin, protamine, or glucagon administration.

Clinical Manifestations of Hypocalcemia

Manifestations of hypocalcemia include paresthesias, confusion, laryngeal stridor (laryngospasm), carpopedal spasm (Trousseau's sign), masseter spasm (Chvostek's sign), and seizures. Biliary colic and bronchospasm have also been described. ECG may reveal cardiac irritability or QT interval prolongation, which may not correlate in severity with the degree of hypocalcemia. Decreased cardiac contractility may result in heart failure, hypotension, or both. Decreased responsiveness to digoxin and β-adrenergic agonists may also occur.

Treatment of Hypocalcemia

10 Symptomatic hypocalcemia is a medical emergency and should be treated immediately with intravenous calcium chloride (3–5 mL of a 10% solution) or calcium gluconate (10–20 mL of a 10% solution). (Ten milliliters of 10% $CaCl_2$ contains 272 mg of Ca^{2+}, whereas 10 mL of 10% calcium gluconate contains only 93 mg of Ca^{2+}.) To avoid precipitation, intravenous calcium should not be given with bicarbonate- or phosphate-containing solutions. Serial ionized calcium measurements are mandatory. Repeat boluses or a continuous infusion (Ca^{2+} 1–2 mg/kg/h) may be necessary. Plasma magnesium concentration should be checked to exclude hypomagnesemia. In chronic hypocalcemia, oral calcium ($CaCO_3$) and vitamin D replacement are usually necessary.

Anesthetic Considerations

Significant hypocalcemia should be corrected preoperatively. Serial ionized calcium levels should be monitored intraoperatively in patients with a history of hypocalcemia. Alkalosis should be avoided to prevent further decreases in [Ca^{2+}]. Intravenous calcium may be necessary following rapid transfusions of citrated blood products or large volumes of albumin solutions. Potentiation of the negative inotropic effects of barbiturates and volatile anesthetics should be expected. Responses to NMBs are inconsistent and require close monitoring with a nerve stimulator.

Disorders of Phosphorus Balance

Phosphorus is an important intracellular constituent. Its presence is required for the synthesis of (1) the phospholipids and phosphoproteins in cell membranes and intracellular organelles, (2) the phosphonucleotides involved in protein synthesis and reproduction, and (3) ATP used for the storage of energy. Only 0.1% of total body phosphorus is in ECF; 85% is in bone and 15% is intracellular.

NORMAL PHOSPHORUS BALANCE

Phosphorus intake averages 800–1500 mg/d in adults. About 80% of that amount is normally absorbed in the proximal small bowel. Vitamin D increases intestinal absorption of phosphorus. The kidneys are the major route for phosphorus excretion and are responsible for regulating total body phosphorus content. Urinary excretion of phosphorus depends on both intake and plasma concentration. Secretion of PTH can augment urinary phosphorus excretion by inhibiting its proximal tubular reabsorption. The latter effect may be offset by PTH-induced release of phosphate from bone.

Plasma Phosphorus Concentration

Plasma phosphorus exists in both organic and inorganic forms. Organic phosphorus is mainly in the form of phospholipids. Of the inorganic phosphorus fraction, 80% is filterable in the kidneys and 20% is protein bound. The majority of inorganic phosphorus is in the form of $H_2PO_4^-$ and HPO_4^{2-} in a 1:4 ratio. By convention, plasma phosphorus is measured as milligrams of elemental phosphorus. Normal plasma phosphorus concentration is 2.5–4.5 mg/dL (0.8–1.45 mmol/L) in adults and up to 6 mg/dL in children. Plasma phosphorus concentration is usually measured during fasting, because a recent carbohydrate intake transiently decreases the plasma phosphorus concentration. Hypophosphatemia increases vitamin D production, whereas hyperphosphatemia depresses it. The latter plays an important role in the genesis of secondary hyperparathyroidism in patients with chronic kidney failure (see Chapter 30).

HYPERPHOSPHATEMIA

Hyperphosphatemia may be seen with increased phosphorus intake (abuse of phosphate laxatives or excessive potassium phosphate administration), decreased phosphorus excretion (renal insufficiency), or massive cell lysis (following chemotherapy for lymphoma or leukemia).

Clinical Manifestations of Hyperphosphatemia

Although hyperphosphatemia itself does not appear to be directly responsible for any functional disturbances, its secondary effect on plasma $[Ca^{2+}]$ can be important. Marked hyperphosphatemia is thought to lower plasma $[Ca^{2+}]$ by precipitation and deposition of calcium phosphate in bone and soft tissues.

Treatment of Hyperphosphatemia

Hyperphosphatemia is generally treated with phosphate-binding antacids such as aluminum hydroxide or aluminum carbonate.

Anesthetic Considerations

Although specific interactions between hyperphosphatemia and anesthesia are generally not described, renal function should be carefully evaluated. Secondary hypocalcemia should also be excluded.

HYPOPHOSPHATEMIA

Hypophosphatemia is usually the result of either a negative phosphorus balance or cellular uptake of extracellular phosphorus (an intercompartmental shift). Intercompartmental shifts of phosphorus can occur during alkalosis and following carbohydrate ingestion or insulin administration. Large doses of aluminum or magnesium-containing antacids, severe burns, inadequate phosphorus supplementation during hyperalimentation, diabetic ketoacidosis, alcohol withdrawal, and prolonged respiratory alkalosis can all produce a negative phosphorus balance and lead to severe hypophosphatemia (<0.3 mmol/dL or <1.0 mg/dL). In contrast to respiratory alkalosis, metabolic alkalosis rarely leads to severe hypophosphatemia.

Clinical Manifestations of Hypophosphatemia

Mild to moderate hypophosphatemia (1.5–2.5 mg/dL) is generally asymptomatic. In contrast, severe hypophosphatemia (<1.0 mg/dL) is often associated with widespread organ dysfunction. Cardiomyopathy, impaired oxygen delivery (decreased

2,3-diphosphoglycerate levels), hemolysis, impaired leukocyte function, platelet dysfunction, encephalopathy, skeletal myopathy, respiratory failure, rhabdomyolysis, skeletal demineralization, metabolic acidosis, and hepatic dysfunction have all been associated with severe hypophosphatemia.

Treatment of Hypophosphatemia

Oral phosphorus replacement is generally preferable to parenteral replacement because of the increased risk of phosphate precipitation with calcium, resulting in hypocalcemia, and also because of the increased risks of hyperphosphatemia, hypomagnesemia, and hypotension. Accordingly, intravenous replacement therapy is usually reserved for instances of symptomatic hypophosphatemia and extremely low phosphate levels (<0.32 mmol/L). In situations where oral phosphate replacement is utilized, vitamin D is required for intestinal phosphate absorption.

Anesthetic Considerations

Anesthetic management of patients with hypophosphatemia requires familiarity with its complications (see above). Hyperglycemia and respiratory alkalosis should be avoided to prevent further decreases in plasma phosphorus concentration. Neuromuscular function must be monitored carefully when **11** NMBs are given. Some patients with severe hypophosphatemia may require mechanical ventilation postoperatively because of muscle weakness.

Disorders of Magnesium Balance

Magnesium is an important intracellular cation that functions as a cofactor in many enzyme pathways. Only 1–2% of total body magnesium stores is present in the ECF compartment; 67% is contained in bone, and the remaining 31% is intracellular. Magnesium has been reported to decrease anesthetic requirements, attenuate nociception, blunt the cardiovascular response to laryngoscopy and intubation, and potentiate NMBs. Suggested mechanisms of action include altering central nervous system neurotransmitter

release, moderating adrenal medullary catecholamine release, and antagonizing the effect of calcium on vascular smooth muscle. Magnesium impairs the calcium-mediated presynaptic release of acetylcholine and may also decrease motor end-plate sensitivity to acetylcholine and alter myocyte membrane potential.

In addition to the treatment of magnesium deficiency, administration of magnesium is utilized therapeutically for preeclampsia and eclampsia, torsades de pointes and digoxin-induced cardiac tachyarrhythmias, and status asthmaticus.

NORMAL MAGNESIUM BALANCE

Magnesium intake averages 20–30 mEq/d (240–370 mg/d) in adults. Of that amount, only 30–40% is absorbed, mainly in the distal small bowel. Renal excretion is the primary route for elimination, averaging 6–12 mEq/d. Magnesium reabsorption by the kidneys is very efficient. Twenty-five percent of filtered magnesium is reabsorbed in the proximal tubule, whereas 50–60% is reabsorbed in the thick ascending limb of the loop of Henle. Factors known to increase magnesium reabsorption in the kidneys include hypomagnesemia, PTH, hypocalcemia, ECF depletion, and metabolic alkalosis. Factors known to increase renal excretion include hypermagnesemia, acute volume expansion, hyperaldosteronism, hypercalcemia, ketoacidosis, diuretics, phosphate depletion, and alcohol ingestion.

Plasma Magnesium Concentration

Plasma $[Mg^{2+}]$ is closely regulated between 1.7 and 2.1 mEq/L (0.7–1 mmol/L or 1.7–2.4 mg/dL) through interaction of the gastrointestinal tract (absorption), bone (storage), and the kidneys (excretion). Approximately 50–60% of plasma magnesium is unbound and diffusible.

HYPERMAGNESEMIA

Increases in plasma $[Mg^{2+}]$ are nearly always due to excessive intake (magnesium-containing antacids or laxatives), renal impairment (GFR < 30 mL/min), or both. Less common causes include adrenal insufficiency, hypothyroidism, rhabdomyolysis, and lithium administration. Magnesium sulfate therapy for preeclampsia and eclampsia can cause hypermagnesemia in the mother as well as in the fetus.

Clinical Manifestations of Hypermagnesemia

Symptomatic hypermagnesemia typically presents with neurological, neuromuscular, and cardiac manifestations, including hyporeflexia, sedation, muscle weakness, and respiratory depression. Vasodilation, bradycardia, and myocardial depression may cause hypotension. ECG signs may include prolongation of the P–R interval and widening of the QRS complex. Marked hypermagnesemia can lead to respiratory and cardiac arrest.

Treatment of Hypermagnesemia

With relatively mild hypermagnesemia, all that is usually necessary is to discontinue source(s) of magnesium intake (most often antacids). In cases of relatively high [Mg^{2+}], and especially in the presence of clinical signs of magnesium toxicity, intravenous calcium can temporarily antagonize most of the effects of clinical toxicity. A loop diuretic in conjunction with intravenous fluid replacement enhances urinary magnesium excretion in patients with adequate renal function. When diuretic administration with intravenous infusion is used to enhance magnesium excretion, serial measurements of [Ca^{2+}] and [Mg^{2+}] should be obtained, a urinary catheter is required, and goal-directed hemodynamic and fluid management should be considered. Dialysis may be necessary in patients with marked renal impairment. In cases of severe magnesium toxicity, ventilatory or circulatory support, or both, may be necessary.

Anesthetic Considerations

Hypermagnesemia requires close monitoring of the ECG, blood pressure, and neuromuscular function. Potentiation of the vasodilatory and negative inotropic properties of anesthetics should be expected. Dosages of nondepolarizing NMBs should be reduced.

TABLE 49–13 **Causes of hypomagnesemia.**

Inadequate intake
    Nutritional

Reduced gastrointestinal absorption
    Malabsorption syndromes
    Small bowel or biliary fistulas
    Prolonged nasogastric suctioning
    Severe vomiting or diarrhea
    Chronic laxative abuse

Increased renal losses
    Diuresis
    Diabetic ketoacidosis
    Hyperparathyroidism
    Hyperaldosteronism
    Hypophosphatemia
    Nephrotoxic drugs
    Postobstructive diuresis

Multifactorial
    Chronic alcoholism
    Protein–calorie malnutrition
    Hyperthyroidism
    Pancreatitis
    Burns

HYPOMAGNESEMIA

Hypomagnesemia is a common and frequently overlooked problem, particularly in critically ill patients, and is often associated with deficiencies of other intracellular components such as potassium and phosphorus. It is commonly found in patients undergoing major cardiothoracic or abdominal operations, and its incidence among patients in intensive care units may exceed 50%. Deficiencies of magnesium are generally the result of inadequate intake, reduced gastrointestinal absorption, and increased renal excretion (Table 49–13). Drugs that cause renal wasting of magnesium include ethanol, theophylline, diuretics, cisplatin, aminoglycosides, cyclosporine, amphotericin B, pentamidine, and granulocyte colony-stimulating factor.

Clinical Manifestations of Hypomagnesemia

Most patients with hypomagnesemia are asymptomatic, but anorexia, weakness, fasciculation, paresthesias, confusion, ataxia, and seizures may be encountered. Hypomagnesemia is frequently associated with both hypocalcemia (impaired PTH secretion) and hypokalemia (due to renal K^+ wasting). Cardiac manifestations include electrical irritability and potentiation of digoxin toxicity; both factors are aggravated by hypokalemia. Hypomagnesemia is associated with an increased incidence of atrial fibrillation. Prolongation of the P–R and QT intervals may also be present.

Treatment of Hypomagnesemia

Asymptomatic hypomagnesemia can be treated orally or intramuscularly. Serious manifestations such as seizures should be treated with intravenous magnesium sulfate, 1–2 g (8–16 mEq or 4–8 mmol) given slowly over 15–60 min.

Anesthetic Considerations

Although no specific anesthetic interactions are described, coexistent electrolyte disturbances such as hypokalemia, hypophosphatemia, and hypocalcemia are often present and should be corrected prior

13 to surgery. Isolated hypomagnesemia should be corrected prior to elective procedures because of its potential for causing cardiac arrhythmias. Moreover, magnesium appears to have intrinsic antiarrhythmic properties and possibly cerebral protective effects (see Chapter 26). It is frequently administered preemptively to lessen the risk of postoperative atrial fibrillation in patients undergoing cardiac surgery.

CASE DISCUSSION

Electrolyte Abnormalities Following Urinary Diversion

A 70-year-old man with carcinoma of the bladder presents for radical cystectomy and ileal loop urinary diversion. He weighs 70 kg and has a 20-year history of hypertension. Preoperative laboratory measurements revealed normal plasma electrolyte concentrations and a blood urea nitrogen (BUN) of 20 mg/dL with a serum creatinine of 1.5 mg/dL. The operation lasts 4 h and is performed under uncomplicated general anesthesia. The estimated blood loss is 900 mL.

Fluid replacement consists of 3500 mL of lactated Ringer's injection and 750 mL of 5% albumin.

One hour after admission to the postanesthesia care unit, the patient is awake, his blood pressure is 130/70 mm Hg, and he appears to be breathing well (18 breaths/min, $Fio_2 = 0.4$). Urinary output has been only 20 mL in the last hour. Laboratory measurements are as follows: Hb, 10.4 g/dL; plasma Na^+, 133 mEq/L; K^+, 3.8 mEq/L; Cl^-, 104 mEq/L; total CO_2, 20 mmol/L; Pao_2, 156 mm Hg; arterial blood pH, 7.29; $Paco_2$, 38 mm Hg; and calculated HCO_3^-, 18 mEq/L.

What is the most likely explanation for the hyponatremia?

Multiple factors tend to promote hyponatremia postoperatively, including nonosmotic antidiuretic hormone (ADH) secretion (surgical stress, hypovolemia, and pain), large evaporative and functional fluid losses (tissue sequestration), and the administration of hypotonic intravenous fluids. Hyponatremia is particularly common postoperatively in patients who have received relatively large amounts of lactated Ringer's injection ($[Na^+]$ 130 mEq/L); the postoperative plasma $[Na^+]$ generally approaches 130 mEq/L in such patients. (Fluid replacement in this patient was appropriate considering basic maintenance requirements, blood loss, and the additional fluid losses usually associated with this type of surgery.)

Why is the patient hyperchloremic and acidotic (normal arterial blood pH is 7.35–7.45)?

Operations for supravesical urinary diversion utilize a segment of bowel (ileum, ileocecal segment, jejunum, or sigmoid colon) that is made to function as a conduit or reservoir. The simplest and most common procedure utilizes an isolated loop of ileum as a conduit: the proximal end is anastomosed to the ureters, and the distal end is brought through the skin, forming a stoma.

Whenever urine comes in contact with bowel mucosa, the potential for significant fluid and electrolyte exchange exists. The ileum actively absorbs chloride in exchange for bicarbonate, and sodium in exchange for potassium or hydrogen ions. When chloride absorption exceeds sodium absorption, plasma chloride concentration increases, whereas plasma bicarbonate concentration decreases—a hyperchloremic metabolic acidosis is established. In addition, the colon absorbs NH_4^+ directly from urine; the latter may also be produced by urea-splitting bacteria. Hypokalemia results if significant amounts of Na^+ are exchanged for K^+. Potassium losses through the conduit are increased by high urinary sodium concentrations. Moreover, a potassium deficit may be present—even in the absence of hypokalemia—because movement of K^+ out of cells (secondary to the acidosis) can prevent an appreciable decrease in extracellular plasma $[K^+]$.

Are there any factors that tend to increase the likelihood of hyperchloremic metabolic acidosis following urinary diversion?

The longer the urine is in contact with bowel, the greater the chance that hyperchloremia and acidosis will occur. Mechanical problems such as poor emptying or redundancy of a conduit—along with hypovolemia—thus predispose to hyperchloremic metabolic acidosis. Preexisting renal impairment also appears to be a major risk factor and probably represents an inability to compensate for the excessive bicarbonate losses.

What treatment, if any, is required for this patient?

The ileal loop should be irrigated with saline—through the indwelling catheter or stent—to exclude partial obstruction and ensure free drainage of urine. Hypovolemia should be considered and treated based on goal-directed hemodynamic and fluid therapy or the response to a fluid challenge (see Chapter 51). A mild to moderate systemic acidosis (arterial pH > 7.25) is generally well tolerated by most patients. Moreover, hyperchloremic metabolic acidosis following ileal conduits is often transient and usually due to urinary stasis. Persistent or more severe acidosis requires treatment with sodium bicarbonate. Potassium replacement may also be required if hypokalemia is present.

Are electrolyte abnormalities seen with other types of urinary diversion?

Procedures employing bowel as a conduit (ileal or colonic) are less likely to result in hyperchloremic metabolic acidosis than those in which bowel functions as a reservoir. The incidence of hyperchloremic metabolic acidosis approaches 80% following ureterosigmoidostomies.

SUGGESTED READING

Awad S, Allison SP, Lobo DN: The history of 0.9% saline. Clin Nutr 2008;27:179.

Bagshaw SM, Townsend DR, McDermid RC: Disorders of sodium and water balance in hospitalized patients. Can J Anesth 2009;56:151.

Chatzizisis YS, Misirli G, Hatzitolios AI, et al: The syndrome of rhabdomyolysis: Complications and treatment. Eur J Intern Med 2008;19:568.

Cooper MS, Gittoes NJL: Diagnosis and management of hypocalcaemia. Brit Med J 2008;336:1298.

Funk G-C, Linder G, Druml W, et al: Incidence and prognosis of dysnatremias present on ICU admission. Intensive Care Med 2010;36:304.

Geerse DA, Bindels AJ, Kuiper MA: Treatment of hypophosphatemia in the intensive care unit. Crit Care 2010;14:R147.

Herrod PJJ, Awad S, Redfern A, et al: Hypo- and hypernatraemia in surgical patients: Is there room for improvement? World J Surg 2010;34:495.

Herroeder S, Schönherr ME, De Hert SG, et al: Magnesium—Essentials for anesthesiologists. Anesthesiology 2010;114:971.

Jacob M, Chappell D, Rehm M: The 'third space'—fact or fiction? Best Pract Res Clin Anaesthesiol 2009;23:145.

Lee R, Weber TJ: Disorders of phosphorus homeostasis. Curr Opin Endocrinol Diabetes Obes 2010;17:561.

Lote C: Regulation and disorders of plasma potassium. Surgery (Oxford) 2007;25:368.

Muller L, Lefrant J-Y: Metabolic effects of plasma expanders. Transfusion Alternatives Transfusion Med 2010;11:10.

O'Hara D, Richardson P: Fluid and electrolyte balance, anaemia and blood transfusion. Surgery (Oxford) 2008;26:383.

Odier C, Nguyen DK, Panisset M: Central pontine and extrapontine myelinolysis: From epileptic and other manifestations to cognitive prognosis. J Neurol 2010;257:1176.

Palmer BF: Managing hyperkalemia caused by inhibitors of the renin-angiotensin-aldosterone system. N Engl J Med 2004;351:585.

Paptistella M, Chappell D, Hofmann-Kiefer K, et al: The role of the glycocalyx in transvascular fluid shifts. Transfusion Alternatives Transfusion Med 2010;11:92.

Pecherstorfer M, Brenner K, Zojer N: Current management strategies for hypercalcemia. Treat Endocrinol 2003;2:273.

Rehm M, Orth V, Scheingraber S, et al: Acid-base changes caused by 5% albumin versus 6% hydroxyethyl starch solution in patients undergoing acute normovolemic hemodilution. Anesthesiology 2000;93:1174.

Rosner MH, Ronco C: Dysnatremias in the intensive care unit. Contrib Nephrol 2010;165:292.

Rueth NM, Murray SE, Huddleston SJ, et al: Severe electrolyte disturbances after hyperthermic intraperitoneal chemotherapy: Oxaliplatin versus mitomycin C. Ann Surg Oncol 2011;18:174.

Sihler KC, Napolitano LM: Complications of massive transfusion. Chest 2010;137:209.

Tavernier B, Faivre S, Bourdon C: Hyperchloremic acidosis during plasma expansion. Transfusion Alternatives Transfusion Med 2010;11:3.

Waters JH, Bernstein CA: Dilutional acidosis following hetastarch or albumin in healthy volunteers. Anesthesiology 2000;93;1184.

50

Acid–Base Management

1. The strong ion difference, P_{CO_2}, and total weak acid concentration best explain acid–base balance in physiological systems.

2. The bicarbonate buffer is effective against metabolic but not respiratory acid–base disturbances.

3. In contrast to the bicarbonate buffer, hemoglobin is capable of buffering both carbonic (CO_2) and noncarbonic (nonvolatile) acids.

4. As a general rule, $Paco_2$ can be expected to increase 0.25–1 mm Hg for each 1 mEq/L increase in $[HCO_3^-]$.

5. The renal response to acidemia is 3-fold: (1) increased reabsorption of the filtered $[HCO_3^-]$, (2) increased excretion of titratable acids, and (3) increased production of ammonia.

6. During chronic respiratory acidosis, plasma $[HCO_3^-]$ increases approximately 4 mEq/L for each 10 mm Hg increase in $Paco_2$ above 40 mm Hg.

7. Diarrhea is a common cause of hyperchloremic metabolic acidosis.

8. The distinction between acute and chronic respiratory alkalosis is not always made, because the compensatory response to chronic respiratory alkalosis is quite variable: plasma $[HCO_3^-]$ decreases 2–5 mEq/L for each 10 mm Hg decrease in $Paco_2$ below 40 mm Hg.

9. Vomiting or continuous loss of gastric fluid by gastric drainage (nasogastric suctioning) can result in marked metabolic alkalosis, extracellular volume depletion, and hypokalemia.

10. The combination of alkalemia and hypokalemia can precipitate severe atrial and ventricular arrhythmias.

11. Changes in temperature affect P_{CO_2}, P_{O_2}, and pH. Both P_{CO_2} and P_{O_2} decrease during hypothermia, but pH increases because temperature does not appreciably alter $[HCO_3^-]$: $Paco_2$ decreases, but $[HCO_3^-]$ is unchanged.

Nearly all biochemical reactions in the body are dependent on maintenance of a physiological hydrogen ion concentration. The latter is tightly regulated because alterations in hydrogen ion concentration are associated with widespread organ dysfunction. This regulation—often referred to as acid–base balance—is of prime importance to anesthesiologists. Changes in ventilation and perfusion and the infusion of electrolyte-containing solutions are common during anesthesia and can rapidly alter acid–base balance.

Our understanding of acid–base balance is evolving. In the past, we focused on the concentration of hydrogen ions [H$^+$], CO$_2$ balance, and the base

1 excess/deficit. We now understand that the strong ion difference (SID), Pco$_2$, and total weak acid concentration (A$_{TOT}$) best explain acid–base balance in physiological systems.

This chapter examines acid–base physiology, common disturbances, and their anesthetic implications. Clinical measurements of blood gases and their interpretation are also reviewed.

Definitions

ACID–BASE CHEMISTRY

Hydrogen Ion Concentration & pH

In any aqueous solution, water molecules reversibly dissociate into hydrogen and hydroxide ions:

$$H_2O \leftrightarrow H^+ + OH^-$$

This process is described by the dissociation constant, K_W:

$$K_W = [H^+] + [OH^-] = 10^{-14}$$

The concentration of water is omitted from the denominator of this expression because it does not vary appreciably and is already included in the constant. Therefore, given [H$^+$] or [OH$^-$], the concentration of the other ion can be readily calculated.

Example: If [H$^+$] = 10^{-8} nEq/L, then [OH$^-$] = 10^{-14} ÷ 10^{-8} = 10^{-6} nEq/L.

Arterial [H$^+$] is normally 40 nEq/L, or 40 × 10^{-9} mol/L. Hydrogen ion concentration is more commonly expressed as pH, which is defined as the negative logarithm (base 10) of [H$^+$] (**Figure 50–1**). Normal arterial pH is therefore –log (40 × 10^{-9}) = 7.40. Hydrogen ion concentrations between 16 and 160 nEq/L (pH 6.8–7.8) are compatible with life.

Like most dissociation constants, K_W is affected by changes in temperature. Thus, the electroneutrality point for water occurs at a pH of 7.0 at 25°C, but at about a pH of 6.8 at 37°C; temperature-related changes may be important during hypothermia (see Chapter 22).

Because physiological fluids are complex aqueous solutions, other factors that affect the

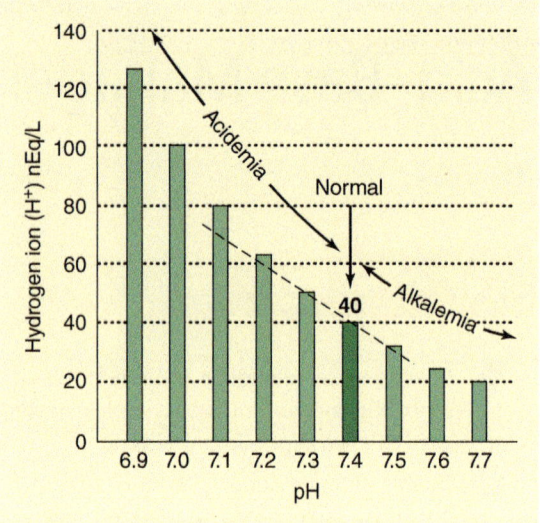

FIGURE 50–1 The relationship between pH and [H$^+$]. Note that between a pH of 7.10 and 7.50, the relationship between pH and [H$^+$] is nearly linear. (Reproduced, with permission, from Narins RG, Emmett M: Simple and mixed acid–base disorders: a practical approach. Medicine 1980;49:161.)

dissociation of water into H$^+$ and OH$^-$ are the SID, the Pco$_2$, and A$_{TOT}$.

Acids & Bases

An acid is usually defined as a chemical species that can act as a proton (H$^+$) donor, whereas a base is a species that can act as a proton acceptor (Brönsted–Lowry definitions). In physiological solutions, it is probably better to use Arrhenius' definitions: An acid is a compound that contains hydrogen and reacts with water to form hydrogen ions. A base is a compound that produces hydroxide ions in water. Using these definitions, the SID becomes important, as other ions in solutions (cations and anions) will affect the dissociation constant for water, and, therefore, the hydrogen ion concentration. A *strong acid* is a substance that readily and almost irreversibly gives up an H$^+$ and increases [H$^+$], whereas a *strong base* avidly binds H$^+$ and decreases [H$^+$]. In contrast, *weak acids* reversibly donate H$^+$, whereas *weak bases* reversibly bind H$^+$; both weak acids and bases tend to have less of an effect on [H$^+$] (for a given concentration of the parent compound) than do strong acids and bases. Biological compounds are either weak acids or weak bases.

For a solution containing the weak acid HA, where

$$HA \leftrightarrow H^+ + A^-$$

a dissociation constant, K, can be defined as follows:

$$K = \frac{[H^+][A^-]}{[HA]} \quad \text{or} \quad [H^+] = \frac{K[HA]}{[A^-]}$$

The negative logarithmic form of the latter equation is called the Henderson–Hasselbalch equation:

$$pH = pK + \log\left(\frac{[A^-]}{[HA]}\right)$$

From this equation, it is apparent that the pH of this solution is related to the ratio of the dissociated anion to the undissociated acid.

The problem with this approach is that it is phenomenological—measure the pH and bicarbonate, and then other variables can be manipulated mathematically. This approach works well with pure water—the concentration of $[H^+]$ must equal $[OH^-]$. But physiological solutions are far more complex. Even in such a complex solution, the $[H^+]$ can be predicted using three variables: the SID, the P_{CO_2}, and A_{TOT}.

Strong Ion Difference

The SID is the sum of all the strong, completely or almost completely dissociated, cations (Na^+, K^+, Ca^{2+}, Mg^{2+}) minus the strong anions (Cl^-, lactate$^-$, etc.) (Figure 50–2). Although we can calculate the SID, because the laws of electroneutrality must be observed, if there is a SID, other unmeasured ions must be present. P_{CO_2} is an independent variable, assuming ventilation is ongoing. The conjugate base of HA is A^- and is composed mostly of phosphates and proteins that do not change independent of the other two variables. A^- plus AH is an independent variable because its value is not determined by any other variable. Note that $[H^+]$ is not a strong ion (water does not completely dissociate), but it can, does, and must change in response to any change in SID, P_{CO_2}, or A_{TOT} to comply with the laws of electroneutrality and conservation of mass. Strong ions cannot be made to achieve electroneutrality, but hydrogen ions, H^+, are created or consumed based on changes in the dissociation of water.

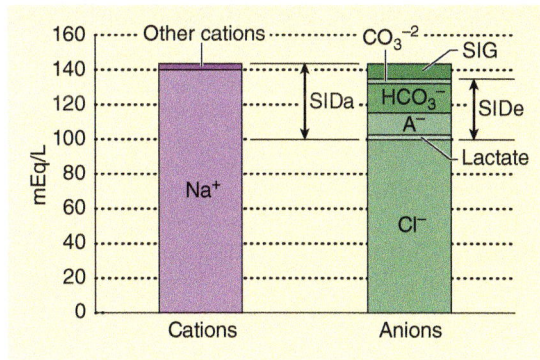

FIGURE 50–2 The strong ion difference (SID). SIDa, apparent strong ion difference. SIDe, effective strong ion difference. The strong ion gap (SIG) is the difference between SIDa and SIDe and represents the anion gap. (Reproduced, with permission, from Greenbaum J, Nirmalan M: Acid-base balance: Stewart's physiochemical approach, Curr Anaesth Crit Care June 2005;16(3):133-135.)

Conjugate Pairs & Buffers

As discussed above, when the weak acid HA is in solution, HA can act as an acid by donating an H^+, and A^- can act as a base by taking up H^+. A^- is therefore often referred to as the conjugate base of HA. A similar concept can be applied for weak bases. Consider the weak base B, where

$$B + H^+ \leftrightarrow BH^+$$

BH^+ is therefore the conjugate acid of B.

A buffer is a solution that contains a weak acid and its conjugate base or a weak base and its conjugate acid (conjugate pairs). Buffers minimize any change in $[H^+]$ by readily accepting or giving up hydrogen ions. It is readily apparent that buffers are most efficient in minimizing changes in the $[H^+]$ of a solution (ie, $[A^-] = [HA]$) when pH = pK. Moreover, the conjugate pair must be present in significant quantities in solution to act as an effective buffer.

CLINICAL DISORDERS

A clear understanding of acid–base disorders and compensatory physiological responses requires precise terminology (Table 50–1). The suffix "-osis" is used here to denote any pathological process that alters arterial pH. Thus, any disorder that tends to reduce pH to a less than normal value is an *acidosis*,

TABLE 50–1 Defining acid–base disorders.

Disorder	Primary Change	Compensatory Response
Respiratory		
Acidosis	↑ Paco$_2$	↑ HCO$_3^-$
Alkalosis	↓ Paco$_2$	↓ HCO$_3^-$
Metabolic		
Acidosis	↓ HCO$_3^-$	↓ Paco$_2$
Alkalosis	↑ HCO$_3^-$	↑ Paco$_2$

whereas one tending to increase pH is termed an *alkalosis*. If the disorder primarily affects [HCO$_3^-$], it is termed *metabolic*. If the disorder primarily affects Paco$_2$, it is termed *respiratory*. Secondary compensatory responses (see below) should be referred to as just that and not as an "-osis." One might therefore refer to a metabolic acidosis with respiratory compensation.

When only one pathological process occurs by itself, the acid–base disorder is considered to be simple. The presence of two or more primary processes indicates a *mixed* acid–base disorder.

The suffix "-emia" is used to denote the net effect of all primary processes and compensatory physiological responses (see below) on arterial blood pH. Because arterial blood pH is normally 7.35–7.45 in adults, the term *acidemia* signifies a pH <7.35, whereas *alkalemia* signifies a pH >7.45.

Compensatory Mechanisms

Physiological responses to changes in [H$^+$] are characterized by three phases: (1) immediate chemical buffering, (2) respiratory compensation (whenever possible), and (3) a slower but more effective renal compensatory response that may nearly normalize arterial pH even if the pathological process remains present.

BODY BUFFERS

Physiologically important buffers in humans include bicarbonate (H$_2$CO$_3$/HCO$_3^-$), hemoglobin (HbH/Hb$^-$), other intracellular proteins (PrH/Pr$^-$), phosphates (H$_2$PO$_4^-$/HPO$_4^{2-}$), and ammonia (NH$_3$/NH$_4^+$). The effectiveness of these buffers in the various fluid compartments is related to their concentration. Bicarbonate is the most important buffer in the extracellular fluid compartment. Hemoglobin, though restricted inside red blood cells, also functions as an important buffer in blood. Other proteins probably play a major role in buffering the intracellular fluid compartment. Phosphate and ammonium ions are important urinary buffers.

Buffering of the extracellular compartment can also be accomplished by the exchange of extracellular H$^+$ for Na$^+$ and Ca^{2+} ions from bone and by the exchange of extracellular H$^+$ for intracellular K$^+$. Acid loads can demineralize bone and release alkaline compounds (CaCO$_3$ and CaHPO$_4$). Alkaline loads (NaHCO$_3$) increase the deposition of carbonate in bone.

Buffering by plasma bicarbonate is almost immediate, whereas that due to interstitial bicarbonate requires 15–20 min. In contrast, buffering by intracellular proteins and bone is slower (2–4 h). Up to 50% to 60% of acid loads may ultimately be buffered by bone and intracellular buffers.

The Bicarbonate Buffer

Although in the strictest sense, the bicarbonate buffer consists of H$_2$CO$_3$ and HCO$_3^-$, CO$_2$ tension (Pco$_2$) may be substituted for H$_2$CO$_3$ because:

$$H_2O + CO_2 \leftrightarrow H_2CO_3 \leftrightarrow H^+ + HCO_3^-$$

This hydration of CO$_2$ is catalyzed by carbonic anhydrase. If adjustments are made in the dissociation constant for the bicarbonate buffer and if the solubility coefficient for CO$_2$ (0.03 mEq/L) is taken into consideration, the Henderson–Hasselbalch equation for bicarbonate can be written as follows:

$$pH = pK' + \left(\frac{[HCO_3^-]}{0.03\ Paco_2} \right)$$

where pK' = 6.1.

Note that its pK' is well removed from the normal arterial pH of 7.40, which means that bicarbonate would not be expected to be an efficient extracellular buffer (see above). The bicarbonate system is, however, important for two reasons: (1) bicarbonate (HCO$_3^-$) is present in relatively high concentrations in extracellular fluid, and (2) more

TABLE 50–2 The relationship between pH and [H⁺].

pH	[H⁺] nEq/L
6.80	158
6.90	126
7.00	100
7.10	79
7.20	63
7.30	50
7.40	40
7.50	32
7.60	25
7.70	20

importantly—$Paco_2$ and plasma $[HCO_3^-]$ are closely regulated by the lungs and the kidneys, respectively. The ability of these two organs to alter the $[HCO_3^-]/Paco_2$ ratio allows them to exert important influences on arterial pH.

A simplified and more practical derivation of the Henderson–Hasselbalch equation for the bicarbonate buffer is as follows:

$$[H^+] = 24 \times \frac{Paco_2}{[HCO_3^-]}$$

This equation is very useful clinically because pH can be readily converted to [H⁺] (Table 50–2). Note that below 7.40, [H⁺] increases 1.25 nEq/L for each 0.01 decrease in pH; above 7.40, [H⁺] decreases 0.8 nEq/L for each 0.01 increase in pH.

Example: If arterial pH = 7.28 and $Paco_2$ = 24 mm Hg, what should the plasma $[HCO_3^-]$ be?

$$[H^+] = 40 + [(40 - 28) \times 1.25] = 55 \text{ nEq/L}$$

Therefore,

$$55 = 24 \times \frac{24}{[HCO_3^-]} \quad \text{and}$$

$$[HCO_3^-] = \frac{(24 \times 24)}{55} = 10.5 \text{ mEq/L}$$

② It should be emphasized that the bicarbonate buffer is effective against metabolic but *not* respiratory acid–base disturbances. If 3 mEq/L of a strong nonvolatile acid, such as HCl, is added to extracellular fluid, the following reaction takes place:

$$3 \text{ mEq/L of } H^+ + 24 \text{ mEq/L of } HCO_3^- \rightarrow H_2CO_3$$
$$+ H_2O + 3 \text{ mEq/L of } CO_2 + 21 \text{ mEq/L of } HCO_3^-$$

Note that HCO_3^- reacts with H⁺ to produce CO_2. Moreover, the CO_2 generated is normally eliminated by the lungs such that $Paco_2$ does not change. Consequently, $[H^+] = 24 \times 40 \div 21 = 45.7$ nEq/L, and pH = 7.34. Furthermore, the decrease in $[HCO_3^-]$ reflects the amount of nonvolatile acid added.

In contrast, an increase in CO_2 tension (volatile acid) has a minimal effect on $[HCO_3]$. If, for example, $Paco_2$ increases from 40 to 80 mm Hg, the dissolved CO_2 increases only from 1.2 mEq/L to 2.2 mEq/L. Moreover, the equilibrium constant for the hydration of CO_2 is such that an increase of this magnitude minimally drives the reaction to the left:

$$H_2O + CO_2 \leftrightarrow H_2CO_3 \leftrightarrow H^+ + HCO_3^-$$

If the valid assumption is made that $[HCO_3^-]$ does not appreciably change, then

$$[H^+] = \frac{(24 \times 80)}{24} = 80 \text{ nEq/L} \quad \text{and} \quad pH = 7.10$$

[H⁺] therefore increases by 40 nEq/L, and because HCO_3^- is produced in a 1:1 ratio with H⁺, $[HCO_3^-]$ also increases by 40 nEq/L. Thus, extracellular $[HCO_3^-]$ increases negligibly, from 24 mEq/L to 24.000040 mEq/L. Therefore, the bicarbonate buffer is not effective against increases in $Paco_2$, and changes in $[HCO_3^-]$ do not reflect the severity of a respiratory acidosis.

Hemoglobin as a Buffer

Hemoglobin is rich in histidine, which is an effective buffer from pH 5.7 to 7.7 (pK_a 6.8). Hemoglobin is the most important noncarbonic buffer in extracellular fluid. Simplistically, hemoglobin may be thought of as existing in red blood cells in equilibrium as a weak acid (HHb) and a potassium salt (KHb). In contrast to the bicarbonate buffer, hemoglobin is capable of buffering both carbonic (CO_2) and noncarbonic (nonvolatile) acids:

$$H^+ + KHb \leftrightarrow HHb + K^+ \quad \text{and}$$

$$H_2CO_3 + KHb \leftrightarrow HHb + HCO_3^-$$

RESPIRATORY COMPENSATION

Changes in alveolar ventilation responsible for the respiratory compensation of $Paco_2$ are mediated by chemoreceptors within the brainstem (see Chapter 23). These receptors respond to changes in cerebrospinal spinal fluid pH. Minute ventilation increases 1–4 L/min for every (acute) 1 mm Hg increase in $Paco_2$. In fact, the lungs are responsible for eliminating the approximately 15 mEq of CO_2 produced every day as a byproduct of carbohydrate and fat metabolism. Respiratory compensatory responses are also important in defending against marked changes in pH during metabolic disturbances.

Respiratory Compensation During Metabolic Acidosis

Decreases in arterial blood pH stimulate medullary respiratory centers. The resulting increase in alveolar ventilation lowers $Paco_2$ and tends to restore arterial pH toward normal. The respiratory response to lower $Paco_2$ occurs rapidly but may not reach a predictably steady state until 12–24 hr; pH is never completely restored to normal. $Paco_2$ normally decreases 1–1.5 mm Hg below 40 mm Hg for every 1 mEq/L decrease in plasma $[HCO_3^-]$.

Respiratory Compensation During Metabolic Alkalosis

Increases in arterial blood pH depress respiratory centers. The resulting alveolar hypoventilation tends to elevate $Paco_2$ and restore arterial pH toward normal. The respiratory response to metabolic alkalosis is generally less predictable than the respiratory response to metabolic acidosis. Hypoxemia, as a result of progressive hypoventilation, eventually activates oxygen-sensitive chemoreceptors; the latter stimulates ventilation and limits the compensatory respiratory response. Consequently, $Paco_2$ usually does not increase above 55 mm Hg in response to metabolic alkalosis. As a general rule, $Paco_2$ can be expected to increase 0.25–1 mm Hg for each 1 mEq/L increase in $[HCO_3^-]$.

RENAL COMPENSATION

The ability of the kidneys to control the amount of HCO_3^- reabsorbed from filtered tubular fluid, form new HCO_3^-, and eliminate H^+ in the form of titratable acids and ammonium ions (see Chapter 29) allows them to exert a major influence on pH during both metabolic and respiratory acid–base disturbances. In fact, the kidneys are responsible for eliminating the approximately 1 mEq/kg per day of sulfuric acid, phosphoric acid, and incompletely oxidized organic acids that are normally produced by the metabolism of dietary and endogenous proteins, nucleoproteins, and organic phosphates (from phosphoproteins and phospholipids). Metabolism of nucleoproteins also produces uric acid. Incomplete combustion of fatty acids and glucose produces keto acids and lactic acid. Endogenous alkali are produced during the metabolism of some anionic amino acids (glutamate and aspartate) and other organic compounds (citrate, acetate, and lactate), but the quantity is insufficient to offset the endogenous acid production.

Renal Compensation During Acidosis

The renal response to acidemia is 3-fold: (1) increased reabsorption of the filtered HCO_3^-, (2) increased excretion of titratable acids, and (3) increased production of ammonia. Although these mechanisms are probably activated immediately, their effects are generally not appreciable for 12–24 hr and may not be maximal for up to 5 days.

A. Increased Reabsorption of HCO_3^-

Bicarbonate reabsorption is shown in Figure 50–3. CO_2 within renal tubular cells combines with water in the presence of carbonic anhydrase. The carbonic acid (H_2CO_3) formed rapidly dissociates into H^+ and HCO_3^-. Bicarbonate ion then enters the bloodstream while the H^+ is secreted into the renal tubule, where it reacts with filtered HCO_3^- to form H_2CO_3.

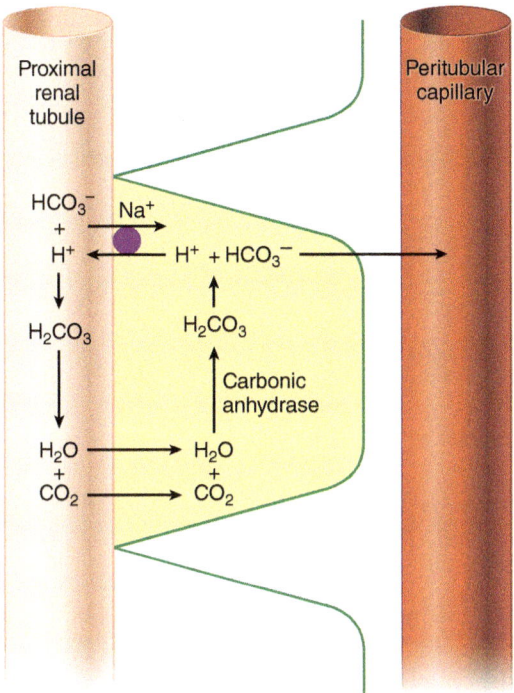

FIGURE 50–3 Reclamation of filtered HCO_3^- by the proximal renal tubules.

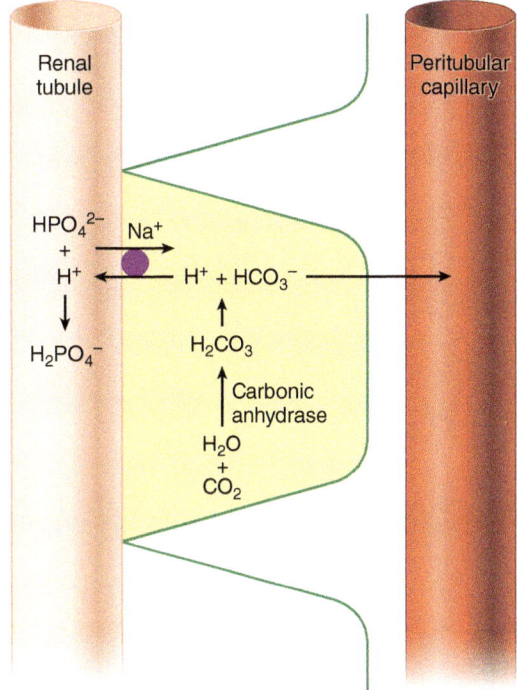

FIGURE 50–4 Formation of a titratable acid in urine.

Carbonic anhydrase associated with the luminal brush border catalyzes the dissociation of H_2CO_3 into CO_2 and H_2O. The CO_2 thus formed can diffuse back into the renal tubular cell to replace the CO_2 originally consumed. The proximal tubules normally reabsorb 80% to 90% of the filtered bicarbonate load along with sodium, whereas the distal tubules are responsible for the remaining 10% to 20%. Unlike the proximal H^+ pump, the H^+ pump in the distal tubule is not necessarily linked to sodium reabsorption and is capable of generating steep H^+ gradients between tubular fluid and tubular cells. Urinary pH can decrease to as low as 4.4 (compared with a pH of 7.40 in plasma).

B. Increased Excretion of Titratable Acids

After all of the HCO_3^- in tubular fluid is reclaimed, the H^+ secreted into the tubular lumen can combine with HPO_4^{2-} to form $H_2PO_4^-$ (**Figure 50–4**); the latter is not readily reabsorbed because of its charge and is eliminated in urine. The net result

is that H^+ is excreted from the body as $H_2PO_4^-$, and the HCO_3^- that is generated in the process can enter the bloodstream. With a pK of 6.8, the $H_2PO_4^-/HPO_4^{2-}$ pair is normally an ideal urinary buffer. When urinary pH approaches 4.4, however, all of the phosphate reaching the distal tubule is in the $H_2PO_4^-$ form; HPO_4^{2-} ions are no longer available for eliminating H^+.

C. Increased Formation of Ammonia

After complete reabsorption of HCO_3^- and consumption of the phosphate buffer, the NH_3/NH_4^+ pair becomes the most important urinary buffer (**Figure 50–5**). Deamination of glutamine within the mitochondria of proximal tubular cells is the principal source of NH_3 production in the kidneys. Acidemia markedly increases renal NH_3 production. The ammonia formed is then able to passively cross the cell's luminal membrane, enter the tubular fluid, and react with H^+ to form NH_4^+. Unlike NH_3, NH_4^+ does not readily penetrate the luminal membrane

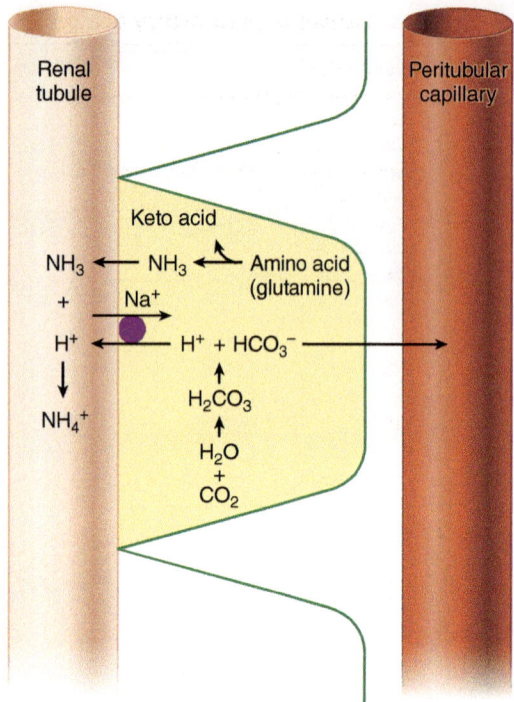

FIGURE 50–5 Formation of ammonia in urine.

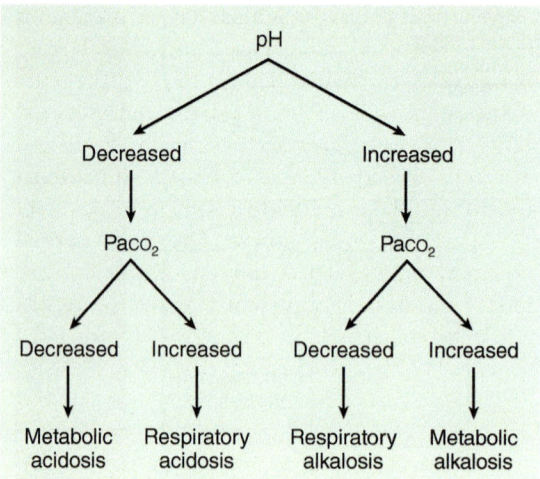

FIGURE 50–6 Diagnosis of simple acid–base disorders.

and is therefore trapped within the tubules. Thus, excretion of NH_4^+ in urine effectively eliminates H^+.

Renal Compensation During Alkalosis

The tremendous amount of HCO_3^- normally filtered and subsequently reabsorbed allows the kidneys to rapidly excrete large amounts of bicarbonate, if necessary (see Chapter 49). As a result, the kidneys are highly effective in protecting against metabolic alkalosis, which therefore generally occurs only in association with concomitant sodium deficiency or mineralocorticoid excess. Sodium depletion decreases extracellular fluid volume and enhances Na^+ reabsorption in the proximal tubule. To maintain neutrality, the Na^+ ion is brought across with a Cl^- ion. As Cl^- ions decrease in number (<10 mEq/L of urine), HCO_3^- must be reabsorbed. Increased H^+ secretion in exchange for augmented Na^+ reabsorption favors HCO_3^- formation with metabolic alkalosis. Similarly, increased mineralocorticoid activity augments aldosterone-mediated Na^+ reabsorption in exchange for H^+ secretion in the distal tubules. The

resulting increase in HCO_3^- formation can initiate or propagate metabolic alkalosis. Metabolic alkalosis is commonly associated with increased mineralocorticoid activity, even in the absence of sodium and chloride depletion.

Base Excess

Base excess is the amount of acid or base (expressed in mEq/L) that must be added for blood pH to return to 7.40 and $Paco_2$ to return to 40 mm Hg at full O_2 saturation and 37°C. Moreover, it adjusts for noncarbonic buffering in the blood. Simplistically, base excess represents the metabolic component of an acid–base disturbance. A positive value indicates metabolic alkalosis, whereas a negative value reveals metabolic acidosis. Base excess is usually derived graphically or electronically from a nomogram originally developed by Siggaard–Andersen and requires measurement of hemoglobin concentration (Figure 50–6).

Acidosis

PHYSIOLOGICAL EFFECTS OF ACIDEMIA

$[H^+]$ is strictly regulated in the nanomole/liter (36–43 nmol/L) range, as H^+ ions have high charge densities and "large" electric fields that can affect the strength of hydrogen bonds that are present on most physiological molecules. Biochemical reactions are very sensitive to changes in $[H^+]$. The overall effects of acidemia seen in patients represent the balance between its direct biochemical effects and the effects of acidemia-induced sympathoadrenal activation. With severe acidosis (pH < 7.20), direct depressant effects predominate. Direct myocardial and smooth muscle depression reduces cardiac contractility and peripheral vascular resistance, resulting in progressive hypotension. Severe acidosis can lead to tissue hypoxia, despite a rightward shift in hemoglobin affinity for oxygen. Both cardiac and vascular smooth muscle become less responsive to endogenous and exogenous catecholamines, and the threshold for ventricular fibrillation is decreased. Progressive hyperkalemia as a result of the movement of K^+ out of cells in exchange for extracellular H^+ is also potentially lethal. Plasma $[K^+]$ increases approximately 0.6 mEq/L for each 0.10 decrease in pH.

Central nervous system depression is more prominent with respiratory acidosis than with metabolic acidosis. This effect is often termed CO_2 **narcosis**. Unlike CO_2, H^+ ions do not readily penetrate the blood–brain barrier.

RESPIRATORY ACIDOSIS

Respiratory acidosis is defined as a primary increase in Pa_{CO_2}. This increase drives the reaction

$$H_2O + CO_2 \leftrightarrow H_2CO_3 \leftrightarrow H^+ + HCO_3^-$$

to the right, leading to an increase in $[H^+]$ and a decrease in arterial pH. For the reasons described above, $[HCO_3^-]$ is minimally affected.

Pa_{CO_2} represents the balance between CO_2 production and CO_2 elimination:

$$Pa_{CO_2} = \frac{CO_2 \text{ production}}{\text{Alveolar ventilation}}$$

CO_2 is a byproduct of fat and carbohydrate metabolism. Muscle activity, body temperature, and thyroid hormone activity can all have major influences on CO_2 production. Because CO_2 production does not appreciably vary under most circumstances, respiratory acidosis is usually the result of alveolar hypoventilation (Table 50–3). In patients

TABLE 50–3 Causes of respiratory acidosis.

Alveolar hypoventilation
　Central nervous system depression
　　Drug-induced
　　Sleep disorders
　　Obesity hypoventilation (Pickwickian) syndrome
　　Cerebral ischemia
　　Cerebral trauma
　Neuromuscular disorders
　　Myopathies
　　Neuropathies
　Chest wall abnormalities
　　Flail chest
　　Kyphoscoliosis
　Pleural abnormalities
　　Pneumothorax
　　Pleural effusion
　Airway obstruction
　　Upper airway
　　　Foreign body
　　　Tumor
　　　Laryngospasm
　　　Sleep disorders
　　Lower airway
　　　Severe asthma
　　　Chronic obstructive pulmonary disease
　　　Tumor
　Parenchymal lung disease
　　Pulmonary edema
　　　Cardiogenic
　　　Noncardiogenic
　　Pulmonary emboli
　　Pneumonia
　　Aspiration
　　Interstitial lung disease
　Ventilator malfunction

Increased CO_2 production
　Large caloric loads
　Malignant hyperthermia
　Intensive shivering
　Prolonged seizure activity
　Thyroid storm
　Extensive thermal injury (burns)

with a limited capacity to increase alveolar ventilation, however, increased CO_2 production can precipitate respiratory acidosis.

Acute Respiratory Acidosis

The compensatory response to acute (6–12 h) elevations in Pa_{CO_2} is limited. Buffering is primarily provided by hemoglobin and the exchange of extracellular H^+ for Na^+ and K^+ from bone and the intracellular fluid compartment (see above). The renal response to retain more bicarbonate is acutely very limited. As a result, plasma $[HCO_3^-]$ increases only about 1 mEq/L for each 10 mm Hg increase in $Paco_2$ above 40 mm Hg.

Chronic Respiratory Acidosis

"Full" renal compensation characterizes chronic respiratory acidosis. Renal compensation is appreciable only after 12–24 hr and may not peak until 3–5 days. During that time, the sustained increase in $Paco_2$ has been present long enough to permit maximal renal compensation. During chronic respiratory acidosis, plasma $[HCO_3^-]$ increases approximately 4 mEq/L for each 10 mm Hg increase in $Paco_2$ above 40 mm Hg.

Treatment of Respiratory Acidosis

Respiratory acidosis is treated by reversing the imbalance between CO_2 production and alveolar ventilation. In most instances, this is accomplished by increasing alveolar ventilation. Measures aimed at reducing CO_2 production are useful only in specific instances (eg, dantrolene for malignant hyperthermia, muscle paralysis for tetanus, antithyroid medication for thyroid storm, and reduced caloric intake in patients receiving enteral or parenteral nutrition). Potential temporizing measures aimed at improving alveolar ventilation (in addition to controlled mechanical ventilation) include bronchodilation, reversal of narcosis, or improving lung compliance (diuresis). Severe acidosis (pH <7.20), CO_2 narcosis, and respiratory muscle fatigue are indications for mechanical ventilation. An increased inspired oxygen concentration is also usually necessary, as coexistent hypoxemia is common. Intravenous $NaHCO_3$ is rarely necessary, unless pH is <7.10 and HCO_3^- is <15 mEq/L. Sodium bicarbonate therapy will transiently increase $Paco_2$:

$$H^+ + HCO_3^- \leftrightarrow CO_2 + H_2O$$

Buffers that do not produce CO_2, such as Carbicarb™ or tromethamine (THAM), are theoretically attractive alternatives; however, there is almost no evidence showing that they have greater efficacy than bicarbonate. Carbicarb™ is a mixture of 0.3 M sodium bicarbonate and 0.3 M sodium carbonate;

buffering by this mixture mainly produces sodium bicarbonate instead of CO_2. Tromethamine has the added advantage of lacking sodium and may be a more effective intracellular buffer.

Patients with a baseline chronic respiratory acidosis require special consideration. When such patients develop acute ventilatory failure, the goal of therapy should be to return $Paco_2$ to the patient's "normal" baseline. Normalizing the patient's $Paco_2$ to 40 mm Hg will produces the equivalent of a respiratory alkalosis (see below). Oxygen therapy must also be carefully controlled, because the respiratory drive in these patients may be dependent on hypoxemia, not $Paco_2$. "Normalization" of $Paco_2$ or relative hyperoxia can precipitate severe hypoventilation.

METABOLIC ACIDOSIS

Metabolic acidosis is defined as a primary decrease in $[HCO_3^-]$. Pathological processes can initiate metabolic acidosis by one of three mechanisms: (1) consumption of HCO_3^- by a strong nonvolatile acid, (2) renal or gastrointestinal wasting of bicarbonate, or (3) rapid dilution of the extracellular fluid compartment with a bicarbonate-free fluid.

A fall in plasma $[HCO_3^-]$ without a proportionate reduction in $Paco_2$ decreases arterial pH. The pulmonary compensatory response in a simple metabolic acidosis (see above) characteristically does not reduce $Paco_2$ to a level that completely normalizes pH but can produce marked hyperventilation (Kussmaul's respiration).

Table 50–4 lists disorders that can cause metabolic acidosis. Note that differential diagnosis of metabolic acidosis may be facilitated by calculation of the anion gap.

The Anion Gap

The anion gap in plasma is most commonly defined as the difference between the major measured cations and the major measured anions:

$$\text{Anion gap} = \text{major plasma cations} - \text{major plasma anions}$$

Or

$$\text{Anion gap} = [Na^+] - ([Cl^-] + [HCO_3^-])$$

TABLE 50–4 Causes of metabolic acidosis.

Increased anion gap
 Increased production of endogenous nonvolatile acids
  Renal failure
  Ketoacidosis
   Diabetic
   Starvation
  Lactic acidosis
  Mixed
   Nonketotic hyperosmolar coma
   Alcoholic
  Inborn errors of metabolism
 Ingestion of toxin
  Salicylate
  Methanol
  Ethylene glycol
  Paraldehyde
  Toluene
  Sulfur
 Rhabdomyolysis

Normal anion gap (hyperchloremic)
 Increased gastrointestinal losses of HCO_3^-
  Diarrhea
  Anion exchange resins (cholestyramine)
  Ingestion of $CaCl_2$, $MgCl_2$
  Fistulas (pancreatic, biliary, or small bowel)
  Ureterosigmoidostomy or obstructed ileal loop
 Increased renal losses of HCO_3^-
  Renal tubular acidosis
  Carbonic anhydrase inhibitors
  Hypoaldosteronism
 Dilutional
  Large amount of bicarbonate-free fluids
   (eg, 0.9% NaCl)
 Total parenteral nutrition (Cl^- salts of amino acids)
 Increased intake of chloride-containing acids
  Ammonium chloride
  Lysine hydrochloride
  Arginine hydrochloride

Some physicians include plasma K^+ in the calculation. Using normal values,

$$\text{Anion gap} = 140 - (104 + 24) = 12 \text{ mEq/L}$$
$$\times (\text{normal range} = 7 - 14 \text{ mEq/L})$$

In reality, an anion gap cannot exist because electroneutrality must be maintained in the body; the sum of all anions must equal the sum of all cations. Therefore,

$$\text{Anion gap} = \text{unmeasured anions}$$
$$- \text{unmeasured cations}$$

"Unmeasured cations" include K^+, Ca^{2+}, and Mg^{2+}, whereas "unmeasured anions" include all organic anions (including plasma proteins), phosphates, and sulfates. Plasma albumin normally accounts for the largest fraction of the anion gap (about 11 mEq/L). The anion gap decreases by 2.5 mEq/L for every 1 g/dL reduction in plasma albumin concentration. **Any process that increases "unmeasured anions" or decreases "unmeasured cations" will increase the anion gap. Conversely, any process that decreases "unmeasured anions" or increases "unmeasured cations" will decrease the anion gap.**

Mild elevations of plasma anion gap up to 20 mEq/L may not be helpful diagnostically during acidosis, but values >30 mEq/L usually indicate the presence of a high anion gap acidosis (below). Metabolic alkalosis can also produce a high anion gap because of extracellular volume depletion, an increased charge on albumin, and a compensatory increase in lactate production. A low plasma anion gap may be encountered with hypoalbuminemia, bromide or lithium intoxication, and multiple myeloma.

High Anion Gap Metabolic Acidosis

Metabolic acidosis with an increased anion gap is characterized by an increase in relatively strong nonvolatile acids. These acids dissociate into H^+ and their respective anions; the H^+ consumes HCO_3^- to produce CO_2, whereas their anions (conjugate bases) accumulate and take the place of HCO_3^- in extracellular fluid (hence the anion gap increases). Nonvolatile acids can be endogenously produced or ingested.

A. Failure to Excrete Endogenous Nonvolatile Acids

Endogenously produced organic acids are normally eliminated by the kidneys in urine (above). Glomerular filtration rates below 20 mL/min (renal failure) typically result in progressive metabolic acidosis from the accumulation of these acids.

B. Increased Endogenous Nonvolatile Acid Production

Severe tissue hypoxia following hypoxemia, hypoperfusion (ischemia), or an inability to utilize oxygen (cyanide poisoning) can result in *lactic acidosis*. Lactic acid is the end product of the anaerobic metabolism of glucose (glycolysis) and can rapidly accumulate under these conditions. Decreased utilization of lactate by the liver, and, to a lesser extent by the kidneys, is less commonly responsible for lactic acidosis; causes include hypoperfusion, alcoholism, and liver disease. Lactate levels can be readily measured and are normally 0.3–1.3 mEq/L. Acidosis resulting from D-lactic acid, which is not recognized by α-lactate dehydrogenase (and not measured by routine assays), may be encountered in patients with short bowel syndromes; D-lactic acid is formed by colonic bacteria from dietary glucose and starch and is absorbed systemically.

An absolute or relative lack of insulin can result in hyperglycemia and progressive *ketoacidosis* from the accumulation of β-hydroxybutyric and acetoacetic acids. Ketoacidosis may also be seen following starvation and alcoholic binges. The pathophysiology of the acidosis often associated with severe alcoholic intoxication and nonketotic hyperosmolar coma is complex and may represent a build-up of lactic, keto, or other unknown acids.

Some inborn errors of metabolism, such as maple syrup urine disease, methylmalonic aciduria, propionic acidemia, and isovaleric acidemia, produce a high anion gap metabolic acidosis as a result of accumulation of abnormal amino acids.

C. Ingestion of Exogenous Nonvolatile Acids

Ingestion of large amounts of salicylates frequently results in metabolic acidosis. Salicylic acid and other acid intermediates rapidly accumulate and produce a high anion gap acidosis. Because salicylates also produce direct respiratory stimulation, most adults develop mixed metabolic acidosis with superimposed respiratory alkalosis. Ingestion of methanol (methyl alcohol) frequently produces acidosis and visual disturbances (retinitis). Symptoms are typically delayed until the slow oxidation of methanol by alcohol dehydrogenase produces formic acid, which is highly toxic to the retina. The high anion gap represents the accumulation of many organic acids, including acetic acid. The toxicity of ethylene glycol is also the result of the action of alcohol dehydrogenase to produce glycolic acid. Glycolic acid, the principal cause of the acidosis, is further metabolized to form oxalic acid, which can be deposited in the renal tubules and result in renal failure.

Normal Anion Gap Metabolic Acidosis

Metabolic acidosis associated with a normal anion gap is typically characterized by hyperchloremia. Plasma $[Cl^-]$ increases to take the place of the HCO_3^- ions that are lost. *Hyperchloremic metabolic acidosis* most commonly results from abnormal gastrointestinal or renal losses of HCO_3^-, or from excessive intravenous administration of 0.9% NaCl solution.

Calculation of the anion gap in urine can be helpful in diagnosing a normal anion gap acidosis.

$$\text{Urine anion gap} = ([Na^+] + [K^+]) - [Cl^-]$$

The urine anion gap is normally positive or close to zero. The principal unmeasured urinary cation is normally NH_4^+, which should increase (along with Cl^-) during a metabolic acidosis; the latter results in a negative urinary anion gap. Impairment of H^+ or NH_4^+ secretion, as occurs in renal failure or renal tubular acidosis (below), results in a positive urine anion gap in spite of systemic acidosis.

A. Increased Gastrointestinal Loss of HCO_3^-

Diarrhea is a common cause of hyperchloremic metabolic acidosis. Diarrheal fluid contains 20–50 mEq/L of HCO_3^-. Small bowel, biliary, and pancreatic fluids are all rich in HCO_3^-. Loss of large volumes of these fluids can lead to hyperchloremic metabolic acidosis. Patients with ureterosigmoidostomies and those with ileal loops that are too long or that become partially obstructed frequently develop hyperchloremic metabolic acidosis. The ingestion of chloride-containing anion-exchange resins (cholestyramine) or large amounts of calcium or magnesium chloride can result in increased absorption of chloride and loss of bicarbonate ions. These nonabsorbable resins bind bicarbonate ions, whereas calcium and magnesium combine with bicarbonate to form insoluble salts within the intestines.

B. Increased Renal Loss of HCO_3^-

Renal wasting of HCO_3^- can occur as a result of failure to reabsorb filtered HCO_3^- or to secrete adequate amounts of H^+ in the form of titratable acid or ammonium ion. These defects are encountered in patients taking carbonic anhydrase inhibitors, such as acetazolamide, and in those with renal tubular acidosis.

Renal tubular acidosis comprises a group of nonazotemic defects of H^+ secretion by the renal tubules, resulting in a urinary pH that is too high for the systemic acidemia. These defects may be a result of a primary renal defect or may be secondary to a systemic disorder. The site of the H^+-secreting defect may be in the distal (type 1) or proximal (type 2) renal tubule. Hyporeninemic hypoaldosteronism is commonly referred to as type 4 renal tubular acidosis. With distal renal tubular acidosis, the defect occurs at a site after most of the filtered HCO_3^- has been reclaimed. As a result, there is a failure to acidify the urine, so that net acid excretion is less than the daily net acid production. This disorder is frequently associated with hypokalemia, demineralization of bone, nephrolithiasis, and nephrocalcinosis. Alkali ($NaHCO_3$) therapy (1–3 mEq/kg/d) is usually sufficient to reverse those side effects. With the less common proximal renal tubular acidosis, defective H^+ secretion in the proximal tubule results in massive wasting of HCO_3^-. Concomitant defects in tubular reabsorption of other substances, such as glucose, amino acids, or phosphates, are common. The hyperchloremic acidosis results in volume depletion and hypokalemia. Treatment involves giving alkali (as much as 10–25 mEq/kg per day) and potassium supplements.

C. Other Causes of Hyperchloremic Acidosis

A *dilutional hyperchloremic acidosis* can occur when extracellular volume is rapidly expanded with a bicarbonate-free fluid, such as normal saline. This is a reason to prefer balanced salt solutions over 0.9% saline for fluid resuscitation. The plasma HCO_3^- decreases in proportion to the amount of fluid infused as extracellular HCO_3^- is diluted. Amino acid infusions (parenteral hyperalimentation) contain organic cations in excess of organic anions and can produce hyperchloremic metabolic acidosis because chloride is commonly used as the anion for the cationic amino acids. Lastly, the administration of excessive quantities of chloride-containing acids, such as ammonium chloride or arginine hydrochloride (usually given to treat a metabolic alkalosis), can cause hyperchloremic metabolic acidosis.

Treatment of Metabolic Acidosis

Several general measures can be undertaken to control the severity of acidemia until the underlying processes are corrected. Any respiratory component

of the acidemia should be corrected. Respiration should be controlled, if necessary; a $Paco_2$ in the low 30s may be desirable to partially return pH to normal. If arterial blood pH remains below 7.20, alkali therapy, usually in the form of $NaHCO_3$ (usually a 7.5% solution), may be necessary. $Paco_2$ may transiently rise as HCO_3^- is consumed by acids (emphasizing the need to control ventilation in severe acidemia). The amount of $NaHCO_3$ given is decided empirically as a fixed dose (1 mEq/kg) or is derived from the base excess and the calculated bicarbonate space (see below). In either case, serial blood gas measurements are mandatory to avoid complications (eg, overshoot alkalosis and sodium overload) and to guide further therapy. Raising arterial pH to >7.25 is usually sufficient to overcome the adverse physiological effects of the acidemia. Profound or refractory acidemia may require acute hemodialysis with a bicarbonate dialysate.

The routine use of large amounts of $NaHCO_3$ in treating cardiac arrest and low flow states is not recommended. Paradoxical intracellular acidosis may occur, particularly when CO_2 elimination is impaired, because the CO_2 formed readily enters cells, but the bicarbonate ion docs not. Alternate buffers that do not produce CO_2, such as Carbicarb™ or tromethamine (THAM), may be theoretically preferable, but are unproven clinically.

Specific therapy for diabetic ketoacidosis includes replacement of the existing fluid deficit (as a result of a hyperglycemic osmotic diuresis) first, as well as insulin, potassium, phosphate, and magnesium. The treatment of lactic acidosis should be directed first at restoring adequate oxygenation and tissue perfusion. Alkalinization of the urine with $NaHCO_3$ to a pH greater than 7.0 increases elimination of salicylate following salicylate poisoning. Treatment options for ethanol or ethylene glycol intoxication include ethanol infusion or fomepizole administration, which competitively inhibit alcohol dehydrogenase and hemodialysis or hemofiltration.

Bicarbonate Space

The bicarbonate space is defined as the volume to which HCO_3^- will distribute when it is given intravenously. Although this theoretically should equal the extracellular fluid space (approximately 25% of body weight), in reality, it ranges anywhere between 25% and 60% of body weight, depending on the severity and duration of the acidosis. This variation is at least partly related to the amount of intracellular and bone buffering that has taken place.

Example: Calculate the amount of $NaHCO_3$ necessary to correct a base deficit (BD) of –10 mEq/L for a 70-kg man with an estimated HCO_3^- space of 30%:

$NaHCO_3 = BD \times 30\% \times$ body weight in L
$NaHCO_3 = -10$ mEq/L $\times$ 30% $\times$ 70 L = 210 mEq

In practice, only 50% of the calculated dose (105 mEq) is usually given, after which another blood gas is measured.

ANESTHETIC CONSIDERATIONS IN PATIENTS WITH ACIDOSIS

Acidemia can potentiate the depressant effects of most sedatives and anesthetic agents on the central nervous and circulatory systems. Because most opioids are weak bases, acidosis can increase the fraction of the drug in the nonionized form and facilitate penetration of the opioid into the brain. Increased sedation and depression of airway reflexes may predispose to pulmonary aspiration. The circulatory depressant effects of both volatile and intravenous anesthetics can also be exaggerated. Moreover, any agent that rapidly decreases sympathetic tone can potentially allow unopposed circulatory depression in the setting of acidosis. Halothane is more arrhythmogenic in the presence of acidosis. Succinylcholine should generally be avoided in acidotic patients with hyperkalemia to prevent further increases in plasma $[K^+]$.

Alkalosis

PHYSIOLOGICAL EFFECTS OF ALKALOSIS

Alkalosis increases the affinity of hemoglobin for oxygen and shifts the oxygen dissociation curve to the left, making it more difficult for hemoglobin to give up oxygen to tissues. Movement of H^+ out of

cells in exchange for the movement of extracellular K^+ into cells can produce hypokalemia. Alkalosis increases the number of anionic binding sites for Ca^{2+} on plasma proteins and can therefore decrease ionized plasma $[Ca^{2+}]$, leading to circulatory depression and neuromuscular irritability. Respiratory alkalosis reduces cerebral blood flow, increases systemic vascular resistance, and may precipitate coronary vasospasm. In the lungs, respiratory alkalosis increases bronchial smooth muscle tone (bronchoconstriction), but decreases pulmonary vascular resistance.

RESPIRATORY ALKALOSIS

Respiratory alkalosis is defined as a primary decrease in $Paco_2$. The mechanism is usually an inappropriate increase in alveolar ventilation relative to CO_2 production. Table 50–5 lists the most common causes of respiratory alkalosis. Plasma $[HCO_3^-]$ usually

TABLE 50–5 Causes of respiratory alkalosis.

Central stimulation
  Pain
  Anxiety
  Ischemia
  Stroke
  Tumor
  Infection
  Fever
  Drug-induced
    Salicylates
    Progesterone (pregnancy)
    Analeptics (doxapram)

Peripheral stimulation
  Hypoxemia
  High altitude
  Pulmonary disease
    Congestive heart failure
    Noncardiogenic pulmonary edema
    Asthma
    Pulmonary embolism
  Severe anemia

Unknown mechanism
  Sepsis
  Metabolic encephalopathies

Iatrogenic
  Ventilator-induced

decreases 2 mEq/L for each 10 mm Hg acute decrease in $Paco_2$ below 40 mm Hg. The distinction between acute and chronic respiratory alkalosis is not always made, because the compensatory response to chronic respiratory alkalosis is quite variable: plasma $[HCO_3^-]$ decreases 2–5 mEq/L for each 10 mm Hg decrease in $Paco_2$ below 40 mm Hg.

Treatment of Respiratory Alkalosis

Correction of the underlying process is the only treatment for respiratory alkalosis. For severe alkalemia (arterial pH >7.60), intravenous hydrochloric acid, arginine chloride, or ammonium chloride may be indicated (see below).

METABOLIC ALKALOSIS

Metabolic alkalosis is defined as a primary increase in plasma $[HCO_3^-]$. Most cases of metabolic alkalosis can be divided into (1) those associated with NaCl deficiency and extracellular fluid depletion, often described as chloride sensitive, and (2) those associated with enhanced mineralocorticoid activity, commonly referred to as chloride-resistant (Table 50–6).

Chloride-Sensitive Metabolic Alkalosis

Depletion of extracellular fluid causes the renal tubules to avidly reabsorb Na^+. Because not enough Cl^- is available to accompany all of the Na^+ ions reabsorbed, increased H^+ secretion must take place to maintain electroneutrality. In effect, HCO_3^- ions that might otherwise have been excreted are reabsorbed, resulting in metabolic alkalosis. Physiologically, maintenance of extracellular fluid volume is therefore given priority over acid–base balance. Because secretion of K^+ ion can also maintain electroneutrality, potassium secretion is also enhanced. Moreover, hypokalemia augments H^+ secretion (and HCO_3^- reabsorption) and will also propagate metabolic alkalosis. Indeed, severe hypokalemia alone can cause alkalosis. Urinary chloride concentrations during a chloride-sensitive metabolic alkalosis are characteristically low (<10 mEq/L).

Diuretic therapy is the most common cause of chloride-sensitive metabolic alkalosis. Diuretics,

TABLE 50–6 Causes of metabolic alkalosis.

Chloride-sensitive
Gastrointestinal
  Vomiting
  Gastric drainage
  Chloride diarrhea
  Villous adenoma
Renal
  Diuretics
  Posthypercapnic
  Low chloride intake
Sweat
  Cystic fibrosis

Chloride-resistant
Increased mineralocorticoid activity
  Primary hyperaldosteronism
  Edematous disorders (secondary hyperaldosteronism)
  Cushing's syndrome
  Licorice ingestion
  Bartter's syndrome
Severe hypokalemia

Miscellaneous
Massive blood transfusion
Acetate-containing colloid solutions
Alkaline administration with renal insufficiency
  Alkali therapy
  Combined antacid and cation-exchange resin therapy
Hypercalcemia
  Milk-alkali syndrome
  Bone metastases
Sodium penicillins
Glucose feeding after starvation

such as furosemide, ethacrynic acid, and thiazides, increase Na^+, Cl^-, and K^+ excretion, resulting in NaCl depletion, hypokalemia, and usually mild metabolic alkalosis. Loss of gastric fluid is also a common cause of chloride-sensitive metabolic alkalosis. Gastric secretions contain 25–100 mEq/L of H^+, 40–160 mEq/L of Na^+, about 15 mEq/L of K^+, and about 200 mEq/L of Cl^-. Vomiting or continuous loss of gastric fluid by gastric drainage (nasogastric suctioning) can result in marked metabolic alkalosis, extracellular volume depletion, and hypokalemia. Rapid normalization of $Paco_2$ after plasma $[HCO_3^-]$ has risen in chronic respiratory acidosis results in metabolic alkalosis (posthypercapnic alkalosis; see above). Infants being fed formulas containing Na^+ without chloride readily develop metabolic alkalosis because of the increased H^+ (or K^+) secretion that must accompany sodium absorption.

Chloride-Resistant Metabolic Alkalosis

Increased mineralocorticoid activity commonly results in metabolic alkalosis, even when it is not associated with extracellular volume depletion. Inappropriate increases in mineralocorticoid activity cause sodium retention and expansion of extracellular fluid volume. Increased H^+ and K^+ secretion takes place to balance enhanced mineralocorticoid-mediated sodium reabsorption, resulting in metabolic alkalosis and hypokalemia. Urinary chloride concentrations are typically greater than 20 mEq/L in such cases.

Other Causes of Metabolic Alkalosis

Metabolic alkalosis is rarely encountered in patients given even large doses of $NaHCO_3$ unless renal excretion of HCO_3^- is impaired. The administration of large amounts of blood products and some plasma protein-containing colloid solution frequently results in metabolic alkalosis. The citrate, lactate, and acetate contained in these fluids are converted by the liver into HCO_3^-. Patients receiving high doses of sodium penicillin (particularly carbenicillin) can develop metabolic alkalosis. Because penicillins act as nonabsorbable anions in the renal tubules, increased H^+ (or K^+) secretion must accompany sodium absorption. For reasons that are not clear, hypercalcemia that results from nonparathyroid causes (milk-alkali syndrome and bone metastases) is also often associated with metabolic alkalosis. The pathophysiology of alkalosis following refeeding is also unknown.

Treatment of Metabolic Alkalosis

As with other acid–base disorders, correction of metabolic alkalosis is never complete until the underlying disorder is treated. When ventilation is controlled, any respiratory component contributing to alkalemia should be corrected by decreasing minute ventilation to normalize $Paco_2$. The treatment of choice for chloride-sensitive metabolic alkalosis is administration of intravenous saline (NaCl) and potassium (KCl). H_2-blocker therapy is useful when excessive loss of gastric fluid is a factor. Acetazolamide may also be useful in edematous patients. Alkalosis associated with primary increases

in mineralocorticoid activity readily responds to aldosterone antagonists (spironolactone). When arterial blood pH is greater than 7.60, treatment with intravenous hydrochloric acid (0.1 mol/L), ammonium chloride (0.1 mol/L), arginine hydrochloride, or hemodialysis should be considered.

ANESTHETIC CONSIDERATIONS IN PATIENTS WITH ALKALEMIA

Respiratory alkalosis seems to prolong the duration of opioid-induced respiratory depression; this effect may result from increased protein binding of opioids. Cerebral ischemia can occur from marked reduction in cerebral blood flow during respiratory alkalosis, particularly during hypotension. **10** The combination of alkalemia and hypokalemia can precipitate severe atrial and ventricular arrhythmias. Potentiation of nondepolarizing neuromuscular blockade is reported with alkalemia, but may be more directly related to concomitant hypokalemia.

DIAGNOSIS OF ACID–BASE DISORDERS

Interpretation of acid–base status from analysis of blood gases requires a systematic approach. A recommended approach follows (Figure 50–6):

1. Examine arterial pH: Is acidemia or alkalemia present?

2. Examine $Paco_2$: Is the change in $Paco_2$ consistent with a respiratory component?

3. If the change in $Paco_2$ does not explain the change in arterial pH, does the change in $[HCO_3^-]$ indicate a metabolic component?

4. Make a tentative diagnosis (see Table 50–1).

5. Compare the change in $[HCO_3^-]$ with the change in $Paco_2$. Does a compensatory response exist (Table 50–7)? Because arterial pH is related to the ratio of $Paco_2$ to $[HCO_3^-]$, both respiratory and renal compensatory mechanisms are always such that $Paco_2$ and $[HCO_3^-]$ change in the same direction.

TABLE 50–7 Normal compensatory responses in acid–base disturbances.

Disturbance	Response	Expected Change
Respiratory acidosis		
Acute	↑ [HCO_3^-]	1 mEq/L/10 mm Hg increase in Pa_{CO_2}
Chronic	↑ [HCO_3^-]	4 mEq/L/10 mm Hg increase in Pa_{CO_2}
Respiratory alkalosis		
Acute	↓ [HCO_3^-]	2 mEq/L/10 mm Hg decrease in Pa_{CO_2}
Chronic	↓ [HCO_3^-]	4 mEq/L/10 mm Hg decrease in Pa_{CO_2}
Metabolic acidosis	↓ Pa_{CO_2}	1.2 × the decrease in [HCO_3^-]
Metabolic alkalosis	↑ Pa_{CO_2}	0.7 × the increase in [HCO_3^-]

A change in opposite directions implies a mixed acid–base disorder.

6. If the compensatory response is more or less than expected, by definition, a mixed acid–base disorder exists.

7. Calculate the plasma anion gap in the case of metabolic acidosis.

8. Measure urinary chloride concentration in the case of metabolic alkalosis.

An alternative approach that is rapid, but perhaps less precise, is to correlate changes in pH with changes in CO_2 or HCO_3. For a respiratory disturbance, every 10 mm Hg change in CO_2 should change arterial pH by approximately 0.08 U in the opposite direction. During metabolic disturbances, every 6 mEq change in HCO_3 also changes arterial pH by 0.1 in the same direction. If the change in pH exceeds or is less than predicated, a mixed acid–base disorder is likely to be present.

MEASUREMENT OF BLOOD GAS TENSIONS & pH

Values obtained by routine blood gas measurement include oxygen and carbon dioxide tensions (Po_2 and Pco_2), pH, [HCO_3^-], base excess, hemoglobin,

and the percentage oxygen saturation of hemoglobin. As a rule, only Po_2, Pco_2, and pH are measured. Hemoglobin and percentage oxygen saturation are measured with a cooximeter. [HCO_3^-] is derived using the Henderson–Hasselbalch equation and base excess from the Siggaard–Andersen nomogram.

Sample Source & Collection

Arterial blood samples are most commonly utilized clinically, though capillary or venous blood can be used if the limitations of such samples are recognized. Oxygen tension in venous blood (normally 40 mm Hg) reflects tissue extraction, not pulmonary function. Venous Pco_2 is usually 4–6 mm Hg higher than $Paco_2$. Consequently, venous blood pH is usually 0.05 U lower than arterial blood pH. Despite these limitations, venous blood is often useful in determining acid–base status. Capillary blood represents a mixture of arterial and venous blood, and the values obtained reflect this fact. Samples are usually collected in heparin-coated syringes and should be analyzed as soon as possible. Air bubbles should be eliminated, and the sample should be capped and placed on ice to prevent significant uptake of gas from blood cells or loss of gases to the atmosphere. Although heparin is highly acidic, excessive amounts of heparin in the sample syringe usually lower pH only minimally, but decrease Pco_2 in direct proportion to percentage dilution and have a variable effect on Po_2.

Temperature Correction

11 Changes in temperature affect Pco_2, Po_2, and pH. Decreases in temperature lower the partial pressure of a gas in solution—even though the total gas content does not change—because gas solubility is inversely proportionate to temperature. Both Pco_2 and Po_2 therefore decrease during hypothermia, but pH increases because temperature does not appreciably alter [HCO_3^-]: $Paco_2$ decreases, but [HCO_3^-] is unchanged. Because blood gas tensions and pH are always measured at 37°C, controversy exists over whether to correct the measured values to the patient's actual temperature. "Normal" values at temperatures other than 37°C are not known. Many clinicians use the measurements at 37°C directly ("α-stat"), regardless of the patient's actual temperature (see Chapter 22).

CASE DISCUSSION

A Complex Acid–Base Disturbance

A 1-month-old male infant with an anorectal malformation undergoes anoplasty. Postoperatively, he is found to be in congestive heart failure resulting from coarctation of the aorta. He is noted to have tachypnea, decreased urinary output, poor peripheral perfusion, hepatomegaly, and cardiomegaly. Following tracheal intubation, the infant is placed on a ventilator (pressure support ventilation, fraction of inspired oxygen [F_{IO_2}] = 1.0). Initial arterial blood gas, hemoglobin, and electrolyte measurements are as follows:

Pa_{CO_2} = 11 mm
pH = 7.47
Pa_{O_2} = 209 mm Hg
Calculated [HCO_3^-] = 7.7 mEq/L
BD = –14.6 mEq/L
Hb = 9.5 g/Dl
[Na^+] = 135 mEq/L
[Cl^-] = 95 mEq/L
[K^+] = 5.5 mEq/L
[Total CO_2] = 8 mEq/L

Note that the [total CO_2] normally measured with electrolytes includes both plasma [HCO_3^-] and dissolved CO_2 in plasma.

What is the acid–base disturbance?

Using the approach described above, the patient clearly has an alkalosis (pH >7.45), which is at least partly respiratory in origin (Pa_{CO_2} <40 mm Hg). Because Pa_{CO_2} has decreased by nearly 30 mm Hg, we would expect [HCO_3^-] to be 18 mEq/L:

$$(40 - 10) \times \frac{2 \text{ mEq/L}}{10} = 6 \text{ mEq/L below 24 mEq/L}$$

In fact, the patient's [HCO_3^-] is nearly 10 mEq/L less than that! The patient therefore also has a mixed acid–base disturbance: primary respiratory alkalosis and primary metabolic acidosis. Note that the difference between the patient's [HCO_3^-] and the [HCO_3^-] expected for a pure respiratory alkalosis roughly corresponds to the base excess.

What are likely causes of these disturbances?

The respiratory alkalosis is probably the result of congestive heart failure, whereas the metabolic acidosis results from lactic acidosis secondary to poor perfusion. The latter is suggested by the calculated plasma anion gap:

$$\text{Anion gap} = 135 - (95 + 8) = 32 \text{ mEq/L}$$

The lactate level was in fact measured and found to be elevated at 14.4 mEq/L. It is probable that fluid overload precipitated the congestive heart failure.

What treatment is indicated?

Treatment should be directed at the primary process, (ie, the congestive heart failure). The patient was treated with diuresis and inotropes.

Following diuresis, the patient's tachypnea has improved, but perfusion still seems to be poor. Repeat laboratory measurements are as follows (F_{IO_2} = 0.5):

Pa_{CO_2} = 23 mm Hg
pH = 7.52
Pa_{O_2} = 136 mm Hg
Calculated [HCO_3^-] = 18 mEq/L
BD = –3.0 mEq/L
Hb = 10.3 g/dL
[Na^+] = 137 mEq/L
[Cl^-] = 92 mEq/L
[K^+] = 3.9 mEq/L
[Total CO_2] = 18.5 mEq/L

What is the acid–base disturbance?

Respiratory alkalosis is still present, whereas the BD seems to have improved. Note that the hemoglobin concentration has increased slightly, but [K^+] has decreased as a result of the diuresis. With the new Pa_{CO_2}, the expected [HCO_3^-] should be 20.6 mEq/L:

$$(40 - 10) \times \frac{2 \text{ mEq/L}}{10} = 3.4 \text{ mEq/L below 24 mEq/L}$$

Therefore, the patient still has metabolic acidosis because the [HCO_3^-] is 2 mEq/L less. Note again that this difference is close to the given BD and that the anion gap is still high:

$$\text{Anion gap} = 137 - (92 + 18) = 27$$

The repeat lactate measurement is now 13.2 mEq/L.

The high anion gap and lactate level explain why the patient is still not doing well and indicate that a new process is masking the severity of the metabolic acidosis (which is essentially unchanged).

Given the clinical course, it is likely that the patient now has a triple acid–base disorder: respiratory alkalosis, metabolic acidosis, and now metabolic alkalosis. The latter probably resulted from hypovolemia secondary to excessive diuresis (chloride-sensitive metabolic alkalosis). Note also that the metabolic alkalosis is nearly equal in magnitude to the metabolic acidosis.

The patient was subsequently given packed red blood cells in saline, and within 24 hr all three disorders began to improve:

Paco$_2$ = 35 mm Hg
pH = 7.51
Pao$_2$ = 124 mm Hg
Calculated [HCO$_3^-$] = 26.8 mEq/L
Base excess = +5.0 mEq/L
Hb = 15 g/dL
[Na$^+$] = 136 mEq/L
[Cl$^-$] = 91 mEq/L
[K$^+$] = 3.2 mEq/L
[Total CO$_2$] = 27 mEq/L
Lactate = 2.7 mEq/L

Outcome

The respiratory alkalosis and the metabolic acidosis have now resolved, and the metabolic alkalosis is now most prominent.

Intravenous KCl replacement and a small amount of saline were judiciously given, followed by complete resolution of metabolic alkalosis. The patient subsequently underwent surgical correction of the coarctation.

SUGGESTED READING

Corey HE: Bench-to-bedside review: Fundamental principles of acid-base physiology. Crit Care 2005;9:184.

Dzierba AL, Abraham P: A practical approach to understanding acid-base abnormalities in critical illness. J Pharm Pract 2011;24:17.

Gunnerson KJ: Clinical review: the meaning of acid-base abnormalities in the intensive care unit – epidemiology. Crit Care 2005;9:508.

Kaplan LJ, Frangos S: Clinical review: acid-base abnormalities in the intensive care unit. Crit Care 2005;9:198.

Kellum JA: Acid-base disorders and strong ion gap. Contrib Nephrol Basel 2007;156:158.

Kraut JA, Madias NE: Metabolic acidosis: pathophysiology, diagnosis and management. Nature Rev Nephrol 2010;6:274.

Morgan TJ: Clinical review: the meaning of acid-base abnormalities in the intensive care unit – effects of fluid administration. Crit Care 2005;9:204.

Morris CG, Low J: Metabolic acidosis in the critically ill: part 1. Classification and pathophysiology. Anaesthesia 2008;63:294.

Morris CG, Low J: Metabolic acidosis in the critically ill: part 2. Causes and treatment. Anaesthesia 2008;63:396.

Fluid Management & Blood Component Therapy

Almost all patients undergoing surgical procedures require venous access for administration of intravenous fluids and medication, and some patients will require transfusion of blood components. The anesthesia provider should be able to assess intravascular volume with sufficient accuracy to correct existing fluid or electrolyte deficits and replace ongoing losses. Errors in fluid and electrolyte replacement or transfusion may result in morbidity or death.

Evaluation of Intravascular Volume

Clinical estimation of intravascular volume must be relied upon because objective measurements of fluid compartment volumes are not practical in the clinical environment. Intravascular volume can be estimated using patient history, physical examination, and laboratory analysis, often with the aid of sophisticated hemodynamic monitoring techniques. Regardless of the method employed, serial evaluations are necessary to confirm initial impressions and to guide fluid, electrolyte, and blood component therapy. Multiple modalities should complement one another, because all parameters are indirect, nonspecific measures of volume; reliance upon any one parameter may lead to erroneous conclusions.

PATIENT HISTORY

The patient history is an important tool in preoperative volume status assessment. Important factors include recent oral intake, persistent vomiting or diarrhea, gastric suction, significant blood loss or wound drainage, intravenous fluid and blood administration, and recent hemodialysis if the patient has kidney failure.

PHYSICAL EXAMINATION

Indications of hypovolemia include abnormal skin turgor, dehydration of mucous membranes, thready peripheral pulses, increased resting heart rate and decreased blood pressure, orthostatic heart rate and blood pressure changes from the supine to sitting or standing positions, and decreased urinary flow rate (Table 51–1). Unfortunately, many medications administered during anesthesia, as well as the neuroendocrine stress response to operative procedures, alter these signs and render them unreliable in the immediate postoperative period. Intraoperatively, the fullness of a peripheral pulse, urinary flow rate, and indirect signs such as the response of blood pressure to positive-pressure ventilation and to the vasodilating or negative inotropic effects of anesthetics, are most often used.

Pitting edema—presacral in the bedridden patient or pretibial in the ambulatory patient—and increased urinary flow are signs of excess extracellular water and likely hypervolemia in patients with normal cardiac, hepatic, and renal function. Late signs of hypervolemia in settings such as congestive heart failure may include tachycardia, elevated jugular pulse pressure, pulmonary crackles and rales, wheezing, cyanosis, and pink, frothy pulmonary secretions.

TABLE 51–1 Signs of fluid loss (hypovolemia).

Sign	Fluid Loss (Expressed as Percentage of Body Weight)		
	5%	10%	15%
Mucous membranes	Dry	Very dry	Parched
Sensorium	Normal	Lethargic	Obtunded
Orthostatic changes	None	Present	Marked
In heart rate			>15 bpm ↑[1]
In blood pressure			>10 mm Hg ↓
Urinary flow rate	Mildly decreased	Decreased	Markedly decreased
Pulse rate	Normal or increased	Increased >100 bpm	Markedly increased >120 bpm
Blood pressure	Normal	Mildly decreased with respiratory variation	Decreased

[1]bpm, beats per minute.

LABORATORY EVALUATION

Several laboratory measurements may be used as surrogates of intravascular volume and adequacy of tissue perfusion, including serial hematocrits, arterial blood pH, urinary specific gravity or osmolality, urinary sodium or chloride concentration, serum sodium, and the blood urea nitrogen (BUN) to serum creatinine ratio. However, these measurements are only indirect indices of intravascular volume, and they often cannot be relied upon intraoperatively because they are affected by many perioperative factors and because laboratory results are often delayed. Laboratory signs of dehydration may include rising hematocrit and hemoglobin, progressive metabolic acidosis (including lactic acidosis), urinary specific gravity greater than 1.010, urinary sodium less than 10 mEq/L, urinary osmolality greater than 450 mOsm/L, hypernatremia, and BUN-to-creatinine ratio greater than 10:1. The hemoglobin and hematocrit are usually unchanged in patients with acute hypovolemia secondary to acute blood loss because there is insufficient time for extravascular fluid to shift into the intravascular space. Radiographic indicators of volume overload include increased pulmonary vascular and interstitial markings (Kerley "B" lines) or diffuse alveolar infiltrates.

HEMODYNAMIC MEASUREMENTS

Hemodynamic monitoring is discussed in Chapter 5. Central venous pressure (CVP) monitoring has been used in patients with normal cardiac and pulmonary function when volume status is difficult to assess by other means or when rapid or major alterations are expected. However, static CVP readings do not provide an accurate or reliable indication of volume status.

Pulmonary artery pressure monitoring has been used in settings where central venous pressures do not correlate with the clinical assessment or when the patient has primary or secondary right ventricular dysfunction; the latter is usually due to pulmonary or left ventricular disease, respectively. Pulmonary artery occlusion pressure (PAOP) readings of less than 8 mm Hg indicate hypovolemia in the presence of confirmatory clinical signs; however, values less than 15 mm Hg may be associated with relative hypovolemia in patients with poor ventricular compliance. PAOP measurements greater than 18 mm Hg are elevated and generally imply left ventricular volume overload. The normal relationship between PAOP and left ventricular end-diastolic volume is altered by the presence of mitral valve disease (particularly stenosis), severe aortic stenosis, or a left atrial myxoma or thrombus, as well as by increased thoracic and pulmonary airway pressures (see Chapters 5, 20, 21, and 22). All PAOP measurements should be obtained at end expiration and interpreted in the context of the clinical setting. Finally, one should recognize that multiple studies have failed to show that pulmonary artery pressure monitoring leads to improved outcomes in critically ill patients, and that echocardiography provides a much more accurate and less invasive estimate of cardiac filling and function.

Intravascular volume status is often difficult to assess, and goal-directed hemodynamic and fluid therapy utilizing arterial pulse contour analysis and estimation of stroke volume variation (eg, LIDCOrapid, Vigileo FloTrak), esophageal Doppler, or transesophageal echocardiography should be considered when accurate determination of hemodynamic and fluid status is important. Stroke volume variation (SVV) is calculated as follows:

$$SVV = SV_{max} - SV_{min}/SV_{mean}$$

The maximum, minimum and mean SV are calculated for a set period of time by the various measuring devices. During spontaneous ventilation the blood pressure decreases on inspiration. During positive pressure ventilation the opposite occurs. Normal SVV is less than 10–15% for patients on controlled ventilation. Patients with greater degrees of SVV are likely to be responsive to fluid therapy. In addition to providing a better assessment of the patient's volume and hemodynamic status than that obtained with CVP monitoring, these modalities avoid the multiple risks associated with central venous and pulmonary artery catheters.

Intravenous Fluids

Intravenous fluid therapy may consist of infusions of crystalloids, colloids, or a combination of both. Crystalloid solutions are aqueous solutions of ions (salts) with or without glucose, whereas colloid solutions also contain high-molecular-weight substances such as proteins or large glucose polymers. Colloid solutions help maintain plasma colloid oncotic pressure (see Chapter 49) and for the most part remain intravascular, whereas crystalloid solutions rapidly equilibrate with and distribute throughout the entire extracellular fluid space.

Controversy exists regarding the use of colloid versus crystalloid fluids for surgical patients. Proponents of colloids justifiably argue that by maintaining plasma oncotic pressure, colloids are more efficient (ie, a smaller volume of colloids than crystalloids is required to produce the same effect) in restoring normal intravascular volume and cardiac output. Crystalloid proponents, on the other hand, maintain that the crystalloid solutions are equally effective when given in appropriate amounts. Concerns that colloids may enhance the formation of pulmonary edema fluid in patients with increased pulmonary capillary permeability appear to be unfounded (see Chapter 23). Several generalizations can be made:

1. Crystalloids, when given in sufficient amounts, are just as effective as colloids in restoring intravascular volume.

2. Replacing an intravascular volume deficit with crystalloids generally requires three to four times the volume needed when using colloids.

3. Surgical patients may have an extracellular fluid deficit that exceeds the intravascular deficit.

4. Severe intravascular fluid deficits can be more rapidly corrected using colloid solutions.

5. The rapid administration of large amounts of crystalloids (>4–5 L) is more frequently associated with tissue edema.

Some evidence suggests that marked tissue edema can impair oxygen transport, tissue healing, and return of bowel function following major surgery.

CRYSTALLOID SOLUTIONS

Crystalloids are usually considered as the initial resuscitation fluid in patients with hemorrhagic and septic shock, in burn patients, in patients with head injury (to maintain cerebral perfusion pressure), and in patients undergoing plasmapheresis and hepatic resection. Colloids may be included in resuscitation efforts following initial administration of crystalloid solutions depending upon anesthesia provider preferences and institutional protocols.

A wide variety of solutions is available (Table 51–2), and choice is according to the type of

TABLE 51–2 Composition of crystalloid solutions.

Solution	Toxicity (mOsm/L)	Na⁺ (mEq/L)	Cl⁻ (mEq/L)	K⁺ (mEq/L)	Ca²⁺ (mEq/L)	Mg²⁺ (mEq/L)	Glucose (g/L)	Lactate (mEq/L)	HCO₃⁻ (mEq/L)	Acetate (mEq/L)	Gluconate (mEq/L)
5% dextrose in water (D₅W)	Hypo (253)–						50				
Normal saline (NS)	Iso (308)	154	154								
D₅ ¼NS	Iso (355)	38.5	38.5				50				
D₅ ½NS	Hyper (432)	77	77				50				
D₅NS	Hyper (586)	154	154				50				
Lactated Ringer's injection (LR)	Iso (273)	130	109	4	3			28			
D₅LR	Hyper (525)	130	109	4	3		50	28			
½NS	Hypo (154)	77	77								
3% S	Hyper (1026)	513	513								
5% S	Hyper (1710)	855	855								
7.5% NaHCO₃	Hyper (1786)	893							893		
Plasmalyte	Iso (294)	140	98	5		3				27	23

fluid loss being replaced. For losses primarily involving water, replacement is with hypotonic solutions, also called maintenance-type solutions. If losses involve both water and electrolytes, replacement is with isotonic electrolyte solutions, also called replacement-type solutions. Glucose is provided in some solutions to maintain tonicity, or prevent ketosis and hypoglycemia due to fasting, or based on tradition. Children are prone to developing hypoglycemia (<50 mg/dL) following 4- to 8-h fasts.

Because most intraoperative fluid losses are isotonic, replacement-type solutions are generally used. The most commonly used fluid is lactated Ringer's solution. Although it is slightly hypotonic, providing approximately 100 mL of free water per liter and tending to lower serum sodium, lactated Ringer's generally has the least effect on extracellular fluid composition and appears to be the most physiological solution when large volumes are necessary. The lactate in this solution is converted by the liver into bicarbonate. **When given in large volumes, normal saline produces a dilutional hyperchloremic acidosis because of its high sodium and chloride content (154 mEq/L): plasma bicarbonate concentration decreases as chloride concentration increases.** Normal saline is the preferred solution for hypochloremic metabolic alkalosis and for diluting packed red blood cells prior to transfusion. Five percent dextrose in water (D_5W) is used for replacement of pure water deficits and as a maintenance fluid for patients on sodium restriction. Hypertonic 3% saline is employed in therapy of severe symptomatic hyponatremia (see Chapter 49). Hypotonic solutions must be administered slowly to avoid inducing hemolysis.

COLLOID SOLUTIONS

The osmotic activity of the high-molecular-weight substances in colloids tends to maintain these solutions intravascularly. Although the intravascular half-life of a crystalloid solution is 20–30 min, most colloid solutions have intravascular half-lives between 3 and 6 h. The relatively greater cost and occasional complications associated with colloids may limit their use. Generally accepted indications for colloids include (1) fluid resuscitation in patients with severe intravascular fluid

deficits (eg, hemorrhagic shock) prior to the arrival of blood for transfusion, and (2) fluid resuscitation in the presence of severe hypoalbuminemia or conditions associated with large protein losses such as burns. For burn patients, colloids are not included in most initial resuscitation protocols (and we strongly recommend that burn surgeons and anesthesia personnel develop a resuscitation protocol and follow it), but may be considered following initial resuscitation with more extensive burn injuries during subsequent operative procedures.

Many clinicians also use colloid solutions in conjunction with crystalloids when fluid replacement needs exceed 3–4 L prior to transfusion. It should be noted that colloid solutions are prepared in normal saline (Cl⁻ 145–154 mEq/L) and thus can also cause hyperchloremic metabolic acidosis (see above). Some clinicians suggest that during anesthesia, maintenance (and other) fluid requirements be provided with crystalloid solutions and blood loss be replaced on a milliliter-per-milliliter basis with colloid solutions (including blood products).

Several colloid solutions are generally available. All are derived from either plasma proteins or synthetic glucose polymers and are supplied in isotonic electrolyte solutions.

Blood-derived colloids include albumin (5% and 25% solutions) and plasma protein fraction (5%). Both are heated to 60°C for at least 10 h to minimize the risk of transmitting hepatitis and other viral diseases. Plasma protein fraction contains α- and β-globulins in addition to albumin and has occasionally resulted in hypotensive reactions. These reactions are allergic in nature and may involve activators of prekallikrein.

Synthetic colloids include dextrose starches and gelatins. Gelatins are associated with histamine-mediated allergic reactions and are not available in the United States. **Dextran** is available as dextran 70 (Macrodex) and dextran 40 (Rheomacrodex), which have average molecular weights of 70,000 and 40,000, respectively. Although dextran 70 is a better volume expander than dextran 40, the latter also improves blood flow through the microcirculation, presumably by decreasing blood viscosity, and is often administered to take advantage of these rheological properties rather than to meet "fluid requirements." Antiplatelet effects are also described for dextrans. Infusions exceeding 20 mL/kg per day can interfere with blood typing, may prolong bleeding time, and have been associated with kidney failure. Dextrans can also be antigenic, and both mild and severe anaphylactoid and anaphylactic reactions are described. Dextran 1 (Promit) may be administered prior to dextran 40 or dextran 70 to prevent severe anaphylactic reactions; it acts as a hapten and binds any circulating dextran antibodies.

Hetastarch (hydroxyethyl starch) is available in multiple formulations, which are designated by concentration, molecular weight, degree of starch substitution (on a molar basis), and ratio of hydroxylation between the C2 and the C6 positions. Thus in some countries a wide variety of formulations are available with concentrations between 6% and 10%, molecular weights between 200 and 670, and degree of molar substitution between 0.4 and 0.7. A greater ratio of C2 versus C6 substitution leads to longer persistence in plasma. The starch molecules are derived from plants. Smaller starch molecules are eliminated by the kidneys, whereas large molecules must first be broken down by amylase. Hetastarch is highly effective as a plasma expander and is less expensive than albumin. Moreover, hetastarch is nonantigenic, and anaphylactoid reactions are rare. Coagulation studies and bleeding times are generally not significantly affected following infusions of older, higher molecular weight formulations up to 1.0 L in adults. Newer, lower molecular weight formulations can safely be given in larger volumes.

Perioperative Fluid Therapy

Perioperative fluid therapy includes replacement of normal losses (maintenance requirements), of preexisting fluid deficits, and of surgical wound losses including blood loss.

NORMAL MAINTENANCE REQUIREMENTS

In the absence of oral intake, fluid and electrolyte deficits can rapidly develop as a result of continued urine formation, gastrointestinal secretions,

TABLE 51–3 Estimating maintenance fluid requirements.[1]

Weight	Rate
For the first 10 kg	4 mL/kg/h
For the next 10 kg	Add 2 mL/kg/h
For each kg above 20 kg	Add 1 mL/kg/h

[1]Example: What are the maintenance fluid requirements for a 25-kg child? Answer: $40 + 20 + 5 = 65$ mL/h.

sweating, and insensible losses from the skin and lungs. Normal maintenance requirements can be estimated from Table 51–3.

PREEXISTING DEFICITS

Patients presenting for surgery after an overnight fast without any fluid intake will have a preexisting deficit proportionate to the duration of the fast. The deficit can be estimated by multiplying the normal maintenance rate by the length of the fast. For the average 70-kg person fasting for 8 h, this amounts to $(40 + 20 + 50)$ mL/h × 8 h, or 880 mL. In fact, the real deficit is less as a result of renal conservation. (After all, how many of us would feel the need to consume nearly 1L of fluid upon awakening after 8 hours of sleep?)

Abnormal fluid losses frequently contribute to preoperative deficits. Preoperative bleeding, vomiting, diuresis, and diarrhea are often contributory. Occult losses (really redistribution; see below) due to fluid sequestration by traumatized or infected tissues or by ascites can also be substantial. Increased insensible losses due to hyperventilation, fever, and sweating are often overlooked.

Ideally, deficits should be replaced preoperatively in surgical patients. The fluids used should be similar in composition to the fluids lost (Table 51–4).

SURGICAL FLUID LOSSES
Blood Loss

One of the most important, yet difficult, tasks of anesthesia personnel is to monitor and estimate blood loss. Although estimates are complicated by

TABLE 51–4 Electrolyte content of body fluids.

Fluid	Na$^+$ (mEq/L)	K$^+$ (mEq/L)	Cl$^-$ (mEq/L)	HCO$_3^-$ (mEq/L)
Sweat	30–50	5	45–55	
Saliva	2–40	10–30	6–30	30
Gastric juice				
High acidity	10–30	5–40	80–150	
Low acidity	70–140	5–40	55–95	5–25
Pancreatic secretions	115–180	5	55–95	60–110
Biliary secretions	130–160	5	90–120	30–40
Ileal fluid	40–135	5–30	20–90	20–30
Diarrheal stool	20–160	10–40	30–120	30–50

occult bleeding into the wound or under the surgical drapes, accuracy is important to guide fluid therapy and transfusion.

The most commonly used method for estimating blood loss is measurement of blood in the surgical suction container and visual estimation of the blood on surgical sponges ("4 by 4's") and laparotomy pads ("lap sponges"). A fully soaked 4 × 4 sponge is said to hold 10 mL of blood, whereas a soaked "lap" holds 100–150 mL. More accurate estimates are obtained if sponges and "laps" are weighed before and after use, which is especially important during pediatric procedures. Use of irrigating solutions complicates estimates, but their use should be noted and an attempt made to compensate. Serial hematocrits or hemoglobin concentrations reflect the ratio of blood cells to plasma, not necessarily blood loss, and rapid fluid shifts and intravenous replacement affect measurements.

Other Fluid Losses

Many surgical procedures are associated with obligatory losses of fluids other than blood. Such losses are due mainly to evaporation and internal redistribution of body fluids. Evaporative losses are most significant with large wounds and are proportional to the surface area exposed and to the duration of the surgical procedure.

Internal redistribution of fluids—often called *third-spacing*—can cause massive fluid shifts and

severe intravascular depletion. Everything related to "third-space" fluid loss is controversial, including whether it actually exists in patients other than those with peritonitis, burns, and similar situations characterized by inflamed or infected tissue. Traumatized, inflamed, or infected tissue can sequester large amounts of fluid in the interstitial space and can translocate fluid across serosal surfaces (ascites) or into bowel lumen. Shifting of intravascular fluid into the interstitial space is especially important; protein-free fluid shift across an intact vascular barrier into the interstitial space is exacerbated by hypervolemia, and pathological alteration of the vascular barrier allows protein-rich fluid shift.

INTRAOPERATIVE FLUID REPLACEMENT

Intraoperative fluid therapy should include supplying basic fluid requirements and replacing residual preoperative deficits as well as intraoperative losses (blood loss, fluid redistribution, and evaporation). Selection of the type of intravenous solution depends on the surgical procedure and the expected blood loss. For minor procedures involving minimal blood loss, dilute maintenance solutions can be used. For all other procedures, lactated Ringer's solution or Plasmalyte is generally used even for maintenance requirements.

Replacing Blood Loss

Ideally, blood loss should be replaced with crystalloid or colloid solutions to maintain intravascular volume (normovolemia) until the danger of anemia outweighs the risks of transfusion. At that point, further blood loss is replaced with transfusions of red blood cells to maintain hemoglobin concentration (or hematocrit) at that level. There are no mandatory transfusion triggers. The point where the benefits of transfusion outweigh its risks must be considered on an individual basis.

Below a hemoglobin concentration of 7 g/dL, the resting cardiac output increases to maintain a normal oxygen delivery. An increased hemoglobin concentration may be appropriate for older and sicker patients with cardiac or pulmonary disease, particularly when there is clinical evidence (eg, a reduced mixed venous oxygen saturation and a persisting tachycardia) that transfusion would be useful.

In settings other than massive trauma, most clinicians administer lactated Ringer's solution or Plasmalyte in approximately three to four times the volume of the blood lost, or colloid in a 1:1 ratio, until the transfusion point is reached. At that time, blood is replaced unit-for-unit as it is lost, with reconstituted packed red blood cells.

The transfusion point can be determined preoperatively from the hematocrit and by estimating **②** blood volume (Table 51–5). Patients with a normal hematocrit should generally be transfused only after losses greater than 10–20% of their blood volume. The exact point is based on the patient's medical condition and the surgical procedure. The amount of blood loss necessary for the hematocrit to fall to 30% can be calculated as follows:

1. Estimate blood volume from Table 51–5.
2. Estimate the red blood cell volume (RBCV) at the preoperative hematocrit ($RBCV_{preop}$).
3. Estimate RBCV at a hematocrit of 30% ($RBCV_{30\%}$), assuming normal blood volume is maintained.
4. Calculate the RBCV lost when the hematocrit is 30%; $RBCV_{lost} = RBCV_{preop} - RBCV_{30\%}$.
5. Allowable blood loss = $RBCV_{lost} \times 3$.

Example

An 85-kg woman has a preoperative hematocrit of 35%. How much blood loss will decrease her hematocrit to 30%?

$$\text{Estimated blood volume} = 65 \text{ mL/kg} \times 85 \text{ kg}$$
$$= 5525 \text{ mL.}$$
$$RBCV_{35\%} = 5525 \times 35\% = 1934 \text{ mL.}$$
$$RBCV_{30\%} = 5525 \times 30\% = 1658 \text{ mL.}$$
$$\text{Red cell loss at 30\%} = 1934 - 1658 = 276 \text{ mL.}$$
$$\text{Allowable blood loss} = 3 \times 276 \text{ mL} = 828 \text{ mL.}$$

Therefore, transfusion should be considered only when this patient's blood loss exceeds 800 mL. Increasingly, transfusions are not recommended until the hematocrit decreases to 24% or lower (hemoglobin <8.0 g/dL), but it is necessary to take into account the rate of blood loss and comorbid conditions (eg, cardiac disease, in which case transfusion might be indicated if only 800 mL of blood is lost).

Clinical guidelines commonly used include: (1) one unit of red blood cells will increase hemoglobin 1 g/dL and the hematocrit 2–3% in adults; and (2) a 10-mL/kg transfusion of red blood cells will increase hemoglobin concentration by 3 g/dL and the hematocrit by 10%.

Replacing Redistributive & Evaporative Losses

Because redistributive and evaporative losses are primarily related to wound size and the extent of surgical dissections and manipulations, procedures can be classified according to the degree of tissue trauma. These additional fluid losses can be replaced

TABLE 51–5 **Average blood volumes.**

Age	Blood Volume
Neonates	
Premature	95 mL/kg
Full-term	85 mL/kg
Infants	80 mL/kg
Adults	
Men	75 mL/kg
Women	65 mL/kg

TABLE 51–6 Redistribution and evaporative surgical fluid losses.

Degree of Tissue Trauma	Additional Fluid Requirement
Minimal (eg, herniorrhaphy)	0–2 mL/kg
Moderate (eg, cholecystectomy)	2–4 mL/kg
Severe (eg, bowel resection)	4–8 mL/kg

according to Table 51–6, based on whether tissue trauma is minimal, moderate, or severe. These values are only guidelines, and actual needs vary considerably from patient to patient.

Transfusion

BLOOD GROUPS

Human red cell membranes are estimated to contain at least 300 different antigenic determinants, and at least 20 separate blood group antigen systems are known. Fortunately, only the ABO and the Rh systems are important in the majority of blood transfusions. Individuals often produce antibodies (alloantibodies) to the alleles they lack within each system. Such antibodies are responsible for the most serious reactions to transfusions. Antibodies may occur "naturally" or in response to sensitization from a previous transfusion or pregnancy.

The ABO System

ABO blood group typing is determined by the presence or absence of A or B red blood cell (RBC) surface antigens: Type A blood has A RBC antigen, type B blood has B RBC antigen, type AB blood has both A and B RBC antigens, and type O blood has neither A nor B RBC antigen present. Almost all individuals not having A or B antigen "naturally" produce antibodies, mainly immunoglobulin (Ig) M, against those missing antigens within the first year of life.

The Rh System

There are approximately 46 Rhesus group red cell surface antigens, and patients with the D Rhesus antigen are considered Rh-positive. Approximately 85% of the white population and 92% of the black population has the D antigen, and individuals lacking this antigen are called Rh-negative. In contrast to the ABO groups, Rh-negative patients usually develop antibodies against the D antigen only after an Rh-positive transfusion or with pregnancy, in the situation of an Rh-negative mother delivering an Rh-positive baby.

Other Red Blood Cell Antigen Systems

Other red cell antigen systems include Lewis, P, Ii, MNS, Kidd, Kell, Duffy, Lutheran, Xg, Sid, Cartright, YK, and Chido Rodgers. Fortunately, with some exceptions (Kell, Kidd, Duffy, and Ss), alloantibodies against these antigens rarely cause serious hemolytic reactions.

COMPATIBILITY TESTING

The purpose of compatibility testing is to predict and to prevent antigen–antibody reactions as a result of red cell transfusions.

ABO–Rh Testing

The most severe transfusion reactions are due to ABO incompatibility; naturally acquired antibodies can react against the transfused (foreign) antigens, activate complement, and result in intravascular hemolysis. The patient's red cells are tested with serum known to have antibodies against A and against B to determine blood type. Because of the almost universal prevalence of natural ABO antibodies, confirmation of blood type is then made by testing the patient's serum against red cells with a known antigen type.

The patient's red cells are also tested with anti-D antibodies to determine Rh status. If the subject is Rh-negative, the presence of anti-D antibody is checked by mixing the patient's serum against Rh-positive red cells. The probability of developing anti-D antibodies after a single exposure to the Rh antigen is 50–70%.

Antibody Screen

The purpose of this test is to detect in the serum the presence of the antibodies that are most commonly associated with non-ABO hemolytic reactions. The test (also known as the indirect Coombs test) requires 45 min and involves mixing the patient's serum with red cells of known antigenic composition; if specific antibodies are present, they will coat the red cell membrane, and subsequent addition of an antiglobulin antibody results in red cell agglutination. Antibody screens are routinely done on all donor blood and are frequently done for a potential recipient instead of a crossmatch (below).

Crossmatch

A crossmatch mimics the transfusion: donor red cells are mixed with recipient serum. Crossmatching serves three functions: (1) it confirms ABO and Rh typing, (2) it detects antibodies to the other blood group systems, and (3) it detects antibodies in low titers or those that do not agglutinate easily.

Type & Crossmatch versus Type & Screen

In the situation of negative antibody screen without crossmatch, the incidence of serious hemolytic reaction with ABO- and Rh-compatible transfusion is less than 1:10,000. Crossmatching, however, assures optimal safety and detects the presence of less common antibodies not usually tested for in a screen. Because of the expense and time involved (45 min), crossmatches are often now performed before the need to transfuse only when the patient's antibody screen is positive, when the probability of transfusion is high, or when the patient is considered at risk for alloimmunization.

EMERGENCY TRANSFUSIONS

When a patient is exsanguinating, the urgent need to transfuse may arise prior to completion of a crossmatch, screen, or even blood typing. If the patient's blood type is known, an abbreviated crossmatch, requiring less than 5 min, will confirm ABO compatibility. **If the recipient's blood type and Rh status is not known with certainty and transfusion must be started before determination, type O Rh-negative (universal donor) red cells may be used.**

BLOOD BANK PRACTICES

Blood donors are screened to exclude medical conditions that might adversely affect the donor or the recipient. Once the blood is collected, it is typed, screened for antibodies, and tested for hepatitis B, hepatitis C, syphilis, and human immunodeficiency virus (HIV). A preservative–anticoagulant solution is added. The most commonly used solution is **CPDA-1,** which contains citrate as an anticoagulant (by binding calcium), phosphate as a buffer, dextrose as a red cell energy source, and adenosine as a precursor for adenosine triphosphate (ATP) synthesis. CPDA-1-preserved blood can be stored for 35 days, after which the viability of the red cells rapidly decreases. Alternatively, use of either AS-1 (Adsol) or AS-3 (Nutrice) extends the shelf-life to 6 weeks.

Nearly all units collected are separated into their component parts (ie, red cells, platelets, and plasma). In other words, whole blood units are rarely available for transfusion in civilian practice. When centrifuged, one unit of whole blood yields approximately 250 mL of packed red blood cells (PRBCs) with a hematocrit of 70%; following the addition of saline preservative, the volume of a unit of PRBCs often reaches 350 mL. Red cells are normally stored at 1–6°C, but may be frozen in a hypertonic glycerol solution for up to 10 years. The latter technique is usually reserved for storage of blood with rare phenotypes.

The supernatant is centrifuged to yield platelets and plasma. The unit of platelets obtained generally contains 50–70 mL of plasma and can be stored at 20–24°C for 5 days. The remaining plasma supernatant is further processed and frozen to yield fresh frozen plasma; rapid freezing helps prevent inactivation of labile coagulation factors (V and VIII). Slow thawing of fresh frozen plasma yields a gelatinous precipitate (cryoprecipitate) that contains high concentrations of factor VIII and fibrinogen. Once separated, this cryoprecipitate can be refrozen for storage. One unit of blood yields about 200 mL of plasma, which is frozen for storage; once thawed, it must be transfused within 24 h. Most platelets are now obtained from donors by apheresis, and a single platelet apheresis unit is equivalent to the amount of platelets derived from 6–8 units of whole blood.

The use of leukocyte-reduced (*leukoreduction*) blood products has been rapidly adopted by many countries, including the United States, in order to decrease the risk of transfusion-related febrile reactions, infections, and immunosuppression.

INTRAOPERATIVE TRANSFUSION PRACTICES

Packed Red Blood Cells

Blood transfusions should be given as PRBCs, which allows optimal utilization of blood bank resources. Surgical patients require volume as well as red cells, and crystalloid or colloid can be infused simultaneously through a second intravenous line for volume replacement.

Prior to transfusion, each unit should be carefully checked against the blood bank slip and the recipient's identity bracelet. The transfusion tubing should contain a 170-μm filter to trap any clots or debris. Blood for intraoperative transfusion should be warmed to 37°C during infusion, particularly when more than 2–3 units will be transfused; failure to do so can result in profound hypothermia. The additive effects of hypothermia and the typically low levels of 2,3-diphosphoglycerate (2,3-DPG) in stored blood can cause a marked leftward shift of the hemoglobin–oxygen dissociation curve (see Chapter 23) and, at least theoretically, promote tissue hypoxia.

Fresh Frozen Plasma

Fresh frozen plasma (FFP) contains all plasma proteins, including most clotting factors. Transfusions of FFP are indicated in the treatment of isolated factor deficiencies, the reversal of warfarin therapy, and the correction of coagulopathy associated with liver disease. Each unit of FFP generally increases the level of each clotting factor by 2–3% in adults. The initial therapeutic dose is usually 10–15 mL/kg. The goal is to achieve 30% of the normal coagulation factor concentration.

FFP may also be used in patients who have received massive blood transfusions (see below) and continue to bleed following platelet transfusions. Patients with antithrombin III deficiency or thrombotic thrombocytopenic purpura also benefit from FFP transfusions.

Each unit of FFP carries the same infectious risk as a unit of whole blood. In addition, occasional patients may become sensitized to plasma proteins. ABO-compatible units should generally be given but are not mandatory. As with red cells, FFP should generally be warmed to 37°C prior to transfusion.

Platelets

Platelet transfusions should be given to patients with thrombocytopenia or dysfunctional platelets in the presence of bleeding. Prophylactic platelet transfusions are also indicated in patients with platelet counts below 10,000–20,000 × 10⁹/L because of an increased risk of spontaneous hemorrhage.

Platelet counts less than 50,000 × 10⁹/L are associated with increased blood loss during surgery. Thrombocytopenic patients often receive prophylactic platelet transfusions prior to surgery or invasive procedures. Vaginal delivery and minor surgical procedures may be performed in patients with normal platelet function and counts greater than 50,000 × 10⁹/L. Administration of a single unit of platelets may be expected to increase the platelet count by 5000–10,000 × 10⁹/L, and with administration of a platelet apheresis unit, by 30,000–60,000 × 10⁹/L.

ABO-compatible platelet transfusions are desirable but not necessary. Transfused platelets generally survive only 1–7 days following transfusion. ABO compatibility may increase platelet survival. Rh sensitization can occur in Rh-negative recipients due to the presence of a few red cells in Rh-positive platelet units. Moreover, anti-A or anti-B antibodies in the 70 mL of plasma in each platelet unit can cause a hemolytic reaction against the recipient's red cells when a large number of ABO-incompatible platelet units is given. Administration of Rh immunoglobulin to Rh-negative individuals can protect against Rh sensitization following Rh-positive platelet transfusions.

Granulocyte Transfusions

Granulocyte transfusions, prepared by leukapheresis, may be indicated in neutropenic patients with bacterial infections not responding to antibiotics. Transfused granulocytes have a very short circulatory life span, so that daily transfusions of 10¹⁰ granulocytes are usually required. Irradiation of these units decreases the incidence of graft-versus-host reactions, pulmonary endothelial damage, and other problems associated with transfusion of leukocytes (see below), but may adversely affect granulocyte function. The availability of granulocyte colony-stimulating factor (G-CSF) and granulocyte-macrophage colony-stimulating factor (GM-CSF) has greatly reduced the use of granulocyte transfusions.

Indications for Procoagulant Transfusions

Blood products can be misused in surgical settings. Use of a transfusion algorithm, particularly for components such as plasma, platelets, and cryoprecipitate, and particularly when the algorithm is guided by appropriate laboratory testing, will reduce unnecessary transfusion of these precious (but dangerous) resources (see Chapter 22). Derived from military experience, there is a trend in major trauma care towards transfusing blood products in equal ratios early in resuscitation in order to preempt or correct trauma-induced coagulopathy. This balanced approach to transfusion of blood products, 1:1:1 (one unit of FFP and one unit of platelets with each unit of PRBCs) is termed damage control resuscitation (see Chapter 39).

Complications of Blood Transfusion

IMMUNE COMPLICATIONS

Immune complications following blood transfusions are primarily due to sensitization of the recipient to donor red cells, white cells, platelets, or plasma proteins. Less commonly, the transfused cells or serum may mount an immune response against the recipient.

1. Hemolytic Reactions

Hemolytic reactions usually involve specific destruction of the transfused red cells by the recipient's antibodies. Less commonly, hemolysis of a recipient's red cells occurs as a result of transfusion of red cell antibodies. Incompatible units of platelet concentrates, FFP, clotting factor concentrates,

or cryoprecipitate may contain small amounts of plasma with anti-A or anti-B (or both) alloantibodies. Transfusions of large volumes of such units can lead to intravascular hemolysis. Hemolytic reactions are commonly classified as either acute (intravascular) or delayed (extravascular).

Acute Hemolytic Reactions

Acute intravascular hemolysis is usually due to ABO blood incompatibility, and the reported frequency is approximately 1:38,000 transfusions. The most common cause is misidentification of a patient, blood specimen, or transfusion unit. These reactions are often severe, and may occur after infusion of as little as 10–15 mL of ABO-incompatible blood. The risk of a fatal hemolytic reaction is about 1 in 100,000 transfusions. In awake patients, symptoms include chills, fever, nausea, and chest and flank pain. In anesthetized patients, an acute hemolytic **4** reaction may be manifested by a rise in temperature, unexplained tachycardia, hypotension, hemoglobinuria, and diffuse oozing in the surgical field. Disseminated intravascular coagulation, shock, and kidney failure can develop rapidly. The severity of a reaction often depends upon the volume of incompatible blood that has been administered.

Management of hemolytic reactions can be summarized as follows:

1. If a hemolytic reaction is suspected, the transfusion should be stopped immediately and the blood bank should be notified.

2. The unit should be rechecked against the blood slip and the patient's identity bracelet.

3. Blood should be drawn to identify hemoglobin in plasma, to repeat compatibility testing, and to obtain coagulation studies and a platelet count.

4. A urinary catheter should be inserted, and the urine should be checked for hemoglobin.

5. Osmotic diuresis should be initiated with mannitol and intravenous fluids.

Delayed Hemolytic Reactions

A delayed hemolytic reaction—also called extravascular hemolysis—is generally mild and is caused by antibodies to non-D antigens of the Rh system or to foreign alleles in other systems such as the Kell, Duffy, or Kidd antigens. Following an ABO and Rh D-compatible transfusion, patients have a 1–1.6% chance of forming antibodies directed against foreign antigens in these other systems. By the time significant amounts of these antibodies have formed (weeks to months), the transfused red cells have been cleared from the circulation. Moreover, the titer of these antibodies subsequently decreases and may become undetectable. Reexposure to the same foreign antigen during a subsequent red cell transfusion, however, triggers an anamnestic antibody response against the foreign antigen. The hemolytic reaction is therefore typically delayed 2–21 days after transfusion, and symptoms are generally mild, consisting of malaise, jaundice, and fever. The patient's hematocrit typically fails to rise, or rises only transiently, in spite of the transfusion and the absence of bleeding. The serum unconjugated bilirubin increases as a result of hemoglobin breakdown.

Diagnosis of delayed antibody-mediated hemolytic reactions may be facilitated by the antiglobulin (Coombs) test. The direct Coombs test detects the presence of antibodies on the membrane of red cells. In this setting, however, this test cannot distinguish between recipient antibodies coated on donor red cells and donor antibodies coated on recipient red cells. The latter requires a more detailed reexamination of pretransfusion specimens from both the patient and the donor.

The treatment of delayed hemolytic reactions is primarily supportive. The frequency of delayed hemolytic transfusion reactions is estimated to be approximately 1:12,000 transfusions. Pregnancy (exposure to fetal red cells) can also be responsible for the formation of alloantibodies to red cells.

2. Nonhemolytic Immune Reactions

Nonhemolytic immune reactions are due to sensitization of the recipient to the donor's white cells, platelets, or plasma proteins; the risk of these reactions may be minimized by the use of leukoreduced blood products.

Febrile Reactions

White cell or platelet sensitization is typically manifested as a febrile reaction. Such reactions are relatively common (1–3% of transfusion episodes) and are characterized by an increase in temperature without evidence of hemolysis. Patients with a history of repeated febrile reactions should receive leukoreduced transfusions only.

Urticarial Reactions

Urticarial reactions are usually characterized by erythema, hives, and itching without fever. They are relatively common (1% of transfusions) and are thought to be due to sensitization of the patient to transfused plasma proteins. Urticarial reactions can be treated with antihistaminic drugs (H_1 and perhaps H_2 blockers) and steroids.

Anaphylactic Reactions

Anaphylactic reactions are rare (approximately 1:150,000 transfusions). These severe reactions may occur after only a few milliliters of blood has been given, typically in IgA-deficient patients with anti-IgA antibodies who receive IgA-containing blood transfusions. The prevalence of IgA deficiency is estimated to be 1:600–800 in the general population. Such reactions require treatment with epinephrine, fluids, corticosteroids, and H_1 and H_2 blockers. Patients with IgA deficiency should receive thoroughly washed packed red cells, deglycerolized frozen red cells, or IgA-free blood units.

Transfusion-Related Acute Lung Injury

Transfusion-related acute lung injury (TRALI) presents as acute hypoxia and noncardiac pulmonary edema occurring within 6 h of blood product transfusion. It may occur as frequently as 1:5000 transfused units, and with transfusion of any blood component, but especially platelets and FFP. It is thought that transfusion of antileukocytic or anti-HLA antibodies results in damage to the alveolar–capillary membrane. Treatment is similar to that for acute respiratory distress syndrome (see Chapter 57), with the important difference that TRALI may resolve within a few days with supportive therapy.

Graft-Versus-Host Disease

This type of reaction may be seen in immunocompromised patients. Cellular blood products contain lymphocytes capable of mounting an immune response against the compromised (recipient) host. Use of special leukocyte filters alone does not reliably prevent graft-versus-host disease; irradiation (1500–3000 cGy) of red cell, granulocyte, and platelet transfusions effectively eliminates lymphocytes without altering the efficacy of such transfusions.

Post-Transfusion Purpura

Rarely, profound thrombocytopenia may occur following blood transfusions. This post-transfusion purpura results from the development of platelet alloantibodies. For unknown reasons, these antibodies also destroy the patient's own platelets. The platelet count typically drops precipitously 5–10 days following transfusion. Treatment includes intravenous IgG and plasmapheresis.

Transfusion-Related Immunomodulation

5 Allogeneic transfusion of blood products may diminish immunoresponsiveness and promote inflammation. Post-transfusion immunosuppression is clearly evident in renal transplant recipients, in whom preoperative blood transfusion improves graft survival. Recent studies suggest that perioperative transfusion may increase the risk of postoperative bacterial infection, cancer recurrence, and mortality, all of which emphasize the need to avoid unnecessary administration of blood products.

INFECTIOUS COMPLICATIONS

Viral Infections

A. Hepatitis

The incidence of post-transfusion viral hepatitis varies greatly, from approximately 1:200,000 transfusions (for hepatitis B) to approximately 1:1,900,000 (for hepatitis C). Most acute cases are anicteric. Hepatitis C is the more serious infection; most cases progress to chronic hepatitis, with cirrhosis developing in 20% of chronic carriers and hepatocellular carcinoma developing in up to 5% of chronic carriers.

B. Acquired Immunodeficiency Syndrome (AIDS)

The virus responsible AIDS, HIV-1, is transmissible by blood transfusion. HIV-2 is a similar, but less virulent virus. All blood is tested for the presence of anti-HIV-1 and anti-HIV-2 antibodies. The requirement for nucleic acid testing by the Food and Drug Administration (FDA) has decreased the risk of transfusion-transmitted HIV to approximately 1:1,900,000 transfusions.

C. Other Viral Infections

Cytomegalovirus (CMV) and Epstein–Barr virus usually cause asymptomatic or mild systemic illness. Some individuals infected with these viruses become asymptomatic infectious carriers; the white cells in blood units from such donors are capable of transmitting either virus. Immunocompromised **6** and immunosuppressed patients (eg, premature infants, organ transplant recipients, and cancer patients) are particularly susceptible to severe transfusion-related CMV infections. Ideally, such patients should receive only CMV-negative units. However, recent studies indicate that the risk of CMV transmission from transfusion of leukoreduced blood products is equivalent to CMV test-negative units. Human T-cell lymphotropic viruses 1 and 2 (HTLV-1 and HTLV-2) are leukemia and lymphoma viruses, respectively, that have been reported to be transmitted by blood transfusion; the former has also been associated with myelopathy. Parvovirus transmission has been reported following transfusion of coagulation factor concentrates and can result in transient aplastic crises in immunocompromised hosts. West Nile virus infection may result in encephalitis with a fatality rate of up to 10%, and transmission of this virus by transfusion has been reported.

Parasitic Infections

Parasitic diseases that can be transmitted by transfusion include malaria, toxoplasmosis, and Chagas' disease. Such cases are very rare.

Bacterial Infections

Bacterial contamination of blood products is the second leading cause of transfusion-associated mortality. The prevalence of positive bacterial cultures in blood products ranges from 1:2000 for platelets to 1:7000 for PRBCs and may be due to transient donor bacteremia or inadequate antisepsis during phlebotomy. The prevalence of sepsis due to blood transfusion ranges from 1:25,000 for platelets to 1:250,000 for PRBCs. Both gram-positive (*Staphylococcus*) and gram-negative (*Yersinia* and *Citrobacter*) bacteria can contaminate blood transfusions and transmit disease. To avoid the possibility of significant bacterial contamination, blood products should be administered over a period shorter than 4 h. Specific bacterial diseases rarely transmitted by blood transfusions from donors include syphilis, brucellosis, salmonellosis, yersiniosis, and various rickettsioses.

MASSIVE BLOOD TRANSFUSION

Massive transfusion is most often defined as the need to transfuse one to two times the patient's blood volume. For most adult patients, that is the equivalent of 10–20 units. The approach to massive transfusion (and to lesser degrees of transfusion) after trauma injury has been greatly influenced by military experience in recent Middle Eastern and Central Asian wars in which outcomes have improved with concurrent transfusion of packed red cells, plasma, and platelets to avoid dilutional coagulopathy (see Chapter 39).

Coagulopathy

7 The most common cause of nonsurgical bleeding following massive blood transfusion is dilutional thrombocytopenia, although clinically significant dilution of coagulation factors may also occur. **Coagulation studies and platelet counts, if readily available, should guide platelet and FFP transfusion.** Although most clinicians will be familiar with "routine" coagulation tests (eg, prothrombin time [PT], activated partial thromboplastin time [aPTT], international normalized ratio [INR], platelet count, fibrinogen), multiple studies show that viscoelastic analysis of whole blood clotting (thromboelastography, rotation thromboelastometry, and Sonoclot analysis) may be more useful in resuscitation, liver transplantation, and cardiac surgical settings.

Citrate Toxicity

Calcium binding by the citrate preservative can rise in importance following transfusion of large volumes of blood or blood products. Clinically
8 important hypocalcemia, causing cardiac

depression, will not occur in most normal patients unless the transfusion rate exceeds 1 unit every 5 min, and intravenous calcium salts should rarely be required in the absence of measured hypocalcemia. Because citrate metabolism is primarily hepatic, patients with hepatic disease or dysfunction (and possibly hypothermic patients) may demonstrate hypocalcemia and require calcium infusion during massive transfusion, as may small children and others with relatively impaired parathyroid–vitamin D function.

Hypothermia

Massive blood transfusion is an absolute indication for warming all blood products and intravenous fluids to normal body temperature. Ventricular arrhythmias progressing to fibrillation often occur at temperatures close to 30°C, and hypothermia can hamper cardiac resuscitation. The use of rapid infusion devices with efficient heat transfer capability has decreased the incidence of transfusion-related hypothermia.

Acid–Base Balance

Although stored blood is acidic due to the citric acid anticoagulant and accumulation of red cell metabolites (carbon dioxide and lactic acid), metabolic acidosis due to transfusion is uncommon because
9 citric acid and lactic acid are rapidly metabolized to bicarbonate by the normal liver. In the situation of massive blood transfusion, acid-base status is largely dependent upon tissue perfusion, rate of blood transfusion, and citrate metabolism. Once normal tissue perfusion is restored, any metabolic acidosis typically resolves, and metabolic alkalosis commonly occurs as citrate and lactate contained in transfusions and resuscitation fluids are converted to bicarbonate by the liver.

Serum Potassium Concentration

The extracellular concentration of potassium in stored blood steadily increases with time. The amount of extracellular potassium transfused with each unit is typically less than 4 mEq per unit. Hyperkalemia can develop regardless of the age of the blood when transfusion rates exceed 100 mL/min. The treatment of hyperkalemia is discussed in

Chapter 49. Hypokalemia is commonly encountered postoperatively, particularly in association with metabolic alkalosis (see Chapters 49 and 50).

Alternative Strategies for Management of Blood Loss During Surgery

AUTOLOGOUS TRANSFUSION

Patients undergoing elective surgical procedures with a high probability for transfusion can donate their own blood for use during that surgery. Collection is usually started 4–5 weeks prior to the procedure. The patient is allowed to donate a unit as long as the hematocrit is at least 34% or hemoglobin at least 11 g/dL. A minimum of 72 h is required between donations to make certain that plasma volume returns to normal. With iron supplementation and erythropoietin therapy, at least 3 or 4 units can usually be collected prior to operation. Some studies suggest that autologous blood transfusions do not adversely affect survival in patients undergoing operations for cancer. Although autologous transfusions likely reduce the risk of infection and transfusion reactions, they are not risk-free. Risks include those of immunological reactions due to clerical errors in collection, labeling, and administration; bacterial contamination; and improper storage. Allergic reactions can occur due to allergens (eg, ethylene oxide) that dissolve into the blood from collection and storage equipment.

BLOOD SALVAGE & REINFUSION

This technique is used widely during cardiac, major vascular, and orthopedic surgery (see Chapter 22). The shed blood is aspirated intraoperatively into a reservoir and mixed with heparin. After a sufficient amount of blood is collected, the red cells are concentrated and washed to remove debris and anticoagulant and then reinfused into the patient. The concentrates obtained usually have hematocrits of 50–60%. To be used effectively, this technique requires blood losses greater than 1000–1500 mL.

Contraindications to blood salvage and reinfusion include septic contamination of the wound and perhaps malignancy. Newer, simpler systems allow reinfusion of shed blood without centrifugation.

NORMOVOLEMIC HEMODILUTION

Acute normovolemic hemodilution relies on the premise that if the concentration of red cells is decreased, total red cell loss is reduced when large amounts of blood are shed; moreover, cardiac output remains normal because intravascular volume is maintained. One or two units of blood are typically removed just prior to surgery from a large-bore intravenous catheter and replaced with crystalloid and colloids so that the patient remains normovolemic but has a hematocrit of 21–25%. The blood that is removed is stored in a CPD bag at room temperature (up to 6 h) to preserve platelet function; the blood is given back to the patient after the blood loss or sooner if necessary.

DONOR-DIRECTED TRANSFUSIONS

Patients can request donated blood from family members or friends known to be ABO compatible. Most blood banks discourage this practice and generally require donation at least 7 days prior to surgery in order to process the donated blood and confirm compatibility. Studies comparing the safety of donor-directed units to that of random donor units have found either no difference, or that random units from blood banks are safer than directed units.

CASE DISCUSSION

A Patient with Sickle Cell Disease

A 24-year-old black woman with a history of sickle cell anemia presents with abdominal pain and is scheduled for cholecystectomy.

What is sickle cell anemia?

Sickle cell anemia is a hereditary hemolytic anemia resulting from the formation of an abnormal hemoglobin (HbS). HbS differs structurally from the normal adult hemoglobin (HbA) only in the substitution of valine for glutamic acid at the sixth position of the β chain. Functionally, sickle hemoglobin has less affinity for oxygen ($P_{50} = 31$ mm Hg) as well as decreased solubility. Upon deoxygenation, HbS readily polymerizes and precipitates inside red blood cells (RBCs), causing them to sickle. Sickle cell patients produce variable amounts (2–20%) of fetal hemoglobin (HbF). It is likely that cells with large amounts of HbF are somewhat protected from sickling. The continuous destruction of irreversibly sickled cells leads to anemia, and hematocrits are typically 18–30% due to the extravascular hemolysis. RBC survival is reduced to 10–15 days, compared with up to 120 days in normal individuals.

What is the difference between sickle cell anemia and sickle cell trait?

When the genetic defect for adult hemoglobin is present on both the maternally and paternally derived chromosomes (No. 11), the patient is homozygous for HbS and has sickle cell anemia (HbSS). When only one chromosome has the sickle gene, the patient is heterozygous and has *sickle cell trait* (HbAS). Patients with the sickle trait produce variable amounts of HbA (55–60%) and HbS (35–40%). Unlike those with HbSS, they are generally not anemic, are asymptomatic, and have a normal life span. Sickling occurs only under extreme hypoxemia or in low-flow states. Sickling is particularly apt to occur in the renal medulla; indeed, many patients with the sickle trait have impaired renal concentrating ability. Some patients with HbAS have been reported to have renal medullary, splenic, and pulmonary infarcts.

What is the prevalence of the sickle cell gene in black Americans?

Sickle cell anemia is primarily a disease of individuals of Central African ancestry. Approximately 0.2–0.5% of African Americans are homozygous for the sickle gene and approximately 8–10% are heterozygous. Sickle cell anemia is found less commonly in patients of Mediterranean ancestry.

What is the pathophysiology?

Conditions favoring the formation of deoxyhemoglobin (eg, hypoxemia, acidosis, intracellular hypertonicity or dehydration, increased 2,3-DPG levels, or increased temperature) can precipitate sickling in patients with HbSS. Hypothermia may also be detrimental because of the associated vasoconstriction (see below). Intracellular polymerization of HbS distorts red cells, makes them less pliable and more "sticky," increasing blood viscosity. Sickling may initially be reversible but eventually becomes irreversible in some cells. Formation of red cell aggregates in capillaries can obstruct tissue microcirculation. A vicious cycle is established in which circulatory stasis leads to localized hypoxia, which, in turn, causes more sickling.

With what symptoms do patients with sickle cell anemia usually present?

Patients with HbSS generally first develop symptoms in infancy, when levels of fetal hemoglobin (HbF) decline. The disease is characterized by both acute episodic crises and chronic and progressive features (Table 51–7). Children display retarded growth and have recurrent infections. Recurrent splenic infarction leads to splenic atrophy and functional asplenism by adolescence. Patients usually die from recurrent infections or kidney failure. Crises are often precipitated by infection, cold weather, dehydration, or other forms of stress. Crises may be divided into three types:

1. **Vasoocclusive crises:** Depending on the vessels involved, these acute episodes can result in micro- or macroinfarctions. Most painful crises are thought to be due to microinfarcts in the various tissues. Clinically, they present as acute abdominal, chest, back, or joint pain. Differentiation between surgical and nonsurgical causes of abdominal pain is difficult. Most patients form pigmented gallstones by adulthood, and many present with acute cholecystitis. Vasoocclusive phenomena in larger vessels can produce thromboses resulting in splenic, cerebral, pulmonary, hepatic, renal, and, less commonly, myocardial infarctions.

TABLE 51–7 **Manifestations of sickle cell anemia.**

Neurological
Stroke
Subarachnoid hemorrhage
Coma
Seizures

Ocular
Vitreous hemorrhage
Retinal infarcts
Proliferative retinopathy
Retinal detachment

Pulmonary
Increased intrapulmonary shunting
Pleuritis
Recurrent pulmonary infections
Pulmonary infarcts

Cardiovascular
Congestive heart failure
Cor pulmonale
Pericarditis
Myocardial infarction

Gastrointestinal
Cholelithiasis (pigmented stones)
Cholecystitis
Hepatic infarcts
Hepatic abscesses
Hepatic fibrosis

Hematological
Anemia
Aplastic anemia
Recurrent infections
Splenic infarcts
Splenic sequestration
Functional asplenia

Genitourinary
Hematuria
Renal papillary necrosis
Impaired renal concentrating ability (isosthenuria)
Nephrotic syndrome
Renal insufficiency
Renal failure
Priapism

Skeletal
Synovitis
Arthritis
Aseptic necrosis of femoral head
Small bone infarcts in hand and feet (dactylitis)
Biconcave ("fishmouth") vertebrae
Osteomyelitis

Skin
Chronic ulcers

2. **Aplastic crisis:** Profound anemia (Hb 2–3 g/dL) can rapidly occur when red cell production in the bone marrow is exhausted or suppressed. Infections and folate deficiency may play a major role. Some patients also develop leukopenia.

3. **Splenic sequestration crisis:** Sudden pooling of blood in the spleen can occur in infants and young children and can cause life-threatening hypotension. The mechanism is thought to be partial or complete occlusion of venous drainage from the spleen.

How is sickle cell anemia diagnosed?

RBCs from patients with sickle cell anemia readily sickle following addition of an oxygen-consuming reagent (metabisulfite) or a hypertonic ionic solution (solubility test). Confirmation requires hemoglobin electrophoresis.

What would be the best way to prepare patients with sickle cell anemia for surgery?

Optimal preoperative preparation is desirable for all patients undergoing surgery. Patients should be well hydrated, infections should be controlled, and the hemoglobin concentration should be at an acceptable level. Preoperative transfusion therapy must be individualized for the patient and to the surgical procedure. Partial exchange transfusions before major surgical procedures are usually advocated, which decrease blood viscosity, increase blood oxygen-carrying capacity, and decrease likelihood of sickling. The goal of such transfusions is generally to achieve a hematocrit of 35–40% with 40–50% normal hemoglobin (HbA).

Are there any special intraoperative considerations?

Conditions that might promote hemoglobin desaturation or low-flow states should be avoided. Every effort must be made to avoid hypothermia, hyperthermia, acidosis, and even mild degrees of hypoxemia, hypotension, or hypovolemia. Generous hydration and a relatively high (>50%) inspired oxygen tension are desirable. The principal compensatory mechanism for impaired tissue oxygen delivery in these patients is increased cardiac output, which should be maintained intra-operatively. Goal-directed hemodynamic monitoring and fluid therapy utilizing arterial pulse wave analysis, esophageal Doppler, or transesophageal echocardiography, or central venous pressure or pulmonary artery pressure monitoring with mixed venous oxygen saturation is often useful. Mild alkalosis may help avoid sickling, but even moderate degrees of respiratory alkalosis may have an adverse effect on cerebral blood flow. Many clinicians also avoid the use of tourniquets.

Are there any special postoperative considerations?

Most perioperative deaths occur in the postoperative period, and the same management principles applied intraoperatively should be utilized in the postoperative period. Hypoxemia and pulmonary complications are major risk factors. Supplemental oxygen, optimal hemodynamic, fluid, and pain and symptom management, and pulmonary physiotherapy and early ambulation all help minimize the risk of these complications.

What is the significance of sickle cell anemia and thalassemia in the same patient?

The combination of HbS and thalassemia, most commonly sickle β-thalassemia, has a variable and unpredictable effect on disease severity. This combination is usually milder in black patients than in those of Mediterranean ancestry.

What is the pathophysiology of thalassemia?

Thalassemia is a hereditary defect in the production of one or more of the normal subunits of hemoglobin. Patients with thalassemia may be able to produce normal HbA but have reduced amounts of α- or β-chain production; the severity of this defect depends on the subunit affected and the degree to which hemoglobin production is affected. Symptoms range from absent to severe. Patients with α-thalassemia produce reduced amounts of α subunit, whereas patients with β-thalassemia produce reduced amounts of the β subunit. The formation of hemoglobins with abnormal subunit composition can alter the red cell membrane and lead to variable degrees of hemolysis as well

as ineffective hematopoiesis. The latter can result in hypertrophy of the bone marrow and often an abnormal skeleton. *Maxillary hypertrophy* may make tracheal intubation difficult. Thalassemias are most common in patients of Southeast Asian, African, Mediterranean, and Indian ancestry.

What is hemoglobin C disease?

Substitution of lysine for glutamic acid at position 6 on the β subunit results in hemoglobin C (HbC). Approximately 0.05% of black Americans carry the gene for HbC. Patients homozygous for HbC generally have only a mild hemolytic anemia and splenomegaly and rarely develop significant complications. The tendency for HbC to crystallize in hypertonic environments is probably responsible for the hemolysis and characteristically produces *target cells* on the peripheral blood smear.

What is the significance of the genotype HbSC?

Nearly 0.1% of black Americans are simultaneously heterozygous for both HbS and HbC (HbSC). These patients generally have a mild to moderate hemolytic anemia. Some patients occasionally have painful crises, splenic infarcts, and hepatic dysfunction. Eye manifestations similar to those associated with HbSS disease are particularly prominent. Females with HbSC have a high rate of complications during the third trimester of pregnancy and delivery.

What is hemoglobin E?

Hemoglobin E is the result of a single substitution on the β chain and is the second most common hemoglobin variant worldwide. It is most often encountered in patients from Southeast Asia. Although oxygen-binding affinity is normal, the substitution impairs production of β chains (similar to β-thalassemia). Homozygous patients have marked microcytosis and prominent target cells, but are not usually anemic and lack any other manifestations.

What is the hematologic significance of glucose-6-phosphate dehydrogenase deficiency?

RBCs are normally well-protected against oxidizing agents. The sulfhydryl groups on

TABLE 51–8 Drugs to avoid in patients with G6PD[1] deficiency.

Drugs that may cause hemolysis
Sulfonamides
Antimalarial drugs
Nitrofurantoin
Nalidixic acid
Probenecid
Aminosalicylic acid
Phenacetin
Acetanilid
Ascorbic acid (in large doses)
Vitamin K
Methylene blue
Quinine[2]
Quinidine[3]
Chloramphenicol
Penicillamine
Dimercaprol
Other drugs
Prilocaine
Nitroprusside

[1]G6PD, glucose-6-phosphate dehydrogenase.
[2]May be safe in patients with A⁻ variant.
[3]Should be avoided because of potential to cause methemoglobinemia.

hemoglobin are protected by reduced glutathione. The latter is regenerated by NADPH (reduced nicotinamide adenine dinucleotide phosphate), which itself is regenerated by glucose metabolism in the hexose monophosphate shunt. Glucose-6-phosphate dehydrogenase (G6PD) is a critical enzyme in this pathway. A defect in this pathway results in an inadequate amount of reduced glutathione, which can potentially result in the oxidation and precipitation of hemoglobin in red cells (seen as *Heinz bodies*) and hemolysis.

Abnormalities in G6PD are relatively common, with over 400 variants described. Clinical manifestations are quite variable, depending on the functional significance of the enzyme abnormality. Up to 15% of black American males have the common, clinically significant, A⁻ variant. A second variant is common in individuals of eastern Mediterranean ancestry, and a third in individuals of Chinese ancestry. Because the locus for the enzyme is on the X chromosome, abnormalities are X-linked traits, with males being primarily affected. G6PD

activity decreases as RBCs age; therefore aging red cells are most susceptible to oxidation. This decay is markedly accelerated in patients with the Mediterranean variant but only moderately so in patients with the A⁻ variant.

Most patients with G6PD deficiency are not anemic but can develop hemolysis following stresses such as viral and bacterial infections, or after administration of certain drugs (Table 51–8). Hemolytic episodes can be precipitated by metabolic acidosis (eg, diabetic ketoacidosis) and may present with hemoglobinuria and hypotension. Such episodes are generally self-limited because only the older population of RBCs is destroyed. Mediterranean variants may be associated with chronic hemolytic anemia of varying severity and may include the classic feature of marked sensitivity to fava beans.

Management of G6PD deficiency is primarily preventive, avoiding factors known to promote or exacerbate hemolysis. Measures aimed at preserving kidney function (see above) are indicated in patients who develop hemoglobinuria.

SUGGESTED READING

Alderson P, Bunn F, Li Wan Po A, et al: Human albumin solution for resuscitation and volume expansion in critically ill patients. Cochrane Database Syst Rev 2011;(10):CD001208. Update in: Cochrane Database Syst Rev 2011;(11):CD001208.

Bolt J, Ince C: The impact of fluid therapy on microcirculation and tissue oxygenation in hypovolemic patients. A review. Intensive Care Med 2010;36:1299.

Brienza N, Giglio MT, Marucci M, et al: Does perioperative hemodynamic optimization protect renal function in surgical patients? A meta-analytic study. Crit Care Med 2009;37:2079.

Canet J, Belda FJ: Perioperative hyperoxia. The debate is only getting started. Anesthesiology 2011;114:1271.

Carson JL, Carless PA, Hebert PC: Transfusion thresholds and other strategies for guiding allogeneic red blood cell transfusion. Cochrane Database Syst Rev 2012;4:CD002042.

Carson JL, Grossman BJ, Kleinman S, et al: For the Clinical Transfusion Medicine Committee of the AABB: Red blood cell transfusion: A clinical practice guideline from the AABB. Ann Intern Med 2012;157:49.

Chowdhury AB, Lobo DN: Fluids and gastrointestinal function. Curr Opin Clin Nutrition Metabolic Care 2011;14:469.

Conte B, L'Hermite J, Ripart J, et al: Perioperative optimization of oxygen delivery. Transfusion Alternatives Transfusion Med 2010;11:22.

Coriat P: Editorial: Should we be more balanced, more 'starched' and more optimized? Transfusion Alternatives in Transfusion Medicine 2010;11:1.

Dalfino L, Giglio MT, Puntillo F, et al: Haemodynamic goal-directed therapy and postoperative infections: Earlier is better. A systematic review and meta-analysis. Crit Care 2011;15:R154.

Giglio MT, Marucci M, Testini M, et al: Goal-directed haemodynamic therapy and gastrointestinal complications in major surgery: A meta-analysis of randomized controlled trials. Br J Anaesth 2009;103:637.

Glance LG, Dick AW, Mukamel DB, et al: Association between intraoperative blood transfusion and mortality and morbidity in patients undergoing noncardiac surgery. Anesthesiology 2011;114:283.

Gurgel ST, do Nascimento Jr P: Maintaining tissue perfusion in high-risk surgical patients: A systematic review of randomized clinical trials. Anesth Analg 2011;112:1384.

Hartog CS, Bauer M, Reinhart K: The efficacy and safety of colloid resuscitation in the critically ill. Anesth Analg 2011;112:156.

Hiltebrand LB, Kimberger O, Arnberger M, et al: Crystalloids versus colloids for goal-directed fluid therapy in major surgery. Crit Care 2009;13:R40.

Inghilleri G: Prediction of transfusion requirements in surgical patients: A review. Transfusion Alternatives Transfusion Med 2009;11:10.

Mayer J, Boldt J, Mengistu AM, et al: Goal-directed intraoperative therapy based on autocalibrated arterial pressure waveform analysis reduces hospital stay in high-risk surgical patients: A randomized, controlled trial. Crit Care 2010;14:R18.

Muller L, Lefrant J-Y: Metabolic effects of plasma expanders. Transfusion Alternatives Transfusion Med 2010;11:10.

Perel P, Roberts I: Colloids versus crystalloids for fluid resuscitation in critically ill patients. Cochrane Database Syst Rev 2011;(3):CD000567.

Reinhart K, Takala J: Hydroxyethyl starches: what do we still know? Anesth Anal 2011;112:507.

Roche AM, Miller TE, Gan TJ: Goal-directed fluid management with trans-oesophageal Doppler. Best Pract Res Clinical Anaesthesiol 2009;23:327.

Senagore AJ, Emery T, Luchtefeld M, et al: Fluid management for laparoscopic colectomy: A prospective, randomized assessment of goal-directed administration of balanced salt solution or hetastarch coupled with an enhanced recovery program. Dis Colon Rectum 2009;52:1935.

Society of Thoracic Surgeons Blood Conservation Guideline Task Force, Ferraris VA, Brown JR, et al: 2011 update to the Society of Thoracic Surgeons and the Society of Cardiovascular Anesthesiologists blood conservation clinical practice guidelines. Ann Thorac Surg 2011;91:944.

Srinivasa S, Taylor MHG, Sammour T, et al: Oesophageal Doppler-guided fluid administration in colorectal surgery: Critical appraisal of published clinical trials. Acta Anaesthesiol Scand 2011;55:4.

Svensen C: Intraoperative fluid losses revisited. Transfusion Alternatives Transfusion Med 2010;11:85.

Tavernier B, Faivre S, Bourdon C: Hyperchloremic acidosis during plasma expansion. Transfusion Alternatives Transfusion Med 2010;11:3.

Vogt KN, Van Koughnett JA, Dubois L, et al: The use of trauma transfusion pathways for blood component transfusion in the civilian population: A systematic review and meta-analysis(*). Transfus Med 2012;22:156.

Thermoregulation, Hypothermia, & Malignant Hyperthermia

1 When there is no attempt to actively warm an anesthetized patient, core temperature usually decreases 1–2°C during the first hour of general anesthesia (phase one), followed by a more gradual decline during the ensuing 3–4 h (phase two), eventually reaching a point of steady state.

2 In the normal, unanesthetized patient the hypothalamus maintains core body temperature within very narrow tolerances, termed the interthreshold range, with the threshold for sweating and vasodilation at one extreme and the threshold for vasoconstriction and shivering at the other.

3 Anesthetics inhibit central thermoregulation by interfering with these hypothalamic reflex responses.

4 Postoperative hypothermia should be treated with a forced-air warming device, if available; alternately (but less satisfactorily) warming lights or heating blankets can be used to restore body temperature to normal.

5 Nearly 50% of patients who experience an episode of malignant hyperthermia (MH) have had at least one previous uneventful exposure to anesthesia during which they received a recognized triggering agent. Why MH fails to occur after every exposure to a triggering agent is unclear.

6 The earliest signs of an MH episode during anesthesia are succinylcholine-induced masseter muscle rigidity (MMR) or other muscle rigidity, tachycardia, and hypercarbia (due to increased CO_2 production).

7 Musculoskeletal diseases associated with a relatively high incidence of MH include central-core disease, multi-minicore myopathy, and King–Denborough syndrome. Duchenne's and other muscular dystrophies, nonspecific myopathies, and osteogenesis imperfecta have been associated with MH-like symptoms in some reports; however, their association with MH is controversial.

8 Treatment of an MH episode is directed at terminating the episode and treating complications such as hyperthermia and acidosis. The mortality rate for MH, even with prompt treatment, ranges from 5% to 30%. First and most importantly, the triggering agent must be stopped; second, dantrolene must be given immediately.

9 Dantrolene, a hydantoin derivative, directly interferes with muscle contraction by inhibiting calcium ion release from the sarcoplasmic reticulum. The dose is 2.5 mg/kg intravenously every 5 min until the episode is terminated (upper limit, 10 mg/kg). Dantrolene should be continued for 24 h after initial treatment.

10 Propofol, thiopental, etomidate, benzodiazepines, ketamine, opiates, droperidol, nitrous oxide, nondepolarizing muscle relaxants, and all local anesthetics are nontriggering agents that are safe for use in MH-susceptible patients.

THERMOREGULATION & HYPOTHERMIA

Hypothermia, usually defined as a body temperature less than 36°C, occurs frequently during anesthesia and surgery. Unintentional perioperative hypothermia is more common in patients at the extremes of age, and in those undergoing abdominal surgery or procedures of long duration, especially with cold ambient operating room temperatures; it will occur in nearly every such patient unless steps are taken to prevent this complication.

Hypothermia reduces metabolic oxygen requirements and can be protective during cerebral or cardiac ischemia. **Nevertheless, hypothermia has multiple deleterious physiological effects** (Table 52–1). In fact, unintended perioperative hypothermia has been associated with an increased mortality rate.

Core temperature is normally the same as the central venous blood temperature (except during periods of relatively rapid temperature change as can occur during extracorporeal perfusion). When there is no attempt to actively warm an anesthetized patient, core temperature usually decreases 1–2°C during the first hour of general anesthesia (phase one), followed by a more gradual decline during the ensuing 3–4 h (phase two), eventually reaching a point of steady state (phase three). With general, epidural, or spinal anesthesia redistribution of heat from warm "central" compartments (eg, abdomen, thorax) to cooler peripheral tissues (eg, arms, legs) from anesthetic-induced vasodilation explains most of the initial decrease in temperature

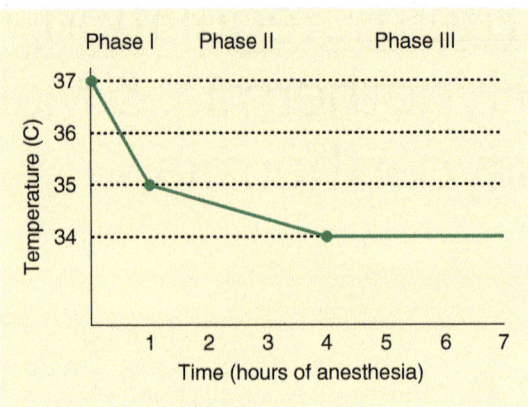

FIGURE 52–1 Unintentional hypothermia during general anesthesia follows a typical pattern: a steep drop in core temperature during the first hour (phase one, redistribution), followed by a gradual decline during the next 3–4 h (phase two, heat loss), eventually reaching a steady state (phase three, equilibrium).

during phase one, with actual heat loss from the patient to the environment being a minor contributor. Continuous heat loss to the environment appears to be primarily responsible for the slower subsequent decline during phase two. At steady state, heat loss equals metabolic heat production (Figure 52–1).

In the normal unanesthetized patient the hypothalamus maintains core body temperature within very narrow tolerances, termed the *interthreshold range,* with the threshold for sweating and vasodilation at one extreme and the threshold for vasoconstriction and shivering at the other. Increasing core temperature a fraction of a degree induces sweating and vasodilation, whereas a minimally reduced core temperature triggers vasoconstriction and shivering. Anesthetic agents inhibit central thermoregulation by interfering with these hypothalamic reflex responses. For example, isoflurane produces a dose-dependent decrease in the threshold temperature that triggers vasoconstriction (3°C decrease for each percent of inhaled isoflurane). Both general and regional anesthetics increase the interthreshold range, albeit by different mechanisms. Spinal and epidural anesthetics, like general anesthetics, lead to hypothermia by causing vasodilation and internal redistribution of heat. The accompanying thermoregulatory

TABLE 52–1 Deleterious effects of hypothermia.

Cardiac arrhythmias and ischemia
Increased peripheral vascular resistance
"Left shift" of the hemoglobin–oxygen saturation curve
Reversible coagulopathy (platelet dysfunction)
Increased postoperative protein catabolism and stress response
Altered mental status
Impaired renal function
Delayed drug metabolism
Impaired wound healing
Increased risk of infection

impairment from regional anesthetics that allows continued heat loss is likely due to altered perception by the hypothalamus of temperature in the anesthetized dermatomes rather than a central drug effect, as with general anesthetics.

Intraoperative Considerations

A cold ambient temperature in the operating room, prolonged exposure of a large wound, and the use of large amounts of room-temperature intravenous fluids or high flows of unhumidified gases can contribute to hypothermia. **Prewarming the patient for half an hour with convective forced-air warming blankets prevents phase one hypothermia by eliminating the central–peripheral temperature gradient.** Methods to minimize phase two hypothermia from heat loss during anesthesia include use of forced-air warming blankets and warm-water blankets, heated humidification of inspired gases, warming of intravenous fluids, and increasing ambient operating room temperature. Passive insulators such as heated cotton blankets or so-called space blankets have limited utility unless virtually the entire body is covered.

Postoperative Considerations

Shivering can occur in postanesthesia care units (PACUs) or critical care units as a result of actual hypothermia or neurological aftereffects of general anesthetic agents. Shivering is also common immediately postpartum. Shivering in such instances represents the body's effort to increase heat production and raise body temperature and may be associated with intense vasoconstriction. Emergence from even brief general anesthesia is sometimes also associated with shivering. Although the shivering can be part of nonspecific neurological signs (posturing, clonus, or the Babinski sign) that are sometimes observed during emergence, shivering is most often associated with hypothermia and volatile anesthetics. Regardless of the mechanism, shivering appears to be more common after longer durations of surgery and the use of greater concentrations of a volatile agent. Occasionally it is intense enough to cause hyperthermia (38–39°C) and metabolic acidosis, both of which promptly resolve when the shivering stops. Both spinal and epidural anesthesia lower the shivering threshold and vasoconstrictive response to hypothermia; shivering may also be encountered in the PACU following regional anesthesia. Other causes of shivering should be excluded, such as sepsis, drug allergy, or a transfusion reaction. Intense shivering may increase oxygen consumption, CO_2 production, and cardiac output. These physiological effects are often poorly tolerated by patients with preexisting cardiac or pulmonary impairment.

Postoperative shivering may increase oxygen consumption as much as fivefold, may decrease arterial oxygen saturation, and may be associated with an increased risk of myocardial ischemia. Although postoperative shivering can be effectively treated with small intravenous doses of meperidine (12.5–25 mg) in adults, the better option is to reduce the likelihood of shivering by maintaining normothermia. Shivering in intubated and mechanically ventilated patients can also be controlled with sedation and a muscle relaxant until normothermia is reestablished and the effects of anesthesia have dissipated.

4 Postoperative hypothermia should be treated with a forced-air warming device, if available; alternately (but less satisfactorily) warming lights or heating blankets can be used to restore body temperature to normal. Hypothermia has been associated with an increased incidence of myocardial ischemia, arrhythmias, increased transfusion requirements, and increased duration of muscle relaxant effects, the latter of which can be especially harmful in the recently extubated patient.

MALIGNANT HYPERTHERMIA

Malignant hyperthermia (MH) is a rare (1:15,000 in pediatric patients and 1:40,000 adult patients) genetic hypermetabolic muscle disease, the characteristic phenotypical signs and symptoms of which most commonly appear with exposure to inhaled general anesthetics or succinylcholine (triggering agents). MH may occasionally present more than an hour after emergence from an anesthetic, and rarely may occur without exposure to known triggering agents. Most cases have been reported in young males; almost none have been reported in infants, and few have been reported in the elderly.

Nevertheless, all ages and both sexes may be affected. The incidence of MH varies greatly from country to country and even among different geographic localities within the same country, reflecting varying gene pools. The upper Midwest appears to have the greatest incidence of MH in the United States.

Pathophysiology

A halogenated anesthetic agent alone may trigger an episode of MH (Table 52–2). In many of the early reported cases, both succinylcholine and a halogenated anesthetic agent were used. However, succinylcholine is less frequently used in modern practice, and about half of the cases in the past decade were associated with volatile anesthetics as the only triggering agents. Nearly 50% of patients who experience an episode of MH have had at least one previous uneventful exposure to anesthesia during which they received a recognized triggering agent. Why MH fails to occur after every exposure to a triggering agent is unclear. Investigations into the biochemical causes of MH reveal an uncontrolled increase in intracellular calcium in skeletal muscle. The sudden release of calcium from sarcoplasmic reticulum removes the inhibition of troponin, resulting in sustained muscle contraction. Markedly increased adenosine triphosphatase activity results in an uncontrolled increase in aerobic and anaerobic metabolism. The hypermetabolic state markedly increases oxygen consumption and CO_2 production, producing severe lactic acidosis and hyperthermia.

One early focus of investigations into the mechanisms of MH has been the gene for the ryanodine (Ryr_1) receptor, located on chromosome 19. Ryr_1 is an ion channel responsible for calcium release from the sarcoplasmic reticulum and it plays an important role in muscle depolarization. Subsequent reports linked MH with mutations involving the sodium channel on chromosome 17. An autosomal recessive form of MH has been associated with the King–Denborough syndrome. Most patients with an episode of MH have a history of relatives with a similar episode or with an abnormal halothane–caffeine contracture test (see below). The complexity of genetic inheritance patterns in families reflects the fact that MH can be caused by mutations of one or more genes on more than one chromosome. To date genetic studies in humans have revealed at least five different chromosomes and more than 180 individual mutations associated with MH. Genetic testing, although available, currently screens for less than 20% of recognized mutations. A patient with a *bona fide* clinical history of MH has about a 30–50% chance of testing positive.

Clinical Manifestations

The earliest signs of MH during anesthesia are succinylcholine-induced masseter muscle rigidity (MMR) or other muscle rigidity, tachycardia, and hypercarbia (due to increased CO_2 production) (Table 52–3). Two or more of these signs greatly increase the likelihood of MH. Tachypnea is prominent when muscle relaxants are not used. Overactivity of the sympathetic nervous system produces tachycardia, arrhythmias, hypertension, and mottled cyanosis. Hyperthermia may be a late sign, but when it occurs, core temperature can rise as much as 1°C every 5 min. Generalized muscle rigidity is not consistently present. Hypertension may be rapidly followed by hypotension if cardiac depression occurs. Dark-colored urine reflects myoglobinemia and myoglobinuria.

Laboratory testing typically reveals mixed metabolic and respiratory acidosis with a marked base deficit, hyperkalemia, hypermagnesemia, and reduced mixed-venous oxygen saturation. Some case reports describe isolated respiratory acidosis early in the course of an episode of MH. Serum ionized calcium concentration is variable: it may initially increase before a later decrease. Patients typically have increased serum myoglobin, creatine

TABLE 52–2 Drugs known to trigger malignant hyperthermia.

Inhaled general anesthetics
Ether
Halothane
Methoxyflurane
Enflurane
Isoflurane
Desflurane
Sevoflurane
Depolarizing muscle relaxant
Succinylcholine

TABLE 52–3 Signs of malignant hyperthermia.

Markedly increased metabolism
Increased CO_2 production
Increased oxygen consumption
Reduced mixed venous oxygen tension
Metabolic acidosis
Cyanosis
Mottling

Increased sympathetic activity
Tachycardia
Hypertension
Arrhythmias

Muscle damage
Masseter spasm
Generalized rigidity
Increased serum creatine kinase
Hyperkalemia
Hypernatremia
Hyperphosphatemia
Myoglobinemia
Myoglobinuria

Hyperthermia
Fever
Sweating

kinase (CK), lactic dehydrogenase, and aldolase levels. When peak serum CK levels (usually 12–18 h after anesthesia) exceed 20,000 IU/L the diagnosis is strongly suspected. It should be noted that succinylcholine administration to some normal patients without MH may cause serum myoglobin and CK levels to increase markedly.

Much of the problem in diagnosing MH arises from its variable presentation. Fever is an inconsistent and often late-presenting sign. An unanticipated doubling or tripling of end-tidal CO_2 (in the absence of a ventilatory change) is one of the earliest and most sensitive indicators of MH. If the patient survives the first few minutes, acute kidney failure and disseminated intravascular coagulation (DIC) can rapidly ensue. Other complications of MH include cerebral edema with seizures and hepatic failure. Most MH deaths are due to DIC and organ failure due to delayed or no treatment with dantrolene.

7 Susceptibility to MH is increased in several musculoskeletal diseases. These include central-core disease, multi-minicore myopathy, and King–Denborough syndrome. The latter syndrome is seen primarily in young boys who exhibit short stature, mental retardation, cryptorchidism, kyphoscoliosis, pectus deformity, slanted eyes, low-set ears, webbed neck, and winged scapulae. Duchenne's and other muscular dystrophies, nonspecific myopathies, heat stroke, and osteogenesis imperfecta have been associated with MH-like symptoms in some reports; however, their association with MH is controversial. Other possible clues to susceptibility include a family history of anesthetic complications, or a history of unexplained fevers or muscular cramps. There are several reports of MH episodes occurring in patients with a history of exercise-induced rhabdomyolysis. Prior uneventful anesthesia procedures and absence of a positive family history are notoriously unreliable predictors of lack of susceptibility to MH. Any patient who develops MMR during induction of anesthesia should be considered potentially susceptible to MH.

Intraoperative Considerations

8 Treatment of an MH episode is directed at terminating the episode and treating complications such as hyperthermia and acidosis. The mortality rate for MH, even with prompt treatment, ranges from 5% to 30%. Table 52-4 illustrates

TABLE 52–4 Protocol for immediate treatment of malignant hyperthermia.

1. Discontinue volatile anesthetic and succinylcholine. Notify the surgeon. Call for help.
2. Mix dantrolene sodium with sterile distilled water and administer 2.5 mg/kg intravenously as soon as possible.
3. Administer bicarbonate for metabolic acidosis
4. Institute cooling measures (lavage, cooling blanket, cold intravenous solutions).
5. Treat severe hyperkalemia with dextrose, 25–50 g intravenously, and regular insulin, 10–20 units intravenously (adult dose).
6. Administer antiarrhythmic agents if needed despite correction of hyperkalemia and acidosis
7. Monitor end-tidal CO_2 tension, electrolytes blood gases, creatine kinase, serum myoglobin, core temperature, urinary output, and color, coagulation status
8. If necessary, consult on-call physicians at the 24-hour MHAUS hotline, **1-800-644-9737**.

Data from the MHAUS protocol available at http://www.mhaus.org/nf/Shop/EmergencyTherapyMHPosterSample.gif.

a standard protocol for management of MH. First and most importantly, the triggering agent must be stopped and dantrolene must be given immediately.

A. Acute Treatment Measures

Volatile agents and succinylcholine must be discontinued immediately. Even trace amounts of anesthetics absorbed by soda lime, breathing tubes, and breathing bags may be detrimental. The patient should be hyperventilated with 100% oxygen to minimize the effects of uncontrolled CO_2 production and increased oxygen consumption.

B. Dantrolene Therapy

The mainstay of therapy for MH is immediate administration of intravenous dantrolene. Dantrolene, a hydantoin derivative, directly interferes with muscle contraction by binding the Ryr_1 receptor channel and inhibiting calcium ion release from the sarcoplasmic reticulum. The dose is 2.5 mg/kg intravenously every 5 min until the episode is terminated (upper limit, 10 mg/kg). Dantrolene is packaged as 20 mg of lyophilized powder to be dissolved in 60 mL of sterile water. Depending on the dose required and drug formulation used, reconstitution can be time consuming. **An assistant may be needed.** A new formulation is available that reconstitutes in about one third the time (20 versus 86 s) required for the older formulation. The effective half-life of dantrolene is about 6 h.

After initial control of symptoms, 1 mg/kg of dantrolene intravenously is recommended every 6 h for 24–48 h to prevent relapse (MH can recur within 24 h of an initial episode). Dantrolene is a relatively safe drug that is also used to decrease temperature in patients with thyroid "storm" and neuroleptic malignant syndrome. Although its use in chronic therapy for spastic disorders has been associated with hepatic dysfunction, the most serious complication following acute administration is generalized muscle weakness that may result in respiratory insufficiency or aspiration pneumonia. Dantrolene can cause phlebitis in small peripheral veins and should be given through a central venous line if one is available. The safety and efficacy of dantrolene therapy mandate its immediate use in this potentially life-threatening situation. Following administration of dantrolene, most patients revert to normal

acid–base status promptly and no further pharmacological treatment is necessary.

C. Correction of Acid–Base/Electrolyte Imbalances

Persisting metabolic acidosis should be treated with intravenous sodium bicarbonate, recognizing that this treatment will worsen the hypercarbia. Hyperkalemia should be treated with glucose, insulin, and diuresis. There is no useful role for intravenous calcium in this setting. Antiarrhythmic agents, vasopressors, and inotropes should be administered, if indicated. Calcium channel blockers should not be given to patients receiving dantrolene because this combination appears to promote hyperkalemia. Furosemide may be used to establish diuresis and prevent acute kidney failure, which may develop as a consequence of myoglobinuria. Dantrolene contains a considerable amount of mannitol (3 g per 20-mg bottle); thus furosemide or bumetanide should be used in preference to mannitol for diuresis.

D. Cooling the Patient

If fever is present, cooling measures should be instituted immediately. Surface cooling with ice packs over major arteries, cold air convection, and cooling blankets are used. Iced saline lavage of the stomach and any open body cavities (eg, in patients undergoing abdominal surgery) should also be instituted. Use of hypothermic cardiopulmonary bypass may be appropriate if other measures fail.

E. Management of the Patient with Isolated Masseter Muscle Spasm

MMR, or trismus, is a forceful contraction of the jaw musculature that prevents full mouth opening. This contrasts with incomplete jaw relaxation, which is a fairly common finding. Both myotonia and MH can cause masseter spasm. The two disorders can be differentiated by the medical history, neurological examination, and electromyography. The historical incidence of MMR following administration of succinylcholine with halothane in pediatric patients at some medical centers was higher than 1%. Isolated MMR occurs in only 15–30% of true MH episodes. Moreover, less than 50% of patients in whom MMR develops prove to be susceptible to MH by muscle testing. In the past, the consensus of clinicians was to assume that any occurrence of MMR was diagnostic of MH and to postpone elective surgery. However, if there is no other sign of MH, and if monitoring and treatment capabilities are readily available, many anesthesiologists now advocate allowing surgery to continue using safe (nontriggering) anesthetic agents. Serum CK levels should be followed for 24 h after an episode of MMR, because an elevation of this enzyme may indicate an underlying myopathy.

Postoperative Considerations

A. Confirmation of the Diagnosis

Patients who have survived an unequivocal episode of MH are considered susceptible; in these patients a muscle biopsy need not be performed for diagnosis. If the diagnosis remains in doubt postoperatively, a fresh biopsy specimen of living skeletal muscle is obtained and exposed to a caffeine, halothane, or combination caffeine–halothane bath. The halothane–caffeine contracture test may have a 10–20% false-positive rate, but the false-negative rate is close to zero. Because of the relative complexity of this test, only a few centers worldwide perform it. If the halothane–caffeine contracture test is positive, genetic counseling and testing of family members are appropriate. Baseline CK may be elevated chronically in 50–70% of people at risk for MH, but the only reliable way to diagnose MH susceptibility is by muscle testing.

Both European and North American MH registries have been established to help physicians identify and treat patients with suspected MH, as well as provide standardization between testing centers. The Malignant Hyperthermia Association of the United States (MHAUS, telephone 1-800-986-4287) operates a 24-hour hotline (1-800-644-9737) and a web site (http://www.mhaus.org).

1. Differential diagnosis—Several disorders may superficially resemble MH (Table 52–5). However, MH is associated with greater degrees of metabolic acidosis and venous desaturation than any of these other conditions. In current practice, the most common condition confused with MH is hypercarbia from CO_2 insufflation for laparoscopy, with or without subcutaneous emphysema. This condition can result in an unexpected increase in end-tidal

TABLE 52–5 Differential diagnosis of hyperthermia in the intraoperative and immediate postoperative periods.

Malignant hyperthermia
Neuroleptic malignant syndrome
Thyroid storm
Pheochromocytoma
Drug-induced hyperthermia
Serotonin syndrome
Iatrogenic hyperthermia
Brainstem/hypothalamic injury
Sepsis
Transfusion reaction

CO_2 with accompanying tachycardia. Surgery and anesthesia can precipitate thyroid storm in undiagnosed or poorly controlled hyperthyroid patients. The signs of thyroid storm include tachycardia, tachyarrhythmias (particularly atrial fibrillation), hyperthermia (often $\geq 40°C$), hypotension, and in some cases congestive heart failure. In contrast to MH, hypokalemia is very common. Also unlike the typical intraoperative presentation of MH, thyroid storm generally develops postoperatively (see Chapter 34). Pheochromocytoma is associated with dramatic increases in heart rate and blood pressure but not with an increase in CO_2 production, end-tidal CO_2, or temperature (see Chapter 34). Cardiac arrhythmias or ischemia may also be prominent. Rarely such patients may have hyperthermia ($>38°C$), which is generally thought to be due to increased heat production from catecholamine-mediated increases in metabolic rate together with decreased heat elimination from intense vasoconstriction. Sepsis shares several characteristics with MH, including fever, tachypnea, tachycardia, and metabolic acidosis (see Chapter 57). Sepsis can be difficult to diagnose if there is no obvious primary site of infection.

Less commonly, drug-induced hyperthermia may be encountered in the perioperative period. In these cases, the drugs appear to markedly increase serotonin activity in the brain, causing hyperthermia, confusion, shivering, diaphoresis, hyperreflexia, and myoclonus. Drug combinations associated with this "serotonin syndrome" include monoamine oxidase inhibitors (MAOIs) and meperidine, and

MAOIs and selective serotonin reuptake inhibitors (SSRIs). Hyperthermia can also be caused by some illicit drugs, including 3,4-methylenedioxymethamphetamine (MDMA or "ecstasy"), "crack" cocaine, amphetamines, phencyclidine (PCP), and lysergic acid diethylamine (LSD).

Iatrogenic hyperthermia is not uncommon, particularly in pediatric patients. Common sources of excessive heat in the operating room include humidifiers on ventilators, warming blankets, heat lamps, and increased ambient temperature. Injuries to the brainstem, hypothalamus, or nearby regions can be associated with marked hyperthermia.

2. Neuroleptic malignant syndrome (NMS)— This syndrome is characterized by hyperthermia, muscle rigidity with extrapyramidal signs (dyskinesia), altered consciousness, and autonomic lability in patients receiving antidopaminergic agents. The syndrome is caused by an imbalance of neurotransmitters in the central nervous system. It can occur either during drug therapy with antidopaminergic agents (eg, phenothiazines, butyrophenones, thioxanthenes, or metoclopramide) or less commonly following the withdrawal of dopaminergic agonists (levodopa or amantadine) in patients with Parkinson's disease. Thus, it appears to involve abnormal central dopaminergic activity, as opposed to the altered peripheral calcium release seen in MH. These differing mechanisms probably explain why nondepolarizing relaxants reverse the rigidity of NMS, but not the rigidity associated with MH.

NMS does not appear to be inherited and typically takes hours to weeks to develop; the majority of episodes develop within 2 weeks of a dose adjustment. Hyperthermia generally tends to be mild, and appears to be proportional to the amount of rigidity. Autonomic dysfunction results in tachycardia, labile blood pressure, diaphoresis, increased secretions, and urinary incontinence. Muscle rigidity can produce dyspnea and respiratory distress and, together with the increased secretions, can promote aspiration pneumonia. CK levels are typically elevated; some patients may develop rhabdomyolysis resulting in myoglobinemia, myoglobinuria, and kidney failure.

Mild forms of NMS promptly resolve after withdrawal of the causative drug (or reinstitution of antiparkinsonian therapy). Initial treatment of more severe forms of NMS should include oxygen therapy and endotracheal intubation for respiratory distress or altered consciousness. Marked muscle rigidity can be controlled with muscle paralysis, dantrolene, or a dopaminergic agonist (amantadine, bromocriptine, or levodopa), depending on the severity and acuity of the syndrome. Resolution of the muscle rigidity usually decreases body temperature.

This syndrome is considered a separate entity from MH; nevertheless some clinicians believe that NMS may predispose patients to MH and recommend that patients with NMS should not receive succinylcholine or a volatile anesthetic. In contrast to patients with NMS, patients susceptible to MH can safely receive phenothiazines.

B. Prophylaxis, Postanesthesia Care, and Discharge

10 Propofol, etomidate, benzodiazepines, ketamine, thiopental, methohexital, opiates, droperidol, nitrous oxide, nondepolarizing muscle relaxants, and all local anesthetics are nontriggering agents that are safe for use in MH-susceptible patients. An adequate supply of dantrolene should always be available wherever general anesthesia is provided. Prophylactic administration of intravenous dantrolene to susceptible patients is not necessary if a nontriggering anesthetic is administered.

For MH-susceptible patients, the consensus is that the vaporizers should be removed from the anesthesia workstation (or fixed in an "off" position) and the machine should be flushed with 10 L/min of fresh gas (air or oxygen) for at least 5 min. This step should reduce concentrations of volatile anesthetics to less than 1 part per million. Additionally, the CO_2 absorbent and circle system (or other anesthetic circuit), hoses should be changed.

MH-susceptible patients who have undergone an uneventful procedure with a nontriggering anesthetic can be discharged from the PACU or ambulatory surgery unit when they meet standard criteria. There are no reported cases of MH-susceptible patients experiencing MH after receiving a nontriggering anesthetic during uneventful surgery.

SUGGESTED READING

Benca J, Hogan K: Malignant hyperthermia, coexisting disorders, and enzymopathies: Risks and management options. Anesth Analg 2009;109:1049.

Kelly FE, Nolan JP: The effects of mild induced hypothermia on the myocardium: A systematic review. Anaesthesia 2010;65:505.

Kim TW, Nemergut ME: Preparation of modern anesthesia workstations for malignant hyperthermia-susceptible patients: A review of past and present practice. Anesthesiology 2011;114:205.

Klingler W, Rueffert H, Lehmann-Horn F, et al: Core myopathies and risk of malignant hyperthermia. Anesth Analg 2009;109:1167.

Mackensen GB, McDonagh DL, Warner DS: Perioperative hypothermia: Use and therapeutic implications. J Neurotrauma 2009;26:342.

Parness J, Bandschapp O, Girard T: The myotonias and susceptibility to malignant hyperthermia. Anesth Analg 2009;109:1054.

Sessler DI: Temperature monitoring and perioperative thermoregulation. Anesthesiology 2008;109:318.

WEB SITES

Association of Anaesthetists of Great Britain & Ireland http://www.aagbi.org/

Malignant Hyperthermia Association of the United States. http://www.mhaus.org/

Nutrition in Perioperative & Critical Care

KEY CONCEPTS

1 The fit, previously well-nourished patient undergoing elective surgery could be fasted for up to a week postoperatively without apparent adverse effect on outcomes, provided that fluid and electrolyte needs are met. On the other hand, it is well established in multiple studies that malnourished patients benefit from nutritional repletion via either enteral or parenteral routes prior to surgery.

2 The indications for total parenteral nutrition (TPN) are narrow, including those patients who cannot absorb enteral solutions (small bowel obstruction, short gut syndrome, etc.); partial parenteral nutrition may be indicated to supplement enteral nutrition (EN), when EN cannot fully provide for nutritional needs.

3 TPN will generally require a venous access line with its catheter tip in the superior vena cava. The line or port through which the TPN solution will be infused should be dedicated to this purpose, if at all possible, and strict aseptic techniques should be employed for insertion and care of the catheter.

4 In the patient with critical illness, discontinuing an EN infusion may require multiple potentially dangerous adjustments in insulin infusions and maintenance of intravenous fluid rates. Meanwhile, the evidence is sparse that EN infusions delivered through an appropriately-sited gastrointestinal feeding tube increases the risk of aspiration pneumonitis.

5 Regardless of whether the TPN infusion is continued, reduced, replaced with 10% dextrose, or stopped, blood glucose monitoring will be needed during all but short, minor surgical procedures.

Issues related to nutrition tend to be far removed from the usual concerns of the surgical anesthesiologist. On the other hand, appropriate nutritional support has been recognized in recent years to be of key importance for favorable outcomes in patients with critical illness, a large fraction of whom will require surgical services. Severe malnutrition causes widespread organ dysfunction and increases perioperative morbidity and mortality rates. Nutritional repletion may improve wound healing, restore immune competence, and reduce morbidity and mortality rates in critically ill patients. This chapter does not provide a complete review of nutrition in the patient undergoing surgery or with critical illness, but rather offers the framework for providing basic nutritional support in such patients. We consider, for example, whether enteral nutrition (EN) or parenteral nutrition (PN) will best meet the needs of an individual patient. This chapter also briefly reviews the conditions under which the ongoing nutritional needs of patients may come into conflict with anesthetic preferences and dogmas, such as the duration that patients must not receive EN before undergoing general anesthesia.

BASIC NUTRITIONAL NEEDS

Maintenance of normal body mass, composition, structure, and function requires the periodic intake of water, energy substrates, and specific nutrients. Nutrients that cannot be synthesized from other nutrients are characterized as "essential." Remarkably, relatively few essential nutrients are required to form the thousands of compounds that make up the body. Known essential nutrients include 8–10 amino acids, 2 fatty acids, 13 vitamins, and approximately 16 minerals.

Energy is normally derived from dietary or endogenous carbohydrates, fats, and protein. Metabolic breakdown of these substrates yields the adenosine triphosphate required for normal cellular function. Dietary fats and carbohydrates normally supply most of the body's energy requirements. Dietary proteins provide amino acids for protein synthesis; however, when their supply exceeds requirements, amino acids also function as energy substrates. The metabolic pathways of carbohydrate, fat, and amino acid substrates overlap, such that some interconversions can occur through metabolic intermediates (see Figure 32–4). Excess amino acids can therefore be converted to carbohydrate or fatty acid precursors. Excess carbohydrates are stored as glycogen in the liver and skeletal muscle. When glycogen stores are saturated (200–400 g in adults), excess carbohydrate is converted to fatty acids and stored as triglycerides, primarily in fat cells.

During starvation, the protein content of essential tissues is spared. As blood glucose concentration begins to fall during fasting, insulin secretion decreases, and counterregulatory hormones, such as glucagon, increase. Hepatic and, to a lesser extent, renal glycogenolysis and gluconeogenesis are enhanced. As glycogen supplies are depleted (within 24 h), gluconeogenesis (from amino acids) becomes increasingly important. Only neural tissue, renal medullary cells, and erythrocytes continue to utilize glucose—in effect, sparing tissue proteins. Lipolysis is enhanced, and fats become the principal energy source. Glycerol from the triglycerides enters the glycolytic pathway, and fatty acids are broken down to acetylcoenzyme A (acetyl-CoA). Excess acetyl-CoA results in the formation of ketone bodies (ketosis). Some fatty acids can contribute to gluconeogenesis.

If starvation is prolonged, the brain, kidneys, and muscle also begin to utilize ketone bodies efficiently. The previously well-nourished patient undergoing elective surgery could be fasted for up to a week postoperatively without apparent adverse effect on outcomes, provided fluid and electrolyte needs are met. The usefulness of nutritional repletion in the immediate postoperative period is not well defined, but likely relates to the degree of malnutrition, number of nutrient deficiencies, and severity of the illness/injury. Moreover, the optimal timing and amount of nutrition support following acute illness remain unknown. On the other hand, malnourished patients may benefit from nutritional repletion prior to surgery.

Modern surgical practice has evolved to an expectation of an accelerated recovery. Accelerated recovery programs generally include early enteral feeding, even in patients undergoing surgery on the gastrointestinal tract, so prolonged periods of postoperative starvation are no longer common practice. All well-nourished patients should receive nutritional support after 5 days of postsurgical starvation, and those with ongoing critical illness or severe malnutrition should be given nutritional support immediately. The malnourished patient presents a different set of issues, and such patients may benefit from both preoperative and early postoperative feeding. Clearly, the healing of wounds requires energy, protein, lipids, electrolytes, trace elements, and vitamins. Depletion of any of these substrates may delay wound healing and predispose to complications, such as infection. Nutrient depletion may also delay optimal muscle functioning, which is important for supporting increased respiratory demands and early mobilization of the patient.

The resting metabolic rate can be measured (but often inaccurately) using indirect calorimetry (known as a metabolic cart) or by estimating energy expenditure using standard nomograms (such as the Harris–Benedict equation), yielding an approximation of daily energy requirements. Alternatively, a simple and practical approach assumes that patients require 25–30 kcal/kg daily. The weight is usually taken as the ideal body weight or adjusted body weight. Even though nutritional requirements can increase greatly above basal levels with certain conditions (eg, burns), the more often relevant reason for determining the daily requirements is to ensure that patients are not unnecessarily overfed. In this regard, obese patients require adjusting the body weight based on the degree of obesity to prevent overfeeding.

HOW TO FEED THE PATIENT

After total parenteral nutrition (TPN) was established as a feasible approach for feeding patients lacking a functional gut, physicians extended the practice of TPN to many circumstances where "logic" and "clinical experience" suggested that it would be better than EN. For example, one such indication was in the patient with acute pancreatitis, where, in the 1970s, many clinicians thought that a period of TPN would put the gut and pancreas at "rest," allowing for resolution of pain and weight loss. Unfortunately, "logic" and "clinical experience" were incorrect. Now, the worldwide consensus expressed in clinical practice guidelines is that patients with acute pancreatitis (and indeed all others with functioning guts) will have worse outcomes **2** if TPN is provided, rather than EN. Today, the indications for TPN are narrow and include patients who cannot absorb enteral solutions (small bowel obstruction, short gut syndrome, etc.); partial PN may be indicated to supplement EN, in cases in which EN cannot fully provide for nutritional needs. In the latter circumstance, recent evidence suggests that the decision to add supplemental PN should be made only after a week's time in previously well-nourished patients. Earlier initiation of supplementary PN in previously well-nourished patients, as had been supported by 2009 European guidelines, resulted in worse outcomes in a large randomized clinical trial; however, these results are not firmly established, as smaller randomized clinical trials have suggested findings to the contrary. The divergent results from these recent trials may be associated with the type of parenteral formulations being used, types of patients being studied, timing of parenteral nutritional administration, and treatment in the control groups. Thus, further studies are needed to better define patients that may benefit from PN, as well as the optimal timing of nutritional support and formulations for feeding. In short, EN should be the primary mode of nutritional support, and PN should

be used when EN is not indicated, not tolerated, or insufficient.

There was a time when nearly every physician who took care of critically ill patients was in the position of frequently ordering TPN for patients. This is no longer the case, given that EN is now so much more widely employed. As a consequence, many hospitals and health systems insist that a nutrition support team take responsibility for those rarer patients who require TPN.

In general, patients with critical illness should undergo whatever initial hemodynamic resuscitation they require before initiation of nutritional support (either EN or PN). Absorption, distribution, and metabolism of nutrients require tissue blood flow, oxygen, and carbon dioxide removal. Adequate tissue blood flow requires an adequately resuscitated patient. Nutrient delivery to ischemic tissues may cause tissue damage by increasing carbon dioxide and oxidant production while consuming energy. Patients with critical illness who require EN will usually require placement of a feeding tube. Feeding tubes may be placed into the stomach in patients with adequate gastric emptying and low risk of aspiration. In patients with delayed gastric emptying or those at high risk of aspiration, feeding tubes are best placed into the small intestine. Ideally, the tip of such tubes will be sited within the small intestine, either by transpyloric placement of a nasoenteral tube or directly into the jejunum during abdominal surgery (via a percutaneous route), reducing the likelihood of gastric distention and regurgitation. Patients who are unable to eat, but require EN over long periods of time, will often undergo percutaneous endoscopic placement of gastrostomy (PEG) tubes (the tips of such tubes can be placed distal to the pylorus). One should confirm that the tips of all feeding tubes are appropriately placed before initiating feeds to reduce the likelihood that EN solutions will be accidentally infused, say, into the tracheobronchial tree or abdominal cavity.

3 TPN will generally require that a venous access line be placed with the catheter tip in the superior vena cava. Peripheral PN can support the nutritional requirements of the patient, but necessitates the use of larger volumes of fluids due to the requirement for lower osmolarities than used with central PN and increases the risk of phlebitis. The line or port through which the TPN solution will be infused should be dedicated to this purpose, if at all possible, and strict aseptic techniques should be employed for insertion and care of the catheter.

COMPLICATIONS OF NUTRITIONAL SUPPORT

Diarrhea is a common problem with enteral feedings and may be related to either hyperosmolarity of the solution or lactose intolerance. Gastric distention is another complication that increases the risk of regurgitation and pulmonary aspiration; the use of duodenal or jejunostomy tubes should decrease the likelihood of gastric distention. Complications of TPN are either metabolic or related to central venous access (Table 53–1). Bloodstream infections associated with central and peripheral venous lines remain a major concern, particularly in the patient with critical illness and immunocompromised states.

Overfeeding with excess amounts of glucose can increase energy requirements and production of carbon dioxide; the respiratory quotient can be >1 because of lipogenesis. Overfeeding can lead to reversible cholestatic jaundice. Mild elevations of serum transaminases and alkaline phosphatase may reflect fatty infiltration of the liver as a result of overfeeding.

SPECIFIC NUTRIENTS

Certain nutrients have been associated with improved outcomes. Surgery and anesthesia are well-recognized inducers of inflammation, producing changes in local (near the wound) and plasma concentrations of neurohormones, cytokines, and other mediators. Many investigators have hypothesized that adverse neurohormonal and inflammatory responses to surgery and anesthesia can be ameliorated through specific diets. Several clinical trials (and a recent meta-analysis) suggest that the addition of "immunomodulating" nutrients

TABLE 53–1 Complications of total parenteral nutrition.

Catheter-related complications
  Pneumothorax
  Hemothorax
  Chylothorax
  Hydrothorax
  Air embolism
  Cardiac tamponade
  Thrombosis of central vein
  Bloodstream infection

Metabolic complications
  Azotemia
  Hepatic dysfunction
  Cholestasis
  Hyperglycemia
    Hyperosmolar coma
    Diabetic ketoacidosis
  Excessive CO_2 production
  Hypoglycemia (due to interruption of infusion)
  Metabolic acidosis or alkalosis
  Hypernatremia
  Hyperkalemia
  Hypokalemia
  Hypocalcemia
  Hypophosphatemia
  Hyperlipidemia
  Pancreatitis
  Fat embolism syndrome
  Anemia
    Iron
  Vitamin D, K, or B-12 deficiency
  Essential fatty acid deficiency
  Hypervitaminosis A
  Hypervitaminosis D

(specifically arginine and "fish" oil) to EN may reduce the risk of infection and reduce the length of hospital stay in high-risk surgical patients. Similarly, current guidelines for perioperative PN also advocate the inclusion of n-3 fatty acids. There is some evidence that inclusion of long-chain n-3 polyunsaturated fatty acids (n-3 PUFAs), long-chain monounsaturated fatty acids (found in olive oil), or medium-chain fatty acids may be preferable to the use of solutions (such as soy bean-derived lipids) that are rich in longer chain n-6 PUFA. However, such solutions (although widely available outside of the United States) are not approved for use in the United States.

In the past, it was customary to individualize TPN solutions for each patient. Currently, there is little evidence that this is necessary, except in patients who cannot handle a sodium load (eg, those with severe heart failure). Adjustments may also be made in patients requiring renal replacement therapy; however, in most cases, this is not necessary. Similarly, except in patients who are already suffering from hepatic encephalopathy, most patients with liver disease can safely receive standard amino acid solutions. Thus, most patients receiving EN and PN can be safely managed with standardized nutritional formulations. Both EN and PN standardized formulations are available in ready-to-use formats that decrease preparation times and reduce contamination risks during formulation.

ENTERAL NUTRITION AND *NIL PER OS* RULES PRIOR TO ELECTIVE SURGERY

Long before the recognition by Mendelsohn of the problem posed by aspiration pneumonitis, anesthesiologists were reluctant to anesthetize patients scheduled for elective surgery if they had not been fasted overnight. Over time, the duration of obligatory time of no solid food *per os* has steadily declined, particularly in infants and young children. In **4** the patient with critical illness, discontinuing an EN infusion may require multiple potentially dangerous adjustments in insulin infusions and maintenance of intravenous fluid rates. Meanwhile, the evidence is sparse that EN infusions delivered through an appropriately sited gastrointestinal feeding tube increases the risk of aspiration pneumonitis. It is also relatively easy to empty the stomach immediately prior to anesthesia and surgery using 5–10 minutes of intermittent suction through a nasogastric tube. Therefore, current guidelines and current published evidence support continuing EN infusions (particularly when they are delivered distal to the pylorus) perioperatively and intraoperatively. Similarly, allowing preoperative patients to consume clear liquids, as desired, up to the time of surgery seems to have no influence on the risk of adverse outcomes from aspiration pneumonitis. Moreover, there is abundant evidence that administering a preoperative carbohydrate "load" to nondiabetic patients shortly before surgery will have the salutary metabolic effect of increasing plasma insulin concentrations and decreasing postoperative insulin resistance. Such preoperative carbohydrate loading is not nearly as commonplace as we believe it should be.

TPN AND SURGERY

Patients who receive TPN often require surgical procedures. Metabolic abnormalities are relatively common, and, ideally, should be corrected preoperatively. For example, hypophosphatemia is a serious and often unrecognized complication that can contribute to postoperative muscle weakness and respiratory failure.

When TPN infusions are suddenly stopped or decreased perioperatively, hypoglycemia may develop. Frequent measurements of blood glucose concentration are therefore required in such instances during general anesthesia. Conversely, if the TPN solution is continued unchanged, excessive hyperglycemia resulting in hyperosmolar nonketotic coma or ketoacidosis (in patients with diabetes) is also possible. The neuroendocrine stress response to surgery frequently aggravates glucose intolerance. Regardless of whether the TPN **5** infusion is continued, reduced, replaced with 10% dextrose, or stopped, blood glucose monitoring will be needed during all but short, minor surgical procedures.

GUIDELINES

American Dietetic Association. Critical illness evidence-based nutrition practice guideline. Available at: http://www.guidelines.gov/content.aspx?id=12818&search=ada+critical+illness+nutrition.

American Gastroenterological Association (AGA) Institute on "Management of Acute Pancreatitis" Clinical Practice and Economics Committee; AGA Institute Governing Board: AGA Institute medical position statement on acute pancreatitis. Gastroenterology. 2007;132:2019.

Braga M, Ljungqvist O, Soeters P, et al: ESPEN Guidelines on Parenteral Nutrition: surgery. Clin Nutr 2009;28:378.

Weimann A, Braga M, Harsanyi L, et al: ESPEN Guidelines on Enteral Nutrition: surgery including organ transplantation. Clin Nutr 2006;25:224.

SUGGESTED READING

Awad S, Lobo DN: Metabolic conditioning to attenuate the adverse effects of perioperative fasting and improve patient outcomes. Curr Opin Clin Nutr Metab Care 2012;15:194-200.

Marik PE, Zaloga GP: Immunonutrition in high-risk surgical patients: a systematic review and analysis of the literature. J Parenter Enteral Nutr 2010;34:378.

Marik PE, Zaloga GP: Meta-analysis of parenteral nutrition versus enteral nutrition in patients with acute pancreatitis. BMJ 2004;328:1407.

Tilg H: Diet and intestinal immunity. N Engl J Med 2012;366:181-183.

Zaloga GP: Parenteral nutrition in adult inpatients with functioning gastrointestinal tracts: assessment of outcomes. Lancet 2006;367:1101.

Anesthetic Complications

1 The rate of anesthetic complications will never be zero. All anesthesia practitioners, irrespective of their experience, abilities, diligence, and best intentions, will participate in anesthetics that are associated with patient injury.

2 Malpractice occurs when four requirements have been met: (1) the practitioner must have a duty to the patient; (2) there must have been a breach of duty (deviation from the standard of care); (3) the patient (plaintiff) must have suffered an injury; and (4) the proximate cause of the injury must have been the practitioner's deviation from the standard of care.

3 Anesthetic mishaps can be categorized as preventable or unpreventable. Of the preventable incidents, most involve human error, as opposed to equipment malfunctions.

4 The relative decrease in death attributed to respiratory rather than cardiovascular damaging events has been attributed to the increased use of pulse oximetry and capnometry.

5 Many anesthetic fatalities occur only after a series of coincidental circumstances, misjudgments, and technical errors coincide (mishap chain).

6 Despite differing mechanisms, anaphylactic and anaphylactoid reactions are typically clinically indistinguishable and equally life-threatening.

7 True anaphylaxis due to anesthetic agents is rare; anaphylactoid reactions are much more common. Muscle relaxants are the most common cause of anaphylaxis during anesthesia.

8 Patients with spina bifida, spinal cord injury, and congenital abnormalities of the genitourinary tract have a very increased incidence of latex allergy. The incidence of latex anaphylaxis in children is estimated to be 1 in 10,000.

9 Although there is no clear evidence that exposure to trace amounts of anesthetic agents presents a health hazard to operating room personnel, the United States Occupational Health and Safety Administration continues to set maximum acceptable trace concentrations of less than 25 ppm for nitrous oxide and 0.5 ppm for halogenated anesthetics (2 ppm if the halogenated agent is used alone).

10 Hollow (hypodermic) needles pose a greater risk than do solid (surgical) needles because of the potentially larger inoculum. The use of gloves, needleless systems, or protected needle devices may decrease the incidence of some (but not all) types of injury.

—Continued next page

Continued—

11 Anesthesiology is a high-risk medical specialty for substance abuse.

12 The three most important methods of minimizing radiation doses are limiting total exposure time during procedures, using proper barriers, and maximizing one's distance from the source of radiation.

1 The rate of anesthetic complications will never be zero. All anesthesia practitioners, irrespective of their experience, abilities, diligence, and best intentions, will participate in anesthetics that are associated with patient injury. Moreover, unexpected adverse perioperative outcomes can lead to litigation, even if those outcomes did not directly arise from anesthetic mismanagement. This chapter reviews management approaches to complications secondary to anesthesia and discusses medical malpractice and legal issues from an American (USA) perspective. Readers based in other countries may not find this section to be as relevant to their practices.

LITIGATION AND ANESTHETIC COMPLICATIONS

All anesthesia practitioners will have patients with adverse outcomes, and in the USA most anesthesiologists will at some point in their career be involved to one degree or another in malpractice litigation. Consequently, all anesthesia staff should expect litigation to be a part of their professional lives and acquire suitably solvent medical malpractice insurance with coverage appropriate for the community in which they practice.

When unexpected events occur, anesthesia staff must generate an appropriate differential diagnosis, seek necessary consultation, and execute a treatment plan to mitigate (to the greatest degree possible) any patient injury. Appropriate documentation in the patient record is helpful, as many adverse outcomes will be reviewed by facility-based and practice-based quality assurance and performance improvement authorities. Deviations from acceptable practice will likely be noted in the practitioner's quality assurance file. Should an adverse outcome lead to litigation, the medical record documents the practitioner's actions at the time of the incident. Often years pass before litigation proceeds to the point where the anesthesia provider is asked about the case in question. Although memories fade, a clear and complete anesthesiology record can provide convincing evidence that a complication was recognized and appropriately treated.

A lawsuit may be filed, despite a physician's best efforts to communicate with the patient and family about the intraoperative events, management decisions, and the circumstances surrounding an adverse event. It is often not possible to predict which cases will be pursued by plaintiffs! Litigation may be pursued when it is clear (at least to the defense team) that the anesthesia care conformed to standards, and, conversely, that suits may not be filed when there is obvious anesthesia culpability. That said, anesthetics that are followed by unexpected death, paralysis, or brain injury of young, economically productive individuals are particularly attractive to plaintiff's lawyers. When a patient has an unexpectedly poor outcome, one should expect litigation irrespective of one's "positive" relationship with the patient or the injured patient's family or guardians.

2 Malpractice occurs when four requirements are met: (1) the practitioner must have a duty to the patient; (2) there must have been a breach of duty (deviation from the standard of care); (3) the patient (plaintiff) must have suffered an injury; and (4) the proximate cause of the injury must have been the practitioner's deviation from the standard of care. A duty is established when the practitioner has an obligation to provide care (doctor–patient relationship). The practitioner's failure to execute that duty constitutes a breach of duty. Injuries can be physical, emotional, or financial. Causation is established; if but for the breach of duty, the patient would not have experienced the injury. When a claim is meritorious, the tort system attempts to compensate the injured patient and/or family members by awarding them monetary damages.

Being sued is stressful, regardless of the perceived "merits" of the claim. Preparation for defense begins before an injury has occurred. Anesthesiology staff should carefully explain the risks and benefits of the anesthesia options available to the patient. The patient grants informed consent following a discussion of the risks and benefits. Informed consent does not consist of handing the patient a form to sign. Informed consent requires that the patient understand the choices being presented. As previously noted, appropriate documentation of patient care activities, differential diagnoses, and therapeutic interventions helps to provide a defensible record of the care that was provided, resistant to the passage of time and the stress of the litigation experience.

When an adverse outcome occurs, the hospital and/or practice risk management group should be immediately notified. Likewise, one's liability insurance carrier should be notified of the possibility of a claim for damages. Some policies have a clause that disallows the practitioner from admitting errors to patients and families. Consequently, it is important to know and obey the institution's and insurer's approach to adverse outcomes. Nevertheless, most risk managers advocate a frank and honest disclosure of adverse events to patients or approved family members. It is possible to express sorrow about an adverse outcome without admitting "guilt." Ideally, such discussions should take place in the presence of risk management personnel and/or a departmental leader.

It must never be forgotten that the tort system is designed to be adversarial. Unfortunately, this makes every patient a potential courtroom adversary. Malpractice insurers will hire a defense firm to represent the anesthesia staff involved. Typically, multiple practitioners and the hospitals in which they work will be named to involve the maximal number of insurance policies that might pay in the event of a plaintiff's victory, and to ensure that the defendants cannot choose to attribute "blame" for the adverse event to whichever person or entity was not named in the suit. In some systems (usually when everyone in a health system is insured by the same carrier), all of the named entities are represented by one defense team. More commonly, various insurers and attorneys represent specific practitioners and institutional providers. In this instance, those involved may deflect and diffuse blame from themselves and focus blame on others also named in the action. One should not discuss elements of any case with anyone other than a risk manager, insurer, or attorney, as other conversations are not protected from discovery. Discovery is the process by which the plaintiff's attorneys access the medical records and depose witnesses under oath to establish the elements of the case: duty, breach, injury, and causation. False testimony can lead to criminal charges of perjury.

Oftentimes, expediency and financial risk exposure will argue for settlement of the case. The practitioner may or may not be able to participate in this decision depending upon the insurance policy. Settled cases are reported to the National Practitioner Data Bank and become a part of the physician's record. Moreover, malpractice suits, settlements, and judgments must be reported to hospital authorities as part of the credentialing process. When applying for licensure or hospital appointment, all such actions must be reported. Failure to do so can lead to adverse consequences.

The litigation process begins with the delivery of a summons indicating that an action is pending. Once delivered, the anesthesia defendant must contact his or her malpractice insurer/risk management department, who will appoint legal counsel. Counsel for both the plaintiff and defense will identify "independent experts" to review the cases. These "experts" are paid for their time and expenses and can arrive at dramatically different assessments of the case materials. Following review by expert consultants, the plaintiff's counsel may depose the principal actors involved in the case. Providing testimony can be stressful. Generally, one should follow the advice of one's defense attorney. Oftentimes, plaintiff's attorneys will attempt to anger or confuse the deponent, hoping to provoke a response favorable to the claim. Most defense attorneys will advise their clients to answer questions as literally and simply as possible, without offering extraneous commentary. Should the plaintiff's attorney become abusive, the defense attorney will object for the record. However, depositions, also known as "examinations before trial," are not held in front of a judge (only the attorneys, the deponent, the court reporter[s], and [sometimes] the videographer are present). Obligatory small talk often occurs among the attorneys and the court reporters. This is natural and should not be a source of anxiety for the defendant, because in most localities, the same plaintiff's and defense attorneys see each other regularly.

Following discovery, the insurers, plaintiffs, and defense attorneys will "value" the case and attempt to monetize the damages. Items, such as pain and suffering, loss of consortium with spouses, lost wages, and many other factors, are included in determining what the injury is worth. Also during this period, the defense attorney may petition the court to grant defendants a "summary judgment," dismissing the defendant from the case if there is no evidence of malpractice elicited during the discovery process. At times, the plaintiff's attorneys will dismiss the suit against certain named individuals after they have testified, particularly when their testimony implicates other named defendants.

Settlement negotiations will occur in nearly every action. Juries are unpredictable, and both parties are often hesitant to take a case to trial. There are expenses associated with litigation, and, consequently, both plaintiff and defense attorneys will try to avoid uncertainties. Many anesthesia providers will not want to settle a case because the settlement must be reported. Nonetheless, an award in excess of the insurance policy maximum may (depending on the jurisdiction) place the personal assets of the defendant providers at risk. This underscores the importance of our advice to all practitioners (not only those involved in a lawsuit) to assemble their personal assets (house, retirement fund, etc.) in a fashion that makes personal asset confiscation difficult in the event of a negative judgment. One should remember that an adverse judgment may arise from a case in which

most anesthesiologists would find the care to meet acceptable standards!

When a case proceeds to trial, the first step is jury selection in the process of *voir dire*—from the French—"to see, to say." In this process, attorneys for the plaintiff and defendant will use various profiling techniques to attempt to identify (and remove) jurors who are less likely to be sympathetic to their case, while keeping the jurors deemed most likely to favor their side. Each attorney is able to strike a certain number of jurors from the pool because they perceive an inherent bias. The jurors will be questioned about such matters as their educational level, history of litigation themselves, professions, and so forth.

Following empanelment, the case is presented to the jury. Each attorney attempts to educate the jurors—who usually have limited knowledge of healthcare (physicians and nurses will usually be struck from the jury)—as to the standard of care for this or that procedure and how the defendants did or did not breach their duty to the patient to uphold those standards. Expert witnesses will attempt to define what the standard of care is for the community, and the plaintiff and defendant will present experts with views that are favorable to their respective cause. The attorneys will attempt to discredit the opponent's experts and challenge their opinions. Exhibits are often used to explain to the jury what should or should not have happened and why the injuries for which damages are being sought were caused by the practitioner's negligence.

After the attorneys conclude their closing remarks, the judge will "charge" the jurors with their duty and will delineate what they can consider in making their judgment. Once a case is in the hands of a jury, anything can happen. Many cases will settle during the course of the trial, as neither party wishes to be subject to the arbitrary decisions of an unpredictable jury. Should the case not settle, the jurors will reach a verdict. When a jury determines that the defendants were negligent and negligence was the cause of the plaintiff's injuries, the jury will determine an appropriate award. If the award is so egregiously large that it is inconsistent with awards for similar injuries, the judge may reduce its amount. Of course, following any verdict, there are numerous appeals that may be filed. It is important to note that appeals typically do not relate to the medical aspects of the case, but are filed because the trial process itself was somehow flawed.

Unfortunately, a malpractice action can take years to reach a conclusion. Consultation with a mental health professional may be appropriate for the defendant when the litigation process results in unmanageable stress, depression, increased alcohol consumption, or substance abuse.

Determining what constitutes the "standard of care" is increasingly complicated. In the United Sates, the definition of "standard of care" is made separately by each state. The standard of care is NOT necessarily "best practices" or even the care that another physician would prefer. Generally, the standard of care is met when a patient receives care that other reasonable physicians in similar circumstances would regard as adequate. The American Society of Anesthesiologists (ASA) has published standards, and these provide a basic framework for routine anesthetic practice (eg, monitoring). Increasingly, a number of "guidelines" have been developed by the multiple specialty societies to identify best practices in accordance with assessments of the evidence in the literature. The increasing number of guidelines proffered by the numerous anesthesia and other societies and their frequent updating can make it difficult for clinicians to stay abreast of the changing nature of practice. This is a particular problem when two societies produce conflicting guidelines on the same topic using the same data. Likewise, the information upon which guidelines are based can range from randomized clinical trials to the opinion of "experts" in the field. Consequently, guidelines do not hold the same weight as standards. Guidelines produced by reputable societies will generally include an appropriate disclaimer based on the level of evidence used to generate the guideline. Nonetheless, plaintiff's attorneys will attempt to use guidelines to establish a "standard of care," when, in fact, clinical guidelines are prepared to assist in guiding the delivery of therapy. However, if deviation from guidelines is required for good patient care, the rationale for such actions should be documented on the anesthesia record, as plaintiff's attorneys will attempt to use the guideline as a *de facto* standard of care.

ADVERSE ANESTHETIC OUTCOMES

Incidence

There are several reasons why it is difficult to accurately measure the incidence of adverse anesthesia-related outcomes. First, it is often difficult to determine whether the cause of a poor outcome is the patient's underlying disease, the surgical procedure, or the anesthetic management. In some cases, all three factors contribute to a poor outcome. Clinically important measurable outcomes are relatively rare after elective anesthetics. For example, death is a clear endpoint, and perioperative deaths do occur with some regularity. But, because deaths attributable to anesthesia are much rarer, a very large series of patients must be studied to assemble conclusions that have statistical significance. Nonetheless, many studies have attempted to determine the incidence of complications due to anesthesia. Unfortunately, studies vary in criteria for defining an anesthesia-related adverse outcome and are limited by retrospective analysis.

Perioperative mortality is usually defined as death within 48 hr of surgery. It is clear that most perioperative fatalities are due to the patient's preoperative disease or the surgical procedure. In a study conducted between 1948 and 1952, anesthesia mortality in the United States was approximately 5100 deaths per year or 3.3 deaths per 100,000 population. A review of cause of death files in the United States showed that the rate of anesthesia-related deaths was 1.1/1,000,000 population or 1 anesthetic death per 100,000 procedures between 1999 and 2005 (Figure 54–1). These results suggest a 97% decrease in anesthesia mortality since the 1940s. However, a 2002 study reported an estimated rate of 1 death per 13,000 anesthetics. Due to differences in methodology, there are discrepancies in the literature as to how well anesthesiology is doing in achieving safe practice. In a 2008 study of 815,077 patients (ASA class 1, 2, or 3) who underwent elective surgery at US Department of Veterans Affairs hospitals, the mortality rate was 0.08% on the day of surgery. The strongest association with perioperative death was the type of surgery (Figure 54–2). Other factors associated with increased risk of death

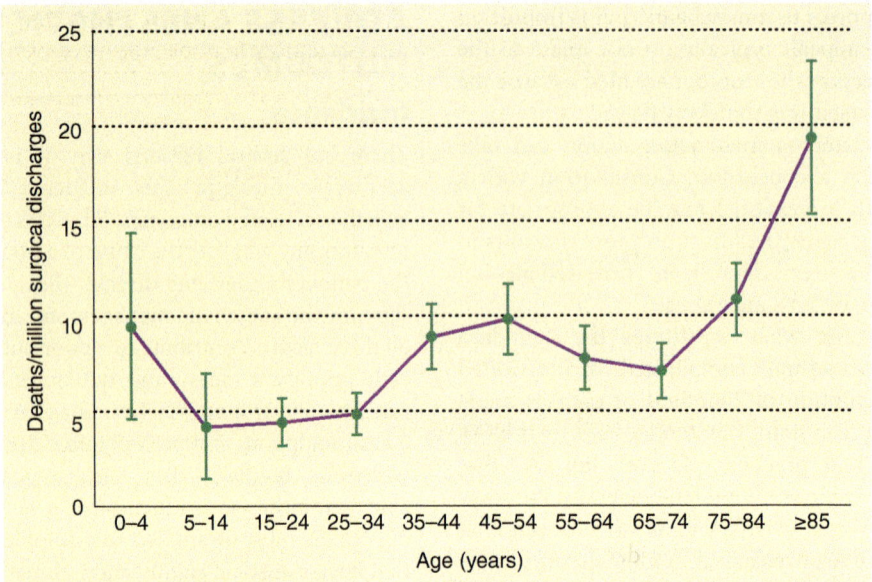

FIGURE 54–1 Annual in-hospital anesthesia-related deaths rates per million hospital surgical discharges and 95% confidence intervals by age, United States, 1999-2005. (Reproduced, with permission, from Li G, Warner M, Lang B, et al: Epidemiology of anesthesia-related mortality in the United States 1999-2005. Anesthesiology 2009;110:759.)

included dyspnea, reduced albumin concentrations, increased bilirubin, and increased creatinine concentrations. A subsequent review of the 88 deaths that occurred on the surgical day noted that 13 of the patients might have benefitted from better anesthesia care, and estimates suggest that death might have been prevented by better anesthesia practice in 1 of 13,900 cases. Additionally, this study reported

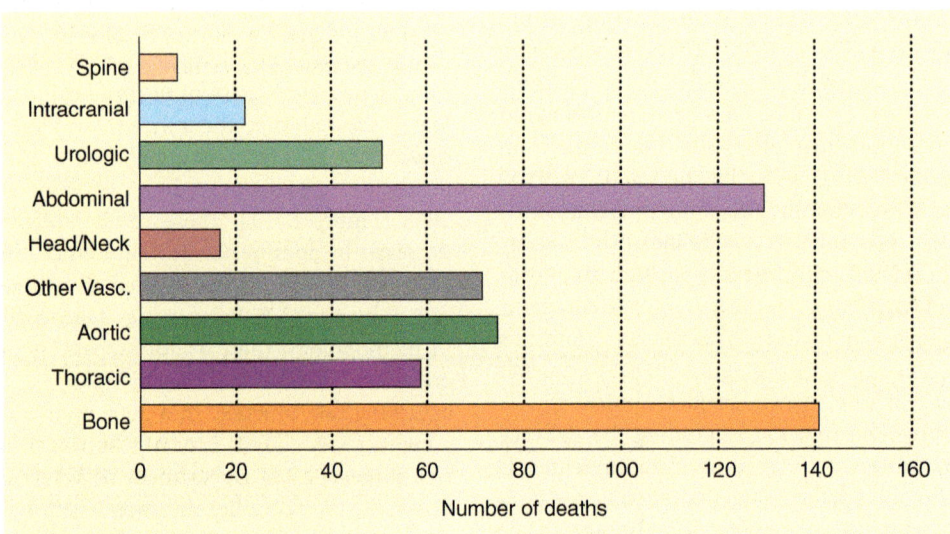

FIGURE 54–2 Total number of deaths by type of surgery in Veterans Affairs hospitals. (Reproduced, with permission, from Bishop M, Souders J, Peterson C, et al: Factors associated with unanticipated day of surgery deaths in Department of Veterans Affairs hospitals. Anesth Analg 2008;107:1924.)

that the immediate postsurgical period tended to be the time of unexpected mortality. Indeed, often missed opportunities for improved anesthetic care occur following complications when "failure to rescue" contributes to patient demise.

American Society of Anesthesiologists Closed Claims Project

The goal of the ASA Closed Claims Project is to identify common events leading to claims in anesthesia, patterns of injury, and strategies for injury prevention. It is a collection of closed malpractice claims that provides a "snapshot" of anesthesia liability rather than a study of the incidence of anesthetic complications, as only events that lead to the filing of a malpractice claim are considered. The Closed Claims Project consists of trained physicians who review claims against anesthesiologists represented by some US malpractice insurers. The number of claims in the database continues to rise each year as new claims are closed and reported. The claims are grouped according to specific damaging events and complication type. Closed Claims Project analyses have been reported for airway injury, nerve injury, awareness, and so forth. These analyses provide insights into the circumstances that result in claims; however, the incidence of a complication cannot be determined from closed claim data, because we know neither the actual incidence of the complication (some with the complication may not file suit), nor how many anesthetics were performed for which the particular complication might possibly develop. Other similar analyses have been performed in the United Kingdom, where National Health Service (NHS) Litigation Authority claims are reviewed.

Causes

3 Anesthetic mishaps can be categorized as preventable or unpreventable. Examples of the latter include sudden death syndrome, fatal idiosyncratic drug reactions, or any poor outcome that occurs despite proper management. However, studies of anesthetic-related deaths or near misses suggest that many accidents are preventable. Of these preventable incidents, most involve human error (Table 54–1), as opposed to equipment

TABLE 54–1 **Human errors that may lead to preventable anesthetic accidents.**

Unrecognized breathing circuit disconnection
Mistaken drug administration
Airway mismanagement
Anesthesia machine misuse
Fluid mismanagement
Intravenous line disconnection

malfunctions (Table 54–2). Unfortunately, some rate of human error is inevitable, and a preventable accident is not necessarily evidence of incompetence. During the 1990s, the top three causes for claims in the ASA Closed Claims Project were death (22%), nerve injury (18%), and brain damage (9%). In a 2009 report based on an analysis of NHS litigation records, anesthesia-related claims accounted for 2.5% of total claims filed and 2.4% of the value of all NHS claims. Moreover, regional and obstetrical anesthesia were responsible for 44% and 29%, respectively, of anesthesia-related claims filed. The authors of the latter study noted that there are two ways to examine data related to patient harm: critical incident and closed claim analyses. Clinical (or critical) incident data consider events that either cause harm or result in a "near-miss." Comparison between clinical incident datasets and closed claims analyses demonstrates that not all critical events generate claims and that claims may be filed in the absence of negligent care. Consequently, closed claims reports must always be considered in this context.

MORTALITY AND BRAIN INJURY

Trends in anesthesia-related death and brain damage have been tracked for many years. In a Closed Claims Project report examining claims in the

TABLE 54–2 **Equipment malfunctions that may lead to preventable anesthetic accidents.**

Breathing circuit
Monitoring device
Ventilator
Anesthesia machine
Laryngoscope

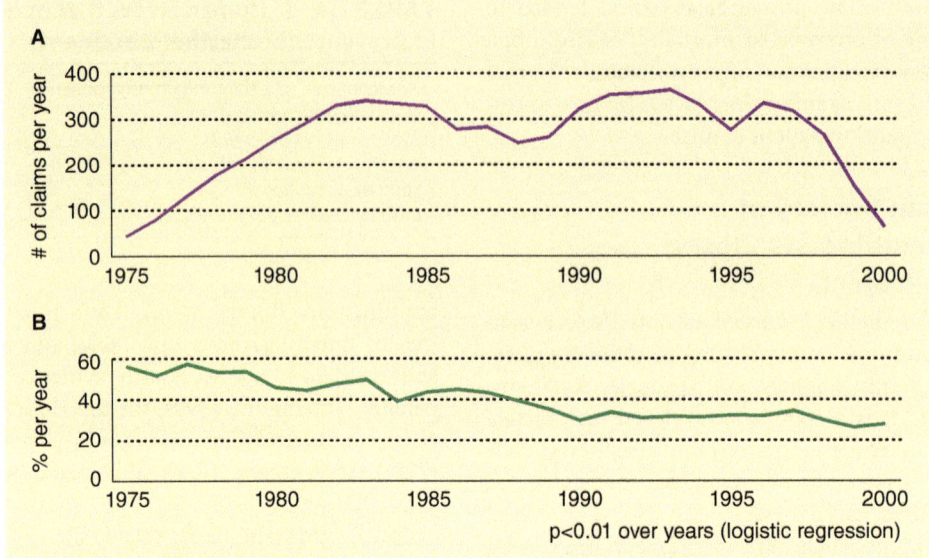

FIGURE 54–3 **A:** The total number of claims by the year of injury. Retrospective data collection began in 1985. Data in this analysis includes data collected through December 2003. **B:** Claims for death or permanent brain damage as percentage of total claims per year by year of injury. (Reproduced, with permission, from Cheney FW, Domino KB, Caplan RA, Posner KL: Nerve injury associated with anesthesia: a closed claims analysis. Anesthesiology 1999;90:1062.)

period between 1975 and 2000, there were 6750 claims (**Figure 54–3A** and **B**), 2613 of which were for brain injury or death. The proportion of claims for brain injury or death was 56% in 1975, but had decreased to 27% by 2000. The primary pathological mechanisms by which these outcomes occurred were related to cardiovascular or respiratory problems. Early in the study period, respiratory-related damaging events were responsible for more than 50% of brain injury/death claims, whereas cardiovascular-related damaging events were responsible for 27% of such claims; however, by the late 1980s, the percentage of damaging events related to respiratory issues had decreased, with both respiratory and cardiovascular events being equally likely to contribute to severe brain injury or death. Respiratory damaging events included difficult airway, esophageal intubation, and unexpected extubation. Cardiovascular damaging events were usually multifactorial. Closed claims reviewers found that anesthesia care was substandard in 64% of claims in which respiratory complications contributed to brain injury or death, but in only 28% of cases in

which the primary mechanism of patient injury was cardiovascular in nature. Esophageal intubation, premature extubation, and inadequate ventilation were the primary mechanisms by which less than optimal anesthetic care was thought to have contributed to patient injury related to respiratory events. The relative decrease in causes of death being attributed to respiratory rather cardiovascular damaging events during the review period was attributed to the increased use of pulse oximetry and capnometry. Consequently, if expired gas analysis was judged to be adequate, and a patient suffered brain injury or death, a cardiovascular event was more likely to be considered causative.

A 2010 study examining the NHS Litigation Authority dataset noted that airway-related claims led to higher awards and poorer outcomes than did nonairway-related claims. Indeed, airway manipulation and central venous catheterization claims in this database were most associated with patient death. Trauma to the airway also generates significant claims if esophageal or tracheal rupture occur. Postintubation mediastinitis should always

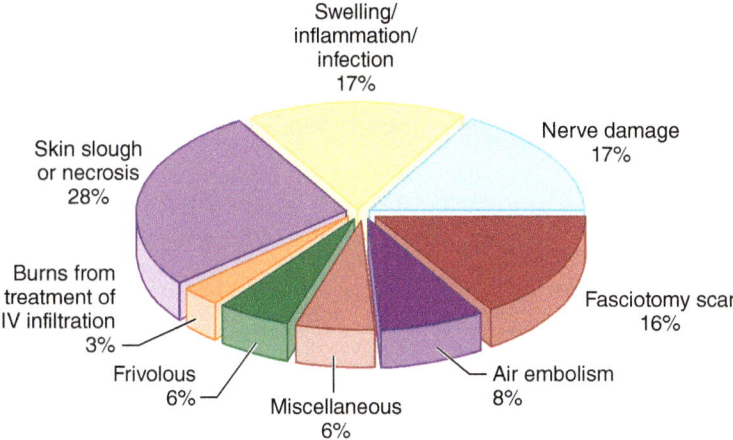

Swelling/
inflammation/
infection
17%

Nerve damage
17%

Skin slough
or necrosis
28%

Fasciotomy scar
16%

Burns from
treatment of
IV infiltration
3%

Frivolous
6%

Miscellaneous
6%

Air embolism
8%

FIGURE 54–4 Injuries related to IV catheters (n = 127). (Reproduced, with permission, from Bhananker S, Liau D, Kooner P, et al: Liability related to peripheral venous and arterial catheterization: a closed claims analysis. Anesth Analg 2009;109:124.)

be considered whenever there are repeated unsuccessful airway manipulations, as early intervention presents the best opportunity to mitigate any injuries incurred.

VASCULAR CANNULATION

Claims related to central venous access in the ASA database were associated with patient death 47% of the time and represented 1.7% of the 6449 claims reviewed. Complications secondary to guidewire or catheter embolism, tamponade, bloodstream infections, carotid artery puncture, hemothorax, and pneumothorax all contributed to patient injury. Although guidewire and catheter embolisms were associated with generally lower level patient injuries, these complications were generally attributed to substandard care. Tamponade claims following line placement were often for patient death. The authors of a 2004 closed claims analysis recommended reviewing the chest radiograph following line placement and repositioning lines found in the heart or at an acute angle to reduce the likelihood of tamponade. Brain damage and stroke are associated with claims secondary to carotid cannulation. Multiple confirmatory methods should be used to ensure that the internal jugular and not the carotid artery is cannulated.

Claims related to peripheral vascular cannulation in the ASA database accounted for 2% of 6849 claims, 91% of which were for complications secondary to the extravasation of fluids or drugs

from peripheral intravenous catheters that resulted in extremity injury (Figure 54–4). Air embolisms, infections, and vascular insufficiency secondary to arterial spasm or thrombosis also resulted in claims. Of interest, intravenous catheter claims in patients who had undergone cardiac surgery formed the largest cohort of claims related to peripheral intravenous catheters, most likely due to the usual practice of tucking the arms alongside the patient during the procedure, placing them out of view of the anesthesia providers. Radial artery catheters seem to generate few closed claims; however, femoral artery catheters can lead to greater complications and potentially increased liability exposure.

OBSTETRIC ANESTHESIA

Both critical incident and closed claims analyses have been reported regarding complications and mortality related to obstetrical anesthesia.

In a study reviewing anesthesia-related maternal mortality in the United States using the Pregnancy Mortality Surveillance System, which collects data on all reported deaths causally related to pregnancy, 86 of the 5946 pregnancy-related deaths reported to the Centers for Disease Control were thought to be anesthesia related or approximately 1.6% of total pregnancy related-deaths in the period 1991–2002. The anesthesia mortality rate in this period was 1.2 per million live births, compared with 2.9 per million live births in the period 1979–1990. The decline in anesthesia-related maternal mortality may be secondary to the decreased use of general anesthesia in parturients, reduced concentrations of bupivacaine in epidurals, improved airway management protocols and devices, and greater use of incremental (rather than bolus) dosing of epidural catheters.

In a 2009 study examining the epidemiology of anesthesia-related complications in labor and delivery in New York state in the period 2002–2005, an anesthesia-related complication was reported in 4438 of 957,471 deliveries (0.46%). The incidence of complications was increased in patients undergoing cesarean section, those living in rural areas, and those with other medical conditions. Complications of neuraxial anesthesia (eg, postdural puncture headache) were most common, followed by systemic complications, including aspiration or cardiac events. Other reported problems related to anesthetic dose administration and unintended overdosages. African American women and those aged 40–55 years were more likely to experience systemic complications, whereas Caucasian women and those aged 30–39 were more likely to experience complications related to neuraxial anesthesia.

ASA Closed Claims Project analyses were reported in 2009 for the period 1990–2003. Four hundred twenty-six claims from this period were compared with 190 claims in the database prior to 1990. After 1990, the proportion of claims for maternal or fetal demise was lower than that recorded prior to 1990. After 1990, the number of claims for maternal nerve injury increased. In the review of claims in which anesthesia was thought to have contributed to the adverse outcome, anesthesia delay, poor communication, and substandard care were thought to have resulted in poor newborn outcomes. Prolonged attempts to secure neuraxial blockade in the setting of emergent cesarean section can contribute to adverse fetal outcome. Additionally, the closed claims review indicated that poor communication between the obstetrician and the anesthesiologist regarding the urgency of newborn delivery was likewise thought to have contributed to newborn demise and neonatal brain injury.

Maternal death claims were secondary to airway difficulty, maternal hemorrhage, and high neuraxial blockade. The most common claim associated with obstetrical anesthesia was related to nerve injury following regional anesthesia. Nerve injury can be secondary to neuraxial anesthesia and analgesia, but also due to obstetrical causes. Early neurological consultation to identify the source of nerve injury is suggested to discern if injury could be secondary to obstetrical rather than anesthesia interventions.

REGIONAL ANESTHESIA

In a closed claims analysis, peripheral nerve blocks were involved in 159 of the 6894 claims analyzed. Peripheral nerve block claims were for death (8%), permanent injuries (36%), and temporary injuries (56%). The brachial plexus was the most common location for nerve injury. In addition to ocular injury, cardiac arrest following retrobulbar block contributed to anesthesiology claims. Cardiac arrest and epidural hematomas are two of the more common damaging events leading to severe injuries related to regional anesthesia. Neuraxial hematomas in both obstetrical and nonobstetrical patients were associated with coagulopathy (either intrinsic to the patient or secondary to medical interventions). In one study, cardiac arrest related to neuraxial anesthesia contributed to roughly one-third of the death or brain damage claims in both obstetrical and nonobstetrical patients. Accidental intravenous injection and local anesthesia toxicity also contributed to claims for brain injury or death.

Nerve injuries constitute the third most common source of anesthesia litigation. A retrospective review of patient records and a claims database showed that 112 of 380,680 patients (0.03%) experienced perioperative nerve injury. Patients with hypertension and diabetes and those who were smokers were at increased risk of developing perioperative nerve injury. Perioperative nerve injuries may result from compression, stretch, ischemia, other traumatic events, and unknown causes. Improper positioning can lead to nerve compression, ischemia, and injury, however not every nerve injury is the result of improper positioning. The care received by patients with ulnar nerve injury was rarely judged to be inadequate in the ASA Closed Claims database. Even awake patients undergoing spinal anesthesia have been reported to experience upper extremity injury. Moreover, many peripheral nerve injuries do not become manifest until more than 48 hr after anesthesia and surgery, suggesting that some nerve damage that occurs in surgical patients may arise from events taking place after the patient leaves the operating room setting.

PEDIATRIC ANESTHESIA

In a 2007 study reviewing 532 claims in pediatric patients aged <16 years in the ASA Closed Claims database from 1973–2000 (Figure 54–5), a decrease in the proportion of claims for death and brain damage was noted over the three decades. Likewise, the percentage of claims related to respiratory events also was reduced. Compared with before 1990, the percentage of claims secondary to respiratory events decreased during the years 1990–2000, accounting for only 23 % of claims in the latter study years compared with 51% of claims in the 1970s. Moreover, the percentage of claims that could be avoided by better monitoring decreased from 63% in the 1970s to 16% in the 1990s. Death and brain damage constitute the major complications for which claims are filed. In the 1990s, cardiovascular events joined respiratory complications in sharing the primary causes of pediatric anesthesia litigation. In the study mentioned above, better monitoring and newer airway management techniques may have reduced the incidence of respiratory events leading to litigation-generating complications in the latter years of the review period. Additionally, the possibility of a claim being filed secondary to death or brain injury is greater in children who are in ASA classes 3, 4, or 5.

In a review of the Pediatric Perioperative Cardiac Arrest Registry, which collects information from about 80 North American institutions that provide pediatric anesthesia, 193 arrests were reported in children between 1998 and 2004. During the study period, 18% of the arrests were "drug related," compared with 37% of all arrests during the years 1994–1997. Cardiovascular arrests occurred most often (41%), with hypovolemia and hyperkalemia being the most common causes. Respiratory arrests (27%) were most commonly associated with laryngospasm. Central venous catheter placement with resultant vascular injury also contributed to some perioperative arrests. Arrests from cardiovascular causes occurred most frequently during surgery, whereas arrests from respiratory causes tended to occur after surgery. The reduced use of halothane seems to have decreased the incidence of arrests secondary to medication administration. However, hyperkalemia and electrolyte disturbances

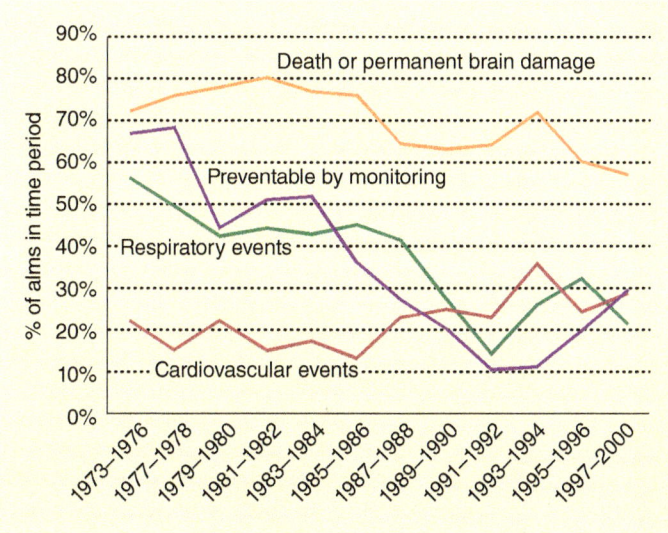

FIGURE 54–5 Trends over time. Outcome, type of event, and prevention by better monitoring. Years are grouped for illustration. (Reproduced, with permission, from Jimenez N, Posner K, Cheney F, et al: An update on pediatric anesthesia liability: a closed claims analysis. Anesth Analg 2007;104:147.)

associated with transfusion and hypovolemia also contribute to sources of cardiovascular arrest in children perioperatively.

A review of data from the Pediatric Perioperative Cardiac Arrest Registry with a focus on children with congenital heart disease found that such children were more likely to arrest perioperatively secondary to a cardiovascular cause. In particular, children with a single ventricle were at increased risk of perioperative arrest. Children with aortic stenosis and cardiomyopathy were similarly found to be at increased risk of cardiac arrest perioperatively.

OUT OF THE OPERATING ROOM ANESTHESIA AND MONITORED ANESTHESIA CARE

Review of the ASA Closed Claims Project database indicates that anesthesia at remote (out of the operating room) locations poses a risk to patients secondary to hypoventilation and excessive sedation. Remote location anesthesia care was more likely than operating room anesthesia care to involve a claim for death (54% vs 29%, respectively). The endoscopy suite and cardiac catheterization laboratory were the most frequent locations from which claims were generated. Monitored Anesthesia Care (MAC) was the most common technique employed in these claims. Overwhelmingly, adverse respiratory events were most frequently responsible for the injury.

An analysis of the ASA Closed Claims Project database focusing on MAC likewise revealed that oversedation and respiratory collapse most frequently lead to claims. Claims for burn injuries suffered in operating room fires were also found in the database. Supplemental oxygen, draping, pooling of flammable antiseptic preparatory solutions, and surgical cautery combine to produce the potential for operating room fires.

EQUIPMENT PROBLEMS

"Equipment problems" is probably a misnomer; the ASA Closed Claims Project review of 72 claims involving gas delivery systems found that equipment *misuse* was three times more common than equipment *malfunction*. The majority (76%) of adverse

TABLE 54–3 **Factors associated with human errors and equipment misuse.**

Factor	Example
Inadequate preparation	No machine checkout or preoperative evaluation; haste and carelessness; production pressure
Inadequate experience and training	Unfamiliarity with anesthetic technique or equipment
Environmental limitations	Inability to visualize surgical field: poor communication with surgeons
Physical and emotional factors	Fatigue; distraction caused by personal problems

outcomes associated with gas delivery problems were either death or permanent neurological damage.

Errors in drug administration also typically involve human error. It has been suggested that as many as 20% of the drug doses given to hospitalized patients are incorrect. Errors in drug administration account for 4% of cases in the ASA Closed Claims Project, which found that errors resulting in claims were most frequently due to either incorrect dosage or unintentional administration of the wrong drug (syringe swap). In the latter category, accidental administration of epinephrine proved particularly dangerous.

Another type of human error occurs when the most critical problem is ignored because attention is inappropriately focused on a less important problem or an incorrect solution (fixation error). Serious anesthetic mishaps are often associated with distractions and other factors (Table 54–3). The impact of most equipment failures is decreased or avoided when the problem is identified during a routine preoperative checkout performed by adequately **5** trained personnel. Many anesthetic fatalities occur only after a series of coincidental circumstances, misjudgments, and technical errors coincide (mishap chain).

Prevention

Strategies to reduce the incidence of serious anesthetic complications include better monitoring and anesthetic techniques, improved education, more comprehensive protocols and standards of practice, and active risk management programs. Better monitoring and anesthetic techniques imply more comprehensive monitoring and ongoing patient assessments and better designed anesthesia equipment and workspaces. The fact that most accidents occur during the maintenance phase of anesthesia—rather than during induction or emergence—implies a failure of vigilance.

Inspection, palpation, percussion, and auscultation of the patient provide important information. Instruments should supplement (but never replace) the anesthesiologist's own senses. To minimize errors in drug administration, drug syringes and ampoules in the workspace should be restricted to those needed for the current specific case. Drugs should be consistently diluted to the same concentration in the same way for each use, and they should be clearly labeled. Computer systems for scanning bar-coded drug labels are available that may help to reduce medication errors. The conduct of all anesthetics should follow a predictable pattern by which the anesthetist actively surveys the monitors, the surgical field, and the patient on a recurrent basis. In particular, patient positioning should be frequently reassessed to avoid the possibility of compression or stretch injuries. When surgical necessity requires patients to be placed in positions where harm may occur or when hemodynamic manipulations (eg, deliberate hypotension) are requested or required, the anesthesiologist should note on the record the surgical request and remind the surgeon of any potential risks to the patient.

QUALITY MANAGEMENT

Risk management and continuous quality improvement programs at the departmental level may reduce anesthetic morbidity and mortality rates by addressing monitoring standards, equipment, practice guidelines, continuing education, quality of care, and staffing issues. Specific responsibilities of peer review committees include identifying (and, ideally, preventing) potential problems, formulating and periodically revising departmental policies, ensuring the availability of properly functioning anesthetic equipment, enforcing standards required

for clinical privileges, and evaluating the appropriateness and quality of patient care. A quality improvement system impartially and continuously reviews complications, compliance with standards, and quality indicators.

AIRWAY INJURY

The daily insertion of endotracheal tubes, laryngeal mask airways, oral/nasal airways, gastric tubes, transesophageal echocardiogram (TEE) probes, esophageal (bougie) dilators, and emergency airways all involve the risk of airway structure damage. Common morbid complaints, such as sore throat and dysphagia, are usually self-limiting, but may also be nonspecific symptoms of more ominous complications.

The most common persisting airway injury is dental trauma. In a retrospective study of 600,000 surgical cases, the incidence of injury requiring dental intervention and repair was approximately 1 in 4500. In most cases, laryngoscopy and endotracheal intubation were involved, and the upper incisors were the most frequently injured. Major risk factors for dental trauma included tracheal intubation, preexisting poor dentition, and patient characteristics associated with difficult airway management (including limited neck motion, previous head and neck surgery, craniofacial abnormalities, and a history of difficult intubation).

Other types of airway trauma are rare. Although there are scattered case reports in the literature, the most comprehensive analysis was performed by the ASA Closed Claims Project. This report describes 266 claims, of which the least serious were temporomandibular joint (TMJ) injuries that were all associated with otherwise uncomplicated intubations and occurred mostly in females younger than age 60 years. Approximately 25% of these patients had previous TMJ disease. Laryngeal injuries included vocal cord paralysis, granuloma, and arytenoid dislocation. Most tracheal injuries were associated with emergency surgical tracheotomy, but a few were related to endotracheal intubation. Some injuries occurred during seemingly easy, routine intubations. Proposed mechanisms include excessive tube movement in the trachea, excessive cuff inflation leading to pressure necrosis, and inadequate relaxation. Esophageal perforations contributed to death in 5 of 13 patients. Esophageal perforation often presents with delayed-onset subcutaneous emphysema or pneumothorax, unexpected febrile state, and sepsis. Pharyngoesophageal perforation is associated with difficult intubation, age over 60 years, and female gender. As in tracheal perforation, signs and symptoms are often delayed in onset. Initial sore throat, cervical pain, and cough often progressed to fever, dysphagia, and dyspnea, as mediastinitis, abscess, or pneumonia develop. Mortality rates of up to 50% have been reported after esophageal perforation, with better outcomes attributable to rapid detection and treatment.

Minimizing the risk of airway injury begins with the preoperative assessment. A thorough airway examination will help to determine the risk for difficulty Documentation of current dentition (including dental work) should be included. Many practitioners believe preoperative consent should include a discussion of the risk of dental, oral, vocal cord, and esophageal trauma in every patient who could potentially need any airway manipulation. If a difficult airway is suspected, a more detailed discussion of risks (eg, emergency tracheotomy) is appropriate. In such cases, emergency airway supplies and experienced help should be available. The ASA algorithm for difficult airway management is a useful guide. After a difficult intubation, one should seek latent signs of esophageal perforation and have an increased level of suspicion for airway trauma. When intubation cannot be accomplished by routine means, the patient or guardian should be informed to alert future anesthesia providers of potential airway difficulty.

Emergent nonoperating room intubations present unique challenges. In a review of 3423 out of the operating room intubations, 10% were considered to be "difficult," and 4% of these intubations were associated with some form of complication, including aspiration, esophageal intubation, or dental injury. In this report, intubation bougies were employed in 56% of difficult intubations. The increased availability of video laryngoscopes and bougies have made emergent intubations less stressful and less likely to be unsuccessful.

PERIPHERAL NERVE INJURY

Nerve injury is a complication of being hospitalized, with or without surgery, regional, or general anesthesia. Peripheral nerve injury is a frequent and vexing problem. In most cases, these injuries resolve within 6–12 weeks, but some are permanent. Because peripheral neuropathies are commonly associated (often incorrectly!) with failures of patient positioning, a review of mechanisms and prevention is necessary.

The most commonly injured peripheral nerve is the ulnar nerve (Figure 54–6). In a retrospective study of over 1 million patients, ulnar neuropathy (persisting for more than 3 months) occurred in approximately 1 in 2700 patients. Of interest, initial symptoms were most frequently noted more than 24 hr after a surgical procedure. Risk factors included male gender, hospital stay greater than 14 days, and very thin or obese body habitus. More than 50% of these patients regained full sensory and motor function within 1 yr. Anesthetic technique was not implicated as a risk factor; 25% of patients with ulnar neuropathy underwent monitored care or lower extremity regional technique. The ASA Closed Claims Project findings support most of these results, including the delayed onset of symptoms and the lack of relationship between anesthesia technique and injury. This study also noted that many neuropathies occurred despite notation of extra padding over the elbow area, further negating compression as a possible mechanism of injury. Finally, the ASA Closed Claims Project investigators found no deviation from the standard of care in the majority of patients who manifested nerve damage perioperatively.

The Role of Positioning

Other peripheral nerve injuries seem to be more closely related to positioning or surgical procedure. They may involve the peroneal nerve, the brachial plexus, or the femoral and sciatic nerves. External pressure on a nerve could compromise its perfusion, disrupt its cellular integrity, and eventually result in edema, ischemia, and necrosis. Pressure injuries are particularly likely when nerves pass through closed compartments or take a superficial course (eg, the

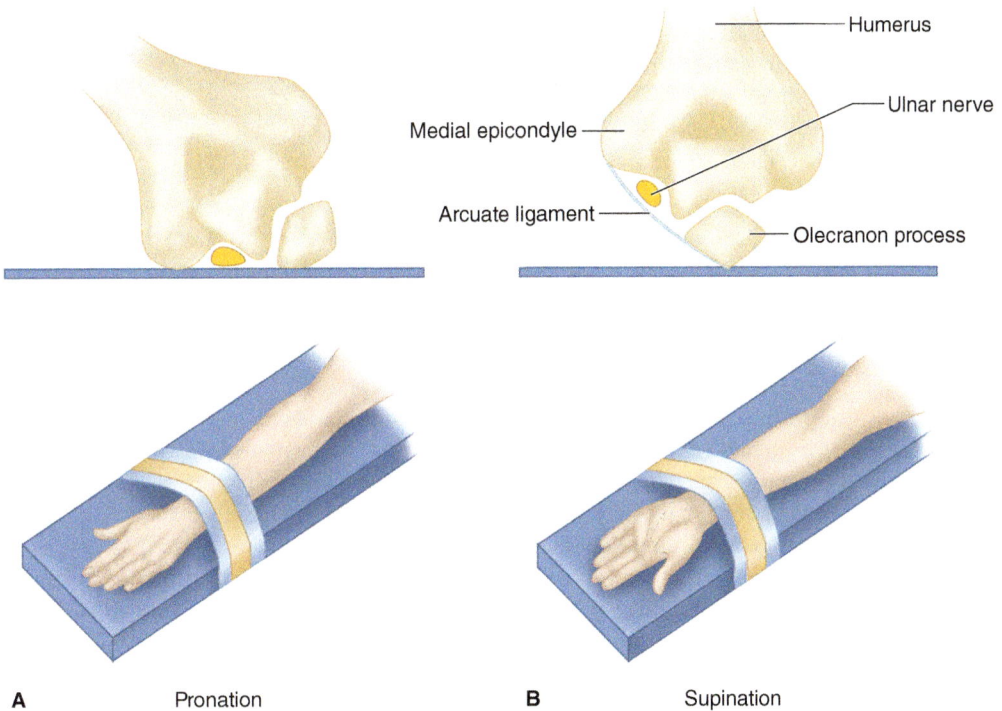

FIGURE 54–6 **A:** Pronation of the forearm can cause external compression of the ulnar nerve in the cubital tunnel. **B:** Forearm supination avoids this problem.

(Modified and reproduced, with permission, from Wadsworth TG: The cubital tunnel and the external compression syndrome. Anesth Analg 1974;53:303.)

peroneal nerve around the fibula). Lower extremity neuropathies, particularly those involving the peroneal nerve, have been associated with such factors as extreme degrees (high) and prolonged (greater than 2 h) durations of the lithotomy position. But, these nerve injuries also sometimes occur when such conditions are not present. Other risk factors for lower extremity neuropathy include hypotension, thin body habitus, older age, vascular disease, diabetes, and cigarette smoking. An axillary (chest) "roll" is commonly used to reduce pressure on the inferior shoulder of patients in the lateral decubitus position. This roll should be located caudad to the axilla to prevent direct pressure on the brachial plexus and large enough to relieve any pressure from the mattress on the lower shoulder.

The data are convincing that some peripheral nerve injuries are not preventable. The risk of peripheral neuropathy should be included in

discussions leading to informed consent. When reasonable, patients with contractures (or other causes of limited flexibility) can be positioned before induction of anesthesia to check for feasibility and discomfort. Final positioning should be evaluated prior to draping. In most circumstances, the head and neck should be kept in a neutral position. Shoulder braces to support patients maintained in a Trendelenberg position should be avoided if possible, and shoulder abduction and lateral rotation should be minimized. The upper extremities should not be extended greater than 90° at any joint. (There should be no continuous external compression on the knee, ankle, or heel.) Although injuries may still occur, additional padding may be helpful in vulnerable areas. Documentation should include information on positioning, including the presence of padding. Finally, patients who complain of sensory or motor dysfunction in the postoperative period should be reassured that this is usually a temporary condition. Motor and sensory function should be documented. When symptoms persist for more than 24 hr, the patient should be referred to a neurologist (or a physiatrist or hand surgeon) who is knowledgeable about perioperative nerve damage for evaluation. Physiological testing, such as nerve conduction and electromyographic studies, can be useful to document whether nerve damage is a new or chronic condition. In the latter case, fibrillations will be observed in chronically denervated muscles.

Complications Related to Positioning

Changes of body position have physiological consequences that can be exaggerated in disease states. General and regional anesthesia may limit the cardiovascular response to such a change. Even positions that are safe for short periods may eventually lead to complications in persons who are not able to move in response to pain. For example, the alcoholic patient who passes out on a hard floor or a park bench may awaken with a brachial plexus injury. Similarly, regional and general anesthesia abolish protective reflexes and predispose patients to injury.

Complications of postural hypotension, the most common physiological consequence of positioning, can be minimized by avoiding abrupt or extreme position changes (eg, sitting up quickly), reversing the position if vital signs deteriorate, keeping the patient well hydrated, and having vasoactive drugs available to treat hypotension. Whereas maintaining a reduced level of general anesthesia will decrease the likelihood of hypotension, light general anesthesia will increase the likelihood that movement of the endotracheal tube during positioning will cause the patient to cough and become hypertensive.

Many complications, including air embolism, blindness from sustained pressure on the globe, and finger amputation following a crush injury, can be caused by improper patient positioning (Table 54–4). These complications are best prevented by evaluating the patient's postural limitations during the preanesthetic visit; padding pressure points, susceptible nerves, and any area of the body that will *possibly* be in contact with the operating table or its attachments; avoiding flexion or extension of a joint to its limit; having an awake patient assume the position

TABLE 54–4 **Complications associated with patient positioning.**

Complication	Position	Prevention
Venous air embolism	Sitting, prone, reverse Trendelenburg	Maintain adequate venous pressure; ligate "open" veins
Alopecia	Supine, lithotomy, Trendelenburg	Avoid prolonged hypotension, padding, and occasional head turning.
Backache	Any	Lumbar support, padding, and slight hip flexion.
Extremity compartment syndromes	Especially lithotomy	Maintain perfusion pressure and avoid external compression.
Corneal abrasion	Any, but especially prone	Taping and/or lubricating eye.
Digit amputation	Any	Check for protruding digits before changing table configuration.
Nerve palsies		
Brachial plexus	Any	Avoid stretching or direct compression at neck, shoulder, or axilla.
Common peroneal	Lithotomy, lateral decubitus	Avoid sustained pressure on lateral aspect of upper fibula.
Radial	Any	Avoid compression of lateral humerus.
Ulnar	Any	Avoid sustained pressure on ulnar groove.
Retinal ischemia	Prone, sitting	Avoid pressure on globe.
Skin necrosis	Any	Avoid sustained pressure over bony prominences.

to ensure comfort; and understanding the potential complications of each position. Monitors must often be disconnected during patient repositioning, making this a time of greater risk for unrecognized hemodynamic derangement.

Compartment syndromes can result from hemorrhage into a closed space following a vascular puncture or prolonged venous outflow obstruction, particularly when associated with hypotension. In severe cases, this may lead to muscle necrosis, myoglobinuria, and renal damage, unless the pressure within the extremity compartment is relieved by surgical decompression (fasciotomy) or in the abdominal compartment by laparotomy.

AWARENESS

A continuing series of media reports have imprinted the fear of awareness under general anesthesia into the psyche of the general population. Accounts of recall and helplessness while paralyzed have made unconsciousness a primary concern of patients undergoing general anesthesia. When unintended intraoperative awareness does occur, patients may exhibit symptoms ranging from mild anxiety to posttraumatic stress disorder (eg, sleep disturbances, nightmares, and social difficulties).

Although the incidence is difficult to measure, approximately 2% of the closed claims in the ASA Closed Claims Project database relate to awareness under anesthesia. Analysis of the NHS Litigation Authority database from 1995–2007 revealed that 19 of 93 relevant claims were for "awake paralysis." Clearly, awareness is of great concern to patients and may lead to litigation. Certain types of surgeries are most frequently associated with awareness, including those for major trauma, obstetrics, and major cardiac procedures. In some instances, awareness may result from the reduced depth of anesthesia that can be tolerated by the patient. In early studies, recall rates for intraoperative events during major trauma surgery have been reported to be as frequent as 43%; the incidence of awareness during cardiac surgery and cesarean sections is 1.5% and 0.4%, respectively. As of 1999, the ASA Closed Claims Project reported 79 awareness claims; approximately 20% of the claims were for awake paralysis, and the remainder

of the claims were for recall under general anesthesia. Most claims for awake paralysis were thought to be due to errors in drug labeling and administration, such as administering paralytics before inducing narcosis. Since the 1999 review, another 71 cases have appeared in the database. Claims for recall were more likely in women undergoing general anesthesia without a volatile agent. Patients with long term substance abuse may have increased anesthesia requirements which if not met can lead to awareness.

Other specific causes of awareness include inadequate inhalational anesthetic delivery (eg, from vaporizer malfunction) and medication errors. Some patients may complain of awareness, when, in fact, they received regional anesthesia or monitored anesthesia care; thus, anesthetists should make sure that patients have reasonable expectations when regional or local techniques are employed. Likewise, patients requesting regional or local anesthesia because they want to "see it all" and/ or "stay in control" often can become irate when sedation dulls their memory of the perioperative experience. In all cases, frank discussion between anesthesia staff and the patient is necessary to avoid unrealistic expectations.

Some clinicians routinely discuss the possibility of intraoperative recall and the steps that will be taken to minimize it as part of the informed consent for general anesthesia. This makes particular sense for those procedures in which recall is more likely. It is advisable to also remind patients who are undergoing monitored anesthesia care with sedation that awareness is expected. Volatile anesthetics should be administered at a level consistent with amnesia. If this is not possible, benzodiazepines (and/or scopolamine) can be used. Movement of a patient may indicate inadequate anesthetic depth. Documentation should include end-tidal concentrations of anesthetic gases (when available) and dosages of amnesic drugs. Use of a bispectral index scale (BIS) monitor or similar monitors may be helpful although randomized clinical trials have failed to demonstrate a reduced incidence of awareness with use of BIS when compared with a group receiving appropriate concentrations of volatile agents. Finally, if there is evidence of intraoperative awareness during postoperative rounds, the practitioner should obtain a detailed account of the experience, answer patient questions, be very empathetic, and refer the patient for psychological counseling if appropriate.

EYE INJURY

A wide range of conditions from simple corneal abrasion to blindness have been reported. Corneal abrasion is by far the most common and transient eye injury. The ASA Closed Claims Project identified a small number of claims for abrasion, in which the cause was rarely identified (20%) and the incidence of permanent injury was low (16%). It also identified a subset of claims for blindness that resulted from patient movement during ophthalmological surgery. These cases occurred in patients receiving either general anesthesia or monitored anesthesia care.

Although the cause of corneal abrasion may not be obvious, securely closing the eye lids with tape after loss of consciousness (but prior to intubation) and avoiding direct contact between eyes and oxygen masks, drapes, lines, and pillows (particularly during monitored anesthesia care, in transport, and in nonsupine positions) can help to minimize the possibility of injury. Adequate anesthetic depth (and, in most cases, paralysis) should be maintained to prevent movement during ophthalmological surgery under general anesthesia. In patients scheduled for MAC, the patient must understand that movement under monitored care is hazardous and, thus, that only minimal sedation may be administered to ensure that he or she can cooperate.

Ischemic optic neuropathy (ION) is a devastating perioperative complication. ION is now the most common cause of postoperative vision loss. Postoperative vision loss is most commonly reported after cardiopulmonary bypass, radical neck dissection, and spinal surgeries in the prone position. Both preoperative and intraoperative factors may be contributory. Many of the case reports implicate preexisting hypertension, diabetes, coronary artery disease, and smoking, suggesting that preoperative vascular abnormalities may play a role. Intraoperative deliberate hypotension and anemia have also been implicated (in spine surgery), perhaps because of their potential to reduce oxygen delivery. Finally, prolonged surgical time in positions that compromise venous outflow (prone, head down, compressed

abdomen) have also been found to be factors in spine surgery. Symptoms are usually present immediately upon awakening from anesthesia, but have been reported up to 12 days postoperatively. Such symptoms range from decreased visual acuity to complete blindness. Analysis of case records submitted to the ASA Postoperative Vision Loss Registry revealed that vision loss was secondary to ION in 83 of 93 cases. Instrumentation of the spine was associated with ION when surgery lasted more than 6 hr and blood loss was more than 1 L. ION can occur in patients whose eyes are free of pressure secondary to the use of pin fixation, indicating that direct pressure on the eye is not required to produce ION.

Increased venous pressure in patients in the Trendelenberg position may reduce blood flow to the optic nerve.

It is difficult to formulate recommendations to prevent this complication because risk factors for ION are often unavoidable. Steps that might be taken include: (1) limiting the degree and duration of hypotension during controlled (deliberate) hypotension, (2) administering a transfusion to severely anemic patients who seem to be at risk of ION, and (3) discussing with the surgeon the possibility of staged operations in high-risk patients to limit prolonged procedures.

Of note, postoperative vision loss can be caused by other mechanisms as well, including angle closure glaucoma or embolic phenomenon to the cortex or retina. Immediate evaluation is advised.

CARDIOPULMONARY ARREST DURING SPINAL ANESTHESIA

Sudden cardiac arrest during an otherwise routine administration of spinal anesthetics is an uncommon complication. The initial published report was a closed claims analysis of 14 patients who experienced cardiac arrest during spinal anesthesia. The cases primarily involved young (average age 36 years), relatively healthy (ASA physical status I–II) patients who were given appropriate doses of local anesthetic that produced a high dermatomal level of block prior to arrest (T4 level). Respiratory insufficiency with hypercarbia due to sedatives was thought to be a potential contributing factor. The average time from induction of spinal anesthesia to arrest was 36 min, and, in all cases, arrest was preceded by a gradual decline in heart rate and blood pressure. Just prior to arrest, the most common signs were bradycardia, hypotension, and cyanosis. Treatment consisted of ventilatory support, ephedrine, atropine, cardiopulmonary resuscitation (average duration 10.9 min), and epinephrine. Despite these interventions, 10 patients remained comatose and 4 patients regained consciousness with significant neurological deficits. A subsequent study concluded that such arrests had little relationship to sedation, but were related more to extensive degrees of sympathetic blockade, leading to unopposed vagal tone and profound bradycardia. Rapid appropriate treatment of bradycardia and hypotension is essential to minimize the risk of arrest. Early treatment of bradycardia with atropine may prevent a downward spiral. Stepwise doses of ephedrine, epinephrine, and other vasoactive drugs should be given to treat hypotension. If cardiopulmonary arrest occurs, ventilatory support, cardiopulmonary resuscitation, and full resuscitation doses of atropine and epinephrine should be administered without delay.

HEARING LOSS

Perioperative hearing loss is usually transient and often goes unrecognized. The incidence of low-frequency hearing loss following dural puncture may be as high as 50%. It seems to be due to cerebrospinal fluid leak, and, if persistent, can be relieved with an epidural blood patch. Hearing loss following general anesthesia can be due to a variety of causes and is much less predictable. Mechanisms include middle ear barotrauma, vascular injury, and ototoxicity of drugs (aminoglycosides, loop diuretics, nonsteroidal antiinflammatory drugs, and antineoplastic agents). Hearing loss following cardiopulmonary bypass is usually unilateral and is thought to be due to embolism and ischemic injury to the organ of Corti.

ALLERGIC REACTIONS

Hypersensitivity (or allergic) reactions are exaggerated immunological responses to antigenic stimulation in previously sensitized persons. The antigen, or

TABLE 54–5 Hypersensitivity reactions.

Type I (immediate)
  Atopy
  Urticaria—angioedema
  Anaphylaxis
Type II (cytotoxic)
  Hemolytic transfusion reactions
  Autoimmune hemolytic anemia
  Heparin-induced thrombocytopenia
Type III (immune complex)
  Arthus reaction
  Serum sickness
  Acute hypersensitivity pneumonitis
Type IV (delayed, cell-mediated)
  Contact dermatitis
  Tuberculin-type hypersensitivity
  Chronic hypersensitivity pneumonitis

allergen, may be a protein, polypeptide, or smaller molecule. Moreover, the allergen may be the substance itself, a metabolite, or a breakdown product. Patients may be exposed to antigens through the respiratory tract, gastrointestinal tract, eyes, skin and from previous intravenous, intramuscular, or peritoneal exposure.

Anaphylaxis occurs when inflammatory agents are released from basophils and mast cells as a result of an antigen interacting with the immunoglobulin (Ig) E. Anaphylactoid reactions manifest themselves in the same manner as anaphylactic reactions, but are not the result of an interaction with IgE. Direct activation of complement and IgG-mediated complement activation can result in similar inflammatory mediator release and activity.

Depending on the antigen and the immune system components involved, hypersensitivity reactions are classically divided into four types (Table 54–5). In many cases, an allergen (eg, latex) may cause more than one type of hypersensitivity reaction. Type I reactions involve antigens that cross-link IgE antibodies, triggering the release of inflammatory mediators from mast cells. In type II reactions, complement-fixing (C1-binding) IgG antibodies bind to antigens on cell surfaces, activating the classic complement pathway and lysing the cells. Examples of type II reactions include hemolytic transfusion reactions and heparin-induced thrombocytopenia. Type III reactions occur when antigen–antibody

(IgG or IgM) immune complexes are deposited in tissues, activating complement and generating chemotactic factors that attract neutrophils to the area. The activated neutrophils cause tissue injury by releasing lysosomal enzymes and toxic products. Type III reactions include serum sickness reactions and acute hypersensitivity pneumonitis. Type IV reactions, often referred to as delayed hypersensitivity reactions, are mediated by $CD4^+$ T lymphocytes that have been sensitized to a specific antigen by prior exposure. Prior TH1 response causes expression of a T-cell receptor protein that is specific for the antigen. Reexposure to the antigen causes these lymphocytes to produce lymphokines—interleukins (IL), interferon (IFN), and tumor necrosis factor-γ (TNF-γ)—that attract and activate inflammatory mononuclear cells over 48–72 hr. Production of IL-1 and IL-6 by antigen-processing cells amplifies clonal expression of the specific sensitized T cells and attracts other types of T cells. IL-2 secretion transforms $CD8^+$ cytotoxic T cells into killer cells; IL-4 and IFN-γ cause macrophages to undergo epithelioid transformation, often producing granuloma. Examples of type IV reactions are those associated with tuberculosis, histoplasmosis, schistosomiasis, and hypersensitivity pneumonitis and some autoimmune disorders, such as rheumatoid arthritis and Wegener's granulomatosis.

1. Immediate Hypersensitivity Reactions

Initial exposure of a susceptible person to an antigen induces $CD4^+$ T cells to lymphokines that activate and transform specific B lymphocytes into plasma cells, producing allergen-specific IgE antibodies (Figure 54–7). The Fc portion of these antibodies then associates with high affinity receptors on the cell surface of tissue mast cells and circulating basophils. During subsequent reexposure to the antigen, it binds the Fab portion of adjacent IgE antibodies on the mast cell surface, inducing degranulation and release of inflammatory lipid mediators and additional cytokines from the mast cell. The end result is the release of histamine, tryptase, proteoglycans (heparin and chondroitin sulfate), and carboxypeptidases. Prostaglandin (mainly prostaglandin

D_2) and leukotriene (B_4, C_4, D_4, E_4, and platelet-activating factor) synthesis is also increased. The combined effects of these mediators can produce arteriolar vasodilatation, increased vascular permeability, increased mucus secretion, smooth muscle contraction, and other clinical manifestations of type I reactions.

Type I hypersensitivity reactions are classified as atopic or nonatopic. Atopic disorders typically affect the skin or respiratory tract and include allergic rhinitis, atopic dermatitis, and allergic asthma. Nonatopic hypersensitivity disorders include urticaria, angioedema, and anaphylaxis; when these reactions are mild, they are confined to the skin (urticaria) or subcutaneous tissue (angioedema), but when they are severe, they become generalized and a life-threatening medical emergency (anaphylaxis). Urticarial lesions are characteristically well-circumscribed skin wheals with raised erythematous borders and blanched centers; they are intensely pruritic. Angioedema presents as deep, nonpitting cutaneous edema from marked vasodilatation and increased permeability of subcutaneous blood vessels. When angioedema is extensive, it can be associated with large fluid shifts; when it involves the pharyngeal or laryngeal mucosa, it can rapidly compromise the airway.

2. Anaphylactic Reactions

Anaphylaxis is an exaggerated response to an allergen (eg, antibiotic) that is mediated by a type I hypersensitivity reaction. The syndrome appears within minutes of exposure to a specific antigen in a sensitized person and characteristically presents as acute respiratory distress, circulatory shock, or both. Death may occur from asphyxiation or irreversible circulatory shock. The incidence of anaphylactic reactions during anesthesia has been estimated at a rate of 1:3500 to 1:20000 anesthetics. Mortality from anaphylaxis can be as frequent as 4% of cases with brain injury, occurring in another 2% of surviving patients. A French study evaluating 789 anaphylactic and anaphylactoid reactions reported that the most common sources of perioperative anaphylaxis were neuromuscular blockers (58%), latex (17%), and antibiotics (15%).

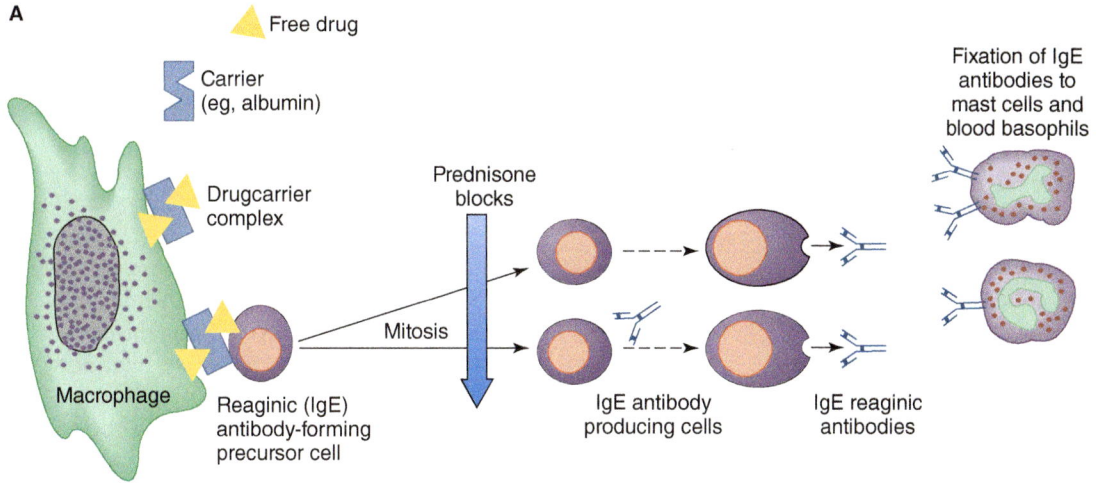

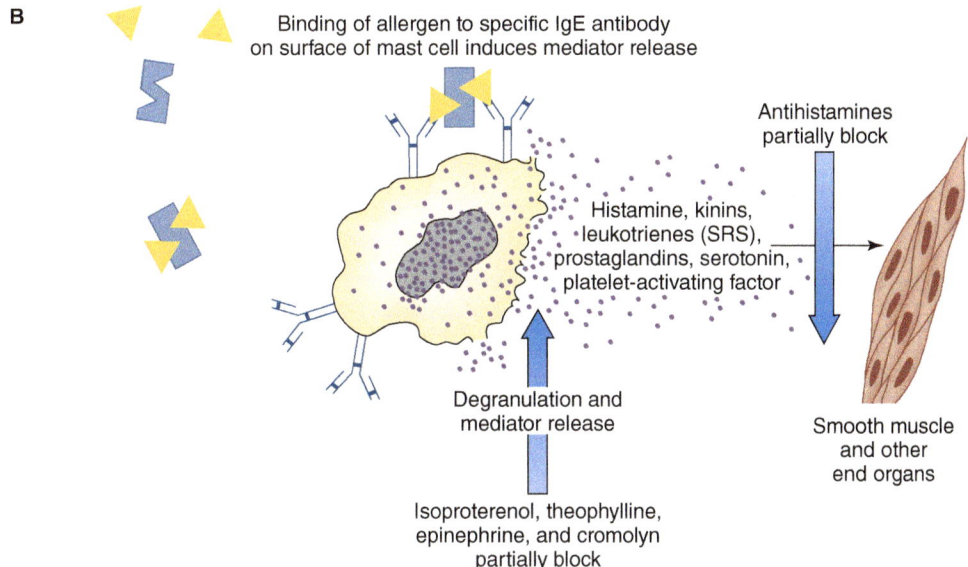

FIGURE 54–7   A: Induction of IgE-mediated allergic sensitivity to drugs and other allergens. **B:** Response of IgE-sensitized cells to subsequent exposure to allergens. Ig, immunoglobulin. (Reproduced, with permission, from Katzung BG [editor]: *Basic & Clinical Pharmacology,* 8th ed. McGraw-Hill, 2001.)

The most important mediators of anaphylaxis are histamine, leukotrienes, basophil kallikrein (BK-A,) and platelet-activating factor. They increase vascular permeability and contract smooth muscle. H_1-receptor activation contracts bronchial smooth muscle, whereas H_2-receptor activation causes vasodilatation, enhanced mucus secretion, tachycardia, and increased myocardial contractility. BK-A cleaves bradykinin from kininogen; bradykinin increases vascular permeability and vasodilatation and contracts smooth muscle. Activation of Hageman factor can initiate intravascular coagulation.

TABLE 54–6 **Clinical manifestations of anaphylaxis.**

Organ System	Signs and Symptoms
Cardiovascular	Hypotension,[1] tachycardia, arrhythmias
Pulmonary	Bronchospasm,[1] cough, dyspnea, pulmonary edema, laryngeal edema, hypoxia
Dermatological	Urticaria,[1] facial edema, pruritus

[1]Key signs during general anesthesia.

Eosinophil chemotactic factor of anaphylaxis, neutrophil chemotactic factor, and leukotriene B$_4$ attract inflammatory cells that mediate additional tissue injury. Angioedema of the pharynx, larynx, and trachea produce upper airway obstruction, whereas bronchospasm and mucosal edema result in lower airway obstruction. Histamine may preferentially constrict large airways, whereas leukotrienes primarily affect smaller peripheral airways. Transudation of fluid into the skin (angioedema) and viscera produces hypovolemia and shock, whereas arteriolar vasodilatation decreases systemic vascular

resistance. Coronary hypoperfusion and arterial hypoxemia promote arrhythmias and myocardial ischemia. Leukotriene and prostaglandin mediators may also cause coronary vasospasm. Prolonged circulatory shock leads to progressive lactic acidosis and ischemic damage to vital organs. Table 54–6 summarizes important manifestations of anaphylactic reactions.

Anaphylactoid reactions resemble anaphylaxis but do not depend on IgE antibody interaction with antigen. A drug can directly release histamine from mast cells (eg, urticaria following high-dose morphine sulfate) or activate complement. Despite differing mechanisms, anaphylactic and anaphylactoid reactions typically are clinically indistinguishable and equally life-threatening. Table 54–7 lists common causes of anaphylactic and anaphylactoid reactions.

Factors that may predispose patients to these reactions include pregnancy, known atopy, and previous drug exposure. Such reactions are more common in younger than older patients. Laboratory identification of patients who have experienced an adverse allergic reaction or who may be particularly

TABLE 54–7 **Causes of anaphylactic and anaphylactoid reactions.**

Anaphylactic reactions against polypeptides	Venoms (Hymenoptera, fire ant, snake, jellyfish) Airborne allergens (pollen, molds, danders) Foods (peanuts, milk, egg, seafood, grain) Enzymes (trypsin, streptokinase, chymopapain, asparaginase) Heterologous serum (tetanus antitoxin, antilymphocyte globulin, antivenin) Human proteins (insulin, corticotropin, vasopressin, serum and seminal proteins) Latex
Anaphylactic reactions against hapten carrier	Antibiotics (penicillin, cephalosporins, sulfonamides) Disinfectants (ethylene oxide, chlorhexidine) Local anesthetics (procaine)
Anaphylactoid reactions	Polyionic solutions (radiocontrast medium, polymyxin B) Opioids (morphine, meperidine) Hypnotics (propofol, thiopental) Muscle relaxants (rocuronium, succinylcholine, cisatracurium) Synthetic membranes (dialysis) Nonsteroidal antiinflammatory drugs Preservatives (sulfites, benzoates) Protamine Dextran Steroids Exercise Idiopathic

Adapted and reproduced, with permission, from Bochner BS, Lichtenstein LM: N Engl J Med 1991;324:1786.

TABLE 54–8 **Treatment of anaphylactic and anaphylactoid reactions.**

Discontinue drug administration
Administer 100% oxygen
Epinephrine (0.01–0.5 mg IV or IM)[1]
Consider intubation
Intravenous fluid bolus
Diphenhydramine (50–75 mg IV)
Ranitidine (150 mg IV)
Hydrocortisone (up to 200 mg IV) or methylprednisolone (1–2 mg/kg)

[1]The dose and route of epinephrine depend on the severity of the reaction. An infusion of 1–5 mcg/min may be necessary in adults.

susceptible is often aided by intradermal skin testing, leukocyte or basophil degranulation testing (histamine release test), or radio-allergosorbent testing (RAST). The latter is capable of measuring the level of drug-specific IgE antibody in the serum. Serum tryptase measurement is helpful in confirming the diagnosis of an anaphylactic reaction. Prophylactic pretreatment with histamine receptor antagonists and corticosteroids decreases the severity of the reaction. Treatment must be immediate and tailored to the severity of the reaction (Table 54–8).

3. Allergic Reactions to Anesthetic Agents

7 True anaphylaxis due to anesthetic agents is rare; anaphylactoid reactions are much more common. Risk factors associated with hypersensitivity to anesthetics include female gender, atopic history, preexisting allergies, and previous anesthetic exposures. Muscle relaxants are the most common cause of anaphylaxis during anesthesia, with an estimated incidence of 1 in 6500 patients. They account for almost 60% of perioperative anaphylactic reactions. In many instances, there was no previous exposure to muscle relaxants. Investigators suggest that over-the-counter drugs, cosmetics, and food products, many of which contain tertiary or quaternary ammonium ions, can sensitize susceptible individuals. A French study found that, in decreasing order of frequency, rocuronium, succinylcholine, and atracurium were most often responsible; this likely reflects the propensity to cause anaphylaxis, together with frequency of use.

Although rarer, hypnotic agents can also be responsible for some allergic reactions. The incidence of anaphylaxis for thiopental and propofol is 1 in 30,000 and 1 in 60,000, respectively. Allergic reactions to etomidate, ketamine, and benzodiazepines are exceedingly rare. True anaphylactic reactions due to opioids are far less common than nonimmune histamine release. Similarly, anaphylactic reactions to local anesthetics are much less common than vasovagal reactions, toxic reactions to accidental intravenous injections, and side effects from absorbed or intravenously injected epinephrine. IgE-mediated reactions to ester-type local anesthetics, however, are well described secondary to reaction to the metabolite, para-aminobenzoic acid, In contrast, true anaphylaxis due to amide-type local anesthetics is very rare; in some instances, the preservative (paraben or methylparaben) was believed to be responsible for an apparent anaphylactoid reaction to a local anesthetic. Moreover, the cross-reactivity between amide-type local anesthetics seems to be low. There are no reports of anaphylaxis to volatile anesthetics.

4. Latex Allergy

The severity of allergic reactions to latex-containing products ranges from mild contact dermatitis to life-threatening anaphylaxis. Latex allergy is the second most common cause of anaphylaxis during anesthesia. Most serious reactions seem to involve a direct IgE-mediated immune response to polypeptides in natural latex, although some cases of contact dermatitis may be due to a type IV sensitivity reaction to chemicals introduced in the manufacturing process. Nonetheless, a relationship between the occurrence of contact dermatitis and the probability of future anaphylaxis has been suggested. Chronic exposure to latex and a history of atopy increases the risk of sensitization. Healthcare workers and patients undergoing frequent procedures with latex items (eg, repeated urinary bladder catheterization, barium enema examinations) should therefore be considered at increased risk. Patients with spina **8** bifida, spinal cord injury, and congenital abnormalities of the genitourinary tract have an increased incidence of latex allergy. The incidence of latex anaphylaxis in children is estimated to be 1 in 10,000. A history of allergic symptoms to latex should be sought in all patients during the preanesthetic interview. Foods that cross-react with latex include mango, kiwi, chestnut, avacado, passion fruit, and banana.

IL-18 and IL-13 single nucleotide polymorphisms may affect the sensitivity of individuals to latex and promote allergic responses.

Anaphylactic reactions to latex may be confused with reactions to other substances (eg, drugs, blood products) because the onset of symptoms can be delayed for more than 1 hr after initial exposure. Treatment is the same as for other forms of anaphylactic reactions. Skin-prick tests, intradermal tests, basophil histamine-release tests, and RAST have been used to evaluate high-risk patients. Preventing a reaction in sensitized patients includes pharmacological prophylaxis and absolute avoidance of latex. Preoperative administration of H_1 and H_2 histamine antagonists and steroids may provide some protection, although their use is controversial. Although most pieces of anesthetic equipment are now latex-free, some may still contain latex (eg, gloves, tourniquets, some ventilator bellows, intravenous injection ports, and older reusable face masks). An allergic reaction has even been documented from inhalation of latex antigen contained within aerosolized glove powder. Manufacturers of latex-containing medical products must label their products accordingly. **Only devices specifically known not to contain latex (eg, polyvinyl or neoprene gloves, silicone endotracheal tubes or laryngeal masks, plastic face masks) can be used in latex-allergic patients.** Rubber stoppers should be removed from drug vials prior to use, and injections should be made through plastic stopcocks, if latex has not been eliminated from containers and injection ports.

5. Allergies to Antibiotics

Many true drug allergies in surgical patients are due to antibiotics, mainly β-lactam antibiotics, such as penicillins and cephalosporins. Although 1% to 4% of β-lactam administrations result in allergic reactions, only 0.004% to 0.015% of these reactions result in anaphylaxis. Up to 2% of the general population is allergic to penicillin, but only 0.01% of penicillin administrations result in anaphylaxis. Cephalosporin cross-sensitivity in patients with penicillin allergy is estimated to be 2% to 7%, but a history of an anaphylactic reaction to penicillin increases the cross-reactivity rate up to 50%. Patients with a prior history of an anaphylactic reaction to penicillin should therefore not receive a cephalosporin. Although imipenem exhibits similar cross-sensitivity, aztreonam seems to be antigenically distinct and reportedly does not cross-react with other β-lactams. Sulfonamide allergy is also relatively common in surgical patients. Sulfa drugs include sulfonamide antibiotics, furosemide, hydrochlorothiazide, and captopril. Fortunately, the frequency of cross-reactivity among these agents is low.

Like cephalosporins, vancomycin is commonly used for antibiotic prophylaxis in surgical patients. Unfortunately, it is associated with adverse reactions. An anaphylactoid-type reaction, "red man syndrome," consists of intense pruritus, flushing, and erythema of the head and upper torso, often with arterial hypotension; this syndrome seems to be related to a rapid rate of administration more than to dose or allergy. Isolated systemic hypotension is a much more frequent side effect and seems to be primarily mediated by histamine release, because pretreatment with H_1 and H_2 antihistamines can prevent hypotension, even with rapid rates of administration.

Immunologic mechanisms are associated with other perioperative pathologies. Transfusion-related lung injury may be secondary to the activity of antibodies in the donor plasma, producing a hypersensitivity reaction that results in lung infiltrates and respiratory failure. IgG antibody formation directed at heparin–PF4 complexes results in platelet activation, thrombosis, and heparin-induced thrombocytopenia.

OCCUPATIONAL HAZARDS IN ANESTHESIOLOGY

Anesthesiologists spend much of their workday exposed to anesthetic gases, low-dose ionizing radiation, electromagnetic fields, blood products,

TABLE 54–9 Relative rate ratios for drug and suicide deaths comparing anesthesiologists with internists before and after January 1, 1987.

		Anesthesiologists (N)	Internists (N)	RR[1]	95% CI
All drug-related deaths	<1987	36	14	2.65	1.42–4.91
	≥1987	55	19	2.87	1.71–4.84
Drug-related suicides	<1987	16	11	1.48	0.69–3.20
	≥1987	32	11	2.88	1.45–5.71
Suicides	<1987	41	33	1.25	0.79–1.97
	≥1987	62	38	1.60	1.07–2.39

CI, confidence interval.

[1]Ratio (RR) of anesthesiologists compared with internists for that time period, RR is adjusted for age, gender, and race.

Reproduced, with permission, from Alexander B, Checkoway H, Nagahama S, Domino K: Cause-specific mortality risks of anesthesiologists. Anesthesiology 2000;93:922.

and workplace stress. Each of these can contribute to negative health effects in anesthesia practitioners. A 2000 paper compared the mortality risks of anesthesiologists and internists. Death from heart disease or cancer did not differ between the groups; however, anesthesiologists had an increased rate of suicides and drug-related deaths (Table 54–9). Anesthesiologists also had a greater chance of death from external causes, such as boating, bicycling, and aeronautical accidents compared with internists. Nevertheless, both anesthesiologists and internists had lower mortality than the general population, likely due to their higher socioeconomic status. Anesthesiologists' access to intravenous opioids likely contributes to a 2.21 relative risk for drug-related deaths compared with that of internists.

1. Chronic Exposure to Anesthetic Gases

9 There is no clear evidence that exposure to trace amounts of anesthetic agents presents a health hazard to operating room personnel. However, because previous studies examining this issue have yielded flawed but conflicting results, the US Occupational Health and Safety Administration continues to set maximum acceptable trace concentrations of less than 25 ppm for nitrous oxide and 0.5 ppm for halogenated anesthetics (2 ppm if the halogenated agent is used alone). Achieving these

low levels depends on efficient scavenging equipment, adequate operating room ventilation, and conscientious anesthetic technique. Most people cannot detect the odor of volatile agents at a concentration of less than 30 ppm. If there is no functioning scavenging system, anesthetic gas concentrations reach 3000 ppm for nitrous oxide and 50 ppm for volatile agents.

Early studies indicated that female operating room staff might be at increased risk of spontaneous abortion compared with other women. It is unclear if other factors related to operating room activity could also contribute to the possibly increased potential for pregnancy loss.

2. Infectious Diseases

Hospital workers are exposed to many infectious diseases prevalent in the community (eg, respiratory viral infections, rubella, and tuberculosis).

Herpetic whitlow is an infection of the finger with herpes simplex virus type 1 or 2 and usually involves direct contact of previously traumatized skin with contaminated oral secretions. Painful vesicles appear at the site of infection. The diagnosis is confirmed by the appearance of giant epithelial cells or nuclear inclusion bodies in a smear taken from the base of a vesicle, the presence of a rise in herpes simplex virus titer, or identification of the virus with antiserum. Treatment is conservative and includes topical application of 5% acyclovir ointment. Prevention involves wearing gloves when contacting oral secretions. Patients at risk of harboring the virus include those suffering from other infections, immunosuppression, cancer, and malnutrition. The risk of this condition has virtually disappeared now that anesthesia personnel routinely wear gloves during manipulation of the airway, which was not the case in the 1980s and earlier.

Viral DNA has been identified in the smoke plume generated during laser treatment of condylomata. The theoretical possibility of viral transmission from this source can be minimized by using smoke evacuators, gloves, and appropriate OSHA approved masks.

More disturbing is the potential of acquiring serious blood-borne infections, such as hepatitis B, hepatitis C, or human immunodeficiency virus (HIV). Although parenteral transmission of these diseases can occur following mucous membrane, cutaneous, or percutaneous exposure to infected body fluids, accidental injury with a needle contaminated with infected blood represents the most common occupational mechanism. The risk of transmission can be estimated if three factors are known: the prevalence of the infection within the patient population, the incidence of exposure (eg, frequency of needlestick), and the rate of seroconversion after a single exposure. The seroconversion rate after a specific exposure depends on several factors, including the infectivity of the organism, the stage of the patient's disease (extent of viremia), the size of the inoculum, and the immune status of the healthcare provider. Rates of seroconversion following a single needlestick are estimated to range between 0.3% and 30%. Hollow (hypodermic) needles pose a greater risk than do solid (surgical) needles because of the potentially larger inoculum. The use of gloves, needleless systems, or protected needle devices may decrease the incidence of some (but not all) types of injury.

The initial management of needlesticks involves cleaning the wound and notifying the appropriate authority within the health care facility. After an exposure, anesthesia workers should report to their institution's emergency or employee health department for appropriate counseling on postexposure prophylaxis options. All OR staff should be made aware of the institution's employee health notification pathway for needle stick and other injuries

Fulminant hepatitis B (1% of acute infections) carries a 60% mortality rate. Chronic active hepatitis (<5% of all cases) is associated with an increased incidence of cirrhosis of the liver and hepatocellular carcinoma. Transmission of the virus is primarily through contact with blood products or body fluids. The diagnosis is confirmed by detection of hepatitis B surface antigen (HBsAg). Uncomplicated recovery is signaled by the disappearance of HBsAg and the appearance of antibody to the surface antigen (anti-HBs). A hepatitis B vaccine is available and is strongly recommended prophylactically for anesthesia personnel. The appearance of anti-HBs after a three-dose regimen indicates successful immunization.

Hepatitis C is another important occupational hazard in anesthesiology; 4% to 8% of hepatitis C infections occur in healthcare workers. Most (50% to 90%) of these infections lead to chronic hepatitis, which, although often asymptomatic, can progress to liver failure and death. In fact, hepatitis C is the most common cause of nonalcoholic cirrhosis in the United States. There is currently no vaccine to protect against hepatitis C infection.

Anesthesia personnel seem to be at a low, but measureable, risk for the occupational contraction of HIV. The risk of acquiring HIV infection following a single needlestick contaminated with blood from an HIV-infected patient has been estimated at 0.4% to 0.5%. Because there are documented reports of transmission of HIV from infected patients to healthcare workers (including anesthesiologists), the Centers for Disease Control and Prevention proposed guidelines that apply to all categories of patient contact. These universal precautions, which are equally valid for protection against hepatitis B or C infection, are as follows:

- No recapping and the immediate disposal of contaminated needles
- Use of gloves and other barriers during contact with open wounds and body fluids
- Frequent hand washing

- Use of proper techniques for disinfection or the disposal of contaminated materials
- Particular caution by pregnant healthcare workers, and no contact with patients by workers who have exudative or weeping skin lesions

3. Substance Abuse

11 Anesthesiology is a high-risk medical specialty for substance abuse. Probable reasons for this include the stress of anesthetic practice and the easy availability of drugs with addiction potential (potentially attracting people at risk of addiction to the field). The likelihood of developing substance abuse is increased by coexisting personal problems (eg, marital or financial difficulties) or a family history of alcoholism or drug addiction.

The voluntary use of nonprescribed mood-altering pharmaceuticals is a disease. If left untreated, substance abuse often leads to death from drug overdose—intentional or unintentional. One of the greatest challenges in treating drug abuse is identifying the afflicted individual, as denial is a consistent feature. Unfortunately, changes evident to an outside observer are often both vague and late: reduced involvement in social activities, subtle changes in appearance, extreme mood swings, and altered work habits. Treatment begins with a careful, well-planned intervention. Those inexperienced in this area would be well advised to consult with their local medical society or licensing authority about how to proceed. The goal is to enroll the individual in a formal rehabilitation program. The possibility that one may lose one's medical license and be unable to return to practice provides powerful motivation. Some diversion programs report a success rate of approximately 70%; however, most rehabilitation programs report a recurrence rate of at least 25%. Long-term compliance often involves continued participation in support groups (eg, Narcotics Anonymous), random urine testing, and oral naltrexone therapy (a long-acting opioid antagonist). Effective prevention strategies are difficult to formulate; "better" control of drug availability is unlikely to deter a determined individual. It is unlikely that education about the severe consequences of substance abuse will bring new information to the potential drug-abusing

physician. There remains controversy regarding the rate at which anesthesia staff will experience recidivism. Many experts argue for a "one strike and you're out" policy for anesthesiology residents who abuse injectable drugs. The decision as to whether a fully trained and certified physician who has been discovered to abuse injectable drugs should return to anesthetic practice after completing a rehabilitation program varies and depends on the rules and traditions of the practice group, the medical center, the relevant medical licensing board, and the perceived likelihood of recidivism. Physicians returning to practice following successful completion of a program must be carefully monitored over the long term, as relapses can occur years after apparent successful rehabilitation. Alcohol abuse is a common problem among physicians and nurses, and anesthesia personnel are no exception. Interventions for alcohol abuse, as is true for injectable drug abuse, must be carefully orchestrated. Guidance from the local medical society or licensing authority is highly recommended.

4. Ionizing Radiation Exposure

The use of imaging equipment (eg, fluoroscopy) during surgery and interventional radiologic procedures exposes the anesthesiologist to the potential **12** risks of ionizing radiation. The three most important methods of minimizing radiation doses are limiting total exposure time during procedures, using proper barriers, and maximizing the distance from the source of radiation. Anesthesiologists who routinely perform fluoroscopic image guided invasive procedures should consider wearing protective eyeware incorporating radiation shielding. Lead glass partitions or lead aprons with thyroid shields are mandatory protection for all personnel who are exposed to ionizing radiation. The inverse square law states that the dosage of radiation varies inversely with the square of the distance. Thus, the exposure at 4 m will be one-sixteenth that at 1 m. The maximum recommended occupational whole-body exposure to radiation is 5 rem/yr. This can be monitored with an exposure badge. The health impact on operating room personnel of exposure to electromagnetic radiation remains unclear.

CASE DISCUSSION

Unexplained Intraoperative Tachycardia & Hypertension

A 73-year-old man is scheduled for emergency relief of an intestinal obstruction from a sigmoid volvulus. The patient had a myocardial infarction 1 month earlier that was complicated by congestive heart failure. His blood pressure is 160/90 mm Hg, pulse 110 beats/min, respiratory rate 22 breaths/min, and temperature 38.8°C.

Why is this case an emergency?

Strangulation of the bowel begins with venous obstruction, but can quickly progress to arterial occlusion, ischemia, infarction, and perforation. Acute peritonitis could lead to severe dehydration, sepsis, shock, and multiorgan failure.

What special monitoring is appropriate for this patient?

Because of the history of recent myocardial infarction and congestive heart failure, an arterial line would be useful. Transesophageal echocardiography and pulse contour analysis monitors of cardiac output could be used. Pulmonary arterial flotation catheters have often been used in the past, but they are associated with significant complications and current evidence does not indicate that their use improves patient outcomes. Large fluid shifts should be anticipated. Furthermore, information regarding myocardial supply (diastolic blood pressure) and demand (systolic blood pressure, left ventricular wall stress, and heart rate) should be continuously available. Central venous pressure may not track left atrial pressure in a patient with significant left ventricular dysfunction.

What cardiovascular medications might be useful during induction and maintenance of general anesthesia?

Drugs causing severe tachycardia or extremes in arterial blood pressure should be avoided.

During the laparotomy, gradual increases in heart rate and blood pressure are noted. ST-segment elevations appear on the electrocardiogram. A nitroglycerin infusion is started. The heart rate is now 130 beats/min, and the blood pressure is 220/140 mm Hg. The concentration of volatile anesthetic is increased, and metoprolol is administered intravenously in 1-mg increments. This results in a decline in heart rate to 115 beats/min, with no change in blood pressure. Suddenly, the rhythm converts to ventricular tachycardia, with a profound drop in blood pressure. As amiodarone is being administered and the defibrillation unit prepared, the rhythm degenerates into ventricular fibrillation.

What can explain this series of events?

A differential diagnosis of pronounced tachycardia and hypertension might include pheochromocytoma, malignant hyperthermia, or thyroid storm. In this case, further inspection of the nitroglycerin infusion reveals a labeling error: although the tubing was labeled "nitroglycerin," the infusion bag was labeled "epinephrine."

How does this explain the paradoxic response to metoprolol?

Metoprolol is a β_1-adrenergic antagonist. It inhibits epinephrine's β_1-stimulation of heart rate, but does not antagonize α-induced vasoconstriction. The net result is a decrease in heart rate, but a sustained increase in blood pressure.

What is the cause of the ventricular tachycardia?

An overdose of epinephrine can cause life-threatening ventricular arrhythmias. In addition, if the central venous catheter was malpositioned, with its tip in the right ventricle, the catheter tip could have stimulated ventricular arrhythmias.

What other factors may have contributed to this anesthetic mishap?

Multiple factors will often combine to create an anesthetic misadventure. Incorrect drug labels are but one example of errors that can result in patient injury. Inadequate preparation, technical failures, knowledge deficits, and practitioner fatigue or distraction can all contribute to adverse outcomes. Careful adherence to hospital policies, checklists, patient identification procedures, and surgical and regional block timeouts can all help to prevent iatrogenic complications.

GUIDELINES

Practice advisory for the prevention of perioperative peripheral neuropathies: a report by the American Society of Anesthesiologists Task Force on prevention of peripheral neuropathies. Anesthesiology 2000;92:1168.

SUGGESTED READING

Alexander B, Checkoway H, Nagahama S, Domino K: Cause-specific mortality risks of anesthesiologists. Anesthesiology 2000;93:922.

Berge E, Seppala M, Lanier W: The anesthesiology community's approach to opioid and anesthetic abusing personnel: time to change course. Anesthesiology 2008;109:762.

Bhananker S, Posner K, Cheney F, et al: Injury and liability associated with monitored anesthesia care. Anesthesiology 2006;104:228.

Bhananker S, Liau D, Kooner P, et al: Liability related to peripheral venous and arterial catheterization; a closed claims analysis. Anesth Analg 2009;109:124.

Bishop M, Souders J, Peterson C, et al: Factors associated with unanticipated day of surgery deaths in Department of Veterans Affairs hospitals. Anesth Analg 2008;107:1924.

Bowdle TA: Drug administration errors from the ASA closed claims project. ASA Newslett 2003;67:11.

Brown RH, Schauble JF, Miller NR: Anemia and hypotension as contributors to perioperative loss of vision. Anesthesiology 1994;80:222.

Bryson E, Silverstein J: Addiction and substance abuse in anesthesiology. Anesthesiology 2008;109:905.

Caplan RA, Ward RJ, Posner K, Cheney FW: Unexpected cardiac arrest during spinal anesthesia: a closed claims analysis of predisposing factors. Anesthesiology 1988;68:5.

Caplan RA, Vistica MF, Posner KL, Cheney FW: Adverse anesthetic outcomes arising from gas delivery equipment: a closed claims analysis. Anesthesiology 1997;87:741.

Chadwick HS: An analysis of obstetric anesthesia cases from the American Society of Anesthesiologists closed claims project database. Int J Obstet Anesth 1996;5:258.

Cheesman K, Brady J, Flood P, Li G: Epidemiology of anesthesia-related complications in labor and delivery, New York state, 2002-2005. Anesth Analg 2009;109:1174.

Cheney FW: The American Society of Anesthesiologists closed claims project: what have we learned, how has it affected practice, and how will it affect practice in the future? Anesthesiology 1999;91:552.

Cheney FW, Posner KL, Caplan RA, Gild WM: Burns from warming devices in anesthesia. Anesthesiology 1994;80:806.

Cheney FW, Domino KB, Caplan RA, Posner KL: Nerve injury associated with anesthesia: a closed claims analysis. Anesthesiology 1999;90:1062.

Cheney F, Posner K, Lee L, et al: Trends in anesthesia-related death and brain damage. Anesthesiology 2006;105:1071.

Cook T, Bland L, Mihai R, Scott S: Litigation related to anaesthesia: an analysis of claims against the NHS in England 1995-2007. Anaesthesia 2009;64:706.

Cook T, Scott S, Mihai R: Litigation related to airway and respiratory complications of anaesthesia: an analysis of claims against the NHS in England 1995-2007. Anaesthesia 2010;65:556.

Coppieters MW, Van De Velde M, Stappaerts KH: Positioning in anesthesiology. Toward a better understanding of stretch-induced perioperative neuropathies. Anesthesiology 2002;97:75.

Cranshaw J, Gupta K, Cook T: Litigation related to drug errors in anaesthesia: an analysis of claims against the NHS in England 1995-2009. Anaesthesia 2009;64:1317.

Crosby E: Medical malpractice and anesthesiology: literature review and role of the expert witness. Can J Anesth 2007;54:227.

Davies J, Posner K, Lee L, et al: Liability associated with obstetric anesthesia. Anesthesiology 2009;110:131.

Domino KB, Posner Kl, Caplan RA, Cheney FW: Awareness during anesthesia: a closed claims analysis. Anesthesiology 1999;90:1053.

Domino KB, Posner KL, Caplan RA, Cheney FW: Airway injury during anesthesia: a closed claims analysis. Anesthesiology 1999;91:1703.

Domino K, Bowdle T, Posner K, et al: Injuries and liability related to central vascular catheters. Anesthesiology 2004;100:1411.

Edbril SD, Lagasse RS: Relationship between malpractice litigation and human errors. Anesthesiology 1999;91:848.

Fisher DM: New York State guidelines on the topical use of phenylephrine in operating rooms. Anesthesiology 2000;92:858.

Fitzgibbon DR, Posner KL, Domino KB, et al: Chronic pain management: American Society of Anesthesiologists Closed Claims Project. Anesthesiology 2004;100:98.

Gayer S: Prone to blindness: answers to postoperative visual loss. Anesth Analg 2011;112:11.

Ghoneim MM: Awareness during anesthesia. Anesthesiology 2000;92:597.

Gild WM, Posner KL, Caplan RA, Cheney FW: Eye injuries associated with anesthesia. Anesthesiology 1992;76:204.

Hawkins J, Chang J, Palmer S, et al: Anesthesia-related maternal mortality in the United States: 1979-2002. Obstet Gynecol 2011;117:69.

Hepner DL, Castells MC: Anaphylaxis during the perioperative period. Anesth Analg 2003;97:1381.

Jimenez N, Posner K, Cheney F, et al: An update on pediatric anesthesia liability: a closed claims analysis. Anesth Analg 2007;104:147.

Lagasse R: Anesthesia safety: model or myth? Anesthesiology 2002;97:1336.

Lagasse R: To see or not to see. Anesthesiology 2006; 105:1971.

Lagasse R: Innocent prattle. Anesthesiology 2009;110:698.

Lee LA: Postoperative visual loss data gathered and analyzed. ASA Newslett 2000;64:25.

Lee L, Posner K, DominoK, et al: Injuries associated with regional anesthesia in the 1980s and 1990s. Anesthesiology 2004;101:143.

Lee L, Posner K, Cheney F, et al: Complications associated with eye blocks and peripheral nerve blocks: an American Society of Anesthesiologists Closed Claims analysis. Reg Anesth Pain Med 2008;33:416.

Lee LA, Rothe S, Posner KL, et al: The American Society of Anesthesiologists Postoperative Visual Loss Registry: analysis of 93 spine surgery cases with postoperative visual loss. Anesthesiology 2006;105:652.

Lesser JB, Sanborn KV, Valskys R, Kuroda M: Severe bradycardia during spinal and epidural anesthesia recorded by an anesthesia information management system. Anesthesiology 2003;99:859.

Levy J, Adkinson N: Anaphylaxis during cardiac surgery: implications for clinicians. Anesth Analg 2008;106:392.

Li G, Warner M, Lang B, et al: Epidemiology of anesthesia related mortality in the United States 1999-2005. Anesthesiology 2009;110:759.

Liang B: "Standards" of anesthesia: law and ASA guidelines. J Clin Anesth 2008;20:393.

Lineberger C: Impairment in anesthesiology: awareness and education. Int Anesth Clin 2008;46:151.

Marco A: Informed consent for surgical anesthesia care: has the time come for separate consent? Anesth Analg 2009;110:280.

Martin L, Mhyre J, Shanks A, et al: 3,423 emergency tracheal intubations at a university hospital: airway outcomes and complications. Anesthesiology 2011;114:42.

Martin JT: Compartment syndromes: concepts and perspectives for the anesthesiologist. Anesth Analg 1992;75:275.

Metzner J, Posner K, Domino K: The risk and safety of anesthesia at remote locations: the US closed claims analysis. Curr Opin Anaesthesiol 2009;22:502.

Monitto C, Hamilton R, Levey E, et al: Genetic predisposition to natural rubber latex allergy differs between health care workers and high risk patients. Anesth Analg 2010;110:1310.

Morray JP, Geiduschek JM, Caplan RA: A comparison of pediatric and adult anesthesia closed malpractice claims. Anesthesiology 1993;78:461.

Newland MC, Ellis SJ, Lydiatt CA, et al: Anesthetic-related cardiac arrest and its mortality. Anesthesiology 2002;97:108.

Pollard JB: Cardiac arrest during spinal anesthesia: common mechanisms and strategies for prevention. Anesth Analg 2001;92:252.

Ramamoorthy C, Haberkern C, Bhananker S, et al: Anesthesia-related cardiac arrest in children with heart disease: data from the pediatric perioperative cardiac arrest (POCA) registry. Anesth Analg 2010;110:1376.

Ranta SOV, Lauila R, Saario J, et al: Awareness with recall during general anesthesia: incidence and risk factors. Anesth Analg 1998;86:1084.

Roh J, Kim D, Lee S, et al: Intensity of extremely low frequency electromagnetic fields produced in operating rooms during surgery at the standing position of anesthesiologists. Anesthesiology 2009;111:275.

Rose G, Brown R: The impaired anesthesiologist: not just about drugs and alcohol anymore. J Clin Anesthesiol 2010;22:379.

Sharma AD, Parmley CL, Sreeram G, Grocott HP: Peripheral nerve injuries during cardiac surgery: risk factors, diagnosis, prognosis, and prevention. Anesth Analg 2000;91:1358.

Silverstein JH, Silva DA, Iberti TJ: Opioid addiction in anesthesiology. Anesthesiology 1993;79:354.

Sprung J, Bourke DL, Contreras MG, et al: Perioperative hearing impairment. Anesthesiology 2003;98:241.

Tait AR: Occupational transmission of tuberculosis: implications for anesthesiologists. Anesth Analg 1997;85:444.

Warner MA, Warner ME, Martin JT: Ulnar neuropathy. Incidence, outcome, and risk factors in sedated or anesthetized patients. Anesthesiology 1994;81:1332.

Warner MA, Warner DO, Harper CM: Lower extremity neuropathies associated with lithotomy positions. Anesthesiology 2000;93:938.

Warner ME, Benenfeld SM, Warner MA, et al: Perianesthetic dental injuries. Anesthesiology 1999;90:1302.

Weinger MB, Englund CE: Ergonomic and human factors affecting anesthetic vigilance and monitoring performance in the operating room environment. Anesthesiology 1990;73:995.

Welch M, Brummett C, Welch T, et al: Perioperative nerve injuries: a retrospective study of 380,680 cases during a 10-year period at a single institution. Anesthesiology 2009;111:490.

Williams EL, Hart WM Jr, Tempelhoff R: Postoperative ischemic optic neuropathy. Anesth Analg 1995;80:1018.

Yuill G, Saroya D, Yuill S: A national survey of the provision for patients with latex allergy. Anaesthesiology 2003;58:775.

Cardiopulmonary Resuscitation

Martin Giesecke, MD and Srikanth Hosur, MBBS, MD

1 Cardiopulmonary resuscitation and emergency cardiac care should be considered any time an individual cannot adequately oxygenate or perfuse vital organs—not only following cardiac or respiratory arrest.

2 Regardless of which transtracheal jet ventilation system is chosen, it must be readily available, use low-compliance tubing, and have secure connections.

3 Chest compressions and ventilation should not be delayed for intubation if a patent airway is established by a jaw-thrust maneuver.

4 Attempts at intubation should not interrupt ventilation for more than 10 s.

5 Chest compressions should be immediately initiated in the pulseless patient.

6 Whether adult resuscitation is performed by a single rescuer or by two rescuers, two breaths are administered every 30 compressions (30:2), allowing 3–4 s for each two breaths. The cardiac compression rate should be 100/min regardless of the number of rescuers.

7 Health care personnel working in hospitals and ambulatory care facilities must be able to provide early defibrillation to collapsed patients with ventricular fibrillation as soon as possible. Shock should be delivered within 3 min ($\pm$ 1 min) of arrest.

8 Lidocaine, epinephrine, atropine, naloxone, and vasopressin, but not sodium bicarbonate, can be delivered via a catheter whose tip extends past the tracheal tube. Dosages 2–2½ times higher than recommended for intravenous use, diluted in 10 mL of normal saline or distilled water, are recommended for adult patients.

9 If intravenous cannulation is difficult, an intraosseous infusion can provide emergency vascular access in children.

10 Because carbon dioxide, but not bicarbonate, readily crosses cell membranes and the blood–brain barrier, the resulting arterial hypercapnia will cause intracellular tissue acidosis.

11 A wide QRS complex following a pacing spike signals electrical capture, but mechanical (ventricular) capture must be confirmed by an improving pulse or blood pressure.

One goal of anesthesiology is to maintain the function of vital organ systems during surgery. It is not surprising, therefore, that anesthesiologists have played a major role in the development of cardiopulmonary resuscitation techniques outside the operating room.

1 Cardiopulmonary resuscitation and emergency cardiac care (CPR-ECC) should be considered any time an individual cannot adequately oxygenate or perfuse vital organs—not only following cardiac or respiratory arrest.

TABLE 55–1 Emergency cardiac care (ECC).

1. Recognition of impending event
2. Activation of emergency response system
3. Basic life support
4. Defibrillation
5. Ventilation
6. Pharmacotherapy

This chapter presents an overview of the American Heart Association (AHA) and the International Liaison Committee on Resuscitation (ILCOR) Year 2010 recommendations for establishing and maintaining the ABCDs of cardiopulmonary resuscitation: Airway, Breathing, Circulation, and Defibrillation (Table 55–1, Figures 55–1 and 55–2). The 2010 CPR-ECC guidelines have been updated with new evidence-based recommendations. Still of import to the layperson are that the pulse should not be checked, and chest compression without ventilation may be as effective as compression with ventilation for the first several minutes. If a lay rescuer is unwilling to perform mouth-to-mouth ventilation, chest compressions alone are preferred to doing nothing. For the health care provider, defibrillation using biphasic electrical current works best and tracheal tube (TT) placement should be confirmed with a quantitative capnographic waveform analysis. More importantly, in the new guidelines, emphasis has been placed on the quality and adequacy of compressions, minimizing interruption time of compressions and the preshock pause (the time taken from the last compression to the delivery of shock).

The sequence of steps in resuscitation has been changed in the 2010 guidelines from *ABC* (airway and breathing first, before compression) to *CAB* (compression first, with airway and breathing treated later). Emphasis has also been placed on physiological monitoring methods to optimize CPR quality and return of spontaneous circulation (ROSC). The rule of tens and multiples can be applied: less than 10 s to check for pulse, less than 10 s to place and secure the airway, target chest compression adequacy to maintain end-tidal pressure of carbon dioxide (P_{ETCO_2}) greater than 10, and target chest compression to maintain arterial diastolic blood pressure greater than 20 and central venous oxygen saturation (S_{CVO_2}) greater than 30.

Changes in drug recommendations are notable for exclusion of atropine in the settings of pulseless electrical activity (PEA) and asystole, addition of the use of chronotropic drug infusions as an alternative to pacing in unstable/symptomatic bradycardia, and recommendation for use of adenosine in the management of wide-complex monomorphic tachycardia.

This chapter is not intended as a substitute for a formal course in either life support without the use of special equipment (Basic Life Support [BLS]) or with the use of special equipment and drugs (Advanced Cardiac Life Support [ACLS]). The recommendations described are for infants, children, and adults; resuscitation of neonates is discussed in Chapter 42.

AIRWAY

Although the *A* of the mnemonic *ABC* stands for *airway,* it should also stand for the initial *assessment* of the patient. Before CPR is initiated, unresponsiveness is established and the emergency response system is activated. During low blood flow states such as cardiac arrest, oxygen delivery to the heart and brain is limited by blood flow rather than by arterial oxygen content; thus, in the new guidelines, greater emphasis is placed on immediate initiation of chest compressions than on rescuer breaths.

The patient is positioned supine on a firm surface. After initiation of chest compressions, the airway is evaluated. The airway is most commonly obstructed by posterior displacement of the tongue or epiglottis. If there is no evidence of cervical spine instability, a head-tilt chin-lift should be tried first (Figure 55–3). One hand (palm) is placed on the patient's forehead applying pressure to tilt the head back while lifting the chin with the forefinger and index finger of the opposite hand. The jaw-thrust may be more effective in opening the airway and is executed by placing both hands on either side of the patient's head, grasping the angles of the jaw, and lifting. Basic airway management is discussed in detail in Chapter 19, and the trauma patient is considered in Chapter 39.

Any vomitus or foreign body visible in the mouth of an unconscious patient should be removed. If the patient is conscious or if the foreign body

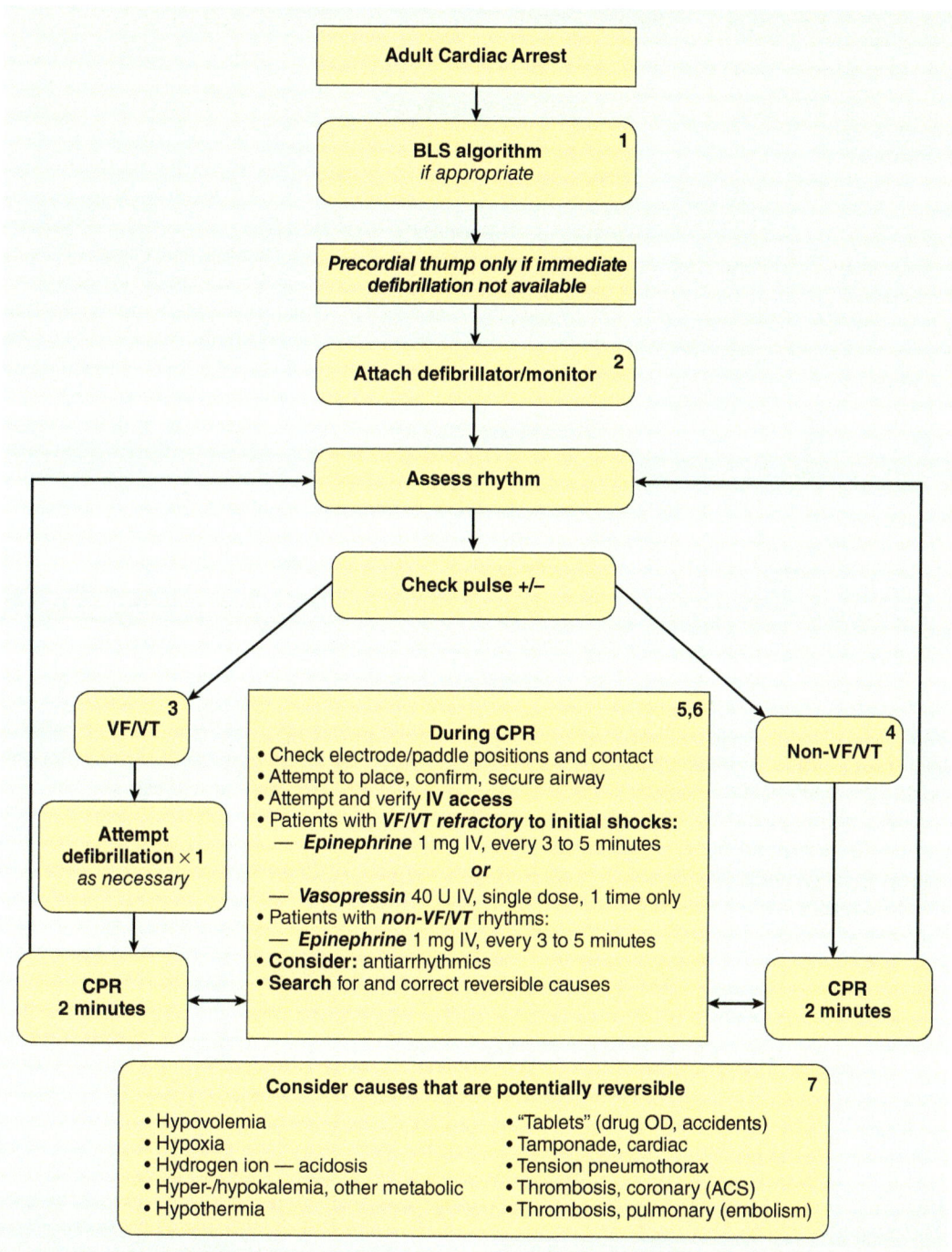

FIGURE 55-1 Universal algorithm for adult emergency cardiac care. BLS, basic life support; VF/VT, ventricular fibrillation and pulseless ventricular tachycardia; CPR, cardiopulmonary resuscitation.

(Data from The American Heart Association BLS and ACLS Guidelines 2010 for cardiopulmonary resuscitation and emergency cardiovascular care. Circulation 2010;122:S685.)

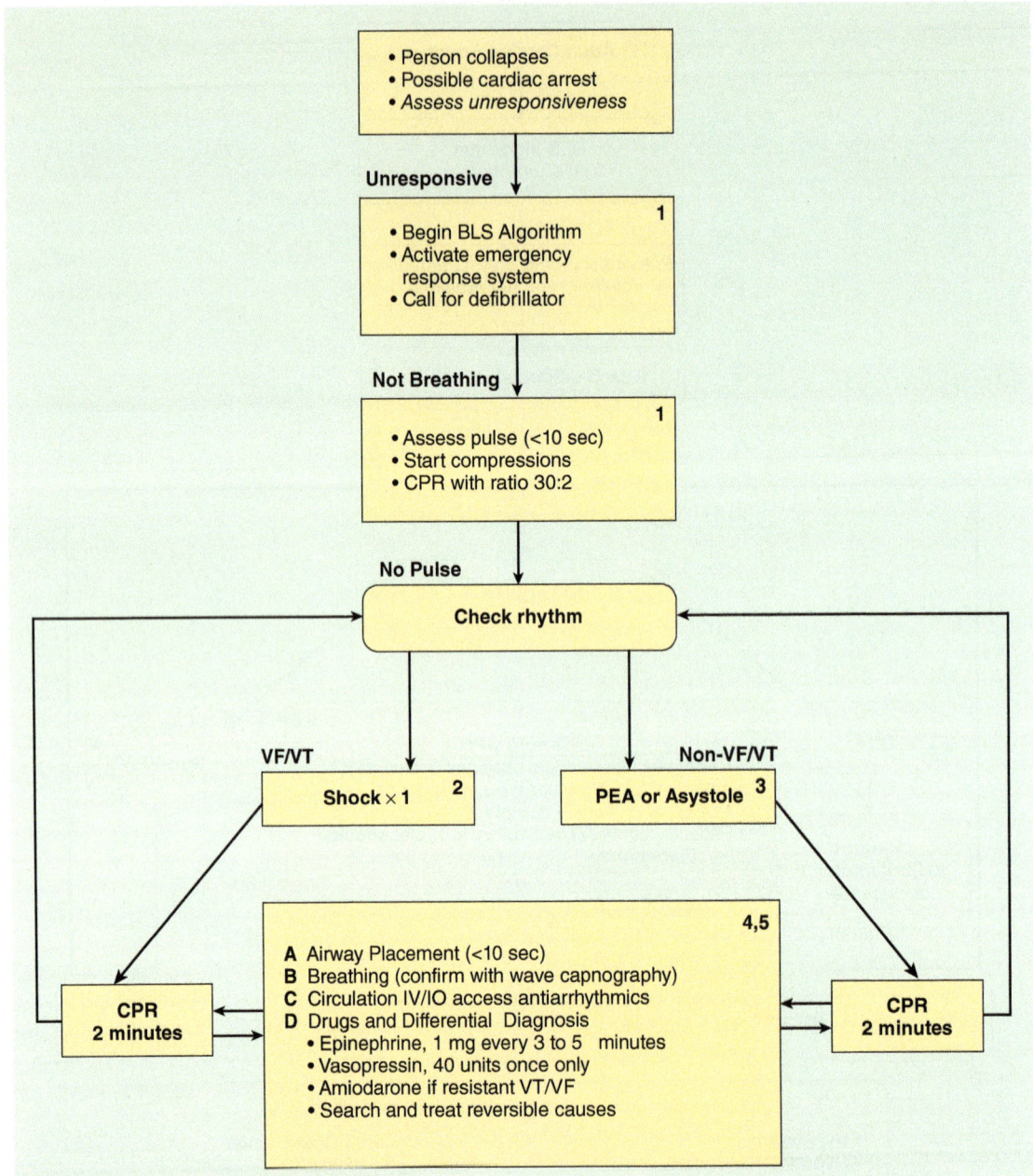

FIGURE 55–2 Comprehensive emergency cardiac care algorithm. BLS, basic life support; VF/VT, ventricular fibrillation and pulseless ventricular tachycardia; PEA, pulseless electrical activity; CPR, cardiopulmonary resuscitation. (Data from The American Heart Association BLS and ACLS Guidelines 2010 for cardiopulmonary resuscitation and emergency cardiovascular care. Circulation 2010;122:S685.)

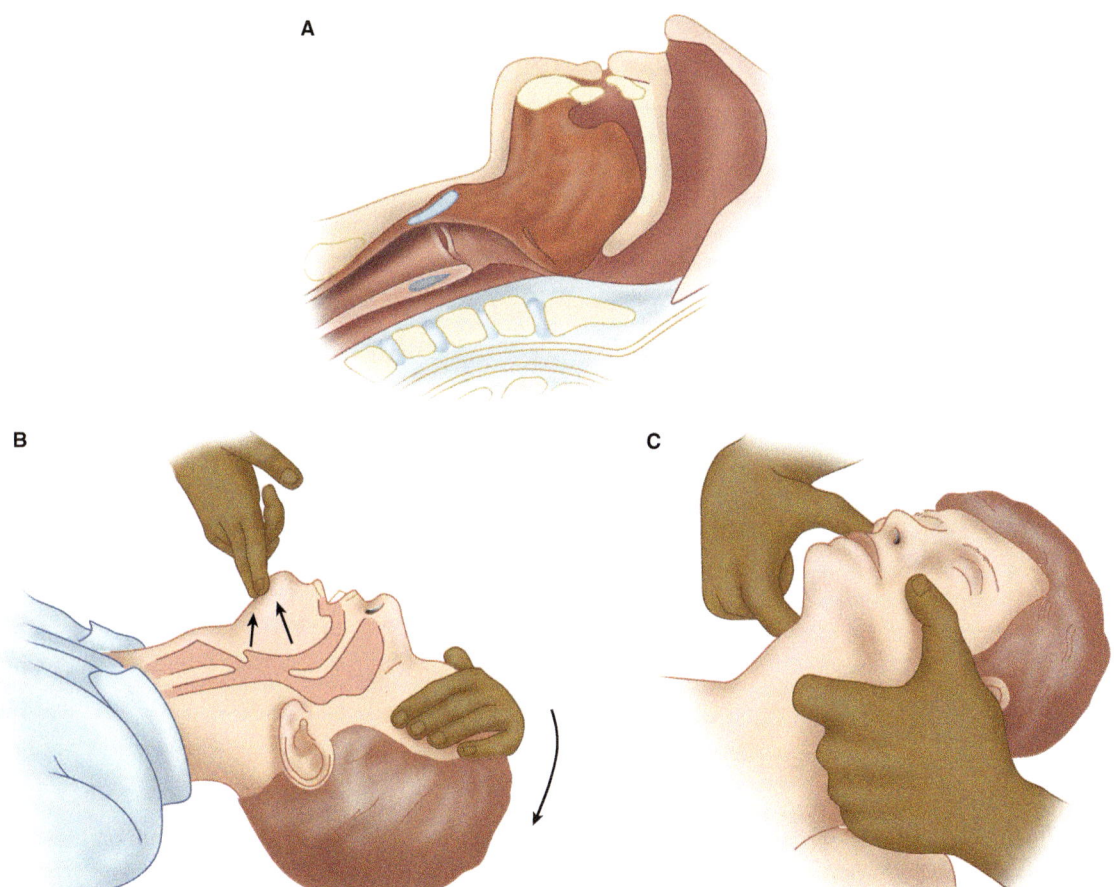

FIGURE 55–3 Loss of consciousness is often accompanied by loss of submandibular muscle tone (**A**). Occlusion of the airway by the tongue can be relieved by a head-tilt chin-lift (**B**) or a jaw-thrust (**C**). In patients with possible cervical spine injury, the angles of the jaw should be lifted anteriorly without hyperextending the neck.

cannot be removed by a finger sweep, the Heimlich maneuver is recommended. This subdiaphragmatic abdominal thrust elevates the diaphragm, expelling a blast of air from the lungs that displaces the foreign body (Figure 55–4). Complications of the Heimlich maneuver include rib fracture, trauma to the internal viscera, and regurgitation. A combination of back blows and chest thrusts is recommended to clear foreign body obstruction in infants (Table 55–2).

If after opening the airway there is no evidence of adequate breathing, the rescuer should initiate assisted ventilation, by inflating the victim's lungs with each breath using mouth-to-mouth, mouth-to-nose, mouth-to-stoma, mouth-to-barrier device, mouth-to-face shield, or mouth-to-mask rescue breathing or by using a bag-mask device (see Chapter 19). Breaths are delivered slowly (inspiratory time of ½–1 s) with a smaller tidal volume [VT] (approximately 700–1000 mL, smaller [400–600 mL] if supplemental O_2 is used) than was recommended in the past.

With positive-pressure ventilation, even with a small VT, gastric inflation with subsequent regurgitation and aspiration are possible. Therefore, as soon as it is feasible, the airway should be secured with a TT, or, if that is not possible, an alternative airway should be inserted. There is inadequate evidence to support the optimal timing of the placement of an artificial airway; however, chest compressions

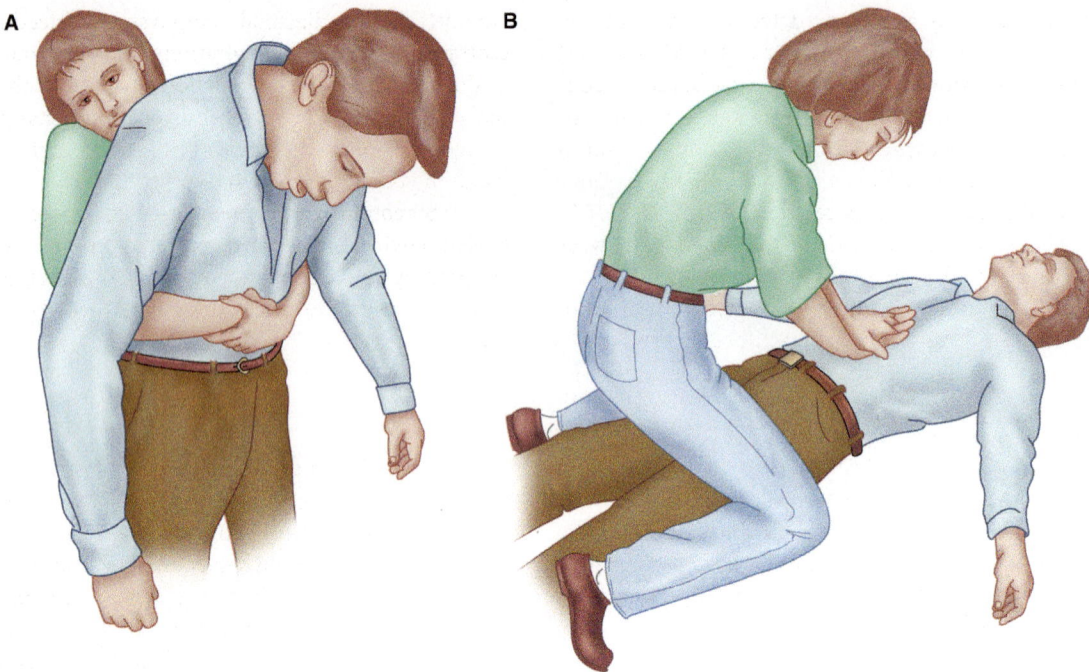

FIGURE 55–4 The Heimlich maneuver can be performed with the victim standing (**A**) or lying down (**B**). The hands are positioned slightly above the navel and well below the xiphoid process and then pressed into the abdomen with a quick upward thrust. The maneuver may need to be repeated.

should not be interrupted for more than 10 seconds to place any airway. Alternative airways include the esophageal–tracheal Combitube (ETC), laryngeal mask airway (LMA), pharyngotracheal lumen airway, King laryngeal tube, and cuffed oropharyngeal airway. The ETC and LMA, along with oral and nasopharyngeal airways, face masks, laryngoscopes, and TTs, are discussed in Chapter 19. Of these, the LMA is increasingly preferred for in-hospital arrests. The 2010 CPR-ECC guidelines recommend a TT as the airway adjunct of choice if personnel skilled in placing it are available.

Independent of which airway adjunct is used, the guidelines state that rescuers must confirm TT

TABLE 55–2 Summary of recommended basic life support techniques.

	Infant (1–12 mo)	Child (>12 mo)	Adult
Breathing rate	20 breaths/min	20 breaths/min	10–12 breaths/min[1]
Pulse check	Brachial	Carotid	Carotid
Compression rate	>100/min	100/min	100/min
Compression method	Two or three fingers	Heel of one hand	Hands interlaced
Compression/ventilation ratio	30:2	30:2	30:2
Foreign body obstruction	Back blows and chest thrusts	Heimlich maneuver	Heimlich maneuver

[1]Decrease to 8–10 breaths/min if the airway is secured with a tracheal tube.

placement with a PETCO$_2$ detector—an indicator, a capnograph, or a capnometric device. The best choice for confirmation of TT placement is continuous capnographic waveform analysis. All confirmation devices are considered adjuncts to clinical conformation techniques (eg, auscultation). Once an artificial airway is successfully placed, *it must be carefully secured with a tie or tape* (25% of airways are displaced during transportation).

Some causes of airway obstruction may not be relieved by conventional methods. Furthermore, tracheal intubation may be technically impossible to perform (eg, severe facial trauma), or repeated attempts may be unwise (eg, cervical spine trauma). In these circumstances, cricothyrotomy or tracheotomy may be necessary. Cricothyrotomy involves placing a large intravenous catheter or a commercially available cannula into the trachea through the midline of the cricothyroid membrane (Figure 55–5). Proper location is confirmed by aspiration of air. A 12- or 14-gauge catheter requires a driving pressure of 50 psi to generate sufficient gas flow (for transtracheal jet ventilation). The catheter must be adequately secured to the skin, as the jet ventilation pressure can otherwise easily propel the catheter out of the trachea.

Various systems are available that connect a high-pressure source of oxygen (eg, central wall oxygen, tank oxygen, or the anesthesia machine fresh gas outlet) to the catheter (Figure 55–6). A hand-operated jet injector or the oxygen flush valve of an anesthesia machine controls ventilation. The addition of a pressure regulator minimizes the risk of barotrauma.

2 Regardless of which transtracheal jet ventilation system is chosen, it must be readily available, use low-compliance tubing, and have secure connections. Direct connection of a 12- or 14-gauge intravenous catheter to the anesthesia circle system does not allow adequate ventilation because of the high compliance of the corrugated breathing tubing and breathing bag. One cannot reliably deliver acceptable ventilation through a 12- or 14-gauge catheter with a self-inflating resuscitation bag.

Adequacy of ventilation—particularly expiration—is judged by observation of chest wall movement and auscultation of breath sounds. Acute complications include pneumothorax, subcutaneous emphysema, mediastinal emphysema, bleeding, esophageal puncture, aspiration, and respiratory acidosis. Long-term complications include tracheomalacia, subglottic stenosis, and vocal cord changes. Cricothyrotomy is not generally recommended in children younger than 10 years of age.

Tracheotomy can be performed in a more controlled environment after oxygenation has been restored by cricothyrotomy. A detailed description of tracheotomy, however, is beyond the scope of this text.

BREATHING

Assessment of spontaneous breathing should immediately follow the opening or the establishment of **3** the airway. Chest compressions and ventilation should not be delayed for intubation if a patent airway is established by a jaw-thrust maneuver. Apnea is confirmed by lack of chest movement, absence of breath sounds, and lack of airflow. Regardless of the airway and breathing methods employed, a specific regimen of ventilation has been proposed for the apneic patient. Initially, two breaths are slowly administered (2 s per breath in adults, 1–1½ s in infants and children). If these breaths cannot be delivered, either the airway is still obstructed and the head and neck need repositioning or a foreign body is present that must be removed.

Mouth-to-mouth or mouth-to-mask (mouth-to-barrier-device) rescue breathing should be instituted in the apneic patient, even in the hospital setting when the crash cart is on its way. Pinching the nose allows formation of an airtight seal between the rescuer's lips and the outside of the victim's mouth. Successful rescue breathing (700–1000 mL V$_T$, 8–10 times per minute in an adult with a secured airway and a ratio of 30 compressions to 2 ventilations if the airway is unsecured) is confirmed by observing the chest rising and falling with each breath and hearing and feeling the escape of air during expiration. The most common cause of inadequate mouth-to-mouth ventilation is insufficient airway control. Mouth-to-mouth-and-nose breathing is more effective in infants and small children than in adults.

A rescuer's exhaled air has an oxygen concentration of only 16–17% and contains significant CO$_2$.

A Locate the cricothyroid membrane.

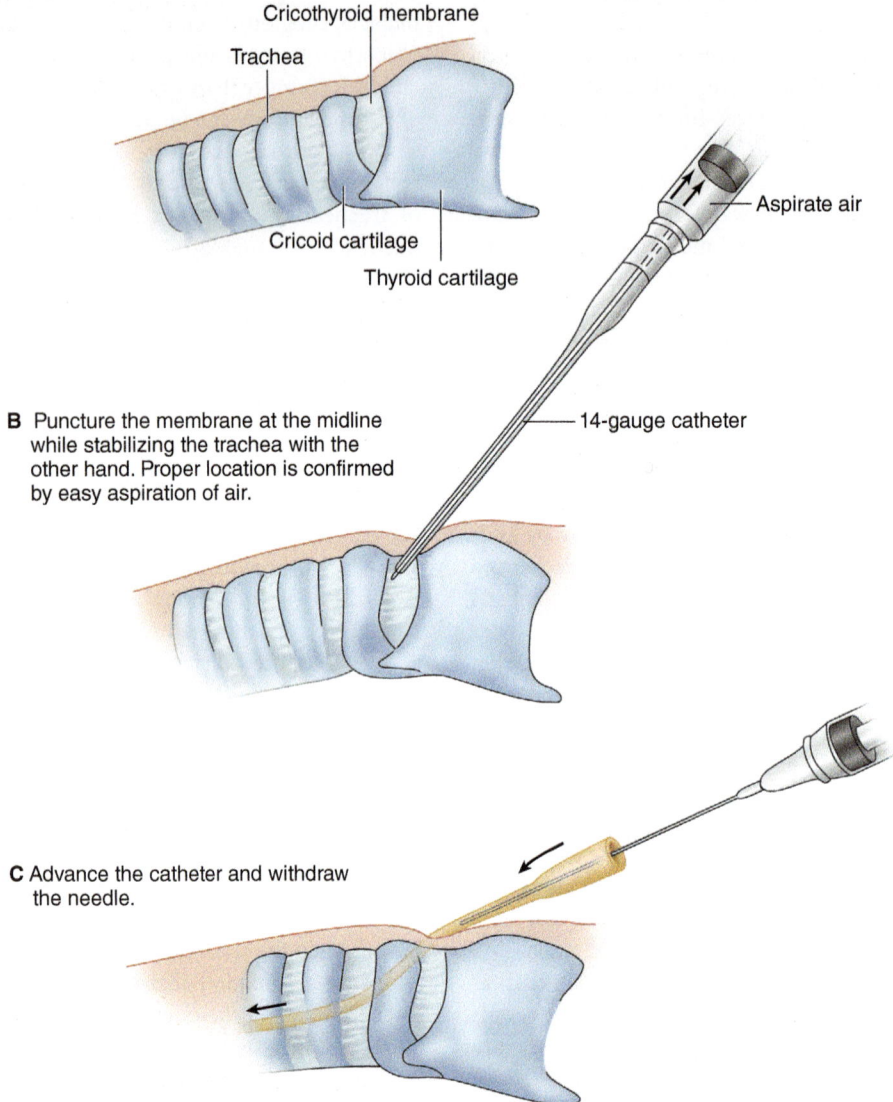

B Puncture the membrane at the midline while stabilizing the trachea with the other hand. Proper location is confirmed by easy aspiration of air.

C Advance the catheter and withdraw the needle.

FIGURE 55–5 Percutaneous cricothyrotomy with a 14-gauge over-the-needle intravenous catheter.

Supplemental oxygen, preferably 100%, should always be used if available. If supplemental oxygen is used, a smaller VT of 400–700 mL is recommended.

Mouth-to-mask or barrier device breathing has a hygienic advantage over mouth-to-mouth breathing as the rescuer's lips form a seal with an intervening device. Devices that avoid mouth-to-mouth contact should be immediately available everywhere in the hospital. Ventilation with a mask may be performed more easily in some patients because the rescuer may be able to adjust the airway or make an airtight seal more effectively. Furthermore, some mouth-to-mask devices allow the delivery of supplemental oxygen.

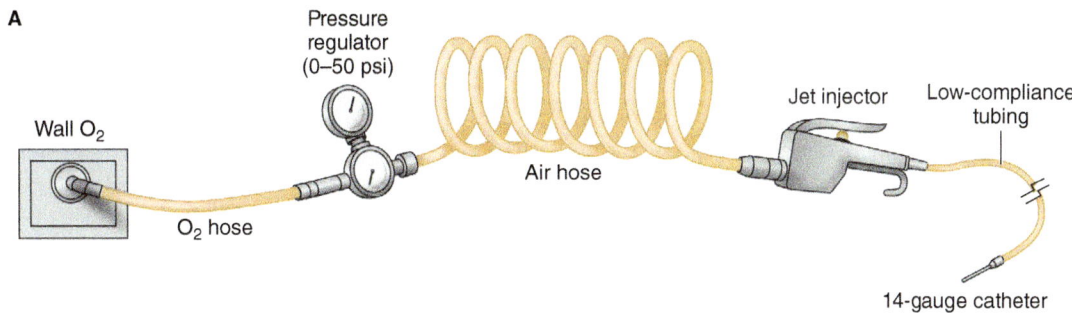

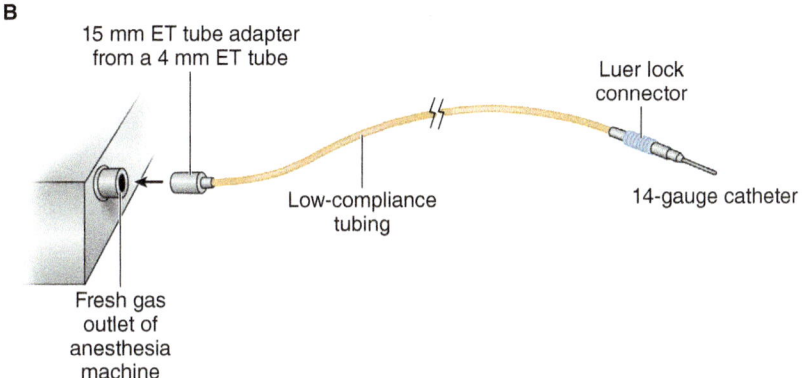

FIGURE 55–6 A,B: Two systems for transtracheal jet ventilation after cricothyrotomy (see Figure 55–5). A jet ventilator and pressure regulator (as shown in A) provide better control of the inspiratory cycle. Both systems use low-compliance tubing and a high-pressure source of oxygen.

A self-inflating bag-valve-mask device is described in Chapter 3 (see the section on Resuscitation Breathing Systems). These devices can be less effective than mouth-to-mask or bag-valve-TT ventilation because of the difficulty inexperienced personnel may have in maintaining an airway and seal with one hand and simultaneously delivering an adequate VT with the other. Use of cricoid pressure to prevent regurgitation during cardiac arrest resuscitation may be considered; however, there are no data to support its efficacy in this circumstance and its routine use is not recommended in the new guidelines.

Tracheal intubation should be attempted as soon as practical. Attempts at intubation should not interrupt ventilation for more than 10 s. After intubation, the patient can be ventilated with a self-inflating bag capable of delivering high oxygen concentrations. Because two hands are now available to squeeze the bag, ventilation should be satisfactory.

A ratio of 8–10 breaths/min in a secure airway should be maintained, as high respiratory rates can impede cardiac output in a cardiac arrest situation.

The ratio of physiological dead space to tidal volume (VD/VT) reflects the efficiency of CO_2 elimination. VD/VT increases during CPR as a result of low pulmonary blood flow and high alveolar pressures. Thus, minute ventilation may need to be increased by 50–100% once circulation is restored as CO_2 from the periphery is brought back to the lungs.

CIRCULATION

Circulation takes precedence over airway and breathing in a cardiac arrest situation. In this scenario, as previously noted, *chest compressions should begin prior to the initial breaths.* Subsequent actions to assess circulation may then vary depending on whether the responder is a lay person or health care provider. Although lay rescuers should assume that an unresponsive patient is in cardiac arrest and need not check pulse; health care providers should assess for presence or absence of a pulse.

After successful delivery of two initial breaths (each 2 s in duration), circulation is rapidly assessed. If the patient has an adequate pulse (carotid artery in an adult or child, brachial or femoral artery in an infant) or blood pressure, breathing is continued at 10–12 breaths/min for an adult or a child older than 8 years, and 20 breaths/min for an infant or a child younger than 8 years of age (Table 55–2). If the patient is pulseless or severely hypotensive, the circulatory system must be supported by a combination of external chest compressions, intravenous drug administration, and defibrillation when appropriate. Initiation of chest compressions is mandated by the inadequacy of peripheral perfusion, and drug choices and defibrillation energy levels often depend on electrocardiographic diagnosis of arrhythmias.

External Chest Compression

Chest compressions force blood to flow either by increasing intrathoracic pressure (thoracic pump) or by directly compressing the heart (cardiac pump). During CPR of short duration, the blood flow is created more by the cardiac pump mechanism; as CPR continues, the heart becomes less compliant and the thoracic pump mechanism becomes more important. As important as the rate and force of compression are for maintaining blood flow, effective perfusion of the heart and brain is best achieved when chest compression consumes 50% of the duty cycle, with the remaining 50% devoted to the relaxation phase (allowing blood return into the chest and heart).

To perform chest compressions in the unresponsive or pulseless patient, the xiphoid process is located and the heel of the rescuer's hand is placed over the lower half of the sternum. The other hand is placed over the hand on the sternum with the fingers either interlaced or extended, but off the chest. The rescuer's shoulders should be positioned directly over the hands with the elbows locked into position and arms extended, so that the weight of the upper body is used for compressions. With a straight downward thrust, the sternum is depressed 1½–2 in.

(4–5 cm) in adults, 1–1½ in. (2–4 cm) in children, and then allowed to return to its normal position. For an infant, compressions ½–1 in. (1½–2½ cm) in depth are made with the middle and ring fingers on the sternum one finger-breadth below the nipple line. Compression and release times should be equal.

6 Whether adult resuscitation is performed by a single rescuer or by two rescuers, two breaths are administered every 30 compressions (30:2), allowing 3–4 s for the two breaths. The cardiac compression rate should be 100/min regardless of the number of rescuers. A slightly higher compression rate of more than 100/min is suggested for infants, with two breaths delivered every 30 compressions.

Assessing the Adequacy of Chest Compressions

Cardiac output can be estimated by monitoring end-tidal CO_2 (P_{ETCO_2} >10 mm Hg, S_{CVO_2} >30%) or arterial pulsations (with an arterial diastolic relaxation pressure >20 mm Hg). Arterial pulsations during resuscitation are not a good measure of adequate chest compression; however, spontaneous arterial pulsations are an indicator of ROSC. There is new emphasis in the 2010 guidelines on physiological parameters, such as P_{ETCO_2}, S_{CVO_2}, and diastolic arterial pressure, to assess the adequacy of chest compressions.

1. P_{ETCO_2}—In an intubated patient, a P_{ETCO_2} greater than 10 mm Hg indicates good-quality chest compressions; a P_{ETCO_2} less than 10 mm Hg has been shown to be a predictor of poor outcomes of CPR (decreased chance of ROSC). A transient increase in P_{ETCO_2} may be seen with administration of sodium bicarbonate; however, an abrupt and sustained rise of P_{ETCO_2} is an indicator of ROSC.

2. **Coronary perfusion pressure (CPP)**—This is the difference between the aortic diastolic pressure and the right atrial diastolic pressure. Arterial diastolic pressure in the radial, brachial, or femoral artery is a good indicator of CPP. Arterial diastolic pressure greater than 20 mm Hg is an indicator of adequate chest compressions.

3. S_{CVO_2}—An S_{CVO_2} less than 30% in the jugular vein is associated with poor outcomes. If the S_{CVO_2} is less than 30%, attempts to improve the quality of CPR, either by improving the quality of compressions or

through administration of medications, should be considered.

DEFIBRILLATION

Ventricular fibrillation develops most commonly in adults who experience nontraumatic cardiac arrest. The time from collapse to defibrillation is the most important determinant of survival. The chances for survival decline 7–10% for every minute without defibrillation (Figure 55–7). Therefore, patients who have cardiac arrest should be defibrillated at the earliest possible moment. Health care personnel working in hospitals and ambulatory care facilities must be able to provide early defibrillation to collapsed patients with ventricular fibrillation as soon as possible. Shock should be delivered within 3 min (±1 min) of arrest.

There is no definite relationship between the energy requirement for successful defibrillation and body size. A shock with too low an energy (current) level will not successfully defibrillate; conversely, too high an energy level may result in functional and morphological injury. Defibrillators deliver energy in either monophasic or biphasic waveforms. Increasingly, biphasic waveforms are recommended for cardioversion as they achieve the same degree of success but with less energy and theoretically less myocardial damage.

In many institutions, automated external defibrillators (AEDs) are available. Such devices are increasingly being used throughout the community by police, firefighters, security personnel, sports marshals, ski patrol members, and airline flight attendants, among others. They are placed in any public location where 20,000 or more people pass by every day. AEDs are technologically advanced, microprocessor-based devices that are capable of electrocardiographic analysis with very high specificity and sensitivity in differentiating shockable from nonshockable rhythms. All AEDs manufactured today deliver some type of biphasic waveform shock. Compared with monophasic shocks, biphasic shocks deliver energy in two directions with equivalent efficacy at lower energy levels and possibly with less myocardial injury. These devices deliver impedance-compensating shocks employing either biphasic truncated exponential (BTE) or rectilinear (RBW) morphology. Biphasic shocks delivering low energy for defibrillation (120–200 joule [J]) have been found to be as or more effective than 200–360 J monophasic damped sine (MDS) waveform shocks. When using AEDs, one electrode pad is placed beside the upper right sternal border, just below the clavicle, and the other pad is placed just lateral to the left nipple, with the top of the pad a few inches below the axilla.

A decrease in time delay between the last compression and the delivery of a shock (the preshock pause) has received special emphasis in the new guidelines. Stacking shocks increases the time to next compression, and it has been noted that the first shock is usually associated with a 90% efficacy. Thus, stacked shocks have been replaced by a recommendation for a single shock, followed by immediate resumption of chest compressions.

For cardioversion of atrial fibrillation (Table 55–3), 120–200 J can be used initially with escalation if needed. For atrial flutter or paroxysmal supraventricular tachycardia (PSVT), an initial energy level of 50–100 J is often adequate. All monophasic shocks should start with 200 J.

Ventricular tachycardia, particularly monomorphic ventricular tachycardia, responds well to shocks at initial energy levels of 100 J. For polymorphic ventricular tachycardia or for ventricular fibrillation, initial energy can be set at 120–200 J,

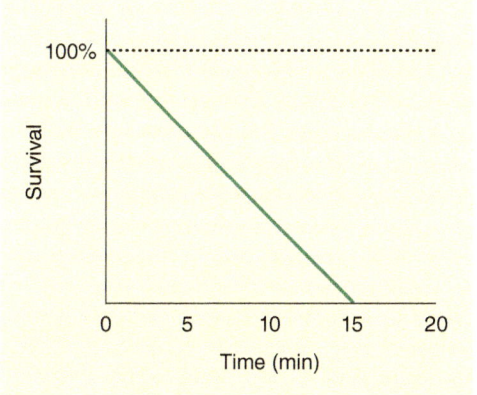

FIGURE 55–7 Success of defibrillation versus time. The chance of successful defibrillation of a patient in ventricular fibrillation decreases 7–10% per minute.

TABLE 55–3 Energy requirements for cardioversion using biphasic truncated exponential (BTE) or rectilinear morphology.[1]

Indications	Shocks (J)
Unstable atrial fibrillation	120–200
Unstable atrial flutter/tachycardia	50–100
Monomorphic ventricular tachycardia	100
Polymorphic ventricular tachycardia or ventricular fibrillation	120–200

depending upon the type of biphasic waveform being used. Stepwise increases in energy levels should be used if the first shock fails, although some AEDs operate with a fixed-energy protocol of 150 J with very high success in terminating ventricular fibrillation (Table 55–3).

Cardioversion should be synchronized with the QRS complex and is recommended for hemodynamically stable, wide-complex tachycardia requiring cardioversion, PSVT, atrial fibrillation, and atrial flutter. Polymorphic VT should be treated as VF with unsynchronized shocks.

Invasive Cardiopulmonary Resuscitation

Thoracotomy and open-chest cardiac massage are not part of routine CPR because of the high incidence of severe complications. Nonetheless, these invasive techniques can be helpful in specific life-threatening circumstances that preclude effective closed-chest massage. Possible indications include cardiac arrest associated with penetrating or blunt chest trauma, penetrating abdominal trauma, severe chest deformity, pericardial tamponade, or pulmonary embolism.

Intravenous Access

Some resuscitation drugs are fairly well absorbed following administration through a TT. Lidocaine, epinephrine, atropine, naloxone, and vasopressin (but *not* sodium bicarbonate) can be delivered via a catheter whose tip extends past the TT. Dosages 2–2½ times higher than recommended for intravenous use, diluted in 10 mL of normal saline or distilled water, are recommended for adult patients. Even though establishing reliable intravenous access is a high priority, it *should not take precedence* over initial chest compressions, airway management, or defibrillation. A preexisting internal jugular or subclavian line is ideal for venous access during resuscitation. If there is no central line access, an attempt should be made to establish peripheral intravenous access in either the antecubital or the external jugular vein. Peripheral intravenous sites are associated with a significant delay of 1–2 min between drug administration and delivery to the heart, as peripheral blood flow is drastically reduced during resuscitation. Administration of drugs given through a peripheral intravenous line should be followed by an intravenous flush (eg, a 20-mL fluid bolus in adults) and/or elevation of the extremity for 10–20 s. Establishing central vein access can potentially cause interruption of CPR but should be considered if an inadequate response is seen to peripherally administered drugs.

If intravenous cannulation is difficult, an intraosseous infusion can provide emergency vascular access in children. The success rate is lower in older children, but even in adults intraosseous cannulas have been successfully placed in the tibia and in the distal radius and ulna. A rigid 18-gauge spinal needle with a stylet or a small bone marrow trephine needle can be inserted into the distal femur or proximal tibia. If the tibia is chosen, a needle is inserted 2–3 cm below the tibial tuberosity at a 45° angle away from the epiphyseal plate (Figure 55–8). Once the needle is advanced through the cortex, it should stand upright without support. Proper placement is confirmed by the ability to aspirate marrow through the needle and a smooth infusion of fluid. A network of venous sinusoids within the medullary cavity of long bones drains into the systemic circulation by way of nutrient or emissary veins. This route is very effective for administration of drugs, crystalloids, colloids, and blood and can achieve flow rates exceeding 100 mL/h under gravity. Much higher flow rates are possible if the fluid is placed under pressure (eg, 300 mm Hg) with an infusion bag. The onset of drug action may be slightly delayed compared with intravenous or tracheal

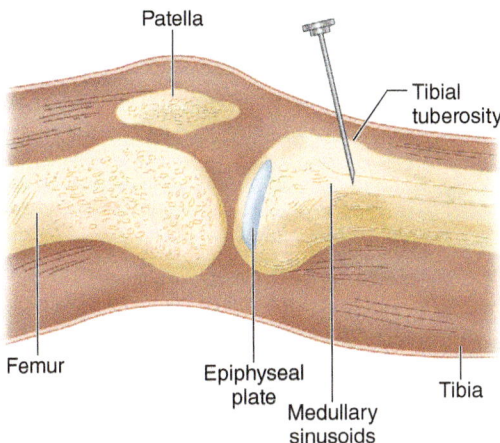

FIGURE 55–8 Intraosseous infusions provide emergency access to the venous circulation in pediatric patients by way of the large medullary venous channels. The needle is directed away from the epiphyseal plate to minimize the risk of injury.

administration. The intraosseous route may require a higher dose of some drugs (eg, epinephrine) than recommended for intravenous administration. The use of intraosseous infusion for induction and maintenance of general anesthesia, antibiotic therapy, seizure control, and inotropic support has been described. (Note that most studies have evaluated the placement of intraosseous access in patients with intact hemodynamics or hypovolemic states, not in cardiac arrest situations.) Because of the risks of osteomyelitis and compartment syndrome, however, intraosseous infusions should be replaced by a conventional intravenous route as soon as possible. In addition, because of the theoretical risk of bone marrow or fat emboli, intraosseous infusions should be avoided if possible in patients with right-to-left shunts, pulmonary hypertension, or severe pulmonary insufficiency.

Arrhythmia Recognition

Successful pharmacological and electrical treatment of cardiac arrest (**Figure 55–9**) depends on definitive identification of the underlying arrhythmia. Interpreting rhythm strips in the midst of a resuscitation situation is complicated by artifacts and variations in monitoring techniques (eg, lead systems, equipment).

Drug Administration

Many of the drugs administered during CPR have been described elsewhere in this text. **Table 55–4** summarizes the cardiovascular actions, indications, and dosages of drugs commonly used during resuscitation.

Atropine is not included as a drug for PEA/asystole in the new CPR-ECC guidelines; however, its use is retained for symptomatic bradycardia. Infusions of chronotropic drugs (eg, dopamine, epinephrine, isoproterenol) can be considered as an alternative to pacing if atropine is ineffective in the setting of symptomatic bradycardia. Calcium chloride, sodium bicarbonate, and bretylium are conspicuously absent from this table. Calcium (2–4 mg/kg of the chloride salt) is helpful in the treatment of documented hypocalcemia, hyperkalemia, hypermagnesemia, or a calcium channel blocker overdose. When used, 10% calcium chloride can be given at 2–4 mg/kg every 10 min. Sodium bicarbonate (0.5–1 mEq/kg) is not recommended in the guidelines and should be considered only in specific situations such as preexisting metabolic acidosis or hyperkalemia, or in the treatment of tricyclic antidepressant or barbiturate overdose. Sodium bicarbonate elevates plasma pH by combining with hydrogen ions to form carbonic acid, which readily dissociates into carbon dioxide and water. Because carbon dioxide, but not bicarbonate, readily crosses cell membranes and the blood–brain barrier, the resulting arterial hypercapnia will cause intracellular tissue acidosis. Although successful defibrillation is not related to *arterial* pH, increased *intramyocardial* carbon dioxide may reduce the possibility of cardiac resuscitation. Furthermore, bicarbonate administration can lead to detrimental alterations in osmolality and the oxygen–hemoglobin dissociation curve. Therefore, effective alveolar ventilation and adequate tissue perfusion are the treatments of choice for the respiratory and metabolic acidosis that accompany resuscitation.

Intravenous fluid therapy with either colloid or balanced salt solutions is indicated in patients with intravascular volume depletion (eg, acute blood loss, diabetic ketoacidosis, thermal burns). Dextrose-containing solutions may lead to a hyperosmotic

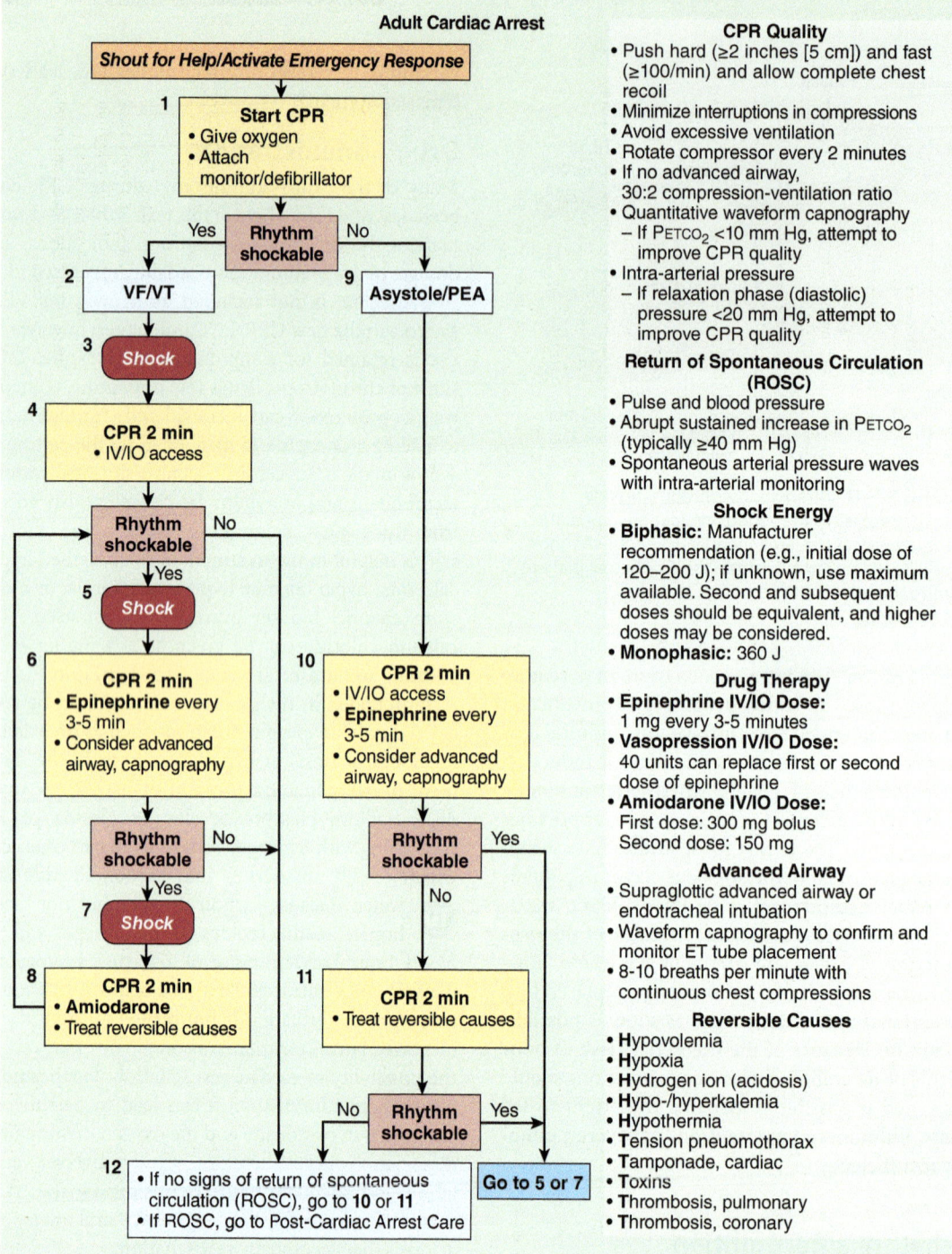

Adult Cardiac Arrest

Shout for Help/Activate Emergency Response

1 **Start CPR**
- Give oxygen
- Attach monitor/defibrillator

Rhythm shockable — Yes / No

2 **VF/VT**

9 **Asystole/PEA**

3 **Shock**

4 **CPR 2 min**
- IV/IO access

Rhythm shockable — No

5 **Shock**

6 **CPR 2 min**
- **Epinephrine** every 3-5 min
- Consider advanced airway, capnography

Rhythm shockable — No

7 **Shock**

8 **CPR 2 min**
- **Amiodarone**
- Treat reversible causes

10 **CPR 2 min**
- IV/IO access
- **Epinephrine** every 3-5 min
- Consider advanced airway, capnography

Rhythm shockable — Yes / No

11 **CPR 2 min**
- Treat reversible causes

Rhythm shockable — No / Yes

12
- If no signs of return of spontaneous circulation (ROSC), go to **10** or **11**
- If ROSC, go to Post-Cardiac Arrest Care

Go to 5 or 7

CPR Quality
- Push hard (≥2 inches [5 cm]) and fast (≥100/min) and allow complete chest recoil
- Minimize interruptions in compressions
- Avoid excessive ventilation
- Rotate compressor every 2 minutes
- If no advanced airway, 30:2 compression-ventilation ratio
- Quantitative waveform capnography
  – If P_{ETCO_2} <10 mm Hg, attempt to improve CPR quality
- Intra-arterial pressure
  – If relaxation phase (diastolic) pressure <20 mm Hg, attempt to improve CPR quality

Return of Spontaneous Circulation (ROSC)
- Pulse and blood pressure
- Abrupt sustained increase in P_{ETCO_2} (typically ≥40 mm Hg)
- Spontaneous arterial pressure waves with intra-arterial monitoring

Shock Energy
- **Biphasic:** Manufacturer recommendation (e.g., initial dose of 120–200 J); if unknown, use maximum available. Second and subsequent doses should be equivalent, and higher doses may be considered.
- **Monophasic:** 360 J

Drug Therapy
- **Epinephrine IV/IO Dose:** 1 mg every 3-5 minutes
- **Vasopression IV/IO Dose:** 40 units can replace first or second dose of epinephrine
- **Amiodarone IV/IO Dose:** First dose: 300 mg bolus Second dose: 150 mg

Advanced Airway
- Supraglottic advanced airway or endotracheal intubation
- Waveform capnography to confirm and monitor ET tube placement
- 8-10 breaths per minute with continuous chest compressions

Reversible Causes
- Hypovolemia
- Hypoxia
- Hydrogen ion (acidosis)
- Hypo-/hyperkalemia
- Hypothermia
- Tension pneuomothorax
- Tamponade, cardiac
- Toxins
- Thrombosis, pulmonary
- Thrombosis, coronary

FIGURE 55–9 Algorithm for treating ventricular fibrillation and pulseless ventricular tachycardia (VF/VT). Pulseless ventricular tachycardia should be treated in the same way as ventricular fibrillation. Note: This figure and Figures 55–1 and 55–2 emphasize the concept that rescuers and health care providers must assume that all unmonitored adult cardiac arrests are due to VF/VT. In each figure, the flow of the algorithm assumes that the arrhythmia is continuing. (Reproduced, with permission, from Neumar RW, Otto CW, Link MS, et al: Part 8: Adult Advanced Cardiovascular Life Support: 2010 American Heart Association Guidelines for Cardiopulmonary Resuscitation and Emergency Cardiovascular Care. Circulation 2012;122(18 Suppl 3): S729-S767.)

TABLE 55–4 Cardiovascular effects, indications, and dosages of resuscitation drugs.[1]

Drug	Cardiovascular Effects	Indications	Initial Dose Adult	Initial Dose Pediatric	Comments
Adenosine	Slows AV nodal conduction	Narrow complex tachycardias, stable supraventricular tachycardia, and wide-complex tachycardias if supraventricular in origin	6 mg over 1–3 s; 12 mg repeat dose	Initial dose 0.1–0.2 mg/kg; subsequent doses doubled to maximum single dose of 12 mg	Recommended as diagnostic or therapeutic maneuver for supraventricular tachycardias; give as rapid IV bolus. Vasodilates, BP may decrease. Theoretical risk of angina, bronchospasm, proarrhythmic action. Drug–drug interaction with theophylline, dipyridamole.
Atropine	Anticholinergic (parasympatholytic). Increases sinoatrial node rate and automaticity; increases AV node conduction	Symptomatic bradycardia, AV block	0.5–1.0 mg repeated every 3–5 min	0.02 mg/kg	Repeat atropine doses every 5 min to a total dose of 3 mg in adults or 0.5 mg in children, 1.0 mg in adolescents. The minimum pediatric dose is 0.1 mg. Do not use for infranodal (Mobitz II) block.
Epinephrine	α-Adrenergic effects increase myocardial and cerebral blood flow. β-Adrenergic effects may increase myocardial work and decrease subendocardial perfusion and cerebral blood flow	VF/VT, electromechanical dissociation, ventricular asystole, severe bradycardia unresponsive to atropine or pacing Severe hypotension	1 mg IV 0.03 mcg/kg/min in an infusion increased to effect	Initial dose 0.01 mg/kg IV; repeat same for subsequent doses or up to 0.1–0.2 mg/kg IV 1 mcg/kg	Repeat doses every 3–5 min as necessary. An infusion of epinephrine (eg., 1 mg in 250 mL D₅W or NS, 4 mcg/mL) can be titrated to effect in adults (1–4 mcg/min) or children (0.1–1 mcg/kg/min). Administration down a tracheal tube requires higher doses (2–2.5 mg in adults, 0.1 mg/kg in children). High-dose epinephrine (0.1 mg/kg) in adults is recommended only after standard therapy has failed.
Lidocaine	Decreases rate of phase 4 depolarization (decreases automaticity); depresses conduction in reentry pathways. Elevates VF threshold. Reduces disparity in action potential duration between normal and ischemic tissue. Reduces action potential and effective refractory period duration	VT that has not responded to defibrillation; premature ventricular contractions. Use only as second-line therapy; thus, consider only if amiodarone is unavailable	1–1.5 mg/kg	1 mg/kg	Doses of 0.5–1.5 mg/kg can be repeated every 5–10 min to a total dose of 3 mg/kg. After infarction or successful resuscitation, a continuous infusion (eg, 1 g in 500 mL D₅W, 2 mg/mL) should be run at a rate of 20–50 mcg/kg/min (2–4 mg/min in most adults). Therapeutic blood levels are usually 1.5–6 mcg/mL.

(continued)

TABLE 55–4 Cardiovascular effects, indications, and dosages of resuscitation drugs.[1] (continued)

Drug	Cardiovascular Effects	Indications	Initial Dose		Comments
			Adult	Pediatric	
Vasopressin	Nonadrenergic peripheral vasoconstrictor; direct stimulation of V_1 receptors	Bleeding esophageal varices; adult shock-refractory VF; hemodynamic support in vasodilatory (septic) shock	40 units IV, single dose, 1 time only	Not recommended	Newly recommended as equivalent to epinephrine in VF and PEA; may be more effective in asystole; used only one time; has a 10–20 min half-life.
Procainamide	Suppresses both atrial and ventricular arrhythmias	AF/flutter; preexcited atrial arrhythmias with rapid ventricular response; wide-complex tachycardia that cannot be distinguished as SVT or VT	20 mg/min until arrhythmia suppressed, hypotension develops, QRS complex increases by >50%, or total dose of 17 mg/kg has infused. In urgent situation, 50 mg/min may be used to maximum of 17 mg/kg. Maintenance infusion, 1–4 mg/min	Loading dose: 15 mg/kg; infusion over 30–60 min; routine use in combination with drugs that prolong QT interval is not recommended	Contraindicated in overdose of tricyclic antidepressants or other antiarrhythmic drugs. Bolus doses can result in toxicity. Should not be used in preexisting QT prolongation or torsades de pointes. Blood levels should be monitored in patients with impaired renal function and when constant infusion >3 mg/min for >24 h.
Amiodarone	Complex drug with effects on sodium, potassium, and calcium channels as well as α- and β-adrenergic blocking properties	SVT with accessory pathway conduction; unstable VT and VF; stable VT, polymorphic VT, wide-complex tachycardia of uncertain origin; AF/flutter with CHF; preexcited AF/flutter; adjunct to electrical cardioversion in refractory PSVTs, atrial tachycardia, and AF	150 mg over 10 min, followed by 1 mg/min for 6 h, then 0.5 mg/min, with supplementary infusion of 150 mg as necessary up to 2 g. For pulseless VT or VF, initial administration is 300 mg rapid infusion diluted in 20–30 mL of saline or dextrose in water	5 mg/kg for pulseless VT/VF; for perfusing tachycardia loading dose, 5 mg/kg IV/IO; maximum dose, 15 mg/kg/d	Antiarrhythmic of choice if cardiac function is impaired, EF <40%, or CHF. Routine use in combination with drugs prolonging QT interval is not recommended. Most frequent side effects are hypotension and bradycardia.
Verapamil	Calcium channel blocking agent used to slow conduction and increase refractoriness in AV node, terminating reentrant arrhythmias that require AV nodal conduction for continuation	Controls ventricular response rate in AF/flutter and MAT; rate control in AF; terminating narrow-complex PSVT	2.5–5 mg IV over 2 min; without response, repeat dose with 5–10 mg every 15–30 min to a max of 20 mg		Use only in patients with narrow-complex PSVT or supraventricular arrhythmia. Do not use in presence of impaired ventricular function or CHF

Diltiazem	Calcium channel blocking agent used to slow conduction and increase refractoriness in AV node, terminating reentrant arrhythmias that require AV nodal conduction for continuation	Slows conduction and increases refractoriness in AV node. May terminate reentrant arrhythmias. Controls ventricular response rate in AF/flutter and MAT	0.25 mg/kg, followed by second dose of 0.35 mg/kg if necessary; maintenance infusion of 5–15 mg/h in AF/flutter	May exacerbate CHF in severe LV dysfunction; may decrease myocardial contractility, but less so than verapamil.
Dobutamine	Synthetic catecholamine and potent inotropic agent with predominant β-adrenergic receptor-stimulating effects that increase cardiac contractility in a dose-dependent manner, accompanied by a decrease in LV filling pressures.	Severe systolic heart failure	5–20 mcg/kg/min	Hemodynamic end points rather than specific dose is goal. Elderly have significantly reduced response. May induce or exacerbate myocardial ischemia with increases in heart rate.
Flecainide	Potent sodium channel blocker with significant conduction-slowing effects	AF/flutter, ventricular arrhythmias and supraventricular arrhythmias without structural heart disease, ectopic atrial heart disease, AV nodal reentrant tachycardia, SVTs associated with an accessory pathway, including preexcited AF	2 mg/kg at 10 mg/min (IV use not approved in the United States)	Should not be used in patients with impaired LV function, or when coronary artery disease is suspected.
Ibutilide	Short-acting antiarrhythmic, prolongs the action potential duration and increases refractory period	Acute conversion or adjunct to electrical cardioversion of AF/flutter of short duration	In patients >60 kg, 1 mg (10 mL) over 10 min; a second similar dose may be repeated in 10 min. In patients <60 kg, initial dose is 0.01 mg/kg	Patients should be monitored for arrhythmias for 4–6 h, and longer in those with hepatic dysfunction.
Magnesium	Hypomagnesemia associated with arrhythmias, cardiac insufficiency, and sudden death; can precipitate refractory VF; can hinder K⁺ replacement	Torsades de pointes with prolonged QT, even with normal serum levels of magnesium	1–2 g in 50–100 mL D₅W over 15 min 500 mg/mL–IV/IO: 25–50 mg/kg; maximum dose: 2 g per dose	Rapid IV infusion for torsades de pointes or suspected hypomagnesemia not recommended in cardiac arrest except when arrhythmia suspected.

(continued)

TABLE 55–4 Cardiovascular effects, indications, and dosages of resuscitation drugs.[1] (continued)

Drug	Cardiovascular Effects	Indications	Initial Dose		Comments
			Adult	Pediatric	
Propafenone	Significant conduction slowing and negative inotropic effects. Nonselective β-adrenergic blocking properties	AF/flutter, ventricular arrhythmias and supraventricular arrhythmias without structural heart disease, ectopic atrial heart disease, AV nodal reentrant tachycardia, SVTs associated with an accessory pathway	2.0 mg/kg at 10 mg/min (IV use not approved in the United States)		Should be avoided with impaired LV function or when CAD suspected.
Sotalol	Prolongs action potential duration and increases cardiac tissue refractoriness. Nonselective β-adrenergic blocking properties	Preexcited AF/flutter, ventricular and supraventricular arrhythmias	1.0–1.5 mg/kg at a rate of 10 mg/min		Limited by need to be infused slowly.

[1]AV, atrioventricular; BP, blood pressure; VF, ventricular fibrillation; VT, ventricular tachycardia; PEA, pulseless electrical activity; AF, atrial fibrillation; SVT, supraventricular tachycardia; CHF, congestive heart failure; PSVT, paroxysmal supraventricular tachycardia; IV/IO, intravenous/intraosseous; EF, ejection fraction; MAT, multifocal atrial tachycardia; LV, left ventricular; CAD, coronary artery disease.

diuresis and may worsen neurological outcome. They should be avoided unless hypoglycemia is suspected. Likewise, administration of free water (eg, D_5W) may lead to cerebral edema.

Emergency Pacemaker Therapy

Transcutaneous cardiac pacing (TCP) is a noninvasive method of rapidly treating arrhythmias caused by conduction disorders or abnormal impulse. TCP is not routinely recommended in cardiac arrest. TCP use may be considered to treat asystole, bradycardia caused by heart block, or tachycardia from a reentrant mechanism. If there is concern about the use of atropine in high-grade block, TCP is always appropriate. If the patient is unstable with marked bradycardia, TCP should be implemented immediately while awaiting treatment response to drugs. The pacer unit has become a built-in feature of some defibrillator models. Disposable pacing electrodes are usually positioned on the patient in an anterior–posterior manner. The placement of the negative electrode corresponds to a V_2 electrocardiograph position, whereas the positive electrode is placed on the left posterior chest beneath the scapula and lateral to the spine. Note that this positioning does not interfere with paddle placement during defibrillation. Failure to capture may be due to electrode misplacement, poor electrode-to-skin contact, or increased transthoracic impedance (eg, barrel-shaped chest, pericardial effusion). Current output is slowly increased until the pacing stimuli obtain electrical and mechanical capture. A wide QRS complex following a pacing spike signals *electrical* capture, but *mechanical* (ventricular) capture must be confirmed by an improving pulse or blood pressure. Conscious patients may require sedation to tolerate the discomfort of skeletal muscle contractions. Transcutaneous pacing can provide effective temporizing therapy until transvenous pacing or other definitive treatment can be initiated. TCP has many advantages over transvenous pacing because it can be used by almost all electrocardiogram providers and can be started quickly and conveniently at the bedside.

Precordial Thump

The precordial thump is to be considered only in witnessed, monitored unstable VT when a defibrillator is not immediately available.

RECOMMENDED RESUSCITATION PROTOCOLS

A resuscitation team leader integrates the assessment of the patient, including electrocardiographic diagnosis, with the electrical and pharmacological therapy (Table 55–5). This person must have a firm grasp of the guidelines for cardiac arrest presented in the CPR-ECC algorithms (Figures 55–9 to 55–13).

TABLE 55–5 Steps for synchronized cardioversion.[1]

1. Consider sedation.
2. Turn on defibrillator (monophasic or biphasic).
3. Attach monitor leads to the patient ("white to right, red to ribs, what's left over to the left shoulder") and ensure proper display of the patient's rhythm.
4. Engage the synchronization mode by pressing the "sync" control button.
5. Look for markers on R waves indicating sync mode.
6. If necessary, adjust monitor gain until sync markers occur with each R wave.
7. Select appropriate energy level.
8. Position conductor pads on patient (or apply gel to paddles).
9. Position paddle on patient (sternum-apex).
10. Announce to team members: "Charging defibrillator—stand clear!"
11. Press "charge" button on apex paddle (right hand).
12. When the defibrillator is charged, begin the final clearing chant. State firmly in a forceful voice the following chant before each shock:
    - *"I am going to shock on three. One, I'm clear."* (Check to make sure you are clear of contact with the patient, the stretcher, and the equipment.)
    - *"Two, you are clear."* (Make a visual check to ensure that no one continues to touch the patient or stretcher. In particular, do not forget about the person providing ventilation. That person's hands should not be touching the ventilatory adjuncts, including the tracheal tube!).
    - *"Three, everybody's clear."* (Check yourself one more time before pressing the "shock" buttons.)
13. Apply 25 lb pressure on both paddles.
14. Press the "discharge" buttons simultaneously.
15. Check the monitor. If tachycardia persists, increase the joules according to the electrical cardioversion algorithm.
16. Reset the sync mode after each synchronized cardioversion because most defibrillators default back to unsynchronized mode. This default allows an immediate defibrillation if the cardioversion produces ventricular fibrillation.

[1]Data from The American Heart Association Guidelines 2010 for cardiopulmonary resuscitation and emergency cardiovascular care. Circulation 2010;122:S706.

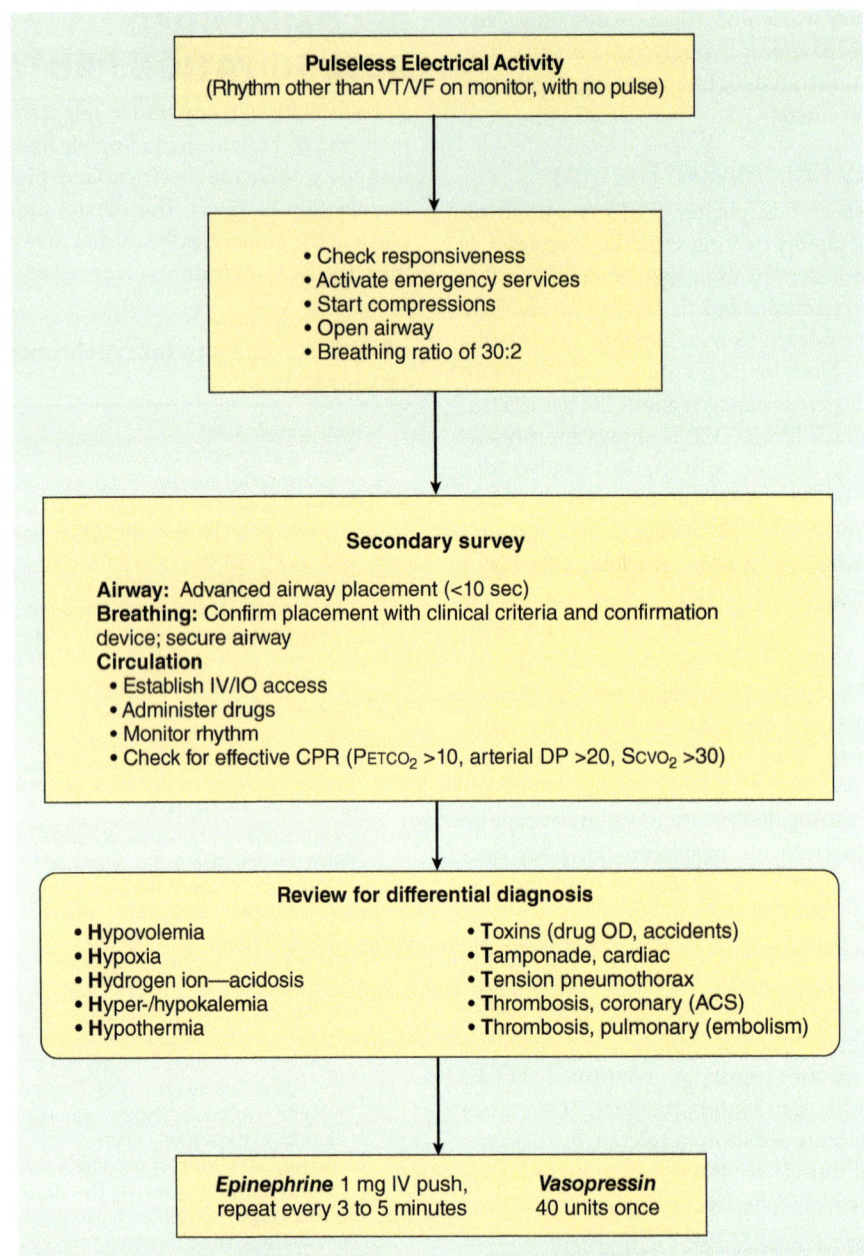

FIGURE 55–10 Pulseless electrical activity algorithm. VF/VT, ventricular fibrillation and pulseless ventricular tachycardia. P$_{ETCO_2}$, end-tidal carbon dioxide; DP, diastolic pressure; S$_{CVO_2}$, central venous oxygen saturation. (Data from the American Heart Association BLS and ACLS Guidelines 2010 for cardiopulmonary resuscitation and emergency cardiovascular care. Circulation 2010.122;S729.)

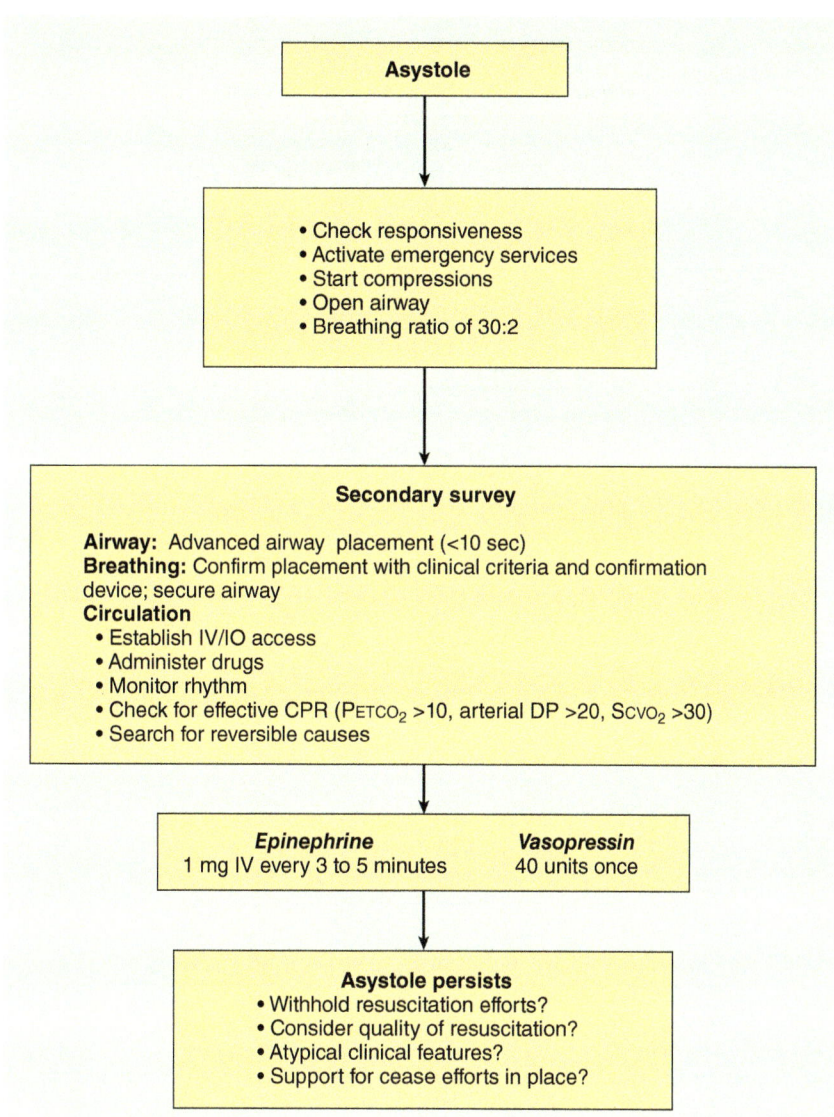

Asystole

- Check responsiveness
- Activate emergency services
- Start compressions
- Open airway
- Breathing ratio of 30:2

Secondary survey

Airway: Advanced airway placement (<10 sec)
Breathing: Confirm placement with clinical criteria and confirmation device; secure airway
Circulation
- Establish IV/IO access
- Administer drugs
- Monitor rhythm
- Check for effective CPR (P_{ETCO_2} >10, arterial DP >20, S_{CVO_2} >30)
- Search for reversible causes

Epinephrine
1 mg IV every 3 to 5 minutes

Vasopressin
40 units once

Asystole persists
- Withhold resuscitation efforts?
- Consider quality of resuscitation?
- Atypical clinical features?
- Support for cease efforts in place?

FIGURE 55–11 Asystole: The silent heart algorithm. VF/VT, ventricular fibrillation and pulseless ventricular tachycardia; P_{ETCO_2}, end-tidal carbon dioxide; DP, diastolic pressure; S_{CVO_2}, central venous oxygen saturation. (Data from The American Heart Association BLS and ACLS Guidelines 2010 for cardiopulmonary resuscitation and emergency cardiovascular care. Circulation 2010:122;S729.)

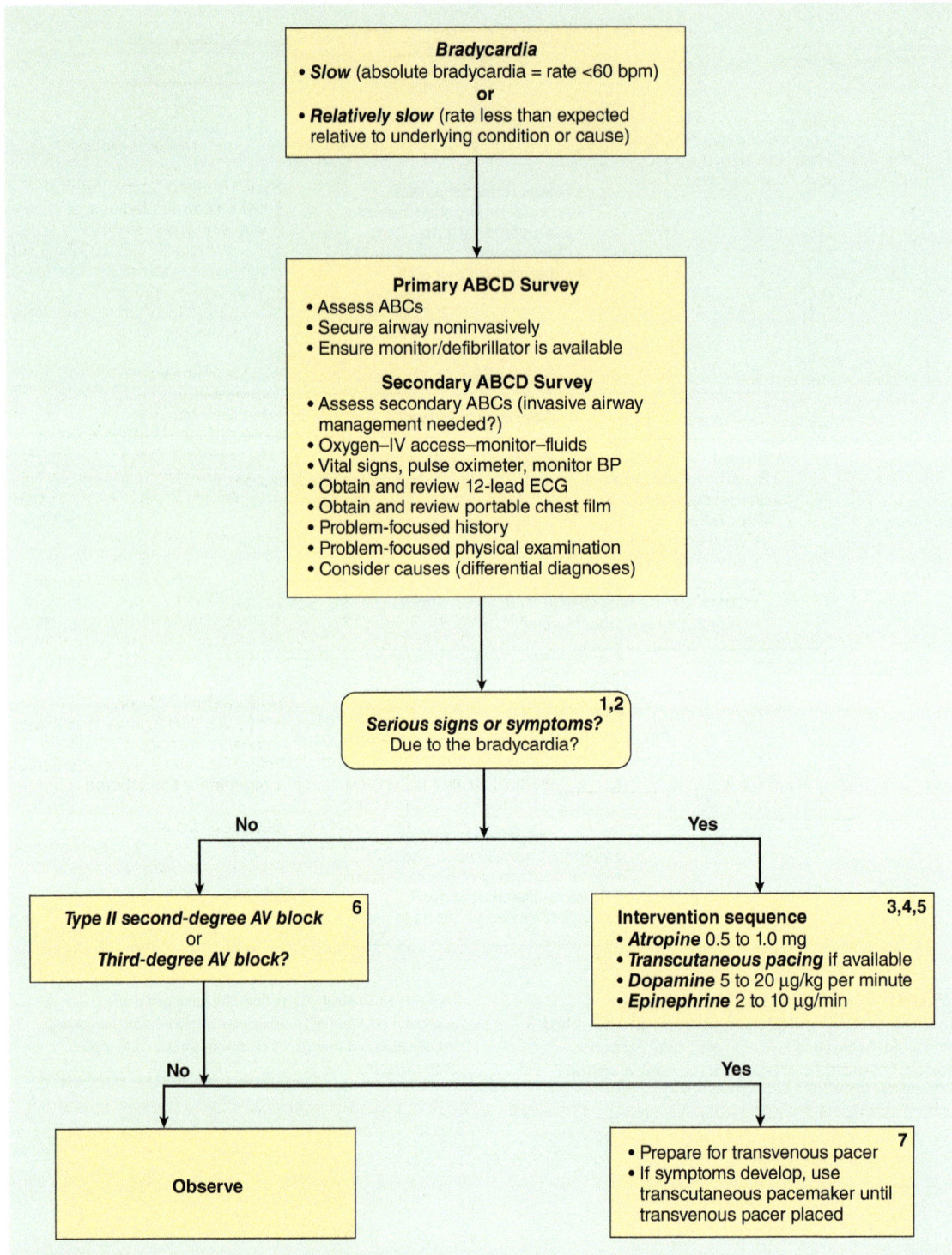

FIGURE 55–12 Bradycardia algorithm. AV, atrioventricular. (Data from The American Heart Association BLS and ACLS Guidelines 2010 for cardiopulmonary resuscitation and emergency cardiovascular care. Circulation 2010:122;S729.)

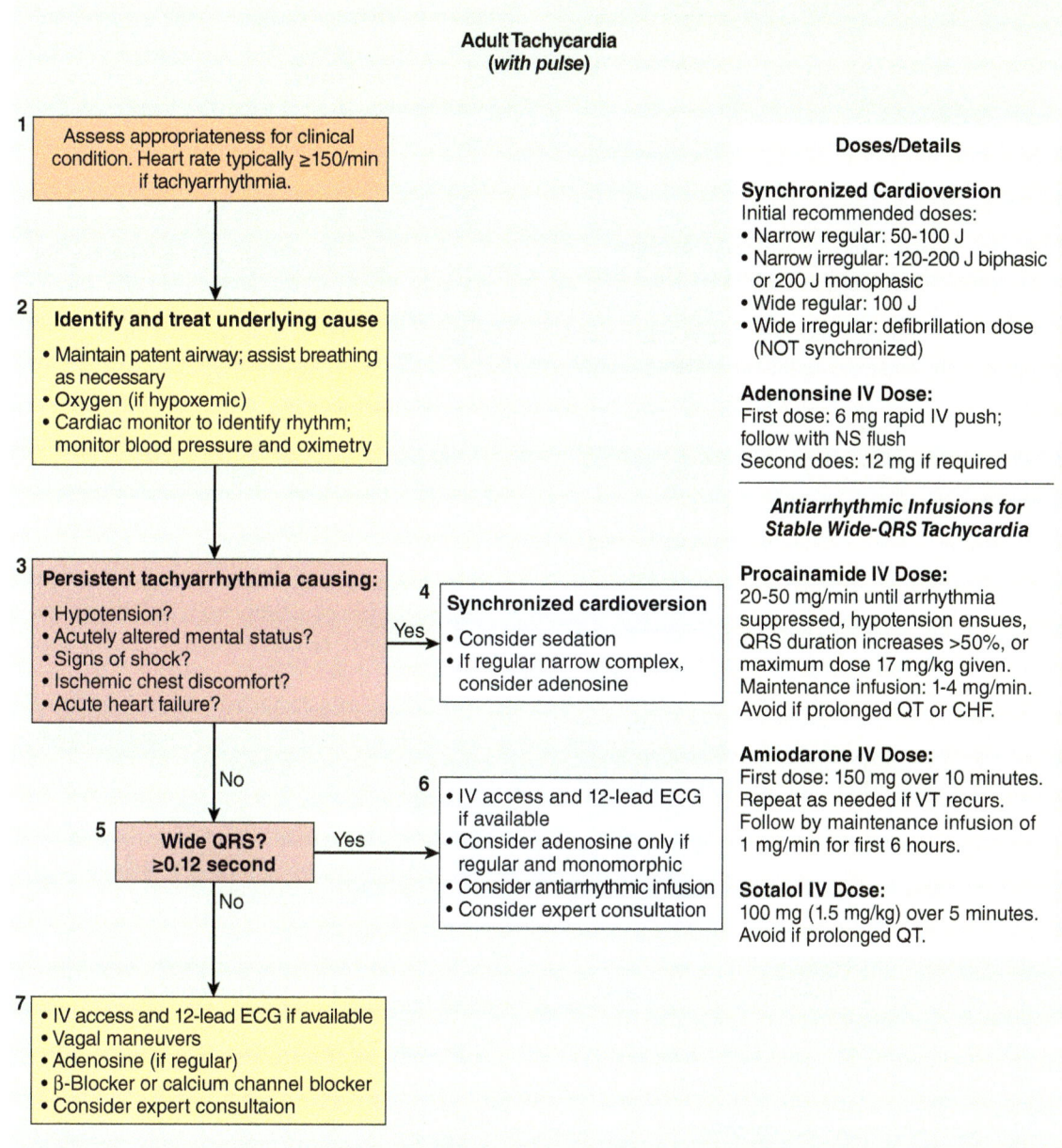

Adult Tachycardia
(with pulse)

1 Assess appropriateness for clinical condition. Heart rate typically ≥150/min if tachyarrhythmia.

2 **Identify and treat underlying cause**
- Maintain patent airway; assist breathing as necessary
- Oxygen (if hypoxemic)
- Cardiac monitor to identify rhythm; monitor blood pressure and oximetry

3 **Persistent tachyarrhythmia causing:**
- Hypotension?
- Acutely altered mental status?
- Signs of shock?
- Ischemic chest discomfort?
- Acute heart failure?

Yes →

4 **Synchronized cardioversion**
- Consider sedation
- If regular narrow complex, consider adenosine

No ↓

5 **Wide QRS?**
≥0.12 second

Yes →

6
- IV access and 12-lead ECG if available
- Consider adenosine only if regular and monomorphic
- Consider antiarrhythmic infusion
- Consider expert consultation

No ↓

7
- IV access and 12-lead ECG if available
- Vagal maneuvers
- Adenosine (if regular)
- β-Blocker or calcium channel blocker
- Consider expert consultaion

Doses/Details

Synchronized Cardioversion
Initial recommended doses:
- Narrow regular: 50-100 J
- Narrow irregular: 120-200 J biphasic or 200 J monophasic
- Wide regular: 100 J
- Wide irregular: defibrillation dose (NOT synchronized)

Adenonsine IV Dose:
First dose: 6 mg rapid IV push; follow with NS flush
Second does: 12 mg if required

Antiarrhythmic Infusions for Stable Wide-QRS Tachycardia

Procainamide IV Dose:
20-50 mg/min until arrhythmia suppressed, hypotension ensues, QRS duration increases >50%, or maximum dose 17 mg/kg given. Maintenance infusion: 1-4 mg/min. Avoid if prolonged QT or CHF.

Amiodarone IV Dose:
First dose: 150 mg over 10 minutes. Repeat as needed if VT recurs. Follow by maintenance infusion of 1 mg/min for first 6 hours.

Sotalol IV Dose:
100 mg (1.5 mg/kg) over 5 minutes. Avoid if prolonged QT.

FIGURE 55-13 Tachycardia overview algorithm. VT, ventricular tachycardia; CHF, congestive heart failure. WPW, Wolff-Parkinson-White syndrome. (Reproduced, with permission, from The American Heart Association BLS and ACLS Guidelines 2010 for cardiopulmonary resuscitation and emergency cardiovascular care. Circulation 2010:122;S729.)

CASE DISCUSSION

Intraoperative Hypotension & Cardiac Arrest

A 16-year-old boy is rushed to the operating room for emergency laparotomy and thoracotomy after suffering multiple abdominal and thoracic stab wounds. In the field, paramedics intubated the patient, started two large-bore intravenous lines, began fluid resuscitation, and inflated a pneumatic antishock garment. Upon arrival in the operating room, the patient's blood pressure is unobtainable, heart rate is 128 beats/min (sinus tachycardia), and respirations are being controlled by a bag-valve device.

What should be done immediately?

Cardiopulmonary resuscitation must be initiated immediately: external chest compressions should be started as soon as the arterial blood pressure is found to be inadequate for vital organ perfusion. Because the patient is already intubated, the location of the tracheal tube should be confirmed with chest auscultation and quantitative waveform capnography (if available, to assist in both confirmation of tube placement as well as to assess the adequacy of CPR) and 100% oxygen should be delivered.

Which CPR sequence best fits this situation?

Pulselessness in the presence of sinus rhythm suggests severe hypovolemia, cardiac tamponade, ventricular rupture, dissecting aortic aneurysm, tension pneumothorax, profound hypoxemia and acidosis, or pulmonary embolism. Epinephrine, 1 mg, should be administered intravenously.

What is the most likely cause of this patient's profound hypotension?

The presence of multiple stab wounds strongly suggests hypovolemia. Abdominal ultrasound can rapidly identify a collapsed vena cava, which is pathognomonic of hypovolemia. Fluids, preferably warmed, should be rapidly administered. Additional venous access can be sought as other members of the operating room team administer fluid through blood pumps or other rapid infusion devices. Five percent albumin or lactated Ringer's solution is acceptable until blood products are available. Activation of a massive transfusion protocol is often indicated.

What are the signs of tension pneumothorax and pericardial tamponade?

The signs of **tension pneumothorax**—the presence of air under pressure in the pleural space—include increasing peak inspiratory pressures, tachycardia and hypotension (decreased venous return), hypoxia (atelectasis), distended neck veins, unequal breath sounds, tracheal deviation, and mediastinal shift away from the pneumothorax.

Pericardial tamponade—cardiac compression from pericardial contents—should be suspected in any patient with narrow pulse pressure; pulsus paradoxus (>10 mm Hg drop in systolic blood pressure with inspiration); elevated central venous pressure with neck vein distention; equalization of central venous pressure, atrial pressures, and ventricular end-diastolic pressures; distant heart sounds; tachycardia; and hypotension. Many of these signs may be masked by concurrent hypovolemic shock.

Fluid administration and properly performed external cardiac compressions do not result in satisfactory carotid or femoral pulsations. What else should be done?

Because external chest compressions are often ineffective in trauma patients, an emergency thoracotomy should be performed as soon as possible to clamp the thoracic aorta, relieve a tension pneumothorax or pericardial tamponade, identify possible intrathoracic hemorrhage, and perform open-chest cardiac compressions. Cross-clamping of the thoracic aorta increases brain and heart perfusion and decreases subdiaphragmatic hemorrhage. Lack of response to cross-clamping is a good predictor of demise.

What is the function of the pneumatic antishock garment, and how should it be removed?

Inflation of the bladders within a pneumatic antishock garment increases arterial blood pressure by elevating peripheral vascular resistance. Functionally, the suit has the same effect as thoracic aorta cross-clamping by decreasing blood flow and hemorrhage in the lower half of the body. Complications of inflating the abdominal section of the pneumatic antishock garment include renal dysfunction, altered lung volumes, and visceral injury during external chest compressions. The suit should be deflated only after restoration of hemodynamic parameters. Even then, deflation should be gradual, as it may be accompanied by marked hypotension and metabolic acidosis caused by reperfusion of ischemic tissues.

GUIDELINES

The American Heart Association in Collaboration with the International Liaison Committee on Resuscitation (ILCOR): Guidelines 2010 for cardiopulmonary resuscitation and emergency cardiovascular care. Circulation 2010;122:S250.

SUGGESTED READING

Adult ACLS. Circulation 2010;122:S729.
Adult BLS. Circulation 2010;122:S685.
Adult CPR overview. Circulation 2010;122:S675.
CPR techniques and devices. Circulation 2010;122:S720.
Electrical therapies: AED, defibrillation, pacing. Circulation 2010;122:S706.
Executive summary ACLS. Circulation 2010;122:S640.

Postanesthesia Care

1. Formerly anesthetized patients should not leave the operating room unless they have a patent airway, have adequate ventilation and oxygenation, and are hemodynamically stable; qualified anesthesia personnel must also be available to attend the transfer.

2. Before the recovering patient is fully responsive, pain is often manifested as postoperative restlessness. Serious systemic disturbances (eg, hypoxemia, respiratory or metabolic acidosis, or hypotension), bladder distention, or a surgical complication (eg, occult intraabdominal hemorrhage) must also be considered in the differential diagnosis of postoperative agitation.

3. Intense shivering causes precipitous rises in oxygen consumption, CO_2 production, and cardiac output. These physiological effects are often poorly tolerated by patients with preexisting cardiac or pulmonary impairment.

4. Respiratory problems are the most frequently encountered serious complications in the postanesthesia care unit (PACU). The overwhelming majority are related to airway obstruction, hypoventilation, and/or hypoxemia.

5. Hypoventilation in the PACU is most commonly due to the residual depressant effects of anesthetic agents on respiratory drive.

6. Obtundation, circulatory depression, or severe acidosis (arterial blood pH < 7.15) is an indication for immediate and aggressive respiratory and hemodynamic intervention, including airway and inotropic support as needed.

7. Following naloxone administration, patients should be observed closely for recurrence of opioid-induced respiratory depression ("renarcotization"), as naloxone has a shorter duration than do most opioids.

8. Increased intrapulmonary shunting from a decreased functional residual capacity relative to closing capacity is the most common cause of hypoxemia following general anesthesia.

9. The possibility of a postoperative pneumothorax should always be considered following central line placement, intercostal blocks, abdominal or chest trauma (including rib fractures), neck dissections, tracheostomy, nephrectomies, or other retroperitoneal or intraabdominal procedures (including laparoscopy), especially if the diaphragm may have been penetrated or disrupted.

10. Hypovolemia is by far the most common cause of hypotension in the PACU.

11. Noxious stimulation from incisional pain, endotracheal intubation, or bladder distention is usually responsible for postoperative hypertension.

Historically, emphasis on specialized nursing care during the immediate postoperative period was prompted by the realization that many early postoperative deaths occurred immediately after anesthesia and surgery and that many of these deaths were preventable. A nursing shortage in the United States following World War II, as well as the experience of providing surgical care to large numbers of battle casualties during the war, contributed to the postwar trend of centralization of immediate postoperative care in the form of recovery rooms, where one or more nurses could pay close attention to several acute postoperative patients at one time. Over the past two decades, the accelerating practice of caring for selected postoperative patients overnight in a postanesthesia care unit (PACU), or the equivalent, has been a response to increasingly complex surgical procedures performed on higher-acuity patients, often in the setting of a shortage of surgical intensive care beds. The success of PACUs in decreasing postoperative morbidity and mortality has been a major influence on the evolution of modern surgical intensive care units.

Another recent transformation in postanesthesia care is related to the shift from inpatient to outpatient surgery. It is estimated that more than 70% of all surgical procedures in the United States are now performed on an outpatient basis. Two phases of recovery may be recognized for outpatient surgery. *Phase 1* is the immediate intensive care level recovery that cares for patients during emergence and awakening from anesthesia and continues until standard PACU criteria are met (see Discharge Criteria below). *Phase 2* is a lower-level care that ensures that the patient is ready to go home. "Fast-tracking" of selected outpatients may allow them to safely bypass phase 1 recovery and go directly to the phase 2 level of care.

In many institutions, the PACU also commonly functions as a more intensely monitored location for perioperative and chronic pain patients undergoing procedures such as single-shot nerve blocks and placement of epidural and peripheral nerve catheters, and for patients undergoing other procedures such as central line placement, electroconvulsive therapy, and elective cardioversion. The PACU must be appropriately staffed and equipped to routinely manage these patients and their potential procedure-related complications. For example, in areas where regional and epidural blocks are administered, Intralipid® should be stocked in anticipation of treating local anesthetic toxicity.

This chapter discusses the essential components of a modern PACU, the general care of patients acutely recovering from anesthesia and surgery, and the respiratory and circulatory complications most commonly encountered in the PACU.

THE POSTANESTHESIA CARE UNIT

At the conclusion of any procedure requiring anesthesia, anesthetic agents are discontinued, monitors are disconnected, and the patient emerging from sedation or anesthesia is taken to the PACU. Following general anesthesia, if an endotracheal tube or laryngeal mask airway (LMA) was utilized, and if ventilation is judged adequate, the endotracheal tube or LMA is usually removed prior to transport. Patients are also routinely observed in the PACU following regional anesthesia and monitored anesthesia care (local anesthesia with sedation). Most procedure guidelines require that a patient be admitted to the PACU following any type of anesthesia, except by specific order of the attending anesthesiologist. After a brief verbal (and in some cases written) "hand off" report to the PACU nurse, the patient is left in the PACU until the major effects of anesthesia have worn off. This period is characterized by a relatively high incidence of potentially life-threatening respiratory and circulatory complications.

The delivery of anesthesia services in areas remote from the main operating room, such as endoscopy, interventional radiology, and magnetic resonance imaging suites is increasingly common. Patients recovering from anesthesia delivered in these areas must receive the same standard of care as patients recovering from anesthesia received in the main operating room. Some institutions have developed "satellite" PACUs to serve each of these remote areas individually, and others have combined their procedural areas into one centralized procedural suite served by a single PACU.

Design

The PACU should be located near the operating rooms and off-site invasive procedure areas. A central location in the operating room area itself is desirable, as it ensures that the patient can be rushed back to surgery, if needed, or that members of the operating room team can quickly respond to urgent or emergent patient care issues. Proximity to radiographic, laboratory, and other intensive care facilities on the same floor is also advantageous. The transfer of critically ill patients in elevators or through long corridors can jeopardize their care because urgent problems may arise along the way.

An open-ward design facilitates observation of multiple patients simultaneously. However, an appropriate number of individually enclosed patient care spaces is required for patients needing isolation for infection control. A ratio of 1.5 PACU beds per operating room is customary, although this number will vary depending on the respective operating room suite's case volume, variety of surgical procedures, and patient acuity. Each patient space should be well-lighted and large enough to allow easy access to patients in spite of poles for intravenous infusion pumps, a ventilator, or radiographic equipment; construction guidelines dictate a minimum of 7 ft between beds and 120 sq ft/patient. Multiple electrical outlets, including at least one with backup emergency power, and at least one outlet each for oxygen and suction, should be present at each bed space.

Equipment

Many PACU incidents leading to serious morbidity or mortality are related to inadequate monitoring. Pulse oximetry (SpO_2), electrocardiogram (ECG), and automated noninvasive blood pressure (NIBP) monitors are mandatory for each space. Although ECG, SpO_2, and NIBP must be utilized for every patient in the initial phase of recovery from anesthesia (phase 1 care), decreased monitoring may be adequate thereafter. Appropriate equipment must be available for those patients requiring invasive arterial, central venous, pulmonary artery, or intracranial pressure monitoring. Capnography is useful for intubated patients and is increasingly employed for extubated patients as well. Temperature-sensitive strips may be used to measure temperature in the PACU but are not sufficiently accurate to document the results of treatment for hypothermia or hyperthermia; mercury or electronic thermometers must be used if an abnormality in temperature is suspected. A forced-air warming device, heating lamp, and/or a warming/cooling blanket should be available.

The PACU must have its own supplies of basic and emergency equipment, separate from that of the operating room, based on the needs of the patient population. This includes airway equipment and supplies, such as oxygen cannulas, a selection of masks, oral and nasal airways, laryngoscopes, endotracheal tubes, LMAs, a cricothyrotomy kit, and self-inflating bags for ventilation. A readily available supply of catheters for vascular cannulation (venous, arterial, central venous) is mandatory. A defibrillation device with transcutaneous pacing capabilities, and an emergency cart with drugs and supplies for advanced life support (see Chapter 55) and infusion pumps, must be present and periodically inspected. Transvenous pacing catheters; pulse generators; and tracheostomy, chest tube, and vascular cut-down trays are typically present, depending on the surgical patient population.

Respiratory therapy equipment for aerosol bronchodilator treatments, continuous positive airway pressure (CPAP), and ventilators should be in close proximity to the recovery room. Immediate availability of a bronchoscope is desirable.

Staffing

Inadequate staffing is often cited as a major contributing factor in PACU mishaps. The PACU should be staffed by nurses specifically trained in the care of adult and/or pediatric patients emerging from anesthesia. They should have expertise in airway management and advanced cardiac life support, as well as problems commonly encountered in surgical patients relating to wound care, drainage catheters, and postoperative bleeding.

Patients in the PACU should be under the medical direction of an anesthesiologist, who must be immediately available to respond to urgent or emergent patient care problems. High-volume tertiary care surgical institutions often have an anesthesiologist assigned full time to the PACU. The management of the patient in the PACU should reflect a coordinated effort involving anesthesiologists, surgeons, nurses, respiratory therapists, and appropriate consultants. The anesthesia team emphasizes management of analgesia, airway, cardiac, pulmonary, and metabolic problems, whereas the surgical team generally manages any problems directly related to the surgical procedure itself. Based on the assumptions that the average PACU stay is 1 hr and that the average inpatient procedure lasts 2–3 hr, a ratio of one recovery nurse for two patients is generally satisfactory. However, staffing for nursing care should be tailored to the unique caseload requirements of each facility. If the operating room schedule regularly includes pediatric patients or frequent short procedures, a ratio of one nurse to one patient is often needed. A charge nurse should be assigned to ensure optimal staffing at all times, including the appropriate response to urgent or emergent patient care problems.

Care of the Patient

EMERGENCE FROM GENERAL ANESTHESIA

Recovery from general or regional anesthesia is a time of great physiological stress. Emergence from general anesthesia should ideally be characterized by a smooth and gradual awakening in a controlled environment. However, problems such as airway obstruction, shivering, agitation, delirium, pain, nausea and vomiting, hypothermia, and autonomic lability are frequently encountered. Patients receiving spinal or epidural anesthesia may experience decreases in blood pressure during transport or recovery; the sympatholytic effects of major conduction blocks prevent compensatory reflex vasoconstriction when patients are moved or when they sit up.

Following an inhalational-based anesthetic, the speed of emergence is directly proportional to alveolar ventilation, but inversely proportional to the agent's blood solubility (see Chapter 8). As the duration of anesthesia increases, emergence also becomes increasingly dependent on total tissue uptake, which is a function of agent solubility, the

average concentration used, and the duration of exposure to the anesthetic. Hypoventilation delays emergence from inhalational anesthesia.

Emergence from an intravenous anesthetic is a function of its pharmacokinetics. Recovery from most intravenous anesthetic agents is dependent primarily on redistribution rather than metabolism and elimination. As the total administered dose increases, however, cumulative effects become clinically apparent in the form of prolonged emergence; the termination of action becomes increasingly dependent on the metabolism or elimination. This is the basis for the concept of a context-sensitive half-time (see Chapter 7). Advanced age or renal or hepatic disease can prolong emergence (see Chapter 9). Short and ultrashort-acting anesthetic agents, such as propofol and remifentanil, significantly shorten emergence, time to awakening, and discharge. Some studies show that the use of a Bispectral Index Scale (BIS) monitor (see Chapter 6) may reduce total drug dosage and shorten recovery and time to discharge. LMA (rather than an endotracheal tube) use may also allow lighter levels of anesthesia that could speed emergence.

The speed of emergence can also be influenced by preoperative medications. Premedication with agents that outlast the procedure (eg, lorazepam) may be expected to prolong emergence. The short duration of action of midazolam makes it a suitable premedication agent for short procedures. The effects of preoperative sleep deprivation or drug ingestion (alcohol, sedatives) can also be additive to those of anesthetic agents and can prolong emergence.

Delayed Emergence

The most frequent cause of delayed emergence (when the patient fails to regain consciousness 30–60 min after general anesthesia) is residual anesthetic, sedative, and analgesic drug effect. Delayed emergence may occur as a result of absolute or relative drug overdose or potentiation of anesthetic agents by prior drug or alcohol ingestion. Naloxone (in 80 mcg increments in adults) and flumazenil (in 0.2 mg increments in adults) will readily reverse the effects of an opioid and benzodiazepine, respectively. Physostigmine (1–2 mg) may partially reverse the effect of other agents. A nerve stimulator can be used to exclude persisting neuromuscular blockade in poorly responsive patients on a mechanical ventilator who have inadequate spontaneous tidal volumes.

Less common causes of delayed emergence include hypothermia, marked metabolic disturbances, and perioperative stroke. A core temperature of less than 33°C has an anesthetic effect and greatly potentiates the actions of central nervous system depressants. Forced-air warming devices are most effective in raising body temperature. Hypoxemia and hypercarbia are readily excluded by pulse oximetry, capnography, and/or blood gas analysis. Hypercalcemia, hypermagnesemia, hyponatremia, and hypoglycemia and hyperglycemia are rare causes of delayed emergence that require laboratory measurements for diagnosis. Perioperative stroke is rare, except after neurological, cardiac, and cerebrovascular surgery (see Chapter 28); diagnosis is facilitated by neurological evaluation and radiological imaging.

TRANSPORT FROM THE OPERATING ROOM TO THE PACU

This seemingly short period may be complicated by the lack of adequate monitoring, medication access, **①** or resuscitative equipment. Formerly anesthetized patients should not leave the operating room unless they have a patent airway, have adequate ventilation and oxygenation, and are hemodynamically stable; qualified anesthesia personnel must attend the transfer. Supplemental oxygen should be administered during transport to patients at risk of hypoxemia. Some studies suggest that transient hypoxemia (Spo$_2$ <90%) may develop in as many as 30% to 50% of otherwise "normal" patients during transport while breathing room air; supplemental oxygen may therefore be advisable for all transported patients, especially if the PACU is not in immediate proximity to the operating room. Unstable patients should remain intubated and should be transported with a portable monitor (ECG, Spo$_2$, and blood pressure) and a supply of emergency drugs.

All patients should be taken to the PACU on a bed or gurney that can be placed in either the head-down (Trendelenburg) or back-up position. The head-down position is useful for hypovolemic patients, whereas the back-up position is useful for patients with underlying pulmonary dysfunction (see Chapters 20 and 23). Patients at increased risk of vomiting or upper airway bleeding (eg, following tonsillectomy) should be transported in the lateral position. This position also helps prevent airway obstruction and facilitates drainage of secretions.

ROUTINE RECOVERY
General Anesthesia

Airway patency, vital signs, oxygenation, and level of consciousness must be assessed immediately upon PACU arrival. Subsequent blood pressure, heart rate, and respiratory rate measurements are routinely made at least every 5 min for 15 min or until stable, and every 15 min thereafter. Pulse oximetry should be monitored continuously in all patients. The occurrence of hypoxemia does not necessarily correlate with the level of consciousness. Neuromuscular function should be assessed clinically (eg, head-lift and grip strength). At least one temperature measurement must also be obtained. Additional monitoring includes pain assessment (eg, numerical or descriptive scales); the presence or absence of nausea or vomiting; and fluid input and output, including urine flow, drainage, and bleeding. After initial vital signs have been recorded, the anesthesia provider should give a brief report to the PACU nurse that includes (1) the preoperative history (including mental status and any communication problems, such as language barriers, deafness, blindness, or mental disability); (2) pertinent intraoperative events (type of anesthesia, the surgical procedure, blood loss, fluid replacement, antibiotic and other relevant medication administration, and any complications); (3) expected postoperative problems; (4) anticipated need for PACU medication administration, such as antibiotics; and (5) postanesthesia orders (analgesia and nausea/vomiting therapy; epidural or perineural catheter care; including the need for acute pain service involvement, administration of fluids or blood products, postoperative ventilation, chest x-ray for follow-up of central venous catheterization, etc.).

All patients recovering from general anesthesia must receive supplemental oxygen and pulse oximetry monitoring during emergence because transient hypoxemia can develop even in healthy patients. A rational decision regarding continuation of supplemental oxygen therapy at the time of PACU discharge can be made based on SpO_2 readings on room air. Arterial blood gas measurements may be obtained to confirm abnormal oximetry readings, but are not necessary in most patients. Oxygen therapy should be carefully controlled in patients with chronic obstructive pulmonary disease and a history of, or potential for, CO_2 retention. Patients should generally be nursed in the back-up position, whenever possible, to optimize oxygenation. However, elevating the head of the bed before the patient is responsive can lead to airway obstruction. In such cases, the oral or nasal airway should be left in place until the patient is awake and able to maintain airway. Deep breathing and coughing should be encouraged periodically.

Regional Anesthesia

Patients who are heavily sedated or hemodynamically unstable following regional anesthesia should also receive supplemental oxygen in the PACU. Sensory and motor levels should be periodically recorded following regional anesthesia to document regression of the block. Precautions in the form of padding or repeated warning may be necessary to prevent self-injury from uncoordinated arm movements following brachial plexus blocks. Blood pressure should be closely monitored following spinal and epidural anesthesia. Bladder catheterization may be necessary in patients who have had spinal or epidural anesthesia for longer than 4 hr.

Pain Control

Moderate to severe postoperative pain is most commonly treated with oral or parenteral opioids. However, perioperative opioid administration is associated with side effects (nausea and vomiting, respiratory depression, pruritis, ileus, and urinary retention) which may have significant adverse effects on postoperative convalescence. In response to this problem, a variety of *opioid sparing* strategies have been increasingly embraced over the past two decades to decrease opioid requirements, and thus opioid-related side effects, while maintaining satisfactory analgesia (see Chapter 47). Preoperative oral administration of nonsteroidal antiinflammatory drugs (NSAIDs), acetaminophen, and gabapentin or pregabalin may significantly reduce postoperative opioid requirements, and these medications may be resumed postoperatively if the patient can continue oral medication. Additional analgesic modalities utilizing local anesthetics, such as intraoperative wound infiltration, postoperative wound catheter infusions, single-shot and continuous catheter peripheral nerve blocks, and continuous epidural infusions, also reduce postoperative opioid analgesic requirements, and thus also reduce opioid-related side effects.

Mild to moderate postoperative pain can be treated orally with acetaminophen, ibuprofen, hydrocodone, or oxycodone. Alternatively, ketorolac tromethamine (15–30 mg in adults) or acetaminophen (15 mg/kg, or 1 g if patient >50 kg) may be administered intravenously.

In situations where moderate to severe postoperative pain is present, or oral analgesia is not possible, parenteral or intraspinal opioids, single-shot or continuous nerve blocks, and continuous epidural analgesia are used, often in combination techniques. Parenteral opioids are most safely administered by titration of small doses. Considerable variability in opioid requirements should be expected in surgical patients recovering in the PACU, and adequate analgesia must be balanced against the risk of excessive sedation and respiratory depression. Opioids of intermediate to long duration, such as hydromorphone 0.25–0.5 mg (0.015–0.02 mg/kg in children) or morphine 2–4 mg (0.025–0.05 mg/kg in children), are most commonly used. Meperidine is most often used in small doses to treat postoperative shivering. Opioid requirements are often markedly increased in patients with a history of chronic pain and chronic opioid therapy, because of opioid tolerance, and in patients with a history of opioid addiction, because of opioid tolerance and psychological dependence. Consultation with a pain specialist is often extremely helpful in these situations.

Analgesic effects of parenteral opioids usually peak within minutes of administration. Maximal respiratory depression, particularly with morphine and hydromorphone, may not occur until 20–30 min later. When the patient is fully awake, patient-controlled analgesia can be instituted for inpatients. Intramuscular administration of opioids is discouraged because delayed and variable onset (10–20 min or longer) and delayed respiratory depression (up to 1 h).

When an epidural catheter is used, epidural bolus administration of fentanyl (50–100 mcg) or sufentanil (20–30 mcg) with 5–10 mL of 0.1% bupivacaine can provide excellent pain relief in adults. Epidural morphine (3–5 mg) may also be used, but delayed respiratory depression with epidural administration of this opioid mandates close monitoring for 24 hr afterward (see Chapter 48).

Agitation

2 Before the recovering patient is fully responsive, pain is often manifested as postoperative restlessness. Serious systemic disturbances (such as hypoxemia, respiratory or metabolic acidosis, or hypotension), bladder distention, or a surgical complication (such as occult intraabdominal hemorrhage) must also be considered in the differential diagnosis of postoperative agitation. Marked agitation may necessitate arm and leg restraints to avoid self-injury, particularly in children. When serious physiological disturbances have been excluded in children, cuddling and kind words from a sympathetic attendant or the parents often calms the pediatric patient. Other contributory factors include marked preoperative anxiety and fear, as well as adverse drug effects (large doses of central anticholinergic agents, phenothiazines, or ketamine). Physostigmine 1–2 mg intravenously (0.05 mg/kg in children) is most effective in treating delirium due to atropine and scopolamine. If serious systemic disturbances and pain are excluded, persistent agitation may require sedation with intermittent intravenous doses of midazolam 0.5–1 mg (0.05 mg/kg in children).

Nausea & Vomiting

Postoperative nausea and vomiting (PONV) is common following general anesthesia, occurring in 30% to 40% of all patients. Moreover, PONV occurs at

TABLE 56–1 **Risk factors for postoperative nausea and vomiting.**

Patient factors
Young age
Female gender, particularly if menstruating on day of surgery or in first trimester of pregnancy
Large body habitus
History of prior postoperative emesis
History of motion sickness

Anesthetic techniques
General anesthesia
Drugs
Opioids
Volatile agents
Nitrous oxide

Surgical procedures
Strabismus surgery
Ear surgery
Laparoscopy
Orchiopexy
Ovum retrieval
Tonsillectomy
Breast surgery

Postoperative factors
Postoperative pain
Hypotension

home within 24 hr of an uneventful discharge (postdischarge nausea and vomiting) in a significant number of ambulatory surgery patients. The etiology of PONV is usually multifactorial and associated with anesthetic and analgesic agents, the type of surgical procedure, and intrinsic patient factors, such as a history of motion sickness. It is also important to recognize that nausea is a common complaint reported at the onset of hypotension, particularly following spinal or epidural anesthesia.

Table 56–1 **lists commonly recognized risk factors for PONV.** An increased incidence of nausea and vomiting is reported following opioid administration and intraperitoneal (especially laparoscopic), breast, and strabismus surgery. The greatest incidence seems to be in young women; nausea may be more common during menstruation. Increased vagal tone manifested as sudden bradycardia commonly precedes, or coincides with, emesis. Propofol anesthesia decreases the incidence of PONV, and a preoperative history of smoking lessens the likelihood of PONV. Selective 5-hydroxytryptamine (serotonin) receptor 3 (5-HT$_3$) antagonists, such as ondansetron 4 mg (0.1 mg/kg in children), granisetron 0.01–0.04 mg/kg, and dolasetron 12.5 mg (0.035 mg/kg in children), are effective in preventing PONV, and, to a lesser extent, in treating established PONV. It should be noted that unlike ondansetron, which is usually effective immediately, dolasetron requires 15 min for onset. An orally disintegrating tablet preparation of ondansetron (8 mg) may be useful for treatment and prophylaxis against postdischarge nausea and vomiting. Metoclopramide, 0.15 mg/kg intravenously, is a less effective alternative to 5-HT$_3$ antagonists. 5-HT$_3$ antagonists are not associated with the acute extrapyramidal (dystonic) manifestations and dysphoric reactions that may be encountered with metoclopramide or phenothiazine-type antiemetics. Transdermal scopolamine is effective, but can be associated with side effects, such as sedation, dysphoria, blurred vision, dry mouth, urinary retention, and exacerbation of glaucoma, particularly in elderly patients. Dexamethasone 4–10 mg (0.10 mg/kg in children), when utilized as an antiemetic, has the additional advantages of providing a varying degree of analgesia and a sense of patient well-being. Moreover, it seems to be effective for up to 24 hr, and, thus, may be useful for postdischarge nausea and vomiting. Oral aprepitant (Emend®) 40 mg may be administered within 3 hr prior to anesthesia induction. Intravenous droperidol 0.625–1.25 mg (0.05–0.075 mg/kg in children), when given intraoperatively, significantly decreases the likelihood of PONV. Unfortunately, droperidol carries a US Food and Drug Administration "black box" warning, indicating that large (5–15 mg) doses can prolong the QT interval and have been associated with fatal cardiac arrhythmias. Nonpharmacological prophylaxis against PONV includes ensuring adequate hydration (20 mL/kg) after fasting, and stimulation of the P6 acupuncture point (wrist). The latter may include application of pressure, electrical current, or injections.

Controversy exists regarding routine PONV prophylaxis for all patients. Because of the cost of treatment of established PONV, it may be cost-effective to provide prophylaxis to all patients in certain populations (eg, outpatients). Clearly, patients with multiple risk factors should receive prophylaxis. In addition, the use of two or three agents that act on differing receptors is more effective than single-agent prophylaxis.

Shivering & Hypothermia

Shivering can occur in the PACU as a result of intraoperative hypothermia or the effects of anesthetic agents, and it is also common in the immediate postpartum period. The most important cause of hypothermia is a redistribution of heat from the body core to the peripheral compartments (see Chapter 6). A relatively cool ambient operating room temperature, prolonged exposure of a large wound, and the use of large amounts of unwarmed intravenous fluids or high flows of unhumidified gases can also be contributory. Nearly all anesthetics, particularly volatile agents and spinal and epidural anesthesia, decrease the normal vasoconstrictive response to hypothermia by decreasing sympathetic tone. Although anesthetic agents also decrease the shivering threshold, shivering commonly observed during or after emergence from general anesthesia represents the body's effort to increase heat production and raise body temperature and may be associated with intense vasoconstriction. Emergence from even brief general anesthesia is sometimes also associated with shivering, and although the shivering can be one of several nonspecific neurological signs (posturing, clonus, or Babinski's sign) that are sometimes observed during emergence, it is most often due to hypothermia. Regardless of the mechanism, its incidence seems to be related to the duration of surgery and the use of a volatile agent. Shivering may occasionally be sufficiently intense to cause hyperthermia (38–39°C) and significant metabolic acidosis, both of which promptly resolve when the shivering stops. Other causes of shivering should be excluded, such as bacteremia and sepsis, drug allergy, or transfusion reaction.

Hypothermia should be treated with a forced-air warming device, or (less satisfactorily) with warming lights or heating blankets, to raise body temperature to normal. Intense shivering causes precipitous rises in oxygen consumption, CO_2 production, and cardiac output. These physiological effects are often poorly tolerated by patients with preexisting cardiac or pulmonary impairment. Hypothermia has been associated with an increased incidence of myocardial ischemia, arrhythmias, increased transfusion requirements due to coagulopathy, and increased duration of muscle relaxant effects. Small intravenous doses of meperidine (10–25 mg) can dramatically reduce or even stop shivering. Intubated and mechanically ventilated patients can also be sedated and given a muscle relaxant until normothermia is reestablished by active rewarming and the effects of anesthesia have dissipated.

Discharge Criteria

A. PACU

All patients must be evaluated by a qualified anesthesia provider prior to discharge from the PACU unless strict discharge criteria are adopted. Standards for discharging patients from the PACU are established by the department of anesthesiology and the hospital medical staff. They may allow PACU nurses to determine when patients may be transferred without the presence of a qualified anesthesia provider if all PACU discharge criteria have been met. Criteria can vary according to whether the patient is going to be discharged to an intensive care unit, a regular ward, the outpatient department (phase 2 recovery), or directly home.

Before discharge, patients should have been observed for respiratory depression for at least 20–30 min after the last dose of parenteral opioid. Other minimum discharge criteria for patients recovering from general anesthesia usually include the following:

1. Easy arousability
2. Full orientation
3. The ability to maintain and protect the airway
4. Stable vital signs for at least 15–30 min
5. The ability to call for help, if necessary
6. No obvious surgical complications (such as active bleeding)

Postoperative pain and nausea and vomiting must be controlled, and normothermia should be reestablished prior to PACU discharge. Scoring systems are widely used. Most assess SpO_2 (or color),

TABLE 56–2 Postanesthetic Aldrete recovery score.[1,2]

Original Criteria	Modified Criteria	Point Value
Color	**Oxygenation**	
Pink	$SpO_2 > 92\%$ on room air	2
Pale or dusky	$SpO_2 > 90\%$ on oxygen	1
Cyanotic	$SpO_2 < 90\%$ on oxygen	0
Respiration		
Can breathe deeply and cough	Breathes deeply and coughs freely	2
Shallow but adequate exchange	Dyspneic, shallow or limited breathing	1
Apnea or obstruction	Apnea	0
Circulation		
Blood pressure within 20% of normal	Blood pressure ± 20 mm Hg of normal	2
Blood pressure within 20% to 50% of normal	Blood pressure ± 20–50 mm Hg of normal	1
Blood pressure deviating >50% from normal	Blood pressure more than ± 50 mm Hg of normal	0
Consciousness		
Awake, alert, and oriented	Fully awake	2
Arousable but readily drifts back to sleep	Arousable on calling	1
No response	Not responsive	0
Activity		
Moves all extremities	Same	2
Moves two extremities	Same	1
No movement	Same	0

[1]Data from Aldrete JA, Kronlik D: A postanesthetic recovery score. Anesth Analg 1970;49:924 and Aldrete JA: The post-anesthesia recovery score revisited. J Clin Anesth 1995;7:89.

[2]Ideally, the patient should be discharged when the total score is 10, but a minimum of 9 is required.

consciousness, circulation, respiration, and motor activity (Table 56–2). The majority of patients can meet discharge criteria within 60 min from the time of PACU arrival. Patients to be transferred to other intensive care areas need not meet all requirements.

In addition to the above criteria, patients receiving regional anesthesia should also be assessed for regression of both sensory and motor blockade. Complete resolution of the block prior to PACU dismissal avoids inadvertent injuries due to motor weakness or sensory deficits; however, many institutions have protocols that allow earlier discharge to appropriately monitored areas, and patients may be discharged with peripheral nerve blocks from single-shot or continuous perineural catheter infusions for the purpose of regional analgesia. Documenting regression of a block is important. Failure of a spinal or epidural block to resolve 6 hr after the last dose of local anesthetic raises the possibility of spinal subdural or epidural hematoma, which should be excluded by prompt radiological imaging and neurologic evaluation.

In some centers, outpatients who meet the above discharge criteria when they come out of the operating room may be "fast-tracked," bypassing the PACU and proceeding directly to the phase 2 recovery area. Similarly, inpatients who meet the same criteria may be transferred directly from the operating room to their ward, if appropriate staffing and monitoring is present.

B. Outpatients

In addition to emergence and awakening, recovery from anesthesia following outpatient procedures includes two additional stages: home readiness (phase 2 recovery) and complete psychomotor recovery. A scoring system has been developed to help assess home readiness discharge (Table 56–3). Recovery of proprioception, sympathetic tone, bladder function, and motor strength are additional criteria following regional anesthesia. For example, intact proprioception of the big toe, minimal orthostatic blood pressure and heart rate changes, and normal plantar flexion of the foot are important signals of recovery following spinal anesthesia. Urination and drinking or eating before discharge are usually no longer required; exceptions include patients with a history of urinary retention and those with diabetes.

All outpatients must be discharged home in the company of a responsible adult who will stay with them overnight (the latter is required if they have received an anesthetic). Patients must be provided with written postoperative instructions on how to obtain emergency help and to perform routine follow-up care. The assessment of home readiness is the responsibility of the qualified anesthesia provider, preferably one who is already familiar with the patient, although authority to discharge a patient

TABLE 56–3 **Postanesthesia discharge scoring system (PADS).[1,2]**

Criteria	Points
Vital signs	
Within 20% of preoperative baseline	2
Within 20% to 40% of preoperative baseline	1
>40% of preoperative baseline	0
Activity level	
Steady gait, no dizziness, at preoperative level	2
Requires assistance	1
Unable to ambulate	0
Nausea and vomiting	
Minimal, treated with oral medication	2
Moderate, treated with parenteral medication	1
Continues after repeated medication	0
Pain: minimal or none, acceptable to patient, controlled with oral medication	
Yes	2
No	1
Surgical bleeding	
Minimal: no dressing change required	2
Moderate: up to two dressing changes	1
Severe: three or more dressing changes	0

[1]Modified from Marshall SI, Chung F: Discharge criteria and complications after ambulatory surgery. Anesth Analg 1999;88:508.
[2]Score ≥ 9 is required for discharge.

home can be delegated to a nurse, if approved discharge criteria are applied.

Home readiness does not imply that the patient has the ability to make important decisions, to drive, or to return to work. These activities require complete psychomotor recovery, which is often not achieved until 24–72 hr postoperatively. All outpatient centers must use some system of postoperative follow-up, preferably phone contact the day after discharge.

Management of Complications

RESPIRATORY COMPLICATIONS

4 Respiratory problems are the most frequently encountered serious complications in the PACU. The overwhelming majority are related to airway obstruction, hypoventilation, or hypoxemia. Because hypoxemia is the final common pathway to serious morbidity and mortality, routine monitoring of pulse oximetry in the PACU leads to earlier recognition of these complications and fewer adverse outcomes.

Airway Obstruction

Airway obstruction in unconscious patients is most commonly due to the tongue falling back against the posterior pharynx (see Chapter 19). Other causes include laryngospasm, glottic edema, secretions, vomitus, a retained throat pack or blood in the airway, or external pressure on the trachea (most commonly from a neck hematoma). Partial airway obstruction usually presents as sonorous respiration. Near-total or total obstruction causes cessation of airflow and an absence of breath sounds and may be accompanied by paradoxic (rocking) movement of the chest. The abdomen and chest should normally rise together during inspiration; however, with airway obstruction, the chest descends as the abdomen rises during each inspiration (paradoxic chest movement). Patients with airway obstruction should receive supplemental oxygen while corrective measures are undertaken. A combined jaw-thrust and head-tilt maneuver pulls the tongue forward and opens the airway, and insertion of an oral or nasal airway often alleviates the problem. Nasal airways may be better tolerated than oral airways by patients emerging from anesthesia and may decrease the likelihood of trauma to the teeth when the patient bites down.

If the above maneuvers fail to reestablish an open airway, laryngospasm should be considered. Laryngospasm is usually characterized by high-pitched crowing noises, but may be silent with complete glottic closure. Spasm of the vocal cords is more apt to occur following airway trauma, repeated instrumentation, or stimulation from secretions or blood in the airway. The jaw-thrust maneuver, particularly when combined with gentle positive airway pressure via a tight-fitting face mask, usually breaks laryngospasm. Insertion of an oral or nasal airway is also helpful in ensuring a patent airway down to the level of the vocal cords. Any secretions or blood in the hypopharynx should be suctioned to prevent

recurrence. Refractory laryngospasm should be treated with a small dose of intravenous succinylcholine (10–20 mg in adults) and positive-pressure ventilation with 100% oxygen. Endotracheal intubation may occasionally be necessary to reestablish ventilation; cricothyrotomy or transtracheal jet ventilation is indicated if intubation is unsuccessful in such instances.

Glottic edema following airway instrumentation is an important cause of airway obstruction in infants and young children because of the relatively small airway lumen. Intravenous corticosteroids (dexamethasone, 0.5 mg/kg, 10 mg dose maximum) or aerosolized racemic epinephrine (0.5 mL of a 2.25% solution with 3 mL of normal saline) may be useful in such cases. Postoperative wound hematomas following thyroid, carotid artery, and other neck procedures can quickly compromise the airway, and opening the wound immediately relieves tracheal compression in most cases. Rarely, gauze packing may be unintentionally left in the hypopharynx following oral surgery and can cause immediate or delayed complete airway obstruction, especially in patients with intermaxillary fixation.

Accidental or intentional decannulation of a fresh tracheostomy is hazardous because the various tissue planes have not yet organized into a well-formed track, thereby often making recannulation very difficult or impossible. In cases of tracheostomy performed within the previous 3–4 weeks, intentional replacement of a tracheostomy cannula should only be performed with a qualified surgeon at the bedside and a surgical tracheostomy instrument set, along with other appropriate airway equipment, immediately available.

Hypoventilation

Hypoventilation, which is generally defined as a $Paco_2$ >45 mm Hg, is common following general anesthesia. In most instances, the hypoventilation is mild, and most cases are undiagnosed. Significant hypoventilation is usually clinically apparent when the $Paco_2$ is >60 mm Hg or arterial blood pH is <7.25. Signs are varied and include excessive somnolence, airway obstruction, slow respiratory rate, tachypnea with shallow breathing, or labored breathing. Mild to moderate respiratory acidosis may cause tachycardia, hypertension, and cardiac irritability (via sympathetic stimulation), but more severe acidosis produces circulatory depression (see Chapter 50. If significant hypoventilation is suspected, assessment and management is facilitated by capnography and/or arterial blood gas measurement.

5 Hypoventilation in the PACU is most commonly due to the residual depressant effects of anesthetics on respiratory drive. Opioid-induced respiratory depression characteristically produces a slow respiratory rate, often with large tidal volumes. Excessive sedation is usually present, but the patient is often responsive and able to breathe on command. Delayed occurrence of respiratory depression have been reported with all opioids. Proposed mechanisms include variations in the intensity of stimulation during recovery and delayed release of the opioid from peripheral compartments, such as skeletal muscle (or possibly the lungs with fentanyl), as the patient rewarms or begins to move.

Causes of residual muscle paralysis in the PACU include inadequate reversal, pharmacological interactions, altered pharmacokinetics (due to hypothermia, altered volumes of distribution, and renal or hepatic dysfunction), and metabolic factors (such as hypokalemia or respiratory acidosis). Regardless of the cause, generalized weakness, dyscoordinated movements ("fish out of water"), shallow tidal volumes, and tachypnea are usually apparent. The diagnosis can be made with a nerve stimulator in unconscious patients; head lift and grip strength can be assessed in awake patients. The ability to sustain a head-lift for 5 sec may be the most sensitive test for assessing the adequacy of reversal.

Splinting due to incisional pain, diaphragmatic dysfunction following upper abdominal or thoracic surgery, abdominal distention, and tight abdominal dressings are other factors that can contribute to hypoventilation. Increased CO_2 production from shivering, hyperthermia, or sepsis can also increase $Paco_2$, even in normal patients recovering from general anesthesia. Marked hypoventilation and respiratory acidosis can result when these factors are superimposed on an impaired ventilatory reserve due to underlying pulmonary, neuromuscular, or neurological disease.

Treatment of Hypoventilation

Treatment should generally be directed at the underlying cause, but marked hypoventilation always requires assisted or controlled ventilation until causal **6** factors are identified and corrected. Obtundation, circulatory depression, and severe acidosis (arterial blood pH <7.15) are indications for immediate and aggressive respiratory and hemodynamic intervention, including airway and inotropic support as needed. Antagonism of opioid-induced depression with large doses of naloxone often results in sudden pain and marked increase in sympathetic tone. The latter can precipitate a hypertensive crisis, pulmonary edema, and myocardial ischemia or infarction. If naloxone is used to reverse opioid-induced respiratory depression, titration in small increments (80 mcg in adults) usually avoids complications by reversal of hypoventilation without significant reversal of analgesia. Following **7** naloxone administration, patients should be observed closely for recurrence of opioid-induced respiratory depression ("renarcotization"), as naloxone has a shorter duration than most opioids. If residual muscle paralysis is present, additional cholinesterase inhibitor may be given. Residual paralysis in spite of a full dose of a cholinesterase inhibitor necessitates controlled ventilation under close observation until spontaneous recovery occurs. Hypoventilation due to pain and splinting following upper abdominal or thoracic procedures should be treated with intravenous or intraspinal opioid administration, intravenous ketorolac, epidural anesthesia, or intercostal nerve blocks.

Hypoxemia

Mild hypoxemia is common in patients recovering from anesthesia when supplemental oxygen is not given. Mild to moderate hypoxemia (Pao_2 50–60 mm Hg) in young healthy patients may be well tolerated initially, but with increasing duration or severity, the initial sympathetic stimulation often seen is replaced with progressive acidosis and circulatory depression. Obvious cyanosis may be absent if the hemoglobin concentration is reduced. Hypoxemia may also be suspected from restlessness, tachycardia, or cardiac irritability (ventricular or atrial). Obtundation, bradycardia, hypotension, and cardiac arrest are late signs. Pulse oximetry facilitates early detection of hypoxemia and must be routinely utilized in the PACU. Arterial blood gas measurements may be performed to confirm the diagnosis and guide therapy.

Hypoxemia in the PACU is usually caused by hypoventilation, increased right-to-left intrapulmonary shunting, or both. A decrease in cardiac output or an increase in oxygen consumption (as with shivering) will accentuate hypoxemia. Diffusion hypoxia (see Chapter 8) is an uncommon cause of hypoxemia when recovering patients are given supplemental oxygen. Hypoxemia due exclusively to hypoventilation is also unusual in patients receiving supplemental oxygen, unless marked hypercapnia or a concomitant increase in intrapulmonary shunting **8** is present. Increased intrapulmonary shunting from a decreased functional residual capacity (FRC) relative to closing capacity is the most common cause of hypoxemia following general anesthesia. The greatest reductions in FRC occur following upper abdominal and thoracic surgery. The loss of lung volume is often attributed to microatelectasis, as atelectasis is often not identified on a chest radiograph. A semi-upright position helps maintain FRC.

Marked right-to-left intrapulmonary shunting ($\dot{Q}s/\dot{Q}_T$ >15%) is usually associated with radiographic findings, such as pulmonary atelectasis, parenchymal infiltrates, or a large pneumothorax. Causes include prolonged intraoperative hypoventilation with low tidal volumes, unintentional endobronchial intubation, lobar collapse from bronchial obstruction by secretions or blood, pulmonary aspiration, or pulmonary edema. Postoperative pulmonary edema most often presents as wheezing within the first 60 min after surgery, and, to a lesser extent, pink frothy fluid in the airway, and may be due to left ventricular failure (cardiogenic), acute respiratory distress syndrome, or relief of prolonged airway obstruction (negative pressure pulmonary edema). In contrast to wheezing associated with pulmonary edema, wheezing due to primary obstructive lung disease, which also often results in large increases in intrapulmonary shunting, is not associated with edema fluid in the airway or infiltrates on the chest **9** radiograph. The possibility of a postoperative pneumothorax should always be considered following central line placement, supraclavicular or

intercostal blocks, abdominal or chest trauma (including rib fractures), neck dissection, tracheostomy, nephrectomy, or other retroperitoneal or intraabdominal procedures (including laparoscopy), especially if the diaphragm may have been penetrated or disrupted. Patients with subpleural blebs or large bullae can also develop pneumothorax during positive-pressure ventilation.

Treatment of Hypoxemia

Oxygen therapy with or without positive airway pressure is the cornerstone of treatment for hypoxemia. Routine administration of 30% to 60% oxygen is usually enough to prevent hypoxemia with even moderate hypoventilation and hypercapnia (conversely, clinical signs of hypoventilation and hypercapnia may be masked by routine oxygen administration). Patients with underlying pulmonary or cardiac disease may require higher concentrations of oxygen; oxygen therapy should be guided by Spo_2 or arterial blood gas measurements. Oxygen concentration must be closely controlled in patients with chronic CO_2 retention to avoid precipitating acute respiratory failure. Patients with severe or persistent hypoxemia should be given 100% oxygen via a nonrebreathing mask or an endotracheal tube until the cause is established and other therapies are instituted; controlled or assisted mechanical ventilation may also be necessary. The chest radiograph (preferably with the patient positioned sitting upright) is valuable in assessing lung volume and heart size and in demonstrating a pneumothorax or pulmonary infiltrates. However, in cases of pulmonary aspiration, infiltrates are usually initially absent. If pneumothorax is suspected, a chest radiograph taken at end-expiration helps highlight the pneumothorax by providing the greatest contrast between lung tissue and adjacent air in the pleural space. In the situation of an intubated patient with hypoxemia, a chest radiograph provides additional usefulness to breath sound assessment in verifying endotracheal tube position, especially when the tube is inadvertently positioned immediately above the carina, with resultant intermittent migration into a main bronchus.

Additional treatment of hypoxemia should be directed at the underlying cause. A chest tube or Heimlich valve should be inserted for any symptomatic pneumothorax or one that is greater than 15% to 20%. An asymptomatic pneumothorax may be aspirated using a intercostal catheter or followed by observation. Bronchospasm should be treated with aerosolized bronchodilator therapy. Diuretics should be given for circulatory fluid overload and cardiac function should be optimized. Persistent hypoxemia in spite of 50% oxygen generally is an indication for positive end-expiratory pressure ventilation or CPAP. Bronchoscopy is often useful in reexpanding lobar atelectasis caused by bronchial plugs or particulate aspiration. In the setting of an intubated patient, secretions or debris must be removed by suction and also by lavage, if necessary, and a malpositioned endotracheal tube must be appropriately repositioned.

CIRCULATORY COMPLICATIONS

The most common circulatory disturbances in the PACU are hypotension, hypertension, and arrhythmias. The possibility that the circulatory abnormality is secondary to an underlying respiratory disturbance should always be considered before any other intervention, especially in children.

Hypotension

Hypotension is usually due to relative hypovolemia, left ventricular dysfunction, or, less commonly, excessive arterial vasodilatation. Hypovolemia is by far the most common cause of hypotension in the PACU. Absolute hypovolemia can result from inadequate intraoperative fluid replacement, continuing fluid sequestration by tissues ("third-spacing"), wound drainage, or hemorrhage. Vasoconstriction during hypothermia with central sequestration of intravascular volume may mask hypovolemia until the patient's temperature begins to rise again; subsequent peripheral vasodilation during rewarming unmasks the hypovolemia and results in delayed hypotension. Relative hypovolemia is often responsible for the hypotension associated with spinal or epidural anesthesia (especially in the setting of concomitant general anesthesia), venodilators, and α-adrenergic blockade: the venous pooling reduces the effective circulating blood volume, despite an otherwise normal intravascular volume (see Chapter 45). Hypotension associated with sepsis and allergic reactions is usually the result of both hypovolemia and vasodilation. Hypotension from a tension pneumothorax or cardiac tamponade is the result of impaired venous return to the right atrium.

Left ventricular dysfunction in previously healthy persons is unusual, unless it is associated with severe metabolic disturbances (hypoxemia, acidosis, or sepsis). Hypotension due to ventricular dysfunction is primarily encountered in patients with underlying coronary artery or valvular heart disease or congestive heart failure and is usually precipitated by fluid overload, myocardial ischemia, acute increases in afterload, or arrhythmias.

Treatment of Hypotension

Mild hypotension during recovery from anesthesia is common and typically does not require intensive treatment. Significant hypotension is often defined as a 20% to 30% reduction in blood pressure below the patient's baseline level and usually requires correction. Treatment depends on the ability to assess intravascular volume. An increase in blood pressure following a fluid bolus (250–500 mL crystalloid or 100–250 mL colloid) generally confirms hypovolemia. With severe hypotension, a vasopressor or inotrope (dopamine or epinephrine) may be necessary to increase arterial blood pressure until the intravascular volume deficit is at least partially corrected. Signs of cardiac dysfunction should be sought in patients with heart disease or cardiac risk factors. Failure of a patient with severe hypotension to promptly respond to initial treatment mandates invasive hemodynamic monitoring, or, better still, echocardiographic examination; manipulations of cardiac preload, contractility, and afterload are often necessary. The presence of a tension pneumothorax, as suggested by hypotension with unilaterally decreased breath sounds, hyperresonance, and tracheal deviation, is an indication for immediate pleural aspiration, even before radiographic confirmation. Similarly, hypotension due to cardiac tamponade, usually following chest trauma or thoracic surgery, often necessitates immediate pericardiocentesis or surgical exploration.

Hypertension

Postoperative hypertension is common in the PACU and typically occurs within the first 30 min after admission. Noxious stimulation from incisional pain, endotracheal intubation, or bladder distention is usually responsible. Postoperative hypertension may also reflect the neuroendocrine stress response to surgery or increased sympathetic tone secondary to hypoxemia, hypercapnia, or metabolic acidosis. Patients with a history of hypertension are likely to develop hypertension in the PACU, even in the absence of an identifiable cause. Fluid overload or intracranial hypertension may also occasionally present as postoperative hypertension.

Treatment of Hypertension

Mild hypertension generally does not require treatment, but a reversible cause should be sought. Marked hypertension can precipitate postoperative bleeding, myocardial ischemia, heart failure, or intracranial hemorrhage. Although decisions to treat postoperative hypertension should be individualized, in general, elevations in blood pressure greater than 20% to 30% of the patient's baseline, or those associated with adverse effects such as myocardial ischemia, heart failure, or bleeding, should be treated. Mild to moderate elevations can be treated with an intravenous β-adrenergic blocker, such as labetalol, esmolol, or metoprolol; an angiotensin-converting enzyme inhibitor, such as enalapril; or a calcium channel blocker, such as nicardipine. Hydralazine and sublingual nifedipine (when administered to patients not receiving β-blockers) may cause tachycardia and myocardial ischemia and infarction. Marked hypertension in patients with limited cardiac reserve requires direct intraarterial pressure monitoring and should be treated with an intravenous infusion of nitroprusside, nitroglycerin, nicardipine, clevidipine, or fenoldopam. The end point for treatment should be consistent with the patient's own normal blood pressure.

Arrhythmias

Respiratory disturbances, particularly hypoxemia, hypercarbia, and acidosis, will commonly be associated with cardiac arrhythmias. Residual effects from anesthetic agents, increased sympathetic nervous system activity, other metabolic abnormalities, and preexisting cardiac or pulmonary disease also predispose patients to arrhythmias in the PACU.

Bradycardia often represents the residual effects of cholinesterase inhibitors, opioids, or β-adrenergic blockers. Tachycardia may represent the effect of an anticholinergic agent; a β-agonist, such as albuterol; reflex tachycardia from hydralazine; and more common causes, such as pain, fever, hypovolemia, and anemia. Anesthetic-induced depression of baroreceptor function makes heart rate an unreliable monitor of intravascular volume in the PACU.

Premature atrial and ventricular beats often represent hypokalemia, hypomagnesemia, increased sympathetic tone, or, less commonly, myocardial ischemia. The latter can be diagnosed with a 12-lead ECG. Premature atrial or ventricular beats noted in the PACU without discernable cause will often also be found on the patient's preoperative ECG, if one is available. Such patients with a preexisting history of extrasystoles may or may not have a history of palpitations or other symptoms, and previous cardiology evaluation often has found no definitive cause. Supraventricular tachyarrhythmias, including paroxysmal supraventricular tachycardia, atrial flutter, and atrial fibrillation, are typically encountered in patients with a history of these arrhythmias and are more commonly encountered following thoracic surgery. The management of arrhythmias is discussed in Chapters 20 and 55.

CASE DISCUSSION

Fever & Tachycardia in a Young Adult Male

A 19-year-old man sustains a closed fracture of the femur in a motor vehicle accident. He is placed in traction for 3 days prior to surgery. During that time, a persistent low-grade fever (37.5–38.7°C orally), mild hypertension (150–170/70–90 mm Hg), and tachycardia (100–126 beats/min) are noted. His hematocrit remains between 30% and 32.5%. Broad-spectrum antibiotic coverage is initiated. He is scheduled for open reduction and internal fixation of the fracture. When the patient is brought into the operating room, vital signs are as follows: blood pressure 162/95 mm Hg, pulse 150 beats/min, respirations 20 breaths/min, and oral temperature 38.1°C. He is sweating and is anxious in spite of intravenous premedication with fentanyl 50 mcg and midazolam 1 mg. On close examination, he is noted to have a slightly enlarged thyroid gland.

Should the surgical team proceed with the operation?

The proposed operation is elective; therefore, significant abnormalities should be diagnosed and properly treated preoperatively, if possible, to make the patient optimally ready for surgery. If the patient had an open fracture, the risk of infection would clearly mandate immediate operation. Even with a closed femoral fracture, cancellations or delays should be avoided because nonoperative treatment potentiates the risks associated with bed rest, including atelectasis, pneumonia, deep venous thrombosis, and potentially lethal pulmonary thromboembolism. In deciding whether to proceed with the surgery, the anesthesia provider must ask the following questions:

1. What are the most likely causes of the abnormalities based on the clinical presentation?
2. What, if any, additional investigations or consultations might be helpful?
3. How would these or other commonly associated abnormalities affect anesthetic management?
4. Are the potential anesthetic interactions serious enough to delay surgery until a suspected cause is conclusively excluded? The tachycardia of 150 beats/min and the low-grade fever therefore require further evaluation prior to surgery.

What are the likely causes of the tachycardia and fever in this patient?

These two abnormalities may reflect one process or separate entities (Tables 56–4 and 56–5). Moreover, although multiple factors can often be simultaneously identified, their relative contribution is often not readily apparent. Fever commonly follows major trauma; contributory factors can include the inflammatory reaction to

TABLE 56–4 Perioperative causes of tachycardia.

Anxiety
Pain
Fever (see Table 56–5)
Respiratory
Hypoxemia
Hypercapnia
Circulatory
Hypotension
Anemia
Hypovolemia
Congestive heart failure
Cardiac tamponade
Tension pneumothorax
Thromboembolism
Drug-induced
Antimuscarinic agents
β-Adrenergic agonists
Vasodilators
Allergy
Drug withdrawal
Metabolic disorders
Hypoglycemia
Thyrotoxicosis
Pheochromocytoma
Adrenal (addisonian) crisis
Carcinoid syndrome
Acute porphyria

TABLE 56–5 Perioperative causes of fever.

Infections
Immunologically mediated processes
Drug reactions
Blood reactions
Tissue destruction (rejection)
Connective tissue disorders
Granulomatous disorders
Tissue damage
Trauma
Infarction
Thrombosis
Neoplastic disorders
Metabolic disorders
Thyroid storm (thyroid crisis)
Adrenal (addisonian) crisis
Pheochromocytoma
Malignant hyperthermia
Neuroleptic malignant syndrome
Acute gout
Acute porphyria

the tissue trauma, superimposed infection (most commonly wound, pulmonary, or urinary), antibiotic therapy (drug reaction), or thrombophlebitis. Infection must be seriously considered in this patient because of the risk of bacteria seeding and infecting the metal fixation device placed during surgery. Although tachycardia is commonly associated with a low-grade fever, it is usually not of this magnitude in a 19-year-old patient. Moderate to severe pain, anxiety, hypovolemia, or anemia may be other contributory factors. Pulmonary fat embolism should also be considered in any patient with long bone fracture, particularly when hypoxemia, tachypnea, or mental status changes are present. Lastly, the possibly enlarged thyroid gland, sweating, and anxious appearance, together with both fever and tachycardia, suggest thyrotoxicosis.

What (if any) additional measures may be helpful in evaluating the fever and tachycardia?

Arterial blood gas measurements and a chest film would be helpful in excluding fat embolism. A repeat hematocrit or hemoglobin concentration measurement would exclude worsening anemia; significant tachycardia may be expected when the hematocrit is below 25% to 27% (hemoglobin <8 g/dL) in most patients. The response to an intravenous fluid challenge with 250–500 mL of a colloid or crystalloid solution may be helpful; a decrease in heart rate after the fluid bolus is strongly suggestive of hypovolemia. Similarly, response of the heart rate to sedation and additional opioid analgesia can be helpful in excluding anxiety and pain, respectively, as causes. Although a tentative diagnosis of hyperthyroidism can be made based on clinical grounds, confirmation requires measurement of serum thyroid hormones; the latter usually requires 24–48 hr in most hospitals. Signs of infection—such as increased inflammation or purulence in a wound, purulent sputum, an infiltrate on the chest film, pyuria, or leukocytosis with premature white cells on a blood smear (shift to the left)—should prompt cultures and a delay of surgery until the results are obtained and correct antibiotic coverage is confirmed.

The patient is transferred to the PACU for further evaluation. A 12-lead ECG confirms sinus tachycardia of 150 beats/min. A chest film is normal. Arterial blood gas measurements on room air are normal (pH 7.44, $Paco_2$ 41 mm Hg, Pao_2 87 mm Hg, and HCO_3^- 27 mEq/L). The hemoglobin concentration is found to be 11 g/dL. Blood for thyroid function tests is sent to the laboratory. The patient is sedated intravenously with midazolam (2 mg) and fentanyl (50 mcg) and is given 500 mL of 5% albumin. He seems to be relaxed and pain free, but the heart rate decreases only to 144 beats/min. The decision is made to proceed with surgery using continuous lumbar epidural anesthesia with 2% lidocaine. Esmolol is administered slowly until his pulse decreases to 120 beats/min, and a continuous esmolol infusion is administered at a rate of 300 mcg/kg/min.

The procedure is completed in 3 1/2 hr. Although the patient did not complain of any pain during the procedure and was given only minimal additional sedation (midazolam, 2 mg), he is delirious upon admission to the PACU. The esmolol infusion is proceeding at a rate of 500 mcg/kg/min. He has also received propranolol, 24 mg intravenously. Estimated blood loss was 500 mL, and fluid replacement consisted of 2 units of packed red blood cells, 1000 mL of hetastarch, and 9000 mL of lactated Ringer's injection. Vital signs are as follows: blood pressure 105/40 mm Hg, pulse 124 beats/min, respirations 30 breaths/min, and rectal temperature 38.8°C. Arterial blood gas measurements are reported as follows: pH 7.37, $Paco_2$ 37 mm Hg, Pao_2 91 mm Hg, and HCO_3^- 22 mEq/L.

What is the most likely diagnosis?

The patient is now obviously in a hypermetabolic state manifested by excessive adrenergic activity, fever, markedly increased fluid requirements, and a worsening mental status. The absence of major metabolic acidosis and lack of exposure to a known triggering agent exclude malignant hyperthermia (see Chapter 52). Other possibilities include a transfusion reaction, sepsis, or an undiagnosed pheochromocytoma. The sequence of events makes the first two unlikely, and the decreasing prominence of hypertension (now replaced with relative hypotension) and increasing fever also make the latter unlikely. The clinical presentation now strongly suggests thyroid storm. He has also received a very large dose of esmolol for several hours and this may be contributing to the relatively low blood pressure despite aggressive fluid administration.

Emergency consultation is obtained with an endocrinologist, who concurs with the diagnosis of thyroid storm and assists with its management. How is thyroid storm managed?

Thyroid storm (crisis) is a medical emergency that carries a 10% to 50% mortality rate. It is usually encountered in patients with poorly controlled or undiagnosed Graves disease. Precipitating factors include (1) the stress of surgery and anesthesia, (2) labor and delivery, (3) severe infection, and, rarely, (4) thyroiditis 1–2 wk following administration of radioactive iodine. Manifestations usually include mental status changes (irritability, delirium, or coma), fever, tachycardia, and hypotension. Both atrial and ventricular arrhythmias are common, particularly atrial fibrillation. Congestive heart failure develops in 25% of patients. Hypertension that often precedes hypotension, heat intolerance with profuse sweating, nausea and vomiting, and diarrhea may be prominent initially. Hypokalemia is present in up to 50% of patients. Levels of thyroid hormones are high in plasma, but correlate poorly with the severity of the crisis. The sudden exacerbation of thyrotoxicosis may represent a rapid shift of the hormone from the protein-bound to the free state or increased responsiveness to thyroid hormones at the cellular level.

Treatment is directed toward reversing the crisis and its complications. Large doses of corticosteroids inhibit the synthesis, release, and peripheral conversion of thyroxine (T_4) to the more active triiodothyronine (T_3). Corticosteroids also prevent relative adrenal insufficiency secondary to the hypermetabolic state. Propylthiouracil is administered to inhibit synthesis of thyroid hormone, and iodide is given to inhibit release of thyroid hormones from the gland. Propranolol

not only antagonizes the peripheral effects of the thyrotoxicosis, but may also inhibit the peripheral conversion of T_4. Combined β_1- and β_2-blockade is preferable to selective β_1-antagonism (esmolol or metoprolol) because excessive β_2-receptor activity is responsible for the metabolic effects. β_2-Receptor blockade also reduces muscle blood flow and may decrease heat production. Supportive measures include surface cooling (cooling blanket), acetaminophen (aspirin is not recommended because it may displace thyroid hormone from plasma carrier proteins), and generous intravenous fluid replacement. Vasopressors are often necessary to support arterial blood pressure.

Ventricular rate control is indicated in patients with atrial fibrillation. Transthoracic echocardiography, transesophageal echocardiography, and hemodynamic monitoring may facilitate management of patients with signs of congestive heart failure or persistent hypotension. β-Adrenergic blockade is contraindicated in patients with congestive heart failure.

Propranolol, dexamethasone, propylthiouracil, and sodium iodide are given; the patient is admitted to the intensive care unit, where treatment is continued. Over the next 3 days, his mental status markedly improves. The T_3 and total thyroxine levels on the day of surgery were both elevated to 250 ng/dL and 18.5 ng/dL, respectively. He was discharged home 6 days later on a regimen of propranolol and propylthiouracil, with a blood pressure of 124/80 mm Hg, a pulse of 92 beats/min, and an oral temperature of 37.3°C.

SUGGESTED READING

Awad IT, Chung F: Factors affecting recovery and discharge following ambulatory surgery. Can J Anesth 2006;53:858.

Baldini G, Bagry H, Aprikian A, et al: Postoperative urinary retention: anesthetic and perioperative considerations. Anesthesiology 2009;110:1139.

Bettelli G: Anaesthesia for the elderly outpatient: preoperative assessment and evaluation, anaesthetic technique and postoperative pain management. Curr Opin Anaesthesiol 2010;23:726.

Buvanendran A, Kroin JS: Multimodal analgesia for controlling acute postoperative pain. Curr Opin Anaesthesiol 2009;22:588.

Buvanendran A, Kroin JS: Multimodal analgesia for controlling acute postoperative pain. Curr Opin Anaesthesiol 2009:22:588.

Capdevila X, Ponrouch M, Morau D: The role of regional anesthesia in patient outcome: ambulatory surgery. Tech Reg Anesth Pain Manag 2008;12:194.

Duncan PG, Shandro J, Bachand R, Ainsworth L: A pilot study of recovery room bypass ("fast-track protocol") in a community hospital. Can J Anesth, 2001; 48:630.

Durkin B, Page C, Glass P: Pregabalin for the treatment of postsurgical pain. Expert Opin Pharmacother 2010;11:2751.

Elvir-Lazo OL, White PF: Postoperative pain management after ambulatory surgery: role of multimodal analgesia. Anesthesiol Clin 2010;28:217.

Franck M, Radtke FM, Apfel CC, et al: Documentation of post-operative nausea and vomiting in routine clinical practice. J Int Med Res 2010;38:1034.

Gupta A: Wound infiltration with local anaesthetics in ambulatory surgery. Curr Opin Anaesthesiol 2010;23:708.

Hanson BS, Søreide E, Warland AM, et al: Risk factors of post-operative urinary retention in hospitalized patients. Acta Anaesthesiol Scand 2011;55:545.

Heitz JW, Witkowski TA, Viscusi ER: New and emerging analgesics and analgesic technologies for acute pain management. Curr Opin Anaesthesiol 2009; 22:608.

Ip HYV, Chung F: Escort accompanying discharge after ambulatory surgery: a necessity or a luxury? Curr Opin Anaesthesiol 2009;22:748.

Jakobsson J: Preoperative single-dose intravenous dexamethasone during ambulatory surgery: update around the benefit versus risk. Curr Opin Anaesthesiol 2010;23:682.

Kaafarani HMA, Itani KMF, Rosen AK, et al: How does patient safety culture in the operating room and post-anesthesia care unit compare to the rest of the hospital? Am J Surg 2009;198:70.

Kehlet H: PROSPECT: evidence-based procedure-specific postoperative pain management. Best Pract Res Clin Anaesthesiol 2007;21:149.

Leskiw U, Weinberg GL: Lipid resuscitation for local anesthetic toxicity: is it really lifesaving? Curr Opin Anaesthesiol 2009;22:667.

Nielsen PR, Rudin Å, Werner MU: Prediction of postoperative pain. Curr Anaesth Crit Care 2007;18:157.

Rawal N: Postdischarge complications and rehabilitation after ambulatory surgery. Curr Opin Anaesthesiol 2008;21:736.

Schug SA, Chong C: Pain management after ambulatory surgery. Curr Opin Anaesthesiol 2009;22:738.

Tang R, Evans H, Chaput A, Kim C: Multimodal analgesia for hip arthroplasty. Orthoped Clin N Am 2009;40:377.

White PF, Tang J, Wender RH, et al: The effects of oral ibuprofen and celecoxib in preventing pain, improving recovery outcomes and patient satisfaction after ambulatory surgery. Anesth Analg 2011;112:323.

Critical Care

1 Brain death criteria can be applied only in the absence of hypothermia, hypotension, metabolic or endocrine abnormalities, neuromuscular blockers, or drugs known to depress brain function.

2 Hyperoxia *and* hypoxia are risk factors, but not the primary causes of retinopathy of prematurity (ROP). Neonates' risk of ROP increases with low birth weight and complexity of comorbidities (eg, sepsis).

3 Pressure control ventilation (PCV) is similar to pressure support ventilation in that peak airway pressure is controlled but is different in that a mandatory rate and inspiratory time are selected. As with pressure support, gas flow ceases when the pressure level is reached; however, the ventilator does not cycle to expiration until the preset inspiration time has elapsed.

4 The disadvantage of conventional PCV is that tidal volume (VT) is not guaranteed (although there are modes in which the consistent delivered pressure of PCV can be combined with a predefined volume delivery).

5 When compared with orotracheal intubation, nasotracheal intubation may be more comfortable for the patient and more secure (fewer instances of accidental extubation).

6 When left in place for more than 2–3 weeks, both orotracheal and nasotracheal tubes predispose patients to subglottic stenosis. If longer periods of mechanical ventilation are necessary, the tracheal tube should generally be replaced by a cuffed tracheostomy tube.

7 The major effect of positive end-expiratory pressure (PEEP) on the lungs is to increase functional residual capacity (FRC). In patients with decreased lung volume, appropriate levels of either PEEP or continuous positive airway pressure (CPAP) will increase FRC and tidal ventilation above closing capacity, will improve lung compliance, and will correct ventilation/perfusion abnormalities.

8 A higher incidence of pulmonary barotrauma is observed with excessive PEEP or CPAP, particularly at levels greater than 20 cm H_2O.

9 Maneuvers that produce sustained maximum lung inflation such as the use of an incentive spirometer can be helpful in inducing cough as well as preventing atelectasis and preserving normal lung volume.

10 While injury from high inspired oxygen concentrations has not been conclusively demonstrated in humans, VT of 12 mL/kg was associated with greater mortality than VT of 6 mL/kg and plateau pressure of less than 30 cm H_2O in patients with acute respiratory distress syndrome.

—Continued next page

Continued—

11 Early elective tracheal intubation is advisable when there are obvious signs of heat injury to the airway.

12 The criteria developed by the Acute Kidney Injury Network are now most often used to stage acute kidney injury (AKI). AKI is diagnosed by documenting an increase in serum creatinine of more than 50%, or an absolute increase of 0.3 mg/dL, and a reduction in urine output to less than 0.5 mL/kg/h for 6 h or longer, with all findings developing over 48 h or less.

13 Age greater than 70 years, corticosteroid therapy, chemotherapy of malignancy, prolonged use of invasive devices, respiratory failure, kidney failure, head trauma, and burns are established risk factors for nosocomial infections.

14 Systemic venodilation and transudation of fluid into tissues result in a relative hypovolemia in patients with sepsis.

Critical care medicine deals with potentially life-threatening illnesses. Anesthesiologists played a major role in developing this multidisciplinary subspecialty. Relative to most other physicians, anesthesiologists have greater expertise in airway management, mechanical ventilation, drug and fluid resuscitation, and advanced monitoring techniques that are central to effective care in critical illness. Moreover, the emphasis in anesthesia on physiology, pathophysiology, and pharmacology, as well as on rapid diagnosis and treatment of acute physiological derangements, provides an excellent foundation for a career in evaluating and treating patients with critical illness. The critical care physician (or "intensivist") also requires broad knowledge that crosses internal medicine, surgery, pediatrics, neurology, emergency medicine, and palliative care. Unlike most subspecialty education, which tends to emphasize a single organ system, intensive care fellowships provide experience in treating patients with systemic inflammatory response syndrome (SIRS) and the related multiple organ dysfunction syndrome (MODS). The American Boards of Anesthesiology, Internal Medicine, Pediatrics, and Surgery, recognizing these requirements, sponsor specialized training for certification in critical care medicine. Clinicians who have such certification are increasingly recognized by multinational corporations and organizations as making important contributions to the outcomes of hospitalized patients.

This chapter provides an abbreviated survey of critical care medicine. Many topics relevant to critical care are covered in other chapters; only important topics not presented elsewhere will be presented.

Economic, Ethical, & Legal Issues in Critical Care

High-quality critical care is very expensive; poor-quality critical care is even more expensive. Intensive care unit (ICU) beds constitute only 10% of all beds in most hospitals yet account for a large fraction of hospital expenditures. If this cost is justified, clear reductions in morbidity or mortality should be readily demonstrable. Unfortunately, confirmatory studies are few and typically flawed by the use of historical controls. A method of reliably identifying those patients who will benefit most from intensive care is needed. Several scoring systems based on the severity of physiological derangements and preexisting health have been used, such as the Acute Physiology and Chronic Health Evaluation (APACHE) and Therapeutic Intervention Scoring System (TISS), but while all reliably identify "sicker" patients none reliably identifies the very sick but recoverable patients for whom intensive care is intended. Survival is generally inversely related to the severity of illness and number of organ systems

ACRONYMS & ABBREVIATIONS

AC	Assist-control (ventilation)
AKI	Acute kidney injury
AMI	Acute myocardial infarction
APACHE	Acute Physiology and Chronic Health Evaluation
APRV	Airway pressure release ventilation
ARDS	Acute respiratory distress syndrome
CMV	Continuous mandatory ventilation
CPAP	Continuous positive airway pressure
CRRT	Continuous renal replacement therapy
EGD	Esophagogastroduodenoscopy
FENa$^+$	Fractional excretion of filtered sodium
F$_{IO_2}$	Fraction of inspired oxygen
FRC	Functional residual capacity
HFJV	High-frequency jet ventilation
HFV	High-frequency ventilation
I:E	Inspiratory:expiratory (ratio)
ILV	Independent lung ventilation
IMV	Intermittent mandatory ventilation
IPAP	Inspiratory positive airway pressure
MMV	Mandatory minute ventilation
MODS	Multiple organ dysfunction syndrome
P$_{plt}$	Plateau pressure
PCV	Pressure control ventilation
PEEP	Positive end-expiratory pressure
PSV	Pressure support ventilation
ROP	Retinopathy of prematurity
RSBI	Rapid shallow breathing index
SIMV	Synchronized intermittent mandatory ventilation
SIRS	Systemic inflammatory response syndrome
TISS	Therapeutic Intervention Scoring System
V$_D$	Volume of distribution
V$_T$	Tidal volume

affected. The Society of Critical Care Medicine has established Project Impact, a system that allows ICUs to compare their outcomes and the care they provide against a national and international network of ICUs.

ETHICAL & LEGAL ISSUES

The high cost of critical care medicine has led to economic constraints being applied by governments and third-party payers. At the same time an increased awareness of ethical and legal issues has changed the practice of critical care medicine.

Decisions about when to initiate or terminate treatment can be difficult. Generally, any treatment that can reasonably be expected to reverse illness or restore health is justified, whereas withholding that treatment requires specific ethical justification. Conversely, if treatment will definitely not reverse a disease process or restore health, then the decision to initiate such treatment may not be justified and may be unethical. Until recently, nearly all patients in the United States—even those who were clearly about to die—received maximal treatment (sometimes contrary to the patient's or family's wishes) for fear of the possible legal repercussions of withholding treatment. "Heroic" measures such as chest compressions, drug resuscitation, and mechanical ventilation were continued until the patient died. These complex decisions must involve the patient (or guardian) and the family and must be consistent with hospital policies and state and federal law.

Fortunately, legal guidelines for arriving at these decisions are available in nearly all states. Although laws vary from state to state, they tend to be similar. The greatest conundrums relate to withholding treatment and discontinuing artificial life-support systems. Competent patients (ie, individuals who have the capacity to understand and make medical decisions) have the right to refuse treatment and the right to have life-support machines or devices turned off (or not initiated) if and when they so request. Most states allow competent individuals to prepare an advance directive, usually either a living will or a durable power of attorney for health care, to prevent needless prolongation of life if they become incompetent (eg, severe mental disability, vegetative state, or irreversible coma). Withholding treatment or discontinuing life support from patients who do not have advance directives or cannot provide their own consent requires permission of the spouse, guardian, next of kin, or an individual to whom the patient has given power of attorney for health care. In some cases, clarification from the courts may be necessary. "Do Not Resuscitate" (DNR) or "Allow Natural Death" (AND) orders have been upheld by the courts for patients in whom resuscitation offers no hope of curing or reversing the disease process responsible for imminent death.

Artificial support of ventilation and circulation complicates legal definitions of death. Until recently, most states required only a determination by a physician that irreversible cessation of ventilatory and circulatory function had occurred. All states have added the concept of brain death to that definition, while some states recognize religious exemptions. In New Jersey, for example, physicians cannot declare brain death "if it would violate the personal religious beliefs of the individual." In addition, although brain death can be established in a pregnant woman, the issue of whether life support can be withdrawn remains subject to both ethical and legal debate. There have been a number of cases of women giving birth to a viable baby weeks or months after having been declared brain dead. These cases involve issues of maternal rights, "fetal rights," and paternal rights and have yet to be resolved.

Brain Death

Brain death is defined as irreversible cessation of all brain function. Spinal cord function below C1 may still be present. Establishing brain death relieves the burden on families of unjustifiable hope and prolonged anxiety; it also prevents waste of medical resources, and potentially allows the retrieval of organs for transplantation.

1 Brain death criteria can be applied only in the absence of hypothermia, hypotension, metabolic or endocrine abnormalities, neuromuscular blockers, and drugs known to depress brain function. A toxicology screen is required if sufficient time since admission (at least 3 days) has not elapsed to exclude a drug effect. Moreover, the patient should be observed long enough to establish with reasonable certainty the irreversible nature of the injury. **Generally accepted clinical criteria for brain death include the following:**

1. Coma
2. Absent motor activity, including no decerebrate or decorticate posturing; spinal cord reflexes may be preserved in some patients

3. Absent brainstem reflexes, including no pupillary, corneal, vestibuloocular (caloric), or gag (or cough) reflexes
4. Absence of ventilatory effort, with the arterial CO_2 tension at least 60 mm Hg or 20 mm Hg above the pretest level.

Repeating the examination (not less than 2 h apart) is optional. In the United States the required number of physician observers varies by state (Florida requires two), as does the level of expertise (Virginia requires a neurologist or neurosurgeon to make the determination). The apnea test should be reserved for last because of its detrimental effects on intracranial pressure. Confirmatory test findings that may be helpful but are not required include an isoelectric electroencephalogram, absence of brainstem auditory evoked potentials, and absence of cerebral perfusion as documented by angiographic, transcranial Doppler, or radioisotopic studies.

Respiratory Care

Respiratory care refers both to the delivery of pulmonary therapy and diagnostic tests and to the allied health profession that has become an integral part of cardiopulmonary diagnostics and critical care. Respiratory therapists' scope of practice encompasses medical gas therapy, delivery of aerosolized medications, airway management, mechanical ventilation, positive airway pressure therapy, critical care monitoring, cardiopulmonary rehabilitation, and the application of various techniques collectively termed *chest physiotherapy*. The latter includes administering aerosols, clearing pulmonary secretions, reexpansion of atelectatic lung, and preserving normal lung function postoperatively or during illness. Diagnostic services may include pulmonary function testing, arterial blood gas analysis, electrocardiography testing, and evaluation of sleep-disordered breathing. The majority of respiratory care procedures are based on clinical practice guidelines developed by the American Association for Respiratory Care using best practice/evidence-based medicine criteria.

MEDICAL GAS THERAPY

The therapeutic medical gases include oxygen at ambient or hyperbaric pressure, helium–oxygen mixtures (heliox), and nitric oxide. Oxygen is made available in high-pressure cylinders, via pipeline systems, from oxygen concentrators, as well as in liquid form. Heliox is occasionally used to partially relieve the increased work of breathing due to partial upper airway obstruction. Nitric oxide is administered as a direct, selective pulmonary vasodilator.

The primary goal of oxygen therapy is to prevent or correct hypoxemia or tissue hypoxia. Table 57–1 identifies classic categories of hypoxia. Oxygen therapy alone may not correct either hypoxemia or hypoxia. Continuous positive airway pressure (CPAP) or positive end-expiratory pressure (PEEP) may be required to recruit collapsed alveoli. Patients with profound hypercapnia may require ventilatory assistance. High concentrations of oxygen may be indicated for conditions requiring removal of entrapped gas (eg, nitrogen) from body cavities or vessels. The short-term inhalation of increased concentrations of oxygen is relatively free of complications.

Supplemental oxygen is indicated for adults, children, and infants (older than 1 month) when Pao_2 is less than 60 mm Hg (8 kPa) or Sao_2 or Spo_2 is less than 90% while at rest breathing room air. In neonates, therapy is recommended if Pao_2 is less than 50 mm Hg (6.7 kPa) or Sao_2 is less than 88% (or capillary Po_2 is less than 40 mm Hg [5.3 kPa]). Therapy may be indicated for patients when clinicians suspect (rather than measure) hypoxemia or hypoxia based on a medical history and physical examination. Patients with myocardial infarction, cardiogenic pulmonary edema, acute lung injury, acute respiratory distress syndrome (ARDS), pulmonary fibrosis, cyanide poisoning, or carbon monoxide inhalation all require supplemental oxygen. Supplemental oxygen is given during the perioperative period because general anesthesia commonly causes a decrease in Pao_2 secondary to increased pulmonary ventilation/perfusion mismatching and decreased functional residual capacity (FRC). Supplemental oxygen should be provided before procedures such as tracheal suctioning or bronchoscopy, which commonly cause arterial desaturation. There is evidence that supplemental oxygen is effective in prolonging survival of patients with chronic obstructive pulmonary disease (COPD) whose resting Pao_2 is lower than 60 mm Hg at sea level. Supplemental oxygen therapy also appears to have a mild beneficial effect on the mean pulmonary arterial pressure and subjective indices of patients' dyspnea.

TABLE 57–1 Classification of hypoxias.[1]

Hypoxia	Pathophysiologic Category	Clinical Example
Hypoxic hypoxia	↓ P_{Barom} or ↓ Fio_2 (<0.21) Alveolar hypoventilation Pulmonary diffusion defect Pulmonary $\dot{V}/\dot{Q}$ mismatch R → L shunt	Altitude, O_2 equipment error Drug overdose, COPD exacerbation Emphysema, pulmonary fibrosis Asthma, pulmonary emboli Atelectasis, cyanotic congenital heart disease
Circulatory hypoxia	Reduced cardiac output Microvascular dysfunction	Severe heart failure, dehydration Sepsis, SIRS
Hemic hypoxia	Reduced hemoglobin content Reduced hemoglobin function	Anemias Carboxyhemoglobinemia, methemoglobinemia
Demand hypoxia Histotoxic hypoxia	↑ Oxygen consumption Inability of cells to utilize oxygen	Fever, seizures Cyanide toxicity, ↑TNF, late sepsis

[1]P_{Barom}, barometric pressure; COPD, chronic obstructive pulmonary disease; $\dot{V}/\dot{Q}$, ventilation/perfusion; R → L, right to left; SIRS, systemic inflammatory response syndrome; TNF, tumor necrosis factor.

AMBIENT OXYGEN THERAPY EQUIPMENT

Classifying Oxygen Therapy Equipment

Oxygen given alone or in a gas can be mixed with air as a partial supplement to patients' tidal or minute volume or serve as the entire source of the inspired volume. This approach provides the basis for classifying devices or systems according to their ability to provide adequate flow levels and a range of fraction of inspired oxygen (F_{IO_2}). Other considerations in selecting therapy include patient compliance, the presence and type of artificial airway, and the need for humidification or an aerosol delivery system.

A. Low-Flow or Variable-Performance Equipment

Oxygen (usually 100%) is supplied at a fixed flow that is only a portion of inspired gas. Such devices are usually intended for patients with stable breathing patterns. As ventilatory demands change, variable amounts of room air will dilute the oxygen flow. Low-flow systems are adequate for patients with

- Minute ventilation less than ~8–10 L/min
- Breathing frequencies less than ~20 breaths/min
- Tidal volumes (V_T) less than ~0.8 L
- Normal inspiratory flow (10–30 L/min).

B. High-Flow or Fixed-Performance Equipment

Inspired gas at a preset F_{IO_2} is supplied continuously at high flow or by providing a sufficiently large reservoir of premixed gas. Ideally, the delivered F_{IO_2} is not affected by variations in ventilatory level or breathing pattern. Profoundly dyspneic and hypoxemic patients may need flows of 100% oxygen in excess of 100 L/min. High-flow systems are indicated for patients who require

- Consistent F_{IO_2}
- Large inspiratory flows of gas (>40 L/min).

1. Variable-Performance Equipment (Table 57–2)

Nasal Cannulas

The nasal cannula is available as either a blind-ended soft plastic tube with an over-the-ear head-elastic or dual-flow with under-the-chin lariat adjustment. Sizes appropriate for adults, children, and infants are available. Cannulas are connected to flowmeters with small-bore tubing and can rapidly be placed on most patients. The tension of attachment should be firm yet comfortable enough to avoid pressure sores on the ears, cheeks, and nose. Patients receiving long-term oxygen therapy most commonly use a nasal cannula. The appliance is usually well tolerated, allowing unencumbered speech, eating, and drinking. Cannulas can be combined with spectacle frames for convenience or to improve acceptance by improving cosmesis. Oxygen-conserving cannulas equipped with inlet reservoirs are available for patients receiving long-term oxygen. Since oxygen flows continuously, approximately 80% of the gas is wasted during expiration.

TABLE 57-2 Oxygen delivery devices and systems.

Device/System	Oxygen Flow Rate (L/min)	F_{IO_2} Range
Nasal cannula	1	0.21–0.24
	2	0.23–0.28
	3	0.27–0.34
	4	0.31–0.38
	5–6	0.32–0.44
Simple mask	5–6	0.30–0.45
	7–8	0.40–0.60
Mask with reservoir	5	0.35–0.50
Partial rebreathing mask-bag	7	0.35–0.75
	15	0.65–1.00
Nonrebreathing mask-bag	7–15	0.40–1.00
Venturi mask and jet nebulizer	4–6 (total flow = 15)	0.24
	4–6 (total flow = 45)	0.28
	8–10 (total flow = 45)	0.35
	8–10 (total flow = 33)	0.40
	8–12 (total flow = 33)	0.50

There are valved reservoir devices that permit storage of incoming oxygen until inspiration occurs.

The actual F_{IO_2} delivered to adults with nasal cannulas is determined by oxygen flow, nasopharyngeal volume, and the patient's inspiratory flow (which depends both on V_T and inspiratory time). Oxygen from the cannula can fill the nasopharynx after exhalation, yet with inspiration, oxygen and entrained air are drawn into the trachea. The inspired percent oxygen increases by approximately 1–2% (above 21%) per liter of oxygen flow with quiet breathing in adults. Cannulas can be expected to provide inspired oxygen concentrations up to 30–35% with normal breathing and oxygen flows of 3–4 L/min. However, levels of 40–50% can be attained with oxygen flows of greater than 10 L/min for short periods. Flows greater than 5 L/min are poorly tolerated because of the discomfort of gas jetting into the nasal cavity and because of drying and crusting of the nasal mucosa.

Data from "normal-breathing subjects" may not be accurate for acutely ill tachypneic patients. Increasing V_T and reducing inspiratory time will dilute the small flow of oxygen. Different proportions of mouth-only versus nose-only breathing and varied inspiratory flow can alter F_{IO_2} by up to 40%. In clinical practice, flow should be titrated according to vital signs, pulse oximetry, and arterial blood gas measurements. Some patients with COPD tend to hypoventilate with even modest oxygen flows, yet are hypoxemic on room air. They may do well with cannula flows of less than 1–2 L/min.

Pediatric-sized nasal cannulas are available. Special cannulas allow babies to nurse and produce less trauma of the face and nose than oxygen masks. Because of the inherently reduced minute ventilation of infants, flow requirements to the cannula must be proportionately reduced. This generally requires a pressure-compensated flowmeter accurate at delivering oxygen flows in the less than 1–3 L/min range. Hypopharyngeal oxygen sampling from infants breathing with cannulas has demonstrated mean F_{IO_2} of 0.35, 0.45, 0.6, and 0.68 with flows of 0.25, 0.5, 0.75, and 1.0 L/min, respectively.

Nasal Mask

The nasal mask is a hybrid of the nasal cannula and a face mask. It can be applied to the face by either an over-the-ear lariat or a headband strap. The lower edge of the mask's flanges rests on the upper lip, surrounding the external nose. Nasal masks have been shown to provide supplemental oxygen equivalent to the nasal cannula under low-flow conditions for adult patients. The primary advantage of the nasal mask over nasal cannulas appears to be patient comfort. The nasal mask does not produce sores around the external nares and dry oxygen is not "jetted" into the nasal cavity. The nasal mask should be considered if it improves patient comfort and compliance.

"Simple" Oxygen Mask

The "simple" or oxygen mask is a disposable lightweight plastic device that covers both nose and mouth. It has no reservoir bag. Masks are fastened to the patient's face by adjustment of an elastic headband; some manufacturers provide a malleable metal nose-bridge adjustment device. The seal is rarely complete: usually there is "inboard" leaking. Thus, patients receive a mixture of oxygen and secondarily entrained room air. This varies depending on the size of the leak, oxygen flow, and breathing pattern. Some brands of the simple mask connect tubing to a standard tapered fitting; others have a small room air–entrainment hole at the connection.

The body of the mask functions as a reservoir for both oxygen and expired carbon dioxide. A minimum oxygen flow of approximately 5 L/min is applied to the mask to limit rebreathing and the resulting increased respiratory work. Wearing any mask appliance for long periods of time is uncomfortable. Speech is muffled and drinking and eating are difficult.

It is difficult to predict delivered F_{IO_2} at specific oxygen flow rates. During normal breathing, it is reasonable to expect an F_{IO_2} of 0.3–0.6 with flows of 5–10 L/min, respectively. Oxygen levels can be increased with smaller V_T or slower breathing rates. With higher flows and ideal conditions, F_{IO_2} may approach 0.7 or 0.8.

Masks lacking oxygen reservoirs may be best suited for patients who require concentrations of oxygen greater than cannulas provide, yet need oxygen therapy for fairly short periods of time. Examples would include medical transport or therapy in the postanesthesia care unit or emergency department. It is not the device of choice for patients with severe respiratory disease who are profoundly hypoxemic, tachypneic, or unable to protect their airway from aspiration.

Masks with Gas Reservoirs

Incorporating a gas reservoir is a logical adaptation to the simple mask. Two types of reservoir mask are commonly used: the partial rebreathing mask and the nonrebreathing mask. Both are disposable, lightweight, transparent plastic under-the-chin reservoirs. The difference between the two relates to use of valves on the mask and between the mask and the bag reservoir. Mask reservoirs commonly hold approximately 600 mL or less of gas volume. The phrase "partial rebreather" is used because "part" of the patient's expired V_T refills the bag. Usually that gas is largely dead space that should not result in significant rebreathing of carbon dioxide.

The nonrebreather uses the same basic system as the partial rebreather but incorporates flap-type valves between the bag and mask and on at least one of the mask's exhalation ports. Inboard leaking is common, and room air will enter during brisk inspiratory flows, even when the bag contains gas. The lack of a complete facial seal and a relatively small reservoir influence the delivered oxygen concentration. The key factor in successful application of the masks is to use a sufficiently high flow of oxygen, so that the reservoir bag is at least partially full during inspiration. Typical minimum flows of oxygen are 10–15 L/min. Well-fitting partial rebreathing masks provide a range of FIO_2 from 0.35 to 0.60 with oxygen flows up to 10 L/min. With inlet flows of 15 L/min or more and ideal breathing conditions, FIO_2 may approach 1.0. Either style of mask is indicated for patients suspected of having significant hypoxemia, with relatively normal spontaneous minute ventilation. Such patients may include victims of trauma, myocardial infarction, or carbon monoxide exposure. Profoundly dyspneic patients with gasping respiration may be served by a fixed-performance, high-flow oxygen system.

2. Fixed-Performance (High-Flow) Equipment

Anesthesia Bag or Bag-Mask-Valve Systems

The basic design follows that of the nonrebreathing reservoir mask but with more "capable" components. Self-inflating bags consist of a roughly 1.5 L bladder, usually with an oxygen inlet reservoir. Anesthesia bags are 1-, 2-, or 3-L non–self-inflating reservoirs with a tailpiece gas inlet. Masks are designed to provide a comfortable leak-free seal for manual ventilation. The inspiratory/expiratory valve systems may vary. The flow to the reservoir should be kept high so that the bags do not deflate substantially. When using an anesthesia bag, operators may frequently have to adjust the oxygen flow and exhaust valve to respond to changing breathing patterns or demands, particularly when maintaining a complete seal between the mask and face is difficult.

The most common systems for disposable and permanent self-inflating resuscitation bags use a unidirectional gas flow. Although these devices offer the potential for a constant FIO_2 greater than 0.9, tailpiece inlet valves will not open for a spontaneously breathing patient. Opening the valves requires negative pressure bag recoil after compression. If this situation is not recognized, clinicians might be misled into thinking the patient is receiving a specific concentration of oxygen when this is not the case.

There are limits to the ability of each system to maintain its fixed-performance characteristics. Delivered FIO_2 can approach 1.0 with either anesthesia or self-inflating bags. Spontaneously breathing patients are allowed to breathe only the contents of the system if the mask seal is tight and the reservoir is adequately maintained.

Failure to maintain an adequate oxygen supply in the reservoir and inlet flow is a concern. The spring-loaded valve of anesthesia bags must be adjusted to prevent overdistention of the bag. Self-inflating bags look the same whether or not oxygen flow to the unit is adequate, and they will entrain room air into the bag, thus lowering the delivered FIO_2.

Air-Entraining Venturi Masks

The gas delivery approach with air-entraining masks is different than with an oxygen reservoir. The goal is to create an open system with high flow about the nose and mouth, with a fixed F_{IO_2}. Oxygen is directed by small-bore tubing to a mixing jet; the final oxygen concentration depends on the ratio of air drawn in through entrainment ports. Manufacturers have developed both fixed and adjustable entrainment selections over an F_{IO_2} range. Most provide instructions for the operator to set a minimum flow of oxygen. Table 57–3 identifies total flow at various inlet flows and F_{IO_2}.

Despite the high-flow concept, F_{IO_2} can vary up to 6% from the anticipated setting. The air-entraining masks are a logical choice for patients who require greater F_{IO_2} than can be provided by devices such as the nasal cannula. Patients with COPD who tend to hypoventilate with a moderate F_{IO_2} are candidates for the Venturi mask. Clinicians providing oxygen therapy with Venturi masks should be aware of the previously mentioned problems involving the mask itself. F_{IO_2} can increase if the air entrainment ports are obstructed by the patient's hands, bed sheets, or water condensate. Clinicians should encourage the patient and caregivers to keep the mask on the face continuously. Interruption of oxygen is a serious problem in unstable patients with hypoxemia and or hypercarbia.

Direct analysis of the F_{IO_2} during air-entrainment mask breathing is difficult to perform accurately. Arterial blood gas analysis and the patient's respiratory rate should guide clinicians as to whether the patient's demands are being met by the mask's flow. If that occurs, then inlet oxygen flows may need to be increased or an alternate device selected.

Air-Entraining Nebulizers

Large-volume, high-output or "all-purpose" nebulizers have been used in respiratory care for many years to provide mist therapy with some control of the F_{IO_2}. These units are commonly placed on patients following extubation for their aerosol-producing properties. Like the air-entraining masks, nebulizers use a pneumatic jet and an adjustable orifice to vary entrained air for varying F_{IO_2} levels. Many commercial devices have an inlet orifice diameter that maximally allows only 15 L/min when the source pressure is 50 psi. This means that on the 100% setting (no air entrainment) output flow is only 15 L/min. Only patients breathing at slow rates and small V_T will receive 100% oxygen. This problem has been addressed by the development of high-flow, high-F_{IO_2} nebulizers. For more common applications that use an F_{IO_2} of 0.3–0.5, room air is entrained, reducing the F_{IO_2} and increasing the total flow output to 40–50 L/min.

Knowledge of the air/oxygen ratio and the input flow rate of oxygen allows the total outflow to be calculated. Nebulizer systems can be applied to the patient with many different devices, including aerosol, tracheostomy dome/collar, face tent, and T-piece adapter. These appliances can all be attached via large-bore tubing to the nebulizer. This open system freely vents inspiratory and expiratory gases around the patient's face or out a distal port of a T-piece adapter. Unfortunately, the lack of any valves allows patients to secondarily entrain room air. It is common practice to use either a reservoir bag before the T-piece or a reservoir tube on the distal side of the T-piece to provide a larger volume of gas than

TABLE 57–3 **Air-entrainment mask input flow versus total flow at varying F_{IO_2}.[1]**

F_{IO_2}	Inlet Oxygen Flow (Minimum)	Total Flow (L/min)
0.24	4	97
0.28	6	68
0.3	6	54
0.35	8	45
0.4	12	50
0.5	12	33
0.7	12	19
0.8	12	16
1.0	12	12

[1]F_{IO_2}, fraction of inspired oxygen.

that coming from the nebulizer. A typical concern of those applying air-entrainment aerosol therapy with controlled oxygen concentration is whether the system will provide adequate flow. Clinicians should observe the mist like a tracer to determine adequacy of flow. When a T-piece is used and the visible mist (exiting the distal port) disappears during inspiration, the flow is inadequate.

Another concern in clinical practice is that excess water in the tubing collects and can obstruct gas flow completely or can offer increased resistance to flow. The latter may increase the FIO_2 above the desired setting. Other complications include bronchospasm or laryngospasm in some patients as a consequence of airway irritation from sterile water droplets (condensate of the aerosol). In such circumstances, a heated (nonaerosol) humidification system should be substituted.

High-Flow Air–Oxygen Systems

Dual air–oxygen flowmeters and air–oxygen blenders are commonly used for oxygen administration as well as freestanding continuous positive airway pressure (CPAP) and "add-on" ventilator systems. These systems differ from the air-entraining nebulizers, as their total output flows do not diminish at FIO_2 greater than 0.4. With these high-flow systems, the total flow to the patient and FIO_2 can be set independently to meet patient needs. This can be done using a large reservoir bag or constant flows in the range of 50 to more than 100 L/min. Clinicians can use a variety of appliances with these systems, including aerosol masks, face tents, or well-fitted nonrebreathing system masks with air–oxygen blenders. Face-sealing mask systems can also be constructed with a reservoir bag and a safety valve to allow breathing if the blender fails. The high flows of gas require use of heated humidifiers of the type commonly used on mechanical ventilators. Humidification offers an advantage for patients with reactive airways. Because of the high flows, such systems are used to apply CPAP or BIPAP for spontaneously breathing patients.

Oxygen Hoods

Although many of the devices previously described have pediatric-sized options, many infants and neonates will not tolerate facial appliances. Oxygen hoods cover only the head, allowing access to the child's lower body while still permitting use of a standard incubator or radiant warmer. The hood is ideal for relatively short-term oxygen therapy for newborns and inactive infants. However, for mobile infants requiring longer term therapy, the nasal cannula, face mask, or full-bed enclosure allow for greater mobility.

Normally, oxygen and air are premixed by an air–oxygen blender and passed through a heated humidifier. Nebulizers should be avoided. Most pneumatic jet-type nebulizers create noise levels (>65 dB) that may cause newborn hearing loss, and cold gas can induce an increase in oxygen consumption. Hoods come in different sizes. Some are simple Plexiglas boxes; others have elaborate systems for sealing the neck opening. There is no attempt to completely seal the system, as a constant flow of gas is needed to remove carbon dioxide (minimum flow >7 L/min). Hood inlet flows of 10–15 L/min are adequate for a majority of patients.

Helium–Oxygen Therapy

Helium–oxygen (heliox) mixtures have a notable, yet limited clinical role. In addition to its uses in industry and deep-sea diving, heliox has a number of medical applications. Helium is premixed with oxygen in several standard blends. The most popular mixture is 79%/21% helium–oxygen, which has a density that is 40% that of pure oxygen. Helium–oxygen mixtures are available in large-sized compressed gas cylinders.

In anesthetic practice, pressures needed to ventilate patients with small-diameter tracheal tubes can be substantially reduced when the 79%/21% mixture is used. Heliox can provide patients with upper airway–obstructing lesions (eg, subglottic edema, foreign bodies, and tracheal tumors) with relief from acute distress until more definitive care can be delivered. The evidence is less convincing in treating lower airway obstruction from COPD or acute asthma. Helium mixtures may also be used as the driving gas for small-volume nebulizers in bronchodilator therapy for asthma. However, with heliox, the nebulizer flow needs to be increased to 11 L/min versus the usual 6–8 L/min with oxygen. Patients' work of breathing can be reduced with heliox as compared to a conventional oxygen/nitrogen gas mixture.

Hyperbaric Oxygen

Hyperbaric oxygen therapy uses a pressurized chamber to expose the patient to oxygen tensions exceeding ambient barometric pressure (at sea level the ambient pressure is 760 mm Hg). With a one-person hyperbaric chamber, 100% oxygen is usually used to pressurize the chamber. Larger chambers allow for the simultaneous treatment of multiple patients and for the presence of medical personnel in the chamber with patients. Multiplace chambers use air to pressurize the chamber, whereas patients receive 100% oxygen by mask, hood, or tracheal tube. Common indications for hyperbaric oxygen include decompression sickness (the "bends"), certain forms of gas embolism, gas gangrene, carbon monoxide poisoning, and treatment of certain wounds.

3. Hazards of Oxygen Therapy

Oxygen therapy can result in both respiratory and nonrespiratory toxicity. Important factors include patient susceptibility, the F_{IO_2}, and duration of therapy.

Hypoventilation

This complication is primarily seen in patients with COPD who have chronic CO_2 retention. These patients develop an altered respiratory drive that becomes at least partly dependent on the maintenance of relative hypoxemia. Elevation of arterial oxygen tension to "normal" can therefore cause severe hypoventilation in these patients. Conversely, stable, spontaneously breathing patients with profound hypercarbia ($Pa_{CO_2} > 80$ mm Hg) who are being supported with supplemental oxygen should not have supplemental oxygen discontinued, even for short intervals. Oxygen therapy can be indirectly hazardous for patients being monitored with pulse oximetry while receiving opioids for pain. Hypoventilation as a consequence of opioids may fail to cause worrisome change in oxygen saturation, despite respiratory rates as infrequent as 2 per minute, delaying the diagnosis.

Absorption Atelectasis

High concentrations of oxygen can cause pulmonary atelectasis in areas of low $\dot{V}/\dot{Q}$ ratios. As nitrogen is "washed out" of the lungs, the lowered gas tension in pulmonary capillary blood results in increased uptake of alveolar gas and absorption atelectasis. If the area remains perfused but nonventilated, the resulting intrapulmonary shunt can lead to progressive widening of the alveolar-to-arterial (A–a) gradient.

Pulmonary Toxicity

Prolonged high concentrations of oxygen may damage the lungs. Toxicity is dependent both on the partial pressure of oxygen in the inspired gas and the duration of exposure. Alveolar rather than arterial oxygen tension is most important in the development of oxygen toxicity. Although 100% oxygen for up to 10–20 h is generally considered safe, concentrations greater than 50–60% are undesirable for longer periods as they may lead to pulmonary toxicity.

Molecular oxygen (O_2) is unusual in that each atom has unpaired electrons. This gives the molecule the paramagnetic property that allows precise measurements of oxygen concentration. Notably, internal rearrangement of these electrons or their interaction with other atoms (iron) or molecules (xanthine) can produce potentially toxic chemical species. Oxygen toxicity is thought to be due to intracellular generation of highly reactive O_2 metabolites (free radicals) such as superoxide and activated hydroxyl ions, singlet O_2, and hydrogen peroxide. A high concentration of O_2 increases the likelihood of generating toxic species. These metabolites are cytotoxic because they readily react with cellular DNA, sulfhydryl proteins, and lipids. Two cellular enzymes, superoxide dismutase and catalase, protect against toxicity by sequentially converting superoxide first to hydrogen peroxide and then to water. Additional protection may be provided by antioxidants and free radical scavengers; however, clinical evidence supporting the use of these agents in preventing pulmonary toxicity is lacking.

In experimental animals oxygen-mediated injury of the alveolar–capillary membrane produces a syndrome that is pathologically and clinically indistinguishable from ARDS. Tracheobronchitis may also be present initially in some patients. Pulmonary O_2 toxicity in newborn infants is manifested as bronchopulmonary dysplasia.

Retinopathy of Prematurity

Retinopathy of prematurity (ROP), formerly termed *retrolental fibroplasia*, is a neovascular retinal disorder that develops in 84% of premature survivors born at less than 28 weeks' gestation. ROP may include disorganized vascular proliferation and fibrosis and may lead to retinal detachment and blindness. ROP resolves in approximately 80% of these cases without visual loss from retinal detachments or scars. ROP was very common in the 1940s–1950s when unmonitored high (>0.5 F_{IO_2}) oxygen was often administered to premature infants. However, it is now known that hyperoxia *and* hypoxia are risk factors, but not the primary causes of ROP. Neonates' risk of ROP increases with low birth weight and complexity of comorbidities (eg, sepsis). In contrast to pulmonary toxicity, ROP correlates better with arterial than with alveolar O_2 tension. The recommended arterial concentrations for premature infants receiving oxygen are 50–80 mm Hg (6.6–10.6 kPa). If an infant requires arterial O_2 saturations of 96%–99% for cardiopulmonary reasons, fear about causing or worsening ROP is not a reason to withhold the oxygen.

Hyperbaric Oxygen Toxicity

The high inspired O_2 tensions associated with hyperbaric O_2 therapy greatly accelerate O_2 toxicity. The risk and expected degree of toxicity are directly related to the pressures used as well as the duration of exposure. Prolonged exposure to O_2 partial pressures in excess of 0.5 atmospheres can cause pulmonary O_2 toxicity. This may present initially with retrosternal burning, cough, and chest tightness and will result in progressive impairment of pulmonary function with continued exposure. Patients exposed to O_2 at 2 atmospheres or greater are also at risk for central nervous system toxicity that may be expressed as behavior changes, nausea, vertigo, muscular twitching, or convulsions.

Fire Hazard

Oxygen vigorously supports combustion. The potential for oxygen enriched gas mixtures to promote fires and explosions is discussed in Chapter 2.

MECHANICAL VENTILATION

Despite early intervention and appropriate respiratory care, patients with critical illness will often require mechanical ventilation. Mechanical ventilation can replace or supplement normal spontaneous ventilation. In most instances, the problem is primarily that of impaired CO_2 elimination (ventilatory failure). In other instances, mechanical ventilation may be used as an adjunct (usually to positive-pressure therapy; see below) in the treatment of hypoxemia. The decision to initiate mechanical ventilation is made on clinical grounds, but certain parameters have been suggested as guidelines (Table 57–4).

Of the two available techniques, positive-pressure ventilation and negative-pressure ventilation, the former has much wider applications and is

TABLE 57–4 Indicators of the need for mechanical ventilation.

Criterion	Measurement
Direct measurement	
Arterial oxygen tension	<50 mm Hg on room air
Arterial CO_2 tension	>50 mm Hg in the absence of metabolic alkalosis
Derived indices	
Pao_2/Fio_2 ratio	<300 mm Hg
PA–ao_2 gradient	>350 mm Hg
V_D/V_T	>0.6
Clinical indices	
Respiratory rate	>35 breaths/min
Mechanical indices	
Tidal volume	<5 mL/kg
Vital capacity	<15 mL/kg
Maximum inspiratory force	>−25 cm H_2O (eg, −15 cm H_2O)

almost universally used. Although negative-pressure ventilation does not require tracheal intubation, it cannot overcome substantial increases in airway resistance or decreases in pulmonary compliance, and it also limits access to the patient.

During positive-pressure ventilation, lung inflation is achieved by periodically applying positive pressure to the upper airway through a tight-fitting mask (noninvasive mechanical ventilation) or through a tracheal or tracheostomy tube. Increased airway resistance and decreased lung compliance can be overcome by manipulating inspiratory gas flow and pressure. The major disadvantages of positive-pressure ventilation are altered ventilation-to-perfusion relationships, potentially adverse circulatory effects, and risk of pulmonary barotrauma and volutrauma. Positive-pressure ventilation increases physiological dead space because gas flow is preferentially directed to the more compliant, nondependent areas of the lungs, whereas blood flow (influenced by gravity) favors dependent areas. Reductions in cardiac output are primarily due to impaired venous return to the heart from increased intrathoracic pressure. Barotrauma is closely related to repetitive high peak inflation pressures and underlying lung disease, whereas volutrauma is related to the repetitive collapse and reexpansion of alveoli.

1. Positive-Pressure Ventilators

Positive-pressure ventilators periodically create a pressure gradient between the machine circuit and alveoli that results in inspiratory gas flow. Exhalation occurs passively. Ventilators and their control mechanisms can be powered pneumatically (by a pressurized gas source), electrically, or by both mechanisms. Gas flow is either derived directly from the pressurized gas source or produced by the action of a rotary or linear piston. This gas flow then either goes directly to the patient (single-circuit system) or, as commonly occurs with operating room ventilators, compresses a reservoir bag or bellows that is part of the patient circuit (double-circuit system).

All ventilators have four phases: inspiration, the changeover from inspiration to expiration, expiration, and the changeover from expiration to inspiration (see Chapter 4). These phases are defined by V_T, ventilatory rate, inspiratory time, inspiratory gas flow, and expiratory time.

Classification of Ventilators

The complexity of modern ventilators defies simple classification. Incorporation of microprocessor technology into the newest generation of ventilators has further complicated this task. Nonetheless, ventilators are most commonly classified according to their inspiratory phase characteristics and their method of cycling from inspiration to expiration.

A. Inspiratory Characteristics

Most modern ventilators behave like flow generators. Constant flow generators deliver a constant inspiratory gas flow regardless of airway circuit pressure. Constant flow is produced by the use of either a solenoid (on–off) valve with a high-pressure gas source (5–50 psi) or via a gas injector (Venturi) with a lower-pressure source. Machines with high-pressure gas sources allow inspiratory gas flow to remain constant despite large changes in airway resistance or pulmonary compliance. The performance of ventilators with gas injectors varies more with airway pressure. Nonconstant flow generators consistently vary inspiratory flow with each inspiratory cycle (such as by a rotary piston); a sine wave pattern of flow is typical.

Constant-pressure generators maintain airway pressure constant throughout inspiration and irrespective of inspiratory gas flow. Gas flow ceases when airway pressure equals the set inspiratory pressure. Pressure generators typically operate at low gas pressures (just above peak inspiratory pressure).

B. Cycling (Changeover from Inspiration to Expiration)

Time-cycled ventilators cycle to the expiratory phase once a predetermined interval elapses from the start of inspiration. V_T is the product of the set inspiratory time and inspiratory flow rate. Time-cycled ventilators are commonly used for neonates and in the operating room.

Volume-cycled ventilators terminate inspiration when a preselected volume is delivered. Many adult ventilators are volume cycled but also have secondary limits on inspiratory pressure to guard against pulmonary barotrauma. If inspiratory pressure exceeds the pressure limit, the machine cycles into expiration even if the selected volume has not been delivered.

Properly functioning volume-cycled ventilators do not deliver the set volume to the patient. A percentage of the set V_T is always lost due to expansion of the breathing circuit during inspiration. Circuit compliance is usually about 3–5 mL/cm H_2O; thus, if a pressure of 30 cm H_2O is generated during inspiration, 90–150 mL of the set V_T is lost to the circuit. Loss of V_T to the breathing circuit is therefore inversely related to lung compliance. For accurate measurement of the exhaled V_T, the spirometer must be placed at the tracheal tube rather than the exhalation valve of the ventilator.

Pressure-cycled ventilators cycle into the expiratory phase when airway pressure reaches a predetermined level. V_T and inspiratory time vary, being related to airway resistance and pulmonary and circuit compliance. A significant leak in the patient circuit can prevent the necessary rise in circuit pressure and machine cycling. Conversely, an acute increase in airway resistance, or decrease in pulmonary compliance, or circuit compliance (kink) causes premature cycling and decreases the delivered V_T. Pressure-cycled ventilators have been most often used for short-term indications (transport).

Flow-cycled ventilators have pressure and flow sensors that allow the ventilator to monitor inspiratory flow at a preselected fixed inspiratory pressure; when this flow reaches a predetermined level (usually 25% of the initial peak mechanical inspiratory flow rate), the ventilator cycles from inspiration into expiration (see the sections on Pressure Support and Pressure Control Ventilation).

C. Microprocessor-Controlled Ventilators

These versatile machines can be set to function in any one of a variety of inspiratory flow and cycling patterns. The microprocessor allows closed-loop control over the ventilator's performance characteristics. Microprocessor-controlled ventilators are the norm in modern critical care units and on newer anesthesia machines.

Ventilatory Modes

Ventilatory mode is defined by the method by which the ventilator cycles from expiration to inspiration as well as whether the patient is able to breathe spontaneously (Table 57–5 and Figure 57–1). Most modern ventilators are capable of multiple ventilatory modes, and some (microprocessor-controlled ventilators) can combine modes simultaneously. Typical ventilatory modes are regulated to deliver a defined V_T or a defined maximal inspiratory pressure. Modern ventilators can provide for breaths that are volume-controlled (machine-initiated inspiration stops when the set volume is delivered), volume-assisted (patient-initiated inspiration stops when the set volume is delivered), pressure-controlled (machine-initiated inspiration at a mandatory inspiratory pressure stops after a defined time has elapsed), pressure-assisted (patient-initiated inspiration at a mandatory inspiratory pressure stops after a defined time has elapsed), or pressure-supported (patient-initiated inspiration continues at a mandatory inspiratory pressure until the inspiratory flow declines to a defined value).

A. Continuous Mandatory Ventilation (CMV)

In this mode, the ventilator cycles from expiration to inspiration after a fixed time interval. The interval determines the ventilatory rate. Typical settings on this mode provide a fixed V_T and fixed rate (and, therefore, minute ventilation) regardless of patient effort, because *the patient cannot breathe spontaneously*. Settings to limit inspiratory pressure guard against pulmonary barotrauma, and indeed CMV can be provided in a pressure-limited (rather than volume-limited) way. Controlled ventilation is best reserved for patients capable of little or no ventilatory effort. Awake patients with active ventilatory effort require sedation, possibly with muscle paralysis.

B. Assist-Control (AC) Ventilation

Incorporation of a pressure sensor in the breathing circuit of AC ventilators permits the patient's inspiratory effort to be used to trigger inspiration.

TABLE 57–5 **Ventilatory modes.**[1]

Mode	I to E Cycling				E to I Cycling		Allows Spontaneous Ventilation	Weaning Mode
	Volume	Time	Pressure	Flow	Time	Pressure		
CMV	+				+			
AC	+				+	+		
IMV	+				+		+	+
SIMV	+				+	+	+	+
PSV				+		+	+	+
PCV			+		+			
MMV							+	
PC-IRV			+		+			
APRV		+			+		+	
HFJV		+			+		+	

[1]CMV, continuous mandatory ventilation; AC, assist-control ventilation; IMV, intermittent mandatory ventilation; SIMV, synchronized intermittent mandatory ventilation; PSV, pressure support ventilation; PCV, pressure control ventilation; MMV, mandatory minute ventilation; IRV, inverse I:E ratio ventilation; APRV, airway pressure release ventilation; HFJV, high-frequency jet ventilation.

A sensitivity control allows selection of the inspiratory effort required. The ventilator can be set for a fixed ventilatory rate, but each patient effort of sufficient magnitude will trigger the set V_T. If spontaneous inspiratory efforts are not detected, the machine functions as if in the control mode. Most often, AC ventilation is used in a volume-limited format, but it can also be provided in a pressure-limited way (see below).

C. Intermittent Mandatory Ventilation (IMV)

IMV allows spontaneous ventilation while the patient is on the ventilator. A selected number of mechanical breaths (with fixed V_T) is given to supplement spontaneous breathing. At high mandatory rates (10–12 breaths/min), IMV essentially provides all of the patient's ventilation; at low rates (1–2 breaths/min), it provides minimal mechanical ventilation and allows the patient to breathe relatively independently. The V_T and frequency of spontaneous breaths are determined by the patient's ventilatory drive and muscle strength. The IMV rate can be adjusted to maintain a desired minute ventilation. IMV has found greatest use as a weaning technique.

Synchronized intermittent mandatory ventilation (SIMV) times the mechanical breath, whenever possible, to coincide with the beginning of a spontaneous effort. Proper synchronization prevents superimposing (stacking) a mechanical breath in the middle of a spontaneous breath, resulting in a very large V_T. As with CMV and AC, settings to limit inspiratory pressure guard against pulmonary barotrauma. The advantages of SIMV include patient comfort, and if used for weaning, the machine breaths provide a backup if the patient becomes fatigued. However, if the rate is too low (4 breaths/min), the backup may be too low, particularly for weak patients who may not be able to overcome the added work of breathing during spontaneous breaths.

IMV circuits provide a continuous supply of gas flow for spontaneous ventilation between mechanical breaths. Modern ventilators incorporate SIMV into their design, but older models must be modified by a parallel circuit, a continuous flow system, or a demand

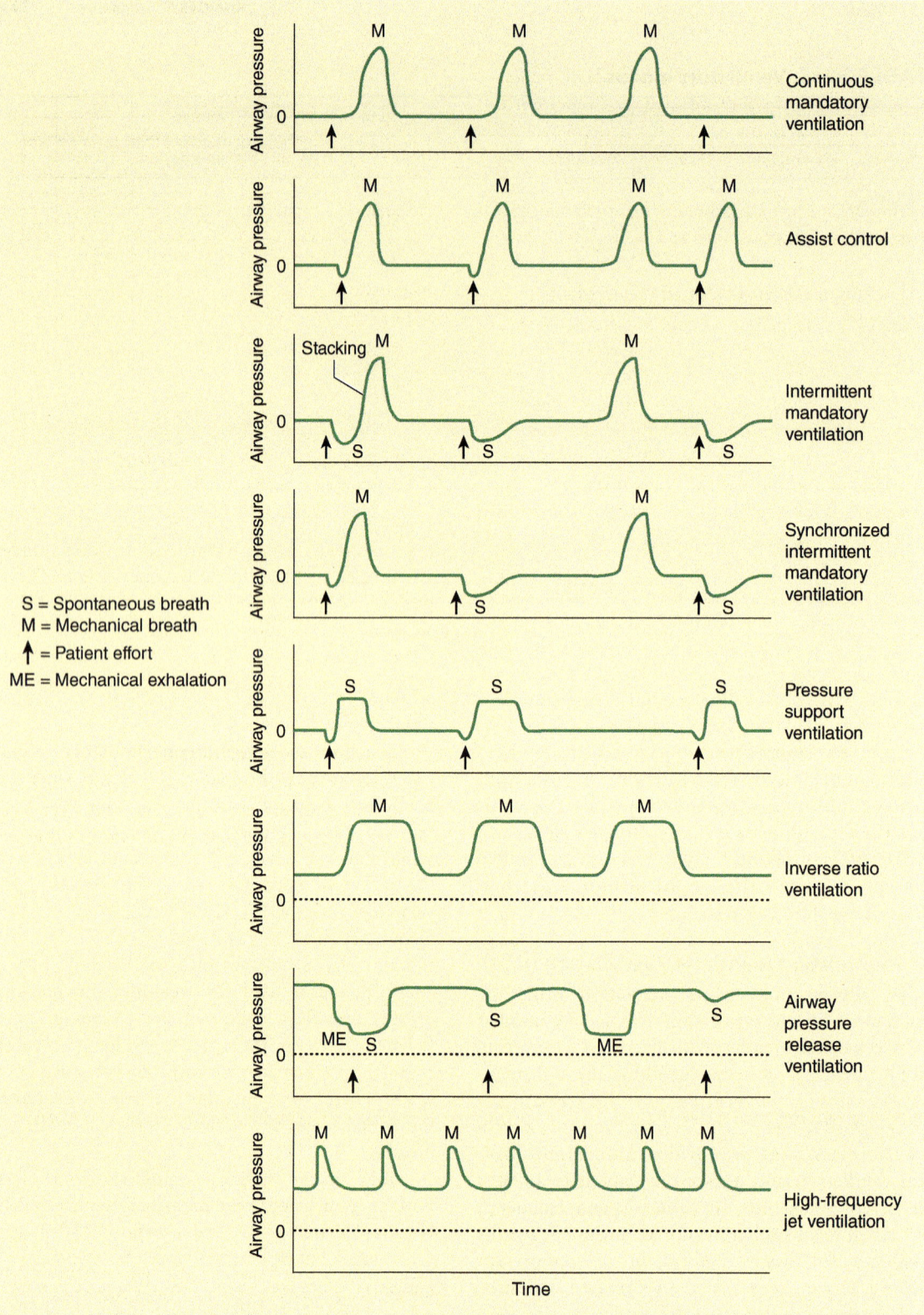

FIGURE 57-1 Airway pressure waveforms of ventilatory modes.

flow valve. Regardless of the system, proper functioning of one-way valves and sufficient gas flow are necessary to prevent an increase in the patient's work of breathing, particularly when PEEP is also used.

The IMV discussion has considered this to be a volume-limited format; however, it can also be provided in pressure-limited format if desired (see below).

D. Mandatory Minute Ventilation (MMV)

With MMV, the patient is able to breathe spontaneously (with pressure support) and also receive SIMV mechanical breaths, while the machine monitors the exhaled minute ventilation. In this mode, the machine continuously adjusts the number of SIMV mechanical breaths so that the sum total of spontaneous and mechanical ventilation equals the desired set minute ventilation. The role of this mode in weaning remains to be defined.

E. Pressure Support Ventilation (PSV)

Pressure support ventilation was designed to augment the VT of spontaneously breathing patients and overcome any increased inspiratory resistance from the tracheal tube, breathing circuit (tubing, connectors, and humidifier), and ventilator (pneumatic circuitry and valves). Microprocessor-controlled machines have this mode, which delivers sufficient gas flow with every inspiratory effort to maintain a predetermined positive pressure throughout inspiration. When inspiratory flow decreases to a predetermined level, the ventilator's feedback (servo) loop cycles the machine into the expiratory phase, and airway pressure returns to baseline (Figure 57–2). The only setting in this mode is inspiratory pressure. The patient determines the respiratory rate and VT varies according to inspiratory gas flow, lung mechanics, and the patient's own inspiratory effort. Low levels of PSV (5–10 cm H_2O) are usually sufficient to overcome any added resistance imposed by the breathing apparatus. Higher levels (10–40 cm H_2O) can function as a standalone ventilatory mode if the patient has sufficient spontaneous ventilatory drive and stable lung mechanics. The principal advantages of PSV are its ability to augment spontaneous VT, decrease the work of breathing, and increase patient comfort. However, if the patient fatigues or lung mechanics change, VT may be inadequate, and there

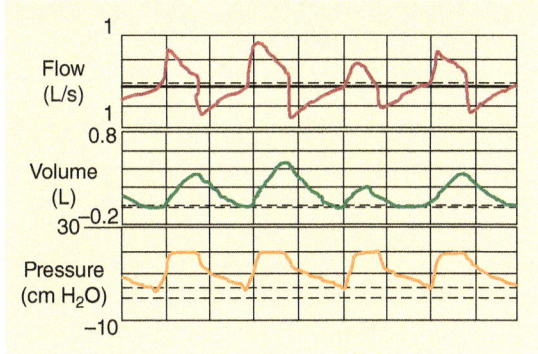

FIGURE 57–2 Pressure support ventilation. The patient initiates a breath; the machine is set to deliver 15 cm H_2O pressure (above 5 cm H_2O of continuous positive airway pressure [CPAP]). When flow ceases, the machine cycles into the expiratory mode.

is no backup rate if the patient's intrinsic respiratory rate decreases or the patient becomes apneic. Pressure support is often used in conjunction with IMV (Figure 57–3). The IMV machine breaths provide backup, and a low level of pressure support is used to offset the increased work of breathing resulting from the breathing circuit and machine.

F. Pressure Control Ventilation (PCV)

3 Pressure control ventilation is similar to PSV in that peak airway pressure is controlled but is different in that a mandatory rate and inspiratory

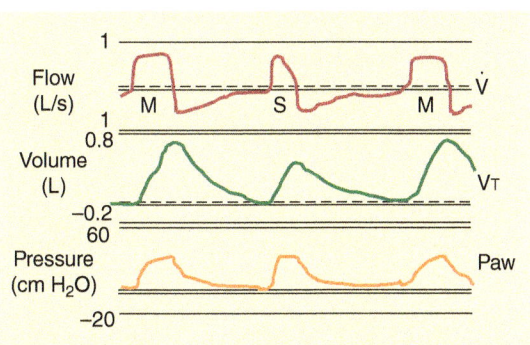

FIGURE 57–3 Intermittent mechanical ventilation with pressure support. M = machine breath → set tidal volume (VT) delivered. S = spontaneous breath, 15 cm of pressure support over 5 cm of PEEP. VT depends on patient effort and lung mechanics. V, flow; Paw, partial airway pressure; PEEP, positive end-expiratory pressure.

time are selected. As with pressure support, gas flow ceases when the pressure level is reached; however, the ventilator does not cycle to expiration until the preset inspiration time has elapsed. PCV may be used in both the AC and IMV modes. In AC, all breaths (either machine initiated or patient initiated) are time cycled and pressure limited. In IMV, machine-initiated breaths are time cycled and pressure limited. The patient may breathe spontaneously between the set rate, and the VT of the spontaneous breaths is determined by the patient's pulmonary muscle strength. The advantage of PCV is that by limiting inspiratory pressure, the risks of barotrauma and volutrauma may be decreased. Also, by extending inspiratory time, better mixing and recruitment of collapsed or flooded alveoli may be achieved, provided adequate PEEP levels are used.

4 The disadvantage of conventional PCV is that VT is not guaranteed (although there are modes in which the consistent delivered pressure of PCV can be combined with a predefined volume delivery). Any change in compliance or resistance will affect the delivered VT. This is a major issue in patients with acute lung injury because if the compliance decreases and the pressure limit is not increased, adequate VT may not be attained. PCV has been used for patients with acute lung injury or ARDS, often with a prolonged inspiratory time or inverse I:E ratio ventilation (IRV) (see below) in an effort to recruit collapsed and flooded alveoli. The disadvantage of using IRV with PCV is that the patient needs to be heavily sedated and often paralyzed to tolerate this particular ventilatory mode.

With PCV, pressure and inspiratory time are preset, whereas airflow and volume are variable and dependent on the patient's resistance and compliance. With volume ventilation, on the other hand, inspiratory time is also preset but flow and VT are also preset, and in this circumstance the inspiratory pressure can be very high.

G. Inverse I:E Ratio Ventilation (IRV)

IRV reverses the normal inspiratory:expiratory time ratio of 1:3 or greater to a ratio of greater than 1:1. This may be achieved by adding an end-inspiratory pause, by decreasing peak inspiratory flow during volume-cycled ventilation (CMV), or by setting an

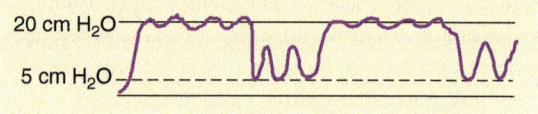

FIGURE 57–4 Airway pressure release ventilation.

inspiratory time such that inspiration is longer than expiration during PCV (PC-IRV). Intrinsic PEEP may be produced during IRV and is caused by air trapping or incomplete emptying of the lung to the baseline pressure prior to the initiation of the next breath. This air trapping increases FRC until a new equilibrium is reached. This mode does not allow spontaneous breathing and requires heavy sedation or neuromuscular blockade. IRV with PEEP is effective for improving oxygenation in patients with decreased FRC.

H. Airway Pressure Release Ventilation (APRV)

APRV or bilevel ventilation is a mode in which a relatively high PEEP is used, despite the patient being allowed to breathe spontaneously. Intermittently, the PEEP level decreases to help augment the elimination of CO_2 (**Figure 57–4**). The inspiratory and expiratory times, high and low PEEP levels, and spontaneous respiratory activity determine minute ventilation. Initial settings include a minimum PEEP of 10–12 cm H_2O and a release level of 5–10 cm H_2O. Advantages of APRV appear to be less circulatory depression and pulmonary barotrauma as well as less need for sedation. This technique appears to be an attractive alternative to PC-IRV for overcoming problems with high peak inspiratory pressures in patients with reduced lung compliance.

I. High-Frequency Ventilation (HFV)

Three forms of HFV are available. High-frequency positive-pressure ventilation involves delivering a small "conventional" VT at a rate of 60–120 breaths/min. High-frequency jet ventilation (HFJV) utilizes a small cannula at or in the airway through which a pulsed jet of high-pressure gas is delivered at a set frequency of 120–600 times/min (2–10 Hz). The jet of gas may entrain air (Bernoulli effect), which may augment VT. High-frequency oscillation employs a driver (usually a piston) that creates to-and-fro gas movement in the airway at rates of 180–3000 times/ min (3–50 Hz).

These forms of ventilation all produce VT at or below anatomic dead space. The exact mechanism of gas exchange is unclear but is probably a combination of effects (including convective ventilation, asymmetrical velocity profiles, Taylor dispersion, pendelluft, molecular diffusion, and cardiogenic mixing). Jet ventilation has found widest use in the operating room. It may be used for laryngeal, tracheal, and bronchial procedures and can be lifesaving in emergency airway management when tracheal intubation and conventional positive-pressure ventilation are unsuccessful (see Chapter 19). In the ICU, HFJV may be useful in managing some patients with bronchopleural and tracheoesophageal fistulas when conventional ventilation has failed. Occasionally, HFJV or high-frequency oscillation is used in patients with ARDS to try to improve oxygenation. Inadequate heating and humidification of inspired gases during prolonged HFV, however, can be a problem. Initial settings for HFJV in the operating room are typically a rate of 120–240 breaths/min, an inspiratory time of 33%, and a drive pressure of 15–30 psi. Mean airway pressure should be measured in the trachea at least 5 cm below the injector to avoid an artifactual error from gas entrainment. Carbon dioxide elimination is generally increased by increasing the drive pressure, whereas adequacy of oxygenation relates to the mean airway pressure. An intrinsic PEEP effect is seen during HFJV at high drive pressures and inspiratory times greater than 40%.

J. Differential Lung Ventilation

This technique, also referred to as independent lung ventilation, may be used in patients with severe unilateral lung disease or those with bronchopleural fistulae. Use of conventional positive-pressure ventilation and PEEP in such instances can aggravate ventilation/perfusion mismatching or, in patients with fistula, result in inadequate ventilation of the unaffected lung. In patients with restrictive disease of one lung, overdistention of the normal lung can lead to worsening hypoxemia or barotrauma. After separation of the lungs with a double-lumen tube,

positive-pressure ventilation can be applied to each lung independently using two ventilators. When two ventilators are used, the timing of mechanical breaths is often synchronized, with one ventilator, the "master," setting the rate for the "slave" ventilator.

2. Care of Patients Requiring Mechanical Ventilation

Tracheal Intubation

Tracheal intubation for mechanical ventilation is most commonly undertaken in ICU patients to manage pulmonary failure. Both nasotracheal and orotracheal intubation appear to be relatively safe for at least 2–3 weeks. When compared with orotracheal intubation, nasotracheal intubation may be more comfortable for the patient and more secure (fewer instances of accidental extubation). Nasal intubation, however, has significant adverse events associated with its use, including nasal bleeding, transient bacteremia, submucosal dissection of the nasopharynx or oropharynx, and sinusitis or otitis media (from obstruction of sinus outflow or of the auditory tubes). Nasal intubation will also generally necessitate use of a smaller diameter tube than orotracheal intubation, and this can make it more difficult to clear secretions and can limit fiberoptic bronchoscopy to use of smaller devices.

Intubation usually can be carried out without the use of sedation or muscle paralysis in agonal and unconscious patients. However, topical anesthesia of the airway and sedation are helpful in patients who still have active airway reflexes. More vigorous and uncooperative patients require varying degrees of sedation; administration of a paralytic agent also greatly facilitates orotracheal intubation. Small doses of relatively short-acting agents are generally used; popular agents include midazolam, etomidate, dexmedetomidine, and propofol. Succinylcholine or a nondepolarizing neuromuscular blocker can be used for paralysis after a hypnotic is given.

The time of tracheal intubation and initiation of mechanical ventilation can be a period of great hemodynamic instability. Hypertension or hypotension and bradycardia or tachycardia may be encountered.

Responsible factors include activation of autonomic reflexes from stimulation of the airway, myocardial depression and vasodilation from sedative-hypnotic agents, straining by the patient, withdrawal of intense sympathetic activity, and reduced venous return due to positive pressure in the airways. Careful monitoring is required during and immediately following intubation.

When left in place for more than 2–3 weeks, both orotracheal and nasotracheal tubes predispose patients to subglottic stenosis. If longer periods of mechanical ventilation are necessary, the tracheal tube should generally be replaced by a cuffed tracheostomy tube. If it is anticipated that a tracheal tube will be required for more than 2 weeks, a tracheostomy may be performed soon after intubation. There is a trend to earlier tracheostomy in victims of trauma, particularly those with major head injuries. While earlier tracheostomy does not reduce mortality, it does tend to reduce the incidence of pneumonia, the duration of mechanical ventilation, and the length of stay.

Initial Ventilator Settings

Depending on the type of pulmonary failure, mechanical ventilation is used to provide either partial or full ventilatory support. For full ventilatory support, CMV, AC, or PCV is generally employed with a respiratory rate of 10–12 breaths/min and a V_T of 8–10 mL/kg; lower V_T (6–8 mL/kg) may be necessary to avoid high peak inflation pressures (>35–40 cm H_2O) and pulmonary barotrauma and volutrauma. High airway pressures that overdistend alveoli (transalveolar pressure >35 cm H_2O) have been shown experimentally to promote lung injury. Likewise, compared with a V_T of 12 mL/kg, a V_T of 6 mL/kg and plateau pressure (P_{plt}) less than 30 cm H_2O have been associated with reduced mortality in patients with ARDS. Partial ventilatory support is usually provided by low SIMV settings (<8 breaths/min), either with or without pressure support. Lower P_{plt} (<20–30 cm H_2O) can help preserve cardiac output, may be less likely to alter normal ventilation/perfusion relationships, and is the current recommendation.

Patients breathing spontaneously on SIMV must overcome the additional resistances of the tracheal tube, demand valves, and breathing circuit of the ventilator. These imposed resistances increase the work of breathing. Smaller tubes (<7.0 mm i.d. in adults) increase resistance and should be avoided whenever possible. The simultaneous use of pressure support of 5–15 cm H_2O during SIMV can compensate for tube and circuit resistance.

The addition of 5–8 cm H_2O of PEEP during positive-pressure ventilation preserves FRC and gas exchange. This "physiological" PEEP is purported to compensate for the loss of a similar amount of intrinsic PEEP (and decrease in FRC) in patients following tracheal intubation. Periodic sigh breaths (large V_T) are not necessary when a PEEP of 5–8 cm H_2O accompanies V_T of appropriate volumes.

Sedation & Paralysis

Sedation and paralysis may be necessary in patients who become agitated and "fight" the ventilator. Repetitive coughing ("bucking") and straining can have adverse hemodynamic effects, can interfere with gas exchange, and may predispose to pulmonary barotrauma and self-inflicted injury. Sedation with or without paralysis may also be desirable when patients continue to be tachypneic despite high mechanical respiratory rates (>16–18 breaths/min).

Commonly used sedatives include opioids (morphine or fentanyl), benzodiazepines (usually midazolam), propofol, and dexmedetomidine. These agents may be used alone or in combination and are often administered by continuous infusion. Nondepolarizing paralytic agents are used in combination with sedation when sedation alone and all other means to ventilate the patient have failed.

Monitoring

Patients on mechanical ventilation require continuous monitoring for adverse hemodynamic and pulmonary effects from positive pressure in the airways. Continuous electrocardiography and pulse oximetry are useful. Direct intraarterial pressure monitoring also allows frequent sampling of arterial blood for respiratory gas analysis (both a convenience and a disadvantage, given the large number of unnecessary laboratory tests that are often performed on patients with critical illness). Accurate recording of fluid intake and output is necessary to assess fluid balance. An indwelling urinary catheter will lead to an increased risk of urinary tract infections and should be avoided when possible, but it is helpful for monitoring urinary output. Central venous (and rarely pulmonary artery) pressure monitoring are used in hemodynamically unstable patients. Frequent chest radiographs are commonly obtained to confirm tracheal tube and central venous catheter positions, evaluate for evidence of pulmonary barotrauma or pulmonary disease, and determine whether there are signs of pulmonary edema.

Airway pressures (baseline, peak, plateau, and mean), inhaled and exhaled V_T (mechanical and spontaneous), and fractional concentration of oxygen should be closely monitored. Monitoring these parameters not only allows optimal adjustment of ventilator settings but helps detect problems with the tracheal tube, breathing circuit, and ventilator. For example, an increasing P_{plt} for a set V_T can indicate worsening compliance. A declining blood pressure and increasing P_{plt} from dynamic hyperinflation (autoPEEP) can be quickly diagnosed by disconnecting the patient from the ventilator. Inadequate suctioning of airway secretions and the presence of large mucus plugs are often manifested as increasing peak inflation pressures (a sign of increased resistance to gas flow) and decreasing exhaled V_T. An abrupt increase in peak inflation pressure together with sudden hypotension strongly suggests a pneumothorax.

3. Discontinuing Mechanical Ventilation

There are two phases to discontinuing mechanical ventilation. In the first, "readiness testing," so-called weaning parameters and other subjective and objective assessments are used to determine whether the patient can sustain progressive withdrawal of mechanical ventilator support. The second phase, "weaning" or "liberation," describes the way in which mechanical support is removed.

Readiness testing should include determining whether the process that necessitated mechanical ventilation has been reversed or controlled. Complicating factors such as bronchospasm, heart failure, infection, malnutrition, metabolic acidosis or

alkalosis, anemia, increased CO_2 production due to increased carbohydrate loads, altered mental status, and sleep deprivation should be adequately treated. Underlying lung disease and respiratory muscle wasting from prolonged disuse often complicate weaning. Patients who fail to wean despite apparent readiness often have COPD or chronic heart failure.

Weaning (or liberation) from mechanical ventilation should be considered when patients no longer meet general criteria for mechanical ventilation (see Table 57–4). In general, this occurs when patients have a pH greater than 7.25, show adequate arterial oxygen saturation while receiving F_{IO_2} less than 0.5, are able to spontaneously breathe, are hemodynamically stable, and have no current signs of myocardial ischemia. Additional mechanical indices have also been suggested (Table 57–6). Useful weaning parameters include arterial blood gas tensions, respiratory rate, and rapid shallow breathing index (RSBI, see below). Intact airway reflexes and a cooperative patient are also mandatory prior to completion of the weaning and extubation unless the patient will retain a cuffed tracheostomy tube. Similarly, adequate oxygenation (arterial oxygen saturation >90% on 40–50% O_2 with <5 cm H_2O of PEEP) is imperative prior to extubation. When the patient is weaned from mechanical ventilation and extubation is planned, the RSBI is frequently used to help predict who can be successfully weaned from mechanical ventilation and extubated. With the patient breathing spontaneously on a T-piece, the V_T (in liters) and respiratory rate (f) are measured:

$$RSBI = \frac{f(\text{breaths/min})}{V_T(L)}$$

TABLE 57–6 Mechanical criteria for weaning/extubation.

Criterion	Measurement
Inspiratory pressure	<−25 cm H_2O
Tidal volume	>5 mL/kg
Vital capacity	>10 mL/kg
Minute ventilation	<10 mL
Rapid shallow breathing index	<100

Patients with an RSBI less than 100 can be successfully extubated. Those with an RSBI greater than 120 should retain some degree of mechanical ventilator support.

The common techniques to wean a patient from the ventilator include SIMV, pressure support, or periods of spontaneous breathing alone on a T-piece or on low levels of CPAP. Mandatory minute ventilation has also been suggested as an ideal weaning technique, but experience with it is limited. Finally, many institutions use "automated tube compensation" to provide just enough pressure support to compensate for the resistance of breathing through an endotracheal tube. Newer mechanical ventilators have a setting that will automatically adjust gas flows to make this adjustment. In practice in adults breathing through conventionally sized tubes (7.5–8.5), the adjustment will typically amount to pressure support of 5 cm H_2O and PEEP of 5 cm H_2O.

Weaning with SIMV

With SIMV the number of mechanical breaths is progressively decreased (by 1–2 breaths/min) as long as the arterial CO_2 tension and respiratory rate remain acceptable (generally <45–50 mm Hg and <30 breaths/min, respectively). If pressure support is concomitantly used, it should generally be reduced to 5–8 cm H_2O. In patients with acid–base disturbances or chronic CO_2 retention, arterial blood pH (>7.35) is more useful than CO_2 tension. Blood gas measurements can be checked after a minimum of 15–30 min at each setting. When an IMV of 2–4 breaths is reached, mechanical ventilation is discontinued if arterial oxygenation remains acceptable.

Weaning with PSV

Weaning with PSV alone is accomplished by gradually decreasing the pressure support level by 2–3 cm H_2O while Vt, arterial blood gas tensions, and respiratory rate are monitored (using the same criteria as for IMV). The goal is to try to ensure a Vt of 4–6 mL/kg and an f of less than 30 with acceptable Pao$_2$ and Paco$_2$. When a pressure support level of 5–8 cm H_2O is reached, the patient is considered weaned.

Weaning with a T-Piece or CPAP

T-piece trials allow observation while the patient breathes spontaneously without any mechanical breaths. The T-piece attaches directly to the tracheal tube or tracheostomy tube and has corrugated tubing on the other two limbs. A humidified oxygen–air mixture flows into the proximal limb and exits from the distal limb. Sufficient gas flow must be given in the proximal limb to prevent the mist from being completely drawn back at the distal limb during inspiration; this ensures that the patient is receiving the desired oxygen concentration. The patient is observed closely during this period; obvious new signs of fatigue, chest retractions, tachypnea, tachycardia, arrhythmias, or hypertension or hypotension should terminate the trial. If the patient appears to tolerate the trial period and the RSBI is less than 100, mechanical ventilation can be discontinued permanently. If the patient can also protect and clear the airway, the tracheal tube can be removed.

If the patient has been intubated for a prolonged period or has severe underlying lung disease, sequential T-piece trials may be necessary. Periodic trials of 10–30 min are initiated and progressively increased by 5–10 min or longer per trial as long as the patient appears comfortable and maintains acceptable arterial blood gas measurements.

Many patients develop progressive atelectasis during prolonged T-piece trials. This may reflect the absence of a normal "physiological" PEEP when the larynx is bypassed by a tracheal tube. If this is a concern, spontaneous breathing trials on low levels (5 cm H_2O) of CPAP can be tried. The CPAP helps maintain FRC and prevent atelectasis.

POSITIVE AIRWAY PRESSURE THERAPY

Positive airway pressure therapy can be used in patients who are breathing spontaneously as well as those who are mechanically ventilated. The principal indication for positive airway pressure therapy is a decrease in FRC resulting in absolute or relative hypoxemia. By increasing transpulmonary distending pressure, positive airway pressure therapy can increase FRC, improve (increase) lung compliance, and reverse ventilation/perfusion mismatching. Improvement in the latter parameter will show as a decrease in venous admixture and an improvement in arterial O_2 tension.

Positive End-Expiratory Pressure

Application of positive pressure during expiration as an adjunct to a mechanically delivered breath is referred to as PEEP. The ventilator's PEEP valve provides a pressure threshold that allows expiratory flow to occur only when airway pressure exceeds the selected PEEP level.

Continuous Positive Airway Pressure

Application of a positive-pressure threshold during both inspiration and expiration with spontaneous breathing is referred to as CPAP. Constant levels of pressure can be attained only if a high-flow (inspiratory) gas source is provided. When the patient does not have an artificial airway, tightly fitting full-face masks, nasal masks, nasal "pillows" (ADAM circuit), or nasal prongs (neonatal) can be used. Because of the risks of gastric distention and regurgitation, CPAP masks should be used only on patients with intact airway reflexes and with CPAP levels less than 15 cm H_2O (less than lower esophageal sphincter pressure in normal persons). Expiratory pressures above 15 cm H_2O require an artificial airway.

CPAP versus PEEP

The distinction between PEEP and CPAP is often blurred in the clinical setting because patients may breathe with a combination of mechanical and spontaneous breaths. Therefore, the two terms are often used interchangeably. In the strictest sense, "pure" PEEP is provided as a ventilator-cycled breath. In contrast, a "pure" CPAP system provides only sufficient continuous or "on-demand" gas flows (60–90 L/min) to prevent inspiratory airway pressure from falling perceptibly below the expiratory level during spontaneous breaths (**Figure 57–5**). Some ventilators with demand valve–based CPAP systems may not be adequately responsive and result in increased inspiratory work of breathing.

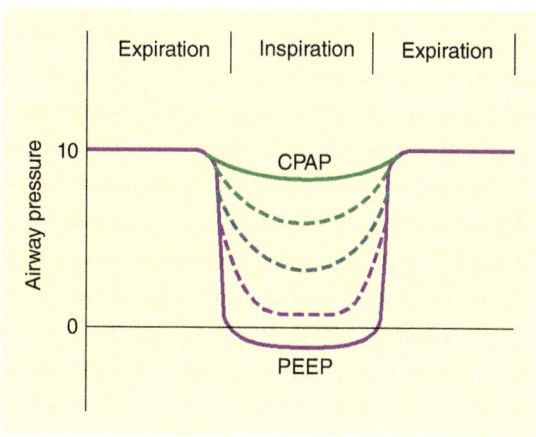

FIGURE 57–5 Airway pressure during positive end-expiratory pressure (PEEP) and continuous positive airway pressure (CPAP). Note that by increasing inspiratory gas flows, PEEP progressively becomes CPAP.

This situation can be corrected by adding low levels of (inspiratory) PSV if in a volume-targeted mode or changing to a pressure-targeted mode. In clinical practice, controlled ventilation, PSV, and CPAP/PEEP support can be delivered by most modern ICU ventilators. Manufacturers have also developed specific devices to deliver bilevel inspiratory positive airway pressure (IPAP) with expiratory positive airway pressure (EPAP) in either a spontaneous or time-cycled fashion. The term *bilevel positive airway pressure* (BiPAP) has become a commonly used phrase, adding to the confusion of airway pressure terminology.

Pulmonary Effects of PEEP & CPAP

The major effect of PEEP and CPAP on the lungs is to increase FRC. In patients with decreased lung volume, appropriate levels of either PEEP or CPAP will increase FRC and tidal ventilation above closing capacity, will improve lung compliance, and will correct ventilation/perfusion abnormalities. The resulting decrease in intrapulmonary shunting improves arterial oxygenation. The principal mechanism of action for both PEEP and CPAP appears to be expansion of partially collapsed alveoli. Recruitment (reexpansion) of collapsed alveoli occurs at PEEP or CPAP levels above the inflection point, defined as the pressure level on

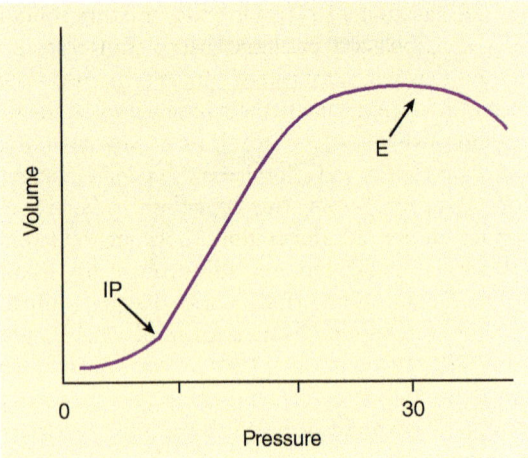

FIGURE 57–6 Pressure–volume curve for pulmonary system (eg, lung, thoracic). Inflection point (IP) above which the majority of alveoli are recruited. E, result of excessive pressure when alveoli are overdistended and pulmonary compliance decreases.

a pressure–volume curve at which collapsed alveoli are recruited (open); with small changes in pressure there are large changes in volume (Figure 57–6). Although neither PEEP nor CPAP decreases total extravascular lung water, studies suggest that they do redistribute extravascular lung water from the interstitial space between alveoli and endothelial cells toward peribronchial and perihilar areas. Both effects can potentially improve arterial oxygenation.

Excessive PEEP or CPAP, however, can overdistend alveoli (and bronchi), increasing dead space ventilation and reducing lung compliance; both effects can significantly increase the work of breathing. By compressing alveolar capillaries, overdistention of normal alveoli can also increase pulmonary vascular resistance and right ventricular afterload.

8 A higher incidence of pulmonary barotrauma is observed with excessive PEEP or CPAP, particularly at levels greater than 20 cm H_2O. Disruption of alveoli allows air to track interstitially along bronchi into the mediastinum (pneumomediastinum). From the mediastinum, air can then rupture into the pleural space (pneumothorax) or the pericardium (pneumopericardium) or can dissect along tissue planes subcutaneously (subcutaneous emphysema) or into the abdomen (pneumoperitoneum or pneumoretroperitoneum). A bronchopleural fistula is the result of failure of an air leak to seal (close). Although barotrauma must be considered in any discussion of CPAP and PEEP, in fact, it may be more clearly associated with higher peak inspiratory pressures that result with increasing level of PEEP or CPAP. Other factors that may increase the risk of barotrauma include underlying lung disease, stacking of breaths (from too frequent breaths or too short expiratory times) so that intrinsic PEEP (dynamic hyperinflation or autoPEEP) develops, large V_T (>10–15 mL/kg), and younger age.

Adverse Nonpulmonary Effects of PEEP & CPAP

Nonpulmonary adverse effects are primarily circulatory and are related to transmission of the elevated airway pressure to the contents of the chest. Fortunately, transmission is directly related to lung compliance; thus, patients with decreased lung compliance (most patients requiring PEEP) are least affected.

Progressive reductions in cardiac output are often seen as mean airway pressure and, secondarily, mean intrathoracic pressure rise. The principal mechanism appears to be intrathoracic pressure–related inhibition of return of venous blood to the heart. Other mechanisms may include leftward displacement of the interventricular septum (interfering with left ventricular filling) because of the increase in pulmonary vascular resistance (increased right ventricular afterload) from overdistention of alveoli, leading to an increase in right ventricular volume. Left ventricular compliance may therefore be reduced; when this occurs, to achieve the same cardiac output may require a higher filling pressure. An increase in intravascular volume will usually at least partially offset the effects of CPAP and PEEP on cardiac output. Circulatory depression is most often associated with end-expiratory pressures greater than 15 cm H_2O.

PEEP-induced elevations in central venous pressure and reductions in cardiac output decrease both renal and hepatic blood flow. Circulating levels of antidiuretic hormone and angiotensin are usually elevated. Urinary output, glomerular filtration, and free water clearance decrease.

Increased end-expiratory pressures, because they impede blood drainage from the brain and blood return to the heart, may increase intracranial pressure in patients whose ventricular compliance is decreased. Therefore, in patients on mechanical ventilation for acute lung injury and who have evidence of increased intracranial pressure, the level of PEEP must be carefully chosen to balance oxygenation requirements against potential adverse effects on intracranial pressure.

Optimum Use of PEEP & CPAP

The goal of positive-pressure therapy is to increase oxygen delivery to tissues, while avoiding the adverse sequelae of excessively increased (>0.5) FIO_2. The latter is best accomplished with an adequate cardiac output and hemoglobin concentration. Ideally, mixed venous oxygen tensions or the arteriovenous oxygen content difference should be followed. The salutary effect of PEEP (or CPAP) on arterial oxygen tension must be balanced against any detrimental effect on cardiac output. Volume infusion or inotropic support may be necessary and should be guided by hemodynamic measurements.

At optimal PEEP the beneficial effects of PEEP exceed any detrimental risks. Practically, PEEP is usually added in increments of 3–5 cm H_2O until the desired therapeutic end point is reached. The most commonly suggested end point is an arterial oxygen saturation of hemoglobin of greater than 88–90% on a nontoxic inspired oxygen concentration (≤50%). Many clinicians favor reducing the inspired oxygen concentration to 50% or less because of the potentially adverse effect of greater oxygen concentrations on the lung. Alternatively, PEEP may be titrated to the mixed venous artery oxygen saturation ($S\bar{v}O_2$ > 50–60%). Monitoring lung compliance and dead space has also been suggested.

OTHER RESPIRATORY CARE TECHNIQUES

Other respiratory care techniques, including administration of aerosolized water or bronchodilators and clearing of pulmonary secretions, preserve or improve pulmonary function.

An aerosol mist is a gas or gas mixture containing a suspension of liquid particles. Aerosolized water may be administered to loosen inspissated secretions and facilitate their removal from the tracheobronchial tree. Aerosol mists are also used to administer bronchodilators, mucolytic agents, or vasoconstrictors (metered-dose inhalers are preferred for administration of bronchodilators). A normal cough requires an adequate inspiratory capacity, an intact glottis, and adequate muscle strength (abdominal muscles and diaphragm). Aerosol mists with or without bronchodilators may induce cough as well as loosen secretions. Instillation of hypertonic saline has been used as a mucolytic and to induce cough. Additional effective measures include chest percussion or vibration therapy and postural drainage of the various lung lobes.

9 Maneuvers that produce sustained maximum lung inflation such as the use of an incentive spirometer can be helpful in inducing cough as well as preventing atelectasis and preserving normal lung volume. Patients should be instructed to inhale approximately 15–20 mL/kg and to hold it for 2–3 s before exhalation.

When thick and copious secretions are associated with obvious atelectasis and hypoxemia, more aggressive measures may be indicated. These include suctioning the spontaneously breathing patient via a nasopharyngeal catheter or flexible bronchoscope, or performing the same two maneuvers through a tracheal tube. When there is atelectasis without retention of secretions, a brief period of CPAP by mask or positive-pressure ventilation through a tracheal tube is often very effective.

Respiratory Failure

Respiratory failure may be defined as impairment of normal gas exchange severe enough to require acute therapeutic intervention. Definitions based on arterial blood gases (see Table 57–1) may not apply to patients with chronic pulmonary diseases. For example, dyspnea and progressive respiratory acidosis may be present in patients with chronic CO_2 retention. Arterial blood gases typically follow one of several patterns in patients with respiratory failure (Figure 57–7). At one extreme, the derangement

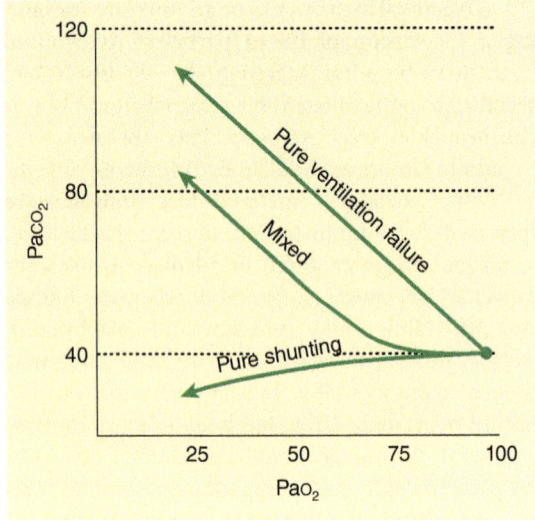

FIGURE 57–7 Arterial gas tension (room air) patterns during acute respiratory failure.

primarily affects oxygen transfer from the alveoli into blood, giving rise to hypoxemia (hypoxic respiratory failure); unless severe ventilation/perfusion mismatching is present, CO_2 elimination in these instances is typically normal or even enhanced. At the other extreme, the disorder primarily affects CO_2 elimination (pure ventilatory failure), resulting in hypercapnia; mismatching of ventilation to perfusion is typically absent or minimal. Hypoxemia, however, can occur with pure ventilatory failure when arterial CO_2 tension reaches 75–80 mm Hg in patients breathing room air (see the alveolar gas equation in Chapter 23). Few patients with respiratory failure display a pattern as "pure" as these extreme examples.

Treatment

Regardless of the disorder, the treatment of respiratory failure is primarily supportive while the reversible components of underlying disease are treated. Hypoxemia is treated with oxygen therapy and positive airway pressure (if FRC is decreased), whereas hypercarbia (ventilatory failure) is treated with mechanical ventilation. Other general measures may include using aerosolized bronchodilators, intravenous antibiotics, and diuretics for fluid

overload, therapy to improve cardiac function, and nutritional support.

PULMONARY EDEMA
Pathophysiology

Pulmonary edema results from transudation of fluid, first from pulmonary capillaries into interstitial spaces and then from the interstitial spaces into alveoli. Fluid within the interstitial space and alveoli is collectively referred to as extravascular lung water. The movement of water across the pulmonary capillaries is similar to what occurs in other capillary beds and can be expressed by the Starling equation:

$$Q = K \times [(Pc' - Pi) - \sigma(\pi c' - \pi i)]$$

where Q is net flow across the capillary; Pc' and Pi are capillary and interstitial hydrostatic pressures, respectively; $\pi c'$ and πi are capillary and interstitial oncotic pressures, respectively; K is a filtration coefficient related to effective capillary surface area per mass of tissue; and σ is a reflection coefficient that expresses the permeability of the capillary endothelium to albumin. Albumin is particularly important in this context because water loss to the interstitium will increase when albumin is also lost to the interstitium. A σ with a value of 1 implies that the endothelium is completely impermeable to albumin, whereas a value of 0 indicates free passage of albumin and other particles/molecules. The pulmonary endothelium normally is partially permeable to albumin, such that interstitial albumin concentration is approximately one half that of plasma; therefore, under normal conditions πi must be about 14 mm Hg (one half that of plasma). Pulmonary capillary hydrostatic pressure is dependent on vertical height in the lung (gravity) and normally varies from 0 to 15 mm Hg (average, 7 mm Hg). Because Pi is thought to be normally about –4 to –8 mm Hg, the forces favoring transudation of fluid (Pc', Pi, and πi) are usually almost balanced by the forces favoring reabsorption ($\pi c'$). The net amount of fluid that normally moves out of pulmonary capillaries is small (about 10–20 mL/h in adults) and is rapidly removed by pulmonary lymphatics, which return it into the central venous system.

The alveolar epithelial membrane is usually permeable to water and gases but is impermeable to albumin (and other proteins). A net movement of water from the interstitium into alveoli occurs only when the normally negative Pi becomes positive (relative to atmospheric pressure). Fortunately, because of the lung's unique ultrastructure and its capacity to increase lymph flow, the pulmonary interstitium usually accommodates large increases in capillary transudation before Pi becomes positive. When this reserve capacity is exceeded, pulmonary edema develops.

Pulmonary edema is often divided into four stages:

Stage I: Only interstitial pulmonary edema is present. Patients often become tachypneic as pulmonary compliance begins to decrease. The chest radiograph reveals increased interstitial markings and peribronchial cuffing.

Stage II: Fluid fills the interstitium and begins to fill the alveoli, being initially confined to the angles between adjacent septa (crescentic filling). Near-normal gas exchange may be preserved.

Stage III: Many alveoli are completely flooded and no longer contain gas. Flooding is most prominent in dependent areas of the lungs. Blood flow through the capillaries of flooded alveoli results in a large increase in intrapulmonary shunting. Hypoxemia and hypocapnia (the latter due to dyspnea and hyperventilation) are characteristic.

Stage IV: Marked alveolar flooding spills into the airways as froth. Gas exchange is compromised due to both shunting and airway obstruction, leading to progressive hypercapnia and severe hypoxemia.

Causes of Pulmonary Edema

Pulmonary edema usually results from either an increase in the net hydrostatic pressure across the capillaries (hemodynamic or cardiogenic pulmonary edema) or an increase in the permeability of the alveolar–capillary membrane (increased permeability edema or noncardiogenic pulmonary edema). If a pulmonary artery catheter is present, the distinction can be based on the pulmonary artery occlusion pressure, which if greater than 18 mm Hg indicates that hydrostatic pressure is involved in forcing fluid across the capillaries into the interstitium and alveoli. The protein content of the edema fluid can also help differentiate the two. Fluid due to hemodynamic edema has a low protein content, whereas that due to permeability edema has a high protein content.

Less common causes of edema include prolonged severe airway obstruction (negative pressure pulmonary edema), sudden reexpansion of a collapsed lung, high altitude, pulmonary lymphatic obstruction, and severe head injury, although the same mechanisms (ie, changes in hemodynamic parameters or capillary permeability) also account for these diagnoses. Pulmonary edema associated with airway obstruction may result from an increase in the transmural pressure across pulmonary capillaries associated with a markedly negative interstitial hydrostatic pressure. Neurogenic pulmonary edema appears to be related to a marked increase in sympathetic tone, which causes severe pulmonary hypertension. The latter can disrupt the alveolar–capillary membrane.

1. Increased Transmural Pressure Pulmonary Edema ("Cardiogenic" Pulmonary Edema)

Significantly increased Pc' can increase extravascular lung water and result in pulmonary edema. As can be seen from the Starling equation, a decrease in πc' may accentuate the effects of any increase in Pc'. Two major mechanisms increase Pc'; namely, pulmonary venous hypertension and a markedly increased pulmonary blood flow. Any elevation of pulmonary venous pressure is transmitted passively backward to the pulmonary capillaries and secondarily increases Pc'. Pulmonary venous hypertension usually results from left ventricular failure, mitral stenosis, or left atrial obstruction. Increases in pulmonary blood flow that exceed the capacity of the pulmonary vasculature will also raise Pc'. Marked increases in pulmonary blood flow can be the result of large left-to-right cardiac or peripheral shunts, hypervolemia (fluid overload), or extremes of anemia or exercise.

Treatment

Management of cardiogenic pulmonary edema involves decreasing the pressure in the pulmonary capillaries. Generally, this includes measures to improve left ventricular function, correct fluid overload with diuretics, or reduce pulmonary blood flow. Pharmacological treatment of acute cardiogenic pulmonary edema has included oxygen, morphine, diuretics (especially loop diuretics), vasodilators such as nitrates or angiotensin-converting enzyme (ACE) inhibitors (although these decrease both preload and afterload), and inotropes such as dobutamine or milrinone. Vasodilators, particularly nitrates, have proved useful. By reducing preload, pulmonary congestion is relieved; by reducing afterload, cardiac output may be improved. Positive airway pressure therapy is also a useful adjunct for improving oxygenation. When pulmonary edema is a consequence of acute coronary ischemia and left ventricular failure, intraaortic balloon counterpulsation or other assist devices may be used.

2. Increased Permeability Pulmonary Edema (Noncardiogenic Pulmonary Edema): Acute Lung Injury & ARDS

Extravascular lung water increases in patients with increased permeability pulmonary edema due to enhanced permeability or disruption of the capillary–alveolar membrane. The protective effect of plasma oncotic pressure is lost as increased amounts of albumin "leak" into the pulmonary interstitium; normal—or even low—capillary hydrostatic pressures are unopposed and result in transudation of fluid into the lungs. Permeability edema is seen with acute lung injury (P:F ratio ≤ 300 [P = Pa_{O_2} and F = F_{IO_2}]) and is often associated with sepsis, trauma, and pulmonary aspiration; when severe (P:F ratio < 200), it is referred to as the acute respiratory distress syndrome (ARDS).

Pathophysiology

Acute lung injury and ARDS represent the pulmonary manifestation of the systemic inflammatory response syndrome (SIRS). Central to the pathophysiology of acute lung injury and ARDS is severe injury of the capillary–alveolar membrane. Regardless of the type of injury, the lung responds to the ensuing inflammatory response in a similar fashion. The released secondary mediators increase pulmonary capillary permeability, induce pulmonary vasoconstriction, and alter vascular reactivity such that hypoxic pulmonary vasoconstriction is abolished. Destruction of alveolar epithelial cells is prominent. Alveolar flooding, with decreased surfactant production (due to loss of type II pneumocytes), result in collapse. The exudative phase of ARDS may persist for a varying period; it is often followed by a fibrotic phase (fibrosing alveolitis), which in some cases leads to permanent scarring.

Clinical Manifestations

The diagnosis of acute lung injury or ARDS requires the exclusion of significant underlying left ventricular dysfunction combined with a P:F ratio of less than 300 (acute lung injury) or less than 200 (ARDS), and the presence of diffuse infiltrates on chest radiograph. The lung is often affected in a nonhomogeneous pattern, although dependent areas tend to be most affected.

Acute lung injury and ARDS are commonly seen in the settings of sepsis or trauma. Patients present with severe dyspnea and labored respirations. Hypoxemia due to intrapulmonary shunting is a universal finding. Although dead space ventilation is increased, arterial CO_2 tension is typically decreased because of a marked increase in minute ventilation. Ventilatory failure may be seen initially in severe cases or may eventually develop due to respiratory muscle fatigue or marked destruction of the capillary–alveolar membrane. Pulmonary hypertension and low or normal left ventricular filling pressures are characteristic hemodynamic findings.

Treatment

In addition to intensive respiratory care, treatment should be directed at reversible processes such as sepsis or hypotension. Hypoxemia is treated with oxygen therapy. Milder cases may be treated with a CPAP mask, but most patients require intubation and at least some degree of mechanical ventilatory support. **Increased P_{plt} pressures (>30 cm H_2O) and high V_T (>6 mL/kg), however, should also be avoided because overdistention of alveoli can induce iatrogenic lung injury, as can high** ⑩ $F_{IO_2}(>0.5)$**.** While injury from high F_{IO_2} has not been conclusively demonstrated in humans, as was previously noted, V_T of 12 mL/kg was associated with greater mortality than V_T of 6 mL/kg and P_{plt} of less than 30 cm H_2O in patients with ARDS. Thus, reduced tidal volumes are associated with the greatest improvement in outcome after ARDS of any intervention subjected to a randomized clinical trial.

If possible, the F_{IO_2} should be maintained at 0.5 or less, primarily by increasing PEEP above the inflection point (see Figure 57–6). Other maneuvers to improve oxygenation include the use of inhaled nitric oxide, inhaled prostacyclin or prostaglandin E_1 (PGE_1), and ventilation in the prone position. These three techniques improve oxygenation in many patients with acute lung injury, but they are not risk free and they have not been associated with an improvement in survival. A recent meta-analysis has concluded that moderate doses of corticosteroids likely improve morbidity and mortality outcomes in ARDS, but the underlying data remain controversial.

Morbidity and mortality from ARDS usually arise from the precipitating cause or from complications rather than from the respiratory failure itself. Among the most common serious complications are sepsis, renal failure, and gastrointestinal hemorrhage. Nosocomial pneumonia is particularly common in patients with a protracted course and is often difficult to diagnose; antibiotics are generally indicated when there is a high index of suspicion (fever, purulent secretions, leukocytosis, and change in chest radiograph). Protected specimen brushings and bronchoalveolar lavage sampling via a flexible bronchoscope may be useful. Breach of mucocutaneous barriers by various catheters, malnutrition, and altered host immunity contribute to a frequent incidence of infection. Kidney failure may result from various combinations of volume depletion, sepsis, or nephrotoxins. Kidney failure substantially increases the mortality rate for ARDS (to >60%).

Prophylaxis for gastrointestinal hemorrhage with sucralfate, antacids, H_2 blockers, or proton pump inhibitors is recommended.

DROWNING & NEAR-DROWNING

Drowning, with or without aspiration of water, is death while submerged in water. Near-drowning, with or without aspiration, is suffocation while submerged with (at least temporary) survival. Survival depends on the intensity and duration of the hypoxia and on the water temperature.

Pathophysiology

Both drowning and near-drowning can occur whether or not inhalation (aspiration) of water occurs. If water does not enter the airways, the patient primarily suffers from asphyxia; however, if the patient inhales water, marked intrapulmonary shunting also takes place. Ninety percent of drowning patients aspirate fluid: fresh water, seawater, brackish water, or other fluids. Although the amount of liquid aspirated is generally small, marked ventilation/perfusion mismatching can result from fluids in the airways and alveoli, reflex bronchospasm, and loss of pulmonary surfactant. Aspiration of gastric contents can also complicate drowning before or after loss of consciousness or during resuscitation.

The hypotonic water aspirated following fresh water drowning is rapidly absorbed by the pulmonary circulation; water cannot usually be recovered from the airways. If a significant amount is absorbed (>800 mL in a 70-kg adult), transient hemodilution, hyponatremia, and even hemolysis may occur. In contrast, aspiration of salt water, which is hypertonic, draws out water from the pulmonary circulation into the alveoli, flooding them. Thus, hemoconcentration and hypernatremia may occasionally occur following saltwater drowning. Hypermagnesemia and hypercalcemia have also been reported following near-drowning in salt water.

Patients who suffer from cold water drowning lose consciousness when core body temperature decreases below 32°C. Ventricular fibrillation occurs at about 28–30°C, but relative to normothermic drowning, the hypothermia has a protective effect on the brain and may improve outcome provided that resuscitation measures are successful.

Clinical Manifestations

Nearly all patients with a true near-drowning episode will have hypoxemia, hypercarbia, and metabolic acidosis. Patients may also suffer from other injuries, such as spine fractures following diving accidents. Neurological impairment is generally related to duration of submersion and severity of asphyxia. Cerebral edema complicates prolonged asphyxia. Acute lung injury and ARDS develop in many patients following resuscitation.

Treatment

Initial treatment of near-drowning is directed at restoring ventilation, perfusion, oxygenation, and acid–base balance as quickly as possible. Immediate measures include establishing a clear and unobstructed airway, administering oxygen, and initiating cardiopulmonary resuscitation. In-line stabilization of the cervical spine is necessary when intubating patients who suffer from near-drowning following a dive. Although salt water can often be drained out of the lungs by gravity, this practice should not delay institution of cardiopulmonary resuscitation; abdominal thrusts may promote aspiration of gastric contents. Resuscitation efforts are always continued until the patient is fully assessed and under treatment in a hospital, particularly following cold water drowning. Complete recovery is possible in such instances even after prolonged periods of asphyxia. Management includes tracheal intubation, positive-pressure ventilation, and PEEP. Bronchospasm should be treated with bronchodilators, electrolyte abnormalities corrected, and acute lung injury and ARDS treated as discussed above. Hypothermia should be corrected gradually over a few hours.

SMOKE INHALATION

Smoke inhalation is the leading cause of death from fires. Affected persons may or may not have sustained a burn. Burn victims who suffer from smoke inhalation have a mortality rate significantly greater than other comparably burned patients without smoke inhalation. Any exposure to smoke in a fire requires a presumptive diagnosis of smoke inhalation until proved otherwise. A suggestive history might include loss of consciousness or disorientation in a patient exposed to a fire, or a burn acquired in a closed space.

Pathophysiology

The consequences of smoke inhalation are complex because they can involve three types of injuries: heat injury to the airways, exposure to toxic gases, and a chemical burn with deposition of carbonaceous particulates in the lower airways. The pulmonary response to smoke inhalation is equally complex and depends on the duration of the exposure, composition of the material that burned, and presence of any underlying lung disease. Combustion of many synthetic materials produces toxic gases such as carbon monoxide, hydrogen cyanide, hydrogen sulfide, hydrogen chloride, ammonia, chlorine, benzene, and aldehydes. When these gases react with water in the airways, they can produce hydrochloric, acetic, formic, and sulfuric acids. Carbon monoxide and cyanide poisoning are common.

After smoke inhalation direct mucosal injury may result in edema, inflammation, and sloughing. Loss of ciliary activity impairs the clearance of mucus and bacteria. Manifestations of acute lung injury and ARDS typically appear 2–3 days after the injury and seem related to the delayed development of SIRS rather than the acute smoke inhalation itself.

Clinical Manifestations

Patients may initially have few if any symptoms after smoke inhalation. Suggestive physical findings include facial or intraoral burns, singed nasal hairs, cough, carbonaceous sputum, and wheezing. The diagnosis usually can be confirmed when flexible bronchoscopy of the upper airway and the tracheobronchial tree reveals erythema, edema, mucosal ulcerations, and carbonaceous deposits. Arterial blood gases initially may be normal or reveal only mild hypoxemia and metabolic acidosis due to carbon monoxide. The chest radiograph is often normal on presentation.

Heat injury to the airways is usually confined to supraglottic structures in the absence of prolonged exposure to steam. Progressive hoarseness and stridor are ominous signs of impending airway obstruction, which may develop over 12–18 h. Fluid resuscitation of any burn injury will frequently aggravate the edema.

Carbon monoxide poisoning is usually defined as greater than 15% carboxyhemoglobin in the blood. The diagnosis is made by cooximetric measurements of arterial blood. Carbon monoxide has 200–300 times the affinity of oxygen for hemoglobin. When a CO molecule combines with hemoglobin to form carboxyhemoglobin, it decreases the affinity of the other binding sites for oxygen, shifting the hemoglobin dissociation curve to the right. The net result is a marked reduction in the oxygen-carrying capacity of blood.

Carbon monoxide dissociates very slowly from hemoglobin with a half-life of approximately 2–4 h. Clinical manifestations result from tissue hypoxia from impaired oxygen delivery. Levels greater than 20–40% carboxyhemoglobin are associated with neurological impairment, nausea, fatigue, disorientation, and shock. Lower levels may also produce symptoms because carbon monoxide also binds cytochrome c and myoglobin. Compensatory mechanisms include increased cardiac output and peripheral vasodilation.

Cyanide toxicity may occur in patients exposed to fumes from fires that contain synthetic materials, particularly those containing polyurethane. The cyanide, which may be inhaled or absorbed through mucosal surfaces and skin, binds the cytochrome system of enzymes and inhibits cellular production of adenosine triphosphate (ATP). Patients present with neurological impairment and lactic acidosis; they typically have arrhythmias, increased cardiac output, and marked vasodilation.

A chemical burn of the respiratory mucosa follows inhalation of large amounts of carbonaceous material, particularly when combined with toxic fumes. Inflammation of the airways results in bronchorrhea and wheezing. Bronchial edema and sloughing of the mucosa lead to obstruction of the lower airways and atelectasis. Progressive ventilation/perfusion mismatching can lead to marked hypoxemia over the course of 24–48 h. Development of the systemic inflammatory response syndrome can lead to acute lung injury or ARDS.

Treatment

Fiberoptic bronchoscopy usually establishes the diagnosis of an inhalation injury. Bronchoscopy is usually carried out with a tracheal tube loaded over the bronchoscope so that intubation can quickly be performed if edema threatens the patency of the airway. Early elective tracheal intubation is advisable when there are obvious signs of heat injury to the airway. Patients with hoarseness and stridor require immediate intubation; emergency cricothyrotomy or tracheostomy is necessary if oral or nasal intubation is unsuccessful.

The presence of clinically important carbon monoxide or cyanide poisoning, as evidenced by obtundation or coma, also requires prompt tracheal intubation and ventilation with oxygen. The diagnosis of carbon monoxide poisoning requires cooximetry: pulse oximeters cannot reliably differentiate between carboxyhemoglobin and oxyhemoglobin. The half-life of carboxyhemoglobin is reduced to 1 h with 100% oxygen; some clinicians advocate hyperbaric oxygen therapy if the patient does not respond to 100% oxygen. The diagnosis of cyanide poisoning is difficult because reliable measurements of cyanide are not readily available (normal levels are <0.1 mg/L). The enzyme rhodanase normally converts cyanide to thiocyanate, which is subsequently eliminated by the kidneys. Treatment for severe cyanide toxicity consists of administering sodium nitrite, 300 mg intravenously as a 3% solution over 3–5 min, followed by sodium thiosulfate, 12.5 g intravenously in the form of a 25% solution over 1–2 min. Sodium nitrite converts hemoglobin to methemoglobin, which has a higher affinity for cyanide than cytochrome oxidase; the cyanide, which is slowly released from cyanomethemoglobin, is converted by rhodanase to the less toxic thiocyanate.

Marked hypoxemia due to intrapulmonary shunting should be managed with tracheal intubation, oxygen therapy, bronchodilators, positive-pressure ventilation, and PEEP. Corticosteroids are ineffective and increase the rate of infections. As with other forms of acute lung injury, nosocomial infectious pneumonias are common.

Acute Myocardial Infarction

Acute myocardial infarction (AMI) is a serious complication of ischemic heart disease, with an overall mortality rate of 25%. More than one half of these deaths occur shortly after onset, usually due to arrhythmias (ventricular fibrillation). With recent advances in interventional cardiology, the in-hospital mortality rate has been reduced to less than 10–15%. Pump (ventricular) failure is now the leading cause of death after AMI in hospitalized patients.

Most myocardial infarctions occur in patients with more than one severely narrowed (>75% narrowing of the cross-sectional area) coronary artery. A transmural infarction occurs in an area distal to a complete occlusion. Patients who die within 24 hours after AMI may demonstrate only coronary atherosclerosis on necropsy examination of the heart. The occlusion is nearly always due to thrombosis at a stenotic atheromatous plaque. Coronary emboli or severe spasm is less commonly the cause. The size and location of the infarct depend on the distribution of the obstructed vessel and whether collateral vessels have formed. Anterior, apical, and septal infarcts of the left ventricle are usually due to thrombosis in the left anterior descending circulation; lateral and posterior left ventricular infarcts result from occlusions in the left circumflex system, whereas right ventricular and posterior–inferior left ventricular infarcts result from thrombosis in the right coronary artery. In contrast, subendocardial (nontransmural, or "non–Q wave") infarctions more often occurs in the setting of reduced myocardial perfusion due to hypotension or intimal hemorrhage, and less commonly follows coronary plaque rupture and thrombosis.

Following brief episodes of severe ischemia, persisting myocardial dysfunction with only a slow and incomplete return of contractility can be observed. This phenomenon of "stunning" is often thought to occur in areas adjacent to infarcted myocardium and can contribute to ventricular dysfunction following AMI. Relief of the ischemia in these areas can restore contractile function, albeit not immediately. Stunning may be observed following aortic cross-clamping during cardiopulmonary bypass and present as a reduced cardiac output upon attempted separation from bypass (see Chapter 22). When severe hypokinesis or akinesis is observed in the setting of severe chronic ischemia, the myocardium in these noninfarcted but poorly contractile areas may be said to be "hibernating." This diagnosis can be confirmed by observing viable tissue with positron emission tomography, or by showing that the hypocontractile myocardium responds to dobutamine during stress echocardiography.

The immediate treatment of AMI is the administration of oxygen, aspirin (160–325 mg), nitroglycerin (sublingual or spray), morphine (2–4 mg intravenously every 5 min) until the pain is relieved, and in most cases of an ST-segment elevation MI (STEMI) movement of the patient to the cardiac catheterization laboratory. The mnemonic "MONA (*m*orphine, *o*xygen, *n*itroglycerin, and *a*spirin) greets all patients" succinctly states this approach. Because the prognosis following AMI is generally inversely proportionate to the extent of necrosis, the focus in management of an evolving myocardial infarction remains on reperfusion. Based on local resources, timing, and anatomic findings during angiography, angioplasty, stenting, or coronary artery bypass surgery may be preferred. Guidelines for treatment of AMI change on a nearly annual basis and are regularly published by the American College of Cardiology/American Heart Association and by the European Society of Cardiology; we strongly recommend that they be consulted.

Patients with ST-segment depression or dynamic T-wave changes (non–Q wave infarction; unstable angina) benefit from antithrombin (heparin) and antiplatelet (aspirin) therapy. All patients without contraindications (such as acute heart failure) should receive β blockers. Other medications and treatments such as ACE inhibitors, statins, and cessation of smoking are the key to secondary prevention. Patients who have recurrent angina should be given nitrates. If angina persists or if there is a contraindication to β blockers, calcium channel blockers should be administered. Persistent or recurrent angina signals the need for angiography, if it has not already been performed.

Intraaortic balloon counterpulsation is usually reserved for hemodynamically compromised patients with refractory ischemia. Temporary pacing following AMI is indicated for Mobitz type II and complete heart block, a new bifascicular block, and bradycardia with hypotension. Emergency treatment of arrhythmias constantly evolves and we recommend that the guidelines for Advanced Cardiac Life Support be followed. In general, ventricular tachycardia, if treated medically is best managed with amiodarone (150 mg intravenous bolus over 10 min). Synchronized cardioversion may be used in patients with ventricular tachycardia and with a pulse. Patients with a stable narrow-complex supraventricular tachycardia should be treated with amiodarone. Patients with paroxysmal supraventricular tachycardia, whose ejection fraction is preserved, should be treated with a calcium channel blocker, a β blocker, or DC cardioversion. Medically unstable hypotensive patients should receive cardioversion.

Patients with ectopic or multifocal atrial tachycardia should not receive DC cardioversion; instead they should be treated with calcium channel blockers, a β blocker, or amiodarone.

Acute Kidney Injury & Failure

Acute kidney injury (AKI) is a rapid deterioration in renal function that is not immediately reversible by altering factors such as blood pressure, intravascular volume, cardiac output, or urinary flow. The hallmark of AKI is azotemia and frequently oliguria. Azotemia may be classified as prerenal, renal, and postrenal. Moreover, the diagnosis of renal azotemia is one of exclusion; thus, prerenal and postrenal causes must always be excluded. However, not all patients with acute azotemia have kidney failure. Likewise, urine output of more than 500 mL/d does not imply that renal function is normal. Basing the diagnosis of AKI on creatinine levels or an increase in blood urea nitrogen (BUN) is also problematic because creatinine clearance is not always a good measure of glomerular filtration rate. The criteria developed by the Acute Kidney Injury Network are now most often used

to stage AKI (see Chapter 30). AKI is diagnosed by documenting an increase in serum creatinine of more than 50%, or an absolute increase of 0.3 mg/dL, and a reduction in urine output to less than 0.5 mL/kg/h for 6 h or longer, with all findings developing over 48 h or less.

PRERENAL AZOTEMIA

Prerenal azotemia results from hypoperfusion of the kidneys; if untreated, it progresses to AKI. Renal hypoperfusion typically the result of decreased arterial perfusion pressure, markedly increased venous pressure, or renal vasoconstriction (Table 57–7). Decreased perfusion pressure is usually associated with the release of norepinephrine, angiotensin II, and arginine vasopressin (or antidiuretic hormone). These hormones constrict cutaneous muscle and splanchnic vasculature and promote salt and water retention. The synthesis of vasodilating prostaglandins (prostacyclin and PGE_2) and nitric oxide in the kidneys and the intrarenal action of angiotensin II

TABLE 57–7 Potentially reversible causes of azotemia.

Prerenal
Decreased renal perfusion
Hypovolemia
Reduced cardiac output
Hypotension
Abdominal compartment syndrome
Increased renal vascular resistance
Neural
Humoral/Pharmacological
Thromboembolic
Postrenal
Urethral obstruction
Bladder outlet obstruction
Neurogenic bladder
Bilateral ureteral obstruction
Intrinsic
Calculi
Tumor
Blood clots
Papillary necrosis
Extrinsic
Abdominal or pelvic tumor
Retroperitoneal fibrosis
Postsurgical (ligation)

TABLE 57–8 Urinary indices in azotemia.

Index	Prerenal	Renal	Postrenal
Specific gravity	>1.018	<0.012	Variable
Osmolality (mmol/kg)	>500	<350	Variable
Urine/plasma urea nitrogen ratio	>8	<3	Variable
Urine/plasma creatinine ratio	>40	<20	Variable
Urine/sodium (mEq/L)	<10	>40	Variable
Fractional excretion of sodium (%)	<1	>3	Variable
Renal failure index	<1	>1	Variable

help maintain glomerular filtration. Use of cyclo-oxygenase inhibitors (eg, ketorolac for postoperative pain control) or ACE inhibitors in the setting of marked prerenal azotemia can precipitate AKI. The diagnosis of prerenal azotemia is usually suspected from the clinical setting and confirmed by urinary laboratory indices (Table 57–8). Treatment of prerenal azotemia is directed at correcting intravascular volume deficits, improving cardiac function, restoring a normal blood pressure, and reversing increases in renal vascular resistance. The hepatorenal syndrome is discussed in Chapter 33.

POSTRENAL AZOTEMIA

Azotemia due to urinary tract obstruction is termed postrenal azotemia. Obstruction of urinary flow from both kidneys is usually necessary for azotemia and oliguria/anuria in these conditions. Complete obstruction eventually develops into AKI and kidney failure, whereas prolonged partial obstruction leads to chronic renal impairment. Rapid diagnosis and relief of acute obstruction usually restore normal renal function, often accompanied by a diuresis. Obstruction may be diagnosed by a physical examination (the upper margin of the bladder can be percussed) or ultrasound (showing a distended bladder) or suggested by a radiograph of the abdomen (revealing bilateral renal calculi), but is definitively diagnosed by demonstrating dilation of the urinary tract proximal to the site of obstruction on imaging studies. Treatment depends on the site of obstruction. Obstruction at the bladder outlet can be relieved with catheterization of the bladder or suprapubic cystostomy, whereas ureteral obstruction requires nephrostomy or ureteral stents.

REVERSIBLE AZOTEMIA VERSUS AKI

It is important to differentiate prerenal and postrenal azotemia from renal azotemia. Exclusion of postrenal azotemia requires physical diagnosis and imaging, whereas exclusion of prerenal azotemia depends on the response to treatments aimed at improving renal perfusion. Diagnosis and treatment may be facilitated by analysis of urine (see Table 57–8); urinary composition in postrenal azotemia is variable and depends on the duration and severity of obstruction. In prerenal azotemia, tubular concentrating ability is preserved and reflected by a low urinary sodium concentration and high urine/serum creatinine ratio. Calculation of the fractional excretion of filtered sodium (FE_{Na^+}) may also be extremely useful in the setting of oliguria:

$$FE_{Na^+} = \frac{\text{Urine sodium/serum sodium}}{\text{Urine creatinine/serum creatinine}} \times 100\%$$

FE_{Na^+} is less than 1% in oliguric patients with prerenal azotemia but typically exceeds 3% in patients with oliguric AKI. Values of 1–3% may be present in patients with nonoliguric AKI. The renal failure index, which is the urinary sodium concentration divided by the urine/plasma creatinine ratio, is a sensitive index for diagnosing kidney failure. The use of diuretics increases urinary sodium excretion and invalidates indices that rely on urinary sodium concentration as a measure of tubular function. Moreover, intrinsic kidney diseases that primarily affect renal vasculature or glomeruli may not affect tubular function and therefore are associated with indices that are similar to prerenal azotemia. Measurement of a 3-h creatinine clearance can estimate the residual glomerular filtration rate but may underestimate the degree of renal impairment if the serum creatinine concentration is still rising.

Etiology of AKI

Causes of AKI are listed in Table 57–9. Up to 50% of cases follow major trauma or surgery; in the majority of instances, ischemia and nephrotoxins are responsible. AKI associated with ischemia is often termed *acute tubular necrosis*. Postischemic acute tubular necrosis follows certain surgical procedures more frequently than others: open abdominal aortic aneurysm resection, cardiac surgery with cardiopulmonary bypass, and operations to relieve obstructive jaundice. Aminoglycosides, amphotericin B, radiographic contrast dyes, cyclosporine, and cisplatin are the most commonly implicated exogenous nephrotoxins. Amphotericin B, contrast dyes, and cyclosporine also appear to produce direct intrarenal vasoconstriction. Hemoglobin and myoglobin are potent nephrotoxins when they are released during intravascular hemolysis and rhabdomyolysis, respectively. Cyclooxygenase inhibitors, particularly nonsteroidal antiinflammatory drugs, may play an important role in at least some patients. Inhibition of prostaglandin

TABLE 57–9 Causes of acute kidney injury.

Renal ischemia
  Hypotension
  Hypovolemia
  Impaired cardiac output
  Abdominal compartment syndrome

Nephrotoxins
  Endogenous pigments
    Hemoglobulin (hemolysis)
    Myoglobin (rhabdomyolysis from crush injury
      and burns)
  Radiographic contrast agents
  Drugs
    Antibiotics (aminoglycosides, amphotericin)
    Nonsteroidal antiinflammatory drugs
    Chemotherapeutic agents (cisplatin, methotrexate)
  Tubular crystals
    Uric acid
    Oxalate
    Sulfonamides
  Heavy metal poisoning
    Organic solvents
    Myeloma protein

Intrinsic kidney disease
  Glomerular disease
  Interstitial nephritis

synthesis by the latter group of agents decreases prostaglandin-mediated renal vasodilation, allowing unopposed renal vasoconstriction. Other factors predisposing to AKI include preexisting renal impairment, advanced age, atherosclerotic vascular disease, diabetes, and dehydration.

Pathogenesis of AKI

The sensitivity of the kidneys to injury may be explained by their very high metabolic rate and ability to concentrate potentially toxic substances. The pathogenesis of AKI is complex and probably has both a vascular endothelial and a renal epithelial (tubular) basis. Inadequate oxygen deliver to the kidney is the likely triggering event, leading to afferent arteriolar constriction, decreased glomerular permeability, increased vascular permeability, altered coagulation, inflammation, leukocyte activation, direct epithelial cell injury, and tubular obstruction from intraluminal debris or edema. All can decrease glomerular filtration. A backleak of filtered solutes through damaged portions of renal tubules may allow reabsorption of creatinine, urea, and other nitrogenous wastes.

Oliguric versus Nonoliguric AKI

AKI is often classified as oliguric (urinary volume <400 mL/d), anuric (urinary volume <100 mL/d), or nonoliguric (urinary volume >400 mL/d). Nonoliguric AKI accounts for up to 50% of cases. Urinary sodium concentrations in patients with nonoliguric AKI are typically lower than those in oliguric patients. In some studies, nonoliguric patients also appear to have a lower complication rate and to require shorter hospitalizations. In another study of AKI patients who required dialysis, nonoliguric AKI patients had a delayed initiation of dialysis, a longer hospital stay, and an increased likelihood of death. It was speculated that it might be possible to convert oliguric AKI into nonoliguric AKI by administering mannitol, furosemide, "renal" doses of dopamine (1–2 mcg/kg/min), or fenoldopam. Theoretically, the resulting increase in urinary output might be therapeutic by preventing tubular obstruction. However, recent studies have found increased mortality in patients with AKI who received diuretics, and a meta-analysis showed no improvement in mortality or decrease in need for dialysis; therefore diuretics should not be routinely administered in AKI.

Treatment of AKI

AKI accounts for approximately 15% of ICU admissions. Despite advances in critical care medicine, the mortality rate for AKI remains approximately 50% and management is primarily supportive. Diuretics continue to be useful for conventional medical indications (eg, pulmonary edema or rhabdomyolysis). AKI due to glomerulonephritis or vasculitis may respond to glucocorticoids. Standard treatment for oliguric and anuric patients includes restriction of fluid, sodium, potassium, and phosphorus. Daily weight measurements help guide fluid therapy. Sodium and potassium intake is limited to 1 mEq/kg/d. Hyponatremia can be treated with water restriction. Hyperkalemia may require administration of an ion-exchange resin (sodium polystyrene), glucose and insulin, calcium gluconate, or sodium bicarbonate. Sodium bicarbonate therapy may also be necessary for metabolic acidosis when the serum bicarbonate level decreases to less than 15 mEq/L. Hyperphosphatemia requires dietary phosphate restriction and phosphate binders such as sevelamer, aluminum hydroxide, calcium carbonate, calcium acetate. The dosages of renally excreted drugs should be adjusted to the estimated glomerular filtration rate or measured creatinine clearance to prevent accumulation.

Renal replacement therapy may be employed to treat or prevent uremic complications (see Table 30–6). A double-lumen catheter placed in the internal jugular, subclavian, or femoral vein is usually used. The high morbidity and mortality rates associated with AKI would seem to argue for early dialysis, but supporting studies are controversial. Dialysis does not appear to hasten recovery but may in fact aggravate kidney injury if hypotension occurs or too much fluid is removed.

Because of concern that intermittent hemodialysis associated with hypotension may perpetuate renal injury, continuous renal replacement therapy (CRRT; continuous venovenous hemofiltration or continuous venovenous hemodialysis, which removes fluid and solutes at a slow controlled rate) has been used in critically ill patients with uremic AKI who do not tolerate the hemodynamic effects of intermittent "standard" hemodialysis. The main problem associated with CRRT is the expense, as the membrane is prone to clot formation and, therefore, must be periodically replaced. Despite this limitation, many experts believe CRRT is the best way to manage uremic ICU patients with AKI. The indications for CRRT are being expanded from oliguria and uremia to metabolic acidosis, fluid overload, and hyperkalemia. Nevertheless, recent clinical trials have failed to show benefit of continuous technique over intermittent hemodialysis in these critically ill patients.

The nutritional management of AKI with uremia continues to evolve, and there is now consensus among nephrologists, intensivists, and nutritionists that nutrition should be provided, and 1.0–1.5 g/kg/d of protein can be given, particularly for patients on CRRT.

Infections & Sepsis

The systemic inflammatory response to infection, termed *sepsis syndrome* (Figure 57–8), does not necessarily indicate the presence of bacteremia. Moreover, the inflammatory response is not unique to severe infections: similar manifestations may be encountered with noninfectious illnesses.

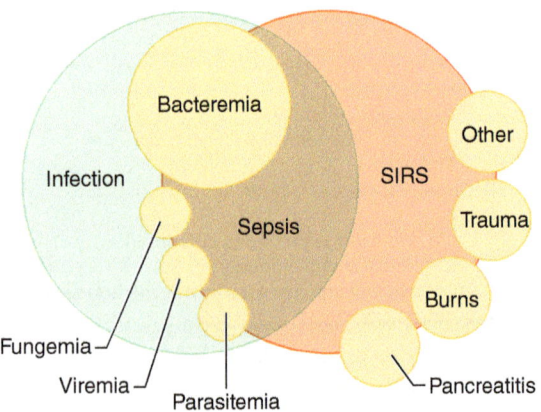

FIGURE 57–8 The relationship among infection, sepsis, and the systemic inflammatory response syndrome (SIRS). (Modified from the American College of Chest Physicians/Society of Critical Care Medicine Consensus Conference: Definitions for sepsis and organ failure and guidelines for the use of innovative therapies in sepsis. Crit Care Med 1992;20:864.)

The use of the term *systemic inflammatory response syndrome* (SIRS) has been suggested by the Society of Critical Care Medicine (SCCM), European Society of Intensive Care Medicine (ESICM), American College of Chest Physicians (ACCP), American Thoracic Society (ATS), and Surgical Infection Society (SIS) (Table 57–10). A combined conference of the preceding long list of societies classified sepsis based on predisposition, insult, infection, response, and organ dysfunction. Severe sepsis exists when these features are associated with organ dysfunction. The term *multiple organ dysfunction syndrome* (MODS) has been suggested to describe dysfunction of two or more organs associated with sepsis. *Septic shock* is defined as acute circulatory failure in a patient with sepsis or, more specifically, systolic blood pressure less than 90 mm Hg that is not responsive to volume resuscitation and requiring vasopressors for life support.

PATHOPHYSIOLOGY OF SIRS

A mild systemic inflammatory response to an injury, infection, or other bodily insult may normally have salutatory effects. However, a marked or prolonged response, such as that associated with severe infections, is often deleterious and can result in widespread organ dysfunction. Although gram-negative organisms account for most cases of infection-related SIRS, many other infectious agents are capable of inducing the same syndrome. These organisms either elaborate toxins or stimulate release of substances that trigger this response. The most commonly recognized initiators are the lipopolysaccharides, which are released by gram-negative bacteria. Lipopolysaccharide is composed of an O polysaccharide, a core, and lipid A. The O polysaccharide distinguishes between different types of gram-negative bacteria, whereas lipid A, an endotoxin, is responsible for the compound's toxicity. The resulting response to endotoxin involves a complex interaction between macrophages/monocytes, neutrophils, lymphocytes, platelets, and endothelial cells that can affect nearly every organ.

The central mechanism in initiating SIRS appears to be the abnormal secretion of cytokines. These low-molecular-weight peptides and

TABLE 57–10 Diagnostic criteria for sepsis.[1–3]

Infection,[4] documented or suspected, and some of the following:
General variables
Fever (core temperature >38.3°C)
Hypothermia (core temperature <36°C)
Heart rate >90/min or >2 SD above the normal value for age
Tachypnea
Altered mental status
Significant edema or positive fluid balance (>20 mL/kg over 24 h)
Hyperglycemia (plasma glucose >120 mg/dL or 7.7 mmol/L) in the absence of diabetes
Inflammatory variables
Leukocytosis (WBC count >12,000/μL)
Leukopenia (WBC count <4000/μL)
Normal WBC count with >10% immature forms
Plasma C-reactive protein >2 SD above the normal value
Plasma procalcitonin >2 SD above the normal value
Hemodynamic variables
Arterial hypotension[5] (SBP <90 mm Hg, MAP <70, or an SBP decrease >40 mm Hg in adults or <2 SD below normal value for age)
$S\bar{v}O_2 > 70\%$[5]
Cardiac index[5] >3.5 L/min per m²
Organ dysfunction variables
Arterial hypoxemia ($PaO_2/FiO_2 < 300$)
Acute oliguria (urine output <0.5 mL/kg/h or 45 mmol/L for at least 2 h)
Creatinine increase > 0.5 mg/dL
Coagulation abnormalities (INR > 1.5 or aPTT > 60 s)
Ileus (absent bowel sounds)
Thrombocytopenia (platelet count < 100,000/μL)
Hyperbilirubinemia (plasma total bilirubin > 4 mg/dL or 70 mmol/L)
Tissue perfusion variables
Hyperlactatemia (>1 mmol/L)
Decreased capillary refill or mottling

[1]Reprinted, with permission, from Levy MM, Fink MP, Marshall JC, et al: 2001 SCCM/ESICM/ACCP/ATS/SIS International Sepsis Definitions Conference. Crit Care Med 2003;31:1250.

[2]WBC, white blood cell; SBP, systolic blood pressure; MAP, mean arterial blood pressure; $S\bar{v}O_2$, mixed venous oxygen saturation; INR, international normalized ratio; aPTT, activated partial thromboplastin time.

[3]Diagnostic criteria for sepsis in the pediatric population are signs and symptoms of inflammation plus infection with hyper- or hypothermia (rectal temperature >38.4°C or <35°C), tachycardia (may be absent in hypothermia patients), and at least one of the following indications of altered organ function: altered mental status, hypoxemia, increased serum lactate level, or bounding pulses.

[4]Infection defined as a pathological process induced by a microorganism.

[5]$S\bar{v}O_2$ >70% (normally, 75–80%) and cardiac index 3.5–5.5 are normal in children; therefore, neither should be used as a sign of sepsis in newborns or children.

glycoproteins function as intercellular mediators regulating such biological processes as local and systemic immune responses, inflammation, wound healing, and hematopoiesis. The most important cytokines released during SIRS are interleukin-6, adrenomedullin, soluble CD_{14}, the adhesion molecule sELAM-1, macrophage inflammatory protein-1α, extracellular phospholipase A_2, and C-reactive protein. The resulting inflammatory response includes release of potentially harmful phospholipids, attraction of neutrophils, and activation of the complement, kinin, and coagulation cascades.

Increased phospholipase A_2 levels release arachidonic acid from cell membrane phospholipids. Cyclooxygenase converts arachidonic acid to thromboxane and prostaglandins, whereas lipoxygenase converts arachidonic acid into leukotrienes (slow-reacting substances of anaphylaxis). Increased phospholipase A_2 and acetyltransferase activities result in the formation of another potent proinflammatory compound, platelet-activating factor. Attraction and activation of neutrophils releases a variety of proteases and free radical compounds that damage vascular endothelium. Activation of monocytes causes them to express increased amounts of tissue factor, which in turn can activate both the intrinsic and extrinsic coagulation cascades.

INFECTIONS IN THE ICU

Infections are a leading cause of death in ICUs. Serious infections may be "community acquired" or subsequent to hospital admission for an unrelated illness. The term *nosocomial infection* describes hospital-acquired infections that develop at least 48 h following admission. The reported incidence of nosocomial infections in ICU patients has ranged between 10% and 50%, but with recent attention to aseptic placement of central venous catheters and earlier removal of bladder catheters the incidence of bloodstream infections has markedly declined. Nearly universal elevation of the head of bed has also led to a marked reduction in ventilator-associated pneumonia.

Strains of bacteria resistant to commonly used antibiotics are often responsible for infections in patients with critical illness. Host immunity plays an important role in determining not only the

course of an infection but also the types of organisms that can cause infection. Thus, organisms that normally do not cause serious infections in immunocompetent patients can produce life-threatening infections in those who are immunocompromised (Table 57–11).

Critically ill patients frequently have abnormal host defenses from advanced age, malnutrition, drug therapy, loss of integrity of mucosal and skin barriers, and underlying diseases. Thus, age greater than 70 years, corticosteroid therapy, chemotherapy of malignancy, prolonged use of invasive devices, respiratory failure, kidney failure, head trauma, and burns are established risk factors for nosocomial infections. Patients with burns involving more than 40% of body surface area have significantly increased risk of mortality from infections. Topical antibiotics delay but do not prevent wound infections. After burns, early removal of the necrotic eschar followed by skin grafting and wound closure appears to reverse immunological defects and reduce infections.

Most nosocomial infections arise from the patient's endogenous bacterial flora. Furthermore, many critically ill patients eventually become colonized with resistant bacterial strains. Infections of the urinary tract account for many nosocomial infections. Urinary infections are usually due to gram-negative organisms and are typically associated with the indwelling catheters or urinary obstruction. Community-acquired and ventilator-associated pneumonias are problems in the ICU. Intravascular catheter-related infections are now relatively rare causes of ICU infections. Surgical site and other wound infections are, however, seen.

Nosocomial pneumonias are usually caused by gram-negative organisms. Gastrointestinal bacterial overgrowth with translocation into the portal circulation and retrograde colonization of the upper airway from the gastrointestinal tract as a result of aspiration are possible mechanisms of entry for these bacteria. Preservation of gastric acidity inhibits overgrowth of gram-negative organisms in the stomach and their subsequent migration into the oropharynx. Tracheal intubation does not provide effective protection because patients commonly aspirate gastric fluid containing bacteria despite a properly

TABLE 57-11   Pathogens commonly associated with serious infections in ICU patients.[1]

Infection or Site	Pathogens	Infection or Site	Pathogens
Pneumonia		**Meningitis**	
Community-acquired (nonimmunocompromised host)	*Streptococcus pneumoniae* *Haemophilus influenzae* *Moraxella catarrhalis* *Mycoplasma pneumoniae* *Legionella pneumophila* *Chlamydia pneumoniae* Methicillin-resistant *Staphylococcus aureus* (MRSA) Influenza virus		*S. pneumoniae* *Neisseria meningitidis* *Listeria monocytogenes* *H. influenzae*
		Neonates	*Escherichia coli* Group B streptococci
Health care–associated	MRSA *Pseudomonas aeruginosa* *Klebsiella pneumoniae* *Acinetobacter* species *Stenotrophomonas* species *L. pneumophila*	Postsurgical or post-trauma	*S. aureus* Enterobacteriaceae *P. aeruginosa*
		Brain abscess	
			Streptococci *Bacteroides* species
		Postsurgical or post-trauma	Enterobacteriaceae *S. aureus*
Immunocompromised host			
Neutropenia	Any pathogen listed above *Aspergillus* species *Candida* species	Immunocompromised or HIV infected	*Nocardia* *Toxoplasma gondii*
		Encephalitis	
Human immunodeficiency virus	Any pathogen listed above *Pneumocystis carinii* *Mycobacterium tuberculosis* *Histoplasma capsulatum* Other fungi Cytomegalovirus		West Nile virus Herpes simplex virus Arbovirus Rabies virus *Bartonella henselae*
		Endocarditis	
Solid organ transplant or bone marrow transplant	Any pathogen listed above (Can vary depending on timing of infection to transplant)		*Streptococcus viridans* *Enterococcus* species *S. aureus* *Streptococcus bovis*
Cystic fibrosis	*H. influenzae* (early) *S. aureus* *P. aeruginosa* *Burkholderia cepacia*	Intravenous drug user, prosthetic valves	MRSA
		Prosthetic valve	*Candida* species
Lung abscess	*Bacteroides* species *Peptostreptococcus* species *Fusobacterium* species *Nocardia* (in immunocompromised patients) Amebic (when suggestive by exposure)	**Catheter-associated bacteremia**	
			Candida species *S. aureus* *Enterococcus* species Enterobacteriaceae *P. aeruginosa*
Empyema		**Pyelonephritis**	
Usually acute	*S. aureus* *S. pneumoniae* Group A streptococci *H. influenzae*		Enterobacteriaceae *E. coli* *Enterococcus* species
		(This group catheter-associated, postsurgical)	*P. aeruginosa* *Acinetobacter* species
Usually subacute or chronic	Anaerobic bacteria Enterobacteriaceae *M. tuberculosis*		

(continued)

TABLE 57-11 Pathogens commonly associated with serious infections in ICU patients.[1] (continued)

Infection or Site	Pathogens	Infection or Site	Pathogens
Peritonitis		**Muscle infection**	
Primary or spontaneous	Enterobacteriaceae S. pneumoniae Enterococcus species Anaerobic bacteria (rare)	Myonecrosis (gas gangrene) Pyomyositis	Clostridium perfringens Other Clostridia species S. aureus
Secondary (bowel perforation)	Enterobacteriaceae Bacteroides species Enterococcus species P. aeruginosa (uncommon)		Group A streptococci Anaerobic bacteria Gram-negative bacteria (rare)
Tertiary (bowel surgery, hospitalized on antibiotics)	P. aeruginosa MRSA Acinetobacter species Candida species	**Septic shock** Community-acquired	S. pneumoniae N. meningitidis H. influenzae Escherichia coli Capnocytophaga (with splenectomy)
Skin structure infections			
Cellulitis	Group A streptococci S. aureus Enterobacteriaceae (diabetics)	Health care–associated	MRSA P. aeruginosa Acinetobacter species Candida species
Decubitus ulcer	Polymicrobial Streptococcus pyogenes Enterococcus species Enterobacteriaceae Anaerobic streptococci P. aeruginosa S. aureus Bacteroides species	Toxic shock syndrome Regional illness or special circumstances	S. aureus Streptococcus species Rickettsial species Ehrlichia species Babesia species B. henselae (immunocompromised hosts)
Necrotizing fasciitis	Streptococcus species Clostridia species Mixed aerobic/anaerobic bacteria		Yersinia pestis Francisella tularensis Leptospira Salmonella enteritidis Salmonella typhi

[1]Reproduced, with permission, from Gabrielli A, Layon AJ, Yu M: *Civetta, Taylor & Kirby's Critical Care,* 4th ed. Lippincott Williams & Wilkins, 2009; Table 104.3, Chapter 104.

functioning cuff; nebulizers and humidifiers can also be sources of infection. Selective decontamination of the gut with nonabsorbable antibiotics may reduce the incidence of infection but does not change outcome. Elevating the head of the bed more than 30° reduces the likelihood of ventilator-associated pneumonia. Enteral nutrition reduces bacterial translocation across the gut and reduces the likelihood of sepsis (see Chapter 53).

Wounds are common sources of sepsis in postoperative and trauma patients; restricting antibiotic prophylaxis to the immediate perioperative time appears to decrease the incidence of postoperative infections in some groups of patients. Although more commonly seen in postoperative patients, intraabdominal infections due to perforated ulcer, diverticulitis, appendicitis, and acalculous cholecystitis can also develop in critically ill nonsurgical patients. Intravascular catheter-related infections are most commonly caused by *Staphylococcus epidermidis, Staphylococcus aureus,* streptococci, *Candida* species, and gram-negative rods. Bacterial sinusitis may be an unrecognized source of sepsis in patients ventilated through nasotracheal tubes. The diagnosis is suspected from purulent drainage and confirmed by imaging and cultures.

SEPTIC SHOCK

The SCCM/ESICM/ACCP/ATS/SIS Consensus Conference defined **septic shock** as sepsis associated with hypotension (systolic blood pressure <90 mm Hg, mean arterial pressure <60 mm Hg, or systemic blood pressure <40 mm Hg from baseline) despite adequate fluid resuscitation. Septic shock is usually characterized by inadequate tissue perfusion and widespread cellular dysfunction. In contrast to other forms of shock (hypovolemic, cardiogenic, neurogenic, or anaphylactic), cellular dysfunction in septic shock is not necessarily related to the hypoperfusion. Instead, metabolic blocks at the cellular and microcirculation levels may contribute to impaired cellular oxidation.

Pathophysiology

An infectious process that induces a severe or protracted SIRS can result in septic shock. In hospitalized patients septic shock most commonly follows gram-negative infections in either the genitourinary tract or the lungs, but identical presentations can be seen with other pathogens. In up to 50% of cases of severe sepsis no organisms can be cultured from blood. Hypotension is due to a decreased circulating intravascular volume resulting from a diffuse capillary leak. Patients may also have myocardial depression. Activation of platelets and the coagulation cascade can lead to the formation of fibrin-platelet aggregates, which further compromise tissue blood flow. Hypoxemia from ARDS accentuates tissue hypoxia. The release of vasoactive substances and formation of microthrombi in the pulmonary circulation increase pulmonary vascular resistance.

Hemodynamic Subsets

The circulation in patients with septic shock is often described as either hyperdynamic or hypodynamic. In reality, both represent the same process, but their expression depends on preexisting cardiac function and intravascular volume and the patient's response. Systemic venodilation and transudation of fluid into tissues result in relative hypovolemia in patients with sepsis. Hyperdynamic septic shock is characterized by normal or elevated cardiac output and profoundly reduced systemic vascular resistance. Decreased myocardial contractility is often demonstrable by echocardiography even in hyperdynamic patients with increased cardiac output. Mixed venous oxygen saturation is characteristically increased in the absence of hypoxemia and likely reflects the increased cardiac output and the cellular metabolic defect in oxygen utilization.

It used to be accepted wisdom that hypodynamic septic shock, characterized by decreased cardiac output with low or normal systemic vascular resistance, was usually seen later in the course of shock. This view is false; hypodynamic shock often occurs early in the course of septic shock. It is more likely to be seen in severely hypovolemic patients and in those with underlying cardiac disease. Myocardial depression is prominent. Mixed venous oxygen saturation is reduced in these patients, and pulmonary hypertension is often prominent. Elevation of pulmonary vascular resistance widens the normal pulmonary artery diastolic-to-wedge pressure gradient; large gradients have been associated with a higher mortality rate. The increase in pulmonary vascular resistance may contribute to right ventricular dysfunction.

Clinical Manifestations

Manifestations of septic shock appear to be primarily related to host response rather than the infective agent. Septic shock classically presents with an abrupt onset of chills, fever, nausea (and often vomiting), decreased mental status, tachypnea, hypotension, and tachycardia. The patient may appear flushed and feel warm (hyperdynamic) or pale with cool and often cyanotic extremities (hypodynamic). In old, debilitated patients and in infants, the diagnosis often is less obvious and hypothermia may be seen.

Leukocytosis with a leftward shift to premature cell forms is typical, but leukopenia can be seen with overwhelming sepsis and is an ominous sign. Progressive metabolic acidosis (usually lactic acidosis) is typically partially compensated by a concomitant respiratory alkalosis. Elevated lactate levels reflect both increased production resulting from poor tissue perfusion and decreased uptake by the liver and kidneys. Hypoxemia may herald the onset of ARDS. Oliguria due to the combination of hypovolemia, hypotension, and a systemic inflammatory insult will often progress to kidney failure. Elevations in serum aminotransferases and bilirubin are due to hepatic dysfunction. Insulin resistance is uniformly present and produces hyperglycemia. Thrombocytopenia is common and is often an early sign of sepsis. Laboratory evidence of disseminated intravascular coagulation (DIC) is often present but is rarely associated with a bleeding diathesis. The latter responds only to control of the sepsis. Stress ulceration of gastric mucosa is common. Respiratory and kidney failure are the leading causes of death in septic patients.

Neutropenic patients (absolute neutrophil count 500/μL) may develop macular or papular lesions that can ulcerate and become gangrenous (ecthyma gangrenosum). These lesions are commonly associated with *Pseudomonas* septicemia but can be caused by other organisms. Perirectal abscesses can develop very quickly in neutropenic patients with few external signs; conscious patients may complain only of perirectal pain.

Treatment

Septic shock is a medical emergency that requires immediate intervention. Treatment is threefold: (1) control and eradication of the infection by appropriate and timely intravenous antibiotics, drainage of abscesses, debridement of necrotic tissues, and removal of infected foreign bodies; (2) maintenance of adequate perfusion with intravenous fluids and inotropic and vasopressor agents; and (3) supportive treatment of complications such as ARDS, kidney failure, gastrointestinal bleeding, and DIC.

Antibiotic treatment usually is initiated before pathogens are identified but only after adequate cultures are obtained (commonly, blood, urine, wounds, and sputum). Pending the results of cultures and tests of antibiotic sensitivity, combination therapy with two or more antibiotics is generally indicated. Typically, the combination of a penicillin/β-lactamase inhibitor or third-generation cephalosporin with an aminoglycoside is used. The choice depends on which organisms are seen with the greatest frequency in one's medical center. Additional diagnostic studies may be indicated (eg, thoracentesis, paracentesis, lumbar puncture, or imaging), depending on the history and physical examination.

Empiric antibiotic therapy in immunocompromised patients should be based on pathogens that are generally associated with the immune defect (see Table 57–11). Vancomycin is added if intravascular catheter-related infection is suspected. Clindamycin or metronidazole may be given to neutropenic patients if a rectal abscess is suspected. Many clinicians initiate therapy for a presumed fungal infection when an immunocompromised patient continues to experience fever despite antibiotic therapy. Granulocyte colony-stimulating factor or granulocyte–macrophage colony-stimulating factor may be used to shorten the period of neutropenia; granulocyte transfusion may occasionally be used in refractory gram-negative bacteremia. Diffuse interstitial infiltrates on a chest radiograph may suggest unusual bacterial, parasitic, or viral pathogens; many clinicians initiate empiric therapy with trimethoprim-sulfamethoxazole and erythromycin in such instances. Nodular infiltrates on a radiograph suggest a fungal pneumonia and may warrant antifungal therapy. Antiviral therapy should be considered in septic patients who are more than 1 month post–bone marrow or solid organ transplantation.

In general, therapy should follow the most recent SCCM/ESICM "surviving sepsis" guidelines. The presence of inadequate perfusion is determined by measurement of blood lactate. "Goal-directed" hemodynamic support is also recommended by many groups. Tissue oxygenation and perfusion are supported with oxygen, intravenous fluids, inotropes, and vasopressors. Central venous pressure is maintained at greater than 8 mm Hg and central venous oxygen saturation is maintained at greater than 70%. Packed red blood cell transfusions are given to keep hemoglobin levels greater than 8 g/dL, especially when central venous pressure and central venous oxygen saturation are below targets. Marked "third-spacing" has long been regarded as characteristic of septic shock, but currently there is debate regarding the existence of the third space and the administration of large volumes of intravenous fluid as to which is cause and which is effect. Colloid solutions more rapidly restore intravascular volume compared with crystalloid solutions but otherwise offer no proven additional benefit. **Vasopressor therapy is generally initiated if hypotension**

(mean arterial pressure <65 mm Hg) or elevated blood lactate levels persist following administration of intravenous fluids. Suggested choices are norepinephrine or dopamine; other positive inotropic drugs (eg, dobutamine) are indicated only when the $S\overline{v}O_2$ falls below 70% despite fluids and vasopressor therapy. Patients with persisting elevations of lactate or persisting low central venous oxygen saturations, despite treatment, should receive a week-long course of steroids (200–300 mg/d of hydrocortisone or the equivalent in divided doses or by infusion). Blood glucose should be controlled with a target value of less than 180 mg/dL. In patients with hypotension that is refractory to norepinephrine plus dopamine or dobutamine, vasopressin may be administered to improve blood pressure. Severe acidosis may decrease the efficacy of inotropes and should therefore generally be corrected (pH > 7.20) with bicarbonate or THAM infusion in patients with refractory hypotension and lactic acidosis. "Renal" doses of dopamine or fenoldopam may increase urinary output but have not been shown to improve or protect kidney function or patient outcomes. Clinical trials of naloxone, opsonins (fibronectin), inhibitors of the coagulation cascade (drotrecogin alfa), and monoclonal antibodies directed against lipopolysaccharide in septic shock have been disappointing.

Gastrointestinal Hemorrhage

Acute gastrointestinal hemorrhage is a common reason for admission to the ICU. Older age (>60 years), comorbid illnesses, hypotension, marked blood loss (>5 units), and recurrent hemorrhage (rebleeding) after 72 h are associated with increased mortality. Management consists of stabilizing the patient with rapid identification of the site of bleeding. Although volume resuscitation is similar, the clinician must attempt to differentiate between upper and lower gastrointestinal bleeding. A history of hematemesis indicates bleeding proximal to the ligament of Treitz. Melena often indicates bleeding proximal to the cecum. Hematochezia (bright red blood from the rectum) indicates either very brisk upper gastrointestinal bleeding (likely to be associated with hypotension) or more commonly lower gastrointestinal bleeding. The presence of maroon stools usually localizes the bleeding to the area between the distal small bowel and the right colon.

Two large-bore intravenous cannulas should be placed, and blood should be sent for laboratory analysis (including hemoglobin, platelet count, prothrombin time, and activated partial thromboplastin time). The patient should also be cross-matched for at least 4 units of red cells. Fluid resuscitation guidelines are discussed in Chapter 51. Serial hemoglobin or hematocrit measurements are useful but may not accurately reflect true blood loss. Intraarterial blood pressure monitoring can be helpful. Central venous cannulation is useful for both venous access and pressure measurements. Placement of a nasogastric tube may help identify an upper gastrointestinal source if bright red blood or "coffee grounds"–appearing material can be aspirated; inability to aspirate blood, however, does not rule out an upper gastrointestinal source.

Upper Gastrointestinal Bleeding

Lavage through a nasogastric tube can help assess the rate of bleeding and facilitate esophagogastroduodenoscopy (EGD). EGD should be performed whenever possible to diagnose the cause of bleeding. Arteriography should be performed if the site of bleeding cannot be visualized with endoscopy. Both EGD and arteriography can also be used therapeutically to stop the bleeding. In unselected patients the more common causes of upper gastrointestinal bleeding, in decreasing order of likelihood, are duodenal ulcer, gastric ulcer, erosive gastritis, and esophageal varices. Erosive gastritis may be due to stress, alcohol, aspirin, nonsteroidal antiinflammatory drugs, and corticosteroids. Less common causes of upper gastrointestinal bleeding include angiodysplasia, erosive esophagitis, Mallory–Weiss tear, gastric tumor, and aortoenteric fistula.

Bleeding from peptic ulcers (gastric or duodenal) can be coagulated via EGD. Surgery is generally indicated for severe hemorrhage (>5 units) and recurrent bleeding. H_2-receptor blockers and proton pump inhibitors are ineffective in stopping hemorrhage but may reduce the likelihood of rebleeding. Selective arteriography of the bleeding vessel allows localized infusion of vasopressin (0.15–0.20 units/min) or embolization.

Erosive gastritis is better prevented than treated. Proton pump inhibitors, H_2-receptor blockers, antacids, and sucralfate are all effective for prevention. In the past some have advocated that all patients with critical illness receive a proton pump inhibitor. However, overuse of proton pump inhibitors is associated with an increased incidence of hospital-acquired pneumonia. Data show that patients who require mechanical ventilation for more than 48 h or who are coagulopathic derive the greatest benefit from prophylaxis. Other groups of patients showing relative benefit from prophylaxis include those with AKI, sepsis, liver failure, hypotension, traumatic brain injury, a history of prior gastrointestinal hemorrhage, recent major surgery, or those receiving large-dose corticosteroid therapy. Once bleeding has begun, there is generally no specific therapy other than embolization or coagulation.

Endoscopic therapy, either with bipolar electrocoagulation or heater probes, is the most effective nonsurgical treatment that reduces blood transfusions, rebleeding, hospital stay, and the need for urgent surgery. Sedation or anesthesia to facilitate these procedures is associated with an increased risk of aspiration. Intravenous vasopressin infusions (0.3–0.8 units/min) are not as effective; concomitant infusion of nitroglycerin with vasopressin can help reduce portal pressure and may reduce the incidence of cardiac complications. Intravenous propranolol can also lower portal venous pressure and may reduce variceal bleeding. Balloon tamponade (Sengstaken–Blakemore, Minnesota, or Linton tubes) may be used as adjunctive therapy but usually requires concurrent tracheal intubation to protect the airway against aspiration.

Lower Gastrointestinal Bleeding

Common causes of lower gastrointestinal bleeding include diverticulosis, angiodysplasia, neoplasms, inflammatory bowel disease, ischemic colitis, infectious colitis, and anorectal disease (hemorrhoids, fissure, or fistula). Rectal examination, anoscopy, and sigmoidoscopy can usually diagnose the more distal lesions. As with EGD, colonoscopy usually allows definitive diagnosis and is often useful therapeutically.

Radionuclide techniques can be used to identify the source of bleeding when colonoscopy cannot be carried out because of inadequate preparation.

Cauterization of the site of bleeding is often possible via colonoscopy. When colonoscopy is unavailable or not possible because of brisk bleeding, selective arteriography can be used to identify the source, which is either embolized or infused with vasopressin. Surgical treatment is reserved for severe or recurrent hemorrhage.

Head Trauma

The diagnosis and management of traumatic brain injury is described in Chapter 39.

End-of-Life Care

In the United States, death is a taboo subject for many, and most people avoid preparing for it until late in their own lives, and some not even then. Many attend to last wills and testaments, estate planning, and taxes, but less than 15% of the adult population is prepared to make advance decisions about restrictions on life-supporting measures. Yet surveys consistently show a strong preference for a dignified, comfortable, and peaceful death at home and a strong wish to avoid dying in a hospital, particularly in an ICU.

The quandary about what to do is particularly vexing when it concerns a surgical patient who sought relief from symptoms, improved functionality, and a better quality of life, but who ends up with a bad outcome requiring ongoing life-supporting measures with little prospect of achieving the goals of the operation.

A substantial number of physicians cannot discuss such difficult situations in a humane, non-adversarial manner or deal with the anger, despair, and other emotions of family members and friends whose expectations have not been met. Good communication skills are the essential foundation. Communications with the family, friends, and all caregivers must be timely, consistent (having only one physician serve as the spokesman has great advantages), accurate, clear to laypersons, advisory without being dictatorial, focused on what is best for the patient, and aligned with the patient's wishes. A gradual stepwise approach over time allows family members and friends time to digest the information; get beyond their normal, initial reactions to the bad news; and make the difficult decision to withdraw intensive support.

Finally, it is important to recognize two ethical principles that are relevant here. The first is the principle of double effect. All medical interventions have potential benefits as well as burdens and risks. If the doses of morphine or sedative drug required to relieve pain and agitation result in unintended side effects, we accept them, even if the result is death. *This is not euthanasia.* The second principle is that withdrawal of medical therapies and interventions is no different from withholding them: both may be done to respect the patient's autonomy. There is a broad religious consensus that heroic measures are not mandated to support a heartbeat at the end of life.

CASE DISCUSSION

An Obtunded Young Woman

A 23-year-old woman is admitted to the hospital obtunded with slow respirations (7 breaths/min). Blood pressure is 90/60 mm Hg and the pulse is 90 beats/min. She was found at home in bed with empty bottles of diazepam, acetaminophen with codeine, and fluoxetine lying next to her.

How is the diagnosis of a drug overdose made?

The presumptive diagnosis of a drug overdose usually must be made from the history, circumstantial evidence, and any witnesses. Signs and symptoms may not be helpful. Confirmation of a suspected drug overdose or poison ingestion usually requires delayed laboratory testing for the suspected agent in body fluids. Intentional overdoses (self-poisoning) are the most common mechanism and typically occur in young adults who are depressed. Ingestion of multiple drugs is common. Benzodiazepines, antidepressants, aspirin, acetaminophen, and alcohol are the most commonly ingested agents.

Accidental overdoses frequently occur in intravenous drug abusers and children. Commonly abused substances include opioids, stimulants (cocaine and methamphetamine), and hallucinogens (phencyclidine [PCP]). Younger children occasionally accidentally ingest caustic household alkali (eg, drain cleaner), acids, and hydrocarbons (eg, petroleum products), in addition to unsecured medications of all types. Organophosphate poisoning (parathion and malathion) usually occurs in adults following agricultural exposure. Overdoses and poisoning less commonly occur as an attempted homicide.

What are appropriate steps in managing this patient?

Regardless of the type of drug or poison ingested, the principles of initial supportive care are the same. Airway patency with adequate ventilation and oxygenation must be obtained. Unless otherwise contraindicated, oxygen therapy (100%) should be administered. Hypoventilation and obtunded airway reflexes require tracheal intubation and mechanical ventilation. Many clinicians routinely administer naloxone (up to 2 mg), dextrose 50% (50 mL), and thiamine (100 mg) intravenously to all obtunded or comatose patients until a diagnosis is established; this may help exclude or treat opioid overdose, hypoglycemia, and Wernicke–Korsakoff syndrome, respectively. The dextrose can be omitted if a glucose determination can be obtained by a fingerstick. In this case, intubation should be performed prior to naloxone because the respiratory depression is likely due to both the codeine and the diazepam.

Blood, urine, and gastric fluid specimens should be obtained and sent for drug screening. Blood is also sent for routine hematological and chemistry studies (including liver function). Urine is usually obtained by bladder catheterization, and gastric fluid can be aspirated from a nasogastric tube; the latter should be placed after intubation to avoid pulmonary aspiration. Alternatively, emesis material may be tested for drugs in conscious persons.

Hypotension should generally be treated with intravenous fluids unless the patient is obviously in pulmonary edema; an inotrope or vasopressor may be necessary in some instances. Seizure activity may be the result of hypoxia or a pharmacological action of a drug (tricyclic antidepressants) or poison. Seizure activity is unlikely in this patient because she ingested diazepam, a potent anticonvulsant.

Should flumazenil be administered?

Flumazenil should generally not be administered to patients who overdose on both a benzodiazepine and an antidepressant and those who have a history of seizures. Reversal of the benzodiazepine's anticonvulsant action can precipitate seizure activity in such instances. Moreover, as is the case with naloxone and opioids, the half-life of flumazenil is shorter than that of benzodiazepines. Thus, it is often preferable to ventilate the patient until the benzodiazepine effect dissipates, the patient regains consciousness, and the respiratory depression resolves.

Should any other antidotes be given?

Because the patient also ingested an unknown quantity of acetaminophen (paracetamol) administration of N-acetylcysteine (NAC; Mucomyst) should be considered. Acetaminophen toxicity is due to depletion of hepatic glutathione, resulting in the accumulation of toxic metabolic intermediates. Hepatic toxicity is usually associated with ingestion of more than 140 mg/kg of acetaminophen. NAC prevents hepatic damage by acting as a sulfhydryl donor and restoring hepatic glutathione levels. If the patient is suspected of having ingested a toxic dose of acetaminophen, an initial dosage of NAC (140 mg/kg orally or by nasogastric tube) should be administered even before plasma acetaminophen levels are obtained; additional doses are given according to the measured plasma level. If the patient cannot tolerate oral or gastric administration of NAC, if the patient is pregnant, or if the risk of hepatotoxicity is high, NAC should be given intravenously.

What measures might limit drug toxicity?

Toxicity might be reduced by decreasing drug absorption or enhancing elimination. Gastrointestinal absorption of an ingested substance can be reduced by emptying stomach contents and administering activated charcoal. Both methods can be effective up to 12 h following ingestion. If the patient is intubated, the stomach is lavaged carefully to avoid pulmonary aspiration. Emesis may be induced in conscious patients with syrup of ipecac 30 mL (15 mL in a child). Gastric lavage and induced emesis are generally contraindicated for patients who ingest caustic substances or hydrocarbons because of a high risk of aspiration and worsening mucosal injury.

Activated charcoal 1–2 g/kg is administered orally or by nasogastric tube with a diluent. The charcoal irreversibly binds most drugs and poisons in the gut, allowing them to be eliminated in stools. In fact, charcoal can create a negative diffusion gradient between the gut and the circulation, allowing the drug or poison to be effectively removed from the body.

Alkalinization of the serum with sodium bicarbonate for tricyclic antidepressant overdose is beneficial because, by increasing pH, protein binding is enhanced; if seizures occur the alkalinization prevents acidosis-induced cardiotoxicity.

What other methods can enhance drug elimination?

The easiest method of increasing drug elimination is forced diuresis. Unfortunately, this method is of limited use for drugs that are highly protein bound or have large volumes of distribution. Mannitol or furosemide with saline may be used. Concomitant administration of alkali (sodium bicarbonate) enhances the elimination of weakly acidic drugs such as salicylates and barbiturates; alkalization of the urine traps the ionized form of these drugs in the renal tubules and enhances urinary elimination. Hemodialysis is usually reserved for patients with severe toxicity who continue to deteriorate despite aggressive supportive therapy.

SUGGESTED READING

Aslakson R, Pronovost PJ: Health care quality in end-of-life care: Promoting palliative care in the intensive care unit. Anesthesiol Clin 2011;29:111.

Chuasuwan A, Kellum JA: Acute kidney injury and its management. Contrib Nephrol 2011;171:218.

Field JM, Hazinski MF, Sayre MR, et al: Part 1: Executive summary: 2010 American Heart Association Guidelines for Cardiopulmonary Resuscitation and Emergency Cardiovascular Care. Circulation 2010;122:S640.

Gabrielli A, Layon AJ, Yu M (Eds): *Civetta, Taylor & Kirby's Critical Care,* 4th ed. Lippincott Williams & Wilkins, 2009.

Legrand M, Paven D: Understanding urine output in critically ill patients. Ann Intensive Care 2011;1:13.

Levy MM, Dellinger, RP, Townsend SR, et al: The Surviving Sepsis Campaign: Results of an international guideline-based performance improvement program targeting severe sepsis. Intensive Care Med 2010;36:222.

Levy MM, Fink MP, Marshall JC, et al: 2001 SCCM/ ESICM/ACCP/ATS/SIS International Sepsis Definitions Conference. Crit Care Med 2003; 31:1250.

Lilly CM, Zuckerman IH, Badawi O, Riker RR: Benchmark data from more than 240,000 adults that reflect the current practice of critical care in the United States. Chest 2011;140:1232-1242.

Patroniti N, Isgrò S, Zanella A: Clinical management of severely hypoxemic patients. Curr Opin Crit Care 2011;17:50.

Peñuelas O, Frutos-Vivar F, Fernández C, et al: Characteristics and outcomes of ventilated patients according to time to liberation from mechanical ventilation. Am J Respir Crit Care Med 2011;184:430.

Tang BM, Craig JC, Eslick GD, et al: Use of corticosteroids in acute lung injury and acute respiratory distress syndrome: A systematic review and meta-analysis. Crit Care Med 2009;37:1594.

Van Norman GA, Jackson S, Rosenbaum SH, Palmer SK: *Clinical Ethics in Anesthesiology: A Case-Based Textbook.* Cambridge Medicine, 2011.

Vincent J-L, Abraham E, Kochanek P, et al (Eds): *Textbook of Critical Care,* 6th ed. Elsevier Saunders, 2011.

WEB SITES

Acute Kidney Injury Network. Available at: http://www. akinet.org/ (Accessed August 9, 2012).

Surviving Sepsis campaign. Available at: http://www. survivingsepsis.org/ (Accessed August 9, 2012).

Safety, Quality, & Performance Improvement

1 In the 1980s, anesthesiologists were recognized for being the first medical specialty to adopt *mandatory* safety-related clinical practice guidelines. Adoption of these guidelines, describing standards for basic monitoring during general anesthesia, was associated with a reduction in the number of patients suffering brain damage or death secondary to ventilation mishaps during general anesthesia.

2 In 1999 the Institute of Medicine of the (U.S.) National Academy of Sciences summarized available safety information in its report, *To Err is Human: Building a Safer Healthcare System*,

which highlighted many opportunities for improved quality and safety.

3 It has long been recognized that quality and safety are closely related to consistency and reduction in practice variation.

4 There is a natural tendency to assume that errors can be prevented by better education or better management of individual workers (ie, to look at errors as individual failures made by individual workers rather than as failures of a system or a process). To reduce errors one changes the system or process to reduce unwanted variation so that random errors are less likely.

PATIENT SAFETY ISSUES

As a profession, anesthesiology has spearheaded efforts to improve patient safety. Some of the first studies to evaluate safety of care focused on provision and sequelae of anesthesia. When spinal anesthesia was virtually abandoned in the United Kingdom (after two patients developed paraplegia following administration of spinal anesthetics), Drs Robert Dripps and Leroy Vandam helped prevent this technique from being abandoned in North America by carefully reporting outcomes of 10,098 patients who received spinal anesthesia. They determined that only one patient (who proved to have a previously undiagnosed spinal meningioma) developed severe, long-term neurological sequelae.

After halothane was introduced into clinical practice in 1954, concerns arose about whether it might be associated with an increased risk of hepatic injury. The National Halothane Study, perhaps the first clinical outcomes study to be performed (long before the term *outcomes research* gained widespread use), demonstrated the remarkable safety of the then relatively new agent compared with the alternatives. It failed, however, to settle the question of whether "halothane hepatitis" actually existed.

1 In the 1980s, anesthesiologists were recognized for being the first medical specialists to adopt *mandatory* safety-related clinical practice guidelines. Adoption of these guidelines was not without controversy, given that for the first time the American Society of Anesthesiologists (ASA) was "dictating" how physicians could practice. The effort resulted in standards for basic monitoring during general anesthesia that included detection of carbon dioxide in exhaled gas. Adoption of these standards was associated with a reduction in the number of patients suffering brain damage or death secondary to ventilation mishaps during general anesthesia. A fortunate associated result was that the cost of medical liability insurance coverage also declined.

In 1984, Ellison Pierce, president of the ASA, created its Patient Safety and Risk Management Committee. The Anesthesia Patient Safety Foundation (APSF), which celebrated its 25th anniversary in 2011, was also Dr Pierce's creation. The APSF continues to spearhead efforts to make anesthesia and perioperative care safer for patients and practitioners. Similarly, through its guidelines, statements, advisories, and practice parameters, the ASA continues to promote safety and provide guidance to clinicians. As Dr Pierce noted, "Patient safety is not a fad. It is not a preoccupation of the past. It is not an objective that has been fulfilled or a reflection of a problem that has been solved. Patient safety is an ongoing necessity. It must be sustained by research, training, and daily application in the workplace."

Meanwhile, other specialties of medicine began to place greater emphasis on quality and safety. In 1999 the Institute of Medicine (IOM) of the (U.S.) National Academy of Sciences summarized available safety information in a report entitled *To Err is Human: Building a Safer Healthcare System*. That document highlighted many opportunities for improved quality and safety in the American health care system. A subsequent IOM report, *Crossing the Quality Chasm: A New Health System for the 21st Century*, explored the way that variation in medical practice reduced quality and safety of health care system. More recently, the Institute for Healthcare Improvement has been "motivating and building the will for change; identifying and testing new models of care in partnership with both patients and health care professionals; and ensuring the broadest possible adoption of best practices and effective innovations," as described on its web site.

QUALITY OF CARE & PERFORMANCE IMPROVEMENT ISSUES

It has long been recognized that quality and safety are closely related to consistency and reduction in practice variation. The quality and safety movement(s) in medicine have their origins in the work of Walter Shewhart and his associate W. Edwards Deming, who popularized the use of statistics and control charts in evaluating the reliability of a process. In manufacturing (where these ideas were initially applied), reducing an error rate reduces the frequency of defective products and increases the customer's satisfaction with the product and the manufacturer. In medicine, reducing the error rate (for everything from accurate timing and delivery of prophylactic antibiotics to ensuring "correct side and site" surgery and regional anesthetic blocks) increases quality and reduces preventable injuries to patients, while also eliminating the additional costs resulting from those errors.

Strategies to Reduce Performance Errors

Both in manufacturing and in medicine, there is a natural tendency to assume that errors can be prevented by better education, better performance, or better management of *individual workers*. In other words, there is a tendency to look at errors as individual failures made by individual workers, rather than as failures of a system or a process. Using the latter point of view (as advocated by Deming), to reduce errors one changes the system or process to reduce unwanted variation so that random errors will be less likely. An outstanding example of this is the universal protocol followed by health care institutions prior to invasive procedures. Adherence to this protocol ensures that the correct procedure is performed on the correct part of the correct patient by the correct physician, that the patient has given informed consent, that all needed equipment and images are available, and that (if needed) the correct prophylactic antibiotic was given at the correct time.

A related example of a simple approach to improve safety and quality of a procedure is the use of a standardized checklist, as described in the popular press by Dr. Atul Gawande. The importance of checklist use is addressed elsewhere in this text, for example, in Chapter 2 in the context of developing a culture of safety in the operating room. Such checklists provide the "script" for the preprocedure universal protocol (Figure 58–1). Studies have shown that the incidence of catheter-related bloodstream infections can be reduced when central venous catheters are inserted after adequate cleansing and disinfection of the operator's hands by an operator wearing a surgical hat and mask, sterile gown, and gloves; using chorhexidine (rather than povidone iodide) skin preparation of the insertion site; and with sterile drapes of adequate size to maintain a sterile field. Studies have also shown that use of all elements in this central line "bundle" is much more likely when a checklist is required prior to every central line insertion; a sample checklist is shown in Figure 58–2.

Benefits of Standardized Checklists

Checklists emphasize two important principles about improving quality and safety in the surgical environment. First, using a checklist requires that a physician *communicate* with other members of the team. Good communication among team members improves quality and prevents errors. It is easy to find examples of good communication strategies. By clearly and forcefully announcing that protamine infusion has been started (after extracorporeal perfusion has been discontinued during a cardiac operation), the anesthesiologist helps prevent the surgeon and perfusionist from making a critical error, such as resuming extracorporeal perfusion without administering additional heparin. By accurately describing the intended surgical procedure (at the time the patient is "posted" on the surgical schedule), the surgeon helps prevent the operating room nurses from making the critical error of not having the necessary instrumentation for the procedure, and helps prevent the anesthesiologist from performing the wrong regional anesthetic procedure. We have selected these examples of good communication because we are aware of adverse patient outcomes that resulted from failure to transfer these specific points of information.

Second, using a checklist underscores the importance of ensuring that every member of the surgical team has a stake in patient safety and good surgical outcomes. The team member who records the checklist "results" is usually not a physician but has the implicit authority to enforce adherence to the checklist. On poorly functioning teams in which there is excessive deference to authority figures, team members may feel that their opinions are not wanted or valued, or may be afraid to bring up safety concerns for fear of retaliation. On well-functioning teams, there is a "flattening" of the hierarchy such that every team member has the authority and every team member feels an obligation to halt the proceedings to prevent potential patient harm.

Quality Assurance Measures

In surgery there are well-recognized indicators of quality, such as having a very low incidence of surgical site infections and of perioperative mortality. However, at present there is no consensus as to the important measurements that can be used to assess quality of anesthesia care. Nevertheless, surrogate anesthesia indicators have been monitored by a variety of well-meaning agencies. Examples include selection and timing of preoperative antibiotics and temperature of patients in the postanesthesia care unit after colorectal surgery. Mindful of the importance of having accurate and relevant outcome measures, the ASA established the Anesthesia Quality Institute in 2009 and charged it with developing and collecting valid quality indicators for anesthetic care that can be used for quality improvement programs. Aggregation of the large amounts of data required for statistical validity is dependent on widespread adoption of electronic medical records (EMR) and anesthesia information management systems (AIMS) (discussed in Chapter 18). Currently these systems are present in a minority of hospitals in the United States. It is our hope that as their use becomes more widespread, the data and indicators that are collected and aggregated will provide greater insight into how quality of anesthesia care may influence clinical outcomes that are important to patients.

Name	Pre-Procedure and Time Out
MRN	**Documentation**
Patient Identification	

Procedure 1: _____

Pre-Procedure Verification	Circle	One	
➤ Patient's identity confirmed using two identifiers	Yes	No	
➤ Procedure confirmed and consistent with documents, e.g. H&P, progress notes	Yes	No	
➤ Procedure site & side verified	Yes	No	NA
➤ Relevant images reviewed/available	Yes	No	NA
➤ Procedure site marked (required for procedures involving laterality, lesions, levels, digits)	Yes	No	NA
➤ Risk/benefits discussed and/or consent form completed	Yes	No	NA

Time Out Verification (Performed immediately prior to the procedure)	Circle	One	
➤ Patient's identity confirmed using two identifiers	Yes	No	
➤ Procedure site and side verified	Yes	No	NA
➤ Correct procedure confirmed	Yes	No	
➤ Correct patient position confirmed	Yes	No	NA
➤ Availability of Implants/special equipment confirmed	Yes	No	NA

Signature & Printed Name or ID of Provider **Performing Procedure**   Date   Time

Signature, Title & Printed Name of Person **Completing Form**   Date   Time

Procedure 2: _____
(to be used for second block or any time patient position is changed (i.e., supine to prone)

Pre-Procedure Verification	Circle	One	
➤ Patient's identity confirmed using two identifiers	Yes	No	
➤ Procedure confirmed and consistent with documents, e.g. H&P, progress notes	Yes	No	
➤ Procedure site & side verified	Yes	No	NA
➤ Relevant images reviewed/available	Yes	No	NA
➤ Procedure site marked (required for procedures involving laterality, lesions, levels, digits)	Yes	No	NA
➤ Risk/benefits discussed and/or consent form completed	Yes	No	NA

Time Out Verification (Performed immediately prior to the procedure)	Circle	One	
➤ Patient's identity confirmed using two identifiers	Yes	No	
➤ Procedure site and side verified	Yes	No	NA
➤ Correct procedure confirmed	Yes	No	
➤ Correct patient position confirmed	Yes	No	NA
➤ Availability of Implants/special equipment confirmed	Yes	No	NA

Signature & Printed Name or ID of Provider **Performing Procedure**   Date   Time

Signature, Title & Printed Name of Person **Completing Form**   Date   Time

Comments: _____

FIGURE 58–1 The "time out" checklist used at the Virginia Commonwealth University Health System before all regional anesthesia procedures. There is space for two separate time outs. An additional time out is performed whenever a patient's position is changed for a second regional block (most commonly for lower extremity surgery). For convenience, the regional anesthesia time out checklist is printed on the reverse of the Consent for Anesthesia acknowledgment form. (Reproduced with permission from Virginia Commonwealth University Health System Authority.)

PATIENT NAME

MRN
(or PATIENT LABEL)

QUALITY DOCUMENT. NOT PART OF THE PERMANENT MEDICAL RECORD.
Return to designated area on your unit.

Intravascular Access Catheter Insertion Checklist

Purpose: To work as a team to decrease patient harm from catheter-related blood stream infections
When: During all central venous catheter insertion or re-wirings
Who: Assistant to complete this form during catheter insertion

1. Date: ______________ Time: ______________ a.m. p.m.

2. Procedure Site: ______________________ ☐ New ☐ Re-wiring

3. Procedure is: ☐ Elective ☐ Emergent

4. Before procedure, did person(s) performing procedure:

➢ Wash hands immediately prior?	☐ Yes	☐ No
➢ Sterilize procedure site (chlorhexidine)?	☐ Yes	☐ No
➢ Drape entire patient in sterile fashion?	☐ Yes	☐ No

5. During procedure, did personnel performing procedure:

➢ Wear sterile gloves?	☐ Yes	☐ No
➢ Wear hat and mask?	☐ Yes	☐ No
➢ Wear sterile gown?	☐ Yes	☐ No
➢ Maintain a sterile field?	☐ Yes	☐ No

6. Did **all** personnel assisting with procedure follow the policy? ☐ Yes ☐ No

7. Procedure stopped at any time due to break in sterile field? ☐ Yes ☐ No

If yes, Corrective Actions Taken:
☐ Person performing procedure applied appropriate barrier, re-prepped and draped the pateint ☐ New checklist initiated
☐ Complete new set up: staff barriers, prep, drape new line ☐ New checklist initiated

☐ Attending/designee paged; problem corrected
☐ Attending/designee paged; problem not corrected

8. After procedure, were:

➢ Sterile dressings applied to the site?	☐ Yes	☐ No
➢ New IV bag & tubing set up?	☐ Yes	☐ No
➢ New stopcocks and access devices used?	☐ Yes	☐ No
➢ All ports closed with sterile dead enders?	☐ Yes	☐ No

9. Comments– Please note any additional corrective actions taken: ______________________________

____

____

STOP The assistant should **STOP** any procedure that does not meet this standard of care. The procedure should not continue until everyone is in compliance. The assistant will contact unit or division leadership immediately for anyone refusing to comply with this policy.

____
Name of Person Performing Procedure (& ID #)
PRINT NAME

____
Assistant Completing Checklist
PRINT NAME

FIGURE 58–2 Mandatory checklist for insertion of central venous catheters in patients who are not currently undergoing anesthesia and surgery at the Virginia Commonwealth University Health System. A similar electronic document is contained within the Anesthesia Information Management electronic record for central venous lines. (Reproduced with permission from Virginia Commonwealth University Health System Authority.)

SUGGESTED READING

Berwick DM: Controlling variation in health care: A consultation from Walter Shewhart. Medical Care 1991;29:1212-1225.

Deming WE: *Out of the Crisis.* MIT Press, 1986.

Dripps RD, Vandam LD: Long-term follow-up of patients who received 10,098 spinal anesthetics: Failure to discover major neurological sequelae. J Am Med Assoc 1954;156:1486.

Gawande A: *The Checklist Manifesto: How to Get Things Right.* Metropolitan Books/Henry Holt, 2009.

Institute of Medicine: *Crossing the Quality Chasm: A New Health System for the 21st Century.* National Academy Press, 2001. Available at http://www.nap.edu/

Institute of Medicine: *To Err Is Human: Building a Safer Healthcare System.* National Academy Press, 2000. Available at http://www.nap.edu/

Maltby JR, Hutter CDD, Clayton KC: The Woolley and Roe case. Brit J Anaesth 2000;84:121.

Pierce EC Jr: The 34th Rovenstine Lecture. 40 years behind the mask: Safety revisited. Anesthesiology 1996;84:965.

Summary of the National Halothane Study. Possible association between halothane anesthesia and postoperative hepatic necrosis. JAMA 1966;197:775.

WEB SITES

American Society of Anesthesiologists Standards, Guidelines, Statements and other Documents. Available at: https://www.asahq.org/For-Healthcare-Professionals/Standards-Guidelines-and-Statements.aspx (accessed August 4, 2012).

Institute for Healthcare Improvement. Available at: www.ihi.org (accessed August 4 2012).

Index

Note: Page numbers followed by *f* and *t* indicate figures and tables, respectively.

Peripheral nerve   **Nerve root**

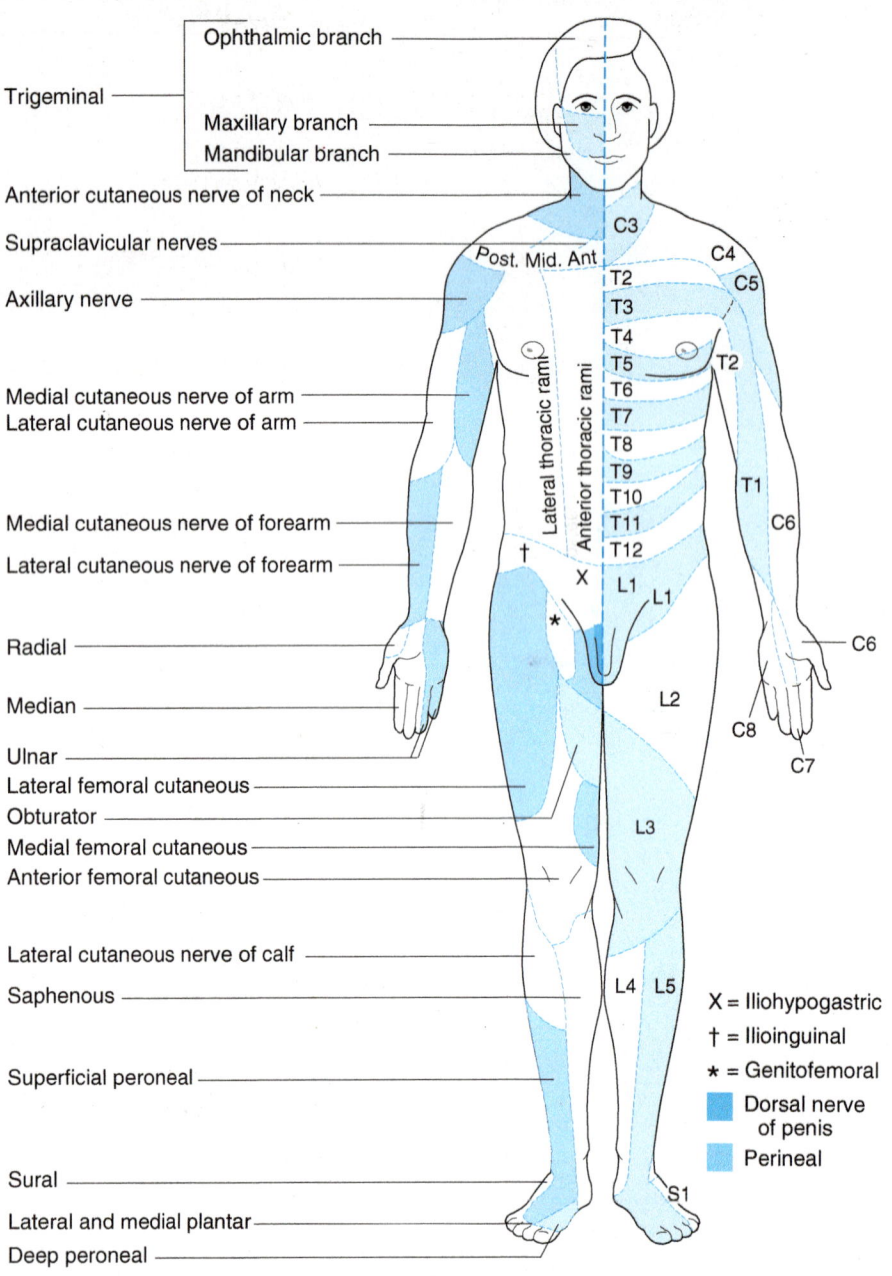

Ophthalmic branch

Trigeminal

Maxillary branch
Mandibular branch

Anterior cutaneous nerve of neck

Supraclavicular nerves

Axillary nerve

Medial cutaneous nerve of arm
Lateral cutaneous nerve of arm

Medial cutaneous nerve of forearm

Lateral cutaneous nerve of forearm

Radial

Median

Ulnar
Lateral femoral cutaneous
Obturator
Medial femoral cutaneous
Anterior femoral cutaneous

Lateral cutaneous nerve of calf

Saphenous

Superficial peroneal

Sural

Lateral and medial plantar

Deep peroneal

Post. Mid. Ant.

Lateral thoracic rami

Anterior thoracic rami

C3
C4
C5
T2
T3
T4
T5   T2
T6
T7
T8
T9
T10   T1
T11   C6
T12
L1   L1
         C6
L2
         C8
         C7

L3

L4   L5
S1

X = Iliohypogastric
† = Ilioinguinal
* = Genitofemoral
■ Dorsal nerve of penis
□ Perineal